ESSENTIALS OF PARAMEDIC CARE

BRYAN E. BLEDSOE, D.O., F.A.C.E.P., EMT-P

Emergency Department Staff Physician
Baylor Medical Center—Ellis County
Waxahachie, Texas
and
Clinical Associate Professor of Emergency Medicine
University of North Texas Health Sciences Center
Fort Worth, Texas

ROBERT S. PORTER, M.A., NREMT-P

Senior Advanced Life Support Educator
Madison County Emergency Medical Services
Canastota, New York
and
Flight Paramedic
AirOne, Onondaga County Sheriff's Department
Syracuse, New York

RICHARD A. CHERRY, M.S., NREMT-P

Clinical Assistant Professor of Emergency Medicine
Assistant Residency Director
SUNY Upstate Medical University
Syracuse, New York

Prentice Hall

Upper Saddle River, New Jersey 07458

Library of Congress Cataloging-in-Publication Data

Bledsoe, Bryan E., 1955-
    Essentials of paramedic care/Bryan E. Bledsoe, Robert S. Porter, Richard A. Cherry.
        p. ; cm.
    Includes bibliographical references and index.
    ISBN 0-13-098792-1
    1. Emergency medicine. 2. Emergency medical technicians. I. Porter, Robert S., 1950-
II. Cherry, Richard A. III. Title.
    [DNLM: 1. Emergency Treatment--methods. 2. Emergencies. 3. Emergency Medical
Services--methods. 4. Physical Examination--methods. WB 105 B646e 2003]
    RC86.7 .B594 2003
    616.02′5--dc21

2002025260

Publisher: Julie Levin Alexander
Executive Assistant and Supervisor: Regina Bruno
Executive Editor: Greg Vis
Managing Development Editor: Lois Berlowitz
Development Editors: Sandra Breuer, Josephine Cepeda,
    John Joerschke, Deborah Parks, and Dan Zinkus
Director of Manufacturing and Production: Bruce Johnson
Managing Production Editor: Patrick Walsh
Production Liaison: Jeanne Molenaar
Production Editor: Lori Dalberg, Carlisle
    Communications, Inc.
Manufacturing Manager: Ilene Sanford
Manufacturing Buyer: Pat Brown
Design Director: Cheryl Asherman
Design Coordinator: Christopher Weigand
Cover Design: Blair Brown
Cover Photography: Andy Sacks/Getty Images Stone
Managing Photography Manager: Michal Heron
Interior Photographers: Michal Heron, Richard Logan, and
    George Dodson
Interior Design: Jill Yutkowitz
Marketing Manager: Tiffany Price
Product Information Manager: Rachele Triano
Printer/Binder: Von Hoffmann Press
Cover Printer: Lehigh Press
Composition: Carlisle Communications, Inc.

Pearson Education LTD.
Pearson Education Australia PTY, Limited
Pearson Education Singapore, Pte. Ltd
Pearson Education North Asia Ltd
Pearson Education Canada, Ltd.
Pearson Educación de Mexico, S.A. de C.V.
Pearson Education -- Japan
Pearson Education Malaysia, Pte. Ltd

Art Acknowledgments

Rolin Graphics, Plymouth, Minnesota

Photo Acknowledgments

All photographs not credited adjacent to the
photograph were photographed on assignment
for Brady/Prentice Hall Pearson Education.

Organizations: We wish to thank the following
organizations for their valuable assistance in
creating the photo program for this edition:

Rockland Paramedic Services
Orangeburg, New York

Technical Advisor: Acknowledgment for
providing technical support during the photo
shoots to:

Rockland Paramedic Services
Orangeburg, New York
Michael Murphy, RN, EMT-P, Assistant Chief
    of Operations
Richard Greer EMT-P
Christopher Westbrook EMT-P
William Oliver EMT-P
Jennifer Legge EMT-P
Gregory Pekera EMT-P
Tara Florida EMT
Craig Sherman EMT

10 9 8 7 6 5 4
ISBN 0-13-098792-1

Notices

It is the intent of the authors and publishers that this textbook be used as part of a formal paramedic education program taught by a qualified instructor and supervised by a licensed physician. The care procedures presented here represent accepted practices in the United States. They are not offered as a standard of care. Paramedic-level emergency care is to be performed only under the authority and guidance of a licensed physician. It is the reader's responsibility to know and follow local care protocols as provided by medical advisors directing the system to which he or she belongs. Also, it is the reader's responsibility to stay informed of emergency care procedure changes.

NOTICE ON DRUGS AND DRUG DOSAGES

Every effort has been made to ensure that the drug dosages presented in this textbook are in accordance with nationally accepted standards. When applicable, the dosages and routes are taken from the American Heart Association's Advanced Cardiac Life Support Guidelines. The American Medical Association's publication *Drug Evaluations,* the *Physician's Desk Reference,* and the Appleton & Lange *Health Professionals Drug Guide 2000* are followed with regard to drug dosages not covered by the American Heart Association's guidelines. It is the responsibility of the reader to be familiar with the drugs used in his or her system, as well as the dosages specified by the medical director. The drugs presented in this book should only be administered by direct order, whether verbally or through accepted standing orders, of a licensed physician.

NOTICE ON GENDER USAGE

The English language has historically given preference to the male gender. Among many words, the pronouns "he" and "his" are commonly used to describe both genders. Society evolves faster than language and the male pronouns still predominate in our speech. The authors have made great effort to treat the two genders equally, recognizing that a significant percentage of paramedics and patients are female. However, in some instances, male pronouns may be used to describe both male and female paramedics and patients solely for the purpose of brevity. This is not intended to offend any readers of the female gender.

NOTICE ON PHOTOGRAPHS

Please note that many of the photographs contained in this book are taken of actual emergency situations. As such, it is possible that they may not accurately depict current, appropriate, or advisable practices of emergency medical care. They have been included for the sole purpose of giving general insight into real-life emergency settings.

DEDICATION

This book is respectfully dedicated to the EMTs and paramedics who toil each day in an environment that is unpredictable, often dangerous, and constantly changing. They risk their lives to aid the sick and the injured, driven only by their love of humanity and their devotion to this profession we call emergency medical services.

We remember the EMS, fire, and law enforcement personnel who have made the ultimate sacrifice for their communities and our nation. May they never be forgotten.

Photo by Ricky Flores/The Journal News/Corbis Sygma

Detailed Contents

Preface

Congratulations on your decision to further your EMS career by undertaking the course of education required for certification as an Emergency Medical Technician-Paramedic! The world of paramedic emergency care is one that you will find both challenging and rewarding. Whether you will be working as a volunteer or paid paramedic, you will find the field of advanced prehospital care very interesting.

This textbook program is derived from Brady's best-selling *Paramedic Care: Principles & Practice* (Volumes 1–5). Ideal for paramedic refresher and abbreviated paramedic programs, this book is based upon the 1998 United States Department of Transportation *EMT-Paramedic: National Standard Curriculum* and is organized into five divisions. The first division, entitled *Introduction to Advanced Prehospital Care,* addresses the fundamentals of paramedic practice, including pathophysiology, pharmacology, medication administration and advanced airway management. The second division, *Patient Assessment,* builds on the assessment skills of the basic EMT with special emphasis on advanced patient assessment at the scene. *Trauma Emergencies,* the third division of the text, discusses advanced prehospital care from the mechanism of injury analysis to shock/trauma resuscitation. The fourth division of the series, *Medical Emergencies,* is the most extensive and addresses paramedic-level care of medical emergencies. Particular emphasis is placed upon the most common medical problems as well as serious emergencies, such as respiratory and cardiovascular emergencies. The last division addresses *Special Considerations/ Operations* including neonatal, pediatric, geriatric, home health care, and specially challenged patients, and incident command, ambulance service, rescue, hazardous material, and crime scene operations.

SKILLS

The psychomotor skills of fluid and medication administration, advanced airway care, ECG monitoring and defibrillation, and advanced medical and trauma patient care are best learned in the classroom, skills laboratory, and then the clinical and field setting. Common advanced prehospital skills are discussed in the text as well as outlined in the accompanying procedure sheets. Review these before and while practicing the skill. It is important to point out that this or any other text cannot teach skills. Care skills are only learned under the watchful eye of a paramedic instructor and perfected during your clinical and field internship.

HOW TO USE THIS TEXTBOOK

Essentials of Paramedic Care is designed to accompany a paramedic education program that includes ample classroom, practical laboratory, in-hospital clinical, and prehospital field experience. These educational experiences must be guided by instructors and preceptors with special training and experience in their areas of participation in your program.

It is intended that your program coordinator will assign reading from the text in preparation for each classroom lecture and discussion section. The knowledge gained from reading this text will form the foundation of the information you will need in order to function effectively as a paramedic in your EMS system. Your instructors will build upon this information to strengthen your knowledge and understanding of advanced prehospital care so that you may apply it in your practice. The in-hospital clinical and prehospital field experiences will further refine your knowledge and skills under the watchful eyes of your preceptors.

The workbook that accompanies this text can also assist in improving classroom performance. It contains information, sample test questions, and exercises designed to assist learning. Its use can be very helpful in identifying the important elements of paramedic education, in exercising the knowledge of prehospital care, and in helping you self-test your knowledge.

Essentials of Paramedic Care presents the knowledge of emergency care in as accurate, standardized, and clear a manner as is possible. However, each EMS system is uniquely different, and it is beyond the scope of this text to address all differences. You must count heavily on your instructors, the program coordinator, and ultimately the program medical director to identify how specific emergency care procedures are applied in your system.

Acknowledgments

CHAPTER CONTRIBUTORS

We wish to acknowledge the remarkable talents and efforts of the following people who contributed to *Essentials of Paramedic Care*. Individually, they worked with extraordinary commitment on this new program. Together, they form a team of highly dedicated professionals who have upheld the highest standard of EMS instruction.

B.E.B., R.S.P., R.A.C.

Beth Lothrop Adams, M.A., R.N., NREMT-P, ALS Coordinator, EHS Programs, Adjunct Assistant Professor, Emergency Medicine, The George Washington University. *Chapters 30, 39, 40*

J. Nile Barnes, B.S., NREMT-P, Associate Professor of EMS Professions, Austin Community College, Austin, Texas and Paramedic, Williamson County (Texas) EMS Department. *Chapter 1*

Brenda Beasley, R.N.; B.S.; EMT-P; EMS Program Director, Calhoun College, Decatur, Alabama. *Chapter 42*

Sandra Bradley, Pleasant Hill, California. *Chapter 45*

Lawrence C. Brilliant, M.D., F.A.C.E.P., Clinical Assistant Professor, Department of Primary Care Education and Community Services, Hahnemann University; Emergency Physician, Doylestown Hospital, Doylestown, Pennsylvania. *Chapter 23, Chapter 28*

Eric C. Chaney, M.S. NREMT-P, Administrator, Office of the State EMS Medical Director, Maryland Institute for Emergency Medical Services Systems, Baltimore, Maryland. *Chapter 1*

Elizabeth Coolidge-Stolz, M.D., Medical Writer, Health Educator, North Reading, Massachusetts. *Chapters 30, 32, 33*

Robert A. De Lorenzo, M.D., F.A.C.E.P.; Lieut. Colonel, Medical Corps, US Army; Brooke Army Medical Center. *Chapters 20, 21*

Kate Dernocoeur, B.S. EMT-P, Lowell, Michigan. *Chapters 1, 9*

Clyde Deschamp, M.Ed., NREMT-P, Chairman and Assistant Professor, Department of Emergency Medical Technology, Director, Helicopter Transport, University of Mississippi Medical Center. *Chapter 37*

James W. Drake, B.S., NREMT-P, Instructor, Department of Emergency Medical Technology, School of Health Related Professions, University of Mississippi Medical Center, Jackson, Mississippi. *Chapter 7*

Robert Elling, M.P.A.; NREMT-P; Professor, American College of Prehospital Medicine; Faculty Member, Institute of Prehospital Emergency Medicine, Hudson Valley Community College, Troy, New York. *Chapter 48*

Robert Feinberg, EMT-P, PA-C, Emergency Medicine, Wayne, Pennsylvania. *Chapter 24*

Joseph P. Funk, M.D., F.A.C.E.P., Peachtree Emergency Associates, Piedmont Hospital, Atlanta, Georgia. *Chapter 8*

Kathleen G. Funk, M.D., F.A.C.E.P., Emergency Medicine Physician, Atlanta, Georgia. *Chapter 8*

Eric W. Heckerson, R.N., M.A., NREMT-P, EMS Coordinator, Mesa Fire Department, Mesa, Arizona. *Chapters 1, 22, 29, 37, 38*

Chris Hendricks, NREMT-P; Field Instructor; Paramedic, Pridemark Paramedics, Boulder, Colorado. *Chapter 46*

Sandra Hultz, B.S., NREMT-P, EMS Instructor, University of Mississippi Medical Center, Jackson, Mississippi. *Chapter 1*

Jeffrey L. Jarvis, M.S., EMT-P, Medical Student, University of Texas Medical Branch, Galveston, Texas. *Chapter 6*

Deborah Kufs, R.N., B.S., C.C.R.N., C.E.N., NREMT-P, Clinical Instructor, Hudson Valley Community College, Institute for Prehospital Emergency Medicine, Troy, New York. *Chapters 35, 43*

Daniel Limmer, EMT-P, Frederick, Maryland. *Chapters 38, 48*

William Marx, D.O.; Associate Professor of Surgery and Critical Care; Director, Surgical Critical Care SUNY Upstate Medical University, Syracuse, New York. *Chapter 26*

Michael O'Keefe, NREMT-P, EMS Training Coordinator, Vermont Department of Health. *Chapter 1*

John M. Saad, M.D., Medical Director of Emergency Services, Navarro Regional Hospital, Corsicana, Texas; Medical Director of Emergency Services, Medical Center at Terrell, Terrell, Texas. *Chapters 34, 36*

John S. Saito, M.P.H., EMT-P, Director, EMS/Paramedic Education, Assistant Professor, Oregon Health Sciences University, School of Medicine, Department of Emergency Medicine, Portland, Oregon. *Chapters 4, 37*

Jo Anne Schultz, B.A., NREMT-P, Paramedic, Lifestar Ambulance Inc., Salisbury, Maryland; Level II Emergency Medical Services Instructor, Maryland Fire and Rescue Institute, University of Maryland; Paramedic Instructor, Maryland Institute of Emergency Medical Services Systems, University of Maryland; ACLS, BTLS, and PALS instructor. *Chapters 5, 36, 41, 47*

Craig A. Soltis, M.D., F.A.C.E.P., Assistant Professor of Clinical Emergency Medicine, Northeastern Ohio Universities College of Medicine; Chairman, Department of Emergency Medicine, Forum Health, Youngstown, Ohio. *Chapters 25, 35*

Marian D. Streger, R.N.; B.S.N.; C.E.N., Cleveland, Ohio. *Chapters 45, 47*

Matthew R. Streger, M.P.A.; NREMT-P; Deputy Commissioner, Cleveland Emergency Medical Services, Cleveland, Ohio. *Chapters 44, 46, 48*

Emily Vacher, Esq., M.P.A., EMT-CC, Associate Director of Judicial Affairs, Syracuse University, Syracuse, New York. *Chapter 2*

Kevin Waddington, EMT-P, MedStar, Fort Worth, Texas. *Chapter 28*

Gail Weinstein, M.A.; EMT-P; Director of Paramedic Training, State University of New York Upstate Medical University, Syracuse, New York. *Chapter 43*

Howard A. Werman, M.D., F.A.C.E.P., Associate Professor of Clinical Emergency Medicine, The Ohio State University College of Medicine and Public Health, Columbus, Ohio; Medical Director, MedFlight of Ohio. *Chapter 27*

Matthew S. Zavarella, B.S.A.S., NREMT-P, CCTEMT-P, Director Prehospital Education, Medical College of Ohio, Toledo, Ohio. *Chapters 4, 32*

DEVELOPMENT AND PRODUCTION

The task of writing, editing, reviewing, and producing a textbook the size of *Essentials of Paramedic Care* is complex. Many talented people have been involved in developing and producing this new program.

First, the authors would like to acknowledge the support of Julie Alexander and Greg Vis. Their belief in us and support of EMS has allowed us to assure that *Essentials of Paramedic Care* will be in the forefront of paramedic education. Special thanks go to Sandra Breuer, who served as Project Coordinator for this new paramedic text. Sandy is a consummate professional. This book, which would not exist without Sandy's dedication and hard work, is as much hers as it is ours. We also thank Josephine Cepeda, John Joerschke, Deborah Parks, and Dan Zinkus, Development Editors for this project. The extraordinary efforts of these exceptionally dedicated editors are deeply appreciated.

The challenges of production were in the very capable hands of Patrick Walsh and Jeanne Molenaar, who skillfully supervised all production stages to create the final product you now hold. In developing our art and photo program we were fortunate to work with yet additional talent, leaders within their professions. Most of the staged photographs are by Michal Heron of New York City, whose commitment to excellence never falters. The new art was drafted by Rolin Graphics of Plymouth, Minnesota.

MEDICAL REVIEW BOARD

Our special thanks to the following physicians for their review of material in our paramedic program. Their reviews were carefully prepared, and we appreciate the thoughtful advice and keen insight each shared with us.

Dr. Robert De Lorenzo, Lieutenant Colonel, Medical Corps, U.S. Army; Associate Clinical Professor of Military and Emergency Medicine, Uniformed Services University of Health Sciences.

Dr. Edward T. Dickinson, Assistant Professor and Director of EMS Field Operations in the Department of Emergency Medicine, University of Pennsylvania School of Medicine in Philadephia.

Dr. Howard A. Werman, Associate Professor, Department of Emergency Medicine, The Ohio State University College of Medicine and Public Health, Columbus, Ohio.

INSTRUCTOR REVIEWERS

The reviewers of *Essentials of Paramedic Care* have provided many excellent suggestions and ideas for improving the text. The quality of the reveiws has been outstanding, and the reviews have been a major aid in the preparation and revision of the manuscript. The assistance provided by these EMS experts is deeply appreciated.

DIVISION 1

Brenda Beasley, RN, BS, EMT-P
EMS Program Director
Calhoun College
Decatur, AL

Tom Blake, MS, EMT-P
Director, Paramedic Associates Degree
    Program
Southern Maine Technical College
South Portland, ME

Alan Brower, RN, NREMT-P
Ricks College Paramedic Program
Rexbury, ID

Kerry Campbell, NREMT-P
Lakeshore Technical College
Cleveland, WI

Albert Dimmitt, Jr.
Penn Valley Community College
Kansas City, MO
Robert Dotterer, BSEd, MEd,
    NREMT-P
Phoenix Fire Department
Phoenix College
Phoenix, AZ

Bill Gentry, MICP
Paramedic Program Coordinator
Northern California Training
    Institute
Sacramento, CA

Blaine Griffiths, BS, NREMT-P
Youngstown State University
Youngstown, OH

Jeffrey Grunow, MSN,
    NREMT-P
Director, Prehospital Education
Carolinas Medical Center
Charlotte, NC

Linda Honeycutt, EMT-P, I/C
HealthStream, Inc.
Nashville, TN

Samuel D. Marciano, MS, EMT-I
Assistant Professor
Erie Community College
Lancaster, NY

Larry W. Masterman, MICP, CEM
Northern California EMS Agency
Redding, CA

Vicki L. May
Houston Community College
Houston, TX

Michael E. Murphy, RN, EMT-P
Deputy Chief
Rockland Paramedic Services
Orangeburg, NY

Gerard Oncale, RN, BSN, CEN,
    REMT-P
EMS Faculty
University of South Alabama
Mobile, AL

Judith Ruple, PhD, RN
Associate Professor
The University of Toledo
Toledo, OH

Larry Ryland
Director of Emergency Medical
    Services
L.B. Wallace College
Andalusia Rescue Squad
Andalusia, AL

John Saito, EMT-P, MPH
EMS/Paramedic Education
Oregon Health Sciences University
Portland, OR

Christopher D. Scott, M. Ed,
    NREMT-P
Paramedic Program Director
Assistant Professor
Springfield College EMSM
Springfield, MA

Brad L. Sparks
Paramedic Program Coordinator
St. Francis Hospital and Health Centers
Indianapolis, IN

Andrew W. Stern, NREMT-P, MPA,
    MA
Senior Paramedic/Flightmedic
Town of Colonie Emergency Medical
    Services
Colonie, NY

Regina M. Twisdale, AS, MICP
Director, School of Paramedic Sciences
Virtua Health/Camden County College
Camden County, NJ

Michael D. Zemany
Director of Education
Mt. Lakes Regional EMS Program
Saranac Lake, NY

DIVISION 2

Linda M. Abrahamson, RN, EMT-P
EMS Education Coordinator
Will Grundy EMS
Silver Cross Hospital
Joliet, IL

Brenda Beasley, RN, BS, EMT-P
EMS Program Director
Calhoun College
Decatur, AL

Jeffery L. Beinke, BS, REMT-P,
    CCEMT-P
Division Chair, Allied Health Sciences
Montgomery Community College
Troy, NC

Ed Carlson, Med, REMT-P
Department of EMS Education
University of South Alabama
Mobile, AL

Chuck Carter, RN, NREMT-P, CEN
Mississippi State Department of
    Health
Division of EMS
Jackson, MS

Claudette Dirzanowski, EMT-P
Certified Instructor/Examiner for the
    State of Texas, AHA, ARC,
    PHTLS
Sweeney Community Hospital and
    Brazosport College
Sweeney, TX

Bob Elling, MPA, REMT-P
Director, Institute of Prehospital
    Emergency Medicine
Hudson Valley Community College
Troy, NY

Joseph J. Mistovich
Chairperson and Associate
    Professor
Department of Health Professions
Youngstown State University
Youngstown, Ohio

Catherine Pattison, RN, MSN, EMT-B
EMS Program Coordinator
Bishop State Community College
Mobile, AL

Steven A. Weinman, RN, BSN, CEN
Instructor, Emergency Department
New York Presbyterian Hospital
New York Cornell Campus
New York, NY

DIVISION 3

Philip Adams, EMT-P, RN, BSN
Paramedic Course Coordinator
Paducah Community College
Paducah, KY

Kim Dickerson, EMT-P, RN
EMS Coordinator
Edison Community College
Fort Myers, FL 33906

Rudy Garrett
Paramedic Training Coordinator
Somerset-Pulaski County EMS
Somerset, KY

Ted S. Goldman, EMT-P
City of Philadelphia Fire
    Department
Director of EMS Programs
Star Technical Institute
Philadelphia, PA

Linda Groarke, MPH/MS, NREMT-P
Paramedic Program Director
Assistant Professor
Natural and Applied Sciences
LaGuardia Community
    College/CUNY
New York, NY

Theresa Jordan, RN, TNS, EMT
Arkansas Emergency Transport
Jacksonville, AR

Scott Kar, M.Ed., NREMT-P
Bevill State Paramedic Program
Sumiton, AZ

David LaCombe, NREMT-P
Center for Research in Medical
    Education
University of Miami School
    of Medicine
Miami, FL

Shelby Louden, BS, EMT-P
Safety and Compliance
    Coordinator
Butler County Joint Vocational
    Schools
Hamilton, OH

Joseph J. Mistovich
Chairperson and Associate
    Professor
Department of Health Professions
Youngstown State University
Youngstown, Ohio

Becky A. Morris, BS, NREMT-P, IC
EMS Department Head
Trenholm State College
Montgomery, AL

John Eric Powell, MS, NREMT-P
Flight Paramedic
UT-Lifestar Aeromedical Service
University of Tennessee Medical
    Center
Level 1 Trauma Facility
Knoxville, TN

Larry Richmond
Mountain Plains Health Consortium
Fort Meade, SD

Captain Michael W. Robinson
EMS Training Coordinator
Baltimore County Fire Department
Baltimore, MD

Tom Rothrock, RN, BSN, CEN,
    PHRN
Flight Nurse, University Medevac
Paramedic Coordinator, Lehigh Valley
    Hospital
Allentown, PA

Andrew W. Stern, NREMT-P,
    MPA, MA
Senior Paramedic/Flightmedic
Town of Colonie Emergency Medical
    Services
Colonie, NY

Michael Tretola, BS, EMT-P
Administrative Coordinator
EMS Institute/Department
    of Emergency Medicine
Catholic Medical Center of Brooklyn
    and Queens, NY

Peter H. Viele, M.S., NREMT-P
Operations Manager
Action Ambulance Service, Inc.
Stoneham, MA

Division 4

John L. Beckman
Fire Fighter/Paramedic Instructor
Lincolnwood Fire Department
Lincolnwood, IL

Mike Coakley
EMS Director
Alabama Fire College
Program in Emergency Medicine
Tuscaloosa, AL

Janice Dorsey, RN, BS
EMS Coordinator, Education
Christ Hospital and Medical Center
Oaklawn, IL

Darren K. Ellenburg, B.S., EMT-P
Assistant Professor, Paramedic
    Education
Northeast State Technical Community
    College
Blountville, TN

Joseph P. Funk, MD, FACEP
Emory University
Department of Emergency Medicine
Atlanta, GA

Mary Gillespie, RN, EMT-P, I/C
Allied Health Division Chair
Davenport College
Grand Rapids, MI

Blaine Griffiths, BSAS, RN, NREMT-P
Youngstown State University
Paramedic Program
Youngstown, OH

J. Scott Hartley, NREMT-P, EMS-I
A.L.S. Affiliates
Omaha, NE

Arthur Hsieh, MA, NREMT-P
Assistant Professor, Emergency Health
    Services Program
Department of Emergency Medicine
George Washington University
Washington, DC

Larry Impson, AS, NREMT-P
Dean of Prehospital Education
METS Inc.
Lodi, CA

Kevin McCoy, CCEMT-P
EMS Administrator/Paramedic
    Instructor
Cherokee Nation EMS
Tahlequah, OK

Robert G. Nixon, BA, EMT-P
Lifecare Medical Training
Walnut Creek, CA

Robert C. Rajsky, MSEd, NREMT-P
Manager of the Department of EMS
    Education
Chair-Southern Tier Regional EMS
    Council
Education Supervisor Erway
    Ambulance
President-Southern Tier ALS

Andria Savary, RN, MSN, ANP,
    EMT-P
Assistant Director
Institute for Emergency Medical
    Services
Northeastern Universtiy
Boston, MA

Andrew Stern, NREMT-P, MPA, MA
Senior Medic/Flightmedic
Town of Colonie Emergency Medical
    Services
Colonie, NY

Eric Stokley, A.A.S., NREMT-P
Program Director
Global Education Services
Lilburn, GA

Dave Tauber, NREMT-P I/C
Executive Director Advanced Life
    Support Institute
Paramedic/Firefighter
Conway, NH

Timothy Walsh, RN, ANP,
    NREMT-P
Assistant Professor
Community College of Rhode Island
Lincoln, RI

Steve Weinman, RN, BSN, CEN
Emergency Department Instructor
New York Hospital–Cornell Medical
    Center
New York, NY

Gail Weinstein
Paramedic Instructor
SUNY Health Science Center
Department of Emergency
    Medicine
Syracuse, NY

Paul A. Werfel, NREMT-P
Director Paramedic Program SUNY
Stony Brook, NY

DIVISION 5

Stanley A. Bell, Jr.
MICP Lead Instructor
Trinitas Hospital Mobile ICU
Elizabeth, NJ

Michael D. Berg, NREMT-P
Medical Liaison Officer
Austin/Travis County EMS
Austin, TX

Robert Carter
Clinical Associate Pediatric Intensive
    Care Unit
Johns Hopkins Children's Center
Paramedic, Baltimore City Fire
    Department
Baltimore, MD

Edna Deacon, EMT
EMT Coordinator Sussex County
    Community College
Mine Hill First Aid Squad President
Newton, NJ

Robert De Lorenzo, MD, FACEP
Lieutenant Colonel, Medical Corps
United States Army
Associate Clinical Professor of
    Military and Emergency Medicine
Uniformed Services University of
    Health Sciences
Bethesda, MD

Robert Dotterer, BSEd, M. Ed
    NREMT-P
Phoenix Fire Department
Phoenix College
Phoenix, AZ

Julie M. Falcone, BS, B.M.
Fire Fighter/Paramedic
Walla Walla Fire Department
Walla Walla, WA

Jonathan Hockman, Paramedic,
    ACLS, EMSIC
Goldrush Consulting
Detroit, MI

Darin Hoggatt, MS, FF/NREMT-P
Clarian Health and Greenwood Fire
    Department
Indianapolis, IN

Tony Hyre, BA, REMT-P
C.E. Officer
West Virginia EMS

James L. Jenkins, Jr.; BA, NREMT-P
Confidential Assistant to the Governor
Office of the Secretary of Public Safety
Virginia Department of Fire Programs
Richmond, VA

Anthony T. Kramer, RN, BSN,
    NREMT-P
Field Service Assistant Professor
Clinical Coordinator, Center for
    Prehospital Education
University of Cincinnati
Cincinnati, OH

Nick Meacher, NREMT-P
Instructor, Public Safety Center
Harrisburg Area Community
    College
York Springs, PA

Steven L. Poffenberger, BS, EMT-P
Paramedic Program Clinical
    Coordinator
Harrisburg Area Community College
Harrisburg, PA

Jackie L. Richey, RN, NREMT-P
Rural/Metro Ambulance
Indianapolis, IN

Captain Michael W. Robinson
EMS Training Coordinator
Baltimore County Fire Department
Baltimore, MD

Michael G. Rubin, BS, NREMT-P
State University of New York at Stony
    Brook
Stony Brook, NY

Daniel L. Sponsler, BS, NREMT-P
Division Chair, Emergency Services
Northwest Technical College
East Grand Forks, MN

Andrew W. Stern, NREMT-P, MPA,
    MA
Senior Paramedic/Flightmedic
Town of Colonie Emergency Medical
    Services
Colonie, NY

Matthew R. Streger, MPA, NREMT-P
Deputy Commissioner
Cleveland Emergency Medical
    Services
Cleveland, OH

Anthony Tucci, EMT-P
Western Berks Ambulance
    Association
West Lawn, PA

Charles N. Zarrelli
Coordinator, EMT Training
Camden County College
Blackwood, NJ

Prehospital emergency personnel, like all health care workers, are at risk for exposure to bloodborne pathogens and infectious diseases. In emergency situations it is often difficult to take or enforce proper infection control measures. However, as a paramedic, you must recognize your high-risk status.

Infection control is designed to protect emergency personnel, their families, and their patients from unnecessary exposure to communicable diseases.

Laws, regulations, and standards regarding infection control include:

* *Centers for Disease Control (CDC) Guidelines.* The CDC has published extensive guidelines regarding infection control. Proper equipment and techniques that should be used by emergency response personnel to prevent or minimize risk of exposure are defined.

* *The Ryan White Act.* The Ryan White Act of 1990 allows emergency personnel to find out if they were exposed to an infectious disease while rendering patient care. Employers are required to name a "designated officer" to coordinate communications with the treating hospital.

* *Americans with Disabilities Act.* This act prohibits discrimination against individuals with disabilities including those with contagious diseases. It guarantees equal employment opportunities and job protection if the infected individual can perform essential job functions and does not pose a threat to the safety and health of patients and coworkers.

* *Occupational Safety and Health Administration (OSHA) Regulations.* OSHA recently enacted a regulation entitled Occupational Exposure to Bloodborne Pathogens that classifies emergency response personnel as being at the greatest risk of occupational exposure to communicable diseases. This regulation requires employers to provide hepatitis B (HBV) vaccinations free of charge, maintain a written exposure control plan, and provide personal protective equipment (PPE). These requirements primarily apply to private employers. Applicability to local and state governmental employees varies by locality. Many states have developed their own OSHA plans.

* *National Fire Protection Association (NFPA) Guidelines.* This is a national organization that has established specific guidelines and requirements regarding infection control for emergency response agencies, particularly fire departments and EMS services.

BODY SUBSTANCE ISOLATION PRECAUTIONS AND PERSONAL PROTECTIVE EQUIPMENT

Emergency response personnel should practice *Body Substance Isolation (BSI)*, a strategy that considers ALL body substances potentially infectious. To achieve this, all emergency personnel should utilize *Personal Protective Equipment (PPE)*. Appropriate PPE should be available on every emergency vehicle. The minimum recommended PPE includes the following:

* *Gloves.* Disposable gloves should be donned by all emergency response personnel BEFORE initiating any emergency care. When an emergency incident involves more than one patient, you should attempt to change gloves between patients. When gloves have been contaminated, they should be removed as soon as possible. To remove gloves, first hook the gloved fingers of one hand under the cuff of the other glove. Then pull that glove off without letting your gloved fingers come in contact with bare skin. Then slide the fingers of the ungloved hand under the remaining glove's cuff. Push that glove off, being careful not to touch the glove's exterior with your bare hand. Always wash hands after gloves are removed, even when the gloves appear intact.

* *Masks and Protective Eyewear.* Masks and protective equipment should be present on all emergency vehicles and used in accordance with the level of exposure encountered. Proper eyewear and masks prevent a patient's blood and body fluids from spraying into your eyes, nose, and mouth. Masks and protective eyewear should be worn together whenever blood spatter is likely to occur, such as arterial bleeding, childbirth, endotracheal intubation, invasive procedures, oral suctioning, and clean-up of equipment that requires heavy scrubbing or brushing. Both you and the patient should wear masks whenever the potential for airborne transmission of disease exists.

* *HEPA Respirators.* Due to the resurgence of tuberculosis (TB), prehospital personnel should protect themselves from TB infection through use of

a high-efficiency particulate air (HEPA) respirator, a design approved by the National Institute of Occupational Safety and Health (NIOSH). It should fit snugly and be capable of filtering out the tuberculosis bacillus. The HEPA respirator should be worn when caring for patients with confirmed or suspected TB. This is especially true when performing "high hazard" procedures such as administration of nebulized medications, endotracheal intubation, or suctioning on such a patient.

* *Gowns.* Gowns protect clothing from blood splashes. If large splashes of blood are expected, such as with childbirth, wear impervious gowns.
* *Resuscitation Equipment.* Disposable resuscitation equipment should be the primary means of artificial ventilation in emergency care. Such items should be used once, then disposed of.

Remember, the proper use of personal protective equipment ensures effective infection control and minimizes risk. Use ALL protective equipment recommended for any particular situation to ensure maximum protection.

Consider ALL body substances potentially infectious and ALWAYS practice body substance isolation.

HANDLING CONTAMINATED MATERIAL

Many of the materials associated with the emergency response become contaminated with possibly infectious body fluids and substances. These include soiled linen, patient clothing, and dressings, and used care equipment, including intravenous needles. It is important that you collect these materials at the scene and dispose of them appropriately to assure your safety as well as that of your patients, their family members, bystanders, and fellow care-givers. Properly dispose of any contaminated materials according to the recommendations outlined below.

* Handle contaminated materials only while wearing the appropriate personal protective equipment.
* Place all blood- or body-fluid-contaminated clothing, linen, dressings and patient care equipment and supplies in properly marked biological hazard bags and assure they are disposed of properly.
* Assure all used needles, scalpels and other contaminated objects that have the potential to puncture the skin are properly secured in a puncture-resistant and clearly-marked sharps container.
* Do not recap a needle after use, stick it into a seat cushion or other object, or leave it lying on the ground. This increases the risk of an accidental needle stick.
* Always scan the scene before leaving to assure all equipment has been retrieved and all potentially infectious material has been bagged and removed.
* Should you be exposed to an infectious disease, have contact with body substances with a route for system entry (such as an open wound on your hand when a glove tears while moving a soiled patient), or receive a needle stick with a used needle, alert the receiving hospital and contact your service's infection control officer immediately.

Following these recommendations will help protect you and the people you care for from the dangers of disease transmission.

ONE LAKE STREET
UPPER SADDLE RIVER, NJ 07458

Dear Paramedic Instructor,

Brady, Your Partner in Education, is pleased to present *Essentials of Paramedic Care,* developed specifically to meet the 1998 U.S. DOT National Standard Curriculum for EMT-Paramedics in shorter courses and refresher programs. Our more comprehensive five-volume series is ideal for longer courses. Either way, Brady provides you with the options you need.

We recognize that for many of you the 1998 curriculum represents a dramatic change in the way your paramedic course will be taught. *Essentials of Paramedic Care* was developed specifically to help both you and your students succeed. Written in a student-friendly, easy-to-understand style, our new text consists of five divisions:

- Division 1: *Introduction to Advanced Prehospital Care*
- Division 2: *Patient Assessment*
- Division 3: *Trauma Emergencies*
- Division 4: *Medical Emergencies*
- Division 5: *Special Considerations/Operations.*

The text is designed to cover all the objectives in the eight modules of the U.S. DOT curriculum. Each division may also be used to help you tailor your course to state and local protocols.

Our complete instructor materials provide everything you need to help get your course up and running. The Instructor's Resource Manual contains lecture outlines and lesson plans that cover the new curriculum, along with student handouts and suggestions for class activities. Brady's PowerPoint Slides on CD-ROM offer a wealth of word slides and images that you can tailor to course needs, and our Test Manager enables you to select questions based on topic area and degree of difficulty.

Essentials of Paramedic Care also offers the latest multimedia technology to enhance and enrich your students' classroom experiences and to help you manage your classes more efficiently. The program's accompanying Companion Website at www.prenhall.com/bledsoe2 contains chapter-by-chapter interactive student quizzes, links to related EMS sites for students, and an online syllabus builder for instructors. Additionally, to accommodate the needs of distance learners, we are pleased to offer Blackboard and CourseCompass options.

We wish you the best of luck.

Sincerely,

Julie Levin Alexander
Vice President and Publisher

BRADY
Your Partner in Education

EMPHASIZING PRINCIPLES

Chapter Objectives with Page References

Each chapter begins with clearly stated **Objectives** that follow the U.S. DOT Paramedic curriculum. Students can refer to these objectives while studying to make sure they understand the material fully. Page references after each objective indicate where relevant content is covered in the chapter.

CHAPTER 7

Medication Administration

Objectives

Part 1: Principles and Routes of Medication Administration
(begins on p. 414)

After reading Part 1 of this chapter, you should be able to:

1. Review the specific anatomy and physiology pertinent to medication administration. (pp. 417–448)
2. Describe the indications, equipment needed, technique used, precautions, and general principles for the following:
   a. inhalation routes of medication administration. (pp. 421–425)
   b. parenteral routes of medication administration. (pp. 432–448)
   c. percutaneous routes of medication administration. (pp. 417–421)
   d. enteral routes of medication administration, including gastric tube administration and rectal administration. (pp. 425–432)
3. Describe the indications, contraindications, side effects, dosages, and routes of administration for medications commonly administered by paramedics. (pp. 417–448)
4. Discuss legal aspects affecting medication administration. (pp. 414–415, 417)
5. Discuss the "six rights" of drug administration and correlate them with the principles of medication administration. (p. 414)
6. Differentiate among the percutaneous routes of medication administration. (pp. 417–421)
7. Discuss medical asepsis and the differences between clean and sterile techniques. (pp. 415–416)
8. Describe uses of antiseptics and disinfectants. (pp. 415–416)
9. Describe the use of body substance isolation (BSI) procedures when administering a medication. (p. 415)

Continued

Content Review

Content Review summarizes important content and gives students a format for quick review.

Key Terms

Reinforcement of **Key Terms** helps students master new terminology.

Key Points

Key Points in the margins help students identify and learn the fundamental principles of paramedic practice.

Content Review

PARENTERAL ROUTES
Intradermal injection
Subcutaneous injection
Intramuscular injection
Intravenous access
Intraosseous infusion

PARENTERAL ROUTES

Parenterally administered drugs can be absorbed locally or systemically. Additionally, depending on the route of administration, their absorption rate may be slow, sustained, or rapid. Parenteral delivery bypasses the digestive tract, thus making the drug's absorption, action, and onset more predictable. Because parenteral routes use hypodermic needles that contact body fluids, the risk of disease transmission is ever present.

Parenteral drug delivery employs the following routes:

- Intradermal injection
- Subcutaneous injection
- Intramuscular injection
- Intravenous access
- Intraosseous infusion

Specific medications require specific routes of parenteral delivery; therefore, you must be competent with every route. In this section we will discuss the specialized equipment, medications, and routes for intradermal, subcutaneous, and intramuscular injections. Because of their complexity, we will discuss intravenous access and intraosseous infusions separately in the following sections.

Whether you are administering a parenteral injection or an IV bolus or infusion, you should explain the entire procedure to the patient to help alleviate his anxiety. Finally, remember that hypoperfusion (hypovolemia or peripheral vascular disease, for instance), may significantly reduce parenteral absorption.

Intradermal Injection

✴ **intradermal** within the dermal layer of the skin.

Using a syringe and hypodermic needle, **intradermal** injections deposit medication into the dermal layer of the skin (*intra-*, within; *derma*, skin). The amount of medication placed in the dermal layer is quite small, typically less than 1 ml (Figure 7-17).

Capillaries in the dermis afford a very slow rate of absorption, with little or no systemic distribution.

Capillaries in the dermis afford a very slow rate of absorption, with little or no systemic distribution. Rather, the bulk of medication remains localized in the area of administration. Intradermal delivery proves useful for allergy testing and tuberculin skin testing and for administering local anesthetics during suturing, wound debridement, and IV establishment.

The forearm and upper back are preferred sites for intradermal injections. They have little hair and are highly visible. Additionally, you should look for sites free of superficial blood vessels, which increase the chance for systemic absorption.

FIGURE 7-17 Intradermal injection.

Epidermis · Dermis · 10°–15° · Subcutaneous tissue · Muscle

Tables and Illustrations

Tables and **illustrations** offer visual support to enhance students' understanding of paramedic principles and practice.

Table 5-1 NORMAL VITAL SIGNS

	Pulse (beats per minute)	Respiration (breaths per minute)	Blood Pressure (average mmHg)	Temperature	
Infancy:					
At birth:	100–180	30–60	60–90 systolic	98°F–100°F	36.7°C–37.8°C
At one year:	100–160	30–60	87–105 systolic	98°F–100°F	36.7°C–37.8°C
Toddler (12 to 36 months)	80–110	24–40	95–105 systolic	96.8°F–99.6°F	36.3°C–37.9°C
Preschool age (3 to 5 years)	70–110	22–34	95–110 systolic	96.8°F–99.6°F	36.3°C–37.9°C
School-age (6 to 12 years)	65–110	18–30	97–112 systolic	98.6°F	37°C
Adolescence (13 to 18 years)	60–90	12–26	112–128 systolic	98.6°F	37°C
Early adulthood (19 to 40 years)	60–100	12–20	120/80	98.6°F	37°C
Middle adulthood (41 to 60 years)	60–100	12–20	120/80	98.6°F	37°C
Late adulthood (61 years and older)	+	+	+	98.6°F	37°C

+ Depends on the individual physical health status.

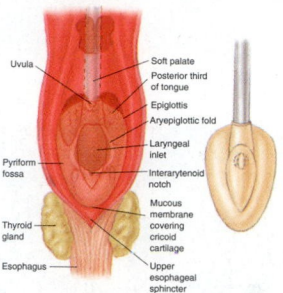

FIGURE 8-37 Laryngeal Mask Airway.

Uvula — Soft palate — Posterior third of tongue — Epiglottis — Aryepiglottic fold — Laryngeal inlet — Pyriform fossa — Interarytenoid notch — Thyroid gland — Mucous membrane covering cricoid cartilage — Esophagus — Upper esophageal sphincter

FIGURE 8-38 Pharyngo-tracheal lumen airway.

PHARYNGO-TRACHEAL LUMEN AIRWAY

* pharyngo-tracheal lumen airway (PtL) is a two tube system.

The **pharyngo-tracheal lumen airway** (PtL) is a two-tube system (Figure 8-38). The first tube is short, with a large diameter; its proximal end is green. A large cuff encircles the tube's lower third. When inflated, the cuff seals the entire oropharynx. Air introduced at this tube's proximal end will enter the hypopharynx. The second tube is long, with a small diameter, and clear. It passes through and extends approximately 10 cm beyond the first tube. This second tube may be inserted blindly into either the trachea or the esophagus. A distal cuff, when inflated, seals off whichever anatomical structure the tube has entered. When the second tube enters the trachea, you will ventilate the patient through it.

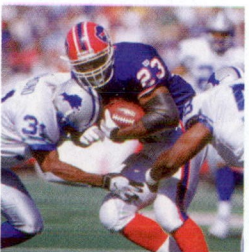

FIGURE 17-26 Contact sports may result in the exchange of great kinetic forces and produce serious injuries. (Allsport NY)

Crush Injuries

Crush injuries are common types of trauma. They may result from mechanisms such as structural collapse as in an explosion, an industrial or agricultural accident where a limb is caught in machinery, or when a limb is caught under a vehicle. These mechanisms direct great force to soft tissues and bones, compressing surfaces together while stretching semifluid soft tissues laterally. The result may be severe tissue disruption and serious associated hemorrhage.

The injury may be further compounded if the crushing pressure remains in place for an extended period of time. The pressure can disrupt blood flow to and through the limb, causing anaerobic metabolism and some tissue death. This causes a build-up of toxins in the blood stream. If blood flow returns to the limb, the blood may carry these toxins back to the central circulation. This acidic and toxic blood may then induce cardiac dysrhythmias or seriously damage the kidneys. Another consequence of the release of the crushing pressure is severe and difficult-to-control hemorrhage. The blood vessels within the limb are severely damaged, and bleeding results from many difficult-to-identify locations. With severe and prolonged crush injury entrapment, prehospital care may include sodium bicarbonate and other medications to combat the effects of acidosis, limit damage, and improve kidney function.

SUMMARY

Blunt trauma accounts for most injury deaths and disabilities. While vehicle crashes are the most frequent cause of blunt trauma, blast injuries, sports injuries, crush injuries, and falls also account for significant mortality and morbidity. Blunt trauma is difficult to assess accurately so you, as the care provider, must look carefully at the mechanism of injury and subtle physical signs to help anticipate serious internal injury. Careful analysis of the mechanism of injury, followed by development of indices of suspicion for injury can help guide you to recognize those patients needing rapid entry into the trauma system and those best served by on-scene care and transport to the nearest appropriate care facility.

End-of-Chapter Summary

Each end-of-chapter **Summary** reviews the main topics covered.

EMPHASIZING PRACTICE

Procedure 11-15   Examining the Knee

11-15a   Palpate the knee.

11-15b   Palpate the patella.

11-15c   Test the collateral ligaments of the knee.

11-15d   Test the cruciate ligaments of the knee.

11-15e   Assess knee flexion and extension.

Anatomical Regions   **669**

Procedure Scans

Newly photographed **Procedure Scans** provide step-by-step visual support on how to perform skills included in the DOT curriculum.

Procedure 11-17   Assessing the Spine

11-17a   Palpate the spine.

11-17b   Test flexion and extension of the head and neck.

11-17c   Test rotation of the head and neck.

11-17d   Assess lateral bending of the head and neck.

11-17e   Assess flexion of the lower spine.

11-17f   Assess lateral bending of the lower spine.

11-17g   Assess spinal extension.

11-17h   Assess spinal rotation.

672 CHAPTER 2   *Physical Exam Techniques*

USES FOR DOCUMENTATION

Content Review

USES FOR PCRs
• Medical
• Administrative
• Research
• Legal

Your PCR will be a valuable resource for a variety of people. They include medical professionals, EMS administrators, researchers, and occasionally, lawyers.

MEDICAL

Hospital staff (nurses and physicians) may need more information from you than they can get before you have to take another call. For example, they may want a chronological account of your patient's mental status from the time you arrived on the scene. Your PCR can tell the emergency department staff of your patient's condition before he arrived at the hospital. It serves as a baseline for comparing assessment findings and detecting trends that indicate improvement or deterioration. The surgical staff will want to know the mechanism of injury and other pertinent findings during your initial assessment of your patient and the scene.

If your patient is admitted to the hospital, the floor or intensive care unit staff may need more information about his original condition than he can remember. In addition, your PCR provides them with information from people at the scene to whom they might not have access—family, bystanders, first responders, or other witnesses. Knowing about the circumstances that led to the event or the mechanism of injury may also help rehabilitation specialists to provide better therapy. Your PCR becomes an important document that helps ensure your patient's continuous effective care (Figure 15-1).

Your PCR is an important document that helps ensure your patient's continuity of care.

＊ **response time** time elapsed from when a unit is alerted until it arrives on the scene.

ADMINISTRATIVE

EMS administrators must gather information for quality improvement and system management. Information regarding **response times,** call location, the use of lights and siren, and date and time is vital to evaluating your system's readiness to respond to life threatening emergencies. It is also essential to providing information of community needs. The quality improvement or quality assurance committee will use PCRs to identify problems with individual paramedics or with the EMS system. In some agencies, the billing department will need to determine which services are billable. Insurance carriers may need to know more about the illness or injury to process the claim. Some states will use your PCR data to allocate funding for regional systems.

Prehospital Care Report

Agency Name	ARLINGTON RESCUE	MILEAGE		USE MILITARY TIMES	
		END	2 4 4 9 6	CALL REC'D	0 7 0 5
Dispatch Information	CARDIAC	BEGIN	2 4 4 7 6	ENROUTE	0 7 0 7
Call Location	124 CYPRUS ST 2ⁿᵈ FLOOR	TOTAL	0 0 0 2 0	ARRIVED AT SCENE	0 7 1 9
CHECK ONE ☐ Residence ☐ Other Work Loc	☐ Health Facility ☐ Roadway ☐ Farm ☐ Recreational ☐ Indus. Facility ☐ Other	LOCATION CODE 0 1 1 2 4		FROM SCENE	0 7 3 8
CALL TYPE AS REC'D	MECHANISM OF INJURY			AT DESTIN	0 7 5 4
☑ Emergency	☐ MVA (✓ seat belt used) ☐ Knife			IN SERVICE	0 8 1 0
☐ Non-Emergency	☐ Fall of ____ feel ☐ Machinery			IN QUARTERS	0 8 3 2
☐ Stand-by	☐ Unarmed assault ☐ GSW				

FIGURE 15-1 The run data in a prehospital care report is vital to your agency's efforts to improve patient care.

Documentation

Covered thoroughly throughout the text, **proper documentation techniques** are critical to ensuring provider protection on the job as well as patient safety during the transition of care.

CALCULATING DOSAGES FOR ORAL MEDICATIONS

The following example illustrates how to calculate the volume of a specific drug dosage:

Example 1. A physician orders you to administer 90 mg of acetaminophen to a pediatric patient. The liquid acetaminophen is packaged as a concentration of 500 mg in 8 ml of solution. How much of the medication will you administer?

Because you cannot see the 90 mg of acetaminophen, you must convert this weight to a volume. To do so you need these facts:

desired dose = 90 mg

dosage on hand = 500 mg

volume on hand = 8 ml

Use the formula to calculate the dosage's volume:

$$\text{volume to be administered} = \frac{\text{volume on hand (8 ml)} \times \text{desired dose (90 mg)}}{\text{dosage on hand (500 mg)}}$$

volume to be administered = $(8 \times 90)/500$

volume to be administered = $720/500$

volume to be administered = 1.44

Administer 1.44 ml of solution to deliver 90 mg of acetaminophen.

Another way to calculate drug dosages is the ratio (fraction) and proportion method. A ratio (fraction) illustrates a relationship between two numbers. A proportion is the comparison of two numerically equivalent ratios. Using the variable x, the above problem can be stated:

$$8/500 \text{ mg} = x \text{ ml}/90 \text{ mg}$$

To solve the problem, cross multiply the numerals:

$$8/500 = x/90$$
$$720/500 = x$$
$$1.44 = x$$
$$x = 1.44 \text{ ml}$$

Math Summary 1

$$x \text{ ml} = \frac{8 \text{ ml} \times 90 \text{ mg}}{500 \text{ mg}}$$

$$x \text{ ml} = \frac{720}{500}$$

$$x \text{ ml} = 1.44$$

Math Summary 2

$$\frac{500 \text{ mg}}{8 \text{ ml}} = \frac{90 \text{ mg}}{x \text{ ml}}$$

$$x \text{ ml} = \frac{720}{500}$$

$$x = 1.44 \text{ ml}$$

CONVERTING PREFIXES

The following example shows how to calculate the volume to be administered when the desired dose, the dosage on hand, and the volume on hand are not all expressed in metric units with the same prefix.

Example 2. A physician orders you to give 250 mg of a drug via IV bolus. The multidose vial contains 2 grams of the drug in 10 ml of solution. How much of the medication should you administer?

Because the desired dose is expressed as *milli*grams, the dosage on hand must be converted from grams to milligrams. In the metric system, 2 grams equal 2000 milligrams. You now know:

desired dose = 250 mg

dosage on hand = 2000 mg

volume on hand = 10 ml

Medical Calculations

Mathematical examples are provided to give students practice in medical calculations, a critical skill in prehospital care.

TEACHING & LEARNING PACKAGE

FOR THE INSTRUCTOR

Instructor's Resource Manual (ISBN 0-13-099513-4)

The Instructor's Resource Manual contains everything needed to teach the 1998 U.S. DOT National Standard Curriculum for Paramedics. It fully covers the DOT curriculum with:

- lecture outlines
- innovative teaching strategies
- suggestions for additional resources
- student activities handouts for reinforcement and evaluation

The manual is also available on disk so instructors can customize resources to their individual needs.

PowerPoint® Presentations on CD-ROM (ISBN 0-13-021590-2)

This CD-ROM offers a comprehensive PowerPoint® presentation that contain word slides and images. The entire presentation can be tailored to your course needs.

Test Manager (ISBN 0-13-041385-2)

The Test Manager contains textbook-based questions in a format that enables instructors to select questions based on topic area and degree of difficulty.

FOR THE STUDENT

Student Workbook (ISBN 0-13-099521-5)

A student workbook with review and practice activities accompanies *Essentials of Paramedic Care*. The workbook includes multiple-choice questions, fill-in-the-blank questions, labeling exercises, case studies, and special projects, along with an answer key with text page references.

ONLINE RESOURCES

Paramedic Care Companion Website: www.prenhall.com/bledsoe2

This free site, tied chapter-by-chapter to the text, reinforces student learning through interactive online study guides, quizzes based on the new curriculum, and links to important EMS-related Internet resources. The *Paramedic Care* Companion Website also allows instructors to create a customized syllabus.

CourseCompass

The comprehensive CourseCompass package includes lecture notes, student activities and exercises, online testing, an electronic gradebook, email/chat communication tools, and a host of other user-friendly course management tools.

**For information on additional media to support the series, please contact your Brady representative:
1-800-638-0220**

INTRODUCTION TO ADVANCED PREHOSPITAL CARE

CHAPTER 1

Introduction to Advanced Prehospital Care

Objectives

Part 1: Introduction to Advanced Prehospital Care (begins on p. 6)

After reading Part 1 of this chapter, you should be able to:

1. Describe the relationship between the paramedic and other members of the allied health professions. (pp. 6–7)
2. Identify the attributes and characteristics of the paramedic. (p. 7)
3. Explain the elements of paramedic education and practice that support its stature as a profession. (pp. 7–8)
4. Define and give examples of the expanded scope of practice for the paramedic. (p. 8)

Part 2: EMS Systems (begins on p. 9)

After reading Part 2 of this chapter, you should be able to:

1. Describe key historical events that influenced the national development of Emergency Medical Services (EMS) systems. (pp. 9–12)
2. Define the following terms: EMS systems (p. 9), licensure (p. 17), certification (p. 17), registration (p. 17), profession (p. 17), professionalism

Continued

(p. 22), health-care professional (p. 18), ethics (p. 22), peer review (p. 22), medical direction (pp. 13–14), protocols (p. 14).

3. Identify national groups important to the development, education, and implementation of EMS as well as the role of national associations, the National Registry of EMTs, and the roles of various EMS standard-setting agencies. (pp. 18–19)

4. Identify the standards (components) of an EMS system as defined by the National Highway Traffic Safety Administration. (p. 12)

5. Differentiate among EMS provider levels: First Responder, Emergency Medical Technician-Basic, Emergency Medical Technician-Intermediate, and Emergency Medical Technician-Paramedic. (pp. 17–18)

6. Describe what is meant by "citizen involvement in the EMS system." (pp. 14–15)

7. Discuss the role of the EMS physician in providing medical direction, prehospital and out-of-hospital care as an extension of the physician, the benefits of on-line and off-line medical direction, and the process for the development of local policies and protocols. (pp. 13–14)

8. Describe the relationship between a physician on the scene, the paramedic on the scene, and the EMS physician providing on-line medical direction. (pp. 13–14)

9. Describe the components of continuous quality improvement and analyze its contribution to system improvement, continuing medical education, and research. (pp. 21–23)

10. Describe the importance, basic principles, process of evaluating and interpreting, and benefits of research. (p. 23)

Part 3: Roles and Responsibilities of the Paramedic (begins on p. 24)

After reading Part 3 of this chapter, you should be able to:

1. Describe the attributes of a paramedic as a health-care professional. (pp. 28–32)

2. Describe the benefits of paramedic continuing education and the importance of maintaining one's paramedic license/certification. (p. 32)

3. List the primary and additional responsibilities of paramedics. (pp. 25–28)

4. Define the role of the paramedic relative to the safety of the crew, the patient, and bystanders. (p. 25)

5. Describe the role of the paramedic in health education activities related to illness and injury prevention. (p. 27)

6. Describe examples of professional behaviors in the following areas: integrity, empathy, self-motivation, appearance and personal hygiene, self-confidence, communications, time management, teamwork and diplomacy, respect, patient advocacy, and careful delivery of service. (pp. 30–32)

7. Identify the benefits of paramedics teaching in their community. (p. 27)

8. Analyze how the paramedic can benefit the health-care system by supporting primary care for patients in the out-of-hospital setting. (p. 26)

9. Describe how professionalism applies to the paramedic while on and off duty. (p. 29)

Continued

Part 4: The Well-Being of the Paramedic (begins on p. 33)

After reading Part 4 of this chapter, you should be able to:

1. Discuss the concept of wellness and its benefits, components of wellness, and role of the paramedic in promoting wellness. (p. 33)
2. Discuss how cardiovascular endurance, weight control, muscle strength, and flexibility contribute to physical fitness. (pp. 33–37)
3. Describe the impact of shift work on circadian rhythms. (p. 47)
4. Discuss the contributions that periodic risk assessments and warning sign recognition make to cancer and cardiovascular disease prevention. (p. 35)
5. Differentiate proper from improper body mechanics for lifting and moving patients in emergency and non-emergency situations. (pp. 35–37)
6. Describe the problems that a paramedic might encounter in a hostile situation and the techniques used to manage the situation. (pp. 50–51)
7. Describe the considerations that should be given to using escorts, dealing with adverse environmental conditions, using lights and siren, proceeding through intersections, and parking at an emergency scene. (pp. 51–52)
8. Discuss the concept of "due regard for the safety of all others" while operating an emergency vehicle. (p. 52)
9. Describe the equipment available in a variety of adverse situations for self-protection, including body substance isolation steps for protection from airborne and bloodborne pathogens. (pp. 38–40, 50, 51–52)
10. Given a scenario where equipment and supplies have been exposed to body substances, plan for the proper cleaning, disinfection, and disposal of the items. (pp. 40–41)
11. Describe the benefits and methods of smoking cessation. (p. 35)
12. Identify and describe the three phases of the stress response, factors that trigger the stress response, and causes of stress in EMS. (pp. 45–47)
13. Differentiate between normal/healthy and detrimental physiological and psychological reactions to anxiety and stress. (pp. 47–48)
14. Describe behavior that is a manifestation of stress in patients and those close to them, and describe how that behavior relates to paramedic stress. (pp. 47–48)
15. Identify and describe the defense mechanisms and management techniques commonly used to deal with stress, the components of critical incident stress management (CISM) and provide example situations where CISM would be beneficial to paramedics. (pp. 47, 49–50)
16. Given a scenario involving a stressful situation, formulate a strategy to help adapt to the stress. (pp. 45–50)
17. Describe the stages of the grieving process (Kübler-Ross) and the unique challenges for paramedics in dealing with themselves, adults, children, and other special populations related to their understanding or experience of death and dying. (pp. 41–45)
18. Given photos of various motor-vehicle collisions, assess scene safety and propose ways to make the scene safer. (pp. 51–52)

Continued

Part 5: Illness and Injury Prevention (begins on p. 52)

After reading Part 5 of this chapter, you should be able to:

1. Describe the incidence, morbidity and mortality, and the human, environmental, and socioeconomic impact of unintentional and alleged unintentional injuries. (pp. 52–53)
2. Identify health hazards and potential crime areas within the community. (pp. 56–57)
3. Identify local municipal and community resources available for physical, socioeconomic crises. (pp. 54–55, 58)
4. List the general and specific environmental parameters that should be inspected to assess a patient's need for preventive information and direction. (pp. 56–58)
5. Identify the role of EMS in local municipal and community prevention programs. (pp. 52, 54–58)
6. Identify the injury and illness prevention programs that promote safety for all age populations. (pp. 56–59)
7. Identify patient situations where the paramedic can intervene in a preventive manner. (pp. 56–59)
8. Document primary and secondary injury prevention data. (pp. 58–59)

Part 6: Ethics in Advanced Prehospital Care (begins on p. 59)

After reading Part 6 of this chapter, you should be able to:

1. Define ethics and morals and distinguish between ethical and moral decisions in emergency medical service. (pp. 60–62)
2. Identify the premise that should underlie the paramedic's ethical decisions in out-of-hospital care. (p. 61)
3. Analyze the relationship between the law and ethics in EMS. (p. 60)
4. Compare and contrast the criteria used in allocating scarce EMS resources. (pp. 67–68)
5. Identify issues surrounding advance directives in making a prehospital resuscitation decision and describe the criteria necessary to honor an advance directive in your state. (pp. 64–65)

FIGURE 1-1 The paramedic is the highest level of prehospital care provider and the leader of the prehospital care team.

INTRODUCTION

Congratulations on your decision to become an EMT-Paramedic. Before you begin this rewarding endeavor, it is important to understand what the job of an EMT-Paramedic in the twenty-first century entails.

Emergency Medical Services (EMS) has made significant advances over the last thirty years. Not that long ago, the ambulance was simply a vehicle that provided rapid, horizontal transportation to the hospital. Today, equipped with the latest in equipment and technology, the ambulance is truly a mobile emergency room. The paramedic of the twenty-first century is a highly trained health care professional.

Emergency Medical Services (EMS) has made significant advances. Roles and responsibilities of the paramedic have advanced accordingly.

Part 1: Introduction to Advanced Prehospital Care

The paramedic is the highest level of prehospital care provider and the leader of the prehospital care team (Figure 1-1). As a member of the **allied health professions,** the paramedic is highly regarded by society.

The paramedic is the highest level of prehospital care provider and the leader of the prehospital care team.

✱ **allied health professions** ancillary health care professions, apart from physicians and nurses.

DESCRIPTION OF THE PROFESSION

The primary task of the paramedic is to provide emergency medical care in an out-of-hospital setting, extending the care of the emergency physician to the patient in the field. To function as a paramedic you must have fulfilled the prescribed requirements of the appropriate licensing or credentialing body. Paramedics may only function under the direction and license of the EMS system's medical director. Because of this, the paramedic must also be approved by the system's medical director before being permitted to practice.

There are many different types of EMS system designs and operations. As a paramedic, you may work for a fire department, private ambulance service, third city service, hospital, police department, or other operation. Regardless of the type of service you work for, as a paramedic you are an essential component in the continuum of care. Furthermore, paramedics often serve as a link between various health resources. While paramedics of the twenty-first century will continue to fill the well-defined and traditional role of 911 response, they will also find themselves taking on a wide variety of additional responsibilities. The emerging roles and responsibilities of the paramedic include public education, health promotion, and participation in injury and illness prevention programs. As a consequence of the need to cut costs, you may be charged with assuring that your patient gets to the appropriate health care facility, which may be a facility other than the hospital emergency department. Thus, the paramedic may begin to function as a facilitator of access to care as well as an individual treatment provider.

Paramedics must always strive toward maintaining high quality health care at a reasonable cost. Nevertheless, you must always be an advocate for your patient and assure that the patient receives the best possible care—without regard to the patient's ability to pay or insurance status.

Paramedics are responsible and accountable to the system medical director, their employer, the public, and their peers. Although this may seem like a difficult standard to meet, if you always act in the best interest of the patient, you will seldom run into problems.

PARAMEDIC CHARACTERISTICS

As a paramedic, you must be a confident leader who can accept the challenge and responsibility of the position. You must have excellent judgment and be able to prioritize decisions so as to act quickly in the best interest of the patient. You must be able to develop rapport with a wide variety of patients so that, for example, you can safely interview hostile patients and communicate with members of diverse cultural groups and the various ages within those groups. Overall, you must be able to function independently at an optimum level in a non-structured, constantly changing environment. The job is never easy and always challenging.

THE PARAMEDIC: A TRUE HEALTH PROFESSIONAL

Despite its relative youth as a profession, the field of emergency medical services is now recognized as an important part of the health care system. As a paramedic, you must never take this status for granted. Instead, you must always strive to earn your acceptance as a health care professional. Consider the completion of your initial paramedic course to be the start of your professional education, not the end. Participate in continuing education programs. Frequently review and practice skills, especially those less frequently used. Participate in routine peer-evaluation and assume an active role in professional and community organizations.

A major step toward the development of EMS as a true health care profession has been to raise the standards of education for prehospital personnel. A significant advance was the 1998 publication by the U.S. Department of Transportation of the revised *EMT-Paramedic: National Standard Curriculum*, which has taken paramedic education to a much higher level. The paramedic course now requires a far more extensive foundation of medical knowledge to underlie the required skills. The 1998 DOT paramedic curriculum is the guideline for this textbook.

You must always be an advocate for your patient and assure that the patient receives the best possible care—without regard to the patient's ability to pay.

Paramedics are accountable to their medical director, their employer, the public, and peers. However, if you always act in the best interest of the patient, you will seldom have problems.

You must be a confident leader—able to function independently at an optimum level in a non-structured, constantly changing environment. The job is never easy and always challenging.

You must always strive to earn your status as a health care professional.

The current EMT-Paramedic National Standard Curriculum provides for a much improved understanding of the pathophysiology of the various illness and injury processes.

Participation in research projects relevant to EMS is an important part of your profession as a paramedic.

As a paramedic, you must actively participate in the design, development, evaluation, and publication of research on topics relevant to your profession. For years, paramedic practice was based on anecdotal data and tradition. Only during the 1990s did we truly begin applying the scientific method to various aspects of prehospital practice. Surprisingly, we found that there was little or no scientific data to support many of our prehospital practices. As a result of research, many traditional EMS treatments have been abandoned or refined. There are still many unanswered questions about paramedic practice, and these can only be answered by sound, ongoing scientific research.

An essential aspect of a health professional is acceptance and adherence to a code of professional ethics and etiquette. The patient is always your primary concern.

Another essential aspect of a health professional is acceptance and adherence to a code of professional ethics and etiquette. The public must feel confident that, for the paramedic, the patient's and public's interests are always placed above personal, corporate, or financial interests. You must never forget that the patient is your primary concern.

EXPANDED SCOPE OF PRACTICE

Paramedics have a very bright future. New technologies and therapies can literally bring the emergency department to the patient. Paramedics must be willing to step up to these expanding roles, or persons from other health care disciplines will fill them. There are many aspects of out-of-hospital care that can provide you with the opportunity to work in an environment other than the typical 911-response vehicle. These include:

- *Critical Care Transport.* Paramedics manage complicated inter-hospital transports—typically from one intensive care unit to another—in specially equipped ambulances or aircraft designed to provide a higher level of care.
- *Primary Care.* In the era of managed care, one goal is to keep patients with non-emergency problems out of the hospital emergency department. As a result, the EMS system has been involved in triaging and directing patients to the proper non-hospital facilities. In many cases, cost-effective, convenient medical care can be provided in the field by paramedics with additional skills.
- *Tactical EMS.* Paramedics accompany specially-trained law enforcement officers on tactical operations such as hostage rescue, drug raids, and similar high-risk emergencies. The tactical paramedic is a member of the operations team but is also trained to provide sophisticated, prolonged, definitive patient care.
- *Industrial Medicine.* Paramedics specially trained in occupational health are used to staff construction sites, oil rigs, and other facilities where unique skills are required. These personnel may also serve as safety officers and inspectors.
- *Sports Medicine.* Many sports teams hire paramedics to complement their trainers. In this role, paramedics participate in pre-game preparation and assume responsibility for injury prevention. They are also trained to deal with injuries specific to the sport, such as orthopedic injuries, with the goal of returning players to action as quickly and safely as possible.

Paramedics are now stepping into new, non-traditional roles because of their unique education and ability to think and work independently.

Paramedics are now stepping into nontraditional roles such as these because of their unique education and ability to think and work independently.

Part 2: EMS Systems

An **emergency medical services (EMS) system** is a comprehensive network of personnel, equipment, and resources established to deliver aid and emergency medical care to the community. An EMS system is comprised of both out-of-hospital and in-hospital components. The out-of-hospital component includes:

- Members of the community who are trained in first aid and CPR
- A communications system that allows public access to emergency services dispatch and allows EMS providers to communicate with each other
- EMS providers, including paramedics
- Fire/rescue and hazardous-materials services
- Public utilities, such as power and gas companies
- Resource centers, such as regional poison control centers

The in-hospital component includes:

- Emergency nurses
- Emergency physicians and specialty physicians
- Ancillary services, such as radiology and respiratory therapy
- Specialty physicians, such as trauma surgeons and cardiologists
- Rehabilitation services

A typical EMS operation begins with citizen activation when someone contacts a 911 dispatch center. EMS dispatch collects essential information and sends out the closest appropriately staffed and equipped unit. In many EMS systems, the dispatcher also provides pre-arrival instructions to caller.

The first EMS provider at the scene may be a police officer, firefighter, lifeguard, teacher, or other community member who has been trained as a First Responder. The First Responder's role is to stabilize the patient until more advanced personnel arrive. The next EMS provider likely to arrive depends on the type of EMS system. In most areas, the dispatcher will send either a **basic life support (BLS)** or an **advanced life support (ALS)** ambulance. Other EMS systems use a "tiered response," sending multiple levels of emergency care personnel to the same incident. In still other areas, ALS personnel respond to every incident regardless of the level of care needed.

Once care has been initiated, EMS providers must quickly decide on the medical facility to which the patient should be transported—based on the type of care needed, transport time, and local protocols. Where specialty centers have been designated (such as pediatric, trauma, and burn centers), it may be necessary to transport the patient to a facility other than the closest hospital. At the receiving medical facility, an emergency nurse or physician assumes responsibility, and the patient is assigned a priority of care. If needed, a surgeon or other specialist will be summoned.

HISTORY OF EMS

There is evidence that emergency medicine has a very long history.

ANCIENT TIMES

Emergency medicine may be traced back to biblical times when it was recorded that a "good Samaritan" provided care to a wounded traveler by the side of a

✳ **emergency medical services (EMS) system** a comprehensive network of personnel, equipment, and resources established for the purpose of delivering aid and emergency medical care to the community.

✳ **basic life support (BLS)** refers to basic life-saving procedures such as artificial ventilation and cardiopulmonary resuscitation (CPR).

✳ **advanced life support (ALS)** refers to advanced life-saving procedures such as intravenous therapy, drug therapy, intubation, and defibrillation.

road. In fact, about 4,000 to 5,000 years ago, Sumerians inscribed clay tablets with some of the earliest medical records. Similar to EMS protocols today, the tablets provided step-by-step instructions for care based on the patient's description of symptoms as well as instructions on how to create and administer medications. The most striking difference between these first "protocols" and EMS today is the absence of a physical exam.

In 1862, the Egyptologist Edwin Smith purchased a papyrus scroll dating to about 1500 B.C.E. It contained 48 medical case histories with data arranged in head-to-toe order and in order of severity, an arrangement very similar to today's patient assessment. One section, the "Book of Wounds," explains the treatment of injuries such as fractures and dislocations.

At about the same time, King Hammurabi of Babylon created a code of laws known today as the "Code of Hammurabi." A section of the code regulated medical fees and penalties based on the social class of the patient. For example, if a surgeon operated successfully on a commoner, he would be paid only half of what his fee would be if he had operated on a rich man. If a surgeon caused the death of a rich man, the surgeon's hand would be cut off, but if a slave died under his care, he only had to replace the slave.

18TH AND 19TH CENTURIES

During the Napoleonic Wars of the early 19th century, one of Napoleon's chief surgeons, Jean Larrey, formed the *ambulance volante,* or "flying ambulance," which focused efforts on providing emergency surgery as close to the battlefield as possible. Though the *ambulance volante* was little more than a covered horse-drawn cart, Larrey is credited with the development of the first prehospital system that used **triage** and transport.

* **triage** a method of sorting patients by the severity of their injuries.

Between 1861 and 1865, during the U.S. Civil War, a nurse named Clara Barton coordinated care for the sick and injured. Defying army leaders, she persisted in going to the front where wounded men suffered and often died from lack of the simplest medical attention. She organized the triage and transport of injured soldiers to improvised hospitals in nearby houses, barns, and churches away from the battlefield.

The first civilian ambulance service was formed about the same time (1865) in Cincinnati, Ohio. Four years later, in 1869, the New York City Health Department Ambulance Service began operating out of Bellevue Hospital. The ambulances of both services were specially designed horse-drawn carts, which were staffed with physician interns from the various hospital wards.

20TH CENTURY

During World War I, a high mortality rate of soldiers was associated with an average evacuation time of 18 hours. As a result, in World War II a system was created in which battlefield ambulance corps transported wounded soldiers from the front lines to the echelons (levels) of care. However, many of the echelons were so far from the battlefield and each other that there were huge delays in patient care. In many cases, it was often days from the injury itself to definitive surgery.

During the Korean and Vietnam conflicts, there were great advances in the patient care delivery system. The wounded soldier was treated on the battlefield when the injury occurred and evacuated by helicopter to a field hospital to receive definitive surgery. In Viet Nam, in many cases, this occurred within 10–20 minutes. Once stabilized and able to be moved (generally within 24–48 hours), the patient would be flown by jet to Clark Air Force Base in the Philippines for further treatment. The decrease in the amount of time to definitive care plus the advances in medical procedures significantly reduced mortality rates.

Throughout history, significant advances in **trauma** care occurred during wartime. However, until the late 1960s, few areas of the U.S. provided adequate civilian prehospital emergency care. Medical care began in the hospital emergency department. Rescue techniques were crude, ambulance attendants poorly educated, and equipment minimal. Police, fire, and EMS personnel had no radio communication. Proper medical direction was not available, and the only interaction between physicians and EMS personnel was at the receiving facility.

Eventually, as costs and demand for additional services forced many rural mortician-operated ambulances to withdraw, local police and fire departments found that they had to provide the ambulance service. In many areas, volunteer ambulance services made up of local, independent EMS provider agencies proliferated. In the urban setting, the increased demand on hospital-based EMS systems resulted in the development of municipal services operated on city, county, or regional levels. However, because they could not communicate with each other, it was impossible to coordinate a response to any but the simplest local calls.

In 1966 the publication of "Accidental Death and Disability: The Neglected Disease of Modern Society" by the National Academy of Sciences, National Resource Council, focused attention on the problem. "The White Paper," as the report was called, spelled out the deficiencies in prehospital emergency care. It suggested guidelines for the development of EMS systems, the training of prehospital emergency medical providers, and the upgrading of ambulances and their equipment. This landmark publication set off a series of federal and private initiatives, including these:

- *1966* Congress passed the National Highway Safety Act, which established the U.S. Department of Transportation (DOT), a cabinet-level department. It provided matching grants to states for emergency medical services and forced them to develop effective EMS systems or risk losing federal highway construction funds. In 1969 the Emergency Medical Technician–Ambulance program was made public. The first paramedic curriculum followed in 1977.
- *1971* The White House gave nearly $9 million to EMS model demonstration projects.
- *1972* The Department of Health, Education, and Welfare funded a $16 million five-state initiative for the development of regional EMS systems. The next year, the Robert Wood Johnson Foundation provided approximately $15 million in grants for establishing regional EMS projects and communication systems.

Then, in 1973 Congress passed the Emergency Medical Services Systems Act, which provided additional funding for a series of projects related to the delivery of trauma care. As a result, the development of regional EMS systems continued from 1974 through 1981. A total of $300 million was allocated to study the feasibility of EMS planning, operations, expansion, and research.

In order to be eligible for this funding, an EMS system had to include the following 15 components: manpower, training, communications, transportation, emergency facilities, critical-care units, public safety agencies, consumer participation, access to care, patient transfer, standardized record keeping, public information and education, system review and evaluation, disaster management plans, and mutual aid. Unfortunately, the designers of this legislation omitted two major components: system financing and **medical direction.** The Emergency Medical Services Systems Act was amended in 1976 and again in 1979, and a total of $215 million was appropriated over a seven-year period toward the establishment of regional EMS systems.

In 1981, the passage of the Consolidated Omnibus Budget Reconciliation Act (COBRA) essentially wiped out federal funding for EMS. The small amount

* **trauma** a physical injury or wound caused by external force or violence.

Content Review

1973 EMSS ACT: 15 COMPONENTS OF EMS SYSTEMS

- Manpower
- Training
- Communications
- Transportation
- Emergency facilities
- Critical care units
- Public safety agencies
- Consumer participation
- Access to care
- Patient transfer
- Standardized record keeping
- Public information and education
- System review and evaluation
- Disaster management plans
- Mutual aid

* **medical direction** medical policies, procedures, and practices that are available to providers either on-line or off-line.

Content Review

**1988 NHTSA:
"10 System Elements"**

- Regulation and policy
- Resources management
- Human resources and training
- Transportation
- Facilities
- Communications
- Trauma systems
- Public information and education
- Medical direction
- Evaluation

✱ **trauma center** medical facility that has the capability of caring for the acutely injured patient. Trauma centers must meet strict criteria to use this designation.

✱ **quality improvement (QI)** an evaluation program that emphasizes service and uses customer satisfaction as the ultimate indicator of system performance.

of funding that remained was placed into state preventive-health and health-services block grants. The National Highway Traffic Safety Administration (NHTSA) attempted to sustain the efforts of the Department of Health and Human Services, but with its other EMS responsibilities and no additional funding, the momentum for continued development was lost.

In 1988, the Statewide EMS Technical Assessment Program was established by the National Highway Traffic Safety Administration (NHTSA). It defines elements necessary to all EMS systems. Briefly, they are:

- *Regulation and policy.* Each state must have laws, regulations, policies, and procedures that govern its EMS system. It also is required to provide leadership to local jurisdictions.
- *Resources management.* Each state must have central control of EMS resources so all patients have equal access to acceptable emergency care.
- *Human resources and training.* A standardized EMS curriculum should be taught by qualified instructors, and all personnel who transport patients in the prehospital setting should be adequately trained.
- *Transportation.* Patients must be safely and reliably transported by ground or air ambulance.
- *Facilities.* Every seriously ill or injured patient must be delivered in a timely manner to an appropriate medical facility.
- *Communications.* A system for public access to the EMS system must be in place. Communication among dispatchers, the ambulance crew, and hospital personnel must also be possible.
- *Trauma systems.* Each state should develop a system of specialized care for trauma patients, including one or more **trauma centers** and rehabilitation programs. It also must develop systems for assigning and transporting patients to those facilities.
- *Public information and education.* EMS personnel should participate in programs designed to educate the public. The programs are to focus on the prevention of injuries and how to properly access the EMS system.
- *Medical direction.* Each EMS system must have a physician as its medical director. This physician delegates medical practice to non-physician caregivers and oversees all aspects of patient care.
- *Evaluation.* Each state must have a **quality improvement** system in place for continuing evaluation and upgrading of its EMS system.

Many EMS providers today fail to realize that each component of the EMS system has gone through many stages of development. Nevertheless, in this technologically advanced country, there are still startling regional differences in the quality of prehospital care.

TODAY'S EMS SYSTEMS

Though EMS systems across the country and the world will vary, certain elements are essential to ensure the best possible patient care.

LOCAL AND STATE-LEVEL AGENCIES

At the municipal and regional levels, an administrative agency manages the local EMS system's resources, developing operational protocols, and establishing standards and guidelines. The agency's planning board should include emergency physicians, the emergency nurse association, the firefighter association, state and local police, and "consumers." It develops a budget and selects a qualified administrative staff. The agency designates who may function within the system and develops policies consistent with existing state requirements and creates a quality assurance or quality improvement program.

State EMS agencies are typically responsible for allocating funds to local systems, sponsoring legislation concerning the prehospital practice of medicine, licensing, and certification, enforcing state EMS regulations, and appointing regional advisory councils.

In essence, EMS is made up of a series of systems within a system. The integration of these systems and the cooperation of all participants help to result in the best quality of emergency care.

MEDICAL DIRECTION

An EMS system must retain a **medical director**—a physician who is legally responsible for all clinical and patient-care aspects of the system. Prehospital medical care provided by non-physicians is considered an extension of the medical director's license; that is, prehospital care providers are the medical director's designated agents, regardless of who their employers may be.

The medical director's role in an EMS system is to:

- Educate and train personnel
- Participate in personnel and equipment selection
- Develop clinical protocols in cooperation with expert EMS personnel
- Participate in quality improvement and problem resolution
- Provide direct input into patient care
- Interface between the EMS system and other health-care agencies
- Advocate within the medical community
- Serve as the "medical conscience" of the EMS system, including advocating for quality patient care

In addition to the responsibilities listed above, the medical director is the ultimate authority for all on-line (direct) and off-line (indirect) medical direction.

On-Line Medical Direction

On-line medical direction occurs when a qualified physician gives direct orders to a prehospital care provider by either radio or telephone (Figure 1-2). Medical direction may be delegated to a mobile intensive care nurse (MICN), a physician assistant (PA), or a paramedic. In all circumstances, ultimate on-line responsibility remains with the medical director.

On-line medical direction offers several benefits to the patient, including immediate medical consultation and use of telemetry to provide instant diagnostic information to the medical director. In most systems, on-line consultations can be recorded for review and quality improvement.

At the emergency scene, the provider with the most knowledge and experience in the delivery of prehospital emergency care should be in charge. When a non-affiliated physician, or **intervener physician,** is on scene and on-line medical direction does not exist, the paramedic should relinquish responsibility to the physician. However, the intervener physician must first identify himself, demonstrate a

* **medical director** a physician who is legally responsible for all of the clinical and patient-care aspects of an EMS system. Also referred to as *medical direction.*

All prehospital care providers are the medical director's designated agents, regardless of who their employer may be.

FIGURE 1-2 The medical director can provide on-line guidance to EMS personnel in the field.

* **on-line medical direction** occurs when a qualified physician gives direct orders to a prehospital care provider by either radio or telephone.

* **intervener physician** a licensed physician, professionally unrelated to patients on scene, who attempts to assist EMS providers with patient care.

willingness to accept responsibility, and document the intervention as required by the local EMS system. If his treatment differs from established protocol, the intervener physician must accompany the patient in the ambulance to the hospital. If an intervener physician is on scene and on-line medical direction does exist, the on-line physician is ultimately responsible. In case of a disagreement, the paramedic must take orders from the on-line physician.

Off-Line Medical Direction

✱ off-line medical direction refers to medical policies, procedures, and practices that medical direction has set up in advance of a call.

Off-line medical direction refers to medical policies, procedures, and practices that a system physician has set up in advance of a call. It includes "prospective medical direction," such as guidelines on the selection of personnel and supplies, training and education, and protocol development. It also includes "retrospective medical direction," such as auditing, peer review, and other quality assurance processes.

✱ protocols the policies and procedures for all components of an EMS system.

Protocols are the policies and procedures of an EMS system. They provide a standardized approach to common patient problems, a consistent level of medical care and a standard for accountability. Based on such protocols, the on-line physician can assist prehospital personnel in interpreting the patient's complaint, understanding assessment findings, and providing the appropriate treatment. Protocols are designed around the four "Ts" of emergency care:

✱ standing orders preauthorized treatment procedures; a type of treatment protocol.

- *Triage.* Guidelines that address patient flow through an EMS system, including how system resources are allocated to meet the needs of patients
- *Treatment.* Guidelines that identify procedures to be performed upon direct order from medical direction and procedures that are pre-authorized protocols called **standing orders**
- *Transport.* Guidelines that address the mode of travel (air vs. ground) based on the nature of the patient's injury or illness, the condition of the patient, the level of care required, and estimated transport time
- *Transfer.* Guidelines that address receiving facilities to ensure that the patient is admitted to the one most appropriate for definitive care

Protocols also are established for special circumstances, such as "Do Not Resuscitate" orders, patients who refuse treatment, sexual abuse, abuse of children or elderly people, termination of CPR, and intervener physicians. Although protocols standardize field procedures, they should allow the paramedic the flexibility to improvise and adapt to special circumstances.

PUBLIC INFORMATION AND EDUCATION

The public is an essential, yet often overlooked, component of an EMS system. EMS should have a plan to educate the public on recognizing an emergency, accessing the system, and initiating basic life support procedures.

Recognizing an emergency can save lives. For example, the American Heart Association (AHA) estimates that over 300,000 cardiac arrests per year occur before the patient reaches the hospital. Such arrests are called "sudden death" because most happen within two hours of the onset of cardiac symptoms. Many patients delay calling for help when symptoms occur. If the patient and bystanders are taught to recognize the emergency and call for help in time, many cases of sudden death could be prevented.

The second aspect of public education is system access. Citizens must know how to activate EMS in an emergency to avoid life-threatening delays. Whether access is by way of 911 or a local seven-digit phone number, the number should be well publicized, and citizens should be taught how to give the necessary information to the emergency medical dispatcher.

Finally, after recognizing an emergency and activating EMS, citizens must know how to provide basic life support assistance, such as cardiopulmonary resuscitation (CPR) and bleeding control after major trauma. Abundant research indicates that a relationship exists between EMS response times and mortality (death) rates of patients. Communities have proven that when many citizens are trained in basic life support—and, there is a rapid advanced life support (ALS) response—a larger number of patients can be successfully resuscitated.

Future public involvement may include bystander defibrillation. With the development of automated external defibrillator (AED) technology, it may soon be possible to place affordable, portable AEDs in the homes of cardiac patients as well as in all public places.

COMMUNICATIONS

The communications network is the heart of a regional EMS system. A communications plan should include:

- *Citizen access.* A well-publicized universal number, such as 911, provides direct citizen access to emergency services. Multiple community numbers add life-threatening minutes to emergency response times. Enhanced 911, or E-911, gives automatic locations of the caller, instant routing of the call to the appropriate emergency service (fire, police, or EMS), and instant callback capability.
- *Single control center* (Figure 1-3). One control center that can communicate with and direct all emergency vehicles within a large

FIGURE 1-3 The ideal communications center can communicate with and control the movement of all emergency units within an EMS system.

geographical area is best. Ideally, all public service agencies should be dispatched from the same communications center.

- *Operational communications capabilities.* With these, EMS dispatch can manage all aspects of system response and assess the system's readiness for the next response. Emergency units can communicate with each other and with other agencies during mutual aid and disaster operations. Hospitals also can communicate with other hospitals in the region to assess specialty capabilities.

- *Medical communications capabilities.* EMS providers can communicate with the receiving facility and, in many areas, transmit ECG telemetry signals to the on-line physician. Hospitals also can communicate with each other to facilitate patient transfer.

- *Communications hardware.* Radios, consoles, pagers, cell phone transmission towers, repeaters, telephone landlines, and other telecommunications equipment are required.

- *Communications software.* This includes radio frequencies and, in many systems, satellite and high-tech computer programs that track ambulances. Procedures, policies consistent with FCC standards and local protocols, and back-up communications plans for disaster operations are essential.

Emergency Medical Dispatcher (EMD)

The **emergency medical dispatcher (EMD)** is crucial to the operation of EMS. EMDs not only send ambulances to the scene, they also make sure that system resources are in constant readiness to respond. EMDs must be both medically and technically trained. The course should be standardized and include certification by a government agency.

EMS Dispatch

Emergency medical dispatching is the nerve center of an EMS system. It should be under the full control of the medical director and the EMS agency. In general, EMS system status management relies on projected call volumes and locations to make strategic placement of ambulances and crews. This method helps to reduce response times. Another management method, "priority dispatching," was first used by the Salt Lake City Fire Department. Using a set of medically approved protocols, EMDs are trained to medically interrogate a distressed caller, prioritize symptoms, select an appropriate response, and give life-saving pre-arrival instructions.

In 1974, the Phoenix Fire Department introduced a pre-arrival instruction program developed by medically trained dispatchers. In that program, callers initiate life-saving first aid with the dispatcher's help while they wait for emergency units to arrive on scene. In 1985, the Seattle EMS system initiated a successful program of instructing callers in CPR. Pre-arrival instruction may result in increased liability, but the liability risk of *not* providing it may far outweigh the risk of providing it.

An effective EMS dispatching system places BLS care on scene within four minutes of onset and ALS care in less than eight minutes.

An effective EMS dispatching system places the first responding units on scene within four minutes of the onset of the emergency. The American Heart Association (AHA) reports that brain resuscitation will not be successful unless there is proper BLS intervention (CPR) within four minutes. Studies also suggest that defibrillation within eight minutes can reverse sudden-death mortality. So, the goal of emergency response is: BLS care in less than four minutes and ALS care in less than eight minutes after the event. High-performance systems meet this standard more than 90 percent of the time.

EDUCATION AND CERTIFICATION

EMS education includes both initial and continuing programs. *Initial education* programs are the original training courses for prehospital providers. *Continuing education* programs include refresher courses for recertification and periodic in-service training.

Initial Education

A paramedic's initial education is completion of a course that follows the most recent "EMT-Paramedic: National Standard Curriculum" published by the U.S. DOT, which establishes the minimum content and sets a nationwide standard for paramedic programs. The National Standard Curriculum is divided into three specific learning domains:

- *Cognitive,* which consists of facts, or information knowledge
- *Affective,* which requires students to assign emotions, values, and attitudes to that information
- *Psychomotor,* which consists of hands-on skills students learn while in laboratory and clinical settings

Once initial education is completed, the paramedic will become either certified or licensed, depending on the state. **Certification** is the process by which an agency or association grants recognition to an individual who has met its qualifications. Many states certify paramedics.

Licensure is a process of occupational regulation. Through licensure, a governmental agency (usually a state agency) grants permission to engage in a given trade or **profession** to an applicant who has attained the degree of competency required to ensure the public's protection. Some states choose to license paramedics instead of certifying them. (Note that there is an unfounded general belief that a licensed professional has greater status than one who is certified or registered. However, a certification granted by a state, conferring a right to engage in a trade or profession, is in fact a license.)

Registration is accomplished by entering your name and essential information within a particular record. Paramedics are registered so that the state can verify the provider's initial certification and monitor recertification. Almost every state has an EMS office that tracks the registration of emergency care providers. While some states track only ALS providers, others maintain registers on the certifications of all provider levels. **Reciprocity** is the process by which an agency grants automatic certification or licensure to an individual who has comparable certification or licensure from another agency. For example, some states grant reciprocity to paramedics who are certified in another state.

Certification Levels

In 1983, because of variations in state and regional EMS terminology, there were as many as 30 levels of prehospital care providers. Since then, the National Registry of EMTs has recognized—and the DOT has developed curricula for—four different levels of providers. They are:

- *First Responder.* Usually the first EMS-trained provider to arrive on scene, the First Responder's role is to stabilize the patient until more advanced EMS personnel arrive. He is trained to perform a general patient assessment and to provide emergency care such as bleeding control, spinal stabilization, and CPR. He also may assist in emergency

* **certification** the process by which an agency or association grants recognition to an individual who has met its qualifications.

* **licensure** the process by which a governmental agency grants permission to engage in a given occupation to an applicant who has attained the degree of competency required to ensure the public's protection.

* **profession** refers to the existence of a specialized body of knowledge or skills.

* **registration** the process of entering your name and essential information within a particular record. In EMS this is done in order for the state to verify the provider's initial certification and to monitor recertification.

* **reciprocity** the process by which an agency grants automatic certification or licensure to an individual who has comparable certification or licensure from another agency.

Content Review

EMS CERTIFICATION LEVELS
- First Responder
- EMT-Basic
- EMT-Intermediate
- EMT-Paramedic

childbirth. In some areas, he is trained in the administration of oxygen and in the use of an automated external defibrillator (AED).

- *Emergency Medical Technician-Basic (EMT-B).* This EMS provider is trained to do all that a First Responder can do, plus perform complex immobilization procedures, restrain patients, and drive and staff ambulances. The EMT-B also may assist in the administration of certain medications and, in some areas, perform an endotracheal intubation.

- *Emergency Medical Technician-Intermediate (EMT-I).* The EMT-I should possess all EMT-B skills and be competent in advanced airway management, intravenous fluid therapy, and certain other advanced skills. In some states, the EMT-I may be trained as a cardiac technician and authorized to administer additional medications.

- *Emergency Medical Technician-Paramedic (EMT-P).* As the most advanced EMS provider, the paramedic is trained in all EMT-I skills, plus advanced patient assessment, trauma management, pharmacology, cardiology, and other medical skills. He should successfully complete advanced cardiac life support (ACLS) and pediatric advanced life support (PALS) courses offered by the American Heart Association. Basic trauma life support (BTLS) or prehospital trauma life support (PHTLS) course completion is also desirable.

In addition to gaining knowledge and skills, paramedics should have or acquire the high regard for human dignity and passion for excellence expected of all **health-care professionals.**

National Registry of EMTs

The National Registry of Emergency Medical Technicians (NREMT) prepares and administers standardized tests for the First Responder, EMT-Basic, EMT-Intermediate, and EMT-Paramedic. It establishes the qualifications for registration and serves as a major tool for reciprocity by providing a process for EMTs to become certified when moving from one state to another. The National Registry also develops and evaluates EMT training programs. Currently, the majority of states use National Registry examinations. Several states instead offer locally developed examinations.

Professional Organizations

Belonging to a professional organization is a good way to keep informed and share ideas. National EMS organizations include:

- National Association of Emergency Medical Technicians (NAEMT)
- National Association of Search and Rescue (NASAR)
- National Association of State EMS Directors (NASEMSD)
- National Association of EMS Physicians (NAEMSP)
- National Flight Paramedics Association (NFPA)
- National Council of State EMS Training Coordinators (NCSEMSTC)

These are just some examples of organizations through which EMS providers can enrich themselves and pursue their particular interests. Such organizations assist in the development of educational programs, operational policies and procedures, and the implementation of EMS. The Joint Review Committee on Educational Programs for the EMT-Paramedic is an example of a standard-setting organization. With input from national professional groups such as the NAEMT, it establishes national standardization within the didactic and clinical portion of paramedic education programs.

Professional Journals

The following is just a partial list of the many journals that are available to keep the paramedic aware of the latest changes in this ever-changing industry as well as offering an opportunity for EMS professionals to write and publish articles:

- *Annals of Emergency Medicine*
- *Emergency Medical Services*
- *Emergency*
- *Journal of Emergency Medical Services*
- *Journal of Emergency Medicine*
- *Journal of Pediatric Emergency Medicine*
- *Journal of Trauma*
- *Prehospital Emergency Care*

PATIENT TRANSPORTATION

Patients who are transported under the direction of an EMS system should be taken to the nearest appropriate medical facility whenever possible. Medical direction should designate that facility, based on the needs of the patient and the availability of services. In some cases, the patient's need for special services (such as care for burns) means designating a facility that is not nearby. At other times, the closest facility will be designated for stabilization of the patient while transfer is arranged. The ultimate authority for this decision remains with on-line medical direction.

Patients may be transported by ground or air. Today, trauma care systems use law enforcement, municipal, hospital-based, private, and military helicopter transport services to transfer patients. Fixed-wing aircraft also are used when patients must be transported long distances, usually more than 200 miles.

All transport vehicles must be licensed and meet local and state EMS requirements. In 1983, the American College of Surgeons Committee on Trauma recommended a standard set of equipment to be carried by providers of BLS services. In 1988, the American College of Emergency Physicians (ACEP) recommended a list of ALS supplies and equipment. These recommendations serve as guidelines for all prehospital EMS systems. Regional standardization of equipment and supplies is most effective in facilitating inter-agency efforts during disaster operations.

In 1974, in response to a request from the DOT, the General Services Administration developed the "KKK-A-1822 Federal Specifications for Ambulances." This was the first attempt at standardizing ambulance design. The act defined the following basic types of ambulances:

- *Type I*. A conventional cab and chassis on which a module ambulance body is mounted, with no passageway between driver's and patient's compartments.
- *Type II*. A standard van, body, and cab form an integral unit. Most have a raised roof.
- *Type III*. A specialty van with forward cab, integral body, and a passageway from driver's compartment to patient's compartment.

Only these certified ambulances may display the registered "Star of Life" symbol as defined by the National Highway Traffic Safety Administration (NHTSA). The word "ambulance" should appear in mirror image on the front so that other drivers can identify the ambulance in their rear-view mirrors.

In 1980, the revision "KKK-A-1822A" aimed at improving ambulance electrical systems by designing a low-amp lighting system to replace antiquated light bars and beacons. In 1985, another revision "KKK-A-1822B" specified changes based on National Institute for Occupational Safety and Health (NIOSH) standards. These include reduced internal siren noise, high engine temperatures, and exhaust emissions; safer cot-retention systems; wider axles; hand-held spotlights; battery conditioners for longer life; and venting systems for oxygen compartments.

All ambulances purchased with federal funds must comply with these criteria. However, some states have adopted their own stricter criteria.

RECEIVING FACILITIES

Not all hospitals are equal in emergency and support service capabilities. So how do you get the right patient to the right facility in an appropriate amount of time? EMS systems categorize hospitals according to their ability to receive and treat emergency patients. EMS coordinators use these categories to quickly identify the most appropriate facility for definitive treatment or life-saving stabilization. Regionalizing available services also helps give all patients reasonable access to the appropriate facility. Burn, trauma, pediatric, psychiatric, perinatal, cardiac, spinal, and poison centers are examples of specialty service facilities that offer high-level care for specific groups of patients in a wide region. Large EMS systems should designate a resource hospital that will coordinate specialty resources and ensure appropriate patient distribution.

To select the appropriate receiving facility for your patient, it is important to know which facilities in your area offer the following services:

- Fully staffed and equipped emergency department
- Trauma care capabilities
- Operating suites available 24 hours a day and seven days a week
- Critical care units, such as post-anesthesia recovery rooms and surgical intensive care units
- Cardiac facilities with on-staff cardiologists
- Neurology department that provides a "stroke team"
- Acute hemodialysis capability
- Pediatric capabilities, including pediatric and neonatal intensive care units
- Obstetric capabilities, including facilities for high-risk delivery
- Radiological specialty capabilities, such as computerized tomography (CT) and magnetic resonance imaging (MRI)
- Burn specialization for infants, children, and adults
- Acute spinal-cord and head-injury management capability
- Rehabilitation staff and facilities
- Clinical laboratory services
- Toxicology, including hazmat decontamination facilities
- Hyperbaric oxygen therapy capability
- Microvascular surgical capabilities for replants
- Psychiatric facilities

Receiving facilities are categorized by the level of care they can provide. For example, the American College of Surgeons categorizes trauma centers by levels:

- *Level I*—provides the highest level of trauma care
- *Level II*—may not have specialty pediatrics or a neurosurgeon on site
- *Level III*—generally does not have immediate surgical facilities available

A fourth designation may be given to specialty referral centers, which offer unique services. They include burn, pediatric, psychiatric, perinatal, cardiac, spinal, and poison centers.

Ideally, all receiving facilities should have the following capabilities: an emergency department with an emergency physician on duty at all times, surgical facilities, a lab and blood bank, x-ray capabilities available around the clock, and critical and intensive care units. They should have a documented commitment to participate in the EMS system, a willingness to receive all emergency patients in transport regardless of their ability to pay, and medical audit procedures to ensure quality care and medical accountability. Finally, receiving facilities should exhibit a desire to participate in multiple-casualty preparedness plans.

MUTUAL AID AND MASS-CASUALTY PREPARATION

Since the resources of any one EMS system can be overwhelmed, a mutual-aid agreement ensures that help is available when needed. Such agreements may be between neighboring departments, municipalities, systems, or states. Cooperation must transcend geographical, political, and historical boundaries.

Each EMS system should have a disaster plan for catastrophes that can overwhelm available resources. There should be a coordinated central management agency, integration of all EMS system components, and a flexible communications system. Frequent drills should test the plan's effectiveness and practicality.

QUALITY ASSURANCE AND IMPROVEMENT

The only acceptable quality of an EMS system is excellence. In 1997, the National Highway Traffic Safety Administration (NHTSA) released a manual called "A Leadership Guide to Quality Improvement for Emergency Medical Services Systems." Its guidelines are based on the following components:

- Leadership
- Information and analysis
- Strategic quality planning
- Human resources development and management
- EMS process management
- EMS system results
- Satisfaction of patients and other stakeholders

A **quality assurance (QA)** program monitors and measures the quality of clinical care delivered to patients through evaluation of objective data such as response times, adherence to protocols, patient survival, and other key indicators. QA programs document the effectiveness of the care provided. They also help to identify problems and selected areas that need improvement. A common complaint about QA programs is that they tend to identify only the problems and therefore focus only on punitive corrective action. Thus, prehospital personnel often view QA programs negatively.

Each EMS system should have a disaster plan that is practiced frequently.

The only acceptable quality of an EMS system is excellence.

Content Review

GUIDELINES FOR QUALITY IMPROVEMENT

- Leadership
- Information and analysis
- Strategic quality planning
- Human resources development and management
- EMS process management
- EMS system results
- Satisfaction of patients and other stakeholders

✱ **quality assurance (QA)** a program designed to maintain continuous monitoring and measurement of the quality of clinical care delivered to patients.

As a result, many EMS systems have taken QA a step further with a **continuous quality improvement (CQI)** program. A CQI program emphasizes customer satisfaction and includes evaluations of such aspects as billing and maintenance. In contrast to QA programs, CQI focuses on recognizing, rewarding, and reinforcing good performance. The dynamic process of CQI includes six basic steps: researching and identifying system-wide problems; elaborating on the probable causes; listing possible solutions; outlining a plan of corrective action; providing the resources and support needed to ensure the plan's success; and re-evaluating results continuously.

In general, EMS quality can be divided into two categories: "take-it-for-granted" quality and service quality.

"Take-It-for-Granted" Quality

People must be able to take it for granted that EMS will respond quickly to a 911 call and act at the highest level of **professionalism,** providing care that is safe, appropriate, and the best that is available.

When considering a new medication, process, or procedure, we must follow set rules before permitting its use in EMS. These rules, often called **rules of evidence,** were developed by Joseph P. Ornato, M.D., Ph.D. They include the following guidelines:

- *There must be a theoretical basis for the change.* That is, the change must make sense based on relevant medical science.
- *There must be ample research.* Any device or medication for patient care must be justified by adequate scientific human research.
- *It must be clinically important.* The device, medication, or procedure must make a significant clinical difference to the patient. For example, a defibrillator may mean the difference between living and dying for some patients, while color-coordinated stretcher linen has little clinical significance.
- *It must be practical, affordable, and teachable.* Some medical devices remain too expensive and too impractical for use in routine prehospital emergency care.

Another way to accomplish "take-it-for-granted" quality improvement is through the ongoing education of personnel. Paramedics can improve their skills by reading, taking classes, soliciting feedback on clinical performance from receiving hospitals, and following up on patients. **Peer review**—the process of EMS personnel reviewing each other's patient reports, emergency care, and interactions with patients and families—is another way for paramedics to improve their knowledge and skills.

Ethics are the standards that govern the conduct of a group or profession. Prehospital providers at all levels have an ethical responsibility to their patients and to the public. The public expects excellence from the EMS system, and we should accept no less than excellence from ourselves.

Service Quality

In the business world, service quality is called "customer satisfaction." This is the kind of quality that individual customers get excited about, feel good about, and tell stories about. These are the little extras that exceed a customer's expectations and elicit thank-you letters. Prime examples of customer satisfaction include patient statements such as: "You fed my cat before we left." "You remembered my name and introduced me to the nurse." "You held my hand." "You seemed like a friend when I needed one."

Customer satisfaction can be created or destroyed with a simple word or deed. A significant part of the way we communicate with one another is through body language and tone of voice. Paramedics who genuinely care about their patients communicate it in many subtle ways. From the patient's perspective this is much more important than IVs, backboards, and ECGs.

Customer satisfaction can be created or destroyed with a simple word or deed.

RESEARCH

The future enhancement of EMS is strongly dependent on the availability of quality research. The current trend of introducing "new and improved" ideas or new "high tech" equipment to existing procedures must be evaluated scientifically. Unfortunately, many EMS protocols and procedures in use today have evolved without clinical evidence of usefulness, safety, or benefit to the patient. One area that will rely heavily on research is funding. As managed care increases its influence, EMS systems will be forced to validate their effectiveness. Restrictions on reimbursement will drive the push for quality EMS research. Outcome studies will also be required to justify funding and assure the future of EMS.

The future enhancement of EMS is strongly dependent on the availability of quality research.

Future EMS research must address the following issues: Which prehospital interventions actually reduce morbidity and mortality? Are the benefits of certain field procedures worth the potential risks? What is the cost-benefit ratio of sophisticated prehospital equipment and procedures? Is field stabilization possible, or should paramedics begin immediate transport in every case?

Paramedics can play a valuable role in data collection, evaluation, and interpretation of research. The components of a research project include the following:

- Identify a problem, explain the reason for the proposed study, and state the hypothesis or a precise question.
- Identify the body of published knowledge on the subject.
- Select the best design for the study, clearly outline all logistics, examine all patient-consent issues, and get them approved through the appropriate investigational review process.
- Begin the study, and collect raw data.
- Analyze and correlate your data in a statistical application.
- Assess and evaluate the results against the original hypothesis or question.
- Write a concise, comprehensive description of the study for publication in a medical journal.

Current EMS practice must be justified by hard clinical data derived from an objective, valid program of ongoing research. EMS providers at all levels share the responsibility for identifying research opportunities, conducting peer review programs, and publishing the results of their projects. As leaders in the prehospital care environment, paramedics should set an example in the development of and participation in research projects.

SYSTEM FINANCING

At present in the U.S., there is a wide variety of EMS system designs. EMS can be hospital-based, fire- or police-department based, a municipal service, a private commercial business, a volunteer service, or some combination. Major differences exist in methods of EMS system finance, too. They range from fully tax-subsidized municipal systems to all-volunteer squads supported solely by contributions.

EMS funding can come from many sources. The most common is fee-for-service revenue, which may be generated from Medicare, Medicaid, private insurance companies, specialty service contracts, or private paying patients. Most of these sources of revenue are referred to as "third-party payers," because payment comes from someone other than the patient. To date, almost all third-party payers require the patient to be transported or the EMS service will not be compensated for a response. Reimbursement may also be based on the level of care the patient receives during transport.

Because of the high costs of health care and complex billing and reimbursement systems, the "Public Utility Model" and the "Failsafe Franchise" are becoming increasingly popular. In these systems, a municipality establishes the design and standards for the contract bid, then periodically—usually every three or four years—holds a wholesale competition open to the market. The provider firm that wins the contract must manage services properly and efficiently throughout the contract term or face severe penalties, usually in the form of fines. The use of models such as these shifts the financial burden of operating an EMS system from the local community to the service franchise.

Part 3: Roles and Responsibilities of the Paramedic

The roles and responsibilities of the paramedic are dramatically different than they were 10 years ago. Today, paramedic emergency care is an enormous responsibility for which you must be mentally, physically, and emotionally prepared. You will be required to have a strong knowledge of **pathophysiology** and of the most current medical technology. You will have to be capable of maintaining a professional attitude while making medical and ethical decisions about severely injured and critically ill patients (Figure 1-4). You will be required to provide not only competent emergency care but also emotional support to your patients and their families.

✳ **pathophysiology** the study of how disease affects normal body processes.

FIGURE 1-4 A paramedic provides emergency medical care to ill and injured patients.

PRIMARY RESPONSIBILITIES

A paramedic's responsibilities include emergency medical care for the patient and a variety of other responsibilities before, during, and after a call.

PREPARATION

Preparation includes making sure that inspection and routine maintenance have been completed on your emergency vehicle and on all equipment. It means restocking medications and intravenous solutions and checking their expiration dates. In addition, you must be very familiar with:

- All local EMS protocols, policies, and procedures
- Communications system hardware (radios) and software (frequency utilization and communication protocols)
- Local geography, including populations during peak utilization times, and alternative routes during rush hours
- Support agencies, including services available from neighboring EMS systems and the methods by which efforts and resources are coordinated

RESPONSE

During an emergency response, remember that personal safety is your number-one priority. If your ambulance crashes en route to an incident because of speeding or running red traffic lights, you will be of no benefit to the patient. Always follow basic safety precautions en route to an incident. Wear a seatbelt, obey posted speed limits, and monitor the road for potential hazards.

You must also get to the scene in a timely manner. Make certain you know the correct location of the incident and, en route, request any additional personnel or services that you think may be needed. Don't wait to ask for such assistance until you get to a chaotic scene. Learn to anticipate potential high-risk situations based on dispatch information and experience. For example, if any of the following is reported to be on scene, you may need to call for assistance:

- Multiple patients
- Motor-vehicle collisions
- Hazardous materials
- Rescue situations
- Violent individuals (patients or bystanders)
- Reported use of a weapon
- Knowledge of previous violence

PATIENT ASSESSMENT AND MANAGEMENT

Your primary responsibilities as a paramedic involve scene size-up and assessment and management of the patient (Figure 1-5). These topics will be discussed fully in subsequent chapters. Keep in mind that your primary concern is the safety of yourself, your crew, the patient, and bystanders.

APPROPRIATE DISPOSITION

As noted earlier, the mode of transport and the selection of receiving facility are critical decisions to be made for your patient. For example, you might opt for

FIGURE 1-5 During the initial assessment of your patient, you will look for and immediately treat any life-threatening conditions.

ground or air transport. You might choose the nearest medical facility or a facility with special treatment capabilities like burn care or hyperbaric oxygen therapy.

Most patients request transportation to the nearest medical facility. However, patients enrolled in managed care programs, such as health maintenance organizations (HMOs) or designated provider groups, may request transport to a facility approved by their group, which may be a facility other than the nearest hospital. Other patients may ask you to transport them to a facility outside of your run area. Even though the requested facility may be appropriate for the patient, there may be an equally appropriate hospital that is closer. Remember, you are responsible for patient care and, therefore, also ultimately responsible for selecting the transport destination. When in doubt, contact on-line medical direction for advice and support.

In some areas, paramedics provide **primary care.** They have well-defined protocols that allow them to treat patients at the scene and transfer them to facilities other than a hospital. For example, a child cuts his arm on a shard of glass. There is a simple two-inch laceration. Instead of transporting the patient to the hospital, using resources that are not needed for this patient, and incurring a costly emergency department fee for the family, the paramedics contact medical direction and request permission to transport the child to a local out-patient center.

Another type of disposition is "treat and release" in which paramedics assess the patient and provide emergency care. If they determine there is no need for further medical attention, they contact medical direction and request orders not to transport. In some systems, paramedics may then contact a specialized dispatch center where an office appointment is made with a local physician.

While disposition systems such as these are not widely accepted, the increasing numbers of people in managed care programs (which generally attempt to achieve optimum care while controlling costs) may change that. Innovative programs such as these are setting standards for the future of EMS.

PATIENT TRANSFER

The managed-care environment has caused many people—both laypersons and health-care providers—to occasionally question whether certain actions that are intended to reduce the cost of medical care are actually in the patient's best interest. For example, to avoid the cost of duplicating equipment and services in a number of facilities that serve the same geographic area, managed care systems have encouraged facilities to specialize and, often, to transfer patients to a facility that can provide the specific care needed.

Occasionally, there may be a question as to whether the transfer of a patient from one facility to another has been approved for cost reasons but may not actually be in the patient's best interest. When you are assigned to transport a patient, you share responsibility—with the receiving and accepting physician—for the treatment and care of the patient. When you are in doubt about the patient's stability for the duration of transport, or about the capabilities of the receiving facility, contact medical direction.

Prior to removing the patient from a hospital, request a verbal report from the primary-care provider (usually a registered nurse or a physician). Also request a copy of essential parts of the patient's chart, including a summary of the patient's past and present medical history. However, if the results of diagnostic tests taken at the facility are not ready when you are prepared to leave, do not delay patient transport. The data can be sent by fax, E-mailed, or telephoned to the receiving facility.

Your first priority during transport is the patient. While en route, contact the receiving facility and provide them with an estimated time of arrival (ETA) and an update on the patient's condition. Upon arrival at your destination, seek out the contact person (usually a registered nurse or physician). Provide that person with an updated patient report, including any treatment or changes in status while en route. All documents provided by the sending facility should be turned over to the receiving care provider along with a copy of your run report. If required by your service, obtain appropriate billing/insurance information at this time.

DOCUMENTATION

Maintaining a complete and accurate written patient care report is essential to the flow of patient information, to research efforts, and to the quality improvement of your EMS system. Documentation will be discussed in detail in Chapter 15.

RETURNING TO SERVICE

Once you have completed patient care, turned the patient over to the hospital staff, and completed all documentation, immediately prepare to return to service (Figure 1-6). Clean and decontaminate the unit, properly discard disposable materials, restock supplies, and replace and stow away equipment. If necessary, refuel the unit on the way back to your station or post. Review the call with crew members, including any problems that may have occurred. Such a dialogue can lead to solutions that enhance the delivery of quality patient care. Finally, the paramedic team leader should check crewmembers for signs of critical incident stress and assist anyone who needs help.

FIGURE 1-6 A paramedic's responsibility does not end with delivering the patient to the emergency department. Documentation, restocking, and a run critique are as important as the call itself.

ADDITIONAL RESPONSIBILITIES

The role of the paramedic involves duties in addition to those associated with emergency response. They may include training civilians in CPR, EMS demonstrations and seminars, teaching first aid classes, organizing prevention programs, and engaging in professional development activities. All involve taking an active role in promoting positive health practices in your community.

COMMUNITY INVOLVEMENT

Prehospital providers should take the lead in helping the public learn how to recognize an emergency, how to provide basic life support (BLS), and how to properly access the EMS system. A successful effort can save lives. Providing educational programs can also encourage positive health practices in the community, such as the American Heart Association's "prudent heart living" campaign. EMS injury prevention projects, such as seat-belt awareness and the proper use of child safety seats, are essential to the reduction of long-term disability and accidental death.

In order to decide what injury prevention projects need to be developed in a community, EMS systems often conduct illness and injury risk surveys. For example, an EMS service reviews run reports for a six-month period and finds they responded to 10 vehicle collisions at railroad crossings. A public safety campaign directed at the safe crossing of railroad tracks may be appropriate. Once an EMS service has identified a problem and target audience, they should seek community agencies—including the local political structure—to assist in the development, promotion, and delivery of the campaign.

Additional benefits of community involvement are the following: It enhances the visibility of EMS, promotes a positive image, and puts forth EMS personnel as positive role models. It also creates opportunities to improve the integration of EMS with other health-care and public safety agencies through cooperative programs.

COST CONTAINMENT

Promoting wellness and preventing illness and injury will be important components of EMS in the future. Some systems have already begun to direct resources toward the development of prevention and wellness programs that decrease the need for emergency services. The theory is to reduce the cost of the services provided to the community by decreasing the burden on the system.

One strategy is to establish protocols that specify the mode of transportation for non-emergency patients. Some systems already operate vans rather than ambulances to transport such patients to and from nursing facilities or from their residences to a doctor's office. Though an additional expense to the system, this service reduces emergency equipment costs and the demand for emergency personnel. The result is a decrease in the overall operating expense, which results in an increase in revenue.

Another strategy being used in many areas of the country is having EMS and hospitals team up to provide an alternative to the emergency department. They transport patients to freestanding outpatient centers or clinics, which ultimately reduces the cost of care to the patient and the system. The development of such alliances will undoubtedly continue. However, caution should be taken to ensure that the patient always receives the appropriate emergency care based on need, not cost.

CITIZEN INVOLVEMENT IN EMS

Citizen involvement in EMS helps to give "insiders" an outside, objective view of quality improvement and problem resolution. Whenever possible, members of the community should be used in the development, evaluation, and regulation of the EMS system. When considering the addition of a new service or the enhancement of an existing one, community members should help to establish what is needed. After all, they are your "customers," and their needs are your priority.

PROFESSIONALISM

A paramedic is a member of the health-care professions. The word *profession* refers to a specialized body of knowledge or skills. Generally self-regulating, a profession will have recognized standards, including requirements for initial and ongoing education. When you have satisfied the initial education requirements as a paramedic, you may then be either certified or licensed. The EMS profession has regulations that ensure that members maintain standards. For the paramedic, these regulations come in the form of periodic recertification with a specified amount of continuing education time.

The term *professionalism* refers to the conduct or qualities that characterize a practitioner in a particular field. Health-care professionals promote quality patient care and pride in their profession, setting and striving for the highest standards and earning the respect of team members and the public. Attaining professionalism requires an understanding of what distinguishes the professional from the non-professional.

PROFESSIONAL ATTITUDES

A commitment to excellence is a daily activity. While on duty, health-care professionals place their patients first; non-professionals place their egos first. True professionals establish excellence as their goal and never allow themselves to become complacent about their performance. They practice their skills to the point of mastery and then keep practicing them to stay sharp and improve. They also take refresher courses seriously, because they know they have forgotten a lot and because they are eager for new information. Non-professionals believe their skills will never fade.

Professionals set high standards for themselves, their crew, their agency, and their system. Non-professionals aim for the minimum standard and can be counted on to take the path of least resistance. Professionals critically review their performance, always seeking ways to improve. Non-professionals look to protect themselves, hide their inadequacies, and place blame on others. Professionals check out all equipment prior to the emergency response. Non-professionals hope that everything will work, supplies will be in place, batteries will be charged, and oxygen levels will be adequate.

A professional paramedic is responsible for acting in a professional manner both on and off duty. Remember, the community you serve will judge other EMS providers, the service you work for, and the EMS profession as a whole by your actions.

Professionalism is an attitude, not a matter of pay. It cannot be bought, rented, or faked. Although it is a young industry, EMS has achieved recognition as a bona fide allied health profession. Gaining professional stature is the result of many hard-working, caring individuals who refused to compromise their standards. Always strive to maintain that level of performance and commitment.

PROFESSIONAL ATTRIBUTES

Leadership

Leadership is an important but often forgotten aspect of paramedic training. Paramedics are the prehospital team leaders (Figure 1-7). They must develop a leadership style that suits their personalities and gets the job done. Although there are many successful styles of leadership, certain characteristics are common to all great leaders. They include:

- Self-confidence
- Established credibility
- Inner strength
- Ability to remain in control
- Ability to communicate
- Willingness to make a decision
- Willingness to accept responsibility for the consequences of the team's actions

FIGURE 1-7 As leader of the EMS team, the paramedic must interact with patients, bystanders, and other rescue personnel in a professional and efficient manner.

The successful team leader knows the members of the crew, including each one's capabilities and limitations. Ask crew members to do something beyond their capabilities and they will question your ability to lead, not their ability to perform.

Integrity

The patient and other members of the health-care team assume that you, as a paramedic, have integrity. The single most important behavior that you will be judged by is honesty. Your work will often put you in the patient's home or in charge of the patient's wallet and other personal possessions, such as jewelry and items left in a vehicle. You must be trustworthy. The easiest way to lose respect is to be dishonest. Additionally, in acting as an agent of the medical director, you are entrusted with carefully following protocols, providing the best possible care, and accurately documenting it.

Empathy

One of the most important components to successful interaction with a patient and family is empathy. To have empathy is to identify with and understand the circumstances, feelings, and motives of others. As a professional, you will often have to place your own feelings aside to deal with others, even when you are having a bad day. Paramedics who act in a professional manner can show empathy by:

- Being supportive and reassuring
- Demonstrating an understanding of the patient's feelings and the feelings of the family
- Demonstrating respect for others
- Having a calm, compassionate, and helpful demeanor

Self-Motivation

You will often work without direct supervision, so it is up to you to be able to motivate yourself and establish a positive work ethic. Examples of a positive work ethic are:

- Completing assigned duties without being asked or told to do so
- Completing all duties and assignments without the need for direct supervision
- Correctly completing all paperwork in a timely manner
- Demonstrating a commitment to continuous quality improvement
- Accepting constructive feedback in a positive manner
- Taking advantage of learning opportunities

Appearance and Personal Hygiene

From the moment you arrive at the scene of an emergency, you are judged by the way you present yourself. Good appearance and personal hygiene are critical. If you have a sloppy appearance, your patient may suspect that your medical care will be sloppy, too. Slang, foul, abusive, or off-color language is not acceptable and will alienate you from your patients. Your appearance, as well as your behavior, are vital to establishing credibility and instilling confidence.

Always wear a clean, pressed uniform. Multiple pagers and holsters with tape hanging from them, or rubber gloves pulled through a belt loop, simply do not give you a professional appearance. Also, avoid wearing an abundance of patches and pins on your uniform. Remember that it is the care you provide, not the patches and pins you wear, that will impress the patient. Keep hair off the collar. If facial hair is allowed, keep it neat and trimmed. A light-colored tee shirt may be worn under your uniform shirt, which should be buttoned up, with only the top collar button open. Jewelry, other than a wedding ring, a watch, or small plain earrings for a female, is unprofessional. Long fingernails that have the potential to puncture protective gloves also should be avoided.

Self-Confidence

The patient and family will not trust you if they sense you do not trust yourself. A lack of self-confidence shows and is the basis of many lawsuits. The easiest way to gain self-confidence is to accurately assess your strengths and limitations, then seek every opportunity to improve any weaknesses. Also, keep in mind that self-confidence does not equal cockiness. When a self-confident paramedic is presented with a complex situation, he will ask for assistance.

Communication

Communication is a skill often underestimated in EMS services. Providing emergency care in the prehospital environment requires constant communication with the patient, family, and bystanders, as well as with other EMS providers and rescuers from other public agencies. Communication skills are discussed in detail in later chapters.

Time Management

The experienced paramedic who plans ahead, prioritizes tasks, and organizes them to make maximum use of time will generally be more effective in the field. A paramedic with good time-management skills is punctual for shifts and meetings and completes tasks such as paperwork and maintenance duties on or ahead of schedule.

Some simple time-management techniques that you can use are making lists, prioritizing tasks, arriving at meetings or appointments early, and keeping a personal calendar. By implementing just one or two of these techniques, you may find your schedule to be more manageable and less stressful.

Teamwork and Diplomacy

The paramedic is a leader. Leadership implies the ability to work with other people—to foster teamwork. Teamwork requires diplomacy, or tact and skill in dealing with people, even when you are under siege from the patient or family. Diplomacy requires the paramedic to place the interests of the patient or team ahead of his own interests. It means listening to others, respecting their opinions, and being open-minded and flexible when it comes to change. A strong leader of any team realizes that he will be successful only if he has the support of all team members. A confident leader will:

- Place the success of the team ahead of personal self-interests
- Never undermine the role or opinion of another team member
- Provide support for members of the team, both on and off duty

- Remain open to suggestions from team members and be willing to change for the benefit of the patient
- Openly communicate with everyone
- Above all, respect the patient, other care providers, and the community you serve

Respect

To respect others is to show—and feel—deferential regard, consideration, and appreciation for them. A paramedic respects all patients, and provides the best possible care to each and every one of them, no matter what their race, religion, sex, age, or economic condition. Showing that you care for a patient's or family member's feelings, being polite, and avoiding the use of demeaning or derogatory language toward even the most difficult patients are simple ways to demonstrate respect.

Patient Advocacy

The paramedic should always be an advocate for the patient.

A paramedic is an advocate for patients, defending them, protecting them, and acting in their best interests. Except when your safety is threatened, you should always place the needs of your patient above your own.

Careful Delivery of Service

Professionalism requires the paramedic to deliver the highest quality of patient care with very close attention to detail. Examples of behaviors that demonstrate a careful delivery of service include:

- Mastering and refreshing skills
- Performing complete equipment checks
- Careful and safe ambulance operations
- Following policies, procedures, and protocols

CONTINUING EDUCATION AND PROFESSIONAL DEVELOPMENT

Only through continuing education and recertification can the public be assured that quality patient care is being delivered consistently. So after you are certified and/or licensed, you have an important responsibility to continue your personal and professional development. Remember, everyone is subject to the decay of knowledge and skills over time. Use this as a rule of thumb: As the volume of calls decreases, training should correspondingly increase. Refresher requirements and courses vary from state to state, but the goal is the same: to review previously learned materials and to receive new information.

The paramedic must continually strive to stay abreast of changes in EMS.

Since EMS is a relatively young industry, new technology and data emerge rapidly. Make a conscious effort to keep up. A variety of journals, seminars, computer news groups, and learning experiences are available to help. So are professional EMS organizations at the local, state, and national levels. Additionally, by participating in activities designed to address work-related issues—such as case reviews and other quality improvement activities, mentoring programs, research projects, multiple-casualty incident drills, in-hospital rotations, equipment in-services, refresher courses, and self-study exercises, you can expect substantial career growth.

Part 4: The Well-Being of the Paramedic

Well-being, or wellness, is a fundamental aspect of top-notch performance in EMS. It includes your physical well-being as well as your mental and emotional well-being.

This section discusses the many elements of well-being. If you listen now and enhance your knowledge later, you stand a good chance of enjoying a long and rewarding career of helping others—all because you helped yourself.

> *Well-being is a fundamental aspect of top-notch performance.*

BASIC PHYSICAL FITNESS

The benefits of achieving acceptable physical fitness are well known. They include a decreased resting heart rate and blood pressure, increased oxygen-carrying capacity, increased muscle mass and metabolism, and increased resistance to illness and injury. Quality of life is enhanced as is self-image. Other benefits are improved mental outlook, reduced anxiety levels, and enhanced ability to maintain sound motor skills throughout life.

CORE ELEMENTS

Core elements of physical fitness are cardiovascular endurance (aerobic capacity), muscular strength, and flexibility. Like a three-legged stool, if any one of the three is deficient, the whole becomes unstable. Each is equally important.

Be careful about plunging into a well-intended effort to get in shape. For example, before starting an exercise or stretching regimen, it can be helpful to measure your current state of fitness. There are various methods of assessing the three core elements of fitness. Many EMS agencies have access to facilities where precise assessment methods—with trained personnel—are available. Take advantage of any information available to you.

Muscular strength is achieved with regular exercise that may be isometric or isotonic. **Isometric exercise** is active exercise performed against stable resistance, where muscles are exercised in a motionless manner. **Isotonic exercise** is active exercise during which muscles are worked through their range of motion. Weight lifting is an obvious way to achieve muscular strength, and it is excellent all-around training for the body. Rotate between training the muscles of your upper body and shoulders, chest and back, and lower body. Do abdominal exercises daily. Take time to get in-depth information about the best approach from a trainer or other knowledgeable person.

Cardiovascular endurance results from exercising at least three days a week vigorously enough to raise your pulse to its target heart rate (Table 1-1). There is no need to become a marathon runner to gain aerobic capacity. Try a brisk walk, or ride a stationary bike while watching TV. Make it a daily habit. Even modest exercise helps. Walking briskly from the outer reaches of the employee parking lot, using stairs whenever possible, and playing actively with your children can all "count" toward physical fitness.

Flexibility seems to be the forgotten element of fitness. Without an adequate range of motion, your joints and muscles cannot be used efficiently or safely. A body builder with tight hamstrings may be as much at risk for back injury as anyone else. To achieve (or regain) flexibility, stretch the main muscle groups regularly. Try to stretch daily. Never bounce when stretching; this causes micro-tears in muscle and connective tissues. Hold a stretch for at least 60 seconds. A side benefit of good flexibility is prevention or reduction of back pain. Stretching is an excellent TV-time activity. If you are interested, consider studying yoga.

Content Review

BASICS OF PHYSICAL FITNESS

- Cardiovascular endurance
- Strength and flexibility
- Nutrition and weight control
- Disease prevention
- Freedom from harmful habits and addictions
- Back safety

---

* **isometric exercise** active exercise performed against stable resistance, where muscles are exercised in a motionless manner.

* **isotonic exercise** active exercise during which muscles are worked through their range of motion.

Table 1-1	FINDING YOUR TARGET HEART RATE

1. Measure your resting heart rate. (You will use this total later).
2. Subtract your age from 220. This total is your estimated maximum heart rate.
3. Subtract your resting heart rate from your maximum heart rate, and multiply that figure by 0.7.
4. Add the figure you just calculated to your resting heart rate.

EXAMPLE: In a 44-year-old woman whose resting heart rate is 52, maximum heart rate would be 176 (220 − 44). Maximum heart rate minus resting heart rate is 124 (176 − 52). Multiply 124 by 0.7 for a value of 86.8. Resting heart rate plus the calculated figure is 138.8 (52 + 86.8). Rounded up, this person's target heart rate is 140 beats per minute.

NUTRITION

Good nutrition is fundamental to your well-being because your food is your fuel. So, in addition to eating balanced meals, you must also eat in moderation, limit fat consumption, and exercise. One key to eating well is to learn the major food groups and eat a variety of foods from them daily:

- *Grains/breads*. 6–11 servings per day, for complex carbohydrates, B vitamins, and fiber
- *Vegetables*. 3–5 servings per day, for fiber, iron, vitamins A and C, and folate
- *Fruits*. 2–4 servings per day, for vitamins A and C, potassium, and fiber
- *Dairy products*. 2–3 servings per day, for calcium, protein, and vitamins A and D
- *Meat/fish*. 2–3 servings per day, for protein, zinc, iron, and B vitamins

Avoid or minimize intake of fat, salt, sugar, cholesterol, and caffeine. For example, you can avoid a dose of fat by eating lean instead of marbled meat. An apple is far more nutritious than a slice of apple pie. In general, aim for a diet that is approximately 40% carbohydrates, 40% protein, and 20% fat. Food portions also have a significant impact on body weight. Even a well planned, healthy diet can result in weight gain if the portions are too large. Note that snacking is a weight-gain trap. Plan to eat low-calorie snacks, and buy them *before* you get hungry. Food labels (Figure 1-8) contain abundant information about nutritional content. Learn to read them. Standardization of food labels has reduced much of the confusion. Be sure to check the serving size to avoid misinterpreting the food's overall nutritional value.

Eating on the run, as EMS providers must often do, can be less detrimental if you plan ahead and carry a small cooler filled with whole-grain sandwiches, cut vegetables, fruit, and other wholesome foods. If you must, stop at a local market instead of the fast-food place next door. Buy fresh fruit, yogurt, and sensible deli selections. They are more nutritious and much cheaper than "fast foods." Monitor your fluid intake. Your body needs plenty of fluids to flush food through your system and eliminate toxins. Fill a "go-cup" with fresh ice water when you stop by the emergency department instead of spending your money on soft drinks.

Nutrition Facts
Serving Size 8 fl oz (240 mL)
Servings Per Container 8

Amount Per Serving	
Calories 110 Calories from Fat 0	

	% Daily Value*
Total Fat 0g	0%
Sodium 0mg	0%
Potassium 450mg	13%
Total Carbohydrate 26g	9%
Sugars 22g	
Protein 2g	

Vitamin C 120%	•	Calcium	2%
Thiamin 10%	•	Niacin	4%
Vitamin B6 6%	•	Folate	15%

Not a significant source of saturated fat, cholesterol, dietary fiber, vitamin A and iron.

* Percent Daily Values are based on a 2,000 calorie diet.

FIGURE 1-8 Example of a standardized food label.

PREVENTING CANCER AND CARDIOVASCULAR DISEASE

Exercising and eating well can help you prevent both cancer and cardiovascular disease. Although for the typically youthful EMS provider, the likelihood of being hit by either of these diseases seems remote, it happens. You can do a lot to prevent it. Minimizing stress through healthy stress management practices, for example, can work wonders. In addition, assess yourself and your family history.

Exercise will improve cardiovascular endurance, help lower blood pressure, and tip the balance of your body composition favorably—all good measures against cardiovascular disease. Know your cholesterol and triglyceride levels, and keep them in check. For women who are menopausal, be informed about the risks and benefits of using hormone replacement therapy (particularly estrogen).

Diet can also do much to minimize the chances of getting certain cancers. Certain foods, such as broccoli and high-fiber foods, can help reduce the incidence of cancer; others, such as charcoal-cooked foods, can increase it. The connection between sun exposure and skin cancer is well known. So, take the precaution of using sunblocks and wear sunglasses and a hat when you can. Watch out for the warning signs of cancer, such as blood in the stools (even in young people, especially men), a changing mole, unexplained weight loss, unexplained chronic fatigue, and lumps.

Be sure to include appropriate periodic risk-assessment screening and self-examination habits in your personal well-being program. That includes tests like mammograms and prostate exams as you gain in years.

HABITS AND ADDICTIONS

Many people who work high-stress jobs overuse and abuse substances such as caffeine and nicotine. These bad habits are rampant in EMS. Each can contribute to long-term diseases such as cancer and cardiovascular disease. Choose a healthier life, and avoid overindulging in these and other harmful substances such as alcohol. For example, smoking cessation programs are usually easily accessed local areas or on the internet. Whatever it takes, the message is clear: get free of addictions, particularly those that threaten your well-being. Substance abuse programs, nicotine patches, 12-step groups—all exist to help you help yourself. But the first step has to be yours.

BACK SAFETY

EMS is a physically demanding endeavor. Of the host of movements needed (scrambling down embankments, climbing ladders or trees, squeezing into narrow spaces, and so on), none will be more frequent than lifting and carrying equipment and patients. To avoid back injury, you must keep your back fit for the work you do. You also must use proper lifting techniques each time you pick up a load, whether the load is heavy or light.

Back fitness begins with conditioning the muscles that support the spinal column. These are the "guy wires" that stabilize the spine, much the way cables help keep telephone poles upright. Note that the muscles of the abdomen are also crucial to overall spinal-column strength and safe lifting. Never perform old-fashioned sit-ups. They can seriously strain your lumbar spine. Instead, use abdominal crunches, which target only the stomach muscles. Consult an exercise coach or trainer for specifics.

Correct posture will minimize the risk of back injury (Figure 1-9). Good nutrition helps to maintain healthy connective tissue and intervertebral discs. Excess weight contributes to disc deterioration. So does smoking. Thus, proper weight

Pay particular attention to keeping your back fit for the work you do. Always use the proper techniques for lifting and moving patients and equipment.

FIGURE 1-9A Correct standing posture.

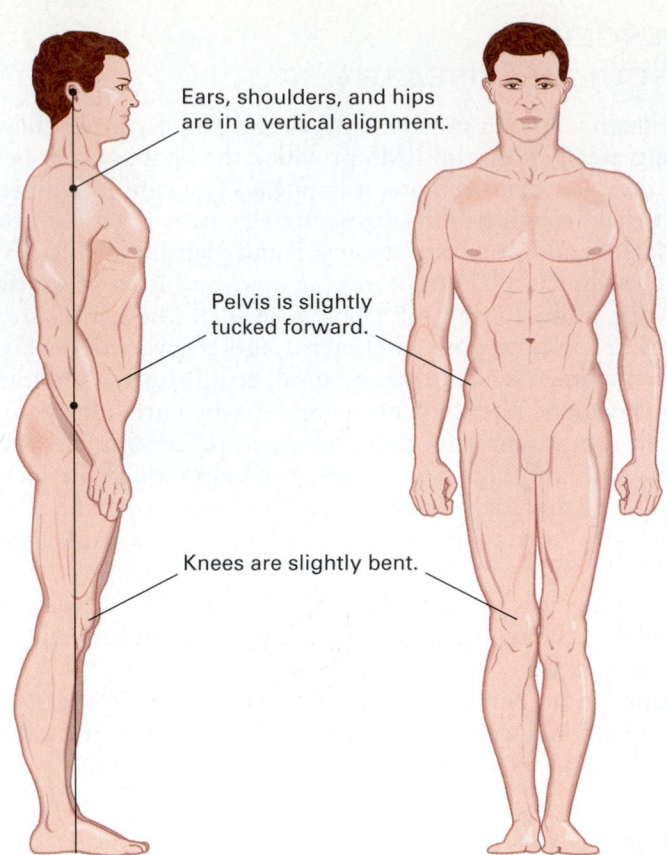

Ears, shoulders, and hips are in a vertical alignment.

Pelvis is slightly tucked forward.

Knees are slightly bent.

FIGURE 1-9B Correct sitting posture. Note the straight line from ear through shoulder and hip and from knee to arch of foot.

Ears, shoulders, and hips are in vertical alignment.

Pelvis is slightly tucked forward.

Weight is evenly distributed on both ischia.

Feet are flat on floor or crossed at ankles.

management and smoking cessation are relevant to back health. Finally, adequate rest gives the spine non-weight-bearing time to nourish discs and repair itself.

Proper lifting techniques should ideally be taught by and practiced with a trainer who understands the variety of challenges faced by EMS providers. Important principles of lifting are as follows:

- Move a load only if you can safely handle it.
- Ask for help when you need it—for *any* reason.
- Position the load as close to your body and center of gravity as possible.
- Keep your palms up whenever possible.
- Do not hurry. Take the time you need to establish good footing and balance. Keep a wide base of support with one foot ahead of the other.
- Bend your knees, lower your buttocks, and keep your chin up. If your knees are bad, do not bend them more than 90 degrees.
- "Lock in" the spine with a slight extension curve, and tighten the abdominal muscles to support spinal positioning.
- Always avoid twisting and turning.
- Let the large leg muscles do the work of lifting, not your back.
- Exhale during the lift. Do not hold your breath.
- Given a choice, push. Do not pull.
- Look where you are walking or crawling. Take only short steps, if you are walking. Move forward rather than backward whenever possible.
- When rescuers are working together as a team to lift a load, only one person should be in charge of verbal commands.

Heed your own body's signals. You are stronger some days than others. Know when you are physically depleted due to exhaustion, lack of food, or minor illness. Use volunteers wisely, and be sure to ask if their backs are strong enough for the job.

Never reach for an item, or attempt to lift it, and twist at the same time. Most back injuries occur because of the cumulative effect of such low-level everyday stresses. Everything you do on behalf of back safety adds up to choices that can mean the difference between a long and rewarding career in EMS, or one shortened by an injury. Be careful!

PERSONAL PROTECTION FROM DISEASE

In recent years the emphasis on infection control has focused on the most devastating diseases, such as HIV/AIDS, hepatitis B, and tuberculosis—and rightly so. Fortunately, there is a lot you can do to minimize your risk of infection. A good first step is to develop a habit of doing the things promoted in this chapter. Eating well, getting adequate rest, and managing stress are among the building blocks of a good defense against infection. In addition, it is a good idea to periodically assess your risk for infection, such as noticing when you are run down or when your hands are dangerously chapped.

✳ infectious disease any disease caused by the growth of pathogenic microorganisms, which may be spread from person to person.

INFECTIOUS DISEASES

Infectious diseases are caused by **pathogens** such as bacteria and viruses, which may be spread from person to person. For example, infection by way of bloodborne

✳ pathogens microorganisms capable of producing disease, such as bacteria and viruses.

Table 1-2 COMMON INFECTIOUS DISEASES

Disease	Mode of Transmission	Incubation Period
AIDS (Acquired Immune Deficiency Syndrome)	AIDS- or HIV-infected blood via intravenous drug use, semen and vaginal fluids, blood transfusions, or (rarely) needle sticks. Mothers also may pass HIV to their unborn children.	Several months or years
Hepatitis B, C	Blood, stool, or other body fluids, or contaminated objects.	Weeks or months
Tuberculosis	Respiratory secretions, airborne or on contaminated objects.	2 to 6 weeks
Meningitis, bacterial	Oral and nasal secretions.	2 to 10 days
Pneumonia, bacterial and viral	Oral and nasal droplets and secretions.	Several days
Influenza	Airborne droplets, or direct contact with body fluids.	1 to 3 days
Staphylococcal skin infections	Contact with open wounds or sores or contaminated objects.	Several days
Chicken pox (varicella)	Airborne droplets, or contact with open sores.	11 to 21 days
German measles (rubella)	Airborne droplets. Mothers may pass it to unborn children.	10 to 12 days
Whooping cough (pertussis)	Respiratory secretions or airborne droplets.	6 to 20 days

* **incubation period** the time between contact with a disease organism and the appearance of the first symptoms.

Treat all blood and other body fluids as if they are infectious, and take appropriate body substance isolation (BSI) precautions whenever you treat a patient.

* **body substance isolation (BSI)** a strict form of infection control that is based on the assumption that all blood and other body fluids are infectious.

pathogens can occur when the blood of an infected person comes in contact with another person's broken skin (cuts, sores, chapped hands) or by way of parenteral contact (stick by a needle or other sharp object). Infection by airborne pathogens can occur when an infected person sneezes or coughs, causing body fluids in the form of tiny droplets to be inhaled or to come in contact with the mucous membranes of another person's eyes, nose, or mouth.

HIV/AIDS, hepatitis B, and tuberculosis are diseases of great concern because they are life threatening. However, one may be exposed to many different infectious diseases. See Table 1-2 for some common ones, their modes of transmission, and **incubation periods.**

Even when someone is carrying pathogens for disease, signs of an illness may not be apparent. For this reason, *you must consider the blood and body fluids of every patient you treat as infectious.* Safeguards against infection are mandatory for all medical personnel. They involve a form of infection control called body substance isolation (BSI).

INFECTION-CONTROL PRACTICES

Body Substance Isolation (BSI)

Body substance isolation (BSI) is a strategy that is based on the assumption that all blood and body fluids are infectious. It dictates that all EMS personnel take

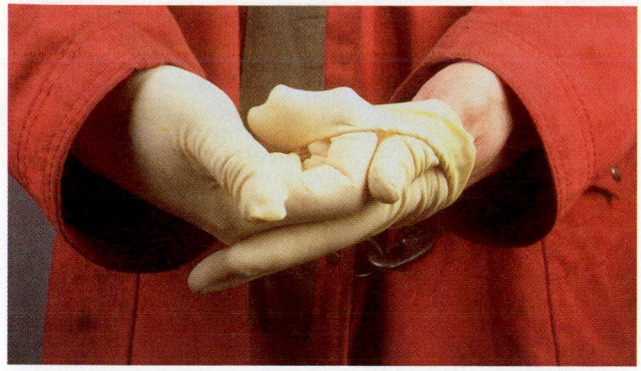

FIGURE 1-10A To remove gloves, first hook the gloved fingers of one hand under the cuff of the other glove. Then pull that glove off without letting your gloved fingers come in contact with bare skin.

FIGURE 1-10B Then slide the fingers of the ungloved hand under the remaining glove's cuff. Push that glove off, being careful not to touch the glove's exterior with your bare hand.

BSI precautions with every patient. To achieve this, appropriate **personal protective equipment (PPE)** should be available in every emergency vehicle. The minimum recommended PPE includes the following:

- *Protective gloves.* Wear disposable protective gloves before initiating any emergency care. When an emergency involves more than one patient, change gloves between patients. When gloves have been contaminated, remove and dispose of them properly as soon as possible (Figure 1-10).

- *Masks and protective eyewear.* These should be worn together whenever blood spatter is likely to occur, such as with arterial bleeding, childbirth, endotracheal intubation and other invasive procedures, oral suctioning, and clean-up of equipment that requires heavy scrubbing or brushing. Both you and your patient should wear masks whenever the potential for airborne transmission of disease exists.

- *HEPA and N-95 respirators.* Due to the resurgence of tuberculosis (TB), you must protect yourself from infection through the use of a high-efficiency particulate air (HEPA) or N-95 respirator. Wear one whenever you care for a patient with confirmed or suspected TB, especially during procedures that involve the airway, such as the administration of nebulized medications, endotracheal intubation, or suctioning.

- *Gowns.* Disposable gowns protect your clothing from splashes. If large splashes of blood are expected, such as with childbirth, wear an impervious gown.

- *Resuscitation equipment.* Use disposable resuscitation equipment as your primary means of artificial ventilation in emergency care.

These garments and equipment will assist you in achieving, to the extent possible, the universal precautions recommended by the Centers for Disease Control. Infectious diseases also are minimized through the use of appropriate work practices and equipment especially engineered to minimize risk. For example, use

✱ **personal protective equipment (PPE)** equipment used by EMS personnel to protect against injury and the spread of infectious disease.

Perhaps the most important infection-control practice is handwashing.

Content Review

HANDWASHING

- Lather with soap and water.
- Scrub for at least 15 seconds.
- Rinse under running water.
- Dry on a clean towel.

Monitor your personal medical history accurately, and be sure to get all appropriate vaccinations, boosters, and screenings on a regular basis.

Infection control includes properly cleaning, disinfecting, sterilizing, or properly discarding all equipment after contact with a patient.

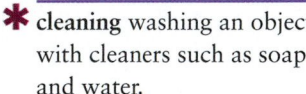

* **cleaning** washing an object with cleaners such as soap and water.

disposable invasive equipment once, then dispose of it properly. Launder reusable clothing with infection control in mind.

Probably the most important infection-control practice is handwashing as soon as possible after every patient contact and decontamination procedure. First remove any rings or jewelry from your hands and arms. Lather your hands vigorously front and back, for at least 15 seconds up to two or three inches above the wrist. Lather and rub between your fingers and in the creases and cracks of your knuckles. Scrub under and around the fingernails with a brush. Rinse well under running water, holding your hands downward so that the water drains off your fingertips. Dry your hands on a clean towel. Plain soap works perfectly well for handwashing. When soap is not available, use an anti-microbial handwashing solution or an alcohol-based foam or towelette.

Vaccinations and Screening Tests

Immunizations against many illnesses are available. Get them. Even "nuisance" illnesses can be avoided if you get vaccinated. Immunizations are available for rubella (German measles), measles, mumps, chicken pox, and other childhood diseases, as well as for tetanus/diphtheria, polio, influenza, hepatitis B, and Lyme disease. Some, such as tetanus, may require booster shots periodically, so monitor your personal medical history well. Also arrange for routine tuberculosis (TB) screenings.

Decontamination of Equipment

Any personal protective equipment (PPE) designed for a single use should be properly disposed of after use. The same is true of medical devices designed for a single use. Such materials should be discarded in a red bag marked with a biohazard seal (Figure 1-11). Needles and other sharp objects should be discarded in properly labeled, puncture-proof containers. Containers should be disposed of according to local guidelines.

Non-disposable equipment that has been contaminated must be cleaned, disinfected, or sterilized:

- **Cleaning** refers to washing an object with soap and water. After caring for a patient, wash your work areas down with approved soaps. Throw away single-use cleaning supplies in a proper biohazard container.

FIGURE 1-11 Dispose of biohazardous wastes in a properly marked bag.

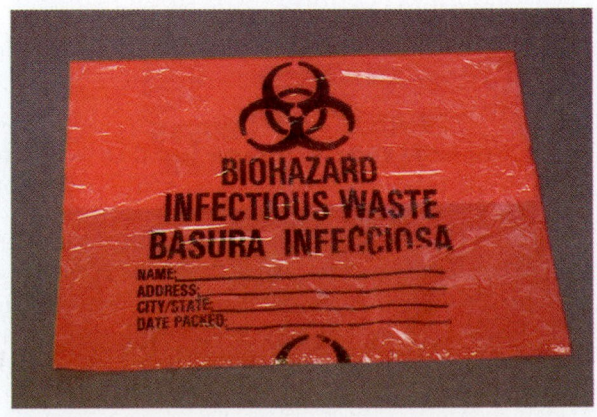

- **Disinfecting** includes cleaning with a disinfecting agent, which should kill many microorganisms on the surface of an object. Disinfect equipment that had direct contact with the intact skin of a patient, such as backboards and splints. Use a commercial disinfectant or bleach diluted in water (one part bleach to 100 parts water, or follow local guidelines).
- **Sterilizing** is the use of a chemical, or a physical method such as pressurized steam, to kill all microorganisms on an object. Items that were inserted into the patient's body (a laryngoscope blade, for example) should be sterilized by heat, steam, or radiation. There are also EPA-approved solutions for sterilization.

If your equipment needs more extensive cleaning, bag it and remove it to an area designated for this purpose. Disposable work gloves worn during cleaning and decontamination should be properly discarded. If your clothing has become contaminated, bag the items and wash them in accordance with local guidelines. After removing contaminated clothing, take a shower before dressing again.

Post-Exposure Procedures

By definition, an **exposure** is any occurrence of blood or body fluids coming in contact with non-intact skin, the eyes or other mucous membranes, or parenteral contact (needle stick). In most areas, an EMS provider who has had an exposure should (Figure 1-12):

- Immediately wash the affected area with soap and water.
- Get a medical evaluation.
- Take the proper immunization boosters.
- Notify the agency's infection-control liaison.
- Document the circumstances surrounding the exposure, including the actions taken to reduce chances of infection.

In general, the EMS provider should cooperate with the incident investigation and comply with all required reporting responsibilities and time frames.

DEATH AND DYING

Paramedics encounter death much more frequently than other people do. They often see it as it happens. This can lead to a sense of cumulative overload, which the paramedic needs to recognize and deal with in a healthy manner.

LOSS, GRIEF, AND MOURNING

A long-standing taboo against discussing death and dying changed when pioneer Elisabeth Kübler-Ross braved the backlash to meet with terminally ill hospital patients to discuss their feelings about death and dying. Before then, it was assumed dying people did not want to talk about the experience. What Kübler-Ross learned is that there are five predictable stages of loss:

- *Denial, or "not me."* This is the inability or refusal to believe the reality of the event. It is a defense mechanism, during which the patient puts off dealing with the inevitable end of life.
- *Anger, or "why me?"* The patient's anger is really frustration related to his inability to control the situation. That anger could focus on anyone or anything.

---

* disinfecting cleaning with an agent that can kill some microorganisms on the surface of an object.

* sterilizing use of a chemical or physical method such as pressurized steam to kill all microorganisms on an object.

* exposure any occurrence of blood or body fluids coming in contact with non-intact skin, mucous membranes, or parenteral contact (needle stick).

Follow your EMS system guidelines on all management and documentation of any exposure to a patient's blood or body fluids.

Content Review

STAGES OF LOSS
- Denial
- Anger
- Bargaining
- Depression
- Acceptance

FIGURE 1-12 A federal regulation called the Ryan White Comprehensive AIDS Resources Emergency (CARE) Act outlines procedures to follow after an occupational exposure to HIV, hepatitis B, diphtheria, meningitis, plague, hemorrhagic fever, rabies, or tuberculosis.

INFECTIOUS DISEASE EXPOSURE PROCEDURE

Airborne Infection Such as TB (Tuberculosis)	Bloodborne Infection Such as HIV (AIDS virus) or HBV (Hepatitus B virus)
You transport a patient who is infected with a life-threatening airborne disease, such as TB, but you are not aware that the patient is infected.	You come into contact with blood or body fluids of a patient, and you wonder if that patient is infected with a life-threatening bloodborne disease such as HIV or HBV.
The medical facility diagnoses the disease in the patient you transported.	You seek immediate medical attention and document the incident for worker's compensation.
The medical facility must notify your designated officer within 48 hours.	You ask your designated officer to determine if you have been exposed to an infectious disease.
Your designated officer notifies you that you have been exposed.	Your designated officer (DO) must gather information and, if DO determines it is warranted, consult the medical facility to which the patient was transported.
Your employer arranges for you to be evaluated and followed up by a doctor or other appropriate health care professional.	The medical facility must gather information and report findings to your designated officer within 48 hours. Your DO notifies you of the findings.

- *Bargaining, or "okay, but first let me . . ."* In the patient's mind, he tries to make a deal to "buy additional time" to put off or change the expected outcome.
- *Depression, or "okay, but I haven't . . ."* The patient is sad and despairing, often mourning things not accomplished and dreams that will not come true. The patient withdraws, or retreats, into a private world, unwilling to communicate with others.
- *Acceptance, or "okay, I'm not afraid."* The patient may come to realize his fate and achieve a reasonable level of comfort with the anticipated outcome. At this stage, the family may need more support than the patient.

A person experiencing any significant loss usually works through these stages, given enough time. Although there is a tendency to progress from one

Given enough time, a person experiencing a significant loss usually works through the five predictable stages: denial, anger, bargaining, depression, and acceptance.

stage to the next in order, both dying patients and their loved ones experience the stages in their own unique ways. They may jump around among the stages, they may go back and forth, or they may never finish them. It is important for you to remain flexible in your expectations, so you can decide how best to help, if asked.

Because paramedics encounter death and dying often, there is a mistaken belief that they handle it better. However, paramedics are human, too. Let yourself deal with death and dying when it occurs. Do not shirk the support of friends and family. Do not try to "tough it out." Use every opportunity to process a specific incident in a healthy manner, through appropriately grieving, losses that have an impact on you.

Grief is a feeling. Mourning is a process. A grieving person feels mostly sadness or distress. A person in mourning is immersed in the process of displaying and ultimately dissipating the feelings of grief. The sense of loss is predictably most intense immediately after the news is received. Although numerous models for the mourning process exist, a good rule of thumb is that after the loss of a close friend or relative, a period of one year of mourning is normal.

Upon initially hearing the news of a death, a person experiences a "paralyzing, totally incapacitating surge of grief that is exactly comparable to the incapacitating pain of an acute eye or testicle blow in that the whole world shrinks down to that acute pain." Typically, the feeling lasts for 5 to 15 minutes. When you deliver the news of a death, remember that a survivor cannot function during this grief spike. After delivering the news, wait until it is past and the survivor is ready and able to receive information and make decisions.

A period of intense feelings that continues for around four to six weeks follows the grief spike. Feelings may include loss, anger, resentment, sadness, and even guilt, depending on the relationship and the circumstances surrounding the death. Gradually, the intensity and immediacy of the loss fades into a phase dominated by a sense of loneliness, which lasts about six months. Finally, a period of recovery ensues. The survivor begins to view the loss more objectively and rediscovers an interest in living. Key to the process of mourning is the passage of significant dates and anniversaries, such as birthdays, holidays, and the monthly (then annual) date when the loss occurred.

How different people cope with difficult moments, such as death, varies. If you are dealing with a child, understand that children's perceptions are different from an adult's. (See Table 1-3 for a summary.) This is true of all the special populations you will encounter, such as the elderly and people with mental disabilities. The elderly, for example, may be particularly concerned about the effects of the loss on other family members, about further loss of their own independence, and about the costs of a funeral and burial. There is a wide variety of responses to death among different peoples and cultures as well. Be flexible, and be ready for anything.

WHAT TO SAY

As "Do Not Resuscitate" orders and other out-of-hospital death situations increase, EMS personnel are more often placed in the position of telling people that someone has died. It would be nice to have a script for those difficult moments, but the reality is that you have to assess the scene and the people in each situation to determine the safest and most compassionate way to deliver the sad news.

In terms of safety, you never know how people will respond, even if you know them. Most people accept the news quietly. However, some allow their grief to flood out of them in very physical ways, such as throwing things, kicking walls, or screaming and running in circles. Before speaking, consciously position yourself between them and the door or other escape route. Remember, initially the grief spike has its grip on the survivors. There is little you can do but

Table 1-3	NEEDS AND EXPECTATIONS OF CHILDREN REGARDING DEATH	
Age Range	**Characteristics**	**Suggestions**
Newborn to age 3	Senses that something has happened in family, and notices that there is much activity in the household. Realizes that people are crying and sad.	Be sensitive to the child's needs. Try to maintain consistency in routines.
	Watch for irritability and changes in eating, sleeping, or other behavioral patterns.	Maintain consistency with significant people in child's life.
Ages 3 to 6	Believes death is a temporary state, and may ask continually when the person will return. Believes in magical thinking, and may feel responsible for the death or it is punishment for own behavior. May be fearful of catching the same illness and die, or may believe that everyone else he loves will die also.	Emphasize that the child was not responsible for the death. Reinforce that when people are sad, they cry, and that crying is normal and natural.
	Watch for changes in behavior patterns with friends and at school, difficulty sleeping, and changes in eating habits.	Encourage the child to talk about and/or draw pictures of his feelings, or to cry.
Ages 6 to 9	May prefer to hide or disguise feelings to avoid looking babyish. Is afraid significant others will die. Seeks out detailed explanations for death, and differences between fatal illness and "just being sick." Has an understanding that death is real, but may believe that those who die are too slow, weak, or stupid. Fantasizes in an effort to make everything the way it was. Denial is most helpful coping skill.	Talk about the normal feelings of anger, sadness, and guilt. Share your own feelings about death. Do not be afraid to cry in front of the child. This and other expressions of loss help to give the child permission to express his feelings.
Ages 9 to 12	Begins to understand the irreversibility of death. May seek details and specifics of the situation, and may need repeated, explicit explanations. Hard-won sense of independence becomes fragile, and may show concern about the practical matters of his lifestyle. May try to act "adult," but then regress to earlier stage of emotional response. When threatened, expresses anger toward the ill/deceased, himself or other survivors.	Set aside time to talk about feelings. Encourage sharing of memories to facilitate grief response.
Ages 12 to 18	Demanding developmental processes are an awkward fit with need to take on different family roles. Retreats to safety of childhood. Feels pressure to act as an adult, while still coping with skills of a child. Suppresses feelings in order to "fit in," leaving teen isolated and vulnerable.	Encourage talking, but respect need for privacy. See if a trusted, reliable friend or adult can provide appropriate support. Locate support group for teens.

give them a safe, private place to get through it. Also, for safety, do not deliver the news to a large group. Ask the primary people (no more than four or five) to step aside with you to a private place. Let them tell the others in their own way.

Find out who is who among the survivors. Do not make assumptions. Then address the closest survivor, preferably in a way that shows compassion. That is, avoid standing above the survivor. Instead, sit or squat so that your eyes are at the same level. If the survivor is alone, call for a friend, neighbor, clergy member, or relative. Wait to tell the survivor the news until that person has arrived.

Introduce yourself by name and function ("My name is Kate. I'm a paramedic with West End Ambulance.) A careful choice of words is helpful. Although it may seem blunt, use the words "dead" and "died," rather than euphemisms which may be misinterpreted or misunderstood. Use gentle eye contact and, if appropriate, the power of touching an arm or holding a hand. Basic elements of your message should include:

- The loved one has died.
- There is nothing more anyone could have done.
- Your EMS service is available to assist the survivors if needed. (Sometimes, medical emergencies occur in survivors in the wake of such stressful news.)
- Information about local procedures for out-of-hospital death, such as the inspection of the scene by the medical examiner or coroner, and so on.

Do not include statements about God's will or relief from pain or any subjective assumption. You do not know the people well enough to know the details about their relationship or their religious preferences.

WHEN IT IS SOMEONE YOU KNOW

Many paramedics are called to serve in small communities, where calls often involve people you know. Elements of this are both rewarding and heart-wrenching. People may be greatly relieved to see a familiar, trusted face among the EMS team. There also is a lot of support for paramedics in small communities because you are there to help others during their most fearful moments. However, being involved when the life of someone you know is threatened—or lost—can have a powerful impact upon your own emotions. If it is too much, you must find a way to manage the stress. Oftentimes, you must grieve as well. Your well-being demands it.

STRESS AND STRESS MANAGEMENT

Many aspects of EMS are stressful. Stress, according to researcher Hans Selye, is "the nonspecific response of the body to any demand." The word **stress** also refers to a hardship or strain, or a physical or emotional response to a stimulus. A person's reactions to stress are individual. They are affected by previous exposure to the stressor, perception of the event, general life experience, and personal coping skills.

A stimulus that causes stress is known as a **stressor.** Stress is usually understood to generate a negative affect, or *distress,* in an individual. There is also "good" stress, which is called *eustress* (for example, seeing a lost loved one for the first time in years). However, even eustress generates physiological and psychological signs and symptoms.

Adapting to stress is a dynamic, evolving process. As a person adapts, he or she develops:

- *Defensive strategies.* While sometimes helpful for the short term, these strategies deny and distort the reality of a stressful situation.
- *Coping.* This is an active process during which a person confronts the stressful situation and changes or adjusts as necessary. Coping may not serve as the best strategy for the long term.
- *Problem-solving skills.* These skills are regarded as the healthiest approach to everyday concerns. Reflected in the ability to analyze a problem and recognize multiple options and potential solutions, mastery generally comes only as a result of extensive experience with similar situations.

* **stress** a hardship or strain; a physical or emotional response to a stimulus.

* **stressor** a stimulus that causes stress.

EMS has abundant stressors, which provide ample opportunities for the development of problem-solving skills. There are administrative stressors, such as waiting for calls, shift work, loud pagers, and inadequate pay. There are scene-related stressors, such as violent and abusive people, flying debris, vomit, loud noises, and chaos. There are emotional and physical stressors, such as fear, demanding bystanders, abusive patients, frustration, exhaustion, hunger or thirst, and lifting heavy objects.

Environmental stress may be in the form of siren noise, inclement weather, confined work spaces, and the frequent urgency of rapid scene responses and life-or-death decisions. In addition, the often difficult world of EMS can strain a paramedic's family relationships and possibly lead to conflicts with supervisors and co-workers. Add this to the common personality traits of paramedics, which include a strong need to be liked and often unrealistically high self-expectations, and the combination can lead to disturbing feelings of guilt or anxiety. All these stressors take a toll on the paramedic.

Your job in managing stress is to learn these things:

- *Your personal stressors.* Each person has an individual list. What is stressful to you may be enjoyable to someone else. What was stressful to you last year may be replaced by new stressors this year.
- *Amount of stress you can take before it becomes a problem.* Stress occurs in a tornado-like continuum. It starts with a few breezes, but it can increase in force until it is whirling out of control. Stopping the "storm" early is key to your well-being. You need to know which stress responses are early indicators for you, so you can deal with them at that point.
- *Stress management strategies that work for you.* Again, this is totally individual. Those who seek personal well-being must become well-versed about personally appropriate options.

If a person piles on stressor after stressor without regard for the consequences, the results are likely to be bad. Stress-related disease is avoidable if you make a habit of doing what is necessary to preserve your personal well-being.

There are three phases of a stress response: alarm, resistance, and exhaustion. At the end comes a period of rest and recovery.

- *Stage I: Alarm.* The alarm phase is the "fight-or-flight" phenomenon. It occurs when the body physically and rapidly prepares to defend itself against a perceived threat. The pituitary gland begins by releasing adrenocorticotropic (stress) hormones. Hormones continue to flood the body via the autonomic nervous system, coordinated by the hypothalamus. Epinephrine and norepinephrine from the adrenal glands increase heart rate and blood pressure, dilate pupils, increase blood sugar and slow digestion, and relax the bronchial tree. This reaction ends when the event is recognized as not dangerous.
- *Stage II: Resistance.* This stage starts when the individual begins to cope with the stress. Over time, an individual may become desensitized or adapted to stressors. Physiological parameters, such as pulse and blood pressure, may return to normal.
- *Stage III: Exhaustion.* Prolonged exposure to the same stressors leads to exhaustion of an individual's ability to resist and adapt. Resistance to all stressors declines. Susceptibility to physical and psychological ailments increase. A period of rest and recovery is necessary for a healthy outcome.

To manage stress, identify your own personal stressors, the amount of stress you can take before it becomes a problem, and what specific stress-management techniques work for you.

Content Review

PHASES OF A STRESS RESPONSE
- Alarm
- Resistance
- Exhaustion

It would be great if we could manage each stressor to the point of recovery before the next one hits, but that is not how it works. Typically, people are still dealing with one stress (or the same ongoing one, such as the chronic stress of shift work) when additional stressors pile on, resulting in cumulative stress. If stress accumulates without intervention, the consequences can be serious.

SHIFT WORK

There will always be shift work in EMS. Because EMS is a 24-hour, 7-days-a-week endeavor, someone has to be functional at all times. This is inherently stressful because of disruptions in the biorhythms of the body, known as **circadian rhythms,** and sleep deprivation.

Circadian rhythms are biological cycles that occur approximately every 24 hours. These include hormonal and body temperature fluctuations, appetite and sleepiness cycles, and other bodily processes. When life patterns disrupt the circadian rhythms, biological effects can be stressful. For example, sleep deprivation is common among people who work at night. The inherent dangers to paramedics are clear. If you have to sleep in the daytime, there are some tips to minimize the stress:

* Sleep in a cool, dark place that mimics the nighttime environment.
* Stick to sleeping at your **anchor time** (times you can rest without interruption), even on days off. Do not try to revert to a daytime lifestyle on days off. For example, if you work 9 p.m. to 5 a.m. and your anchor time is 8 a.m. to 12 noon, then go to bed "early" on days off and on workdays sleep from 8 a.m. to 3 p.m.
* Unwind appropriately after a shift in order to rest well. Do not eat a heavy meal or exercise right before bedtime.
* Post a "day sleeper" sign on your front door, turn off the phone's ringer, and lower the volume of the answering machine.

SIGNS OF STRESS

A variety of factors can trigger a stress response. They include the loss of something valuable, injury or the threat of injury, poor health or nutrition, general frustration, and ineffective coping mechanisms. Remember, each individual is susceptible to different stressors and therefore has a different constellation of signs and symptoms.

These signs and symptoms (Table 1-4) are a blessing in a way, because they are the body's way of warning that corrective stress management is needed. The warnings typically are mild at first, but left uncorrected they will build in intensity until you are forced to rest. If it means having a heart attack or collapsing, that is what the body will do. So, pay attention. If you catch a warning sign of excessive stress early and manage it, there is no need to reach the extreme endpoint commonly referred to as **burnout.**

COMMON TECHNIQUES FOR MANAGING STRESS

There are two main groups of defense mechanisms and techniques for managing stress: beneficial and detrimental. Detrimental techniques may provide a temporary sense of relief, but they will not cure the problem. They only make things worse. They include substance abuse (alcohol, nicotine, illegal and prescription drugs), overeating or other compulsive behaviors, chronic complaining, freezing out or cutting off others and the support they could give you, avoidance behaviors, and dishonesty about your actual state of well-being ("I'm just fine!").

✳ circadian rhythms physiological phenomena that occur at approximately 24-hour intervals.

✳ anchor time set of hours when a night-shift worker can reliably expect to rest without interruption.

✳ burnout occurs when coping mechanisms no longer buffer stressors, which can compromise personal health and well-being.

Table 1-4	WARNING SIGNS OF EXCESSIVE STRESS
Physical	**Cognitive**
Nausea/vomiting	Confusion
Upset stomach	Lowered attention span
Tremors (lips, hands)	Calculation difficulties
Feeling uncoordinated	Memory problems
Diaphoresis (profuse sweating), flushed skin	Poor concentration
Chills	Difficulty making decisions
Diarrhea	Disruption in logical thinking
Aching muscles and joints	Disorientation, decreased level of awareness
Sleep disturbances	Seeing an event over and over
Fatigue	Distressing dreams
Dry mouth	Blaming someone
Shakes	
Headache	
Vision problems	
Difficult, rapid breathing	
Chest tightness or pain, heart palpitations, cardiac rhythm disturbances	
Emotional	**Behavioral**
Anticipatory anxiety	Change in activity
Denial	Hyperactivity, hypoactivity
Fearfulness	Withdrawal
Panic	Suspiciousness
Survivor guilt	Change in communications
Uncertainty of feelings	Change in interactions with others
Depression	Change in eating habits
Grief	Increased or decreased food intake
Hopelessness	Increased smoking
Feeling overwhelmed	Increased alcohol intake
Feeling lost	Increased intake of other drugs
Feeling abandoned	Being overly vigilant to environment
Feeling worried	Excessive humor
Wishing to hide	Excessive silence
Wishing to die	Unusual behavior
Anger	Crying spells
Feeling numb	
Identifying with victim	

It is far better for you to spend your energy on beneficial, or healthy, techniques that serve to dissipate the accumulation of stress and promote actual recovery. In situations where your stress response threatens your ability to handle the moment, you can:

- *Use controlled breathing.* Focus attention on your breathing. Take in a deep breath through your nose. Then exhale forcefully but steadily through your mouth, so that you can hear the air rush out. Press all the air out of your lungs with your abdomen. Do this two or more times, until you feel steadier. This technique helps to reduce your adrenaline levels and slow your heart rate, so you can do your job appropriately.

- *Reframe.* Mentally reframe interfering thoughts, such as "I can't do this" or "I'm scared." Be sure to deal with the thoughts later, or they will continue to interfere with the performance of your duties.

- *Attend to the medical needs of the patient.* Even if you know the people involved, do not let those relationships interfere with your responsibilities as an EMS provider. Later, when it is appropriate to do so, address your stress about the call.

For long-term well-being, one of the best stress management techniques is to take care of yourself—physically, emotionally, and mentally. Remember that regular exercise does not have to be extreme. Do something that you enjoy and find relaxing. At stressful times, pay especially close attention to your diet. If you smoke, make it a goal to quit.

Create a non-EMS circle of friends, and renew old friendships or activities. Take a vacation or a few days off. Say "no!" to the next offer of an overtime shift. Listen to music, meditate, and learn positive thinking. Try the soothing techniques of guided imagery and progressive relaxation. Some paramedics have even quit EMS for a while. In general, you can make many choices. The key principle is to generate positive options for yourself, and keep choosing them until you have recovered.

> *For long-term well-being, the best stress-management technique is to take care of yourself; that is, eat properly, exercise regularly, and take time off!*
>

CRITICAL INCIDENT STRESS MANAGEMENT (CISM)

Uniquely stressful situations that arise in EMS are known as **critical incidents**, or events that have a powerful emotional impact which can cause acute stress reactions. Such events are not common, even by EMS standards. They include:

* **critical incident** an event that has a powerful emotional impact on a rescuer that can cause an acute stress reaction.

- Injury or death of an infant or child
- Injury or death of someone known to EMS personnel
- Injury, death, or suicide of an EMS worker
- Extreme threat to an EMS worker
- Disasters, or multiple-casualty incidents (especially when most of the victims are dead)
- Injury or death of a civilian caused by EMS operations
- Incidents that draw unusual media attention
- Prolonged incidents
- Other significant events

A critical incident can impact a single crew or an entire agency. It also tends to generate intense, rapid-onset stress responses. Critical incident stress

> *Critical incidents will affect you, so take advantage of your EMS system's critical incident stress management (CISM) services.*
>

critical incident stress management (CISM) a system of related interventions usually performed by regional, non-partisan, multi-disciplinary teams composed of EMS peers and specifically trained mental health workers.

is managed by a system of related interventions called **critical incident stress management (CISM)**. These interventions are best performed by regional, non-partisan, multi-disciplinary teams composed of EMS peers (fire, police, EMTs, dispatchers, and so on) in combination with specifically trained mental health workers. The components of CISM are:

- *Pre-incident stress training.* For all EMS personnel in the service area (fire, police, EMS, dispatchers, and so on), pre-incident education occurs during initial education and in subsequent training sessions.
- *On-scene support.* Techniques for reducing crisis-induced stress on scene include regular rest intervals, replacement of food and fluids, limiting exposure to the incident, and changing assignments.
- *Advice to command staff* during a large-scale incident.
- *Initial discussion.* This is a spontaneous, post-call, initial airing of crew responses. It is a process of simply talking about the incident. It is not intended as a critique. A trained member of a CISM team is present who can provide excellent emotional support during discussions.

defusing a short, informal type of debriefing held within hours of a critical incident.

- *Defusing.* Held two to four hours, but not more than 12 hours, post-event, a **defusing** is a short, informal meeting that provides a chance for crews to vent their feelings about the incident. A CISM-trained peer usually conducts it.

demobilization establishment and staffing of a transition point with the object of providing crews time to regroup between a large-scale critical stress situation and going off duty or back to regular duty.

- *Demobilization.* **Demobilization** is an on-scene CISM service in which a site is established and staffed as a transition point between a large-scale situation and going off duty or back to regular duty. What goes on is not a critique, but rather a chance to give crews time to regroup before reentering everyday life.
- *Critical incident stress debriefing.* The **critical incident stress debriefing (CISD)** is a formal, structured, carefully planned intervention. It is done 24 to 72 hours post-event by a trained CISM team, including mental health providers and peer supporters.

critical incident stress debriefing (CISD) a process used to help rescuers work through their responses to a critical incident within 24 to 72 hours after the event.

- *Follow-up services.* Sometimes, the CISM team follows up with additional meetings to allow a safe environment for crews to grapple with ongoing reactions to the situation.
- *Special debriefings to non-emergency community groups.*
- *Spouse and family education and support.*
- *Individual consultations.*

GENERAL SAFETY CONSIDERATIONS

The topic of scene safety is vast and requires career-long attention. Considering the many problems that can occur, it is impressive how few injuries there are. Your risks include violent people, environmental hazards, structural collapse, motor vehicles, and infectious disease. Many of these hazards can be minimized with protective equipment, such as helmets, body armor, reflective tape for night visibility, footwear with ankle support, and BSI precautions against infectious disease. Whatever protective equipment you have should be used.

INTERPERSONAL RELATIONS

Safety issues that arise in out-of-hospital care often stem from poor interpersonal relations. Paramedics are public ambassadors of health care. Interpersonal safety begins with effective communication. If you can build a rapport with the strangers you have been sent to serve, you will gain their trust. Suspicious, angry, upset people are far more likely to be defensive and inflict harm than those who see a reason to trust what you are doing.

Building rapport depends on the ability to put your personal prejudices aside. Everyone has prejudices. But as a representative of an institution far greater than yourself, you must never allow them to interfere with appropriate patient and bystander management. In fact, go beyond curbing prejudice, and challenge yourself to treat every person you meet with dignity and respect.

You can begin by taking time to pay attention to the rich array of cultural diversity and learning to see those differences as valuable and positive. In particular, learn about the different cultural backgrounds of people in your area and how to work with them effectively. For example, although you may like a lot of eye contact, understand that it is regarded as more polite in several cultures to avoid eye contact. Therefore, someone showing you esteem might avoid eye contact with you. This is not wrong. It is just different. Listen well to the stories of other people and see what you can learn. When a person can accept differences easily, it becomes easier to work toward win-win situations on the streets.

Treat every person you meet with dignity and respect, no matter what their race, sex, age, religion, economic background, or present condition.

ROADWAY SAFETY

Roadways are unsafe places. There are good books, classes, and mentors to help you become aware of the various roadway hazards. Learn the principles of:

- Safely following an emergency escort vehicle
- Intersection management, when traffic is moving in several directions
- Noting hazardous conditions, such as spilled hazardous materials (gasoline, industrial chemicals, and so on), downed power lines, and proximity to moving traffic; also noting adverse environmental conditions
- Evaluating the safest parking place when arriving at a roadway incident
- Safely approaching a vehicle in which someone is slumped over the wheel
- Patient compartment safety—in particular, bracing yourself against sudden deceleration or swerving to avoid roadway hazards; and making a habit of hanging on consistently, especially when changing positions
- Safely using emergency lights and siren

One of the greatest hazards in EMS is the motor vehicle. Be sure to obey roadway laws and follow all driving safety guidelines.

An ambulance escort can create additional hazards. Inexperienced ambulance operators often follow the escort vehicle too closely and are unable to stop when the escort does. Inexperienced operators also may assume that other drivers know the ambulance is following an escort. In fact, other drivers do not know and often pull out in front of the ambulance just after the escort vehicle passes.

Multiple-vehicle responses can be just as dangerous, especially when responding vehicles travel in the same direction close together. When two vehicles approach the same intersection at the same time, not only may they fail to yield to each other, but other drivers may yield for the first vehicle only, not the second one. Extreme caution must be taken when approaching intersections.

Certain equipment is intended to promote your safety on roadways. For example, to be visible to oncoming drivers, who may have dirty, smeared, pitted windshields and may not be sober, wear reflective tape and orange or lime-green safety vests. In fact, you also may be issued other protective gear, especially if you are in the fire service. Using respiratory protection, gloves, boots, turnout coat and pants (or coveralls), and other specialty safety equipment is the mark of an aware, professional paramedic. Ask non-medical personnel to set out flares or cones, if needed. Leave some emergency lights flashing, although be careful not to blind oncoming drivers.

To park safely at a roadway incident, make it a habit to scan each individual setting. Notice curves, hilltops, volume, and the speed of surrounding traffic. Ideally, park in the front of a crash site on the same side of the street. This facilitates access to the patient compartment and equipment, and it protects you from traffic coming from behind. However, when responding to an incident such as "person slumped behind wheel," maintain the defensive advantage by staying behind the vehicle, and use spotlights to "blind" the person until you know there are no hostile intentions. Walk to the vehicle with cautious alertness until you are sure it is not a trap.

The use of seatbelts in the front of an ambulance should be an obvious habit, both for safety and for role modeling. Less obvious is the use of safety restraints in the patient compartment. An improper assumption is that the paramedic is too busy attending the patient and passengers to wear a seatbelt. However, buckling into a seatbelt for a safer ride is, in fact, possible during much or most of ambulance transport times. Death and major disability is common when someone is in the patient compartment during a crash. For your well-being, wear a seatbelt whenever possible, even "in back."

Because ambulances represent help and hope, it is doubly tragic when a paramedic crew is involved in a motor-vehicle crash caused by the misuse of lights and siren. Lights and siren are tools, not toys. They are the paramedic's means for gaining quick access to people in dire need. Those who misuse the mandate to operate them chip away at the public's trust in EMS. Whether using lights and siren or not, in most states, the paramedic has a legal responsibility to drive with "due regard for the safety of all others." As a professional, you are obligated to study and use safe driving practices at all times.

Part 5: Illness and Injury Prevention

How often do EMS crews respond to incidents that could easily have been prevented? How often have you thought to yourself "I wish there was something I could have done" in the wake of senseless circumstances surrounding an accidental injury or illness? But what if EMS personnel asked questions before an incident occurred? How many injuries could be prevented? How many lives could be saved? This section focuses on these questions and discusses illness and injury prevention as a paramedic's crucial duty and responsibility.

EPIDEMIOLOGY

Injury is one of our nation's most important health problems.

Injury is one of our nation's most important health problems. Consider the following facts offered by the U.S. Department of Transportation:

- Injury surpassed stroke as the third leading cause of death in the United States, and it is the leading cause of death in people ages 1 to 44.
- Injuries that are unintentional result in nearly 70,000 deaths and millions of nonfatal injuries each year. The leading causes of death from unintentional injuries are motor-vehicle collisions, fires, burns, falls, drownings, and poisonings.
- The estimated lifetime cost of injuries will exceed $114 billion.
- For every one death caused by injury, there are an estimated 19 hospitalizations and 254 emergency department visits.

Injuries result from interaction with potential hazards in the environment, which means that they may be predictable and preventable.

Though many people believe that injuries "just happen," evidence shows that injuries result from interaction with potential hazards in the environment.

Thus, it has been suggested that "MVAs" (motor vehicle accidents) should be called "MVCs" (motor vehicle collisions), since driving drunk or at 80 mph and crashing is no accident. In other words, many injuries may be predictable and preventable. The study of the factors that influence the frequency, distribution, and causes of injury, disease, and other health-related events in a population is called **epidemiology.**

Concepts related to epidemiology that you should know include **years of productive life,** a calculation made by subtracting the age at death from 65. (For example, in a liability suit concerning the death of a 45-year-old, a jury might assess damages based on the deceased's loss of 20 years as a wage-earner.) Another concept is **injury,** which refers to the intentional or unintentional damage to a person resulting from acute exposure to thermal, mechanical, electrical, or chemical energy or from the absence of such essentials as heat and oxygen. An accident is an *unintentional injury,* but an injury that is purposefully inflicted either on oneself (e.g., suicide) or on another person (e.g., homicide) is an *intentional injury.* Intentional injuries make up about a third of all injury deaths. Other categories of intentional injury include rape, assault, and domestic, elder, and child abuse.

Other concepts related to epidemiology include **injury risk,** which is a real or potentially hazardous situation that puts people in danger of sustaining injury. As medical professionals, EMS providers should assess every scene and situation for injury risk and maintain statistics as part of an **injury-surveillance program,** or the ongoing systematic collection, analysis, and interpretation of injury data essential to the planning, implementation, and evaluation of public health practice.

An injury-surveillance program must also include a component for the timely dissemination of data to those who need to know. The final link in the injury-surveillance chain is the application of these data to prevention and control. **Teachable moments** occur shortly after an injury when the patient and observers remain acutely aware of what has happened and may be more receptive to teaching about how similar injury or illness could be prevented in the future.

By becoming involved in injury prevention, EMS providers can focus on **primary prevention,** or keeping an injury from ever occurring. Medical care and rehabilitation activities that help to prevent further problems from occurring are referred to, respectively, as **secondary prevention** and **tertiary prevention.**

PREVENTION WITHIN EMS

Even armed with the best equipment and technology, EMS providers cannot save every life. However, by working as partners in public health and safety, members of the EMS community can go beyond their normal daily routine and work with the public to prevent avoidable illness and injury.

EMS providers are widely distributed in the population, often reflecting the composition of their communities. They are often considered to be champions of the health-care consumer and are welcome in schools and other community institutions. Medical personnel are high-profile role models and, as such, can have a significant impact on the reduction of injury rates. In rural areas, EMS providers are sometimes the most medically educated individuals, often looked upon for advice and direction. Essentially, the more than 600,000 EMS providers in the United States comprise a great arsenal in the war to prevent injury and disease.

* **epidemiology** the study of factors that influence the frequency, distribution, and causes of injury, disease, and other health-related events in a population.

* **years of productive life** age at death subtracted from 65.

* **injury** intentional or unintentional damage to a person resulting from exposure to mechanical or any other form of energy or from absence of essentials such as heat or oxygen.

* **injury risk** a situation that puts people in danger of injury.

* **injury-surveillance program** ongoing systematic collection, analysis, and interpretation of injury data important to public health practice.

* **teachable moment** the time shortly after an injury when patients and observers may be more receptive to teaching about how similar injuries may be prevented in the future.

* **primary prevention** keeping an injury or illness from ever occurring.

* **secondary prevention** medical care after an injury or illness that helps to prevent further problems from occurring.

* **tertiary prevention** rehabilitation after an injury or illness that helps to prevent further problems from occurring.

The more than 600,000 EMS providers in the United States comprise a great arsenal in the war to prevent injury and disease.

ORGANIZATIONAL COMMITMENT

EMS organizational commitment is vital to the development of prevention activities.

Content Review

ORGANIZATIONAL COMMITMENT

- Protect EMS providers
- Provide initial and continuing education
- Collect and distribute illness and injury data
- Empower EMS personnel

EMS organizational commitment is vital to the development of prevention activities in the following areas:

- *Protection of EMS providers.* The leadership of EMS agencies must assure that policies are in place to promote response, scene, and transport safety. The appropriate body substance isolation (BSI) and personal protective equipment (PPE) should be issued to protect against exposure to bloodborne and airborne pathogens as well as environmental hazards. An overall commitment to safety and wellness should be emphasized and supported.

- *Education of EMS providers.* A "buy-in" from employees at every level is key to the success of any prevention program. EMS managers have the responsibility of instructing employees in the fundamentals of primary prevention. Public and private sector specialty groups may be called upon for specific training (Figure 1-13). EMS providers should also have the skills and training necessary to defend against violent patients or other hostile attackers. Classes in on-scene survival techniques should be commonplace in every EMS agency.

- *Data collection.* Monitoring and maintaining records of patient illnesses and injuries is essential in determining trends and in developing and measuring the success of prevention programs. Each agency should contribute data to local, regional, state, and national systems that track such information.

- *Financial support.* An agency's internal budget should reflect support for prevention strategies as a priority. If necessary, support must be sought from outside the organization. Large corporations

FIGURE 1-13 Training in specialized safety procedures should be available to you.

are often willing to donate funds in exchange for stand-by coverage at an event or company function. State highway safety offices can offer funding for traffic-related projects, such as those involving child safety seats, seat belts, and drunk driving. Advertising agencies may contribute billboards for safety messages and public service announcements. Partnerships with local hospitals can result in advertising safety messages in newsletters and flyers. Community groups such as Mothers against Drunk Driving (MADD) and junior auxiliaries also are great resources for initiating community and school programs.

- *Empowerment of EMS providers.* Frontline personnel are the ultimate factor in achieving success in a prevention program. Managers should identify, encourage, and foster, and reward employee interest, support, and involvement. In addition, managers should rotate assignment to prevention programs and provide salary for off-duty injury prevention activities.

EMS PROVIDER COMMITMENT

Illness and injury prevention should begin at home and be carried over into the workplace. The priority for EMS providers is to protect themselves from harm. Employers have an obligation to provide a safe environment. Written guidelines and policies should promote wellness and safety among employees, emphasizing the following areas (Part 4 of this chapter provided more information on the points listed):

- Body substance isolation precautions
- Physical fitness
- Stress management
- Seeking professional care and counseling
- Driving safely

SCENE SAFETY

Safety is always your first priority. Once your unit is dispatched to a call, evaluate the dispatch information prior to arrival. Focus your attention on response and equipment needed. Upon arrival, park the unit in the safest and most convenient place to load the patient as well as to leave the scene. Consider traffic, road conditions, and all other possible hazards. Directing traffic is primarily the responsibility of local law enforcement agencies. The safest method for traffic control at serious vehicle collisions is to stop all traffic and reroute it to different roads. This is for the safety of patients, bystanders, and rescue personnel.

Safety is always your first priority.

Note that if you are called to an area with potential health hazards, such as an industrial park or a chemical plant or an area with high crime rates, approach the scene with caution. Be sure to protect yourself appropriately. If you do not have adequate protection or are not specifically trained to control specific hazards, never enter a hazardous scene. Call in specialized teams, such as a hazardous materials crew, if necessary. Law enforcement agencies should be contacted for any violent, potentially violent, or dangerous scene, including those involving domestic abuse or other crimes.

If the scene is safe to enter, be sure to wear reflective clothing to provide added protection on the scene. With BSI precautions in place, approach patients with your safety in mind. Determine the mechanisms of injury (forces that caused injury) or the nature of illness. Treat the patient according to protocol.

After patient care is addressed and a transport decision is made, make sure your unit is secure before departure. Have your partner check the outside of the unit to make certain that all doors are secured. The patient should be secured on an ambulance stretcher with at least three straps and shoulder straps if available. If a family member is allowed to accompany the patient, that person should be placed in the passenger seat in the front compartment with vehicle restraints in place.

PREVENTION IN THE COMMUNITY

EMS has a responsibility to prevent injury and illness not only among EMS workers but also among members of the public.

As a component of healthcare, EMS has a responsibility to not only prevent injury and illness among EMS workers, but also to promote prevention among the members of the public.

AREAS OF NEED

Infants and Children

Each year, nearly 290,000 infants are born weighing less than 5.5 pounds (2,500 grams), often as a result of inadequate prenatal care. Low birth weight is a key indicator of poor health at the time of birth. Babies born too small or too soon are far more likely to die in the first year of life. Annually, over 4,000 die of low birth weight and prematurity. Among those who survive, an estimated 2% to 5% have a disability, and one quarter of the smallest survivors (born weighing less than 1,500 grams) have serious disabilities such as mental retardation, cerebral palsy, seizure disorders or blindness.

One of every three deaths among children in the United States results from an injury. The number of injuries, of course, far exceeds the number of deaths. The most common causes of fatal injuries in children include motor-vehicle collisions, pedestrian or bicycle injuries, burns, falls, and firearms. Injuries generally can be classified into intentional events (such as shootings and assaults), unintentional events (such as motor-vehicle collisions), and alleged unintentional events (such as suspicious injury patterns that suggest possible abuse).

In motor-vehicle collisions, young children are easily thrown on impact. Because a young child's head is large in proportion to the body, unrestrained children tend to fly head first into the windshield or out of the car when a collision occurs. The back seat is the best seat for children 12 years old or younger. In this location, the properly restrained child is least likely to sustain injuries in a crash. Car safety seats and seat belts can prevent most severe injuries to passengers of all ages if they are used correctly. Air bags are designed to save people's lives when used with seat belts, and they can protect drivers and passengers who are correctly buckled.

Infants and toddlers are commonly injured by cars backing up in driveways or parking lots. Children between the ages of five and nine who are struck by cars typically dart out in front of traffic. Children riding bicycles can be injured when they collide with cars or other fixed objects or when they are thrown from the bicycle. The most serious bicycle-related injuries are head injuries, which can cause death or permanent brain damage.

Falls are the most frequent cause of injury to children younger than six years old. About 200 children die from falls each year. Fire and burn injuries occur in the highest numbers in the very young. Most are caused by scalding from a hot liquid such as when children grab pot handles and spill the contents.

In this modern age of media and the internet, children and young adults are bombarded with an incredible amount of information and are often faced with some of the same stressors as adults. Sometimes those stressors become overwhelming. One of the most troubling recent trends is the number of violent acts among young people, occurring in the form of self-destructive behavior, gang violence, and assaults. In addition, firearm injury is becoming more common as a result of the accessibility of handguns to children. Injuries and deaths occur when children and adolescents take guns to school. The number of firearm deaths has doubled since 1953. About 15% of all firearm-related deaths are unintentional, often resulting from improper handling and lack of safety mechanisms.

Geriatric Patients

Falls account for the largest number of preventable injuries for persons over 75 years of age. As a result of slower reflexes, failing eyesight and hearing, and arthritis, the elderly are at increased risk of injury from falls. Falls frequently result in fractures since the bones become weaker and more brittle with age.

The aging process also places the elderly at greater risk for serious head injury as well as other injuries. Although many geriatric patients are completely coherent, many others suffer from some degree of dementia. Alzheimer's disease is merely one of the mental conditions that can affect the elderly. The associated confusion can contribute to dangerous behaviors such as wandering away from home or into a roadway.

Motor-Vehicle Collisions

As noted earlier, EMS and law enforcement have long referred to vehicular collisions as motor-vehicle accidents (MVAs). However, the term motor-vehicle collision (MVC) more accurately reflects the fact that no collision is an accident: something caused the crash to occur. Such crashes are responsible for over half of all deaths from unintentional injuries. Alcohol use is a factor in about half of all motor-vehicle fatalities.

Work and Recreation Hazards

In the workplace, back injuries account for 22% of all disabling injuries. Injuries to the eyes, hands, and fingers are responsible for another 22%. Even the quietest office setting can be hazardous. Never underestimate the potential dangers in an area that appears to be safe. Copy machines, electrical cords, faulty wiring, and shoddy building construction can be hazardous.

Sports injuries are commonly seen in persons of all ages due to the increased popularity and participation in outdoor recreational activities. Football, soccer, baseball, as well as running, hiking, and biking are among popular sports that can result in fractures, dislocations, sprains, and strains.

Medications

When an illness or injury occurs and treatment is sought, medications are often part of the treatment regimen. These medications are occasionally taken improperly (too much or not enough), or they are taken by others, sometimes causing serious medical problems. Medications of any kind should be taken only by those for whom they are prescribed. They should be stored according to label directions. They should also be continued until the prescription is completed. Following the physician's, the pharmacist's, and the label directions is imperative.

Early Discharge

Managed-care organizations such as HMOs and insurance companies often mandate shorter hospital stays and early discharges from the hospital, urgent care centers, and other out-patient facilities. Such policies often result in more patients who are at home sooner with illnesses that are less completely treated. These patients may call upon 911 for supportive care and intervention.

IMPLEMENTATION OF PREVENTION STRATEGIES

The following is a list of prevention strategies that you should be able to implement:

Content Review

PREVENTION STRATEGIES

- Preserve the safety of the response team
- Recognize scene hazards
- Document findings
- Engage in on-scene education
- Know community resources
- Conduct a community needs assessment

- *Preserve the safety of the response team.* Always remember that your first priority is your safety and the safety of your fellow crew members. The next priorities are the patient and, finally, bystanders. Do what you can and what is within your training to maintain a safe and secure working area. Do not hesitate to contact back-up units and law enforcement personnel if necessary.

- *Recognize scene hazards.* Size up the scene for potential risks or dangers before entering. Be aware of your surroundings. Is there anyone or anything that could cause harm to you, your crew, or the patient? Does the mechanism that injured the patient still pose a threat to the rescuers? Are there any hazardous materials in the area? Has any crime been committed? Are there structural risks? Are there temperature extremes for which you are unprepared? Call for the appropriate assistance.

- *Document findings.* Document your patient-care findings at the end of every call. Note that EMS patient forms often can be designed to include specific data on injury prevention in order to benefit researchers and implement future prevention programs. Such a form should include space to describe scene conditions at the time of EMS arrival, the mechanism of injury, and any risks that were overcome. If protective devices were used (or not used) during the emergency, these should be documented, too. (See Figure 1-14 for an example.)

- *Engage in on-scene education.* Take advantage of a teachable moment to decrease future emergency responses. Remain objective, nonjudgmental, and nonthreatening. Inform your listeners of how they can prevent the recurrence of a similar emergency and, if needed, instruct them on the use of protective devices.

- *Know your community resources.* Determine what your patient's needs are and how you may assist him. Your patient may require a referral to an outside agency such as a prenatal clinic, a social service organization that offers food, shelter, clothing, mental health resources or counseling, or other services. Your system may also allow for referral or transportation to a clinic, urgent care, or alternative form of health care. Be aware of the presence of both licensed and unlicensed day care centers in your area. Encourage parents to provide pre-existing consent for treatment and transport in case of illness or injury at a day care facility. Follow local protocol to report suspected abuse situations. Consider developing a social service resource guide for your organization to provide solutions and ideas for these and other situations.

- *Conduct a community needs assessment.* Conducting a needs assessment will assist in identifying community priorities. Consider the following:
  - Childhood and flu immunizations
  - Prenatal and well-baby clinics
  - Elder-care clinics

FIGURE 1-14 Documentation of primary and secondary injury prevention data.

- Defensive driving classes
- Workplace safety courses
- Health clinics (co-sponsored by local hospitals or health-care organizations)
- Prevention information on your agency's internet website

The population served and its ethnic, cultural, and religious makeup may affect the needs and approaches that are most appropriate. Also consider community members who are learning disabled or physically challenged. These are just a few of the ideas that may be appropriate for your organization.

Part 6: Ethics in Advanced Prehospital Care

When asked what the most difficult part of the job is, most paramedics do not say "ethics." Nonetheless, a significant percentage of advanced life support calls do pose possible ethical conflicts, for example regarding refusal of care, choice of hospital destination, and advance directives. So, whether or not you are consciously thinking about ethics, you are almost certain to be called upon to decide what is the ethical thing to do from time to time in the course of your work.

OVERVIEW OF ETHICS

Ethics and morals are closely related concepts. **Morals** are generally considered to be social, religious, or personal standards of right and wrong. **Ethics** more often refers to the rules or standards that govern the conduct of members of a particular group or profession. Both ethics and morals address a question Socrates asked: "How should one live?"

RELATIONSHIP OF ETHICS TO LAW AND RELIGION

Ethics and the law have a great deal in common, but they are distinct. In general, laws have a much narrower focus. Laws frequently describe what is wrong in the eyes of society. Ethics goes beyond what is wrong and examines what is right, or good. As a result, the law frequently has little or nothing to say about ethical problems. In fact, laws themselves can be unethical, for example laws that once perpetuated racial segregation. Even though ethics and the law are different, ethical discussions can sometimes benefit from techniques developed in the law. In particular, the law emphasizes impartiality, consistency, and methods to identify and balance conflicting interests.

Just as ethics differs from the law, it also differs from religion. In a pluralistic society such as ours, ethics must be understood by and apply to people who hold a broad range of religious beliefs or no religious beliefs at all. Thus ethics cannot derive from a single religion. It is true, however, that religion can enhance and enrich one's ethical principles and values.

MAKING ETHICAL DECISIONS

There are many approaches to determining how a medical professional should behave. One is to say that each person must decide how to behave and whatever decision that person makes is okay. This is known as *ethical relativism*. However, people typically do not find ethical relativism satisfactory. For example, no reasonable person would say that it was acceptable for the Nazis to behave as they did. A similar approach is to say, "Just do what is right." This sounds fine, but different people have different beliefs about what is "right." Even the Golden Rule—"Do unto others as you would have them do unto you"—is not a sufficient guideline. What happens when the care provider's desires and values differ from the patient's? It becomes clear that reason and logic must be used and emotion must be excluded as much as possible from the decision-making process.

Reason must be used and emotion must be excluded as much as possible from the decision-making process.
🗝

CODES OF ETHICS

Over the years, a number of organizations have drafted codes of ethics for the members of their organizations. The American Medical Association has a code of ethics for physicians. The American College of Emergency Physicians has a code of ethics specifically for emergency physicians. The American Nurses Association and Emergency Nurses Association both have codes for practitioners in their fields. In 1948, the World Medical Association adopted the "Oath of Geneva." The National Association of EMTs adopted a code of ethics for EMTs in 1978.

Most codes of ethics address broad humanitarian concerns and professional etiquette. Few provide solid guidance on the kind of ethical problems commonly faced by practitioners. For example, a paramedic is expected to work in an uncontrolled environment that is sometimes dangerous. A person who is unwilling to enter a scene until every risk has been totally eliminated is not acting in accordance with the expectations of the profession. Conversely, a paramedic is expected to refrain from entering a hazardous area until the risks have been made manageable. Common sense should help in resolving conflicts such as these.

THE FUNDAMENTAL QUESTIONS

The single most important question a paramedic has to answer when faced with an ethical challenge is "What is in the patient's best interest?" Usually the answer is obvious, but not always. For example, what is in the best interest of a terminally ill patient who goes into cardiac arrest—to resuscitate, or not to start resuscitation in order to prevent further suffering?

A paramedic must be very cautious in accepting a family's description of what a patient desires. The family is often under a great deal of stress when the paramedic encounters them. The paramedic must also realize that the family may not agree with the patient's desires. They may be led to substitute their own desires for the patient's.

Under ideal circumstances, a written statement describing the patient's desires will be available. In many states, such a statement (which meets other specified state and local requirements) is required by law before a paramedic may elect not to start resuscitation efforts. In less extreme circumstances, the patient may state verbally what he wishes you to do and not do. It may sometimes be difficult for a paramedic to agree or to comply with a patient's wishes, but as long as the patient is competent and the desires are consistent with good practice, the paramedic is obligated to respect the patient's wishes.

The single most important question a paramedic has to answer when faced with an ethical challenge is "What is in the patient's best interest?"

FUNDAMENTAL PRINCIPLES

A common approach to resolving problems in **bioethics** today is to employ four fundamental principles or values. These principles are beneficence, nonmaleficence, autonomy, and justice.

* **Beneficence** is related to a more familiar term, *benevolence*. Both come from Latin and concern doing good. However, *benevolence* means the desire to do good (usually the main reason people become paramedics), whereas *beneficence* means actually doing good (the paramedic's obligation to the patient).

* **Nonmaleficence** means *not* doing harm. (*Maleficence* means doing harm, the opposite of *beneficence*.) Few medical interventions are without risk of harm. Under the principle of nonmaleficence, however, the paramedic is obligated to minimize that risk as much as possible. This includes, for example, making the scene safe and protecting the patient from impaired or unqualified health-care providers. The Latin phrase, *primum non nocere*, which means "first, do no harm," sums up nonmaleficence very well.

* **Autonomy** refers to a competent adult patient's right to determine what happens to his own body, including treatment for medical illnesses and injuries. Under ordinary conditions, a patient must give consent before the paramedic can begin treatment. There are, of course, exceptions to this (see the discussion of consent later in this chapter and in Chapter 2), but the implication is that the paramedic must be truthful in describing to the patient his condition and the risks and benefits of treatment. It also implies respect for the patient's privacy.

* **Justice** refers to the paramedic's obligation to treat all patients fairly, without regard to sex, race, ability to pay, or cultural background, among other conditions.

* **bioethics** ethics as applied to the human body.

* **beneficence** the principle of doing good for the patient.

* **nonmaleficence** the obligation not to harm the patient.

First, do no harm (primum non nocere).

* **autonomy** a competent adult patient's right to determine what happens to his own body.

* **justice** the obligation to treat all patients fairly.

RESOLVING ETHICAL CONFLICTS

The paramedic needs to have a system for resolving ethical conflicts. One such method of resolving ethical issues is illustrated in the following scenario:

You represent your service at the regional EMS coordinating agency. The head nurse for the emergency department of a large hospital mentions how recent cutbacks in support staff have led to difficulty retrieving patients' medical records in a timely manner. This has led to a number of difficulties in treating patients. As a result, the ED was considering asking incoming ambulances to give patients' names and dates of birth on the radio. This would give the ED staff additional time to search for the patient's medical records.

You consider the issue's ethical aspects. First, you identify the problem: Is it justifiable to breach patient confidentiality in order to expedite the retrieval of medical records? Second, you list the possible actions that might be taken in this situation:

- Provide all patients' names and dates of birth on the radio.
- Continue, as now, to identify patients only by age and sex.
- Provide selected patients' names and dates of birth on the radio.

To reason out an ethical problem, first state the action in a universal form. Then list the implications or consequences of the action. Finally, compare them to relevant values, as follows:

1. *State the action in a universal form. Describe what should be done, who should do it, and under what conditions.* For example, EMS (who) will volunteer names and dates of birth for all patients (what) on the radio (condition).

2. *List the implications, or consequences, of the action.* Positive consequences: The ED will be able to get records sooner for patients who have records at that hospital. There will be no change for most patients because hospital records are often irrelevant to emergency care. The ED admitting staff may be able to admit patients more quickly. Negative consequences: Patients' names and dates of birth will be broadcast to thousands of people listening with scanners. Long term, people with scanners will learn more about patients who go to the hospital via EMS. Because private information may be broadcast, patients may become reluctant to call EMS. Conceivably, there may be more burglaries at homes of patients who use EMS.

3. *Compare the consequences to relevant values.* A list of values that pertain to this case might include: beneficence, nonmaleficence, autonomy, and confidentiality. That is, if EMS provided names and dates of birth for all patients on the radio, what would be the benefit to the patient (beneficence)? A few patients might be cared for sooner because their records arrived sooner. Most patients will see no benefit because they have no records at that hospital or time is not a significant issue (such as for a laceration that requires sutures). Autonomy suffers under this arrangement because the patient is not given the opportunity to consent (or decline). The patient's name and date of birth go out over the air without his permission. And, in this case, nonmaleficence and confidentiality are intertwined. There is potential for harm to the patient and to future patients who lose faith in the EMS system's ability to maintain privacy.

Since the possible consequences of providing all patients' names and dates of birth on the radio are not compatible with the values we consider important and relevant, you must go back and test another action using this same method.

What about the second option, simply to continue the current policy of identifying all patients over the radio only by age and sex? The consequences might be that people listening to scanners can learn about patients EMS is transporting but not their identities, and a few patients may get delayed care because their records do not arrive quickly enough. A comparison with relevant values reveals that patient confidentiality and patient confidence in EMS are unchanged, but the patients who might benefit from earlier arrival of their records may be suffering.

What about the third option, to provide names and dates of birth of selected patients, for example, those in serious condition whose treatment must not be delayed? A comparison with relevant values shows that there is potential benefit for selected patients, a breach of confidentiality for those patients, but no breach of confidentiality any other patients. So, the scenario may conclude as follows:

> The third option sounds closer to being acceptable, but you wonder if there is a way to further limit loss of confidentiality. You suggest revising the rule to read, "EMS broadcasts the names and dates of birth of selected patients who (1) *meet predetermined criteria, (2) when there is no other private means of communication available.*" This strictly limits the loss of confidentiality to patients who may benefit from it and encourages both EMS and the ED to find other less public means of identifying patients. For example, having someone at the scene telephone the ED to relay the patient's name and date of birth privately.

The method described above is useful when you come upon a new ethical problem and time is not an issue. In situations where time is limited, an abbreviated method can sometimes be used. First, ask yourself whether the current problem is similar to other problems for which you have already formulated a rule. If the answer is yes, follow that rule. If the answer is no, analyze the potential action against three tests suggested by Iserson: the impartiality test, the universalizability test, and the interpersonal justifiability test:

- *Impartiality test*—asks whether you would be willing to undergo this procedure or action if you were in the patient's place. This is really a version of the Golden Rule (Do unto others as you would have them do unto you), which helps to reduce the possibility of bias.

- *Universalizability test*—asks whether you would want this action performed in all relevantly similar circumstances, which helps the paramedic to avoid shortsightedness.

- *Interpersonal justifiability test*—asks whether you can defend or justify your actions to others. It helps to ensure that an action is appropriate by asking the paramedic to consider whether other people would think the action reasonable.

When there is little time to consider a new ethical problem, these three questions can help a paramedic navigate murky waters, allowing him to find an acceptable solution in a short time.

ETHICAL ISSUES IN CONTEMPORARY PARAMEDIC PRACTICE

The preceding discussion described principles and methods for dealing with ethical issues. The following discussion is meant to help you apply those principles to several commonly encountered situations as well as some less common situations you may face.

RESUSCITATION ATTEMPTS

Consider the following scenario:

> You are leaving the emergency department in your ambulance when a woman jumps out of a window of the hospital and lands on the road in front of you. Your partner stops the vehicle, and you grab your kit. As you reach the patient, a breathless aide runs out the door and says, "Don't do anything! She's got a DNR order!" How does this affect the care you administer? Your instincts say, treat her now and let the hospital sort things out later if she survives.

In this case, your instincts are probably steering you in the right direction for a number of reasons. First, state law requires that you see the order and verify its legitimacy in some manner. In this case, the order is not available for you to see so you are under no legal obligation to withhold care.

Second, if the patient is alive (as she appears to be), even a valid DNR order would not prevent you from assessing the patient and administering basic care, including comfort care.

Third, the principle of nonmaleficence says do no harm. Refraining from helping her might cause irreversible harm, perhaps death. The principle of beneficence also urges you to help the patient. The potential conflict arises when you consider autonomy. The competent patient of legal age has a right to determine what happens to her body, but you are unable to verify her wishes regarding resuscitation.

The conclusion of the scenario is as follows:

> You and your partner go ahead and assess the patient. She responds to verbal stimuli by moaning, her airway is open, ventilations are adequate, and she has several lacerations and apparent fractures. Since you are literally in front of the hospital, you limit your interventions to quick immobilization on a spine board with bleeding control and oxygen by mask. You rapidly move her to the ED and turn her over to the team there.
>
> Later you discover that she had originally been admitted for evaluation of new-onset seizures. When the doctors told her she might have a brain tumor, she signed a DNR form. Fortunately, no tumor was found and her prognosis is actually quite good. The trauma team finds no life-threatening injuries from her fall and expects her to be able to begin psychiatric treatment before she leaves the hospital. This additional information makes you very glad you decided to go ahead with treatment.

More and more states are passing laws or regulations allowing prehospital personnel to withhold certain treatment when the patient has a DNR order. A valid order consists of a written statement describing interventions a particular patient does not wish to have that is recognized by the authorities of that state. (See Chapter 2 for legal aspects of DNR orders.)

Paramedics spend a great deal of time and energy learning how to assess and treat patients with life-threatening problems. It becomes difficult, then, for a paramedic to watch someone die without doing something to try to stop it. You must nonetheless respect the patient's wishes when a competent patient has clearly communicated what he really wants. DNR orders make this easier because they typically must be signed or approved by a physician, increasing the likelihood that the decision was thoroughly thought through.

When there is no such order, however, it becomes more difficult for the paramedic to determine what the patient's wishes truly are. Family members may be able to describe the patient's desires, but they can have conflicts of interest that make their statements less credible. For example, the patient may have accepted his impending death before his family has. They may want you to attempt resuscitation when that was clearly against the patient's expressed wishes. A less common situation is one in which the patient wishes all resuscitation efforts, but the family does not because they do not wish to prolong their own suffering or they have other less noble motivations.

The general principle for paramedics to follow in cases such as these is: "When in doubt, resuscitate." This usually satisfies the principles of beneficence and nonmaleficence, admittedly perhaps at the expense of autonomy, but one of the biggest advantages to this approach is that, unlike the alternative, it is not irreversible. If you refrain from attempting resuscitation, it is certain that the patient will die. If you attempt resuscitation, there is no guarantee the patient will survive, but the patient can be removed from life-sustaining equipment later if that is deemed appropriate. Another advantage is that there will be more time later to sort out competing interests.

The general principle for paramedics to follow is "When in doubt, resuscitate."

What about not attempting resuscitation when the situation appears futile? This option may appear attractive at first glance. After a little investigation, though, the issue becomes much more complex. How would a reasonable person or society define "futile"? Except at the extreme ends of the spectrum, there is no consensus on what constitutes a futile attempt at resuscitation. In addition, there is the issue of who would actually make the decision that a resuscitation attempt is futile in a particular case. Is it the experienced paramedic who has seen very few lives saved under similar circumstances or the new paramedic who is still excited about the prospect of saving lives every day? How can it be fair to have such wide disparities in such an important decision? Clearly, the concept of futility does not provide a useful guide for whether or not to attempt resuscitation.

Another related topic is what to do when an advance directive is presented to you after you have begun resuscitation. Once you have verified the validity of the order and the identity of the patient, you are obligated ethically (and perhaps legally, depending on your state) to cease resuscitation efforts. This can be a very difficult situation for you emotionally, but you have an obligation to respect the patient's autonomy and stop doing something to him that he did not want. Follow your local protocols regarding procedures for cessation of resuscitation efforts.

CONFIDENTIALITY

Consider this scenario:

You are called at one o'clock in the morning to a local hotel for a man reported to be unresponsive (but breathing) at the front desk. When you arrive, one of the guests at the hotel meets you and tells you he found the clerk slumped over in his chair, apparently unconscious, with what smelled like alcohol on his breath.

You approach the patient. His skin appears normal, and he is moving air well. He does not respond when you call him by the name on his name plate, Howard. He has a strong, regular radial pulse that is within normal limits. You do not smell anything except for a faint minty odor. When you shake his shoulder and call his name again, he opens his eyes, looks around, and asks, "Who are you?"

You explain to Howard that you were called by a concerned guest who could not wake him up. Howard says he is fine now and does not want to go to a hospital. He is alert and oriented to person, place, and time. He denies any complaints, takes no medications, and has no past medical history. His vital signs are within normal limits. He denies any alcohol intake or use of any other drugs. The physical exam is unremarkable.

By your protocols and standard operating procedures, you have no reason to attempt to force the patient to go to a hospital. You complete the appropriate documentation for a refusal of transport and are leaving the lobby when the guest who called 911 stops you. "Aren't you going to take him to the hospital?" he asks. No, you reply, he does not want to go. "But what if there's a fire in the hotel and he's passed out and unable to help guests evacuate?"

This makes you stop and think, and you begin to weigh the rights of the hotel guests against the rights of your patient.

Your obligation to the patient is to maintain as confidential the information you obtained as a result of your participation in this medical situation. If you reported his condition to hotel management, what would you report? You have found no objective evidence that he is under the influence of alcohol or drugs. Depending on the state you are in, you may actually have a legal obligation to maintain confidentiality under circumstances such as these. On the other hand, what if there is an emergency in which the desk clerk's assistance is needed and he is unable to provide it? That is a conceivable but unlikely possibility. There is no clear and present danger that would require you to report.

There are a number of reasons to respect confidentiality in general. In an emergency, a patient assumes that he can be honest with these strangers who have come to help him because they will protect his privacy. If that trust was violated without sufficient cause, patients might very well be embarrassed or humiliated. This would undermine the public's trust in EMS. If word got around that private information was being made public, patients might not be forthcoming in giving their medical histories, potentially leading to disastrous consequences. For example, a man who had recently taken sildenafil (Viagra) for erectile dysfunction might deny taking it before you give him nitroglycerin. That drug interaction is potentially serious, possibly even fatal.

There are nonetheless times when it is appropriate and necessary to breach confidentiality. Every state has laws requiring the reporting of certain health facts such as births, deaths, particular infectious diseases, child neglect and abuse, and elder neglect and abuse. These last requirements have the most applicability to EMS. They are considered justifiable reasons to breach confidentiality because, in the eyes of society, the benefit to someone who is defenseless (protection from harm and perhaps even death) and to the public (a safer environment for children and the elderly) outweighs the right to privacy of a particular person. A valid court order is also considered a reasonable justification for breaching confidentiality. So is a clear threat by a patient to a specific person, as well as informing other health-care professionals who will care for the patient.

Clearly, patient confidentiality is an important principle, but not an inviolable one. When determining whether it is appropriate to breach confidentiality, take into account the probability of harm, the magnitude of the expected harm, and alternative methods of avoiding harm that do not require encroaching on confidentiality.

In the scenario above, factors do not justify breaching confidentiality. The person who called 911 for emergency assistance, however, is under no such obligation. The scenario comes to an end as follows:

> You inform the hotel guest that you are unable to discuss the case with anyone because of confidentiality. However, you point out, the guest is not under the same obligation. He replies, "OK, you may not be able to do anything about it, but I'm calling the manager!"

CONSENT

Consider this scenario:

> Bob, a 58-year-old male, has been having crushing substernal pain radiating to his left arm for several hours. He also is pale, sweaty, and nauseated. He denies shortness of breath. His condition remains unchanged after you give him oxygen and nitroglycerin. When you ask Bob which hospital he wants to go to, he tells you, "I'm not going to any hospital." Surprised, you find it difficult to understand why someone in this much pain would not want to go to a hospital. You try to enlist the help of relatives over the telephone (Bob lives alone), but they are unable to persuade the patient. He has no regular physician, so that option is not available to you. Finally, you decide to try on-line medical direction. While you are waiting for the physician to come to the phone, you wonder: If the patient continues to refuse, can you force him to go? How can you act in the best interest of a patient who refuses to accept what you feel certain is best for him?

A competent patient of legal age has the fundamental right to decide what health care he will receive and will not receive. This is at the core of patient autonomy. To exercise this right, a patient must have the information necessary to make an informed decision, the mental faculties to weigh the risks and benefits of various treatment options, and the freedom from restraints that might hamper his ability to exercise his options (such as threats).

It is sometimes appropriate to use the doctrine of implied consent to force the patient to go to the hospital. For the paramedic to use this approach, the patient must be unable to give consent. Typically, the doctrine is invoked when the patient is unable to communicate, but it also can be employed when the patient is incapacitated because of drugs, illness, or injury. In this scenario, however, the patient shows no signs of being incapacitated. He is alert and oriented, making judgments and answering questions in a manner completely compatible with competence. The fact that the patient refuses something you recommend does not, in itself, indicate that he is incompetent.

Before you leave the patient, you must not only do the things you need to do to protect yourself legally, but you must also assure yourself that the patient truly understands the issues at hand and is able to make an informed decision. As difficult as it may be for you, if the patient is able to do these things, you may have to accept the patient's desires and leave him.

ALLOCATION OF RESOURCES

Paramedics do not usually think of themselves as guardians of finite resources, but occasionally they are. The most obvious example of this is when there are more patients present than the paramedic is able to manage, such as in a multiple-casualty incident (MCI). While learning how to provide emergency medical care for multiple patients at the same scene, you might ask: What are the ethics of triage?

There are several possible approaches to consider in parceling out scarce resources. Patients could all receive the same amount of attention and resources (true parity). They could receive resources based on need. Or they could receive what someone has determined they've earned.

The civilian method of triage, where the most seriously injured patients receive the most care, is based on need. This is intended to produce the most good for the most people. However, other methods of triage are in use. Military triage, for example, has traditionally concentrated on helping the least seriously injured because this approach produces the greatest number of soldiers who can return to duty. When the President or Vice President visits a town or city, there is typically an ambulance dedicated for the dignitary's use if needed. The ambulance is not to be used for anyone else. Because these officials are so important and because so many others need them, the typical order of care is changed.

A controversy exists in emergency medicine as to whether or not celebrities should be treated ahead of others. The argument for doing so typically emphasizes the disorder brought to the ED by the presence of a celebrity and the need to get the person out of the ED as quickly as possible to restore normal operation. The argument against takes the position that giving preferential treatment to a celebrity is an affront to justice and fairness.

All of these methods have their proponents for different situations. The key to resolving the issue of allocation of scarce resources is to examine the competing theories in light of the circumstances at hand.

OBLIGATION TO PROVIDE CARE

Those who provide emergency care have a special obligation to help all those in need. Many other health-care professionals are free to pick and choose their patients, accepting only those who have health insurance or who can themselves pay for the services delivered by the health-care professional. This is not the case in emergency medicine. Paramedics, like other emergency professionals, are obligated to provide medical care for those in need without regard to ability to pay. They also have an ethical obligation to prevent and report instances of patient "dumping," where those without insurance are transferred against their will to public or charity hospitals.

A particular issue arises regarding the patient who is a member of a managed care organization such as a health maintenance organization (HMO). The HMO may insist that the patient be treated at a particular facility with which it has a contract. This must not be allowed to interfere with the patient's emergency care. The paramedic, like every other member of the EMS system, has an obligation to act in the patient's best interest, even when that goes against the HMO's economic interests.

Another situation is offering assistance when off duty. Although only two states require paramedics, among others, to stop and render help when they come upon someone in need of emergency care, there is still a strong ethical obligation to do so. This does not extend to situations where the paramedic would put himself in danger (such as, getting into a car teetering on the edge of a cliff), if assisting would interfere with important duties owed to others (such as leaving young children unattended in a car), or when someone else is already providing assistance. In return, society offers limited liability in the form of Good Samaritan statutes in every state in the United States (as discussed in Chapter 2).

TEACHING

When patients call for EMS, they generally expect to receive care from qualified, credentialed individuals. EMS systems with students working in them should make sure students are clearly identified by the uniform they wear. The paramedic acting as preceptor should also, when appropriate, inform patients of the presence of a student and request the patient's consent before the student performs a procedure. This sounds more cumbersome than it actually is. Patients who are unable to consent obviously do not fall into this category. Implied consent is invoked in this case. Patients who are able to consent are frequently very understanding of the student's need for experience. As long as the preceptor stresses that he is overseeing the student, the vast majority of patients usually consent.

Another issue related to students is how many attempts they should be allowed in order to perform procedures such as intravenous placement and endotracheal intubation before the preceptor steps in. Factors to consider include the student's skill level, the anticipated difficulty of the procedure, and the relative importance of the procedure. It is important to have a limit, at least initially, for the number of times a student will be allowed to attempt a procedure. Such a number will need to be decided by each system in consultation with the medical director.

PROFESSIONAL RELATIONS

As a health-care professional, the paramedic answers to the patient. As a physician extender, the paramedic answers to a physician medical director. As an employee (or volunteer), the paramedic answers to the EMS system. These competing interests can sometimes make life difficult. Each can lead to ethical challenges.

In general, there are three potential sources of conflict between paramedics and physicians. One possibility is a case in which a physician orders something the paramedic believes is contraindicated. For example, suppose a physician ordered a paramedic to transport a critical blunt-trauma patient without attempting any intravenous access, either at the scene or en route during the anticipated 45-minute transport. This order would run counter to standard medical practice.

A different situation arises when the physician orders something the paramedic believes is medically acceptable but not in the patient's best interests. For example, imagine you are transporting a patient with stable vital signs who is complaining of abdominal pain. In accordance with your protocols, you and your partner have each tried twice to start an IV line without success. The patient's veins are some of the worst you have ever seen, and you have no expectation that you will be successful on further attempts. The patient experienced considerable pain with each attempt and is now crying, asking you not to try any more. The physician, however, insists you continue attempts to gain access.

A third potential source of conflict is the situation in which the physician orders something the paramedic believes is medically acceptable but morally wrong. For example, say you are ordered to stop CPR on a young male found in cardiac arrest after blunt trauma. His initial rhythm of asystole has remained unchanged, and you know it is almost always associated with death. Nonetheless, although there is a very slim chance of recovery for the patient if you continue your resuscitation efforts, you would not be able to live with yourself if you did not at least try.

In each of the three cases, it is certainly appropriate for the paramedic to start by confirming the order and asking the physician to repeat it. If the order is confirmed, the medic would be prudent to ask the physician for an explanation, given the controversial nature of the orders. The next steps will depend on the physician's explanation, the patient's condition, the need for the intervention in the judgment of the paramedic, the feasibility of performing the intervention (like gaining IV access), and the amount of time available to discuss the issue.

Ultimately, the paramedic must determine for himself how the patient's interests are best served. This typically does not lead to conflict, but on occasion the paramedic may run into situations like the ones described above. In these cases, the medic must consider the competing interests of beneficence, non-maleficence, autonomy, and justice; the roles of the physician and the paramedic; the relative confidence (or lack thereof) the paramedic has in his own medical and ethical judgment; how far the paramedic is willing to go as an advocate for his patient; and the degree of risk acceptable to the paramedic in contravening physician orders.

It is important for the paramedic to understand that no matter what decision he makes, he will have to defend it. The explanation that he was just following the doctor's orders (or, conversely, just doing what he felt was right) will not be sufficient in and of itself. A paramedic is expected to be more than a robot. He is expected to simultaneously be a physician extender, working under a physician's license, and a clinician with the ability and independence to recognize and question inappropriate orders. The paramedic should also understand that he is not expected to act in ways he feels are immoral. On the other hand, if the individual's morals are significantly out of step with the expectations of the profession, he needs to reconsider his profession.

Disagreements with physician orders happen rarely. Usually they are the result of poor communication (such as, saying one thing while meaning another or static interfering with the radio transmission) or lack of sufficient information. Conflicts with physicians that reach the level in the examples above are fortunately rare. When they happen, the paramedic must be willing to be an advocate for the patient and act in the patient's best interests.

RESEARCH

EMS research is only in its infancy, but it will clearly become more important and more common as the field establishes the foundation necessary to introduce, modify, and justify field interventions. As this occurs, paramedics will become instrumental in implementing research protocols and gathering data. It is essential that a paramedic participating in a research project understand the importance of gaining expressed patient consent or following federal, state, and local regulations regarding implied consent.

The goal of patient care is to improve the patient's condition. The goal of research, on the other hand, is to help future. The two goals are not the same, so patients must be protected from untoward outcomes as much as possible.

One very important way of protecting the patient is by gaining the patient's expressed consent. There are several difficulties with this. One is the concern that a patient experiencing an emergency may not be able to truly consent because of the emotional pressures he is feeling. This pressure may occur in spite of the paramedic's best efforts to explain matters calmly and impartially.

Another concern is with the patient who is unable to consent. An excellent example of this occurs in cardiac arrest research. By the very nature of the problem being studied, the investigators will be unable to gather consent from the patient. In this case, the federal government has strict rules, for example, about community notification before the study begins and gaining consent from the patient or an appropriate family member as soon as possible after a patient is entered into the study. A paramedic participating in such a study needs to be familiar with these rules and their implications.

Although many interventions have been tested and found to be life saving, there are unfortunately documented instances of patients denied treatment for life-threatening conditions in the name of research in the United States (e.g., the Tuskegee syphillis research project in which treatment for the disease was withheld). The paramedic has an obligation to prevent such things from happening in EMS research.

SUMMARY

This is an exciting time for EMS and prehospital medicine. The paramedic of the twenty-first century is a true health-care professional who can provide a significant impact on health care.

EMS has evolved over many years. Today, a comprehensive EMS system provides a continuum of care from First Responder to hospital and rehabilitative staff, from the mechanic who maintains the ambulance fleet to the emergency physician. It is a total team effort. The paramedic is the leader of the prehospital emergency medical team. You must undertake the responsibility of preparing yourself to do the job and of continually updating your knowledge and skills. The best paramedics are those who make a commitment to excellence.

As a paramedic, you must attend first to your own well-being in order to maintain the health and fitness to help others and to be a positive role model. Additionally, each member of EMS shares the responsibility of promoting wellness and preventing illness and injury among co-workers and in the community.

As a paramedic, you also have the responsibility to behave ethically by acquiring a foundation in ethical values and having a system for making ethical decisions.

The best paramedics are those who make a commitment to excellence.

CHAPTER 2

Medical/Legal Aspects of Advanced Prehospital Care

Objectives

After reading this chapter, you should be able to:

1. Differentiate legal, ethical, and moral responsibilities. (p. 74)
2. Describe the basic structure of the legal system and differentiate civil and criminal law. (pp. 74-75)
3. Differentiate licensure and certification. (p. 77)
4. List reportable problems or conditions and to whom the reports are to be made. (p. 77)
5. Define:
   Abandonment (p. 88); Advance directives (pp. 90–92); Assault (pp. 84, 88); Battery (pp. 84, 88); Breach of duty (p. 79); Confidentiality (pp. 83–84); Consent (expressed, implied, informed, involuntary) (pp. 84–87); Do not resuscitate orders (p. 91); Duty to act (p. 79); Emancipated minor (p. 86); False imprisonment (p. 89); Immunity (pp. 78, 81); Liability (pp. 74, 78–82); Libel (p. 84); Minor (p. 86); Negligence (pp. 78–81); Proximate cause (pp. 80–81); Scope of practice (pp. 76–77); Slander (p. 84); Standard of care (p. 79); Tort (p. 75)

Continued

INTRODUCTION

To practice competent prehospital care today, paramedics must become familiar with the legal issues they are likely to encounter in the field. As a paramedic, you must be prepared to make the best medical decisions and the most appropriate legal decisions. This chapter addresses general legal principals in addition to specific laws and legal concepts that affect the paramedic's daily practice.

Note that since laws vary from state to state, and protocols can vary from county to county, the information contained in this chapter cannot be used as a substitute for competent legal advice. Just like the practice of medicine, the practice of law involves some art, some science, and is always heavily dependent on the unique facts present in each situation. If you are faced with a specific legal question, you must rely on the advice of your attorney.

LEGAL DUTIES AND ETHICAL RESPONSIBILITIES

Your best protection from liability is to perform systematic assessments, provide appropriate medical care, and maintain accurate and complete documentation.

As a paramedic, you have specific legal duties. Failure to perform your job appropriately can result in civil or criminal liability. Your best protection from **liability** (legal responsibility) is to perform a systematic patient assessment, provide the appropriate medical care, and maintain accurate and complete documentation of all incidents.

A paramedic also is responsible for meeting ethical standards. Ethical standards are not laws. They are principles that identify desirable conduct by members of a particular group. Your ethical responsibilities include:

- Promptly respond to the needs of every patient.
- Treat all patients and their families with courtesy and respect.
- Maintain mastery of your skills and medical knowledge.
- Participate in continuing education and refresher training.
- Critically review your performance, and seek improvement.
- Report honestly and with respect for patient confidentiality.
- Work cooperatively and with respect for other emergency professionals.

In addition you will encounter moral issues. Morality concerns right and wrong as governed by individual conscience. Always strive to meet the highest legal, ethical, and moral standards when providing patient care.

THE LEGAL SYSTEM

Sources of Law

In the United States, there are four primary sources of law: constitutional law, common law, legislative (or statutory) law, and administrative (or regulatory) law.

Constitutional law is based on the Constitution of the United States, which sets forth our basic governmental structures and protects people against governmental abuse. For example, the Fourth Amendment protects people from unreasonable searches and seizures.

Common law, also referred to as "case" or "judge-made" law, originated with the English legal system and is derived from society's acceptance of customs and norms over time. Common law changes and grows over the years. As a part of common law, precedents set by the courts are generally followed by other courts.

Legislative law (or statutory law) does not come from court decisions. It is created by law-making or legislative bodies. Statutes are enacted at the federal, state, and local levels by the legislative branches of government. Examples of legislative bodies include the U.S. Congress, state assemblies, city councils, and district boards. Legislative law takes precedence over common-law decisions.

Administrative law (or regulatory law) is enacted by an administrative or governmental agency at either the federal or state level. Administrative agencies, such as the Occupational Safety and Health Administration (OSHA), will take a statute enacted by a legislative body and will produce rules and regulations necessary to implement it. The agency is given the authority to make regulations based on that statute, enforce rules, regulations, and statutes under its authority, and hold administrative hearings to carry out penalties for any violations of its rules.

Categories of Law

The United States has two general categories of law: civil law and criminal law. **Criminal law** deals with crime and punishment. It is an area of law in which the federal, state, or local government will prosecute an individual on behalf of society for violating laws meant to protect society. Homicide, rape, and burglary are examples of criminal wrongs. Violations of criminal laws are punished by imprisonment, a fine, or combination of the two.

Civil law deals with noncriminal issues, such as personal injury, contract disputes, and matrimonial issues. In civil litigation, which involves conflicts between two or more parties, the *plaintiff* (person initiating the litigation) will seek to recover damages from the *defendant* (person against whom the complaint is made). **Tort** law, which is a branch of civil law, deals with civil wrongs committed by one individual against another (rather than against society). Tort law claims include negligence, medical malpractice, assault, battery, and slander.

Note that the United States has a *federal court system* and a *state court system*. The federal court system was created by the U.S. Constitution. Generally, only cases that involve a question of federal law or cases in which the parties are citizens of different states will be heard in a federal court. The state court system is the location for most of the cases in which a paramedic may become involved. In *trial courts*, a judge or jury determines the outcome of individual cases. *Appellate courts* hear appeals of decisions by trial courts or other appeals courts. The decisions of appellate courts may set precedents for later cases.

✱ **criminal law** division of the legal system that deals with wrongs committed against society or its members.

✱ **civil law** the division of the legal system that deals with noncriminal issues and conflicts between two or more parties.

✱ **tort** a civil wrong committed by one individual against another.

ANATOMY OF A CIVIL LAWSUIT

If you have ever been served with legal papers, you know that being sued or even being called to testify at a trial can be very unsettling. A basic understanding of the legal system can help. The following is a brief description of the components of a civil lawsuit:

- *Incident.* For example, a person is driving on a road and fails to see a stop sign. When he passes through the intersection, he hits another car and that driver sustains several injuries.

- *Investigation.* The injured driver's attorney makes a preliminary inquiry into the facts and circumstances surrounding the incident to determine if the case has merit.

- *Filing of the complaint.* The injured driver (now called the "plaintiff") commences the lawsuit by filing a complaint with the court. The complaint contains information such as the names of the parties, the legal basis for the claim, and the damages sought by the plaintiff. A copy of the complaint is served on the defendant.

- *Answering the complaint.* The defendant's attorney then prepares an answer, which addresses each allegation made in the complaint. The answer is then filed with the court, and a copy is given to the plaintiff's attorney.

- *Discovery.* Before any lawsuit appears in front of a judge or jury, both parties to an action participate in pre-trial discovery. This is the stage of the lawsuit when all relevant information about the incident is shared so that parties can prepare trial strategies. Discovery may include:
  – *An examination before trial,* which is also called a "deposition," allows a witness to answer questions under oath with a court stenographer present.

Content Review

COMPONENTS OF A CIVIL LAWSUIT

- Incident
- Investigation
- Filing of complaint
- Answering complaint
- Discovery
- Trial
- Decision
- Appeal
- Settlement

– *An interrogatory,* used by either side, is a set of written questions that requires written responses.
– *Requests for document production* entitles each side to request relevant documents, including the patient care report, records of the receiving hospital, any subsequent medical records, police records, and other records necessary to help prove or defend the lawsuit.

• *Trial.* A trial will be commenced at the lowest level of court in the state. In many states, they are called "superior" courts. At the trial, each side will be given the opportunity to present all relevant evidence and testimony from witnesses.

• *Decision.* After deliberations, the judge or jury determines the guilt or liability of the defendant and then decides the amount of damages to award the plaintiff.

• *Appeal.* After the jury's decision is entered by the court, either party may be entitled to an appeal. Generally, grounds for an appeal are limited to errors of law made by the court. Appeals will not be heard at the lower-level court, but by the higher-level appellate court.

• *Settlement.* This can occur at any stage of the lawsuit. Generally, the defendant will offer the plaintiff an amount of money that is less than the amount for which he is being sued. The plaintiff may then agree to accept the reduced amount on the condition, for example, that he will no longer pursue the case.

LAWS AFFECTING EMS AND THE PARAMEDIC

Most of the laws that affect EMS and paramedics are state laws. Although these laws vary from state to state, they share common principles.

Scope of Practice

The range of duties and skills paramedics are allowed and expected to perform is called the **scope of practice.** Usually, the scope of practice is set by state law or regulation and by local medical direction. Often, a state will have a general "medical practice act" that governs the practice of medicine and all health-care professionals. These acts prescribe how and to what extent a physician may delegate authority to a paramedic. As you learned in Chapter 1, paramedics may function only under the direct supervision of a licensed physician through a delegation of authority. Generally, paramedics should follow orders given by on-line and off-line medical direction. However, you should not blindly follow orders that you know are medically inappropriate.

Circumstances in which an order from medical direction may be legitimately refused include: when you are ordered to provide a treatment that is beyond the scope of your training and inconsistent with established protocols or procedures, and when you are ordered to administer a treatment that you reasonably believe would be harmful to the patient. For example, imagine that a paramedic is en route to the hospital with a 200-pound (100 kg) patient who is having 15 multifocal premature ventricular contractions (PVCs) per minute. The treatment protocol for such a condition is to administer 1.0 to 1.5 mg/kg of lidocaine, or 100 to 150 mg to a 200-pound patient. The on-line physician orders the paramedic to administer 1 gram (1000 mg) of lidocaine. The paramedic knows this amount of medication would seriously harm the patient. What should he do? He should first raise the concern with the physician. If the physician still insists, the paramedic should refuse to follow the order and document the incident thoroughly on the patient care report.

✳ scope of practice range of duties and skills paramedics are allowed and expected to perform.

You may function as a paramedic only under the direct supervision of a licensed physician through a delegation of authority.

In addition, every EMS system should have a policy in place to guide paramedics in dealing with intervener physicians (on-scene licensed physicians who are professionally unrelated to the patient and who are attempting to assist with patient care). Generally, such a policy requires that certain conditions be met before the paramedic should allow the intervener physician to assume control of patient care. That is, the physician must be properly identified to the paramedic, licensed to practice medicine in the state, willing to accept the responsibility of continuing medical care until the patient reaches the hospital, and willing to document the intervention as required by the local EMS system.

Licensure and Certification

Other laws that directly affect the paramedic's ability to practice relate to certification and licensure requirements. *Certification* refers to the recognition granted to an individual who has met predetermined qualifications to participate in a certain activity. It is usually given by a certifying agency (not necessarily a government agency) or professional association. For example, after completing an approved paramedic program in New York State, a student who passes an approved written and practical examination will become a certified New York State paramedic.

Licensure is a process used to regulate occupations. Generally, a governmental agency, such as a state medical board, grants permission to an individual who meets established qualifications to engage in a particular profession or occupation. Certification or licensure, or perhaps both, may be required by your state or local authorities for you to practice as a paramedic.

Most states have laws that govern paramedic practice and set forth the requirements for certification, licensure, recertification, and relicensure. It is your responsibility to understand fully the EMS laws and regulations in your state.

Motor-Vehicle Laws

As with other EMS-related laws, motor-vehicle laws vary from state to state. Generally, there are special motor-vehicle laws that govern the operation of emergency vehicles and the equipment they carry. These laws apply to areas such as vehicle maintenance and use of the siren and emergency lights. It is important that you become familiar with the laws of your state. Keep up to date with local regulations, too.

Mandatory Reporting Requirements

Each state enacts different laws designed to protect the public. For example, most states have laws that require a health-care worker to report to local authorities any suspected spousal abuse, child abuse and neglect, or abuse of the elderly. In many states, violent crimes, such as sexual assault, gunshot wounds, and stab wounds must be reported to law enforcement. Emergencies that threaten public health, such as animal bites and communicable diseases, also must be reported to the proper authorities. The content of such reports and to whom they must be made is set by law, regulation, or policy. Become familiar with the circumstances under which you are required to make a report. If you fail to make a required report, you may be criminally and civilly liable for your inaction.

Content Review

COMMONLY MANDATED REPORTS
- Spouse abuse
- Child abuse and neglect
- Elder abuse
- Sexual assault
- Gunshot and stab wounds
- Animal bites
- Communicable diseases

Legal Protection for the Paramedic

In addition to the laws that protect patients, legislative bodies have enacted laws to protect paramedics. For example, some jurisdictions have enacted laws that criminally punish a person who commits assault or battery against a paramedic while he is providing medical care. Others have laws prohibiting the obstruction of paramedic activity.

Immunity, or exemption from legal liability, is another form of protection. Governmental immunity is a judicial doctrine that prohibits a person from bringing a lawsuit against a government without its consent. However, most states today have waived their immunity rights, and courts are becoming increasingly likely to strike down the ones that still exist. This type of liability protection, even if allowed under law, generally serves to protect only the government agency, not the individual paramedic. Therefore, you should not rely on governmental immunity to protect you from claims of negligence.

* **immunity** exemption from legal liability.

Virtually every state has **Good Samaritan laws,** which provide immunity to people who assist at the scene of a medical emergency. Though these laws vary from state to state, generally, they protect a person from liability if that person acts in good faith, is not negligent (most states will cover acts of simple negligence but not ones of gross negligence), acts within his scope of practice, and does not accept payment for services. The Good Samaritan laws of many states have been expanded to protect both paid and volunteer prehospital personnel.

* **Good Samaritan laws** laws that provide immunity to certain people who assist at the scene of a medical emergency.

As a paramedic, you should also become familiar with local laws and regulations governing the use of physical restraints for dangerous or violent patients. There also may be regulations governing entry into restricted areas such as military installations, nuclear power plants, and sites with hazardous materials. Since the laws affecting paramedic practice vary from state to state, your agency should obtain the advice of an attorney in order to minimize potential exposure to liability.

Other laws are designed to protect the paramedic in the event of exposure to bloodborne or airborne pathogens. For example, the Ryan White Comprehensive AIDS Resources Emergency Act (Ryan White CARE Act) requires hospitals and EMS agencies to create a notification system to provide information and assist the paramedic when an exposure occurs. This law allows the paramedic who has been exposed to certain diseases (such as hepatitis B, AIDS, and tuberculosis) access to medical records to determine if the patient has tested positive for, or is exhibiting signs and symptoms of, an infectious disease. The Ryan White CARE Act is a federal law, but many states have enacted similar or even more comprehensive laws to protect paramedics who may have been exposed to infectious diseases. It is important for each agency to appoint an infection control officer and for this individual to implement protocols and an appropriate infection control plan.

LEGAL ACCOUNTABILITY OF THE PARAMEDIC

As a paramedic, you are required to provide a level of care to your patients that is consistent with your education and training and equal to that of any other competent paramedic with equivalent training. You also are expected to perform your duties in a reasonable and prudent manner, as any other paramedic would in a similar situation. Any deviation from this standard might open you to allegations of negligence and liability for any resulting damages.

NEGLIGENCE AND MEDICAL LIABILITY

Negligence is defined as a deviation from accepted standards of care recognized by law for the protection of others against the unreasonable risk of harm. It can result in legal accountability and liability. In the health-care professions, negligence is synonymous with malpractice.

* **negligence** deviation from accepted standards of care recognized by law for the protection of others against the unreasonable risk of harm.

Components of a Negligence Claim

In a negligence claim against a paramedic, the plaintiff must establish and prove four particular elements in order to prevail: a duty to act, a breach of that duty, actual damages to the patient or other individual, and proximate cause (causation of damages).

First, the plaintiff must establish that the paramedic had a **duty to act.** That is, he must prove that the paramedic had a formal contractual or informal legal obligation to provide care. Note that the act of voluntarily assuming care of a patient may imply that there was a duty to act, which creates a continuing duty to act. For example, in some states if an off-duty paramedic witnesses a person choking, he may be under no legal duty to act. However, if that paramedic initiates care, then he has a duty to continue care. The rationale behind this rule is if bystanders see that a victim is being helped, they may walk away. If the paramedic rendering assistance walks away after initiating treatment, but not completing it, the patient may actually be left in a worse condition than if the paramedic never tried to help.

Duties that are expected of the paramedic include:

- Duty to respond to the scene and render care to ill or injured patients
- Duty to obey federal, state, and local laws and regulations
- Duty to operate the emergency vehicle reasonably and prudently
- Duty to provide care and transportation to the expected standard of care
- Duty to provide care and transportation consistent with the paramedic's scope of practice and local medical protocols
- Duty to continue care and transportation through to appropriate conclusions

Second, the plaintiff must prove there was a **breach of duty** by the paramedic. A paramedic always must exercise the degree of care, skill, and judgment that would be expected under like circumstances by a similarly trained, reasonable paramedic in the same community. The **standard of care** specific to the paramedic's practice is generally established by court testimony and referenced to published codes, standards, criteria, and guidelines applicable to the situation. A breach of duty may occur by **malfeasance, misfeasance,** or **nonfeasance:**

- *Malfeasance,* or the performance of a wrongful or unlawful act by the paramedic. For example a paramedic commits malfeasance if he assaults a patient.
- *Misfeasance,* or the performance of a legal act in a manner that is harmful or injurious. For example, a paramedic commits misfeasance when he inadvertently intubates a patient's esophagus, fails to confirm tube placement, and leaves the tube in place.
- *Nonfeasance,* or the failure to perform a required act or duty. For example, it would be an act of nonfeasance to fail to fully immobilize a collision patient who is complaining of neck and back pain.

In some cases, negligence may be so obvious that it does not require extensive proof. Unlike criminal cases, which require proof "beyond a reasonable doubt," civil cases require only a proof of guilt by a "preponderance of evidence." In most cases, the burden of proving negligence rests on the plaintiff. As

* **duty to act** a formal contractual or informal legal obligation to provide care.

* **breach of duty** an action or inaction that violates the standard of care expected from a paramedic.

Always exercise the degree of care, skill, and judgment expected under like circumstances by a similarly trained, reasonable paramedic in the same community.

* **standard of care** the degree of care, skill, and judgment that would be expected under like or similar circumstances by a similarly trained, reasonable paramedic in the same community.

* **malfeasance** a breach of duty by performance of a wrongful or unlawful act.

* **misfeasance** a breach of duty by performance of a legal act in a manner that is harmful or injurious.

* **nonfeasance** a breach of duty by failure to perform a required act or duty.

a result, when it is difficult to do so, a plaintiff may sometimes invoke the doctrine of *res ipsa loquitur,* which is Latin for "the thing speaks for itself."

To support a claim of *res ipsa loquitur,* the complainant must prove that the damages would not have occurred in the absence of somebody's negligence, the instruments causing the damages were under the defendant's control at all times, and the patient did nothing to contribute to his own injury. After the doctrine of *res ipsa loquitur* is invoked in court, the burden of proof shifts from the plaintiff to the defendant.

For example, a classic situation in which *res ipsa loquitur* might be used occurs when a patient has an appendectomy and wakes to find that a surgical instrument has been left inside his abdomen. To prove negligence in this case, the plaintiff's attorney would show that the damage would not have occurred without the physician's negligence, that the surgical instrument was under the physician's control at all relevant times, and that the patient did not contribute to the injury. Many cases in which *res ipsa loquitur* would be successful are settled out of court.

Another situation in which little proof is required occurs when the paramedic violates a statute and injury to a plaintiff results. Some laws state that if a statute is violated and an injury resulted, a person will be guilty of *negligence per se,* or automatic negligence. For example, if a paramedic, who is driving in non-emergency mode, fails to stop at a red light and hits a pedestrian, the paramedic's negligence is obvious. He violated vehicle and traffic statutes that prohibit a vehicle from running a red light, and he is therefore guilty of *negligence per se.*

After a duty to act and a breach of that duty have been proven, **actual damages** is the third required element of proof in a negligence claim. That is, the plaintiff must prove that he was actually harmed in a way that can be compensated by the award of damages. This is an essential component. A lawsuit cannot be won if the paramedic's action caused no ill effects. The plaintiff must prove that he suffered compensable physical, psychological, or financial damage such as medical expenses, lost wages, lost future earnings, conscious pain and suffering, or wrongful death.

In addition, the plaintiff may seek punitive (punishing) damages. These are awarded only when a defendant commits an act of gross negligence or willful and wanton misconduct. An act of ordinary negligence, such as accidentally allowing an IV to infiltrate, will not support an award of punitive damages. If punitive damages are awarded to the plaintiff, most insurance policies will not cover them. Therefore, the paramedic may become personally liable for any punitive damages awarded to the plaintiff.

Finally, to prove negligence, the plaintiff must show that the paramedic's action or inaction was the **proximate cause** of the damages; that is, the action or inaction of the paramedic immediately caused or worsened the damage suffered by the plaintiff. For example, a cardiac patient who breaks his arm during an ambulance collision while en route to the hospital will likely be able to prove that his injuries resulted from the incident; that is, the collision was the proximate cause of his injuries. However, a patient with a sprained wrist who happens to suffer a stroke while in the ambulance would have difficulty proving the ambulance ride was the proximate cause of the stroke.

Proximate cause may also be thought of in terms of "foreseeability." To show the existence of proximate cause, the plaintiff needs to prove that the damage to the patient was reasonably foreseeable by the paramedic. This is usually established by expert testimony. For example, imagine that a paramedic negligently crashes into a telephone pole with the ambulance. As a result, two people are injured—the patient who was in the back of the ambulance and, two blocks away, a baby who was dropped by his mother when the loud crash startled her. It should be easy for the patient to prove proximate cause, because it was reasonably foreseeable that an ambulance crash could hurt passengers. However, if the woman who dropped her baby sued the paramedic, she probably would not be able to establish proximate cause. Although the crash was the reason her baby was injured, it was not a foreseeable injury resulting from the ambulance crash.

Defenses to Charges of Negligence

If you are accused of negligence, you may be able to avoid liability if you can establish a defense to the plaintiff's claim. The following is a list of potential defenses to negligence:

- *Good Samaritan laws.* If the paramedic can establish that his actions were protected by a Good Samaritan law, liability may be avoided. Note that such laws generally do not protect providers from acts of gross negligence, reckless disregard, or willful or wanton conduct, and they do not prohibit the filing of lawsuits.

- *Governmental immunity.* These laws do not offer much protection for the individual paramedic accused of negligence. Though governmental immunity laws vary from state to state, the current legal trend is toward limiting this type of protection.

- *Statute of limitations.* This is a law that sets the maximum time period during which certain actions can be brought in court. After the time limit is reached, no legal action can be brought regardless of whether or not a negligent act occurred. Statutes of limitations vary from state to state, so carefully review the laws in your state. Note that they may vary for different negligent acts and for cases involving children.

- *Contributory or comparative negligence.* Some state laws will reduce or eliminate a plaintiff's award of damages if the plaintiff is found to have caused or worsened his own injury. For example, imagine that a patient involved in a car crash complained of neck pain but refused to let the paramedics properly immobilize his spine. The paramedics explained the risks of refusing treatment, but the patient signed a "release-from-liability" form anyway. Later, the patient learns that he has permanent spinal-cord damage and sues the paramedics for negligence. Many courts will find that the paramedics were not negligent because, by refusing necessary treatment, the patient contributed to the exacerbation of his own injury.

To protect yourself against claims of negligence, you should receive appropriate education, training, and continuing education; receive appropriate medical direction, both on-line and off-line; always prepare accurate, thorough documentation; have a professional attitude and demeanor at all times; always act in good faith, and use your own common sense. In addition, it is essential for all paramedics to be covered by liability insurance. Although many employers and agencies carry coverage, it is a good idea to obtain your own because your agency's coverage may be inadequate.

It is essential for all paramedics to be covered by liability insurance.

SPECIAL LIABILITY CONCERNS

Medical Direction

If a paramedic makes a mistake in the field and is sued by the injured patient, it is possible that the patient will also sue the paramedic's medical director and the on-line physician. The on-line physician may be liable to a patient for giving the paramedic medically incorrect orders or advice, for the refusal to authorize the administration of a medically necessary medication, or for directing an ambulance to take a patient to an inappropriate medical facility.

A paramedic's medical director may be liable to the patient for the negligent supervision of the paramedic. In order for the patient to be successful in this type of claim, he would have to prove that the physician breached a duty to supervise the paramedic and that breach was the proximate cause of the patient's injuries. Examples include: the medical director's failure to establish medication protocols or standing orders consistent with the current standards of medical practice for the paramedic to use in the field; the medical director observed and then failed to correct a paramedic's poor intubation technique; or the medical director received complaints of inappropriate care by a paramedic and then failed to effectively investigate and resolve the problem.

Borrowed Servant Doctrine

As a paramedic, you may find yourself in the position of supervising other emergency care providers, such as EMT-Basics or EMT-Intermediates. When doing so, it will be your responsibility to make sure they perform their duties in a professional and medically appropriate manner. Depending on the degree of supervision and the amount of control you have, you may be liable for any negligent act they commit. This is called the "borrowed servant" doctrine. For it to apply, the paramedic accused of negligence must have taken the employees of another employer under his control and exercised supervisory powers over them.

Civil Rights

In addition to suing you for negligence, a patient may be able to sue you under certain circumstances for violating his civil rights if you fail to render care for a discriminatory reason. As a paramedic, you may not withhold medical care for reasons such as race, creed, color, gender, national origin, or in some cases, ability to pay. Also, all patients should be provided with appropriate care regardless of their status, condition, or disease (including AIDS/HIV, tuberculosis, and other communicable diseases).

Off-Duty Paramedics

Liability also may arise in a situation in which an off-duty paramedic renders assistance at the scene of an illness or injury. Generally, any person who provides basic emergency first aid to another person would be protected from liability under a Good Samaritan law. However, when the off-duty paramedic provides advanced life support, a problem may arise. In most states, paramedics cannot practice advanced skills unless they are practicing within an EMS system. To perform paramedic skills and procedures that require delegation from a physician while off-duty may constitute the crime of practicing medicine without a license. Learn the law in your jurisdiction.

PARAMEDIC-PATIENT RELATIONSHIPS

The relationship you establish with your patient is a very important one. Not only must you provide the best medical care, you also have legal and ethical duties to protect the patient's privacy and treat him with honesty, respect, and compassion.

CONFIDENTIALITY

All records related to the emergency care rendered to a patient must be kept strictly confidential. Keeping patient **confidentiality** means that any medical or personal information about a patient—including medical history, assessment findings, and treatment—will not be released to a third party without the express permission of the patient or legal guardian. However, there are specific circumstances under which a patient's confidential information may be released:

- *Patient consents to the release of his records.* A patient may request a copy of his medical records for any reason. If the patient is a child, consent for release of medical records must be obtained from the child's parent or other legal guardian. The request should be accepted only if it is in writing, specifically authorizes the agency to release the records, and contains the patient's signature (or other authorized signature). If the request so directs, it is permissible to forward the records to the patient's physician, insurance company, attorney, or any other party the patient specifies. Be sure your agency retains a copy of the consent document.

- *Other medical care providers have a need to know.* For example, it is not a breach of patient confidentiality to discuss the patient's condition with on-line medical direction or to give a patient report to an emergency department nurse upon arrival at the hospital. This is permitted because it allows medical care appropriate for the patient to be continued. It is not acceptable, however, to discuss confidential patient information with medical providers who have no responsibility for the patient's care.

- *EMS is required by law to release a patient's medical records.* Records may be requested by a court order that is signed by a judge, or they may be requested by *subpoena* (a command to appear at a certain time and place to give testimony). When an agency receives a court order or subpoena, it is good practice to consult with an attorney to make sure the order is valid and for assistance with compliance. Failure to comply with a court order or subpoena may result in severe penalties.

- *There are third-party billing requirements.* For EMS agencies that bill patients for services, it is generally necessary to release certain confidential information to receive reimbursement from private insurance companies, Medicaid, or Medicare. If possible, the agency should obtain patient authorization for this purpose.

The law provides penalties for the breach of confidentiality. The improper release of information may result in a lawsuit against the paramedic for defamation (libel or slander), breach of confidentiality, or invasion of privacy. If found guilty, the paramedic may be responsible for paying money damages to the patient.

Defamation

Defamation occurs when a person makes an intentional false communication that injures another person's reputation or good name. A patient may sue a paramedic for defamation if the paramedic communicates an untrue statement about a patient's character or reputation without legal privilege or consent. Defamation can occur in written form or through verbal statements.

Libel is the act of injuring a person's character, name, or reputation by false statements made in writing or through the mass media with malicious intent or reckless disregard for the falsity of those statements. Allegations of libel can be avoided by completing an accurate, professional, and confidential patient care report. Do not use slang and value-loaded words or phrases in your report (for example, do not refer to a patient as "stupid" or use any derogatory race-based terms). Since many states consider the patient care report part of the public record, never write anything on it that could be considered libelous.

Slander is the act of injuring a person's character, name, or reputation by false or malicious statements spoken with malicious intent or reckless disregard for the falsity of those statements. An allegation of slander can be avoided by limiting oral reporting of a patient's condition to appropriate personnel only. Note that many EMS systems record ambulance-hospital radio transmissions, and scanners, which give the public access to EMS transmissions, are common in the United States. Therefore, information transmitted over the radio should be limited to essential matters of patient care. In most cases, the patient's name and insurance status should not be transmitted over the radio.

Invasion of Privacy

A paramedic may be accused of invasion of privacy for the release of confidential information, without legal justification, regarding a patient's private life, which might reasonably expose the patient to ridicule, notoriety, or embarrassment. That includes, for example, the release of information regarding HIV status or other sensitive medical information. The fact that released information is true is not a defense to an action for invasion of privacy.

CONSENT

By law, you must get a patient's consent before you can provide medical care or transport. **Consent** is the granting of permission to treat. More accurately, it is the granting of permission to touch. It is based on the concept that every adult human being of sound mind has the right to determine what should be done with his own body. Touching a patient without appropriate consent may subject you to charges of assault and battery.

A patient must be **competent** in order to give or withhold consent. A competent adult is one who is lucid and able to make an informed decision about medical care. He understands your questions and recommendations, and he understands the implications of his decisions made about medical care. Although there is no absolute test for determining competency, keep the following factors in mind when making a determination: the patient's mental status, the patient's ability to respond to questions, statements regarding the patient's competency from family or friends, evidence of impairment from drugs or alcohol, or indications of shock.

Informed Consent

Conscious, competent patients have the right to decide what medical care to accept. However, for consent to be legally valid, it must be **informed consent,** or consent given based on full disclosure of information. That is, a patient must understand the nature, risks, and benefits of any procedures to be performed. So, before providing medical care, you must explain the following to the patient in a manner he can understand:

- Nature of the illness or injury
- Nature of the recommended treatments
- Risks, dangers, and benefits of those treatments
- Alternative treatment possibilities, if any, and the related risks, dangers, and benefits of accepting each one
- Dangers of refusing treatment, including transport

Informed consent must be obtained from every competent adult before treatment may be initiated. Conscious, competent patients may revoke consent at any time during care and transport. In most states, a patient must be 18 years of age or older in order to give or withhold consent. Generally, a child's parent or legal guardian must give informed consent before treatment of the child can begin.

Expressed, Implied, and Involuntary Consent

There are three more types of consent: expressed, implied, and involuntary. **Expressed consent** is the most common. It occurs when a person directly grants permission to treat—verbally, non-verbally, or in writing. Often, the act of a patient requesting an ambulance is considered an expression of a desire to be treated. However, just because the patient consents to a ride to the hospital does not mean he has consented to all types of treatment (such as the initiation of an IV and/or the administration of medications). You must obtain consent for each treatment you plan to provide. Consent from the patient does not always need to be granted verbally. It may be expressed by allowing care to be rendered.

Unconscious patients cannot grant consent. When treating them or any patient who requires emergency intervention but is mentally, physically, or emotionally unable to grant consent, treatment depends on **implied consent** (sometimes called "emergency doctrine"). That is, it is assumed that the patient would want life-saving treatment if he were able to give informed consent. Implied consent is effective only until the patient no longer requires emergency care or until the patient regains competence.

Occasionally, a court will order patients to undergo treatment, even though they may not want it. This is called **involuntary consent**. It is most commonly encountered with patients who must be held for mental-health evaluation or as directed by law enforcement personnel who have the patient under arrest. It also is used on occasion to force patients to undergo treatment for a disease that threatens the community at large (tuberculosis, for example). Law-enforcement personnel often will accompany patients who are undergoing court-ordered treatment.

Consent issues also can arise when a paramedic is called by law-enforcement officials to treat a sick or injured prisoner or arrestee. The officers may tell you that they have the legal authority to give consent to treatment for the patient simply because the patient is in police custody. However, a competent adult in police custody does not necessarily lose the right to make medical decisions for himself. In fact, many prisoners have successfully sued health-care providers for rendering treatment without consent. Generally, forced treatment is limited to emergency treatment necessary to save life or limb or treatment ordered by the court. Be sure that you are familiar with your local protocols and laws on this issue.

* **expressed consent** verbal, non-verbal, or written communication by a patient that he wishes to receive medical care.

* **implied consent** consent for treatment that is presumed for a patient who is mentally, physically, or emotionally unable to grant consent. Also called *emergency doctrine*.

* **involuntary consent** consent to treatment granted by the authority of a court order.

Special Consent Situations

In the case of a **minor** (depending on state law, this is usually a person under the age of 18), consent should be obtained from a parent, legal guardian, or court-appointed custodian. The same is true of a mentally incompetent adult. If a responsible person cannot be located, and if the child or mentally incompetent adult is suffering from an apparent life-threatening injury or illness, treatment may be rendered under the doctrine of implied consent.

Generally, an **emancipated minor** is considered an adult. This is a person under 18 years of age who is married, pregnant, a parent, a member of the armed forces, or financially independent and living away from home. As an adult, an emancipated minor may legally give informed consent. Anyone else under the age of 18 may not grant informed consent.

Withdrawal of Consent

A competent adult may withdraw consent for any treatment at any time. However, refusal must be informed. That is, the patient must understand the risks of not continuing treatment or transport to the hospital in terms he can fully understand. A common example of a patient withdrawing consent occurs after a hypoglycemic patient regains full consciousness with the administration of dextrose. The patient should be encouraged—*but may not be forced*—to go to the emergency department. If he is competent, the patient may refuse transport. In such cases, advanced life support measures, such as IV fluids, which were initiated when the patient was unconscious, should be discontinued. The patient also should complete a release-from-liability form (Figure 2-1).

Sometimes patients choose to accept one recommended treatment, but refuse others. For example, a patient involved in a motor-vehicle crash may refuse to be fully immobilized but ask to be transported to the hospital. It is very important for you to do everything in your power to be sure he understands why spinal precautions are necessary and what may happen if they are not taken. If a competent adult continues to refuse care, be sure to thoroughly document his reason for refusal and your attempts to convince him to change his mind. Have the patient and a witness sign a release-from-liability form.

REFUSAL OF TREATMENT AND TRANSPORTATION

I, THE UNDERSIGNED HAVE BEEN ADVISED THAT MEDICAL ASSISTANCE ON MY BEHALF IS NECESSARY AND THAT REFUSAL OF SAID ASSISTANCE AND TRANSPORTATION MAY RESULT IN DEATH, OR IMPERIL MY HEALTH. NEVERTHELESS, I REFUSE TO ACCEPT TREATMENT OR TRANSPORT AND ASSUME ALL RISKS AND CONSEQUENCES OF MY DECISION AND RELEASE GOLD CROSS AMBULANCE COMPANY AND ITS EMPLOYEES FROM ANY LIABILITY ARISING FROM MY REFUSAL.

_____
SIGNATURE OF PATIENT

_____
WITNESSED BY

_____
DATE SIGNED

FIGURE 2-1 Example of a "release-from-liability" form.

Refusal of Service

Not every EMS run results in the transportation of a patient to a hospital. Emergency care should always be offered to a patient, no matter how minor the injury or illness may be. However, often, the patient will refuse. If this occurs, you must:

- Be sure that the patient is legally permitted to refuse care; that is, the patient must be a competent adult.
- Make multiple and sincere attempts to convince the patient to accept care.
- Enlist the help of others, such as the patient's family or friends, to convince the patient to accept care.
- Make certain that the patient is fully informed about the implications of his decision and the potential risks of refusing care.
- Consult with on-line medical direction.
- Have the patient and a disinterested witness, such as a police officer, sign a release-from-liability form.
- Advise the patient that he may call you again for help if necessary.
- Attempt to get the patient's family or friends to stay with the patient.
- Document the entire situation thoroughly and accurately on your patient care report.

Remember, the refusal of care must be informed. That is, the patient must be told of and understand all possible risks of refusal. Decisions not to transport should involve medical direction. It is a good idea to put the patient directly on the phone with the on-line physician. If all efforts fail, be sure to thoroughly document the reasons for refusal and your efforts to change the patient's mind. If an on-line physician was involved, it is a good idea to obtain his signature on your patient care report.

Problem Patients

As a paramedic, you will occasionally encounter a "problem patient," one who is violent, a victim of a drug overdose, an intoxicated adult or minor, or an ill or injured minor with no adult available to provide consent for medical treatment. Such a patient can present you with a medical–legal dilemma. For example, consider the patient who has allegedly taken an overdose of medication. Concerned family members may panic and activate the EMS system. However, upon your arrival at the scene, you find the patient alert, oriented, denying that he has taken any medication, and refusing to give consent for treatment or transport.

In a case such as this, attempt to develop trust and some rapport with the patient. If he continues to refuse, and remains alert and oriented, a refusal form should be completed and witnessed by a police officer. If the patient will not sign the form, have a police officer or family member sign it, indicating that the patient verbally refused care. If, however, the situation becomes dangerous, or you have reason to suspect the patient has tried to injure himself, police officers or family members should consider legal measures to force the patient to receive treatment.

The intoxicated person who refuses treatment and transport also poses a problem for the paramedic. Every effort should be made to encourage the patient to accept care and transport to the hospital. If the patient refuses, explain to him in a calm and detailed manner the implications of refusal. However, if you determine that the patient cannot understand the nature of his illness or the consequences of his refusal, then he may not refuse treatment because he is not competent to do so. Involve law enforcement at this point. If the patient is competent to make such a decision, then have him sign a refusal form. Your conversation with the patient and his refusal should be witnessed by a disinterested third party such as a police officer.

Regardless of the type of problem patient, always document the encounter in detail. Your records should include a description of the patient, the results of any physical examination (or reasons for the lack of one), important statements made by the patient and other persons at the scene, and the names and addresses of any witnesses. If you are going to include an important statement from the patient or witnesses in your patient care report, put the exact statement in quotation marks.

Ideally, a police officer should respond to the scene of all problem patients and should either sign the patient care report as a witness or, if the paramedic's safety is at risk, accompany the patient and paramedic to the emergency department.

Involve the police and document in detail any encounter with a "problem patient."

LEGAL COMPLICATIONS RELATED TO CONSENT

There are many legal complications related to consent to treatment. If the paramedic does not obtain the proper consent to treat or fails to continue appropriate treatment, he may be liable for damages based on a tort cause of action, such as abandonment, assault, battery, or false imprisonment.

Abandonment

✱ abandonment termination of the paramedic-patient relationship without assurance that an equal or greater level of care will continue.

Abandonment is the termination of the paramedic-patient relationship without providing for the appropriate continuation of care while it is still needed and desired by the patient. You cannot initiate patient care and then discontinue it without sufficient reason. You cannot turn the care of a patient over to personnel who have less training than you without creating potential liability for an abandonment action. For example, a paramedic who has initiated advanced life support should not turn the patient over to an EMT-Basic or an EMT-Intermediate for transport.

Abandonment can occur at any point during patient contact, including in the field or in the hospital emergency department. Physically leaving a patient unattended, even for a short time, may also be grounds for a charge of abandonment. If, for example, you leave a patient at a hospital without properly turning over his care to a physician or nurse, you may be liable for abandonment. It is always a good idea to have the nurse or physician to whom you have passed responsibility for patient care sign your patient care report.

Assault and Battery

✱ assault an act that unlawfully places a person in apprehension of immediate bodily harm without his consent.

✱ battery the unlawful touching of another individual without his consent.

Failure to obtain appropriate consent before treatment could leave the paramedic open to allegations of assault and battery. **Assault** is defined as unlawfully placing a person in apprehension of immediate bodily harm without his consent. For example, your patient states that he is scared of needles and refuses to let you start an IV. If you then show him an IV catheter and bring it toward his arm as if to start an IV, you may be liable for assault.

Battery is the unlawful touching of another individual without his consent. It would be battery to actually start an IV on a patient who does not consent to such treatment. A paramedic can be sued for assault and battery in both criminal and civil contexts.

False Imprisonment

False imprisonment may be charged by a patient who is transported without consent or who is restrained without proper justification or authority. It is defined as intentional and unjustifiable detention of a person without his consent or other legal authority, and may result in civil or criminal liability. Like assault and battery, a charge of false imprisonment can be avoided by obtaining appropriate consent.

This is a particular problem with psychiatric patients. In most cases, you can avoid allegations of false imprisonment by having a law enforcement officer apprehend the patient and accompany you to the hospital. If no officer is available, you should attempt to consult with medical direction and carefully judge the risks of false imprisonment against the benefits of detaining and treating the patient. You should determine whether medical treatment is immediately necessary and whether the patient poses a threat to himself or to the public when you are making your decision to treat or transport.

✱ **false imprisonment** intentional and unjustifiable detention of a person without his consent or other legal authority.

REASONABLE FORCE

If it is safe to do so, you may use a reasonable amount of force to control an unruly or violent patient. The definition of **reasonable force** depends on the amount of force necessary to ensure that the patient does not cause injury to himself, you, or others. Excessive force can result in liability for the paramedic. Force used as punishment will be considered assault and battery for which the patient may be able to recover damages and the paramedic may face criminal charges. When you believe it is necessary to use force, involve law enforcement if possible.

The use of restraints may be indicated for a combative patient. Restraints must conform to your local protocols. Restraining devices typically used by EMS providers include straps, jackets, and restraining blankets. In this circumstance, an EMS team's goal is to use the least amount of force necessary to safely control the patient while causing him the least amount of discomfort. If the use of restraints is indicated, involve law enforcement officials.

✱ **reasonable force** the minimal amount of force necessary to ensure that an unruly or violent person does not cause injury to himself or others.

PATIENT TRANSPORTATION

The transportation of patients to a health-care facility is an integral part of the patient-care continuum. During transportation to a health-care facility, be sure to maintain the same level of care as was initiated at the scene. This means that if you, as a paramedic, initiate advanced emergency care procedures, you must either ride with the patient to the hospital or ensure that another paramedic will accompany the patient. If you fail to do so, and the patient is harmed as a result, you may be liable for abandonment.

One of the greatest areas of potential liability for paramedics is emergency vehicle operations. It is essential that you become familiar with your state and local laws. The laws that provide exceptions from driving rules and regulations may allow you, for example, to drive at a rate of speed in excess of a posted speed limit, but if you are negligent at any time during the operation of your vehicle, you will not be protected from liability.

Another issue that will arise is patient choice of destination. If you work in a small area with only one hospital, you are not likely to encounter difficulties. However, many paramedics work in areas that have many hospitals and medical

During transport of a patient to a health-care facility, be sure to maintain the same level of care as was initiated at the scene.

centers to choose from. Over the past few years, increasing numbers of lawsuits involving facility selection have been brought by patients. Some have sued paramedics themselves, claiming negligence based on the failure to transport to the nearest or most appropriate hospital.

An additional issue you may need to address involves the patient's insurance company protocols. In some situations, it may be appropriate to respect a patient's choice of facility based on his insurance company's facility-choice protocols. Local restrictions by insurance companies and health-care maintenance organizations may determine under what conditions and to what facilities patient transport may be authorized and paid for. While most areas are not yet being confronted with restrictions on service provision, it may be only a matter of time. However, never put patient care in jeopardy by transporting to a less appropriate facility because of insurance concerns.

In general, facility selection should be based on patient request, patient need, and facility capability. Local written protocols, the paramedic, on-line medical direction, and the patient should all play a role in facility selection. The patient's preference, however, should be honored unless the situation or the patient's condition dictates otherwise.

RESUSCITATION ISSUES

Advances in medical technology have saved and prolonged thousands of lives. However, in some instances, the use of sophisticated medical technology may only prolong pain, suffering, and death. When a person is seriously injured or gravely ill, family members must make difficult decisions regarding the medical care to be provided, including the use or withdrawal of life-support systems.

Generally, you are under obligation to begin resuscitative efforts when summoned to the scene of a patient who is unresponsive, pulseless, and apneic (not breathing). There are times, however, when you will determine that resuscitation is not indicated. This occurs with patients who have a valid Do Not Resuscitate (DNR) order, with patients who are obviously dead (decapitated, for example), with patients with obvious tissue decomposition or extreme dependent lividity (gravitational pooling of blood in dependent areas of the body), or with a patient who is at a scene that is too hazardous to enter.

Always follow your state laws, local protocols, and medical direction. The role of medical direction should be clearly delineated and included in your agency's protocols. If you are authorized to determine that resuscitative efforts are not indicated, be sure to thoroughly document your decision and the criteria upon which it was based.

ADVANCE DIRECTIVES

To improve communication between patients, their family members, and physicians regarding such matters, the federal government enacted the Patient Self-Determination Act of 1990. This act requires hospitals and physicians to provide patients and their families with sufficient information to make informed decisions about medical treatment and the use of life-support measures, including cardiopulmonary resuscitation (CPR), artificial ventilation, nutrition, hydration, and blood transfusions.

Patients and their families are therefore more likely than ever to have prepared a written statement of the patient's own preference for future medical care, or an **advance directive.** An advance directive is a document created to ensure that certain treatment choices are honored when a patient is unconscious

* **advance directive** a document created to ensure that certain treatment choices are honored when a patient is unconscious or otherwise unable to express his choice of treatment.

or otherwise unable to express his choice of treatments. They come in a variety of forms. The most common encountered in the field are: living wills, durable powers of attorney for health care, and Do Not Resuscitate orders.

The types of advance directives recognized in each state are governed by state law and local protocols. Medical direction must establish and implement policies for dealing with advance directives in the field. Those policies should clearly define the obligations of a paramedic who is caring for a patient with an advance directive. They should also provide for reasonable measures of comfort to the patient and emotional support to the patient's family and loved ones. Some states do not allow paramedics to honor living wills in the field, but do allow them to honor valid Do Not Resuscitate orders. Be sure you are familiar with your state law and local policies.

Living Will

A **living will** is a legal document that allows a person to specify the kinds of medical treatment he wishes to receive should the need arise. For example, many states allow patients to include in living wills their wishes concerning dying in a hospital or at home, receiving CPR, and donation of their organs and other body parts. In addition, patients with prolonged illnesses sometimes invoke the right to choose a person who may make health-care decisions for them in the event that their mental functions become impaired. They might formalize this decision by way of a special notation in a living will. (They may also do this through execution of a document called a "Durable Power of Attorney for Health Care" or "Health Care Proxy.") Living wills, once signed and witnessed, are effective until they are revoked by the patient.

Be sure you know your local protocols concerning living wills. If any question arises on scene, contact medical direction for instructions.

> * **living will** a legal document that allows a person to specify the kinds of medical treatment he wishes to receive should the need arise.

Do Not Resuscitate Orders

A **Do Not Resuscitate (DNR) order** is a common type of advance directive. Usually signed by the patient and his physician, the DNR order is a legal document that indicates to medical personnel which, if any, life-sustaining measures should be taken when the patient's heart and respiratory functions have ceased. DNR orders generally direct EMS personnel to withhold CPR in the event of a cardiac arrest. When you honor a DNR order, do not simply pack up your equipment and leave the scene. You still may have the patient's family and loved ones to attend to. Provide emotional support as appropriate.

DNR orders pose a particular problem in the field. Paramedics are often called to nursing homes or residences where they find a patient in cardiac arrest and in need of resuscitation. As a rule, you are legally obligated to attempt resuscitation. If a physician has written a specific order to avoid it, the paramedics should not have been summoned. Even so, people tend to panic and will call for help. Valid DNR orders should be honored as your protocols allow. Note, however, that if there is any doubt as to the patient's wishes, resuscitation should be initiated.

Occasionally, you may be requested to treat a patient as a "slow code" or "chemical code only." This is not legally permitted. Cardiac resuscitation is an all-or-nothing proposition. Treating a cardiac arrest with only medications would mean abandoning airway management and defibrillation. To do so, even at the request of the family, amounts to negligence and must be avoided.

> * **Do Not Resuscitate (DNR) order** legal document, usually signed by the patient and his physician, that indicates to medical personnel which, if any, life-sustaining measures should be taken when the patient's heart and respiratory functions have ceased.

Potential Organ Donation

Over the past few years, advances in medicines have led to an increased number of organ transplants. As organs and tissues are in very high demand and short supply, many EMS systems are now becoming a vital link in the organ procurement and transplant process. Some have developed protocols that specifically address organ viability after a patient's death. These include providing circulatory support through IV fluids and CPR and ventilatory support via endotracheal tube. Whether or not your EMS has protocols in place for potential organ donation, it is important for you to consult with on-line medical direction when you have identified a patient as a potential donor.

DEATH IN THE FIELD

Whether you arrive at the scene of a patient who has died prior to your arrival or you make an authorized decision to terminate resuscitative efforts, a death in the field must be appropriately dealt with and thoroughly documented. Follow state and local protocols and contact medical direction for guidance.

CRIME AND ACCIDENT SCENES

Preserve evidence at a crime scene whenever possible.

You may be called to treat a patient at a crime scene. You must not sacrifice patient care to preserve evidence or to become involved in detective work. You can best assist investigating officers by properly treating the patient and by doing your best to avoid destroying any potential evidence. As a paramedic, your responsibilities at a crime scene include the following:

- If you believe a crime may have been committed on scene, immediately contact law enforcement if they are not already involved.
- Protect yourself and the safety of other EMS personnel. This should always be your primary consideration. You will not be held liable for failing to act if a scene is not safe to enter.
- Once a crime scene has been deemed safe, initiate patient contact and medical care.
- Do not move or touch anything at a crime scene unless it is necessary to do so for patient care. Observe and document the original placement of any items moved by your crew. If the patient's clothing has holes made by a gunshot or a stabbing, leave them intact if possible. If the patient has an obvious mortal wound, such as decapitation, try not to touch the body at all. Do your best to protect any potential evidence.
- If you need to remove items from the scene, such as an impaled weapon or bottle of medication, be sure to document your actions and notify investigating officers.

Treat the scene of an accident in the same way. Ensure your own safety and the safety of your crew and treat your patients as medically indicated.

DOCUMENTATION

The treatment of your patient does not end until you have properly documented the entire incident. A complete patient care report is your best protection in a malpractice action. In fact, a well-written report may actually discourage a plaintiff from filing a malpractice case in the first place. In general, a plaintiff's attorney will request copies of all medical records, including the paramedic's report, before filing a lawsuit. If the paramedic's report is sloppy, incomplete, or otherwise not well written, this may encourage the plaintiff to sue.

A well-documented patient care report has the following characteristics:

- *It is completed promptly after patient contact.* It should be made in the course of business, not long after the event. Any delay could cause you to forget important observations or treatments. If possible, a copy of the completed report should be left with the emergency department staff before you leave the hospital. This copy will become part of the patient's permanent medical records. Note: never delay patient care to attend to a patient care report.

- *It is thorough.* The main purpose is not simply to record patient data, it also is meant to support the diagnosis and treatment that you provided to the patient. All actions, procedures, and administered medications should be documented. Remember: "If you didn't write it down, you didn't do it."

- *It is objective.* Avoid the use of emotional and value-loaded words. They are irrelevant and also may be the cause of a libel suit.

- *It is accurate.* Be precise, avoiding abbreviations and jargon that are not commonly understood. Try to limit your report to information that you have personally seen or heard. If you document something that you do not have personal knowledge of, indicate the source of your information. Document your observations, not your assumptions, and do not draw a medical conclusion that you are not competent to make. For example, you cannot conclusively diagnose a patient as having pneumonia. You can, however, report your suspicion of pneumonia and document consistent findings.

- *It maintains patient confidentiality.* Follow your agency's policies regarding the release of patient information. Whenever possible, patient consent should be obtained prior to release of information.

Intentional alteration of a medical record amounts to an admission of guilt by the paramedic. If a patient care report is found to be incomplete or inaccurate, a written amendment should be attached with the date and time the amendment was written, not the date of the original report. Send a copy of the addendum to the receiving hospital to become a part of the patient's medical records. Medical records need to be maintained for a period prescribed by state law. Become familiar with the record retention requirements in your state.

A patient care report should never be altered.

ʃUMMARY

It is in your best interest to learn and follow all state laws and local protocols related to your practice as a paramedic. Also be sure to receive good training and keep current by pursuing continuing education, reading industry journals, and obtaining recertification or relicensure as required by state law. Always act in good faith and use your common sense. High-quality patient care and high-quality documentation are always your best protection from liability.

CHAPTER 3

Anatomy and Physiology

Objectives

Part 1: The Cell and the Cellular Environment (begins on p. 96)

After reading Part 1 of this chapter, you should be able to:

1. Describe the structure and function of the normal cell. (pp. 96–100)
2. List types of tissue. (p. 100)
3. Define organs, organ systems, the organism, and system integration. (pp. 100–104)
4. Discuss the cellular environment (fluids and electrolytes), including osmosis and diffusion. (pp. 104–113)
5. Discuss acid-base balance and pH. (pp. 113–116)

Part 2: Body Systems (begins on p. 116)

After reading Part 2 of this chapter, you should be able to:

1. Describe the anatomy and physiology of the integumentary system, including the skin, hair, and nails. (pp. 116–119)
2. Describe the anatomy and physiology of the hematopoietic system, including the components of the blood, and discuss hemostasis, the

Continued

hematocrit, and hemoglobin. (pp. 119–130)

3. Describe the anatomy and physiology of the musculoskeletal system, including bones, joints, skeletal organization, and muscular tissue and structure. (pp. 130–152)

4. Describe the anatomy and physiology of the head, face, and neck and their relation to the physiology of the central nervous system. (pp. 153–166)

5. Describe the anatomy and physiology of the spine, including the cervical, thoracic, lumbar, and sacral spine and the coccyx. (pp. 166–172)

6. Describe the anatomy and physiology of the thorax, including its skeletal and muscular structure and the organs and vessels contained within it. (pp. 172–177).

7. Describe the anatomy and physiology of the nervous system, including the neuron, the central nervous system (brain and spine), and the peripheral nervous system (somatic, autonomic, sympathetic, and parasympathetic divisions). (pp. 177–195)

8. Describe the anatomy and physiology of the endocrine system, including the glands and other organs with endocrine activity. (pp. 195–206)

9. Describe the anatomy and physiology of the cardiovascular system, including the heart and the circulatory system. (pp. 206–220)

10. Describe the physiology of perfusion. (pp. 220–226)

11. Describe the anatomy of the respiratory system (upper and lower airway and pediatric airway) and the physiology of the respiratory system (respiration and ventilation and measures of respiratory function). (pp. 226–240)

12. Describe the anatomy and physiology of the abdomen, including its divisions and the organs and vessels contained within it. (pp. 240–243)

13. Describe the anatomy and physiology of the digestive system, including the digestive tract and the accessory organs of digestion, and also the spleen. (pp. 243–246)

14. Describe the anatomy and physiology of the urinary system, including the kidneys, ureters, urinary bladder, and urethra. (pp. 246–252)

15. Describe the anatomy and physiology of the female reproductive system, the menstrual cycle, and the pregnant uterus. (pp. 253–259)

16. Describe the anatomy and physiology of the male reproductive system. (pp. 259–260)

INTRODUCTION

An understanding of basic human anatomy and physiology is fundamental to paramedic practice. Part 1 of this chapter presents an overview of organization of human body systems, including:

- The cell
- Tissues
- Organs
- Organ systems
- The organism
- System integration
- Fluids and electrolytes
- Acid-base balance

Part 2 describes the major body systems:

- The integumentary system
- The blood
- The musculoskeletal system
- The head, face, and neck
- The spine and thorax
- The nervous system
- The endocrine system
- The cardiovascular system
- The respiratory system
- The abdomen
- The digestive system and spleen
- The urinary system
- The reproductive system

Part 1: The Cell and the Cellular Environment

THE NORMAL CELL

✱ **cell** the basic structural unit of all plants and animals. A membrane enclosing a thick fluid and a nucleus. Cells are specialized to carry out all of the body's basic functions.

The fundamental unit of the human body is the **cell** (Figure 3-1). It contains all necessary components to turn essential nutrients into energy, remove waste products, reproduce, and carry on other essential life functions.

There are two kingdoms of cells: *prokaryotes* and *eukaryotes*. Prokaryotes are the cells of lower plants and animals such as blue-green algae and bacteria. Their structure is very simple, with an indistinct nucleus that is not encased in a membrane, and containing no other internal structures. Eukaryotes are the cells of higher plants and animals such as most algae, fungi, protozoa—and humans.

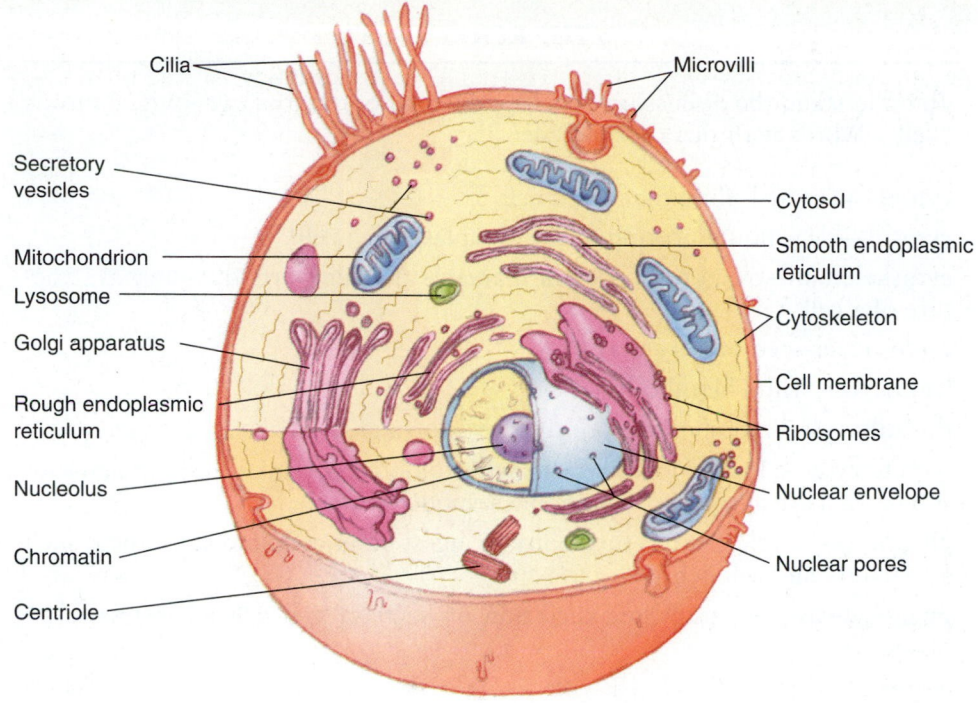

Cilia

Microvilli

Secretory
vesicles

Cytosol

Mitochondrion

Smooth endoplasmic
reticulum

Lysosome

Cytoskeleton

Golgi apparatus

Cell membrane

Rough endoplasmic
reticulum

Ribosomes

Nucleolus

Nuclear envelope

Chromatin

Nuclear pores

Centriole

FIGURE 3-1   The cell.

Eukaryotes are, of course, more complex than prokaryotes. The cell structure discussed on the following pages relates to the eukaryotes.

CELL STRUCTURE

A cell is something like a small, self-sustaining city. Within the cell, specialized structures perform specific functions. In a normal cell, all the structures and functions work together to maintain a normal, balanced environment. Each cell has three main elements: the cell membrane, the cytoplasm, and the organelles.

The Cell Membrane

The **cell membrane** (sometimes called the *plasma membrane*) is the outer covering that encircles and protects the cell.

The membrane is selectively permeable, or **semipermeable,** which means that it allows certain substances to pass from one side to another but does not allow others to pass. Vital functions of the cell membrane, made possible by its selective permeability, include electrolyte and fluid balance and the transfer of enzymes, hormones, and nutrients into and out of the cell. These functions will be discussed in greater detail later.

Without the cell membrane, the interior contents of a cell would become exposed to the extracellular environment and quickly die. That is why the bacterial cellular membrane is the site targeted by many antibiotic drugs—because destroying the cell membrane kills the cell.

THE ROOT CYT

To understand the discussion of cells, take note of the root *cyt*—which means "cell." Words with this root include:

cytoplasm—thick fluid that fills a cell.

cytosol—clear liquid portion of the cytoplasm in a cell.

cytoskeleton—structure of protein filaments that supports the internal structure of a cell.

erythrocyte—red blood cell.

leukocyte—white blood cell.

thrombocyte—blood cell responsible for clotting; also called a *platelet*.

lymphocyte—a type of leukocyte, or white blood cell, that attacks foreign substances as part of the body's immune response.

phagocyte—a cell that has the ability to ingest other cells and substances such as bacteria and cell debris.

phagocytosis—ingestion and digestion of bacteria and other substances by phagocytes.

monocyte—white blood cell with a single nucleus; the largest normal blood cell.

granulocyte—white cell with multiple nuclei that has the appearance of a bag of granules.

cytokine—protein produced by a white blood cell that instructs neighboring cells to respond in a genetically preprogramed fashion.

cytotoxin—substance that is poisonous to cells.

cytotoxic—poisonous (toxic) to cells.

The Cytoplasm

✱ **cytoplasm** the thick fluid, or *protoplasm,* that fills a cell.

Cytoplasm is the thick, viscous fluid that fills and gives shape to the cell, also called *protoplasm.* The clear liquid portion of the cytoplasm is called *cytosol.* Substances dissolved in the cytosol are mainly electrolytes, proteins, glucose (sugar), and lipids (fatty substances). Structures of various sizes and functions are dispersed throughout the cytosol.

The Organelles

✱ **organelles** structures that perform specific functions within a cell.

Structures that perform specific functions within the cell are called **organelles**. Six of the most important organelles are the *nucleus,* the *endoplasmic reticulum,* the *Golgi apparatus, mitochondria, lysosomes,* and *peroxisomes.* A brief discussion of a few of their functions provides an idea of the complex activity that takes place within a cell.

✱ **nucleus** the organelle within a cell that contains the DNA, or genetic material; in the cells of higher organisms, the nucleus is surrounded by a membrane.

- *Nucleus.* The **nucleus** contains the genetic material, deoxyribonucleic acid (DNA), and the enzymes necessary for replication of DNA. DNA determines our inherited traits and also plays a critical ongoing role within our bodies. DNA must be constantly copied and transferred to the cells.

- *Endoplasmic reticulum.* The endoplasmic reticulum is a network of small channels that has both rough and smooth portions. Rough endoplasmic reticulum functions in the synthesis (building) of proteins. Smooth endoplasmic reticulum functions in the synthesis of lipids, some of which are used in the formation of cell membranes, and carbohydrates.

- *Golgi apparatus.* The Golgi apparatus is located near the nucleus of most cells. It performs a variety of functions including synthesis and packaging of secretions such as mucus and enzymes.

- *Mitochondria.* The mitochondria are the energy factories, sometimes called the "powerhouses," of the cells. They convert essential nutrients into energy sources, often in the form of **adenosine triphosphate (ATP).**

- *Lysosomes.* Lysosomes contain digestive enzymes. Their functions include protection against disease and production of nutrients, breaking down bacteria and organic debris that has been taken into the cells and releasing usable substances such as sugars and amino acids.

- *Peroxisomes.* Peroxisomes are similar to lysosomes. Especially abundant in the liver, they absorb and neutralize toxins such as alcohol.

✳ adenosine triphosphate (ATP) a high-energy compound present in all cells, especially muscle cells; when split by enzyme action it yields energy. Energy is stored in ATP.

A wide variety of other structures and functions exist within the cell. Within the nucleus, for example, there are one or more smaller organelles called *nucleoli* (plural of *nucleolus*). Another component of the nucleus is *chromatin* (tangles of chromosome filaments containing DNA). Additional organelles exist in the cytoplasm (cytosol) outside the nucleus, including the *cytoskeleton* (a structure of protein filaments that supports the internal structure of the cell), *ribosomes* (granular structures that manufacture proteins—some float free, others attach to the surface of the endoplasmic reticulum, which creates the "rough" endoplasmic reticulum), *vesicles* (which play a role in transferring and storing secretions from the rough endoplasmic reticulum and Golgi complex), and *centrioles* (which play a role in cell division). On the surface of some cells are *microvilli* (folds on the cell surface), and, on some cells, whiplike *cilia* and *flagella* (which move fluids across cell surfaces and move cells through the surrounding extracellular fluid).

CELL FUNCTION

All the cells of the human body have the same general structure and contain the same genetic material but, through a process called *differentiation,* or *maturation,* cells become specialized. Eventually, cells perform specific functions that are different from the functions performed by other cells. There are seven major functions of cells:

- *Movement* is performed by muscle cells. Skeletal muscles move arms and legs. The smooth muscle around blood vessels causes them to dilate or constrict as necessary. Other smooth muscle moves food and wastes through the digestive tract. Cardiac muscle causes the chambers of the heart to contract. (See Muscle Tissue in the next section.)

- *Conductivity* is the function of nerve cells that creates and transmits an electrical impulse in response to a stimulus.

- *Metabolic absorption* is a function of cells of the intestines and kidneys, which take in nutrients that pass through the body.

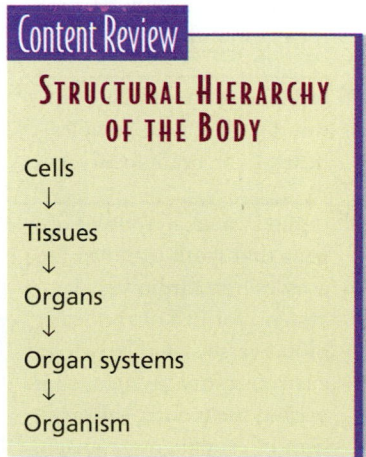

Content Review

STRUCTURAL HIERARCHY OF THE BODY

Cells
↓
Tissues
↓
Organs
↓
Organ systems
↓
Organism

tissue a group of cells that perform a similar function.

epithelial tissue the protective tissue that lines internal and external body tissues. Examples: skin, mucous membranes, the lining of the intestinal tract.

muscle tissue tissue that is capable of contraction when stimulated. There are three types of muscle tissue: *cardiac* (myocardium, or heart muscle), *smooth* (within intestines, surrounding blood vessels), and *skeletal*, or *striated* (allows skeletal movement). Skeletal muscle is mostly under voluntary, or conscious, control; smooth muscle is under involuntary, or unconscious, control; cardiac muscle is capable of spontaneous, or self-excited, contraction.

connective tissue the most abundant body tissue; it provides support, connection, and insulation. Examples: bone, cartilage, fat, blood.

nerve tissue tissue that transmits electrical impulses throughout the body.

organ a group of tissue functioning together. Examples: heart, liver, brain, ovary, eye.

organ system a group of organs that work together. Examples: the cardiovascular system, formed of the heart, blood vessels, and blood; the gastrointestinal system, comprising the mouth, salivary glands, esophagus, stomach, intestines, liver, pancreas, gall bladder, rectum, and anus.

- *Secretion* is performed by glands that produce substances such as hormones, mucus, sweat, and saliva.
- *Excretion* is a function all cells perform as they break down nutrients and expel wastes.
- *Respiration* is the function by which cells take in oxygen, which is used to transform nutrients into energy.
- *Reproduction* is the process by which cells enlarge, divide, and reproduce themselves, replacing dead cells and enabling new tissue growth and healing of wounds. Some cells, such as nerve cells, cannot reproduce—so that, for instance, a severed spinal cord cannot repair itself.

TISSUES

Tissue refers to a group of cells that perform a similar function. The following are the four basic types of tissue:

- **Epithelial tissue** lines internal and external body surfaces and protects the body. In addition, certain types of epithelial tissue perform specialized functions such as secretion, absorption, diffusion, and filtration. Examples of epithelial tissue are skin, mucous membranes, and the lining of the intestinal tract.
- **Muscle tissue** has the capability of contraction when stimulated. There are three types of muscle tissue (see figure 3-42 in the Musculoskeletal System section later in this chapter).
  — *Cardiac muscle* is tissue that is found only within the heart. It has the unique capability of spontaneous contraction without external stimulation.
  — *Smooth muscle* is the muscle found within the intestines and encircling blood vessels. Smooth muscle is generally under the control of the involuntary, or autonomic, component of the nervous system.
  — *Skeletal muscle* is the most abundant muscle type. It allows movement and is mostly under voluntary control.
- **Connective tissue** is the most abundant tissue in the body. It provides support, connection, and insulation. Examples of connective tissue include bones, cartilage, and fat. Blood is also sometimes classified as connective tissue.
- **Nerve tissue** is tissue specialized to transmit electrical impulses throughout the body. Examples of nerve tissue include the brain, spinal cord, and peripheral nerves.

ORGANS, ORGAN SYSTEMS, AND THE ORGANISM

A group of tissues functioning together is an **organ**. For example, the pancreas consists of epithelial tissue, connective tissue, and nervous tissue. Together, these tissues perform the essential functions of the pancreas. These functions include production of certain digestive enzymes and regulation of glucose metabolism.

A group of organs that work together is referred to as an **organ system**. The following are important organ systems:

- *Cardiovascular System.* The cardiovascular system consists of the heart, blood vessels, and blood. It transports nutrients and other essential elements to all parts of the body.

- *Respiratory System.* The respiratory system consists of the lungs and associated structures. It provides oxygen to the body, while removing carbon dioxide and other waste products.

- *Gastrointestinal System.* The gastrointestinal system consists of the mouth, salivary glands, esophagus, stomach, intestines, liver, pancreas, gall bladder, rectum, and anus. It takes in complex nutrients and breaks them down into a form that can be readily used by the body. It also aids in the elimination of excess wastes.

- *Genitourinary System.* The genitourinary system consists of the kidneys, ureters, bladder, and urethra. It is important in the elimination of various waste products. It also plays a major role in the regulation of water, electrolytes, blood pressure, and other essential body functions.

- *Reproductive System.* The reproductive system provides for reproduction of the organism. In the female, it consists of the ovaries, fallopian tubes, uterus, and vagina. In the male, it consists of the testes, prostate, seminal vesicles, vas deferens, and penis.

- *Nervous System.* The nervous system consists of the brain, spinal cord, and all of the peripheral nerves. It controls virtually all bodily functions and is the seat of intellect, awareness, and personality.

- *Endocrine System.* The endocrine system is a control system closely associated with the nervous system. It consists of the pituitary gland, pineal gland, pancreas, testes (male), ovaries (female), adrenal glands, thyroid gland, and parathyroid glands. There is evidence that other organs—such as the heart, kidney, and intestines—have endocrine functions. As noted earlier, the endocrine system exerts its effects through the release of chemical messengers called hormones.

- *Lymphatic System.* The lymphatic system is often considered a part of the cardiovascular system. It consists of the spleen, lymph nodes, lymphatic channels, thoracic duct, and the lymph fluid itself. It is important in fighting disease, in filtration, and in removing waste products of cellular metabolism.

- *Muscular System.* The muscular system is responsible for movement, posture, and heat production. It consists, primarily, of the skeletal muscles.

- *Skeletal System.* The skeletal system consists of the bones, cartilage, and associated connective tissue. It provides for support, protection, and movement. The bone marrow is the site for production of various blood cells, including the red blood cells and certain types of white blood cells.

The sum of all cells, tissues, organs, and organ systems is the **organism.** The failure of any component, from the cellular level to the organ-system level, can result in the development of a serious medical emergency.

✱ **organism** the sum of all the cells, tissues, organs, and organ systems of a living being. Examples: the human organism, a bacterial organism.

The failure of any component of an organism—from the cellular level to the organ system level—can result in a serious medical emergency.

SYSTEM INTEGRATION

The human body is not just a static structure of bones and cavities and tubes. It is a dynamic organization in which cells, tissues, organs, and organ systems perform functions essential to the preservation of the organism. **Homeostasis** is the term for the body's natural tendency to keep the internal environment and metabolism steady and normal. At the cellular level, the body will strive to maintain a very constant environment, because cells do not tolerate extreme environmental fluctuations.

A significant amount of energy is needed to maintain the order that is evident in the structures (**anatomy**) and functions (**physiology**) of the organism. Potential energy is stored in the biochemical bonds of cells and tissues in plants and animals, and the kinetic energy necessary to maintain homeostasis is obtained by the breaking of those bonds. Food provides energy substrates such as sugar, fats, and proteins which, when broken down, produce the energy for the maintenance of homeostasis. **Metabolism** is the term used to refer to the building up (*anabolism*) and breaking down (*catabolism*) of biochemical substances to produce energy.

The body's cells interact and intercommunicate, rather like a multi-cellular "social" organism. Communication between the cells consists of electrochemical messages. When something interferes with the normal sending or receiving of these messages, a disease process can begin or advance.

Many intercellular messages are conveyed by substances secreted by various body glands. *Endocrine glands,* sometimes called ductless glands (including the pituitary, thyroid, parathyroid, adrenal glands, the Islets of Langerhans in the pancreas, the testes, and the ovaries), secrete hormones directly into the circulatory system, where they travel to the target organ or tissue. *Exocrine glands* secrete substances such as sweat, saliva, mucus, and digestive enzymes onto the epithelial surfaces of the body (the skin or linings of body cavities and organs) via ducts.

Several types of signaling take place among cells. *Endocrine signaling* (via hormones distributed throughout the body) is one mode of intercellular communication. *Paracrine signaling* (non-endocrine, non-hormonal) involves secretion of chemical mediators by certain cells that act only on nearby cells. In *autocrine signaling*, cells secrete substances that may act upon themselves. In *synaptic signaling*, cells secrete specialized chemicals called neurotransmitters, such as norepinephrine, acetylcholine, serotonin, and dopamine, that transmit signals across synapses, the junctions between neurons.

These chemical signals—in the form of hormones and neurotransmitters—are received by various kinds of receptors. Receptors can be nerve endings, sensory organs, or proteins that interact with, and then respond to the chemical signals and other stimuli. Many of the medications administered by paramedics act upon these receptors. *Chemoreceptors* respond to chemical stimuli. Chemoreceptors within the brain respond to increasing levels of CO_2 in the cerebrospinal fluid, stimulating respiratory centers in the brainstem to increase the rate and depth of respirations. *Baroreceptors* respond to pressure changes. Baroreceptors in the arch of the aorta and in the carotid sinuses along the carotid artery sense changes in blood pressure, which then cause the cardiac centers in the medulla to alter the heart rate. *Alpha and beta adrenergic receptors* on the surfaces of cells in the bronchi, heart, and blood vessels respond to neurotransmitters and medications, resulting in a variety of cardiovascular and respiratory responses.

As the above examples demonstrate, when normal intercellular communication is interrupted and normal metabolism is disturbed, the body will respond in various ways to compensate and attempt to restore the normal metabolism, i.e., homeostasis.

Each organ system plays a role in maintaining homeostasis. An example is the body's response to the accumulation of cellular carbon dioxide that occurs

---

✱ **homeostasis** the natural tendency of the body to maintain a steady and normal internal environment.

✱ **anatomy** the structure of an organism; body structure.

✱ **physiology** the functions of an organism; the physical and chemical processes of a living thing.

✱ **metabolism** the total changes that take place during physiological processes.

When something interferes with the electrochemical messages cells send to each other, a disease process can begin or advance.

When normal metabolism is disturbed the body attempts to restore normal metabolism, i.e., homeostasis.

during exercise. The respiratory system immediately attempts to return the internal environment to its normal state by increasing the respiratory rate and depth to eliminate excess carbon dioxide—which is why runners pant.

The organization of the human body is very complex, with constant interactions occurring within and among the systems to maintain homeostasis. When disease interrupts these interactions, it can cause both local effects (at the specific site of the illness or injury) and systemic effects (throughout the body). When this happens, body cells and systems will respond to restore normal conditions.

To understand how human systems interact, physiologists sometimes view them from an engineering perspective. Various body systems respond to *inputs,* or stressors, that may be sensed by other systems. The system receiving the input responds in some fashion, creating an *output.* The portion of the system creating the output, be it a cell or an organ, is known as the *effector.* For example, consider a large laceration to an extremity with severe blood loss. The drop in blood pressure resulting from the blood loss is sensed by the baroreceptors, which in turn cause messages to be sent from the cardiac center in the medulla to the heart, resulting in an increase in the rate and strength of contractions in an attempt to restore normal blood pressure. By definition, the input would be the drop in pressure sensed by the baroreceptors; the effector would be the heart, which increased its rate in response to signals from the medulla; and the output would be the resultant increase in blood pressure.

This kind of feedback is essential for maintaining stability within a system and homeostasis for the organism. When the output of a system corrects the situation that created the input, it is said to loop, or feedback on the input, and a **negative feedback loop** exists—"negative" because the feedback negates the input caused by the original stressor. To elaborate on the example of the baroreceptors, the output or increase in blood pressure resulting from the increased heart rate feeds back on, or cancels out, the original input (low blood pressure), and the heart (effector) no longer has to maintain an elevated rate. This particular feedback loop is known as the baroreceptor reflex mechanism.

Unfortunately, the grim reality of this model is that blood loss often overwhelms the heart's ability to respond with an increased rate. At that point, the system has lost the ability to compensate, and, as a paramedic, you must intervene by administering fluids and taking other necessary therapeutic measures. When the outputs of effector organs are ineffective in correcting the input condition, *decompensation* is said to have occurred.

In the case of decompensation, the feedback system doesn't or can't restore homeostasis. The opposite problem can also occur when the feedback system goes too far and overcompensates for the original problem. To prevent this, it is important for the body to have some way to stop the output—to restore the heart rate to normal, because the inability to control the pulse rate would cause instability in the cardiovascular system and danger to the organism. In fact, the body does have numerous means of controlling or halting output.

Biological systems generally employ negative feedback loops to maintain stability. Positive feedback systems do exist in human physiology. (Positive feedback enhances, rather than negates, the effects of input.) An example would be some short-lived positive feedback loops involved in follicular (egg) development in females. However, these loops work in conjunction with negative feedback loops to maintain stability.

Feedback activity must be orchestrated and synchronized to maintain homeostasis. Two systems work together to maintain homeostasis and to integrate the responses of different systems: the nervous system and the endocrine system. They are functionally and anatomically coupled to allow for this integration. For example, the pituitary gland of the endocrine system is joined with the hypothalamus of the nervous system by a stalk-like structure called the infundibulum. This allows for rapid communication between these two body control systems.

Content Review

EFFECTS OF DISEASE
- Local (at the site of the illness or injury)
- Systemic (throughout the body)

---

* **negative feedback loop** body mechanisms that work to reverse, or compensate for, a pathophysiological process, (or to reverse any physiological process, whether pathological or nonpathological).

Content Review

CONTROL SYSTEMS
- Nervous system
- Endocrine system

There are important temporal differences in the responses of these two systems. Nervous system response is generally rapid in onset but short-lived. An example is the baroreceptor reflex mechanism, mentioned earlier, which is primarily mediated by the nervous system. Conversely, endocrine responses generally take longer—that is, they have a slower onset of action but a longer duration. For example, the pituitary gland secretes anti-diuretic hormone (ADH) in response to low blood pressure. ADH acts on the renal (kidney) tubules, causing water to be reabsorbed into the blood instead of being eliminated from the body. This causes an increase in intravascular fluid volume that compensates for the decrease in intravascular volume caused by the blood loss. All these responses are stimulated by pathological alterations or events.

THE CELLULAR ENVIRONMENT: FLUIDS AND ELECTROLYTES

Many pathological conditions, both medical and traumatic, adversely affect the fluid and electrolyte balance of the body. Certain disease processes, such as diabetic ketoacidosis and heat emergencies, are associated with certain electrolyte abnormalities. Severe derangements in fluid and electrolyte status can result in death. For this reason, as a paramedic, you need to have a good understanding of the fluids and electrolytes present in the human body.

WATER

Water is the most abundant substance in the human body. In fact, water accounts for approximately 60 percent of the total body weight (the average for all ages). The total amount of water in the body at any given time is referred to as the **total body water (TBW)**. In an adult weighing 70 kilograms (154 pounds), the amount of total body water would be approximately 42 liters (11 gallons) (Figure 3-2).

Water is distributed into various compartments of the body (Table 3-1). These compartments are separated by cell membranes. The largest compartment is the *intracellular compartment*. This compartment contains the **intracellular fluid (ICF)**, which is all of the fluid found inside body cells. Approximately 75 percent of all body water is found within this compartment. The *extracellular compartment* contains the remaining 25 percent of all body water. It contains the **extracellular fluid (ECF)**, all of the fluid found outside the body cells.

There are two divisions within the extracellular compartment. The first contains the **intravascular fluid**—the fluid found outside of cells and within the circulatory system. It is essentially the same as the blood plasma. The remaining compartment contains the **interstitial fluid**—all the fluid found outside of the cell membranes, yet not within the circulatory system. For example, minute amounts of fluid are found in the synovial fluid that lubricates the joints, the aqueous humor of the eye, secretions including saliva, gastric juices, bile, and so on.

Total body water and its distribution vary with age and physiological condition. At birth, an infant's TBW is about 75–80 percent of its body weight, compared to the 65 percent TBW of the average adult. Infants have a higher TBW for two reasons. First, infants have less fat than adults. (Fat does not absorb water, so the less fat in the body, the more water.) Second, water is essential for the high rates of metabolism that are necessary to promote growth in the infant. The TBW slowly decreases to approximately 70–75 percent by age one. Diarrhea is especially worrisome in the infant, because it can mean the loss of a significant percentage of TBW. In addition, body systems that compensate for fluid loss are still immature, so that infants can rapidly become dangerously dehydrated and subject to electrolyte imbalances. By late childhood the TBW decreases to 65–70 percent.

Some fluid and electrolyte derangements can result in death.

* **total body water (TBW)** the total amount of water in the body at a given time.

* **intracellular fluid (ICF)** the fluid inside the body cells.

* **extracellular fluid (ECF)** the fluid outside the body cells. Extracellular fluid is comprised of intravascular fluid and interstitial fluid.

* **intravascular fluid** the fluid within the circulatory system; blood plasma.

* **interstitial fluid** the fluid in body tissues that is outside the cells and outside the vascular system.

FIGURE 3-2 Percentage of total body weight due to water as distributed into various fluid compartments.

15% of body weight. Extracellular fluid (4.5% intravascular; 10.5% interstitial)

45% of body weight: Intracellular fluid

60% of body weight: Total body water

By early adulthood, the TBW of males and females begins to differ. In adult males, TBW constitutes approximately 65–70 percent of the body weight, while in adult females the average TBW is 60–65 percent. The gender difference is the result of hormonal differences that result in the male's greater muscle mass and the female's greater percentage of body fat.

As the human body ages, the loss of muscle mass, increased percentage of fat, and the body's decreasing ability to regulate fluid levels lowers the TBW to around 45–55 percent. Due to a decreasing ability to regulate electrolytes and fluid levels, the elderly, like the very young, are at high risk for dehydration and disorders related to electrolyte imbalances.

Hydration

Water is the universal **solvent.** That is, most substances dissolve in water. When they do, various chemical changes take place. For this reason, the water content

✱ **solvent** a substance that dissolves other substances, forming a solution.

Water is the universal solvent. Water is crucial to virtually all of the body's biochemical processes.

Table 3-1	BODY FLUID COMPARTMENTS	
Compartment	**Percentage of Total Body Water**	**Volume in 70 kg Adult**
Intracellular fluid	75.0%	31.50 L
Extracellular fluid	25.0%	10.50 L
Interstitial fluid	17.5%	7.35 L
Intravascular fluid	7.5%	3.15 L

The Cellular Environment: Fluids and Electrolytes **105**

of the body is crucial to virtually all of the body's biochemical processes. Normally, the total volume of water in the body, as well as the distribution of fluid in the three body compartments, remains relatively constant. This occurs despite wide fluctuations in the amount of water that enters and is excreted from the body on a daily basis. The water coming into the body is referred to as intake. The water excreted from the body is referred to as output. To maintain relative homeostasis, the intake must equal the output, as shown below.

Intake
digestive system:
liquids	1,000 ml
food (solids)	1,200 ml
metabolic sources:	300 ml

TOTAL: 2,500 ml

Output
lungs (water vapor):	400 ml
kidneys (urine):	1,500 ml
skin (perspiration):	400 ml
intestines (feces):	200 ml

TOTAL: 2,500 ml

Several mechanisms work to maintain a relative balance between input and output. For example, as explained earlier, when the fluid volume drops, the pituitary gland secretes antidiuretic hormone (ADH), which causes the kidney tubules to reabsorb more water into the blood and to excrete less urine. This process helps to restore the fluid volume to normal values.

Thirst also regulates fluid intake. The sensation of thirst normally occurs when body fluids decrease, stimulating the person to take in more fluids orally. Conversely, when too many fluids enter the body, the kidneys are activated and more urine is excreted, thus eliminating excess fluid. The body also maintains fluid balance by shifting water from one body space to another.

Dehydration Dehydration is an abnormal decrease in the total body water and can result from several factors:

- *Gastrointestinal losses* result from prolonged vomiting, diarrhea, or malabsorption disorders.
- *Increased insensible loss* is loss of water through normal mechanisms that is difficult to detect or measure (e.g., perspiration, water vapor from the lungs, saliva). These can be increased in fever states, during hyperventilation, or with high environmental temperatures.
- *Increased sweating* (also called perspiration or diaphoresis) can result in significant fluid loss. This can occur with many medical conditions or high environmental temperatures.
- *Internal losses* (commonly called "third space" losses) are losses of fluid into various body fluid compartments. In this situation, fluid is typically lost from the intravascular compartment into the interstitial compartment, effectively taking it out of the circulating volume. This can occur with peritonitis, pancreatitis, or bowel obstruction. It can also occur in poor nutritional states where there is not enough protein in the vascular system to retain water.
- *Plasma losses* occur from burns, surgical drains and fistulas, and open wounds.

✳ **dehydration** excessive loss of body fluid.

Content Review

SOME CAUSES OF DEHYDRATION
- Vomiting
- Diarrhea
- Perspiration
- Peritonitis
- Malnutrition
- Burns
- Open wounds

Dehydration rarely involves only the loss of water. More commonly, there is also a loss of electrolytes. At the hospital, fluid replacement will be based on both fluid and electrolyte deficits, once the patient's electrolyte abnormalities are determined through laboratory testing.

Clinically, the dehydrated patient will exhibit dry mucous membranes and poor skin **turgor.** There often is excessive thirst. As it becomes more severe, dehydration will be accompanied by an increased pulse rate, decreased blood pressure, and orthostatic hypotension (increased pulse and decreased blood pressure on rising from a supine position). In infants, the anterior fontanelle may be sunken and the diaper may be dry or reveal the presence of highly concentrated (dark yellow, strong-smelling) urine. The absence of tears in a crying infant, a capillary refill time greater than two seconds, dry mucosa, and a decrease in urinary output are signs that indicate severe dehydration. The treatment for dehydration is replacement of fluid.

Overhydration **Overhydration** can occur as well. The major sign of overhydration is edema. Patients with heart disease may manifest overhydration much earlier than patients without heart disease. In severe cases of overhydration, overt heart failure may be present. Treatment is directed at removing the excessive fluid.

ELECTROLYTES

Dehydration usually involves loss of both water and electrolytes.

* turgor normal tension in a cell; the resistance of the skin to deformation. (In a normally hydrated person, the skin, when pinched, will quickly return to its normal formation. In a dehydrated person, the return to normal formation will be slower.)

* overhydration the presence of retention of an abnormally high amount of body fluid.

HOW TO READ CHEMICAL NOTATION

To describe chemical substances and reactions, scientists use chemical notation, a kind of "shorthand."

Every chemical element has a one- or two-letter abbreviation. Just four elements—hydrogen, oxygen, carbon, and nitrogen—make up over 99% of the body's atoms. These are called the "major elements." Nine "trace elements" account for the remaining less-than-1%.

Major Element	Symbol	Percent	Trace Element	Symbol
Hydrogen	H	62.0%	Calcium	Ca
Oxygen	O	26.0%	Chlorine	Cl
Carbon	C	10.0%	Iodine	I
Nitrogen	N	1.5%	Iron	Fe
			Magnesium	Mg
			Phosphorus	Ph
			Potassium	K
			Sodium	Na
			Sulfur	S

An *atom* is the smallest particle of an element. A *molecule* is a combination of atoms. The notation for a molecule combines the notations of the included elements. A subscript number after an element indicates the number of atoms of that element. If there is just one atom, there is no number. For example:

NaCl (Sodium chloride, or table salt. A sodium chloride molecule has 1 sodium atom and 1 chlorine atom.)

H_2O (Water. A water molecule has 2 hydrogen atoms and 1 oxygen atom.)

H_2CO_3 (Carbonic acid. A carbonic acid molecule has 2 hydrogen, 1 carbon, and 3 oxygen atoms.)

(continued)

Ions

Each atom is made up of even smaller particles: electrons (that have a negative electrical charge), protons (that have a positive electrical charge) and neutrons (that are uncharged). Protons and neutrons are in the inner core, or nucleus, of the atom while electrons occupy outer orbits around the nucleus. Sometimes an atom of an element can lose one or more of its outer electrons or can capture one or more extra electrons from another element.

An *ion* is an atom that has lost one or more negatively charged electrons and now has a positive charge, or an atom that has gained one or more electrons and now has a negative charge. A superscript plus ($^+$) indicates a positively charged cation. A superscript minus ($^-$) indicates a negatively charged anion. For example:

Na^+ (A sodium ion has lost an electron and has a positive charge.)

Ca^{++} (A calcium ion has lost two electrons and has a double positive charge.)

Cl^- (A chloride ion has gained an electron and has a negative charge.)

Electrolytes are substances that form ions when they break down, or dissociate, in water. Remember that the body and its blood are mostly water. The ions formed by dissociation of electrolytes in the body's fluids is a major factor in body metabolism.

Chemical Reactions

Notations for chemical reactions use a plus sign ($+$) to indicate substances that are combined and an arrow ($\rightarrow$) to show the direction of the reaction. The reactants are usually on the left, the product of the reaction on the right.

$$2H + O \rightarrow H_2O$$

(2 hydrogen atoms + 1 oxygen atom → 1 water molecule)

In some circumstances, a reaction may be reversible. That is, separate elements may synthesize (combine), or the synthesized substance may dissociate (break down) into separate components. A two-directional arrow ($\leftrightarrow$) shows that a reaction is reversible and can be read in either direction.

$$CO_2 + H_2O \leftrightarrow H_2CO_3$$

Read as: (carbon dioxide + water → carbonic acid) or
(carbonic acid → water + carbon dioxide).

Notice that no atoms are gained or lost in a chemical reaction. In the example above, the two oxygen atoms in CO_2 and the single oxygen atom in H_2O combine to equal the three oxygen atoms in H_2CO_3. The hydrogen and carbon atoms are also equal on both sides of the reaction.

Up and down arrows ($\uparrow \downarrow$) are used to indicate an increase or decrease in the substance that follows the arrows. For example:

$\uparrow H^+$ (an increase in hydrogen ions)

$\downarrow CO_2$ (a decrease in carbon dioxide)

The various chemical substances present throughout the body can be classified either as electrolytes or non-electrolytes. **Electrolytes** are substances that **dissociate** into electrically charged particles when placed into water. The charged particles are referred to as **ions**. Ions with a positive charge are called **cations,** while ions with a negative charge are called **anions.**

An example of this would be the dissociation of the drug sodium bicarbonate when placed into water. Sodium bicarbonate is a neutral salt. When placed into water, it dissociates into two charged particles, as shown below.

$$NaHCO_3 \rightarrow Na^+ + HCO_3^-$$

sodium bicarbonate → sodium cation + bicarbonate anion

neutral salt → cation + anion

Sodium bicarbonate is an example of an electrolyte that is taken into the body as a medication. However, there are many naturally occurring electrolytes present in the body.

The most frequently occurring cations include:

- *Sodium* (Na^+). Sodium is the most prevalent cation in the extracellular fluid. It plays a major role in regulating the distribution of water because water is attracted to and moves with sodium. In fact, it is often said that "water follows sodium." Sodium is also important in the transmission of nervous impulses. An abnormal increase in the relative amount of sodium in the body is called *hypernatremia,* while an abnormal decrease is referred to as *hyponatremia.*
- *Potassium* (K^+). Potassium is the most prevalent cation in the intracellular fluid. It is also important in the transmission of electrical impulses. An abnormally high potassium level is called *hyperkalemia,* while an abnormally low potassium level is referred to as *hypokalemia.*
- *Calcium* (Ca^{++}). Calcium has many physiological functions. It plays a major role in muscle contraction as well as nervous impulse transmission. An abnormally increased calcium level is called *hypercalcemia,* while an abnormally decreased calcium level is called *hypocalcemia.*
- *Magnesium* (Mg^{++}). Magnesium is necessary for several biochemical processes that occur in the body and is closely associated with phosphate in many processes. An abnormally increased magnesium level is called *hypermagnesemia*; an abnormally decreased magnesium level is called *hypomagnesemia.*

The most frequently occurring anions include:

- *Chloride* (Cl^-). Chloride is an important anion. Its negative charge balances the positive charge associated with the cations. It also plays a major role in fluid balance and renal function. Chloride has a close association with sodium.
- *Bicarbonate* (HCO_3^-). Bicarbonate is the principle **buffer** of the body. This means that it neutralizes the highly acidic hydrogen ion (H^+) and other organic acids. (Buffering will be discussed in more detail later in this chapter.)
- *Phosphate* (HPO_4^-). Phosphate is important in body energy stores. It is closely associated with magnesium in renal function. It also acts as a buffer, primarily in the intracellular space, in much the same manner as bicarbonate.

* **electrolyte** a substance that, in water, separates into electrically charged particles.

* **dissociate** separate; break down. For example, sodium bicarbonate, when placed in water, dissociates into a sodium cation and a bicarbonate anion.

* **ion** a charged particle; an atom or group of atoms whose electrical charge has changed from neutral to positive or negative by losing or gaining one or more electrons. (In an atom's normal, non-ionized state, its positively charged protons and negatively charged electrons balance each other so that the atom's charge is neutral.)

* **cation** an ion with a positive charge—so called because it will be attracted to a cathode, or negative pole.

* **anion** an ion with a negative charge—so called because it will be attracted to an anode, or positive pole.

* **buffer** a substance that tends to preserve or restore a normal acid-base balance by increasing or decreasing the concentration of hydrogen ions.

Many other compounds carry negative charges. Among these are some of the proteins, certain organic acids, and other compounds. Electrolytes are usually measured in *milliequivalents* per liter (mEq/L).

Non-electrolytes are molecules that do not dissociate into electrically charged particles. These include glucose, urea, proteins, and similar substances.

OSMOSIS AND DIFFUSION

As discussed earlier, the various fluid compartments are separated by cell membranes. These membranes are semipermeable, allowing the passage of certain materials while restricting the passage of others. Compounds with small molecules, such as water (H_2O), pass readily through the membrane; larger compounds, such as proteins, are restricted. This selective movement of fluids results from the presence of pores (openings) in the membrane. Electrolytes do not pass as readily as water through the membrane. This is due not so much to their size as to their electrical charge.

When solutions on opposite sides of a semipermeable membrane are equal in concentration, the relationship is said to be **isotonic.** When the concentration of a given solute (dissolved substance) is greater on one side of the membrane than on the other, it is said to be **hypertonic.** When the concentration is less on one side of the cell membrane, as compared to the other, it is referred to as **hypotonic.** This difference in concentration is known as the **osmotic gradient.**

The natural tendency of the body is to keep the balance of electrolytes and water equal on both sides of the cell membrane. This is an example of homeostasis. If one side of a cell membrane has an increased quantity of a given electrolyte (is hypertonic), there will be a shift of the electrolyte from that side and a shift of water from the other side to restore balance in concentration—the balanced state.

The tendency of molecules to move from an area of higher concentration to an area of lower concentration is referred to as **diffusion** and does not require energy (Figure 3-3). The diffusion of a solute (usually an electrolyte) across a cell

✱ **isotonic** equal in concentration of solute molecules; solutions may be isotonic to each other.

✱ **hypertonic** having a greater concentration of solute molecules; one solution may be hypertonic to another.

✱ **hypotonic** having a lesser concentration of solute molecules; one solution may be hypotonic to another.

✱ **osmotic gradient** the difference in concentration between solutions on opposite sides of a semipermeable membrane.

✱ **diffusion** the movement of molecules through a membrane from an area of greater concentration to an area of lesser concentration.

FIGURE 3-3 Diffusion is the movement of a substance from an area of greater concentration to an area of lesser concentration.

Osmosis

Interstitial fluid ... 1

30% Solute concentration

20% Solute concentration

Intracellular fluid

Interstitial fluid ... 2

25% Solute concentration

H_2O

25% Solute concentration

Intracellular fluid

H_2O

FIGURE 3-4   Osmosis is the movement of water from an area of higher WATER concentration to an area of lesser WATER concentration. Because water is a solvent, it moves from an area of lower SOLUTE concentration to an area of higher SOLUTE concentration.

membrane from the area of higher concentration to the area of lower concentration continues until the natural balance is again attained. This movement from an area of higher concentration to an area of lower concentration is termed a movement *with the osmotic gradient.*

Water also moves across the cell membrane so as to dilute the area of increased electrolyte concentration. The movement of water is more rapid than the movement of electrolytes. This form of diffusion (the passage of any solvent, usually water, through a membrane) is referred to as **osmosis** (Figure 3-4). It occurs in the direction opposite to the direction of solute movement. For example, if a semipermeable membrane separates solutions of water and sodium, and if the concentration of sodium is two times higher on one side of the membrane than on the other, then two things will occur. Sodium will diffuse from the area of higher concentration (the hypertonic side) to the area of lesser concentration (the hypotonic side). Concurrently, water will diffuse in the opposite direction. That is, water will leave the hypotonic side and diffuse across the membrane to the hypertonic side. These actions will continue until the concentration of water and sodium on both sides has equalized.

In addition to diffusion, two other mechanisms—active transport and facilitated diffusion—can transport substances across cell membranes. **Active transport** is the movement of a substance across the cell membrane *against the osmotic gradient* (that is, toward the side that already has more of the substance).

For example, the body requires cells of the myocardium to be negatively charged on the inside of the cells as compared to the outside. However sodium, with its positive charge, tends to diffuse passively into the cell. This would destroy the negative charge inside the cell. In order to maintain the desired negative charge, sodium ions are actively pumped out of the cell, while potassium ions are pumped into the cell, by a mechanism known as the sodium-potassium pump. (Sodium and potassium ions are both positive, but more sodium ions are pumped out of the cell than potassium ions are pumped in, creating the desired negative charge inside the cell.)

Active transport is faster than diffusion, but it requires the expenditure of energy, which diffusion does not. Proteins are moved across the cell membrane in a similar fashion.

✱ **osmosis** the passage of a solvent such as water through a membrane.

✱ **active transport** movement of a substance through a cell membrane against the osmotic gradient; that is, from an area of lesser concentration to an area of greater concentration, opposite to the normal direction of diffusion.

facilitated diffusion diffusion of a substance such as glucose through a cell membrane that requires the assistance of a "helper," or carrier protein.

osmolality the concentration of solute per kilogram of water. *See also* osmolarity.

osmolarity the concentration of solute per liter of water (often used synonymously with *osmolality*).

osmotic pressure the pressure exerted by the concentration of solutes on one side of a membrane that, if hypertonic, tends to "pull" water (cause osmosis) from the other side of the membrane.

oncotic force a form of osmotic pressure exerted by the large protein particles, or colloids, present in blood plasma. In the capillaries, the plasma colloids tend to pull water from the interstitial space across the capillary membrane into the capillary. Oncotic force is also called *colloid osmotic pressure*.

hydrostatic pressure blood pressure or force against vessel walls created by the heart beat. Hydrostatic pressure tends to force water out of the capillaries into the interstitial space.

filtration movement of water out of the plasma across the capillary membrane into the interstitial space.

Certain molecules can move across the cell membrane by another process known as **facilitated diffusion.** Glucose is an example of such a molecule. Facilitated diffusion requires the assistance of "helper proteins," parts of a membrane transport system, on the surface of the cell membrane. These proteins, once activated, bind to the glucose molecule. Following binding, the protein changes its configuration and transports the glucose molecule to the inside of the cell, where it is released. Depending on the substance being transported, facilitated diffusion may or may not require energy.

Water Movement between Intracellular and Extracellular Compartments

The mechanisms by which water and solutes move across cell membranes, as described above, assure that the **osmolality** of body water, both within and outside the cells, is normally in equilibrium. (The term *osmolality* refers to the concentration of solute per kilogram of water; a related term, **osmolarity,** refers to the concentration of solute per liter of water. The terms are often used interchangeably.) Sodium, the most abundant ion in the extracellular fluid, is responsible for the osmotic balance of the extracellular space. Potassium plays the same role in the intracellular space.

Generally, the osmolality of intracellular fluid does not change very rapidly. However, when there is a change in the osmolality of extracellular fluid, water will move from the intracellular to the extracellular compartment, or vice versa, until osmotic equilibrium is regained.

Water Movement between Intravascular and Interstitial Compartments

Within the extracellular compartment, movement of water between the plasma in the intravascular space and the interstitial space is primarily a function of forces at play in the capillary beds.

In general, the movement of water and solutes across a cell membrane is governed by **osmotic pressure.** Osmotic pressure is the pressure exerted by the concentration of solutes on one side of a semipermeable membrane, such as a cell membrane or the thin wall of a capillary. Osmotic pressure can be thought of as a "pull" rather than a "push," because a hypertonic concentration of solutes tends to pull water from the other side of the membrane.

Generally, this is a two-way street as solutes move out of a space while water moves into the space to balance the concentration of solutes on both sides of the membrane. However, there is a somewhat different osmotic mechanism that operates between the plasma inside a capillary and the interstitial space outside the capillary. Blood plasma generates **oncotic force,** which is sometimes called *colloid osmotic pressure.* Plasma proteins are colloids, large particles that do not readily move across the capillary membrane. They tend to remain within the capillary. At the same time, there is very little water in the interstitial space. The small amount of water that does get into the interstitial space is usually taken up by the lymph system. Therefore, since there is little water outside the capillary, and because plasma proteins do not readily move outside the capillary, the forces governing movement of water between the capillary and the interstitial space are almost all on one side, governed by the plasma on the inside of the capillary.

Another force inside the capillaries is **hydrostatic pressure,** which is the blood pressure, or force against the vessel walls, created by contractions of the heart. Hydrostatic pressure does tend to force some water out of the plasma and across the capillary wall into the interstitial space, a process that is called **filtration.** Hydrostatic pressure (a force that favors filtration, pushing water out of the capillary) and oncotic force (a force opposing filtration, pulling water into the capillary) together are responsible for **net filtration,** which is described in *Starling's hypothesis:*

Net filtration = (Forces favoring filtration) − (Forces opposing filtration)

Net filtration in a capillary is normally zero. It works this way: As plasma enters the capillary at the arterial end, hydrostatic pressure forces water to cross the capillary membrane into the interstitial space. This loss of water increases the relative concentration of plasma proteins. By the time the plasma reaches the venous end of the capillary, the oncotic force exerted by the increased concentration of plasma proteins is great enough to pull the water from the interstitial space back into the capillary. The outcome is that water is retained in the intravascular space and does not remain in the interstitial space.

ACID-BASE BALANCE

Acid-base balance is a dynamic relationship that reflects the relative concentration of hydrogen ions (H^+) in the body. Hydrogen ions are acidic and the concentration of these within the body must be maintained within fairly strict limits. Any deviation in the hydrogen ion concentration adversely affects all of the biochemical events that occur in the body. The hydrogen ion concentration is dynamic, changing from second to second.

THE pH SCALE

The total number of hydrogen ions present in the body at any given time is very high. Because of this, the **pH** system of measurement is used. The pH scale is inversely related to hydrogen ion concentration. That is, the greater the hydrogen ion concentration, the lower the pH. The lower the hydrogen ion concentration, the higher the pH.

The pH scale is logarithmic, each number representing a value ten times that of its neighboring number, so that pH 6 represents a hydrogen ion concentration 10 times as great as that represented by pH 7. The following formula represents pH:

$$pH = \log \frac{1}{[H^+]}$$

The pH scale ranges from 1 to 14. A pH of 1 means that only hydrogen ions are present. A pH of 14 means that there are virtually no hydrogen ions present. The pH of water is 7.0, which is a neutral pH. The pH of the body is normally 7.35 to 7.45 (Table 3-2).

Because hydrogen ions are acidic, a pH below 7.35 is referred to as **acidosis.** A substance that produces negatively charged ions that can neutralize the positively charged hydrogen ions (or other acids) is called an alkali or a base. An excess of alkaline (base) substances or a deficit of acids will produce a pH above 7.45, which is referred to as **alkalosis.** In humans, a variation of only 0.4 of a pH unit in either direction from normal (6.9 or 7.8) can be fatal.

BODILY REGULATION OF ACID-BASE BALANCE

The body is constantly producing hydrogen ions (acids) through metabolism and other biochemical processes. To maintain the acid-base balance, these hydrogen ions must be constantly eliminated from the body. There are three major mechanisms to remove hydrogen ions from the body. The fastest mechanism is often referred to as the *buffer system* or the *bicarbonate buffer system.*

✱ **net filtration** the total loss of water from blood plasma across the capillary membrane into the interstitial space. Normally, hydrostatic pressure forcing water out of the capillary is balanced by oncotic force pulling water into the capillary for a net filtration of zero.

✱ **pH** abbreviation for *potential of hydrogen.* A measure of relative acidity or alkalinity. Since the pH scale is inverse to the concentration of acidic hydrogen ions, the lower the pH the greater the acidity and the higher the pH the greater the alkalinity. A normal pH range is 7.35 to 7.45.

✱ **acidosis** a high concentration of hydrogen ions; a pH below 7.35.

✱ **alkalosis** a low concentration of hydrogen ions; a pH above 7.45.

Content Review

THREE MECHANISMS OF HYDROGEN ION REMOVAL
- Bicarbonate buffer system
- Respiration
- Kidney function

Table 3-2 — THE pH SCALE AND HYDROGEN ION CONCENTRATIONS

pH		Example	H^+ Concentration*	
Acidic	0	Hydrochloric acid	10^{-0}	(1.0)
	1	Stomach secretions	10^{-1}	(0.1)
	2	Lemon juice	10^{-2}	(0.01)
	3	Cola drinks	10^{-3}	(0.001)
	4	White wine	10^{-4}	(0.0001)
	5	Tomato juice	10^{-5}	(0.00001)
	6	Coffee, urine, saliva	10^{-6}	(0.000001)
Neutral	7	Distilled water	10^{-7}	(0.0000001)
Basic	8	Blood, semen	10^{-8}	(0.00000001)
	9	Bile	10^{-9}	(0.000000001)
	10	Bleach	10^{-10}	(0.0000000001)
	11	Milk of magnesia	10^{-11}	(0.00000000001)
	12	Ammonia water	10^{-12}	(0.000000000001)
	13	Drain opener	10^{-13}	(0.0000000000001)
	14	Lye	10^{-14}	(0.00000000000001)

*Hydrogen ion concentrations are expressed in moles per liter, a quantity based on molecular weight.

The two components of the bicarbonate buffer system are bicarbonate ion (HCO_3^-) and carbonic acid (H_2CO_3). These two compounds are in equilibrium with hydrogen ion (H^+), as follows: In some circumstances hydrogen ion will combine with bicarbonate ion to produce carbonic acid. In other circumstances, carbonic acid will dissociate into bicarbonate ion and hydrogen ion:

$$H^+ + HCO_3^- \leftrightarrow H_2CO_3$$

hydrogen ion + bicarbonate ion ↔ carbonic acid

In a healthy individual, for every molecule of carbonic acid, there are 20 molecules of bicarbonate ion. Any change in this 20:1 ratio is immediately corrected without significant change in the total body pH. This occurs in the following manner: An increase in hydrogen ion (acidosis) is corrected as the excess hydrogen ions combine with bicarbonate ions to form carbonic acid. (Thus an increase in hydrogen ion leads to an increase in carbonic acid—driving the equation above to the right.) Conversely, when there is a deficit in hydrogen ions (alkalosis), carbonic acid will dissociate into bicarbonate ion and hydrogen ion. (Thus a decrease in hydrogen ion leads to a decrease in carbonic acid—driving the equation above to the left.) (Figure 3-5)

$$\text{Increased Acid:} \uparrow H^+ + HCO_3^- \rightarrow \uparrow H_2CO_3$$
$$\text{Decreased Acid:} \downarrow H^+ + HCO_3^- \rightarrow \downarrow H_2CO_3$$

Carbonic acid is a weak acid that is better tolerated by the body than pure hydrogen ion. However, the body carries this reaction further. Any increase in carbonic acid must also be eliminated.

The elimination of excess carbonic acid takes place as follows: Carbonic acid is unstable and will eventually dissociate into carbon dioxide and water. This

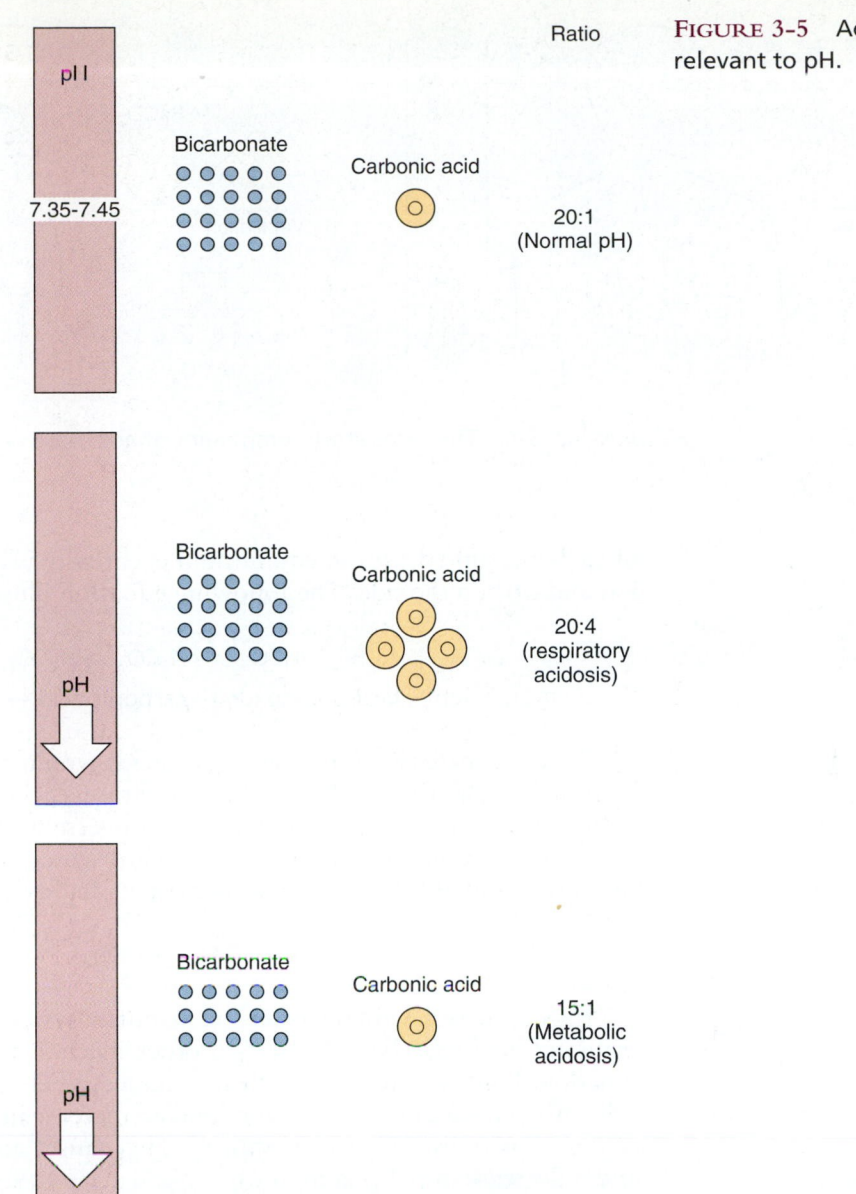

Ratio

FIGURE 3-5 Acid-base ratios relevant to pH.

pH

7.35-7.45

Bicarbonate

Carbonic acid

20:1
(Normal pH)

Bicarbonate

Carbonic acid

20:4
(respiratory
acidosis)

pH

Bicarbonate

Carbonic acid

15:1
(Metabolic
acidosis)

pH

normally slow process is speeded by the blood's erythrocytes, which contain an enzyme called *carbonic anhydrase*. Carbonic anhydrase causes carbonic acid to be converted to carbon dioxide and water very rapidly—so rapidly that carbonic acid exists for only a fraction of a second before it is converted into carbon dioxide and water. Most buffering of acid in the body occurs in the erythrocytes.

The enzyme also works in a reverse fashion, which allows carbon dioxide and water to be quickly converted into carbonic acid. The reaction proceeds in accordance with *LeChetalier's Principle*. Given an excess of carbon dioxide on the right hand side of the equilibrium, a stress is placed on it such that it must shift to the left, which is sometimes referred to as a mass action effect. The net effect of this is the generation of more hydrogen ion, and acidosis. The clinical application of this is that when a patient is said to hypoventilate, that is, retain CO_2, then the accumulation (stress) of increased CO_2 forces the equilibrium to shift to the left, causing what is known as respiratory acidosis. So, with the aid

Acid-Base Balance **115**

FIGURE 3-6   The respiratory component of acid-base balance.

of carbonic anhydrase, an equilibrium eventually is attained between hydrogen ion and carbon dioxide. The following equation illustrates this relationship.

$$H^+ + HCO_3^- \leftrightarrow H_2CO_3 \leftrightarrow H_2O + CO_2$$

hydrogen ion + bicarbonate ion $\leftrightarrow$ carbonic acid $\leftrightarrow$ water + carbon dioxide

Thus an increase in hydrogen ion (acid) would result in an increase in carbonic acid. With the aid of carbonic anhydrase, carbonic acid would quickly dissociate into water and carbon dioxide. Conversely (since the reaction can move in either direction), an increase in CO_2 causes an increase in hydrogen ion concentration and a decrease in pH (increase in acidity), as shown below.

$$\uparrow H^+ \leftrightarrow \uparrow CO_2$$

In conjunction with the bicarbonate buffer system described above, the body regulates acid-base balance by two other mechanisms, respiration and kidney function. Increased respirations cause increased elimination of CO_2, which results in a decrease in hydrogen ions and an increase in pH. Conversely, decreased respirations cause CO_2 to be retained. This causes an increase in hydrogen ions and a decrease in pH (Figure 3-6).

The kidneys also can regulate the pH by altering the concentration of bicarbonate ion (HCO_3^-) in the blood. Increased elimination of HCO_3^- results in a lowered pH. (There is less bicarbonate ion to combine with and eliminate hydrogen ion.) Conversely retention of HCO_3^- causes an increase in pH. (There is more bicarbonate ion to combine with and eliminate hydrogen ion.) In addition, the kidneys affect the acid-base balance by removing or retaining various chemicals. Normally, the kidneys remove larger metabolic acids, excreting them in the urine, resulting in an increase in pH.

Part 2: Body Systems

THE INTEGUMENTARY SYSTEM

The protective envelope we call the skin is a complex structure. Understanding how it is put together and how it functions will help you appreciate the importance of injuries to it and the value of their proper care.

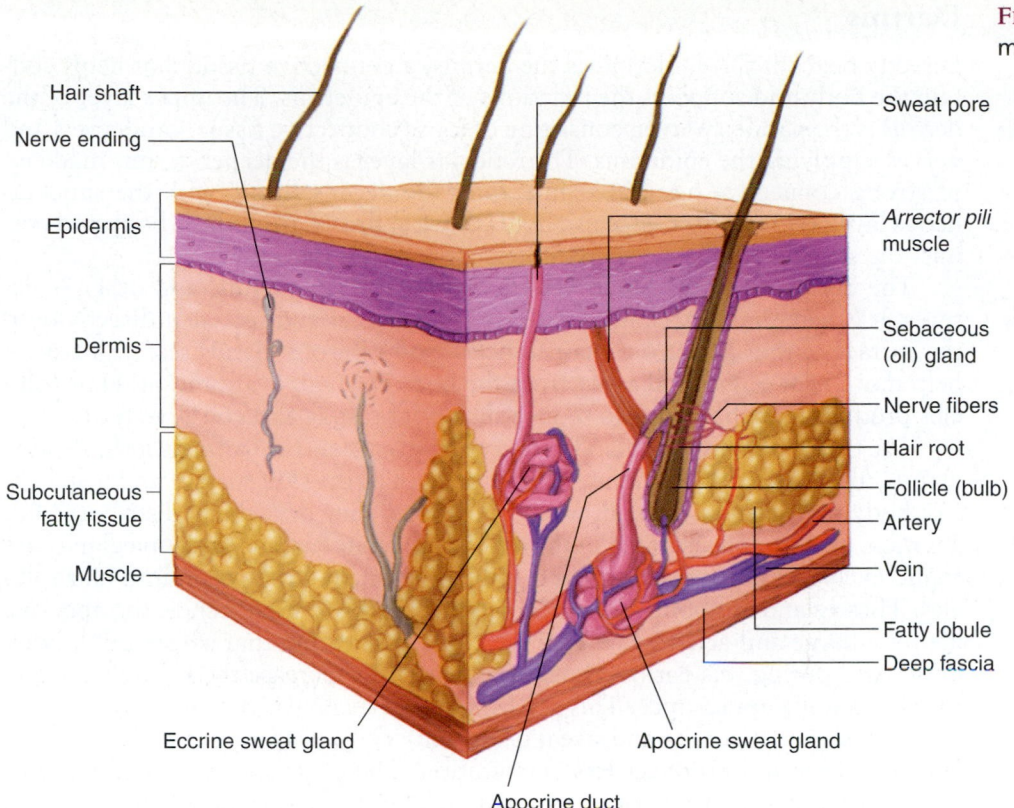

FIGURE 3-7 Layers and major structures of the skin.

Hair shaft

Nerve ending

Epidermis

Dermis

Subcutaneous fatty tissue

Muscle

Sweat pore

Arrector pili muscle

Sebaceous (oil) gland

Nerve fibers

Hair root

Follicle (bulb)

Artery

Vein

Fatty lobule

Deep fascia

Eccrine sweat gland

Apocrine sweat gland

Apocrine duct

THE SKIN

The epidermis, dermis, and subcutaneous tissue layers comprise what is commonly known as the skin (Figure 3-7). Each of these layers performs functions essential to helping the body maintain homeostasis and each plays an important role in the wound repair process.

Epidermis

The outermost skin layer is the **epidermis.** It is generated by a layer of cells just above the dermis (stratum germinativum). These cells divide rapidly, generating a movement of cells upward toward the epidermal surface. As the epidermis contains no vasculature, the further these cells are pushed away from the dermis, the less circulation they receive, and they eventually die. As they die, they flatten and interlock, providing a firm and secure barrier around the body (stratum corneum). The outermost cells are eventually abraded or washed away and then replaced, allowing the epidermis to maintain its thickness. It normally takes 2 weeks for a cell to move from the dermal border to the surface of the epidermis and another 2 to 4 weeks until it is abraded away. This outward movement of cells helps the body resist invasion by bacteria.

A waxy substance called **sebum** lubricates the surface of the epidermis. This lubrication acts much like oil on leather. It keeps the outer layers of the skin flexible, strong, and resistant to penetration by water. The epidermis is also responsible for the pigmentation that protects the skin from the harmful effects of ultraviolet radiation. The thickness of the epidermis varies greatly, depending on the amount of abrasion and pressure it receives. On the soles of the feet, it is very thick and strong, while over the eye it is microscopic in thickness and very delicate.

Content Review

LAYERS OF THE SKIN
- Epidermis
- Dermis
- Subcutaneous tissue

✱ **epidermis** outermost layer of the skin comprised of dead or dying cells.

✱ **sebum** fatty secretion of the sebaceous gland that helps keep the skin pliable and waterproof.

Dermis

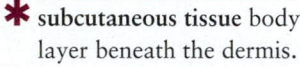

dermis true skin, also called the corium; it is the layer of tissue producing the epidermis and housing the structures, blood vessels, and nerves normally associated with the skin.

sebaceous glands glands within the dermis secreting sebum.

sudoriferous glands glands within the dermis that secrete sweat.

Directly beneath the epidermis is the **dermis**, a connective tissue that helps contain the body and supports the functions of the epidermis. The upper layer of the dermis is the papillary layer, consisting of loose connective tissue, capillaries, and nerves supplying the epidermis. The reticular layer is the deeper dermis made up of strong connective tissue that integrates the dermis firmly with the subcutaneous layer below. This tissue also holds the skin firmly around the body and permits the stretching and flexibility necessary for articulation.

The dermis contains blood vessels, nerve endings, glands, and other structures. It is here that **sebaceous glands** produce sebum and secrete it directly onto the surface of the skin or into hair follicles. **Sudoriferous glands** secrete sweat to help move heat out of and away from the body through evaporation. Hair follicles produce hair that helps to reduce surface abrasion and conserve heat.

The two types of sweat glands are *eccrine glands* and *apocrine glands*. Eccrine glands, also known as merocrine glands, open onto the skin surface and help control body temperature through water excretion. They are widely distributed but are most heavily concentrated in the axilla and genital areas. Apocrine glands are found exclusively in the armpits and genital region, and they open into hair follicles. These glands respond to emotional stress. During adolescence, the apocrine glands enlarge and actively increase the axillary sweating that causes adult body odor. Also during this period, the sebaceous glands increase their activity, giving the skin an oily appearance. This predisposes the teenager to acne problems.

As we age, sebaceous and sweat gland activity decreases. As a result, the skin becomes drier and produces less perspiration. The epidermis thins and flattens, and the dermis loses some of its vascularity. The skin wrinkles as it loses turgor. In warmer climates, the skin can become thickened, yellowed, and furrowed and take on a weather-beaten appearance. Elderly people develop a variety of spots on the thin skin of the backs of their hands and forearms. Whitish, depigmented marks are known as pseudoscars. Purple spots (purpura) caused by minor capillary bleeding may appear and fade after a few weeks.

In the dermis are several resident body cells responsible for initiating the attack on invading organisms, foreign materials, and damaged cells, and for beginning the repair of damaged tissue. The macrophages and lymphocytes (types of white blood cells) begin the inflammation response by killing invading bodies and triggering a call for other, similiar cells. Mast cells control the microcirculation to tissues and respond to the initial invasion, increasing capillary flow and permeability. Fibroblasts lay down and repair protein strands to strengthen the wound site and begin restoring the skin's integrity.

Subcutaneous Tissue

subcutaneous tissue body layer beneath the dermis.

Subcutaneous tissue is the body layer beneath the dermis. It is rich in fatty or adipose tissue, which helps it absorb the forces of trauma, protecting the tissues and vital organs beneath. Because of its fatty content, heat moves outward through the subcutaneous tissue three times more slowly than through muscles or other layers of the skin; hence it is of great value in conserving body temperature. The body directs blood below the subcutaneous tissue to conserve heat and above it through the dermis when it is necessary to radiate heat.

THE HAIR

Hair is a tactile sensory organ, while also playing a role in sexual stimulation and attraction. It covers the entire body except the palms, soles, and parts of the sex organs. Hair develops from the base of the hair follicle, where it is nourished by

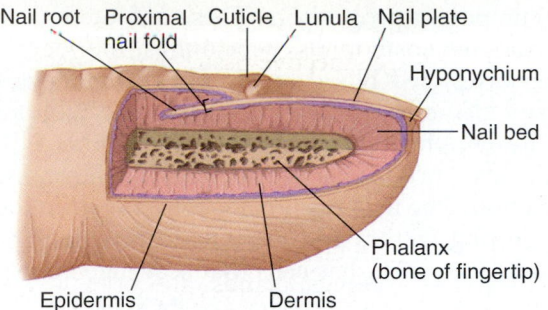

Nail root Proximal Cuticle Lunula Nail plate
         nail fold

Hyponychium

Nail bed

Phalanx
(bone of fingertip)

Epidermis   Dermis

FIGURE 3-8   The nail.

the papilla, a vast capillary network. An involuntary arrector pili muscle fiber attaches to the base of the hair shaft. When these arrectores pilorum contract, the hair stands erect and goose bumps appear on the skin.

The two types of hair are vellus and terminal. Vellus hair is short, fine, and lacking pigment (similar to "peach fuzz"). Terminal hair is coarser, thicker, and pigmented. It appears on the eyebrows and scalp, in the armpits and groin of both sexes, and on the faces and bodies of males.

With aging the hair turns gray from a decrease in pigmentation and its growth declines. A transition from terminal to vellus hair on the scalp causes baldness in both men and women. The opposite occurs in the nares and ears of men, where terminal hair replaces vellus hair. Both genders generally experience a decrease in body hair as they age. Loss of the lateral third of the eyebrow is also normal in the elderly.

THE NAILS

Nails are found at the most distal ends of fingers and toes and are primarily for protection. Nails are strong yet flexible and provide a sharp edge for scratching, scraping, and clawing. They are made up of the nail plate, the nail bed, the proximal nail fold, and the nail root (Figure 3-8). The angle between the proximal nail fold and the nail plate should be less than 180°. Fingernails grow approximately 0.1 mm daily, slightly faster in the summertime. The nail plate lies on a highly vascular nail bed that gives the nail a pink appearance. Nail edges should be smooth and rounded. The nail plates should be smooth, flat, or slightly curved and should feel hard and uniformly thick. As we age, nail growth diminishes because of decreased peripheral circulation. The nails, especially the toenails, become hard, thick, brittle, and yellowish.

THE BLOOD

The **hematopoietic system** consists of blood (both cells and plasma), bone marrow, the liver, the spleen, and the kidneys. The cellular components of blood are formed by the differentiation of a **pluripotent stem cell** in a process termed **hematopoiesis.** In the fetus, hematopoiesis occurs first outside of the bone marrow (*extramedullary hematopoiesis*) in the liver, spleen, lymph nodes, and thymus. By the fourth month, the developing bone marrow begins to produce blood cells (*intramedullary hematopoiesis*). After birth, the bone marrow is the primary site of blood cell production and extramedullary hematopoiesis greatly diminishes, occurring mostly in the liver and spleen. By adulthood, hematopoiesis occurs exclusively in the bone marrow unless a pathological state exists.

In hematopoiesis, the stem cell reproduces to maintain a constant population of cells. Some stem cells then further differentiate into myeloid multipotent stem

✱ **hematopoietic system** body system having to do with the production and development of blood cells, consisting of the bone marrow, liver, spleen, kidneys, and the blood itself.

Content Review

HEMATOPOIETIC SYSTEM COMPONENTS
- Bone marrow
- Liver
- Spleen
- Kidneys
- Blood

✱ **pluripotent stem cell** a cell from which the various types of blood cells can form.

✱ **hematopoiesis** the process through which pluripotent stem cells differentiate into various types of blood cells.

cells that, in turn, differentiate into unipotent progenitors. These unipotent progenitors ultimately mature into basophils, eosinophils, neutrophils, monocytes (types of white blood cells), erythrocytes (red blood cells), and thrombocytes (platelets.) Pluripotent stem cells may also differentiate into common lymphoid stem cells that ultimately mature into lymphocytes (another type of white cell). The kidney, and to a lesser extent the liver, produce **erythropoietin,** the hormone responsible for red blood cell production. The liver also removes toxins from the blood and produces many of the clotting factors and proteins in plasma. The spleen, an important part of the immune system, has cells that scavenge abnormal blood cells and bacteria.

Blood volume normally remains relatively constant at about six percent of total body weight. With an average of 80–85 milliliters of blood per kilogram of body weight, a person who weighs 75 kilograms has approximately 6 liters of blood. The body can easily handle up to about one-half liter of lost blood or fluid. An example is routine blood donations where healthy donors tolerate the blood loss without complication.

The major determinants of the blood volume are red cell mass and plasma volume. Red blood cells remain confined to the intravascular compartment. If their destruction remains constant, then only changes in the rate of production can alter the size of the circulating red cell mass. The plasma volume on the other hand can rapidly change due to fluid shifts between the intravascular and extravascular space. These fluid shifts help to preserve circulating blood volume in the event of acute hemorrhage. Other compensatory mechanisms include vasoconstriction, tachycardia, and increased cardiac contractility to maintain adequate tissue perfusion until significant losses overwhelm these measures. When these compensatory measures fail, the patient enters decompensated shock. Fortunately, young healthy individuals' bodies can compensate for loss of as much as 25–30 percent of blood volume.

COMPONENTS OF BLOOD

Blood consists of liquid, or plasma, and of formed elements—red blood cells, white blood cells, and platelets.

Plasma

Plasma is a thick, pale yellow fluid that is 90–92 percent water and 6–7 percent proteins. Fats, carbohydrates, electrolytes, gases, and certain chemical messengers comprise the remaining 2–3 percent. Plasma transports the cellular components of blood and dissolved nutrients throughout the body and, at the same time, transports waste products from cellular metabolism to the liver, kidneys, and lungs, where they can be removed from the body.

Most plasma components can move back and forth across the capillary membranes to the interstitial fluid. However, plasma proteins, such as albumin, are large molecules and have great difficulty diffusing across the membranes. This is fortunate, since they remain in the plasma to help retain water in the capillaries. As noted earlier, this is known as *oncotic force,* or *colloid osmotic pressure.* Plasma proteins perform many other functions, including clotting of blood, dismantling of clots, buffering of the blood's acid/base balance, transporting hormones and regulating their effects, and providing a source of energy.

Electrolytes are also found in the plasma. (As noted earlier, these are chemical substances that dissociate into charged particles in water.) They are essential for nerve conduction, muscle contraction, and water balance. They can easily diffuse across capillary membranes based on their concentration gradients. Carbohydrates

* erythropoietin the hormone responsible for red blood cell production.

Content Review

COMPONENTS OF BLOOD

- Plasma
- Formed elements
  - Red blood cells
  - White blood cells
  - Platelets

* plasma thick, pale yellow fluid that makes up the liquid part of the blood.

in plasma are generally in the form of glucose, the primary energy source for all body tissues. Glucose is especially important to brain cells as they cannot obtain energy from fat metabolism. (Glucose cannot diffuse across most cell membranes without assistance from the hormone insulin.) Plasma also performs a role in gas transport. In addition to being carried by red blood cells, carbon dioxide and oxygen are dissolved and transported in plasma.

Red Blood Cells

The primary function of blood is to transport oxygen from the lungs to the tissues. At rest, the body consumes about 4 ml of oxygen per kilogram of body weight every minute. Because it stores little oxygen, the body would quickly succumb to anoxia without the continued transport provided by the blood.

The red blood cell (RBC), or **erythrocyte**, is a biconcave disc that does not have a nucleus when mature (Figure 3-9). It contains **hemoglobin** molecules that transport oxygen. Hemoglobin comprises four subunits of *globin,* each bonded to a *heme* (iron containing) molecule. Each globin subunit can bind with one oxygen molecule; thus, each complete hemoglobin molecule can carry up to four oxygen molecules. When all four subunits are carrying an oxygen molecule, the hemoglobin is 100 percent saturated. When fully saturated, each gram of hemoglobin can transport 1.34 milliliters of oxygen.

Oxygen Transport The effectiveness of oxygen transport depends on many factors. Red blood cell mass (the number of red blood cells present) is obviously a factor in oxygen transport. The greater the number of red blood cells, the greater will be the potential oxygen carrying capacity. The percentage of oxygen bound to hemoglobin increases as the **pO$_2$** increases. This is illustrated in the oxygen-hemoglobin dissociation curve (Figure 3-10). Normal pO$_2$ is approximately 95 mmHg. Based on this, the oxygen-hemoglobin dissociation curve indicates that normal oxygen saturation is about 97 percent. Hemoglobin's affinity for oxygen is also a factor in oxygen transport. Several factors affect oxygen affinity, including pH, **pCO$_2$**, concentration of 2,3-DPG, and temperature.

The lower the pH (that is, the more acidic the blood), the more readily hemoglobin will release oxygen. This shifts the oxygen-hemoglobin dissociation curve to the right. In contrast, alkalosis makes hemoglobin bind to oxygen more tightly. This shifts the oxygen-hemoglobin dissociation curve to the left (Figure 3-11). The pCO$_2$ is directly related to the pH. Thus, in the lungs, as pCO$_2$ decreases with diffusion of CO$_2$ into the alveoli, the quantity of oxygen that binds with the hemoglobin increases. The opposite effect occurs when the

Red blood cells

FIGURE 3-9 Red blood cells.

✻ **erythrocyte** red blood cell.

✻ **hemoglobin** oxygen-bearing molecule in the red blood cells. It is made up of iron-rich red pigment called *heme* and a protein called *globin.*

✻ **pO$_2$** partial pressure of oxygen; (*partial pressure* is the pressure exerted by a given component of a gas containing several components).

✻ **pCO$_2$** partial pressure of carbon dioxide; (*partial pressure* defined—see pO$_2$).

FIGURE 3-10 The oxygen-hemoglobin dissociation curve.

FIGURE 3-11 Effects of pH, increased carbon dioxide, temperature, and 2,3-DPG on the oxygen-hemoglobin dissociation curve.

blood reaches the tissues. There, waste CO_2 from the tissues diffuses into the blood, causing the hemoglobin to give up more oxygen to the tissues. This is called the **Bohr effect**.

Except for hemoglobin, the most abundant chemical in red blood cells is **2,3-diphosphoglycerate (2,3-DPG)**. During prolonged periods of hypoxia, the level of 2,3-DPG increases. This shifts the oxygen-hemoglobin dissociation curve to the right and can increase the pO_2 in the plasma as much as 10 percent more than it otherwise would have been. However, the increased 2,3-DPG makes it more difficult for oxygen to combine with hemoglobin in the lungs. This effect casts doubt on whether 2,3-DPG's effect in hypoxia is as beneficial as was once thought.

An elevation in the body temperature causes a shift to the right of the oxygen-hemoglobin dissociation curve and a decrease in hemoglobin's affinity for blood. Conversely, a fall in body temperature causes hemoglobin to bind oxygen more tightly. During periods of hyperthermia and pyrexia (fever), hemoglobin's decreased affinity for oxygen enhances oxygenation of the peripheral tissues and end organs.

Exercise has several effects on oxygen affinity. First, exercise causes the production and release of carbon dioxide and other acids, especially from the large muscles. It also increases body temperature. Thus, both a decrease in pH and an increase in body temperature will cause hemoglobin to release oxygen more readily. This serves to enhance peripheral tissue oxygenation during strenuous exercise and work.

Importantly, other substances can compete with oxygen for hemoglobin's binding sites. The greater a substance's affinity for the binding sites, the more readily the substance will bind with hemoglobin. The classic example is carbon monoxide (CO). Carbon monoxide has 210–250 times oxygen's affinity for hemoglobin and competes for the same binding sites. In carbon monoxide poisoning, when CO binds to one of the hemoglobin molecule's four binding sites, the hemoglobin molecule is altered so that the remaining three oxygen molecules are held more tightly. This inhibits oxygen release in the peripheral tissues, contributing to hypoxia, acidosis, and eventually shock.

Red Blood Cell Production Red blood cell production is termed **erythropoiesis**. Erythropoietin, a hormone produced primarily by the kidney, stimulates the bone marrow's production of erythrocytes. Erythropoietin is secreted when the renal cells sense hypoxia. This in turn stimulates the bone marrow to increase RBC production, resulting in increased red cell mass. Although a relatively slow process, this effectively increases the oxygen carrying capacity of blood, thereby increasing oxygen delivery to the tissues.

The red blood cell lives approximately 120 days. Hemorrhage, **hemolysis** (destruction of the RBC), or **sequestration** of the RBCs by the liver or spleen may significantly reduce its life span. Hemorrhage may occur outside the body or be

* **Bohr effect** phenomenon in which a decrease in pCO_2/acidity causes an increase in the quantity of oxygen that binds with the hemoglobin; conversely, an increase in pCO_2/acidity causes the hemoglobin to give up a greater quantity of oxygen.

* **2,3-diphosphoglycerate (2,3-DPG)** chemical in the red blood cells that affects hemoglobin's affinity for oxygen.

* **erythropoiesis** the process of producing red blood cells.

* **hemolysis** destruction of red blood cells.

* **sequestration** the trapping of red blood cells by an organ such as the spleen.

hidden within a body cavity such as the peritoneum, retroperitoneum, or GI tract. Hemolysis may occur within the circulatory system in sickle cell disease and in rare autoimmune anemias. The spleen and liver contain specialized scavenger cells called macrophages (a type of white blood cell) that can remove damaged or abnormal red blood cells from the circulation.

Laboratory Evaluation of Red Blood Cells and Hemoglobin Red blood cells (RBCs) are quantified or measured and reported in two ways: red blood cell count and hematocrit. The red blood cell count is the total number of RBCs reported in millions per cubic millimeter (mm^3) of blood. Normal values vary with age and sex but in general run between 4.2 and 6.0 million/mm^3.

The **hematocrit** is the packed cell volume of red blood cells per unit of blood (Figure 3-12). This measurement is obtained by placing a sample of blood in a centrifuge and spinning it at high speed so that the cellular elements separate from the plasma. The red blood cells are the heaviest blood component since they carry the iron-containing pigment hemoglobin. They are forced to the bottom of the tube. Above the red blood cells are the white blood cells. On the top of the specimen is the plasma, which consists primarily of water. The RBCs' column height is divided by the blood's total column height (cellular component plus plasma) and reported as a percentage. Normal values range between 40 and 52 percent, with females generally running a few percentage points below males.

Another way to determine the status of the red blood cell is to measure the concentration of hemoglobin present. This is typically expressed as the number of grams of hemoglobin present per deciliter of whole blood. The hemoglobin concentration will decrease in two ways. First, when the number of red blood cells present is below normal, the hemoglobin will also be below normal. In some cases, the red blood cell volume can be normal, but the amount of hemoglobin present may be decreased. In emergency medicine, it is commonplace to measure the hemoglobin in addition to the hematocrit (H&H). Both values indicate red blood cell volume and capability. The normal hemoglobin in a man is 12.0–15.0 g/dl; for females, it is 10.5–14.0 g/dl.

White Blood Cells

White blood cells, called **leukocytes** or white corpuscles, circulate through the bloodstream and tissues, providing protection from foreign invasion. White blood cells (WBCs) are extremely mobile, traveling through the blood stream to wherever they are needed in order to fight infection.

A large population of leukocytes does not move freely within the blood stream but instead is attached to the blood vessels' walls. These *marginated* leukocytes may quickly return to the circulating pool in response to stress, corticosteroids, seizures, epinephrine, and exercise. This process is called *demargination*. Marginated leukocytes that attach more firmly to the vascular lining through *adhesion* may then leave the blood vessels by *diapedesis*. This enables the leukocytes to squeeze between the cells lining the blood vessels and to follow chemical signals (**chemotaxis**) to the infection site. There, they may engulf and destroy an invader by **phagocytosis** (Figure 3-13). Others stimulate either chemical or immune responses to fight infection.

Healthy people have from 5,000 to 9,000 white blood cells per microliter of blood. An infection can increase that number to more than 16,000. An increase in the white blood cell number is a classic sign of bacterial infection. White blood cells originate in the bone marrow from undifferentiated stem cells. Through a process termed **leukopoiesis**, these stem cells respond to specific growth factors that allow them to differentiate into three main-blasts (immature forms): myeloblasts, monoblasts, and lymphoblasts.

FIGURE 3-12 Hematocrit, including plasma.

Plasma: 54%

Red cells: 45%

Hematocrit

* **hematocrit** the packed cell volume of red blood cells per unit of blood.

* **leukocyte** white blood cell.

* **chemotaxis** the movement of white blood cells in response to chemical signals.

* **phagocytosis** process in which white blood cells engulf and destroy an invader.

* **leukopoiesis** the process through which stem cells differentiate into the white blood cells' immature forms.

Content Review

WHITE BLOOD CELL
–BLASTS
• Myeloblasts
• Monoblasts
• Lymphoblasts

FIGURE 3-13 White blood cells engulfing and destroying an invader in the process called phagocytosis.

White cell

Invading particle

Invading particle ingested by white cell

＊ **major basic protein (MBP)** a larvacidal peptide.

White blood cells are categorized as *granulocytes, monocytes,* or *lymphocytes* (Figure 3-14).

Granulocytes Granulocytic white blood cells, so named for the granules they contain, form from stem cells that differentiate in the bone marrow in response to hormonal stimulation. These cells mature through several stages from myeloblast to promyelocyte, myelocyte, metamyelocyte, band form, and mature form (Figure 3-15). Their mature forms are classified by the type of stain they absorb. *Basophils* absorb basic stains and have blue granules. *Eosinophils* absorb acidic stains and contain red granules. *Neutrophils* absorb neither acidic nor basic stains well and contain pale blue and pink granules.

Basophils Basophils are granulocytes that primarily function in allergic reactions. Within their granules they store all of the histamine in the circulating blood. In response to an allergic stimulus, the cells degranulate, releasing histamines that cause vasodilation, bronchoconstriction, rhinorrhea, increased vascular permeability, and increased neutrophil and eosinophil chemotaxis. Basophils also contain heparin, which breaks down blood clots.

Eosinophils Eosinophils are highly specialized members of the granulocytic series. They can inactivate the chemical mediators of acute allergic reactions, thereby modulating the anaphylactic response. They also contain **major basic protein (MBP)**, which they release in conjunction with an antibody response shown to fight parasitic infections.

FIGURE 3-14 Types of white blood cells.

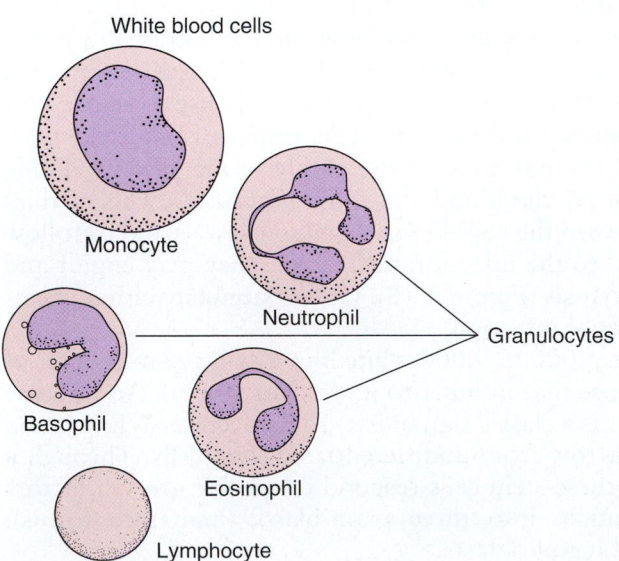

White blood cells

Monocyte

Neutrophil

Granulocytes

Basophil

Eosinophil

Lymphocyte

MYELOBLAST

PROMYELOCYTE (PROGRANULOCYTE)

BASOPHILIC MYELOCYTE	NEUTROPHILIC MYELOCYTE	EOSINOPHILIC MYELOCYTE
BASOPHILIC METAMYELOCYTE	NEUTROPHILIC METAMYELOCYTE	EOSINOPHILIC METAMYELOCYTE
BASOPHILIC BAND	NEUTROPHILIC BAND	EOSINOPHILIC BAND
BASOPHILIC SEGMENTED	NEUTROPHILIC SEGMENTED	EOSINOPHILIC SEGMENTED
BASOPHIL	**NEUTROPHIL**	**EOSINOPHIL**

FIGURE 3-15   Granulocyte maturation.

Neutrophils   The neutrophils' primary function is to fight infection. They leave the blood stream by diapedesis and engulf and kill microorganisms that have invaded the body. Once they have phagocytized the microorganism, primary and secondary granules within the neutrophil fuse with the phagosome, and the organism is killed and digested. In severe infections the total neutrophil count may rise rapidly, with immature (band) forms apparent on the peripheral blood smear under microscopic examination. If the neutrophil count is low (**neutropenia**), the body cannot mount an appropriate response to infection, and the infection may overwhelm the body's defenses and kill the individual. Neutropenia may result from primary bone marrow disorders that decrease production, from overwhelming infection, viral syndrome, autoimmune disease, or drugs, and from nutritional deficiencies.

✱ **neutropenia** a low neutrophil count.

Monocytes Monocytes are unique in that after their initial phase of maturation they are released into the circulation and can remain there as circulating monocytes or migrate to distant sites to further mature into free or fixed tissue macrophages. Macrophages, the "garbage collectors" of the immune system, engulf both foreign invaders and dead neutrophils. They also can attack tumor cells and participate in tissue repair. Monocytes and macrophages also secrete growth factors to stimulate production of granulocytes and red blood cells. Some macrophages are fixed within tissues, residing in the liver, spleen, lungs, and lymphatic system. These cells are part of the reticuloendothelial system. They remove foreign matter, cellular debris, and proteins from the blood. After engulfing foreign proteins or infectious agents, these fixed macrophages of the reticuloendothelial system can stimulate lymphocyte production in an immune response against these agents.

Lymphocytes Lymphocytes are the primary cells involved in the body's immune response. They are located throughout the body in the circulating blood as well as in other tissues such as lymph nodes, circulating in lymph fluid, bone marrow, spleen, liver, lungs, intestine, and skin. Lymphocytes are characteristically small, round, white blood cells containing no granules on staining. However similar they may appear, these cells are highly specialized. They contain surface receptor sites specific to a single antigen (foreign protein) and stand ready to initiate the immune response to rid the body of that particular substance or infectious agent.

Immunity The two basic subpopulations of lymphocytes are T cells and B cells. T cells mature in the thymus gland, located in the mediastinum, and then migrate throughout the body. They are responsible for developing *cell-mediated immunity*, also called *cellular immunity*. Once an antigen activates them, they generate other cells called effector cells that are responsible for delayed-type hypersensitivity reactions, tumor suppression, graft rejection (organ transplant rejections), and defense against intracellular organisms. B cells produce antibodies to combat infection, which is termed *humoral immunity*. They originate in the bone marrow and then migrate to peripheral lymphatic tissues. There they can be exposed to antigens from invading organisms and respond by producing the specific antibodies necessary to defend against them. Some of these B cells' lines are maintained and give the body a "memory" of the previous infection. When the body is subsequently exposed to the same antigen or infection, it generates a rapid response to quickly overwhelm the infection.

Autoimmune Disease Autoimmune disease occurs when the body makes antibodies against its own tissues. These antibodies may be limited to specific organs, such as the thyroid, as occurs in *Hashimoto's thyroiditis*. Or, they may involve virtually every tissue type as in the antinuclear antibodies of *systemic lupus erythematosis (SLE)* that attack the body's cell nuclei. Several anemias result from autoimmunity. Mechanisms for the development of autoimmune disease include genetic factors and viral infections.

Alterations in Immune Response Several factors can alter the body's immune response. For example, patients who receive an organ transplant must take drugs that inhibit cellular immunity and prevent graft rejection. If they do not, the T cells will recognize the new organ as "not self" and begin the process of attacking it. This is called rejection. Unfortunately, organ recipient immunosuppressed patients are at risk for infections from many different organisms including bacteria, viruses, fungi, and protozoa. Human immunodeficiency virus (HIV) effectively destroys cell-mediated immunity by selectively attacking and ultimately killing T cells. This also leaves the patient at risk for opportunistic infections against which the body cannot defend itself, ultimately killing him. Patients who have cancer are often immunocompromised by the disease itself or by chemotherapy agents that also attack the bone marrow. These agents decrease leukocyte

✱ **autoimmune disease** condition in which the body makes antibodies against its own tissues.

production to extremely low levels, leaving the body defenseless against infection. As a paramedic, you must protect your immunosuppressed patients from undue exposure to infection by good hand-washing technique, correct IV technique, and proper wound care. If you have an infection, you must take precautions not to transmit it to your patients. If the infection is highly contagious, as in influenza or chicken pox, you may have to work in a non-patient-care setting.

Inflammatory Process The **inflammatory process** is a nonspecific defense mechanism that wards off damage from microorganisms or trauma. It attempts to localize the damage while destroying the source, at the same time facilitating repair of the tissues. Causes of the inflammatory process may be an infectious agent, trauma, chemical, or immunologic. After local tissue injury occurs, the damaged tissues release chemical messengers that attract white blood cells (chemotaxis), increase capillary permeability, and cause vasodilation. If bacteria are present, responding neutrophils or macrophages will phagocytize them and tissue repair begins. The greater capillary permeability and vasodilation allows increased blood flow to the area and enables fluid to leak out of the capillaries. The process of local inflammation results in redness, warmth, swelling, and usually pain. The pain serves as a reminder against overuse, allowing time for rest and repair. Systemic inflammation is an inflammatory reaction, often in response to a bacterial infection. Fever is a common symptom and likely occurs in response to chemical mediators that macrophages release in response to the infectious agent. These chemical mediators act on the brain and lead to stimulation of the sympathetic nervous system, which causes vasoconstriction, heat conservation, and fever. The macrophages also release factors that stimulate the release of leukocytes from the bone marrow, leading to an elevated white blood cell count.

Platelets

Platelets, or **thrombocytes,** are small fragments of large cells called *megakaryocytes*. Like the other blood cells described so far, megakaryocytes come from an undifferentiated stem cell in the bone marrow. The hormone *thrombopoietin* stimulates these stem cells to differentiate through several stages into megakaryocytes, which then mature and break up into platelets, small fragments without nuclei. The normal number of platelets ranges from 150,000 to 450,000 per microliter of blood. As they function to form a plug at an initial bleeding site and also secrete factors important in clot formation, too few platelets, a condition called *thrombocytopenia*, can lead to bleeding problems and blood loss. Too many platelets, *thrombocytosis*, may cause abnormal clotting, plugs in vessels, and emboli that may travel to the extremities, heart, lungs, or brain. Platelets survive from seven to ten days and are removed from circulation by the spleen.

Platelets are activated when they contact injured tissue. This contact stimulates an enzyme within the platelet, causing the surface to become "sticky," which in turn leads the platelets to aggregate and form a plug. Platelets also adhere to the damaged tissue to keep the plug in place. As the platelets aggregate, they release chemical messengers that also activate the blood clotting system.

HEMOSTASIS

Hemostasis—from *hemo* (blood) and *stasis* (standing still)—is the term used to describe the combined three mechanisms that work to prevent or control blood loss. These mechanisms include:

- Vascular spasms
- Platelet plugs
- Stable fibrin blood clots (coagulation)

FIGURE 3-16 Clot formation.

Broken Blood Vessel Wall

Blood vessel wall

Red blood cell

Platelet

Clot Formation

Fibrin

Activated platelet

When a blood vessel tears, the smooth muscle fibers (*tunica media*) in the vessel walls contract. This causes vasoconstriction and reduces the size of the tear. Less blood flows through the constricted area, effectively limiting blood loss, and the smaller tear makes it easier for a platelet plug to develop and stop blood loss. At any tear in a blood vessel, platelets aggregate and adhere to collagen, a connective tissue that supports the blood vessels. This forms a platelet plug, which acts much like bubble gum stuck into a hole. The plug is unstable, however, and would permit the vessel to bleed again if not for the formation of a stable fibrin clot. This process, blood coagulation, is initiated in part by the platelet plug (Figure 3-16).

Due to the smoothness of the *tunica intima,* the blood vessels' innermost lining, blood normally flows through the vessels without frictional damage to cells or platelets. Damage to cells or to the vessel lining, however, starts the coagulation cascade. This cascade, or sequence of events, can be activated either by damage to vessels (extrinsic pathway) or by trauma to blood from turbulence (intrinsic pathway). Either results in the cascade's progression to a clot. Most clotting proteins are produced in the liver and circulate in an inactive state. The best known of these are *prothrombin* and *fibrinogen*. The damaged cells send out a chemical message that activates a specific clotting factor. This activates each protein in turn, until a stable fibrin clot forms. To completely stop the bleeding, the coagulation cascade relies on the platelet plug and the clotting factors to interact. Once the bleeding stops, the inflammatory and healing processes can begin. The coagulation cascade can be summarized thus (Figure 3-17):

FIGURE 3-17 The coagulation cascade.

Extrinsic Pathway

Tissue damage

↓

Platelet aggregation

↓

Chemicals that activate

Intrinsic Pathway

Platelet damage

↓

Platelet aggregation

↓

Chemicals that activate

Common Pathway

Prothrombin activator

↓ Ca^{++}

Activates prothrombin, converting it to thrombin

↓

Thrombin

↓ Ca^{++}

Activates fibrinogen, converting it to fibrin clot (traps more platelets)

↓

Fibrinolysis

Produces plasminogen activator

↓

plasmin ⟶ dismantles the clot

1. a. *Intrinsic pathway.* Platelets release substances that lead to the formation of prothrombin activator

   or

   b. *Extrinsic pathway.* Tissue damage causes platelet aggregation and the formation of prothrombin activator.

2. *Common pathway.* The prothrombin activator, in the presence of calcium, converts prothrombin to thrombin.

3. *Thrombin.* In the presence of calcium, thrombin converts fibrinogen to stable fibrin, which then traps blood cells and more platelets to form a clot.

The development of a clot does not end the coagulation cascade. What the body can do it usually can undo, given sufficient time. Once a fibrin clot is formed, it releases a chemical called *plasminogen*. Plasminogen is converted to *plasmin* and is then capable of dismantling, or lysing, a clot through the process of **fibrinolysis**. A clot's dismantling generally takes from hours to days. By that time, scarring has begun.

Thrombosis (clot formation), when it occurs in coronary arteries or cerebral vasculature, may lead to heart attack and stroke. To stimulate or speed fibrinolysis and thus breakdown clots, medical researchers have developed several thrombolytic agents. These agents may help reestablish blood flow to these vital organs, limiting or preventing tissue death, and thus helping to prevent the patient's disability or death. Thrombolytics are effective only against blockages whose components include a fibrin clot.

Patients who lack certain clotting factors can have bleeding disorders that may complicate their assessment and treatment. Other patients take medications that

✶ **fibrinolysis** the process through which plasmin dismantles a blood clot.

✶ **thrombosis** clot formation, which is extremely dangerous when it occurs in coronary arteries or cerebral vasculature.

decrease the effectiveness of platelets or the coagulation cascade. Recall that an enzyme on a platelet membrane makes the membrane sticky. Certain medications such as aspirin, dipyridamole (Persantine), and ticlopidine (Ticlid) irreversibly alter the enzyme, thus decreasing the platelets' ability to aggregate and initiate the coagulation cascade. Other medications such as heparin and warfarin (Coumadin) cause changes within the clotting cascade that prevent clot formation. Heparin, in conjunction with antithrombin III (a naturally occurring thrombin inactivator), rapidly inactivates thrombin, which then prevents formation of the fibrin clot. Warfarin (Coumadin) blocks vitamin K activity necessary to generate the activated forms of clotting factors II, VII, IX, and X, effectively interrupting the clotting cascade.

Vitamin K (AquaMEPHYTON) enhances clotting. Certain byproducts of tobacco smoking (especially in females on birth control pills) also enhance clotting. Relative or complete immobility, trauma, polycythemia (high red blood cell count), and cancer may also lead to increased clotting as blood becomes relatively stagnant. This allows platelet activation to begin, which leads to clotting. To counteract the effects of decreased activity, many patients take aspirin or other antiplatelet inhibitors and wear compressive stockings to facilitate venous drainage from the lower extremities.

THE MUSCULOSKELETAL SYSTEM

The musculoskeletal system is a complex arrangement of levers and fulcrums, powered by biochemical motors, that provides motion and support for the body. It consists of two distinct subsystems, the skeleton and the muscles. The skeleton is the human body's superstructure, while the muscles supply the power of motion to this superstructure, the organs, and the other body components. These subsystems also produce body heat, store essential salts and energy sources, and create the majority of blood cells for transporting oxygen and combating disease.

The musculoskeletal system is covered by the skin and subcutaneous tissue. These elements protect the skeleton and muscles, as well as other body systems, from trauma, fluid loss, infection, and fluctuations in body temperature. The skin also provides some cushioning for the skeletal components, as on the soles of the feet during walking.

SKELETAL TISSUE AND STRUCTURE

As the body's living framework, the skeleton has a structure and design that permits it to perform a variety of functions and to repair itself as needed within limits. The skeleton is a complex, living system of cells, salt deposits, protein fibers, and other specialized elements. Besides giving the body its structural form, the skeleton serves four other important purposes:

- It protects the vital organs.
- It allows for efficient movement despite the forces of gravity.
- It stores many salts and other materials needed for metabolism.
- It produces the red blood cells used to transport oxygen.

Although the skeleton is not often thought of as alive, it is exactly that. Its cells live within a matrix of protein fibers and salt deposits. These living cells constantly change the structure and dynamics of the human frame. In fact, 20 percent of the total bone mass (salts, protein fiber, and bone cells) is replaced each year by the remodeling process.

Some 20 percent of the total bone mass is replaced each year by the remodeling process.

Bone Structure

The structure of a typical bone consists of numerous aligned cylinders of bone. Minute blood vessels travel lengthwise along the bone through small tubes, called **haversian canals**. These blood vessels are surrounded by layers of salts deposited in collagen fibers. Bone cells called **osteocytes** are trapped within the matrix and maintain the collagen and the calcium, phosphate, carbonate, and other salt crystals. Other bone cells, osteoblasts and osteoclasts, deposit or dissolve these salt deposits as necessary. **Osteoblasts** lay down new bone in areas of stress during growth and during the bone repair cycle. **Osteoclasts** dissolve bone structures that are not carrying the pressures of articulation and support or when the body requires more salts for electrolyte balance. These three types of bone cells maintain a dynamic and efficient structure for supporting and moving the body.

A continuous blood supply brings oxygen and nutrients to the bones and removes carbon dioxide and waste products from them. The blood vessels enter and exit the bone shaft through **perforating canals** and distribute blood to both the bone tissue and the structures located within the medullary canal of the shaft and bone ends. As with any other body tissue, bone tissue becomes ischemic and will eventually die if the blood supply is reduced or cut off. The bone does not show evidence of such degeneration for quite some time, and certainly not during prehospital emergency care. However, the long-term effects of **devascularization** may be devastating.

The long bones, such as those of the forearm (humerus) and thigh (femur), best demonstrate the organization of bone tissue into structural body elements (Figure 3-18). The major areas and tissues of the long bones include the diaphysis, the epiphysis, the metaphysis, the medullary canal, the periosteum, and the articular cartilage.

The Diaphysis The **diaphysis** is the central portion or shaft of the long bone. It consists of a very dense and relatively thin layer of compact bone. Because of its tubular structure, the diaphysis efficiently supports weight yet is relatively light. While the design of the bone shaft enables it to carry weight well, lateral forces may cause the shaft to break rather easily.

The Epiphysis Toward the ends of the long bone, its structure changes. The bone's diameter increases dramatically, and the underlying thin, hard, compact bone of the shaft changes to a network of skeletal fibers and strands. This network, called the **epiphysis**, spreads the stresses and pressures of weight bearing over a larger surface. The tissue of the epiphysis in cross-section resembles a rigid bony sponge and is called spongy or **cancellous** bone. Covering this network of fibers is a very thin layer of compact bone supporting the surface that meets and moves against another bone, the **articular surface**.

The Metaphysis The **metaphysis** is an intermediate region between the epiphysis and diaphysis. It is where the diaphysis's hollow tube of compact bone makes the transition to the bone-fiber honeycomb of the epiphysis's cancellous bone. In this region is the **epiphyseal plate**, also called the *growth plate*. During childhood, cartilage is generated here and the plate widens. Osteoblasts from the end of the diaphysis deposit salts within the cartilage's collagen matrix to create new bone tissue. This results in the lengthening of the infant's and then the child's bone. During the growth period, the epiphyseal plate is also weaker than the rest of the bone and associated joints and is thus a frequent site of fractures in pediatric patients.

* **haversian canals** small perforations of the long bones through which the blood vessels and nerves travel into the bone itself.

* **osteocyte** bone-forming cell found in the bone matrix that helps maintain the bone.

* **osteoblast** cell that helps in the creation of new bone during growth and bone repair.

* **osteoclast** bone cell that absorbs and removes excess bone.

* **perforating canals** structures through which blood vessels enter and exit the bone shaft.

* **devascularization** loss of blood vessels from a body part.

* **diaphysis** hollow shaft found in long bones.

* **epiphysis** end of a long bone, including the epiphyseal, or growth plate and supporting structures underlying the joint.

* **cancellous** having a lattice-work structure, as in the spongy tissue of a bone.

* **articular surface** surface of a bone that moves against another bone.

* **metaphysis** growth zone of a bone, active during the development stages of youth. It is located between the epiphysis and the diaphysis.

* **epiphyseal plate** area of the metaphysis where cartilage is generated during bone growth in childhood; *growth plate*.

FIGURE 3-18 The internal anatomy of a long bone.

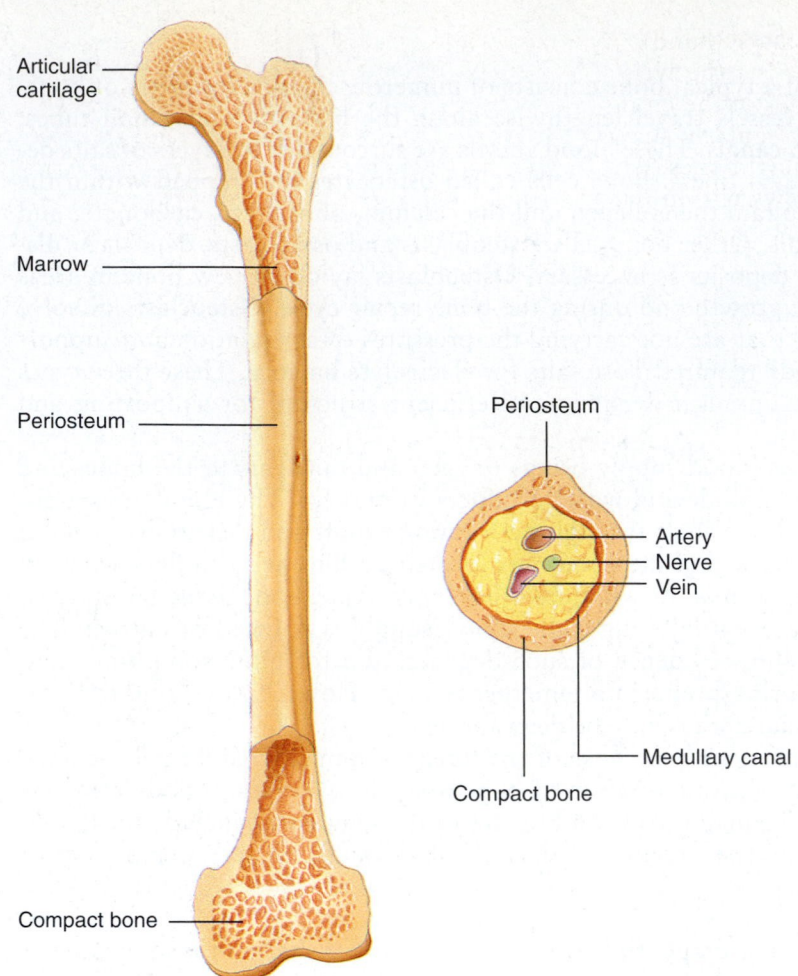

Articular cartilage

Marrow

Periosteum

Periosteum

Artery
Nerve
Vein

Medullary canal

Compact bone

Compact bone

✳ **medullary canal** cavity within a bone that contains the marrow.

✳ **yellow bone marrow** tissue that stores fat in semi-liquid form within the internal cavities of a bone.

✳ **red bone marrow** tissue within the internal cavity of a bone responsible for manufacture of erythrocytes and other blood cells.

✳ **periosteum** the tough exterior covering of a bone.

✳ **cartilage** connective tissue providing the articular surfaces of the skeletal system.

Bones are classified according to their general shape.

The Medullary Canal The chamber formed within the hollow diaphysis and the cancellous bone of the epiphysis is called the **medullary canal.** The central medullary canal is filled with **yellow bone marrow** that stores fat in a semi-liquid form. The fat is a readily available energy source the body can use quickly and easily. **Red bone marrow** fills the cancellous bone chambers of the larger long bones, the pelvis, and the sternum. It is responsible for the manufacture of erythrocytes and other blood cells.

The Periosteum A tough fibrous membrane called the **periosteum** covers the exterior of the diaphysis. With extensive vasculature and innervation, it transmits sensations of pain when the bone fractures and then initiates the bone repair cycle. Blood vessels and nerves penetrate both the periosteum and compact bone by traveling through the small perforating canals. Tendons intermingle with the collagen fibers of the periosteum and with the collagen fibers of the bony matrix to form strong attachments.

Cartilage A layer of connective tissue called **cartilage** is a continuous collagen extension of the underlying bone and covers a portion of the epiphyseal surface. It is a smooth, strong, and flexible material that functions as the actual surface of articulation between bones. Cartilage is very slippery and somewhat compressible. It permits relatively friction-free joint movement and absorbs some of the shock associated with activity, such as walking.

Bones are classified according to their general shape. Those as described above are considered long bones and include the humerus, radius, ulna, tibia, fibula, metacarpals (hand), metatarsals (foot), and phalanges (fingers and toes). The bones of the wrists and ankles, the carpals and tarsals, are short bones. The bones of the cranium, sternum, ribs, shoulder, and pelvis are classified as flat. Irregularly shaped bones include the bones of the vertebral column and the facial bones. Another special type of bone is the **sesamoid bone,** a bone that grows within tendinous tissue; one example is the kneecap, also called the patella.

Joint Structure

Bones move at, and are held together by, a relatively sophisticated structure called a **joint.**

Types of Joints There are three basic types of joints, which are classified by the amount of movement they permit.

Synarthroses are immovable joints, such as the sutures of the skull or the juncture between jaw and the teeth (which is called a gomphosis). **Amphiarthroses** are joints that allow some very limited movement. Examples include the joints between the vertebrae and between the sacrum and the ilium of the pelvis. **Diarthroses,** or **synovial joints,** permit relatively free movement. Such joints include the elbow, knee, shoulder, and hip.

Diarthroses are divided into three categories of joints based on the movements they allow (Figure 3-19). These include:

- *Monaxial joints*
  Hinge joints permit bending in a single plane. Examples include the knees, elbows, and fingers.
  Pivot joints are characterized by the articulation between the atlas (the first cervical vertebrae) and the axis of the spine. They allow the head to rotate through a wide range of motion.

- *Biaxial joints*
  Condyloid, or gliding, joints provide movement in two directions. They are located at the joints of carpal bones in the wrist and between the clavicle and sternum.
  Ellipsoidal joints provide a sliding motion in two planes, as between the wrist and the metacarpals.
  Saddle joints allow for movement in two planes at right angles to each other. Examples are the joints at the bases of the thumbs.

- *Triaxial joints*
  Ball-and-socket joints permit full motion in a cone of about 180 degrees and allow a limb to rotate. Examples include the hip and shoulder.

These joints permit various types of motion. **Flexion/extension** is the bending motion that reduces/increases the angle between articulating elements. **Adduction/abduction** is the movement of a body part toward/away from the midline. **Rotation** refers to a turning along the axis of a bone or joint. **Circumduction** refers to movement through an arc of a circle.

Ligaments Ligaments are bands of connective tissue that hold bones together at joints. They stretch and permit motion at the joint while holding the bone ends firmly in position. The ends of the ligaments attach to the joint ends of each of the associated bones. Ligaments surround the articular region and cross it at many oblique angles. This arrangement ensures that the joint is held together firmly but flexibly enough to permit movement through a designed range of motion.

✳ **sesamoid bone** bone that forms in a tendon.

✳ **joint** area where adjacent bones articulate.

Content Review

TYPES OF JOINTS
- Synarthroses—immovable
- Amphiarthroses—very limited movement
- Diarthroses (synovial joints)—relatively free movement:
  –Monaxial
  –Biaxial
  –Triaxial

✳ **synarthorsis** joint that does not permit movement

✳ **amphiarthrosis** joint that permits a limited amount of independent motion.

✳ **diarthrosis** a synovial joint.

✳ **synovial joint** joint that permits the greatest degree of independent motion.

✳ **flexion** bending motion that reduces the angle between articulating elements.

✳ **extension** bending motion that increases the angle between articulating elements.

✳ **adduction** movement of a body part toward the midline.

✳ **abduction** movement of a body part away from the midline.

✳ **rotation** a turning along the axis of a bone or joint.

✳ **circumduction** movement at a synovial joint where the distal end of a bone describes a circle but the shaft does not rotate; movement through an arc of a circle.

✳ **ligaments** connective tissue that connects bone to bone and holds joints together.

Bone

Ligaments

Synovial membrane

Joint cavity

Articular cartilage

Bone

| Ball and socket joint | Condyloid joint | Gliding joint | Hinge joint | Pivot joint | Saddle joint |

FIGURE 3-19   Types of joints.

Joint Capsule The ligaments surrounding a joint form what is known as the **joint capsule** or *synovial capsule* (Figure 3-20). This chamber holds a small amount of fluid to lubricate the articular surfaces. This oily, viscous substance, known as **synovial fluid,** assists joint motion by reducing friction. Its lubrication reduces friction to about one fifth that of two pieces of ice sliding together. Small sacs filled with synovial fluid, known as **bursae,** are also located between tendons and ligaments or cartilage in the elbows, knees, and other joints to reduce friction and absorb shock. Synovial fluid flows into and out of the articular cartilage as the joint undergoes pressure and movement. The cartilage acts like a sponge, pushing out fluid as it is compressed and drawing in fluid when it is relaxed. This movement of synovial fluid circulates oxygen, nutrients, and waste products to and from the joint cartilage.

SKELETAL ORGANIZATION

The human skeleton is made up of approximately 206 bones (Figure 3-21). These bones form two major divisions, the axial and the appendicular skeletons.

The **axial skeleton** consists of the bones of the head, thorax, and spine. These bones form the axis of the body, protect the elements of the central nervous system, and make up the thoracic cage, which is the dynamic housing for respiration. The components of the axial skeleton will be discussed under the headings, "The Head, Face, and Neck" and "The Spine and Thorax."

✱ **joint capsule** the ligaments surround a joint; *synovial capsule.*

✱ **synovial fluid** substance that lubricates synovial joints.

✱ **bursae** sacs containing synovial fluid that cushion adjacent structures; singular *bursa.*

✱ **axial skeleton** bones of the head, thorax, and spine.

FIGURE 3-20 Structure of a joint.

Bone

Tendon

Synovial membrane

Bursa

Joint cavity

Articular cartilage

Bone

Joint capsule

FIGURE 3-21 The human skeleton.

Skull — Cranium

Face

Hyoid

Sternum

Ribs

Vertebra column

Sacrum

Clavicle

Scapula

Humerus

Radius

Ulna

Pelvis

Carpals

Metacarpals

Phalanges

Femur

Patella

Tibia

Fibula

Tarsals

Metatarsals

Phalanges

FIGURE 3-22 Bones and joints of the hand and wrist.

Distal interphalangeal joint (DIP)

Proximal interphalangeal joint (PIP)

Metacarpophalangeal joint (MCP)

Wrist (radiocarpal) joint

Distal phalanx

Middle phalanx

Proximal phalanx

Metacarpal

Carpals

Radius

✱ **appendicular skeleton** bones of the extremities, shoulder girdle, and pelvis (excepting the sacrum).

The **appendicular skeleton** consists of the bones of the upper and lower extremities, including both the shoulder girdle and the pelvis, and excepting the sacrum. These bones provide the structure for the extremities and permit the major articulations of the body. Extremity long bones are similar in design and structure. Both upper and lower extremities are affixed to the axial skeleton and articulate with joints supported by several bones. Each of these extremities has a single long bone proximally and paired bones distally. The terminal member, the hand or foot, is made up of numerous bones with differing purposes, yet parallel designs.

The Extremities

The extremities are the arms and legs, including the wrists and hands, elbows, shoulders, ankles and feet, knees, hips, and pelvis.

Wrists and Hands The radius and ulna articulate with the carpal bones at the wrist, or radiocarpal joint (Figure 3-22). The carpals articulate with the metacarpals. The metacarpals articulate with the proximal phalanges at the metacarpophalangeal (MCP) joint. The proximal phalanges articulate with the middle phalanges at the proximal interphalangeal (PIP) joint. The middle phalanges articulate with the distal phalanges at the distal interphalangeal (DIP) joint. Movement at the wrist includes flexion, extension, radial deviation, and ulnar deviation. Movement at the MCP, PIP, and DIP joints includes flexion and extension. The MCP joints also allow abduction (spreading the fingers out) and adduction (bringing them back together). The major flexor muscles are the flexor carpi radialis and flexor

Triceps brachii

Brachioradialis

Extensor
carpi
radialis

Extensor
carpi
ulnaris

Flexor
carpi
ulnaris

Extensor
digitorum

Adductor
pollicis

Radius

Humerus

Coracobrachialis

Biceps brachii

Brachialis

Pronator teres

Brachioradialis

Flexor carpi
radialis

Palmaris
longus

Flexor carpi
ulnaris

Flexor
digitorum
superficialis

Pronator
quadratus

FIGURE 3-23   Muscles of the arm.

carpi ulnaris (Figure 3-23). The major extensor muscles are the extensor carpi radialis longus, extensor carpi radialis brevis, and extensor carpi ulnaris.

Elbows The lateral and medial epicondyles (large rounded edges) of the distal humerus, the olecranon process of the proximal ulna, and the proximal radius comprise the elbow joint (Figure 3-24). Between the olecranon process and skin lies a bursa. The ulnar nerve (funny bone) extends through the groove between the olecranon process and the medial epicondyle. The elbow is a hinge joint, allowing flexion and extension. The major flexor muscles are the biceps (Figure 3-25). The

FIGURE 3-24   The elbow.

FIGURE 3-25   Elbow flexors.

FIGURE 3-26   Elbow
extensors.

Triceps
brachii

Posterior

major extensor muscles are the triceps (Figure 3-26). Just below the elbow, the relationship of the radius and ulna to the pronator and supinator muscles allows the forearm to supinate (turn palm up) and pronate (turn palm down) (Figure 3-27).

Shoulders   The shoulder girdle consists of articulations between the clavicle and the scapula and between the scapula and the head of the humerus (Figure 3-28). The sternoclavicular joint, which joins the clavicle and the manubrium, is the only bony link between the upper extremity and the axial skeleton. Movement at this joint is largely passive and occurs as a result of active movements of the scapula. The distal clavicle articulates with the acromion, or acromion process, of the scapula at the acromioclavicular (AC) joint. The clavicle acts as a strut, keeping the upper limb away from the thorax and permitting a greater range of motion. The AC joint also helps provide stability to the upper limb, reducing the need for muscle energy to keep the shoulder in its proper alignment.

The glenohumeral joint is a ball-and-socket joint that allows flexion, extension, internal and external rotation, abduction, and adduction. It has the greatest range of motion of any joint in the body and as a result is the most frequent site for dislocation. The head of the humerus (ball) fits into the glenoid

Pronator
teres

Supinator

Pronator
teres

Radius

Ulna

Radius

Pronator
quadratus

FIGURE 3-27   Pronator-supinator muscles.

cavity (socket) of the scapula. The proximal humerus has two rounded protrusions called the greater and lesser tubercles. The biceps tendon runs through the bicipital groove between the greater and lesser tubercles and is easily palpable on the lateral surface of the shoulder. The glenohumeral joint is encapsulated and reinforced by the tendons and four muscles that make up the rotator cuff and by the large deltoid muscle (Figures 3-29 and 3-30). The muscles of the rotator cuff include the supraspinatus, the infraspinatus, the teres minor, and the subscapularis muscles.

Jugular notch

Manubrium

Angle

Sternum

Body

Xiphoid
process

Clavicle: Articulates with
the manubrium, the superior
part of the sternum, forming
the sternoclavicular joint.

Acromion process

Coracoid process

Head of humerus

Greater tubercle

Lesser tubercle

Bicipital groove

Glenohumeral joint:
Margin of glenoid cavity.

Scapula

Shaft of humerus

Lateral epicondyle

Capitulum

Trochlea

Medial epicondyle

FIGURE 3-28   The shoulder girdle.

Coracoacromial ligament

Acromioclavicular ligament

Acromion

Subacromial bursa

Tendon of
infraspinatus muscle

Glenohumeral ligaments

Glenoid fossa

Glenoid labrum

Articular capsule

Teres minor muscle

Clavicle

Coracoclavicular
ligament

Coracoid process

Subcoracoid bursa

Coracohumeral
ligament (cut)

Tendon of *biceps
brachii muscle*

Subscapular bursa

Subscapularis muscle

FIGURE 3-29   Shoulder girdle
ligaments.

141

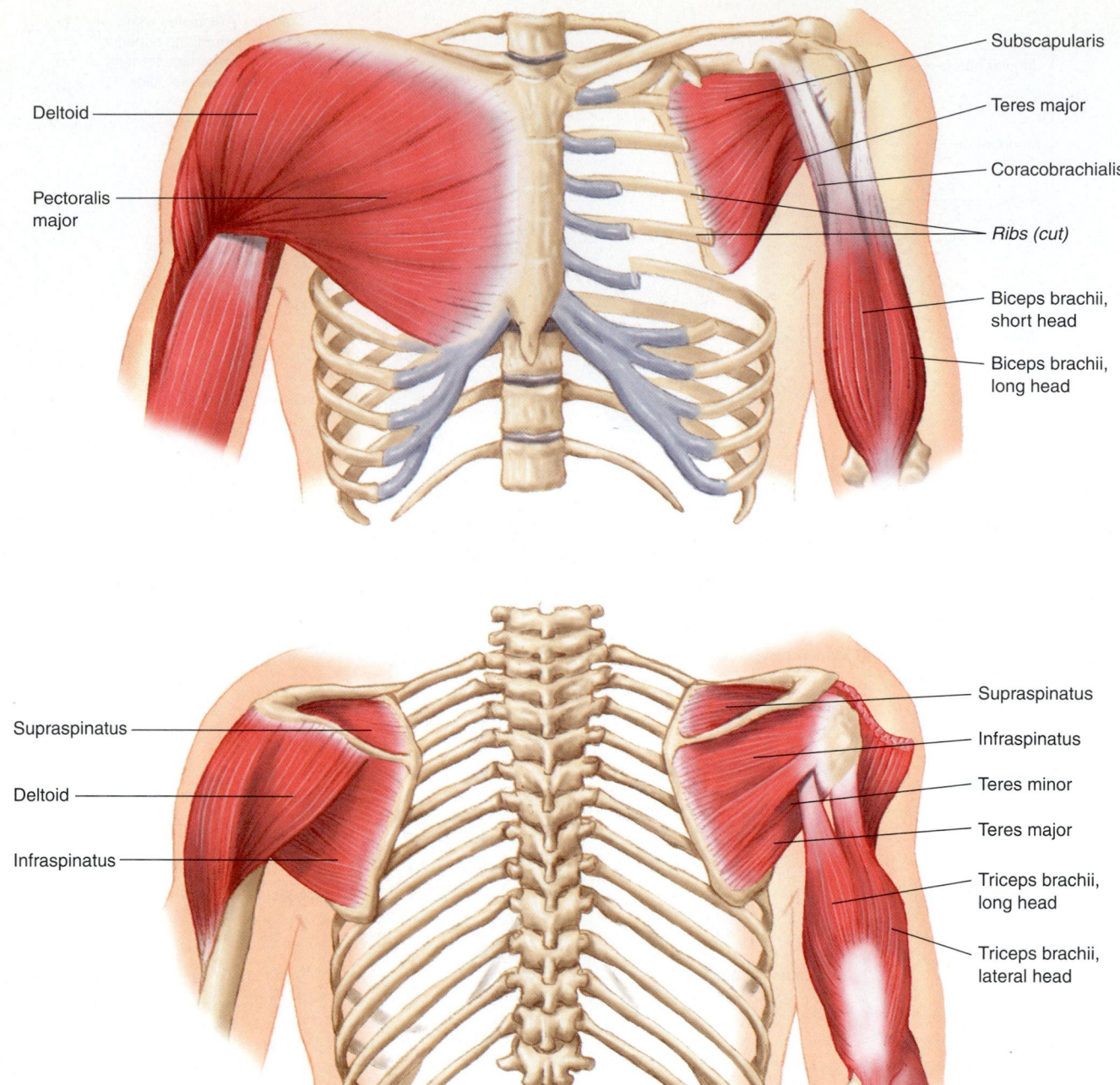

Deltoid

Pectoralis
major

Subscapularis

Teres major

Coracobrachialis

Ribs (cut)

Biceps brachii,
short head

Biceps brachii,
long head

Supraspinatus

Deltoid

Infraspinatus

Supraspinatus

Infraspinatus

Teres minor

Teres major

Triceps brachii,
long head

Triceps brachii,
lateral head

FIGURE 3-30 Shoulder muscles.

Ankles and Feet The foot comprises seven tarsal bones, five metatarsal bones, and fourteen phalanges (Figure 3-31). The talus, the calcaneus (heel), and the other tarsals articulate in a system of joints that allows inversion (lifting the inside of the foot) and eversion (lifting the outside of the foot). The most distal tarsals articulate with the metatarsals, which articulate with the proximal phalanges at the metatarsophalangeal joints.

FIGURE 3-31   Bones of the foot.

14 Phalanges

5 Metatarsal bones

First cuneiform

Second cuneiform

Third cuneiform

Navicular

Cuboid

7 Tarsal bones

Talus

Calcaneus

At the ankle joint, the distal tibia (medial malleolus) and the distal fibula (lateral malleolus) articulate with the talus (Figure 3-32). Ligaments stretching from each malleolus to the foot itself hold the ankle joint together. The strong Achilles tendon, which inserts on the calcaneus (heel), also helps maintain the ankle's integrity. Movement in the ankle is limited to dorsiflexion (raising the foot) and plantar flexion (lowering the foot). The major dorsiflexor muscle is the tibialis anterior (Figure 3-33). The major plantar flexor is the gastrocnemius (calf muscle) (Figure 3-34).

Knees The knee joint involves the distal femur, the proximal tibia, and the patella (Figure 3-35). The distal femur and the proximal tibia meet at this joint and are cushioned by the lateral meniscus and the medial meniscus, which form a cartilaginous surface for pain-free movement. The joint capsule contains synovial fluid. Several ligaments surround the knee joint and help maintain its integrity. The medial and lateral collateral ligaments provide side-to-side stability and are easily palpable. The anterior and posterior cruciate ligaments, which give the knee front-to-back stability, lie deep within the joint capsule and are not palpable.

FIGURE 3-32   The foot and ankle.

FIGURE 3-33   The dorsiflexors.

FIGURE 3-34   The plantar flexors.

The knee is a modified hinge joint, allowing flexion and extension, with some rotation during flexion. The major flexors are a group of three muscles (biceps femoris, semimembranosus, and semitendinosus) known as the hamstrings (Figure 3-36). The major extensors are a group of four muscles (vastus lateralis, vastus intermedius, vastus medialis, and rectus femoris) known as the quadriceps (Figure 3-37). The femur can rotate on the tibia slightly. The patella lies deep in the middle of the quadriceps tendon, which inserts on the tibial tuberosity below the knee. Concave areas at each side of the patella and below it contain synovial fluid.

Lateral condyle

Anterior cruciate ligament

Fibular (lateral) collateral ligament

Lateral meniscus

Cut tendon

Tibia

Tibial (medial) collateral ligament

Fibula

Patellar surface

Posterior cruciate ligament

Medial condyle

Synovial membrane

Medial meniscus

Joint capsule

Gastrocnemius muscle

Soleus muscle

Tibialis posterior muscle

Knee extensor muscles

Femur

Extensor tendon

Suprapatellar bursa

Patella

Prepatellar bursa

Fat pad

Lateral meniscus

Patellar ligament

Tibia

FIGURE 3-35   The knee.

Sartorius

Gracilis

Biceps femoris, short head

Hamstrings {
Semimembranosus
Semitendinosus
Biceps femoris, long head
}

Sartorius

FIGURE 3-36   The knee flexors.

Gluteus medius

Iliacus

Psoas major

} Iliopsoas

Tensor fasciae latae

Pectineous

Adductor longus

Gracilis

Vastus intermedius

Sartorius

Rectus femoris (cut)

Vastus lateralis

Vastus medialis

Patella

Patellar ligament

FIGURE 3-37   The knee extensors. (The vastus intermedius is behind the rectus femoris.)

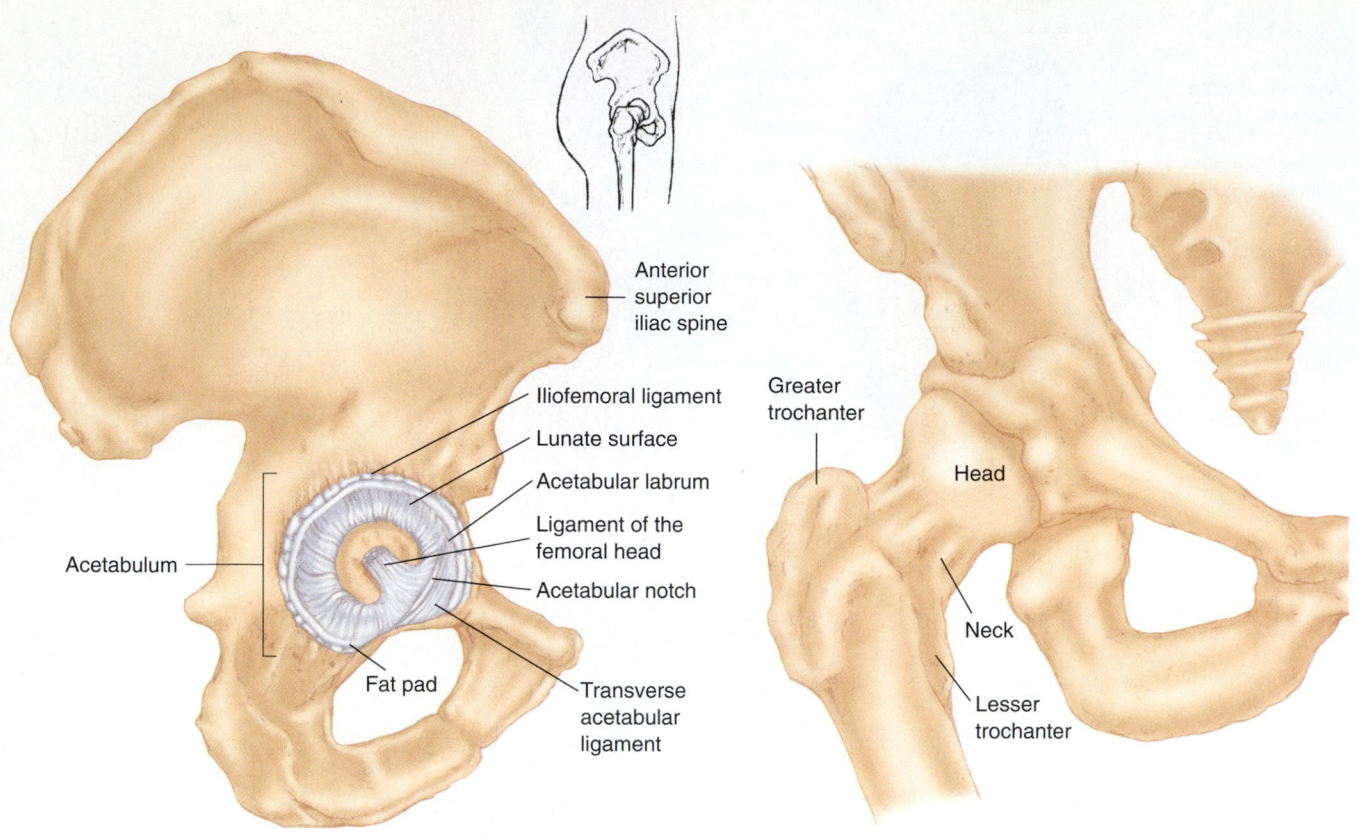

Labels on figure:

Anterior superior iliac spine

Iliofemoral ligament

Lunate surface

Acetabular labrum

Ligament of the femoral head

Acetabular notch

Acetabulum

Fat pad

Transverse acetabular ligament

Greater trochanter

Head

Neck

Lesser trochanter

FIGURE 3-38   The hip joint.

Hips and Pelvis The hip is the juncture of the lower extremities with the pelvis. The pelvis is a strong skeletal structure consisting of two symmetrical structures called the inominates. The sacrum of the spine is posterior to and joined to the inominates. Each inominate is constructed from one large flat bone, the ilium, the two irregular bones, the ischium and the pubis, all fused together.

The hip joint involves the head of the proximal femur (ball) and the acetabulum (socket) of the ischium (Figure 3-38). Although the hip is a ball-and-socket joint like the shoulder, the two are very different. While the shoulder has a wide range of motion, the hip joint is restricted by many large ligaments, a bony ridge in the pelvis, and capsular fibers. Hip flexion, the most important movement, occurs via the iliopsoas muscle group (Figure 3-39). Other movements, though much more limited in range than the shoulder, include extension, abduction, adduction, and internal and external rotation.

A number of muscle groups control these movements. One of these is the gluteus, a series of adductor muscles and lateral rotators (Figure 3-40). Three bursa in the hip play an important role in pain-free movement. The iliopectineal bursa sits just anterior to the hip joint. The trochanteric bursa lies just to the side and behind the greater trochanter. The ischiogluteal bursa resides under the ischial tuberosity.

BONE AGING

The bones, like all other body tissues, evolve during fetal development and after birth. Bone initially forms in the embryo as loose cartilaginous tissue. Before birth, the skeletal structure is predominantly cartilage, with very little ossified

FIGURE 3-39 The hip flexors.

Iliopsoas

Iliacus Psoas major

Sartorius

Pectineus

Adductor brevis

Adductor longus

Adductor magnus

Gracilis

Gluteus maximus

Gluteus minimus

Gluteus medius

FIGURE 3-40 The gluteus muscles.

bone evident. This is one reason that infants are highly flexible yet unable to support themselves. Ossified bone begins to appear along the long bone shafts and then extends to the epiphyseal plates. It also develops within the epiphyses and grows outward to form the articular surfaces. Over time, the bone formation becomes complete to the epiphyseal plate, and the epiphysis is fully formed. The epiphyseal plate continues to generate cartilage, with the shaft and epiphyses growing from it. As the young adult reaches full height and the end of skeletal growth, the epiphyseal plates narrow, become bony, and cease to produce cartilage.

Associated with bone development and aging is the transition from flexible, cartilaginous bone to firm, strong, and fully ossified bone. Bones of the young child remain flexible and do not reach maximum strength until early adulthood. While each bone matures at a different time, almost all maturation is complete by 18 to 20 years of age.

Around the age of 40, the body begins to lose its ability to maintain the bone structure. It is unable to rebuild the collagen matrix and the deposition of salt crystals is reduced from what it was in earlier years. The effects of these changes appear very slowly. They include a very gradual diminution of bone strength, an increase in bone brittleness, a progressive loss of body height, and some curvature of the spine. The incidence of bone fractures also increases, especially at the high stress points of the lumbar spine and the femur's surgical neck.

Age-related changes in the skeletal system also affect other body systems. For example, the cartilage of the costal-condral joints and the costal bones (the ribs) becomes less flexible, which leads to shallower, more energy-consuming respirations. Also, the intravertebral disks lose water content and become less flexible, more prone to herniation, and narrower, thus shortening the trunk.

MUSCULAR TISSUE AND STRUCTURE

More than 600 muscle groups make up the muscular system (Figure 3-41). As you might expect, a large number of EMS calls involve injuries to this extensive system. Injuries to it may result from excessive forces indirectly expressed to the muscles and their attachments or from direct trauma, either blunt or penetrating.

There are three types of muscle tissue within the body—cardiac, smooth, and skeletal (Figure 3-42). Of these, the most specialized is the cardiac muscle comprising the myocardium. It contracts rhythmically on its own (automaticity), emitting an electrical impulse in the process (excitability), and passing that impulse along to the other cells of the myocardium (conductivity). In this way, the heart provides its lifelong rhythmic contraction and pumping. Cardiac muscle can also be classified according to its structure, which combines characteristics of both skeletal and smooth muscle and is thus called smooth-striated.

The second muscle type is smooth, or involuntary, muscle, which is not under conscious control but functions at the direction of the autonomic nervous system. These muscles are found in the arterial and venous blood vessels, the bronchioles, the bowel, and many other organs. Smooth muscle contracts to reduce (or relaxes to expand) the lumen (diameter) of the vasculature, airways, or digestive tract. Smooth muscles have the ability to contract over a wide lateral distance, enabling them to accommodate great changes in length, such as those that occur during filling and evacuation of the bladder and contraction and dilation of the arterioles.

The final type of muscle tissue is skeletal (also called striated or voluntary). We have conscious control over these muscles, which are associated with the mobility of the extremities and the body in general. Skeletal muscles are also controlled by the nerves of the somatic nervous system. The skeletal muscles are the largest component of the muscular system, comprising between 40 and 50 percent of the body's total weight. They are the type of muscle most commonly traumatized.

Bones of the young child remain flexible and do not reach maximum strength until maturation, which is usually completed by 18 to 20 years of age.

After approximately the age of 40, the body begins to lose the ability to maintain bone structure.

Content Review

TYPES OF MUSCLE
- Cardiac muscle
- Smooth muscle
- Skeletal muscle

FIGURE 3-41
The muscular system (posterior view).

sternocleidomastoid

trapezius

teres minor

teres major

deltoid

latissimus dorsi

triceps

olecranon

lumbodorsal fascia

gluteus maximus

iliotibial band

biceps femoris

semitendinosus

semimembranous

gastrocnemius

soleus

Achilles tendon

FIGURE 3-41 CONTINUED
The muscular system (anterior view).

temporalis

orbicularis oculi

obicularis oris

masseter

sternocleidomastoid

trapezius

deltoid

pectoralis major

serratus anterior

biceps brachii

brachioradialis

flexor carpi

extensor carpi

intercostals

external oblique

internal oblique

rectus abdominis

aponeurosis

adductor longus

rectus femoris

sartorius

quadriceps femoris

peroneus longus

tibalis anterior

gastrocnemius

soleus

150

FIGURE 3-42 Three types of muscle.

Skeletal muscle

Cardiac muscle

Smooth muscle

Skeletal muscles lie directly beneath a protective layer of skin and subcutaneous fat. Because of their hunger for oxygen during activity, they have a more than ample supply of blood vessels. Individual muscle cells layer together to form a muscle fiber, many fibers layer together to form a muscle **fasciculus,** and fasciculi layer together to form a muscle body, such as the triceps. A muscle body has a strength of about 50 pounds of lift for each square inch of cross-sectional area.

Skeletal muscles attach to the bones at a minimum of two locations. These attachment points are called the origin and the insertion, depending upon how the bones move with contraction. The point of attachment that remains stationary as the muscle contracts is the **origin,** while the attachment to the moving bone is the **insertion.**

Muscles usually pair, one on each side of a joint. This configuration is essential because muscles can actively contract, not lengthen. One muscle moves the extremity in one direction by contraction, while the opposing (and relaxed) muscle stretches. The opposing muscle can then in turn contract, stretching the first muscle and moving the extremity in the opposite direction. This arrangement, called **opposition,** permits the straightening (extension) and then bending (flexion) of the limbs.

With several muscles attached to a joint with different origins and insertions, the body enjoys a wide variety of motions. In the shoulder, for example, the humerus can travel through several types and ranges of motion. These include

✱ **fasciculus** small bundle of muscle fibers.

✱ **origin** attachment of a muscle to a bone that does not move (or experiences the least movement) when the muscle contracts.

✱ **insertion** attachment of a muscle to a bone that moves when the muscle contracts.

✱ **opposition** pairing of muscles that permits extension and flexion of limbs.

The Musculoskeletal System **151**

FIGURE 3-43 How muscle attaches to bone.

Muscle

Bone

Tendon

Ligament

Bone

moving the extremity away from the body (abduction) and toward the body (adduction), turning the humerus (rotation) through about 60 degrees, and circling the entire extremity (circumduction) through a 180-degree arc.

Tendons are specialized bands of connective tissue that accomplish the attachment of muscle to bone at the insertion and, in some cases, at the origin (Figure 3-43). These very fibrous ribbons, actually parts of the muscles, are extremely strong and do not stretch. They are so strong that in some instances they will break an area of bone loose rather than tear. The Achilles tendon demonstrates the strength of this particular tissue. It can be felt as the band posterior to the malleoli of the ankle. This tendon is the muscle-controlled cord that allows a person to lift the entire body weight when standing on the toes.

The forearm demonstrates the sophistication of the muscle-tendon relationship. As the muscles controlling finger flexion contract, you can feel them tensing in the dorsal forearm. You can also visualize and palpate tendon movement in the distal forearm and wrist as the fingers flex and extend. It is easy to appreciate the damage a deep transverse laceration can cause to the underlying connective tissues and their control of distal skeletal structures. Tendons are often classified by the action they perform when the muscle associated with them contracts—for example, flexor or extensor, abductor or adductor, etc.

The muscle tissue is responsible not only for the body's movement but also for the production of heat energy. A chemical reaction between oxygen and simple sugars produces the energy of motion. Heat, water, and carbon dioxide are by-products of this reaction. More than half the energy created by muscle motion is heat that helps maintain body temperature. The body then excretes water in the urine or sweat, expels carbon dioxide through respiration, and dissipates excess heat through the skin via radiation or convection. The body must constantly meet the requirements of muscle tissues for oxygen and nutrients and eliminate the waste products of those tissues, including heat.

Muscles are found in a condition of slight contraction called **tone.** Even while the body is at rest, the central nervous system sends some limited impulses to the muscle fibers causing a few to contract. These impulses give the muscles firmness and assure that they are ready to contract when the need arises. Muscle tone may be very significant in a well-conditioned athlete or absent (flaccid muscle tone) in someone with peripheral motor nerve disruption.

✱ **tone** state of slight contraction of muscles that gives them firmness and keeps them ready to contract.

THE HEAD, FACE, AND NECK

THE HEAD

The head is made up of three structures that cover the brain: the scalp, the cranium, and the meninges. Each of these structures provides essential protection from the environment and from trauma.

The Scalp

The scalp is a strong and flexible mass of skin, fascia (bands of connective tissue), and muscular tissue that is able to withstand and absorb tremendous kinetic energy. The scalp is also extremely vascular in order to help maintain the brain at the body's core temperature. Scalp hair further insulates the brain from environmental temperatures and, to a lesser degree, from trauma.

The scalp is only loosely attached to the skull and is made up of the overlying skin and a number of thin layers of muscle and connective tissue underneath. Directly beneath the skin and covering the most superior surface of the head is a fibrous connective tissue sheet called the **galea aponeurotica**. Connected anteriorly to it and covering the forehead is a flat sheet of muscle, the frontal muscle. Connected posteriorly and covering the posterior skull surface is the occipitalis muscle. Laterally, the auricularis muscles cover the areas above the ears and between the lateral brow ridge and the occiput. A layer of loose connective tissue beneath these muscles and the galea and just above the periosteum is called the areolar tissue. It contains emissary veins that permit venous blood to flow from the dural sinuses into the venous vessels of the scalp. These emissary veins also exist in the upper reaches of the nasal cavity. These veins become potential routes for infection in scalp wounds or nasal injuries. A helpful way to remember the layers of skin protecting the scalp is the mnemonic SCALP: S—skin; C—connective tissue; A—aponeurotica; L—layer of subaponeurotica (areolar) tissue; P—the periosteum of the skull (the pericranium).

> ✳ **galea aponeurotica** connective tissue sheet covering the superior aspect of the cranium.

The Cranium

The bony structure supporting the head and face is the skull. It can be subdivided into two components, the facial bones that form the skeletal base for the face and the vault for the brain, called the **cranium** (Figure 3-44). The cranium actually consists of several bones fused together at pseudo-joints called **sutures**. These bony plates are constructed of two narrow layers of hard compact bone, separated by a layer of cancellous bone. The plates form a strong, light, rigid, and spherical container for the brain. The cranium is, therefore, quite effective in protecting its contents from the direct effects of trauma. This vault, however, provides very little space for internal swelling or hemorrhage. Any expanding lesion within the cranium results in an increase in **intracranial pressure** (ICP). This reduces cerebral perfusion and can severely damage the delicate brain tissue.

> ✳ **cranium** vault-like portion of the skull encasing the brain.
>
> ✳ **sutures** pseudo-joints that join the various bones of the skull to form the cranium.
>
> ✳ **intracranial pressure (ICP)** pressure exerted on the brain by the blood and cerebrospinal fluid.

The cranial bones form regions that are helpful in describing the cerebral structures beneath. The anterior or frontal bone begins at the brow ridge and covers the upper and anterior surface of the brain. The parietal bones, one on either side, begin just behind the lateral brow ridge and form the skull above the external portions (pinnae) of the ears. The occipital bone forms the posterior and inferior aspect of the cranium, extending to and forming the foramen magnum. The temporal bones form the lateral cranial surfaces anterior to the ears, while the ethmoid and sphenoid bones, which are very irregular in shape, form the portion of the cranium concealed and protected by the facial bones.

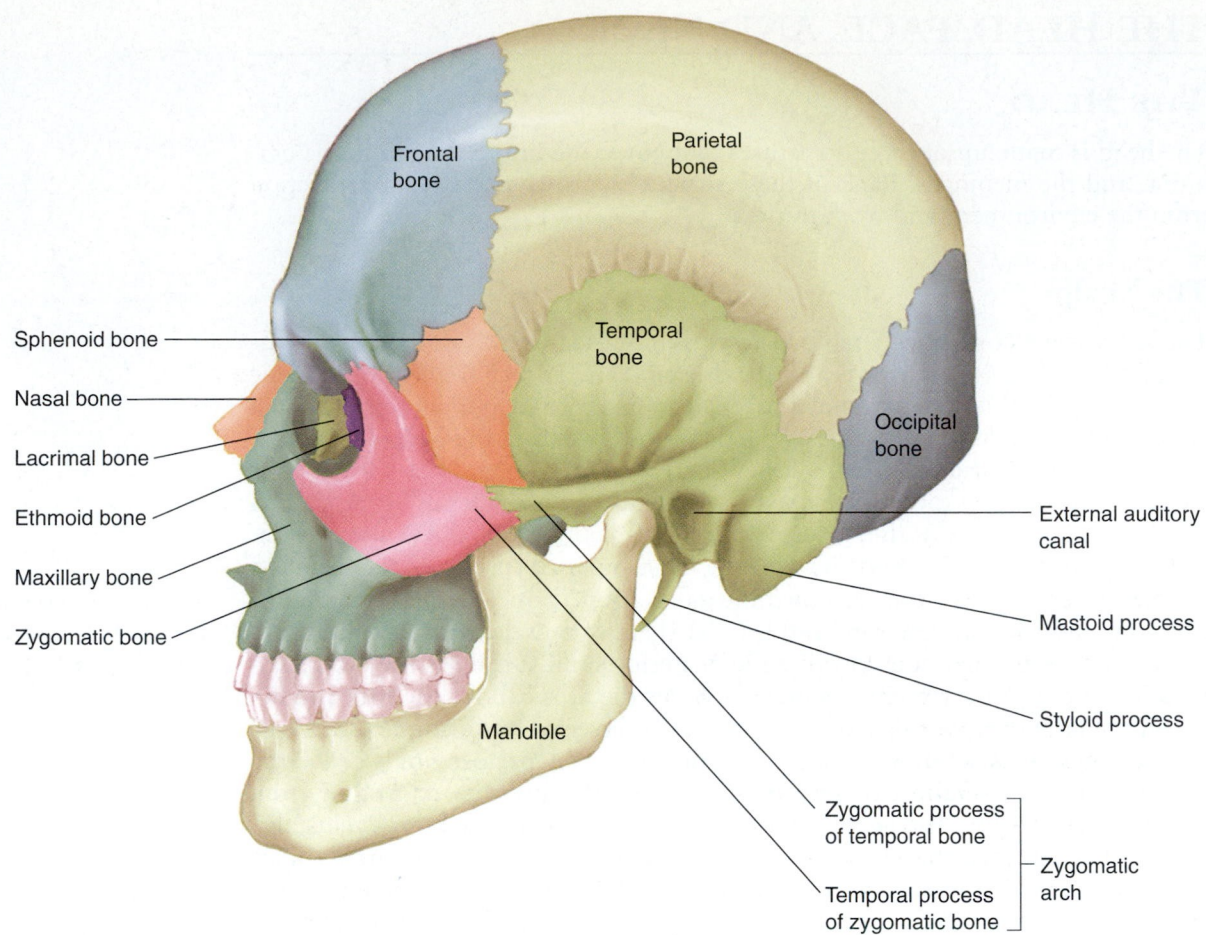

FIGURE 3-44   Bones of the human skull.

Labels in figure:
Frontal bone
Parietal bone
Temporal bone
Occipital bone
Sphenoid bone
Nasal bone
Lacrimal bone
Ethmoid bone
Maxillary bone
Zygomatic bone
External auditory canal
Mastoid process
Styloid process
Mandible
Zygomatic process of temporal bone
Temporal process of zygomatic bone
Zygomatic arch

The base of the skull consists of portions of the occipital, temporal, sphenoid, and ethmoid bones. This area is important in cases of trauma because the openings, or foramina, for blood vessels, the spinal cord, the auditory canal, and the cranial nerves pass through it. These openings weaken the area, leaving it prone to fracture with serious trauma.

Other anatomic points of interest within the cranium are the cribriform plate and the foramen magnum. The cribriform plate is an irregular portion of the ethmoid bone and a portion of the base of the cranium. It and the remainder of the base of the cranium have rough surfaces against which the brain may abrade, lacerate, or contuse during severe deceleration. The foramen magnum is the largest opening in the skull. It is located at the base of the skull where it meets the spinal column and is where the spinal cord exits the cranium.

The Meninges

The final protective mechanisms for the brain and the spinal cord are the **meninges** (Figure 3-45). They are a group of three tissues between the cranium and the brain and the spinal column and cord. The outermost layer is the **dura mater** (tough mother), a tough connective tissue that provides protection for the central nervous system. The dura mater is actually two layers. The outer layer is the cranium's inner periosteum. The dural layer is made up of tough, continuous connective tissue that extends into the cranial cavity where it forms partial struc-

✳ **meninges** three membranes that surround and protect the brain and spinal cord. They are the dura mater, pia mater, and arachnoid membrane.

✳ **dura mater** tough layer of the meninges firmly attached to the interior of the skull and interior of the spinal column.

FIGURE 3-45 The meninges and skull.

tural divisions (the falx cerebri and the tentorium cerebelli). Above the dura mater lie some of the larger arteries that provide blood flow to the surface of the brain. Between the dural layers lie the dural sinuses, major venous drains for the brain.

The meningeal layer closest to the brain and spinal cord is the **pia mater** (tender mother). It is a delicate tissue, covering all the convolutions of the brain and cord. Although more delicate when compared to the dura mater, the pia mater is still more substantial than brain and spinal cord tissue. The pia mater is a highly vascular tissue with large vessels that supply the superficial areas of the brain.

Separating the two layers of mater is a stratum of connective tissue called the **arachnoid membrane.** It covers the inner dura mater and suspends the brain in the cranial cavity with collagen and elastin fibers. The arachnoid membrane gets its name from its web-like appearance (arachnoid, meaning "spider-like"). Beneath the arachnoid membrane is the subarachnoid space, which is filled with cerebrospinal fluid. This region provides cushioning for the brain when the head is subjected to strong forces of acceleration or deceleration.

✳ **pia mater** inner and most delicate layer of the meninges. It covers the convolutions of the brain and spinal cord.

✳ **arachnoid membrane** middle layer of the meninges.

Cerebrospinal Fluid

Cerebrospinal fluid is a clear, colorless solution of water, proteins, and salts surrounding the central nervous system that absorbs the shock of minor acceleration and deceleration. The brain constantly generates cerebrospinal fluid in the largest two of four spaces (or ventricles) within the substance of the brain. The fluid circulates through the ventricles, then through the subarachnoid space, where it is returned to the venous circulation through the dural sinuses. The cerebrospinal fluid provides buoyancy for the brain and actually floats it in a near-weightless environment within the cranial cavity. This fluid also is a medium through which nutrients and waste products such as oxygen, proteins, salts, and carbon dioxide are diffused into and out of the brain tissue.

✳ **cerebrospinal fluid** fluid surrounding and bathing the brain and spinal cord (the elements of the central nervous system).

The Brain

The brain occupies about 80 percent of the interior of the cranium. It is made up of three major structures essential to human function—the cerebrum, cerebellum, and the brainstem.

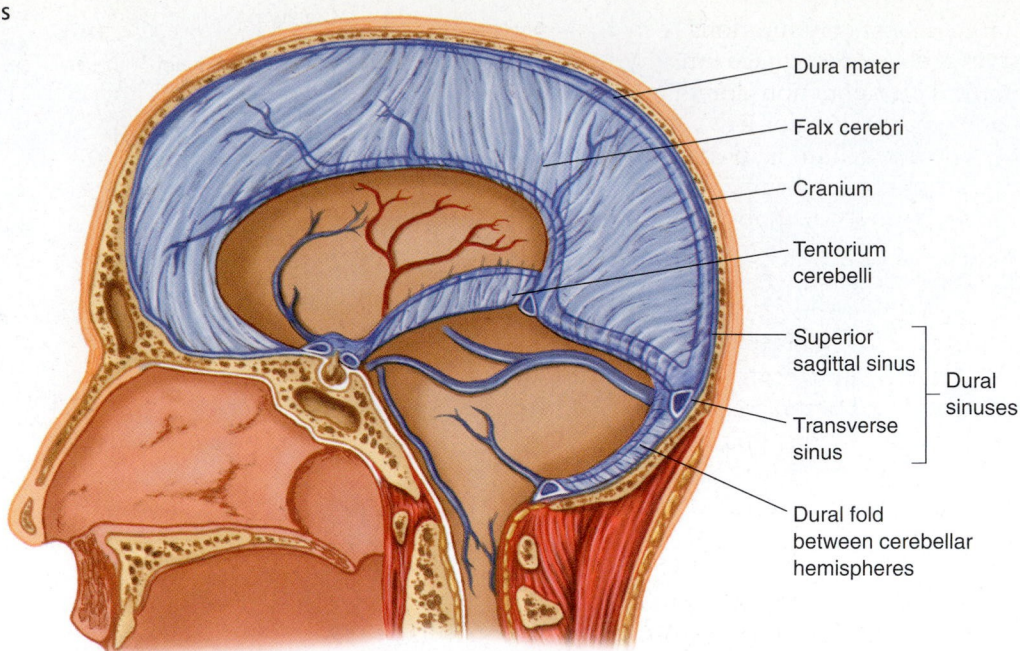

FIGURE 3-46 The partitions extending into the skull, the falx cerebri and tentorium cerebellum.

Dura mater

Falx cerebri

Cranium

Tentorium cerebelli

Superior sagittal sinus

Transverse sinus

Dural sinuses

Dural fold between cerebellar hemispheres

✱ **cerebrum** largest part of the brain. It consists of two hemispheres separated by a deep longitudinal fissure. It is the seat of consciousness and the center of the higher mental functions such as memory, learning, reasoning, judgment, intelligence, and emotions.

The crossing of nerve impulses from one side of the body to the other takes place just below the medulla oblongata.

The **cerebrum** is the largest element of the nervous system and occupies most of the cranial cavity. It consists of an exterior cortex of gray matter (cell bodies) and is the highest functional portion of the brain. The central portion of the cerebrum is predominantly white matter, mostly communication pathways (axons). The cerebrum is the center of conscious thought, personality, speech, motor control, and of visual, auditory, and tactile (touch) perception. The cerebrum is regionalized into lobes roughly lying beneath the bones of the cranium (and given the same names). The frontal region is anterior and determines personality. The parietal region, which is superior and posterior, directs motor and sensory activities as well as memory and emotions. The occipital region, which is posterior and inferior, is responsible for sight. Laterally, the temporal regions are the centers for long-term memory, hearing, speech, taste, and smell.

A structure called the falx cerebri divides the cerebrum into right and left hemispheres. A dural partition, the falx cerebri extends into the cranial cavity from the interior and superior surface of the cranium (Figure 3-46). Corresponding to the falx cerebri is a fissure in the cerebrum called the central sulcus. This fissure physically splits the cerebrum into the left and right hemispheres, each of which controls (for the most part) the activities of the opposite side of the body. The crossing of nerve impulses from one side to the other takes place just below the medulla oblongata. The tentorium cerebelli is a similar fibrous sheet within the occipital region, running at right angles to the falx cerebri. It separates the cerebrum from the cerebellum. The brainstem perforates the tentorium through an opening called the tentorium incisura.

The oculomotor nerve (CN-III), which controls pupil size, travels along the tentorium. It is likely to be compressed as intracranial pressure rises or the brain is displaced due to edema, a growing mass, or hemorrhage. This compression causes pupillary disturbances that manifest most commonly on the same side as the problem. If the pressure is great enough, it may affect both sides and both pupils may dilate and fix.

The left cerebral hemisphere is identified as the dominant hemisphere in most of the population, excepting a few left-handed individuals. It is responsible for mathematical computations (occipital region) and writing (parietal region) and is the center for language interpretation (occipital region) and speech (frontal region). The right, non-dominant cerebral hemisphere processes nonverbal imagery (occipital region).

The **cerebellum** is located directly under the tentorium. It lies posterior and inferior to the cerebrum. The cerebellum "fine tunes" motor control and allows the body to move smoothly from one position to another. Additionally, it is responsible for balance and maintenance of muscle tone.

The **brainstem** is an important central processing center and the communication junction among the cerebrum, spinal cord, cranial nerves, and cerebellum. It includes the midbrain, the pons, and the medulla oblongata. The **midbrain** makes up the upper portion of the brainstem and consists of the hypothalamus, thalamus, and associated structures. The **hypothalamus** controls much of endocrine function, the vomiting reflex, hunger, thirst, kidney function, body temperature, and emotions. The **thalamus** is the switching center between the pons and the cerebrum and is a critical element in the **reticular activating system (RAS)**, the system that establishes consciousness. This region also provides the major tracts, or pathways, for the optic and olfactory nerves.

The **pons** acts as the communication interchange between the various components of the central nervous system—the cerebellum, the cerebrum, midbrain, and the spinal cord. It is a bulb-shaped structure directly above the medulla oblongata and appears to be responsible for the sleep component of the reticular activating system.

The last nervous system structure still within the cranial vault is the **medulla oblongata.** It is recognizable as a bulge in the very top of the spinal cord. The medulla contains three important centers—the respiratory center, the cardiac center, and the vasomotor center. The cardiac center regulates the rate and strength of cardiac contractions. The vasomotor center controls the distribution of blood and maintains blood pressure. The respiratory center controls respiratory depth, rate, and rhythm.

In order to maintain its advanced functioning, the brain has a high metabolic rate. Though the brain accounts for only 2 percent of the body's total weight, it receives about 15 percent of the cardiac output and consumes about 20 percent of the body's oxygen. It requires this circulation whether it is at rest or engaged in active thought. Further, this blood supply must be constant because the brain has no stored energy sources. It needs constant supplies of glucose, thiamine (to help metabolize glucose), and oxygen and relies almost solely on aerobic metabolism. If the blood supply stops, unconsciousness follows within 10 seconds, and brain death will ensue within 4 to 6 minutes.

CNS Circulation

Four major arterial vessels provide blood flow to the brain. The first two are the internal carotid arteries. These vessels divide from the common carotid at the carotid sinus and then enter the cranium through its base. The two posterior vessels, the vertebral arteries, ascend along and through the vertebral column. They then enter the base of the skull, where they join and form a singular basilar artery.

The internal carotid and basilar arteries interconnect through the circle of Willis in the base of the brain. This structure is an arterial circle that assures good circulation to the brain, even if one of the large feeder vessels is obstructed. Various arteries branch out from the circle of Willis and supply the substance of the brain itself.

Venous drainage occurs initially through bridging veins that drain the surface of the cerebrum. They "bridge" with the dural sinuses (large, thin-walled veins). These ultimately drain into the internal jugular veins and then into the superior vena cava.

* **cerebellum** portion of the brain located dorsally to the pons and medulla oblongata. It plays an important role in the fine control of voluntary muscular movements.

* **brainstem** the part of the brain connecting the cerebral hemispheres with the spinal cord. It is comprised of the medulla oblongata, the pons, and the midbrain.

* **midbrain** portion of the brain connecting the pons and cerebellum with the cerebral hemispheres.

* **hypothalamus** portion of the brain important for controlling certain metabolic activities, including the regulation of body temperature.

* **thalamus** switching station between the pons and the cerebrum in the brain.

* **reticular activating system (RAS)** a series of nervous tissues keeping the human system in a state of consciousness.

* **pons** process of tissue responsible for the communication interchange between the cerebellum, the cerebrum, midbrain, and the spinal cord.

* **medulla oblongata** lower portion of the brainstem containing the respiratory, cardiac, and vasomotor centers.

Though the brain accounts for only 2 percent of the body's total weight, it consumes about 20 percent of the body's oxygen.

Blood-Brain Barrier

The capillaries of the brain are special in that their walls are thicker and not as permeable as those found elsewhere in the body. They do not permit the interstitial flow of proteins and other materials as freely as do other body capillaries. This assures that many substances found in the circulatory system, such as some hormones, do not affect the central nervous system cells. Lymphatic circulation is also lacking in the brain and is replaced by the cerebrospinal fluid flow system. This results in a very special and protected environment for central nervous system cells. If frank blood seeps into the central nervous system tissue, it acts as an irritant, initiating an inflammatory response, resulting in edema.

Cerebral Perfusion Pressure

Cerebral perfusion is exceptionally critical and depends on many factors. Primarily, the pressure within the cranium (intracranial pressure or ICP) resists blood flow and good perfusion to the central nervous system tissue. Usually the pressure is less than 10 mmHg and does not significantly impede blood flow as long as the mean arterial blood pressure (MAP is the diastolic blood pressure plus one third the pulse pressure) is at least 50 mmHg. The pressure moving blood through the cranium is the **cerebral perfusion pressure (CPP)**. This is calculated as the mean arterial pressure (MAP) minus the intracranial pressure (ICP). Changes in ICP are met with compensatory changes in blood pressure to assure adequate cerebral perfusion pressure and cerebral blood flow. This compensating reflex is called **autoregulation.**

Since the cranium is a fixed vault for the structures of the brain, its volume and the pressure within are shared by the occupants. Any expanding mass (tumor), hemorrhage, or edema within the cranium will displace some other occupant such as the cerebrospinal fluid or blood, since they are the only readily movable media. This displacement maintains the intracranial pressure very effectively, up to a point. When the volumes of cerebrospinal fluid and venous blood are reduced to their limits, however, the intracranial pressure begins to rise. Autoregulation then raises the blood pressure to assure there is enough differential (CPP) to provide good cerebral perfusion. However, this increase in blood pressure causes the intracranial pressure to rise still higher and cerebral blood perfusion to diminish even more. As this cycle of increasing intracranial pressure and increasing blood pressure continues, brain injury and death are close at hand.

Cranial Nerves

The cranial nerves are nerve roots originating within the cranium and along the brainstem. They comprise 12 distinct pathways that account for some of the more important senses, innervate the facial area, and control significant body functions (see figure 3-72 in the Nervous System section later in this chapter.).

Ascending Reticular Activating System

The ascending reticular activating system is a tract of neurons within the upper brainstem, the pons, and the midbrain that is responsible for the sleep-wake cycle. It is a complex control system that monitors the amount of stimulation the body receives and regulates important bodily functions such as respiration, heart rate, and peripheral vascular resistance. Injury to the midbrain may result in unconsciousness or coma, while injury to the pons may result in a protracted waking state.

* **cerebral perfusion pressure (CPP)** the pressure moving blood through the brain.

$$CPP = MAP - ICP$$

* **autoregulation** process that controls blood flow to the brain tissue by causing alterations in the blood pressure.

FIGURE 3-47 The facial bones.

Lacrimal bone

Zygomatic bone

Maxillary bone

Inferior nasal concha

Mandible

Nasal bones

Vomer

THE FACE

Facial bones make up the anterior and inferior structures of the head and include the zygoma, maxilla, mandible, and nasal bones (Figure 3-47). The **zygoma** is the prominent bone of the cheek. It protects the eyes and the muscles controlling eye and jaw movement. The **maxilla** comprises the upper jaw, supports the nasal bone, and provides the lower border of the orbit. The nasal bone is the attachment for the nasal cartilage as it forms the shape of the nose. The last of the facial bones is the **mandible,** or jawbone. It resembles two horizontal "L's," which join anteriorly and hinge underneath the posterior zygomatic arch. Besides forming the beginning of the airway and the alimentary canal, the facial bones form supporting and protective structures for several sense organs, including the tongue (taste), eye (sight), and olfactory nerve (smell).

The facial region, like most other areas of the body, is covered with skin that serves to protect the tissue underneath from trauma and against adverse environmental effects. In the facial region, the skin is very flexible and relatively thin. It also has a very good vascular supply and hemorrhages freely when injured. Beneath the skin is a minimal layer of subcutaneous tissue and, beneath that, are the many small muscles that control facial expression and the movements of the mouth, eyes, and eyelids.

Circulation for the facial area is provided by the external carotid artery as it branches into the facial, temporal, and maxillary arteries. The facial artery crosses the mandible, then travels up and along the nasal bone. The maxillary artery runs under the mandible and zygoma, then provides circulation to the cheek area. The temporal artery runs anterior to the ear just posterior to the zygoma. Each major artery has an associated vein paralleling its path.

✱ **zygoma** the cheekbone.

✱ **maxilla** bone of the upper jaw.

✱ **mandible** the jawbone.

The most important cranial nerves traversing this area are the trigeminal (CN-V) and the facial (CN-VII). The trigeminal nerve provides sensation for the face and some motor control over eye movement as well as enabling the chewing process. The facial nerve provides motor control to the facial muscles and contributes to the sensation of taste.

The nasal cavity is formed by the juncture of the ethmoid, nasal, and maxillary bones. It is a channel running posteriorly with a bony septum dividing it into left and right chambers and plates protruding medially from the lateral sides. These plates, called turbinates, form support for the vascular mucous membranes that serve to warm, humidify, and collect particulate matter from the incoming air. The lower border of the nasal cavity is formed by the bony hard palate and then, posteriorly, by the more flexible cartilaginous soft palate. The soft palate moves upward to close off the opening of the posterior nasal cavity during swallowing. The nasal bone lies anterior and inferior to the eyes and provides a base for the nasal cartilage. The nasal cartilage defines the shape of the nose and divides the nostrils and their openings, which are called the **nares.**

The oral cavity is formed by the concave shape of the maxillary bone, the palate, and the upper teeth meeting the mandible and the lower teeth. The floor of the chamber consists of musculature and connective tissue that span the mandible and support the tongue. The tongue is a large muscle that occupies much of the oral cavity, provides the taste sensation, and moves food between the teeth during chewing (mastication) and propels the chewed food posteriorly, then inferiorly during swallowing. The tongue connects with the hyoid bone, a free floating U-shaped bone located inferiorly and posteriorly to the mandible. The mandible articulates with the temporal bone at the temporomandibular joint, under the posterior zygoma, and is moved by the masseter muscles. The lip muscles (obicularis oris) are responsible for sealing the mouth during chewing and swallowing.

Special structures are found in and around the oral cavity. Salivary glands provide saliva, the first of the digestive juices. These glands are located just anterior and inferior to the ear, under the tongue, and just inside the inferior mandible. Specialized lymphoid nodules, the tonsils, are located in the posterior wall of the pharynx.

Prominent cranial nerves serving the oral area include the hypoglossal, the glossopharyngeal, the trigeminal, and the facial nerves. The hypoglossal nerve (CN-XII) directs swallowing and tongue movement. The glossopharyngeal nerve (CN-IX) controls saliva production and taste. The trigeminal nerve (CN-V) carries sensations from the facial region and assists in chewing control. The facial nerve (CN-VII) controls the muscles of facial expression and taste.

Posterior and inferior to the oral cavity is a collection of soft tissue called the pharynx. The process of swallowing begins in the pharynx once the bolus of food has been propelled back and down by the tongue. The epiglottis moves downward while the larynx moves up, sealing the lower airway opening. The food or liquid moves into the esophagus where a peristaltic wave begins its trip to the stomach. This area is of great importance because it maintains the critical segregation of materials between the digestive tract and the airway.

Sinuses are hollow spaces within the bones of the cranium and face that lighten the head, protect the eyes and nasal cavity, and help produce the resonant tones of the voice. They also strengthen this region against the forces of trauma.

* **nares** the openings of the nostrils.

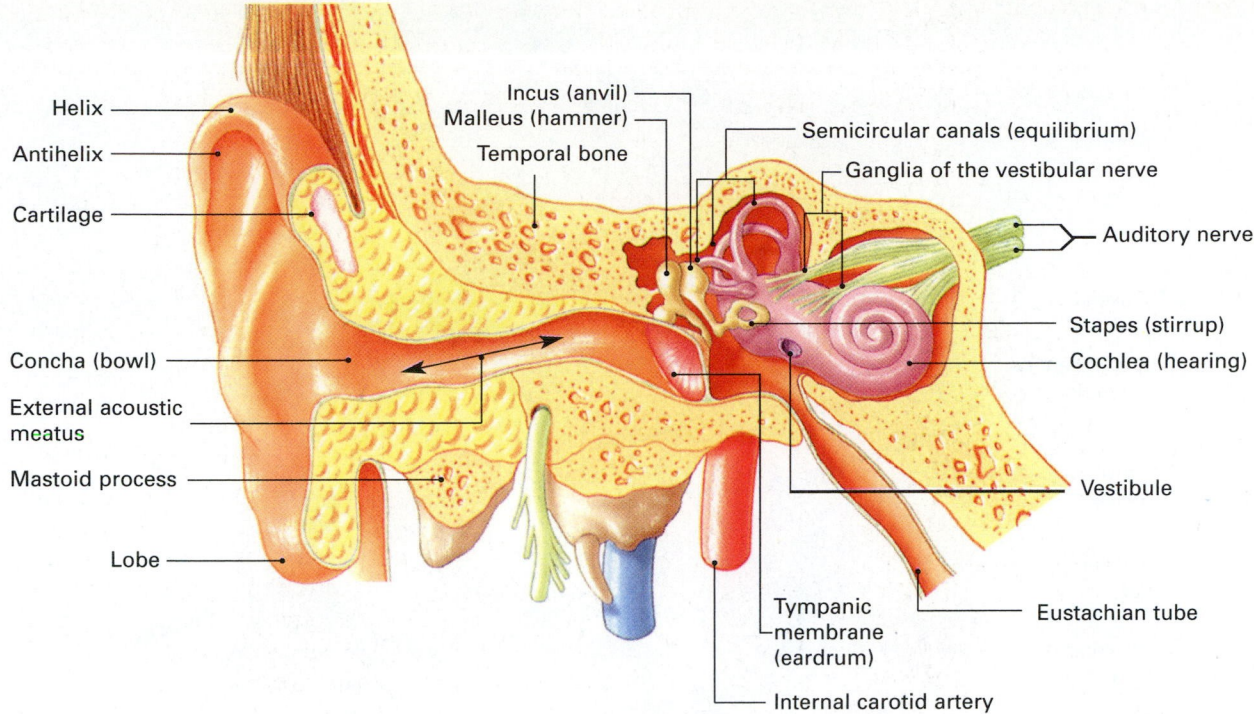

Helix
Antihelix
Cartilage

Incus (anvil)
Malleus (hammer)
Temporal bone

Semicircular canals (equilibrium)
Ganglia of the vestibular nerve
Auditory nerve

Concha (bowl)
External acoustic meatus
Mastoid process
Lobe

Stapes (stirrup)
Cochlea (hearing)

Vestibule

Tympanic membrane (eardrum)
Internal carotid artery

Eustachian tube

FIGURE 3-48   The anatomy of the ear.

The Ear

The outer, visible portion of the ear is termed the **pinna.** It is composed of cartilage and has a poor blood supply. It connects to the external auditory canal, which leads to the eardrum. The external auditory canal contains glands that secrete wax (cerumen) for protection. The ear's important structures are interior and exceptionally well protected from nearly all trauma (Figure 3-48). Only trauma involving great pressure differentials (e.g., blast and diving injuries) or basilar skull fractures are likely to damage this area.

The ear provides the body with two very useful functions, hearing and positional sense. The middle and inner ear contain the structures needed for hearing. Hearing occurs when sound waves cause the tympanic membrane (eardrum) to vibrate. The eardrum transmits the vibrations through three very small bones (the ossicles) to the cochlea, the organ of hearing. These vibrations stimulate the auditory nerve, which in turn transmits the signal to the brain.

The **semicircular canals** are responsible for sensing position and motion. They are three hollow, fluid-filled rings set at different angles. When the head moves, fluid in these rings shifts. Small cells with hairlike projections sense the motion and signal the brain to help maintain balance. This positional sense is present even when the eyes are closed. If injury or illness disturbs this area, it transmits excess signals to the brain. Patients then experience a continuous moving sensation known as vertigo.

✱ **pinna** outer, visible portion of the ear.

✱ **semicircular canals** the three rings of the inner ear. They sense the motion of the head and provide positional sense for the body.

Fovea

Central artery
and vein

Optic
nerve

Orbital
fat

Posterior
chamber

Retina

Sclera

Bony orbit

Anterior
chamber

Cornea

Edge of
pupil

Visual
axis

Lens

Iris

Conjunctiva

FIGURE 3-49   The anatomy of the eye.

The Eye

The eyes provide much of the input we use to interact with our environment. Although they are placed prominently on the face, the eyes are well protected from trauma by a series of facial bones. The frontal bones project above the globe of the eye, while the nasal bones and cartilage protect medially. The bone of the cheek, or zygoma, completes the physical protection both laterally and inferiorly. These bones collectively form the eye socket or **orbit.** The soft tissue of the eyelid and the eyelashes give additional protection to the critical ocular surface.

The eye is a spherical globe, filled with liquid (Figure 3-49). Its major compartment (the posterior chamber) contains a crystal-clear gelatinous fluid called **vitreous humor.** Lining the posterior of the compartment is a light- and color-sensing tissue known as the **retina.** Images focused on the retina are transmitted to the brain via the optic nerve. The lens separates the posterior and anterior chambers. The lens is responsible for focusing light and images on the retina by

✱ **orbit** the eye socket.

✱ **vitreous humor** clear watery fluid filling the posterior chamber of the eye. It is responsible for giving the eye its spherical shape.

✱ **retina** light- and color-sensing tissue lining the posterior chamber of the eye.

the action of small muscles that change its thickness. A fluid called **aqueous humor,** which is similar to vitreous humor, fills the anterior chamber. The anterior chamber also contains the **iris,** the muscular and colored portion of the eye that regulates the amount of light reaching the retina. Light enters the eye through the dark opening in the center of the iris called the **pupil.**

By examining the eye, you can easily identify several of its components such as the colored iris and the central black pupil. Bordering the iris is the **sclera,** the white and vascular area that forms the remaining, underlying surface of the exposed eye. The **cornea,** a very thin, clear, and delicate layer, covers both the pupil and iris. Continuous with the cornea and extending out to the eyelid's interior surface is the **conjunctiva,** another delicate, smooth layer that slides over itself and the cornea when the eye closes or blinks.

The eye is bathed in **lacrimal fluid,** which is produced by almond-shaped lacrimal glands located along the brow ridge just lateral and superior to the eyeball. Lacrimal fluid flows through lacrimal ducts and then over the cornea. Because the cornea does not have blood vessels, the fluid provides crucial lubrication, oxygen, and nutrients. If injury or some other mechanism—for example, a contact lens left in an unconscious patient's eye—prevents this fluid from reaching the cornea, the surface of the eye may be damaged. The lacrimal fluid is drained from the eye into the lacrimal sac, located along the medial orbit, and empties then into the nose.

The last major functional elements of the eye are the muscles that move them and their controlling cranial nerves. These small muscles are attached to the eyeball in the region of the conjunctival fold and are hidden within the eye socket and under the zygomatic arch. The oculomotor (CN-III), trochlear (CN-IV), and abducens (CN-VI) nerves control these muscles, which in turn control the eye's motion. The oculomotor nerve controls pupil dilation, conjugate movement (movement of the eyes together), and most of the eye's travel through its normal range of motion. The trochlear nerve moves the eye downward and inward, while the abducens nerve is responsible for eye abduction (outward gaze).

The Mouth

The lips mark the entrance to the mouth and play a role in the articulation of speech. The mouth houses the tongue, the gums (gingiva), and the teeth (Figure 3-50). The roof of the mouth is formed by the hard palate and the soft palate. The uvula is the peninsular extension of the soft palate that hangs in the back of the mouth. The oral cavity, lined with buccal (cheek/mouth) mucosa, is rich in mucous membranes. The parotid glands, just in front of the ears, and the submandibular glands, just beneath the mandible, secrete digestive enzymes and saliva into the oral cavity (Figure 3-51). The sublingual glands secrete enzymes just beneath the tongue. You can easily palpate these glands under the chin.

The tongue, a large, mobile muscle covered by mucous membranes, has many functions. It helps in chewing by keeping food on the teeth, and it assists in swallowing by moving the food into the oropharynx. It also contains the taste buds and is essential in forming words when we speak.

A highly vascular mucosa lines the gingiva, giving it a pink color. The teeth are anchored in bony sockets; only their white enamel-covered crowns are visible. An adult normally has 32 permanent teeth, including incisors, canines, premolars, and molars. The pharynx consists of three distinct areas: the nasopharynx (behind the nasal cavity), the oropharynx (back of the throat), and the laryngopharynx (just above the epiglottis). At the back of the throat on either side, the tonsils help separate the oropharynx (food processing) from the nasopharynx (air passage).

* **aqueous humor** clear fluid filling the anterior chamber of the eye.

* **iris** pigmented portion of the eye. It is the muscular area that constricts or dilates to change the size of the pupil.

* **pupil** dark opening in the center of the iris through which light enters the eye.

* **sclera** the "white" of the eye.

* **cornea** thin, delicate layer covering the pupil and the iris.

* **conjunctiva** mucous membrane that lines the eyelids.

* **lacrimal fluid** liquid that lubricates the eye.

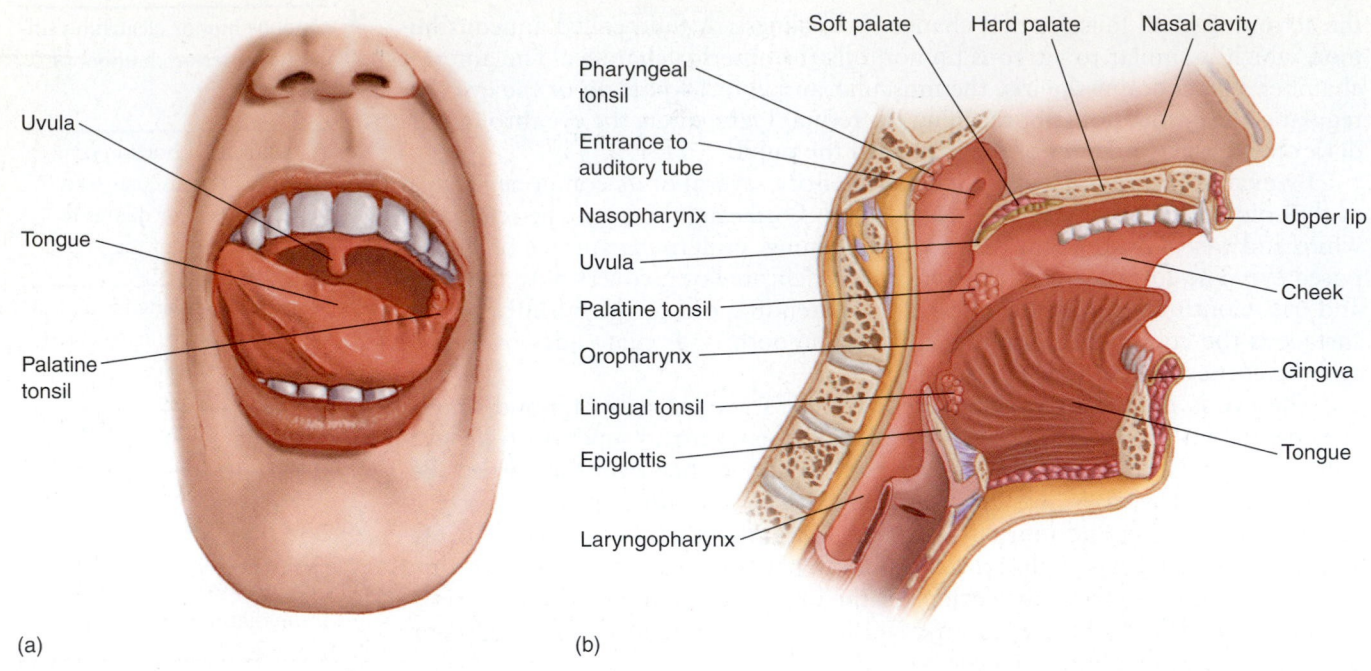

(a)

(b)

FIGURE 3-50 The mouth.

FIGURE 3-51 The salivary glands.

FIGURE 3-52 The neck.

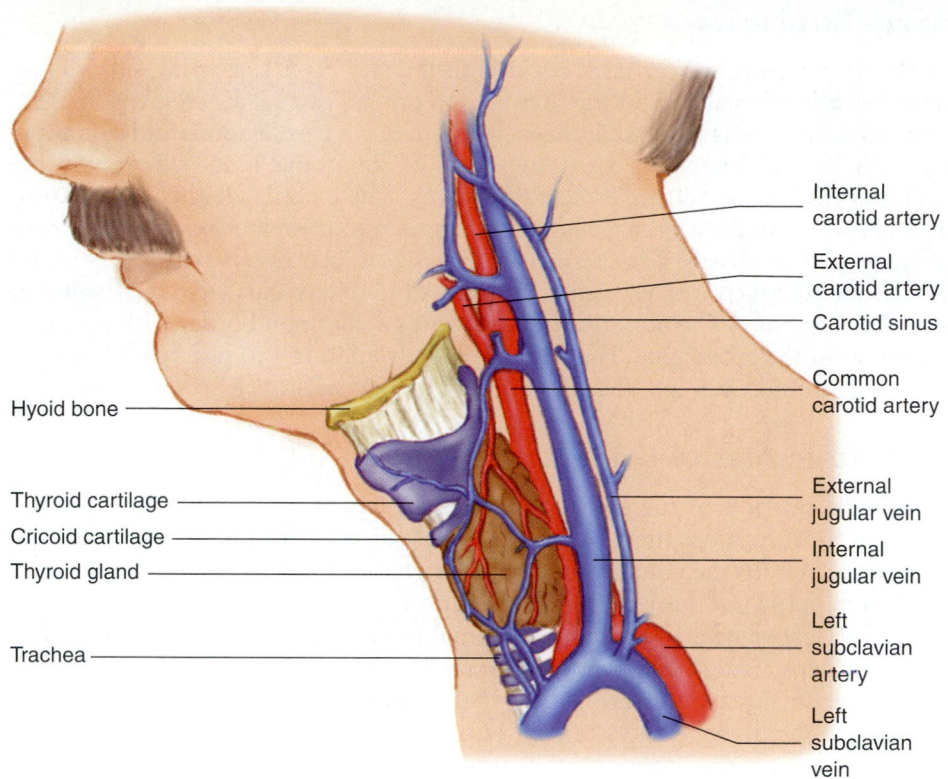

Internal
carotid artery

External
carotid artery

Carotid sinus

Common
carotid artery

External
jugular vein

Internal
jugular vein

Left
subclavian
artery

Left
subclavian
vein

Hyoid bone

Thyroid cartilage

Cricoid cartilage

Thyroid gland

Trachea

THE NECK

The neck (Figure 3-52) is the region that links the head to the rest of the body. Traveling through this anatomic area are blood for the facial region and brain, air for respiration, food for digestion, and neural communications to sense the body and its environment and to control both the voluntary and involuntary muscles and glands of the body. The neck also contains some of the important muscles used to provide head and shoulder movement as well as the thyroid and parathyroid glands of the endocrine system.

Vasculature of the Neck

The major blood vessels traversing the neck are the carotid arteries and the jugular veins. The carotid arteries arise from the brachiocephalic artery on the right and the aorta on the left. They travel upward and medially along the trachea and split into internal and external carotid arteries at about the level of the larynx's upper border. At this split are the carotid bodies and carotid sinuses, which are responsible for monitoring carbon dioxide and oxygen levels in the blood and the blood pressure respectively. The jugular veins are paired on each side of the neck. The internal jugular vein runs in a sheath with the carotid artery and vagus nerve, while the external jugular vein runs superficially just lateral to the trachea. The jugular veins join the brachiocephalic veins just beneath the clavicles.

Airway Structures

The airway structures of the neck begin with the larynx. It is a prominent hollow cylindrical column made up of the thyroid and cricoid cartilages, atop the trachea. The thyroid opening is covered during swallowing by a cartilaginous and soft tissue flap, the epiglottis. The vocal cords, two folds of connective tissue sitting atop the opening of the larynx, further protect the airway. These cords vibrate with air passage and form sounds; they may also close in spasm to prevent foreign bodies from entering the lower airway. The cricoid cartilage is a circular ring between the thyroid cartilage and the trachea. The trachea is a series of C-shaped cartilages that maintain the tracheal opening. The posterior trachea shares a common border with the anterior surface of the esophagus. The trachea extends inferiorly to just below the sternum, where it bifurcates into the left and right mainstem bronchi at the carina.

Other Structures of the Neck

The cervical portion of the spinal column traverses the neck and provides the skeletal support for both the head and neck. It is also an attachment point for the ligaments that hold the column together and give it its strength and for the tendons that support and move the head and shoulders.

The cervical spine also contains the spinal cord. The spinal cord is the critical conduit for nervous signals between the brain and the body, and injury to it can be serious, even life threatening. From the spinal cord and between each vertebral junction, the peripheral nerve roots branch out. These structures direct signals to and receive signals from the limbs, internal organs, and sensory structures of the body. (The anatomy of the cervical spine is addressed in detail later in this chapter.)

Other structures within the neck include the esophagus, cranial nerves, thoracic duct, thyroid and parathyroid glands, and brachial plexus. The esophagus is a smooth muscle tube located behind the trachea that carries food and liquid to the stomach. Its anterior border is continuous with the posterior border of the trachea. Some cranial nerves, including the glossopharyngeal (CN-IX) and the vagus (CN-X), traverse the neck. The vagus nerve is essential for many parasympathetic activities including speech, swallowing, and cardiac, respiratory, and visceral function. The glossopharyngeal nerve innervates the carotid bodies and carotid sinuses, monitoring blood oxygen levels and blood pressure.

> *** lymphatic system** a network of valveless vessels that drains fluid, called lymph, from the body tissues. Lymph nodes help filter impurities en route to the subclavian vein and thence to the heart.

The **lymphatic system** helps drain fluid from the head and face and assists in fighting infection. A long chain of lymph nodes runs along the side of the neck, behind the ears, and under the chin (Figure 3-53). They are palpable when congested with infectious products. (The lymphatic system is discussed further in the Cardiovascular System section, later in this chapter.) The right and left thoracic ducts deliver lymph to the venous system at the juncture of the jugular and subclavian veins.

The thyroid gland sits over the trachea just below the cricoid cartilage and controls the rate of cellular metabolism as well as the systemic levels of calcium. The brachial plexus is a network of nerves in the lower neck and shoulder responsible for lower arm and hand function. Lastly, numerous muscles (including the sternocleidomastoid, platysma, and upper trapezius), fascia, and soft tissues are found in the neck.

THE SPINE AND THORAX

THE SPINE

The spine consists of a supporting skeletal structure, the vertebral column, and a central nervous system pathway, the spinal cord. These are important functional elements both for body posture and movement and for communication among the body's many systems. The vertebral column provides skeletal support

FIGURE 3-53 The lymph nodes of the head and neck.

Posterior auricular
Occipital
Superficial cervical
Posterior cervical
Supraclavicular

Preauricular
Tonsillar
Submental
Submandibular
Deep cervical chain

for and permits movement of the head, assists in maintaining the shape of the thoracic cage, supports the upper body, and forms the posterior aspect of the pelvis. The spinal cord, contained and protected within the vertebral column, is the main communication conduit of the central nervous system. It is responsible for transmitting messages from the brain to the body organs and tissues and from the sensory nerves in the organs, skin, and other tissues back to the brain.

The Vertebral Column

The vertebral column is a hollow skeletal tube made up of 33 irregular bones, called **vertebrae.** This column attaches to the head, to the bones of the rib cage, and to the pelvis. It provides the central skeletal support structure and a major portion of the axial skeleton. At the same time, the vertebrae provide a protective container for the spinal cord. Several components with differing functions may make up the structure of each individual vertebra.

The major weight-bearing component of a vertebra is the **vertebral body.** It is a cylinder of skeletal tissue made up of cancellous bone surrounded by a layer of hard, compact bone. It lies anterior to the other components of the vertebra.

The size of the vertebral body varies with its location along the spinal column (Figure 3-54). The first two cervical vertebrae (C-1 and C-2) do not have vertebral bodies because of their specialized functions. Below C-1 and C-2, the size of the vertebral bodies increases progressively as you move down the spine because the vertebral column is supporting an increasing portion of the upper body's weight. The lumbar spine has the strongest and largest vertebral bodies due to the weight they bear. Because of the fused nature of the sacrum and coccyx, these regions have no discernable bodies.

A component of the vertebra posterior to the vertebral body is the **spinal canal,** which is the opening, or foramen, that accommodates the spinal cord. This

✱ **vertebrae** the 33 bones making up the vertebral column; singular *vertebra.*

✱ **vertebral body** short column of bone that forms the weight-bearing portion of a vertebra.

✱ **spinal canal** opening in the vertebrae that accommodates the spinal cord.

The Spine and Thorax **167**

FIGURE 3-54 Changing dimensions of the vertebral column.

Front view of vertebral column

Vertebrae from above

* **pedicles** thick, bony struts that connect the vertebral bodies with the spinous and transverse processes and help make up the opening for the spinal canal.

* **laminae** posterior bones of a vertebra that help make up the foramen, or opening, of the spinal canal.

* **transverse process** bony outgrowth of the vertebral pedicle that serves as a site for muscle attachment and articulation with the ribs.

* **spinous process** prominence at the posterior part of a vertebra.

opening is formed by small fused bony structures that are joined together to create a ring. The lateral structures of the ring are called **pedicles**, while the two posterior structures are called **laminae**. The inferior surface of the pedicle contains a notch, called the intervertebral foramen. This notch permits the exit of a peripheral nerve root and spinal vein and the entrance of a spinal artery on each side of the spinal canal and at each vertebral junction.

At the juncture of the pedicle and lamina on each side of a vertebra, there is a bony outgrowth called the **transverse process.** There is also a bony outgrowth where the laminae join, which is called the **spinous process.** The spinous process is the posteriorly and inferiorly oriented bony protrusion that you can feel along the spine.

The spinous and transverse processes are points of attachment for ligaments and tendons. Ligaments hold the vertebrae firmly together and in place while they permit limited motion. The tendons attach muscles to the vertebral column and permit these muscles to move the spine, other bones, and the body. This attachment of muscles and capsule of ligaments protects and strengthens the vertebral column against the forces of trauma.

Between the vertebral bodies are cartilaginous **intervertebral disks.** These disks are formed of a strong yet somewhat flexible outer cover called the annulus fibrosus and a soft and gelatinous inner region called the nucleus pulposus. The intervertebral disks accommodate some motion of the adjacent vertebrae, limit bone wear, and absorb shock along the length of the spinal column. The intervertebral disks make up about 25 percent of the total length of the spinal column, and their degeneration accounts for much of the height loss associated with advancing age.

The elements of the spinal column also have numerous articular surfaces. These surfaces are found on the vertebral bodies, the pedicles, and on the transverse and spinous processes. The articular surfaces enable the spinal column to move around the spinal cord without compressing it, permit articulation with the skull and ribs, and make possible the formation of the rigid, immobile joint of the pelvis.

The vertebral bodies are held firmly together by strong ligaments to assure that the spinal foramen safely accommodates the spinal cord and that the body has a reasonable range of motion. The anterior longitudinal ligament travels along the anterior surfaces of the vertebral bodies. It provides the major stability of the spinal column and resists hyperextension. The posterior longitudinal ligament travels along the posterior surfaces of the vertebral bodies, within the spinal canal. This ligament helps to prevent hyperflexion; when it is disrupted, the result is, frequently, a spinal cord injury. Other ligaments encapsulate the spinous processes (interspinous ligaments) and the transverse processes. These ligaments strengthen and stabilize the column against excessive lateral bending, rotation, and flexion.

Divisions of the Vertebral Column

The vertebral column is divided into five regions: the cervical, the thoracic, the lumbar, the sacral, and the coccygeal (Figure 3-55). Each region is unique in its design and function and has a curve that reverses the curve of the spinal section(s) adjacent to it. The individual vertebrae of the column are identified by the first letter of their region and numbered from superior to inferior. For example, the most inferior of the seven cervical vertebrae is identified as C-7.

Cervical Spine The cervical spine consists of seven cervical vertebrae located between the base of the skull and the shoulders. The cervical spine is the sole skeletal support for the head, which weighs about 16 to 22 pounds.

The first two cervical vertebrae have a unique relationship with the head and each other that permits rotation to left and right and nodding of the head. The first cervical vertebra, C-1, is called the atlas (after the Greek god who held up the world) and supports the head. It is securely affixed to the occiput and permits nodding but does not accommodate any twisting or turning motion. It and the next vertebra, C-2, differ from most vertebrae in not having discernable vertebral bodies. Vertebra C-2, called the axis, has a small bony tooth, called the odontoid process or dens, that projects upward. This projection provides a pivotal point around which the atlas and head can rotate from side to side.

The remaining cervical vertebrae permit some rotation as well as flexion, extension, and lateral bending. The range of motion provided by the cervical spine is greater than allowed by any other portion of the spinal column, while the portion of the spinal cord traveling through the region is most critical to life functions. The last cervical vertebra (C-7) is quite noticeable as its spinous process is pronounced and can be felt as the first bony prominence along the spine and just above the shoulders.

Thoracic Spine The thoracic spine consists of 12 thoracic vertebrae. The first rib articulates individually with the first thoracic vertebra at two locations, with

✱ intervertebral disk cartilaginous pad between vertebrae that serves as a shock absorber.

Content Review

DIVISIONS OF THE VERTEBRAL COLUMN

- Cervical spine
- Thoracic spine
- Lumbar spine
- Sacral spine
- Coccygeal spine

The range of motion provided by the cervical spine is the greatest allowed by any region, yet the chord in this region is critical to life functions.

FIGURE 3-55 Divisions of the veretebral column.

Spinal Curves

Cervical

Thoracic

Lumbar

Sacral

Vertebral regions

Cervical

Thoracic

Lumbar

Sacral

Coccygeal

the transverse process and with the vertebral body. The next nine ribs articulate with the transverse process and the superior portion of the vertebral body as well as with the inferior portion of the vertebral body that is adjacent (superior) to it. This system of fixation limits rib movement and increases the strength and rigidity of the thoracic spine. The last two ribs articulate only with the vertebral bodies, which permits greater movement and flexibility.

Because the thoracic spine supports more of the human body than the cervical spine, the thoracic vertebral bodies are larger and stronger. The spinous and transverse processes are also larger and more prominent because they are associated with the musculature holding the upper body erect and with the movement of the thoracic cage during respiration.

Lumbar Spine The five bones of the lumbar spine each carry the weight of the head, neck, and thorax above them. They also bear the forces of bending and lifting above the pelvis. The vertebral bodies are largest in this region of the spinal column, and the intervertebral disks are also the thickest and bear the greatest stress. The lumbar pedicles and lamina are also thick, while the transverse and spinous processes are shorter and stouter than those in the thoracic spine. The spinal foramen is largest in the lumbar region.

Sacral Spine The sacral spine consists of five sacral vertebrae that fuse into the posterior plate of the pelvis. This plate, in conjunction with the two innominate bones of the pelvis, protects the urinary and reproductive organs and attaches the pelvis and lower extremities to the axial skeleton. The articulation with the pelvis occurs at the sacroiliac joint on the lateral surface of the sacrum. This joint is very strong and permits no movement. The upper body balances on the sacrum.

Coccygeal Spine The coccygeal spine is made up of three to five fused verte-brae that represent the residual elements of a tail. They comprise the short skele-tal end of the vertebral column.

The vertebral column curves through each region of the spine. The cervical and lumbar regions of the spine demonstrate concave curves, while the thoracic and sacral regions represent convex curves. These curves both strengthen the spine and permit a greater range of supported motion.

The Spinal Meninges

The spinal meninges are similar to those covering and protecting the structures within the cranium. They consist of the dura mater, the arachnoid, and the pia mater. The meninges cover the entire spinal cord and the peripheral nerve roots as they leave the spinal column. However, the spinal meninges are not as strongly secured to the spinal column as the meninges are to the cranium. The dura mater is firmly attached to the base of the skull and to a collagen fiber called the coc-cygeal ligament at the top of the sacrum. These attachments and the dura mater's attachments associated with each pair of peripheral nerve roots help position the cord centrally within the spinal canal yet permit the column to move around the cord (Figure 3-56).

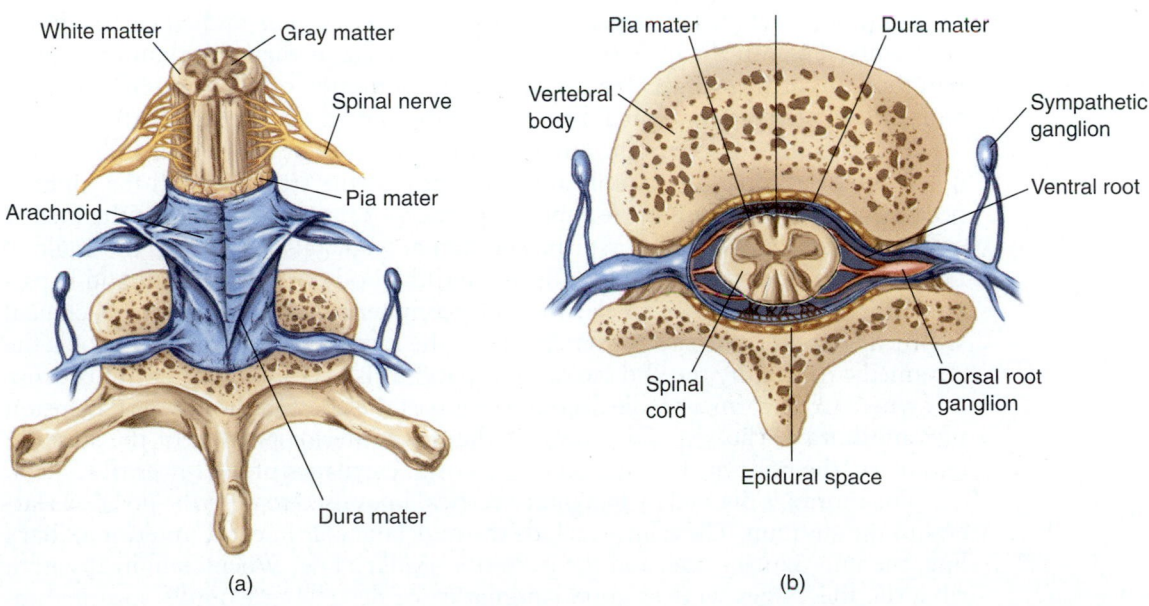

FIGURE 3-56 Structural protection of the spinal cord.

As it does in the brain, cerebrospinal fluid bathes the spinal cord by filling the subarachnoid space. The fluid provides a medium for the exchange of nutrients and waste products and absorbs the shocks of sudden movements. Cerebrospinal fluid is produced in the ventricles of the brain and then circulates through the ventricles and through the arachnoid space of the spinal meninges. The fluid is absorbed by specialized cells (the arachnoid villi) in the lower portion of the lumbar meninges, a region called the spinal cistern.

The distance between the spinal cord and the interior of the vertebral foramen varies in the different spinal regions. The region with the closest tolerance between the cord and the interior surfaces of the spinal foramen is the thoracic spine, where movement of the spinal column is most limited. Although this region is injured only infrequently, just a slight displacement into the vertebral foramen is likely to cause spinal cord injury. The greatest spacing between the cord and the interior of the vertebral column is found in upper lumbar and upper cervical (C-1 and C-2) regions.

Injuries to the mid- or lower lumbar regions do not endanger the spinal cord because the cord ends at the L-1 level in mature adults. Injury to the lumbar spine can, however, damage the peripheral nerve roots there. The vertebral foramen below L-1 is filled with cerebrospinal fluid and is where the fluid may be most safely removed for diagnostic testing (spinal tap).

THE THORAX

The thoracic cage is the chamber that moves air in and out and where oxygen and carbon dioxide are exchanged to support the body's metabolism. It consists of the thoracic skeleton, diaphragm, and associated musculature. It is also the location of the heart, major blood vessels, and other important structures essential for body function. It contains the trachea, bronchi, and lungs, and the mediastinum. Finally, the dynamics of the chest, respiration, are controlled by a series of centers in the brain and blood vessels.

The Thoracic Skeleton

The thoracic skeleton is defined by 12 pairs of C-shaped ribs, which articulate posteriorly with the thoracic spine and then extend in an anterior and inferior direction (Figure 3-57). The upper seven pairs join the sternum at their cartilaginous endpoints. The 8th through 10th ribs have cartilage at their distal anterior ends that join the cartilage of the 7th rib at the inferior margin of the sternum. The 11th and 12th ribs are often termed the floating ribs and have no anterior attachment.

The sternum completes the anterior bony structure of the thorax and is made up of three sections: the manubrium, the body of the sternum, and the xiphoid process. The manubrium is the superior portion of the sternum and is the medial endpoint of the clavicle and first rib. The sternal angle (also known as the angle of Louis) is the junction of the manubrium and the body of the sternum and is palpable through the skin as an elevation or prominence. This structure has clinical significance as it is the site of attachment of the second rib and quickly allows the paramedic to identify the 2nd intercostal space. This location is important because it is where to perform a needle decompression of the chest in the event of a tension pneumothorax. The xiphoid process is the most inferior portion of the sternum and meets the body at the junction of the costal cartilages of the lower ribs.

The thorax is divided by imaginary vertical lines used to describe positions lateral to the sternum. These lines include the midclavicular line, the anterior axillary line, the mid-axillary line, and the posterior axillary line. When combined with a rib level, these lines serve as good landmarks for describing wounds, locating underlying structures, and for identifying locations to perform procedures. The space

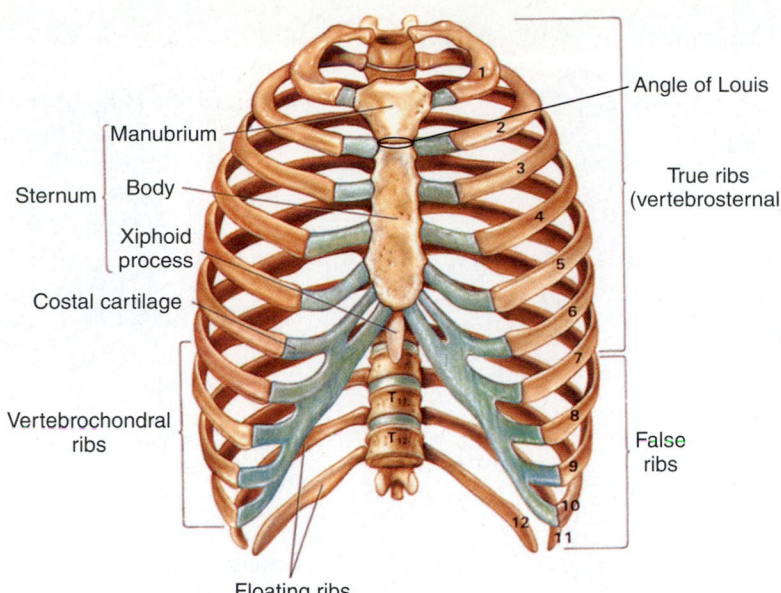

FIGURE 3-57 Skeletal components of the thorax.

Manubrium

Sternum — Body

Xiphoid process

Costal cartilage

Vertebrochondral ribs

Floating ribs

Angle of Louis

True ribs (vertebrosternal)

False ribs

just inferior to each rib is called an intercostal space and is given the number of the rib above it. For example, the anterior axillary line extends from the anterior margin of the axilla (armpit) inferiorly along the thoracic wall. Its intersection with the 5th intercostal space is generally used in the emergency department to place a thoracostomy tube in patients with pneumothorax or hemothorax. It is not frequently used for prehospital needle decompression because this site is often obscured by the patient's arms or by immobilization devices and blankets.

The thoracic inlet is the superior opening in the thorax. It is narrow in comparison to the thoracic outlet, and is defined by the curvature of the first rib, with its posterior attachment at the first thoracic vertebra and ending anteriorly, at the manubrium. The thoracic outlet is formed posteriorly by the 12th vertebra, laterally by the curvature of the 12th rib, and extends anteriorly and superiorly along the costal margin to the **xiphisternal joint**.

✱ **xiphisternal joint** union between xiphoid process and body of the sternum.

The Diaphragm

The diaphragm is a muscular, dome-like structure that separates the abdominal cavity from the thoracic cavity. It is affixed to the lower border of the rib cage, while its central and superior margin may extend to the level of the 4th intercostal space anteriorly and the 6th intercostal space posteriorly during maximal expiration. This superior positioning may allow penetrating wounds of the lower half of the thorax to penetrate the diaphragm and enter the abdominal cavity. The aorta, esophagus, and inferior vena cava exit the thoracic cavity through separate openings in this structure. The diaphragm is a major muscle of respiration, contracting to displace the floor of the thoracic cavity downward during inspiration and relaxing and moving upward with expiration.

Associated Musculature

The chest wall musculature along with the shoulder musculature, clavicles, scapula, and humerus provide additional protection to the vital structures within the upper thorax (Figure 3-58). The clavicles articulate laterally with the acromion process of the scapula. The scapula covers the posterior and lateral aspects of the first six ribs and articulates with the humerus to complete the shoulder girdle.

Ribs and
sternum
elevate

Diaphragm
contracts

Ribs
raised

External
intercostal
muscles
active

Diaphragm
contracts
and moves
downward

Ribs
lowered

Internal
intercostal
muscles
active

Diaphragm
relaxes
and moves
upward

Inspiration   Expiration

FIGURE 3-58   The diaphragm and muscles of the chest change its volume to effect respirations.

Chest wall muscles between the ribs, called the intercostal muscles, along with the diaphragm and the sternocleidomastoid muscles are the major muscles of respiration. The sternocleidomastoid muscles raise the upper rib and sternum and, with the sternum, the anterior attachments of the next nine ribs. The intercostal muscles contract to further elevate the ribs and increase the anterior-posterior dimension of the thorax. Simultaneously, the diaphragm, which forms the floor of the thorax, contracts and flattens to further increase the volume of the thoracic cavity. As the thoracic volume increases, the pressure within it becomes less than atmospheric. Air rushes in through the tracheobronchial tree and into the alveoli to equalize this pressure gradient, filling the lungs.

As the musculature relaxes, the diaphragm again intrudes upward into the thoracic cavity, the ribs and sternum move inferiorly, and the ribs move closer together in an inferior and posterior direction. This decreases the thoracic volume and increases the intrathoracic pressure. When the pressure within the thorax exceeds that of the surrounding atmosphere, air rushes out. Therefore exhalation in the resting state is largely a passive activity aided by the elastic recoil of the lungs. Gravity helps facilitate this action with downward displacement of the ribs in either the upright or supine position. This changing of volume to move air in and out is called the bellows effect.

The changing volume and pressure within the thoracic cage also assist with the pumping of blood to and venous return from the systemic circulation. The decreased intrathoracic pressure of inspiration helps move venous blood toward the thorax and heart, while the increased pressure of expiration helps move arterial blood away from the heart and thorax. The changing intrathoracic pressure affects the blood pressure and pulse strength. Normally, the systolic blood pressure and pulse strength fall during inspiration and rise during expiration.

The diaphragm is the primary muscle of respiration. The intercostal muscles are recruited to increase the depth of respiration. As the rate, depth, and work of respiration increase due to exercise or stress from trauma or infection, more ac-

Normal inspiration is an active process, while normal expiration is a passive process.

cessory muscles of ventilation are recruited. These include the sternocleidomastoid and scalene muscles of the neck for inspiration and the anterior abdominal muscles to aid in forceful exhalation. The rhomboid muscles lift, abduct, and rotate the scapulae to help lift the upper chest with inspiration. The cough reflex, important to keeping the airways clear and alveoli expanded, depends on the addition of the latissimus dorsi muscles located along the posterior and lateral thoracic wall and the erector spinae muscles along the spine to allow for forceful contraction of the thorax.

Trachea, Bronchi, and Lungs

Contained within the thoracic cavity are the tracheobronchial tree and the lungs. The trachea is the hollow and cartilage-supported respiratory pathway through which air moves in and out of the thorax and lungs. It enters through the thoracic inlet and divides into the right and left mainstem bronchi at the carina, located in the upper central thorax. The right and left mainstem bronchi extend for about 3 centimeters and enter their respective lungs at the **pulmonary hilum.** The pulmonary hilum is also where the pulmonary arteries enter and the pulmonary veins exit the lungs and is the sole point of fixation of the lung in the thoracic cage. The bronchi then further divide into bronchioles, which ultimately terminate in the alveoli. The lungs contain millions of these tiny "grape" shaped alveoli, which are the basic unit of structure and function in the lungs.

> ✳ **pulmonary hilum** central medial region of the lung where the bronchi and pulmonary vasculature enter the lung.

Each lung occupies one side of the thoracic cavity and is divided into lobes. The right lung has three lobes, the upper, middle and lower. The left lung has two lobes, the upper and lower. The left upper lobe contains the cardiac notch against which the heart rests. The lower section of the left upper lobe (the lingula), projects around the lateral border of the heart and corresponds to the middle lobe of the right lung.

The lungs are covered by the visceral pleura, a smooth membrane that lines the exterior of the lungs. It folds over on itself at the pulmonary hilum and then lines the inside of the thoracic cavity, becoming the parietal pleura. This dual layer forms a potential space called the pleural space. It contains a small amount of serous (pleural) fluid for lubrication and permits the lungs to expand and contract easily. This dual layer also creates the seal that causes the lungs to expand and contract with the changing volume of the thoracic cavity.

> *The layers of the pleura and the small volume of fluid between them cause the lungs to move with the thoracic cage.*
>
>

The trachea, bronchi, and lungs are discussed further in the Respiratory System section later in this chapter.

Mediastinum and Heart

The mediastinum (Figure 3-59) is the central space within the thoracic cavity bounded laterally by the lungs, inferiorly by the diaphragm, and superiorly by the thoracic outlet. The heart is located within and fills most of the mediastinum. (The heart is discussed in detail in the Cardiovascular System section, later in this chapter.) Through the mediastinum, the great vessels (see the next section) traverse to and from the heart, and the trachea and esophagus enter the thorax. The esophagus then courses anterior to the aorta before exiting through the diaphragm at the thoracic outlet (esophageal hiatus or foramen).

The vagus nerve, which provides parasympathetic innervation of thoracic and abdominal viscera, enters the thorax bilaterally through the thoracic inlet and traverses the mediastinum giving branches to the larynx, esophagus, trachea, bronchi, and heart. The vagus nerve then exits the thorax through the esophageal opening in the diaphragm to innervate the abdominal viscera. The phrenic nerve (originating from the 3rd, 4th, and 5th cervical nerve roots) also enters the thorax through the thoracic inlet and traverses the thorax to innervate the diaphragm.

FIGURE 3-59 Structures of the mediastinum and thorax.

Right pleural cavity

Bronchus of lung

Esophagus

Tissue of mediastinum

Aorta

Pulmonary artery

Left pleural cavity

Pulmonary vein

Superior vena cava

Right atrium

Right ventricle

Aorta

Visceral pericardium

Parietal pericardium

Pericardial cavity

Left ventricle

Left atrium

The thoracic duct (part of the lymphatic system) also traverses the thorax from the thoracic outlet where it enters through the aortic opening in the diaphragm. It typically crosses the midline from the right side of the aorta in the posterior mediastinum at the level of the 5th thoracic vertebra and then ascends above the level of the left clavicle before arching back downward to empty into the left internal jugular vein. The thoracic duct carries most of the body's lymphatic drainage (all but the right side of the head, neck, thorax, and right upper extremity).

Great Vessels

The **great vessels** are those large arteries and veins that enter and leave the heart and are found in the mediastinum. They are the aorta, the superior and inferior vena cava, the pulmonary arteries, and the pulmonary veins. Injury to these large vascular structures can lead to significant blood loss and death if the condition is not quickly recognized and repaired. The aorta, which is fixed at three positions within the thorax, is not only susceptible to penetrating injury, but also to blunt injury by rapid deceleration or shear forces. It is fixed at the annulus where it attaches to the heart, at the **ligamentum arteriosum** near the bifurcation of the pulmonary artery, and at the aortic hiatus where it passes through the diaphragm and enters the abdomen.

Other major vessels that branch from the great vessels in the upper thorax include the subclavian arteries and veins, the common carotid arteries, and the innominate artery (which is the first large branch off the aortic arch dividing into the right common carotid and right subclavian). The internal mammary vessels are inferior branches of the subclavians running along the anterior surface of the pleura, posterior to the costochondral (rib-cartilage) junction. They are often harvested for coronary artery bypass grafts. The intercostal arteries are branches of the thoracic aorta (except for the first two, which arise from branches of the sub-

✱ great vessels the large arteries and veins located in the mediastinum that enter and exit the heart; the aorta, superior and inferior vena cava, pulmonary arteries, and pulmonary veins.

✱ ligamentum arteriosum cord-like remnant of a fetal vessel connecting the pulmonary artery to the aorta at the aortic isthmus.

clavian) that run along the lower margins of the ribs along with the intercostal nerves. Finally, the bronchial arteries (one right and two left) are usually branches of the thoracic aorta that nourish the non-respiratory tissues of the lung.

Esophagus

The esophagus enters the thorax through the thoracic inlet with and just posterior to the trachea. It continues the length of the mediastinum and exits through the esophageal hiatus of the diaphragm. It is a muscular tube that is contiguous with the posterior wall of the trachea and conducts food and drink from the oral pharynx to the stomach. It moves food and liquid toward the stomach through a rhythmic muscular contraction called peristalsis. During vomiting, peristalsis reverses and propels the emesis up the esophagus.

THE NERVOUS SYSTEM

The nervous system is the body's principal control system. This network of cells, tissues, and organs regulates nearly all bodily functions via electrical impulses transmitted through nerves, all of which are highly susceptible to hypoxia (oxygen deficiency). The endocrine system is closely related to the nervous system. It exerts bodily control via hormones. You will learn more about this system later in this chapter. A third system, the circulatory system, assists in regulatory functions by distributing hormones and other chemical messengers.

The nervous system consists of two main divisions—the central nervous system and the peripheral nervous system. The **central nervous system** consists of the brain and the spinal cord. The **peripheral nervous system** is somewhat more complex. As you look at Figure 3-60, note that the peripheral nervous system is divided into two major subdivisions—the **somatic nervous system,** which governs voluntary functions (those we control consciously), and the **autonomic nervous system** which has two subdivisions—the **sympathetic nervous system** and the **parasympathetic nervous system.** These two subdivisions of the autonomic nervous system work together to carry out involuntary physiological processes such as regulation of blood pressure, heart rate, and digestion.

You will learn more about these divisions of the nervous system as you continue through the next pages. As you read, it will be helpful if you think of the nervous system as a "living computer." The central nervous system is the central processing unit and the various divisions of the peripheral nervous system carry on the input and output processes.

FUNDAMENTAL UNIT: THE NEURON

The fundamental unit of the nervous system is the nerve cell, or **neuron.** The neuron includes the *cell body* (soma), containing the nucleus; the *dendrites,* which transmit electrical impulses to the cell body; and the *axons,* which transmit electrical impulses away from the cell body (Figure 3-61).

The transmission of impulses in the nervous system resembles the conduction of electrical impulses through the heart. In its resting state, the neuron is positively charged on the outside and negatively charged on the inside. When electrically stimulated, sodium rapidly surges into the cell and potassium rapidly leaves it so that there is no longer a difference in electrical charge between the inside and the outside. This "depolarization," or loss of the charge difference, is subsequently transmitted down the neuron at an extremely high rate of speed.

The neuron joins with other neurons at junctions called *synapses* (Figure 3-62). The neurons never come into direct contact with each other at these synapses.

The nervous system is the body's principal control system.

* **central nervous system** the brain and the spinal cord.

* **peripheral nervous system** part of the nervous system that extends throughout the body and is composed of the cranial nerves arising from the brain and the peripheral nerves arising from the spinal cord. Its subdivisions are the somatic and the autonomic nervous systems.

* **somatic nervous system** part of the nervous system controlling voluntary bodily functions.

* **autonomic nervous system** part of the nervous system controlling involuntary bodily functions. It is divided into the sympathetic and the parasympathetic systems.

* **sympathetic nervous system** division of the autonomic nervous system that prepares the body for stressful situations. Sympathetic nervous system actions include increased heart rate and dilation of the bronchioles and pupils. Its actions are mediated by the neurotransmitters epinephrine and norepinephrine.

* **parasympathetic nervous system** division of the autonomic nervous system that is responsible for controlling vegetative functions. Parasympathetic nervous system actions include decreased heart rate and constriction of the bronchioles and pupils. Its actions are mediated by the neurotransmitter acetylcholine.

* **neuron** nerve cell; the fundamental component of the nervous system.

FIGURE 3-60 Overview of the nervous system.

FIGURE 3-61 Anatomy of a neuron.

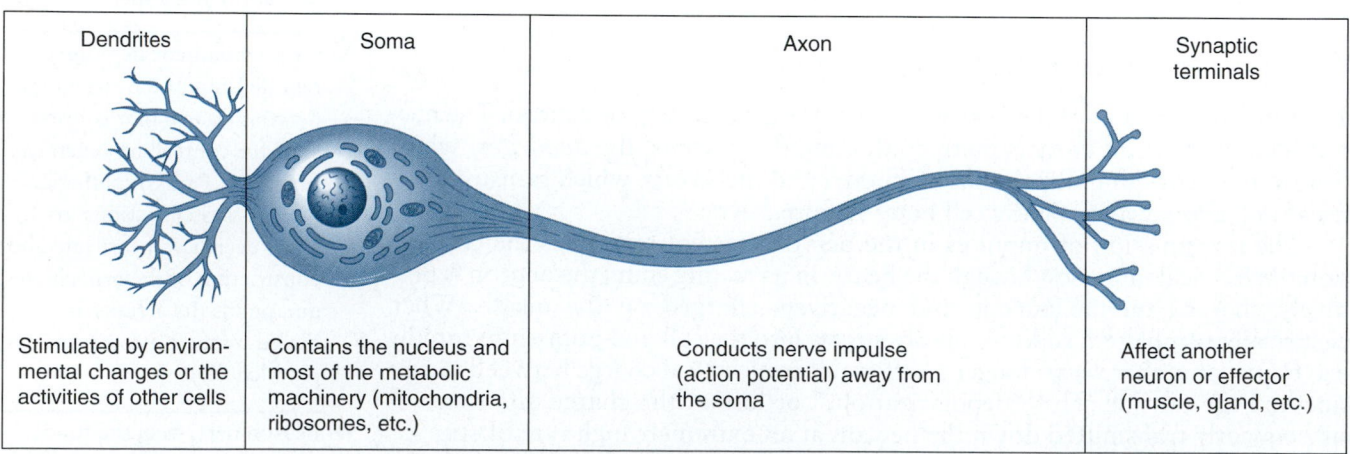

Dendrites	Soma	Axon	Synaptic terminals
Stimulated by environmental changes or the activities of other cells	Contains the nucleus and most of the metabolic machinery (mitochondria, ribosomes, etc.)	Conducts nerve impulse (action potential) away from the soma	Affect another neuron or effector (muscle, gland, etc.)

FIGURE 3-62 The synapse: (a) electron micrograph, (b) schematic.

Instead, upon reaching the synapse, the axon causes the release of a chemical **neurotransmitter.** This neurotransmitter, either acetylcholine or norepinephrine, then crosses the gap between the axon of the depolarized neuron and the dendrite of the adjacent neuron. The neurotransmitter stimulates the post-synaptic membrane of the connecting nerve. Acetylcholine is the neurotransmitter of the parasympathetic and voluntary (somatic) nervous systems. Norepinephrine is found in the synaptic terminals of sympathetic nerves. (See the later description of the divisions of the peripheral nervous system.)

✱ neurotransmitter a substance that is released from the axon terminal of a presynaptic neuron upon excitation and that travels across the synaptic cleft to either excite or inhibit the target cell. Examples include acetylcholine, norepinephrine, and dopamine.

THE CENTRAL NERVOUS SYSTEM

Knowledge of the anatomy and physiology of the central nervous system—the brain and the spinal cord—is essential to understanding and treating nervous system emergencies. Note that the basic structures of the central nervous system and some of the related terminology were presented earlier in the chapter under the headings "The Head, Face, and Neck" and "The Spine and Thorax."

Content Review

CENTRAL NERVOUS SYSTEM
- Brain
- Spinal cord

Protective Structures

Most of the central nervous system is protected by bony structures. The brain lies within the cranial vault, protected by the skull. Covered by the scalp, the cranium consists of the bones of the head, excluding the facial bones. Bones composing the cranium include two single bones—the frontal and occipital bones—and a series of paired bones—the parietals, temporals, sphenoids, and ethmoids (Figure 3-63; also review Figure 3-44).

The spinal cord is housed inside and is protected by the "spinal canal" formed by the vertebrae of the spinal column (Review Figure 3-54).

Protective membranes called the *meninges* cover the entire central nervous system. There are three layers of meninges that pad, or cushion, the brain and spinal cord (Figure 3-64). The durable, outermost layer is referred to as the *dura mater.* The middle layer is a web-like structure known as the *arachnoid membrane.* The innermost layer, directly overlying the central nervous system, is

FIGURE 3-63   The bones of the skull.

Frontal bone

Ethmoid bone

Sphenoid bone

Foramen ovale

Temporal bone

Foramen spinosum

Parietal bone

Occipital bone

Sella turcica

Foramen rotundum

Foramen lacerum

Foramen magnum

Jugular foramen

Hypoglossal canal

White matter

Gray matter

Spinal nerve

Arachnoid membrane

Pia mater

Dura mater

(a)

Skin of scalp

Periosteum

Bone of skull

Epidural space

Dura mater

Subdural space

Arachnoid membrane

Subarachnoid space

Pia mater

Lobe of brain

(b)

FIGURE 3-64   The meninges: (a) posterior view of the spinal cord showing the meningeal layers; (b) the meninges of the brain.

called the *pia mater*. The space between the pia mater and the arachnoid membrane is referred to as the subarachnoid space, while the space between the dura mater and the arachnoid membrane is called the subdural space. The space outside the dura mater is called the epidural space. Both the brain and the spinal cord are bathed in *cerebrospinal fluid,* a watery, clear fluid that acts as a cushion to protect these organs from physical impact.

The Brain

The brain is the largest part of the central nervous system. The following information provides a general profile of the brain's anatomy and physiology.

Divisions of the Brain Filling the cranial vault, the brain is divided into six major parts: the cerebrum, the diencephalon (which includes the thalamus and hypothalamus), the mesencephalon (midbrain), the pons, the medulla oblongata, and the cerebellum (Figure 3-65).

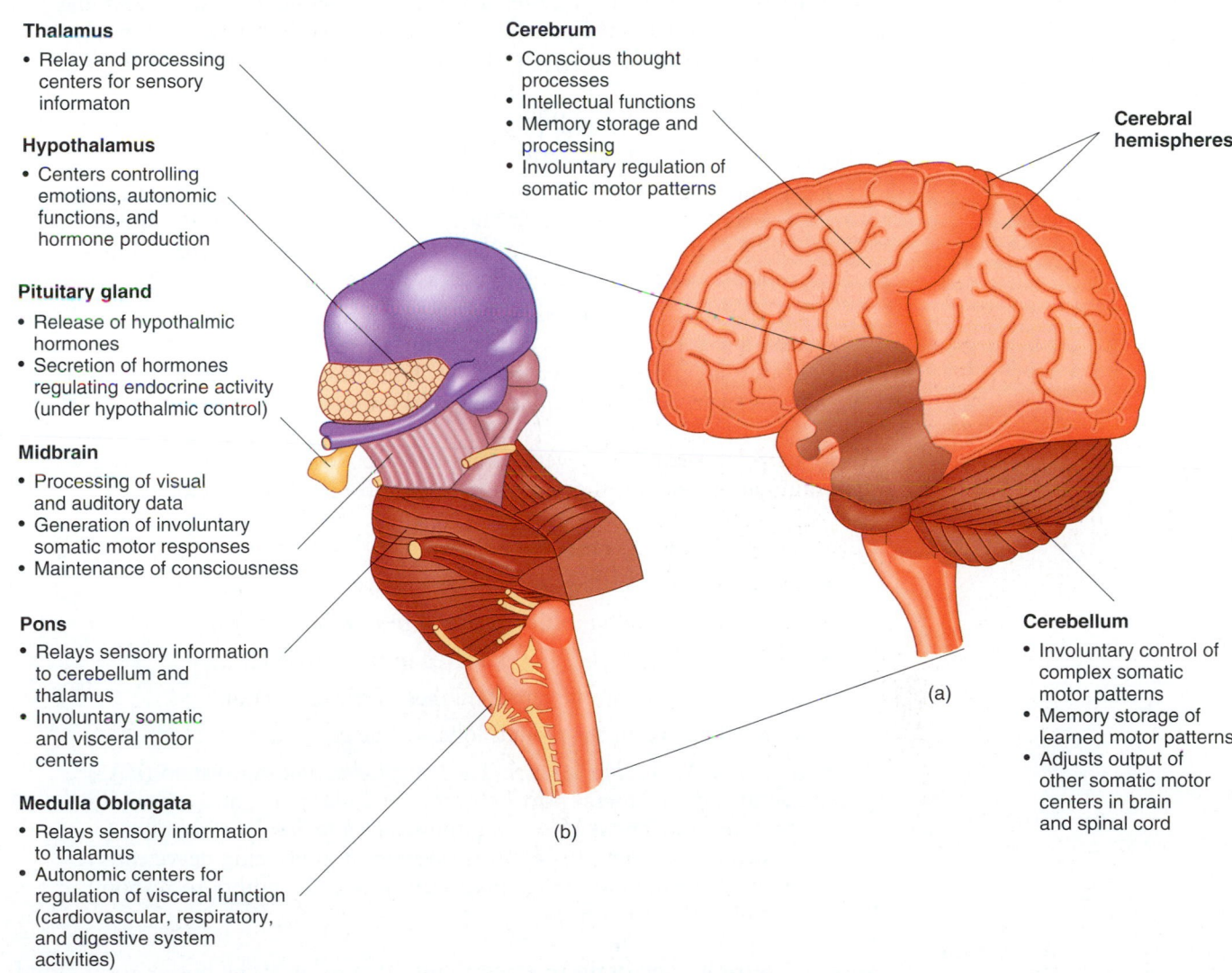

Thalamus
- Relay and processing centers for sensory informaton

Hypothalamus
- Centers controlling emotions, autonomic functions, and hormone production

Pituitary gland
- Release of hypothalmic hormones
- Secretion of hormones regulating endocrine activity (under hypothalmic control)

Midbrain
- Processing of visual and auditory data
- Generation of involuntary somatic motor responses
- Maintenance of consciousness

Pons
- Relays sensory information to cerebellum and thalamus
- Involuntary somatic and visceral motor centers

Medulla Oblongata
- Relays sensory information to thalamus
- Autonomic centers for regulation of visceral function (cardiovascular, respiratory, and digestive system activities)

Cerebrum
- Conscious thought processes
- Intellectual functions
- Memory storage and processing
- Involuntary regulation of somatic motor patterns

Cerebral hemispheres

Cerebellum
- Involuntary control of complex somatic motor patterns
- Memory storage of learned motor patterns
- Adjusts output of other somatic motor centers in brain and spinal cord

(a)

(b)

FIGURE 3-65   The human brain: (a) superficial view of the brain; (b) components of the brainstem.

The cerebrum and diencephalon constitute the *forebrain*.

- *Cerebrum*. The cerebrum is in the anterior and middle area of the cranium. Containing two hemispheres, it is joined by a structure called the *corpus callosum*. The cerebrum governs all sensory and motor actions. It is the seat of intelligence, learning, analysis, memory, and language. The *cerebral cortex* is the outermost layer of the cerebrum.
- *Diencephalon*. Covered by the cerebrum, the diencephalon is sometimes called the *interbrain*. Inside it are the *thalamus, hypothalamus* (which is connected to the pituitary gland), and the *limbic system*. This area is responsible for many involuntary actions such as temperature regulation, sleep, water balance, stress response, and emotions. It plays a major role in regulating the autonomic nervous system.

The mesencephalon (midbrain), pons, and the medulla oblongata collectively form the *brainstem*. The brainstem and the cerebellum together constitute the *hindbrain*.

- *Mesencephalon,* or *midbrain*. The mesencephalon, located between the diencephalon and the pons, is responsible for certain aspects of motor coordination. The mesencephalon is the major region controlling eye movement.
- *Pons*. Between the midbrain and the medulla oblongata, the pons contains connections between the brain and the spinal cord.
- *Medulla Oblongata*. The medulla oblongata is located between the pons and the spinal cord. It marks the division between the spinal cord and the brain. Located here are major centers for controlling respiration, cardiac activity, and vasomotor activity.
- *Cerebellum*. The cerebellum is located in the posterior fossa of the cranial cavity. It consists of two hemispheres closely related to the brainstem and higher centers. The cerebellum coordinates fine motor movement, posture, equilibrium, and muscle tone.

Areas of Specialization Several areas of specialization are recognized within the brain and have clinical application (Figure 3-66). These include:

- *Speech*. Located in the temporal lobe of the cerebrum.
- *Vision*. Located in the occipital cortex of the cerebrum.
- *Personality*. Located in the frontal lobes of the cerebrum.
- *Balance and Coordination*. Located in the cerebellum.
- *Sensory*. Located in the parietal lobes of the cerebrum.
- *Motor*. Located in the frontal lobes of the cerebrum.
- *Reticular Activating System*. The **reticular activating system (RAS)** operates in the lateral portion of the medulla, pons, and especially the midbrain. The RAS sends impulses to and receives impulses from the cerebral cortex. It is a diffuse system of interlacing nerve cells responsible for maintaining consciousness and the ability to respond to stimuli (Figure 3-67).

Vascular Supply The brain receives about 20 percent of the body's total blood flow per minute. Blood flow to the brain is provided by two systems. The *carotid system* is anterior, while the *vertebrobasilar system* is posterior. Both join at the

Somatic motor association
area (premotor cortex)

Primary motor cortex
(precentral gyrus)

Primary sensory
cortex
(postcentral gyrus)

FRONTAL LOBE

PARIETAL LOBE

Prefrontal cortex

Somatosensory
association area

Visual association area

OCCIPITAL LOBE

Visual cortex

Auditory association area

Olfactory cortex

Auditory cortex

TEMPORAL LOBE

FIGURE 3-66   External anatomy of the brain.

Circle of Willis before entering the structures of the brain (Figure 3-68). The system is designed so that interruption of any part will not cause significant loss of blood flow to the tissues. Venous drainage of the brain is through the venous sinuses and the internal jugular veins.

Besides blood flow, cerebrospinal fluid bathes the brain and spinal cord. Several chambers within the brain, called ventricles, contain most of the intracranial volume of this fluid.

Thalamus

RAS

Midbrain

Pons

Reticular formation

Medulla

Spinal cord

Cerebellum

FIGURE 3-67   The reticular activating system (RAS), which sends and receives messages from various parts of the brain.

FIGURE 3-68 An interior view of the brain showing the Circle of Willis, which is formed by the anterior and posterior communicating arteries.

Anterior communicating artery

Internal carotid artery

Anterior cerebral artery

Posterior communicating artery

Middle cerebral artery

Circle of Willis

Basilar artery

Vertebral artery

The Spinal Cord

✱ **spinal cord** central nervous system pathway responsible for transmitting sensory input from the body to the brain and for conducting motor impulses from the brain to the body muscles and organs.

The **spinal cord** is the central nervous system (CNS) pathway responsible for transmitting sensory input from the body to the brain and for conducting motor impulses from the brain to the body muscles and organs. Through this pathway, the brain monitors and controls most body functions. Additionally, the spinal cord acts as a reflex center, intercepting sensory signals and initiating short-circuited (reflex) signaling to muscle bodies as needed. If this pathway is compromised, control of the body below the injury is lost.

In the fetus, the cord fills the entire length of the vertebral column. However, the growth of cord does not keep pace with the growth of the vertebral column. This discrepancy means that, as a person grows, the peripheral nerve roots are pulled into the spinal foramen. The sheath of the dura below L-2 is thus filled with numerous strands of peripheral nerves. The resulting structure resembles the tail of a horse and is called the cauda equina (Latin for horse's tail). In the adult, the spinal cord extends from the base of the brain (the medulla oblongata) to approximately the L-1 or L-2 level.

Like all central nervous system tissue, the spinal cord constantly needs oxygenated blood. This blood is supplied through paired spinal arteries that branch off the vertebral, cervical, thoracic, and lumbar arteries. These spinal arteries travel through intervertebral foramina, then split into anterior and posterior arteries. On the surface of the spinal cord there are numerous interconnections (anastomoses) between the arteries to provide a better chance for adequate circulation in case of vascular blockage or injury.

✱ **anterior medial fissure** deep crease along the ventral surface of the spinal cord that divides the cord into right and left halves.

✱ **posterior medial sulcus** shallow longitudinal groove along the dorsal surface of the spinal cord.

✱ **gray matter** areas in the central nervous system dominated by nerve cell bodies; the central portion of the spinal cord.

Anatomically, the spinal cord is a long cylinder divided into left and right halves by the **anterior medial fissure** and by the **posterior medial sulcus**. In cross section, the central part of the cord has a butterfly or "H" shape and appears gray in color. This **gray matter** is made up largely of neural cell bodies and plays an important role in the reflex system.

The remaining areas, or **white matter,** then form three bundles or columns of myelinated (covered with a protein sheath) nerve fibers on each side of the cord around the gray matter: the anterior white column, the lateral white column, and the posterior white column. This white matter is composed of nerve cell pathways, called axons. It contains bundles of axons that transmit signals upward to the brain in what are called **ascending tracts** and bundles that transmit signals downward to the body in what are called **descending tracts.** These tracts are paired, one ascending and one descending on each side, and injury may affect either or both.

A thorough discussion of organization and functions of the ascending and descending spinal tracts is beyond the scope of this textbook. However, knowing the functions of some motor and sensory pathways can aid you in recognizing spinal cord injury.

The important ascending (sensory) tracts or fasciculi include the fasciculus gracilis, fasciculus cutaneous, and the spinothalamic tracts. The fasciculus gracilis and fasciculus cutaneous carry sensory impulses of light touch, vibration, and positional sense from the skin, muscles, tendons, and joints to the brain. They are located on the posterior portion of the cord (posterior columns). Their injury causes disruption on the ipsilateral (same side) of the body because the left to right switching occurs at the medulla. The spinothalamic tracts include both lateral and anterior tracts. The anterior pathway conducts pain and temperature, while the lateral pathway conducts touch and pressure sensation. These pathways cross as they enter the cord, hence injury results in contralateral (opposite side) deficits.

The important descending (motor) spinal nerve tract is the corticospinal tract. It is responsible for voluntary and fine muscle movement on the ipsilateral side of the body. This pathway lies on the posterior and lateral portions of the cord. Two other descending tracts are the reticulospinal and rubrospinal tracts. The reticulospinal tract consists of three sub-tracts, one lateral, one medial, and one anterior. It is thought to be involved with sweating and the muscular activity associated with posturing. The rubrospinal tracts are lateral pathways that affect and control fine motor function of the hands and feet. Injury affects the ipsilateral side of the body with both of these pathways.

Spinal Nerves

Spinal nerves are the peripheral nerve roots that branch in pairs from the spinal cord (Figure 3-69). They travel through the intervertebral foramina and have both sensory and motor components. They provide the largest part of the innervation of the skin, muscles, and internal organs.

There are 31 pairs of spinal nerve roots. The first pair exits the spinal column between the skull and the first cervical vertebra. Each of the next seven pairs exits just below one of the cervical vertebrae and is identified as C-2 through C-8. (While there are only seven cervical vertebrae, there are eight cervical spinal nerves.) There are twelve pairs of thoracic nerves, five lumbar, five sacral, and one coccygeal. Each of these pairs originates just below the vertebra with whose name it is identified. Each spinal nerve pair has two dorsal and two ventral roots. The ventral roots carry motor impulses from the cord to the body, while the dorsal roots carry sensory impulses from the body to the cord. (C-1 and Co [coccygeal]-1 do not have dorsal [sensory] roots.)

The nerve roots often converge in a cluster of nerves called a plexus (Table 3-3). A plexus (or braiding) permits peripheral nerve roots to rejoin and function as a group. The cervical plexus, made up of the first five cervical nerve roots, innervates the neck and produces the phrenic nerve. The phrenic nerve (consisting of peripheral nerve roots C-3 through C-5) is responsible for diaphragm control. The brachial plexus joins the nerves controlling the upper extremity (C-5 through T-1). The lumbar and sacral plexuses control the innervation of the lower extremity.

* **white matter** material that surrounds gray matter in the spinal cord; made up largely of axons.

* **ascending tracts** bundles of axons along the spinal cord that transmit signals from the body to the brain.

* **descending tracts** bundles of axons along the spinal cord that transmit signals from the brain to the body.

* **spinal nerves** 31 pairs of nerves that originate along the spinal cord from anterior and posterior nerve roots.

FIGURE 3-69 The spinal cord and spinal nerves.

Lesser occipital nerve
Greater auricular nerve
Transverse cervical nerve
Supraclavicular nerve
Phrenic nerve

Axillary nerve
Musculocutaneous nerve
Thoracic nerves
Median nerve
Radial nerve
Ulnar nerve

Iliohypogastric nerve
Genitofemoral nerve
Ilioinguinal nerve
Lateral femoral cutaneous nerve
Obturator nerve
Femoral nerve
Gluteal nerves — Superior / Inferior
Sciatic nerve
Saphenous nerve

Cervical plexus
Brachial plexus
Lumbosacral plexus
Lumbar plexus
Sacral plexus

C_1 C_2 C_3 C_4 C_5 C_6 C_7 C_8 T_1 T_2 T_3 T_4 T_5 T_6 T_7 T_8 T_9 T_{10} T_{11} T_{12} L_1 L_2 L_3 L_4 L_5 S_1 S_2 S_3 S_4 S_5 Co_1

Dorsal root
Dorsal root ganglion
White matter
Central canal
Posterior median sulcus
Spinal nerve
Ventral root
Gray matter
Anterior median sulcus
C_3

T_3
T_{12}
L_2

Table 3-3 — SPINAL NERVE PLEXUSES

Plexus	Origin	Nerve	Control	Result of Injury
Cervical	C-1 to C-5	phrenic	diaphragm	respiratory paralysis
Brachial	C-5 to C-8, T-1	axillary	deltoid/skin of shoulder	deltoid muscle paralysis
		radial	triceps/forearm	wristdrop
		median	flexor muscles, forearm, arm	decreased usage
		musculocutaneous	flexor muscles of arm	decreased usage
		ulnar	wrist/hand	claw hand; inability to spread fingers
Lumbar	T-12 to L-4	femoral	lower abdomen, gluteus, thighs	inability to extend leg, flex hip
		obturator	abductor muscles medial thigh	decrease in usage
Sacral	L-4 to 5-3	sciatic	lower extremity	decreased usage

FIGURE 3-70 The dermatomes. Each dermatome corresponds to a spinal nerve.

The sensory components of the spinal nerves innervate specific and discrete areas of the body surface. These areas are called **dermatomes** and are distributed from the occiput of the head to the heel of the foot and buttocks (Figure 3-70). Key locations to recognize for assessment include the collar region (C-3), the little finger (C-7), the nipple line (T-4), the umbilicus (T-10), and the small toe (S-1).

The motor components of the spinal nerve roots also innervate discrete tissues and muscles of the body in regions called **myotomes**. However, as the body grows and matures, some muscles merge and their control is not as specific as it is with the dermatomes. Key myotomes for neurologic evaluation include arm extension (C-5), elbow extension (C-7), small finger abduction (T-1), knee extension (L-3), and ankle flexion (S-1). Evaluation of areas controlled by both dermatomes and myotomes can help you identify the spinal cord region associated with an injury.

The spinal cord also performs some primary processing functions, speeding body responses and helping the brain maintain balance and muscle tone. These responses, called reflexes, occur as special neurons in the cord, called interneurons, intercept sensory signals (Figure 3-71). For example, if you touch a hot stove, the severe pain sends an intense signal to the brain. This strong signal simultaneously triggers an interneuron in the spinal cord to direct a signal to the flexor muscles telling them to contract. The limb withdraws without waiting for the signal sent to the brain to reach it, be processed, and trigger a command to be sent back to the limb. The speed of this reflex action reduces the seriousness of injury. Other reflexes help stabilize the body if it stands in one position for a length of time. As the

✱ **dermatome** topographical region of the body surface innervated by one nerve root.

✱ **myotome** muscle and tissue of the body innervated by a spinal nerve root.

FIGURE 3-71 The reflex response.

To brain

Painful stimulus

Extensors stimulated

Extensors inhibited

Flexors inhibited

Flexors stimulated

stretch receptors report the body is moving, the interneurons signal muscles to counteract the movement to help maintain position. This again reduces the body's reaction time and allows the body to stand or maintain a steady position.

The spinal nerves can be further subdivided according to the division of the autonomic nervous system they serve and to their spinal origin. The parasympathetic nervous system controls rest and regenerative functions and consists of the peripheral nerve roots branching from the sacral region and the cranial nerves (predominantly the vagus nerve). The parasympathetic nervous system's major tasks are to slow the heart and increase digestive system activity; the system also plays a role in sexual stimulation. The sympathetic nervous system adjusts the body's metabolic rate to waking activity, provides "fight-or-flight" functions, and branches from nerves originating in the thoracic and lumbar regions. This system decreases organ and digestive activity through vasoconstriction, constricts the venous blood vessels, and affects the body's metabolic rate through the release of the adrenal hormones norepinephrine and epinephrine. In shock, the sympathetic nervous system causes systemic vasoconstriction to reduce the venous blood volume and increase peripheral vascular resistance. It also increases the heart rate to increase cardiac output in response to dropping preload and blood pressure.

THE PERIPHERAL NERVOUS SYSTEM

Consisting of the cranial and the peripheral nerves, the peripheral nervous system has both voluntary and involuntary components. The twelve pairs of **cranial nerves** originate in the brain and supply nervous control to the head, neck, and certain thoracic and abdominal organs (Figure 3-72). The peripheral nerves, as described previously, originate in the spinal cord and supply nervous control to the periphery.

The four categories of peripheral nerves are:

- *Somatic Sensory.* These afferent nerves transmit sensations involved in touch, pressure, pain, temperature, and position (proprioception).
- *Somatic Motor.* These efferent fibers carry impulses to the skeletal (voluntary) muscles.

✳ **cranial nerves** twelve pairs of nerves that extend from the lower surface of the brain.

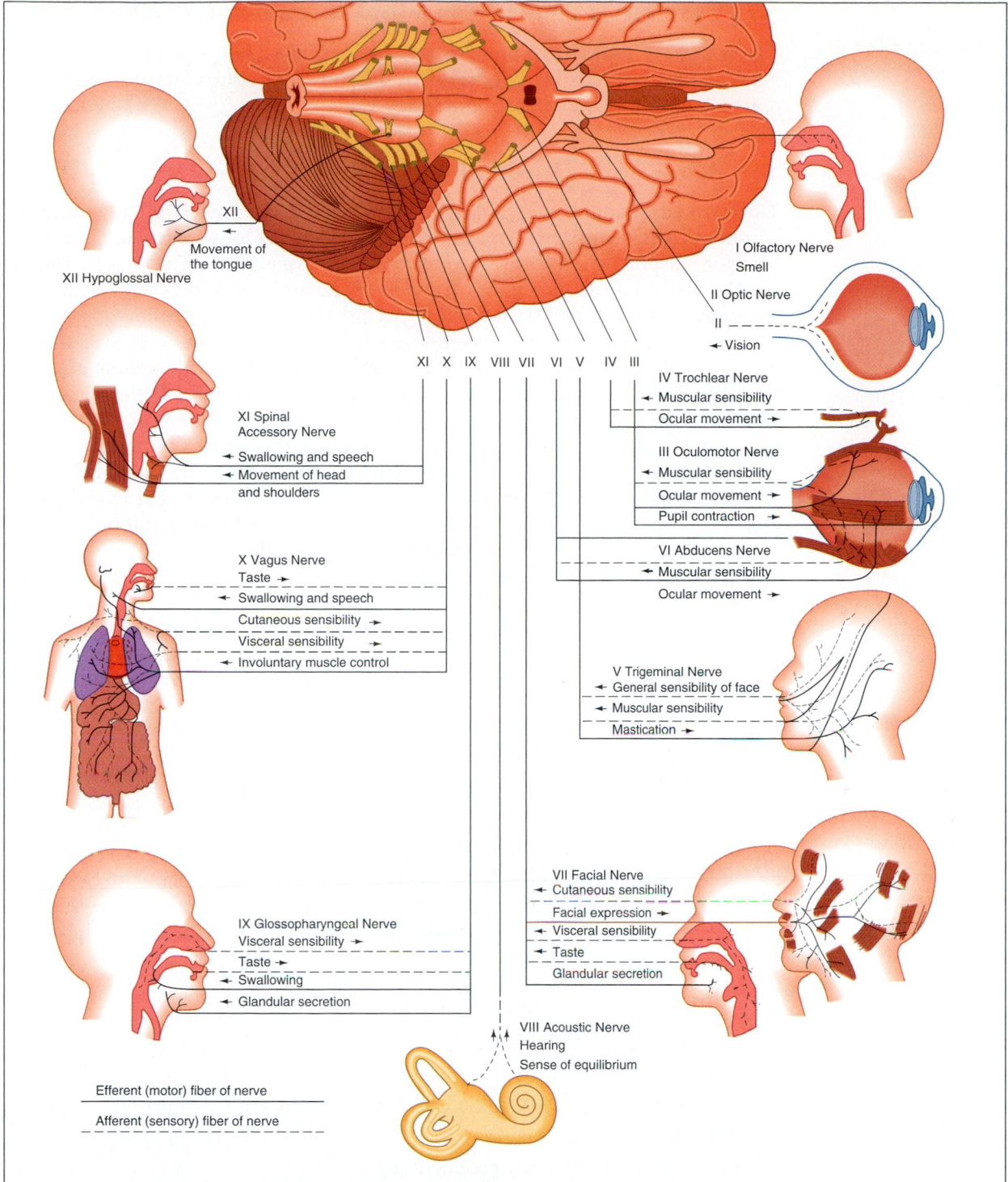

FIGURE 3-72   The cranial nerves.

- *Visceral (Autonomic) Sensory.* These afferent tracts transmit sensations from the visceral organs. Sensations such as a full bladder or the need to defecate are mediated by visceral sensory fibers.
- *Visceral (Autonomic) Motor.* These efferent fibers exit the central nervous system and branch to supply nerves to the involuntary cardiac muscle and smooth muscle of the viscera (organs) and to the glands.

The Somatic (Voluntary) Nervous System

The voluntary component of the peripheral nervous system, often called the somatic nervous system, is responsible for the conscious control of movement, primarily controlling the skeletal muscles.

The Autonomic (Involuntary) Nervous System

The involuntary component of the peripheral nervous system, commonly called the autonomic nervous system, is responsible for the unconscious control of many body functions, including those governed by the smooth muscle, cardiac muscle, and the glands. There are two functional divisions of the autonomic nervous system—the sympathetic nervous system and the parasympathetic nervous system.

✳ **autonomic ganglia** groups of autonomic nerve cells located outside the central nervous system.

The autonomic nervous system arises from the central nervous system. The nerves of the autonomic nervous system exit the central nervous system and subsequently enter specialized structures called **autonomic ganglia.** In the autonomic ganglia, the nerve fibers from the central nervous system interact with nerve fibers that extend from the ganglia to the various target organs. Autonomic nerve fibers that exit the central nervous system and terminate in the autonomic ganglia are called **pre-ganglionic nerves.** Autonomic nerve fibers that exit the ganglia and terminate in the various target tissues are called **post-ganglionic nerves.** The ganglia of the sympathetic nervous system are located close to the spinal cord, while the ganglia of the parasympathetic nervous system are located close to the target organs (Figure 3-73).

✳ **pre-ganglionic nerves** nerve fibers that extend from the central nervous system to the autonomic ganglia.

The sympathetic and parasympathetic systems are antagonistic. In their normal state, they exist in balance with each other. During stress, the sympathetic system dominates. During rest, the parasympathetic system dominates.

✳ **post-ganglionic nerves** nerve fibers that extend from the autonomic ganglia to the target tissues.

The Sympathetic Nervous System The sympathetic nervous system, often referred to as the "fight-or-flight" system, prepares the body for stressful situations. It is located near the thoracic and lumbar part of the spinal cord.

Pre-ganglionic nerves leave the spinal cord through the spinal nerves and end in the sympathetic ganglia. There are two types of sympathetic ganglia: sympathetic chain ganglia and collateral ganglia (Figure 3-74). In addition, special pre-ganglionic sympathetic nerve fibers innervate the adrenal medulla. Post-ganglionic nerves that exit the sympathetic chain ganglia extend to several peripheral target tissues of the sympathetic nervous system. When stimulated, these fibers have several effects. They include:

- Stimulation of secretion by sweat glands
- Constriction of blood vessels in the skin
- Increase in blood flow to skeletal muscles
- Increase in the heart rate and force of cardiac contractions
- Bronchodilation
- Stimulation of energy production

The collateral ganglia are located in the abdominal cavity. Nerves leaving the collateral ganglia innervate many of the organs of the abdomen. Stimulation of these fibers causes several conditions. They include:

- Reduction of blood flow to abdominal organs
- Decreased digestive activity
- Relaxation of smooth muscle in the wall of the urinary bladder
- Release of glucose stores from the liver

FIGURE 3-73 Components of the autonomic nervous system.

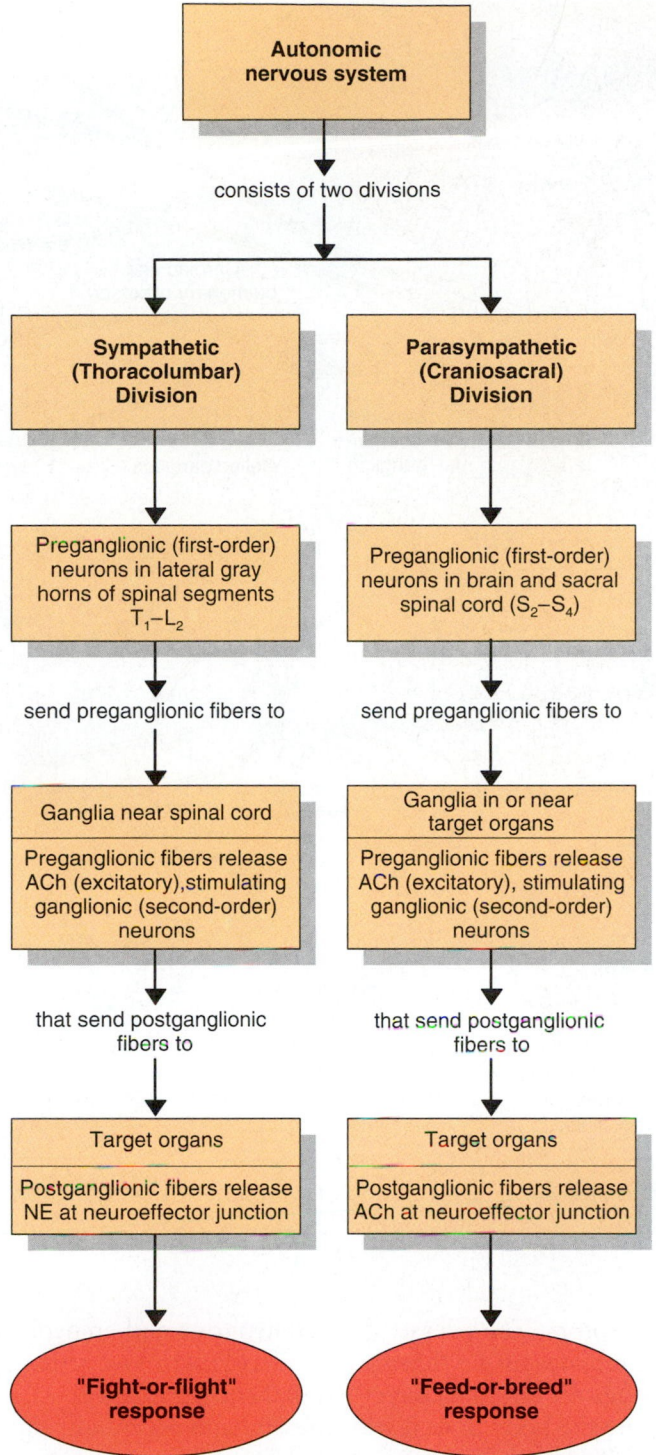

Sympathetic nervous system stimulation also results in direct stimulation of the adrenal medulla, the inner portion of the adrenal gland (Figure 3-75). The adrenal medulla in turn releases the hormones norepinephrine (noradrenalin) and epinephrine (adrenalin) into the circulatory system. Approximately 80 percent of the hormones released by the adrenal medulla are epinephrine, while norepinephrine constitutes the remaining 20 percent. Once released, these hormones are carried throughout the body where they cause their intended effects by acting on hormone

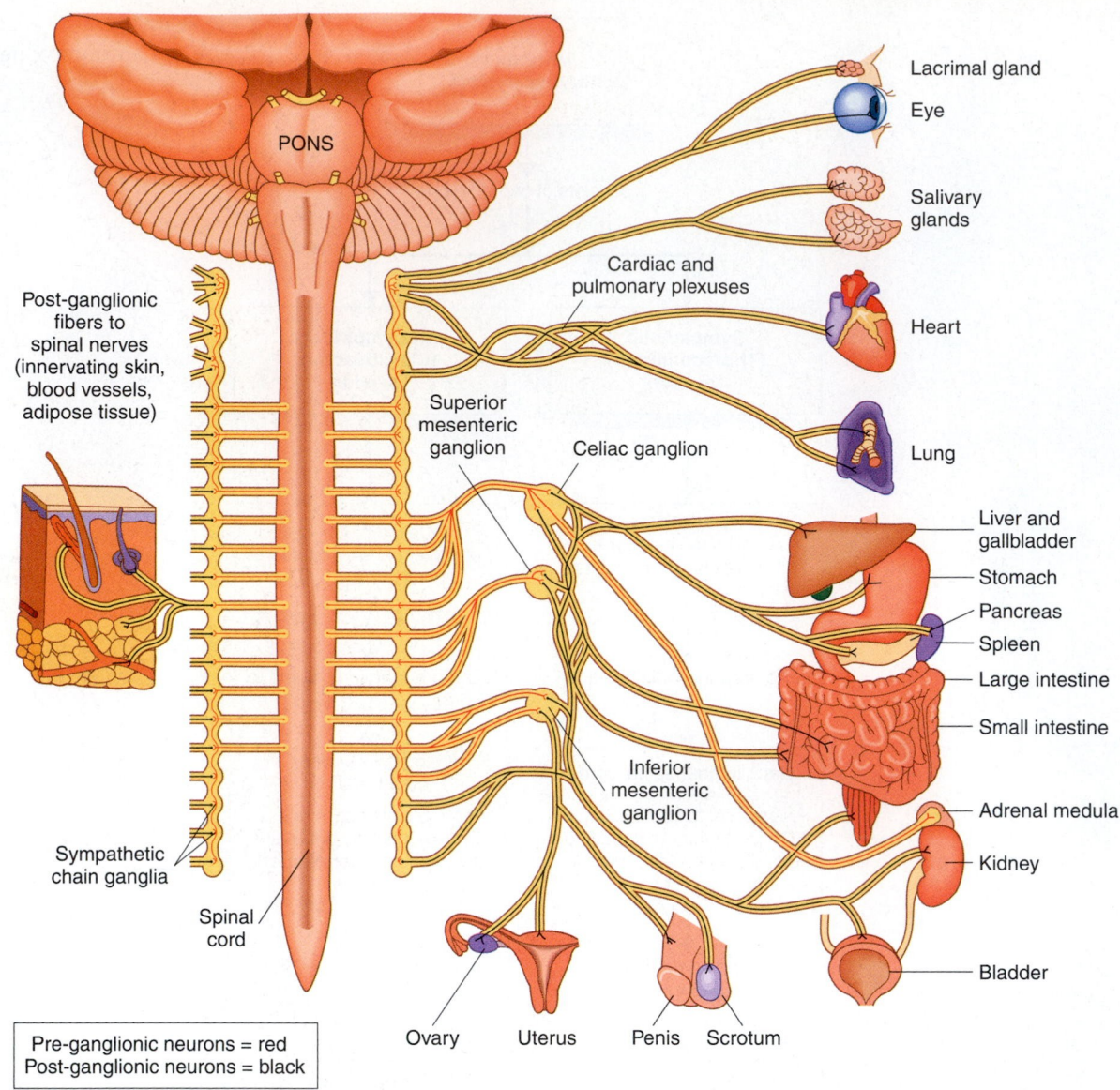

PONS

Post-ganglionic
fibers to
spinal nerves
(innervating skin,
blood vessels,
adipose tissue)

Lacrimal gland

Eye

Salivary
glands

Cardiac and
pulmonary plexuses

Heart

Superior
mesenteric
ganglion

Celiac ganglion

Lung

Liver and
gallbladder

Stomach

Pancreas

Spleen

Large intestine

Small intestine

Inferior
mesenteric
ganglion

Adrenal medula

Kidney

Sympathetic
chain ganglia

Spinal
cord

Bladder

Ovary   Uterus   Penis   Scrotum

Pre-ganglionic neurons = red
Post-ganglionic neurons = black

FIGURE 3-74   Distribution of sympathetic post-ganglionic fibers.

receptors. The release of norepinephrine and epinephrine by the adrenal medulla stimulates tissues that are not innervated by sympathetic nerves. In addition, it prolongs the effects of direct sympathetic stimulation. All of these effects serve to prepare the body to deal with stressful and potentially dangerous situations.

Sympathetic stimulation ultimately results in the release of the hormone norepinephrine from post-ganglionic, presynaptic nerves. The norepinephrine subsequently crosses the synaptic cleft and interacts with adrenergic receptors on the postsynaptic nerves. Shortly thereafter, the norepinephrine is either taken up by the presynaptic neuron for reuse or broken down by enzymes present within the synapse (Figure 3-76). Sympathetic stimulation also results in the release of the hormones epinephrine and norepinephrine from the adrenal medulla. In addition, both epinephrine and norepinephrine interact with specialized adrenergic receptors on the membranes of the target organs. These receptors are located throughout the body. Once stimulated by the appropriate hormone, they cause a response in the organ or organs they control.

FIGURE 3-75 Organization of the sympathetic division of the autonomic nervous system.

FIGURE 3-76 Physiology of an adrenergic synapse. Norepinephrine is released from the presynaptic nerve and stimulates receptors on the postsynaptic nerve. Subsequently, the norepinephrine is either taken up by the presynaptic nerve or deactivated by enzymes in the synapse.

Content Review

TYPES OF SYMPATHETIC RECEPTORS

- Adrenergic
  - alpha₁ (α₁)
  - alpha₂ (α₂)
  - beta₁ (β₁)
  - beta₂ (β₂)
- Dopaminergic

Content Review

CRANIAL NERVES CARRYING PARASYMPATHETIC FIBERS

- III
- VII
- IX
- X

The two known types of sympathetic receptors are the *adrenergic receptors* and the *dopaminergic receptors*. The adrenergic receptors are generally divided into four types. These four receptors are designated alpha₁ (α_1), alpha₂ (α_2), beta₁ (β_1), and beta₂ (β_2). The α_1 receptors cause peripheral vasoconstriction, mild bronchoconstriction, and stimulation of metabolism. The alpha₂ receptors are found on the presynaptic surfaces of sympathetic neuro-effector junctions. Stimulation of alpha₂ receptors is inhibitory. These receptors serve to prevent over-release of norepinephrine in the synapse. When the level of norepinephrine in the synapse gets high enough, the alpha₂ receptors are stimulated and norepinephrine release is inhibited. Stimulation of beta₁ receptors causes increases in heart rate, cardiac contractile force, and cardiac automaticity and conduction. Stimulation of beta₂ receptors causes vasodilation and bronchodilation. Dopaminergic receptors, although not fully understood, evidently cause dilation of the renal, coronary, and cerebral arteries.

The Parasympathetic Nervous System The parasympathetic nervous system, sometimes called the "feed-or-breed" system, is responsible for controlling vegetative functions, such as normal heart rate and blood pressure.

The parasympathetic nervous system arises from the brain stem and the sacral segments of the spinal cord. The pre-ganglionic neurons of the parasympathetic nervous system are typically much longer than those of the sympathetic nervous system, because the ganglia are located close to the target tissues. Parasympathetic nerve fibers that leave the brain stem travel within four of the cranial nerves including the oculomotor nerve (III), the facial nerve (VII), the glosso-pharyngeal nerve (IX), and the vagus nerve (X). These fibers synapse in the parasympathetic ganglia with short post-ganglionic fibers that then continue to their target tissues. Postsynaptic fibers innervate much of the body, including the intrinsic eye muscles, the salivary glands, the heart, the lungs, and most of the organs of the abdominal cavity. The sacral segment of the parasympathetic nervous system forms distinct pelvic nerves that innervate ganglia in the kidneys, bladder, sex organs, and the terminal portions of the large intestine (Figure 3-77). Stimulation of the parasympathetic nervous system results in the following conditions:

- Pupillary constriction
- Secretion by digestive glands
- Reduction in heart rate and cardiac contractile force
- Bronchoconstriction
- Increased smooth muscle activity along the digestive tract

These and other functions facilitate the processing of food, energy absorption, relaxation, and reproduction (Figure 3-78).

All pre-ganglionic and post-ganglionic parasympathetic nerve fibers use acetylcholine as a neurotransmitter. Acetylcholine, when released by presynaptic neurons, crosses the synaptic cleft and activates receptors on the postsynaptic neurons or on the neuroeffector junction. Acetylcholine is also the neurotransmitter for the somatic nervous system and is present in the neuromuscular junction. Acetylcholine is very short-lived. Within a fraction of a second after its release, it is deactivated by another chemical called acetylcholinesterase. Acetic acid and choline, which are produced when acetylcholine is deactivated, are taken back up by the presynaptic neuron (Figure 3-79).

The parasympathetic system has two main types of ACh receptors, nicotinic and muscarinic. Knowing these receptors' locations and functions will greatly simplify learning the functions of drugs in this class. Nicotinic$_N$ (neuron) receptors are found in all autonomic ganglia, where acetylcholine serves as the presynaptic neurotransmitter of both the parasympathetic and sympathetic nervous systems. Nicotinic$_M$ (muscle) receptors are found at the neuromuscular junction and initiate muscular contraction as part of the somatic nervous system. Muscarinic receptors

Ganglionic (second – order) neurons

Target organs

N III — Ciliary ganglion → Intrinsic eye muscles (pupil and lens shape)

N VII — Sphenopalatine and submandibular ganglia → Nasal glands, tear glands, and salivary glands

N IX — Otic ganglion → Parotid salivary gland

N X — Intramural ganglia → Visceral organs of head, neck, thoracic cavity, and most of abdominopelvic cavity

Parasympathetic division of ANS

Preganglionic (first –order) neurons in brain stem

Preganglionic (first–order) neurons in spinal cord segments S$_2$-S$_4$

Pelvic nerves — Intramural ganglia → Visceral organs in lower abdominopelvic cavity

FIGURE 3-77 Organization of the parasympathetic division of the autonomic nervous system.

are found in many organs throughout the body and are primarily responsible for promoting the parasympathetic response. Table 3-4 summarizes the locations and actions of the muscarinic receptors.

THE ENDOCRINE SYSTEM

There are eight major glands in the endocrine system: the hypothalamus, pituitary gland, thyroid gland, parathyroid glands, thymus, pancreas, adrenal glands, and gonads. The pineal gland is also an endocrine gland, but much of its function remains unclear. In addition to the endocrine glands, many body tissues have been found to have endocrine function. These include the kidneys, heart, placenta, and parts of the digestive tract.

The endocrine glands are located throughout the body (Figure 3-80). Although Figure 3-80 shows an adult, remember that the thymus is primarily active during childhood, when it plays a role in maturation of the immune system. By adulthood, the thymus is so small that it is not visualized on chest X-rays. The hormones secreted by endocrine glands, their target tissues, and their effects are listed in Table 3-5.

Content Review

ENDOCRINE GLANDS
- Hypothalamus
- Pituitary
- Thyroid
- Parathyroid
- Thymus
- Pancreas
- Adrenals
- Gonads
- Pineal

Sphenopalatine ganglion
Lacrimal gland
Eye
N III
Ciliary ganglion
N VII
Submandibular ganglion
N IX
Otic ganglion
Salivary glands
Vagus (N X)
Heart
Cardiac Plexus
Lung
Celiac Plexus
Liver and gallbladder
Stomach
Pancreas
Spleen
Large intestine
Hypogastric plexus
Small intestine
Pelvic nerves
Rectum
Kidney
Spinal cord
Bladder
Ovary
Uterus
Penis
Scrotum

Preganglionic neurons = red
Postganglionic neurons = black

FIGURE 3-78 Distribution of the parasympathetic post-ganglionic fibers.

Postsynaptic terminal
Synaptic vesicles
Synaptic cleft
Presynaptic terminal
Diffusion of transmitter
Action potential
ACH

Choline
Acetic acid
ATP
Acetyl-cholinesterase
Pi + ADP
ACH

FIGURE 3-79 Physiology of a cholinergic synapse. Acetylcholine is released from the presynaptic nerve and stimulates receptors on the postsynaptic nerve. Subsequently, acetylcholinesterase breaks down the acetylcholine and the presynaptic nerve fiber takes up the products.

Table 3-4   LOCATION AND EFFECT OF MUSCARINIC RECEPTORS

Organ	Functions	Location
Heart	Decreased heart rate Decreased conduction rate	Sinoatrial node Atrioventricular node
Arterioles	Dilation Dilation Dilation	Coronary Skin and mucosa Cerebral
GI Tract	Relaxed Increased Increased salivation Increased secretion	Sphincters Motility Salivary glands Exocrine glands
Lungs	Bronchoconstriction Increased mucus production	Bronchiole smooth muscle Bronchial glands
Gallbladder	Contraction	
Urinary bladder	Relaxation Contraction	Urinary sphincter Detrusor muscle
Liver	Glycogen synthesis	
Lacrimal glands	Secretion (increased tearing)	Eye
Eye	Contraction for near vision Constriction	Ciliary muscle Pupil
Penis	Erection	

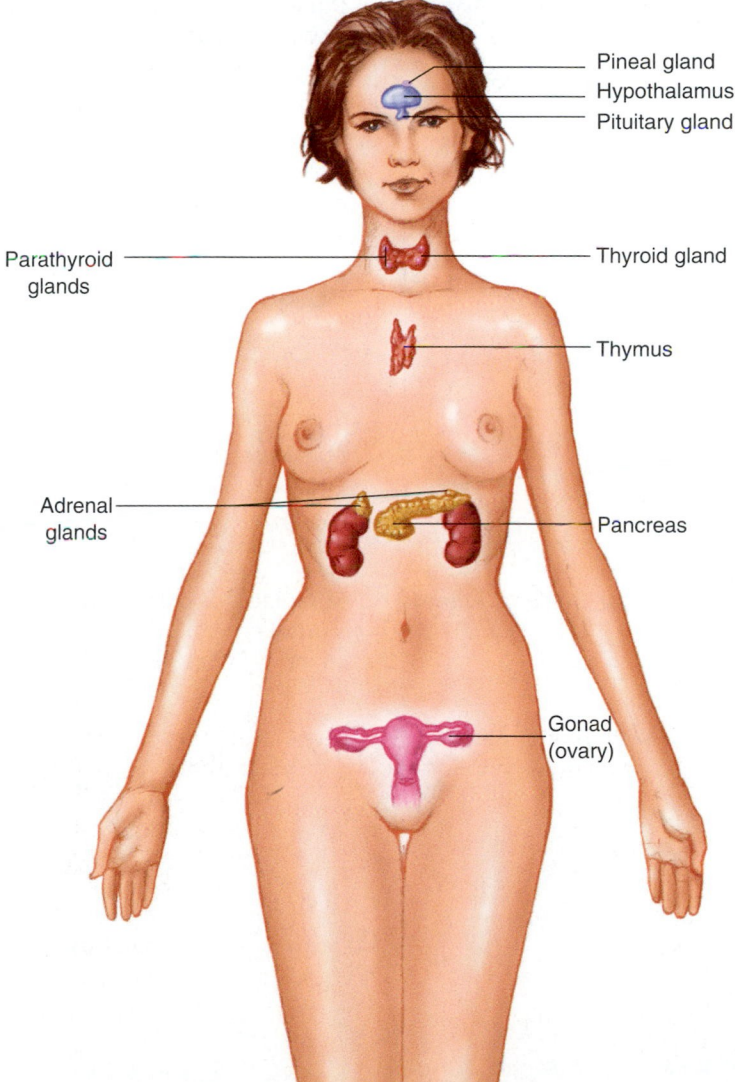

FIGURE 3-80 The major glands of the endocrine system.

Pineal gland
Hypothalamus
Pituitary gland

Parathyroid glands

Thyroid gland

Thymus

Adrenal glands

Pancreas

Gonad (ovary)

Table 3-5 ENDOCRINE SYSTEM: GLANDS, HORMONES, TARGET TISSUES, HORMONE EFFECTS

Gland and Major Hormone(s)	Target Tissues	Major Hormone Effect(s)
Hypothalamus		
Growth hormone releasing hormone, GHRH	Anterior pituitary	Stimulates release of growth hormone
Growth hormone inhibiting hormone, GHIH (or somatostatin)	Anterior pituitary	Suppresses release of growth hormone
Corticotropin releasing hormone, CRH	Anterior pituitary	Stimulates release of adrenocorticotropin
Thyrotropin releasing hormone, TRH	Anterior pituitary	Stimulates release of thyroid-stimulating hormone
Gonadotropin releasing hormone, GnRH	Anterior pituitary	Stimulates release of luteinizing hormone and follicle-stimulating hormone
Prolactin releasing hormone, PRH	Anterior pituitary	Stimulates release of prolactin
Prolactin inhibiting hormone, PIH	Anterior pituitary	Suppresses release of prolactin
Posterior pituitary gland		
Antidiuretic hormone, ADH	Kidneys	Stimulates increased reabsorption of water into blood volume
Oxytocin	Uterus and breasts of females, kidneys	Stimulates uterine contractions and milk release
Anterior pituitary gland		
Growth hormone, GH	All cells, especially growing cells	Stimulates body growth in childhood; causes switch to fats as energy source
Adrenocorticotropic hormone, ACTH	Adrenal cortexes	Stimulates release of corticosteroidal hormones cortisol and aldosterone
Thyroid-stimulating hormone, TSH	Thyroid	Stimulates release of thyroid hormones thyroxine and triiodothyronine
Follicle-stimulating hormone, FSH	Ovaries or Testes	FSH stimulates development of sex cells (ovum or sperm)
Luteinizing hormone, LH	Ovaries or Testes	LH stimulates release of hormones (estrogen, progesterone or testosterone)
Prolactin, PRL	Mammary glands	Stimulates production and release of milk
Thyroid gland		
Thyroxine, T_4	All cells	Stimulates cell metabolism
Triiodothyronine, T_3	All cells	Stimulates cell metabolism
Calcitonin	All cells	Stimulates calcium uptake by bones, decreasing blood calcium level
Parathyroid glands		
Parathyroid hormone, PTH	Bone, intestine, kidneys	Stimulates calcium release from bone, calcium uptake from GI tract, calcium reabsorption in kidney, all increasing blood calcium level
Thymus		
Thymosin	White blood cells, primarily T lymphocytes	Stimulates reproduction and functional development of T lymphocytes

Gland and Major Hormone(s)	Target Tissues	Major Hormone Effect(s)
Pancreas		
Glucagon	All cells, particularly in liver, muscle, and fat	Stimulates hepatic glycogenolysis and gluconeogenesis, increasing blood glucose level
Insulin	All cells, particularly in liver, muscle, and fat	Stimulates cellular uptake of glucose, increased rate of synthesis of glycogen, proteins, and fats, decreasing blood glucose level
Somatostatin	Alpha and Beta cells in the pancreas	Suppresses secretion of glucagon and insulin within islets of Langerhans
Adrenal medulla		
Epinephrine (or adrenaline)	Muscle, liver, cardiovascular system	Stimulates features of "Fight-or-Flight" response to stress
Norepinephrine	Muscle, liver, cardiovascular system	Stimulates vasoconstriction
Adrenal cortex		
Glucocorticoids		
Cortisol	Most cells, particularly white blood cells (cells responsible for inflammatory and immune responses)	Stimulates glucagon-like effects, acts as anti-inflammatory and immunosuppressive agent
Mineralocorticoids		
Aldosterone	Kidneys, blood	Contributes to salt and fluid balance by stimulating kidneys to increase potassium excretion and decrease sodium excretion, increasing blood volume
Androgenic hormones		
Estrogen	Most cells	See effects under Gonads (Ovaries and Testes)
Progesterone	Uterus	
Testosterone	Most cells	
Ovaries		
Estrogen	Most cells, particularly those of female reproductive tract	Stimulates development of secondary sexual characteristics, plays role in maturation of egg prior to ovulation
Progesterone	Uterus	Stimulates uterine changes necessary for successful pregnancy
Testes		
Testosterone	Most cells, particularly those of male reproductive tract	Stimulates development of secondary sexual characteristics, plays role in development of sperm cells
Pineal gland		
Melatonin	Exact action unknown	Releases melatonin in response to light, may help determine daily, lunar, and reproductive cycles, may affect mood

HYPOTHALAMUS

The *hypothalamus* is located deep within the cerebrum of the brain. Hypothalamic cells act both as nerve cells, or neurons, and as gland cells. The hypothalamus is the junction, or connection, between the central nervous system and the endocrine system. As neurons, many hypothalamic cells receive messages from the autonomic nervous system—peripheral nerves that, among other functions, detect internal conditions such as blood pressure or blood glucose level and convey that information to the central nervous system through nerve impulses. Some hypothalamic cells respond by producing nerve impulses that travel to cells in the posterior pituitary gland. Other hypothalamic cells respond as gland cells by producing and releasing hormones into the stalk of tissue that connects the hypothalamus and the anterior pituitary gland.

In response to impulses from the autonomic nervous system, the hypothalamus—and other organs of the endocrine system—can release the hormones that promote homeostasis:

- *Growth hormone releasing hormone (GHRH)*
- *Growth hormone inhibiting hormone (GHIH)*
- *Corticotropin releasing hormone (CRH)*
- *Thyrotropin releasing hormone (TRH)*
- *Gonadotropin releasing hormone (GnRH)*
- *Prolactin releasing hormone (PRH)*
- *Prolactin inhibiting hormone (PIH)*

As you can see in Table 3-5, most hypothalamic hormones, including thyrotropin releasing hormone (TRH) and growth hormone releasing hormone (GHRH), stimulate secretion of pituitary hormones that rouse yet another endocrine gland or body tissue to increased activity. For example, in response to TRH the anterior pituitary releases thyroid stimulating hormone, and thyroid stimulating hormone then acts upon the thyroid gland to increase thyroid activity.

The pair of hypothalamic hormones—growth hormone releasing hormone (GHRH) and growth hormone inhibitory hormone (GHIH)—demonstrate a major trait of endocrine function: Many hormonal activities are driven not by one hormone, but rather by two hormones with opposing effects. GHRH stimulates secretion of growth hormone, and GHIH suppresses secretion of growth hormone. The actual amount of growth hormone secreted by the anterior pituitary depends on the net amount of stimulation (Figure 3-81).

FIGURE 3-81 Regulation by hormone pairs. The net level of stimulation created by the opposing actions of growth hormone releasing hormone (GHRH) and growth-hormone inhibitory hormone (GHIH) determines the amount of growth hormone (GH) secreted by the anterior pituitary.

PITUITARY GLAND

The *pituitary gland* is only about the size of a pea. It is divided into posterior and anterior pituitary lobes. These tissues have different embryonic origins and different functional relationships with the hypothalamus. The *posterior pituitary gland* responds to nerve impulses from the hypothalamus, whereas the *anterior pituitary gland* responds to hypothalamic hormones that travel down the stalk that connects the anterior pituitary and hypothalamus. As you look at the target tissues of the anterior pituitary in Table 3-5, you will understand why physiologists once thought of the pituitary gland as the "master gland." Its hormones have a direct impact on endocrine glands throughout the body. The term isn't used much anymore, because the dependence of the pituitary on the hypothalamus has been made clear.

As noted above, the pituitary gland has two lobes, the posterior and the anterior.

Posterior Pituitary

The posterior pituitary produces two hormones:

- *Antidiuretic hormone (ADH)*—causes retention of body water
- *Oxytocin*—causes uterine contraction and lactation

Antidiuretic hormone (ADH), also known as vasopressin, causes the kidneys to increase water reabsorption. This retention of water, or antidiuretic effect, results in increased circulating blood volume and decreased urine volume. Increased secretion of ADH is part of the homeostatic mechanism that can counteract losses of blood volume up to about 25 percent. Clinically, you will see increased ADH secretion in early shock states associated with dehydration or hemorrhage. Note that the opposite effect, decreased secretion of ADH, occurs after ingestion of alcohol and when there is a significant rise in circulating blood volume.

Although it is unlikely that a disorder in ADH secretion will present as a medical emergency, you should understand such endocrine dysfunction when patients discuss their medical histories. *Diabetes insipidus,* a disorder marked by large volumes of urine, is caused by inadequate ADH secretion relative to blood volume. The resultant reduction of blood volume, or diuretic effect, appears as excessive urine production. In a 24-hour period, the kidneys normally produce 1 to 1.5 liters of urine. In diabetes insipidus, it is not uncommon for urine output to increase to almost 20 liters per day. You can remember the characteristic urine presentation of diabetes insipidus by remembering that dilute urine has an insipid, or neutral, odor (and taste).

Oxytocin, the natural form of the drug Pitocin, stimulates uterine contraction and lactation in women who have just delivered a baby. Oxytocin actually causes the "letdown" of milk by stimulating contractile cells within the mammary glands. An infant suckling at the breast stimulates receptors in the nipples that causes the release of oxytocin from the posterior pituitary. This, in turn, causes discharge of milk so that the infant can feed. Following delivery, it is recommended that the infant be placed on the breast to suckle, thus stimulating the release of oxytocin. In addition to stimulating milk letdown, the oxytocin stimulates uterine contraction, which can help minimize post-partum bleeding.

In both sexes, oxytocin has a mild antidiuretic effect, which is similar to that of ADH due to their chemical similarity. The relationship between oxytocin and ADH has direct application to emergency medicine. Women in preterm labor are often given an IV fluid bolus in an attempt to suppress uterine contractions without the use of drugs. This works in the following way: The administration of IV fluid bolus causes an increase in circulating blood volume, which is detected by autonomic nerves in the kidneys. An impulse is sent through the hypothalamus to the posterior pituitary, where it causes decreased secretion of ADH. This inhibition of ADH secretion in turn triggers decreased secretion of oxytocin, which contributes to the observed increase in urine production and, one hopes, the goal of suppression of preterm labor.

Anterior Pituitary

Because almost all of the anterior pituitary hormones regulate other endocrine glands, disorders directly involving the anterior pituitary are rarely a factor in endocrine emergencies. Table 3-5 lists the six hormones secreted by the anterior pituitary, as well as target tissues and hormone effects. As you can see, five of the six hormones regulate the activity of target glands, while the sixth affects almost all cells:
Five anterior pituitary hormones affect target glands.

- *Adrenocorticotropic hormone (ACTH)*—targets the adrenal cortexes
- *Thyroid-stimulating hormone (TSH)*—targets the thyroid
- *Follicle-stimulating hormone (FSH)*—targets the gonads, or sex organs
- *Luteinizing hormone (LH)*—also targets the gonads
- *Prolactin (PRL)*—targets the mammary glands of women

The sixth anterior pituitary hormone has a broader effect.

- *Growth hormone (GH)*—targets almost all body cells.

GH has its most significant effects in children because it is the primary stimulant of skeletal growth. In adults, GH has several physiologic effects, but the most significant is metabolic. GH causes adipose cells to release their stored fats into the blood and causes body cells to switch from glucose to fats as the primary energy source. The net effect is that the body uses up fat stores and conserves its sugar stores.

THYROID GLAND

The two lobes of the *thyroid gland* are located in the neck anterior to and just below the cartilage of the larynx, with one lobe on either side of the midline. The two lobes are connected by a small isthmus, or band of tissue, that crosses the trachea at the level of the cricoid cartilage. The thyroid produces three hormones:

- *Thyroxine (T_4)*—stimulates cell metabolism
- *Triiodothyronine (T_3)*—stimulates cell metabolism
- *Calcitonin*—lowers blood calcium levels

The thyroid is composed of tiny hollow sacs called follicles, which are filled with a thick fluid called *colloid*. The hormones *thyroxine (T_4)* and *triiodothyronine (T_3)* are produced within the colloid. When stimulated by the pituitary hormone TSH or by environmental conditions such as cold, the thyroid gland releases these hormones to increase the general rate of cell metabolism.

The thyroid gland also contains perifollicular cells called C cells which produce a different hormone, *calcitonin*. Calcitonin lowers blood calcium levels by increasing uptake of calcium by bones and inhibiting breakdown of bone tissue. Parathyroid hormone has the opposite, or antagonistic, effect on the blood calcium level, which is covered in the following discussion of the parathyroid glands.

Disorders of excessive or deficient production of thyroid hormones T_4 and T_3, are called hyperthyroidism and hypothyroidism respectively.

PARATHYROID GLANDS

Each *parathyroid gland* is very small, with a maximum diameter of 5 mm and weight of only 35–40 mg. Normally, four parathyroid glands are located on the posterior lateral surfaces of the thyroid, one pair above the other. Sometimes there are more than four parathyroid glands, but only rarely are there fewer. The parathyroid glands secrete:

- *Parathyroid hormone (PTH)*—increases blood calcium levels

PTH increases blood calcium levels through actions on three different target tissues. In bone, the primary target, PTH causes release of calcium into the blood. In the intestines, PTH converts Vitamin D into its active form, causing increased absorption of calcium. In the kidneys, PTH causes increased reabsorption of calcium. PTH is the antagonist of calcitonin, and the balance of PTH and calcitonin determines the level of blood calcium. The parathyroid glands rarely cause clinical problems. However, they can be accidentally damaged or removed during surgery or they may be damaged if the thyroid gland is irradiated. In either case, the loss of parathyroid function may result in hypocalcemia, low blood calcium levels.

THYMUS GLAND

The *thymus* is in the mediastinum just behind the sternum. It is fairly large in children but shrinks into a small remnant of fat and fibrous tissue in adults. Although the thymus is usually considered a lymphatic organ on the basis of its anatomy, its most important function is as an endocrine gland: During childhood, it secretes

- *Thymosin*—promotes maturation of T lymphocytes

Thymosin is critical to maturation of T lymphocytes, the cells responsible for cell-mediated immunity. The T of T lymphocyte stands for thymus.

PANCREAS

The *pancreas,* located in the upper retroperitoneum behind the stomach and between the duodenum and spleen, is composed of both endocrine and exocrine tissues. The exocrine tissues, known as acini, secrete digestive enzymes essential to digestion of fats and proteins into a duct that empties into the small intestine.

The microscopic clusters of endocrine tissue found within the pancreas are known as *islets of Langerhans.* Although there are one to two million islets interspersed throughout the pancreas, they comprise only about two percent of its total mass. The three most important types of endocrine cells in the islets of Langerhans are termed *alpha (α), beta (β),* and *delta (δ)* (Figure 3-82). Each type produces and secretes a different hormone. In addition, the islets contain a much smaller number of cells called polypeptide cells. These cells produce pancreatic polypeptide (PP), the function of which is still unclear.

The alpha and beta cells produce two hormones essential for homeostasis of blood glucose:

- *Glucagon*—increases blood glucose
- *Insulin*—decreases blood glucose

FIGURE 3-82 The internal anatomy of the pancreas.

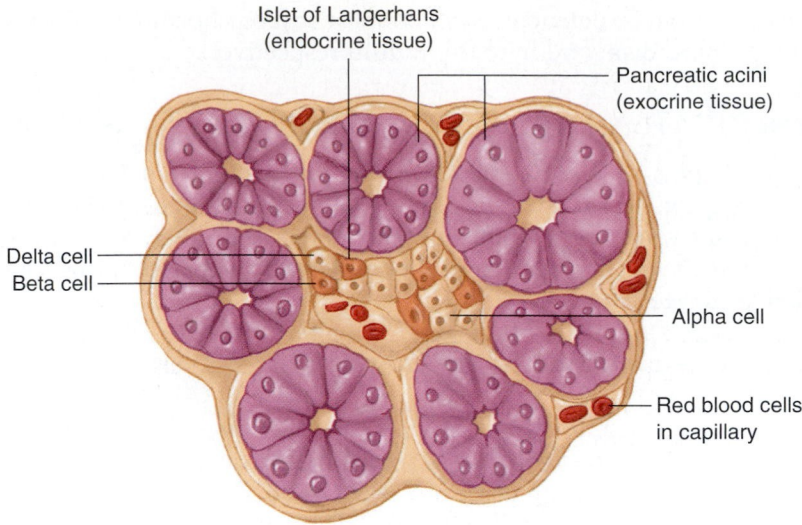

Islet of Langerhans
(endocrine tissue)

Pancreatic acini
(exocrine tissue)

Delta cell

Beta cell

Alpha cell

Red blood cells
in capillary

Approximately 25 percent of islet tissue is made up of alpha cells. Alpha cells produce the hormone *glucagon*. When blood glucose level falls, alpha cells increase secretion of glucagon. Glucagon stimulates breakdown of glycogen, the complex carbohydrate that is the storage form of glucose, into individual glucose molecules that are released into the blood. This process, called **glycogenolysis,** takes place in more than one tissue, but activity in the liver is by far the most important in raising blood glucose level.

The liver is the largest and heaviest of the internal organs and so it has many cells that can contain glycogen. In addition, liver cells have the greatest capacity to store glycogen—liver cells can store 5 to 8 percent of their weight as glycogen. Compare this with the capacity of skeletal muscle (1 to 3 percent), another important storage tissue in the body. In addition to stimulating glycogenolysis, the hormone glucagon also stimulates liver breakdown of body proteins and fats with subsequent chemical conversion to glucose. This second process, which produces glucose from non-sugar sources, is called **gluconeogenesis.** Both processes contribute to homeostasis by raising the blood glucose level.

Beta cells make up about 60 percent of islet tissue, and they produce the hormone *insulin*. Insulin is the antagonist of glucagon: Insulin lowers the blood glucose level by increasing the uptake of glucose by body cells. In addition, insulin promotes energy storage in the body by increasing the synthesis of glycogen, protein, and fat. Because the liver removes circulating insulin within 10 to 15 minutes from time of secretion, it must be secreted constantly to sustain an appropriate balance of glucagon and insulin—a balance that results in a steady supply of glucose for immediate use as an energy source and for appropriate energy storage. Loss of functional beta cells leads to increased blood glucose levels as seen in diabetes.

Delta cells, which comprise about 10 percent of islet tissue, produce *somatostatin*. This hormone acts within islets to inhibit secretion of glucagon and insulin. Somatostatin also retards nutrient absorption from the intestines, although its mechanisms of action in the gut are poorly understood. As you look at Table 3-5, note that somatostatin is the same substance as growth-hormone inhibiting hormone (GHIH).

ADRENAL GLANDS

The paired *adrenal glands* are located on the superior surface of the kidneys. Each gland has two distinct anatomical divisions with different functions. The inner portion of the adrenal gland is called the *adrenal medulla,* and its cells be-

* glycogenolysis the breakdown of glycogen to glucose, primarily by liver cells.

* gluconeogenesis conversion of protein and fat to form glucose.

have both as nerve cells and as gland cells. The adrenal medulla is intimately related to the sympathetic component of the autonomic nervous system. When sympathetic nerves carry an impulse into the adrenal medulla, its cells respond by secreting the catecholamine hormones *epinephrine* (or adrenalin) and *norepinephrine* into the bloodstream. The outer portion of the adrenal gland is called the *adrenal cortex*, and it consists of endocrine tissue. The adrenal cortex secretes three classes of steroidal hormones that differ only slightly in chemical structure but have very distinct effects in the body:

- *Glucocorticoids*, of which *cortisol* is by far the most important, account for 95 percent of adrenocortical hormone production. Like glucagon, they increase the blood glucose level by promoting gluconeogenesis and decreasing glucose utilization as an energy source. If you recall that cortisone is a commonly used medical glucocorticoid, you will realize that this class of hormones also inhibits inflammatory reactions and immune-system responses, as well as potentiates the effects of catecholamines. The anterior pituitary hormone that promotes release, ACTH, is secreted in response to stress, trauma, or serious infection.
- *Mineralocorticoids*, of which *aldosterone* is the most important, contribute to salt and fluid balance in the body by regulating sodium and potassium excretion through the kidneys.
- *Androgenic* hormones have the same effects as those secreted by gonads, and they will be covered in that discussion.

You may see disorders related to deficient or excessive secretion of adrenal hormones present as medical emergencies.

GONADS

Some differences in the *gonads* are obvious: Ovaries produce eggs, whereas testes produce sperm cells. However, the gonads of both sexes share one vital function: They are the endocrine glands chiefly responsible for the sexual maturation of puberty and any subsequent reproduction.

Ovaries

The *ovaries*, or female gonads, are paired organs about the size of an almond that are located in the pelvis on either side of the uterus. Under the regulation of the anterior pituitary hormones FSH and LH, the ovaries produce:

- *Estrogen*
- *Progesterone*

The hormone *estrogen* promotes the development and maintenance of secondary female sexual characteristics. Estrogen also plays a role in the egg development that precedes ovulation during each menstrual cycle. *Progesterone* is familiarly known as the "hormone of pregnancy" because it is necessary for implantation of the fertilized egg and maintenance of the uterine lining throughout pregnancy. Estrogen also serves to protect the female against heart disease. When estrogen levels fall at menopause, the female's risk of developing heart disease quickly increases to the level of the male's. In addition, the ovaries produce small amounts of *testosterone*, which influences some body changes associated with puberty.

Testes

The male gonads, or *testes,* are located outside of the abdominal cavity in the scrotum. Under the regulation of the anterior pituitary hormones FSH and LH, the testes produce:

- *Testosterone*

The hormone *testosterone* promotes the development and maintenance of secondary male sexual characteristics and plays a role in development of sperm.

PINEAL GLAND

The *pineal gland* is located in the roof of the thalamus in the brain. Its function has remained somewhat elusive. However, it has been shown that the pineal gland releases the hormone *melatonin* in response to changes in light. For example, melatonin production is lowest during daylight hours and highest in the dark of the night. Because of this, the pineal is felt to help determine day-length and lunar cycles and plays a role in controlling the reproductive "biological clock." Melatonin may affect a person's mood. The pineal gland has been implicated in "seasonal affective disorder (SAD)," which is characterized by severe depression during the winter months. Further research will help clarify the role of melatonin.

OTHER ORGANS WITH ENDOCRINE ACTIVITY

We have discussed the principal glands of the endocrine system. Many tissues not considered part of the endocrine system have important endocrine functions. There are organs in other systems that secrete hormones directly into the blood. The placenta can be considered an endocrine gland because of its secretion of *human chorionic gonadotropin (hCG)* throughout gestation. It is the early secretion of hCG that is detected by at-home pregnancy tests. In the digestive tract, gastric and intestinal mucosa produce the hormones *gastrin* and *secretin,* both of which regulate digestive function.

Additionally, there are hormone-producing cells in the atrial walls of the heart. *Atrial natriuretic hormone (ANH)* is secreted by certain atrial cells in response to increased stretching of the atrial walls due to abnormally high blood volume or blood pressure. The hormone ANH is an antagonist to ADH and inhibits secretion of aldosterone, thus contributing to a homeostatic reduction in blood volume by increasing urine production.

The kidneys also have some endocrine function. Certain kidney cells will react to a decrease in blood volume or blood pressure by releasing the enzyme *renin.* Renin acts on *angiotensinogen,* converting it to *angiotensin I.* In the lungs, angiotensin I is converted to *angiotensin II* by *angiotensin-converting enzyme (ACE).* Angiotensin II stimulates the adrenal production of aldosterone, which causes water retention by the kidneys. This leads to increased blood volume and blood pressure. In addition to renin, the kidneys secrete the hormone erythropoietin that stimulates the production of red blood cells by the bone marrow.

THE CARDIOVASCULAR SYSTEM

The cardiovascular system's two major components are the heart and the peripheral blood vessels.

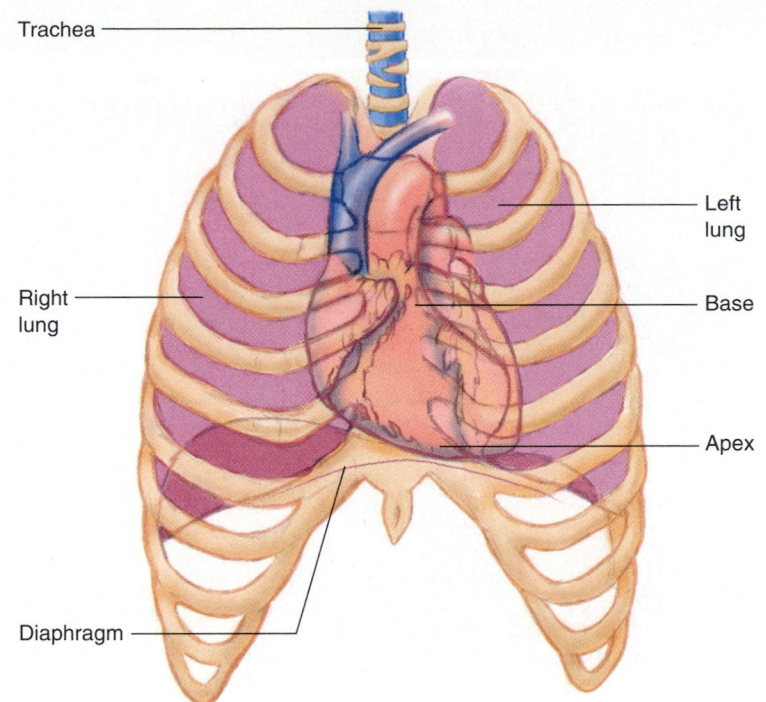

FIGURE 3-83 Location of the heart within the chest.

Trachea

Left lung

Right lung

Base

Apex

Diaphragm

ANATOMY OF THE HEART

The *heart* is a muscular organ, approximately the size of a closed fist. It is in the center of the chest in the mediastinum, anterior to the spine and posterior to the sternum (Figure 3-83). Approximately two-thirds of the heart's mass is to the left of the midline, with the remainder to the right. The bottom of the heart, or *apex*, is just above the diaphragm, left of the midline. The top of the heart, or *base*, lies at approximately the level of the second rib. The great vessels connect to the heart through the base.

Tissue Layers

The heart consists of three tissue layers: endocardium, myocardium, and pericardium (Figure 3-84). The *endocardium* is the innermost layer. It lines the heart's chambers and is bathed in blood. The *myocardium* is the thick middle layer of the heart. Its cells are unique in that they physically resemble skeletal muscle but have electrical properties similar to smooth muscle. These cells also contain specialized structures that help to rapidly conduct electrical impulses from one muscle cell to another, enabling the heart to contract.

The *pericardium* is a protective sac surrounding the heart. It consists of two layers, visceral and parietal. The *visceral pericardium*, also called the *epicardium*, is the inner layer, in contact with the heart muscle itself. The *parietal pericardium* is the outer, fibrous layer. In the pericardial cavity, between these two layers, is about 25 milliliters of pericardial fluid, a straw-colored lubricant that reduces friction as the heart beats and changes position. Certain disease processes and injuries can increase the amount of fluid in this sac, compressing the heart and decreasing cardiac output.

FIGURE 3-84 Layers of the heart.

Myocardium
Visceral pericardium (epicardium)
Pericardial cavity
Lung
Parietal pericardium
Pleural cavity
Pleura
Endocardium
Diaphragm

Chambers

The heart contains four chambers (Figure 3-85). The *atria*, the two superior chambers, receive incoming blood. The *ventricles*, the two larger, inferior chambers, pump blood out of the heart. The right and left atria are separated by the *interatrial septum*. The ventricles are separated by the *interventricular septum*. Both septa contain fibrous connective tissue as well as contractile muscle. The walls of the atria are much thinner than those of the ventricles and do not contribute significantly to the heart's pumping action.

FIGURE 3-85 The chambers of the heart.

Interatrial septum
Left atrium
Right atrium
Right ventricle
Left ventricle
Interventricular septum

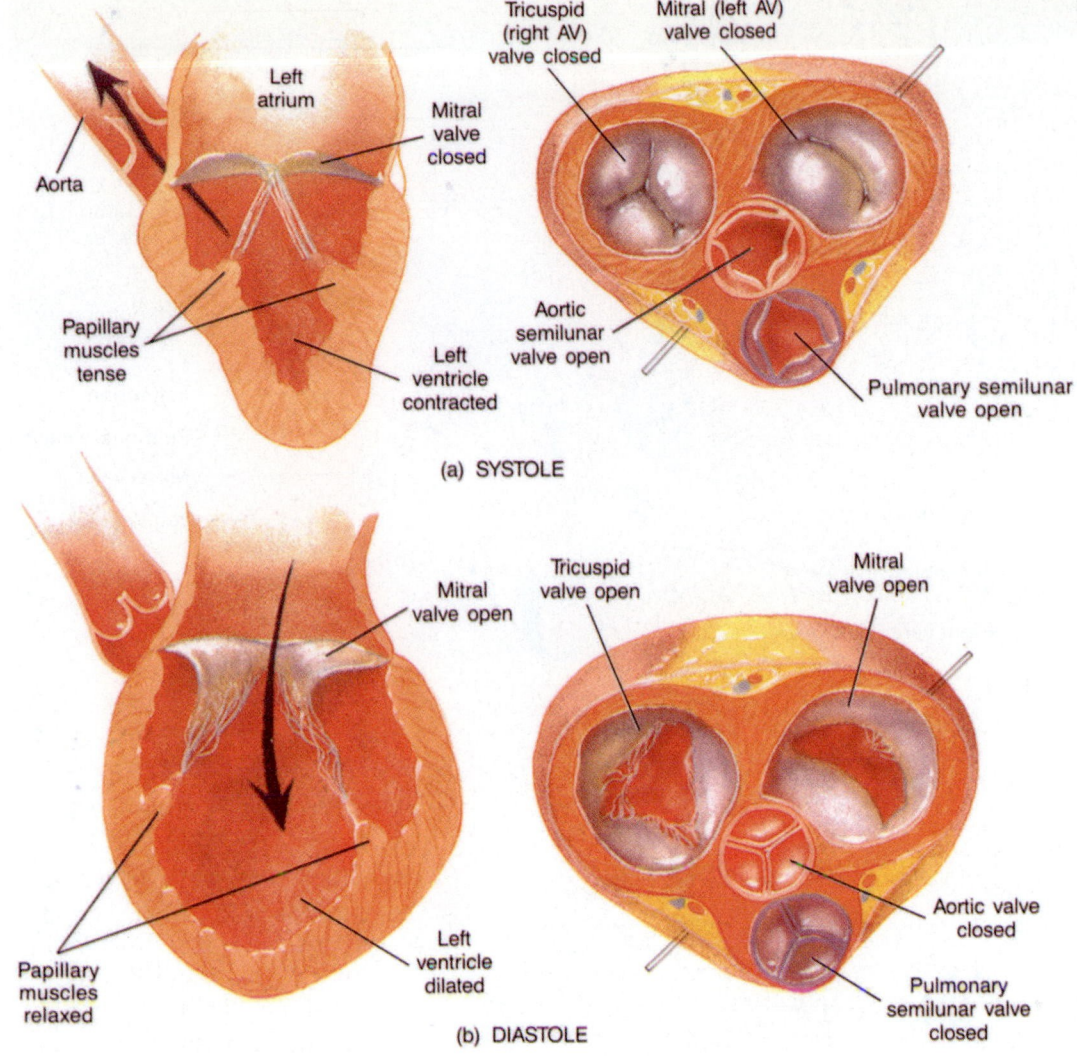

Left atrium

Aorta

Papillary muscles tense

Mitral valve closed

Left ventricle contracted

Tricuspid (right AV) valve closed

Mitral (left AV) valve closed

Aortic semilunar valve open

Pulmonary semilunar valve open

(a) SYSTOLE

Mitral valve open

Papillary muscles relaxed

Left ventricle dilated

Tricuspid valve open

Mitral valve open

Aortic valve closed

Pulmonary semilunar valve closed

(b) DIASTOLE

FIGURE 3-86   The valves of the heart.

Valves

The heart contains two pairs of valves, the *atrioventricular valves* and the *semilunar valves,* made of endocardial and connective tissue (Figure 3-86). The atrioventricular valves control blood flow between the atria and the ventricles. The right atrioventricular valve is called the *tricuspid valve* because it has three leaflets, or cusps. The left atrioventricular valve, called the *mitral valve*, has two leaflets. These valves are connected to specialized *papillary muscles* in the ventricles. When relaxed, these papillary muscles open the valves and allow blood flow between the two chambers. Specialized fibers called *chordae tendoneae* connect the valves' leaflets to the papillary muscles. They prevent the valves from prolapsing into the atria and allowing backflow during ventricular contraction.

The semilunar valves regulate blood flow between the ventricles and the arteries into which they empty. The left semilunar valve, or aortic valve, connects the left ventricle to the aorta. The right semilunar valve, or pulmonic valve, connects the right ventricle to the pulmonary artery. These valves permit one-way movement of blood and prevent backflow.

FIGURE 3-87 Blood flow through the heart.

Superior vena cava

Aorta

Pulmonary trunk

Left pulmonary arteries

Left pulmonary veins

Left atrium

Pulmonary valve

Mitral valve

Left ventricle

Right atrium

Tricuspid valve

Right ventricle

Inferior vena cava

Blood Flow

The right atrium receives deoxygenated blood from the body via the superior and inferior venae cavae (Figure 3-87). The *superior vena cava* receives deoxygenated blood from the head and upper extremities, the *inferior vena cava* from the areas below the heart. The right atrium pumps this blood through the tricuspid valve and into the right ventricle. The right ventricle then pumps the deoxygenated blood through the pulmonic valve to the *pulmonary artery* and on to the lungs. (The pulmonary artery is the only artery in the body that carries deoxygenated blood.)

After the blood circulates through the lungs and becomes oxygenated, it returns to the left atrium via the *pulmonary veins*. (The pulmonary veins are the only veins in the body that carry oxygenated blood.) The left atrium sends this oxygenated blood through the mitral valve and into the left ventricle. Finally the left ventricle pumps the blood through the aortic valve to the aorta, which feeds the oxygenated blood to the rest of the body. Intracardiac pressures are higher on the left than on the right because the lungs offer less resistance to blood flow than the systemic circulation. Thus, the left myocardium is thicker than the right.

The major vessels of the body all branch off of the aorta, which has three main parts. The *ascending aorta* comes directly from the heart. The *thoracic aorta* curves inferiorly and goes through the chest (or thorax). The *abdominal aorta* goes through the diaphragm and enters the abdomen.

FIGURE 3-88 The coronary circulation: (a) anterior; (b) posterior.

Coronary Circulation

Although the endocardium is bathed in blood, the heart does not receive its nutrients from the blood within its chambers but from the *coronary arteries* (Figure 3-88). The coronary arteries originate in the aorta, just above the leaflets of the aortic valve. The main coronary arteries lie on the surface of the heart, and small penetrating arterioles supply the myocardial muscle. The *left coronary artery* supplies the left ventricle, the interventricular septum, part of the right ventricle, and the heart's conduction system. Its two major branches are the *anterior descending artery* and the *circumflex artery*.

The *right coronary artery* supplies a portion of the right atrium and right ventricle and part of the conduction system. Its two major branches are the *posterior descending artery* and the *marginal artery*. (Although the blood supply to most people's hearts follows this pattern, anatomical variants do exist.) The coronary vessels receive blood during diastole, when the heart relaxes, because the aortic valve leaflets cover the coronary artery openings (*ostia*) during systole, when the heart contracts.

Blood drains from the left coronary system via the *anterior great cardiac vein* and the *lateral marginal veins*. These empty into the *coronary sinus*. The right coronary artery empties directly into the right atrium via smaller cardiac veins.

Many **anastomoses** (communications between two or more vessels) among the various branches of the coronary arteries allow *collateral circulation*. Collateral circulation is a protective mechanism that provides an alternative path for blood flow in case of a blockage somewhere in the system. This is analogous to a river's developing small tributaries to reach a larger body of water.

✱ **anastomosis** communication between two or more vessels.

FIGURE 3-89   Relation of
blood flow to cardiac
contractions.

Pulmonic
valve
closed

Aortic
valve
closed

Mitral
valve
open

Tricuspid
valve
open

Aortic
valve
open

Pulmonic
valve
open

Mitral
valve
closed

Tricuspid
valve
closed

DIASTOLIC PHASE   SYSTOLIC PHASE

CARDIAC PHYSIOLOGY

The Cardiac Cycle

Although the heart's right and left sides perform different functions, they act as a unit. The right and left atria contract at the same time, filling both ventricles to their maximum capacities. Both ventricles then contract at the same time, ejecting blood into the pulmonary and systemic circulations. The pressure of the contraction closes the tricuspid and mitral valves and opens the aortic and pulmonic valves at the same time.

The **cardiac cycle** is the sequence of events that occurs between the end of one heart contraction and the end of the next. To evaluate heart sounds and read electrocardiographs, you must thoroughly understand the pumping action of the cardiac cycle (Figure 3-89). **Diastole,** the first phase of the cardiac cycle, is the relaxation phase. This is when ventricular filling begins. Blood enters the ventricles through the mitral and tricuspid valves. The pulmonic and aortic valves are closed.

During the second phase, **systole,** the heart contracts. The atria contract first, to finish emptying their blood into the ventricles. Atrial systole is relatively quick and occurs just before ventricular contraction; in healthy hearts, this atrial "kick" boosts cardiac output. The pressure in the ventricles now increases until it exceeds the pressure in the aorta and pulmonary artery. At this point blood flows out of the ventricles through the pulmonic and aortic valves and into the arteries. The pressure also closes the mitral and tricuspid valves and, if working properly, prevents backflow of blood into the atria. When pressures in the artery exceed the pressures in the ventricles, the valves close and diastole begins again.

Nervous Control of the Heart

The sympathetic and parasympathetic components of the autonomic nervous system work in direct opposition to one another to regulate the heart. In the heart's normal state the two systems balance. In stressful situations, however, the sympathetic system becomes dominant, while during sleep the parasympathetic system dominates. The sympathetic nervous system innervates the heart through the *cardiac plexus,* a network of nerves at the base of the heart (Figure 3-90).

The sympathetic nerves arise from the thoracic and lumbar regions of the spinal cord, then leave the spinal cord and form the sympathetic chain, which runs along the spinal column. The cardiac plexus arises in turn from ganglia in the sympathetic chain and innervates both the atria and ventricles. The chemical

* **cardiac cycle** the period of time from the end of one cardiac contractions to the end of the next.

* **diastole** the period of time when the myocardium is relaxed and cardiac filling and coronary perfusion occur.

* **systole** the period of the cardiac cycle when the myocardium is contracting.

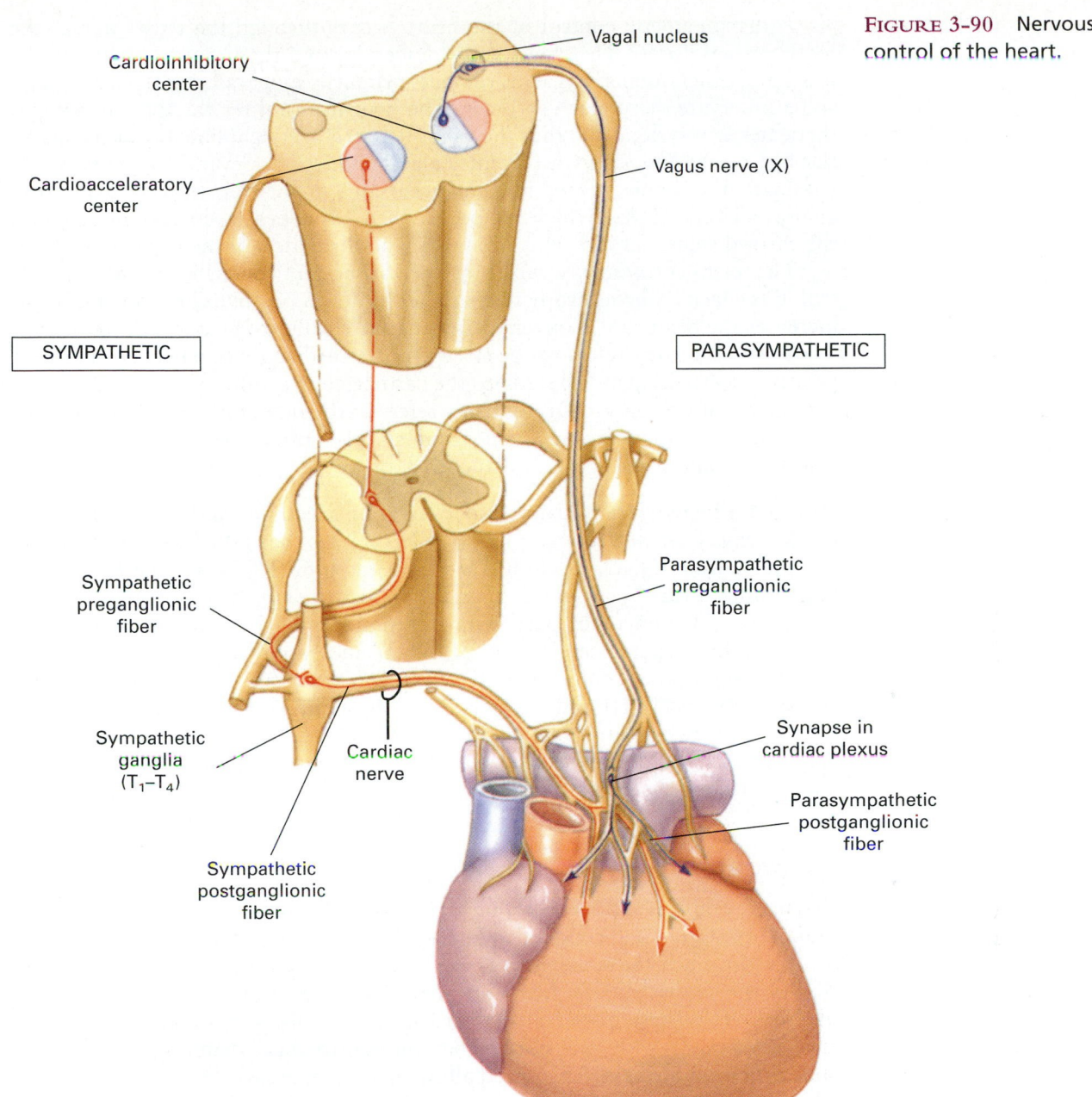

FIGURE 3-90 Nervous control of the heart.

Vagal nucleus

Cardioinhibitory center

Cardioaccelerstory center

Vagus nerve (X)

SYMPATHETIC

PARASYMPATHETIC

Parasympathetic preganglionic fiber

Sympathetic preganglionic fiber

Sympathetic ganglia (T_1–T_4)

Cardiac nerve

Synapse in cardiac plexus

Parasympathetic postganglionic fiber

Sympathetic postganglionic fiber

neurotransmitter for the sympathetic nervous system, and thus for the cardiac plexus, is norepinephrine. Its release increases heart rate and cardiac contractile force, primarily through its actions on beta receptors.

As noted earlier, the sympathetic nervous system has two principal types of receptors, alpha and beta. Alpha receptors are located in the peripheral blood vessels and are responsible for vasoconstriction. Beta$_1$ receptors, primarily located in the heart, increase the heart rate and contractility. Beta$_2$ receptors, principally located in the lungs and peripheral blood vessels, cause bronchodilation and peripheral vasodilation. Medications specific to these various receptors cause different physiological effects. For instance, beta blockers slow the heart rate and lower blood pressure by blocking the beta$_1$ receptors, whose job is to increase heart rate and contractility.

Parasympathetic control of the heart occurs through the *vagus nerve* (the tenth cranial nerve). The vagus nerve descends from the brain to innervate the heart and other organs. Vagal nerve fibers primarily innervate the atria, although some innervate the upper ventricles. The neurotransmitter for the parasympathetic nervous system, and thus the vagus nerve, is acetylcholine. Its release slows the heart rate and slows atrioventricular conduction. Several maneuvers can stimulate the vagus nerve, including Valsalva maneuver (forced expiration against a closed glottis, which can occur when lifting heavy objects), pressure on the carotid sinus (carotid sinus massage), and distention of the urinary bladder.

The terms *chronotropy, inotropy,* and *dromotropy* describe autonomic control of the heart. **Chronotropy** refers to heart rate. A positive chronotropic agent increases the heart rate. Conversely, a negative chronotropic agent decreases the heart rate. **Inotropy** refers to the strength of a cardiac muscular contraction. A positive inotropic agent strengthens the cardiac contraction, while a negative inotropic agent weakens it. **Dromotropy** refers to the rate of nervous impulse conduction. A positive dromotropic agent speeds impulse conduction, while a negative dromotropic agent slows conduction.

Role of Electrolytes Cardiac function, both electrical and mechanical, depends heavily on electrolyte balances. Electrolytes that affect cardiac function include sodium (Na^+), calcium (Ca^{++}), potassium (K^+), chloride (Cl^-), and magnesium (Mg^{++}). Sodium plays a major role in depolarizing the myocardium. Calcium takes part in myocardial depolarization and myocardial contraction. Hypercalcemia can result in increased contractility, whereas hypocalcemia is associated with decreased myocardial contractility and increased electrical irritability. Potassium influences repolarization. Hyperkalemia decreases automaticity and conduction, whereas hypokalemia increases irritability. New research is also investigating the roles of magnesium and chloride in the cardiac cycle.

Electrophysiology

The heart comprises three types of cardiac muscle: atrial, ventricular, and specialized excitatory and conductive fibers. The atrial and ventricular muscle fibers contract in much the same way as skeletal muscle, with one major difference. Within the cardiac muscle fibers are special structures called **intercalated discs** (Figure 3-91). These discs connect cardiac muscle fibers and conduct electrical impulses quickly—400 times faster than the standard cell membrane—from one muscle fiber to the next. This speed allows cardiac muscle cells to function physiologically as a unit. That is, when one cell becomes excited, the action potential spreads rapidly across the entire group of cells, resulting in a coordinated contraction. This functional unit is a **syncytium.**

The heart has two syncytia—the *atrial syncytium* and the *ventricular syncytium.* The atrial syncytium contracts from superior to inferior, so that the atria express blood to the ventricles. The ventricular syncytium, on the other hand, contracts from inferior to superior, expelling blood from the ventricles into the aorta and pulmonary arteries. The syncytia are separated from one another by the fibrous structure that supports the valves and physically separates the atria from the ventricles. The only way an impulse can be conducted from the atria to the ventricles is through the *atrioventricular (AV) bundle.* Cardiac muscle functions according to an "all-or-none" principle. That is, if a single muscle fiber becomes *depolarized,* the action potential will spread through the whole syncytium. Stimulating a single atrial fiber will thus completely depolarize the atria, and stimulating a single ventricular fiber will completely depolarize the ventricles.

✳ **chronotropy** pertaining to heart rate.

✳ **inotropy** pertaining to cardiac contractile force.

✳ **dromotropy** pertaining to the speed of impulse transmission.

✳ **intercalated discs** specialized bands of tissue inserted between myocardial cells that increase the rate in which the action potential is spread from cell to cell.

✳ **syncytium** group of cardiac muscle cells that physiologically function as a unit.

Cardiocytes

Nucleus

Mitochondrion

Intercalated discs

Cardiac Depolarization

Understanding **cardiac depolarization** is essential to interpreting electrocardiograms (ECGs). Normally, an ionic difference exists on the two sides of a cell membrane. The cell's sodium-potassium pump expels sodium (Na^+) from the cell. This leaves more negatively charged anions inside the cell than positively charged cations. Thus, the inside of the cell is more negatively charged than the outside. This difference, called the **resting potential,** can be measured experimentally by placing one probe inside the cell and another outside the cell and determining the difference in millivolts. The resting potential in a myocardial cell is approximately 290 mV (Figure 3-92).

When the myocardial cell is stimulated, the membrane surrounding the cell changes instantaneously to allow sodium ions to rush into the cell, bringing with them their positive charge. This charge is so strong that it gives the inside of the cell a positive charge approximately 120 mV greater than the outside. This influx of sodium and change of membrane polarity is the **action potential.** After the influx of sodium, a slower influx of calcium ions (Ca^{++}) through the calcium channels increases the positive charge inside the cell. Once depolarization occurs in a muscle fiber, it is transmitted throughout the entire syncytium, via the intercalated

✱ **cardiac depolarization** a reversal of charges at a cell membrane so that the inside of the cell becomes positive in relation to the outside; the opposite of the cell's resting state in which the inside of the cell is negative in relation to the outside.

✱ **resting potential** the normal electrical state of cardiac cells.

✱ **action potential** the stimulation of myocardial cells, as evidenced by a change in the membrane electrical charge, that subsequently spreads across the myocardium.

discs, until the entire muscle mass is depolarized. Contraction of the muscle follows depolarization.

The cell membrane remains permeable to sodium for only a fraction of a second. Thereafter, sodium influx stops and potassium escapes from inside the cell. This returns the charge inside the cell to normal (negative). In addition, sodium is actively pumped outside the cell, allowing the cell to **repolarize** and return to its normal resting state.

* **repolarization** return of a cell to its pre-excitation resting state.

Cardiac Conductive System

The cardiac conductive system stimulates the ventricles to depolarize in the proper direction. As mentioned earlier, the atria contract from superior to inferior, the ventricles from inferior to superior. If the depolarization impulse originated in the atria and spread passively to the ventricles, then the ventricles would depolarize from superior to inferior and would be ineffective. The cardiac conduction system, therefore, must initiate an impulse, spread it through the atria, transmit it quickly to the apex of the heart, and thence stimulate the ventricles to depolarize from inferior to superior. To do this, the conduction system relies on specialized conductive fibers comprising muscle cells that transmit the depolarization potential through the heart much faster than can regular myocardial cells.

To accomplish their task, the cells of the cardiac conductive system have the important properties of excitability, conductivity, automaticity, and contractility.

- **Excitability** The cells can respond to an electrical stimulus, like all other myocardial cells.
- **Conductivity** The cells can propagate the electrical impulse from one cell to another.
- **Automaticity** The individual cells of the conductive system can depolarize without any impulse from an outside source. This property is also called self-excitation. Generally, the cell in the cardiac conductive system with the fastest rate of discharge, or automaticity, becomes the heart's pacemaker. As a rule, the highest cell in the conductive system has the fastest rate of automaticity. Normally, this cell is in the sinoatrial (SA) node, high in the right atrium; however, if one pacemaker cell fails to discharge and depolarize, then the cell with the next fastest rate becomes the pacemaker.
- **Contractility** Since the cells of the cardiac conductive system are specialized cardiac muscle cells, they retain the ability to contract.

✱ **excitability** ability of the cells to respond to an electrical stimulus.

✱ **conductivity** ability of the cells to propagate the electrical impulse from one cell to another.

✱ **automaticity** pacemaker cells' capability of self-depolarization.

✱ **contractility** ability of muscle cells to contract, or shorten.

Internodal atrial pathways connect the SA node to the AV node (Figure 3-93). These internodal pathways conduct the depolarization impulse to the atrial muscle mass and through the atria to the AV junction. The AV junction (the "gatekeeper") slows the impulse and allows the ventricles time to fill. Then, the impulse passes through the AV junction into the AV node and on to the AV fibers, which conduct the impulse from the atria to the ventricles. In the ventricles the AV fibers form the *bundle of His*.

The bundle of His subsequently divides into the right and left bundle branches. The *right bundle branch* delivers the impulse to the apex of the right ventricle. From there the *Purkinje system* spreads it across the myocardium. The *left bundle branch* divides into *anterior and posterior fascicles* that also

SA node

AV node

Interventricular septum

Right bundle branch

Purkinje system

Internodal atrial pathways

AV junction

Bundle of His

Left bundle branch

Purkinje fibers

FIGURE 3-93 The cardiac conductive system.

ultimately terminate in the Purkinje system. At the same time that the impulse is transmitted to the right ventricle, the Purkinje system spreads it across the mass of the myocardium. Repolarization predominantly occurs in the opposite direction.

Each component of the conductive system has its own intrinsic rate of self-excitation:

SA node = 60–100 beats per minute

AV node = 40–60 beats per minute

Purkinje system = 15–40 beats per minute

ANATOMY OF THE PERIPHERAL CIRCULATION

The peripheral circulation (Figure 3-94) transports oxygenated blood from the heart to the tissues and subsequently transports deoxygenated blood back to the heart. Oxygenated blood leaves the heart via the arterial system, while deoxygenated blood returns via the venous system. (As noted earlier, the exceptions to this rule are the pulmonary artery and the pulmonary veins.)

A capillary wall consists of a single layer of cells. The walls of arteries and veins, however, comprise several layers (Figure 3-95). The arteries' and veins' innermost lining, the *tunica intima,* is a single cell layer thick. The middle layer, the *tunica media,* consists of elastic fibers and muscle. It gives blood vessels their strength and recoil, which results from the difference in pressure inside and outside the vessel. The tunica media is much thicker in arteries than in veins. The outermost lining is the *tunica adventitia,* a fibrous tissue covering. It gives the vessel strength to withstand the pressures generated by the heart's contractions. The cavity inside a vessel is the *lumen.*

The vessels' diameters vary significantly and are directly related to the amount of blood they can transport. The larger the diameter, the greater the blood flow. In fact, according to **Poiseuille's law** the blood flow through a vessel is directly proportional to the fourth power of the vessel's radius. For example, a vessel with a relative radius of 1 would transport 1 ml per minute of blood at a pressure difference of 100 mmHg. If the vessel's radius were increased to 4, keeping the pressure difference constant, the flow would increase to 256 ml (4^4) per minute.

✱ **Poiseuille's law** a law of physiology stating that blood flow through a vessel is directly proportional to the radius of the vessel to the fourth power.

The Arterial System

The *arterial system,* which carries oxygenated blood from the heart, functions under high pressure. The larger arterial vessels are the *arteries.* The arteries branch into smaller structures called *arterioles,* which control blood flow to various organs by their degree of resistance. The arterioles continue to divide until they become *capillaries,* which are the connection points between the arterial and venous systems. The vascular system and the tissues are able to exchange gases, fluids, and nutrients through the very thin capillary walls.

The Venous System

The *venous system* transports blood from the peripheral tissues back to the heart. It functions under low pressure with the aid of surrounding muscles and one-way valves within the veins. Blood enters the venous system through the capillaries, which drain into the *venules.* The venules, in turn, drain into the *veins,* the veins into the venae cavae, and the venae cavae into the atria.

MAJOR ARTERIES

Internal carotid
External carotid
Common carotid
Subclavian
Innominate
Axillary
Pulmonary
Aorta
Brachial
Radial
Ulnar
Common iliac
Palmar arches
Digital
Deep femoral
Femoral
Popliteal
Anterior tibial
Peroneal
Posterior tibial
Dorsal pedis
Arcuate

MAJOR VEINS

External jugular
Internal jugular
Innominate
Brachial
Cephalic
Axillary
Basilic
Antecubital
Volar digital
Subclavian
Venae cavae
Splenic artery and vein
Right gastric artery and vein
Hepatic artery and vein
Renal artery and vein
Mesenteric arteries and veins
Common iliac
Great saphenous
Femoral
Popliteal
Peroneal
Posterior tibial
Anterior tibial
Dorsal venous arch

FIGURE 3-94   The circulatory system.

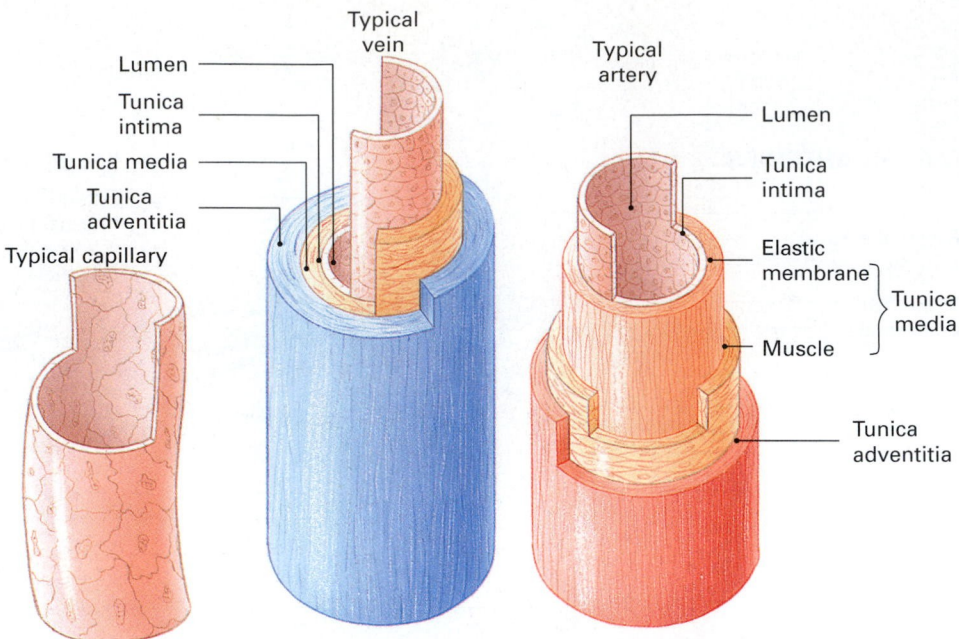

FIGURE 3-95 The layers of the peripheral arteries.

The Lymphatic System

The *lymphatic system* is a network of valveless vessels that drains fluid, called lymph, from the body tissues and delivers it to the subclavian vein (Figure 3-96). Lymph nodes in the neck, the axilla, and the groin help filter impurities en route to the heart. The lymph system plays an important role in the body's immune system. It also plays an important role in our circulatory system.

When arterial blood flows into a capillary bed, hydrostatic pressure pushes fluid across the capillary membrane into the tissues. As the blood flows through the capillary bed, this pressure diminishes. Plasma proteins in the capillaries create an oncotic pressure gradient that draws fluid back into the blood stream. On the venous side of the capillary bed, the oncotic pressure drawing fluid in is greater than the hydrostatic pressure pushing fluid out. The net effect is that fluid returns to the capillary for its return to the heart. In a perfect system, whatever fluid enters the tissues at one end of the capillary bed should return to the circulation at the other end. In reality, some fluid usually remains in the tissues. The lymph system acts as an auxiliary drainage system, collecting the remaining fluid from the tissues and returning it to the heart.

THE PHYSIOLOGY OF PERFUSION

As discussed earlier, all body cells require a constant supply of oxygen and other essential nutrients, while waste products, such as carbon dioxide, must be constantly removed. It is the circulatory system, in conjunction with the respiratory

All body cells require a constant supply of oxygen and other nutrients.

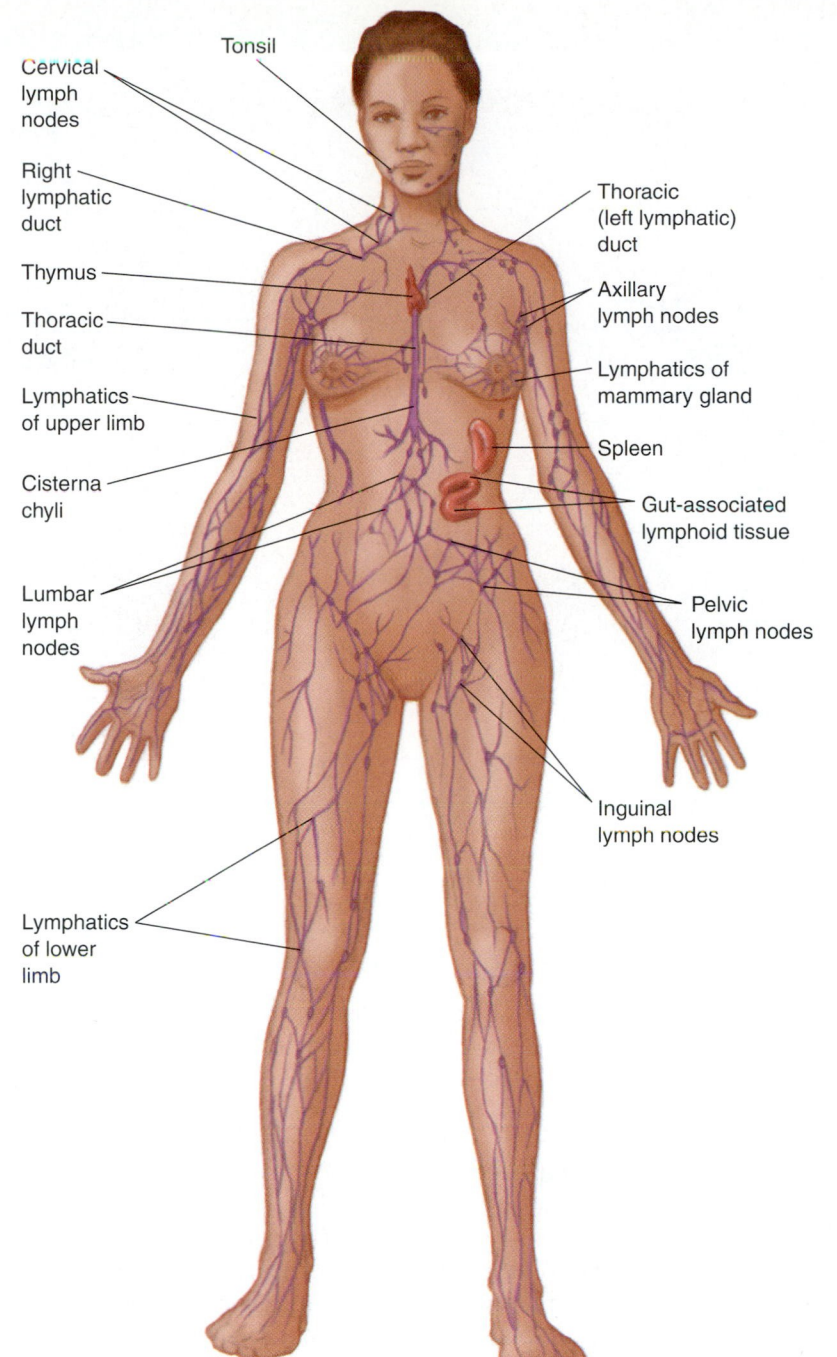

FIGURE 3-96 The lymphatic system.

Tonsil

Cervical lymph nodes

Right lymphatic duct

Thymus

Thoracic duct

Lymphatics of upper limb

Cisterna chyli

Lumbar lymph nodes

Lymphatics of lower limb

Thoracic (left lymphatic) duct

Axillary lymph nodes

Lymphatics of mammary gland

Spleen

Gut-associated lymphoid tissue

Pelvic lymph nodes

Inguinal lymph nodes

and gastrointestinal systems, that provides the body's cells with these essential nutrients and removal of wastes. This is accomplished by the passage of blood through the capillaries, the small vessels that interface with body cells, while oxygen and carbon dioxide, nutrients and wastes, are exchanged by movement across the capillary walls and cell membranes. This constant and necessary passage of blood through the body's tissues is called **perfusion.** Inadequate perfusion of body tissues is **hypoperfusion,** which is commonly called *shock.*

✳ perfusion the supplying of oxygen and nutrients to the body tissues as a result of the constant passage of blood through the capillaries.

✳ hypoperfusion inadequate perfusion of the body tissues, resulting in an inadequate supply of oxygen and nutrients to the body tissues. Also called *shock.*

The Cardiovascular System **221**

FIGURE 3-97 Components of the circulatory system.

Pump

Container

Volume (blood within circulatory system)

Components of the Circulatory System

Perfusion is dependent on a functioning and intact circulatory system. The three components of the circulatory system are listed below. A derangement in any one of these can adversely affect perfusion (Figure 3-97).

- The pump (heart)
- The fluid (blood)
- The container (blood vessels)

The Pump The heart is the pump of the cardiovascular system. It receives blood from the venous system, pumps it to the lungs for oxygenation, and then pumps it to the peripheral tissues. The normal ventricle ejects about two-thirds of the blood it contains at the end of diastole. This ratio is the **ejection fraction.** The amount of blood ejected by the heart in one contraction is referred to as the **stroke volume.** Each time the ventricle pumps blood into the aorta, it generates a pressure wave along the major arteries, which we feel as a pulse. Stroke volume varies between 60 and 100 ml, with the average being 70 ml. Three factors affect stroke volume: preload, cardiac contractile force, and afterload.

Preload is the amount of blood delivered to the heart during diastole (when the heart fills with blood between contractions). Preload depends on venous return. The venous system is a capacitance, or storage system. That is, it can be contracted or expanded, to some extent, as needed to meet the physiological demands of the body. When additional oxygenated blood is required, the venous capacitance is reduced, thus increasing the amount of blood delivered to the heart. The greater the preload, the greater the stroke volume.

✱ **ejection fraction** ratio of blood pumped from the ventricle to the amount remaining at the end of diastole.

✱ **stroke volume** the amount of blood ejected by the heart in one cardiac contraction.

Content Review

FACTORS AFFECTING STROKE VOLUME
- Preload
- Cardiac contractility
- Afterload

✱ **preload** the pressure within the ventricles at the end of diastole, commonly called the *end-diastolic volume.*

Preload also affects **cardiac contractile force.** The greater the volume of pre-load, the more the ventricles are stretched. The greater the stretch, up to a certain limit, the greater will be the subsequent cardiac contraction. This phenomenon (known as **Starling's law of the heart**) can be illustrated through the example of a rubber band. The more the rubber band is stretched, the greater will be its velocity when released. Myocardial muscle, however, has its limits. If stretched too far, it will not contract properly and will weaken. Think of blowing up a tire. The tension in the walls increases as you put more air in the tire. If you were to put too much air in the tire, the tire would break or bulge from the side. If either of these happened, the tension in the wall would decrease, and if you filled the tire again it would not perform as well as before.

In addition, cardiac contractile force is affected by the circulating hormones called catecholamines (epinephrine and norepinephrine) controlled by the sympathetic nervous system. Catecholamines enhance cardiac contractile force by action on the beta-adrenergic receptors on the surface of the cells.

Finally, stroke volume is affected by afterload. **Afterload** is the resistance against which the ventricle must contract. This resistance must be overcome before ventricular contraction can result in ejection of blood. Afterload is determined by the degree of peripheral vascular resistance, which depends on the amount of vasoconstriction present. (The arterial system can be expanded and contracted to meet the metabolic demands of the body.) An increase in peripheral vascular resistance will decrease stroke volume, and conversely, a decrease in peripheral vascular resistance will allow stroke volume to increase.

The amount of blood pumped by the heart in one minute is referred to as the **cardiac output.** It is a function of stroke volume (milliliters per beat) and heart rate (beats per minute). Cardiac output is usually expressed in liters per minute. It can be defined by this equation:

stroke volume (ml/b) × heart rate (bpm) = cardiac output (ml/min)

Since the average stroke volume is 70 ml and the normal heart rate is about 70 beats per minute, the average cardiac output is 4900 milliliters per minute (rounded to 5000 ml/min or 5 liters per minute).

The foregoing equation illustrates the factors that can affect cardiac output. An increase in stroke volume or an increase in heart rate can increase cardiac output. Conversely, a decrease in stroke volume (in turn governed by preload, contractile force, and afterload) or a decrease in heart rate can decrease cardiac output.

Blood pressure, the tension exerted by blood against the arterial walls, is dependent upon both cardiac output and peripheral vascular resistance.

blood pressure = cardiac output × peripheral vascular resistance

Peripheral vascular resistance is the pressure against which the heart must pump. Since the circulatory system is a closed system, increasing either cardiac output or peripheral vascular resistance will increase blood pressure. Likewise, a decrease in cardiac output or a decrease in peripheral vascular resistance will decrease blood pressure.

The body does its best to keep the blood pressure relatively constant by employing compensatory mechanisms and negative feedback loops to regulate the elements of the above formula. As noted earlier, baroreceptors in the carotid sinuses and in the arch of the aorta closely monitor blood pressure. If blood pressure increases, the baroreceptors send signals to the brain that cause the blood pressure to return to its normal values. This is accomplished by decreasing the heart rate, decreasing the preload, or decreasing peripheral vascular resistance.

The baroreceptors are also stimulated if the blood pressure falls. The heart rate is increased, as is the strength of the cardiac contractions. There is also arteriolar constriction, venous constriction (which results in decreased container size),

* **cardiac contractile force** force of the strength of a contraction of the heart.

* **Starling's law of the heart** law of physiology stating that the more the myocardium is stretched, up to a certain limit, the more forceful the subsequent contraction will be.

* **afterload** the resistance against which the heart must pump.

* **cardiac output** the amount of blood pumped by the heart in one minute.

* **blood pressure** the tension exerted by blood against the arterial walls.

* **peripheral vascular resistance** the resistance of the vessels to the flow of blood: increased when the vessels constrict, decreased when the vessels relax.

and overall increased peripheral vascular resistance. Also, the adrenal medulla (the inner portion of the adrenal gland) is stimulated. This results in the secretion of epinephrine and norepinephrine, which further enhance the response.

The Fluid Blood is the fluid of the cardiovascular system. It is a viscous fluid; that is, it is thicker and more adhesive than water. As a result, blood flows more slowly than water. Blood, which consists of the plasma and the formed elements (red cells, white cells, and platelets), transports oxygen, carbon dioxide, nutrients, hormones, metabolic waste products, and heat.

An adequate amount of blood is required for perfusion. Since the cardiovascular system (the heart and blood vessels) is a closed system, the volume of blood present must be adequate to fill the container, as described below.

The Container Blood vessels (arteries, arterioles, capillaries, venules, and veins) serve as the container of the cardiovascular system. The blood vessels can be thought of as a continuous, closed, and pressurized pipeline by which blood moves throughout the body. While the heart functions as the pump of the circulatory system, the blood vessels—under the control of the autonomic nervous system—can regulate blood flow to different areas of the body by adjusting their size as well as by selectively rerouting blood through the microcirculation.

While the arteries and veins, like the heart, are subject to direct stimulation from sympathetic portions of the autonomic nervous system, the microcirculation (comprised of the small vessels: the arterioles, capillaries, and venules) is primarily responsive to local tissue needs. The capability of some vessels in the capillary network to adjust their diameter permits the microcirculation to selectively supply undernourished tissue, while temporarily bypassing tissues with no immediate need. Capillaries have a sphincter at the origin of the capillary (between arteriole and capillary), called the *pre-capillary sphincter,* and another at the end of the capillary (between capillary and venule), called the *post-capillary sphincter.* The pre-capillary sphincter responds to local tissue conditions, such as acidosis and hypoxia, and opens as more arterial blood is needed. The post-capillary sphincter opens when blood is to be emptied into the venous system.

Blood flow through the vessels is regulated by two factors: peripheral vascular resistance and pressure within the system. Peripheral vascular resistance, as noted earlier, is the resistance to blood flow. Vessels with larger inside diameters offer less resistance, while vessels with smaller inside diameters offer greater resistance. Peripheral vascular resistance is governed by three factors—the length of the vessel, the diameter of the vessel, and blood viscosity.

There is very little resistance to blood flow through the aorta and arteries, but a significant change in peripheral resistance occurs at the arterioles and precapillary sphincters. This is because the inside diameter of the arteriole is much smaller, as compared to that of the aorta and arteries. Additionally, the arteriole has the ability to make a pronounced change in its diameter, as much as fivefold. It tends to do this in response to local tissue needs and autonomic nervous signals.

Contraction of the venous side of the vascular system results in decreased capacitance and increased cardiac preload. The arterial system, on the other hand, provides systemic vascular resistance. An increase in arterial tone increases resistance, which increases blood pressure.

Oxygen Transport

Oxygen is brought into the body via the respiratory system. During inspiration, approximately 500 to 800 ml of atmospheric air is taken in through the upper and lower airways, coming to rest in the alveoli of the lungs.

Surrounding the alveoli are capillaries that are perfused by the pulmonary circulation. The blood that comes into the pulmonary capillaries is oxygen-

The precapillary sphincter responds to local tissue demands such as acidosis and hypoxia.

Content Review

MAJOR FUNCTIONS OF PERFUSION
- Oxygen transport
- Waste removal

depleted blood that was returned from the body to the right atrium of the heart, then pumped by the right ventricle of the heart into the pulmonary arteries and thence into the pulmonary capillaries.

The air in the alveoli contains a concentration of about 13.6 percent oxygen. This is less than the 21 percent concentration of oxygen in atmospheric air because of various factors, including the fact that some air always remains in the alveoli from earlier respirations and oxygen is constantly being absorbed from this air. Nevertheless, alveolar air is far richer in oxygen than blood that enters the pulmonary capillaries.

Another way of stating this is that the *partial pressure of oxygen* present in air in the alveoli of the lungs is greater than the partial pressure of oxygen in the blood within the pulmonary circulation. (In a mix of gases, the portion of the total pressure exerted by each component of the mix is known as the partial pressure of that component.) For this reason, oxygen from the alveoli diffuses across the alveolar-capillary membrane and into the bloodstream—from the area of greater partial pressure to the area of lower partial pressure.

The red blood cells "pick up" this oxygen while passing through the pulmonary capillary bed. Oxygen binds to the hemoglobin molecule of the red blood cells, which serve as the primary carriers of oxygen within the bloodstream. Normally, between 95 and 100 percent of the hemoglobin is saturated with oxygen. The oxygen-enriched blood then circulates back to the heart through the venous side of the pulmonary circulation. Passing through the left atrium and into the left ventricle, the oxygen-enriched blood is pumped throughout the body via the systemic circulation.

Upon reaching capillaries throughout the body, the oxygen-rich blood interfaces with the tissues. The tissues contain cells that are oxygen-deficient as a result of normal metabolic activity. Since the partial pressure of oxygen is greater in the bloodstream than in the cells, oxygen will diffuse from the red blood cells across the capillary wall-cell membrane barrier, into the cells and tissues.

Overall, the movement and utilization of oxygen in the body is dependent upon the following conditions:

- Adequate concentration of inspired oxygen
- Appropriate movement of oxygen across the alveolar/capillary membrane into the arterial bloodstream
- Adequate number of red blood cells to carry the oxygen
- Proper tissue perfusion
- Efficient off-loading of oxygen at the tissue level

The dependence on this set of conditions for oxygen movement and utilization is known as the Fick Principle.

Waste Removal

The waste products of cellular metabolism are expelled from the cells and carried away by the blood. Carbon dioxide leaves the bloodstream during the oxygen-carbon dioxide exchange, which occurs through the alveolar/capillary membranes. Carbon dioxide is ultimately eliminated by exhalation from the lungs. Some cellular waste products are expelled into the interstitial fluid and picked up by the lymphatic system. These ultimately flow through the lymph channels into the thoracic duct. The thoracic duct empties the waste products into the venous side of the circulatory system. Other wastes are cleansed from the blood by the kidneys and excreted as urine. Finally, some cellular waste products are emptied into the gastrointestinal system and expelled in the feces.

There is some local control of both tissue perfusion and waste removal. When the amounts of metabolic waste products (such as lactic acid) increase, the tissues subsequently become acidotic. This local acidosis causes nearby precapillary sphincters to relax, thus opening the capillaries and increasing perfusion of the affected tissues. This provides increased capacity for waste elimination and response to local metabolic demands.

THE RESPIRATORY SYSTEM

The respiratory system provides a passage for oxygen, a gas necessary for energy production, to enter the body and for carbon dioxide, a waste product of the body's metabolism, to exit. This gas exchange, called **respiration,** requires a patent, open airway as well as adequate respiratory function. Many pathologic processes can inhibit respiration. To understand the interventions that you will use to maintain adequate airway and ventilatory function, you must thoroughly understand the anatomy of the upper and lower airway.

UPPER AIRWAY ANATOMY

The upper airway extends from the mouth and nose to the larynx (Figure 3-98). It includes the nasal cavity, oral cavity, and pharynx. The larynx joins the upper and lower airways.

* respiration the exchange of gases between a living organism and its environment.

Content Review

UPPER AIRWAY COMPONENTS
- Nasal cavity
- Oral cavity
- Pharynx

FIGURE 3-98 Anatomy of the upper airway.

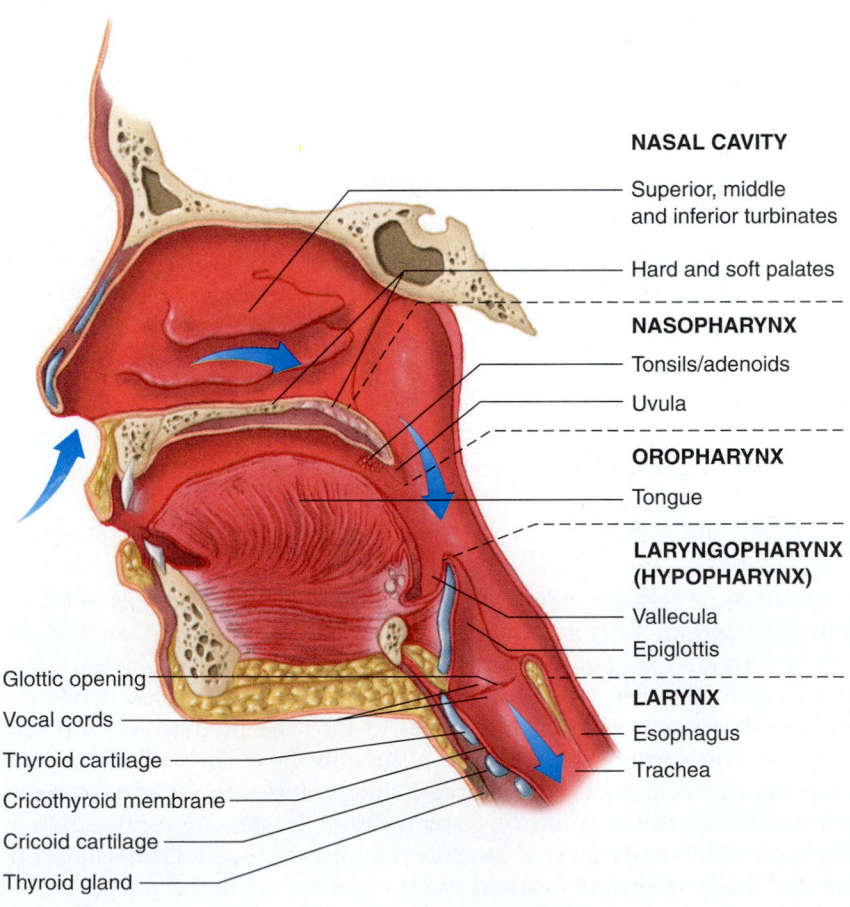

NASAL CAVITY

Superior, middle and inferior turbinates

Hard and soft palates

NASOPHARYNX

Tonsils/adenoids

Uvula

OROPHARYNX

Tongue

LARYNGOPHARYNX (HYPOPHARYNX)

Vallecula

Epiglottis

LARYNX

Esophagus

Trachea

Glottic opening

Vocal cords

Thyroid cartilage

Cricothyroid membrane

Cricoid cartilage

Thyroid gland

The Nasal Cavity

The nasal cavity is the most superior part of the airway. The maxillary, frontal, nasal, ethmoid, and sphenoid bones comprise the lateral and superior walls of the nasal cavity. The hard palate forms the floor of the nasal cavity. The cartilaginous and highly vascular **nasal septum** separates the right and left nasal cavities.

Several different structures connect with the nasal cavity. These include the sinuses, the eustachian tubes, and the nasolacrimal ducts. The **sinuses** are air-filled cavities that are lined with a mucous membrane. There are four pairs of sinuses: the ethmoid sinuses, the frontal sinuses, the maxillary sinuses, and the sphenoid sinuses. The sinuses, named for the bone where they are contained, help reduce the overall weight of the head and are thought to assist in heating, purifying, and moistening the inhaled air. The sinuses help trap bacteria entering the nasal cavity. Because of this, they can become infected. Fractures of the upper sinuses (sphenoids) can occasionally cause cerebrospinal fluid (CSF) to leak from the cranial cavity into the nasal cavity. Clinically this presents with clear fluid draining from the nose (rhinorrhea) and can provide a direct route for the transmission of pathogens to the brain and associated structures.

The **eustachian tubes,** or auditory tubes, connect the ear with the nasal cavity and allow for equalization of pressure on each side of the tympanic membrane. Swallowing can assist in equalizing this pressure. The **nasolacrimal ducts** drain tears and debris the eyes into the nasal cavity. This can cause the nose to run when someone cries.

Air enters the nasal cavity through the external **nares** (nostrils). Nasal hairs just inside the external nares initially filter the incoming air. The air then proceeds into the nasal cavity, where it strikes three bony projections, the superior, middle, and inferior turbinates, or conchae. These shelf-like structures, which are parallel to the nasal floor, serve as conduits into the sinuses, increase the surface area of the nasal cavity, and cause turbulent airflow. This turbulence helps to filter the air by depositing airborne particles on the **mucous membrane** lining the nasal cavity. Hairlike fibers called cilia propel those trapped particles to the back of the pharynx, where they are swallowed.

Because the mucous membrane is covered with **mucus** and has a rich blood supply, it also immediately warms and humidifies the air entering the nose. By the time the air reaches the lower airway, it is at body temperature (37°C), 100% humidified, and virtually free of airborne particles. Air proceeds from the nasal cavity through internal nares into the nasopharynx. The tissue of the nasal cavity is extremely delicate and vascular. Because of this, it is susceptible to trauma.

The Oral Cavity

The cheeks, the hard and soft palates, and the tongue form the mouth, or oral cavity. The lips that surround the mouth's opening are fleshy folds of skin. Behind the lips lie the gums and teeth, normally numbering 32 in the adult. Significant force is required to avulse (dislodge) or fracture the teeth. Broken or dislodged teeth can potentially obstruct the airway. The hard palate anteriorly and the soft palate posteriorly form the top of the oral cavity and separate it from the nasal cavity.

The tongue, a large muscle on the bottom of the oral cavity, is the most common airway obstruction. It attaches to the mandible and the hyoid bone through a series of muscles and ligaments. The U-shaped hyoid bone is located just beneath the chin. The hyoid bone is unique. It is the only bone in the axial skeleton that does not articulate with any other bone. Instead, it is suspended by ligaments from the styloid process of the temporal bone and serves to anchor the tongue and larynx, as well as to support the trachea.

✳ nasal septum cartilage that separates the right and left nasal cavities.

✳ sinus air cavity that conducts fluids from the eustachian tubes and tear ducts to and from the nasopharynx.

✳ eustachian tube a tube that connects the ear with the nasal cavity.

✳ nasolacrimal duct narrow tube that carry into the nasal cavity tears and debris that have drained from the eye.

✳ nare nostril.

✳ mucous membranes tissues lining body cavities that communicate with the air; usually contains mucus-secreting cells.

✳ mucus slippery secretion that lubricates and protects airway surfaces.

pharynx a muscular tube that extends vertically from the back of the soft palate to the superior aspect of the esophagus.

Content Review

REGIONS OF THE PHARYNX
- Nasopharynx
- Oropharynx
- Laryngopharynx

gag reflex mechanism that stimulates retching, or striving to vomit, when the soft palate is touched.

vallecula depression between the epiglottis and the base of the tongue.

endotracheal intubation passing a tube into the trachea to protect and maintain the airway and to permit medication administration and deep suctioning.

larynx the complex structure that joins the pharynx with the trachea.

The Pharynx

The **pharynx** is a muscular tube that extends vertically from the back of the soft palate to the superior aspect of the esophagus. It allows the air to flow into and out of the respiratory tract and food and liquids to pass into the digestive system. It contains several openings, including the internal nares, the mouth, the larynx, and the esophagus.

The pharynx is divided into three regions: the nasopharynx, the oropharynx, and the laryngopharynx (hypopharynx). The nasopharynx is the uppermost region, extending from the back of the nasal opening to the plane of the soft palate. The oropharynx extends from the plane of the soft palate to the hyoid bone. The adenoids, lymphatic tissue in the mouth and nose, filter bacteria. Either hypertrophy or swelling of the adenoids from infection may make them large enough to obscure your view. The laryngopharynx extends posteriorly from the hyoid bone to the esophagus and anteriorly to the larynx. The laryngopharynx is especially important in airway management.

Because the mouth and pharynx serve dual purposes for respiration and digestion, a number of mechanisms help prevent accidental blockage. To prevent foreign material from entering the trachea and lungs, sensitive nerves activate the body's cough and swallowing mechanisms as well as the **gag reflex.**

Located anteriorly in the hypopharynx is the epiglottis, a leaf-shaped cartilage that prevents food from entering the respiratory tract during swallowing. Just anterior and superior to the epiglottis is the **vallecula,** a fold formed by the base of the tongue and the epiglottis. It is an important landmark for **endotracheal intubation.** A series of ligaments and muscles connect the epiglottis to the hyoid bone and mandible. Immediately behind the hypopharynx are the fourth and fifth cervical vertebral bodies.

The Larynx

The **larynx** is the complex structure that joins the pharynx with the trachea (Figure 3-99). Lying midline in the neck, it is attached to and lies just inferior to the hyoid bone and anterior to the esophagus. It consists of the thyroid and cricoid cartilage (both considered tracheal cartilage), glottic opening, vocal cords, arytenoid cartilage, pyriform fossae, and cricothyroid membrane.

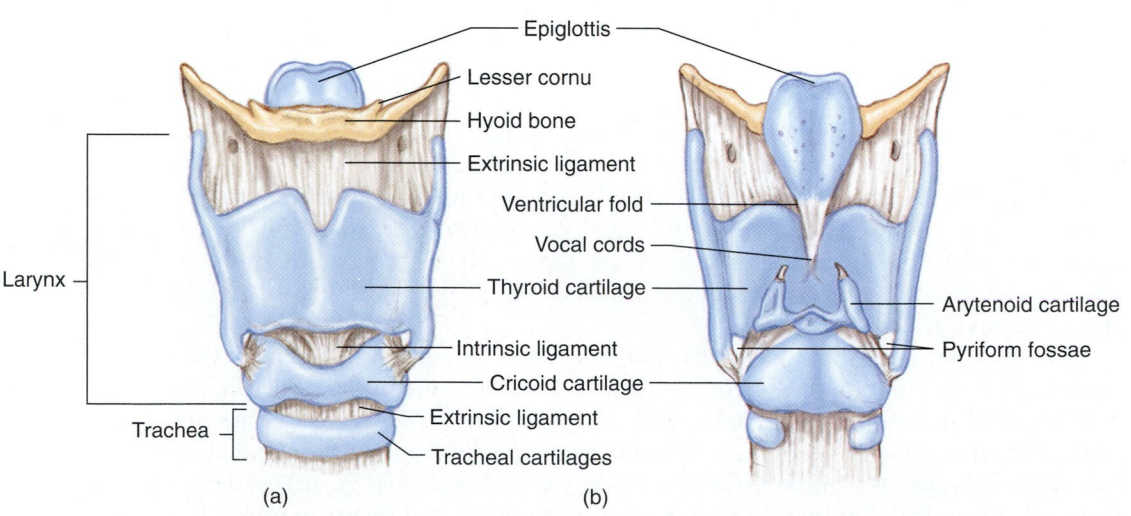

Epiglottis	
Lesser cornu	
Hyoid bone	
Extrinsic ligament	
Ventricular fold	
Vocal cords	
Thyroid cartilage	Arytenoid cartilage
Intrinsic ligament	Pyriform fossae
Cricoid cartilage	
Extrinsic ligament	
Tracheal cartilages	

Larynx

Trachea

(a)   (b)

FIGURE 3-99   Internal anatomy of the upper airway.

The main laryngeal cartilage is the shield-shaped thyroid cartilage. Larger in males than in females, the thyroid cartilage forms the anterior prominence called the Adam's apple. The arytenoid cartilage, which forms a pyramid-shaped attachment for the vocal cords posteriorly, is an important landmark for endotracheal intubation. Posteriorly, smooth muscle closes a gap in the thyroid cartilage. Directly behind the Adam's apple, the thyroid cartilage houses the glottic opening, the narrowest part of the adult trachea, which is bordered by the vocal cords. The patency of the glottic opening, or **glottis**, depends heavily on muscle tone. On either side of the glottic opening are the pyriform fossae, recesses that form the lateral borders of the larynx. The thyrohyoid membrane attaches the upper end of the thyroid cartilage to the hyoid bone.

Within the laryngeal cavity lie the true vocal cords, white bands of cartilage that regulate the passage of air through the larynx and produce voice by contraction of the laryngeal muscles. The vocal cords can also close together to prevent foreign bodies from entering the airway. The passage of an endotracheal tube between the vocal cords interferes not only with the creation of sound, but also with the protective function of coughing.

Beneath the thyroid cartilage is the cricoid cartilage, which forms the inferior border of the larynx. Often it is considered the first tracheal ring. Unlike the thyroid and other tracheal cartilages, whose posterior surfaces are open and not fused, the cricoid cartilage forms a complete ring. The esophagus lies behind the cricoid cartilage, so pressure applied in a posterior direction to the anterior cricoid cartilage occludes the esophagus (**Sellick's maneuver**), thus inhibiting vomiting and subsequent **aspiration** during airway management. In children, the cricoid cartilage is the narrowest part of the laryngeal airway. The fibrous **cricothyroid membrane** connects the inferior border of the thyroid cartilage with the superior aspect of the cricoid cartilage. It is the site for surgical airway techniques.

A mucous membrane lines most of the larynx. Rich with nerve endings from the vagus nerve, it is so sensitive that any irritation sparks a cough, or forceful exhalation of a large volume of air. First, air is drawn into the respiratory passageways. Next, the glottic opening shuts tightly, trapping the air within the lungs. Then the abdominal and thoracic muscles contract, pushing against the diaphragm and increasing intrathoracic pressure. The vocal cords suddenly open, and a burst of air forces foreign particles out of the lungs. The laryngeal mucous membrane is so sensitive that its stimulation by a laryngoscope or endotracheal tube can cause bradycardia (slow pulse rate), hypotension (low blood pressure), and decreased respiratory rate.

Other structures proximate to the larynx and of particular interest when you perform surgical airways are the thyroid gland, carotid arteries, and jugular veins. The thyroid gland is a "bow-tie" shaped endocrine gland located in the neck. It is highly vascular and lies inferior to the cricoid cartilage. It contains two lobes, one on each side of the trachea. These lobes are joined in the middle by the isthmus that extends across the trachea. The carotid arteries run closely along the trachea. Several branches of the carotid arteries cross the trachea. Likewise, the jugular veins lie very close to the trachea. Several branches of the jugular veins, such as the superior thyroid vein, cross the trachea.

LOWER AIRWAY ANATOMY

The lower airway extends from below the larynx to the alveoli (Figure 3-100). This is where the respiratory exchange of oxygen and carbon dioxide occurs. Helpful landmarks are the fourth cervical vertebra at the posterior superior border, and the xiphoid process anterior inferiorly, though the posterior lung extends beyond this inferiorly.

✱ **glottis** lip-like opening between the vocal cords.

✱ **Sellick's maneuver** pressure applied in a posterior direction to the anterior cricoid cartilage that occludes the esophagus.

✱ **aspiration** inhaling foreign material, such as vomitus, into the lungs.

✱ **cricothyroid membrane** membrane between the cricoid and thyroid cartilages of the larynx.

Content Review

LOWER AIRWAY COMPONENTS

- Trachea
- Bronchi
- Alveoli
- Lung parenchyma
- Pleura

FIGURE 3-100 Anatomy of the lower airway.

The Trachea

As air enters the lower airway from the upper airway, it first enters and then passes through the **trachea.** The trachea is a 10–12 centimeter-long tube that connects the larynx to the two mainstem bronchi. It contains cartilaginous, C-shaped, open rings that form a frame to keep it open. The trachea is lined with respiratory epithelium containing cilia and mucus-producing cells. The mucus traps particles that the upper airway did not filter. The cilia then move the trapped particulate matter up into the mouth where it is swallowed or expelled.

The Bronchi

At the carina, the trachea divides, or bifurcates, into the right and left mainstem **bronchi.** The right mainstem bronchus is almost straight, while the left mainstem bronchus angles more acutely to the left. Because of this, the right mainstem is often the site of aspirated foreign bodies. In addition, when an endotracheal tube is inserted too far, it tends to enter the right mainstem bronchus, thus ventilating only the right lung. Mainstem bronchi enter the lung tissue at the hilum, and then divide into the secondary and tertiary bronchi. The secondary and tertiary bronchi ultimately branch into the bronchioles, or small airways.

The bronchioles are encircled with smooth muscle that contains beta$_2$ (β_2) adrenergic receptors. When stimulated, these beta$_2$ receptors relax the bronchial smooth muscle, thus increasing the airway's diameter. This bronchodilation can increase the amount of air transported through the bronchiole. Conversely,

✱ **trachea** 10–12 cm-long tube that connects the larynx to the mainstem bronchi.

✱ **bronchi** tubes from the trachea into the lungs.

FIGURE 3-101 Anatomy of the alveoli.

Smooth muscle

Elastin fibers

Alveoli

Capillaries

parasympathetic receptors, when stimulated, cause the bronchial smooth muscles to contract, thus reducing the diameter of the bronchiole. This bronchoconstriction can inhibit the movement of air through the bronchiole.

After approximately 22 divisions, the bronchioles turn into the respiratory bronchioles. These structures contain only muscular connective tissue and have a limited capacity for gas exchange. The respiratory bronchioles terminate at the alveoli.

The Alveoli

The respiratory bronchioles divide into the alveolar ducts, which terminate in balloon-like clusters of **alveoli** called alveolar sacs (Figure 3-101). The alveoli contain an alveolar membrane that is only one or two cell layers thick. Because of this, the alveoli comprise the key functional unit of the respiratory system. Most oxygen and carbon dioxide gas exchanges take place here, although limited gas exchange may occur in the alveolar ducts and respiratory bronchioles. The alveoli become thinner as they expand. This facilitates diffusion of oxygen and carbon dioxide.

The alveoli's surface area is massive, totaling more than 40 square meters—enough to cover half of a tennis court. These hollow structures resist collapse largely because of the presence of surfactant, a chemical that decreases their surface tension and makes it easier for them to expand. Alveolar collapse (**atelectasis**) can occur if surfactant is insufficient or if the alveoli are not inflated. No gas exchange takes place in atelectatic alveoli.

The Lung Parenchyma

The alveoli are the terminal end of the respiratory tree and the functional units of the lungs. As such, they are the core of the lung **parenchyma.** The lung parenchyma is arranged in two pulmonary lobules that form the anatomic division of the lungs. These lobules are further organized into lobes. The right lung has three lobes, the upper lobe, the middle lobe, and the lower lobe. The left lung, which shares thoracic space with the heart, has only two lobes, the upper lobe and the lower lobe.

✳ **alveoli** microscopic air sacs where most oxygen and carbon dioxide gas exchanges take place.

✳ **atelactasis** alveolar collapse.

✳ **parenchyma** principle or essential parts of an organ.

The Pleura

Membranous connective tissue called **pleura** covers the lungs. The pleura consists of two layers, visceral and parietal. The visceral pleura envelopes the lungs and does not contain nerve fibers. In contrast, the parietal pleura lines the thoracic cavity and does contain nerve fibers. The potential space between these two layers, called the pleural space, usually holds a small amount of fluid that reduces friction between the pleural layers during respiration. Occasionally, the pleura can become inflamed, causing significant pain with respiration. This condition, called pleurisy, is a common cause of chest pain, particularly in cigarette smokers.

THE PEDIATRIC AIRWAY

The pediatric airway is fundamentally the same as an adult's, but you will need to know the differences in relative size and position of some components. The airway is smaller in all aspects, particularly the diameters of the openings and passageways.

In the pharynx, the jaw is smaller and the tongue relatively larger, resulting in greater potential airway encroachment (Figure 3-102). The epiglottis is much floppier and rounder ("omega" shaped). The dental (alveolar) ridge and teeth are softer and more fragile than an adult's and potentially more subject to damage from airway maneuvers.

The larynx lies more superior and anterior in children and is funnel-shaped because the cricoid cartilage is undeveloped. Before the age of ten, the cricoid cartilage is the narrowest part of the airway. Most significantly, even a small foreign body or a limited degree of swelling in the pediatric airway can be life threatening. Because of this, young children tend to suffer more problems related to the

FIGURE 3-102 Anatomy of the pediatric airway.

Relatively greater proportion of soft tissue

Larynx more superior and anterior

Epiglottis rounder and floppier

Loosely attached mucous membranes

Smaller jaw

Cricoid cartilage — narrowest part of the pediatric airway

trachea than do older children. A common example is croup (laryngotracheo-bronchitis), a viral infection that causes the soft tissues below the glottis to swell. This can reduce the diameter of the airway, potentially causing serious problems.

The ribs and the cartilage of the pediatric thoracic cage are softer and more pliable. This lack of rigidity lessens the thoracic wall's and accessory muscles' ability to assist lung expansion during inspiration. As a result, infants and children tend to rely more on their diaphragms for breathing. Always pay close attention to these differences when treating pediatric patients, especially those with respiratory complaints.

PHYSIOLOGY OF THE RESPIRATORY SYSTEM

Just as successful airway management requires a firm understanding of airway anatomy, a good outcome for these patients requires a working knowledge of the mechanics of oxygenation and ventilation. Your knowledge of normal respiratory physiology will lay the groundwork for your comprehension of important pathophysiology and will help you to determine which actions will assure optimal patient care.

Respiration and Ventilation

Respiration is the exchange of gases between a living organism and its environment. Pulmonary, or external, respiration occurs in the lungs when the respiratory gases are exchanged between the alveoli and the red blood cells in the pulmonary capillaries through the capillary membranes (Figure 3-103). Cellular, or internal, respiration, on the other hand, occurs in the peripheral capillaries. It is the exchange of the respiratory gases between the red blood cells and the various body tissues. Cellular respiration in the peripheral tissue produces carbon dioxide (CO_2). The blood picks up this waste product in the capillaries and transports it as bicarbonate ions through the venous system to the lungs. While respiration describes the process of gas exchange in the lungs and peripheral tissues, **ventilation** is the mechanical process that moves air into and out of the lungs. Ventilation is necessary for respiration to occur.

The Respiratory Cycle Nothing within the lung parenchyma makes it contract or expand. Pulmonary ventilation, therefore, depends upon changes in pressure within the thoracic cavity. These changes occur in a respiratory cycle involving coordinated interaction among the respiratory system, the central nervous system, and the musculoskeletal system.

The thoracic cavity is a closed space, opening to the external environment only through the trachea. The diaphragm separates the thoracic cavity from the abdomen. When the diaphragm contracts, it draws downward, away from the thoracic cavity, thus enlarging it. Likewise, when the muscles between the ribs, or intercostal muscles, contract, they draw the ribcage upward and outward, away from the thoracic cavity, further increasing its volume.

The respiratory cycle begins when the lungs have achieved a normal expiration and the pressure inside the thoracic cavity equals the atmospheric pressure. At this point, respiratory centers in the brain communicate with the diaphragm by way of the phrenic nerve, signaling it to contract and thus initiate the respiratory cycle. As the size of the thorax increases in relation to the volume of air it holds, pressure within the thorax decreases, becoming lower than atmospheric pressure. This negative intrathoracic pressure invites air into the thorax through the airway. Because the visceral and parietal pleura remain in contact with each other under normal circumstances, the highly elastic lungs immediately assume the thoracic cavity's internal contour. These combined factors move air into the lungs (inspiration). At the same time, the alveoli inflate

* **ventilation** the mechanical process that moves air into and out of the lungs.

FIGURE 3-103 Diffusion of gases across an alveolar membrane.

In quiet breathing

500 ml
of inspired air

Contains: 20.94% Oxygen
79.01% Nitrogen
0.04% Carbon dioxide

150 ml
occupies the
conducting pathways
"Dead space"

350 ml (together
with 150 ml of air
previously contained
in conducting pathways)
reach the Alveoli

Expired air

Contains: 16.4% Oxygen
79.6% Nitrogen
4.0% Carbon dioxide

O_2

CO_2

Oxygenated blood
circulated
back to the heart

Deoxygenated
blood from the heart

with the lungs. They become thinner as they expand, allowing oxygen and carbon dioxide to diffuse across their membranes.

When the pressure in the thoracic cavity again reaches that of the atmosphere, the alveoli are maximally inflated. Pulmonary expansion stimulates microscopic stretch receptors in the bronchi and bronchioles. These receptors signal the respiratory center by way of the vagus nerve to inhibit inspiration, and the air influx stops. This process is primarily protective, as it prevents overinflation of the lungs.

At the end of inspiration, the respiratory muscles now relax, thus decreasing the size of the chest cavity, and in turn increasing the intrathoracic pressure. The naturally elastic lungs recoil, forcing air out through the airway (expiration) until intrathoracic and atmospheric pressure are equal once again. Normal expiration is a passive process, while inspiration is an active process, using energy. In respiratory inadequacy, when this process fails to provide satisfactory gas exchange, the patient may use accessory respiratory muscles such as the strap muscles of his neck and his abdominal muscles to augment his efforts to expand the thoracic cavity.

Pulmonary Circulation Respiration also requires an intact circulatory system. In fact, during each cardiac cycle, the heart pumps as much blood to the lungs as it pumps to the peripheral tissues. In the capillaries, these cells take oxygen from red blood cells coming from the arterial system and give up carbon dioxide to

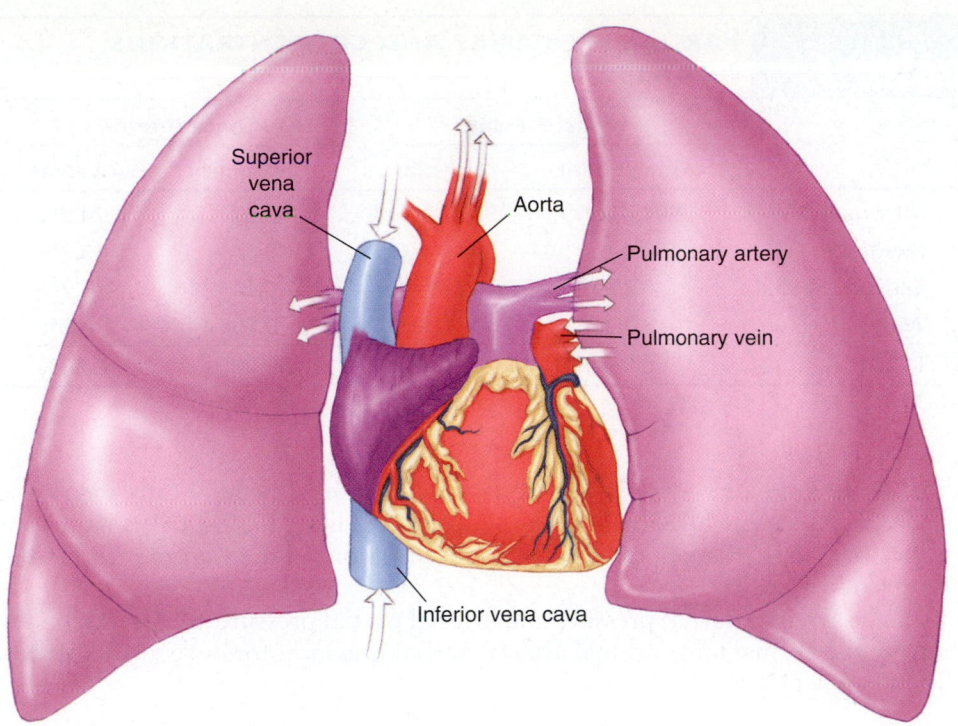

FIGURE 3-104 Pulmonary circulation.

Superior vena cava

Aorta

Pulmonary artery

Pulmonary vein

Inferior vena cava

blood returning to the venous system. The venous system carries this deoxygenated blood to the right side of the heart, and the right ventricle pumps it into the pulmonary artery (Figure 3-104).

The pulmonary artery immediately branches into the right and the left pulmonary arteries, each supplying its respective lung. In turn, both branches quickly fan into smaller arteries that end in the pulmonary capillaries. These capillaries are spread over the surfaces of the alveoli, where the red blood cells exchange carbon dioxide for oxygen. The pulmonary capillaries recombine into larger veins, eventually terminating in the pulmonary vein. The pulmonary vein empties the oxygenated blood into the left atrium of the heart. Finally, the heart transports the oxygenated blood through the left ventricle and into the systemic arterial system via the aorta and its tributaries.

The lungs themselves receive little of their blood supply from the pulmonary arteries or veins. Instead, bronchial arteries that branch from the aorta supply most of their blood. Bronchial veins return this blood from the lungs to the superior vena cava.

Measuring Oxygen and Carbon Dioxide Levels

You can determine the amount of oxygen and carbon dioxide in the blood by measuring their partial pressures. **Partial pressure** is the pressure exerted by each component of a gas mixture. In other words, the partial pressure of a gas is its percentage of the mixture's total pressure. The partial pressure of oxygen at normal atmospheric pressure, for example, is the percentage of oxygen in atmospheric air (21%) multiplied by the atmospheric pressure at sea level (760 torr, or 14.7 pounds per square inch):

$$0.21 \times 760 \text{ torr} = 159.6 \text{ torr}$$

(Note that torr and mmHg are the same measures of pressure.) Earth's atmosphere consists of four major respiratory gases: nitrogen (N_2), oxygen (O_2), carbon

✱ **partial pressure** the pressure exerted by each component of a gas mixture.

Table 3-6 — PARTIAL PRESSURES AND CONCENTRATIONS OF GASES

	Partial Pressure		Concentration	
	Atmospheric	Alveolar	Atmospheric	Alveolar
Nitrogen	597.0 torr	569.0 torr	78.62%	74.9%
Oxygen	159.0 torr	104.0 torr	20.84%	13.7%
Carbon Dioxide	0.3 torr	40.0 torr	0.04%	5.2%
Water	3.7 torr	47.0 torr	0.50%	6.2%
TOTAL	760.0 torr	760.0 torr	100.00%	100.0%

dioxide (CO_2), and water (H_2O). Although nitrogen is metabolically inert, it is needed to inflate gas-filled body cavities such as the chest. Table 3-6 lists these four respiratory gases' partial pressures and concentrations in the environment and in the alveoli.

Since alveolar partial pressure and arterial partial pressure are essentially the same in the normal lung, normal arterial partial pressures for oxygen and carbon dioxide may be expressed:

Oxygen (PaO_2) = 100 torr (average = 80–100)

Carbon dioxide ($PaCO_2$) = 40 torr (average = 35–45)

* **PA** alveolar partial pressure.

* **Pa** arterial partial pressure.

Alveolar partial pressures are abbreviated **PA** (PAO_2 and $PACO_2$) while arterial partial pressures are abbreviated **Pa** (PaO_2 and $PaCO_2$). Because these values are usually the same, however, they typically appear as the shortened notations PO_2 and PCO_2.

* **diffusion** movement of a gas from an area of higher concentration to an area of lower concentration.

Diffusion **Diffusion** is the movement of a gas from an area of higher concentration to an area of lower concentration, attempting to reach equilibrium. Diffusion transfer gases between the lungs and the blood and between the blood and the peripheral tissues. The rate of diffusion of a gas across the pulmonary membranes depends on the gas's solubility in water. For example, carbon dioxide is 21 times more soluble in water than oxygen and readily crosses the pulmonary capillary membranes. In the peripheral tissues, the gradient (direction of diffusion) for CO_2 is from the tissue, where its concentration is high, to the capillary blood, where its concentration is low.

In the lungs, oxygen dissolves in water at the alveolar membrane and leaves the area of higher concentration, the alveoli, and enters the area of lower concentration, the venous blood in the pulmonary capillaries. Concurrently, carbon dioxide leaves the area of higher concentration, the arterial blood, and enters the area of lower concentration, the alveoli. The blood returns from the pulmonary vein to the heart and then moves into the systemic circulation.

Oxygen Concentration in the Blood Oxygen diffuses into the blood plasma, where most of it combines with hemoglobin and is measured as oxygen saturation (SaO_2). The remainder is dissolved in the blood and is measured as the PaO_2. Hemoglobin approaches 100% saturation when the PaO_2 of dissolved oxygen reaches 90–100 torr. Each gram of saturated hemoglobin carries 1.34 milliliters of oxygen. Oxygen saturation is the ratio of the blood's actual oxygen content to its total oxygen-carrying capacity:

Oxygen saturation = O_2 content/O_2 capacity $\times$ 100(%)

The hemoglobin molecule carries the vast majority of oxygen in the blood (approximately 97%). Very little oxygen dissolves in the plasma. Since partial pressure measurements detect only the amount of oxygen dissolved in the plasma and do not always reflect the total oxygen saturation, they can be misleading. For example, a patient who has suffered carbon monoxide poisoning cannot transport enough oxygen to the peripheral tissues since carbon monoxide displaces oxygen from the hemoglobin molecule. But an arterial blood gas sample might reveal a normal or high PaO_2. This would indicate that adequate oxygen was reaching the blood. In fact, however, an inadequate amount of hemoglobin would be available to transport the oxygen to the peripheral tissues, thus resulting in peripheral hypoxia.

Several factors can affect oxygen concentrations in the blood:

- *Decreased hemoglobin concentration* (anemia, hemorrhage)
- *Inadequate alveolar ventilation* due to low inspired-oxygen concentration, respiratory muscle paralysis, and pulmonary conditions such as emphysema, asthma, or pneumothorax
- *Decreased diffusion across the pulmonary membrane* when diffusion distance increases or the pulmonary membrane changes; for example, when fluid enters the space between the alveolar membrane and the pulmonary capillary membrane, as in pneumonia, chronic obstructive pulmonary disease (COPD), or pulmonary edema (swelling).
- *Ventilation/perfusion mismatch* occurs when a portion of the alveoli collapses, as in atelectasis. Blood travels past these collapsed alveoli without oxygenation (shunting), without carbon dioxide, and without oxygen uptake. This can result from **hypoventilation,** which can occur secondary to pain or inability to inspire (traumatic asphyxia). When the lung collapses, as in **pneumothorax, hemothorax,** or a combination of the two, less surface area is available for gas exchange. Alternatively, a ventilation/perfusion mismatch can occur when blood is prevented from reaching the alveolar capillary membranes but alveolar ventilation remains adequate. This occurs when a blood clot travels to or is formed in the pulmonary arterial system, a condition known as pulmonary thromboembolism.

You can correct oxygen derangements by increasing ventilation, administering supplemental oxygen, using intermittent positive pressure ventilation (IPPV), or administering drugs to correct underlying problems such as pulmonary edema, asthma, or **pulmonary embolism.** The emergency being treated determines the desired fractional concentration of oxygen (**FiO$_2$**) to be delivered. It is crucial to remember not to withhold oxygen from any patient whose clinical condition indicates its need.

Carbon Dioxide Concentration in the Blood The blood transports carbon dioxide mainly in the form of bicarbonate ion (HCO_3^-). It carries approximately 70% as bicarbonate and approximately 20% combined with hemoglobin. Less than 7% is dissolved in the plasma. Several factors influence carbon dioxide's concentration in the blood, including increased CO_2 production and/or decreased CO_2 elimination:

- *Hyperventilation lowers CO$_2$ levels* and can be the result of an increased respiratory rate or deeper respiration, both of which increase the minute volume. (We will discuss minute volume more completely later.)

✴ **hypoventilation** reduction in breathing rate and depth.

✴ **pneumothorax** accumulation of air or gas in the pleural cavity.

✴ **hemothorax** accumulation in the pleural cavity of blood or fluid containing blood.

✴ **pulmonary embolism** blood clot that travels to the pulmonary circulation and hinders oxygenation of the blood.

✴ **FiO$_2$** concentration of oxygen in inspired air.

- *Increased CO_2 production* can be caused by:
  —Fever
  —Muscle exertion
  —Shivering
  —Metabolic processes resulting in the formation of metabolic acids
- *Decreased CO_2 elimination* (increased CO_2 levels in the blood) resulting from decreased alveolar ventilation is commonly caused by hypoventilation due to:
  —Respiratory depression by drugs
  —Airway obstruction
  —Impairment of the respiratory muscles
  —Obstructive diseases such as asthma and emphysema

✱ **hypercarbia** excessive pressure of carbon dioxide in the blood.

Increased CO_2 levels (**hypercarbia**) are usually treated by increasing the rate and/or volume of ventilation and by correcting the underlying cause.

Regulation of Respiration

Respiratory Rate The number of times a person breathes in one minute, the **respiratory rate,** is unique in that both voluntary and involuntary nervous system mechanisms control it. We do not ordinarily need to make a conscious effort to breathe; our brains automatically regulate this function. However, we can voluntarily override our involuntary respirations until physical and chemical mechanisms signal the nervous system's respiratory centers to provide involuntarily impulses and correct any breathing irregularities.

✱ **respiratory rate** the number of times a person breathes in one minute.

Nervous Impulses from the Respiratory Center The main respiratory center lies in the *medulla oblongata* in the brainstem. Various neurons within the medulla initiate impulses that result in respiration. A rise in the frequency of these impulses increases the respiratory rate. Conversely, a decrease in their frequency decreases the respiratory rate. The medulla is connected to the respiratory muscles primarily via the vagus nerve. This is an involuntary pathway. If the medulla fails to initiate respiration, an additional control center in the pons, called the *apneustic center,* assumes respiratory control to ensure the continuation of respirations. A third center, the *pneumotaxic center,* also in the pons, controls expiration.

Stretch Receptors During inspiration, the lungs become distended, activating stretch receptors. As the degree of stretch increases, these receptors fire more frequently. The impulses they send to the brainstem inhibit the medullary cells, decreasing the inspiratory stimulus. Thus, the respiratory muscles relax, allowing the elastic lungs to recoil and expel air from the body. As the stretch decreases, the stretch receptors stop firing. This process, called the *Hering-Breuer reflex,* prevents overexpansion of the lungs.

Chemoreceptors Other involuntary respiration controls include central chemical receptors in the medulla and peripheral chemoreceptors in the carotid bodies and in the arch of the aorta. These chemoreceptors are stimulated by decreased PaO_2, increased $PaCO_2$, and decreased pH. (The pH scale expresses the degree of acidity or alkalinity. A lower pH indicates greater acidity; a higher pH indicates greater alkalinity. The general principles of pathophysiology chapter discusses pH in greater detail.) Cerebrospinal fluid (CSF) pH is the primary control of respiratory center stimulation. The CSF pH responds very quickly to changes in arterial PCO_2. Any increase in PCO_2 will decrease CSF pH, which will in turn stimulate the central chemoreceptors to increase respiration. Conversely, low $PaCO_2$ levels will raise CSF pH, in turn decreasing chemoreceptor stimulation and slowing respiratory activity. Because $PaCO_2$ is inversely related to CSF pH, $PaCO_2$ is seen as the normal neuroregulatory control of respirations. Additionally, any increase in the arterial $PaCO_2$ stimulates the peripheral chemoreceptors to signal the brainstem to increase respiration, thus speeding CO_2 elimination from the body.

Hypoxic Drive The body also constantly monitors the PaO_2 and the pH. In fact, **hypoxemia** (decreased partial pressure of oxygen in the blood) is a profound stimulus of respiration in a normal individual. People with chronic respiratory disease such as emphysema and chronic bronchitis tend to retain CO_2 and, therefore, have a chronically elevated $PaCO_2$. Chemoreceptors in the periphery eventually become accustomed to this chronic condition, and the central nervous system stops using $PaCO_2$ to regulate respiration. This activates a default mechanism called **hypoxic drive,** which increases respiratory stimulation when PaO_2 falls and inhibits respiratory stimulation when PaO_2 climbs. High-volume oxygen administration to people with this condition can cause respiratory arrest. Because high-flow oxygen can quickly double or even triple the PaO_2, peripheral chemoreceptors stop stimulating the respiratory centers, causing **apnea.** (Although this is a potential threat, it is never appropriate to withhold oxygen from a patient for whom oxygen therapy is indicated; if the respiratory effort becomes inadequate, ventilatory assistance will be necessary.)

Measures of Respiratory Function

The respiratory rate is the number of respiratory cycles per minute, normally 12–20 breaths per minute in adults, 18–24 in children, and 40–60 in infants. Several factors affect respiratory rate:

- Fever—increases rate
- Emotion—increases rate
- Pain—increases rate
- Hypoxia (inadequate tissue oxygenation)—increases rate
- Acidosis—increases rate
- Stimulant drugs—increase rate
- Depressant drugs—decrease rate
- Sleep—decreases rate

Paramedics must fully understand ventilatory mechanics and capacities for the average adult's respiratory system. This knowledge will enable you to adapt your mechanical ventilation techniques to your patient's size, lung compliance, need for hyperventilation, or other individual requirements. It is especially crucial in situations that call for advanced mechanical ventilator skills. Respiratory capacities and measurements with which you must be familiar include:

- *Total Lung Capacity (TLC).* This is the maximum lung capacity—the total amount of air contained in the lung at the end of maximal inspiration. In the average adult male, this volume is approximately 6 liters.
- *Tidal Volume (V_T).* The tidal volume is the average volume of gas inhaled or exhaled in one respiratory cycle. In the adult male this is approximately 500 ml (5–7 ml/kg).
- *Dead Space Volume (V_D).* The dead space volume is the amount of gas in the tidal volume that remains in air passageways unavailable for gas exchange. It is approximately 150 ml in the adult male. Anatomic dead space includes the trachea and bronchi. Obstructions or diseases such as chronic obstructive pulmonary disease or atelectasis can cause physiologic dead space.

✱ hypoxemia decreased blood oxygen level.

✱ hypoxic drive mechanism that increases respiratory stimulation when blood oxygen falls and inhibits respiratory stimulation when blood oxygen climbs.

✱ apnea absence of breathing.

✱ total lung capacity maximum lung capacity.

✱ tidal volume average volume of gas inhaled or exhaled in one respiratory cycle.

- *Alveolar Volume (V_A).* The alveolar volume is the amount of gas in the tidal volume that reaches the alveoli for gas exchange. It is the difference between tidal volume and dead-space volume (approximately 350 ml in the adult male):

$$V_A = V_T - V_D$$

- *Minute Volume (V_{min}).* The minute volume is the amount of gas moved in and out of the respiratory tract in one minute:

$$V_{min} = VT \times \text{respiratory rate}$$

- *Alveolar Minute Volume (V_{A-min}).* The alveolar minute volume is the amount of gas that reaches the alveoli for gas exchange in one minute:

$$V_{A-min} = (V_T - V_D) \times \text{respiratory rate}$$

or

$$V_{A-min} = V_A \times \text{respiratory rate}$$

- *Inspiratory Reserve Volume (IRV).* The inspiratory reserve volume is the amount of air that can be maximally inhaled after a normal inspiration.
- *Expiratory Reserve Volume (ERV).* The expiratory reserve volume is the amount of air that can be maximally exhaled after a normal expiration.
- *Residual Volume (RV).* The residual volume is the amount of air remaining in the lungs at the end of maximal expiration.
- *Functional Residual Capacity (FRC).* The functional residual capacity is the volume of gas that remains in the lungs at the end of normal expiration:

$$FRC = ERV + RV$$

- *Forced Expiratory Volume (FEV).* The forced expiratory volume is the amount of air that can be maximally expired after maximum inspiration.

THE ABDOMEN

The abdominal cavity is bound by the diaphragm, superiorly; the pelvis, inferiorly; the vertebral column, the posterior and inferior ribs, and the back muscles (psoas and paraspinal muscles), posteriorly; the muscles of the flank, laterally; and the abdominal muscles, anteriorly (Figure 3-105). The cavity is divided into three spaces: the **peritoneal space** (containing those organs or portions of organs covered by the abdominal (peritoneal) lining); the **retroperitoneal space** (containing those organs posterior to the peritoneal lining); and the **pelvic space** (containing the organs within the pelvis). Anatomic landmarks of this area include the centrally located umbilicus (the navel), the xiphoid process (tip of the sternum) at the upper and central abdominal border, the bony ridges of the pelvis (the iliac crests) inferiorly and laterally, and the pubic prominence inferiorly.

The abdomen is divided into four subregions by imaginary vertical and horizontal lines intersecting at the umbilicus (naval) and forming the right and left upper and lower quadrants. The right upper quadrant contains the gallbladder, right kidney, most of the liver, some small bowel, a portion of the ascending and transverse colon, and a small portion of the pancreas. The left upper quadrant

---

✳ **minute volume** amount of gas inhaled and exhaled in one minute.

✳ **peritoneal space** division of the abdominal cavity containing those organs or portions of organs covered by the peritoneum.

✳ **retroperitoneal space** division of the abdominal cavity containing those organs posterior to the peritoneal lining.

✳ **pelvic space** division of the abdominal cavity containing those organs located within the pelvis.

Serratus anterior
Internal intercostals
External intercostals
Tendinous inscriptions
External oblique
Rectus abdominus

Latissimus dorsi
Erector spinae
Quadratus lumborum
Psoas
Transversus abdominus
Internal oblique
External oblique
Rectus abdominus
Linea alba

FIGURE 3-105 Muscles protecting the organs of the abdominal cavity.

a. Anterior view of the trunk, showing superficial and deep members of the oblique and rectus groups.

b. Diagrammatic sectional view through the abdominal region.

contains the stomach, spleen, left kidney, most of the pancreas, and a portion of the liver, small bowel, and transverse and descending colon. The right lower quadrant contains the appendix, and portions of the urinary bladder, small bowel, ascending colon, rectum, and female genitalia. The left lower quadrant contains the sigmoid colon and portions of the urinary bladder, small bowel, descending colon, rectum, and female genitalia.

The major structures within the abdomen include the digestive tract, the accessory organs of digestion, the spleen, the structures and organs of the urinary system, and the female reproductive organs. (The male reproductive organs, or genitalia, are considered to be part of the urinary system. The female reproductive organs are separate from the urinary system, and include the reproductive organs within the abdomen as well as the external genitalia.)

ABDOMINAL VASCULATURE

The abdominal contents are supplied with blood via the abdominal aorta, which travels along and to the left of the spinal column. It sends forth many branches to discrete organs and the bowel (Figure 3-106). The abdominal aorta bifurcates at the upper sacral level into two large iliac arteries. These eventually become the femoral arteries as they traverse and then exit the pelvis. The attachment of these arteries to the pelvic structure is quite firm and may result in their tearing if the pelvis is fractured and displaced. The inferior vena cava is located along the spinal column and collects venous blood from the lower extremities and the abdomen, relatively parallel to the arterial system, returning it to the heart. The abdomen also houses a special circulatory system, the portal system. This venous subsystem collects venous blood and the fluid and nutrients absorbed by the bowel and transports them to the liver. The liver detoxifies the fluid, stores excess nutrients, adds nutrients when they are deficient, and then sends the blood/nutrient/fluid mixture into the inferior vena cava, just below the heart. There it mixes with venous blood and is circulated through the heart and then the rest of the body.

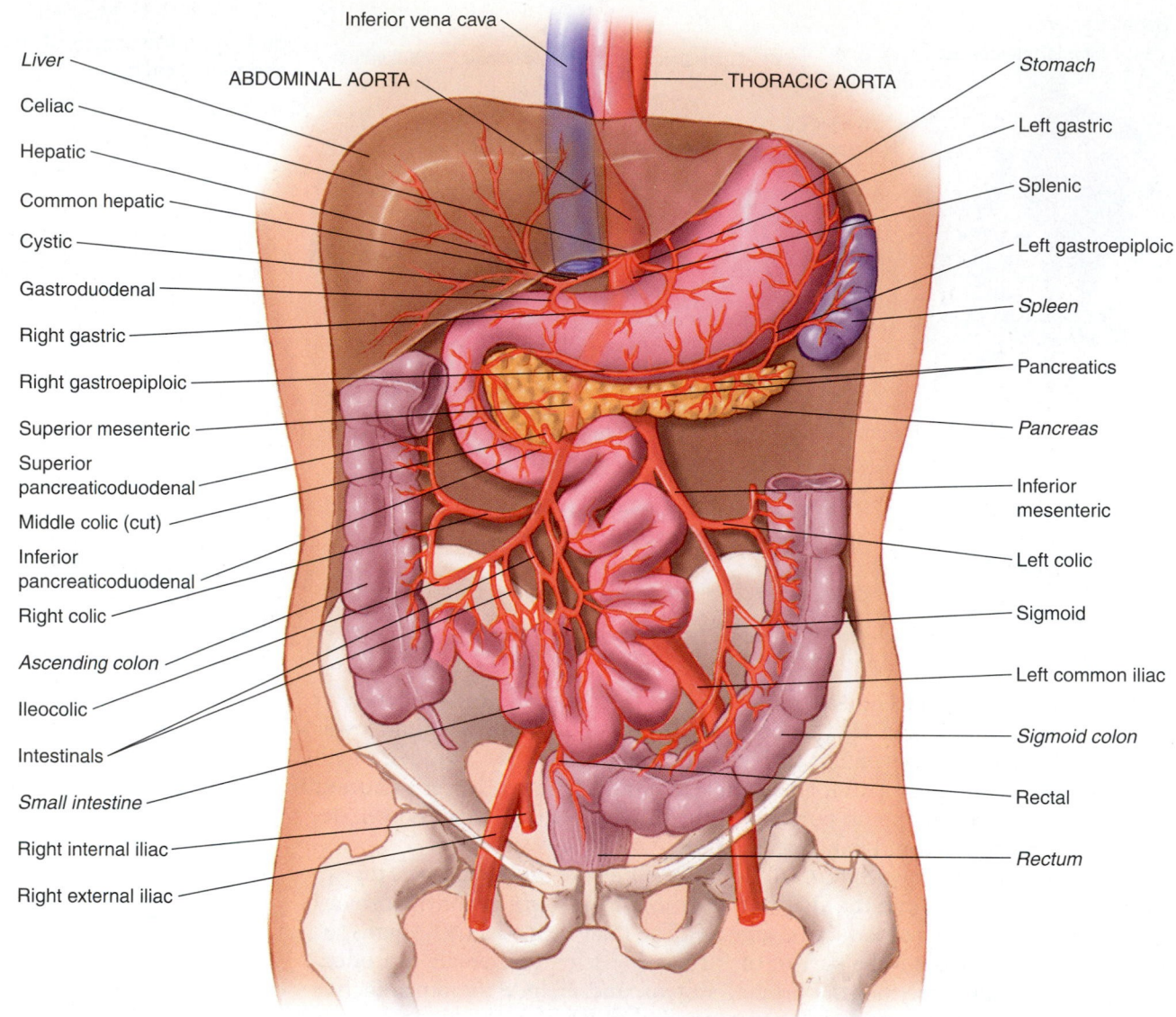

Inferior vena cava

Liver

ABDOMINAL AORTA

Celiac

Hepatic

Common hepatic

Cystic

Gastroduodenal

Right gastric

Right gastroepiploic

Superior mesenteric

Superior pancreaticoduodenal

Middle colic (cut)

Inferior pancreaticoduodenal

Right colic

Ascending colon

Ileocolic

Intestinals

Small intestine

Right internal iliac

Right external iliac

THORACIC AORTA

Stomach

Left gastric

Splenic

Left gastroepiploic

Spleen

Pancreatics

Pancreas

Inferior mesenteric

Left colic

Sigmoid

Left common iliac

Sigmoid colon

Rectal

Rectum

FIGURE 3-106 The abdominal arteries.

THE PERITONEUM

Many of the abdominal organs are covered by a serous membrane called the **peritoneum** (Figure 3-107). This tissue resembles the pleura of the lungs and functions in a similar manner. The parietal peritoneum covers the most of the interior surface of the anterior and lateral abdominal cavity, while the visceral peritoneum covers the individual organs. A small amount of fluid is found between the peritoneal layers and permits free movement of the bowel during digestion.

The digestive tract is restrained and prevented from tangling by a structure called the **mesentery.** The mesentery is a double fold of peritoneum containing blood vessels, lymphatic vessels, nerves, and fatty tissue. It suspends the bowel from the posterior abdominal wall. An additional fold of mesentery, called the omentum, also covers, insulates, and protects the anterior surface of the abdomen. The thickness of the omentum varies with the size and percentage of body fat of the patient. It may be several inches thick in the obese patient or very narrow in the thin and muscular patient.

✳ **peritoneum** fine fibrous tissue surrounding the interior of most of the abdominal cavity and covering most of the small bowel and some of the abdominal organs.

✳ **mesentery** double fold of peritoneum that supports the major portion of the small bowel, suspending it from the posterior abdominal wall.

FIGURE 3-107   Reflections of the peritoneum.

Liver
Diaphragm
Lesser omentum
Stomach
Pancreas
Duodenum
Mesenteries
Large intestine
Greater omentum
Parietal peritoneum
Large intestine
Rectum
Small intestine
Uterus
Urinary bladder

Most of the abdominal structures are covered by peritoneum, excepting the kidneys, duodenum, pancreas, urinary bladder, the posterior portions of the ascending and descending colon, and the rectum. Most of the major vascular structures within the abdomen are also retroperitoneal. An organ's relation to the peritoneum becomes important in trauma because irritation of the peritoneum (peritonitis) presents with more apparent signs and symptoms than does hemorrhage or the release of other fluids into the retroperitoneal space.

The abdominal cavity is a dynamic place. The diaphragm moves up and down, displacing the abdominal contents with each breath. With deep expiration, the central portion of the diaphragm moves as far upward as the 4th intercostal space, anteriorly (the nipple line), and the 7th intercostal space (the inferior tips of the scapulae), posteriorly. (The edge of the diaphragm attaches to the border of the rib cage.) During forced and maximal expiration, the diaphragm moves as much as 3 inches (9 cm) inferiorly. This movement displaces the abdominal contents up and down with each breath.

Additionally, the volume of substance within the hollow organs varies—an empty (10 mL) versus a distended (500 mL) bladder or a full (1.5 L) versus an empty stomach. The digestive tract is also suspended from the back of the abdominal cavity and is permitted some movement as it digests food. This dynamic movement becomes an important consideration when anticipating abdominal injury due to blunt or penetrating trauma

THE DIGESTIVE SYSTEM

The digestive system includes the digestive tract and the accessory organs of digestion (Figure 3-108). The digestive tract (also called the *alimentary canal*) is the muscular tube that physically and chemically breaks down and absorbs the fluids and nutrients from the food we eat. The accessory organs of digestion include the liver, gallbladder, and pancreas. These organs prepare and store digestive enzymes and perform other important body functions.

The Digestive System

ORGANS OF THE DIGESTIVE SYSTEM

Parotid gland
Pharynx
Tongue
Teeth
Sublingual gland
Submaxillary gland
Larynx
Trachea
Esophagus

Stomach
Spleen
Bile ducts
Liver
Cardiac sphincter
Gallbladder
Cystic duct
Common bile duct
Splenic flexure
Hepatic flexure
Pancreas
Ascending colon
Pyloric sphincter
Ileocecal valve
Duodenum
Cecum
Ileum
Appendix
Descending colon
Transverse colon
Sigmoid colon
Rectum
Anus

LIVER, STOMACH, AND PANCREAS

Liver
Gallbladder
Pancreas
Stomach
Duodenum

LARGE INTESTINE

Esophagus
Duodenum
Diaphragm
Stomach
Hepatic flexure
Splenic flexure
Ascending colon
Transverse colon
Ileocecal valve
Descending colon
Cecum
Appendix
Rectum
Sigmoid colon
Anus

SMALL INTESTINE

Ascending colon
Duodenum
Transverse colon
Jejunum
Cecum
Descending colon
Sigmoid colon
Ileum

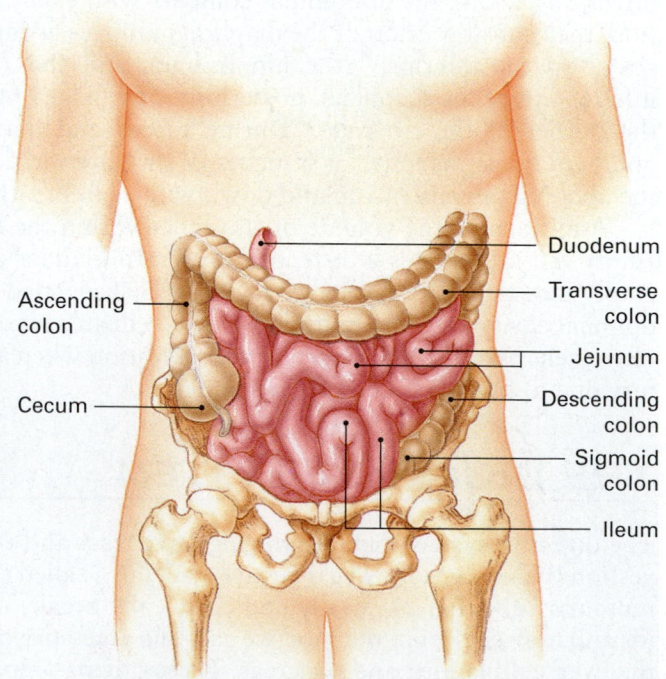

FIGURE 3-108   The digestive tract and accessory organs.

244

THE DIGESTIVE TRACT

The **digestive tract** is a thin, 25-foot-long hollow muscular tube responsible for churning the material to be digested, for excreting digestive juices to be mixed with it, and for absorbing nutrients and then water. Abdominal components of the digestive tract consist of the stomach, the small bowel (duodenum, jejunum, and ileum), the large bowel (or colon), the rectum, and the anus. These structures fill the anterior and lateral aspects of the abdominal cavity, except for the area occupied by the liver.

The esophagus enters the abdomen through the hiatus of the diaphragm (just posterior to the xiphoid process) and then deposits its contents into the stomach. The stomach is a J-shaped muscular container that mixes the ingested material with hydrochloric acid and enzymes (both produced in the gastric wall) into a thick fluid called **chyme.** The acid released by the stomach increases the gastric acidity (pH) to between 1.5 and 2.0. This is a very acidic fluid that would damage the stomach and the initial lining of the small bowel if not for the continuous production of a protective mucus. The stomach is highly variable in size, depending upon the amount of material it contains. It can distend to hold as much as 1.5 liters of food after a large meal.

Chyme is released in small boluses into the first component of the small bowel, the duodenum. The duodenum is approximately 1 foot in length and is where the digesting material is mixed with bile from the liver (stored in the gallbladder) and pancreatic digestive juices. These agents raise the pH of the chyme (returning it towards neutral) and help release the nutrients it contains.

The digesting food is propelled along the small and large bowel by waves of contraction called **peristalsis.** The muscles of the digestive tract constrict the bowel's lumen behind a mass of food, then progressively constrict the lumen in the direction of desired movement. The resulting rhythmic constriction moves the digesting material through the tract. As chyme enters the next two segments of the small bowel (the jejunum and the ileum), the mixing decreases and the nutrients, released by the physical and chemical digestion processes, are absorbed, directed to the liver for detoxification, and then released into the circulatory system.

As the food continues its travel through the digestive tract, it arrives at the large bowel. Here masses of bacteria assist in releasing vitamins and fluid from the digesting food while the large bowel absorbs most of the remaining fluid content. The water serves to hydrate the body while the digestive juices are re-absorbed and reprocessed to rejoin the digestive process upstream again. The large bowel ascends superiorly along the right side of the abdomen (ascending colon), traverses the abdomen just below the liver and stomach (transverse colon), then descends along the left lateral abdomen (descending colon). It aligns with the rectum through the S-shaped sigmoid colon where the end waste products of the digestive process (feces) await excretion (defecation) through the terminal valve, the anus.

ACCESSORY ORGANS OF DIGESTION

The liver is a vascular structure responsible for detoxifying the blood, removing damaged or aged erythrocytes, and storing glycogen and other important agents for body metabolism. The liver also assists in the osmotic regulation of fluids in the blood and plays a role in the clotting process. Finally, the liver detoxifies materials absorbed by the digestive system and either stores or releases nutrients to assure the body's metabolic needs are met. It is located in the right upper quadrant, just below the diaphragm and extends into the medial portion of the left upper quadrant. It is the largest abdominal organ, accounting for 2.5 percent of total body weight. It receives about 25 percent of cardiac output and holds the greatest blood reserve of any body organ. The lower portion of its mass can

* **digestive tract** internal passageway that begins at the mouth and ends at the anus; also called the *alimentary canal*.

* **chyme** semifluid mixture of ingested food and digestive secretions found in the stomach and small intestine.

* **peristalsis** wavelike muscular motion of the esophagus and bowel that moves food through the digestive system.

occasionally be palpated just below the margin of the rib cage. It is suspended in its location by several ligaments including the ligamentum teres, and connects to the omentum inferiorly. The liver is a solid organ but is rather delicate in nature. It is contained within a fibrous capsule (visceral peritoneum) that serves to retard hemorrhage and helps hold the liver together if injured by blunt trauma. When injured, the liver will regenerate to some degree but will not function as efficiently as before the injury.

The gallbladder is a small hollow organ located behind and beneath the liver. It receives bile (a waste product from the reprocessing of red blood cells) from the liver and stores it until it is needed during digestion of fatty foods. It then constricts and sends bile through the bile duct and into the duodenum. Bile helps the body by emulsifying (breaking apart and suspending) ingested fats that would otherwise remain as clumps during the digestive process.

The other accessory digestive organ is the pancreas. It is responsible for the production of glucagon and insulin, hormones responsible for the regulation of blood glucose levels and the transport of glucose across cell membranes. The pancreas also produces very powerful digestive enzymes that help return the pH of the chyme toward normal and break down proteins. These enzymes enter the duodenum through the common bile duct. Like the liver, the pancreas is a solid, though delicate, organ, encapsulated in a serous membrane. It is located in the medial and lower portion of the left upper quadrant and extends into the medial portion of the right upper quadrant. The duodenum wraps around the right pancreatic border. If the cells of the pancreas are damaged, the pancreatic enzymes become active and begin to "self-digest" pancreatic tissue. If these enzymes are released into the retroperitoneal space, they will also damage surrounding tissue.

THE SPLEEN

The spleen is not an accessory organ of digestion but rather a part of the immune system. It is a very vascular organ about the size of the palm of the hand and is located behind the stomach and lateral to the kidney in the left upper quadrant. The spleen performs some immunological functions and also stores a large volume of blood. It is the most fragile abdominal organ, though well protected in its location by the rib cage, spine, and **flank** and back muscles. The spleen, however, can be injured during blunt trauma, especially with impacts affecting the left flank and, when injured, it bleeds heavily.

✳ flanks the part of the back below the ribs and above the hip bones.

THE URINARY SYSTEM

The urinary system contains four major structures, the kidneys, ureters, urinary bladder, and urethra (Figure 3-109). First we will discuss the structures and functions of the urinary system, focusing on the kidneys. Then we will cover the additional structures of the male genitourinary system.

THE KIDNEYS

✳ kidney an organ that produces urine and performs other functions related to the urinary system.

✳ nephron a microscopic structure within the kidney that produces urine.

The left kidney lies in the upper abdomen behind the spleen, and the right kidney lies behind the liver. These locations correspond to the left and right areas of the small of the back, or the flanks. A healthy **kidney** in a young adult is about the size of a fist and contains about one million **nephrons,** the microscopic structures that produce urine. With aging comes a normal loss of nephrons—ten percent per decade of life after age 40—so you should always be alert to the possibility of compromised kidney function in elderly patients.

Renal artery   Renal vein

Adrenal gland

Outline of
lowest rib

Right kidney

Abdominal aorta

Right ureter

Inferior
vena cava

Urinary bladder

Urethra

FIGURE 3-109 Anatomy of the urinary system, posterior view.

Gross and Microscopic Anatomy of the Kidney

The renal artery and vein, as well as nerves, lymphatic vessels, and the ureter, pass into the kidney through the notched region called the **hilum.** The tissue of the kidney itself is visibly divided into an outer region, the **cortex,** and an inner region, the **medulla.** Medullary tissue is divided into fan-shaped regions, or **pyramids.** Each pyramid ends in a portion of tissue called the **papilla,** which projects into the hollow space of the **renal pelvis** (Figure 3-110). The spaces of the pelvis come together at the origin of the ureter. Urine forms in the cortical and medullary tissue of the kidney and leaves the kidney through the renal pelvis and ureter.

The functional unit of the kidney, the nephron, forms urine (Figure 3-111). Each nephron consists of a tubule divided into structurally different portions and capillaries that form a complex net of vessels covering the surface of the tubule. Blood that has entered the kidney through the renal artery flows through successively smaller vessels until it reaches a **glomerulus,** a cluster of capillaries surrounded by **Bowman's capsule,** the cup-shaped, hollow structure that is the first part of the nephron. Water and chemical substances enter the tubule through Bowman's capsule. After passage through successive parts of the tubule—the

* **hilum** the notched part of the kidney where the ureter and other structures join kidney tissue.

* **cortex** the outer tissue of an organ such as the kidney.

* **medulla** the inner tissue of an organ such as the kidney.

* **pyramids** the visible tissue structures within the medulla of the kidney.

* **papilla** the tip of a pyramid; it juts into the hollow space of the kidney.

* **renal pelvis** the hollow space of the kidney that junctions with a ureter.

* **glomerulus** a tuft of capillaries from which blood is filtered into a nephron.

* **Bowman's capsule** the hollow, cup-shaped first part of the nephron tubule.

The Urinary System **247**

FIGURE 3-110 Cross section of the kidney.

Hilum

Papilla

Artery

Vein

Pelvis

Medulla

Cortex

Pyramid

Renal capsule

Ureter

FIGURE 3-111 Anatomy of the nephron.

Distal tubule

Artery

Arteriole

Bowman's capsule

Glomerulus

Proximal tubule

Vein

Collecting duct

Decending limb Loop of Henle

Venule

Ascending limb Loop of Henle

proximal tubule, descending loop of Henle, ascending loop of Henle, and distal tubule—urine drips into the **collecting duct** before entering the renal pelvis and ureter.

Kidney Physiology

The physiology of the kidneys is one of the most complex topics in human physiology. Its explanation often requires several book chapters. The following is a brief overview.

Overview of Nephron Physiology Forming and eliminating urine are the basis for two of the kidneys' major functions: (1) maintaining blood volume with proper balance of water, electrolytes, and pH and (2) retaining key compounds such as glucose while excreting wastes such as urea. A third function, controlling arterial blood pressure, relies both on urine formation and on a second mechanism that does not involve urine production. Last, kidney cells regulate erythrocyte development, but this process does not involve urine formation in any way.

Urine is produced through the interactions among capillary blood flowing over the nephron tubule, the fluid flowing inside the tubule, and the capillary and tubular cells themselves. Three general processes are involved in formation of urine: **glomerular filtration, reabsorption** of substances from the renal tubule into blood, and **secretion** of substances from blood into the renal tubule.

The first step in urine formation is filtration of blood. As blood flows through the capillaries of the glomerulus, water and numerous chemical materials are filtered out of the blood and into Bowman's capsule. Normally, the only blood elements that are not freely filtered into the capsule are blood cells and the plasma proteins, all of which are too large to pass through the pores formed by cell junctions in the capillary walls. Consequently, the fluid formed in the capsule—the **filtrate**—roughly resembles blood plasma except for the absence of proteins.

The rate at which blood is filtered, the **glomerular filtration rate (GFR)**, averages 180 liters/day, the equivalent of 60 complete passages of blood plasma through the glomerular filters. This remarkable efficiency underlies the kidneys' ability to excrete toxic or foreign substances such as urea or drug metabolites so quickly that the substances do not accumulate in the blood.

Filtration is a nonselective process based primarily on molecular size (electrical charge is a secondary factor), and it is essential to urine formation. In contrast, reabsorption of substances into the blood and secretion of substances into the renal tubule are highly selective processes. Almost all elements of filtrate are handled independently of the other elements. The processes of reabsorption and secretion are essential to forming urine with the correct composition and volume to compensate for current body conditions, that is, to maintain homeostasis.

Reabsorption and secretion involve intercellular transport, the movement of a molecule across a cell membrane to either enter or exit a cell. Like other intercellular transport processes, they occur in one of three ways: **simple diffusion,** facilitated diffusion, or active transport. Both simple and facilitated diffusion are passive processes: neither requires the cell to spend energy. In simple diffusion, molecules small enough to pass through a cell membrane randomly move into and out of the cell. Because net movement is always from the region of higher concentration to that of lower concentration, simple diffusion leads toward equalization of molecular concentration on both sides of the membrane. Water molecules always move by simple diffusion. **Osmosis** is the process in which water molecules move so that the concentrations of particles dissolved in water (or

* **proximal tubule** the part of the tubule beyond Bowman's capsule.

* **descending loop of Henle** the part of the tubule beyond the proximal tubule.

* **ascending loop of Henle** the part of the tubule beyond the descending loop of Henle.

* **distal tubule** the part of the tubule beyond the ascending loop of Henle.

* **collecting duct** the larger structure beyond the distal tubule into which urine drips.

* **glomerular filtration** the removal from blood of water and other elements, which enter the nephron tubule.

* **reabsorption** the movement of a substance from a nephron tubule back into the blood.

* **secretion** the movement of a substance from the blood into a nephron tubule.

* **filtrate** the fluid produced in Bowman's capsule by filtration of blood.

* **glomerular filtration rate (GFR)** the volume per day at which blood is filtered through capillaries of the glomerulus.

* **simple diffusion** the random motion of molecules from an area of high concentration to an area of lower concentration.

* **osmosis** the diffusion pattern of water in which molecules move to equalize concentrations on both sides of a membrane.

osmolarity) approach equivalence on both sides of a membrane. A solution with a higher concentration than another solution is **hyperosmolar** to the other; a solution with a lower, more dilute concentration is **hypo-osmolar** to the other.

In **facilitated diffusion,** molecules still move from the region of higher concentration to that of lower concentration. However, a molecule-specific carrier in the membrane acts as a tunnel and speeds the molecules' movement through the membrane. The body cells' normal handling of glucose is an example of this process. When insulin binds to a glucose-specific carrier in the cell membrane, glucose can pass into the cell ten times faster than when insulin is not bound to the carrier.

Active transport is the only process that can produce a net movement of molecules from a region of lower concentration to one of higher concentration. This uphill movement against the concentration gradient is possible because energy is spent to drive the action of the molecule-specific carrier in the membrane. Active transport processes are vital to renal tubular physiology because they allow for the precise balance of reabsorption and secretion that results in independent, homeostatic handling of electrolytes and other substances such as glucose.

Tubular Handling of Water and Electrolytes Tubular handling of water and electrolytes including sodium (Na^+), potassium (K^+), hydrogen (H^+), and chloride (Cl^-) is the basis for control of blood volume and maintenance of electrolyte balance, including pH. As you recall, Na^+ is the dominant cation in the body's extracellular fluids, including blood, whereas K^+ is the dominant cation in intracellular fluid. Appropriate retention of Na^+ in the body, along with osmotic retention of water, is key to maintaining blood volume. Selective retention of K^+ and H^+, along with anions such as Cl^-, maintains the balance of blood electrolytes and blood pH.

Filtrate formed in Bowman's capsule enters the proximal tubule (review Figure 3-111). The cells of the proximal tubule have an extensive brush border that maximizes contact between cell membrane and filtrate. They also have high concentrations of molecule-specific carriers in their membranes and maintain a high level of metabolic activity, producing energy that can support active transport. Under normal conditions, about 65 percent of filtered Na^+ and Cl^- is reabsorbed in the proximal tubule, along with osmotic reabsorption of about the same percentage of filtered water. Reabsorption takes place by both passive and active transport processes. Much of the active Na^+ reabsorption is coupled with secretion of H^+ into the tubule; H^+ secretion raises the pH of the arterial-derived blood flowing in capillaries surrounding the tubule. Further handling of H^+ as the filtrate moves through the tubule determines the pH both of the venous blood leaving the kidneys and of the urine excreted from the body.

As filtrate moves through the next part of the nephron, the loop of Henle, its volume and composition change further. Simple diffusion is the dominant process in the first part of the loop. By the time filtrate has moved through the descending limb of the loop, roughly another 20 percent of the filtrate's original water load has been reabsorbed. The cells of the second, ascending limb of the loop of Henle are normally virtually impermeable to water; however, passive and active reabsorption of significant amounts of electrolytes occurs in the same part of the tubule. This reabsorption of electrolytes without reabsorption of water produces a relatively dilute fluid that may exit the collecting duct as dilute urine. Healthy kidneys can produce urine with an osmolarity as low as one-sixth the osmolar concentration of blood plasma, an action termed **diuresis.** A number of hormones alter tubular handling of water and electrolytes (Table 3-7). Some increase the permeability of the distal tubule, collecting duct, or both, so that far more water is reabsorbed. **Antidiuresis,** the result of this hormonal activity, can form a very concentrated urine with an osmolarity as high as four times that of plasma.

Table 3-7	HORMONES THAT AFFECT TUBULAR HANDLING OF WATER AND KEY ELECTROLYTES	
Hormone	**Target Tissue**	**Effect(s)**
Aldosterone	Distal tubule, collecting duct	Increase in reabsorption of Na^+, Cl^-, and water
		Increase in secretion of K^+
Angiotensin II	Proximal tubule	Increase in reabsorption of Na^+, Cl^-, and water
		Increase in secretion of H^+
Antidiuretic Hormone (ADH)	Distal tubule, collecting duct	Increase in reabsorption of water
Atrial Natriuretic Hormone (ANH)	Distal tubule, collecting duct	Decrease in reabsorption of Na^+ and Cl^-

Note: Aldosterone, ADH, and ANH are discussed in detail in "Endocrinology," Chapter 30; angotensin II is discussed in "Cardiology," Chapter 28.

Table derived from Arthur C. Guyton and John E. Hall, *Textbook of Medical Physiology,* 9th ed. (Philadelphia: W.B. Saunders Company, 1996).

The ability of healthy kidneys to handle significant swings in water and electrolyte intake is remarkably large. Studies have shown that an individual can increase his sodium intake to ten times the average amount or decrease it to roughly one-tenth the average, and the kidneys will still compensate properly. Blood volume and sodium content will change only modestly from their baseline, normal levels.

Tubular Handling of Glucose and Urea Glucose and urea represent substances that the kidneys handle in opposite fashion. Critical substances such as glucose are retained in the body, and wastes such as urea are excreted.

Glucose is freely filtered into Bowman's capsule as an element of filtrate. Normally, glucose is completely reabsorbed through an active transport process by the time filtrate leaves the proximal tubule. The body's absolute retention of glucose is usually maintained until the blood glucose level reaches about 180 mg/dL; above that level, glucose begins to be lost in urine. This pattern, in which glucose is completely reabsorbed until a ceiling, or threshold level of blood glucose is reached, is due to saturation of the active-transport process responsible for reabsorption of glucose. At excessively high blood glucose levels, so much glucose enters the filtrate that the proximal tubule's transport capacity to reabsorb it is insufficient. When this occurs, as in uncontrolled diabetes mellitus type I, the body loses not only glucose but also large amounts of water through **osmotic diuresis.**

Urea, a waste product, is also freely filtered into Bowman's capsule. However, tubular handling of this small molecule is very different from that of glucose. Urea is passively reabsorbed throughout most of the tubule, and about half of the filtered load will remain in urine. Thus, the kidneys' ability to excrete urea efficiently depends on the glomerular filtration rate, or GFR. If blood passes through the glomerular capillaries at an adequate rate, the net result of filtration and passive reabsorption will keep the blood level from rising toward a toxic level. The blood urea nitrogen test, or BUN, directly measures blood concentration of urea and is an indirect indicator of GFR. **Creatinine,** another waste product of metabolism, has larger molecules than urea and is not reabsorbed. Because all of the filtered creatinine will be eliminated in urine, the blood concentration of creatinine is a direct indicator of GFR.

Control of Arterial Blood Pressure The kidneys regulate systemic arterial blood pressure in several ways. Over the long term, they control the body's balance of water and electrolytes, thus maintaining blood volume at a healthy level.

✱ **osmotic diuresis** greatly increased urination and dehydration that results when high levels of glucose cannot be reabsorbed into the blood from the kidney tubules and the osmotic pressure of the glucose in the tubules also prevents water reabsorption.

✱ **creatinine** a waste product caused by metabolism within muscle cells.

BUN and creatinine are both important indications of renal function.

renin an enzyme produced by kidney cells that plays a key role in controlling arterial blood pressure.

In addition, juxtaglomerular cells, specialized cells adjacent to glomerular capillary cells, respond to low blood pressure by releasing an enzyme called **renin.** Within seconds of its release renin produces significant amounts of the active hormone angiotensin I. As angiotensin I flows through the lungs, angiotensin converting enzyme (ACE) produces angiotensin II, the powerful vasoconstrictor that immediately raises arterial blood pressure. Angiotensin II acts both on kidney tubular cells (Table 3-7) and on adrenal cells, causing the latter to secrete aldosterone. The renin-angiotensin system has an important role in maintenance of blood pressure, as noted earlier.

erythropoietin a hormone produced by kidney cells that stimulates maturation of red blood cells.

Control of Erythrocyte Development The kidneys produce 90 percent of the body's **erythropoietin,** a hormone that regulates the rate at which erythrocytes mature in bone marrow. The exact mechanism that produces erythropoietin is unclear. The impact of renal tissue death, however, is clear and profound; the nonkidney sources of erythropoietin can produce only about one-third to one-half the red cell mass (measured as hematocrit) needed by the body.

THE URETERS

ureter a duct that carries urine from kidney to urinary bladder.

Urine drains from the renal pelvis into the **ureter,** the long duct that runs from the kidney to the urinary bladder (review Figure 3-109). Each ureter is about 25 cm long, and like the kidney, is located in the retroperitoneum of the abdomen. A thin muscular layer in the ureters' walls limits their ability to distend in response to internal pressure. The ureters' nerves derive from renal, gonadal, or hypogastric nerve trunks. The microscopic structure of the ureters and the nature of their nerve supply are important in understanding the symptoms caused by kidney stones caught in a ureter.

THE URINARY BLADDER

urinary bladder the muscular organ that stores urine before its elimination from the body.

The **urinary bladder,** the anteriormost organ in the pelvis of both men and women, stores urine. The muscular bladder usually contains at least a small amount of urine, which produces its roughly spherical shape. The bladder neck, through which urine passes during urination, is held in place by ligaments. In women, connective tissue loosely attaches the bladder's posterior wall to the anterior vaginal wall. In men, the bladder's wall bladder is structurally continuous with the prostate gland.

THE URETHRA

urethra the duct that carries urine from the urinary bladder out of the body; in men, it also carries reproductive fluid (semen) to the outside of the body.

The **urethra** is the duct that carries urine from the bladder to the exterior of the body. In women, the urethra is only about 3 to 4 cm long and opens to the external environment via a small orifice just anterior to that of the vagina. In men, the urethra is about 20 cm long and ends at the tip of the penis. The female urethra's shortness is probably one reason the female urinary system is more vulnerable to bacterial infection from environmental (largely skin) sources. Because the male urethra carries both urine and male reproductive fluid, it can be an entry way for sexually transmitted diseases.

THE REPRODUCTIVE SYSTEM

It is important to have an understanding of both the female and the male reproductive systems.

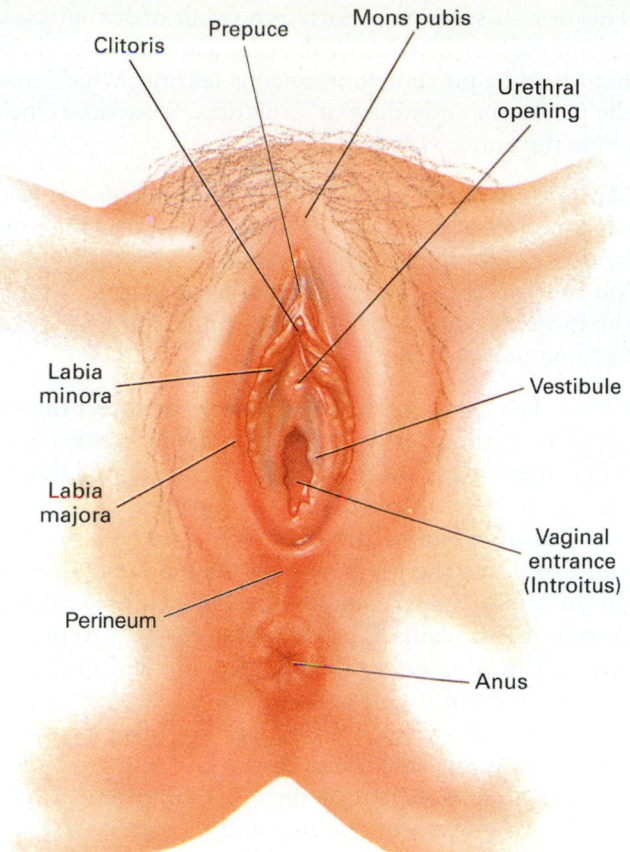

FIGURE 3-112 The vulva.

Clitoris
Prepuce
Mons pubis
Urethral opening
Labia minora
Vestibule
Labia majora
Vaginal entrance (Introitus)
Perineum
Anus

THE FEMALE REPRODUCTIVE SYSTEM

The most important female reproductive organs are internal and are located within the pelvic cavity. These include the ovaries, fallopian tubes, uterus, and vagina, which are essential to reproduction. The external genitalia have accessory functions, in that they protect body openings and play an important role in sexual functioning.

The External Genitalia

The female external genitalia are known collectively as the *vulva*, or *pudendum* (Figure 3-112). These external genitalia consist of highly-vascular tissues that protect the entrance to the birth canal. They include the perineum, mons pubis, labia, and clitoris.

   The external genital organs begin to mature and take adult proportions during adolescence. Puberty also marks the appearance of breast buds, pubic hair, and the first period (menarche). The age in which sexual development occurs varies among individuals. As women grow older, ovarian function diminishes, menstrual periods cease, and pubic hair becomes gray and sparse. The labia and clitoris become smaller; the vagina narrows and shortens and its lining (the mucosa) becomes thin, pale, and dry. The ovaries and uterus decrease in size.

Perineum The **perineum** is a roughly diamond-shaped, skin-covered muscular tissue that separates the vagina and the anus. These tissues form a sling-like structure supporting the internal pelvic organs and are able to stretch during childbirth.

✱ **perineum** muscular tissue that separates the vagina and the anus.

This area is sometimes torn as a result of sexual assault or during childbirth. An *episiotomy*, or incision of the perineum, may be done to facilitate delivery of the baby and to prevent spontaneous tearing, which may cause significant injury to the perineum and adjacent structures. Sometimes the term *perineum* is used to include the entire vulvar area.

✱ mons pubis fatty layer of tissue over the pubic symphysis.

Mons Pubis The **mons pubis** is a fatty layer of tissue over the pubic symphysis, the junction of pubic bones. During puberty, the hormone estrogen causes fat to be deposited under the skin, giving it a mound-like shape. This serves as a cushion that protects the pubic symphysis during intercourse. Also during puberty, the mons becomes covered with pubic hair and its sebaceous and sweat glands become more active.

✱ labia structures that protect the vagina and urethra, including the *labia majora* and the *labia minora*.

Labia The **labia** are the structures that protect the vagina and the urethra. There are two distinct sets of labia. The labia majora are located laterally, while the labia minora are more medial. Both sets of labia are subject to injury during trauma to the vulvar area, such as occurs with sexual assault.

The *labia majora* are two folds of fatty tissue that arise from the mons pubis and extend to the perineum, forming a cleft. During puberty, pubic hair grows on the lateral surface, and sebaceous glands on the hairless medial surface begin to secrete lubricants. The labia majora serve to protect the inner structures of the vulva. The *labia minora,* lying medially within the labia majora, are two smaller, thinner folds of highly vascular tissue, well supplied with nerves and sebaceous glands, which secrete lubricating fluid. During sexual arousal the labia minora become engorged with blood.

The area protected by the labia minora is called the *vestibule*. The vestibule contains the urethral opening and the external opening of the vagina called the vaginal orifice, or *introitus*. The secretions of two pairs of glands (Skene and Bartholin) lubricate these structures during sexual stimulation. Located within the vestibule is the *hymen*. It is a thin fold of mucous membrane that forms the external border of the vagina, partly closing it.

✱ clitoris highly innervated and vascular erectile tissue anterior to the labia minora.

Clitoris The **clitoris** is highly innervated and richly vascular erectile tissue that lies anterior to the labia minora. This cylindrical structure is a major site of sexual stimulation and orgasm in women. The *prepuce* is a fold of the labia minora that covers the clitoris.

The Internal Genitalia

The internal female reproductive organs are the vagina, the uterus, the fallopian tubes, and the ovaries (Figures 3-113 and 3-114).

✱ vagina canal that connects the external female genitalia to the uterus.

Vagina The **vagina** is an elastic canal made up primarily of smooth muscle, 9 to 10 centimeters in length, that connects the external genitalia to the uterus. It lies between the urethra/bladder and the anus/rectum. Lined with mucous membrane, the vagina extends up and back from the vaginal orifice to the lower end of the uterus (cervix). The vaginal walls are crisscrossed with ridges that allow it to stretch during childbirth, allowing passage of the fetus. The vagina's primary blood supply is the vaginal artery. The pudendal nerve innervates the lower third of the vagina and the external genitalia. The vagina has three functions:

- It is the female organ of copulation and receives the penis during sexual intercourse.
- Often called the birth canal, it forms the final passageway for the infant during childbirth.
- It provides an outlet for menstrual blood and tissue to leave the body.

Fimbriae of
fallopian tube

Rectum

Cervix of uterus

Vagina

Anus

Fallopian tube

Ovary

Uterus

Urinary bladder

Symphysis pubis

Urethra

Clitoris

Labium minor

Labium major

Vaginal orifice

FIGURE 3-113 Cross-sectional anatomy of the female reproductive system.

Uterus The **uterus** is a hollow, thick-walled, muscular, inverted-pear-shaped organ that connects with the vagina. It lies in the center of the pelvis and is flexed forward between the bladder and rectum above the vagina. Approximately 7.5 centimeters (three inches) long and 5 centimeters (two inches) wide, the uterus is held loosely in position by ligaments, peritoneal folds, and the pressure of adjacent abdominal structures. The primary function of the uterus is to provide a site for fetal development. During pregnancy, the uterus stretches to a size capable of containing the fetus, placenta, and the associated membranes and amniotic fluid. At term, the gravid uterus measures approximately 40 centimeters (16 inches) in length. The uterus has an extensive blood supply, primarily from the uterine arteries which are branches of the internal iliac artery. The autonomic nervous system innervates the uterus. In a non-pregnant state, the uterine cavity is flat and triangular.

The uterus has two major parts: the *body* (or corpus) and the *cervix,* or neck. The upper two-thirds of the uterus forms the body and is comprised of smooth muscle layers. The lower third is the cervix.

The rounded uppermost portion of the body of the uterus is the *fundus,* which lies above the point where the fallopian tubes attach. Measurement of fundal height (distance from the symphysis pubis to the fundus) may be used to estimate gestational age during pregnancy. The fundal height measured in centimeters is generally comparable to the weeks of gestation. For instance, if the fundal height is 30 centimeters, the gestational age is about 30 weeks. This method of assessing uterine size is most accurate from 22 to 34 weeks.

The body of the uterus has three layers of tissue that make up the uterine wall. The innermost layer or lining is called the **endometrium.** Each month, stimulated by estrogen and progesterone, the endometrium builds up in preparation for the implantation of a fertilized ovum. If fertilization does not occur, the lining degenerates

✱ **uterus** hollow organ in the center of the abdomen that provides the site for fetal development.

✱ **endometrium** the inner layer of the uterine wall where the fertilized egg implants.

The Reproductive System **255**

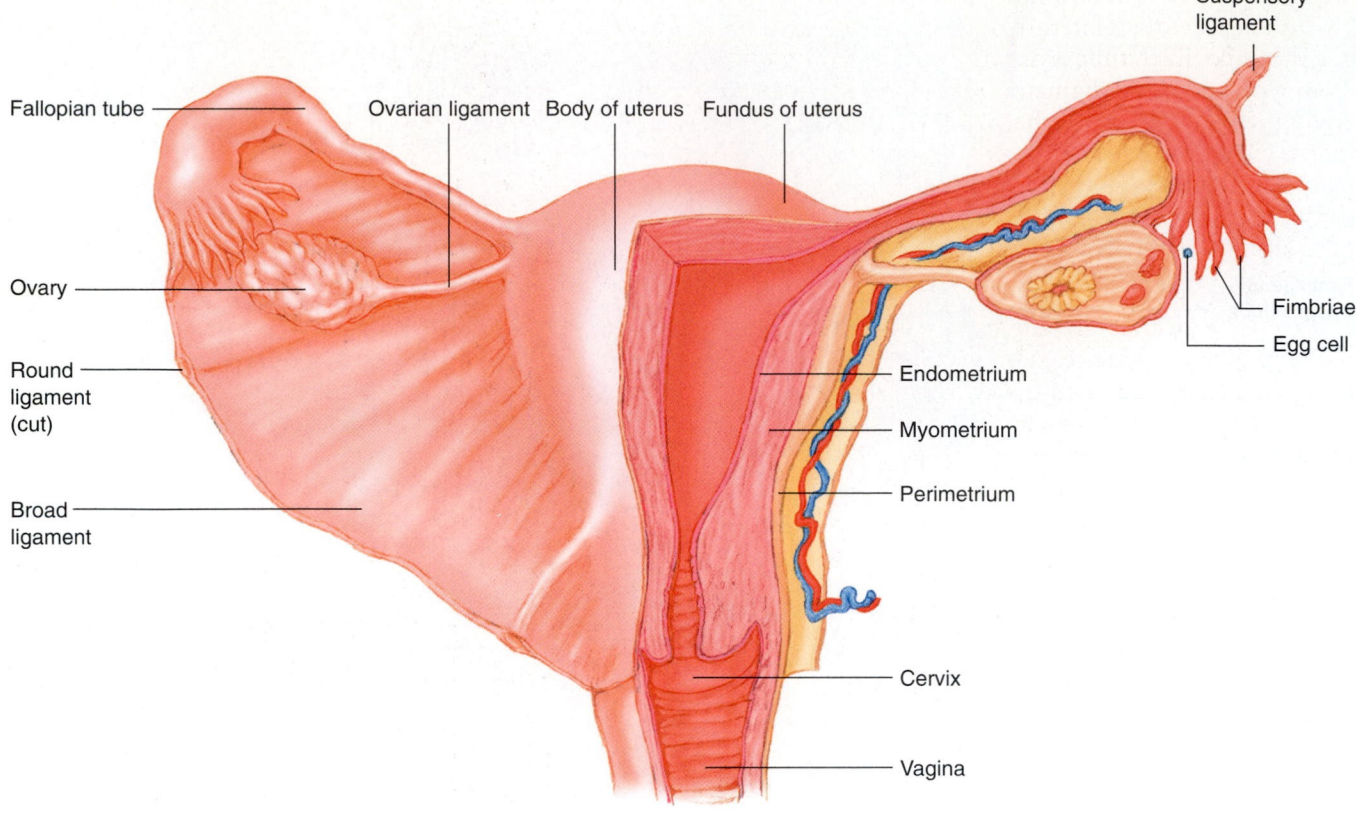

Fallopian tube

Ovary

Round ligament (cut)

Broad ligament

Ovarian ligament   Body of uterus   Fundus of uterus

Suspensory ligament

Fimbriae

Egg cell

Endometrium

Myometrium

Perimetrium

Cervix

Vagina

FIGURE 3-114   The uterus, fallopian tubes, and ovaries.

✱ myometrium the thick middle layer of the uterine wall made up of smooth muscle fibers.

✱ perimetrium the serosal peritoneal membrane which forms the outermost layer of the uterine wall.

and sloughs off. This sloughing of the uterine lining is referred to as the *menses*, or menstrual period.

The thick middle layer of the uterine wall, called the **myometrium** is made up of three distinct layers of smooth muscle fibers. In the outer layer, primarily over the fundus, the fibers run longitudinally, which allows expulsion of the fetus following cervical dilation. The middle (and thicker) layer is made up of figure-eight patterns of interlaced muscle fibers which surround large blood vessels. The contraction of these fibers helps control post-delivery bleeding. The myometrial fibers also contract during menstruation to maximize the sloughing of the endometrium. It has been suggested that menstrual cramps are due to fatigue of the myometrial fibers. The innermost layer of the myometrium is comprised of circular smooth muscle fibers that form sphincters at the point of fallopian tube attachment and at the internal opening of the cervix.

The outermost layer of the uterine wall is a serous membrane called the **perimetrium** that partially covers the corpus of the uterus. The perimetrium, which is a layer of the visceral peritoneum that lines the abdominal cavity and abdominal organs, does not extend to the cervix. The most significant aspect of this partial coverage is that it allows surgical access to the uterus without the risk of infection that is associated with peritoneal incisions.

The cervix, or neck of the uterus, extends from the narrowest portion of the uterus to connect with the vagina. That distance forms the cervical canal and is only approximately 2.5 centimeters (1 inch) in length. Elasticity characterizes the cervix. During labor, it dilates to a diameter of approximately 10 centimeters to allow delivery of the fetus.

Fallopian Tubes The two **fallopian tubes**, also called uterine tubes, are thin flexible tubes that extend laterally from the uterus and curve up and over each ovary on either side. Each tube is approximately 10 centimeters (4 inches) in length and about 1 centimeter in diameter (about the size of a pencil lead), except at its ovarian end which is trumpet-shaped. Each fallopian tube has two openings, a fimbriated (fringed) end that opens into the abdominal cavity in the area adjacent to the ovaries and a minute opening into the uterus. The function of the tubes is to conduct the egg from the space around the ovaries into the uterine cavity via peristalsis (wavelike muscular contractions). Fertilization usually occurs in the distal third of the fallopian tube.

Ovaries The **ovaries** are the primary female gonads, or sex glands. Almond-shaped, the ovaries are situated laterally on either side of the uterus in the upper portion of the pelvic cavity. They have two functions One function is the secretion of the hormones estrogen and progesterone in response to stimulation from follicle stimulating hormone (FSH) and luteinizing hormone (LH) secreted from the anterior pituitary gland. The second function of the ovaries is the development and release of eggs (ova) for reproduction.

The Menstrual Cycle

The female undergoes a monthly hormonal cycle, generally every 28 days, that prepares the uterus to receive a fertilized egg. The onset of the menstrual cycle, that is, the onset of ovulation at puberty, establishes female sexual maturity. This onset, known as **menarche**, usually begins between the ages of 10 and 14. At first, the periods are irregular. Later they become more regular and predictable. The length of the menstrual cycle may vary from 21 to 32 days. A "normal" menstrual cycle is what is normal for the woman in question. Because of this, it is important to inquire as to the normal length of the patient's menstrual cycle. Regardless of the length of the menstrual cycle, the period of time from ovulation to menstruation is always 14 days. Any variance in cycle length occurs during the pre-ovulatory phase.

From puberty to menopause, the female sex hormones (estrogen and progesterone) control the ovarian-menstrual cycle, pregnancy, and lactation. These hormones are not produced at a constant rate, but rather their production surges and diminishes in a cyclical fashion. The secretion of estrogen and progesterone by the ovaries is controlled by the secretion of FSH and LH.

The Proliferative Phase The first two weeks of the menstrual cycle, known as the proliferative phase, are dominated by estrogen, which causes the uterine lining (endometrium) to thicken and become engorged with blood. In response to a surge of LH at approximately day 14, **ovulation** (release of an egg) takes place.

At birth, each female's ovary contains some 200,000 ova within immature ovarian follicles known as graafian follicles. This is the female's lifetime supply of ova, which are gradually "used up" through ovulation during her lifetime.

In response to FSH and increased estrogen levels, once during every menstrual cycle, a follicle reaches maturation and ruptures, discharging its egg through the ovary's outer covering into the abdominal cavity. The ruptured follicle, under the influence of LH, develops the corpus luteum, a small yellowish body of cells, which produces progesterone during the second half of the menstrual cycle. If the egg is not fertilized, the corpus luteum will atrophy about 3 days prior to the onset of the menstrual phase. If the egg is fertilized, the corpus luteum will produce progesterone until the placenta takes over that function.

The cilia (fine, hairlike structures) on the fimbriated ends of the fallopian tubes draw the egg into the tube and sweep it toward the uterus. If the woman has had sexual intercourse within approximately 24 hours of ovulation, fertilization

* **fallopian tubes** thin tubes that extend laterally from the uterus and conduct eggs from the ovaries into the uterine cavity.

* **ovaries** the primary female sex glands that secrete estrogen and progesterone and produce eggs for reproduction.

* **menarche** the onset of menses, usually occurring between ages 10 and 14.

* **ovulation** the release of an egg from the ovary.

may take place. If the egg is fertilized, it normally implants in the thickened lining of the uterus, where the fetus subsequently develops. If it is not fertilized, it passes into the uterine cavity and is expelled.

The Secretory Phase The stage of the menstrual cycle immediately surrounding ovulation is referred to as the secretory phase. If the egg is not fertilized, the woman's estrogen level drops sharply while the progesterone level dominates. Uterine vascularity increases during this phase in anticipation of implantation of a fertilized egg.

The Ischemic Phase If fertilization doesn't occur, estrogen and progesterone levels fall. Vascular changes cause the endometrium to become pale and small blood vessels to rupture.

The Menstrual Phase During the menstrual phase, the ischemic endometrium is shed, along with a discharge of blood, mucus, and cellular debris. This is known as **menstruation**. A "normal" menstrual cycle depends upon the regular pattern in the individual woman. The first day of the menstrual cycle is the day on which bleeding begins and the menstrual flow usually lasts from 3 to 5 days, although this varies from woman to woman. An average blood loss of about 50 ml is common. The absence of a menstrual period in any woman in the child-bearing years (generally ages 12 to 55) who is sexually active and whose periods are usually regular should raise the suspicion of pregnancy.

Some women regularly experience marked physical signs and symptoms immediately prior to the onset of their menstrual period. These are collectively known as **premenstrual syndrome (PMS)**. Although you may hear crude jokes made about PMS, there is no denying the reality of the physical changes that accompany the changing hormonal levels. It is not uncommon for women to report breast tenderness or engorgement, transient weight gain or bloating as a result of fluid retention, excessive fatigue, and/or cravings for specific foods. Women who are prone to migraine headaches may see them increase during the premenstrual period. Other women may have only minimal physical symptoms, but are more affected by emotional responses such as irritability, anxiety, or depression. The severity of PMS varies with each individual and may require treatment focused on relief of symptoms.

Menopause, the cessation of menses, marks the cessation of ovarian function and the cessation of estrogen secretion. Menstrual periods generally continue to occur until a woman is 45 to 55, at which time they begin to decline in frequency and length until they ultimately stop. The end of reproductive life is also known as the "climacteric," which is derived from Greek meaning "critical time of life." Occasionally, physicians use the term surgical menopause, which means that a woman's periods have stopped because of surgical removal of her uterus, ovaries, or both. The decrease in estrogen levels causes many women to experience hot flashes, night sweats, and mood swings during menopause. It is not uncommon for hormone replacement therapy (oral estrogen, or estrogen and progesterone) to be prescribed to help relieve these complaints and to provide other health benefits associated with continuing adequate levels of these hormones.

The Pregnant Uterus

The dynamics of pregnancy greatly affect the anatomy of the female abdominal cavity (Figure 3-115). The uterus and its contents grow rapidly from the time of conception until delivery and are well protected during the first trimester (3 months) of pregnancy. During the second trimester (12 to 24 weeks), the progressive enlargement of the uterus displaces most of the abdominal contents upward as the growing uterus rises out of the pelvis and its upper border extends

* **menstruation** sloughing of the uterine lining (endometrium) if a fertilized egg is not implanted. It is controlled by the cyclical release of hormones. Menstruation is also called a *period*.

* **premenstrual syndrome (PMS)** a variety of signs and symptoms, such as weight gain, irritability, or specific food cravings associated with the changing hormonal levels that precede menstruation.

* **menopause** the cessation of menses and ovarian function resulting from decreased secretion of estrogen.

3 Months

8 Months

Placenta

Umbilical cord

Amniotic sac

Uterus

Placenta

Cervix

Umbilical cord

Pubic bone

Vagina

Bladder

Cervix

FIGURE 3-115 The pregnant uterus.

above the umbilicus. By 32 weeks and until the end of the pregnancy, the uterus fills the abdominal cavity to the level of the lower rib margin. This enlarging mass in the abdomen also increases the intra-abdominal pressure and displaces the diaphragm upward. This displacement reduces lung capacity at the same time that the physiologic changes of pregnancy increase the tidal volume.

Pregnancy also affects the maternal physiology by raising the circulatory volume by about 45 percent and, by the third trimester, raising the cardiac rate by about 15 beats per minute and the cardiac output by up to 40 percent. The increase in the vascular volume is accompanied by a less significant increase in the number of erythrocytes. The result is a relative anemia that becomes an important consideration with aggressive fluid resuscitation for the mother in shock. In the last trimester of pregnancy, the uterus is significant in both size and weight and may compress the vena cava, reducing venous return to the heart and inducing a temporary hypotension in the supine patient (supine hypotensive syndrome). Finally, the developing fetus means there are now two lives to protect when the mother suffers any trauma, especially involving the abdomen.

THE MALE REPRODUCTIVE SYSTEM

As noted earlier, the male reproductive organs are considered to be part of the urinary system (Figure 3-116). Like the female reproductive system, the male reproductive system includes both external and internal genitalia.

The Testes The **testes** are the primary male reproductive organs. They produce both the hormones responsible for sexual maturation and sperm cells, male sex cells. The testes lie outside of the abdomen in a muscular sac called the scrotum. Normal scrotal temperature is about 2–3°C lower than abdominal temperature, which is critical for development of sperm.

The Epididymis and Vas Deferens Sperm cells pass from the testis into the **epididymis,** a small sac where they are stored. Each testis with its paired epididymis is palpable inside the scrotum. Sperm are channeled from the epididymis into the **vas deferens,** a muscular duct that carries them into the pelvis

✳ **testes** primary male reproductive organs that produce hormones responsible for sexual maturation and sperm; singular *testis.*

✳ **epididymis** small sac in which sperm cells are stored.

✳ **vas deferens** duct that carries sperm cells to the urethra for ejaculation.

The Reproductive System **259**

FIGURE 3-116 Anatomy of
the male genitourinary system.

Opening:
Vas deferens

Seminal vesicle

Ejaculatory duct

Prostate

Vas deferens

Epididymis

Scrotal sac

Urinary bladder

Urethra

Penile erectile
tissue

Prepuce

Glans

Testis

and through the substance of the prostate gland to its opening into the urethra. Sperm cells mix with special fluid before passing into the urethra for ejaculation, elimination from the body.

The vas deferens passes through an opening in the inguinal ligament known as the *inguinal canal*. The testicular blood supply also runs through this opening, an anatomical weak point that is the site of male hernias.

✱ prostate gland gland that surrounds the male urinary bladder neck and is a major source of the fluid that combines with sperm to form semen.

The Prostate Gland The **prostate gland** surrounds the male urinary bladder neck, and the first part of the urethra runs through its tissue. The prostate gland is a major source of the fluid that combines with sperm to form semen, the ejaculated male reproductive fluid. In emergency care, the prostate is probably most important in its role as part of the urinary system. Because the first part of the urethra passes through the prostate, enlargement of the prostate can narrow or obstruct the urethra and block urine flow.

✱ penis male organ of copulation.

The Penis The **penis** is the male organ of copulation. Its spongy internal tissues fill with blood to produce penile erection. The skin covering the end of the penis, the *foreskin,* is often surgically removed in infancy through circumcision; the difference in appearance is noticeable.

The male genital organs begin to mature and take adult proportions during adolescence. Puberty also marks a noticeable increase in the size of the testes. As in the female, the actual age in which sexual development occurs will vary widely. As men grow older, the penis decreases in size and the testes hang lower in the scrotum. The pubic hair becomes gray and sparse.

SUMMARY

An understanding of human anatomy and physiology is basic to paramedic practice. This begins with an understanding of the basic organization of the human body, beginning with the cell and moving on to more complex structures: the tissues, organs, organ systems, and system integration within the organism itself.

Also critical is an understanding of the important body systems including the integumentary system; the blood; the musculoskeletal system; the head, face, and neck; the spine and thorax, the nervous, endocrine, cardiovascular, and respiratory systems; the abdomen, digestive system, and spleen, and the urinary and reproductive systems.

CHAPTER 4

General Principles of Pathophysiology

Objectives

Continued

Part 2: The Body's Defenses against Disease and Injury (begins on p. 295)

After reading Part 2 of this chapter, you should be able to:

1. Define the characteristics of the immune response. (pp. 299–302)
2. Discuss induction of the immune system. (pp. 300–302)
3. Describe the inflammation response and its systemic manifestations. (pp. 302–307)
4. Discuss the role of mast cells, the plasma protein system, and cellular components plus resolution and repair as part of the inflammation response. (pp. 303–307)

5. Discuss hypersensitivity. (pp. 308–309)
6. Describe deficiencies in immunity and inflammation. (pp. 309–311)
7. Describe homeostasis as a dynamic steady state. (p. 313)
8. Describe neuroendocrine regulation. (pp. 313–317)
9. Discuss the interrelationships between stress, coping, and illness. (pp. 317–318)

INTRODUCTION

As a paramedic, you will assess your patient (noting the patient's complaints, signs, and symptoms) and plan a course of treatment. If you understand basic human physiology (how the body functions normally) and pathophysiology (how the body functions in the presence of disease or injury), you will be far more able to understand the probable causes of common assessment findings and, consequently, far more able to choose effective treatments.

General principles of pathophysiology are presented in this chapter. Before reading this chapter, be familiar with the fundamentals of anatomy and normal physiology as presented in Chapter 3—especially the sections on the cell and cellular environment.

This chapter is divided into two parts:

Part 1: How Normal Body Processes Are Altered by Disease and Injury
Part 2: The Body's Defenses against Disease and Injury

Part 1: How Normal Body Processes Are Altered by Disease and Injury

PATHOPHYSIOLOGY

* **pathology** the study of disease and its causes.

* **pathophysiology** the study of how diseases alter normal physiology.

Keep in mind that our understanding of pathophysiology, as a consequence of basic science and clinical outcomes research, is constantly expanding. This has resulted in changes and improvements in how we care for patients.

In shock, many physiological changes occur before the classic signs, hypotension and rapid pulse, become evident. Therefore, you must treat for shock promptly based on the mechanism of injury and early, subtle signs and symptoms, without waiting for the classic signs to appear.

Pathology, from the root *patho* meaning "disease," is the study of disease and its causes. **Pathophysiology** is the study of how diseases alter the normal physiological processes of the human body. The concept "disease" may include both medical illness and injury.

As a paramedic, you should realize that our understanding of pathophysiology, as a consequence of basic science and clinical outcomes research, is constantly expanding. This has resulted in many changes and improvements in how we care for patients.

One example of this is the assessment and management of shock. From the origin of EMS until the mid 1980s, emergency department and EMS personnel depended on hypotension with tachycardia (low blood pressure with an accelerated pulse rate) as the primary indicators of shock in trauma and medical patients. Basic scientific research has revealed the pathophysiology of shock to be a cellular event, with many compensatory mechanisms occurring before a patient actually presents with hypotension and tachycardia. A patient with this combination of vital signs has already been in shock for an undetermined amount of time without any intervention, and will probably not have a good outcome. Clinical research validated what had been deduced from basic scientific research, and the standard of care shifted from using the presence of hypotension and tachycardia to using the mechanism of injury and earlier, more subtle clinical signs and symptoms as the catalysts for responding to shock before it has advanced beyond the stage where it can be effectively reversed.

In this chapter, we will discuss the elements of physiology and pathophysiology: more about the cell (its function and environment), the role of genetics, the interplay and integration of systems to maintain homeostasis, and the impact of system disorders that result in stress, disease, and death. You will confirm, as you read, that an understanding of the cell is critical to an understanding of all these topics.

HOW CELLS RESPOND TO CHANGE AND INJURY

Keep in mind the concept of homeostasis: the body's tendency to maintain a constantly balanced environment and to correct or compensate for any change that upsets the balance. In this section, we will look at a variety of mechanisms by which cells respond to change and potential or actual injury.

CELLULAR ADAPTATION

Cells, tissues, organs, and even entire organ systems can adapt to both normal and injurious (pathological) conditions. For example, the growth of the uterus during pregnancy is a response to a normal change in condition. Dilation of the left ventricle after a myocardial infarction is an example of response to a pathological condition.

Adaptation to external stressors results in alterations in structure and function at the cellular level. These alterations are classified as atrophy, hypertrophy, hyperplasia, metaplasia, and dysplasia.

Many of these cellular adaptations are successful, at least in the short run, but may also be part of the process of a disease. Therefore, it is sometimes hard to distinguish an adaptive change that is a successful response to a functional demand from one that is pathological in nature.

> **Content Review**
>
> **CELLULAR ADAPTIONS**
> Atrophy
> Hypertrophy
> Hyperplasia
> Metaplasia
> Dysplasia

Atrophy

The size of an individual cell is generally determined by its workload. The cell's size will be sufficient to meet the demands placed on it by the body without wasting energy or vital nutrients. If demands decrease, cell size will also decrease to meet the demands efficiently, using minimal energy and nutrients. The cell will use less oxygen and ATP, due to its decrease in size, and the number of organelles within the cytoplasm will decrease. The process of decreasing size and increasing efficiency is known as **atrophy.**

In addition to a decrease in workload, a variety of other causes of atrophy have been identified. Atrophy may occur as a result of disuse, lack of stimulation, lack of nervous impulses, decreased nutrient supply, ischemia (lack of oxygen), or a decreased vascular (blood) supply.

Atrophy generally affects the cells found in skeletal muscle, the heart, the brain, and sex organs.

✱ **atrophy** a decrease in cell size resulting from a decreased workload.

Hypertrophy

When there is an increase in workload, a cell will often respond, in the opposite direction from atrophy, as **hypertrophy.** Hypertrophy is an increase in the size of the cell and its functional mass, including an increase in the number of organelles. The increased functional mass allows the cell to meet the increased demand. Hypertrophy of the myocardium (heart muscle) gradually occurs in response to aerobic exercise. When the heart enlarges as a consequence of a pathological event, such as after an AMI (acute myocardial infarction, or heart attack), the term applied is **dilation.** In a dilated state, the heart muscle cells have increased in size, often with a decrease in the force of contraction.

It is thought that cells that undergo hypertrophy are those that must enlarge in mass because they are unable to increase their numbers through division as in hyperplasia, described below. Hypertrophy most commonly affects cells of the heart and kidneys (enlarged heart, enlarged kidney).

✱ **hypertrophy** an increase in cell size resulting from an increased workload.

✱ **dilation** enlargement. In reference to the heart, an abnormal enlargement resulting from pathology.

Hyperplasia

Another type of response to an increased workload is **hyperplasia.** Hyperplasia is an increase in the number of cells through cell division. Cell division and duplication also includes duplication of the genetic material (DNA) and the nucleus in a process called **mitosis.** Cells capable of undergoing hyperplasia include epithelial, glandular, and epidermal cells. Others, such as skeletal, cardiac, and nerve tissues, cannot divide by mitosis and therefore cannot undergo hyperplasia.

Hyperplasia is very commonly seen along with hypertrophy, because the demand placed on cells in a specific area often affect cells and tissues throughout the body, some of which respond through hypertrophy and others of which respond through hyperplasia.

Metaplasia

Sometimes, damaged or destroyed cells of one type are replaced by cells of another type in a process called **metaplasia.** Metaplasia often involves replacement of one type of epithelial cell with another type of epithelial cell.

This process can be seen in chronic inflammation or irritation of the respiratory tract from inhalation of irritants, commonly cigarette smoke. The irritants in the smoke will damage and destroy the ciliated columnar epithelial cells of the trachea and larger airways. The response by the body will be to replace these cells with stratified squamous epithelial cells. The squamous epithelium is less likely to be damaged by the carcinogens in the smoke. However, the squamous epithelial cells do not secrete mucus or have cilia, thus causing loss of a vital protective mechanism. In addition, the stratified squamous epithelial cells have a higher tendency to become malignant (cancerous).

Metaplasia is reversible if the causative factor is removed in time. If the person stops smoking before a malignancy (cancer) develops, the body will replace the stratified squamous cells with normal ciliated columnar cells.

Dysplasia

The last adaptive mechanism of cellular response is **dysplasia.** Dysplasia is an abnormal change in cell size, shape, and appearance due to some type of external stressor. (Dysplasia is related to hyperplasia and is often called abnormal or atypical hyperplasia.)

With dysplasia, the external stressor is usually chronic inflammation due to chronic irritation of the tissue. The changes seen result from the irritation and inflammation of the cells. As a result, there is cellular proliferation to protect underlying cells. If the irritant is removed early on, then the cellular changes are often reversible.

Dysplastic cells have a high tendency to cause malignant (cancerous) changes if they are present for an extended period of time. For example, dysplasia of the female cervix potentially leads to cervical cancer.

CELLULAR INJURY

In addition to the cellular adaptations just described, there is an enormous variety of cellular responses to injury or insult. In this section, we will discuss the seven most common mechanisms of cellular injury—hypoxia, chemicals, infectious agents, immunologic/inflammatory reactions, physical agents, nutritional factors, and genetic factors—and provide examples of the ways cells respond to these types of injury in the effort to restore homeostasis.

Content Review

FORMS OF CELLULAR INJURY

Hypoxia
Chemicals
Infectious agents
Inflammatory reactions
Physical agents
Nutritional factors
Genetic factors

Hypoxic Injury

The most common cause of cellular injury is **hypoxia,** or oxygen deficiency. Hypoxia can have various causes, usually a deficit in the respiratory or cardiovascular system. Such causes include an inadequate amount of oxygen being taken into the lungs (as from a lack of oxygen in the environment, an occluded airway, or inadequate respiration), a condition that prevents oxygen in the lungs from passing into the bloodstream (as with emphysema), inadequate pumping of blood throughout the body (as in congestive heart failure), or by a blockage in the arterial system that prevents oxygenated blood from reaching the cells (as in myocardial infarction or stroke). A blockage or reduction of the delivery of oxygenated blood to the cells is known as **ischemia.**

Ischemia can also result if there is a deficiency of red blood cells to carry the oxygenated hemoglobin, a deficiency in hemoglobin in the blood, or a lack of available binding sites as occurs in patients with carbon monoxide poisoning. As the cell becomes progressively more ischemic, the intracellular metabolism becomes *anaerobic* (without oxygen). With anaerobic metabolism, there is a marked decrease in cellular ATP production and an increase in the production of harmful acids, primarily lactic acid. The cell and some of its organelles then begin to swell due to increased levels of sodium that result from the breakdown of the sodium-potassium ATPase pump. In those cells that use fats as their primary sources of energy, fat may accumulate within the cells, worsening the swelling.

If oxygen is supplied to the cell in time, the injury is reversible. But if oxygen is not supplied, the cell begins to break down and the cell membrane ruptures, releasing lysosomes and digestive enzymes into the extracellular environment. As a result, the cellular injury has progressed from reversible to irreversible. The result is the cellular and tissue death called *infarction.*

Chemical Injury

Cellular injury due to chemical products is very common. Deadly chemicals can be found under our sink, in our walls, in our work environment, and everywhere around us. Harmful chemical agents include heavy metals such as lead, carbon monoxide, ethanol (alcohol), drugs (misused medicinal drugs as well as street drugs), and insecticides, among others. Some, such as cyanide, cause cell damage and death within minutes. Others, such as common air pollutants, cause injury through prolonged exposure.

Children make up a large percentage of the population affected by chemicals. From accidental ingestion of poisons, such as cleaning products, to ingestion of lead-based-paint chips, to ingestion of ethanol products, children lead the way. However, persons of all ages can suffer injury from chemical agents.

Chemicals can damage the body in many ways. Injuries to the cells cause disruption of the cellular membrane resulting in enzymatic reactions, alteration of coagulation, and eventually death of the cell.

Infectious Injury

Infectious, or disease-causing, agents are a common cause of cellular injury. A healthy person harbors many microorganisms (living things so tiny they are invisible to the naked eye) in various body sites. These include bacteria, viruses, fungi, and parasites. The vast majority are harmless, some even useful to their human hosts. Only a few cause infection or disease. Those that do are known as **pathogens.**

The body has a variety of entry-blocking barriers and mechanisms that ward off most pathogens. The chief barrier is the skin. Mucous secretions trap

* **hypoxia** oxygen deficiency.

* **ischemia** a blockage in the delivery of oxygenated blood to the cells.

Patients suffering a heart attack should be thought of as having myocardial ischemia. Myocardial infarction is irreversible, and we hope to intervene before this occurs.

* **pathogen** a microorganism capable of producing infection or disease.

pathogens and are another important barrier. Normal bacteria, enzymes, gastric acids, and other body substances destroy many pathogens. Coughing, sneezing, vomiting, and elimination of urine and feces also rid the body of pathogens.

When a pathogen does succeed in invading the body, three things can happen: First, it may multiply and spread, overwhelming the body's defenses. Second, the body and the pathogen may battle to a draw, producing a chronic infection that is kept in check but is not destroyed by the body. Third, the body's defenses, with or without the assistance of medical treatment, may defeat and destroy the pathogen.

The greater the number of body cells invaded or destroyed by a pathogen, the greater the risk of serious or permanent damage to the body. An example would be a localized infection of the hand as compared with widespread peritonitis of the abdominal cavity.

The degree of damage or injury that can be created by a pathogen depends on its numbers, its virulence (or pathogenicity), and the body's ability to contain or destroy it. Virulence is dependent on three factors: first, the pathogen's ability to invade and destroy cells; second, its ability to produce toxins; and third its ability to produce hypersensitivity (allergic) reactions.

Immunologic/Inflammatory Injury

Protective responses of the body can cause cell injury and even death. The body's responses to cell injury are inflammation and immune responses in which the body attacks invading foreign substances. Sometimes an exaggerated immune response called *hypersensitivity* (allergy), or even a life-threatening *anaphylactic* response, may develop. Any immune response, whether mild or severe, not only attacks foreign cells, it also tends to injure healthy body cells in the same area, in particular damaging or interfering with the function of the cell membrane. Once the foreign cells are destroyed, the injured body cells will generally begin to repair themselves.

Immunological responses will be discussed in greater detail later in this chapter.

Injurious Physical Agents

Cellular damage can be caused by physical agents. Extreme variances in temperature, whether hot or cold, can cause injury to the epidermis and underlying tissue, as from a burn or frostbite. Electrical burns, including lightning injuries, cause severe cellular damage. Hyperthermia and hypothermia (exposure to unusually warm or cool environmental temperatures) can also cause cell damage by altering body temperature, breathing patterns, and so on.

Other physical agents that can cause cellular damage include atmospheric pressure changes (for example in a blast injury or deep-sea-diving injury), exposure to ionizing radiation (X-rays, nuclear radiation), illumination (eyestrain from fluorescent lighting, skin cancers from ultraviolet radiation), noise (hearing impairment), and mechanical stresses (blunt or penetrating trauma, irritation to the skin, repetitive-motion injuries, over-exertion back injuries).

Injurious Nutritional Imbalances

Atherosclerosis is a disease almost solely limited to developed countries that have drifted away from a balanced agrarian diet.

Improper nutrition contributes to one of the most widely publicized forms of cellular injury: atherosclerosis caused by the deposition of lipid, cholesterol, and calcium inside arteries. Many nutritionists identify excessive intake of saturated fats and cholesterol as major contributing causes. Others place the blame on excessive carbohydrate (glucose) intake, which triggers increased insulin secretion, which in turn stimulates production of cholesterol by the liver. Whatever the underlying causes, the result is a narrowing diameter of the arteries, which decreases the amount of oxygenated blood that reaches target cells, increasing the risk of ischemia to vital organs such as the heart and brain.

Problems other than atherosclerosis can also be caused or exacerbated by nutritional imbalances. In diabetic patients, an imbalance between insulin levels and carbohydrate intake causes complex, often severe metabolism problems.

While excessive intake of nutrients may cause problems such as those mentioned above, insufficient intake of nutrients can cause other problems. The cells require proteins, carbohydrates, lipids, vitamins, and minerals for their metabolism and survival. Deficient intake of any of these nutrients can cause cellular damage and illness.

More commonly in less-developed countries, less commonly in the United States, malnutrition and starvation lead to cellular injury and diseases such as beriberi, scurvy, and rickets, which are all caused by vitamin deficiencies in the diet.

Injurious Genetic Factors

Genes, the basic units of heredity, are composed of DNA. A large number of genes attach to form double-stranded helical molecules of DNA. Molecules of DNA are carried on long threadlike strands called *chromosomes.* The DNA resides in the nucleus of the cells. Some cellular dysfunctions are caused by genetic predisposition, either defective genes or altered chromosomes that the person is born with. Genetic cell injuries can involve alterations to the nucleus or the cell membrane, the shape of the cell, the receptors on the cell membrane, or the transport mechanisms that carry substances across the cell membrane.

A person's genetic makeup is determined at conception, and the interaction of genes and environmental factors determine that person's development. Some diseases are mainly environmental, for example invasion of the body by bacteria. Other diseases are mainly genetic, for example sickle cell disease, which is due to a genetic defect. Many diseases result from the combined effects of environmental and genetic factors, including certain metabolic disorders such as diabetes.

Manifestations of Cellular Injury

There are two aspects of the metabolism that takes place within cells: anabolism and catabolism. **Anabolism** is the constructive or "building up" phase of metabolism—the processes in which the cell takes in non-living substances from the blood and the extracellular environment and converts them into the living cytoplasm of the cell. **Catabolism** is the destructive, or "breaking down," phase of metabolism—the processes in which the cell converts complex substances into simpler substances, usually with an accompanying release of energy.

When cells are injured, metabolism goes awry. A chief consequence is that substances, not all of which are in the cells normally, *infiltrate* or *accumulate* in the cells to an abnormal degree. This can occur from one of three causes: (1) Endogenous substances (substances normally found in the cells) are anabolized (produced) in excess; (2) endogenous substances are not properly catabolized (broken down); or (3) harmful exogenous substances (substances from outside the cell, such as heavy metals, mineral dusts, or microorganisms) are taken into and remain in the cells.

When the cells attempt to catabolize the accumulated substances, excessive amounts of metabolites (products of catabolism) are excreted into the extracellular environment. Large numbers of phagocytes (specialized white blood cells) migrate to the area to ingest the excreted metabolites, and this causes swelling of the tissues, as may be seen in enlargement of the liver or spleen.

✱ **anabolism** the constructive phase of metabolism in which cells convert nonliving substances into living cytoplasm.

✱ **catabolism** the destructive phase of metabolism in which cells break down complex substances into simpler substances with release of energy.

A variety of substances can accumulate in the cells, including water, lipids, carbohydrates, glycogen, proteins, pigments, calcium, and urate, causing a variety of effects from diabetic disorders to moles and skin color changes to arthritic conditions. Regardless of the type or agent of injury, among the most commonly seen effects of cell injury and accumulation are cellular swelling and fatty change.

Cellular swelling, resulting from a permeable or damaged cellular membrane, is the most frequent result of cellular injury. The cellular swelling is caused by an inability to maintain stable intra- and extracellular fluid and electrolyte levels (which will be explained in more detail later).

Another response that frequently accompanies cellular swelling is the **fatty change,** in which lipids (small fat vesicles) invade the area of injury. Fatty change with swelling is an ominous sign of impending cellular destruction. The fatty deposits commonly occur in vascular organs such as the kidney and heart, but most commonly in the liver. These deposits begin to cause disruption of the cellular membrane and metabolism and interfere with the vital functions of the affected organs. If the injury does not involve the circulatory system, cellular damage may be contained in the immediate area. If the circulatory system is involved, chemical mediators and lysosomes from the local injury response can enter into the circulatory system, potentially causing systemic injury.

Systemic signs and symptoms of cellular injury include general feelings of fatigue and malaise, an altered appetite (increased or decreased hunger), fever associated with the inflammatory response, an increased heart rate associated with fever, and pain. Laboratory blood chemistry tests may reveal a high leukocyte (white blood cell) count, resulting from the immune response, as well as the presence of certain cellular enzymes indicating specific sites of cellular injury, such as the skeletal muscle, bone, heart, brain, liver, kidney, or pancreas.

CELLULAR DEATH: APOPTOSIS AND NECROSIS

Cellular death leads to one of two processes: apoptosis or necrosis. If the cellular injury or insult is confined to a local region, **apoptosis** may occur. Apoptosis is the body's way of ridding itself of destroyed or nonfunctional cells. It occurs as a result of both normal and pathological tissue changes. The word is Greek, meaning "falling apart." Simply stated, the injured cell releases digestive enzymes that will engulf and destroy itself. By eliminating damaged and dead cells, apoptosis allows tissues to repair and possibly regenerate.

The other process that may follow cellular death is **necrosis.** Unlike apoptosis, necrosis is always a pathological process. Four types of necrotic cell change may occur: coagulative, liquefactive, caseous, and fatty. *In coagulative necrosis,* the transparent viscous albumin of the cell becomes firm and opaque, like a cooked egg white. It generally results from hypoxia and commonly occurs in the kidneys, heart, and adrenal glands. In *liquefactive necrosis,* the cells become liquid and contained in walled cysts. This is common in the ischemic death of neurons and brain cells. In *caseous necrosis,* common in tubercular lung infection, incompletely digested cells take on a cottage-cheese-like consistency. In *fatty necrosis,* commonly occurring in the breast and abdominal structures, fatty acids combine with calcium, sodium, and magnesium ions to create soaps (a process called *saponification*). The dead tissue is opaque and white.

Gangrenous necrosis refers to tissue death over a wide area. *Dry gangrene* results from coagulative necrosis and affects the skin, most commonly of the lower extremities, turning it dry, shrunken, and black. *Wet gangrene* results from liquefactive necrosis and usually affects internal organs. *Gas gangrene* is the result of a bacterial infection of injured tissue, generating gas bubbles in the cells. By attacking red blood cells, gas gangrene can cause death from shock.

---

* **cellular swelling** swelling of a cell caused by injury to or change in permeability of the cell membrane with resulting inability to maintain stable intra- and extracellular fluid and electrolyte levels.

* **fatty change** a result of cellular injury and swelling in which lipids (fat vesicles) invade the area of injury; occurs most commonly in the liver.

* **apoptosis** response in which an injured cell releases enzymes that engulf and destroy itself; one way the body rids itself of damaged and dead cells.

* **necrosis** cell death; a pathological cell change. Four types of necrotic cell change are *coagulative, liquefactive, caseous,* and *fatty. Gangrenous necrosis* refers to tissue death over a wide area.

Content Review

RESULTS OF CELL DEATH

Apoptosis (usually normal)
Necrosis (always pathological)
– Coagulative
– Liquefactive
– Caseous
– Fatty
Gangrenous necrosis (over a wide area)
– Dry gangrene
– Wet gangrene
– Gas gangrene

There are several key differences between apoptosis and necrosis. In apoptosis, cells shrink. In necrosis, cells swell and rupture. Apoptosis appears to be a form of normal bodily housekeeping. Destroyed cells are cleared away and digested by phagocytes, permitting repair and regeneration. Necrosis is always pathological. Dead cells take on a different physical form (becoming hardened or liquefied) and destroy or interfere with normal physiological processes. Apoptosis has specificity. It occurs in scattered, single cells. Necrosis lacks specificity. It will destroy not only the injured cells but also neighboring cells.

FLUIDS AND FLUID IMBALANCES

Many pathological conditions adversely affect the body's fluid and electrolyte balances.

WATER

Body fluids are mostly water, which is distributed into various compartments. The main compartments are intracellular and extracellular (fluid inside and outside of the body cells). Extracellular fluid is further divided into intravascular (fluid that is part of the blood, mostly plasma) and interstitial (fluid that is neither in the cells nor in the vascular system). Fluid in the interstitial space is generally absorbed into the lymphatic system, which returns it to the vascular system. Fluid moves between body compartments by the mechanisms of osmosis and diffusion.

As described in Chapter 3, movement of water in and out of the vascular system is governed by hydrostatic pressure (blood pressure)—which tends to force water out of the capillaries into the interstitial space—and the counter-effect of oncotic force exerted by the large proteins in the plasma—which tends to pull interstitial fluid back into the capillaries. In a healthy person, net filtration of fluid in and out of the capillaries is zero.

EDEMA

Edema is the accumulation of water in the interstitial space, caused by a disruption in the forces that normally keep net filtration at zero. Four mechanisms commonly result in accumulation of water in the interstitial space: (1) a decrease in plasma oncotic force resulting from a decrease in plasma proteins; (2) increased hydrostatic pressure, which may result from venous obstruction, thrombophlebitis, or other causes; (3) increased capillary permeability resulting from mechanisms of inflammation and immune response; and (4) lymphatic channel obstruction, which can result from infection or surgical removal.

Edema can be localized or generalized. There may be local swelling at an injury site or within organ systems such as the lungs or heart or within body areas such as the abdomen or the feet. Edema is not only a sign of an underlying disease or injury. Edema itself causes problems, interfering with the movement of nutrients and wastes between tissues and capillaries and diminishing capillary blood flow. Edema affecting organs such as the brain, lung, heart, or larynx can be life threatening. Little can be done to treat edema in the prehospital setting except elevation of edematous limbs.

* **edema** excess fluid in the interstitial space.

INTRAVENOUS THERAPY

Intravenous (IV) therapy is the introduction of fluids and other substances into the venous side of the circulatory system. It is used to replace blood lost through hemorrhage, for electrolyte or fluid replacement, and for introduction of medications directly into the vascular system.

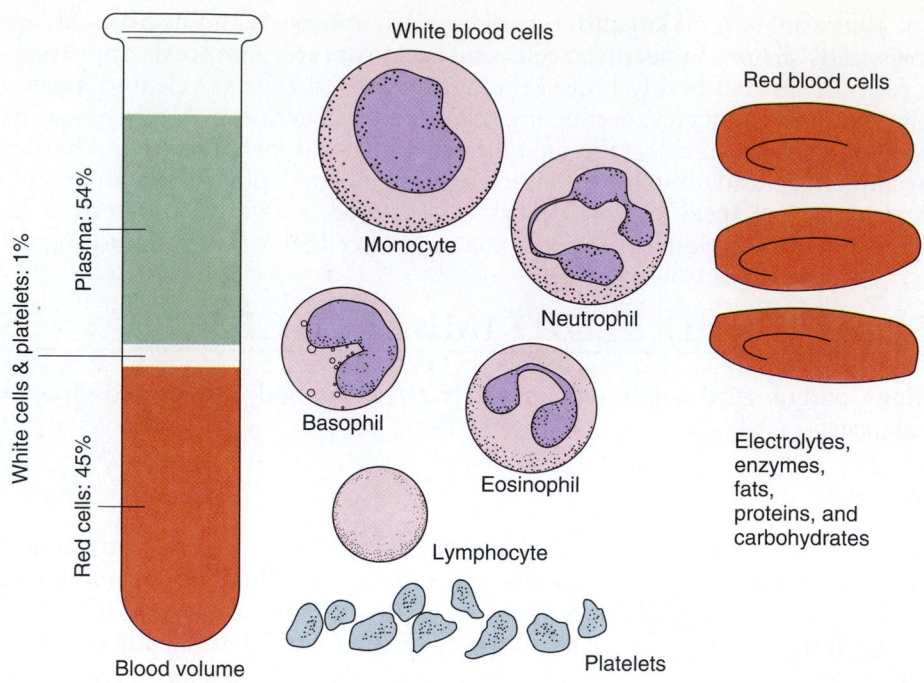

FIGURE 4-1 Blood components.

Blood and Blood Components

To understand IV therapy, it is necessary to understand the function of blood and its components. The blood is the fluid of the cardiovascular system. An adequate amount of blood is required for the transport of nutrients, oxygen, hormones, and heat. Blood consists of the liquid portion, or plasma, and the formed elements, or blood cells (Figure 4-1).

Plasma Plasma is made up of approximately 92 percent water, 6–7 percent proteins, and a small portion consisting of electrolytes, lipids, enzymes, clotting factors, glucose, and other dissolved substances.

Formed Elements The formed elements include the red blood cells, or **erythrocytes;** the white blood cells, or **leukocytes;** and the platelets, or **thrombocytes.** More than 99 percent of the blood cells are erythrocytes. Erythrocytes contain hemoglobin and are responsible for transporting oxygen to the body's peripheral cells. **Hemoglobin** is an iron-based compound that binds with oxygen in the pulmonary (lung) capillaries and transports the oxygen to the peripheral tissues where it can be unloaded and taken into the cells. Factors such as pH (to be discussed later in this chapter) and oxygen concentration affect the amount of oxygen that can be transported by hemoglobin.

The leukocytes are responsible for immunity and fighting infection. The thrombocytes play a major role in blood clotting. The viscosity (thickness) of the blood is determined by the ratio of plasma to formed elements. The greater the proportion of formed elements within the plasma, the greater the viscosity.

The plasma can be separated from the formed elements by centrifugation. That is, blood can be placed in a test tube inside a centrifuge and spun at high speed. The heavier cells, the erythrocytes, will be forced to the bottom of the tube, leaving the plasma portion at the top. Usually, the erythrocytes will account for approximately 45 percent of the blood volume. The percentage of blood occupied by erythrocytes is referred to as the **hematocrit** (Figure 4-2).

Fluid Replacement

The most desirable fluid for blood loss replacement is whole blood. There are several reasons for this. First, blood contains hemoglobin, which can transport oxygen. In addition, it is the most natural replacement. However, even in the hospital setting, the routine use of whole blood is not practical (Table 4-1). Blood is a precious commodity, and it must be conserved so that it can benefit the most people. Because of this, blood is often fractionated, or separated into parts. The red cells are packaged separately as packed red blood cells. The white cells are used for other purposes. Plasma is packaged as fresh frozen plasma for use when plasma or clotting factors are needed. Thus, with the exception of true hemorrhagic shock (resulting from blood loss), where whole blood is the fluid of first choice, packed red blood cells are now more frequently used than whole blood.

Before blood, or blood products, can be administered to a patient, they must be typed and cross-matched to prevent a severe allergic reaction. The exception to this is fresh frozen plasma, which does not require cross-matching. If there is not adequate time for typing and cross-matching, O-negative blood (type O, Rh negative), the universal donor, can be administered.

FIGURE 4-2 The percentage of the blood occupied by the red blood cells is termed the hematocrit.

Transfusion Reaction

Blood and blood products are not used in the field. However, on occasion, you may be called upon to transport a patient with blood infusing. Because of this, you must be able to recognize the signs and symptoms of a transfusion reaction. Transfusion reactions occur when there is a discrepancy between the blood type of the patient and the blood type of the blood being transfused. In addition to the ABO and Rh types, there are many minor types that can cause a transfusion reaction. Common signs and symptoms of a transfusion reaction include fever, chills, hives, hypotension, palpitations, tachycardia, flushing of the skin, headaches, loss of consciousness, nausea, vomiting, or shortness of breath.

If a transfusion reaction is suspected, IMMEDIATELY stop the transfusion and save the substance being transfused. A rapid IV fluid infusion should be started to prevent renal damage. Quickly assess the patient's mental status. Administer oxygen and contact medical direction. The medical direction physician may request the administration of mannitol (Osmotrol), diphenhydramine (Benadryl), or furosemide (Lasix). These drugs are used to maintain renal function, which is often severely compromised during a transfusion reaction.

Be alert for signs and symptoms of transfusion reaction. If they occur, immediately stop the transfusion.

Table 4-1	RESUSCITATION FLUIDS			
	Resuscitation Fluid Used			
Diagnosis	**1st Choice**	**2nd Choice**	**3rd Choice**	**4th Choice**
Hemorrhagic Shock	Whole blood	Packed RBCs	Plasma or plasma substitute	Lactated Ringer's or normal saline
Shock Due to Plasma Loss (Burns)	Plasma	Plasma substitute	Lactated Ringer's or normal saline	—
Dehydration	Lactated Ringer's or normal saline	—	—	—

In addition to overt reaction, you must always be alert for signs of fluid overload and congestive heart failure secondary to transfusion. This is evidenced by increased dyspnea, pulmonary congestion, edema, and altered mental status. If fluid overload is suspected, stop the infusion and start a crystalloid solution at a TKO (to keep open) rate. Administer oxygen and contact the medical direction physician.

Intravenous Fluids

Intravenous fluids are the most common products used in prehospital care for fluid and electrolyte therapy. Intravenous fluids occur in two general forms—colloids and crystalloids.

Colloids Colloids contain proteins, or other high-molecular-weight molecules, that tend to remain in the intravascular space for an extended period of time. In addition, as described earlier, colloids have oncotic force (colloid osmotic pressure), which means they tend to attract water into the intravascular space from the interstitial space and the intracellular space. Thus, a small amount of a colloid can be administered to a patient with a greater-than-expected increase in intravascular volume. The following are examples of colloids:

* *Plasma protein fraction (Plasmanate)* is a protein-containing colloid. The principal protein present is **albumin,** which is suspended along with other proteins in a saline solvent.
* *Salt-poor albumin* contains only human albumin. Each gram of albumin holds approximately 18 milliliters of water in the bloodstream.
* *Dextran* is not a protein, but a large sugar molecule with osmotic properties similar to albumin. It comes in two molecular weights: 40,000 and 70,000 Daltons. Dextran 40 has 2–2.5 times the colloid osmotic pressure of albumin.
* *Hetastarch (Hespan),* like dextran, is a sugar molecule with osmotic properties similar to protein. It does not appear to share many of dextran's side-effects.

Colloid replacement therapy, at present, does not have a role in prehospital care except under rare circumstances. The colloid products are expensive and have a short shelf life.

Crystalloids Crystalloids are the primary compounds used in prehospital intravenous fluid therapy. There are multiple fluid preparations. It is often helpful to classify them according to their **tonicity** relative to plasma:

* *Isotonic solutions* have electrolyte composition similar to the blood plasma. When placed into a normally hydrated patient, they will not cause a significant fluid or electrolyte shift. Examples: normal saline (0.9% sodium chloride, also written as 0.9% NaCl), lactated Ringer's.
* *Hypertonic solutions* have a higher solute concentration than the cells. These fluids will tend to cause a fluid shift out of the interstitial space and intracellular compartment into the intravascular space when administered to a normally hydrated patient. Later, there will be a diffusion of solute in the opposite direction. Examples: plasmanate, dextran.
* *Hypotonic solutions* have a lower solute concentration than the cells. When administered to a normally hydrated patient, they will cause a movement of fluid from the intravascular space into the interstitial space and intracellular compartment. Later, solutes will move in an opposite direction. Example: 5% dextrose in water (D_5W).

---

* **colloids** substances, such as proteins or starches, consisting of large molecules or molecule aggregates that disperse evenly within a liquid without forming a true solution.

* **albumin** a protein commonly present in plant and animal tissues. In the blood, albumin works to maintain blood volume and blood pressure and provides colloid osmotic pressure, which prevents plasma loss from the capillaries.

* **crystalloids** substances capable of crystallization. In solution, unlike colloids, they can diffuse through a membrane, such as a capillary wall.

* **tonicity** solute concentration or osmotic pressure relative to the blood plasma or body cells.

Intravenous replacement fluids should be chosen based on the needs of the patient and the patient's underlying problem. This is typically guided by laboratory studies obtained in the hospital. However, these studies are not available in the prehospital setting. Hemorrhage occurs so fast that there is usually not time for a significant fluid shift to occur between the intravascular space and interstitial/intracellular spaces. Because of this, isotonic replacement fluids, such as lactated Ringer's and normal saline, should be used. (See Figure 4-3)

Certain conditions, such as gastroenteritis (characterized by diarrhea, vomiting, and fever) can cause a patient to lose water more rapidly than sodium. These patients will have a deficit in total body water (TBW) due to reduced water intake, excessive water loss, or a combination of both. When water is lost in this manner, the level of sodium in the serum can increase, resulting in hypernatremia (elevated sodium levels). Patients with hypernatremia primarily need water. Because of this, hypotonic intravenous solutions, such as 0.45% sodium chloride (half-normal saline) are often chosen, because they provide the needed water with less sodium. However, it is important to point out that, even in cases of hypernatremia, initial fluid replacement therapy should be with an isotonic solution until adequate blood pressure and adequate tissue perfusion have been restored.

Some replacement fluids contain a single element, such as sodium chloride or dextrose, while others contain multiple elements. Solutions such as lactated Ringer's are designed so that the concentration of electrolytes is very similar to that of the plasma. As a result, these solutions are referred to as balanced salt solutions.

The most commonly used solutions in prehospital care are lactated Ringer's solution, 0.9% sodium chloride (normal saline), and 5% dextrose in water (D_5W).

- *Lactated Ringer's* is an isotonic electrolyte solution of sodium chloride, potassium chloride, calcium chloride, and sodium lactate in water.
- *Normal saline* is an electrolyte solution of sodium chloride in water. It is isotonic with the extracellular fluid.
- D_5W is a hypotonic glucose solution used to keep a vein open and to supply calories necessary for cell metabolism. While it will have an initial effect of increasing the circulatory volume, glucose molecules rapidly diffuse across the vascular membrane. Water follows the glucose into the interstitial space, resulting in an increase in interstitial water.

Both lactated Ringer's solution and normal saline are used for fluid replacement, because their administration causes an immediate expansion of the circulatory volume. However, as was noted earlier, due to the movement of electrolytes and water, two-thirds of either of these solutions is lost into the interstitial space within one hour.

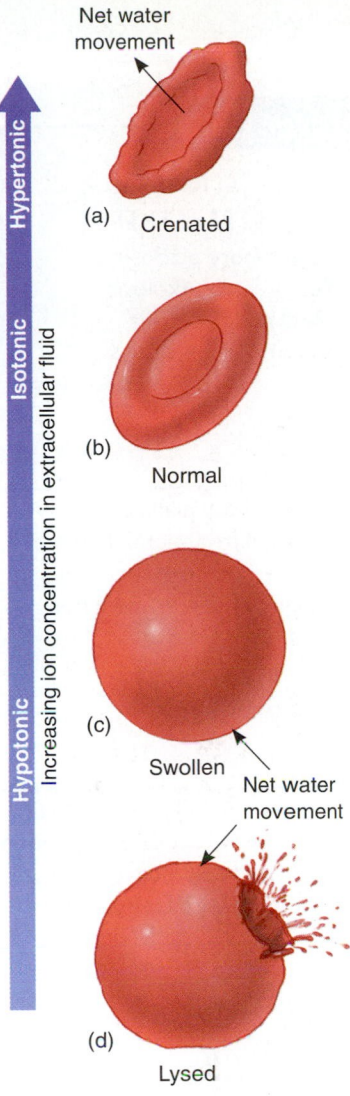

(a) Crenated

(b) Normal

(c) Swollen — Net water movement

(d) Lysed

FIGURE 4-3 The effects of hypertonic, isotonic, and hypotonic solutions on red blood cells.

The three most commonly used fluids in prehospital care are lactated Ringer's, normal saline, and D_5W.

ACID–BASE DERANGEMENTS

An increase in hydrogen ion (as occurs, for example, in cardiac arrest) triggers an alteration in acid-base balance. Hydrogen ion is immediately combined with bicarbonate ion. This combination results in the formation of carbonic acid, which then dissociates into carbon dioxide and water with the assistance of carbonic anhydrase. Carbon dioxide is eliminated by the lungs, and water is eliminated through the kidneys. Any change in a component of this equation affects the other components. For example:

$$\uparrow H^+ + HCO_3^- \rightarrow \uparrow H_2CO_3 \rightarrow H_2O + \uparrow CO_2$$

Conversely, if the amount of carbon dioxide is increased, the equation is driven in the other direction, resulting in an increase in hydrogen ion (acid).

$$\uparrow CO_2 + H_2O \rightarrow \uparrow H_2CO_3 \rightarrow \uparrow H^+ + HCO_3^-$$

Both types of acid-base derangements, alkalosis and acidosis, can be divided into two categories based on the underlying causes. Changes in the concentration of CO_2 result from changes in respiratory function. Thus, an acidosis caused by retained CO_2 is referred to as *respiratory acidosis*. An alkalosis caused by the excess removal of CO_2 is called *respiratory alkalosis*. However, if acidosis results from the production of metabolic acids, such as lactic acid, then *metabolic acidosis* is said to exist. If an alkalosis is caused by the excess elimination of hydrogen ion, it is termed *metabolic alkalosis*.

Respiratory Acidosis

Respiratory acidosis is caused by the retention of CO_2. This can result from impaired ventilation due to problems occurring either in the lungs or in the respiratory center of the brain. The CO_2 level is increased and the pH is decreased.

$$\downarrow RESPIRATION = \uparrow CO_2 + H_2O \rightarrow \uparrow H_2CO_3 \rightarrow \uparrow H^+ + HCO_3^-$$

Treatment is directed at improving ventilation.

Respiratory Alkalosis

Respiratory alkalosis results from increased respiration and excessive elimination of CO_2. This can occur with anxiety or following ascent to a high altitude. The CO_2 level is decreased and the pH is increased.

$$\uparrow RESPIRATION = \downarrow CO_2 + H_2O \rightarrow \downarrow H_2CO_3 \rightarrow \downarrow H^+ + HCO_3^-$$

Treatment, if required, consists of increasing the CO_2 level by emotionally supporting the patient and coaching him to reduce his respiratory rate.

Metabolic Acidosis

Metabolic acidosis results from the production of metabolic acids such as lactic acid, which consume bicarbonate ion. In addition, it can result from dehydration (as from diarrhea, vomiting) diabetes, and medication usage. The pH is decreased, and the CO_2 level is normal.

$$\uparrow H^+ + HCO_3^- \rightarrow \uparrow H_2CO_3 \rightarrow H_2O + \uparrow CO_2$$

In addition to treating the underlying cause, treatment includes ventilation, which causes the elimination of CO_2 and, subsequently, hydrogen ion (Figure 4-4). On rare occasions, an IV bolus of sodium bicarbonate ($NaHCO_3$) may be required.

Metabolic Alkalosis

Metabolic alkalosis occurs much less frequently than metabolic acidosis. It is usually caused by the administration of **diuretics,** loss of chloride ions associated with prolonged vomiting, or the overzealous administration of sodium bicarbonate. The pH is increased and the CO_2 level is normal.

$$\downarrow H^+ + HCO_3^- \rightarrow \downarrow H_2CO_3 \rightarrow H_2O + \downarrow CO_2$$

Treatment consists of correcting the underlying cause.

✶ respiratory acidosis acidity caused by abnormal retention of carbon dioxide resulting from impaired ventilation.

✶ respiratory alkalosis alkalinity caused by excessive elimination of carbon dioxide resulting from increased respirations.

✶ metabolic acidosis acidity caused by an increase in acid, often because of increased production of acids during metabolism or from causes such as vomiting, diarrhea, diabetes, or medication.

✶ metabolic alkalosis alkalinity caused by an increase in plasma bicarbonate resulting from causes including diuresis, vomiting, or ingestion of too much sodium bicarbonate.

✶ diuretic an agent that increases urine secretion and elimination of body water.

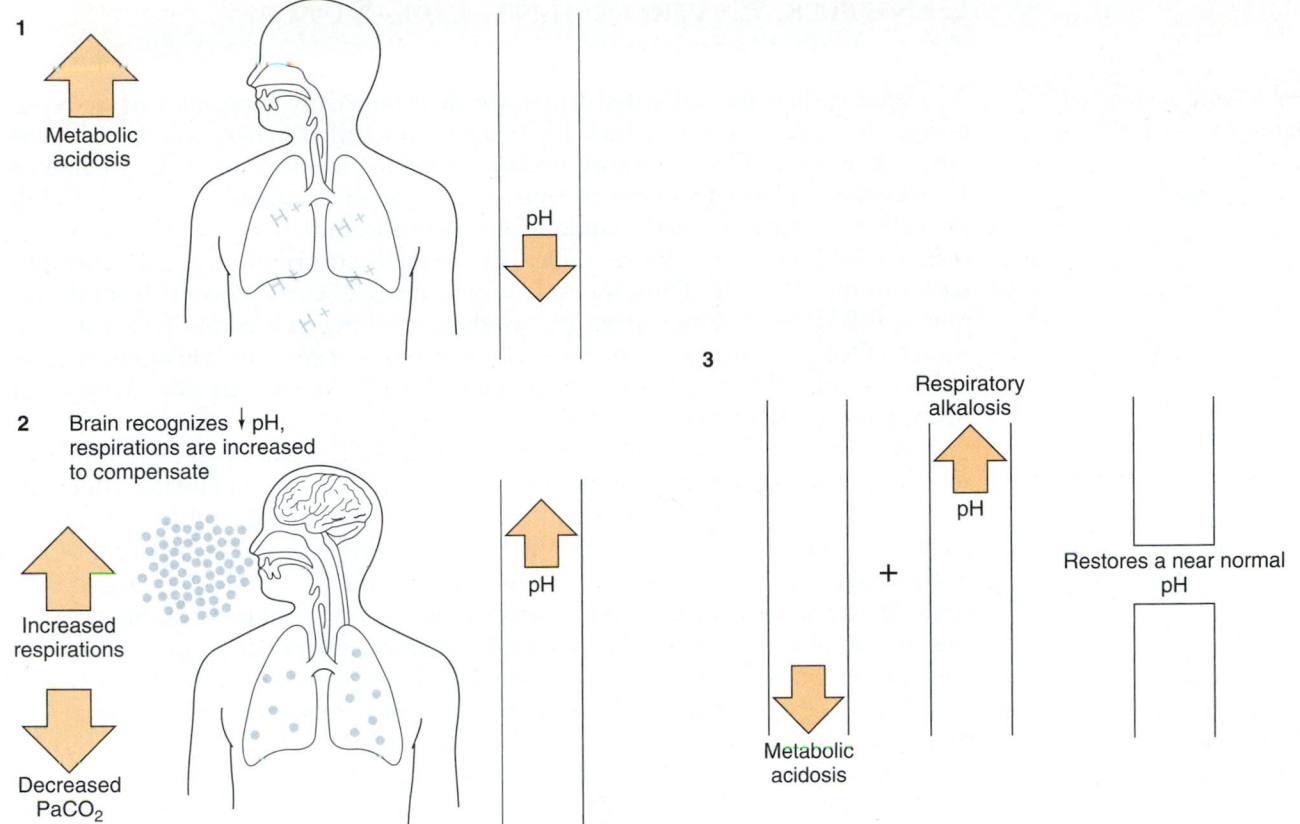

1 Metabolic acidosis

pH

2 Brain recognizes ↓ pH, respirations are increased to compensate

Increased respirations

Decreased PaCO₂

pH

3 Respiratory alkalosis

pH

+

Metabolic acidosis

Restores a near normal pH

FIGURE 4-4   Compensation for metabolic acidosis begins with an increase in respirations.

Usually, both a respiratory and a metabolic component are present in an acid-base derangement. The type of acid-base derangement present can only be determined by arterial blood gas studies. These, of course, are only available in the hospital setting. Arterial blood gases report the pH, $PaCO_2$, PaO_2, bicarbonate concentration, and oxygen saturation.

GENETICS AND OTHER CAUSES OF DISEASE

When we think of disease, we are likely to think first of infections caused by pathogens, including bacteria, viruses, fungi, and parasites. In recent years, great strides have been made in the medical treatment of infectious diseases, but many diseases result from genetic causes, which have been far more difficult to identify and treat. The picture is additionally complicated by the fact that many diseases result from a combination of genetic and environmental factors (including life-style factors) as well as factors such as age and gender.

Even a family history of a particular disease does not necessarily mean that the disease has a purely genetic origin, because families also share environmental and life-style factors that may cause or contribute to the family disease. While family history points to the possibility of genetic causes, these cannot be confirmed, much less treated, until scientists are able to make definitive identifications of the defective genes or chromosomes that cause or contribute to particular diseases.

At present, there is increasing progress in identifying and understanding genetic and other non-infectious causes of disease. Many promising advances toward gene therapies (the replacement of defective genes with normal genes) and other therapies for diseases have been made.

GENETICS, ENVIRONMENT, LIFE-STYLE, AGE, AND GENDER

As noted earlier, our inherited traits are determined by molecules of deoxyribonucleic acid, or DNA, which form structures called genes, which reside on larger structures called chromosomes within the nuclei of all our cells. We inherit our genetic structure from our parents. Every one of a person's somatic cells (all the cells except the sex cells) contains 46 chromosomes. The sex cells, however, contain only 23 chromosomes each. The sex cells contribute these 23 chromosomes to the offspring. Thus, the offspring receives 23 chromosomes from the father and 23 chromosomes from the mother, resulting in a total of 46 chromosomes. Occasionally one or more of a person's genes or chromosomes is abnormal, and this may cause a congenital disease (one we are born with) or a propensity toward acquiring a disease later in life.

Some diseases are thought to be purely genetic. For example, cystic fibrosis, which affects mainly people of European origin, and sickle cell disease, which affects mainly people of African origin, are known to be caused by disorders of single genes. They affect different populations to a different degree because of the evolutionary history of those populations. A genetic disease may be caused by a single defective gene or by several defective genes or chromosomes. Single-gene causes are, obviously, easier for medical researchers to identify and potentially devise treatments for than are other, more complex genetic causes of disease.

Other diseases are caused by a combination of genetic and environmental factors and are called *multifactorial disorders*. For example, Type II (adult-onset) diabetes has a very high correlation with family history of the disease. However, it is also affected by environmental and life-style factors such as a high-fat or high carbohydrate diet and lack of exercise, which results in obesity, and with age. (There is a higher incidence of Type II diabetes in overweight people, and the disease tends to appear in middle age or later.) Heart disease, which is highly correlated with family history and age, also has a gender/hormonal factor: Women appear to be somewhat protected from heart disease before menopause, when their bodies are still producing estrogen. Following menopause, women quickly "catch up" with men in the development of heart disease. Estrogen replacement therapy following menopause may afford prolonged protection against heart disease.

Clinical practitioners and epidemiologists study disease, respectively, from the point of view of their effects on individuals and from the point of view of their effects on populations as a whole.

Content Review

CAUSATIVE ANALYSIS OF DISEASE

Clinical Factors:
Host
Agent
Environment

Epidemiological Factors:
Incidence
Prevalence
Mortality

- *Effects on Individuals.* Physicians and other clinical practitioners study the effects of diseases on individuals, and find it instructive to view the development of diseases as products of the interactions among three factors: *host, agent,* and *environment.* This establishes a framework for determining how one, or a combination of these factors, may precipitate a disease state. Genetic predisposition, gender, and ethnic origin are determinants related to the host. These may interact with a specific agent, in a specific type of environment, to cause illness. The agent may be a bacterium, toxin, gunshot, or other pathophysiological process. The environment may be defined by the local climate, socioeconomic or demographic features, culture, religion, and associated factors. Determination of how the host, agent, and environment interact may yield solutions to curing a disease process. Injury and trauma are now being viewed as "diseases," in the sense of how the interaction of host, agent, and environment may contribute to an understanding of what, heretofore, have been perceived as social problems.

- *Effects on Populations.* Epidemiologists, who study the effects of diseases on populations, generally report disease data with three basic measures: *incidence, prevalence,* and *mortality. Morbidity,* a term commonly used in discussing disease statistics, can be more precisely reported as incidence and prevalence. Incidence is the number of new cases of the disease that are reported in a given period of time, usually one year. Prevalence is the proportion of the total population who are affected by the disease at a given point in time. (Prevalence is higher than incidence, as those who acquire the disease each year are added to those who already have the disease.) *Mortality* is the rate of death from the disease.

Epidemiologists and clinical practitioners are now collaborating to study risk factors, such as the relationship between smoking and lung cancer. Risk factor analysis is both statistical and complex. Although the correlation of smoking to lung cancer is extremely high, not everyone who smokes develops lung cancer, and not everyone who develops lung cancer has been a smoker. Risk factor analysis would compare the number of smokers to non-smokers among lung cancer cases, the pack/year (number of packs per day × number of years) history of the smokers with lung cancer, factors that might have aggravated or mitigated the effects of smoking, and so on.

FAMILY HISTORY AND ASSOCIATED RISK FACTORS

It is important for those who have a family history of a particular disease not to conclude that acquiring the disease is their destiny and there is nothing they can do about it. This is not always true. Most diseases with a genetic component that come on during adulthood also have associated risk factors that can be modified to prevent, delay, or reduce the impact of the disease.

Consider the variety of possible risk factors for disease: People who live in less-developed countries are often at higher risk for disease from microorganisms flourishing in their water supply and disease transmission caused by poor sanitation. Physical conditions commonly seen in larger U.S. cities as well as rural areas, such as inadequate housing, poor nutrition, and little or no medical attention, potentiate disease transmission. Chemical factors such as smoke, smog, illicit drug use, occupational chemical exposure, and additives in our food are causative agents for a variety of diseases.

Personal habit is among the most publicized—and controllable—causes of disease in our society. For example, predisposing factors for cardiovascular disease include smoking, alcohol consumption, inactivity, and obesity. Unfortunately, changes in individual life style often occur only after a disease has already manifested itself. As we age, the predisposing factors and causative agents take their toll. The body's ability to defend itself against disease decreases due to the effects of aging on our immunological system and other compensatory mechanisms.

Following is a discussion of some of the most common diseases in which both genetics and other risk factors play a role. You will notice, as you read, that the causation of various diseases varies widely, and that while the causes are known for some diseases, the causes of other diseases are still not clearly understood.

Immunologic Disorders

A number of immunologic disorders, such as rheumatic fever, allergies, and asthma, are more prevalent among those with a family history of the disorder but also involve other risk factors.

Rheumatic fever is an inflammatory reaction to an infection but is not an infection itself. There seems to be a hereditary factor, but inadequate nutrition and crowded living conditions are contributing factors.

Allergies often have a family-history factor (and some allergies can be passed from the mother to the fetus during pregnancy). However, allergic reactions are triggered by exposure to allergens and can usually be controlled by avoiding or reducing the presence of allergens as well as with medication.

Asthma sufferers may inherit the propensity for airway-narrowing in response to various stimuli, but other triggering factors may be identified and, perhaps, controlled, including stress, overexertion, exposure to cold air, and stimuli such as pollens, dust mites, cockroach detritus, and smoke.

Cancer

A wide variety of family-history and environmental factors are included among the risk factors for cancer. Some kinds of cancer, such as breast and colorectal cancer, tend to cluster in families and seem to have a combination of genetic and environmental causes. Others, such as lung cancer, are more strongly identified with environmental causes.

For *breast cancer,* the greatest risk factor is age, with the majority occurring after age 60 and the greatest risk after age 75. A history of breast cancer in a first-degree relative (mother, sister, or daughter) increases the risk by two or three times. Some progress has been made in identifying genes for certain breast cancers. Life-style factors such as lack of exercise and obesity may contribute slightly to the incidence of breast cancer, but this has not been proven.

As with breast cancer, *colorectal cancer* risk factors include age (with the incidence rising after age 40 and peaking between 60 and 75) and family history (incidence in a first-degree relative increases the risk by two or three times). There are gender factors, with rectal cancer being more common in men and colon cancer more common in women. Diet may also be a risk factor, although recent studies have failed to confirm a link between a high-fat, low-fiber diet and colorectal cancer. (However, a high-fat, low-fiber diet has been positively linked to heart disease and other health problems.)

The causes of *lung cancer* are overwhelmingly environmental. Smoking has been identified as the main cause of 90 percent of lung cancers in men and 70 percent of lung cancers in women. Lung cancer can also be caused by inhaling substances such as asbestos, arsenic, and nickel, usually in the workplace.

Endocrine Disorders

The most common endocrine disorder is *diabetes mellitus,* which is a leading cause of blindness, heart disease, kidney failure, and premature death. The causes of diabetes are complex and still not well understood.

There are two major types of diabetes: Type I and Type II. Type I diabetes usually occurs before age 40, sometimes in childhood. Although it is less prevalent than Type II diabetes (accounting for about 20 percent of diabetes cases), it is more severe. In the Type I diabetic, the pancreas produces no or almost no insulin, which is required for the cellular utilization of glucose, the body's chief source of energy. Type I diabetics must take insulin daily. There is some association of Type I diabetes with family history (siblings of Type I diabetics have a 6 percent risk compared to 0.3 percent in the general population), and medical researchers have pinpointed some possible genetic factors. Other causative factors may include autoimmunity disorders and viral infections that invade the pancreas and destroy the insulin-producing cells.

Type II diabetes accounts for about 80 percent of all diabetes cases. It usually occurs after age 40 and the incidence increases with age. It clusters much more strongly in families than does Type I diabetes (siblings have a 10–15 percent risk). In contrast to Type I diabetes, in which there is a total lack of insulin, Type II diabetes is associated with a decreased insulin receptor response or a decrease in insulin production. Diet and exercise may also be factors, since the majority of Type II diabetics are obese. Type II diabetes can often be controlled with diet and exercise or with oral medications.

Hematologic Disorders

Hereditary coagulation disorders have been studied by geneticists and physicians in great detail. There are many causes of hereditary hematological disorders such as gene alteration and histocompatibility (tissue interaction) dysfunctions.

Hemophilia is a bleeding disorder that is caused by a genetic clotting factor deficiency. It can be mild, but if severe it can cause not only serious bruising but bleeding into the joints, which can lead to crippling deformities. A slight bump on the head can cause bleeding within the skull, often resulting in brain damage and death. The heredity is sex-linked (associated with the sex chromosomes), inherited through the mother and affecting male children almost exclusively. There is no cure, but administration of concentrated clotting factors can improve the condition.

Hemochromatosis is another genetic disorder, but this time caused by a histocompatibility complex dysfunction. It is marked by an excessive absorption and accumulation of iron in the body, causing weight loss, joint pain, abdominal pain, palpitations, and testicular atrophy in males. It is treated by removing blood from the body at intervals.

Not all blood disorders are genetic. Environmental factors, for example, can cause *anemia* (reduction in circulating red blood cells). For example, some antihypertensive medications and other drugs may cause a drug-induced hemolytic (red-blood-cell-destroying) anemia.

Cardiovascular Disorders

The cardiovascular system can be greatly affected by genetic disorders. Disorders such as *prolongation of the QT interval* (a delay between depolarization and repolarization of the ventricles as revealed in an electrocardiogram) and *mitral-valve prolapse* (an upward ballooning of the valve between the left ventricle and atrium that allows blood to regurgitate back into the atrium when the ventricle contracts) tend to cluster in families.

The American Heart Association lists heredity as a major risk factor for cardiovascular disease. Those with parents who have *coronary artery disease* (deposits on the walls of the coronary arteries that reduce blood flow to the heart muscle) have an approximately five-fold risk of developing the disease. This is why it is important to ask about family history of congenital heart disease (CHD), hypertension, and stroke when assessing patients with possible cardiovascular disease. However, environmental factors, such as a diet high in saturated fats and cholesterol (or a diet high in carbohydrates) and lack of exercise, also play a large role in cardiovascular disease.

Hypertension (high blood pressure) is a major risk factor, not only for cardiac disease but also for stroke and kidney disease. Studies of family history show that approximately 20 to 40 percent of the causation of hypertension is genetic. The remaining causative factors, then, are environmental, and may include high sodium ingestion, lack of physical activity, stress, and obesity.

Not all cardiac disorders have a genetic component. For example, *cardiomyopathy* (disease affecting the heart muscle), is thought to occur secondary to other causes such as infectious disease, toxin exposure, connective tissue disease, or nutritional deficiencies, which may be partially or totally environmental.

Renal Disorders

Renal (kidney) failure is caused by a variety of factors (primarily hypertension) which may eventually require a patient to receive dialysis treatment several times a week. As the location of dialysis treatment shifts from medical centers to homes and community satellite centers, EMS personnel are increasingly being called to deal with the complications of dialysis. These include problems with vascular access devices (shunts, fistulas), localized infection and sepsis, and electrolyte abnormalities (hyperkalemia), which can result in cardiac arrest.

As dialysis treatment shifts from medical centers to homes and community centers, EMS personnel are increasingly being called to deal with complications of dialysis.

Rheumatic Disorders

Gout is a condition that may have both genetic and environmental causes. It is characterized by severe arthritic pain caused by deposit of crystals in the joints, most commonly the great toe. The crystals form as the result of an abnormally high level of uric acid in the blood that may be caused when the kidneys do not excrete enough uric acid or by high production of uric acid. High production of uric acid may be caused by a hereditary metabolic abnormality. Although the underlying cause may be genetic, attacks of gout can be triggered by environmental factors such as trauma, alcohol consumption, ingestion of certain foods, stress, or other illnesses. Patients with gout also have a tendency to develop *kidney stones*.

Gastrointestinal Disorders

Gastrointestinal disorders have a variety of causes, and the causes of some are not known. *Lactose intolerance,* for example, is usually identified by the inability of the patient to tolerate milk and some other dairy products. The patient lacks lactase, the enzyme that usually breaks down lactose in the digestive tract. This enzyme deficiency may be congenital (inborn) or may develop later on.

Crohn's disease is a chronic inflammation of the wall of the digestive tract that usually affects the small intestine, the large intestine, or both. The cause is not known, but medical researchers have focused on immune system dysfunction, infection, and diet as the major probabilities. A similar disorder is ulcerative colitis, in which the large intestine becomes inflamed and develops ulcers. As with Crohn's disease, the cause is not known, but an overactive immune response is suspected, and heredity seems to play a role.

Peptic ulcers develop when the normal protective structures and mechanisms, such as mucous production, break down and areas in the lining of the stomach or duodenum are inflamed by stomach acid and digestive juices. Environmental factors, bacterial infection (by *Helicobacter pylori*), diet, stress, and alcohol consumption, are thought to play roles in the development of peptic ulcers. Many medications, particularly non-steroidal anti-inflammatory medications, are associated with ulcer formation.

Cholecycstits is an inflammation of the gallbladder that usually results from blockage by a gallstone. There may be a genetic predisposition for gallstone formation. Gallstones are more prevalent in women and in some groups such as Native Americans and Mexican Americans. Other risk factors include age, a high-fat diet, and obesity.

Obesity can be defined as being more than 20 percent over the ideal body weight. Obesity has both an environmental and familial risk transmission. Research has shown that children whose parents are obese have a much-increased chance of developing obesity. Environmental factors such as proper nutrition and exercise may not be modeled or taught by obese parents, but there also seems to be a genetic factor to many cases of obesity. Obesity has been linked to, or defined as a cause for, diseases such as hypertension, heart disease, and vascular diseases.

Neuromuscular Disorders

Diseases of the nervous and muscular systems also have a variety of causes. *Huntington's disease* (which results in uncontrollable jerking and writhing movements) and muscular dystrophy (which results in progressive muscle weakness) are both known to be caused by genetic defects.

Multiple sclerosis (which affects the nerves of the eye, brain, and spinal cord) seems to have some hereditary factor with clustering among close relatives. Its exact cause is unknown, but it seems to result when the virus-triggered autoimmune response begins to attack the myelin sheath that protects the nerves.

Alzheimer's disease is thought to cause about 50 percent of dementias, or progressive mental deterioration. Its cause is unknown, but it does cluster strongly in families and appears to be either caused or influenced by specific gene abnormalities.

Psychiatric Disorders

Genetic and biological causes of psychiatric disorders are being studied and increasingly understood. An example is *schizophrenia*, which affects about one percent of the population worldwide and is more prevalent than Alzheimer's disease, diabetes, or multiple sclerosis. The schizophrenic loses contact with reality and suffers from hallucinations, delusions, abnormal thinking, and disrupted social functioning. People who develop schizophrenia are now thought to be "biologically vulnerable" to the disease, but what makes them vulnerable is not fully understood. The cause may be a genetic predisposition or some problem that occurs before, during, or after birth or a viral infection of the brain.

Another common psychiatric disorder is *manic-depressive illness,* also called *bipolar disorder,* in which the person experiences alternating periods of depression and mania or excitement. It can be mild or severe enough to interfere with the patient's ability to work or function socially. Manic-depressive illness affects about twice as many people as schizophrenia. It is believed to be hereditary, but the exact gene deficit has not yet been discovered.

HYPOPERFUSION

All body cells require a constant supply of oxygen and other essential nutrients, while waste products, such as carbon dioxide, must be constantly removed. It is the circulatory system, in conjunction with the respiratory and gastrointestinal systems, that provides the body's cells with these essential nutrients and removal of wastes. This is accomplished by the passage of blood through the capillaries, the small vessels that interface with body cells, while oxygen and carbon dioxide, nutrients and wastes are exchanged by movement across the capillary walls and cell membranes. This constant and necessary passage of blood through the body's tissues is called *perfusion.*

Many disease processes have a genetic cause.

All body cells require a constant supply of oxygen and other nutrients.

There is some local control of both tissue perfusion and waste removal. When the amounts of metabolic waste products (such as lactic acid) increase, the tissues subsequently become acidotic. This local acidosis causes nearby precapillary sphincters to relax, thus opening the capillaries and increasing perfusion of the affected tissues. This provides increased capacity for waste elimination and response to local metabolic demands.

Inadequate perfusion of body tissues is **hypoperfusion,** which is commonly called shock. Shock occurs first at a cellular level. If allowed to progress, the tissues, organs, organ systems, and ultimately the entire organism is affected. Hypoperfusion is a condition that is progressive (that is, it triggers a self-worsening cycle of pathophysiological events) and fatal if not corrected. It can occur for many reasons, such as trauma, fluid loss, myocardial infarction, infection, allergic reaction, spinal cord injury, and other causes.

Although causes differ, all forms of shock have the same underlying pathophysiology at the cellular and tissue levels. As discussed in the next section, shock may be triggered by anything that affects one or more of these components of the cardiovascular system: the pump (the heart), the fluid (the blood), or the container (the blood vessels).

THE PATHOPHYSIOLOGY OF HYPOPERFUSION

Causes of Hypoperfusion

Hypoperfusion (shock) is almost always a result of inadequate cardiac output. A number of factors can decrease effective cardiac output. These include:

Content Review

PHYSIOLOGICAL CLASSIFICATIONS OF SHOCK

Inadequate pump (cardiogenic)

Inadequate fluid (hypovolemic)

Inadequate container (distributive/neurogenic)

- Inadequate pump
  - Inadequate preload
  - Inadequate cardiac contractile strength
  - Inadequate heart rate
  - Excessive afterload
- Inadequate fluid
  - Hypovolemia (abnormally low circulating blood volume)
- Inadequate container
  - Dilated container without change in fluid volume (inadequate systemic vascular resistance)
  - Leak in container

Occasionally, hypoperfusion can develop even when cardiac output is adequate. This can happen when cell metabolism is so excessive that the body cannot increase perfusion enough to meet the cells' metabolic requirements. It can also happen when abnormal circulatory patterns develop, so that circulating blood is bypassing critical tissues.

As mentioned earlier, the conditions that lead to hypoperfusion can result from a number of underlying causes, such as infection, trauma and hemorrhage, loss of plasma through burns, severe cardiac dysrhythmia, central nervous system dysfunction, and many others. But the outcome is always the same: inadequate delivery of oxygen and essential nutrients to, and removal of wastes from, all the tissues of the body, especially the critical tissues (brain, heart, kidneys).

Shock at the Cellular Level

Shock is a complex phenomenon. The causes vary. The signs and symptoms vary. At the simplest level, however, shock is inadequate tissue perfusion. Additionally, all types of shock have this in common: The ultimate outcome is impairment of cellular metabolism. Two characteristics of impaired cellular metabolism in any type of shock are impaired oxygen use and impaired glucose use.

Impaired Use of Oxygen One characteristic of any type of shock is that the cells are either not receiving enough oxygen or are unable to use it effectively. This may be caused by hypoperfusion resulting from reduced cardiac function, inadequate blood volume, or vasodilation (pump, fluid, or container problems). It may result from insufficient red cells to carry the oxygen, from fever that increases cellular oxygen demand, or chemical disruption of cellular metabolism.

When the cells don't receive enough oxygen or cannot use it effectively, they change from **aerobic metabolism** to **anaerobic metabolism,** a far less efficient means of producing energy—as explained below.

The primary energy source for the cells is glucose, taken into the cell with the aid of insulin. Glucose does not provide energy until it is broken down inside the cell. The first stage of glucose breakdown, called glycolysis, is anaerobic (does not require oxygen). Glycolysis produces pyruvic acid but yields very little energy. Thus, by itself, glycolysis is an inefficient utilization of glucose. Therefore, in a normal state of metabolism, a second stage of glucose breakdown is required. During this second stage, which is aerobic (requires oxygen), pyruvic acid is further degraded into carbon dioxide, water, and energy in a process termed the Krebs or citric acid cycle. The energy yield of this second-stage aerobic process is much higher than from the first-stage anaerobic process (Figure 4-5).

During shock, or any condition in which the cells do not receive adequate oxygen or cannot use it effectively, glucose breakdown can only complete the first-stage, anaerobic process of glycolysis and cannot enter into the second-stage, aerobic, citric acid cycle. This causes an accumulation of the end product of glycolysis, pyruvic acid. In these cases, pyruvic acid is quickly degraded to lactic acid. If oxygen is promptly restored to the cells, lactic acid will be reconverted to pyruvic acid. However, if time elapses and the cellular hypoxia is not corrected, lactic acid and other metabolic acids will accumulate. One outcome is that the acidic condition of the blood reduces the ability of hemoglobin in red blood cells to bind with and carry oxygen, which compounds the problem of cellular oxygen deprivation.

The energy that is produced during glucose breakdown is in the form of the chemical adenosine triphosphate (ATP), which is essential to all the metabolic processes in the cells. As just noted, the amount of energy, or ATP, produced during first-stage, anaerobic glycolysis is very small. Without oxygen, when the process of glucose breakdown stops after glycolysis (during which very little energy has been produced), cellular stores of ATP are used up much faster than they can be replaced, so that all of the processes of cellular metabolism are gravely impaired.

Because of changes to the internal cell and because blood flow has been slowed by the decreased pumping action and vasodilation, sludging of the blood occurs. This further impedes blood flow. Thus, the normal diffusion of nutrients and wastes in and out of the cells is disrupted and the balance of the cellular electrolytes is altered. Lysosomes, the organelles that assist in digestion of nutrients, are normally enclosed by a membrane that prevents the digestive enzymes from damaging other cell components. Now the lysosomes rupture, releasing the lysosomal enzymes into the cell. The sodium-potassium pumping mechanism fails, changing the electrical charge of the cells' internal environment. There is an increase in sodium and water (since water follows sodium)

Content Review

CHARACTERISTICS OF IMPAIRED CELLULAR METABOLISM IN SHOCK
Impaired use of oxygen
Impaired use of glucose

* **aerobic metabolism** the second stage of metabolism, requiring the presence of oxygen, in which the breakdown of glucose (in a process called the Krebs or citric acid cycle) yields a high amount of energy. *Aerobic* means "with oxygen."

* **anaerobic metabolism** the first stage of metabolism, which does not require oxygen, in which the breakdown of glucose (in a process called glycolysis) produces pyruvic acid and yields very little energy. *Anaerobic* means "without oxygen."

(A) Stage one: Anaerobic metabolism

Glucose

Small amount
of energy

Pyruvic
acid

Lactic acid

No oxygen

Anaerobic metabolism
(without oxygen)

(B) Stage two: Aerobic metabolism

Glucose

Energy

Aerobic metabolism
(with oxygen)

Oxygen

FIGURE 4-5 Glucose breakdown. (A) Stage one, glycolysis, is anaerobic (does not require oxygen). It yields pyruvic acid, with toxic by-products such as lactic acid, and very little energy. (B) Stage two is aerobic (requires oxygen). In a process called the Krebs or citric acid cycle, pyruvic acid is degraded into carbon dioxide and water, which produces a much higher yield of energy.

inside the cells, causing cellular edema. The cell membrane then ruptures, allowing lysosomal enzymes and other cellular contents to leak into the interstitial spaces. Cellular death soon follows.

Impaired Use of Glucose The same factors that reduce delivery of oxygen to the cells also reduce delivery of glucose to the cells. In addition, uptake of glucose by the cells may be disrupted by fever, cell damage, or the presence of bacteria, toxins, histamine, or other substances produced or activated by the body's immune and inflammatory responses to disease or injury. Compensatory mechanisms activated by shock may also be responsible for substances that inhibit glucose uptake, including catecholamines and the hormones cortisol and growth hormone.

Glucose that is prevented from entering the cells remains in the blood, resulting in a condition of high serum glucose, or hyperglycemia. Since glucose is the substance from which cells produce energy, the consequences of reduced glucose delivery and uptake are critical.

In the absence of an adequate supply of glucose, certain body cells can create fuel for energy production by converting other substances to glucose. One source is glycogen, the form of glucose that cells store and hold in reserve. Cells convert glycogen to glucose in a process called *glycogenolysis*. However, there is very little stored glycogen in cells other than the liver, kidneys, and muscles. When glycogen reserves are depleted, which typically occurs in four to eight hours, the cells will then derive energy from the breakdown of fats (*lipolysis*) and from the conversion of non-carbohydrate substrates, such as amino acids from proteins, to glucose (*gluconeogenesis*). The energy costs of glycogenolysis and lipolysis are high and contribute to the failure of cells. But the depletion of proteins in gluconeogenesis will ultimately cause organ failure.

In addition, the anaerobic breakdown of proteins produces ammonia, which is toxic to the cells, and urea, which leads to uric acid, which is also toxic to cells. Finally, when cellular metabolism is impaired, the waste products of metabolism build up in the cells, further impairing cell function and damaging cell membranes.

Impaired use of oxygen and glucose soon leads to cellular death. Cellular death will ultimately lead to tissue death; tissue death will lead to organ failure; and organ failure will lead to death of the individual.

Compensation and Decompensation

Usually, the body is able to compensate for any of the changes described above. However, when the various compensatory mechanisms fail, shock develops and may progress.

Compensation In shock, the fall in cardiac output, detected as a decrease in arterial blood pressure by the baroreceptors, activates several body systems that attempt to reestablish a normal blood pressure—a process known as *compensation*. The sympathetic nervous system stimulates the adrenal gland of the endocrine system to secrete the catecholamines epinephrine and norepinephrine. These chemicals profoundly affect the cardiovascular system, causing an increased heart rate, increased cardiac contractile strength, and arteriolar constriction—all of which serve to elevate the blood pressure.

Another compensatory mechanism, the *renin-angiotensin system,* aids the body in maintaining an adequate blood pressure. When the renin-angiotensin system is activated by a fall in blood pressure, the enzyme *renin* is released from the kidneys into the systemic circulation. Renin acts on a specialized plasma protein called *angiotensin* to produce a substance called *angiotensin I.* Angiotensin I is converted to *angiotensin II* by an enzyme found in the lungs called *angiotensin converting enzyme (ACE).* Angiotensin II is a potent vasoconstrictor. As angiotensin II causes the diameter of the vascular container to decrease, the blood pressure increases. Angiotensin II also stimulates the production of aldosterone, a hormone secreted by the adrenal cortex (outer layer of the adrenal gland) which, in turn, stimulates the kidneys to reabsorb sodium, and, subsequently, water (as noted earlier, "water follows sodium") into peritubular capillaries. The intravascular volume is maintained and elimination of water by the kidneys is reduced.

Another endocrine response by the pituitary gland results in the secretion of anti-diuretic hormone (ADH), which also causes the kidneys to reabsorb water, creating an additive effect to that of aldosterone.

The spleen, capable of storing over 300 ml of blood, can expel up to 200 ml of blood into the venous circulation, consequently increasing blood volume, preload, cardiac output, and blood pressure in response to a sudden drop in blood pressure.

Some passive compensatory responses also occur, with beneficial fluid shifts taking place as a result of simple diffusion. With volume loss, the hydrostatic pressure in capillary beds is reduced, and water from the interstitial spaces diffuses into the capillaries.

All of the forementioned mechanisms work to compensate for the shock state, and may be able to restore normal circulatory volume—if excessive bleeding is managed and the shock state has not progressed too far. In this case, the patient is said to be in **compensated shock.**

Once normal circulatory function and blood pressure are reestablished, the blood pressure will "feed back" on all of the compensatory mechanisms so that all systems can return to normal. In this way, negative feedback loops work to maintain stability by "signaling" the systems to cease the compensatory responses. In this way, stability and homeostasis are maintained.

Decompensation If the conditions causing shock are too serious, or progress too rapidly, compensatory mechanisms may not be able to restore normal function. In those cases, *decompensation* is said to occur, and the patient is in a state of **decompensated shock,** also called **progressive shock.** During decompensated or progressive shock, medical intervention may still be able to correct the condition.

Cellular death will ultimately lead to tissue death, tissue death to organ failure, and organ failure to death of the individual.

Content Review

THE STAGES OF SHOCK
Compensated
Decompensated (progressive)
Irreversible

✱ **compensated shock** early stage of shock during which the body's compensatory mechanisms are able to maintain normal perfusion.

✱ **decompensated shock** advanced stages of shock when the body's compensatory mechanisms are no longer able to maintain normal perfusion; also called **progressive shock.**

Since all of the "responding" systems have a point at which they can no longer sustain their action, i.e., a limited duration of action, the shock state may progress to a condition where correction, either by the body's own compensatory mechanisms or through medical intervention, is no longer possible. This condition is known as **irreversible shock.**

A critical factor in the downward spiral of decompensation is cardiac depression. The compensatory mechanisms that increase heart rate and contractile strength create a greatly increased demand for oxygen by the myocardium. When arterial blood pressure has fallen sufficiently, however, coronary blood flow is reduced below the level necessary to adequately perfuse the myocardium. The heart is weakened and cardiac output falls even further.

Depression of the vasomotor center of the brain is another consequence of reduced blood pressure. In early shock, as previously discussed, the sympathetic nervous system is stimulated to cause release of catecholamines that support the function of the circulatory system. But when blood pressure falls to a certain point, in the late stages of shock, reduced blood supply to the vasomotor center results in a slowing, then stoppage, of sympathetic activity.

Metabolic wastes, products of anaerobic metabolism, are released into the slower-flowing blood. The blood in the capillary beds becomes acidic, causing formation of minute blood clots ("sludged" blood), which further slows the flow of blood. And a more generalized, systemic acidosis develops, causing further deterioration of cells and tissues, including the capillary walls.

Capillary cells, like other cells, suffer from lack of oxygen and other nutrients, as well as from the ravages of acidosis. This begins to cause permeability of the capillaries and leakage of fluid into the interstitial spaces. This is another self-perpetuating process, as the decreased circulating volume and anaerobic metabolism cause further cell hypoxia and increased permeability.

Cellular deterioration progresses to tissue deterioration, which progresses to organ failure. (See Multiple Organ Dysfunction Syndrome, later in the chapter.) Medical intervention may save the patient if initiated early enough, but when enough damage has been done to cells, tissues, and organs, no known treatment can help the patient to recover. Medical therapies may support function for awhile, but death becomes inevitable.

> *The hallmark of decompensated shock is a fall in blood pressure.*
>

TYPES OF SHOCK

Shock is usually classified according to the cause. Some newer terminology classifies shock as *cardiogenic* (caused by impaired pumping power of the heart), *hypovolemic* (caused by decreased blood or water volume), *obstructive* (caused by an obstruction that interferes with return of blood to the heart, such as a pulmonary embolism, cardiac tamponade, or tension pneumothorax), and *distributive* (caused by abnormal distribution and return of blood resulting from vasodilation, vasopermeability, or both, as in neurogenic, anaphylactic, or septic shock).

Another, more familiar terminology classifies shock as *cardiogenic, hypovolemic, neurogenic, anaphylactic,* and *septic.* The following discussion of types of shock uses these classifications.

Although all types of shock ultimately have the same effects on the body's cells, tissues, and organs, it is important to try to identify the underlying cause, because correcting the cause is the most important element in reversing the condition and saving the patient's life. Many of the treatments that you, as a paramedic, will provide for the shock patient will be the same, no matter what the cause or type of shock is, but some differ in important ways. For example, providing IV fluid boluses, which may be appropriate to support circulating volume in the hypovolemic patient, would not be indicated for the patient in cardiogenic shock with pulmonary edema.

> *Try to identify the underlying cause of shock, because correcting the cause is the most important element in reversing the condition and saving the patient's life.*

Cardiogenic Shock

An inability of the heart to pump enough blood to supply all body parts is referred to as **cardiogenic shock.** Cardiogenic shock is usually the result of severe left ventricular failure secondary to acute myocardial infarction or congestive heart failure. The reduced blood pressure that accompanies this form of shock aggravates the situation by decreasing coronary artery perfusion. With decreased coronary perfusion, the heart muscle becomes even more damaged, thus establishing a vicious cycle that ultimately results in complete pump failure.

During cardiogenic shock, as noted earlier, the activation of compensatory mechanisms can actually worsen the situation. When the peripheral resistance increases in an attempt to maintain blood pressure, the myocardial workload increases. This, in turn, increases the myocardial oxygen demand, further aggravating myocardial ischemia and infarction. Cardiac output is further depressed and ejection fraction (the percentage of blood in the ventricle that is ejected with each beat) is decreased.

While the most common cause of cardiogenic shock is severe left ventricular failure, a number of other factors can have the same result. These include chronic progressive heart disease such as cardiomyopathy, rupture of the papillary heart muscles or interventricular septum, and end-stage valvular disease (mitral stenosis or aortic regurgitation).

Most patients who experience cardiogenic shock will have normal blood volume. However, some patients will be hypovolemic from an excessive use of prescribed diuretics or the severe diaphoresis that accompanies some acute cardiac events. Patients may also experience relative hypovolemia (neurogenic shock) from the vasodilatory (vessel dilation) effects of drugs such as nitroglycerin.

Evaluation and Treatment A major difference between cardiogenic and other types of shock is the presence of pulmonary edema (excess fluid in the lungs), which will probably result in a complaint of difficulty breathing. There may be diminished lung sounds as fluid enters the interstitial spaces of the lungs. As fluid levels rise, wheezes, crackles, or rales may be heard. A productive cough may develop, characterized by white- or pink-tinged foamy sputum. Cyanosis (a dusky blue-gray skin color) is typical, resulting from the decreased diffusion of oxygen across the alveolar/capillary interface, decreasing oxygen delivery to cells that are already hypoxic because of decreased blood pressure and perfusion. Other signs of shock include altered mentation (resulting from reduced perfusion of the brain) and oliguria (diminished urination resulting from compensatory mechanisms that stimulate reabsorption of water by the kidneys to enhance circulating volume).

Treatment of cardiogenic shock includes the supportive measures that should be provided for shock of any origin: Assure an open airway, administer oxygen and assist ventilations if necessary (to support oxygenation of myocardial and other body cells), and keep the patient warm (because impaired cellular metabolism is no longer producing enough energy to keep body temperature normal).

In cardiogenic shock, when pulmonary edema is present, elevate the patient's head and shoulders so that gravity can help isolate fluid and create a clear area where oxygen exchange from the alveoli can take place.

A peripheral intravenous line should be established with normal saline at a TKO rate to provide access for medications, but fluid administration should be kept to a minimum to avoid aggravating the edema. (Some patients with chronic heart failure may be on diuretics and suffering dehydration however, requiring some fluid support.) Since the heart rate may vary from bradycardic (abnormally slow) to tachycardic (abnormally fast), monitoring the heart rate is important. Atropine administration or application of an external pacer may be recommended to manage bradycardia, while extreme tachycardia may be treated by sedation and cardioversion (a type of electric shock) if the patient is awake.

* **cardiogenic shock** shock caused by insufficient cardiac output; the inability of the heart to pump enough blood to perfuse all parts of the body.

Most patients with cardiogenic shock have a normal or increased blood pressure.

Provide supportive measures for shock of any origin: Assure an open airway, administer oxygen, assist ventilations, and keep the patient warm.

Dopamine may be administered to elevate the blood pressure but it will also increase heart rate. Dobutamine may be administered to increase contractile force with little effect on the heart rate. Follow local protocols.

Hypovolemic Shock

Shock due to a loss of intravascular fluid volume is referred to as **hypovolemic shock**. Possible causes of hypovolemic shock include:

- Internal or external hemorrhage (This type of hypovolemic shock is also known as hemorrhagic shock.)
- Traumatic injury
- Long bone or open fractures
- Severe dehydration from vomiting or diarrhea
- Plasma loss from burns
- Excessive sweating
- Diabetic ketoacidosis with resultant **osmotic diuresis**

Hypovolemic shock can also be due to internal third-space loss. Such a condition can occur with bowel obstruction, peritonitis, pancreatitis, or liver failure resulting in ascites (accumulation of fluid within the abdominal cavity).

Evaluation and Treatment The signs of hypovolemic shock are considered the "classic" signs of shock. The mental status becomes altered, progressing from anxiety to lethargy or combativeness to unresponsiveness. The skin becomes pale, cool, and clammy (sweaty). The blood pressure may be normal during compensated shock, but then begins to fall. The pulse may be normal in the beginning, then become rapid, finally slowing and disappearing. As the kidneys continue to reabsorb water, urination decreases. Cardiac dysrhythmias may develop in late shock, deteriorating to asystole (absence of heartbeat).

Provide supportive treatment for hypovolemic shock: airway assurance, oxygen, assisted ventilations if necessary. Control any severe bleeding. Keep the patient warm. An IV bolus of crystalloid solution (such as normal saline or lactated Ringer's) should be started for fluid replacement. Application of the pneumatic anti-shock garment (PASG) may also be part of your local protocols.

Neurogenic Shock

Neurogenic shock results from injury to either the brain or the spinal cord, resulting in an interruption of nerve impulses to the arteries. The arteries lose tone and dilate, causing a relative hypovolemia. There has been no loss of fluid, but the container has been enlarged. With this inappropriate vasodilation, a disproportionate amount of blood collects in the capillary bed. This reduces venous return, cardiac output, and arterial blood pressure. Sympathetic nerve impulses to the adrenal glands are lost, which prevents the release of catecholamines and their compensatory effects. With injury high in the cervical spine, there may be interruption of impulses to the peripheral nervous system, causing paralysis and loss of sensation. The respiratory and cardiac centers of the brain may also be affected.

The usual cause of neurogenic shock is central nervous system injury. Neurogenic shock is most commonly due to an injury that has resulted in severe spinal cord injury or total transection of the cord (which may be called *spinal shock*) or injury or deprivation of oxygen or glucose to the medulla of the brain.

Evaluation and Treatment The vasodilation in neurogenic shock causes warm, red skin, and sweat gland malfunction causes dry skin—in contrast to the cool, pale, sweaty skin associated with hypovolemic shock. Because of the lack of compensatory stimulation from catecholamine release, the patient will have a low blood pressure and a slow pulse even in the early stages—again, in contrast to hypovolemic shock.

Treatment for neurogenic shock or spinal shock is similar to treatment for other types of shock and includes support of the airway, oxygenation, ventilation, maintenance of body temperature, and intravenous access. Spinal shock is characterized by hypotension, reflex bradycardia, and warm, dry skin. Because these symptoms signal a likelihood of spinal injury, cervical spine stabilization must be established on first patient contact, and the patient must be immobilized to a backboard as quickly as possible. A thorough search for other causes of shock (e.g., internal hemorrhage) must be made before concluding that a patient's hypotension is due to spinal shock alone. Treatment of spinal shock should include intravenous fluids (especially if there has been blood or fluid loss) and medications that increase the blood pressure by increasing peripheral vascular resistance. These include norepinephrine (Levophed) and dopamine (Intropin).

Anaphylactic Shock

When a foreign substance enters the body, the immune system responds to rid the body of the invader. (See the discussion of immunity later in this chapter.) This usually happens with no noticeable effects, and the person is not even aware that an immune response is taking place. Some foreign substances (antigens) provoke an exaggerated immune response (allergic response) that will cause noticeable symptoms such as a rash (as from contact with poison ivy) or swollen, irritated airway passages (as with hay fever). In rare cases, an allergic response is very severe and life threatening. This kind of severe allergic response is called **anaphylaxis,** or **anaphylactic shock.**

* **anaphylaxis** a life-threatening allergic reaction; also called **anaphylactic shock.**

An anaphylactic reaction usually occurs very rapidly. Signs and symptoms most often appear within a minute or less, but occasionally may appear an hour or more after exposure. Generally, the faster the reaction develops, the more severe it is likely to be. Death can occur before the patient can get to a hospital, so prompt intervention is critical. This is a situation when the paramedic at the scene can make the difference between life and death.

Anaphylactic reactions can be triggered by a variety of substances, including foods (especially nuts, eggs, shellfish), venoms, aspirin or non-steroidal anti-inflammatory drugs (NSAIDS), hormones (animal-derived insulin), preservatives, and others. The most rapid and severe reactions are usually caused by substances injected directly into the circulation, which is one reason that penicillin injections and hymenoptera stings (e.g., from bees, wasps, hornets) are the most common causes of fatal anaphylactic reactions.

Evaluation and Treatment Because the immune responses involved in anaphylaxis can affect different body systems, the signs and symptoms can vary widely. For example:

- Skin
  - Flushing
  - Itching
  - Hives
  - Swelling
  - Cyanosis
- Respiratory system
  - Breathing difficulty
  - Sneezing, coughing
  - Wheezing, stridor
  - Laryngeal edema
  - Laryngospasm

- Cardiovascular system
  - Vasodilation
  - Increased heart rate
  - Decreased blood pressure
- Gastrointestinal system
  - Nausea, vomiting
  - Abdominal cramping
  - Diarrhea
- Nervous system
  - Altered mental status
  - Dizziness
  - Headache
  - Seizures
  - Tearing

The patient may present with an altered mental status that can progress to unresponsiveness, so gather a brief history as soon as possible, including previous allergic reactions and any information about what the patient may have ingested or been exposed to that could have caused the present reaction. Be sure the patient is no longer in contact with the allergen; if a stinger is in the skin, scrape it away with a finger nail or scalpel blade.

Since laryngeal edema is often a problem, protecting the patient's airway will be your first concern. Administer oxygen by nonrebreather mask or, as necessary, by endotracheal intubation. The anaphylactic response causes depletion of circulatory volume by promoting capillary permeability and leaking of fluid into interstitial spaces, so establish an IV of crystalloid solution (normal saline or lactated Ringer's) for volume support.

The primary treatment for anaphylaxis is pharmacological. In addition to oxygen, epinephrine is usually administered (if the patient has a history of anaphylaxis, he may be carrying a prescribed spring-loaded epinephrine injector), as are antihistamines (diphenhydramine), corticosteroids (methylprednisolone, hydrocortisone, dexamethasone), and vasopressors (dopamine, norepinephrine, epineprine). Occasionally an inhaled beta agonist (albuterol) may be required. Follow local protocols.

Septic Shock

* **septic shock** shock that develops as the result of infection carried by the bloodstream, eventually causing dysfunction of multiple organ systems.

Septic shock begins with *septicemia* (also called *sepsis*), an infection that enters the bloodstream and is carried throughout the body. The person may have septicemia for some time before septic shock develops, but eventually toxins released by the invading organism overcome the compensatory mechanisms. Unless it is corrected, septic shock will cause the dysfunction of more than one organ system, resulting in multiple organ dysfunction syndrome (discussed in the next section).

Evaluation and Treatment The signs and symptoms of septic shock are progressive. In the beginning, cardiac output is increased, but toxins causing vasodilation may prevent an increase in blood pressure. The person may seem to be sick, but not alarmingly so. By the last stages, toxins have increased permeability of the blood vessels to the point where great amounts of fluid are lost from the vasculature and blood pressure falls drastically.

Signs and symptoms can vary widely as the patient progresses from early to late stages of septic shock. Some patients may have a high fever, but others, especially the elderly or the very young may have no fever or may even be hypothermic. The skin can be flushed, if fever is present, or very pale and cyanotic in the late stages.

The most susceptible organ system is the lungs and respiratory system, so the patient may present with breathing difficulty and altered lung sounds. The brain may be infected, resulting in altered mental status. Suspicion of septic shock is usually based on a history of recent infection or illness.

Treatment includes administration of high-flow oxygen by nonrebreather mask or endotracheal intubation, as necessary. An IV of crystalloid solution (normal saline or lactated Ringer's) should be established, and dopamine may be administered to support the blood pressure. The heart rhythm must be monitored and medications administered to correct any dysrhythmias. Follow local protocols. In the hospital, antibiotic therapy will be initiated.

MULTIPLE ORGAN DYSFUNCTION SYNDROME

In the 1970s, a syndrome of multiple organ failure began to be noticed in hospital intensive care units. Medical advances were allowing patients to survive serious illness and trauma—only to die later of complications of the original disease or injury. The syndrome was described in 1975 as *multi-system organ failure*. In 1991, the American College of Chest Physicians and the Society of Critical Care Medicine named it **multiple organ dysfunction syndrome (MODS)**.

MODS is the progressive impairment of two or more organ systems resulting from an uncontrolled inflammatory response to a severe illness or injury. Sepsis and septic shock are the most common causes of MODS, with MODS being the end stage. (The progression from infection to sepsis to septic shock to MODS is known as systemic inflammatory response syndrome, or SIRS).

Actually, MODS can result from any severe disease or injury that triggers a massive systemic inflammatory response—including trauma, burns, surgery, circulatory shock, acute pancreatitis, acute renal failure, and others. Risk factors include age (>65), malnutrition, and preexisting chronic disease such as cancer or diabetes. With a mortality rate of 60–90 percent, MODS is the major cause of death following sepsis, trauma, and burn injuries.

Pathophysiology of MODS

MODS occurs in two stages. In primary MODS, organ damage results directly from a specific cause such as ischemia or inadequate perfusion resulting from an episode of shock, trauma, or major surgery. There are stress and inflammatory responses (discussed in detail later in this chapter) to this initial injury, but they may be mild and not readily detectable. However, during this response, neutrophils and macrophages (cells that attack and destroy bacteria, protozoa, foreign cells, and cell debris) as well as mast cells (cells that produce histamine and other components of allergic response) are thought to be "primed" by cytokines (proteins released during an inflammatory or immune response).

The next time there is an insult, such as an additional injury or ischemia or infection—even though the insult may be mild—the primed cells are activated, producing an exaggerated inflammatory response, known as secondary MODS.

Now the inflammatory response enters a self-perpetuating cycle. As inflammatory mediators are released by the injured organ, they enter the circulation, activating inflammatory responses in organ systems throughout the body. These mediators, especially cytokines such as tumor necrosis factor (TNF) and interleukin 1 (IL-1), damage the endothelium (cells that line the blood vessels, the heart, and various body cavities). Gram-negative bacteria, if present, release endotoxins that also damage endothelial cells. The injured endothelial cells release factors that aggravate the inflammation and cause vasodilation. The injured epithelium becomes permeable, allowing leakage of fluid into interstitial spaces,

* **multiple organ dysfunction syndrome (MODS)** progressive impairment of two or more organ systems resulting from an uncontrolled inflammatory response to a severe illness or injury.

Content Review

PROGRESSION TO MODS

Infection
↓
Sepsis
↓
Septic shock
↓
MODS
↓
Death (if not corrected early)

and loses much of its anticoagulation function, which allows formation of tiny blood clots (thrombi) in the microvasculature.

The secondary insult also triggers an exaggerated neuroendocrine response. Catecholamine release causes many of the manifestations of MODS, including tachycardia, increased metabolic rates, and increased oxygen consumption. Release of a variety of hormones contributes to the hypermetabolism and release of endorphins contributes to vasodilation. Additionally, plasma protein systems are activated: specifically, the complement system, the coagulation system, and the kallikrein-kinin system. Plasma proteins are key mediators of the inflammatory response. When activated, each of these systems triggers a cascade of responses with the overall result of increased vasodilation, vasopermeability, cardiovascular instability, endothelial damage, and clotting abnormalities.

As a result of the release of the inflammatory mediators and toxins and the plasma protein cascades, a massive immune/inflammatory and coagulation response develops. Vascular changes (vasodilation, increased capillary permeability, selective vasoconstriction, and microvascular thrombi) continue and worsen. Two metabolites that are released have opposing vascular effects: Prostacyclin, also called prostaglandin I_2 (PGI_2) is a vasodilator, while thromboxane A_2 (TXA_2) is a vasoconstrictor. They are released in differing amounts within different organ tissues, contributing to a maldistribution of blood flow to organs and organ systems.

As noted earlier, the release of catecholamines stimulates hypermetabolism within the body cells, which in turn creates a greatly increased oxygen demand. Because of lung damage, hypoxemia, and hypoperfusion, a severe oxygen supply/demand imbalance develops. As the cells switch from aerobic to anaerobic metabolism, fuel supplies within the cells (ATP and glucose) are used up faster than they can be replenished. Without adequate ATP, the cells lose their ability to operate the sodium-potassium pump, which is essential to cardiac function. The myocardium is profoundly weakened. Cellular lysosomes begin to break down, releasing lysosomal enzymes which damage the cell membrane and the surrounding cells. Large amounts of lactic acid are released, contributing to acidosis, which further damages the cells. The overall response is similar to that seen in septic and anaphylactic shock, except on a larger scale.

Clinical Presentation of MODS

The cumulative effects of MODS at the cellular and tissue levels begin to cause the breakdown of organ systems: The organs that fail first are not necessarily the organs where the initial insult occurred, and there is a lag time between the initial insult and the onset of organ failure. Dysfunction may develop in the pulmonary, gastrointestinal, hepatic, renal, cardiovascular, hematologic, and immune systems. There is decreased cardiac function and myocardial depression, caused by the factors discussed earlier, possibly abetted by release of myocardial depressant factor (MDF) and a decrease in beta-adrenergic receptors in the heart. The smooth muscle of the vascular system fails with consequent release of capillary sphincters and increased vasodilation.

MODS will usually develop over a period of two, three, or more weeks.

MODS does not occur in one intense crisis. It will usually develop over a period of two, three, or more weeks. There is no specific therapy for MODS, and the only chance of rescuing the patient from its self-perpetuating spiral toward death is early recognition and initiation of supportive measures. For this reason, it is important to understand how MODS usually presents in the first 24 hours after initial resuscitation.

Survival from MODS is dependent on early recognition and supportive care.

Although MODS will usually be detected in the hospital rather than the out-of-hospital setting, there may be occasions when a patient who has not been hospitalized or has returned home from the hospital is the subject of a call to EMS, or when a patient being transported by EMS from one facility to another is suffering from MODS.

The most common presentation of MODS over time is as follows:

24 Hours after Resuscitation

- Low-grade fever
- Tachycardia (rapid heart rate)
- Dyspnea (breathing difficulty)
- Altered mental status
- General hypermetabolic, hyperdynamic state

Within 24 to 72 Hours

- Pulmonary (lung) failure begins

Within 7 to 10 Days

- Hepatic (liver) failure begins
- Intestinal failure begins
- Renal (kidney) failure begins

Within 14 to 21 days

- Renal and hepatic failure intensify
- Gastrointestinal collapse
- Immune system collapse

After 21 Days

- Hematologic (blood system) failure begins
- Myocardial (heart muscle) failure begins
- Altered mental status resulting from encephalopathy (brain infection)
- Death

Part 2: The Body's Defenses Against Disease and Injury

As discussed so far in this chapter, the human body is vulnerable to attack by a variety of diseases and foreign invaders as well as to injury. The major focus of Part 2 will be the body's chief defenses against disease, invaders, and injury—the immune response and the inflammatory response—and the interactions between the immune and inflammatory responses.

In Part 2, we will also examine hypersensitivity, or allergic and anaphylactic responses; that is, what happens when the immune system over-responds to invasive agents to the extent that the body is actually harming itself. Immune deficiencies will also be discussed, including acquired immunodeficiency syndrome, or AIDS.

Finally, we will discuss the interrelationships between stress and disease, including the body's use of the neuroendocrine and immune systems to regulate the stress response. Psychological responses to stress, including various coping mechanisms, are also described.

SELF-DEFENSE MECHANISMS

In Chapter 3, normal body anatomy and physiology were discussed (the normal cell and its environment: fluids and electrolytes, the acid-base balance). In Part 1 of this chapter we discussed how the body may be attacked or injured (cellular injury, infection, genetic and other causes of disease, hypoperfusion, and multiple organ dysfunction syndrome). In the next sections, we will discuss how the body defends itself from infection and injury.

It is important to keep in mind that the body has powerful ways of defending and healing itself (restoring homeostasis) and that medical intervention is needed only when, on occasion, these natural defense mechanisms are unequal to the task and become overwhelmed.

INFECTIOUS AGENTS

Bacteria

Bacteria are single-cell organisms that consist of internal cytoplasm surrounded by a rigid cell wall. Bacteria are prokaryotic cells which, unlike the eukaryotic cells of the human body, lack an organized nucleus and other intracellular organelles. Bacteria can reproduce independently, but they need a host to supply food and other support. Inside the body, they achieve this by binding to host cells.

Bacteria can be cultured and identified readily in most hospital laboratories. Many bacteria are categorized according to their appearance under the microscope after staining with several dyes referred to as *Gram stains*. Some bacteria stain blue, while others stain red. Bacteria that stain blue are referred to as *Gram-positive* bacteria. They are somewhat similar to each other in their structure. Bacteria that stain red are referred to as *Gram-negative* bacteria. They are also somewhat similar to each other in their structure.

Bacteria can cause many of the common infections in medicine, including middle ear infections in children, many cases of tonsillitis, and meningitis. (These kinds of infections can also be caused by viruses, which are discussed in the next section.) Most bacterial infections respond to treatment with drugs called **antibiotics.** Once administered, antibiotics kill or inhibit the growth of invading bacteria. As mentioned earlier, the bacterial cell membrane is the site of action for many antibiotics. Once the cell membrane is broken down, phagocytes (cells that ingest and destroy pathogens and other foreign and abnormal substances) can begin to destroy the bacterium. A variety of antibiotic drugs have been developed with mechanisms of action tailored to different types of bacteria. However, the broad variety of infectious bacteria, and their ability to develop resistance to drugs, makes developing antibiotics to battle them a difficult job.

Some bacteria protect themselves by forming a capsule outside the cell wall that protects the organism from digestion by phagocytes. Some bacteria, such as *Mycoplasmic* bacteria, have no protective capsule but rely on other mechanisms to survive and attack the body. *Mycobacterium tuberculosis,* which has no protective capsule, can actually survive and be transported by phagocytes. Other bacteria simply multiply faster than the body's defense systems can respond. Still others overpower the body's defenses by producing enzymes and toxins that attack and injure cells and produce hypersensitivity reactions.

Simple infection is not the only consequence of a bacterial invasion. Many bacteria release poisonous chemicals, or *toxins*. There are two types of toxins produced by bacteria: exotoxins and endotoxins. **Exotoxins** are proteins secreted and released by the bacterial cell during its growth. They travel throughout the body via the blood or lymph, ultimately causing problems. For example, botulism toxin, released by the bacterium *Clostridium botulinum,* blocks the release

Content Review

INFECTIOUS AGENTS

Bacteria
Viruses
Fungi
Parasites
Prions

* **bacteria** (singular *bacterium*) single-cell organisms with a cell membrane and cytoplasm but no organized nucleus. They bind to the cells of a host organism to obtain food and support.

* **antibiotics** substances that destroy or inhibit microorganisms, tiny living bodies invisible to the naked eye. (*Antibiotic* means "destructive to life.")

* **exotoxins** toxic (poisonous) substances secreted by bacterial cells during their growth.

of cholingeric neurotransmitters at neuromuscular junctions and elsewhere in the autonomic nervous system, causing systemic paralysis. Another example is tetanus, which is caused by the bacterium *Clostridium tetani*. The actual infection by the bacteria themselves is mild and may be limited, for example, to the site of a puncture wound in the foot. Yet, on entering the body, the bacteria release their toxin, *tetanospasmin*. This toxin then travels through the blood to the skeletal muscles, causing the spastic rigidity classically seen in tetanus.

Endotoxins are complex molecules that are contained in the cell walls of certain gram-negative bacteria. Endotoxins can be released during the destruction of the bacterial cell by phagocytes or even when the bacterial cell is attacked by an antibiotic, so that antibiotics cannot control the endotoxic effects of bacteria. When released, endotoxins trigger the inflammatory process and produce fever. In the bloodstream, they can cause widespread clotting within the blood vessels, capillary damage, and hypotension, as well as respiratory distress and fever—a condition known as endotoxin shock. Endotoxins can survive even when the cell that produced them is dead.

Depending on their amount and site of release, the effects of toxins can be local or systemic. When a bacterial organism enters the circulatory system, its released toxins can spread throughout the body. The systemic spread of toxins through the bloodstream is known as **septicemia**, or *sepsis*, and is a grave medical illness.

The body encounters the bacterial invasion and release of enzymes and toxins through activation of the immune system. The immune system will mobilize foreign-cell-destroying macrophages (a type of white blood cell) to the site of infection in an attempt to rid the body of the foreign pathogen. As the macrophages attempt to destroy the bacteria, they release substances known as pyrogens. Pyrogens are responsible for causing the increase in temperature known as fever. Pyrogens act on the thermoregulation center in the hypothalamus to cause the increased body temperature, which is thought to aid in the destruction of pathogens.

Viruses

Most infections are caused by **viruses**. Viruses are much smaller than bacteria and can only be seen with an electron microscope. In addition, they cannot grow without the assistance of another organism. In fact, viruses are referred to as *intracellular parasites*, since they must invade the cells of the organism they infect.

A virus has no organized cellular structure except a protein coat (capsid) surrounding the internal genetic material, deoxyribonucleic acid (DNA) or ribonucleic acid (RNA). With no organized cellular structure or cellular organelles, viruses are incapable of metabolism. Once inside a cell, they take over, using the various cellular enzymes to replicate and produce more viruses, which decreases synthesis of macromolecules vital to the host cell.

Some viruses develop a coating in addition to the capsid, called an envelope. The envelope and the protein capsid allow the virus to resist destruction by the phagocytes of the immune system. However, since viruses cannot reproduce outside a host cell, if the virus does not find a host cell, it will die.

The symptoms of a virus may not be readily apparent because it is hidden within the host cell. After replication is complete, the virus will sometimes destroy the host cell. In other cases, a virus will remain dormant within a cell for months or years. An example is the *varicella zoster virus*, which causes childhood chickenpox and may then remain dormant, only to cause shingles in the adult decades later. Some viruses form a long-term symbiotic relationship with the host cell, resulting in a persistent but unapparent infection.

Viruses do not produce toxins, but they can still cause very serious illnesses. Some viruses are capable of altering the host cell to induce a malignancy (cancer). Others, such as the *human immunodeficiency virus (HIV)*, which causes

* **endotoxins** molecules in the walls of certain gram-negative bacteria that are released when the bacterium dies or is destroyed, causing toxic (poisonous) effects on the host body.

* **septicemia** the systemic spread of toxins through the bloodstream. Also called *sepsis*.

* **virus** an organism much smaller than a bacterium, visible only under an electron microscope. Viruses invade and live inside the cells of the organisms they infect.

AIDS, can proliferate, attacking cells of the immune system and destroying its ability to ward off infections of all types.

Unlike bacteria, viruses are very difficult to treat. Once a virus infects a cell, it can only be killed by destroying the infected cell. Drugs have not yet been developed that can selectively destroy cells infected by viruses while leaving uninfected cells unharmed. This partially explains the dilemma facing researchers trying to find a cure for AIDS. An additional problem is that some viruses mutate (change) frequently, which is why a new flu vaccine must be developed for every flu season. Fortunately, most viral illnesses are mild and fairly self-limiting. (Because viral agents must spread from cell to cell, the immune system is eventually able to "catch" them outside a host cell and destroy them.) Even so, at present, viruses usually cannot be treated with more than symptomatic care.

Other Agents of Infection

Other biological agents that cause human infection include *fungi* (the plural of *fungus*) and parasites.

Fungi, which includes yeasts and molds, are more like plants than animals. Fungi rarely cause human disease other than minor skin infections such as athlete's foot and some common vaginal infections. Fungus infections are called *mycoses*. Patients with an impaired immune system, such as HIV patients or patients with organ transplants, suffer fungal infection more commonly than healthy people. In such patients, the fungi can invade the lungs, blood, and several organs. Treatment of complicated, deep fungal infections has proven difficult, even in the hospital setting.

Parasites range in size from protozoa (single-cell animals not much larger than bacteria) to large intestinal worms. Parasites tend to be more common in developing nations than in the United States. Treatment depends upon the organism and the location.

Prions are the most recently recognized classification of infectious agents. Initially thought to be slow acting viruses, prions differ from viruses in that they are smaller, are made entirely of proteins, and do not have protective capsids.

For more about infectious diseases, see Chapter 37.

THREE LINES OF DEFENSE

There are three chief lines of self-defense against infection and injury. One involves anatomical barriers. The other two—the inflammatory response and the immune response—rely on actions of the leukocytes (white blood cells). Each line of defense can be characterized as external or internal, nonspecific or specific (Table 4-2)—characterizations you may want to keep in mind as you read the following sections and compare the ways these defenses protect the body.

Before an infectious agent can attack the body, it has to get past the body's natural anatomical barrier, the epithelium (the skin and the mucous membranes that line the respiratory, gastrointestinal, and genitourinary tracts). The epithelium is more than just a physical barrier; it also provides a chemical defense against infection. The sebaceous glands of the skin secrete fatty and lactic acids, which attack bacteria and fungi. Sweat, tears, and saliva secreted by other glands contain bacteria-attacking enzymes. Various mechanical responses also work to

Content Review

THREE LINES OF DEFENSE
Anatomic barriers
Inflammatory response
Immune response

Table 4-2	THREE LINES OF DEFENSE AGAINST INFECTION AND INJURY			
	External	**Internal**	**Nonspecific**	**Specific**
Anatomical Barriers	External		Nonspecific	
Inflammatory Response		Internal	Nonspecific	
Immune Response		Internal		Specific

Table 4-3	**CHARACTERISTICS OF THE INFLAMMATORY AND IMMUNE RESPONSES**	
	Inflammatory Response	**Immune Response**
Speed	Fast	Slow
Specificity	Nonspecific	Specific
Duration (Memory)	Transient (no memory)	Long-term (memory)
Involving Which Plasma Systems	Multiple plasma protein systems (complement, coagulation, kinin systems)	One plasma protein system (immunoglobulin)
Involving Which Cell Type	Multiple cell types (granulocytes, monocytes, macrophages)	One blood cell type (lymphocytes)

get rid of invading substances. For example, the invader may be coughed or sneezed out of the respiratory tract, flushed out of the urinary tract, or eliminated from the gastrointestinal tract by vomiting or diarrhea.

The anatomical defenses are *external* and *nonspecific*. They are considered external because they prevent substances from penetrating the skin or the coverings of internal passageways. They are nonspecific because they defend against all invaders, such as foreign bodies, chemicals, or microorganisms, without targeting any specific type of invader.

If an invading foreign body, chemical, or microorganism penetrates the anatomical barriers and begins to attack internal cells and tissues, two other lines of defense are triggered: the inflammatory response and the immune response. These twin responses of the immune system have contrasting characteristics of speed, specificity, duration (memory), and of the plasma systems and cell types that are involved in the response (Table 4-3).

The *inflammatory response,* or *inflammation,* begins within seconds of injury or invasion by a pathogen. As noted earlier, it is nonspecific, attacking any invader by surrounding it with cells and fluids to isolate, destroy, and eliminate it. Inflammation is mediated by multiple plasma protein systems, especially the complement system, the coagulation system, and the kinin system (which will be explained later) and involves a variety of cell types as it attacks the invader.

The *immune response* develops more slowly (one type of response requires a second exposure after priming by the first exposure to the invader). The immune response is specific, in that it will develop a specialized response for each different invader. It is mediated by just one plasma protein system (immunoglobulin) and attacks the invader mainly with a single cell type (lymphocytes, which are one type of leukocyte, or white blood cell).

Inflammation and the immune response interact in many ways. We will discuss the immune response first, because understanding the immune response is necessary for understanding some parts of the inflammatory response.

THE IMMUNE RESPONSE

HOW THE IMMUNE RESPONSE WORKS: AN OVERVIEW

Most viruses, bacteria, fungi, and parasites—as well as noninfectious substances such as pollens, foods, venoms, drugs, and others that may enter the body—have proteins on their surface called **antigens**. The immune system detects these antigens as being foreign, or "non-self" and responds to produce substances called **antibodies** that combine with antigens to control or destroy them. This is known

✱ **antigen** a marker on the surface of a cell that identifies it as "self" or "non-self."

✱ **antibody** a substance produced by B lymphocytes in response to the presence of a foreign antigen that will combine with and control or destroy the antigen, thus preventing infection.

* **immune response** the body's reactions that inactivate or eliminate foreign antigens.

* **immunity** a long-term condition of protection from infection or disease.

* **natural immunity** inborn protection against infection or disease.

* **acquired immunity** protection from infection or disease that is (a) developed by the body after exposure to an antigen or (b) transferred to the person from an outside source.

* **lymphocyte** a type of leukocyte, or white blood cell, that attacks foreign substances as part of the body's immune response.

* **B lymphocytes** white blood cells that, in response to the presence of an antigen, produce antibodies that attack the antigen, develop a memory for the antigen, and confer long-term immunity to the antigen.

* **humoral immunity** the long-term immunity to an antigen provided by antibodies produced by B lymphocytes.

* **T lymphocytes** white blood cells that do not produce antibodies but, instead, attack antigens directly.

* **cell-mediated immunity** the short-term immunity to an antigen provided by T lymphocytes, which directly attack the antigen but do not produce antibodies or memory for the antigen.

* **immunogens** antigens that are able to trigger an immune response.

as the **immune response.** As part of this process, *memory cells* "remember" the antigen and will trigger an even faster and more effective response to destroy the same antigen if it enters the body again. Such long-term protection against specific foreign substances is known as **immunity.**

CHARACTERISTICS OF THE IMMUNE RESPONSE AND IMMUNITY

The immune response and immunity can be classified as natural versus acquired immunity or humoral versus cell-mediated immunity.

Natural versus Acquired Immunity

Natural immunity is not generated by the immune response. It is inborn, part of the genetic makeup of the individual or the species. For example, dogs are naturally immune to measles and humans are naturally immune to canine distemper. (Some diseases such as leukemia, however, can affect more than one species.)

Acquired immunity develops as an outcome of the immune response. Acquired immunity can be either active or passive. *Active acquired immunity* is generated by the immune system after exposure to an antigen. *Passive acquired immunity* is transferred to a person from an outside source. For example, a mother may transfer antibodies to the fetus. Or antibodies may be administered as an immune serum against an invader such as rabies, tetanus, or snake venom. Active acquired immunity is long-lasting. Passive acquired immunity is temporary.

Humoral versus Cell-Mediated Immunity

A special type of leukocyte (white blood cell) is the **lymphocyte.** Lymphocytes (20 to 35 percent of all leukocytes) are responsible for several critical immune functions, including recognizing foreign antigens, producing antibodies, and developing memory.

As lymphocytes mature, they become one of several types, including B lymphocytes and T lymphocytes. **B lymphocytes** do not attack antigens directly. Instead, they produce the antibodies (immunoglobulins) that attack antigens. B lymphocytes also develop memory, and confer long-term immunity to specific antigens. This type of immunity is called **humoral immunity.** (*Humor* refers to the blood and other fluids of the body; *humoral immunity* refers to the long-lasting antibodies and memory cells present in the blood and lymph.)

T lymphocytes do not produce antibodies. Instead, they recognize the presence of a foreign antigen and attack it directly. This type of immunity is called **cell-mediated immunity.**

INDUCTION OF THE IMMUNE RESPONSE

The immune response must be triggered, or induced. The following sections discuss the role of antigens, immunogens, and blood groups.

Antigens and Immunogens

Antigens that can trigger the immune response are called **immunogens.** Not every antigen is an immunogen. That is, not every antigen is capable of triggering the immune response. For example, the immune response is not triggered by antigens present on various helpful bacteria in our bodies.

What makes a molecule an antigen is a chemical structure that is capable of reacting with immune system components, such as antibodies and T lymphocytes. However, having this chemical structure, the ability to *react* once the immune system has been triggered, is not enough to *trigger* the immune system in the first place. In order to be immunogenic—able to trigger an immune response—an antigen must have additional characteristics.

Characteristics of Antigenic Immunogenicity

- Sufficient foreignness
- Sufficient size
- Sufficient complexity
- Presence in sufficient amounts

Normally, the immune system is not triggered by self antigens. In fact, the immune system does not just "tolerate" self antigens, it actively protects them through suppression of the immune system.

Blood Group Antigens

HLA antigens do not exist on the surface of erythrocytes (red blood cells), but other antigens, known as the blood group antigens, do. There are more than 80 of these red cell antigens that have been grouped into a number of different blood group systems. The two groups that trigger the strongest immune response are the Rh system and the ABO system.

The Rh System The **Rh blood group** is named for the rhesus monkey in which it was first identified. One of several antigens in this group is known as Rh antigen D, or the **Rh factor.** Rh factor is present in about 85 percent of North Americans (Rh positive), but absent in about 15 percent (Rh negative).

Incompatibility between Rh positive and Rh negative blood can cause harmful immune responses. For example, if a patient with Rh negative blood receives a transplant of Rh positive blood, a primary immune response is triggered. A second transfusion of Rh positive blood may cause a severe transfusion reaction.

Hemolytic disease of the newborn may result from Rh incompatibility between mother and fetus. Problems will usually not occur in a first pregnancy where the mother is Rh negative and the fetus is Rh positive, because few fetal erythrocytes cross the placental barrier to the mother. However, a significant number of fetal erythrocytes do enter the mother's bloodstream at birth when the placenta separates from the uterus. These may (depending on several factors) activate a primary immune response and development of Rh antibodies. If the fetus in her next pregnancy is also Rh positive, the mother's Rh antibodies can cross the placenta and destroy the red blood cells of the fetus. This is actually a rare occurrence. Rh incompatibility occurs in only about ten percent of pregnancies. Since not all such incompatibilities produce Rh antibodies in the mother, only about five percent of women ever have babies with hemolytic disease, even after numerous pregnancies.

The ABO System The **ABO blood group** consists of only two antigens, named A and B. Persons with blood type A carry only A antigens on their red blood cells. Those with blood type B carry only B antigens. Those with blood type AB carry both, and those with blood type O carry neither.

An immune response will be activated in a person with type A blood who receives a transfusion of type B blood, which is recognized as non-self. The same will happen when a person with type B blood receives type A blood. People with type O blood are known as *universal donors,* because type O blood has no antigens that will trigger an immune response in any other group. Those with type AB blood are known as *universal recipients,* because they

All immunogens are antigens, but not all antigens are immunogens. In other words, only some antigens are capable of triggering an immune response.

✱ **Rh blood group** a group of antigens discovered on the red blood cells of rhesus monkeys that is also present to some extent in humans.

✱ **Rh factor** an antigen in the Rh blood group that is also known as antigen D. About 85% of North Americans have the Rh factor (are Rh positive) while about 15% do not have the Rh factor (are Rh negative). Rh positive and Rh negative blood are incompatible; that is, a person who is Rh negative can experience a severe immune response if Rh positive blood is introduced, as through a transfusion or during childbirth.

✱ **ABO blood group** two antigens known as A and B. A person may have either (type A or type B), both (type AB), or neither (type O). An immune response will be activated whenever a person receives blood containing A or B antigen if this antigen is not already present in his own blood.

have both types of antigens and will not produce antibodies in response to any other blood groups.

Mother-fetus ABO incompatibility is more common than Rh incompatibility, occurring in about 20 to 25 percent of pregnancies, but only 10 percent of ABO incompatibilities will result in hemolytic disease of the infant.

INFLAMMATION

INFLAMMATION CONTRASTED TO THE IMMUNE RESPONSE

Inflammation, also called the *inflammatory response,* is the body's response to cellular injury. It differs from the immune response in many ways. (Review Tables 4-2 and 4-3.) As you read the following sections, keep in mind that:

* The immune response develops *slowly;* inflammation develops *swiftly.*
* The immune response is *specific* (targets specific antigens); inflammation is *nonspecific* (it attacks all unwanted substances in the same way). In fact, inflammation is sometimes called "the nonspecific immune response."
* The immune response is *long-lasting* (memory cells will remember an antigen and trigger a swift response on reexposure, even years later); inflammation is *temporary,* lasting only until the immediate threat is conquered—usually only a few days to two weeks.
* The immune response involves *one type of white blood cell* (lymphocytes); inflammation involves *platelets and many types of white cells* (the granulatory cells called neutrophils, basophils, and eosinophils; the monocytes that mature into macrophages).
* The immune response involves *one type of plasma protein* (immunoglobulins, also called antibodies); inflammation involves *several plasma protein systems* (complement, coagulation, and kinin).

However, the immune response and inflammation are interdependent. For example, macrophages that are developed during the inflammatory response must ingest antigens before helper T cells can recognize them and trigger the immune response. Conversely, IgE antibody produced by B cells during an immune response can stimulate mast cells to activate inflammation.

Although inflammation differs from the immune response in many ways, inflammation and the immune response are both considered to be part of the body's immune system.

HOW INFLAMMATION WORKS: AN OVERVIEW

Inflammation is somewhat easier to understand than the immune response, because we have all observed it. The immune response is often hidden; your body's immune system may be knocking out an infectious antigen without your ever being aware of it. However, if you cut your finger, you will probably be acutely aware of the inflammatory process. You will actually see the redness and swelling and feel the pain. You may observe the formation of pus. As days go by, you will see the progress of wound healing and, perhaps, scar formation.

This is not to say that inflammation is simple; in its way, it is as complex as the immune response. There are several phases to inflammation. After each phase, healing may take place, and that will be the end of it. If healing doesn't take place, inflammation moves into its next phase. However, healing is the goal of all the phases.

* **inflammation** the body's response to cellular injury; also called the *inflammatory response.* In contrast to the immune response, inflammation develops swiftly, is nonspecific (attacks all unwanted substances in the same way) and is temporary, leading to healing.

Phases of Inflammation

Phase 1: Acute inflammation → healing
(If healing doesn't take place, moves to phase 2)

Phase 2: Chronic inflammation → healing
(If healing doesn't take place, moves to phase 3)

Phase 3: Granuloma formation

Phase 4: Healing

During each phase, the components of inflammation work together to perform four functions.

The Four Functions of Inflammation (During all Phases)

- Destroy and remove unwanted substances
- Wall off the infected and inflamed area
- Stimulate the immune response
- Promote healing

ACUTE INFLAMMATORY RESPONSE

Acute inflammation is triggered by any injury, whether lethal or nonlethal, to the body's cells. As discussed earlier in this chapter, cell injury can result from causes such as hypoxia, chemicals, infectious agents (bacteria, viruses, fungi, parasites), trauma, heat extremes, radiation, nutritional imbalances, genetic factors, and even the injurious effects of the immune and inflammatory responses themselves. When cells are injured, the acute inflammatory response begins within seconds. (Figure 4-6).

> **Content Review**
>
> **FOUR FUNCTIONS OF INFLAMMATION**
> Destroy and remove unwanted substances
> Wall off the infected and inflamed area
> Stimulate the immune response
> Promote healing

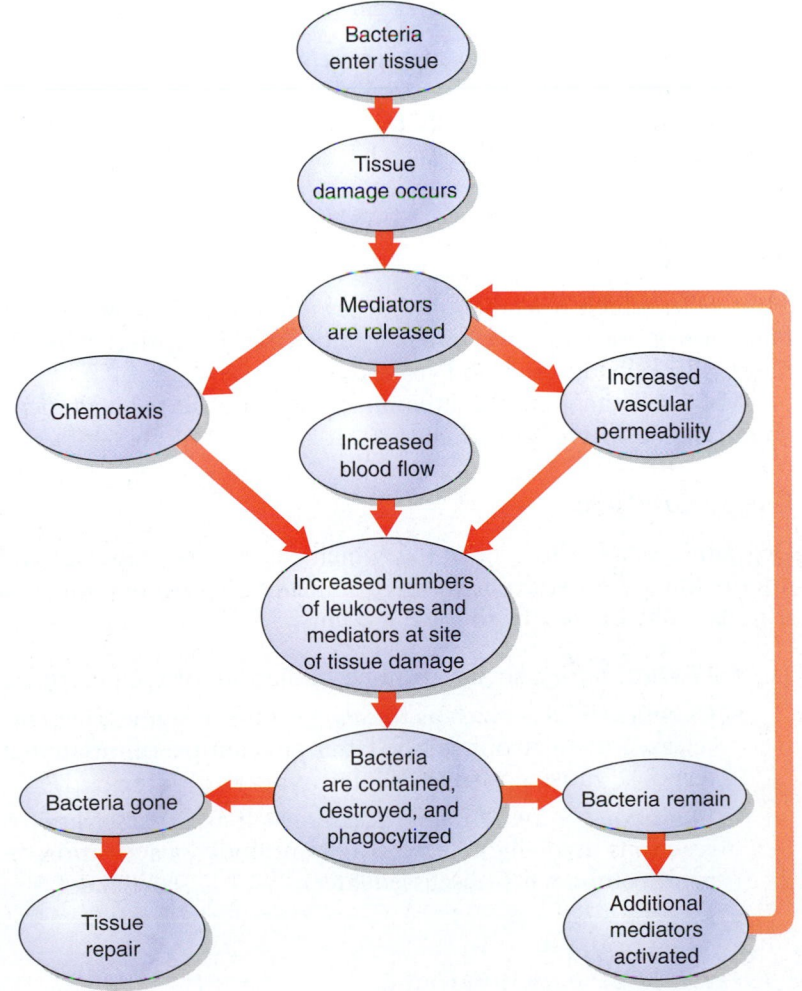

FIGURE 4-6 The inflammatory response.

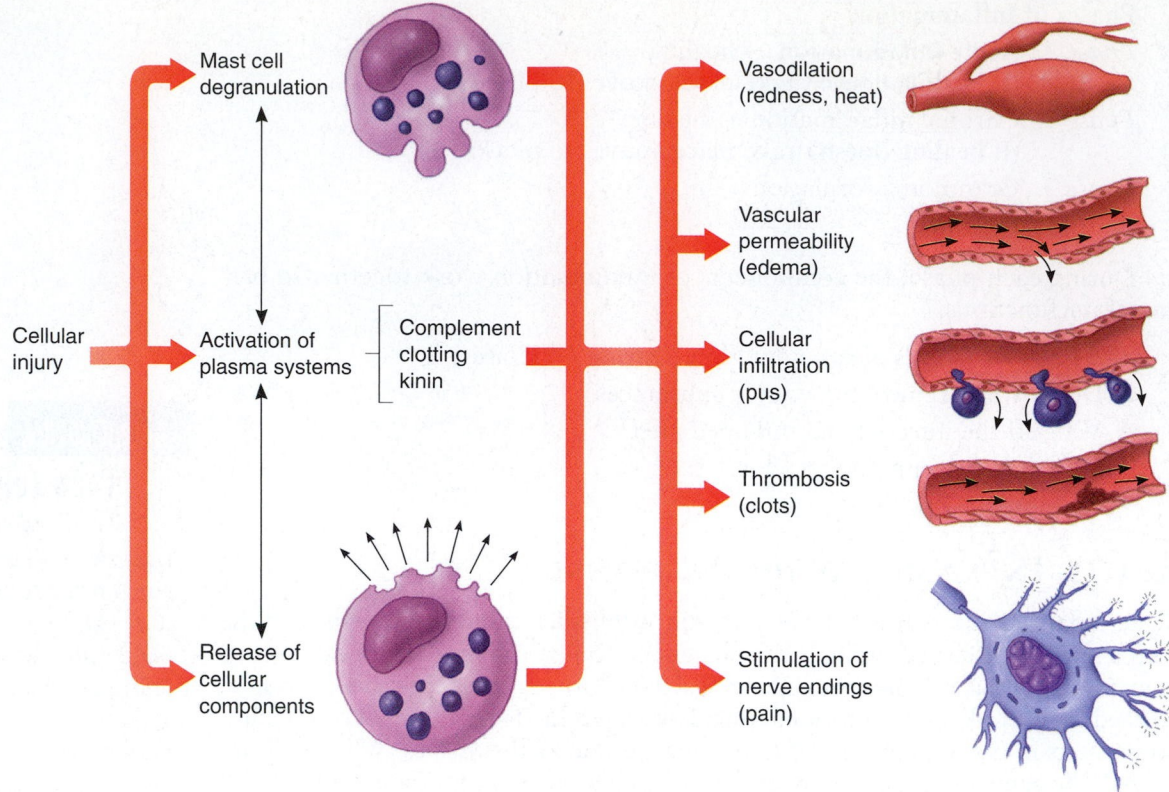

FIGURE 4-7   The acute inflammatory response.

The basic mechanics are always the same: (1) Blood vessels contract and dilate to move additional blood to the site. Then, (2) vascular permeability increases so that (3) white cells and plasma proteins can move through the capillary walls and into the tissues to begin the tasks of destroying the invader and healing the injury site (Figure 4-7).

MAST CELLS

Mast cells, which resemble bags of granules, are the chief activators of the inflammatory response. They are not blood cells. Instead, they reside in connective tissues just outside the blood vessels.

Mast cells activate the inflammatory response through two functions: *degranulation* and *synthesis* (Figure 4-8).

Degranulation

Degranulation is the process by which mast cells empty granules from their interior into the extracellular environment. This occurs when the mast cell is stimulated by one of the following events:

- *Physical injury,* such as trauma, radiation, or temperature extremes
- *Chemical agents,* such as toxins, venoms, enzymes, or a protein released by neutrophils (the latter an example of inflammatory response causing further cellular injury)
- *Immunologic and direct processes,* such as hypersensitivity (allergic) reactions involving release of IgE antibody or activation of complement components (discussed later)

✱ **mast cells** large cells, resembling bags of granules, that reside near blood vessels. When stimulated by injury, chemicals, or allergic responses, they activate the inflammatory response by degranulation (emptying their granules into the extracellular environment) and synthesis (construction of leukotrines and prostaglandins).

Content Review

MAST CELL FUNCTIONS
Degranulation
Synthesis

✱ **degranulation** the emptying of granules from the interior of a mast cell into the extracellular environment.

Cause: Mast cell stimulated by:
- Physical injury (e.g., trauma, radiation, temperature extremes)
- Chemical agent (e.g., toxin, venom, enzyme, neutrophil-produced protein)
- Immunologic process (e.g., allergic reaction/IgE antibody, activated complement)

Plasma membrane

Granules

Result: Degranulation
(release of histamine, serotonin, and chemotactic factors)

Result: Synthesis
(construction of leukotrienes and prostaglandins)

Nucleus

FIGURE 4-8   Mast cell degranulation and synthesis.

During degranulation, biochemical agents in the mast cell granules are released, notably vasoactive amines and chemotactic factors.

Vasoactive Amines Histamine is a vasoactive amine (organic compound) released during degranulation of mast cells. The effect of vasoactive amines is the constriction of the smooth muscle of large vessel walls and dilation of the post-capillary sphincter, resulting in increased blood flow at the injury site.

Basophils (a type of white blood cell) also release histamine, with the same effect. Additionally, **serotonin**, released by platelets, can have effects of both vasoconstriction and vasodilation that may affect blood flow to the affected site.

Chemotactic Factors Another consequence of degranulation of mast cells is the release of various **chemotactic factors.** Chemotactic factors are chemicals that attract white cells to the site of inflammation. This attraction of white cells is called **chemotaxis.**

Synthesis

When stimulated, mast cells synthesize, or construct, two substances that play important roles in inflammation: leukotrienes and prostaglandins.

Leukotrienes, also known as *slow-reacting substances of anaphylaxis (SRS-A),* have actions similar to histamines—vasoconstriction and increased permeability—as well as chemotaxis. However, they are more important in the later stages of inflammation because they promote slower and longer-lasting effects

✱ **histamine** a substance released during the degranulation of mast cells and also released by basophils that, through constriction and dilation of blood vessels, increases blood flow to the injury site and also increases the permeability of vessel walls.

✱ **serotonin** a substance released by platelets that, through constriction and dilation of blood vessels, affects blood flow to an injured or affected site.

✱ **chemotactic factors** chemicals that attract white cells to the site of inflammation, a process called **chemotaxis.**

✱ **leukotrienes** also called *slow-reacting substances of anaphylaxis (SRS-A);* substances synthesized by mast cells during inflammatory response that cause vasoconstriction, vascular permeability, and chemotaxis.

* prostaglandins substances synthesized by mast cells during inflammatory response that cause vasoconstriction, vascular permeability, and chemotaxis and also cause pain. Prostaglandins also act to control inflammation by suppressing release of histamines and lysosomal enzymes.

* fibroblasts cells that secrete collagen, a critical factor in wound healing.

* pus a liquid mixture of dead cells, bits of dead tissue, and tissue fluid that may accumulate in inflamed tissues.

* granuloma a tumor or growth that forms when foreign bodies that cannot be destroyed by macrophages are surrounded and walled off.

than histamines. Like leukotrienes, **prostaglandins** cause increased vasoconstruction, vascular permeability, and chemotaxis. They are also the substances that cause pain. In addition, they control inflammation by suppressing release of histamine and lysosomal enzymes from some white cells.

SYSTEMIC RESPONSES OF ACUTE INFLAMMATION

The three chief manifestations of acute inflammation are fever, leukocytosis (proliferation of circulating white cells), and an increase in circulating plasma proteins.

Endogenous pyrogen is a fever-causing chemical that is identical to IL-1 and is released by neutrophils and macrophages. It is released after the cell engages in phagocytosis or is exposed to a bacterial endotoxin or is exposed to an antigen-antibody complex. Fever can have both beneficial and harmful effects. On one hand, an increase in temperature can create an environment that is inhospitable to some invading microorganisms. On the other hand, fever may increase susceptibility of the infected person to the effects of endotoxins associated with some gram-negative bacterial infections.

In some infections, the number of circulating leukocytes, especially neutrophils, increases. Several components of the inflammatory response stimulate production of neutrophils, including a component of the complement system. Phagocytes produce a factor that induces production of granulocytes, including neutrophils, eosinophils, and basophils.

Plasma proteins called *acute phase reactants*, mostly produced in the liver, increase during inflammation. Their synthesis is stimulated by various interleukins. Many of these act to inhibit and control the inflammatory response.

CHRONIC INFLAMMATORY RESPONSES

Defined simply, chronic inflammation is any inflammation that lasts longer than two weeks. It may be caused by a foreign object or substance that persists in the wound, for example a splinter, glass, or dirt. Or it may accompany a persistent bacterial infection. This can occur because some microorganisms have cell walls with a high lipid or wax content that resist phagocytosis. Other microorganisms can survive inside a macrophage. Still others produce toxins that persist even after the bacterium is dead, continuing to incite inflammatory responses. Inflammation can also be prolonged by the presence of chemicals and other irritants.

During chronic inflammation, large numbers of neutrophils—the phagocytes that were first on the scene during acute inflammation—degranulate and die. Now, the neutrophils are replaced by components that have taken longer to develop, and there is a large infiltration of lymphocytes from the immune response and of macrophages that have matured from monocytes. In addition to attacking foreign invaders, macrophages produce a factor that stimulates **fibroblasts,** cells that secrete collagen, a critical factor in wound healing.

As neutrophils, lymphocytes, and macrophages die, they infiltrate the tissues, sometimes forming a cavity that contains these dead cells, bits of dead tissue, and tissue fluid, a mixture called **pus.** Enzymes present in pus eventually cause it to self-digest, and it is removed through the epithelium or the lymph system.

Occasionally, when macrophages are unable to destroy the foreign invader, a **granuloma** will form to wall off the infection from the rest of the body. The granuloma is formed as large numbers of macrophages, other white cells, and fibroblasts are drawn to the site and surround it. Cells decay within the granuloma, and the released acids and lysosomes break the cellular debris down to basic components and fluid. The fluid eventually diffuses out of the granuloma, leaving a hollow, hard-walled structure buried in the tissues. Some granulomas persist for the life of the individual. Granuloma formation is common in leprosy and tuberculosis, which are caused by mycobacteria, bacteria that resist destruction by phagocytes.

Tissue repair and possible scar formation are the final stages of inflammation and will be discussed in more detail later.

LOCAL INFLAMMATORY RESPONSES

All of the manifestations observed at the local inflammation site result from (1) vascular changes and (2) exudation. Redness and heat result from vascular dilation and increased blood flow to the area. Swelling and pain result from the vascular permeability that permits infiltration of exudate into the tissues.

Exudate has three functions:

- To dilute toxins released by bacteria and the toxic products of dying cells
- To bring plasma proteins and leukocytes to the site to attack the invaders
- To carry away the products of inflammation, e.g., toxins, dead cells, pus

The composition of exudate varies with the stage of inflammation and the type of injury or infection. Early exudate (serous exudate) is watery with few plasma proteins or leukocytes, as in a blister. In a severe or advanced inflammation, the exudate may be thick and clotted (fibrinous exudate) as in lobar pneumonia. In persistent bacterial infections, the exudate contains pus (purulent, or suppurative, exudate), as with cysts and abscesses. If bleeding is present, the exudate contains blood (hemorrhagic exudate).

The lesions (infected areas or wounds) that result from inflammation vary, depending on the organ affected. In myocardial infarction, cellular death results in the replacement of dead tissue by scar tissue. An infarction of brain tissue may result in liquefactive necrosis, in which the dead cells liquefy and are contained in walled cysts. In the liver, destroyed cells result in the regeneration of liver cells.

Keep in mind that inflammation can only occur in vascularized tissues (tissues to which blood can flow). When perfusion is cut off, as in a gangrenous limb or a limb distal to a tourniquet, inflammation cannot take place—and without inflammation, healing cannot take place.

RESOLUTION AND REPAIR

Healing begins during acute inflammation and may continue for as long as two years. The best outcome is **resolution,** the complete restoration of normal structure and function. This can happen if the damage was minor, there are no complications, and the tissues are capable of *regeneration* through the proliferation of the remaining cells. If resolution is not possible, then **repair** takes place with scarring being the end result. This happens if the wound is large, an abscess or granuloma has formed, or fibrin remains in the damaged tissues.

Both resolution and repair begin in the same way, with the *debridement,* or "cleaning up," of the site. Debridement involves phagocytosis of dead cells and debris and dissolution of fibrin cells (scabs). After debridement, there is a draining away of exudate, toxins, and particles from the site, and vascular dilation and permeability are reversed. At this point, either regeneration and resolution or repair and scar formation will take place. Minor wounds with little tissue loss, like paper cuts, close and heal easily, while more extensive wounds require more complex processes of sealing, filling, and contracting the wound.

> **Content Review**
>
> **OUTCOMES OF HEALING**
> Resolution – complete restoration of normal structure
> Repair – scar formation

* **resolution** the complete healing of a wound and return of tissues to their normal structure and function; the ending of inflammation with no scar formation.

* **repair** healing of a wound with scar formation.

VARIANCES IN IMMUNITY AND INFLAMMATION

Sometimes the immune and inflammatory systems work "too well" and sometimes not well enough. Hypersensitivity reactions are an example of the former, immune deficiency diseases an example of the latter.

HYPERSENSITIVITY

Immune responses are normally protective and helpful. **Hypersensitivity,** however, is an exaggerated and harmful immune response. The word *hypersensitivity* is often used as a synonym for *allergy*. However, *hypersensitivity* is also used as an umbrella term for allergy and two other categories of harmful immune response, which are defined as follows:

> **Three Types of Hypersensitivity**
>
> * **Allergy**—an exaggerated immune response to an environmental antigen, such as pollen or bee venom
> * **Autoimmunity**—a disturbance in the body's normal tolerance for self antigens, as in hyperthyroidism or rheumatic fever
> * **Isoimmunity** (also called *alloimmunity*)—an immune reaction between members of the same species, commonly of one person against the antigens of another person, as in the reaction of a mother to her infant's Rh negative factor or in transplant rejections

The exact cause of such pathological immune responses is not known, but at least three factors seem to be involved: (1) the original insult (exposure to the antigen); (2) the person's genetic makeup, which determines susceptibility to the insult; and (3) an immunological process that boosts the response beyond normal bounds.

Hypersensitivity reactions are classified as **immediate hypersensitivity reactions** or **delayed hypersensitivity reactions,** depending on how long it takes the secondary reaction to appear after reexposure to an antigen. The swiftest immediate hypersensitivity reaction is *anaphylaxis,* a severe allergic response that usually develops within minutes of reexposure. (Review anaphylactic shock earlier in this chapter. Also see Volume 3 Chapter 6 on allergies and anaphylaxis.)

Mechanisms of Hypersensitivity

Usually, when a hypersensitivity reaction takes place, inflammation is triggered that results in destruction of healthy tissues. Four mechanisms, or types, of hypersensitivity that cause this destructive reaction have been identified.

> **Mechanisms of Hypersensitivity Reaction**
>
> * Type I—IgE-mediated allergen reactions
> * Type II—tissue-specific reactions
> * Type III—immune complex-mediated reactions
> * Type IV—cell-mediated reactions

In reality, hypersensitivity reactions are not so easy to categorize. Most involve more than one type of mechanism.

Type I—IgE Reactions IgE is the immunoglobulin most involved in allergic reactions. The first exposure to the allergen (antigen that causes allergic reaction)

✱ hypersensitivity an exaggerated and harmful immune response; an umbrella term for allergy, autoimmunity, and isoimmunity.

✱ allergy exaggerated immune response to an environmental antigen.

✱ autoimmunity an immune response to self antigens, which the body normally tolerates.

✱ isoimmunity an immune response to antigens from another member of the same species, for example Rh reactions between a mother and infant or transplant rejections; also called *alloimmunity.*

✱ immediate hypersensitivity reaction a swiftly occurring secondary hypersensitivity reaction (one that occurs after reexposure to an antigen). Immediate hypersensitivity reactions are usually more severe than delayed reactions. The swiftest and most severe such reaction is anaphylaxis.

✱ delayed hypersensitivity reaction a hypersensitivity reaction that takes place after the elapse of some time following reexposure to an antigen. Delayed hypersensitivity reactions are usually less severe than immediate reactions.

Content Review

FOUR TYPES OF HYPERSENSITIVITY REACTIONS

Type I – IgE reactions
Type II – Tissue-specific reactions
Type III – Immune-complex mediated reactions
Type IV – cell-mediated tissue reactions

stimulates B lymphocytes to produce IgE antibodies. These bind to receptors on mast cells in the tissues near blood vessels. On reexposure, the allergen binds to the IgE on the mast cell, which causes degranulation of the mast cell, release of histamine, and triggering of the inflammatory response.

Type II—Tissue-Specific Reactions Most tissues contain tissue-specific antigens, so called because they exist on the cells of only some body tissues. An immune response against one of these will affect only the organs or tissues that present that particular antigen.

Type III—Immune-Complex-Mediated Reactions These result from antigen-antibody complexes, or immune complexes, formed when antibody meets and binds to a specific antigen. The immune complexes generally circulate for a time before being deposited in vessel walls or other tissues. For this reason, which organs are affected may have very little connection with where or how the antigen or the immune complex originated.

Type IV—Cell-Mediated Tissue Reactions Types I, II, and III hypersensitivity reactions are mediated by antibody. Type IV reactions are activated directly by T Cells and do not involve antibody. There are two cell-mediated mechanisms. One involves Td cells, which produce lymphokine that activates other cells such as macrophages. The other involves Tc cells that directly attack and destroy antigen-bearing cells and their toxins.

DEFICIENCIES IN IMMUNITY AND INFLAMMATION

Immune deficiency disorders result from impaired function of some component of the immune system, including phagocytes, complement, and lymphocytes (T cells and B cells), with lymphocyte dysfunction being the primary cause. Immune deficiency can be congenital (inborn) or acquired (after birth). The most common manifestations of immune deficiency are recurrent infections, because the body's ability to ward off invaders has been damaged.

Congenital Immune Deficiencies

Congenital, or primary, immune deficiency develops if the development of lymphocytes in the fetus or embryo is impaired or halted. Different immune-deficiency diseases may develop, depending on whether the T cells, the B cells, or both have been affected.

In the *DiGeorge syndrome,* there is a lack or partial lack of thymus development, resulting in a severe decrease in T cell production and function. *Bruton agammaglobulinemia* is caused by impaired development of B cell precursors, resulting in B cells that cannot produce IgM or IgD antibodies. In *bare lymphocyte syndrome,* lymphocytes and macrophages are unable to produce Class I or Class II HLA antigens, which disrupts the ability of cells to recognize self or nonself substances, resulting in severe infections that are usually fatal before age five.

Sometimes there is a defect that depresses the function of just a small portion of the immune system. For example, in *Wiskott-Aldrich syndrome,* IgM antibody production is reduced. *Selective IgA deficiency* is the most common immune deficiency. IgA is the antibody present in mucous membranes. People with IgA deficiency frequently suffer from sinus, lung, and gastrointestinal infections.

Some immune system deficiencies cause a decreased ability to respond to one particular antigen. For example, in *chronic mucocutaneous candidiasis,* the T lymphocytes are unable to respond against candida infections.

Acquired Immune Deficiencies

Acquired, or secondary, immune deficiencies develop after birth and do not result from genetic factors. They can be caused by or associated with pregnancy, infections, and diseases such as diabetes or cirrhosis. The elderly are more prone to acquired immune deficiencies than the young. Among the factors that can severely affect immune function are nutritional deficiencies, medical treatment, trauma, and stress. Of special interest is the fatal acquired immune disorder AIDS.

Nutritional Deficiencies Critical deficits in calorie or protein ingestion can lead to depression of T cell production and function. Complement activity, neutrophil chemotaxis, and the ability of neutrophils to kill bacteria are also seriously affected by starvation. Zinc deficiencies and vitamin deficiencies can affect both B cell and T cell function.

Iatrogenic Deficiencies Iatrogenic deficiencies are those that are caused by medical treatment. Some drugs depress blood cell formation in the bone marrow. Others trigger immune responses that destroy granulocytes. Immunosuppressive drugs administered in the treatment for transplants, cancer, or autoimmune diseases suppress B and T cell function and antibody production. Radiation treatment for cancer exacerbates this effect. Surgery and anesthesia also can suppress B and T cell function, with severely depressed white cell levels persisting for several weeks after surgery. Surgical removal of the spleen depresses humor response against encapsulated bacteria, depresses IgM levels, and decreases the levels of opsonins.

Deficiencies Caused by Trauma Burn victims are especially susceptible to bacterial infection. Not only has the normal barrier presented by the skin been disrupted, but thermal burns also appear to decrease neutrophil function, complement levels, and other immune functions while increasing immunosuppressive functions, which further depress immune function.

Deficiencies Caused by Stress It has long been suggested that persons undergoing emotional stress (major stresses such as divorce, but also minor stresses such as studying for final exams) are more prone to illness. The speculation was that stress has deleterious effects on immune function. Research into the possible mechanisms of stress-induced immune deficiency are just getting underway. (Stress and susceptibility to disease will be discussed later in the chapter.)

AIDS AIDS is an acronym for *acquired immunodeficiency syndrome*, which has become the best known acquired immune deficiency disorder. AIDS is a syndrome of disorders that develop from infection with **HIV**, the *human immunodeficiency virus*.

HIV is a retrovirus; that is, it carries its genetic information in RNA rather than DNA molecules. As a retrovirus, HIV infects target cells by binding to receptors on their surfaces, then inserting the HIV RNA into the cell. There, the RNA is converted into DNA and becomes part of the infected cell's genetic material. HIV can remain dormant inside the host cell for years; however, once the cell is activated (and the mechanism by which this occurs is not fully understood), HIV proliferates, kills the host cell, and can then infect other cells. The result is a pervasive breakdown of the immune defenses, making the body vulnerable to a wide variety of infections and disorders.

HIV can infect anybody, male or female, homosexual or heterosexual, mostly through the exchange of body fluids during sexual intercourse or through injection. In the United States, most cases to date have involved homosexual men and intravenous drug users. However, preventive measures (safe sex practices, including use of condoms, and clean-needle programs) have reduced the incidence of HIV/AIDS among homosexual populations and drug users. An increasing pro-

***AIDS** *acquired immunodeficiency syndrome*, a group of signs, symptoms, and disorders that often develop as a consequence of HIV infection.

***HIV** *human immunodeficiency virus*, a virus that breaks down the immune defenses, making the body vulnerable to a variety of infections and disorders.

portion of new patients are females who have acquired the infection during heterosexual intercourse. In other parts of the world, HIV/AIDS occurs equally among men and women.

The possibility of acquiring HIV/AIDS by contact with patients or accidental needle sticks fostered something of a panic among health care workers when AIDS first spread so alarmingly in the United States in the 1970s. Following recommendations by OSHA, universal precautions (body substance isolation practices) have been widely adopted—including the use of disposable gloves, protective eyewear, masks, and gowns, as appropriate, to avoid contact with any body fluids, along with improved techniques for handling needles and other sharps. These measures have proved effective in reducing the fear of HIV/AIDS infection and also in making such infections very rare among health care workers.

Until recently, more than 90 percent of those with AIDS have died within five years of the development of severe symptoms. This picture has improved somewhat in developed nations with the initiation of treatments involving multiple chemotherapies (treatment "cocktails") that have shown success in prolonging life, greatly improving feelings of health and well-being, and suppressing measurable blood levels of HIV.

It is not yet known if such treatments can eradicate HIV and cure AIDS. One fear is that the treatments suppress but do not totally destroy the HIV virus, which "hides" somewhere in the body, waiting to proliferate at some later date. Another fear is that HIV will develop strains that are resistant to the treatments that appear to be successful in the short term. Nevertheless, the success of these treatments has caused the first feelings of optimism since AIDS was identified. Preventive measures have also helped to greatly reduce the number of new cases reported in the United States. In some parts of the world, however, including Africa and Asia, HIV/AIDS is still spreading at an extremely alarming rate, with seriously inadequate reporting, prevention, and treatment.

Universal precautions, including body substance isolation practices, have been effective in relieving fears of HIV/AIDS infection and in making such infections very rare among health care workers.

Replacement Therapies for Immune Deficiencies

Advances have been made in the treatment of immune deficiencies through the use of replacement therapies, such as those listed below.

Replacement Therapies

- *Gamma globulin therapy*—Gamma globulin is administered to individuals with B cell deficiencies that cause immunoglobulin (antibody) deficiencies.

- *Transplantation and transfusion*—HLA-matched bone marrow is transplanted into patients suffering *severe combined immune deficiencies (SCID)*, which is caused by a lack of the stem cells from which T cells and B cells develop. In patients who lack a thymus or have a defective thymus, fetal thymus tissue may be transplanted. Enzyme deficiencies that cause SCID have been treated with transfusions of red blood cells that contain the needed enzyme. Other substances have been transfused into individuals to help restore T cell function and reactivity against certain antigens.

- *Gene therapy*—Therapies involving identification of defective genes that are responsible for immune disorders, and replacement of these defective genes with cloned normal genes, are in the early stages of development and use.

STRESS AND DISEASE

Stress is a word that is used a lot in modern life. You might have a stressful job, or feel stressed out by too many demands on your job, or be going through a lot of emotional stress in connection with a personal relationship. In some situations, you may be acutely aware of some of the physiological components of stress, for example sweaty palms and a pounding heart just before you have to get up and give a speech. If so, you already have a basic understanding of stress that can help you grasp the physiological and medical concepts of stress and how stress is related to disease.

CONCEPTS OF STRESS

Today, it is commonly understood that mind and body interact. It was not always so. In fact, the concept that psychological states influence physiological states—and particularly that there is a cause-effect relationship between stress and disease—date primarily from the work of Hans Selye, an Austrian-born Canadian physician and educator, in the 1940s.

> *Mind and body interact. There is a cause-and-effect relationship between stress and disease.*
>
>

General Adaptation Syndrome

Dr. Selye was not studying stress when he made his discovery. Instead, he was trying to identify a new sex hormone. He was injecting ovarian extracts into laboratory rats when he discovered the following triad of physiological effects:

Triad of Stress Effects

- Enlargement of the cortex (outer portion) of the adrenal gland
- Atrophy of the thymus gland and other lymphatic structures
- Development of bleeding ulcers of the stomach and duodenum

Dr. Selye soon discovered that this triad of effects was not a response only to the ovarian extracts. The same effects occurred when he subjected the rats to other stimuli, such as cold, surgical injury, and restraint. He concluded that the triad of effects was not specific to any particular stimulus but comprised a nonspecific response to any noxious stimulus, or stressor. (**Stress** is generally defined as a state of physical and/or psychological arousal to a stimulus. Dr. Selye originally intended to use the word *stress* for the stimulus, or cause, but through a mistranslation of his work, *stress* came to mean the arousal, or effect. Dr. Selye then coined the word **stressor** for the stimulus/cause.)

Because the same responses occurred to a wide array of stimuli, Dr. Selye named it the **general adaptation syndrome (GAS).** Later, he identified three stages in the development of GAS:

Stages of GAS

- *Stage I, Alarm*—The sympathetic nervous system is aroused and mobilized in the "fight or flight" response syndrome. Pupils dilate, heart rate increases, bronchial passages dilate. In addition, blood glucose levels rise, digestion slows, blood pressure rises, and the flow of blood to the skeletal muscles increases. At the same time, the endocrine system is aroused, resulting in secretion by the pituitary and adrenal glands of hormones that enhance the body's readiness to meet the challenge.
- *Stage II, Resistance, or Adaptation*—The person begins to cope with the situation. Sympathetic nervous system responses and circulating

* **stress** a state of physical or psychological arousal to stimulus.

* **stressor** the stimulus or cause of stress.

* **general adaptation syndrome (GAS)** a sequence of stress response stages: stage I, alarm; stage II, resistance or adaptation; stage III, exhaustion.

> **Content Review**
>
> **GENERAL ADAPTATION SYNDROME (GAS)**
>
> Stage I – Alarm
> Stage II – Resistance, or adaptation
> Stage III – Exhaustion

hormones return to normal. In most situations, this is the last stage; the stress is resolved. If the stress is very severe or prolonged, however, stress is not resolved and stage III occurs.

- *Stage III, Exhaustion*—This is the stage sometimes known as "burnout." During this stage, the triad of physiological effects described by Dr. Selye occurs. The person can no longer cope with or resolve the stress, and physical illness may ensue.

The stages of GAS begin with **physiological stress,** defined by Dr. Selye as a chemical or physical disturbance in the cells or tissue fluid produced by a change, either in the external environment of within the body itself, that requires a response to counteract the disturbance. Selye identified three components of physiological stress: (1) the stressor that initiates the disturbance, (2) the chemical or physical disturbance the stressor produces, and (3) the body's counteracting (adaptational) response.

Psychological Mediators and Specificity

Since Dr. Selye defined GAS, others who have studied adaption to stress have refined the concept. For example, more attention has been paid to the psychological mediators of stress. Experiments have shown that there isn't a direct correlation between stressor and response. People react differently to the same stressor. One person may take in stride the same situation that greatly upsets another person, and the degree of physiological response may be governed more by the psychological, or emotional, or social response to the stressor than to the stressor itself. In particular, research has demonstrated pituitary gland and adrenal cortex sensitivity to emotional/psychological/social influences.

Another way in which recent research has diverged from Dr. Selye's original hypotheses regards specificity. Dr. Selye postulated that the triad of physiological responses he identified were nonspecific; the same for any stressor. It is now thought that, while the triad of responses he identified may occur in response to a wide variety of stressors, the total body response to different stressors must be specific, that is targeted toward correction of the specific disturbance. For example, the body reacts to cold by shivering, to heat through vasodilation and sweating.

Homeostasis as a Dynamic Steady State

An older definition of homeostasis states that the body maintains itself at a "constant" composition. More recently, homeostasis has been described as a **dynamic steady state.** This takes into account the concept of **turnover,** the continual synthesis and breakdown of all body substances (e.g., fats, proteins). Thus, the internal environment of the body is always changing, not constant, but the net effect of all the changes is the dynamic (always changing), yet steady (tending always toward normal balance) state.

Stressors cause a series of reactions that alter the dynamic steady state. Usually, there is a return to normal, which may be rapid or slow. If a disturbance in the dynamic steady state, for example a high blood glucose level, is prolonged and a causative stressor is no longer present, it is considered a sign of disease.

STRESS RESPONSES

Alteration of the immune system is the ultimate outcome of a stress response that resists quick and successful adaption. The interactions of psychological, neurological/endocrine, and immunological factors that lead to this outcome are known as **psychoneuroimmunologic regulation.**

* **physiological stress** a chemical or physical disturbance in the cells or tissue fluid produced by a change in the external environment or within the body.

* **dynamic steady state** homeostasis; the tendency of the body to maintain a net constant composition although the components of the body's internal environment are always changing.

* **turnover** the continual synthesis and breakdown of body substances that results in the dynamic steady state.

* **psychoneuroimmunological regulation** the interactions of psychological, neurological/endocrine, and immunological factors that contribute to alteration of the immune system as an outcome of a stress response that is not quickly resolved.

FIGURE 4-9 The stress response: effects on the sympathetic nervous, endocrine, and immune systems.

The **stress response** is initiated by a stressor. The input of the stressor into the central nervous system, as mediated by the person's psychological response, leads to production of corticotropin-releasing factor (CRF) from the hypothalamus, which in turn stimulates responses by the sympathetic nervous system and the endocrine system (neuroendocrine regulation), which then affect the immune system. This chain of events is outlined in Figure 4-9 and described in the next sections.

Neuroendocrine Regulation

As mentioned above, when a person encounters a stressor and has a psychological response to the stressor, the sympathetic nervous system is stimulated by *corticotropin-releasing factor (CRF)*. In turn this stimulates release of catecholamines, cortisol, and other hormones.

Catecholamines Sympathetic nervous system stimulation results in the release of norepinephrine (noradrenalin), and epinephrine (adrenalin), which constitute the category of hormones called *catecholamines*. The nerves of the sympathetic nervous system exit the spine at the thoracic and lumbar levels, and norepinephrine is released into the synaptic spaces (the spaces between the presynaptic ganglia and the postsynaptic nerves).

Content Review

HORMONES PRODUCED IN RESPONSE TO STRESS

Catecholamines
  (norepinephrine and
  epinephrine)
Cortisol
Beta endorphins
Growth hormone
Prolactin

Additionally, sympathetic nervous system stimulation results in direct stimulation of the adrenal medulla, the inner portion of the adrenal gland. The adrenal medulla, in turn, releases the norepinephrine and epinephrine into the circulatory system. Approximately 80 percent of the hormones released by the adrenal medulla are epinephrine, while norepinephrine constitutes the remaining 20 percent. Once released, these hormones are carried throughout the body where their effects (preparing the body to deal with stressful situations) act on hormone receptors.

Both epinephrine and norepinephrine interact with specialized adrenergic receptors on the membranes of target organs. These receptors are located throughout the body. Once stimulated by the appropriate hormone, they cause a response in the organ or organs they control.

The adrenergic receptors are generally divided into four types, designated alpha 1 (α_1), alpha 2 (α_2), beta 1 (β_1), and beta 2 (β_2). The α_1 receptors cause peripheral vasoconstriction, mild bronchoconstriction, and stimulation of metabolism. The α_2 receptors are found on the pre-synaptic surfaces of sympathetic neuro-effector junctions. Stimulation of α_2 receptors is inhibitory. These receptors serve to prevent over-release of norepinephrine in the synapse. When the level of norepinephrine in the synapse gets high enough, the α_2 receptors are stimulated and norepinephrine release is inhibited. Stimulation of β_1 receptors causes increases in heart rate, cardiac contractile force, and cardiac automaticity and conduction. Stimulation of β_2 receptors causes vasodilation and bronchodilation.

All of the effects of the catecholamines prepare the body to "fight or flee" in response to a stressor. Their physiological effects are summarized in Table 4-4.

Table 4-4	PHYSIOLOGICAL EFFECTS OF CATECHOLAMINES
Organ	**Effects**
Brain	Increased blood flow
	Increased glucose metabolism
Cardiovascular system	Increased contractile force and rate
	Peripheral vasoconstriction
Pulmonary system	Increased ventilation
	Bronchodilation
	Increased oxygen supply
Liver	Increased glucose production
	Increased gluconeogenesis
	Increased glycogenolysis
	Decreased glycogen synthesis
Gastrointestinal and genitourinary tracts	Decreased protein synthesis
Muscle	Increased glycogenolysis
	Increased contraction
	Increased dilation of skeletal muscle vasculature
Skeleton	Decreased glucose uptake and utilization (insulin release decreased)
Adipose (fatty) tissue	Increased lipolysis
	Increased fatty acids and glycerol
Skin	Decreased blood flow
Lymphoid tissue	Increased protein breakdown (shrinkage of lymphoid tissue)

Cortisol Cortisol is another hormone produced in response to stress. The corticotropin-releasing factor (CRF) that stimulates the sympathetic nervous system, as discussed above, simultaneously stimulates the anterior pituitary gland to produce *adrenocorticotropic hormone (ACTH),* which in turn stimulates the adrenal cortex to produce a variety of steroid hormones, primarily cortisol.

One of the primary functions of cortisol is the stimulation of gluconeogenesis. It enhances the elevation of blood glucose by other hormones and also inhibits peripheral uptake and oxidation of glucose by the cells. Because of these functions, it has the overall effect of elevating blood glucose.

Cortisol also affects protein metabolism—increasing synthesis of proteins in the liver but increasing breakdown of proteins in the muscle, lymphoid tissue, fatty tissues, skin, and bone. The breakdown of proteins results in increased blood levels of amino acids. Cortisol also promotes lipolysis (fat breakdown) in the extremities and lipogenesis (fat synthesis and deposition) in the face and trunk.

Cortisol acts as an immunosuppressant by inhibiting protein synthesis, including synthesis of immunoglobulins (antibodies). Additionally, it reduces the numbers of lymphocytes, eosinophils, and macrophages in the blood. In large amounts, cortisol can cause lymphoid atrophy. Through a series of actions, cortisol diminishes the actions of helper T cells, which results in a decrease in B cells and antibody production. It inhibits production of interleukin-1 and interleukin-2 and, consequently, blocks cell-mediated immunity and generation of fever. It inhibits the accumulation of leukocytes at the site of inflammation and inhibits release of substances that are critical in the inflammatory response, including kinins, prostaglandins, and histamine. Cortisol also inhibits fibroblast proliferation during inflammatory response, which in turn causes poor wound healing and increased susceptibility to wound infection.

In the gastrointestinal tract, cortisol increases gastric secretions, occasionally enough to cause ulcer formation. Cortisol also suppresses the release of sex hormones, including testosterone and estradiol.

Cortisol—produced in response to stress—has harmful immunosuppressive actions, yet seems to have a little-understood beneficial effect in protecting against stress.

The immunosuppressive actions of cortisol seem clearly harmful, yet its production in response to stress indicates that it is beneficial in protecting against stress. Its beneficial effects in stress, however, are not well understood. It has been suggested that its promotion of gluconeogenesis helps assure an adequate source of glucose as energy for body tissues, especially nerve tissues. Pooled amino acids from protein breakdown may promote protein synthesis in some cells. Its depressive influence on inflammatory responses may play a role in decreasing peripheral blood flow and redirecting blood to critical organs or sites of injury. Suppression of immune function may also help prevent tissue damage that results from prolonged immune responses.

Role of the Immune System

During a stress response, as noted earlier, there is a complex interaction among the nervous and endocrine systems and the immune system. As a consequence, a variety of immune-related disorders are associated with stress.

The specific mechanisms by which stress leads to immune-related disorders is the subject of ongoing research but is not yet well understood. However, research points to the substances that serve as communicators between the cells of the nervous system, the endocrine system, and the immune system—including hormones, neurotransmitters, neuropeptides, and cytokines—as the pathways of cause and effect.

The pathway is not a straight line. The directional arrows of cause and effect move forward, backward, and in circles. Many components of the immune system can be affected by the factors produced by the neuroendocrine system. Conversely, immune system products can affect components of the neuroendocrine system. Here are two examples:

- *Pathway 1: central nervous system to immune system*—The central nervous system *stimulates* the hypothalamus to produce CRF → which *stimulates* the pituitary gland to produce ACTH → which *stimulates* the adrenal gland to secrete cortisol → which *suppresses* the development of macrophages, T cells, B cells, and natural killer (NK) cells, a lymphocyte specially adapted to recognize and kill virally-infected cells and malignant cells.
- *Pathway 2: immune system to central nervous system*—During immune system response, macrophages secrete cytokines → which stimulate the hypothalamus to secrete CRF (which begins Pathway 1 again).

The above are only two examples of the many pathways and interactions that take place among the nervous, endocrine, and immune systems.

The suppression of immune system function that is caused by stress-related products of the sympathetic nervous and endocrine systems—especially catecholamines and cortisol—has been linked to a number of immune-mediated diseases, as listed in Table 4-5.

STRESS, COPING, AND ILLNESS INTERRELATIONSHIPS

Research has shown that the ability to cope with stress has significant effects on associated illnesses. Those who cope positively with stress have a reduced chance of becoming ill in the first place and a better chance of getting better or getting

Table 4-5	STRESS- AND IMMUNE-RELATED DISEASES AND CONDITIONS	
Target Organ	**Diseases and Conditions**
Cardiovascular system	Coronary artery disease Hypertension Stroke Dysrhythmias
Muscles	Tension headaches Muscle-related backaches
Connective tissues	Rheumatoid arthritis
Pulmonary system	Asthma Hay fever
Immune system	Immunosuppression or immune deficiency
Gastrointestinal system	Ulcer Irritable bowel syndrome Ulcerative colitis
Genitourinary system	Diuresis Impotence
Skin	Eczema Acne
Endocrine system	Diabetes mellitus
Central nervous system	Fatigue Depression Insomnia

better faster if they do become ill. Conversely, those who don't cope as well with stress have a greater chance of becoming ill or of prolonging the course of illness or of not surviving an illness.

Physiological stress is caused by events that directly affect the body, such as a burn, extreme cold, or starvation. *Psychological stress* consists of the unpleasant emotions caused by life events, such as taking exams or a divorce. The effects that these stresses will have on the body depend on the individual's ability to cope with them. Some people are "thrown" by events others would perceive as relatively minor, such as a traffic jam or a sprained ankle. Others can take in stride events that others would find very difficult, such as loss of a job or a long term disability.

The effects of stress, including the degree to which stress causes or affects illness, are moderated by the type, duration, and severity of the stressor in combination with the individual's perception and ability to cope with it. Stressors that are the most likely to have a negative effect on immunity and disease have been characterized as those that are not only undesirable but also are uncontrollable and that overtax the person's ability to cope.

Effective and ineffective coping has been seen to have potentially different effects in healthy persons, symptomatic persons (those who already have some manifestations of disease), and persons who are undergoing medical treatment.

Potential Effects of Stress Based on Effectiveness of Coping

- *In a healthy person:*
  Effective coping → Transient effects, return to normal function
  Ineffective coping → Significant stress effects, illness

- *In a symptomatic person:*
  Effective coping → Little or no effect on symptoms
  Ineffective coping → Exacerbation of symptoms, illness

- *In a person undergoing medical treatment:*
  Effective coping → Person does not perceive the treatment itself as

  stressful → Treatment is more likely to have a positive effect on symptoms and the course of illness

  Ineffective coping → Person perceives the treatment itself as

  stressful → Treatment is more likely to have a negative effect on symptoms and the course of illness

Because of the importance of coping ability in the interplay between stress and illness, attention is increasingly being paid to providing counseling and support systems—including family members, friends, and other support networks—to assist persons who are ill or in stressful life situations. There is recognition that supporting the patient's ability to cope is a critical adjunct to medical treatment itself.

Summary

Pathophysiology is the study of how disease and injury alter normal physiology (body processes). The cell is the basic unit of life. The cells exist in an environment of fluids and electrolytes. When something interferes with normal cell function or the normal cell environment or normal cell intercommunication, disease can begin or advance.

Cells can be injured in a variety of ways, including hypoxia, chemicals, infectious agents, immunological/inflammatory injuries, and others. Diseases can be caused by genetic factors, environmental factors, or a combination of factors (multifactorial diseases).

The body responds to cellular injury in a variety of ways to restore homeostasis, the body's normal dynamic steady state. Cells can adapt through atrophy, hypertrophy, hyperplasia, metaplasia, and dysplasia. Negative feedback mechanisms work to correct, or compensate for, shock—if shock has not progressed too far.

Perfusion of the tissues is necessary to provide essential nutrients to the cells (especially oxygen and glucose) and to remove wastes. Inadequate perfusion, called hypoperfusion or shock, can be caused by a problem in any of the three parts of the cardiovascular system (the heart, the blood vessels, or the blood), sometimes abetted by problems with the respiratory or gastrointestinal system in which the normal intake and transfer of oxygen and glucose may be interrupted. If not corrected, shock continues in a downward spiral toward irreversible shock, possible multiple organ dysfunction syndrome (MODS), and death.

The body's chief means of self defense is the immune system and the immune and inflammatory responses, which work to attack and destroy infectious agents and other unwanted invaders. Occasionally, the immune response system works "too well," as in hypersensitivity reactions, or not well enough, as in immune deficiency disorders. Stress can also contribute to disease through the interactions of the nerve, endocrine, and immune systems.

CHAPTER 5

Life-Span Development

Objectives

After reading this chapter, you should be able to:

INTRODUCTION

People change over the span of a lifetime. Changes in vital signs, body systems, and psychosocial development can necessitate adjustments in your treatment of patients. For example, drug dosages are based on body size, weight, and ability of the patient to process the drug.

Many changes can be associated with development stages. The stages discussed in this chapter are *infancy* (birth to 12 months), *toddlerhood* (12 to 36 months), *preschool age* (3 to 5 years), *school age* (6 to 12 years), *adolescence* (13 to 18 years), *early adulthood* (20 to 40 years), *middle adulthood* (41 to 60 years), and *late adulthood* (61 years and older).

INFANCY

PHYSIOLOGICAL DEVELOPMENT

Vital Signs

The greatest vital signs changes occur in the pediatric patient (Table 5-1). At birth, the heart rate ranges from 100 to 180 beats per minute but settles to around 120 after the first 30 minutes. An at-birth respiratory rate of 30 to 60 will drop to 30 to 40 after the first few minutes.

Unlike heart and respiratory rates that decrease with age, blood pressure tends to increase with age. An average systolic blood pressure of 60 to 90 at birth rises to a range of 87 to 105 at 12 months.

The younger the child, the more rapid are the pulse and respiratory rates.

Table 5-1	NORMAL VITAL SIGNS			
	Pulse (beats per minute)	Respiration (breaths per minute)	Blood Pressure (average mmHg)	Temperature
Infancy:				
At birth:	100–180	30–60	60–90 systolic	98°F–100°F	36.7°C–37.8°C
At one year:	100–160	30–60	87–105 systolic	98°F–100°F	36.7°C–37.8°C
Toddler (12 to 36 months)	80–110	24–40	95–105 systolic	96.8°F–99.6°F	36.3°C–37.9°C
Preschool age (3 to 5 years)	70–110	22–34	95–110 systolic	96.8°F–99.6°F	36.3°C–37.9°C
School-age (6 to 12 years)	65–110	18–30	97–112 systolic	98.6°F	37°C
Adolescence (13 to 18 years)	60–90	12–26	112–128 systolic	98.6°F	37°C
Early adulthood (19 to 40 years)	60–100	12–20	120/80	98.6°F	37°C
Middle adulthood (41 to 60 years)	60–100	12–20	120/80	98.6°F	37°C
Late adulthood (61 years and older)	+	+	+	98.6°F	37°C

+ Depends on the individual physical health status.

FIGURE 5-1 Infants double their weight by 4 to 6 months old and triple it by 9 to 12 months.

The infant's head is equal to 25% of total body weight.

Weight

Normal birth weight of an infant usually is between 3.0 and 3.5 kg. Because of the excretion of extracellular fluid in the first week of life, the infant's weight usually drops by 5% to 10%; however, infants usually exceed their birth weight by the second week. During the first month, infants grow at approximately 30 grams per day, and they should double their birth weight by 4 to 6 months and triple it at 9 to 12 months (Figure 5-1). The infant's head is equal to 25% of total body weight.

Growth charts are good for comparing physical development to the norm, but parents should keep in mind that every child develops at his own rate.

Cardiovascular System

As newborns make the transition from fetal to pulmonary circulation in the first few days of life, several important changes occur. Shortly after birth, the *ductus venosus,* a blood vessel that connects the umbilical vein and the inferior vena cava in the fetus, constricts. As a result, blood pressure changes and the *foramen ovale,* an opening in the interatrial septum of the fetal heart, closes. The *ductus arteriosus,* a blood vessel that connects the pulmonary artery and the aorta in the fetus, also constricts after birth. Once it is closed, blood can no longer bypass the lungs by moving from the pulmonary trunk directly into the aorta.

These changes lead to an immediate increase in systemic vascular resistance and a decrease in pulmonary vascular resistance. Although the constriction of the ductus arteriosus may be functionally complete within 15 minutes, the permanent closure of the foramen ovale may take from 30 days to one year. The left ventricle of the heart will strengthen throughout the first year.

(You may wish to note that in an adult, the ductus venosus becomes a fibrous cord called the *ligamemtum venosum,* which is superficially embedded in the wall of the liver. Also, in an adult, the site of the foramen ovale is marked by a depression called the *fossa ovalis,* and the ductus arteriosus is represented by a cord called the *ligamentum arteriosum.*)

Pulmonary System

The first breath an infant takes must be forceful, because until that moment the lungs have been collapsed. Fortunately, the lungs of a full-term fetus continuously secrete surfactant. Surfactant is a chemical that reduces the surface tension that tends to hold the moist membranes of the lungs together. After the first powerful breath begins to expand the lungs, breathing becomes easier.

An infant's airway is shorter, narrower, less stable, and more easily obstructed than at any other stage in life.

In general, an infant's airway is shorter, narrower, less stable, and more easily obstructed than at any other stage in life. The infant is primarily a "nose breather" until at least four weeks of age; therefore, it is important for the nasal passages to stay clear. A common complaint in infants less than 6 months of age is nasal congestion. This occurs because, as mentioned, young infants are obligate nasal breathers. Even a mild nasal obstruction, as occurs with a viral upper respiratory infection, can cause difficulty breathing, especially during feeding.

An infant's lung tissue is fragile and prone to *barotrauma* (an injury caused by a change in atmospheric pressure). Because of this, prehospital personnel must be careful when applying mechanical ventilation with a bag-valve-mask unit. There are fewer alveoli with decreased collateral ventilation. In addition, the accessory muscles for breathing are immature and susceptible to early fatigue, so they cannot sustain a rapid respiratory rate over a long period of time. Breathing becomes ineffective at rates higher than 60 breaths per minute because air moves only in the upper airway, never reaching the lungs. Rapid respiratory rates also lead to rapid heat and fluid loss.

The chest wall of the infant is less rigid than an adult's, and the ribs are positioned horizontally, causing diaphragmatic breathing. So when you assess respiratory rate and effort in an infant, it is important to observe the abdomen rise and fall. An infant needs less pressure and a lower volume of air for ventilation than an adult does, but the infant has a higher metabolic rate and a higher oxygen-consumption rate than an adult.

Renal System

Usually, the newborn's kidneys are not able to produce concentrated urine, so the baby excretes a relatively dilute fluid with a specific gravity that rarely exceeds 1.0. (Specific gravity is the weight of a substance compared to an equal amount of water. For comparisons, water is considered to have a specific gravity of 1.0.) For this reason, the newborn can easily become dehydrated and develop a water and electrolyte imbalance.

Immune System

During pregnancy, certain antibodies pass from the maternal blood into the fetal bloodstream. As a result, the fetus acquires some of the mother's active immunities against pathogens. Thus, the fetus is said to have naturally acquired passive immunities, which may remain effective for six months to a year after birth. A breast-fed baby also receives antibodies through the breast milk to many of the diseases the mother has had.

Nervous System

Sensation is present in all portions of the body at birth, so a young infant feels pain but lacks the ability to localize it and isolate a response to it. As nerve connections develop, the response to pain becomes much more localized. In addition, motor and sensory development are most advanced in the cranial nerves at birth, because of their life-sustaining function and protective reflexes. Since the cranial nerves control such things as blinking, sucking, and swallowing, the infant has strong, coordinated sucking and gag reflexes. The infant also will have well flexed extremities, which move equally when the infant is stimulated.

Reflexes The infant has several reflexes that disappear over time. These include the Moro, palmar, rooting, and sucking reflexes. The **Moro reflex,** which is sometimes referred to as the "startle reflex," is the characteristic reflex of newborns. When the baby is startled, he throws his arms wide, spreading his fingers and then grabbing instinctively with the arms and fingers. The reflex should be brisk and symmetrical. An asymmetric Moro reflex (in which one arm does not respond exactly like the other) may imply a paralysis or weakness on one side of the body.

The **palmar grasp** is a strong reflex in the full-term newborn. It is elicited by placing a finger firmly in the infant's palm. The palmar grasp weakens as the hand becomes less continuously fisted. Sometime after two months, it merges into the voluntary ability to release an object held in the hand.

The **rooting reflex** causes the hungry infant to turn his head to the right or left when a hand or cloth touches his cheek. If the mother's nipple touches either side of the infant's face, above or below the mouth, the infant's lips and tongue tend to follow in that direction. Stroking the infant's lips causes a sucking movement, or the **sucking reflex,** in the infant. Both the rooting and sucking reflexes should be present in all full-term babies and are most easily elicited before a feeding. They usually last until the infant is three or four months old; however, the rooting reflex may persist during sleep for seven or eight months.

✳ **Moro reflex** occurring when a newborn is startled, arms are thrown wide, fingers spread, and a grabbing motion follows. Also called *startle reflex.*

✳ **palmar grasp** a reflex in the newborn, which is elicited by placing a finger firmly in the infant's palm.

✳ **rooting reflex** occurring when an infant's cheek is touched by a hand or cloth, the hungry infant turns his head to the right or left.

✳ **sucking reflex** occurring when an infant's lips are stroked.

Fontanelles Fontanelles allow for compression of the head during childbirth and for rapid growth of the brain during early life. They are diamond-shaped soft spots of fibrous tissue at the top of the infant's skull where three or four bones will eventually fuse together. The fibrous tissue is strong and, generally, can protect the brain adequately from injury. The posterior fontanelle usually closes in 2 or 3 months, and the anterior one closes between 9 and 18 months. You may wish to note that the fontanelles, especially the anterior one, may be used to provide an indirect estimate of hydration. Normally, the anterior fontanelle is level with the surface of the skull, or slightly sunken. With dehydration, the anterior fontanelle may fall below the level of the skull and appear sunken.

Sleep A newborn usually sleeps for 16 to 18 hours daily, with periods of sleep and wakefulness evenly distributed over a 24-hour period. Sleep time will gradually decrease to 14 to 16 hours per day, with a 9 to 10 hour period at night. Infants usually begin to sleep through the night within two to four months. The normal infant is easily aroused.

Musculoskeletal System

The developing infant's extremities grow in length from growth plates, which are located on each end of the long bones. The infant also has *epiphyseal plates,* or secondary bone-forming centers that are separated by cartilage from larger (or parent) bones. As each epiphysis grows, it becomes part of the larger bone. Bones grow in thickness by way of deposition of new bone on existing bone. Factors affecting bone development and growth include nutrition, exposure to sunlight, growth hormone, thyroid hormone, genetic factors, and general health. Muscle weight in infants is about 25% of the entire musculoskeletal system.

Other Developmental Characteristics

Expect rapid changes during an infant's first year of life. At about two months of age, he is able to track objects with his eyes and recognize familiar faces. At about three months of age, he can move objects to his mouth with his hands and display primary emotions with distinct facial expressions (such as a smile or a frown). At four months of age, he drools without swallowing and begins to reach out to people. By five months, he should be sleeping through the night without waking for a feeding, and he should be able to discriminate between family and strangers. Teeth begin to appear between five and seven months of age.

At six months, the baby can sit upright in a high chair and begin to make one-syllable sounds, such as "ma," "mu," "da," and "di." At seven months, he has a fear of strangers and his moods can quickly shift from crying to laughing. At eight months, the infant begins to respond to the word "no," he can sit alone, and he can play "peek-a-boo." At nine months, he responds to adult anger.

At about nine months old, the baby begins to pull himself up to a standing position, and explores objects by mouthing, sucking, chewing, and biting them. At 10 months, he pays attention to his name and crawls well. At 11 months, he attempts to walk without assistance and begins to show frustration about restrictions. By 12 months, he can walk with help, and he knows his own name.

PSYCHOSOCIAL DEVELOPMENT

Family Processes and Reciprocal Socialization

The psychosocial development of an individual begins at birth and develops as a result of instincts, drives, capacities, and interactions with the environment. A key component of that environment is the family. The interactions babies have with their families help them to grow and change and help their families do the same. This is called "reciprocal socialization," a model that recognizes the child's active role in its own development.

Raising a baby requires a lot of hard work, but studies show that healthy, happy, and self-reliant children are the products of stable homes in which parents give a great deal of time and attention to their children.

Crying A newborn's only means of communication is through crying. While every cry may seem the same to a stranger, most mothers quickly learn to notice the differences in a basic cry, an anger cry, and a pain cry.

Attachment Infants have their own unique timetables and paths to becoming attached to their parents. **Bonding** is initially based on **secure attachment,** or an infant's sense that his needs will be met by his caregivers. Secure attachment is consistent with healthy development, and leads to a child who is bold in his explorations of the world and competent in dealing with it. It is important for this sense of security to develop within the first six months of an infant's life.

When an infant is uncertain about whether or not his caregivers will be responsive or helpful when needed, another type of attachment develops. It is called **anxious resistant attachment.** It leads to a child who is always prone to separation anxiety, causing him to be clinging and anxious about exploring the world.

A third type of attachment is called **anxious avoidant attachment.** It occurs when the infant has no confidence that he will be responded to helpfully when he seeks care. In fact, the infant expects to be rebuffed. This causes him to attempt to live without the love and support of others. The most extreme cases result from repeated rejection or prolonged institutionalization and can lead to a variety of personality disorders from compulsive self-sufficiency to persistent delinquency.

Trust vs. Mistrust Some psychologists believe that human life progresses through a series of stages, each marked by a crisis that needs to be resolved. Each of the crises involves a conflict between two opposing characteristics. From birth to approximately $1\frac{1}{2}$ years of age, the infant goes through the stage called **trust vs. mistrust.** According to psychologists, the infant wants the world to be an orderly, predictable place where causes and effects can be anticipated. When this is true, the infant develops trust based on consistent parental care. When an infant begins life with irregular and inadequate care, he develops anxiety and insecurity, which have a negative effect on family and other relationships important to the development of trust. This may lead to feelings of mistrust and hostility, which may in turn develop into antisocial or even criminal behavior.

Scaffolding

Infants learn in many ways from their parents and others around them. One way they learn—from infancy and throughout their school years—is through **scaffolding,** or building on what they already know. For example, parents or caregivers usually talk to infants as a natural part of caring for them. With scaffolding, the dialogue is maintained just above the level where the child can perform activities independently. As the baby learns, the parent or caregiver changes the nature of the dialogues so that they continue to support the baby but also give him responsibility for the task. In this way, infants continue to build on what they know.

Temperament

An infant may be classified as an easy child, a difficult child, or slow-to-warm-up child. An **easy child** is characterized by regularity of bodily functions, low or moderate intensity of reactions, and acceptance of new situations. A

* **bonding** the formation of a close personal relationship (as between mother and child), especially through frequent or constant association.

* **secure attachment** a type of bonding that occurs when an infant learns that his caregivers will be responsive and helpful when needed.

* **anxious resistant attachment** a type of bonding that occurs when an infant learns to be uncertain about whether or not his caregivers will be responsive or helpful when needed.

* **anxious avoidant attachment** a type of bonding that occurs when an infant learns that his caregivers will not be responsive or helpful when needed.

* **trust vs. mistrust** refers to a stage of psychosocial development that lasts from birth to about $1\frac{1}{2}$ years of age.

* **scaffolding** a teaching/learning technique in which one builds on what has already been learned.

* **easy child** an infant, who can be characterized by regularity of bodily functions, low or moderate intensity of reactions, and acceptance of new situations.

✱ **difficult child** an infant, who can be characterized by irregularity of bodily functions, intense reactions, and withdrawal from new situations.

✱ **slow-to-warm-up child** an infant, who can be characterized by a low intensity of reactions and a somewhat negative mood.

Parental-separation reactions in an infant include protest, despair, and withdrawal.

🗝️

---

difficult child is characterized by irregularity of bodily functions, intense reactions, and withdrawal from new situations. A **slow-to-warm-up child** is characterized by a low intensity of reactions and a somewhat negative mood.

Situational Crisis and Parental-Separation Reactions

Infants who have good relationships with their parents usually follow a predictable sequence of behaviors when they experience a situational crisis (a crisis caused by a particular set of circumstances), such as being separated from parents. The first stage of parental-separation reaction is protest; the second stage is despair; and the last is detachment or withdrawal.

Protest may begin immediately upon separation and continue for about one week. Loud crying, restlessness, and rejection of all adults show how distressed the infant is. In the second stage, despair, the infant's behavior suggests growing hopelessness marked by monotonous crying, inactivity, and steady withdrawal. In the final stage, detachment or withdrawal, the infant displays renewed interest in its surroundings, even though it is usually a remote, distant kind of interest. This phase is apathetic and may persist even if the parent reappears.

TODDLER AND PRESCHOOL AGE

PHYSIOLOGICAL DEVELOPMENT

Vital signs for toddlers (12 to 36 months, Figure 5-2) and preschool age children (3 to 5 years old, Figure 5-3) are not the same as an infant's. The heart rate for toddlers ranges from 80 to 110 beats per minute. Respiratory rate ranges from 24 to 40 breaths per minute. Systolic blood pressure ranges from 95 to 105 mmHg. For preschoolers, heart rate ranges from 70 to 110 beats per minute, respiratory rate from 22 to 34 breaths per minute, and systolic blood pressure from 75 to 110 mmHg. Normal temperature for both ranges from 96.8°F to 99.6°F (36.3°C to 37.9°C). In addition, the rate of weight gain is slowing dramatically. The average toddler or preschooler gains approximately 2.0 kg per year.

Changes in body systems include the following:

FIGURE 5-2   A toddler beginning to stand and walk on his own.

Remember that toddlers and preschool age children have immature chest muscles and cannot sustain an excessively rapid respiratory rate for long.

🗝️

- *Cardiovascular system.* The capillary beds are now better developed and assist in thermoregulation of the body more efficiently. Hemoglobin levels approach normal adult levels at this point.

- *Pulmonary system.* The terminal airways continue to branch off from the bronchioles and alveoli increase in number, providing more surfaces for gas exchange to take place in the lungs. It is still important to remember that children have immature chest muscles and cannot sustain an excessively rapid respiratory rate for long. They will tire quickly and respiratory rate will decrease, indicating the onset of ventilatory failure.

- *Renal system.* The kidneys are well developed by the toddler years. Specific gravity and other characteristics of urine are similar to what would be found in an adult.

- *Immune system.* By this point in life, the passive immunity born with the infant is lost, and the child becomes more susceptible to minor respiratory and gastrointestinal infections. This occurs at the same time the child is being exposed to the infections of other children in day care and preschool. Fortunately, the toddler and preschooler will develop their own immunities to common pathogens as they are exposed to them.

- *Nervous system.* The brain is now at 90% of adult weight. Myelination (the development of the covering of nerves) has increased, which allows for effortless walking as well as other basic skills. Fine motor skills, including the use of hands and fingers in grasping and manipulating objects, begin developing at this stage.
- *Musculoskeletal system.* Both muscle mass and bone density increase during this period.
- *Dental system.* All of the primary teeth have erupted by the age of 36 months.
- *Senses.* Visual acuity is at 20/30 during the toddler years. Hearing reaches maturity at 3 to 4 years old.

FIGURE 5-3   In the preschool-age child, exploratory behavior accelerates.

In addition, though children are physiologically capable of being toilet trained by the age of 12 to 15 months, they are not psychologically ready until 18 to 30 months of age. So, it is important not to rush toilet training. Children will let their parents know when they are ready. The average age for completion of toilet training is 28 months.

The average age for completion of toilet training is 28 months.

PSYCHOSOCIAL DEVELOPMENT

Cognition

Children begin to use actual words at about 10 months, but they do not begin to grasp that words "mean" something until they are about one year of age. Usually, by the time they are three or four years old, they have mastered the basics of language, which they will continue to refine throughout their childhood. Between 18 and 24 months, they begin to understand cause and effect. Between the ages of 18 and 24 months, they develop separation anxiety, becoming clinging and crying when a parent leaves. Between 24 and 36 months, they begin to develop "magical thinking" and engage in play-acting, such as playing house and similar activities.

By the age of three or four, children have mastered the basics of language.

Between the ages of 18 and 24 months, children develop separation anxiety.

Play

Exploratory behavior accelerates at this stage. The child is able to play simple games and follow basic rules, and he begins to display signs of competitiveness. Play provides an emotional release for youngsters, because it lacks the right-or-wrong, life-and-death feelings that may accompany interactions with adults. Therefore, observations of children at play may uncover frustrations otherwise unexpressed.

Sibling Relationships

While there are many positive aspects to growing up with siblings, there also may be negative ones, which can lead to sibling rivalry. The first-born child often finds it very difficult to share the attention of his parents with a younger sibling. If the older child must also help care for the younger ones, he may become even more frustrated. While first-born children usually maintain a special relationship with parents, they also are expected to exercise more self-control and show more responsibility when interacting with younger siblings. Younger children often see only the apparent privileges extended to the older children, such as later bedtimes and more freedom to come and go. Still, when asked if they would be happier if their siblings did not exist, most prefer to keep them around.

Peer-Group Functions

Peers, or youngsters who are similar in age (within 12 months of each other), are very important to the development of toddler and school-age children. In fact, peer groups actually become more important as childhood progresses. Peers provide a source of information about other families and the outside world. Interaction with peers offers opportunities for learning skills, comparing oneself to others, and feeling part of a group.

Parenting Styles and Their Effects

* **authoritarian** a parenting style that demands absolute obedience without regard to a child's individual freedom.

* **authoritative** a parenting style that emphasizes a balance between a respect for authority and individual freedom.

* **permissive** a parenting style that takes a tolerant, accepting view of a child's behavior.

There are three basic styles of parenting: **authoritarian**, **authoritative**, and **permissive:**

- *Authoritarian* parents are demanding and desire instant obedience from a child. No consideration is given to the child's view, and no attempt is made to explain why. Frequently, the child is punished for even asking the reason for some decision or directive. This parenting style often leads to children with low self esteem and low competence. Boys are often hostile and girls are often shy.
- *Authoritative* parents respond to the needs and wishes of their children. While they believe in parental control, they attempt to explain their reasons to the child. They expect mature behavior and will enforce rules, but they still encourage independence and actualization of potential. These parents believe that both they and children have rights and try to maintain a happy balance between the two. This parenting style usually leads to children who are self-assertive, independent, friendly, and cooperative.
- *Permissive* parents take a tolerant, accepting view of their children's behavior, including aggressive behavior and sexual behavior. They rarely punish or make demands of their children, allowing them to make almost all of their own decisions. They may be either "permissive-indifferent" or "permissive-indulgent" parents, but it is very difficult to make the distinction. This parenting style may lead to impulsive, aggressive children who have low self-reliance, low self-control, low maturity, and lack responsible behavior.

Divorce and Child Development

Nearly half of today's marriages end in divorce. As a result of divorce, a child's physical way of life often changes (a new home, for example, or a reduced standard of living). The child's psychological life is also touched. The effects on the child's development, however, depend greatly on the child's age, his cognitive and social competencies, the amount of dependency on his parents, how the parents interact with each other and the child, and even the type of day care. Toddlers and preschoolers commonly express feelings of shock, depression, and a fear that their parents no longer love them. They may feel they are being abandoned. They are unable to see the divorce from their parents' perspective, and therefore believe the divorce centers on them. The parent's ability to respond to a child's needs greatly influences the ultimate effects of divorce on the child.

Television

Virtually every family has at least one television in the home. Most children watch television for several hours each day, many with few, if any, parental restrictions. Television violence increases levels of aggression in toddlers and preschoolers, and it increases passive acceptance of the use of aggression by others. Parental screening of the television programs children watch may be effective in avoiding these outcomes.

Modeling

Toddlers and preschool age children begin to recognize sexual differences, and, through **modeling,** they begin to incorporate gender-specific behaviors they observe in parents, siblings, and peers.

* modeling a procedure whereby a subject observes a model perform some behavior and then attempts to imitate that behavior. Many believe it is the fundamental learning process involved in socialization.

SCHOOL AGE

PHYSIOLOGICAL DEVELOPMENT

Between the ages of 6 and 12 years, a child's heart rate is between 65 and 110 beats per minute, respiratory rate is between 18 to 30 breaths per minute, and systolic blood pressure ranges from 97 to 112 mmHg. Body temperature is approximately 98.6°F (37°C). The average child of this age gains 3 kg per year and grows 6 cm per year. In most children, vital signs reach adult levels during this period of time, but their lymph tissues are proportionately larger than those of an adult. In addition, brain function increases in both hemispheres, and primary teeth are being replaced by permanent ones.

Vital signs in most children reach adult levels during the school-age years.

PSYCHOSOCIAL DEVELOPMENT

School-age children (Figure 5-4) have developed decision-making skills, and usually are allowed more self-regulation, with parents providing general supervision. Parents spend less time with school-age children than they did with toddlers and preschoolers.

The development of a self-concept occurs at this age. School-age children have more interaction with both adults and other children, and they tend to compare themselves to others. They are beginning to develop self-esteem, which tends to be higher during the early years of school than in the later years. Often self-esteem is based on external characteristics and may be affected by popularity with peers, rejection, emotional support, and neglect. Negative self-esteem can be very damaging to further development.

As children mature, moral development begins when they are rewarded for what their parents believe to be right and punished for what their parents believe to be wrong. With cognitive growth, moral reasoning appears and the control of the child's behavior gradually shifts from external sources to internal self-control. According to one theory, there are three levels of moral development

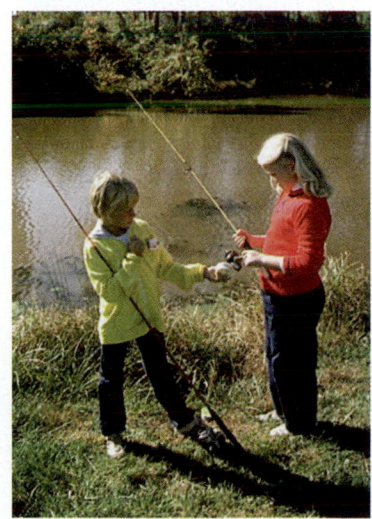

FIGURE 5-4 School-age children are allowed more self-regulation and independence as they grow older.

✳ pre-conventional reasoning the stage of moral development during which children respond mainly to cultural control to avoid punishment and attain satisfaction.

✳ conventional reasoning the stage of moral development during which children desire approval from individuals and society.

✳ post-conventional reasoning the stage of moral development during which individuals make moral decisions according to an enlightened conscience.

pre-conventional reasoning, **conventional reasoning**, and **post-conventional reasoning**, each level having two stages:

- *Pre-conventional reasoning.* Stage one is punishment and obedience; that is, children obey rules in order to avoid punishment. There is no concern about morals. Stage two is individualism and purpose; that is, children obey the rules but only for pure self-interest. They are aware of fairness to others but only as it pertains to their own satisfaction.

- *Conventional reasoning.* In stage three, children are concerned with interpersonal norms, seeking the approval of others and developing the "good boy" or "good girl" mentality. They begin to judge behavior by intention. In stage four, they develop the social system's morality, becoming concerned with authority and maintaining the social order. They realize that correct behavior is "doing one's duty."

- *Post-conventional reasoning.* Stage five is concerned with community rights as opposed to individual rights. Children at this level believe that the best values are those supported by law because they have been accepted by the whole society. They believe that if there is a conflict between human need and the law, individuals should work to change the law. Stage six is concerned with universal ethical principles, such as that an informed conscience defines what is right, or people act not because of fear, approval, or law, but from their own standards of what is right or wrong.

According to this theory, individuals will move through the levels and stages of moral development throughout school age and young adulthood and at their own rates.

Both males and females reach reproductive maturity during adolescence.

ADOLESCENCE

PHYSIOLOGICAL DEVELOPMENT

Vital signs in adolescents (12 to 18 years old) are as follows: heart rate is between 60 and 90 beats per minute, respiratory rate is between 12 and 26 breaths per minute, and systolic blood pressure is between 112 and 138 mmHg. Body temperature is approximately 98.6°F (37°C). In addition, the adolescent usually experiences a rapid two- to three-year growth spurt, beginning distally with enlargement of the feet and hands followed by enlargement of the arms and legs. The chest and trunk enlarge in the final stage of growth. Girls are usually finished growing by the age of 16 and boys by the age of 18. In late adolescence, the average male is taller and stronger than the average female.

At this age, both males and females reach reproductive maturity (Figure 5-5). Secondary sexual development occurs, with noticeable development of the external sexual organs. Pubic and axillary hairs appear and, mostly in males, vocal quality changes. In females, menstruation has begun, breasts and the ductile system of the mammary glands develops, and there is increased deposition of adipose tissue in the subcutaneous layer of the breasts, thighs, and buttocks. In addition, in the female, endocrine system changes include the release of *follicle-stimulating hormone (FSH)*, *luteinizing hormone (LH)*,

FIGURE 5-5 Children reach reproductive maturity during adolescence.

and *gonadrotropin,* which promotes estrogen and progesterone production. In the male, gonadrotropin promotes testosterone production.

Muscle mass and bone growth are nearly complete at this stage. Body fat decreases in early adolescence and increases later. Females require 18% to 20% body fat in order for menarche, or the first menstruation, to occur. Blood chemistry is nearly equal to that of an adult, and skin toughens through sebaceous gland activity. (You may wish to note that a disorder of the sebaceous glands is responsible for acne, which is common in adolescence. In acne, the glands become overactive and inflamed, ducts become plugged, and small red elevations containing blackheads or pimples appear.)

PSYCHOSOCIAL DEVELOPMENT

Family

Adolescence can be a time of serious family conflicts as the adolescent strives for autonomy and parents strive for continued control. The many biological changes that occur at this stage cause inner conflict in both the adolescent and parents. Privacy becomes extremely important at this stage of life and, because of modesty, the adolescent prefers that parents not be present during physical examinations. It also is likely that when a patient history is being taken, questions asked in the presence of parents or guardians may not be answered honestly.

Children experience an increase in idealism during adolescence. They believe that adults should be able to live up to their expectations, which of course they cannot always do, which leads to disappointment.

The many biological changes that occur in adolescence cause inner conflict in both the adolescent and parents.

Development of Identity

At this age, adolescents are trying to achieve more independence. They take "time out" to experiment with a variety of identities, knowing that they do not have to assume responsibility for the consequences of those identities. As they attempt to develop their own identity, self-consciousness and peer pressure increase. They become interested in the opposite sex, and they find this somewhat embarrassing. They really do not know how to handle this increased interest. They want to be treated like adults and do not know how to achieve this.

How well and how fast adolescents progress through the various stages of identity development depends on how well they are able to handle crises. Minority adolescents tend to have more identity crises than others. In general, anti-social behavior usually peaks at around the eighth or ninth grade.

Body image is a great concern at this point in life. Peers continually make comparisons, and certainly the media lead to unrealistic ideas of what the "perfect" body should look like. This is a time when eating disorders are common. It also is a time when self-destructive behaviors begin, such as use of tobacco, alcohol, and illicit drugs. Depression and suicide are more common at this age group than in any other.

Adolescents want to be treated like adults.

Depression and suicide are more common during adolescence than in any other age group.

Ethical Development

As adolescents develop their capacity for logical, analytical, and abstract thinking, they begin to develop a personal code of ethics. Just as they get disappointed when adults do not live up to their expectations, they tend to get disappointed in anyone who does not meet their personal code of ethics.

EARLY ADULTHOOD

Between the ages of 20 and 40 years, heart rate averages 70 beats per minute, respiratory rate averages between 12 and 20 breaths per minute, blood pressure averages 120/80 mmHg, and body temperature averages 98.6°F (37°C). This is the period of life during which adults develop life-long habits and routines.

Peak physical condition occurs between the ages of 19 and 26 years of age, when all body systems are at optimal performance levels. At the end of this period, the body begins its slowing process. Spinal disks settle, leading to a decrease in height. Fatty tissue increases, leading to weight gain. Muscle strength decreases, and reaction times level off and stabilize. Accidents are a leading cause of death in this age group.

The highest levels of job stress occur at this point in life, the time in which the young adult strives to find his place in the world. Love develops, both romantic and affectionate. Childbirth is most common in this age group, with new families providing new challenges and stress. In spite of all this, this period is not associated with psychological problems related to well-being.

> *Peak physical condition occurs between the ages of 19 and 26 years of age, when all body systems are at optimal performance levels.*
>

> *Accidents are a leading cause of death in early adulthood.*
>

MIDDLE ADULTHOOD

Between the ages of 41 and 60 years, average vital signs are as follows: heart rate, 70 beats per minute; respiratory rate between 12 to 20 breaths per minute; blood pressure at 120/80 mmHg; and body temperature averages 98.6°F (37°C).

The body still functions at a high level with varying degrees of degradation based on the individual. There are usually some vision and hearing changes during this period. Cardiovascular health becomes a concern, with cardiac output decreasing and cholesterol levels increasing. Cancer often strikes this age group, weight control becomes more difficult, and for women in the late 40s to early 50s, menopause commences.

Adults in this age group are more concerned with the "social clock" and become more task oriented as they see the time for accomplishing their life-time goals recede. Still, they tend to approach problems more as challenges than as threats. This is also the time of life for "empty-nest syndrome," or the time after the last offspring has left home. Some women feel depression or a sense of loss and purposelessness at this time, feelings that are made worse by aging and menopause. Sometimes a father also becomes depressed, but the syndrome seems to affect mothers to a greater extent. Many parents, however, view the period after children have left home as a time of increased freedom and opportunity for self fulfillment. Unfortunately, adults in this age group often find themselves burdened by financial commitments for elderly parents, as well as for young adult children.

> *Cardiovascular health becomes a concern during middle adulthood.*
>
>

* **maximum life span** the theoretical, species-specific, longest duration of life, excluding premature or "unnatural" death.

* **life expectancy** based on the year of birth, the average number of additional years of life expected for a member of a population.

LATE ADULTHOOD

Maximum life span is the theoretical, species-specific, longest duration of life, excluding premature or "unnatural" death. For human beings, maximum life span is approximately 120 years. **Life expectancy,** which is based on the year of birth, is defined as the average number of additional years of life expected for a member of a population. Human beings almost always die of disease or accident before they reach their biological limit.

PHYSIOLOGICAL DEVELOPMENT

Vital Signs

At 61 years of age and older, vital signs—heart rate, respiratory rate, and blood pressure—depend on the individual's physical health status. Body temperature still averages 98.6°F (37°C).

Cardiovascular System

During late adulthood, the cardiovascular system changes in ways that affect its overall function. The walls of the blood vessels thicken, causing increased peripheral vascular resistance and reduced blood flow to organs. There is decreased baroreceptor sensitivity and, by 80 years of age, there is approximately a 50% decrease in vessel elasticity.

In addition, the heart tends to show disease in the heart muscle, heart valves, and coronary arteries. Increased workload causes cardiomegaly (enlargement), mitral and aortic valve changes, and decreased myocardial elasticity. The myocardium is less able to respond to exercise, and the SA node and other cells responsible for producing heartbeats become infiltrated with fibrous connective tissue and fat. Pacemaker cells diminish, resulting in arrhythmia. Because of prolonged contraction time, decreased response to various medications that would ordinarily stimulate the heart, and increased resistance to electrical stimulation, the heart also becomes less able to contract. Tachycardia (abnormally rapid heart action) is not well tolerated.

Functional blood volume decreases in late adulthood. Decreases also can be expected in platelet count and the number of red blood cells (RBCs), which can lead to poor iron levels.

Respiratory System

The trachea and large airways increase in diameter in late adulthood, and enlargement of the end units of the airway results in a decreased surface area of the lungs. Decreased elasticity of the lungs leads to an increase in lung volume and to a reduction in surface area. The decreased elasticity also causes the chest to expand and the diaphragm to descend. The end of the ribs calcifies to the breastbone, producing stiffening of the chest wall, which increases the workload of the respiratory muscles.

These changes lead to an increased likelihood for older adults to develop lung disease and progressive declines in lung function. Metabolic changes also may lead to decreased lung function, and because of life-long exposure to pollutants, diffusion through alveoli is diminished. Coughing also becomes ineffective because of a weakened chest wall and bone structure. Of all the factors that influence lung function, smoking continues to produce the greatest amount of disability.

Endocrine System

During this stage of life, there is a decrease in glucose metabolism and insulin production. The thyroid shows some diminished triiodothyronine (T3) production, cortisol (from the adrenal cortex) is diminished by 25%, the pituitary gland is 20% less effective, and reproductive organs atrophy in women.

At 61 years of age and older, vital signs—heart rate, respiratory rate, and blood pressure—depend on the individual's physical health status.

During late adulthood, the cardiovascular system changes in ways that affect its overall function.

Changes in the respiratory system lead to an increased likelihood for older adults to develop lung disease and progressive declines in lung function.

Gastrointestinal System

One way the gastrointestinal system is affected at this stage of life is by way of tooth loss. Age-related dental changes do not necessarily lead to loss of teeth. Usually tooth loss is caused by cavities or periodontal disease, both of which may be prevented by good dental hygiene. With age, the location of cavities in teeth changes and an increasing amount of root cavities and cavities around existing sites of previous dental work are seen. Tooth loss can lead to changes in diet, an increased chance of malnutrition, and serious vitamin and mineral deficiencies.

This is also true when the individual has false teeth, which do not completely restore normal chewing ability and can reduce taste sensation. In addition, alterations in swallowing are more common in older people without teeth because they tend to swallow larger pieces of food. Swallowing takes 50% to 100% longer, probably because of subtle changes in the swallowing mechanism. Peristalsis is decreased and the esophageal sphincter is less effective.

In general, the gastrointestinal system shows less age-associated change in function than other body systems. Stomach contractions appear to be normal, but it does take longer to empty liquids from the stomach. The amount of stomach acid secretions decrease, probably because of the loss of the cells that produce gastric acid. There is usually a small amount of atrophy to the lining of the small intestine. In the large intestine, expect to see atrophy of the lining, changes in the muscle layer, and blood vessel abnormalities. Approximately one of every three people over 60 has diverticula, or outpouchings, in the lining of the large intestine resulting from increased pressure inside the intestine. Weakness in the bowel wall also may be a contributing factor.

The number of some opiate receptors increase with aging, which may lead to significant constipation when narcotics are ingested. Changes may occur in the metabolism and in absorption of some sugars, calcium, and iron. Highly fat-soluble compounds such as vitamin A appear to be absorbed faster with age. The activity of some enzymes such as lactase—which aids in the digestion of some sugars, particularly those found in dairy products—appears to decrease. The absorption of fat also may change, and the metabolism of specific compounds, including drugs, can be significantly prolonged in elderly people.

Renal System

With aging, there is a 25% to 30% decrease in kidney mass. About 50% of nephrons are lost and abnormal glomeruli are more common. Reduced kidney function leads to a decreased clearance of some drugs and decreased elimination. The kidney's hormonal response to dehydration is reduced as is the ability to retain salt under conditions when it should be conserved. The ability of the kidneys to modify vitamin D to a more active form may also lessen.

The Senses

Taste buds diminish during this stage of life, which leads to a loss of taste sensation. Smell declines rapidly after the age of 50 and the parts of the brain involved in smell degenerate significantly so that by age 80, the detection of smell is almost 50% poorer than it was at its peak. Since taste and smell work together to make enjoyment of food possible, appetite often declines. Response to painful stimuli is diminished as is kinesthetic sense, or the ability to sense movement.

Visual acuity and reaction time is diminished, and there are actual changes in the organs of hearing. The ear canal atrophies, the eardrum thickens, and there may be degenerative and even arthritic changes in the small joints connecting the bones in the middle ear. Significant changes take place in the inner ear. These changes in structure significantly affect hearing. Hearing loss for pure tones, which increases with age in men and women, is called "presbycusis." With presbycusis, higher frequencies become less audible than lower frequencies. Pitch discrimination plays an important role in speech perception so, with age, speech discrimination declines. When exposed to loud background noise or indistinct speech, older people hear less, but at the same time, they may be very sensitive to loud sounds.

Nervous System

With aging, there is a decrease of neurotransmitters and a loss of neurons in the cerebellum, which controls coordination, and the hippocampus, which is involved in some aspects of memory function. The sleep-wake cycle also is disrupted, causing older adults to have sleep problems.

PSYCHOSOCIAL DEVELOPMENT

While disease may reduce physical and mental capabilities, the ability to learn and adjust continues throughout life, greatly influenced by interests, activity, motivation, health, and income (Figure 5-6). However, there is a **terminal-drop hypothesis** that there is a decrease in cognitive functioning over a five-year period prior to death. The individual may or may not be aware of diffuse changes in mood, mental functioning, or the way his body responds.

✱ **terminal-drop hypothesis** a theory that death is preceded by a five-year period of decreasing cognitive functioning.

Housing

While most older adults would rather stay in their own homes, it is not always possible because home-care services are not affordably available in all communities as a viable alternative to nursing homes. Home-care services usually provide assistance with household chores such as preparing meals, cleaning and laundry, and performing personal care tasks such as feeding and bathing. Health-care services in the home are provided by nurses and physical or speech therapists. In order to be eligible for these services under Medicare, the patient must be home-bound, need an intensive level of services, and be expected to benefit from such services over a reasonable amount of time. Home-care services are usually time-limited.

An alternative to home-care services is "assisted living," or living in a facility that offers a combination of home care and nursing home facilities. There is a greater sense of control, independence, and privacy because the older adult has more choices while still being in an institutional setting. Bedrooms and bathrooms can be locked by residents, but dining and recreational facilities are usually shared.

About 95% of older adults live in communities, from simple groupings of homes where mostly older adults live to a relatively new type of living arrangement called the "continuing-care retirement community." The appeal of these communities is that future health-care needs are covered in a setting that is an attractive residential campus where cultural and recreational activities are available. Entrance fees to this type of community may be as much as $250,000, plus monthly fees which average $1000.

Challenges

One of the major challenges for the older adult is maintaining a sense of self-worth. Senior citizens are commonly seen as "over the hill," less intelligent than younger adults, and certainly less able to care for themselves. Many older adults

FIGURE 5-6 The ability to learn and adjust continues throughout life.

It is not until adults reach the age of 40 that ill health—as opposed to accidents, homicide, and suicide—becomes the major cause of death.

are forced into retirement because they are seen as less productive. In reality, although older workers may have slowed down a bit, they are often more concerned with producing quality work than younger workers. Another problem older adults face at this stage of life is a feeling of declining well-being. It is not until adults reach the age of 40 that ill health—as opposed to accidents, homicide, and suicide—becomes the major cause of death. Arteriosclerotic heart disease is the major killer after the age of 40 in all age, sex, and racial groups.

Financial Burdens

The duration of each state in the life cycle, and the ages of family members for each stage, will vary from family to family. Obviously, this will have an effect on the financial status of families. For example, a couple who completes their family while in their early adult years will have a different life-style when their last child leaves home than a couple with a "change-of-life" child. Late children can cause serious economic problems for retirees on fixed incomes who are trying to meet the staggering costs of education.

Retirement brings about changes for both spouses, but it seems to be particularly stressful for those wives who are not prepared emotionally or financially.

Retirement usually means a decrease in income and in the standard of living, which can be very difficult to handle.

A decreasing level of interest in work is natural as one grows older, but it has a severe impact on the income of older people. Almost 22% of all older people live in households below the poverty level. More than 50% of all single women above the age of 60 live at or below the poverty level. Older women in the United States make up the single poorest group in our society.

Dying Companions or Death

Whether it is the death of a companion or one's own impending death, fear and grief seem to have a great deal in common. Grief not only follows death, but when there is advance warning, grief may well precede death. Frequently, the death or impending death of a companion leads us to fear for our own lives. Psychiatrist Elisabeth Kübler-Ross believes that regardless of whether it is one's own death or the death of a companion, everyone must go through certain emotions. While the five stages in her theory may sometimes overlap, everyone must deal with each of the stages of death before the grieving process ends. (Review Chapter 1 for Kübler-Ross's five stages.)

Note: Human physiological and psychosocial development will be discussed in more detail in later chapters.

SUMMARY

The changes that take place during the span of a lifetime are innumerable. At some stages, the changes seem to occur almost daily. It is only through experience with patients at all of the various stages of life that you will come to feel comfortable dealing with each of them. Remember that no matter what the stage of development, patience and a sincere desire to help a patient will help you to make the right decisions about emergency care.

CHAPTER 6

General Principles of Pharmacology

Please refer to the *Drug Guide for Paramedics* that accompanies this program as a special supplement.

Objectives

Part 1: Basic Pharmacology (begins on p. 340)

After reading Part 1 of this chapter, you should be able to:

1. Describe important historical trends in pharmacology. (p. 340)
2. Differentiate among the chemical, generic (nonproprietary), official (USP), and trade (proprietary) names of a drug. (pp. 340–341)
3. List the four main sources of drug products. (p. 341)
4. List the authoritative sources for drug information. (pp. 341–342)
5. List legislative acts controlling drug use and abuse in the United States. (pp. 343–344)
6. Differentiate among Schedule I, II, III, IV, and V substances and list examples of substances in each schedule. (p. 343)
7. Discuss standardization of drugs. (p. 344)
8. Discuss special considerations in drug treatment with regard to pregnant, pediatric, and geriatric patients. (pp. 346–348)
9. Discuss the paramedic's responsibilities and scope of management pertinent to the administration of medications. (pp. 344–346)
10. Review the specific anatomy and physiology pertinent to pharmacology. (pp. 348–360)
11. List and describe general properties of drugs. (pp. 355–357)
12. List and describe liquid and solid drug forms. (p. 354)
13. List and differentiate routes of drug administration. (pp. 352–354)
14. Differentiate between enteral and parenteral routes of drug administration. (pp. 353–354)
15. Describe mechanisms of drug action. (pp. 355–357)

Continued

Part 2: Drug Classifications (begins on p. 360)

After reading Part 2 of this chapter, you should be able to:

INTRODUCTION

The use of herbs and minerals to treat the sick and injured has been documented as long ago as 2,000 B.C. Ancient Egyptians, Arabs, and Greeks probably passed formulations down through generations by word of mouth for centuries until they were finally recorded in pharmacopeias. By the end of the Renaissance, pharmacology was a distinct and growing discipline, separate from medicine. During the seventeenth and eighteenth centuries, tinctures of opium, coca, and digitalis were available. The related concept of vaccination with biologic extracts began in 1796 with Edward Jenner's smallpox inoculations. By the nineteenth century, atropine, chloroform, codeine, ether, and morphine were in use. The discoveries of animal insulin and penicillin in the early twentieth century dramatically changed the treatment of endocrine/metabolic and infectious diseases. Now, at the start of the twenty-first century, recombinant DNA technology has produced human insulin and tissue plasminogen activator (tPA). These drugs have markedly changed the treatment of diabetes and cardiovascular disease.

Presently in the United States, the Food and Drug Administration (FDA) is allowing many previously prescription-only drugs to become available over the counter. This is due in part to a growing consumer awareness in health care and also in part to consumer marketing by the pharmaceutical industry. The industry is actively seeking drugs that appeal widely to the consumer for treatments and cures. Pharmaceutical research to limit aging or increase the life span is growing rapidly. The federal government also offers incentives to pharmaceutical companies to research drugs for rare diseases. These so-called "orphan drugs" are often expensive to investigate and have a limited sales potential, making them less profitable to develop and manufacture than others.

General principles of pharmacology are presented in this chapter, which is divided into two parts:

Part 1: Basic Pharmacology
Part 2: Drug Classifications

Part 1: Basic Pharmacology

Part 1 concerns the basics of pharmacology. Drug names (including chemical, generic, official, and brand names) will be explained. The sources of drugs, reference materials for drugs, components of a drug profile, and legal considerations will be described. A major focus of Part 1 will be the safe and effective administration of medications, including the "six rights" (right medication, dose, time, route, patient, and documentation) as well as special considerations in medication administration for pregnant, pediatric, and geriatric patients. Finally, basic concepts of pharmacology, specifically pharmacokinetics and pharmacodynamics, will be examined.

✱ **drug** chemical used to diagnose, treat, or prevent disease.

✱ **pharmacology** the study of drugs and their interactions with the body.

NAMES

Drugs are chemicals used to diagnose, treat, or prevent disease. **Pharmacology** is the study of drugs and their actions on the body. To study and converse about pharmacology, health care professionals must have a systematic method for naming drugs. The most detailed name for any drug is its chemical description, which states its chemical composition and molecular structure. Ethyl-1-methyl-4-phenylisonipecotate hydrochloride, for example, is a chemical name. A generic name is usually suggested by the manufacturer and confirmed by the United States Adopted Name Council. It becomes the Federal Drug Administration's (FDA) official name when listed in the *United States Pharmacopeia* (USP), the official standard for information about pharmaceuticals in the United States. In the case of ethyl-1-methyl-4-phenylisonipecotate hydrochloride, the generic name is meperidine hydrochloride, USP. To foster brand loyalty among its customers, the manufacturer gives the drug a brand name (sometimes called a trade name or proprietary name)—in our example, Demerol. The brand name is a proper name and should be capitalized. Most manufacturers also register the name as a trademark, so the stylized ® or ™ may follow the name, as in Demerol®. Another example is the widely prescribed sedative Valium:

- *Chemical Name:* 7-chloro-1, 3-dihydro-1-methyl-5-phenyl-2H-1, 4-benzodiazepin-2-one
- *Generic Name:* diazepam
- *Official Name:* diazepam, USP
- *Brand Name:* Valium®

SOURCES

The four main sources of drugs are plants, animals, minerals, and the laboratory (synthetic). Plants may be the oldest source of medications; primitive people probably used them directly as "herbal" medicines. Indirectly, plant extracts such as gums and oils have long been a source of medications. Examples include the purple foxglove, a source of digitalis (a glycoside), and deadly nightshade, a source of atropine (an alkaloid). Animal extracts are another important source of drugs. For many years the primary sources of insulin for treating diabetes mellitus were the extracts of bovine (cow) and porcine (pig) pancreas. Minerals are inorganic sources of drugs such as calcium chloride and magnesium sulfate. Synthetic drugs are created in the laboratory. They may provide alternative sources of medications for those found in nature, or they may be entirely new medications not found in nature.

REFERENCE MATERIALS

Obtaining information on drugs can be difficult. Using multiple sources of information about drugs is usually a good idea. Every book about drugs, including this one, has a disclaimer regarding doses and current uses, referring the reader to local medical direction for the final word. Using multiple sources and comparing the authors' statements about a drug may lead you to the best available information. EMS providers generally like small, short guides that they can carry in a shirt pocket. These usually include important details about drugs that out-of-hospital providers administer along with a long list of commonly prescribed drugs and their classes. These EMS guides will be useful if you clearly understand the drugs used in your system and have a working knowledge of commonly prescribed drug classes.

Drug inserts, the printed fact sheets that drug manufacturers supply with most medications, contain information prescribed by the United States Food and Drug Administration. The *Physician's Desk Reference*, a compilation of these drug inserts, also includes three indices and a section containing photographs of

It is helpful to carry a pharmaceutical reference in paramedic response vehicles.

drugs. It is among the most popular references, but it contains only factual information and must be interpreted by informed readers. The American Hospital Formulary Service annually publishes *Drug Information* as a service to the American Society of Health System Pharmacists. It contains an authoritative listing of monographs on virtually every drug used in the United States. A less bulky reference to keep in an ambulance might be one of the many drug guides for nurses. They contain information on hundreds of drugs in a format much like the EMS drug guides, but they also offer information on commonly prescribed drugs rather than only on emergency drugs. Also popular is the *Monthly Prescribing Reference*. Designed to assist physicians in prescribing medications, it can also help them determine which medications are available for treating specific diseases. Its information about new medications is especially useful. Most hospitals also maintain a listing of drugs, or formulary, that profiles the particular drugs they have available. The American Medical Association also publishes a useful reference, the *AMA Drug Evaluation*. The World Wide Web (WWW) provides an enormous amount of information, but you must be especially cautious when using it as a source, because it allows anyone with a computer to be a publisher, with no requirement for accuracy.

COMPONENTS OF A DRUG PROFILE

A drug's profile describes its various properties. As a paramedic student, you will become familiar with drug profiles as you study specific medications. A typical drug profile will contain the following information:

- *Names.* These most frequently include the generic and trade names, although the occasional reference will include chemical names.
- *Classification.* This is the broad group to which the drug belongs. Knowing classifications is essential to understanding the properties of drugs.
- *Mechanism of Action.* The way in which a drug causes its effects; its pharmacodynamics.
- *Indications.* Conditions that make administration of the drug appropriate (as approved by the Food and Drug Administration).
- *Pharmacokinetics.* How the drug is absorbed, distributed, and eliminated; typically includes onset and duration of action.
- *Side effects/adverse reactions.* The drug's untoward or undesired effects.
- *Routes of administration.* How the drug is given.
- *Contraindications.* Conditions that make it inappropriate to give the drug. Unlike when the drug is simply not indicated, a contraindication means that a predictable harmful event will occur if the drug is given in this situation.
- *Dosage.* The amount of the drug that should be given.
- *How supplied.* This typically includes the common concentrations of the available preparations; many drugs come in different concentrations.
- *Special considerations.* How the drug may affect pediatric, geriatric, or pregnant patients.

Drug profiles may also include other components, such as its interactions with other drugs or with foods, when appropriate.

LEGAL

Knowing and obeying the laws and regulations governing medications and their administration will be an important part of your career. These laws and regulations come from three distinct authorities: federal law, state laws and regulations, and individual agency regulations.

Federal Drug legislation in the United States has been aimed primarily at protecting the public from adulterated or mislabeled drugs. The *Pure Food and Drug Act of 1906*, enacted to improve the quality and labeling of drugs, named the United States Pharmacopeia as this country's official source for drug information. The *Harrison Narcotic Act of 1914* limited the indiscriminate use of addicting drugs by regulating the importation, manufacture, sale, and use of opium, cocaine, and their compounds or derivatives. *The Federal Food, Drug and Cosmetic Act of 1938* empowered the Food and Drug Administration (FDA) to enforce and set premarket safety standards for drugs. In 1951, the *Durham-Humphrey Amendments* to the 1938 act (also known as the prescription drug amendments) required pharmacists to have either a written or verbal prescription from a physician to dispense certain drugs. It also created the category of over-the-counter medications. The *Comprehensive Drug Abuse Prevention and Control Act* (also known as the Controlled Substances Act) of 1970 is the most recent major federal legislation affecting drug sales and use. It repealed and replaced the Harrison Narcotic Act.

The federal government strictly regulates controlled substances because of their high potential for abuse. Since not all drugs cause the same level of physical or psychological dependence, they do not all need to be regulated in the same way. To accommodate their differences, the Controlled Substance Act of 1970 created five schedules of controlled substances, each with its own level of control and record keeping requirements (Table 6-1). Most emergency medical services administer only a few controlled substances, usually a narcotic analgesic such as morphine sulfate and a benzodiazepine anticonvulsant such as diazepam.

The majority of the remaining drugs provided by an EMS are prescription drugs—those whose use the FDA has designated sufficiently dangerous to require

Know and obey the laws and regulations governing medications and their administration.

Content Review

DRUG LAWS AND REGULATIONS

- Federal law
- State laws and regulations
- Individual agency regulations

Table 6-1	SCHEDULES OF DRUGS ACCORDING TO THE CONTROLLED SUBSTANCES ACT OF 1970.	
Schedule	**Description**	**Examples**
Schedule I	High abuse potential; may lead to severe dependence; no accepted medical indications; used for research, analysis or instruction only	Heroin, LSD, mescaline
Schedule II	High abuse potential; may lead to severe dependence; accepted medical indications	Opium, cocaine, morphine, codeine, oxycodone, methadone, secobarbital
Schedule III	Less abuse potential than Schedule I and II; may lead to moderate or low physical dependence or high psychological dependence; accepted medical indications	Limited opioid amounts or combined with noncontrolled substances: Vicodin, Tylenol with codeine
Schedule IV	Low abuse potential compared to Schedule III; limited psychological and/or physical dependence; accepted medical indications	Diazepam, lorazepam, phenobarbital
Schedule V	Lower abuse potential compared to Schedule IV; may lead to limited physical or psychological dependence; accepted medical indications	Limited amounts of opioids; often for cough or diarrhea

the supervision of a health care practitioner (physician, dentist, and in some states, nurse practitioner or certified physician's assistant). For emergency medical services this means the physician medical director is in effect prescribing the drugs in advance, based on the assessments and judgments of EMS providers in the field.

Over-the-counter (OTC) medications are generally available in small doses and, when taken as recommended, present a low risk to patients. Of the few OTC drugs that EMS providers administer, acetaminophen and aspirin are probably the most common. Although laws vary from state to state, they still require most EMS providers to obtain a physician's order (either written, verbal, or standing) to administer OTC drugs.

Federal drug laws require that certain substances be appropriately secured, distributed, and accounted for. Because of the complexity of this issue and the large variability of drugs used in EMS systems across the country, specific answers to these concerns are not practical here. Consult your local protocols, laws, and most importantly, medical director for guidance in this area.

State State laws vary widely. Some states have legislated which medications are appropriate for paramedics to give, while others have left those decisions to local control. Local control varies as well. In some areas, regional EMS authorities set the local standards; in others the individual medical directors and department directors do. In all cases, however, the physician medical director can delegate to paramedics the authority to administer medications, either by written, verbal, or standing order. You must know the laws of the state where you practice.

Local In each community, local leaders are responsible for ensuring public safety. Local EMS agencies have the responsibility to create local policies and procedures to ensure the public well being. An excellent example of a local procedure protecting the patient (and thereby the individual EMS provider and agency) would be a requirement to use a pulse oximeter whenever a patient is sedated or paralyzed. While this requirement would not have the force of law, it would locally help to ensure that local EMS providers do not overlook hypoxia in these patients.

Standards Because some generic drugs affect patients differently than their brand name counterparts, standardization of drugs is a necessity. Despite FDA standards, drugs sold or distributed by various manufacturers may have biological or therapeutic differences. An **assay** determines the amount and purity of a given chemical in a preparation in the laboratory (in vitro). While two generically equivalent preparations may contain the same amount of a given chemical (drug), they may have different therapeutic effects. This relative therapeutic effectiveness of chemically equivalent drugs is their **bioequivalence.** Bioequivalence is determined by a **bioassay,** which attempts to ascertain the drug's availability in a biological model (in vivo). Again, the *United States Pharmacopeia* (USP) is the official standard for the United States.

PATIENT CARE: THE SAFE AND EFFECTIVE ADMINISTRATION OF MEDICATIONS

Paramedics are responsible for the standard of care for patients in their charge. They are, therefore, personally responsible—legally, morally, and ethically—for the safe and effective administration of medications. The following guidelines will help you to meet that responsibility:

- Know the precautions and contraindications for all medications you administer.
- Practice proper technique.

Consult local protocols, laws, and, medical direction for guidance in securing and distributing controlled substances.

* **assay** test that determines the amount and purity of a given chemical in a preparation in the laboratory.

* **bioequivalence** relative therapeutic effectiveness of chemically equivalent drugs.

* **bioassay** test to ascertain a drug's availability in a biological model.

- Know how to observe and document drug effects.
- Maintain a current knowledge in pharmacology.
- Establish and maintain professional relationships with other health care providers.
- Understand the pharmacokinetics and pharmacodynamics.
- Have current medication references available.
- Take careful drug histories including:
  - Name, strength, and daily dose of prescribed drugs
  - Over-the-counter drugs
  - Vitamins
  - Herbal medications
  - Folk-medicine or folk-remedies
  - Allergies
- Evaluate the compliance, dosage, and adverse reactions.
- Consult with medical direction when appropriate.

SIX RIGHTS OF MEDICATION ADMINISTRATION

No pharmacology chapter would be complete without discussing the six rights of medication administration. They include the right medication, the right dose, the right time, the right route, the right patient, and the right documentation.

Right Medication When following a physician's verbal medication order, repeat the order back to him to confirm that you both intend the same thing for the patient. Inspect the label on the drug at least three times before giving the medication to the patient: first, as you remove the medication from the drug box or cabinet; second, as you draw the medication into the syringe or dole the tablet into a cup; third, immediately before you administer the medication. Failure to confirm the medication name is one of the most common medication administration errors. If you have any question about a drug, do not administer it without confirmation. Showing the medication container to your partner and asking for confirmation is an easy way to further ensure that you are giving the right drug.

Right Dose To reduce medication errors, many drugs come in unit **dose packaging.** That is, the package contains a single dose for a single patient. Dosages of many emergency drugs, however, are based on patient weight, so a prefilled syringe may not contain the exact amount a patient needs. You will have to calculate the correct dose. One good practice for identifying potential medication errors is to consider the number of unit dose packages needed for a single dose. If your calculations tell you to open ten vials for one dose of medication, prudence requires you to check the calculation and dose carefully. The package may contain a unit dose of the wrong medication, or you may have miscalculated.

Right Time While paramedics usually give medications in urgent and emergent situations rather than on a schedule, timing can still be very important. Giving nitroglycerin tablets too soon may precipitate hypotension; if epinephrine is not repeated on time during cardiac arrest it may not help to lower the threshold for defibrillation. Take care to give medications punctually and to document their administration promptly.

Right Route You often will have to choose from among several treatments for a particular problem. In these cases, knowing the principles of pharmacokinetics can help greatly in giving your patient the medication via the right route. For example, your knowledge that you should administer epinephrine intravenously rather than subcutaneously to the patient in anaphylactic shock because his blood is being shunted away from the skin will guide you to the proper administration route.

Content Review

SIX RIGHTS OF MEDICATION ADMINISTRATION
- Right medication
- Right dose
- Right time
- Right route
- Right patient
- Right documentation

✱ **dose packaging** medication packages contain a single dose for a single patient.

Right Patient As the paramedic's role in health care expands, you will find yourself caring for more people than just "the patient in the back of the truck." You will deal with multiple patients, and the potential for giving medication to the wrong patient will be real. You will have to identify patients by name before administering medications.

Right Documentation The drugs you administer in the field do not stop affecting your patients when they enter the hospital. As a result, you must completely document all of your care, especially any drugs you have administered, so that long after you have gone on to your next call, other providers will know what drugs your patient has had.

SPECIAL CONSIDERATIONS

Pregnant Patients Any time you administer drugs to a woman of childbearing years, you must consider the possibility that she is pregnant. Treating pregnant patients clearly means treating two patients. Although emphasis appropriately seems to center on the mother during care, you must understand that many drugs that affect the mother also affect the fetus. A drug's possible benefits to the mother must clearly outweigh its potential risks to the fetus. For example, some situations such as cardiac arrest justify giving the mother medications that may harm the fetus because the drug's possible harm to the fetus is clearly outweighed by the fetus's certain death if the mother dies.

Pregnancy presents two particular pharmacological problems: changes in the mother's anatomy and physiology, and the potential for drugs to harm the fetus. Because the mother is supporting the fetus entirely, her heart rate, cardiac output, and blood volume will increase. This altered maternal physiology can affect the onset and duration of action of many medications. During the first trimester of pregnancy the ingestion of some drugs (**teratogenic drugs**) may potentially deform, injure, or kill the fetus. During the last trimester, drugs administered to the mother may pass through the placenta to the fetus. Some of these drugs will have unwanted effects on the fetus. Others may not be metabolized and/or excreted, possibly resulting in toxic accumulations. Additionally, a breast-feeding mother's milk may pass some drugs to her infant.

Under some conditions, of course, the health and safety of mother and fetus demand the use of drugs during the pregnancy. Examples include pregnancy-induced diabetes, hypertension, and seizure disorders. To help health care providers determine when drugs are needed during pregnancy, the FDA has developed the classification system shown in Table 6-2. Always consult medical direction for any questions about drug safety in pregnancy.

Pediatric Patients Several physiological factors affect pharmacokinetics in newborns and young children. These patients' absorption of oral medications is less than an adult's due to various differences in gastric pH, gastric emptying time, and low enzyme levels. A newborn's skin is thinner than an older patient's and is therefore more permeable to topically administered drugs. This can result in unexpected toxicity. Older children still have less gastric acid than adults do, but their gastric emptying times reach an adult's around the sixth to eighth month of life. Because children up to a year old have diminished plasma protein concentrations, drugs that bind to proteins have higher **free drug availability.** That is, a greater proportion of the drug will be available in the body to cause either desired or undesired effects. Water distribution is different in the neonate as well. Neonates have a much higher proportion of extracellular fluid (nearly 80 percent) than adults (50–55 percent). This higher amount of water means a greater volume and, with less than expected protein binding, may require higher drug doses. The premature infant is especially susceptible to drugs penetrating the *blood-brain barrier* because his immature connective tissues form a weaker obstacle.

✳ **teratogenic drug** medication that may deform or kill the fetus.

Children are not "small adults." Drug dosages must consider the various physiological differences.

✳ **free drug availability** proportion of a drug available in the body to cause either desired or undesired effects.

Table 6-2 FDA PREGNANCY CATEGORIES

Category	Description
A	Adequate studies in pregnant women have not demonstrated a risk to the fetus in the first trimester or later trimesters.
B	Animal studies have not demonstrated a risk to the fetus, *but* there are no adequate studies in pregnant women. OR Adequate studies in pregnant women have not demonstrated a risk to the fetus in the first trimester and there is no risk in the last trimester, *but* animal studies have demonstrated adverse effects.
C	Animal studies have demonstrated adverse effects, *but* there are no adequate studies in pregnant women; however, benefits may be acceptable despite the potential risks. OR No adequate animal studies or adequate studies of pregnant women have been done.
D	Fetal risk has been demonstrated. In certain circumstances, benefits could outweigh the risks.
X	Fetal risk has been demonstrated. This risk outweighs any possible benefit to the mother. Avoid using in pregnant or potentially pregnant patients.

The newborn's metabolic rates may be much lower than an adult's, but they rise rapidly and by a few years of age may triple an adult's. These metabolic rates then decline steadily until early adolescence, when they reach adult levels. A newborn's low metabolic rate and incompletely developed hepatic system put him at higher risk for toxic interactions. Neonates' metabolic pathways also are different from an adult's, meaning that some drugs will not have the expected effect or may have other, unexpected effects. Finally, the neonatal renal and hepatic systems' immaturity delays elimination of many drugs and their metabolites. Dosing schedules may have to be adjusted to accommodate longer half-lives until these systems mature at about six months to one year of age.

With all of these factors, a pediatric patient's drug function can differ radically from an adult's. Pediatric drug dosages must be individualized to minimize the risks of toxicity. Body surface area and weight are the two most common factors in calculating dosages. The Broselow tape gives a good approximation for children of average height/weight ratio. It bases its calculations on the child's height (length), and assumes the child's weight is at the fiftieth percentile for his height (Figure 6-1). The Broselow tape primarily addresses drugs administered in the critical care setting.

Geriatric Patients Significant changes in pharmacokinetics may also occur in patients older than about 60 years. They may absorb oral medications slower due to decreased gastrointestinal motility. Decreased plasma protein concentration may alter distribution of drugs in their systems, leaving drugs free that would otherwise have been protein bound. Body fat increases and muscle mass decreases with age; therefore, lipid soluble drugs may have greater deposition, thereby lowering the amount of available drug. Absorption and distribution of intramuscular injections may alter if volumes are inappropriate for the remaining muscle mass. Because the liver primarily handles biotransformation, depressed liver function in an aging patient may delay or prolong drug action. The aging process may also slow elimination by the renal system.

Older patients are also more likely to be on multiple medications or to have multiple underlying disease processes. Various medication interactions can have

Use caution when administering medications to older patients because they are apt to be on multiple medications.

FIGURE 6-1   A Broselow tape is useful for calculating drug dosages for pediatric patients.

a severe impact on patients. For example, sildenafil (Viagra) and nitroglycerin given together may cause severe hypotension. Underlying diseases may affect therapeutics in unexpected ways. Congestive heart failure, for instance, may cause congestion of the gastrointestinal tract's vasculature, delaying the absorption of oral medications. The congestive heart failure patient may also have compromised renal function, delaying his elimination of drugs.

PHARMACOLOGY

Pharmacology is the study of drugs and their interactions with the body. Drugs do not confer any new properties on cells or tissues; they only modify or exploit existing functions. They may be given for their local action (in which case systemic absorption of the drug is discouraged) or for systemic action. Although generally given for a specific effect, drugs tend to have multiple actions at multiple sites, so they must be thought of in terms of their systemic effects rather than in terms of an isolated single effect. Pharmacology's two major divisions are pharmacokinetics and pharmacodynamics. You have already learned that **pharmacokinetics** addresses how drugs are transported into and out of the body. **Pharmacodynamics** deals with their effects once they reach the target tissues.

PHARMACOKINETICS

Strictly defined, pharmacokinetics is the study of the basic processes that determine the duration and intensity of a drug's effect. These four processes are absorption, distribution, biotransformation, and elimination.

Review of Physiology of Transport

Pharmacokinetics is dependent upon the body's various physiological mechanisms that move substances across the body's compartments. These mechanisms can be broken down into two broad categories based on their energy requirements and

✱ **pharmacokinetics** how drugs are transported into and out of the body.

✱ **pharmacodynamics** how a drug interacts with the body to cause its effects.

Content Review

PHARMACOKINETIC PROCESSES
- Absorption
- Distribution
- Biotransformation
- Elimination

then further classified. A mechanism is referred to as **active transport** if it requires the use of energy to move a substance. This energy is achieved by the breakdown of high-energy chemical bonds found in chemicals such as ATP (adenosine triphosphate). ATP is broken down into ADP (adenosine diphosphate) liberating a considerable amount of biochemical energy. A common example of an active transport mechanism is the sodium-potassium (Na^+-K^+) pump. This is a protein pump that actively moves potassium ions into the cell and sodium ions out of the cell. Because this movement goes *against* the ions' concentration gradients, it must use energy.

Large molecules, such as glucose and most of the amino acids, do not readily pass through the cell membrane because of their size. These molecules are moved across the cell membrane with the help of special "carrier" proteins found on the surface of the target cells. These large molecules are "carried" across the cell membrane in a special transport process called **carrier-mediated diffusion** or **facilitated diffusion.** Once the molecule to be transported binds with the carrier protein, the configuration of the cell membrane changes, allowing the large molecule to enter the target cell. Insulin, an important hormone secreted by the endocrine pancreas, can increase the rate of carrier-mediated glucose transport from 10- to 20-fold. This is the principle mechanism by which insulin controls glucose use in the body.

Most drugs travel through the body by means of **passive transport,** the movement of a substance without the use of energy. This requires the presence of concentration gradients in a solution. Diffusion and osmosis are forms of passive transport. **Diffusion** involves the movement of solute in the solution, while osmosis involves the movement of the solvent (usually water). In diffusion, the solute's molecules or ions move *down* their concentration gradients from an area of higher concentration to an area of lower concentration. Conversely, in osmosis the solvent's molecules move *up* the concentration gradient from an area of low solute concentration to an area of higher solute concentration. Another way of looking at this is to think of osmosis as simply the diffusion of solvent from an area of high *solvent* concentration to an area of low *solvent* concentration. A final type of passive transport is **filtration.** This is simply the movement of molecules across a membrane down a *pressure* gradient, from an area of high pressure to an area of lower pressure. This pressure typically results from the hydrostatic force of blood pressure.

Absorption

When a drug is administered to a patient it must find its way to the site of action. If a drug is given orally or injected into any place except the blood stream, its absorption into the blood stream is the first step in this process. (Since drugs given intravenously or intra-arterially enter directly into the blood stream no absorption needs to occur.) Several factors affect a drug's absorption. The body absorbs most drugs faster when they are given intramuscularly than when they are given subcutaneously. This is because muscles are more vascular than subcutaneous tissue. Of course, anything that slows blood flow will delay absorption. Shock and hypothermia are just two examples. Conversely, processes such as fever and hyperthermia increase peripheral blood flow and speed absorption.

Drugs given orally (enterally) must first survive the digestive processes before being absorbed across the mucosa of the gastrointestinal system. If a drug is not soluble in water, it will have difficulty being absorbed. Time-released medications take advantage of this with an enteric coating that slowly releases the medication. Some drugs have an enteric coating that will not dissolve in the more acidic environment of the stomach, but will dissolve in the alkaline environment of the duodenum. This allows a drug that would irritate the stomach or be destroyed by stomach acid to be passed through the stomach into the duodenum and absorbed there. Besides being able to survive stomach acid, a drug must also be somewhat lipid (fat) soluble in order to cross the cells' lipid two-layered (bilayered) membranes. Many drugs

* **active transport** requires the use of energy to move a substance.

* **carrier mediated diffusion** or **facilitated diffusion** process in which carrier proteins transport large molecules across the cell membrane.

* **passive transport** movement of a substance without the use of energy.

* **diffusion** movement of solute in a solution from an area of higher concentration to an area of lower concentration.

* **osmosis** movement of solvent in a solution from an area of lower solute concentration to an area of higher solute concentration.

* **filtration** movement of molecules across a membrane from an area of higher pressure to an area of lower pressure.

✳ **ionize** to become electrically charged or polar.

✳ **bioavailability** amount of a drug that is still active after it reaches its target tissue.

ionize, or become electrically charged or polar following administration. Generally speaking, ionized drugs do not absorb across the membranes of cells (lipid bilayers), but fortunately, most drugs do not fully ionize. Instead they reach an equilibrium between their ionized and non-ionized forms, and the non-ionized form can be absorbed. A drug's pH also affects the extent to which it ionizes. A drug that is a weak acid will ionize much more substantially in an alkaline environment than in an acidic environment; conversely, an alkaline drug will ionize more readily in an acidic environment than in an alkaline environment. For example, aspirin (an acidic drug) does not dissociate well in the stomach (an acidic environment) and is therefore readily absorbed there.

The nature of the absorbing surface and the blood flow to the administration site also affect drug absorption. The rate of absorption is directly related to the amount of surface area available for absorption. The greater the area, the faster the absorption. Much of the gastrointestinal system has multiple invaginations, or folds, that increase its surface area. Also, the greater the blood flow is to an area, the faster will be the rate of absorption. Again, the GI tract has a rich vascular system with many capillaries that perfuse its absorbing surfaces, allowing nutrients (and drugs) to diffuse into the blood stream.

Finally, the drug's concentration affects its absorption. Because drugs diffuse in the body, the higher their concentration, the more rapidly the body will absorb them. This principle is frequently used when giving a "loading dose" of a drug and following it with a "maintenance infusion." The loading dose is typically a larger dose of the same concentration of the drug. On occasion, a more concentrated solution of the drug is used as the loading dose. Regardless, the desired effect is to rapidly raise the amount of the drug in the system to a therapeutic level. This is typically followed by a continuous infusion of the drug at a lower concentration, or slower administration rate, to keep it at the therapeutic level.

Bioavailability is the measure of the amount of a drug that is still active after it reaches its target tissue. This is the bottom line as far as absorption is concerned. The goal of administering a drug is to assure sufficient bioavailability of the drug at the target tissue in order to produce the desired effect, after considering all of the absorption factors.

Distribution

Once a drug has entered the blood stream, it must be distributed throughout the body. Most drugs will pass easily from the blood stream, through the interstitial spaces, into the target cells. Some drugs, however, will bind to proteins found in the blood, most commonly albumin, and remain in the body for a prolonged time. They thus have a sustained release from the blood stream and a prolonged period of action. The therapeutic effects of a drug are primarily due to the unbound portion of the drug in the blood. A drug that is bound to plasma proteins cannot cross membranes and reach the target cells. Thus, only the unbound drug is in equilibrium with the target cells and can cross the cell membranes.

Changing the blood stream's pH can affect the protein-binding action of a drug. Tricyclic antidepressants (TCAs), for instance, are strongly bound to plasma proteins. Making the blood more alkaline increases protein-binding of the TCA molecules. Therefore, in addition to supportive therapy, serious overdoses of TCAs are treated by administering sodium bicarbonate. Sodium bicarbonate makes the blood more alkaline (raises the pH) causing increased binding of the TCA to serum proteins. Cumulatively, this decreases the amount of free drug in the blood, thus decreasing the adverse effects. Sodium bicarbonate administration also facilitates elimination of the drug through the urine.

The presence of other serum protein binding drugs can also affect drug-protein binding. For example, the drug warfarin (Coumadin) is highly protein-bound (99 percent). Its therapeutic effects are due to the one percent of the drug that is unbound and circulating in the blood stream. Aspirin molecules bind to the same binding site on the serum proteins as do warfarin molecules. Thus, when aspirin is administered to a patient on warfarin, it displaces some of the protein-bound warfarin, increasing the amount of free (unbound) warfarin in the blood. Even if it displaces only one percent of the total warfarin, it effectively doubles the available warfarin. This can lead to unwanted side-effects such as hemorrhage.

Albumin is one of the chief proteins in the blood that is available for binding with drugs. When albumin levels are low (hypoalbuminemia), as occurs in malnutrition, drugs that are normally protein bound rise to much greater blood levels than anticipated. For example, consider a patient who has been taking warfarin without difficulty. If he develops hypoalbuminemia, his normal dose of warfarin will result in much more of the drug being available in the body, possibly leading to dangerous bleeding.

Certain organs exclude some drugs from distribution. For example, the tight junctions of the capillary endothelial cells in the central nervous system (CNS) vasculature form a **blood-brain barrier.** These cells are packed together so tightly that only non-protein-bound, highly lipid-soluble drugs can cross into the CNS. The so-called **placental barrier** can likewise prevent drugs from reaching a fetus, although it is not the solid barrier that its name implies. The fetus is exposed to almost every drug that the mother takes. But because any drug must traverse the maternal blood supply and cross the capillary membranes into the placenta (fetal) circulation, delivering drugs to a fetus requires them to be lipid soluble, non-ionized and non-protein-bound. This may slow some drugs or reduce their placental transfer to benign levels.

Other drugs are deposited in specific tissues. Fatty tissue, for example, can serve as a drug depot, or reservoir. Because blood flow is lower in fatty areas than in muscular areas, fatty tissue is a relatively stable depot; it can neither absorb nor release a large amount of drug in a short time. Similarly, bones and teeth can accumulate high amounts of drugs that bind to calcium, especially tetracycline antibiotics.

Biotransformation

Like other chemicals that enter the body, drugs are metabolized, or broken down into different chemicals (metabolites). The special name given to the **metabolism** of drugs is **biotransformation.** Biotransformation has one of two effects on most drugs: 1) it can transform the drug into a more or less active metabolite, or 2) it can make the drug more water soluble (or less lipid soluble) to facilitate elimination. Some drugs, such as lidocaine, are totally metabolized before elimination, others only partially, and still others not at all. The body will transform some molecules of most drugs and eliminate others without transformation. Protein-bound drugs are not available for biotransformation. Some so-called **prodrugs** (or parent drugs) are not active when administered, but biotransformation converts them into active metabolites.

Many biotransformation processes occur in the liver. The endoplasmic reticula of hepatocytes (liver cells) contain microsomal enzymes that perform much of the metabolizing. (Smaller quantities of these enzymes are also found in the kidney, lung, and GI tract.) Because the blood supply from the GI tract passes through the liver via the portal vein, all drugs absorbed in the GI tract pass through the liver before moving on through the systemic circulation. The first pass through the liver may partially or completely inactivate many drugs. This **first-pass effect** is why some drugs cannot be given orally but instead must be given intravenously to bypass the GI tract and prevent first-pass hepatic metabolism. It also is why drugs that can be given either orally or intravenously may require a much higher oral dose than IV dose. Because we can observe the extent of first-pass metabolism, we can predict how much to increase a dose of an oral medication to deliver an effective amount of the drug into the general circulation.

* **blood-brain barrier** tight junctions of the capillary endothelial cells in the central nervous system vasculature through which only non-protein-bound, highly lipid-soluble drugs can pass.

* **placental barrier** biochemical barrier at the maternal/fetal interface that restricts certain molecules.

* **metabolism** the body's breaking down chemicals into different chemicals.

* **biotransformation** special name given to the metabolism of drugs.

* **prodrug (parent drug)** medication that is not active when administered, but whose biotransformation converts it into active metabolites.

* **first-pass effect** the liver's partial or complete inactivation of a drug before it reaches the systemic circulation.

* oxidation the loss of hydrogen atoms or the acceptance of an oxygen atom. This increases the positive charge (or lessens the negative charge) on the molecule.

* hydrolysis the breakage of a chemical bond by adding water, or by incorporating a hydroxyl (OH⁻) group into one fragment and a hydrogen ion (H⁺) into the other.

The liver's microsomal enzymes react with drugs in two ways: phase-I, or nonsynthetic reactions; and phase-II, or synthetic reactions. *Phase-I reactions* most often **oxidize** the parent drug, although they may reduce it or **hydrolyze** it. These nonsynthetic reactions make the drug more water soluble to ease excretion. A number of drugs and chemicals increase the activity of, or induce, the microsomal enzyme that causes phase-I reactions. This means that more enzyme is produced and drugs will be metabolized more rapidly. Because the microsomal enzymes are nonspecific, they can be induced by one drug or chemical and then biotransform other drugs or chemicals. *Phase-II reactions,* which are also called conjugation reactions, combine the prodrug or its metabolites with an endogenous (naturally occurring) chemical, usually making the drug more polar and easier to excrete.

Elimination

Whether they are unchanged or metabolized before elimination, most drugs (toxins and metabolites) are excreted in the urine. Some are excreted in the feces or in expired air.

Renal excretion occurs through two major processes: glomerular filtration and tubular secretion. Glomerular filtration is a function of glomerular filtration pressure, which in turn results from blood pressure and blood flow through the kidneys. Conditions that affect blood pressure and blood flow can affect renal elimination. Specialized transport systems in the walls of the proximal kidney tubules secrete drugs into the urine. These "pumps" are active transport systems and require energy in the form of adenosine triphosphate (ATP) to function. Some are specialized and transport only specific chemicals, while others can transport a range of similar chemicals. When drugs compete for the same pump, toxicity or other unwanted effects can result; however, combinations of some drugs can take advantage of this specialization to prolong their circulation. For example, probenecid blocks renal tubular pumps and competes for them with many antibiotics, among them penicillin, ampicillin, and oxacillin. Probenecid thus is sometimes given with those antibiotics to increase and prolong their blood levels.

The same factors that affect absorption at any other site also affect reabsorption in the renal tubules. Of particular concern is the urine pH. Lipid soluble and non-ionized molecules are readily reabsorbed. Changing the urine pH (usually by administering sodium bicarbonate to make it more alkaline) can affect the reabsorption in the renal tubules. For example, if a drug becomes ionized in a more alkaline environment, then making the urine more alkaline will interfere with reabsorption and cause more of the drug to be excreted. Some drugs and their metabolites can be eliminated in the expired air. This is the basis of the breath test that police use to determine a driver's blood alcohol level. Ethanol is released in the expired air in proportion to its concentration in the blood stream. Although the liver degrades most ingested ethanol, exhalation releases a measurable quantity. Drugs also can be excreted in the feces. In enterohepatic circulation, if a drug (or its metabolites) is excreted into the intestines from bile, the body may reabsorb the drug and experience a sustained effect. Additionally, drugs may be excreted through sweat, saliva, and breast milk. Excretion through sweat glands is rarely a significant mechanism for elimination. Excretion through mammary glands becomes a concern when nursing mothers take medications.

Drug Routes

The route of a drug's administration clearly has an impact on the drug's absorption and distribution. The route's impact on biotransformation and elimination may not be so clear. The blood stream will more quickly absorb and distribute

Content Review

DRUG ROUTES
- Enteral
- Parenteral

water soluble drugs if given in more vascular compartments than if given in less vascular compartments. Oral or nasogastric administration of alkaline drugs may allow the gastric acids to neutralize the drug and prevent its absorption. The liver's first-pass effect may biotransform some orally administered drugs and degrade them almost immediately.

Enteral Routes **Enteral routes** deliver medications by absorption through the gastrointestinal tract, which goes from the mouth to the stomach and on through the intestines to the rectum. They may be oral, orogastric/nasogastric, sublingual, buccal, or rectal.

- *Oral (PO).* The oral route is good for self-administered drugs. Most home medications are administered by this route. The drug must be able to tolerate the acidic gastric environment and be absorbed. Few emergency drugs are administered through this route.
- *Orogastric/nasogastric tube (OG/NG).* This route is generally used for oral medications when the patient already has the tube in place for other reasons.
- *Sublingual (SL).* This is a good route for self-administration and excellent absorption from the sublingual capillary bed without the problems of gastric acidity or absorption.
- *Buccal.* Absorption through this route between the cheek and gum is similar to sublingual absorption.
- *Rectal (PR).* This route is usually reserved for unconscious or vomiting patients or patients who cannot cooperate with oral or IV administration (small children).

Parenteral Routes Broadly defined, **parenteral** denotes any area outside of the gastrointestinal tract; however, additional, specific criteria apply to parenteral drug administration. Parenteral routes typically use needles to inject medications into the circulatory system or tissues. Consequently, some forms of parenteral drug delivery afford the most rapid drug delivery and absorption.

- *Intravenous (IV).* With its rapid onset, this is the preferred route in most emergencies.
- *Endotracheal (ET).* This is an alternative route for *selected* medications in an emergency.
- *Intraosseous (IO).* The intraosseous route delivers drugs to the medullary space of bones. Most often used as an alternative to IV administration in pediatric emergencies, it also sees limited use in adults.
- *Umbilical.* Both the umbilical vein and umbilical artery can provide an alternative to IV administration in newborns.
- *Intramuscular (IM).* The intramuscular route allows a slower absorption than IV administration, as the drug passes into the capillaries.
- *Subcutaneous (SC, SQ, SubQ).* This route is slower than the IM route, because the subcutaneous tissue is less vascular than the muscular tissue.
- *Inhalation/Nebulized.* This route, which offers very rapid absorption, is especially useful for delivering drugs whose target tissues are in the lungs.
- *Topical.* Topical administration delivers drugs directly to the skin.

* **enteral route** delivery of a medication through the gastrointestinal tract.

* **parenteral route** delivery of a medication outside of the gastrointestinal tract, typically using needles to inject medications into the circulatory system or tissues.

Most emergency medications are given intravenously to avoid drug degradation in the liver.

- *Transdermal.* For drugs that can be absorbed through the skin, the transdermal route allows slow, continuous release.
- *Nasal.* Useful for delivering drugs directly to the nasal mucosa, the nasal route has an expanding role in delivering systemically acting drugs.
- *Instillation.* Instillation is similar to topical administration, but places the drug directly into a wound or an eye.
- *Intradermal.* For allergy testing, intradermal administration delivers a drug or biologic agent between the dermal layers.

Drug Forms

Drugs come in many forms. Solid forms, generally given orally, include:

- *Pills.* Drugs shaped spherically to be easy to swallow.
- *Powders.* Although they are not as popular as they once were, some powdered drugs are still in use.
- *Tablets.* Powders compressed into a disklike form.
- *Suppositories.* Drugs mixed with a waxlike base that melts at body temperature, allowing absorption by rectal or vaginal tissue.
- *Capsules.* Gelatin containers filled with powders or tiny pills; the gelatin dissolves, releasing the drug into the gastrointestinal tract.

Liquid drugs are usually solutions of a solid drug dissolved in a solvent. Some can be given parenterally, while others must be given enterally.

- *Solutions.* The most common liquid preparations. Generally water based; some may be oil based.
- *Tinctures.* Prepared using an alcohol extraction process; some alcohol usually remains in the final drug preparation.
- *Suspensions.* Preparations in which the solid does not dissolve in the solvent; if left alone, the solid portion will precipitate out.
- *Emulsions.* Suspensions with an oily substance in the solvent, even when well mixed globules of oil separate out of the solution.
- *Spirits.* Solution of a volatile drug in alcohol.
- *Elixirs.* Alcohol and water solvent, often with flavorings added to improve the taste.
- *Syrups.* Sugar, water, and drug solutions.

Some drugs come in a gaseous form. The most common drug supplied this way is oxygen. Paramedics may also find nitrous oxide (N_2O) used as an inhaled analgesic in ambulances and emergency departments.

Drug Storage

Certain guidelines should dictate the manner in which drugs are stored; their properties may be altered by the environment in which they are stored. While some EMS units are parked in heated stations, others are kept outdoors and exposed to the elements. EMS systems must consider the storage requirements of all drugs and diluents when deciding operational issues such as vehicle design and posting policies (as occurs in system status management). This rapidly becomes a clinical issue because the actual potency of most medications is altered if they are not stored in proper conditions. Examples of variables to consider when determining the proper method of drug storage include temperature, light, moisture and shelf-life.

PHARMACODYNAMICS

When we consider a drug's pharmacodynamics, or effects on the body, we are specifically interested in its mechanisms of action and the relationship between its concentration and its effect.

Actions of Drugs

Drugs can act in four different ways. They may bind to a receptor site, change the physical properties of cells, chemically combine with other chemicals, or alter a normal metabolic pathway. Each of these actions involves a physio-chemical interaction between the drug and a functionally important molecule in the body.

Drugs that Act by Binding to a Receptor Site Most drugs operate by binding to a **receptor.** Almost all drug receptors are protein molecules on the surfaces of cells. They are part of the body's normal regulatory stimulation/inhibition function, and can be stimulated or inhibited by chemicals. Each different receptor's name generally corresponds to the drug that stimulates it. For example, if an opiate stimulates the receptor, then the receptor is an opioid receptor. When multiple drugs stimulate the same receptor, standard practice is to use the generic name.

The force of attraction between a drug and a receptor is their **affinity.** The greater the affinity, the stronger the bond. Different drugs may bind to the same type of receptor site, but the strength of their bond may vary. The binding site's shape determines its receptivity to other chemicals, whether they are drugs or endogenous substances. These binding sites are relatively specific—a nonopiate drug generally will not affect an opiate binding site, although occasionally a drug with a similar receptor binding site will unexpectedly cross react. Receptors can also have subtypes. At least five subtypes of adrenergic receptors, for example, are important to paramedic practice.

A drug's pharmacodynamics also involve its ability to cause the expected response, or **efficacy.** Just as different drugs may have different affinities for a site, they may also have different efficacies; that is, drug A may cause a stronger response than drug B. Affinity and efficacy are not directly related. Drug A may cause a stronger response than drug B, even though drug B binds to the receptor site more strongly than drug A.

When a drug binds with its specific type of receptor, a chemical change occurs that ultimately leads to the drug's effect. In most cases, drugs will either stimulate or inhibit the cell's normal biochemical actions. In fact, a drug cannot impart a new function to a cell. Some drugs may interact with a receptor and directly result in the desired effect. Other drugs, however, may interact with a receptor and cause the release or production of a second compound. This secondary compound, or **second messenger,** includes such compounds as calcium or cyclic adenosine monophosphate (cAMP). Cyclic AMP is the most common second messenger. It has a multitude of effects inside the cell. These secondary messengers are particularly important in the endocrine system, as they principally occur in endocrine glands. Once cAMP is formed inside the cell, it activates still other enzymes, usually in a cascading action. That is, the first enzyme activates another enzyme, which activates a third enzyme, and so forth. This is important in that it amplifies the action so that even a small

* **receptor** specialized protein that combines with a drug resulting in a biochemical effect.

* **affinity** force of attraction between a drug and a receptor.

* **efficacy** a drug's ability to cause the expected response.

* **second messenger** chemical that participates in complex cascading reactions that eventually cause a drug's desired effect.

amount of a drug (or hormone) acting on the cell surface can initiate a powerful, cascading, activating force for the entire cell.

The number of receptors on a target cell usually does not remain constant on a daily basis, or even from minute to minute. This is because the receptor proteins are often destroyed during the course of their function. At other times, they are either reactivated or remanufactured by the protein-manufacturing mechanism of the cell. Binding of a drug (or hormone) to a target cell receptor causes the number of receptors to decrease. This process is **down-regulation** of the receptors. It results in a decreased responsiveness of the target cell to the drug or hormone as the number of available active receptors decreases. In other cases, but less commonly, a drug (or hormone) can cause the formation of more receptors than normal. This process, **up-regulation,** increases the target tissue's sensitivity to the particular drug or hormone.

Chemicals that stimulate a receptor site generally fall into two broad categories, agonists and antagonists. **Agonists** bind to the receptor and cause it to initiate the expected response. **Antagonists** bind to a site but do not cause the receptor to initiate the expected response. Some drugs, **agonist-antagonists** (also called **partial agonists**), may do both. Nalbuphine (Nubain), for instance, stimulates some of the opioid agonists' analgesic properties but partially blocks others such as respiratory depression.

Receptor-mediated drug actions work like a lock (the receptor) and key (the agonist). If you put the key in the lock and turn it, the lock will open. An antagonist is like a key that fits into the lock but will not turn and cannot open the lock. Target tissues generally have many receptors, so to take the analogy another step, imagine that to get maximal effect a single key (agonist) must move around and open many doors (trigger many biochemical responses). An agonist-antagonist would be a key that unlocks and opens a door but gets stuck in the lock. That is, the drug will cause the expected effect, but that drug will also block another drug from triggering the same receptor. This **competitive antagonism** is considered *surmountable* because a sufficiently large dose of the agonist can overcome the antagonism.

Noncompetitive antagonism can also occur. Continuing the lock, key, and door analogy, imagine the door is barred. This antagonism would be *insurmountable*; no amount of agonist could overcome it. Noncompetitive antagonism occurs because the binding of the antagonist at a different site causes a deformity of the binding site that actually prevents the agonist from fitting and binding. **Irreversible antagonism** may also occur when a competitive antagonist permanently binds with a receptor site. When this occurs, no amount of agonist will stimulate the receptor. For the effects of such an antagonist to wear off, the body must create new receptors.

Two drugs may appear to be antagonists while actually acting independently. This physiologic antagonism can occur when one drug's effects counteract another's. While neither agent chemically affects the other, their net effect is antagonistic. An example of a receptor, agonist, antagonist, and agonist-antagonist can be described using an opiate receptor. These receptors occur naturally in the brain and respond to natural endorphins. Morphine sulfate acts as an agonist. It binds to the opiate receptor and causes the expected response of pain relief. Naloxone (Narcan) acts as an antagonist. It will bind to the opiate receptor, but will not initiate the pain relief. It will prevent morphine sulfate from binding to the site and thus effectively blocks the morphine and its response. If the patient is given nalbuphine (Nubain), an agonist-antagonist, it will bind to the opiate receptor and relieve pain, but it is less efficacious than morphine. The nalbuphine blocks morphine from the receptor like an antagonist, but stimulates the receptor on its own like an agonist, although to a lesser extent.

---

* **down-regulation** binding of a drug or hormone to a target cell receptor that causes the number of receptors to decrease.

* **up-regulation** a drug causes the formation of more receptors than normal.

* **agonist** drug that binds to a receptor and causes it to initiate the expected response.

* **antagonist** drug that binds to a receptor but does not cause it to initiate the expected response.

* **agonist-antagonist (partial agonist)** drug that binds to a receptor and stimulates some of its effects but blocks others.

* **competitive antagonism** one drug binds to a receptor and causes the expected effect while also blocking another drug from triggering the same receptor.

* **noncompetitive antagonism** the binding of an antagonist causes a deformity of the binding site that prevents an agonist from fitting and binding.

* **irreversible antagonism** a competitive antagonist permanently binds with a receptor site.

Drugs that Act by Changing Physical Properties Some drugs change the physical properties of a part of the body. Drugs that change the osmotic balance across membranes are good examples of this type of drug action. The osmotic diuretic mannitol (Osmotrol), for instance, increases urine output by increasing the blood's osmolarity, or osmotic "pull." This increased osmolarity triggers the normal regulatory systems to decrease water reabsorption in the renal tubules, thereby reducing the total amount of water in the body.

Drugs that Act by Chemically Combining with Other Substances Drugs that participate in chemical reactions that change the chemical nature of their substrates (the chemical or substance on which a drug acts) play a large role in paramedic practice. For example, isopropyl alcohol, which is often used to disinfect skin before percutaneous needle insertion for phlebotomy or IV cannulation, denatures the proteins on the surface of bacterial cells. This ruptures the cells, destroying the bacteria. The antacids are another example. They act by chemically neutralizing the hydrochloric acid in the stomach. Sodium bicarbonate given intravenously chemically neutralizes some of the acids in the blood stream, effectively making the blood more alkalotic.

Drugs that Act by Altering a Normal Metabolic Pathway Some anticancer and antiviral drugs are chemical analogs of normal metabolic substrates. In a process that has been dubbed a counterfeit incorporation mechanism, these drugs can be incorporated into the products of metabolism of cancer cells. Since these drugs are not really the expected substrate, the anticipated product either will not form or, if formed, will be substantially or completely inactive.

Responses to Drug Administration

When a drug is administered, a response is obviously anticipated. The actual response may be the one desired, or it may be an unintended **side effect**. Most, if not all, drugs have at least some minor side effects. Because our knowledge of pharmacology and physiology has not yet arrived at the point where we can engineer the perfect drug, we must weigh the need for the desired response against the dangers of side effects. In essence, every time we give a medication, we must carefully weigh the risks against the benefits. Although undesirable, side effects are predictable. Iatrogenic responses, on the other hand, are not predicted. In general, the term *iatrogenic* refers to a disease or response induced by the actions of a care provider. Derived from the Greek *iatros* (physician) and *gennan* (to produce), it literally means *physician produced*. Negligence is not the only cause of iatrogenic responses. Some common unintended adverse responses to drugs include:

- *Allergic reaction.* Also known as hypersensitivity; this effect occurs as the drug is antigenic and activates the immune system, causing effects that are normally more profound than seen in the general population.

- *Idiosyncrasy.* A drug effect that is unique to the individual; different than seen or expected in the population in general.

- *Tolerance.* Decreased response to the same amount of drug after repeated administrations.

- *Cross tolerance.* Tolerance for a drug that develops after administration of a different drug. Morphine and other opioid agents are common examples. Tolerance for one agent implies tolerance for others as well.

- *Tachyphylaxis.* Rapidly occurring tolerance to a drug. May occur after a single dose. This typically occurs with sympathetic agonists, specifically decongestant and bronchodilation agents.

 side effect unintended response to a drug.

Always weigh the need for a drug's desired response against the dangers of its side effects.

- *Cumulative effect.* Increased effectiveness when a drug is given in several doses.
- *Drug dependence.* The patient becomes accustomed to the drug's presence in his body and will suffer from withdrawal symptoms upon its absence. The dependence may be physical or psychological.
- *Drug interaction.* The effects of one drug alter the response to another drug.
- *Drug antagonism.* The effects of one drug block the response to another drug.
- *Summation.* Also known as an additive effect. Two drugs that both have the same effect are given together, analogous to $1+1=2$.
- *Synergism.* Two drugs that both have the same effect are given together and produce a response greater than the sum of their individual responses, analogous to $1+1=3$.
- *Potentiation.* One drug enhances the effect of another. A common example is promethazine (Phenergan) enhancing the effects of morphine.
- *Interference.* The direct biochemical interaction between two drugs; one drug affects the pharmacology of another drug.

Drug-Response Relationship

To have its optimal desired or therapeutic effects, a drug must reach appropriate concentrations at its site of action. The magnitude of the response therefore depends on the dosage and the drug's course through the body over time. Factors that can affect the drug's concentration may be pharmaceutical (the dosage form's disintegration and the drug's dissolution), pharmacokinetic (the drug's absorption, distribution, metabolism, and excretion), or pharmacodynamic (drug-receptor interaction). To predict how the drug will affect different people, a **drug-response relationship** thus correlates different amounts of drug to the resultant clinical response.

Most of the information needed to describe drug-response relationships comes from **plasma-level profiles,** which describe the lengths of onset, duration, and termination of action, as well as the drug's minimum effective concentration and toxic levels. The **onset of action** is the time from administration until a medication reaches its **minimum effective concentration** (the minimum level of drug necessary to cause a given effect). The length of time the amount of drug remains above this level is its **duration of action. Termination of action** is measured from when the drug's level drops below the minimum effective concentration until it is eliminated from the body.

The ratio of a drug's lethal dose for 50 percent of the population (LD_{50}) to its effective dose for 50 percent of the population (ED_{50}) is its **therapeutic index** (TI) or LD_{50}/ED_{50}. The therapeutic index represents the drug's margin of safety. As the range between effective dose and lethal dose decreases, the value of TI decreases; that is, it becomes closer to one. TI values of close to one indicate a very small margin of safety. In other words, the effective dose and lethal dose of a drug whose TI value is close to one are nearly the same. This drug would be very difficult to effectively dose without causing toxicity.

The last component of the drug-response relationship, the **biologic half-life,** is the time the body takes to clear one half of the drug. Although the rates of metabolism and excretion both affect it, a drug's half-life ($t_{1/2}$) is independent of its concentration. For example, if the concentration of a drug were 500 μg/dl after administration and 250 μg/dl in 10 minutes, then its half-life would be 10 minutes. After another 10 minutes, 125 μg/dl would remain.

---

* drug-response relationship correlation of different amounts of a drug to clinical response.

* plasma-level profile describes the lengths of onset, duration, and termination of action, as well as the drug's minimum effective concentration and toxic levels.

* onset of action the time from administration until a medication reaches its minimum effective concentration.

* minimum effective concentration minimum level of drug needed to cause a given effect.

* duration of action length of time the amount of drug remains above its minimum effective concentration.

* termination of action time from when the drug's level drops below its minimum effective concentration until it is eliminated from the body.

* therapeutic index ratio of a drug's lethal dose for 50 percent of the population to its effective dose for 50 percent of the population.

* biologic half-life time the body takes to clear one half of a drug.

Factors Altering Drug Response

Different individuals may have different responses to the same drug given. Factors that alter the standard drug-response relationship include the following:

- *Age.* The liver and kidney functions of infants are not yet fully developed, so the response to drugs may be altered. Likewise, as we age, the functions of these organs begins to deteriorate. As a result, infants and the elderly are most susceptible to having an altered response to a drug.

- *Body mass.* The more body mass a person has, the more fluid is potentially available to dilute a drug. A given amount of drug will cause a higher concentration in a person with little body mass than in a much larger person. Thus, most drug dosages are stated in terms of body mass. For example, the standard dose of lidocaine for a patient in cardiac arrest is 1.5 mg/kg. A 100 kg patient will receive 150 mg of lidocaine, while a 50 kg patient will receive only 75 mg.

- *Sex.* Most differences in drug response due to sex result from the relative body masses of men and women. The different distribution and amounts of body fat also affect the amounts of drug available at any given time.

- *Environmental milieu.* Various stimuli in a patient's environment affect his response to a given drug. This is most clearly seen with drugs affecting mood or behavior. The same dose of an antianxiety medication such as diazepam (Valium) will have different effects, depending on the patient's mood or surroundings. For example, if the patient were afraid of heights, his usual dose of diazepam would not be likely to help him remain calm while rappelling from the top of a tall building. Surrounding conditions may also affect the distribution or elimination of a drug. Heat, for example, causes vasodilation and increases perspiration, both of which may alter the rate at which the body distributes and eliminates a drug.

- *Time of administration.* If a patient takes a drug immediately after eating, its absorption will be different than if he took the same drug before breakfast in the morning. Some drugs may cause nausea if taken on an empty stomach and must therefore be taken only after eating.

- *Pathologic state.* Several disease states alter the drug-response relationship. Most notable are renal and hepatic dysfunctions, both of which may lead to excess accumulation of a drug in the body. Renal failure is likely to decrease elimination of drugs, while hepatic failure may decrease or inhibit their metabolism, prolonging their duration of action. Acid-base disturbances may alter a drug's solubility or the extent to which it ionizes, thus changing its absorption rate.

- *Genetic factors.* Genetic traits such as the lack of specific enzymes or lowered basal metabolic rate alter drug absorption or biotransformation and thus modify the patient's response.

- *Psychological factors.* A patient's mental state can also affect his response to a drug. The best known example of this is the placebo effect. Essentially, if a patient believes that a drug will have a given effect, then he is much more likely to perceive that the effect has occurred.

Content Review

FACTORS AFFECTING DRUG-RESPONSE RELATIONSHIP

- Age
- Body mass
- Sex
- Environment
- Time of administration
- Pathology
- Genetics
- Psychology

Drug Interactions

Drug interactions occur whenever two or more drugs are available in the same patient. The interaction can increase, decrease, or have no effect on their combined actions. Any number of variables may cause these drug-drug interactions, including:

- One drug could alter the rate of intestinal absorption.
- The two drugs could compete for plasma protein binding, resulting in one's accumulation at the other's expense.
- One drug could alter the other's metabolism, thus increasing or decreasing either's bioavailability.
- One drug's action at a receptor site may be antagonistic or synergistic to another's.
- One drug could alter the other's rate of excretion through the kidneys.
- One drug could alter the balance of electrolytes necessary for the other drug's expected result.

In addition to drug-drug interactions, other types of interactions are possible. They include a drug's effects on the rate of absorption of food and nutrients, alteration of enzymes, and food-initiated alteration of drug excretion. Alcohol consumption and smoking may also cause interactions with drugs. Finally, some drugs are incompatible with each other. As an example, catecholamines such as epinephrine will precipitate in an alkaline solution such as sodium bicarbonate.

Part 2: Drug Classifications

Part 2 begins with a discussion of how drugs are classified, that is, how drugs are organized into groups with common characteristics, most often according to the body system affected. The remainder of Part 2 discusses drugs and sub-groups of drugs that are included in the following major classifications:

- Drugs used to affect the nervous system
- Drugs used to affect the cardiovascular system
- Drugs used to affect the respiratory system
- Drugs used to affect the gastrointestinal system
- Drugs used to affect the eyes
- Drugs used to affect the ears
- Drugs used to affect the endocrine system
- Drugs used to treat cancer
- Drugs used to treat infectious diseases and inflammation
- Drugs used to affect the skin
- Drugs used to supplement the diet
- Drugs used to treat poisoning and overdoses

CLASSIFYING DRUGS

The enormous amount of material that you must learn about pharmacology can easily become overwhelming. The best way to surmount this challenge is to break the information into manageable groups. Drugs can be classified many ways. You will often find them listed by the body system they affect, by their mechanism of action, or by their indications. Drugs also can be classified by source or by chemical class. Understanding the properties of drug classes (or the model drug of a class) can increase your understanding of drugs and quicken your learning of new drugs.

Grouping medications according to their uses is a very practical way of classifying them. For example, one class of drugs is used to treat heart dysrhythmias, another to treat hypertension. While the specific dosing regimens and contraindications vary among medications within any class, their general properties are consistent. If you understand those general principles, learning the specific information about individual medications becomes much easier. Thinking in terms of prototypical medications usually helps to describe each classification. A **prototype** is a drug that best demonstrates the class's common properties and illustrates its particular characteristics.

In the rest of this chapter we will look at specific classifications of medications that as a paramedic you will commonly either administer or encounter. Even though you may not frequently administer medications from every classification, knowing how they work remains important. It will help you to understand the implications of medications your patients may be taking themselves or getting from another caregiver. An example often cited to demonstrate the importance of understanding the classes of medications, even those that you will rarely administer, is the patient who has taken an overdose of tricyclic antidepressants. Based on your knowledge of this classification, you will know to increase your index of suspicion for hypotension and abnormal cardiac rhythms.

✱ **prototype** drug that best demonstrates the class's common properties and illustrates its particular characteristics.

DRUGS USED TO AFFECT THE NERVOUS SYSTEM

The two major divisions of the nervous system are the central nervous system and the peripheral nervous system (Figure 6-2). The *central nervous system* includes the brain and spinal cord; all nerves that originate and terminate within either the brain or the spinal cord are considered central. The *peripheral nervous*

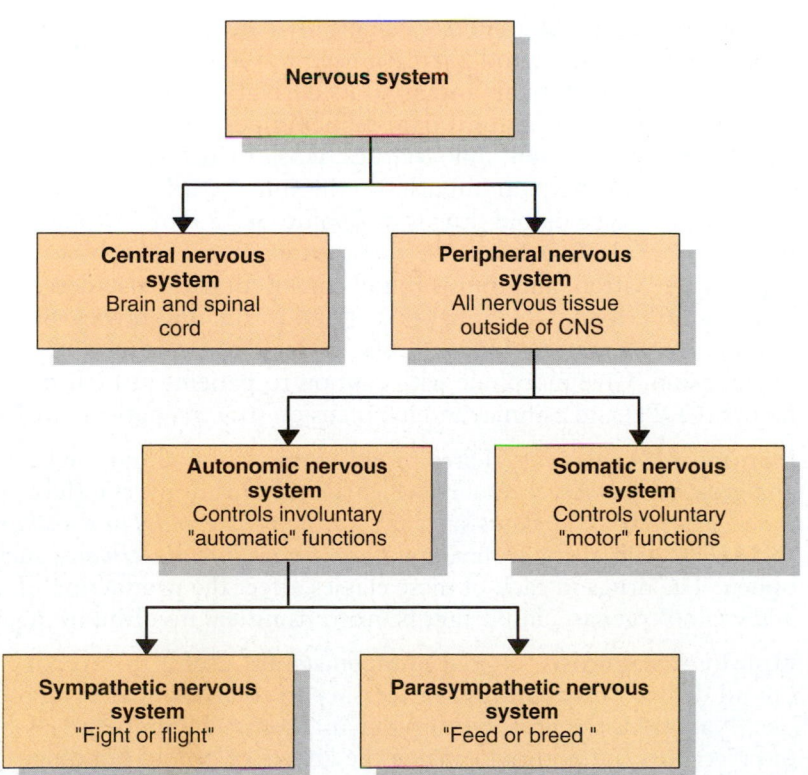

FIGURE 6-2 Functional organization of the autonomic nervous system.

system comprises everything else. If a neuron originates within the brain and terminates outside of the spinal cord, it is part of the peripheral nervous system, which in turn consists of the somatic nervous system and the autonomic nervous system. The *somatic nervous system* controls voluntary, or motor, functions. The *autonomic nervous system,* which controls involuntary, or automatic, functions, is further divided into the sympathetic and parasympathetic nervous systems. The two major groupings of medications used to affect the nervous system are those that affect the central nervous system and those that affect the autonomic nervous system.

CENTRAL NERVOUS SYSTEM MEDICATIONS

Many pathologic conditions involve the central nervous system (CNS). As a result, a great number of drugs have been developed to affect the CNS, including analgesics, anesthetics, drugs to treat anxiety and insomnia, anticonvulsants, stimulants, psychotherapeutic agents (antidepressants and antimanic agents), and drugs used to treat specific nervous system disorders such as Parkinson's disease. Obviously, this is a very broad classification with many different types of agents. Having a firm grasp on the basic physiology involved will help you to understand the various drugs you encounter.

Analgesics and Antagonists

Analgesics are medications that relieve the sensation of pain. The distinction between **analgesia,** the absence of the sensation of *pain,* and **anesthesia,** the absence of *all* sensation, is important. Where an analgesic decreases the specific sensation of pain, an anesthetic prevents all sensation, often impairing consciousness in the process. A frequently used class of medications, analgesics are available by prescription or over the counter. The two basic subclasses of analgesics are opioid agonists and their derivatives and nonopioid derivatives. Opioid antagonists, which we also discuss in this section, reverse the effects of opioid analgesics; **adjunct medications** enhance the effects of other analgesics.

Opioid Agonists An opioid is chemically similar to opium, which is extracted from the poppy plant and has been used for centuries for its analgesic and hallucinatory effects. Opium and all of its derivatives effectively treat pain because of their similarity to natural pain-reducing peptides called *endorphins.* Endorphins and, by extension, opioid drugs, work by decreasing the sensory neurons' ability to propagate pain impulses to the spinal cord and brain.

The prototype opioid drug is morphine. Several of morphine's effects make it useful for clinical practice. At therapeutic doses, morphine causes analgesia, euphoria, sedation, and miosis (pupil constriction). It also decreases cardiac preload and afterload, which makes it useful in treating myocardial infarction and pulmonary edema. At higher doses, it may cause respiratory depression and hypotension. Give morphine with caution to patients at high risk for respiratory failure (COPD and asthma) and hypotension (trauma patients with hypovolemia).

Nonopioid Analgesics Three broad types of nonopioid medications also have analgesic properties, several of which also share antipyretic (fever fighting) properties. These are *salicylates* such as aspirin, *nonsteroidal anti-inflammatory drugs (NSAIDS)* such as ibuprofen, and *para-aminophenol derivates* such as acetaminophen. The drugs in each of these classes affect the production of prostaglandins and cyclooxygenase, important neurotransmitters involved in the pain response.

Opioid Antagonists Opioid antagonists are useful in reversing the effects of opioid drugs. This typically is necessary to treat respiratory depression. Nalaxone (Narcan) is the prototype opioid antagonist. It competitively binds with opioid receptors but without causing the effects of opioid bonding. It is commonly

* **analgesic** medication that relieves the sensation of pain.

* **analgesia** the absence of the sensation of pain.

* **anesthesia** the absence of all sensations.

* **adjunct medication** agent that enhances the effects of other drugs.

Give morphine with caution to patients at high risk for respiratory failure and hypotension.

used to treat overdoses of heroin and other opioid derivatives; however, it has a shorter half-life than most opioid drugs so repeated doses may be necessary to prevent its unwanted side effects.

Adjunct Medications Adjunct medications are given concurrently with other drugs to enhance their effects. While they may have only limited or no analgesic properties by themselves, combined with a true analgesic they either prolong or intensify its effect. Examples of adjunct medications are benzodiazepines (diazepam [Valium], lorazepam (Ativan), midazolam [Versed]), antihistamines (promethazine [Phenergan]) and caffeine. We will discuss many of these agents in separate sections.

Opioid Agonist–Antagonists An opioid agonist-antagonist displays both agonistic and antagonistic properties. Pentazocine (Talwin) is the prototype for this class. Nalbuphine (Nubain) is commonly used in field care. It is an agonist because, like opioids, it decreases pain response, and it is an antagonist because it has fewer respiratory depressant and addictive side effects. Butorphanol (Stadol) is another common opioid agonist-antagonist.

Anesthetics

Unlike analgesics, an **anesthetic** induces a state of anesthesia, or loss of sensation to touch or pain. Anesthetics are useful during unpleasant procedures such as surgery or electrical cardioversion. At low levels of anesthesia, patients may have a decreased sensation of pain but remain conscious. **Neuroleptanesthesia,** a type of anesthesia that combines this effect with amnesia, is useful in procedures that require the patient to remain alert and responsive.

Anesthetics as a group tend to cause respiratory, central nervous system (CNS), and cardiovascular depression. Different agents affect these systems to different degrees and are typically chosen for their ability to produce the desired effect with minimal side effects. Anesthetic agents are rarely used singly; rather, several different agents are typically given together to achieve a balanced anesthetic result. For example, intubating a conscious patient requires his natural gag reflex to be inhibited. Neuromuscular blocking agents such as succinylcholine are used to induce paralysis. Because this would be a terribly frightening and potentially painful procedure, antianxiety, amnesic, and analgesic agents are also given to produce the desired anesthetic effect.

Anesthetics are given either by inhalation or injection. The gaseous anesthetics given by inhalation include halothane, enflurane, and nitrous oxide. The first clinically useful anesthetic was ether, a gas. Its discovery marked a new generation in surgical care, but it is very flammable. The modern gaseous anesthetics are much less volatile, while still decreasing consciousness and sensation as required. These drugs, by some as yet unidentified mechanism, hyperpolarize neural membranes, making depolarization more difficult. This decreases the firing rates of neural impulses and, therefore, the propagation of action potentials through the nervous system, thus reducing sensation. These effects appear to depend upon the gases' solubility. The rate of onset of anesthesia further depends on several additional factors including cardiac output, inhaled concentration of gas, pulmonary minute volume, and end organ perfusion. Because these gases clear mostly through the lungs, respiratory rate and depth affect the duration of their effect. While halothane is the prototype of inhaled anesthetics, nitrous oxide is the only medication in this class with which you are likely to have much involvement.

Most anesthetics used outside the operating room are given intravenously. This gives them a considerably faster onset and shorter duration, making them much more useful in emergency care. Paramedics primarily use these agents to assist with intubation in rapid sequence intubation. They include several pharmacologic classes including ultra-short acting barbiturates (thiopental [Pentothal] and methohexital [Brevital]), benzodiazepines (diazepam [Valium] and

✱ **anesthetic** medication that induces a loss of sensation to touch or pain.

✱ **neuroleptanesthesia** anesthesia that combines decreased sensation of pain with amnesia while the patient remains conscious.

midazolam [Versed]), and opioids (fentanyl [Sublimaze], remifentanil [Ultiva]). We discuss barbiturates' and benzodiazepines' mechanisms of action in the section on antianxiety and sedative-hypnotics.

Anesthetics are also given locally to block sensation for procedures such as suturing and most dentistry. These agents are injected into the skin around the nerves that innervate the area of the procedure. They decrease the nerve's ability to depolarize and propagate the impulse from this area to the brain. Cocaine's first clinical use was as a topical anesthetic of the eye in 1884. The current prototype of this class is lidocaine (Xylocaine). It is frequently mixed with epinephrine. The epinephrine causes local vasoconstriction, decreasing bleeding and systemic absorption of the drug.

Antianxiety and Sedative-Hypnotic Drugs

Antianxiety and sedative-hypnotic drugs are generally used to decrease anxiety, induce amnesia, and assist sleeping and as part of a balanced approach to anesthesia. **Sedation** refers to a state of decreased anxiety and inhibitions. **Hypnosis** in this context refers to the instigation of sleep. Sleep may be categorized as either rapid-eye-movement (REM) or non-rapid-eye-movement (non-REM). REM sleep is characterized by rapid eye movements and lack of motor control. Most dreaming is thought to occur during REM sleep. Insomnia, or difficulty sleeping, typically presents with increased latency (the period of time between lying down and going to sleep) or awakening during sleep.

The two main pharmacologic classes within this functional class are benzodiazepines and barbiturates. Alcohol is also in this functional class. Benzodiazepines and barbiturates work in similar ways. Benzodiazepines are frequently prescribed for oral use and are relatively safe and effective for treating general anxiety and insomnia. Barbiturates, which have broader general depressant activities and a higher potential for abuse, are used much less frequently than benzodiazepines. Before the release of benzodiazepines in the 1960s, however, barbiturates were the drug of choice for treating anxiety and insomnia.

Both benzodiazepines and barbiturates hyper-polarize the membrane of central nervous system neurons, which decreases their response to stimuli. Gamma-aminobutyric acid (GABA) is the chief inhibitory neurotransmitter in the central nervous system. GABA receptors are dispersed widely throughout the CNS on proteins that make up chloride ion channels in the cell membrane. When GABA combines with these receptors, the channel "opens" and chloride, which is more prevalent outside of the cell, diffuses through the channel. As chloride is an anion, or negative ion, it makes the inside of the cell more negative than the outside. This hyper-polarizes the membrane and makes it more difficult to depolarize. Depolarization therefore requires a larger stimulus to cause the cell to fire. Both benzodiazepines and barbiturates increase the GABA receptor-chloride ion channel complexes' potential for binding with GABA, and both are dose dependent. At low doses, they decrease anxiety and cause sedation. As the dose increases, they induce sleep (hypnosis) and, at higher doses, anesthesia. Because benzodiazepines only increase the effectiveness of GABA, the amount of GABA present limits their effects. This actually makes benzodiazepines much safer than barbiturates, which at high doses can actually mimic GABA's effects and thus can have unlimited effects. Benzodiazepines and barbiturates are also useful in treating convulsions.

Just as opiates have an antagonist in naloxone (Narcan), benzodiazepines have an antagonist in flumazenil (Romazicon). Flumazenil competitively binds with the benzodiazepine receptors in the GABA receptor-chloride ion channel complex without causing the effects of benzodiazepines. This reverses the sedation from benzodiazepines, but it can occasionally have untoward consequences, specifically if a patient depends upon benzodiazepines for seizure con-

✳ sedation state of decreased anxiety and inhibitions.

✳ hypnosis instigation of sleep.

trol, is withdrawing from alcohol, or is taking tricyclic antidepressants. In these cases, the patient may develop seizures following the administration of flumazenil.

Antiseizure or Antiepileptic Drugs

Seizures are a state of hyperactivity of either a section of the brain (partial seizure) or all of the brain (generalized seizure). They may or may not be accompanied by convulsions. Therefore, although the medications in this functional class may be called anticonvulsants, they are more appropriately referred to as antiseizure or antiepileptic drugs. The goal of seizure management is to balance eliminating the seizures against the side effects of the medications used to treat them. Controlling seizures is a life-long process for most patients and requires diligent compliance with medication dosing regimens.

Partial (or focal) seizures erupt from a specific focus and are described in terms of alterations in consciousness or behavior. These may be further divided into simple or complex partial seizures based upon the specific area of the brain in which the focus is located. Complex partial seizures are also known as psychomotor seizures and are characterized by repetitive motions.

Generalized seizures involve both hemispheres of the brain and are described in terms of visible motor activity. Grand mal seizures involve periods of muscle rigidity (tonic stage) followed by spasmodic twitching (clonic stage) and then flaccidity and a gradual return to consciousness (postictal stage). Petit mal seizures are also generalized but do not have obvious convulsions. They involve brief losses of consciousness that may occur hundreds of times a day. They are also called absence seizures and are treated differently than other types of seizures. Finally, status epilepticus is a life-threatening condition characterized by uninterrupted grand mal seizures lasting more than 30 minutes or by two or more tonic-clonic seizures without an intervening lucid interval. The preferred therapy for each type of seizure differs.

Seizures are treated through several general mechanisms. The most common is direct action on the sodium and calcium ion channels in the neural membranes. Phenytoin (Dilantin) and carbamazepine (Tegretol) both inhibit the influx of sodium into the cell, thus decreasing the cell's ability to depolarize and propagate seizures. Valproic acid and ethosuximide act similarly, but they interact with calcium channels in the hypothalmus, where absence seizures typically begin. These two drugs are particularly useful because they are specific to hyperactive neurons and therefore have few side effects. Other medications such as benzodiazepines and barbiturates interact with the GABA receptor-chloride ion channel complex, as explained in the section on antianxiety and sedative-hypnotic drugs.

Antiseizure medications comprise several phamacologic classes, including benzodiazepines (diazepam [Valium] and lorazepam (Ativan]), barbiturates (phenobarbitol [Luminal]), hydantoins (phenytoin [Dilantin], fosphenytoin [Cerebyx]), succinimides (ethosuximide [Zarontin]), and miscellaneous medications such as valproic acid (Depakote). Table 6-3 lists the preferred medication for treating each type of seizure.

Central Nervous System Stimulants

Stimulating the central nervous system is desirable in certain circumstances such as fatigue, drowsiness, narcolepsy, obesity, and attention deficit hyperactivity disorder. Broadly, two techniques may accomplish this:

- Increasing the release or effectiveness of excitatory neurotransmitters
- Decreasing the release or effectiveness of inhibitory neurotransmitters

The goal of seizure management is to balance eliminating the seizures against the side effects of the medications used to treat them.

Table 6-3	ANTISEIZURE MEDICATIONS
Type of Seizure	**Drug of Choice**
Partial Seizures	Phenytoin
	Carbamazepine
Grand Mal	Carbamazepine
	Phenytoin
	Phenobarbitol
Absence	Valproic acid
	Ethosuximide

Within the functional class of CNS stimulants are three pharmacologic classes, amphetamines, methylphenidates, and methylxanthines.

The amphetamines also include methamphetamine and dextroamphetamine. These drugs all increase the release of excitatory neurotransmitters including norepinephrine and dopamine. Norepinephrine is the primary cause of these drugs' effects, which include an increased wakefulness and awareness as well as a decreased appetite. Amphetamines' most common uses, therefore, are treating drowsiness and fatigue and suppressing the appetite. Most of amphetamines' side effects result from overstimulation; they include tachycardia and other dysrhythmias, hypertension, convulsions, insomnia, and occasionally psychoses with hallucinations and agitation. Examples of this class include amphetamine sulfate (the prototype) and Dexedrine.

Methylphenidate, marketed as Ritalin, is the most commonly prescribed drug for attention deficit hyperactivity disorder (ADHD). While it is chemically different than the amphetamines, its pharmacologic mechanism of action is similar. Also, like the amphetamines, it has a high abuse potential and is therefore listed as a Schedule II controlled substance. While treating hyperactivity with a stimulant may seem odd, it is quite effective. Frequently, the cause of inappropriate behavior in a child with ADHD is his inability to concentrate or focus. Ritalin's stimulant effects increase this ability, and the unwanted behavior often diminishes.

The methylxanthines include caffeine, aminophylline, and theophylline. While caffeine, the prototype drug in this class, has few clinical uses, it is frequently ingested in coffee, colas, and chocolates. Theophylline's relaxing effects on bronchial smooth muscle make it helpful in treating asthma. The methylxanthines' mechanism of action is unclear, but it seems to block adenosine receptors. Adenosine is an endogenous neurotransmitter which is used clinically for certain types of tachycardias. Because methylxanthines block the adenosine receptors, larger than normal doses may be needed to achieve the desired result. This class's side effects are similar to the amphetamines', but they have a much lower potential for abuse and are not controlled drugs.

Psychotherapeutic Medications

* psychotherapeutic medication drug used to treat mental dysfunction.

Psychotherapeutic medications treat mental dysfunction. Unlike other disease states, we do not thoroughly understand the pathophysiology of mental dysfunction; therefore, we base much of our pharmacologic treatment of these conditions on our limited knowledge and on clinical correlation (scientific observation that these medications are indeed effective, even if we do not fully understand their mechanism). Medications are typically only one tactic in a balanced strategy for treating mental illness. Depending on the specific disorder, physicians will use other treatments such as psychotherapy and electroconvulsive therapy in conjunction with pharmaceutical interventions.

While we do not completely understand these diseases' specific pathologies, they seem to involve the monoamine neurotransmitters in the central nervous system. These neurotransmitters (norepinephrine, dopamine, serotonin) have been implicated in the control and regulation of emotions. Imbalances in these neurotransmitters, especially dopamine, appear to be at least involved with, if not responsible for, most mental disease. Regulating these and other excitatory and inhibitory neurotransmitters forms the basis for psychopharmaceutical therapy. Schizophrenia appears to be related to an increased release of dopamine, so treatment is aimed at blocking dopamine receptors. Depression seems to be related to inadequate amounts of these neurotransmitters, so treatment is aimed at increasing their release or duration.

The major diseases treated with psychotherapeutic medications are schizophrenia, depression, and bipolar disorder. *The Diagnostic and Statistical Manual,* fourth edition (DSM-IV), published by the American Psychiatric Association, gives schizophrenia's chief characteristics as a lack of contact with reality and disorganized thinking. Its many different manifestations include delusions, hallucinations (auditory more frequently than visual), disorganized and incoherent speech, and grossly disorganized or catatonic behavior. Schizophrenia is typically treated with antipsychotic medications, frequently in conjunction with medications from other classes such as antianxiety drugs or antidepressants. **Extrapyramidal symptoms** (EPS), a common side effect of antipsychotic medications, include muscle tremors and parkinsonism-like effects. As a result, antipsychotic medications are also known as **neuroleptic** (literally, *affecting the nerves*) drugs.

The two chief pharmaceutical classes of antipsychotics and neuroleptics are phenothiazines and butyrophenones. Both have been mainstays of psychiatry since the mid-1950s and are considered traditional antipsychotic drugs. Medications in this group block dopamine, muscarinic acetylcholine, histamine, and alpha$_1$ adrenergic receptors in the central nervous system. These medications' therapeutic effects appear to come from blocking the dopamine receptors; their side effects are fairly well understood to originate in blocking the other receptors. The phenothiazines' and butyrophenones' mechanisms of action are the same; they differ only in potency and pharmacokinetics. The distinction between potency and strength is important. Strength refers to the drug's concentration, while potency is the amount of drug necessary to produce the desired effect. While the phenothiazines are considered low-potency and the butyrophenones are considered high-potency, they both produce the same effect. The differences in potency and pharmacokinetics determine which class of medication will be prescribed. Chlorpromazine (Thorazine) is the prototype phenothiazine; haloperidol (Haldol) is the prototype of the butyrophenones.

Since the phenothiazines' and the butyrophenones' mechanisms of action are identical, their common side effects are also similar: extrapyramidal symptoms from cholinergic blockade in the basal ganglia of the cerebral hemispheres; orthostatic hypotension from blockage of alpha$_1$ adrenergic receptors; sedation; and sexual dysfunction. Treatment for these side effects typically involves modifying the drug dose. Diphenhydramine (Benadryl), an antihistamine with anticholinergic properties, is indicated for treating acute dystonic reactions (manifestations of EPS), which often present with tongue and neck spasm. Patients with a newly prescribed antipsychotic may experience these effects and contact EMS. Fortunately, treatment with diphenhydramine is effective and rapid. Orthostatic hypotension is treated in the usual fashion described in Chapter 19 on hemorrhage and shock.

Other medications used to treat psychotic conditions are considered atypical antipsychotics. While their mechanisms of action are similar to those of the traditional antipsychotics, the atypical antipsychotics block more specific receptors.

Content Review

MAJOR DISEASES TREATED WITH PSYCHOTHERAPEUTIC MEDICATIONS
- Schizophrenia
- Depression
- Bipolar disorder

✱ **extrapyramidal symptoms (EPS)** common side effects of antipsychotic medications, include muscle tremors and parkinsonism-like effects.

✱ **neuroleptic** antipsychotic (literally, *affecting the nerves*).

Content Review

MAJOR CLASSES OF ANTIPSYCHOTIC MEDICATIONS
- Phenothiazines
- Butyrophenones

This specificity allows them to function much like traditional antipsychotics, but without causing the prominent extrapyramidal symptoms. These drugs include clozapine (Clozaril) and risperidone (Risperdal).

Another functional class of psychotherapeutic medications includes the antidepressants. The DSM-IV characterizes major depressive episodes as causing significantly depressed mood, loss of interest in things that normally give the patient pleasure, weight loss or gain, sleeping disturbances, suicide attempts, feelings of hopelessness and helplessness, loss of energy, agitation or withdrawal, and an inability to concentrate. While the specific pathology of this disease is not yet known, it appears to be related to an insufficiency of monoamine neurotransmitters (norepinephrine and serotonin). Thus, the pharmaceutical interventions for this disease appear to increase the number of neurotransmitters released in the brain. The several ways of doing this include increasing the amount of neurotransmitter produced in the presynaptic terminal, increasing the amount of neurotransmitter released from the presynaptic terminal, and blocking the neurotransmitter's reuptake (reabsorption by the presynaptic terminal). This results in a net increase in the neurotransmitter. The antidepressants comprise three pharmacologic classes: tricyclic antidepressants, selective serotonin reuptake inhibitors, and monoamine oxidase inhibitors.

Tricyclic antidepressants (TCAs) are frequently used in treating depression because they are effective, relatively safe, and have few significant side effects when taken in therapeutic dosages. TCAs act by blocking the reuptake of norepinephrine and serotonin, thus extending the duration of their action (Figure 6-3). Unfortunately, they also have anticholinergic properties that cause many side effects including blurred vision, dry mouth, urinary retention, and tachycardia. Another frequent side effect, orthostatic hypotension, is likely due to the alpha$_1$ adrenergic blockade. This is commonly seen when patients try to stand up too quickly and become dizzy. Additionally, because TCAs can lower the seizure threshold, patients with existing seizure disorders are at risk for convulsions. Unfortunately, when taken in overdose, TCAs can have very significant cardiotoxic effects that make them a favored means of attempting suicide among depressed patients. These effects include myocardial infarction and dysrhythmias. Partly because of this potential for overdose, TCAs have fallen behind the newer selective serotonin reuptake inhibitors as the drug of choice for depression. Overdoses of these medications also frequently cause marked hypotension. Treatment of TCA overdoses is primarily supportive, with sodium bicarbonate given to increase the excretion of TCAs by alkalanizing the urine. The prototype tricyclic antidepressant, imipramine (Tofranil), was also the first one on the mar-

FIGURE 6-3 Effects of TCAs on reuptake of serotonin and norepenephrine.

(a) Neurotransmission without TCA

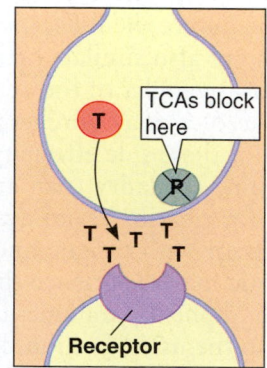

(b) Neurotransmission with TCA

ket. Other common examples include amitriptyline (Elavil), desipramine (Norpramin), and nortriptyline (Pamelor).

Selective serotonin reuptake inhibitors (SSRIs) are a recent addition to the antidepressants. The prototype, fluoxetine (Prozac), is the most widely prescribed antidepressant in the United States. These drugs' antidepressant effects are comparable to the TCAs', but because the SSRIs selectively block the reuptake of serotonin, they do not affect dopamine or norepinephrine. Nor do they block histaminic or cholinergic receptors, thus avoiding many of the TCAs' side effects. The primary adverse reactions to SSRIs are sexual dysfunction, headache, and nausea. Other selective serotonin reuptake inhibitors include sertraline (Zoloft) and paroxetine (Paxil).

A third pharmacologic class of psychotherapeutic medications includes the monoamine oxidase inhibitors (MAOIs). The monoamine neurotransmitters are thought to be insufficient in depression. Monoamine oxidase, an enzyme, metabolizes monoamines into inactive metabolites. MAOIs inhibit monoamine oxidase and block the monoamines' breakdown, thus increasing their availability. Monoamine oxidase is also present in the liver and has a significant role in metabolizing foods that contain tyramine, a substance that increases the release of norepinephrine. The MAOIs' major side effect is hypertensive crisis brought on by the consumption of foods rich in tyramine such as cheese and red wine. By inhibiting monoamine oxidase, these drugs also decrease the body's ability to inactivate tyramine; they therefore promote the release of norepinephrine, a potent vasopressor. Because of this and other unwanted side effects, MAOIs are not commonly used anymore; rather, they are reserved for treating depression that is refractory to TCAs and SSRIs. The prototype of this class is phenelzine (Nardil).

Patients with bipolar disorder (manic depression) exhibit cyclic swings from mania to depression with periods of normalcy in between. According to the DSM-IV the manic phases of this disease are characterized by hyperactivity, thoughts of grandeur or inflated self-esteem, decreased need for sleep, increased goal-oriented behavior, increased productivity, flight of ideas (moving from thought to thought with little connection between them), distractibility, and increased risk taking. Lithium is the drug of choice for the management of bipolar disorder. It is frequently given in conjunction with benzodiazepines or antipsychotics. Lithium's mechanism of action is unknown, but it effectively decreases the signs of mania without causing sedation. Adverse reactions include headache, dizziness, fatigue, nausea, and vomiting. Recently, two antiseizure medications—carbamazepine (Tegretol) and valproic acid (Depakote)—have proven successful in treating bipolar disorder.

Drugs Used to Treat Parkinson's Disease

Parkinson's disease is a nervous disorder caused by the destruction of dopamine-releasing neurons in the *substantia nigra,* a part of the basal ganglia, which is a specialized area of the brain involved in controlling fine movements. Dysfunction of parts of the basal ganglia causes the extrapyramidal symptoms (EPS) often seen as a side effect of antipsychotic medications.

Parkinson's disease is characterized by dyskinesia (dysfunctional movements) such as involuntary tremors, unsteady gait, and postural instability. Severe cases also involve bradykinesia (slow movements) and akinesia (the absence of movement). In the later stages, patients frequently present with psychological impairment including dementia, depression, and impaired memory. Parkinson's is a progressive disease that usually begins in middle age with subtle signs and progresses to a state of incapacitation. While no treatments can cure Parkinson's or even slow

Lithium, widely used in the treatment of bipolar disorder, has a very low therapeutic index.

its progression, treating the symptoms can return some function to the patient. The goal in treating these patients is to restore their ability to function without causing unacceptable side effects. Some remarkably effective drugs are available. Unfortunately, they usually are effective for only several years. After that, signs and symptoms return and often are more severe than before treatment began.

The medications that are effective in treating Parkinson's disease are also effective in treating the extrapyramidal side effects (EPS) of antipsychotics. This is because fine motor control is based in part on a balance between inhibitory and excitatory neurotransmitters. In the basal ganglia, dopamine, an inhibitory transmitter, opposes acetylcholine, an excitatory neurotransmitter. Parkinson's disease and the medications that cause EPS both decrease the number of presynaptic terminals that release dopamine in the basal ganglia. This allows the excitatory stimulus of acetylcholine to dominate, ultimately impeding fine motor control.

Pharmacologic therapy for Parkinson's disease seeks to restore the balance of dopamine and acetylcholine. This may be done either by increasing the stimulation of dopamine receptors or by decreasing the stimulation of acetylcholine receptors. Drugs can do this either through dopaminergic effects or through anticholinergic effects. Dopaminergic effects increase the release of dopamine from the neuron, directly stimulate the dopamine receptors, or decrease the breakdown of however much dopamine is being released. Anticholinergic effects prevent acetylcholine's effects either by reducing the amount of the neurotransmitter released or by directly blocking the acetylcholine receptors.

Dopamine cannot be given directly to Parkinson's disease patients because it cannot cross the blood-brain barrier and consequently would be ineffective in treating the disease while still causing many side effects. The drug of choice in treating Parkinson's disease, therefore, is levodopa, an inactive drug that readily crosses the blood-brain barrier. Levodopa is absorbed by the dopamine-releasing neuron terminals, where the enzyme decarboxylase metabolizes it into dopamine, thus increasing the amount of dopamine available for release. Levodopa is very effective and reduces symptoms in the vast majority of patients. As previously mentioned, however, symptoms will return within a period of years as the disease progresses. Levodopa's side effects include nausea, vomiting, and ironically, for unknown reasons, dyskinesias. Because it is converted to dopamine, levodopa may also have cardiovascular effects, including tachycardias and hypertension.

When given alone, levodopa is metabolized primarily outside of the brain, where it is ineffective. To prevent this, Sinemet, the most popular anti-Parkinson preparation available, combines levodopa with an inactive ingredient, carbidopa. While carbidopa by itself produces no effects, it prevents levodopa's conversion into dopamine in the periphery. Because carbidopa does not cross the blood-brain barrier, however, levodopa can still be metabolized in the CNS. This decreases the incidence of cardiovascular side effects and enables lower doses of levodopa to be effective. Sinemet's side effects are essentially those of levodopa by itself. Nausea and vomiting, stimulated from within the CNS, remain problematic.

Another dopaminergic medication, amantadine (Symmetrel), promotes the release of dopamine from those dopamine-releasing neurons that remain unaffected by the disease. It has a rapid onset but generally becomes ineffective in less than a year. While it can be effective alone, it is usually given in conjunction with Sinemet or levodopa. Several other medications such as bromocriptine directly stimulate the dopamine receptors instead of attempting to increase the amount of dopamine released.

One additional dopaminergic approach is to decrease the breakdown of dopamine after it has been released. The enzyme responsible for breaking down monoamines such as norepinephrine, dopamine, and serotonin is monoamine oxidase. (We have previously described monoamine oxidase inhibitors in our discussion of their role in depression.) One monoamine oxidase inhibitor, selegiline (Carbex), is specific for monoamine oxidase type B. This MAO-B enzyme is involved only in the breakdown of dopamine. (MAO-A is responsible for breaking down norepinephrine and serotonin.) By selectively inhibiting the breakdown of dopamine, selegiline increases the amount available for binding with dopamine receptors, thus promoting the dopamine-acetylcholine balance. This selective blockage avoids increased norepinephrine levels that can lead to undesired tachycardia and hypertension.

As opposed to dopaminergic medications, which act on the dopamine side of the dopamine-acetylcholine balance, anticholinergic medications act on the acetylcholine side to block the acetylcholine receptors. The prototype anticholinergic, atropine, was initially used in this context with success, but it also had the typical peripheral anticholinergic side effects of blurred vision, dry mouth, and urinary hesitancy. More recently developed medications affect the CNS more than they do the peripheral nervous system. The prototype centrally acting anticholinergic medication is benztropine (Cogentin). Another example is diphenhydramine (Benadryl), which is more frequently administered for its antihistaminic properties.

AUTONOMIC NERVOUS SYSTEM MEDICATIONS

The **autonomic nervous system** is the part of the nervous system that controls involuntary (automatic) actions. Many medications used in prehospital care directly affect the autonomic nervous system. It is essential that you have a good understanding of this aspect of the nervous system and the ways in which emergency medications affect it.

The two functional divisions of the autonomic nervous system are the sympathetic nervous system and the parasympathetic nervous system. The sympathetic nervous system allows the body to function under stress. It is often referred to as the fight-or-flight aspect of the nervous system. The parasympathetic nervous system, on the other hand, primarily controls vegetative functions such as digestion of food. It is often referred to as the feed-or-breed or the rest-and-repose aspect of the nervous system. The parasympathetic nervous system and the sympathetic nervous system work in constant opposition to control organ responses. For example, the sympathetic nervous system stimulates specific receptors in the heart that increase the heart rate. At the same time, the parasympathetic nervous system stimulates specific receptors that decrease the heart rate. The net result is the resting heart rate. When the body's physiologic needs dictate an increased heart rate, the sympathetic stimuli dominate the parasympathetic effects. Conversely, when the body needs to rest (with a decreased heart rate), the parasympathetic stimuli predominate.

Basic Anatomy and Physiology

The autonomic nervous system arises from the central nervous system. The nerves of the autonomic nervous system exit the central nervous system and subsequently enter specialized structures called **autonomic ganglia.** In the autonomic ganglia, the nerve fibers from the central nervous system interact with nerve fibers that extend from the ganglia to the various target organs. Autonomic nerve fibers that exit the central nervous system and terminate in the autonomic ganglia are called **pre-ganglionic nerves.** Autonomic nerve fibers that exit the ganglia and terminate in the various target tissues are called **post-ganglionic nerves.** The ganglia of the sympathetic nervous system are located close to the spinal cord, while the ganglia of the parasympathetic nervous system are located close to the target organs (Figure 3-73, page 191).

* **autonomic nervous system** the part of the nervous system that controls involuntary actions.

* **autonomic ganglia** groups of autonomic nerve cells located outside the central nervous system.

* **pre-ganglionic nerves** nerve fibers that extend from the central nervous system to the autonomic ganglia.

* **post-ganglionic nerves** nerve fibers that extend from the autonomic ganglia to the target tissues.

No actual physical connection exists between two nerve cells or between a nerve cell and the organ it innervates. Instead, there is a space, or synapse, between nerve cells. The space between a nerve cell and the target organ is a **neuroeffector junction.** Specialized chemicals called **neurotransmitters** conduct the nervous impulse between nerve cells or between a nerve cell and its target organ.

Neurotransmitters are released from presynaptic neurons and subsequently act on postsynaptic neurons or on the designated target organ. When released by the nerve ending, the neurotransmitter travels across the synapse and activates membrane receptors on the adjoining nerve or target tissue. The neurotransmitter is then either deactivated or taken back up into the presynaptic neuron.

The two neurotransmitters of the autonomic nervous system are acetylcholine and norepinephrine. Acetylcholine is utilized in the pre-ganglionic nerves of the sympathetic nervous system and in both the pre-ganglionic and post-ganglionic nerves of the parasympathetic nervous system. Norepinephrine is the post-ganglionic neurotransmitter of the sympathetic nervous system. Synapses that use acetylcholine as the neurotransmitter are **cholinergic** synapses. Synapses that use norepinephrine as the neurotransmitter are **adrenergic** synapses.

The anatomy and physiology of the autonomic nervous system were discussed in detail in Chapter 3.

Drugs Used to Affect the Parasympathetic Nervous System

The parasympathetic system uses acetylcholine as a neurotransmitter. Acetylcholine released by presynaptic neurons activates receptors on the postsynaptic neurons or on the neuroeffector junction.

Receptors that are specialized for acetylcholine are termed cholinergic receptors. Medications that stimulate them are known as cholinergics (**parasympathomimetics**), and those that block them are known as anticholinergics or cholinergic blockers (**parasympatholytics**).

Cholinergics Cholinergic drugs act either directly or indirectly. Direct-acting cholinergics (also called cholinergic esters) simulate the affects of ACh by directly binding with the cholinergic receptors. Drugs in this class generally produce the same effects as cholinergic stimulation, mostly focused on the muscarinic receptors. Their adverse effects are related primarily to decreased heart rate, decreased peripheral vascular resistance resulting in hypotension and excessive salivation, urination, defecation, and sweating. Vomiting and abdominal cramps may also occur. The acronym SLUDGE (salivation, lacrimation, urination, defecation, gastric motility, emesis) is helpful for remembering these effects.

The prototype direct-acting cholinergic is bethanechol (Urecholine). Its pharmacokinetics make it a good clinical substitute for acetylcholine. It is not broken down by cholinesterase, the enzyme responsible for destroying acetylcholine, and therefore it has a longer duration of action. Most of its effects are on muscarinic receptors in the urinary bladder and gastrointestinal tract. It may be given orally or subcutaneously. Thus, it is used primarily to increase micturition (urination) and peristalsis. Adverse effects are rare but related to its parasympathomimetic effects. Another direct-acting cholinergic medication, pilocarpine, is used as a topical treatment for glaucoma.

Indirect-acting cholinergic drugs affect acetylcholinesterase. By inhibiting its actions in degrading acetylcholine, they prolong the cholinergic response. These drugs affect both muscarinic and nicotinic receptors and therefore have little specificity. Their uses are limited primarily to treating myasthenia gravis, some types of poisoning, and glaucoma as well as for reversing nondepolarizing neuromuscular blockade.

The two basic types of indirect-acting cholinergic drugs are reversible inhibitors and irreversible inhibitors. Both types bind with cholinesterase (ChE), acting as a substitute for ACh. In doing so, they prevent ChE from destroying ACh. The difference between the reversible and irreversible inhibitors is how long they remain bound with cholinesterase. The reversible inhibitors remain bound with cholinesterase much longer than acetylcholine but eventually release it. The irreversible inhibitors, too, will eventually release cholinesterase, but they remain bound for so long that, from a practical standpoint, they can be considered irreversible.

Neostigmine (Prostigmin) is the prototype reversible cholinesterase inhibitor. It is used to treat myasthenia gravis, an illness characterized by muscle weakness and progressive fatigue. This illness is an autoimmune disease that destroys the nicotinic$_M$ receptors at the neuromuscular junction. With fewer of these receptors, muscles cannot be stimulated as well and weakness occurs. Neostigmine treats the symptoms of myasthenia gravis by blocking the degradation of ACh, thereby prolonging its effects and increasing motor strength. Its primary side effects are due to the stimulation of muscarinic receptors and include the SLUDGE responses. Fortunately, these responses may be treated effectively with a cholinergic blocker. Neostigmine can also reverse a nondepolarizing neuromuscular blockade. This use is fairly uncommon, however, because such blockades typically are administered only intentionally as part of anesthesia or before intubation.

Physostigmine (Antilirium) is another reversible cholinesterase inhibitor. Its mechanism is similar to neostigmine's, with their primary difference being in their pharmacokinetics. While neostigmine is poorly absorbed across the cell membrane, physostigmine crosses rapidly and therefore has a shorter onset and may be given in lower doses. Physostigmine's chief use is for reversing overdoses of atropine, an anticholinergic drug that blocks muscarinic receptors.

Irreversible cholinesterase inhibitors have only one clinical function, the treatment of glaucoma, and only one drug, echothiophate (Phospholine Iodide), has been approved for that purpose. Cholinesterase inhibitors, however, are very useful as insecticides (organophosphates), and unfortunately, their mechanism of action is also very attractive for makers of chemical weapons. They are the chief component in nerve gases such as VX and sarin. They cause extensive stimulation of cholinergic receptors, ultimately resulting in the SLUDGE response. Toxic levels may also affect nicotinic$_M$ receptors, leading to paralysis. Treatment for such toxic exposures involves drugs such as high doses of atropine or pralidoxime (Protopam, 2-PAM) to block the effects of the accumulating acetylcholine. Pralidoxime can encourage irreversible cholinesterase inhibitors to release cholinesterase.

Anticholinergics Anticholinergic agents oppose the parasympathetic (cholinergic) nervous system. Just as there are multiple types of cholinergic receptors, there are multiple classes of cholinergic receptor antagonists. We will discuss agents that selectively block muscarinic and nicotinic receptors as well as nonselective blockers (ganglionic blockers). A special subclass of nicotinic receptors is neuromuscular blocking drugs.

Muscarinic Cholinergic Antagonists Cholinergic antagonists block the effects of acetylcholine almost exclusively at the muscarinic receptors. They are often called anticholinergics or parasympatholytics. They work by competitively binding with muscarinic receptors without stimulating them. As a result, these receptors cannot bind with acetylcholine.

The prototype anticholinergic drug is atropine, which is widely used to block muscarinic receptors and is commonly administered in the field. Found in the

Content Review

TYPES OF PARASYMPATHETIC ACETYLCHOLINE RECEPTORS
- Muscarinic
- Nicotinic
  – Nicotinic$_N$ (neuron)
  – Nicotinic$_M$ (muscle)

EFFECTS OF ATROPINE OVERDOSE

- Hot as hell
- Blind as a bat
- Dry as a bone
- Red as a beet
- Mad as a hatter

plant *Atropa belladonna,* atropine is one of several drugs classified as belladonna alkaloids (scopolamine is also in this classification). Readily absorbed through both enteral and parenteral routes, it has therapeutic effects at dose dependent levels at most sites with muscarinic receptors. At low doses, atropine decreases secretion from salivary and bronchial glands as well as from the sympathetically innervated sweat glands. At moderate doses, it increases heart rate and causes mydriasis (dilated pupils) and blurry vision. At higher doses, it decreases gastric motility and stomach acid secretion. Atropine is also useful in reversing overdoses of muscarinic agonists (cholinergics or cholinesterase inhibitors). Its side effects, which are predictable, include dry mouth, blurred vision and photophobia, urinary retention, increased intraocular pressure, tachycardia, constipation, and anhidrosis (decreased sweating), which may cause hyperthermia. A helpful mnemonic for remembering the effects of atropine overdose is "hot as hell, blind as a bat, dry as a bone, red as a beet, mad as a hatter."

Scopolamine is another belladonna anticholinergic. Its actions are similar to atropine's, but unlike atropine, scopolamine causes sedation and antiemesis. Thus, its primary purpose is to prevent motion sickness. It is available as a transdermal patch.

Several synthetic medications mimic the effects of the belladonna alkaloids while minimizing their side effects. Ipratropium bromide (Atrovent), an inhaled anticholinergic, is effective in treating asthma because it relaxes the bronchial smooth muscle and causes bronchodilation. It is frequently administered along with an inhaled beta-adrenergic agonist. Because it is inhaled and has little systemic effect, ipratropium bromide avoids many of atropine's side effects.

Other anticholinergic drugs include dicyclomine (Bentyl) and benztropine (Cogentin).

Nicotinic Cholinergic Antagonists Nicotinic cholinergic antagonists block acetylcholine only at nicotinic sites. They include ganglionic blocking agents that block the nicotinic$_N$ receptors in the autonomic ganglia and neuromuscular blocking agents that block nicotinic$_M$ receptors at the neuromuscular junction.

Ganglionic Blocking Agents Ganglionic blockade is produced by competitive antagonism with acetylcholine at the nicotinic$_N$ receptors in the autonomic ganglia. This can, in effect, turn off the entire autonomic nervous system. The two drugs in this class are trimethaphan (Arfonad) and mecamylamine (Inversine). Both are used to treat hypertension. The adverse effects of ganglionic blockade include signs associated with antimuscarinic drugs like atropine—dry mouth, blurred vision, urinary retention, and tachycardia. Other adverse effects arising from the vasodilation and decreased preload caused by sympathetic blockage include profound hypotension, with orthostatic hypotension even more evident. Trimethaphan is administered primarily for hypertensive crisis when other treatments are ineffective. These agents are almost never used anymore because they are not selective and many superior agents are available.

Neuromuscular Blocking Agents Neuromuscular blockade produces a state of paralysis without affecting consciousness. Imagine how terrifying it would be to be fully conscious and aware but completely paralyzed, unable to move or breathe. Neuromuscular blockade is caused by competitive antagonism of nicotinic$_M$ receptors at the neuromuscular junction. This is useful during surgery as part of anesthesia and during electroconvulsive therapy for depression. These agents are most often used in the field to facilitate intubation.

Neuromuscular blocking agents are either depolarizing or nondepolarizing, depending on their mechanism of action. Most are nondepolarizing; only one depolarizing drug, succinylcholine (Anectine), is commonly used in the clinical setting. Tubocurarine, while not frequently used clinically, is the oldest neuromuscular blocker and the prototype nondepolarizing agent. It produces neuromuscular blockade by binding with the nicotinic$_M$ receptor sites without causing muscle depolarization. Succinylcholine acts in the same manner, but like acetylcholine, it does cause muscle depolarization when it binds with the nicotinic$_M$ receptor. It is useful as a neuromuscular blocker because, in contrast to ACh, which rapidly separates from the receptor, it remains bound, preventing the muscle's repolarization. Several nondepolarizing agents are available; the specific agent chosen depends on its rate of onset and duration of action. Succinylcholine has the shortest onset and duration of action because it has a naturally occurring enzyme, pseudocholinesterase, which degrades it.

Ganglionic Stimulating Agents Nicotinic$_N$ receptors reside at the ganglia of both the parasympathetic and sympathetic nervous systems. The alkaloid nicotine stimulates these receptors. Nicotine is found in tobacco and, although it has no therapeutic uses, is of interest for two reasons. Historically, nicotine, along with muscarine, led to a much better understanding of the autonomic nervous system's specific receptors. Also it is one of the most abused drugs in the world.

Nicotine may cause a variety of responses, most of which are dose related. At low doses, like those from smoking, nicotine causes excitation at the autonomic ganglia. This affects both the parasympathetic and sympathetic nervous systems. The parasympathetic response causes increased salivation, peristalsis, and secretion of gastric acid. The sympathetic response causes the release of norepinephrine and epinephrine. These lead to increases in heart rate, myocardial contractility, vasoconstriction, and blood pressure, all of which increase the heart's workload. Sympathetic stimulation also increases awareness and suppresses fatigue and appetite.

Drugs Used to Affect the Sympathetic Nervous System

Medications that stimulate the sympathetic nervous system are **sympathomimetics.** Medications that inhibit the sympathetic nervous system are called **sympatholytics.** Some medications are pure alpha agonists, while others are pure alpha antagonists. Some medications are pure beta agonists, while others are pure beta antagonists. Medications such as epinephrine stimulate both alpha and beta receptors. Other medications, such as the bronchodilators, are termed beta selective, since they act more on beta$_2$ receptors than on beta$_1$ receptors.

The sympathetic nervous system releases norepinephrine from post-ganglionic end terminals and epinephrine from the adrenal medulla. These neurotransmitters bind with adrenergic receptors. (Epinephrine is also called adrenalin because of its release from the adrenal medulla; hence the term *adren*-ergic). There are two main types of adrenergic receptors, each with two subtypes. These receptors' effects depend primarily on their locations. Table 6-4 describes the chief locations and primary actions of each receptor.

The primary clinical purpose for medications that stimulate alpha$_1$ receptors is peripheral vasoconstriction. Constriction of the arterioles increases afterload, while constriction of venules increases preload (decreasing venous capacitance or 'pooling'). Both of these effects increase systolic and diastolic blood pressure and represent the chief therapeutic indication for alpha$_1$ agonists. Stimulation of alpha$_1$ receptors locally may be useful in combination with local anesthetics. The main reason to add the alpha$_1$ agonist in this context is to cause local vasoconstriction so that the systemic absorption of the anesthetic will decrease, and its duration will increase. Alpha$_1$ agonists are also useful topically to decrease nasal congestion caused by dilation and engorgement of nasal blood vessels. The primary adverse responses to alpha$_1$ agonist agents are hypertension and local tissue necrosis. If a medication with significant alpha$_1$ properties infiltrates the surrounding tissue or distal body parts such as fingers, toes, earlobes or nose, inadequate local blood flow due to profound vasoconstriction will likely kill the tissue. Also, alpha$_1$ stimulation may cause reflex bradycardia due to the feedback

✳ **sympathomimetic** drug or other substance that causes effects like those of the sympathetic nervous system (also called adrenergic).

✳ **sympatholytic** drug or other substance that blocks the actions of the sympathetic nervous system (also call antiadrenergic).

Table 6-4 LOCATION OF ADRENERGIC RECEPTORS AND EFFECTS OF STIMULATION

Receptor	Response to Stimulation	Location
Alpha 1 (α_1)	Constriction	Arterioles
	Constriction	Veins
	Mydriasis	Eye
	Ejaculation	Penis
Alpha 2 (α_2)	Presynaptic terminals inhibition*	
Beta 1 (β_1)	Increased heart rate	Heart
	Increased conductivity	
	Increased automaticity	
	Increased contractility	
	Renin release	Kidney
Beta 2 (β_2)	Bronchodilation	Lungs
	Dilation	Arterioles
	Inhibition of contractions	Uterus
	Tremors	Skeletal muscle
Dopaminergic	Vasodilation (increased blood flow)	Kidney

*Stimulation of α_2 adrenergic receptors inhibits the continued release of norepinephrine from the pre-synaptic terminal. It is a feedback mechanism that limits the adrenergic response at that synapse. These receptors have no other identified peripheral effects.

mechanism that regulates blood pressure. As baroreceptors detect a rise in blood pressure, heart rate decreases to compensate.

Alpha$_1$ antagonism is indicated almost exclusively for controlling hypertension. By preventing the peripheral vasoconstriction of alpha$_1$ stimulation, these agents decrease blood pressure. They are also useful in treating local tissue necrosis caused by infiltration of alpha$_1$ agonists. Injecting alpha$_1$ antagonists into the area surrounding the infiltration prevents tissue death from excessive vasoconstriction. The effects of pheochromocytoma, a tumor of the adrenal medulla that causes the release of large amounts of catecholamine, may be treated with an alpha$_1$ blocker. The most common adverse effects of alpha$_1$ antagonism are orthostatic hypotension and reflex tachycardia. Just as alpha$_1$ stimulation may increase blood pressure and cause a baroreceptor-mediated bradycardia, the hypotension from alpha$_1$ blockage may lead to reflex tachycardia from the same mechanism. Other side effects include nasal congestion and inhibition of ejaculation. These agents may also increase blood volume. This is ironic, since their primary indication is hypertension. As another feedback mechanism detects hypotension, the kidneys begin to reabsorb sodium and water to increase blood volume. This is typically addressed by use of a diuretic concomitant with the alpha$_1$ antagonist.

Beta$_1$ stimulation increases heart rate, contractility, and conduction. Its primary indications are cardiac arrest and hypotension resulting from inadequate pumping. During cardiac arrest, beta$_1$ activation may stimulate contractions or increase the force of any existing contractions. Even if the heart is only fibrillating, these agents may increase the effectiveness of electrical defibrillation. In cardiogenic shock, when the heart is not pumping with enough force to overcome the afterload created by peripheral vascular resistance, beta$_1$ agonists can adequately increase the contractions' force. The chief adverse effects of beta$_1$ agonists include tachycardia, dysrhythmias, and chest pain from increasing work load.

Beta$_1$ antagonists are among the most frequently prescribed medications in the United States. Their most common use is to control blood pressure. By blocking the effects of beta$_1$ stimulation, they decrease heart rate (choronotropy) and

Phentolamine (Regitine), an alpha antagonist, can be used to help minimize tissue necrosis following extravasation of an alpha$_1$ agonist such as dopamine or norepinephrine.

contractility (inotropy). These agents are also effective in treating supraventricular tachycardias because they decrease the rate of impulse generation at the SA node (negative chronotropic effects) while also slowing conductivity through the AV node (negative dromotropic effects). Blocking beta$_1$ stimulation also helps treat angina pectoris and reduces the recurrence of myocardial infarction. Its main adverse effects are symptomatic bradycardia, hypotension, and AV block.

Beta$_2$ agonists are used to treat asthma and other conditions with excessive narrowing of the bronchioles. By stimulating beta$_2$ receptors in the lungs, these agents relax the bronchial smooth muscle and cause bronchodilation. Beta$_2$ agonists can also cause uterine smooth muscle relaxation, which may help to suppress preterm labor. Their primary adverse effects are muscle tremors and "bleed over" effects on unintended beta$_1$ stimulation such as tachycardias.

While beta$_2$ blockade serves no clinically useful purpose, nonselective beta blockers have side effects of beta$_2$ blockade. Chief among these is bronchoconstriction and inhibition of glycogenolysis, the release of stored glycogen by the liver and skeletal muscles. Beta$_2$ stimulation causes glycogenesis. Antagonizing the beta$_2$ receptors can inhibit this release. While this is not typically a problem for most people, it can be very problematic for diabetics. It not only makes hypoglycemia more likely but also masks one of its common early warning signs, tachycardia.

Adrenergic Agonists Drugs that stimulate the effects of adrenergic receptors work either directly, indirectly, or through a combination of the two. The direct acting agents bind with the receptor and cause the same response as the normal neurotransmitter. In fact, most of the drugs in this category either are synthetically produced versions of the naturally occurring neurotransmitter or are derivatives of those synthetically produced versions. The indirect acting agents stimulate the release of epinephrine from the adrenal medulla and of norepinephrine from the presynaptic terminals. In turn, the epinephrine and norepinephrine stimulate the adrenergic receptors. The mixed actions of direct-indirect acting medications combine these mechanisms.

The most frequently used adrenergic agents are chemically and functionally similar to the endogenous neurotransmitters. These drugs, which are called catecholamines, include norepinephrine, epinephrine, and dopamine. Synthetic catecholamines are also available. They include dobutamine and isoproterenol. Noncatecholamine adrenergic agents, including ephedrine, phenylephrine, and terbutaline, also affect the adrenergic receptors and have useful clinical applications.

Almost all of the drugs in this section act on more than one type of receptor. Their specificity varies and is important in determining their uses. Table 6-5 lists their actions on various receptors.

Adrenergic Antagonists Unlike most adrenergic agonists, the majority of available adrenergic antagonists are remarkably selective in which receptor they affect. This selectivity, however, occurs only at therapeutic doses. At higher doses, most agents lose their selectivity and begin affecting other receptors as well.

The two basic subcategories of alpha adrenergic antagonists are "noncompetitive, long-acting" and "competitive, short-acting." They differ chiefly in the stability of their bond with the receptor. The prototype noncompetitive, long-acting alpha antagonist is phenoxybenzamine (Dibenzyline). The prototype competitive, short-acting antagonist is prazosin (Minipress). Prazosin also is the prototype for all alpha adrenergic antagonists. Phentolamine (Regitine) is an important nonselective alpha antagonist because of its effects in reversing tissue necrosis caused by catecholamine infiltration.

Beta adrenergic antagonists are more commonly referred to as beta-blockers. Propranolol (Inderal) is the prototype beta-blocker. It is a nonselective antagonist, which means that it blocks both beta$_1$ and beta$_2$ receptors. It is used to treat tachycardia, hypertension, and angina, all results of beta$_1$ blockade. Because it is

Content Review

COMMON CATECHOLAMINES
- Natural
  - Epinephrine
  - Norepinephrine
  - Dopamine
- Synthetic
  - Isoproterenol
  - Dobutamine

Table 6-5 ADRENERGIC RECEPTOR SPECIFICITY

Medication	Receptor				
	Alpha$_1$	Alpha$_2$	Beta$_1$	Beta$_2$	Dopaminergic
Phenylephrine	✔				
Norepinephrine	✔	✔	✔		
Ephedrine	✔	✔	✔	✔	
Epinephrine	✔	✔	✔	✔	
Dobutamine			✔		
Dopamine*			✔		✔
Isoproterenol			✔	✔	
Terbutaline				✔	

*Receptor specificity is dose-dependent. The higher the dose, the less dopaminergic effects are seen.

nonselective, it also has the side effects of beta$_2$ blockade—bronchoconstriction and inhibited glycogenolysis. Propranolol was the first clinically employed beta-blocker, but its use has declined since the development of more selective beta$_1$ antagonists. The prototype of these cardioselective beta-blockers is metoprolol (Lopressor). At normal doses, metoprolol is selective for only beta$_1$ receptors; therefore, it does not cause propranolol's problematic side effects for asthmatics and diabetics. Atenolol (Tenormin) is another commonly used cardioselective beta-blocker.

Skeletal Muscle Relaxants Skeletal muscle relaxants are used to treat muscle spasm from injury and muscle spasticity from CNS injuries or diseases such as multiple sclerosis. Treatment can involve centrally acting agents or direct acting agents.

The centrally acting muscle relaxants' mechanism is not clear, but it appears to be associated with general sedation. The prototype centrally acting skeletal muscle relaxant is baclofen (Lioresal), which is indicated in the treatment of spasticity. While baclofen is effective in the treatment of muscle spasticity, it is generally ineffective in muscle spasm. Several drugs are effective in treating muscle spasm, including cyclobenzaprine (Flexeril) and carisoprodol (Soma).

The prototype of the direct acting muscle relaxants is dantrolene (Dantrium). Unlike the centrally acting agents, dantrolene's mechanism is well understood. It decreases the release of calcium from the sarcoplasmic reticulum in response to action potentials propagated from the neuromuscular junction. This calcium is required for the cross-bridge binding of the actin and myosin filaments in the muscle fibers responsible for contraction. Dantrolene is indicated for treating the spasticity associated with multiple sclerosis and cerebral palsy. It is also indicated for treating malignant hyperthermia, which is on rare occasion seen with some anesthetics and succinylcholine. This hyperthermia results from muscular contractions. Since dantrolene decreases these contractions, the heat that they generate also decreases. Dantrolene is not effective in treating muscle spasm.

DRUGS USED TO AFFECT THE CARDIOVASCULAR SYSTEM

Cardiovascular drugs have traditionally comprised one of the largest parts of the paramedic's pharmacologic "tool box." While this is changing with the expansion of paramedic practice, cardiovascular care (and agents used in that care) remains an important and integral part of a paramedic's knowledge base.

Table 6-6 ANTIDYSRHYTHMIC CLASSIFICATIONS AND EXAMPLES

General Action	Class	Prototype	ECG Effects
Sodium Channel Blockers	IA	Quinidine, procainamide*, disopyramide	Widened QRS, prolonged QT
	IB	Lidocaine*, phenytoin, tocainide, mexiletine	Widened QRS, prolonged QT
	IC	Flecainide*, propafenone	Prolonged PR, widened QRS
	I (Misc.)	Moricizine*	Prolonged PR, widened QRS
Beta Blockers	II	Propranolol*, acebutolol, esmolol	Prolonged PR, bradycardias
Potassium Channel Blockers	III	Bretylium*, amiodarone	Prolonged QT
Calcium Channel Blockers	IV	Verapamil*, diltiazem	Prolonged PR, bradycardias
Miscellaneous		Adenosine, digoxin	Prolonged PR, bradycardias

* prototype

CLASSES OF CARDIOVASCULAR DRUGS

The drugs used to treat cardiovascular disease generally fall into the two broad functional classifications of antidysrhythmics and antihypertensives.

Antidysrhythmics

Antidysrhythmic drugs (Table 6-6) are used to treat and prevent abnormal cardiac rhythms. Used inappropriately, these medications can also cause dysrhythmias or deterioration in existing rhythms.

✱ antidysrhythmic drug used to treat and prevent abnormal cardiac rhythms.

Sodium Channel Blockers (Class I) All of the medications in this general class affect the sodium influx in phases 0 and 4 of fast potentials. This slows the propagation of impulses down the specialized conduction system of the atria and ventricles, although it does not affect the SA or AV node.

Class IA drugs include quinidine (Quinidex), procainamide (Pronestyl), and disopyramide (Norpace). In addition to slowing conduction, these drugs also decrease the repolarization rate. This widens the QRS complex and prolongs the QT interval. Quinidine is the prototype for this class, but procainamide is administered more frequently in emergency medicine. Procainamide is indicated in the treatment of atrial fibrillation with rapid ventricular response and ventricular dysrhythmias. Quinidine has a similar mechanism of action, but it also has anticholinergic properties that may induce unintended tachycardias.

Class IB drugs include lidocaine (Xylocaine), phenytoin (Dilantin), tocainide (Tonocard) and mexiletine (Mexitil). Unlike Class IA drugs, Class IB drugs increase the rate of repolarization. They also reduce automaticity in ventricular cells, which makes them effective in treating rhythms originating from ectopic ventricular foci. Lidocaine is the drug of choice for treating ventricular tachycardia and ventricular fibrillation. While lidocaine was once used prophlactically for patients with myocardial infarction, its use is now limited to life-threatening dysrhythmias. When given in overdose, lidocaine has significant CNS side effects including tinnitus, confusion, and convulsions.

Class IC drugs include flecainide (Tambocor) and propafenone (Rythmol). They decrease conduction velocity through the atria and ventricles as well as through the bundle of His and the Purkinje network. Like the Class IA drugs, they delay ventricular repolarization. Both of these medications, which are

Content Review

Antidysrhythmics are routinely classified in the Vaughn-Williams and Singh Classification System.

- I: Na$^+$ channel blockers
  - –1A
  - –1B
  - –1C
- II: Beta blockers
- III: K$^+$ channel blockers
- IV: Miscellaneous

administered orally, are given to prevent recurrence of ventricular dysrhythmias, but both also have prodysrhythmic properties; that is, they are likely to cause dysrhythmias as well as treat them. They also depress myocardial contractility and are therefore reserved for potentially lethal ventricular dysrhythmias that do not respond to any other conventional therapy.

Moricizine (Ethmozine) has additional properties that exclude it from the other Class I subclasses. It blocks sodium influx during fast potential depolarization, thereby decreasing conduction velocity, but it can also depress myocardial contractility. Like the Class IC drugs, it is reserved for the treatment of ventricular dysrhythmias refractory to other conventional therapy.

Beta-Blockers (Class II) The drugs in this class, propranolol (Inderal), acebutolol (Sectral) and esmolol (Brevibloc) are all beta adrenergic antagonists. Propranolol is nonselective, while acebutolol and esmolol are both selective for the $beta_1$ receptors in the heart. Of the many beta-blockers, these are the only ones approved for the treatment of dysrhythmias. They are indicated in the treatment of tachycardias resulting from excessive sympathetic stimulation. The $beta_1$ receptor in the heart is attached to the calcium channels. Blocking the $beta_1$ receptors thus blocks the calcium channel and prevents the gradual influx of calcium in phase 0 of the slow potential. As a result, the effects of beta blocker therapy on dysrhythmias are almost identical to those of calcium channel blockers. Propranolol is the prototype Class II drug. Because it is nonselective, it also blocks the effect of $beta_2$ receptors, which leads to many of its side effects.

Potassium Channel Blockers (Class III) Potassium channel blocking drugs are also known as antiadrenergic medications because of their complex actions on sympathetic terminals. They include bretylium (Bretylol) and amiodarone (Cordarone); Bretylium is the prototype. They act on the potassium channels in the fast potentials. By blocking the efflux of potassium, bretylium prolongs repolarization and the effective refractory period. It is indicated in the treatment of ventricular fibrillation and refractory ventricular tachycardia. It causes an initial release, then an inhibition, of norepinephrine at the sympathetic end terminals. This delayed repolarization prolongs the QT interval; consequently, bretylium's primary and frequent side effect is hypotension.

Calcium Channel Blockers (Class IV) Calcium channel blockers' effect on the heart is almost identical to that of beta blockers. They decrease SA and AV node automaticity, but most of their usefulness arises from decreasing conductivity through the AV node. They effectively slow the ventricular conduction of atrial fibrillation and flutter, and they can terminate supraventricular tachycardias originating from a reentrant circuit. Verapamil (Calan) and diltiazem (Cardizem) are the only two calcium channel blockers that affect the heart. Verapamil is the prototype. Their chief side effect is hypotension and bradycardia.

Miscellaneous Antidysrhythmics Adenosine (Adenocard) and digoxin (Lanoxin) are both effective antidysrhythmics. Magnesium is the drug of choice in *torsade de pointes*, a type of polymorphic ventricular tachycardia. We will briefly discuss each.

Adenosine does not fit any of the previous categories. It is an endogenous nucleoside with a very short half-life (about 10 seconds). It acts on both potassium and calcium channels, increasing potassium efflux and inhibiting calcium influx. This results in a hyperpolarization that effectively slows the conduction of slow potentials such as those found in the SA and AV node. It has little effect on the fast potentials in the ventricles and is not particularly effective on ventricular tachycardias or atrial fibrillation or flutter. Because of its short half-life its side effects are short lived, but they can be alarming. They include facial flushing, shortness of breath, chest pain, and marked bradycardias. Adenosine must be given as a rapid IV push, as the drug is rapidly metabolized. Doses should be increased in patients taking adenosine blockers such as aminophylline or caffeine. They should be decreased in patients taking adenosine uptake inhibitors like dipyridamole (Persantine) and carbamazepine (Tegretol).

Digoxin (Lanoxin) is a paradoxical drug. Its many effects on the heart make it both an effective antidysrhythmic and a potent prodysrhythmic (generator of dysrhythmias). While we do not clearly understand its specific actions on the heart's electrical activity, we do understand its effects. Digoxin decreases the intrinsic firing rate in the SA node, whereas it decreases conduction velocity in the AV node. Both of these effects are due to its increasing the strength of the parasympathetic effects on the heart. In the Purkinje fibers and ventricular myocardial cells, it decreases the effective refractory period and increases automaticity, both of which may explain its ability to increase ventricular dysrhythmias. To compound this, by depressing SA node activity, digoxin makes ectopic ventricular beats more likely to assume the pacing activity of the heart. Its side effects include bradycardias, AV blocks, PVCs, ventricular tachycardia, ventricular fibrillation, and atrial fibrillation. Actually, there are few dysrhythmias that digoxin does not produce. In addition, digoxin has a very narrow therapeutic index, meaning that it is difficult to find a patient's effective dose without producing side effects. Digoxin also increases cardiac contractility. It is indicated for atrial fibrillation with rapid ventricular conduction and chronic treatment of congestive heart failure.

Magnesium is the drug of choice in *torsade de pointes,* a polymorphic ventricular tachycardia, and in other ventricular dysrhythmias refractory to other therapy. Its mechanism of action is not known, but it may act on the sodium or potassium channels or on $Na^+K^+ATPase$.

Antihypertensives

Hypertension affects more than 50 million people in the United States alone and is a major contributor to coronary artery disease, stroke, and blindness. Fortunately, available drugs can effectively manage blood pressure in the vast majority of patients with limited side effects. Multiple studies have shown conclusively that controlling blood pressure decreases both morbidity and mortality. Blood pressure is equal to cardiac output times the peripheral vascular resistance:

$$blood\ pressure = cardiac\ output \times peripheral\ vascular\ resistance$$

Cardiac output is equal to the heart rate times the stroke volume:

$$cardiac\ output = heart\ rate \times stroke\ volume$$

Antihypertensive agents can manipulate each of these factors. The primary determinant of peripheral vascular resistance is the diameter of peripheral arterioles, which are affected by alpha$_1$ receptors. Heart rate is affected by both muscarinic receptors of the parasympathetic nervous system and beta$_1$ receptors of the sympathetic nervous system; however, hypertension control typically manipulates only beta$_1$ receptors. Stroke volume is affected by contractility and volume. Recall that Starling's Law says that preload and stroke volume are proportionate; that is, as preload increases stroke volume increases (up to a point) and as preload decreases stroke volume decreases. Drugs that affect blood volume control hypertension by manipulating preload.

Several pharmacologic classes of medications are used to control blood pressure. The major approaches to dealing with hypertension are diuretics, beta blockers and other antiadrenergic drugs, angiotensin converting enzyme (ACE) inhibitors, calcium channel blockers and direct vasodilators. Of these, diuretics and beta blockers are the most frequently prescribed, and they are effective in many patients. The remaining agents are used when diuretics or beta blockers are contraindicated or when those approaches are not effective, although ACE inhibitors

* **antihypertensive** drug used to treat hypertension.

are gaining increasing popularity. Often, physicians must prescribe multiple drugs to manage hypertension effectively. In these cases, they will pick one drug from two or more classes that complement each other. For example, a physician might prescribe a diuretic with a beta-blocker.

Diuretics Diuretics reduce circulating blood volume by increasing the amount of urine. This reduces preload to the heart, which in turn reduces cardiac output. The main categories of diuretics include loop diuretics (high ceiling diuretics), thiazides, and potassium sparing diuretics. They all affect the reabsorption of sodium and chloride and create an osmotic gradient that decreases the reabsorption of water. These classes differ according to which area of the nephron they affect. In general, the earlier in the nephron the drug works, the more sodium and water will be affected. Almost all electrolytes and other small particles in the blood are filtered through the glomerulus. Most sodium and water (approximately 65 percent) is reabsorbed in the proximal convoluted tubule. Another 20 percent is reabsorbed in the thick portion of the ascending loop of Henle, while only about 1–5 percent is recaptured in the distal convoluted tubule and collecting duct. Therefore, a drug that decreases sodium reabsorption in the proximal convoluted tubule will cause the kidneys to excrete more water than will a drug that works on the distal convoluted tubule.

Loop diuretics profoundly affect circulating blood volume. In fact, they decrease blood volume so well that they are typically considered excessive for treating moderate hypertension. They are, however, one of the primary tools in treating left ventricular heart failure (congestive heart failure). Their use for hypertension is typically because other diuretics have failed. Furosemide (Lasix) is the prototype of this class. Furosemide blocks sodium reabsorption in the thick portion of the ascending loop of Henle (hence, the name *loop diuretic*). In doing so, it decreases the pull of water from the tubule and into the capillary bed, thus decreasing fluid volume. Furosemide's main side effects are hyponatremia, hypovolemia, hypokalemia, and dehydration. Because the decrease in volume is most noticeable as decreased preload, orthostatic hypotension is a problem. Reflex tachycardia may also occur as the baroreceptors detect a decreased blood pressure and attempt to compensate by increasing heart rate. This happens in individuals with hypertension because the homeostatic 'thermostat' has been set too high. In other words, the body believes that what is actually hypertension is normal and tries to maintain a higher blood pressure than is healthy. This reflex tachycardia is frequently treated with concurrent administration of a loop diuretic with a beta$_1$ blocker. Hypokalemia is frequently treated by increasing dietary potassium intake (bananas are rich in potassium) or by prescribing potassium supplements. An unexplained side effect of loop diuretics is ototoxicity (tinnitus and deafness). Administering loop diuretics slowly can decrease ototoxicity.

Thiazides have a mechanism similar to loop diuretics. The main difference is that the thiazides' mechanism affects the early part of the distal convoluted tubules and therefore cannot block as much sodium from reabsorption. Thiazides are often the drugs of choice in hypertension treatment because they can decrease fluid volume sufficiently to prevent hypertension but not so much that they promote hypotension. The prototype thiazide is hydrochlorothiazide (HydroDIURIL). This class has essentially the same side effects as loop diuretics. One important distinction is that thiazides depend on the glomerular filtration rate, while loop diuretics do not. Thus, loop diuretics may be preferred for patients with renal disease.

Potassium sparing diuretics have a slightly different mechanism than other diuretics. Although they still affect sodium absorption, they do so by inhibiting either the effects of aldosterone on the distal tubules (as does spironolactone) or the specific sodium-potassium exchange mechanism (as does triamterene).

Loop diuretics, particularly furosemide (Lasix), play a major role in the emergency treatment of CHF and acute pulmonary edema.

Acting so late in the nephritic loop, these agents are not very potent diuretics. In fact, they are rarely used alone but instead are typically administered in conjunction with either a loop diuretic or a thiazide diuretic. They are useful as adjuncts to other diuretics because they not only decrease sodium reabsorption (although in small volumes) but also increase potassium reabsorption. This helps to limit the other diuretics' hypokalemic effects. Spironolactone (Aldactone) is the prototype potassium sparing diuretic.

While not used in the treatment of hypertension, osmotic diuretics are important because they alter the reabsorption of water in the proximal convoluted tubule. To do this, they use an osmotically large sugar molecule that is freely filtered through the glomerulus and pulls water after it. Mannitol (Osmitrol), the prototype osmotic diuretic, is used to treat increased intracranial and intraocular pressure.

Adrenergic Inhibiting Agents Inhibiting the effects of adrenergic stimulation can also control hypertension. Several broad mechanisms accomplish this: beta adrenergic antagonism, centrally acting alpha adrenergic antagonism, adrenergic neuron blockade, alpha$_1$ blockade, and alpha/beta blockade.

Beta Adrenergic Antagonists From Table 6-4 in our earlier discussion of beta$_1$ blockers, you will recall that most beta$_1$ receptors are in the heart but some also exist in the juxtaglomerular cells of the kidney. Selective beta$_1$ blockade is useful in treating hypertension for several reasons. It decreases contractility, thereby directly decreasing cardiac output. It also reduces reflex tachycardia by inhibiting sympathetically induced compensatory increases in heart rate. Finally, it represses renin release from the kidneys, which in turn inhibits the vasoconstriction activated by the renin-angiotensin-aldosterone system. The prototype selective beta$_1$ blocker is metropolol (Lopressor); the prototype nonselective beta blocker is propranolol (Inderal). The section on beta$_1$ blockers discussed these agents' side effects.

Centrally Acting Adrenergic Inhibitors Centrally acting adrenergic inhibitors reduce hypertension by inhibiting CNS stimulation of adrenergic receptors. In effect, they are CNS alpha$_2$ agonists. Recall that alpha$_2$ receptors are located on the presynaptic end terminals in the sympathetic nervous system. When stimulated, they inhibit the release of norepinephrine to counterbalance sympathetic stimulation. By increasing the stimulation of alpha$_2$ receptors in the section of the CNS responsible for cardiovascular regulation, centrally acting adrenergic inhibitors decrease the sympathetic stimulation of both alpha$_1$ and beta$_2$ receptors. The net effect is to decrease heart rate and contractility by decreasing release of norepinephrine at beta$_1$ receptors and to promote vasodilation by decreasing norepinephrine release at alpha$_1$ receptors at vascular smooth muscle. The prototype drug in this category is clonidine (Catapres). While it does have some side effects, notably drowsiness and dry mouth, clonidine is a relatively safe and frequently prescribed antihypertensive agent. Methyldopa (Aldomet) is another centrally acting antihypertensive with a mechanism similar to clonidine.

Peripheral Adrenergic Neuron Blocking Agents Like the centrally acting adrenergic inhibitors, peripheral adrenergic neuron blocking agents work indirectly to decrease stimulation of adrenergic receptors. They do this by decreasing the amount of norepinephrine released from sympathetic presynaptic terminals. These agents are no longer commonly used.

The prototype of this class is reserpine (Serpalan). Reserpine has two actions that decrease the amount of norepinephrine released. First, it decreases the synthesis of norepinephrine. Second, it exposes norepinephrine in the terminal vesicles to monoamine oxidase, an enzyme that destroys it. This decreases stimulation of alpha$_1$ receptors, resulting in peripheral vasodilation, and of beta$_1$ receptors, resulting in decreased heart rate and contractility. The decreased peripheral vascular resistance and cardiac output in turn lower blood pressure.

Beta blockers have proven to decrease both short-term and long-term mortality associated with acute MI.

Reserpine also decreases synthesis of several CNS neurotransmitters (serotonin and other catecholamines). This causes reserpine's primary adverse effect, depression. Reserpine, therefore, is not frequently used as an antihypertensive. Additional side effects include gastrointestinal cramps and increased stomach acid production. Other drugs with similar actions include guanethidine (Ismeline) and guanadrel (Hylorel).

Alpha₁ Antagonists This chapter's section on drugs affecting the sympathetic nervous system discusses the alpha₁ receptor antagonists in detail. Only their specific action will be repeated here. The prototype selective alpha₁ antagonist is prazosin (Minipress). It decreases blood pressure by competitively blocking the alpha₁ receptors, thereby inhibiting the sympathetically mediated increases in peripheral vascular resistance. By causing the arterioles to dilate, prazosine directly decreases afterload. By causing the venules to dilate, it promotes venous pooling, which decreases preload. The decreased afterload and preload help to lower blood pressure. Terazosin (Hytrin) is another drug with similar properties.

Combined Alpha/Beta Antagonists Labetalol (Normodyne) and carvedilol (Coreg) competitively bind with both alpha₁ and beta₁ receptors, increasing their antihypertensive actions. Hypertension is treated by decreasing alpha₁ mediated vasoconstriction, which, again, decreases both preload and afterload. Beta₁ blockade decreases heart rate, contractility, and renin release from kidneys. By blocking the release of renin, which promotes vasoconstriction, these agents decrease peripheral vascular resistance even further. Labetalol is commonly used to treat hypertensive crisis and is rapidly replacing the use of sublingual nifedipine (Procardia) for this purpose.

Angiotensin Converting Enzyme (ACE) Inhibitors

Agents in this class interrupt the renin-angiotensin-aldosterone system (RAAS) by preventing the conversion of angiotensin I to angiotensin II. Angiotensin II is one of the most potent vasoconstrictors yet discovered. By decreasing the amount of circulating angiotensin II, peripheral vascular resistance can be decreased, which leads to a decrease in blood pressure.

The juxtaglomerular apparatus in the kidneys releases renin in response to decreases in blood volume, sodium concentration, and blood pressure. Renin acts as an enzyme to convert the inactive protein angiotensinogen into angiotensin I. Neither angiotensinogen nor angiotensin I has much pharmaceutical effect, but angiotensin-converting enzyme (ACE) almost immediately converts angiotensin I in the blood into angiotensin II. (ACE is found in the lumen of almost all vessels and is found in the lungs in very high concentrations.) Angiotensin II causes both systemic and local vasoconstriction, with more pronounced effects on arterioles than on venules. It also lessens water loss by decreasing renal filtration secondary to renal vasoconstriction. Finally, angiotensin II also increases the release of aldosterone, a corticosteroid produced in the adrenal cortex. Aldosterone in turn increases sodium and water reabsorption in the distal convoluted tubule of the nephrons.

Angiotensin converting enzyme inhibitors are very effective in treating hypertension and have also seen success in managing heart failure and renal failure. ACE inhibitors block the conversion of angiotensin I to angiotensin II, thereby providing a host of beneficial effects for patients with hypertension. These include a rapid decrease in arteriolar constriction, which lowers peripheral vascular resistance and afterload. While it does cause some dilation of the venules, this effect is limited. Because of the limited decrease in preload, orthostatic hypotension, common in other antihypertensives, is not a significant concern with ACE inhibitors. These agents also appear to be effective in preventing some of the untoward structural changes in the heart and blood vessels that angiotensin II causes over time.

The prototype ACE inhibitor is captopril (Capoten). Captopril acts like all ACE inhibitors to prevent hypertension. Its main advantage is the absence of side effects common to other antihypertensives. It does not interfere with beta receptors, so it does not decrease the ability to exercise or respond to hemorrhage. It does not cause potassium loss like many diuretics, and it does not cause depression or drowsiness. Because it has no effect on sexual desire or performance, it is much more attractive to many patients who might not comply with other medications. Other common ACE inhibitors include enalapril (Vasotec) and lisinopril (Zestril). These medications are all taken orally. For intravenous use in hypertensive crisis, enalaprilat (Vasotec I.V.) is available.

The most dangerous side effect of ACE inhibitors is pronounced hypotension after the first dose. This can be minimized by reducing initial doses, and it does not reoccur. The main adverse effects of continual use are a persistent cough and angioedema.

In addition to their role in the treatment of hypertension, ACE inhibitors play an important role in the treatment of CHF by decreasing afterload.

Angiotensin II Receptor Antagonists

This recently developed classification of antihypertensive drugs also acts on the renin-angiotensin-aldosterone system. Angiotensin II receptor antagonists achieve the same effects as the ACE inhibitors without the side effects of cough or angioedema. The prototype of this new class is losartan (Cozaar).

Calcium Channel Blocking Agents

We have already discussed two calcium channel blockers, verapamil and diltiazem, in the section on antidysrhythmics. Another structural subclass of calcium channel blockers is the dihydropyridines. The prototype dihydropyridine is nifedipine (Procardia, Adalat). Nifedipine, as well as the other members of the dihydropyridines, differ from verapamil and diltiazem in that they do not affect the calcium channels of the heart at therapeutic doses. Rather, they act only on the vascular smooth muscle of the arterioles. These agents act by blocking the calcium channels in the arterioles. Calcium, which is required for muscle contraction, is released from sarcoplasmic reticulum upon activation by an action potential. When it enters the muscle cell through calcium channels, muscle contraction ensues. Blocking the calcium channels prevents the arterioles' smooth muscle from contracting and therefore dilates these vessels. When this occurs, peripheral vascular resistance decreases and blood pressure falls as a result of lower afterload. Because nifedipine has little effect on veins, it does not cause a corresponding drop in preload and consequently avoids orthostatic hypotension. While nifedipine does not affect the cardiac electrical conduction system, it is effective in dilating the coronary arteries and arterioles and thereby helps to increase coronary perfusion. The primary indications for nifedipine are angina pectoris and chronic treatment of hypertension. Its primary side effects include reflex tachycardia (responding to baroreceptor response to decreased blood pressure), facial flushing, dizziness, headache, and peripheral edema. It has been used commonly for the emergent reduction of blood pressure in the field; however, labetalol is replacing it.

Nifedipine was used extensively for emergent reduction of blood pressure. Now, other agents, such as labetalol, are preferred.

Direct Vasodilators

We have already discussed several drugs that cause vasodilation. Two specific classes of vasodilators are those that dilate arterioles and those that dilate both arterioles and veins. All of these drugs are used to decrease blood pressure.

Selective dilation of arterioles causes a decrease in peripheral vascular resistance or afterload. This is the resistance that the heart must overcome in order to eject blood. Decreasing peripheral vascular resistance lowers blood pressure, increases cardiac output, and reduces cardiac workload. On the other hand, dilating the veins increases capacitance and decreases preload, the amount of blood in the heart prior to contraction. Starling's law tells us that as preload increases, so do stroke volume and cardiac output (up to a point). By decreasing preload, venodilators decrease both blood pressure and cardiac output.

Hydralizine (Apresoline) is the prototype for the selective arteriole dilators. It is effective in decreasing peripheral vascular resistance and afterload and thus lowering blood pressure. Its primary side effects are reflex tachycardia and increased blood volume. Both occur as a compensatory mechanism to lowered blood pressure, and both have the effect of increasing cardiac workload. As a result, hydralazine is almost always prescribed in conjunction with a beta blocker and a diuretic. It is frequently used in the treatment of pregnancy-induced hypertension.

Minoxidil (Loniten) is another selective arteriole dilator with properties similar to those of hydralazine. One side effect deserves comment. It produces hypertrichosis (excessive hair growth) in about 80 percent of those taking it. While this is particularly irritating when it occurs all over a patient's body, it can become a therapeutic effect when the drug is applied as a topical ointment. Minoxidil is marketed in this form as Rogaine for promoting hair growth in men.

Unlike hydralazine, sodium nitroprusside (Nipride) acts on both arterioles and veins. It is the fastest acting antihypertensive available and is the drug of choice in hypertensive emergencies. It is very potent and is given via controlled IV infusion. Its effects are almost immediate and end within minutes of drug cessation; therefore, blood pressure must be carefully and continuously monitored during infusion, preferably in the ICU. Sodium nitroprusside has several significant side effects. Obviously, hypotension can be a problem when this medication is not carefully administered. Because cyanide and thyocyanate are byproducts of nitroprusside metabolism, other adverse effects include cyanide poisoning and thyocyanate toxicity.

Ganglionic Blocking Agents   Ganglionic blocking agents are nicotinic$_N$ antagonists. The prototype is trimethaphan (Arfonad). Since nicotinic$_N$ receptors exist at the ganglia of both the sympathetic and the parasympathetic nervous systems, competitive antagonism of these receptors turns off the entire autonomic nervous system, obviously not a very selective approach. When this happens, the effects on each organ system are determined by the predominant autonomic tone (the division of the ANS that normally has the greater influence on that organ). Because the arteries and veins have predominant sympathetic control, they dilate in response to trimethaphan administration. This reduces both preload and afterload, and blood pressure drops. Trimethaphan also directly affects vascular smooth muscle, causing dilation and the release of histamine, which is also a vasodilator. Mecamylamine (Inversine) is the other ganglionic blocking drug available in the United States, although it is not commonly used anymore.

Cardiac Glycosides   The cardiac glycosides occur naturally in the foxglove plant. The two drugs in the class, digoxin (Lanoxin) and digitoxin (Crystodigin), are chemically related. These drugs are also known as digitalis glycosides. Digoxin is the prototype. One of the ten most frequently prescribed medications in the country, it is indicated for heart failure and some types of dysrhythmias. Digoxin's mechanism of action is complex. It blocks the effects of Na$^+$K$^+$ATPase, an enzyme responsible for returning ion flow to normal levels after muscle depolarization. By interfering with this sodium-potassium pump, digoxin increases the intracellular levels of sodium. Because sodium is also involved in a reciprocal exchange with calcium, a build up of intracellular sodium leads to a similar build up of intracellular calcium. These elevated levels of intracellular calcium increase the strength of muscle contraction and are the basis for digoxin's primary indication. Digoxin reduces the symptoms of congestive heart failure by increasing myocardial contractility and cardiac output. This diminishes the dilation of the heart's chambers frequently seen in left heart failure because it enables the heart to effectively pump blood out of its ventricles, thus decreasing the engorgement typical of this condition. Increasing cardiac output decreases the sympathetic discharge mediated by baroreceptor reflexes, resulting in reduced afterload. Furthermore, digoxin indirectly lessens preload by increasing renal blood flow, which results in higher glomerular filtration and decreased blood volume. Digoxin also has antidysrhythmic effects, which we discuss more thoroughly in the section on antidysrhythmic medications.

While digoxin effectively treats the symptoms of heart failure, it also is potentially dangerous. Its therapeutic index is very small, and the individual variability is large. This leads to toxicity in some individuals even though they have normal digoxin levels. Digoxin's chief adverse effects are dysrhythmias. In fact, digoxin frequently induces some of the same dysrhythmias it is used to treat. Other side effects include fatigue, anorexia, nausea and vomiting, and blurred vision with a yellowish haze and halos around dark objects.

Other Vasodilators and Antianginals The drugs discussed in this section have vasodilatory properties that are useful in reducing blood pressure, but they are most commonly used to treat angina. The three basic types of angina pectoris (chest pain) are stable (exertional) angina; unstable angina; and variant, or Prinzmetal's, angina. Stable and unstable angina have the same pathophysiology and differ only by causation: stable angina occurs after exercise as a result of increased myocardial oxygen demand; unstable angina occurs without exertion. Both result from an imbalance between myocardial supply and demand. A buildup of plaque (atherosclerosis) along the walls of coronary arteries decreases these vessels' diameter and, as a result, the amount of blood flow to the heart. The same imbalance causes Prinzmetal's angina but it results from vasospasm instead of plaque buildup. The medications discussed in this section all either increase oxygen supply or decrease oxygen demand.

In addition to their previously discussed use as antihypertensives and antidysrhythmics, calcium channel blockers have a role in the treatment of angina. The three calcium channel blockers most frequently used for this purpose are verapamil (Calan, Isoptin), diltiazem (Cardizem), and nifedipine (Procardia). Recall that calcium is an integral part of both depolarization and muscle contraction. The effects of blocking its entry into the cells are twofold. All of these agents directly affect vascular smooth muscle, leading to dilation of the arterioles and, to a lesser degree, of the venules. This arterial dilation decreases peripheral vascular resistance and, as a result, afterload, which in turn directly decreases the workload of the heart and myocardial oxygen demand. Verapamil and diltiazem also reduce SA and AV node conductivity, which can decrease reflex tachycardia and dysrhythmias. Nifedipine has relatively few effects on the heart and, thus, has limited antidysrhythmic properties. The calcium channel blockers are effective in all forms of angina. A primary side effect of these agents is hypotension.

Organic nitrates are potent vasodilators used to treat all forms of angina. First used clinically in 1879, nitroglycerin (Nitrostat) is the oldest of these drugs and is the category's prototype. Other agents include isosorbide (Isordil, Sorbitrate) and amyl nitrite. Nitroglycerin acts on vascular smooth muscle via a complex series of events to decrease intracellular calcium, thus causing vasodilation. Nitroglycerin primarily dilates veins rather than arterioles. This decreases preload and thus decreases myocardial workload, which is its primary antianginal effect. In Prinzmetal's angina, nitroglycerin reverses coronary artery spasm and increases oxygen supply.

Nitroglycerin is very lipid soluble, which allows it to cross membranes easily. Because of this, it is readily absorbed and can be administered via sublingual, buccal, and transdermal routes. The primary concern with nitroglycerin is orthostatic hypotension, a side effect more common in the presence of right ventricular failure. Other common side effects include headache and reflex tachycardia. Headache is frequently used as an indicator of the effectiveness of nitroglycerin, which rapidly loses its potency when exposed to light. While orthostatic hypotension is a serious concern with the administration of nitroglycerin, this condition typically responds well to fluid infusions.

Nitroglycerin is effective in the management of angina pectoris as it decreases cardiac work.

Hemostatic Agents

✱ **hemostasis** the stoppage of bleeding.

Hemostasis is the stoppage of bleeding. It is a series of events in response to a tear in a blood vessel. Damage to the vessel's intima (innermost layer) exposes the underlying collagen and triggers a release of two naturally occurring substances, adenosine diphosphate (ADP) and thromboxane A_2 (TXA_2). Both ADP and TXA_2 stimulate the aggregation of platelets and vasoconstriction. The vasoconstriction decreases the flow of blood past the tear, thus allowing the newly "sticky" platelets to form a plug that temporarily occludes the bleeding.

While this plug effectively halts bleeding for the short term, it must be reinforced to continue the stoppage until the tear can be permanently repaired. Stabilizing the plug requires a complex cascade of events involving the activation of naturally occurring factors and ending with the conversion of prothrombin into thrombin. The thrombin then converts fibrinogen into fibrin, a strand-like substance that attaches to the vessel's surface and contracts in a mesh web over the platelet plug to form a blood clot. Several of the factors involved need vitamin K to carry out their functions. A vitamin K deficiency inhibits clotting and makes uncontrolled bleeding more likely. Conversely, limiting the clotting cascade to the immediate area of the vessel injury is important for obvious reasons. The protein antithrombin III is key in this process. Antithrombin III binds with several of the factors needed for clotting, thus inhibiting their ability to coagulate.

Once the vessel has been permanently repaired, the fibrin mesh must be broken down. This process, called fibrinolysis, involves another cascading system that ends with the activation of plasminogen into plasmin, which in turn breaks up the clot. Tissue plasminogen activator, a substance in the tissue, activates this last conversion.

Content Review

DRUGS USED TO TREAT THROMBI
- Antiplatelets
- Anticoagulants
- Thrombolytics

Thrombi (blood clots that obstruct vessels or heart cavities) are the primary pathology in several clinical conditions, including myocardial infarction, stroke, and pulmonary embolism. Drugs can effectively treat the causes of these conditions by decreasing platelet aggregation (antiplatelet drugs), interfering with the clotting cascade (anticoagulants) or directly breaking up the thrombus (thrombolytics).

✱ **antiplatelet** drug that decreases the formation of platelet plugs.

Antiplatelets Antiplatelet drugs decrease the formation of platelet plugs. The prototype antiplatelet drug is aspirin. Aspirin inhibits cyclooxygenase, an enzyme needed for the synthesis of thromboxane A_2 (TXA_2). Remember that TXA_2 causes platelets to aggregate and promotes local vasoconstriction. By inhibiting TXA_2, aspirin decreases the formation of platelet plugs and potential thrombi. Aspirin, as well as other antiplatelet and anticoagulant drugs, has no effect on existing thrombi; it only curbs the formation of new thrombi. Aspirin is indicated in the acute treatment of developing myocardial infarction. It is also useful in preventing the reoccurrence of MI and of ischemic stroke following transient ischemic attacks (TIAs).

One of aspirin's primary side effects is bleeding. Aspirin also may lead to an increase in gastric ulcers, which are a frequent source of gastrointestinal hemorrhage. By both stimulating the development of a potential source of bleeding as well as blocking an important mechanism for stopping that bleeding, aspirin can cause dangerous blood loss. Other antiplatelet drugs include dipyridamole (Persantine), Abciximab (ReoPro) and ticlopidine (Ticlid).

✱ **anticoagulant** drug that interrupts the clotting cascade.

Anticoagulants Anticoagulants interrupt the clotting cascade. The two main types of anticoagulants are parenteral and oral. The prototype parenteral anticoagulant is heparin, a substance derived from the lungs of cattle or the intestines of pigs. Its primary mechanism of action is to enhance antithrombin III's ability to inhibit the clotting cascade. Because heparin is very polar, it is very poorly absorbed and must be given parenterally. Heparin injections and infusions are indicated in treating and preventing deep vein thrombosis, pulmonary embolism, and some forms of stroke. Heparin also is used frequently in conjunction with thrombolytics to treat myocardial infarction. Finally, it is used to keep rubber-capped IV catheters (Hep-Locks) free from clots. As you would expect, bleeding is heparin's primary side effect. Other untoward effects include thrombocytopenia (decreased platelet counts) and allergic reactions. Heparin is measured in units rather than milligrams. A unit is that amount of heparin necessary to keep 1 ml of sheep plasma from clotting for one hour. Using this measurement is necessary because heparin's potency varies greatly when measured in milligrams.

Protamine sulfate is available as a heparin antagonist. Protamine can reverse the effects of heparin in the presence of dangerous and unintended bleeding by binding with heparin. This prevents heparin from binding with antithrombin III and enhancing its anticlotting abilities.

The prototype oral anticoagulant is warfarin (Coumadin). Warfarin's history serves as a useful reminder of its primary side effect. Warfarin was first developed as a rat poison that killed through uncontrolled bleeding. After noticing that a patient who attempted suicide by ingesting warfarin did not, in fact, die, its clinical use was investigated. Needless to say, this drug's primary side effect is bleeding.

Warfarin prevents coagulation by antagonizing the effects of vitamin K, which is needed for the synthesis of multiple factors involved in the clotting cascade. It is prescribed for chronic use to prevent thrombi in high risk patients such as those who have hip replacements or artificial heart valves or those who are in atrial fibrillation. Because warfarin easily crosses the placental barrier and has dangerous *teratogenic* (capable of causing malformations) properties, it is contraindicated in pregnant patients. It also interacts adversely with many other medications. Like heparin, warfarin may lead to bleeding. In cases of overdose, you may give vitamin K as an antidote.

Thrombolytics Thrombolytics act directly on thrombi to break them up. The several available thrombolytics share a similar mechanism of action. The prototype drug of this class is streptokinase (Streptase). Other thrombolytics include alteplase (tPA), reteplase (Retavase) and anistreplase (Eminase). These medications all dissolve clots effectively; they differ primarily in their administration and risk of bleeding side effects.

Streptokinase, which is derived from the streptococci bacterium, is the oldest available thrombolytic. Its mechanism of action is to promote plasminogen's conversion to plasmin. Since plasmin dissolves the fibrin mesh of clots, it can directly treat the cause of most myocardial infarctions and some strokes, as opposed to antiplatelet agents and anticoagulants, which can only prevent potential future thrombi. Streptokinase also breaks down fibrinogen, the precursor to fibrin. While this action does not serve a clinical purpose (the problematic clot has already been formed), it does play an important role in streptokinase's chief side effect, bleeding. Other side effects include allergic reaction, hypotension, and fever.

Alteplase (Activase) is produced by recombinant DNA technology that is identical to the naturally occurring tissue plasminogen activator (hence its common name, tPA).

The window of opportunity for thrombolytic therapy is limited. Because of this, some EMS systems administer thrombolytics in the prehospital setting. Many have chosen to use retaplase (Eminase) because of its ease of administration (two 10-unit boluses administered 30 minutes apart).

Antihyperlipidemic Agents

Elevated levels of low-density lipoproteins (LDLs) have been clearly indicated as a causative factor in coronary artery disease. Lipoproteins are essentially transport mechanisms for lipids (triglycerides and cholesterol). Because lipids are insoluble

✳ thrombolytic drug that acts directly on thrombi to break them down.

in plasma, the body coats them in a plasma-soluble shell in order to transport them to their target destinations. Lipoproteins are categorized as very low-density (VLDL), low-density (LDL), intermediate-density (IDL), and high-density (HDL). Low-density lipoproteins contain most of the cholesterol in the blood and are required for transporting cholesterol from the liver to the peripheral tissues. Conversely, high-density lipoproteins (HDLs) carry cholesterol from the peripheral tissues to the liver, where it is broken down.

HDLs have been described as good cholesterol because they lower blood cholesterol levels and decrease the risk of coronary artery disease (CAD). LDLs are known as bad cholesterol because they increase blood cholesterol levels and the risk of CAD. As blood cholesterol levels increase, fatty plaque is deposited under the arteries' endothelial tissues. Atherosclerosis then develops, and coronary arteries decrease in diameter. Coronary vasoconstriction in turn reduces blood flow to the heart and, in times of increased myocardial oxygen demand, may lead to angina. Also, newly deposited plaque is often unstable. Typically, the plaque is under the endothelial tissues, which cap the plaque deposits. As the deposits age, the cap usually becomes fairly stable. In some cases, however, the cap breaks open and exposes the plaque to the blood. When this happens, platelet aggregation and coagulation begin. If the developing clot breaks free of the vessel, it becomes a thrombus and may completely occlude a coronary artery, leading to myocardial infarction.

The goal in lowering LDL levels is to prevent atherosclerosis and subsequent CAD. While raising HDL levels would help accomplish this, no pharmaceutical means of doing so currently exists. By far, the best way to lower LDL levels remains dietary modification. If this is not sufficient, several classifications of **antihyperlipidemic** medications may be used. The most common are drugs that inhibit hydroxymethylglutaryl coenzyme A (HMG CoA) reductase. The liver must have HMG CoA to synthesize cholesterol. By inhibiting this enzyme, HMG CoA agents lower LDL levels; however, they also increase the number of LDL receptors in the liver, causing a further uptake of LDL.

Five HMG CoA reductase inhibitors are available. Because the names of all five end in –*statin,* these agents are also known as statins. They include lovastatin (Mevacor) and simvastatin (Zocor). Lovastatin is the HMG CoA reductase inhibitors' prototype. Overall, these drugs are well tolerated. Their chief side effects are headache, rash, and flushing. In rare cases, they may cause hepatotoxicity and lead to liver failure.

Bile acid-binding resins can also reduce LDL levels. Inert substances that have no direct biologic activity, these agents pass straight through the GI system without being absorbed and are excreted in feces. They are useful, however, in that they indirectly increase the number of LDL receptors in the liver by binding with bile acids, thus decreasing their availability. Because the liver needs cholesterol to synthesize bile acids, it must have more cholesterol to compensate for the decrease in bile acids. The body therefore increases the LDL receptors on the liver. As more LDLs remain in the liver, their levels in the blood drop. Since the body does not absorb bile acid-binding agents, they have no systemic effects. Their chief untoward effect is constipation. Cholestyramine (Questran) is the prototype.

DRUGS USED TO AFFECT THE RESPIRATORY SYSTEM

Drugs that affect the respiratory system are useful for several purposes. The most obvious is the treatment of asthma, but this class also includes cough suppressants, nasal decongestants, and antihistamines.

* **anithyperlipidemic** drug used to treat high blood cholesterol.

Table 6-7   DRUGS USED IN THE TREATMENT OF ASTHMA

Mechanism of Action	Medication
Bronchodilators	
Nonspecific agonists	Epinephrine
	Ephedrine
Beta$_2$ specific agonists	
Inhaled (short acting)	Albuterol (Ventolin, Proventil)
	Metaproterenol (Alupent)
	Terbutaline (Brethine)
	Bitolterol (Tornalate)
Inhaled (long-acting)	Salmeterol (Serevent)
Methylxanthines	Theophylline (Theo-Dur, Slo-Bid)
	Aminophylline
Anticholinergics	Atropine
	Ipratropium (Atrovent)
Anti-inflammatory agents	
Glucocorticoids	
Inhaled	Beclomethasone (Beclovent)
	Flucticasone (Flovent)
	Triamcinolone (Azmacort)
Oral	Prednisone (Deltasone)
Injected	Methyprednisolone (Solu-Medrol)
	Dexamethasone (Decadron)
Leukotriene Antagonists	Zafirlukast (Accolate)
	Zileuton (Zyflo)
Mast-Cell Membrane Stabilizer	Cromolyn (Intal)

ANTIASTHMATIC MEDICATIONS

Asthma is a common disease that decreases pulmonary function and may limit daily activities. It typically presents with shortness of breath, wheezing, and coughing. Its basic pathophysiology has two components, bronchoconstriction and inflammation. Typically a response to some sort of allergen sets both of these processes in motion. Common culprits include pet dander, mold, and dust. In patients with existing asthma, cold air, tobacco smoke, or other pollutants may bring on acute episodes of shortness of breath.

The response to asthma typically begins with an allergen's binding to an antibody on mast cells. This causes the mast cell membrane to rupture and release its contents, including histamine, leukotrines, and prostaglandins. These cause immediate bronchoconstriction followed by a slower inflammatory response that can lead to mucus plugs and a further decrease in airway size. The inflammation may in turn cause a hyperreactivity to stimuli, and allergens that might not normally produce dyspnea may lead to an acute attack.

Drug treatment of asthma aims to relieve bronchospasm and decrease inflammation. Specific approaches are categorized as beta$_2$ selective sympathomimetics, nonselective sympathomimetics, methylxanthines, anticholinergics, glucocorticoids, and leukotriene antagonists. Cromolyn (Nasalcrom), a frequently used anti-inflammatory agent, does not fit neatly into any of those categories. Table 6-7 summarizes these agents.

Beta$_2$ Specific Agents Drugs that are selective for beta$_2$ receptors are the mainstay in treating asthma induced shortness of breath. Albuterol (Proventil, Ventolin) is the prototype of this class. In general, these agents relax bronchial

Drug treatment of asthma aims to relieve bronchospasm and decrease inflammation.

smooth muscle, which results in bronchodilation and relief from bronchospasm. Agents from this class are first line therapy for acute shortness of breath and may also be used daily for prophylaxis. Most are administered via metered dose inhaler or nebulizer. Albuterol and terbutaline may both be taken orally, and terbutaline may be given by injection. These medications' beta$_2$ specificity is not absolute; some patients may experience beta$_1$ effects such as tachycardia or dysrhythmias. Patients may also experience tremors resulting from the stimulation of beta$_2$ receptors in smooth muscles. Overall, these agents are very safe.

Early pharmacological intervention in asthma is important in order to minimize inflammation.

Nonselective Sympathomimetics Medications that stimulate both beta$_1$ and beta$_2$ receptors, as well as alpha receptors are rarely used to treat asthma because they have the undesired effects of increased peripheral vascular resistance and increased risks for tachycardias and other dysrhythmias. Nonselective drugs include epinephrine, ephedrine, and isoproterenol. Epinephrine is the only nonselective sympathomimetic in common use today, due to the availability of selective agents. It may be given subcutaneously for patients who have severe bronchospasm that does not respond to other treatments.

Methylxanthines The methylxanthines are CNS stimulants that have additional bronchodilatory properties. While they were once first-line therapy for asthma, now they are used only when other drugs such as beta$_2$ specific agents are ineffective. We do not know the methylxanthines' specific action, but they may block adenosine receptors. The prototype methylxanthine, theophylline, is taken orally. Aminophylline, an IV medication, is rapidly metabolized into theophylline and, therefore, has identical effects. These agents' chief side effects are nausea, vomiting, insomnia, restlessness, and dysrhythmias. Aminophylline is still used occasionally in the emergency treatment of acute asthma attacks.

Anticholinergics Ipratropium (Atrovent) is an atropine derivative given by nebulizer. Because stimulating the muscarinic receptors in the lungs results in constriction of bronchial smooth muscle, ipratropium, a muscarinic antagonist, causes bronchodilation. Ipratropium is inhaled and, therefore, has no systemic effects. Ipratropium and beta$_2$ agonists like albuterol act along different pathways, so their concurrent administration has an additive effect. Ipratropium's most common side effect is dry mouth. It results from the local effects of the drug that remains in the oropharynx after administration.

Glucocorticoids Glucocorticoids have anti-inflammatory properties. They lower the production and release of inflammatory substances such as histamine, prostaglandins, and leukotrienes, and they reduce mucus and edema secondary to decreasing vascular permeability. These drugs may be inhaled or taken orally, or they may be given intravenously in emergencies. The prototype inhaled glucocorticoid is beclomethasone; the prototype oral glucocorticoid is prednisone. Primarily preventative, they are taken on a regular schedule as opposed to the as-needed administration of the beta$_2$ agonists. An injectable glucocorticoid (methylprednisolone) is available for use secondary to beta$_2$ agonists in emergencies. When inhaled, glucocorticoids cause few side effects. Those are due mostly to direct exposure on the oropharynx, and gargling after taking the drug can decrease them. Likewise, side effects from the intravenous administrations of methylprednisolone in emergencies are not likely. Given orally or intravenously over long periods, however, glucocorticoids may have profound side effects, including adrenal suppression and hyperglycemia.

Another anti-inflammatory agent used to prevent asthma attacks is cromolyn (Intal), an inhaled powder. While it is not a glucocorticoid, its actions are similar. While the inhaled glucocorticoids are relatively safe, cromolyn is even safer. In fact, it is the safest of all antiasthma agents. Its only side effects are coughing or wheezing due to local irritation caused by the powder. Cromolyn is often used for preventing asthma in adults and children. It is also a useful prophylaxis before activities known to cause shortness of breath such as exercise or mowing grass.

Leukotriene Antagonists **Leukotrienes** are mediators released from mast cells upon contact with allergens. They contribute powerfully to both inflammation and bronchoconstriction. Consequently, agents that block their effects are useful in treating asthma. Leukotriene antagonists can either block the synthesis of leukotrienes or block their receptors. Zileuton (Zyflo) is the prototype of those that block the synthesis of leukotrienes. Zafirlukast (Accolate) is the prototype of those that block their receptors.

* **leukotriene** mediator released from mast cells upon contact with allergens.

DRUGS USED FOR RHINITIS AND COUGH

Rhinitis (inflammation of the nasal lining) comprises a group of symptoms including nasal congestion, itching, redness, sneezing, and rhinorrhea (runny nose). Either allergic reactions or viral infections such as the common cold may cause it. Drugs that treat the symptoms of rhinitis and cold are commonly found in over-the-counter remedies. In addition, nasal decongestants, antihistamines, and cough suppressants are available in prescription medications. Although manufacturers of cold medications often combine several drugs in one product intended to treat multiple symptoms, we will discuss each class separately.

Nasal Decongestants Nasal congestion is caused by dilated and engorged nasal capillaries. Drugs that constrict these capillaries are effective nasal decongestants. The main pharmacologic classification in this functional category is alpha$_1$ agonists. Alpha$_1$ agonists may be given either topically or orally. The chief examples of these agents, phenylephrine, pseudoephedrine, and phenylpropanolamine, can be administered either as a mist or in drops. Topical administration reduces systemic effects but has the undesired local effect of rebound congestion, a form of tolerance. Rebound congestion occurs after long term use (greater than seven consecutive days). As the drug wears off, congestion becomes progressively worse. This effect ends when the patient stops taking the drug; however, the longer the patient has been using the drug, the more unpleasant stopping becomes.

Nasal decongestants, when overused, can elevate both the pulse rate and the blood pressure.

Antihistamines Antihistamines arrest the effects of histamine by blocking its receptors. **Histamine** is an endogenous substance that affects a wide variety of organ systems. It is noted for its role in allergic reaction. In the vasculature, histamine binds with H$_1$ receptors to cause vasodilation and increased capillary permeability. In the lungs, H$_1$ receptors cause bronchoconstriction. In the gut, H$_2$ receptors cause an increase in gastric acid release. Histamine also acts as a neurotransmitter in the central nervous system. Histamine is synthesized and stored in two types of granulocytes; tissue-bound mast cells and plasma-bound basophils. Both types are full of secretory granules, which are vesicles containing inflammatory mediators such as histamine, leukotrienes, and prostaglandins, among others. When these cells are exposed to allergens, they develop antibodies on their surfaces. On subsequent exposures, the antibodies bind with their specific allergen. The secretory granules then migrate toward the cell's exterior and fuse with the cell membrane. This causes them to release their contents. While some available medications stabilize this membrane to prevent the release of these substances, the traditional antihistamines work by antagonizing the histamine receptors.

* **histamine** an endogenous substance that affects a wide variety of organ systems.

Commonly thought of as a nuisance, histamines are useful in our immune systems. Only when our immune systems overreact do allergies such as hay fever or cedar fever send us running for the antihistamines. The typical symptoms of allergic reaction include most of those associated with rhinitis. Severe allergic reactions (anaphylaxis) may cause hypotension. While histamines play a major role in mild and moderate allergic reactions, their part in anaphylaxis is minimal; therefore, antihistamines are at best only a secondary drug for treating anaphylaxis. (Epinephrine is the drug of choice.)

Just as there are H_1 and H_2 histamine receptors, there are H_1 and H_2 histamine receptor antagonists. When most people refer to antihistamines, they are thinking of H_1 receptor antagonists. These agents were in popular use long before the discovery of the H_2 receptors. (We discuss H_2 receptor antagonists in the section on drugs used to treat peptic ulcer disease.) The chief side effect of antihistamines is sedation, which the early antihistamines all caused to some degree. Now a second generation of antihistamines that do not cause sedation is available.

The first-generation antihistamines comprise several chemical subclasses. Examples include alkylamines (chlorpheniramine [Chlor-Trimeton]), ethanolamines (diphenhydramine [Benadryl], clemastine (Tavist)), and phenothiazines (promethazine [Phenergan]). While the different classes of agents have the same actions, they differ in the degree of sedation they cause and in their ability to block other, nonhistamine, receptors. Several antihistamines also have significant anticholinergic properties. In fact, some are used specifically for their anticholinergic effects, notably promethazine and dimenhydrinate (Dramamine), which are used to reduce motion sickness. Other than the sedation that first generation antihistamines cause, these agents' primary side effects are constipation and the effects of muscarinic blockade, such as dry mouth. Because they can thicken bronchial secretions, antihistamines should not be used in patients with asthma.

The second generation antihistamines include terfenadine (Seldane), loratadine (Claritin), cetirizine (Zyrtec), and fexofenadine (Allegra). These agents' actions are similar to the first generation's, with the notable exception that they do not cross the blood-brain barrier and therefore do not cause sedation. In addition, their H_1 receptor antagonism is more pronounced, and their anticholinergic actions are greatly diminished. Terfenadine was used widely until the FDA removed it from the market because it had rare but significant side effects of cardiac dysrhythmias in patients with liver dysfunction or taking certain medications. Terfenadine's manufacturer is now marketing fexofenadine (Allegra) as a replacement.

Cough Suppressants Coughing is a complex reflex that depends on functions in the CNS, the PNS, and the respiratory muscles. It is a defense mechanism that aids the removal of foreign particles like smoke and dust. A productive cough is one in which these particles are actually being coughed up. In general, treating a productive cough is not appropriate, as it is performing a useful function. An unproductive cough, on the other hand, usually results from an irritated oropharynx and can be troublesome. The three classifications of cough suppressants include one that is supported by evidence and two that are not. **Antitussive** medications suppress the stimulus to cough in the central nervous system. This functional class includes two specific pharmacologic types, opioids and nonopioids. The two most common opioid antitussives are codeine and hydrocodone. Both inhibit the stimulus for coughing in the brain but also produce varying degrees of euphoria. The doses required for cough suppression are not high enough to cause euphoria, but these drugs still have the potential for abuse. The nonopioid antitussives, in contrast, do not have the potential for abuse. Dextromethoraphan is the leading drug in this class. While it is almost never given alone, it is the most common antitussive used in over-the-counter combination products for treating cold and flu symptoms. Diphenhydramine (Benadryl) is also used as a nonopioid antitussive, although its mechanism of action is not clear. Finally, the locally acting anesthetic benzonatate (Tessalon) depresses the cough stimulus by directly reducing oropharyngeal irritation. **Expectorants** are intended to increase the productivity of cough, and **mucolytics** make mucus more watery and, therefore, easier to cough up; however, little data supports the effectiveness of either of these approaches to cough suppression.

Because they can thicken bronchial secretions, you should not use antihistamines in patients with asthma.

In general, treating a productive cough is not appropriate, as the cough is performing a useful function.

* antitussive medication that suppresses the stimulus to cough in the central nervous system.

* expectorant medication intended to increase the productivity of cough.

* mucolytic medication intended to make mucus more watery.

DRUGS USED TO AFFECT THE GASTROINTESTINAL SYSTEM

The main purposes of drug therapy in the gastrointestinal system are to treat peptic ulcers, constipation, diarrhea, and emesis, and to aid digestion.

DRUGS USED TO TREAT PEPTIC ULCER DISEASE

Peptic Ulcer Disease (PUD) is characterized by an imbalance between factors in the gastrointestinal system that increase acidity and those that protect against acidity. PUD may manifest as indigestion, heartburn, or more seriously, as perforated ulcers. If the imbalance becomes too severe, parts of the lining of the GI system may be eaten away, exposing the tissue and vasculature underneath to the highly acidic environment of the stomach or duodenum. The GI system's structure fits its function. Many mucus-lined folds surround the GI lumen. The cells of these folds secrete acids needed to help break down foods; they secrete protective mucus that prevents the acid from injuring the underlying tissue; and finally, they secrete bicarbonates, which buffer the effects of acids on the GI system's absorbing surfaces. To absorb the digested nutrients and supply the mucus producing cells of the lumen wall with oxygen, the entire GI system is very vascular. If the protective lining covering these vessels is removed, hemorrhage may occur.

Several pathologic factors oppose the GI system's defenses. Contrary to popular belief, the most common cause of peptic ulcer disease is not stress or alcohol, but the *Helicobacter pylori* bacterium. *H. pylori* infests the space between the endothelial cells and the mucus lining of the stomach and duodenum. It can remain there for decades, protected against the acid environment by the mucus layer. While we are still uncertain how this bacteria promotes ulcers, it apparently decreases the body's ability to produce the protective mucus lining. *H. pylori* by itself, however, does not cause ulcers. Many people remain infected for years and years without signs of PUD. Evidently, predisposing and contributing factors combine with *H. pylori* to cause ulceration. Some of these factors include smoking and long-term use of nonsteroidal anti-inflammatory drugs (NSAIDs) like aspirin and acetaminophen.

The approaches to treating PUD include antibiotics and drugs that block or decrease the secretion of gastric acid. Most often they are used in conjunction with each other. First, and most effective, are antibiotics. When the *H. pylori* infection is eliminated, the signs of PUD resolve and recurrence is low. Typically, three antibiotics will be utilized to assure elimination of the bacteria and prevent resistance. Common medications for this purpose include bismuth (Pepto-Bismol), metronidazole (Flagyl), amoxicillin (Amoxil), and tetracycline (Achromycin V).

Drugs that block or decrease the secretion of gastric acid include H_2 receptor antagonists (H_2RAs), proton pump inhibitors, and anticholinergic agents. Mucosal protectants and antacids are also used.

H_2 receptors occur throughout the gut on the membranes of the parietal cells lining the GI lumen. When stimulated with histamine, they increase the action of H^+, K^+ ATPase, an enzyme that exchanges potassium for hydrogen, leading to increased gastric acid secretion. Acetylcholine and prostaglandin receptors appear along with H_2 receptors. Stimulating the ACh receptors (muscarinic receptors) increases gastric acid secretion; stimulating the prostaglandin receptors inhibits it.

H_2 Receptor Antagonists H_2RA agents block the H_2 receptors in the gut. This inhibits gastric acid secretion and helps return the balance between protective and aggressive factors. Four approved H_2RAs are in use: cimetidine (Tagamet), ranitidine (Zantac), famotidine (Pepcid), and nizatidine (Axid Pulvules). Cimetidine is the oldest of these and serves as the prototype. These agents' primary therapeutic use is for ulcers, gastroesophageal reflux, heartburn or acid indigestion, and preventing aspiration pneumonia during anesthesia. Most of these agents have few significant side effects, with the exception of cimetidine, which may lead to decreased libido, impotence, and CNS effects in some patients. While these agents could technically be called antihistamines, that name by tradition is reserved for the H_1 antagonists. The H_2RAs have no effect on the H_1 receptors and are of no value in allergic reaction.

Proton Pump Inhibitors Proton pump inhibitors act directly on the K^+, H^+ ATPase enzyme that secretes gastric acid. Omeprazole (Prilosec) and lansoprazole (Prevacid) are examples. Omeprazole is the prototype. These agents irreversibly block this enzyme, which means that the body must produce new enzyme in order to begin secreting acid again. This gives proton pump inhibitors a long duration of effect. Side effects are minor and rare, occurring in less than one percent of patients. They include diarrhea and headache.

Antacids Antacids are alkalotic compounds used to increase the gastric environment's pH. Most available products are either aluminum, magnesium, calcium, or sodium compounds. They are used in conjunction with other approaches to PUD and are available over the counter for relief of acid indigestion and heartburn.

Anticholinergics While it might seem that all muscarinic blocking agents would be effective in decreasing gastric acid secretion, most atropine-like drugs produce too many unwanted effects and, therefore, are not used. The one exception is pirenzepine (Gastrozepine), because of its ability to selectively block the ACh receptors in the gut.

DRUGS USED TO TREAT CONSTIPATION

Laxatives decrease the firmness of stool and increase the water content. While an uninformed public frequently uses these agents unnecessarily, they are effective in some situations, specifically with patients for whom excessive strain is inappropriate. These patients include those with recent episiotomy, hemorrhoids, colostomies, or cardiovascular disease (for whom excessive straining may decrease heart rate).

Laxatives are traditionally grouped into four categories based on their mechanism of action: bulk-forming, surfactant, stimulant, and osmotic. The bulk-forming agents such as methylcellulose (Citrucel) and psyllium (Metamucil) produce a response almost identical to normal dietary fiber intake. Fiber is undigestible and unabsorbable; therefore, it remains in the lumen of the GI system and is passed more or less intact in stool. Most water absorption takes place in the colon. Fiber (or bulk-forming laxatives) in the colon absorbs water, leading to a softer, more bulky stool. Fiber can also provide nutrients for bacteria living in the colon. These bacteria feed and provide even more bulk. The enlarged stool stimulates stretch receptors in the colonic wall, which increases peristalsis. Softening the stool also lessens strain on defecation.

The **surfactant** laxatives include docusate sodium (Colace). They decrease surface tension, which increases water absorption into the feces. They also increase water secretion and limit its reabsorption by the intestinal wall.

Stimulant laxatives increase motility. Like the surfactant laxatives, they also increase water secretion and decrease its absorption. The prototype stimulant laxative is phenolphthalein (Ex-Lax, Correctol). Bisacodyl (Bisacolax) is another example.

The osmotic laxatives are poorly absorbed salts that increase the feces' osmotic pull, thereby increasing their water content. Magnesium hydroxide, the active ingredient in Milk of Magnesia, is the prototype of this class.

* **antacid** alkalotic compound used to increase the gastric environment's pH.

* **laxative** medication used to decrease stool's firmness and increase its water content.

Content Review

CATEGORIES OF LAXATIVES
- Bulk-forming
- Stimulant
- Osmotic
- Surfactant

* **surfactant** substance that decreases surface tension.

DRUGS USED TO TREAT DIARRHEA

Diarrhea is the abnormally frequent passage of soft, liquid stool. It is a symptom of an underlying disease, usually a bacterial infection. It may be caused by an increased gastric motility (the stool does not stay in the colon long enough to have much water absorbed), increased water secretion, or decreased water absorption. While it is a nuisance, diarrhea is often a helpful process because it increases the expulsion of the offending agent. It is usually self-correcting and does not need to be treated. When treatment is necessary, either specific or nonspecific agents may be used. A specific agent directly treats the cause, usually a bacteria. As you would expect, antibiotics are a common specific antidiarrheal medication.

DRUGS USED TO TREAT EMESIS

Emesis is a complex process that involves different parts of the brain as well as receptors and muscles in the stomach and inner ear. The two involved parts of the brain include the vomiting center in the medulla and the chemoreceptor trigger zone (CTZ). The vomiting center stimulates vomiting directly, while the CTZ does so indirectly.

The vomiting center is stimulated by H_1 and ACh receptors in the pathway between itself and the inner ear, by sensory input from the eyes and nose (unpleasant or disturbing sights and smells), and by other parts of the brain in response to anxiety or fear. The CTZ stimulates the vomiting center in response to stimuli from serotonin receptors in the stomach and blood-borne substances such as opioids and ipecac.

Stimulating emesis is rarely desired, but it can be useful in treating certain types of overdoses or poisonings. Ipecac is the drug of choice when stimulating emesis is indicated. It stimulates the CTZ which, in turn, stimulates the vomiting center.

Antiemetics Unlike causing emesis, preventing emesis is frequently desirable. **Antiemetics** are indicated in conjunction with chemotherapy, which may cause violent nausea and vomiting. Antiemetics are also indicated in the prophylactic treatment of motion sickness.

Multiple transmitters are involved in the vomiting reflex. They include serotonin, dopamine, acetylcholine, and histamine. Drugs that interfere with any of these transmitters can decrease or prevent nausea and vomiting. This functional class includes several pharmacologic subclasses: serotonin antagonists, dopamine antagonists, anticholinergics and cannabinoids.

Serotonin Antagonists The prototype serotonin antagonist is ondansetron (Zofran). It blocks the serotonin receptors in the CTZ, the stomach, and the small intestines. It is very effective in the treatment of nausea and vomiting associated with chemotherapy, and unlike the dopamine antagonists, it does not cause extrapyramidal effects like dystonia and ataxia. Its most common side effects are headache and diarrhea.

Dopamine Antagonists Both phenothiazines and butyrophenones effectively block dopamine receptors in the CTZ. (This chapter's section on psychotherapeutic medications discusses both of these medications at length.) The phenothiazines include prochlorperazine (Compazine) and promethazine (Phenergan), while the butyrophenones include haloperidol (Haldol) and droperidol (Inapsine). Agents from both classes cause side effects of extrapyramidal effects and sedation. Another dopamine antagonist, metoclopramide (Reglan) is neither a phenothiazine nor a butyropenone. It is unique in that it blocks both serotonin and dopamine receptors in the CTZ.

Ipecac is the drug of choice when stimulating emesis is indicated.

* **antiemetic** medication used to prevent vomiting.

Many of the antiemetics used in emergency care can cause extrapyramidal symptoms. Always be alert for these.

Cannabinoids The cannabinoids are derivatives of tetrahydrocannabinol (THC) and are effective antiemetics used to treat chemotherapy-induced nausea and vomiting. The two available agents are dronabinol (Marinol) and nabilone (Cesamet). Because both agents are essentially the same as THC (the active ingredient in marijuana), their side effects include euphoria similar to that of marijuana. While those effects may be desirable for some, they may be intensely unpleasant for others.

DRUGS USED TO AID DIGESTION

Several drugs are available to aid the digestion of carbohydrates and fats. These agents are similar to endogenous digestive enzymes released into the duodenum in response to vagal stimulation. Occasionally, supplemental enzymes are necessary for patients whose vagal stimulus has been surgically severed or whose duodenum has been bypassed. Two of these drugs are pancreatin (Entozyme) and pancrelipase (Viokase). Their chief side effects are nausea, vomiting, and abdominal cramping.

DRUGS USED TO AFFECT THE EYES

Ophthalmic drugs are used to treat conditions involving the eyes, primarily glaucoma and trauma. In addition, some ophthalmic agents are used in diagnosing and examining the eyes.

Glaucoma is a degenerative disease that effects the optic nerve. Its causative factors are not clear; however, correlations are known between it and several risk factors including intraocular pressure, race (its rate is three times higher among African-Americans than among whites), and age. The medications used to treat glaucoma are all aimed at reducing intraocular pressure (IOP). Beta blockers and cholinergics are the most common. Beta blockade decreases IOP by an unknown mechanism. Timolol (Timoptic) and betaxolol (Betoptic) are examples of this class. Pilocarpine (Isopto Carpine) is the prototype cholinergic drug for treating glaucoma. It stimulates muscarinic receptors in the eye to cause miosis (pupil constriction) and ciliary muscle contraction, which indirectly lowers IOP. Drugs from these classes are given topically. Beta blockers have few side effects, while pilocarpine causes blurred vision and local irritation.

Some diagnostic procedures call for causing mydriasis (pupil dilation) and cycloplegia (paralysis of the ciliary muscles used to focus vision). The two pharmacologic approaches to doing this involve anticholinergics or adrenergic agonists. In this functional class, atropine solutions such as Atropisol and scopolamine solutions such as Isopto Hyoscine are typical anticholinergics; phenylephrine solution (AK-Dilate) is the class's principal adrenergic agonist. This chapter's sections on anticholinergics and adrenergic agonists discuss these pharmacologic classes in more detail.

Tetracaine (Pontocaine) is a local anesthetic of the ester class. (It is related to cocaine, another ester, but not to lidocaine, an amide.) It is used to decrease pain and sensation in the eye from trauma or during ophthalmic procedures.

If tetracaine is administered in the field, remind the patient not to rub his eyes, as he can worsen the injury.

DRUGS USED TO AFFECT THE EARS

Most drugs used to treat conditions involving the ear are aimed at eliminating underlying bacterial or fungal infections or at breaking up impacted ear wax. Chloramphenicol (Chloromycetin Otic) and gentamicin sulfate otic solution (Garamycin) are common antibiotics; carbamide peroxide (Auro Ear Drops) and carbamide peroxide and glycerin (Ear Wax Removal System) are both used to treat ear wax. Finally, several drugs are available to treat swimmer's ear, an inflammation/irritation of the external ear. They include isopropyl alcohol (Auro-Dri Ear Drops) and boric acid and isopropyl alcohol (Aurocaine 2).

Some drugs that are used for other purposes have ototoxic (harmful to the organs or nerves that produce hearing or balance) properties if taken in overdose or administered too quickly. The most common ototoxic symptom is tinnitus, or ringing in the ears. Drugs with ototoxic properties include aspirin and other NSAIDs, some antibiotics (including erythromycin and vancomycin), and the diuretic furosemide (Lasix).

DRUGS USED TO AFFECT THE ENDOCRINE SYSTEM

The endocrine system and nervous system together are chiefly responsible for the regulatory activities that maintain homeostasis. The nervous system, with its direct connections between nerves and organs, may be thought of as a "wired" system, while the endocrine system, which releases hormones directly into the bloodstream, may be thought of as "wireless." The endocrine system comprises the following glands: pituitary (anterior and posterior lobes), pineal, thyroid, parathyroid, thymus, adrenal, pancreas, ovaries, and testes. Of these, the pituitary is commonly referred to as the master gland because of its role in controlling the other endocrine glands. (The hypothalmus in turn controls many of the pituitary's functions.) Once in the bloodstream, the hormones from these glands circulate widely throughout the body. To be effective, however, they must bind with very specific receptors. This discussion will focus on the pharmacologic actions of drugs that affect the various endocrine glands.

DRUGS AFFECTING THE PITUITARY GLAND

The pituitary gland has a posterior and an anterior lobe. Anteror pituitary-like drugs are used to treat abnormal growth: dwarfism, acromegaly, and gigantism. The two posterior pituitary hormones are oxytocin and antidiuretic hormone. Oxytocin is discussed in the section on drugs affecting labor and delivery. Antidiuretic hormone (ADH) promotes water retention. ADH analogs are used to treat diabetes insipidus and nocturnal enuresis (bedwetting). At higher doses, ADH can cause vasoconstriction and increased blood pressure; hence its other name, vasopressin. Vasopressin (Pitressin), desmopressin (Stimate), and lypressin (Diapid) are all available to reverse ADH deficiency.

DRUGS AFFECTING THE PARATHYROID AND THYROID GLANDS

The parathyroid glands are primarily responsible for regulating calcium levels. Hypoparathyroidism leads to decreased levels of calcium and Vitamin D. Treatment, therefore, is through calcium and Vitamin D supplements. Hyperparathyroidism leads to high levels of calcium. Because it usually results from tumors, the treatment of choice is surgical removal of all or part of the parathyroid glands.

The thyroid gland produces thyroid hormones, which play a vital role in regulating growth, maturation, and metabolism. Hypothyroidism can occur in children or adults. When it develops in children, it is known as cretinism and manifests itself as dwarfism and mental retardation with characteristic features. Because most growth and maturation in adults is complete, adult onset of hypothyroidism appears as decreased metabolic rate, weight gain, fatigue, and bradycardia. In some cases, myxedema (facial puffiness) may be present. Treatment is aimed at thyroid hormone replacement. The prototype drug, levothyroxine (Synthroid), is also the most commonly used. A synthetic analogue of T_4 (thyroxine), one of the thyroid hormones, levothyroxine generally has no significant side effects when taken in therapeutic doses. Overdose may lead to thyrotoxicosis or thyroid storm. Thyrotoxicosis is a condition in which hyperthyroidism causes an increase in thyroid hormones. Thyroid storm is a severe form of thyrotoxicosis where the manifestations of the disease increase to life-threatening proportions. Thyroid storm is characterized by tachycardic dysrhythmias, angina, hypertension, and hyperthermia.

Goiters are enlargements of the thyroid gland. They are typically caused by insufficient dietary iodine. In developed countries, goiter is much rarer than in undeveloped countries and is most commonly caused by Hashimoto's disease, a chronic autoimmune disease. Treatment of goiters is aimed at supplementing the inadequate iodine.

Hyperthyroidism is caused by excessive release of thyroid hormones, typically as a result of tumors. The most common cause of hyperthyroidism in the United States is Grave's Disease. It presents with tachycardia, hypertension, hyperthermia, nervousness, insomnia, increased metabolic rate, and weight loss. In severe cases, exophthalmos (protrusion of the eyeballs) may occur. Treatment is typically surgical removal of all or part of the thyroid gland. Radioactive iodine (^{131}I) may also be given for radiation therapy. Propylthiouracil (PTU) may be given alone or as adjunct therapy to surgery or radiation in treating hyperthyroidism.

DRUGS AFFECTING THE ADRENAL CORTEX

The adrenal cortex synthesizes and secretes three classes of hormones: glucocorticoids, mineralocorticoids, and androgens. The glucocorticoids and mineralocorticoids are referred to collectively as corticosteroids, adrenocortiocoids, or corticoids. As their name implies, glucocorticoids increase the production of glucose by enhancing carbohydrate metabolism, promoting gluconeogenesis, and reducing peripheral glucose utilization. The most important glucocorticoid is cortisol. The mineralocorticoids regulate salt and water balance. The primary mineralocorticoid is aldosterone. The androgens are important hormones in regulating sexual maturation and development.

Two diseases typify the disorders associated with the adrenal cortex: Cushing's disease and Addison's disease. Cushing's disease is characterized by hypersecretion of adrenocorticotropic hormone, an anterior pituitary tropic hormone that increases the synthesis of corticoids, leading to excessive glucocorticoid secretion. Common signs and symptoms include hyperglycemia, obesity, hypertension, and electrolyte imbalances. Addison's disease is characterized by hyposecretion of corticoids as a result of damage to the adrenal gland. Common signs and symptoms include hypoglycemia, emaciation, hypotension, hyperkalemia, and hyponatremia.

Treatment of Cushing's disease is typically surgical. Symptomatic pharmacologic intervention with an antihypertensive (potassium sparing diuretics such as spironolactone [Aldactone] or ACE inhibitors such as captopril [Capoten]) may be necessary. Drugs that may inhibit the synthesis of corticosteroids (antiadrenals) may also be used as an adjunct to surgery or radiation. In high doses, the antifungal agent ketoconazole (Nizoral) is an effective temporary antiadrenal drug. At such doses, however, it may cause liver dysfunction.

Treatment of Addison's disease is aimed at replacement therapy. Cortisone (Cortistan) and hydrocortisone (SoluCortef) are the drugs of choice. Occasionally, a specific mineralocorticoid is necessary. Fludrocortisone (Florinef Acetate) is the only mineralocorticoid available.

DRUGS AFFECTING THE PANCREAS

Diabetes mellitus is the most important disease involving the pancreas. Diabetes mellitus (as opposed to diabetes insipidus, which involves inadequate ADH secretion) involves inappropriate carbohydrate metabolism. Traditionally, the term diabetes used alone refers to diabetes mellitus, of which the two main types are, logically, type I and type II. Type I diabetes is also known as insulin-dependent diabetes mellitus, or IDDM. It results from an inadequate release of insulin from the beta cells of the pancreatic islets. Patients with type I diabetes rely on insulin replacement therapy to survive. Because IDDM typically manifests itself at an early age (usually before 30 years) it is also commonly called juvenile onset diabetes. Most diabetics have type II diabetes, which is also referred to as non-insulin-dependent diabetes mellitus (NIDDM) or adult onset diabetes. It results from a decreased responsiveness to insulin and a lack of synchronization between insulin release and blood glucose levels. Type II diabetes typically begins later in life (after 40 years) and almost always occurs in patients with obesity. Because they have functioning beta cells that release insulin, type II diabetics usually do not depend on insulin replacement. Gestational diabetes, a third type, occurs transitionally during pregnancy. Gestational diabetes is a form of stress-induced diabetes in which the mother cannot effectively manage her blood glucose levels during pregnancy without medical intervention. Gestational diabetes resolves itself within hours to days after delivery.

The two main substances involved with regulating blood glucose are insulin and glucagon. Both are secreted from the pancreas and both are used to manage diabetes. Secreted from the beta cells of the pancreatic islets of Langerhans in response to increased blood glucose levels, **insulin** increases cellular transport of glucose, potassium, and amino acids. It also converts glucose into glycogen for storage in the liver and in skeletal muscle. Finally, insulin promotes cell growth and division.

* **insulin** substance that decreases blood glucose level.

Glucagon, too, is secreted from the pancreatic islets, but by alpha cells rather than by the insulin-producing beta cells. Glucagon's actions are the direct opposite of insulin's; it increases both glycogenolysis (glycogen breakdown into glucose) and gluconeogenesis (the synthesis of glucose from glycerol and amino acids). So, while insulin decreases blood glucose levels, glucagon increases them.

* **glucagon** substance that increases blood glucose level.

Patients with either type I or type II diabetes may experience both hyperglycemia and hypoglycemia. While hyperglycemia more often results from the disease, hypoglycemia is a common side effect of treatment. The main intervention for patients with IDDM is insulin replacement therapy. Several insulin preparations are available. The most effective therapy for patients with NIDDM is usually weight loss through diet modification and exercise. When this is not effective, oral hypoglycemic agents and, occasionally, insulin are used. Finally, glucagon and diazoxide (both can be considered hyperglycemic agents) are occasionally used for treating emergency hypoglycemia.

Always consider glucagon in the hyperglycemic patient when an IV cannot be started.

Insulin Preparations Insulin comes from one of three sources. Initially, it came from either beef or pork intestines. Now, recombinant DNA technology has made human insulin available (that is, insulin synthesized with a human RNA template, not harvested directly from humans). Insulin preparations differ primarily in their onset and duration of action and in their incidence of allergic reaction. Insulin preparations may be short acting, intermediate acting, or long acting, depending on their onset and duration of action. (Table 6-8 lists insulin preparations.)

Insulin is also classified as natural (regular) or modified. As their name suggests, the natural insulins are used as they occur in nature. The other insulin preparations have been modified to increase their duration of action and thus decrease the frequency of their administration. All insulin preparations are given subcutaneously, with the exception of regular insulin, which may also be given

Table 6-8	INSULIN PREPARATIONS		
Classification	**Trade Name**	**Source**	
Rapid Acting			
Lispro Insulin	Humalog	Human	
Regular Insulin	Humulin R	Human	
	Novolin R	Human	
	Velosulin BR	Human	
	Regular Iletin I	Beef/Pork	
	Regular Iletin II	Pork	
Intermediate Acting			
NPH Insulin	NPH Iletin I	Beef/Pork	
	Pork NPH Iletin II	Pork	
	Humulin N	Human	
	Novolin N	Human	
Lente	Lente Iletin I	Beef/Pork	
	Lente Iletin II (Pork)	Pork	
	Humulin L	Human	
	Novolin L	Human	
Long Acting			
Ultralente	Humulin U	Human	
	Ultralente		
Combination Products			
NPH/Regular 70%/30%	Humulin 70/30	Human	
	Novolin 70/30	Human	
NPH/Regular 50%/50%	Humulin 50/50	Human	

Diabetic ketoacidosis (DKA) is best treated by a continuous insulin infusion accompanied by frequent checks of the blood glucose levels.

intravenously. Insulin is not available as an oral medication because the digestive enzymes would rapidly render it inactive; therefore, IDDM patients must take multiple injections every day of their lives. This may discourage compliance in some patients.

The modified insulin preparations include NPH (neutral protamine Hagedorn) insulin, which is regular insulin attached to a large protein designed to delay absorption, and the lente series, which is attached to zinc. Two preparations of lente insulin are available by themselves, lente and ultralente. A third, semilente insulin, is available only in a combination product with other insulins.

Insulin preparations are used for life-long replacement therapy in IDDM and for emergency treatment of hyperglycemia and hyperkalemia in nondiabetics. (Recall that insulin also increases potassium uptake by cells and is therefore useful in lowering potassium levels). These preparations' primary side effect is unintended hypoglycemia. Because beta$_2$ adrenergic blockers can hide the effects of hypoglycemia, patients may not recognize this condition's signs until they cannot care for themselves. Also, beta blockers decrease the release of glucagon, so these patients' hypoglycemia may be even worse. Insulin preparations derived from beef or pork, as well as the lentes, may lead to allergic reactions. The natural human insulin preparations do not have this effect.

Oral Hypoglycemic Agents Oral hypoglycemic agents are used to stimulate insulin secretion from the pancreas in patients with NIDDM. These agents are ineffective in people with type I diabetes since those patients cannot secrete insulin. This functional class comprises four pharmacologic classes: sulfonylureas, biguanides, alpha-glucosidase inhibitors, and thiazolidinediones. The sulfonylureas were the first class of oral hypoglycemics available and as such are also known as first-generation or second-generation oral hypoglycemics, depending on when they were released. Drugs in this class include tolbutamide (Orinase), chlorpropamide (Diabinese), glipizide (Glucotrol) and glyburide (Micronase). They work by increasing insulin secretion from the pancreas and may also increase tissue response to insulin. Their major side effect is hypoglycemia.

The only agent in the biguanide class is metformin (Glucophage). It decreases glucose synthesis and increases glucose uptake. It does not stimulate the release of insulin from the pancreas and therefore does not cause hypoglycemia. Its primary side effects are nausea, vomiting, and decreased appetite.

Alpha-glucosidase inhibitors include acarbose (Precose) and miglitol (Glyset). They work by delaying carbohydrate metabolism, which moderates the increase in blood glucose that occurs after meals. These agents' primary side effects are flatulence, cramps, diarrhea, and abdominal distention resulting from colonic bacteria feeding on the increased number of carbohydrates remaining in fecal matter.

Thiazolidinediones are a new class of oral hypoglycemic agents unrelated to the others. The only drug in this class is troglitazone (Rezulin). It works by promoting tissue response to insulin and thus making the available insulin more effective). Troglitazone has no major side effects.

Hyperglycemic Agents Two hyperglycemic agents, glucagon and diazoxide (Proglycem), act to increase blood glucose levels. Glucagon is indicated for the emergency treatment of patients with hypoglycemia. It will frequently be given intramuscularly to hypoglycemic patients in whom an IV line is unobtainable. Occasional side effects are nausea and vomiting and, rarely, allergic reactions. Diazoxide (Proglycem) inhibits insulin release and is typically used only for patients with hyperinsulin secretion resulting from pancreatic tumors; it is more commonly used for hypertension. It is not indicated for treating diabetes-induced hypoglycemia.

$D_{50}W$ (50% dextrose in water) is a sugar solution given intravenously for acute hypoglycemia. Its primary side effect is local tissue necrosis if infiltration occurs.

Dilute $D_{50}W$ to $D_{25}W$ for administration to pediatric patients.

DRUGS AFFECTING THE FEMALE REPRODUCTIVE SYSTEM

The main groups of drugs affecting the female reproductive system are estrogens, progestins, oral contraceptives, drugs affecting uterine contraction, and those used to treat infertility.

Estrogens and Progestins Estrogens are produced in females by the ovaries and the ovarian follicles, and in pregnancy, the placenta. Outside of pregnancy, the ovaries are the principal source of estrogens. The principal ovarian estrogen is estradiol, of which there are many commercial preparations. The principal indication for estrogen is replacement therapy in postmenopausal women. After menopause, estrogen levels drop significantly and have been indicated as a major increased risk factor for osteoporosis and coronary artery disease. Hormone replacement therapy with estrogen has been shown to reverse these risk factors and increase life expectancy; however, it is not without its own risks. There is much debate about the increased chances of breast cancer associated with hormone replacement therapy. Unfortunately, the data on this issue are conflicting, and no conclusive answer is currently possible. Side effects include nausea, fluid retention, and breast tenderness. The nausea usually diminishes after several months of therapy. Estrogen is also administered in cases of delayed puberty in girls as a result of hypogonadism.

The progestins' principal noncontraceptive use is to counteract the untoward effects of estrogen on the endometrium in hormone replacement therapy for postmenopausal women. They are also used to treat amenorrhea, endometriosis, and dysfunctional uterine bleeding.

Oral Contraceptives Oral contraception is an effective means of preventing pregnancy. All oral contraceptives' primary mechanism of action is the prevention of ovulation, which makes the endometrium less favorable for implantation and promotes the development of a thick mucus plug that blocks access to sperm through the cervix. These contraceptives are either a combination of estrogen and progestin or, in the case of "mini-pills," progestin only. They may also be classified based on their administration cycle as monophasic, biphasic, or triphasic. These classes differ in how they alter the dose of estrogen or progestin throughout the menstrual cycle. Many different preparations are available, although they all work in similar fashion. In general, these drugs are well tolerated and have few side effects. The oral contraceptives' chief side effects are unintended pregnancy (in less than three percent of users), thromboembolism (this risk is much lower with the newer low-estrogen dose preparations), hypertension and abnormal uterine bleeding. They are in wide use and are one of the most widely prescribed drug classes. They are the second most popular means of birth control after surgical sterilization (male and female combined).

Uterine Stimulants and Relaxants Drugs that increase uterine contraction (uterine stimulants) are oxytocics (oxytocin means rapid birth). Drugs that relax the uterus or inhibit uterine contraction are tocolytics.

The primary indications for administration of an oxytocic are to induce labor and to treat severe postpartum hemorrhage. Oxytocin is available commercially as Pitocin and Syntocinon. The uterus becomes increasingly sensitive to oxytocin throughout gestation, progressing from relatively insensitive before pregnancy to very sensitive around the time of labor. Oxytocin's chief side effect, water retention, is rarely significant and only so if large volumes of fluid have been administered without careful ongoing assessment. Ergonovine (Ergotrate), a derivative of a rye fungus, is a powerful uterine stimulant. It increases both the force and duration of contraction. Because of this increased duration, ergonovine is only used in the treatment of postpartum hemorrhage.

The tocolytics relax uterine smooth muscle by stimulating the beta$_2$ receptors in the uterus. The two beta$_2$ agonists commonly used for this purpose are terbutaline (Brethine) and ritodrine (Yutopar). Terbutaline's primary use is to treat asthma, but it is commonly used to delay labor even though the FDA does not currently approve it for that purpose. Both agents decrease both the force and frequency of contraction. Their chief side effects are the same as those of the other beta$_2$ agonists used to treat asthma: tremors and tachycardia. Occasionally, hyperglycemia may result from glycogenolysis in the liver.

Infertility Agents A number of conditions may cause infertility, which is the inability to become pregnant, and medications can treat only some of them. Most infertility drugs are developed for women and promote maturation of ovarian follicles. Clomiphene (Clomid), urofollitropin (Metrodin) and menotropins (Pergonal) are all within this class, although they each act by a different mechanism. These agents' side effects include ovarian enlargement or cysts, abdominal pain, and menstrual irregularities.

DRUGS AFFECTING THE MALE REPRODUCTIVE SYSTEM

Drugs that affect the male reproductive system include those that treat testosterone deficiency and benign prostatic hyperplasia. Testosterone replacement therapy may be indicated in testosterone deficiency caused by cryptorchidism (failure of one or both of the testes to descend during puberty), orchitis (testicular inflammation), or orchidectomy (testicular removal). It is also used in delayed puberty.

Preparations include testosterone enanthate, methyltestosterone (Metandren), and fluoxymesterone (Halotestin).

Benign prostatic hyperplasia is an enlarged prostate. This is a common but problematic age-related disease. By the age of 70, close to 75 percent of men will have symptoms severe enough to seek therapy. These symptoms may include urinary hesitancy and retention. Treatment has traditionally been surgery, but several drugs are available, including finasteride (Proscar), which interferes with the production of an enzyme involved with prostate growth. Side effects may include rash, breast tenderness, headache, impotence, and decreased libido.

DRUGS AFFECTING SEXUAL BEHAVIOR

For centuries, cultures have searched for drugs that would increase libido and sexual potency. Ironically, the reverse has most commonly been found. The largest category of drugs affecting sexual behavior do so as a side effect of their intended purpose. Many drug classifications decrease libido in both sexes and inhibit erection and ejaculation. Examples include antihypertensives (betablockers, centrally acting alpha antagonists, and diuretics) and antianxiety/antipsychotic medications (benzodiazepines, phenothiazines, MAO inhibitors, and tricyclic antidepressants).

Many drugs are purported to increase libido. The most notable of these is cantharis (Spanish fly). Despite common belief, no evidence indicates that cantharis actually increases sexual appetite. Indeed, it can produce some very dangerous side effects. Hallucinogens such as LSD and marijuana, as well as alcohol, are also commonly believed to heighten sexuality. Any such effect from these agents is likely an indirect result of decreased inhibitions or anxiety. These drugs all have very different effects, depending on each individual's unique physiology, expectations before use, and surrounding circumstances. They have no proven direct physiologic effect on sexual gratification.

Levodopa (L-dopa), an anti-Parkinson's drug, has demonstrated increased libido and improved erectile ability as a side effect of treatment. Whether this results directly from increased autonomic stimulation or indirectly from improved self-esteem achieved in therapy, any improvement seems to be only temporary. Finally, sildenafil (Viagra) was approved in 1998 for pharmacologic therapy in patients with erectile dysfunction. Sildenafil acts by relaxing vascular smooth muscle, which increases blood flow to the corpus cavernosum, the sponge-like tissue on the sides of the penis responsible for erection. This drug is unique in that it has no effect in the absence of sexual stimulation. Other drugs used to treat impotence have caused prolonged and painful erections (priapism). The chief side effect of sildenafil is seen when it is used in combination with nitrates. The combined effect of relaxing vascular smooth muscle may lead to a dangerously decreased preload, which may lower blood pressure and lead to myocardial infarction. Prehospital personnel should be aware of this important interaction. If you are called on to treat a patient with chest pain who has taken sildenafil recently, do not give him nitroglycerin or any other nitrate.

If you treat a patient with chest pain who has taken sildenafil recently, do not give him nitroglycerin or any other nitrate.

DRUGS USED TO TREAT CANCER

Drugs used to treat cancer are called **antineoplastic** agents. A detailed discussion of the many different antineoplastic agents is beyond the scope of this text; however, this section will briefly overview their main classes and prototype drugs.

✱ **antineoplastic agent** drug used to treat cancer.

Cancer involves the modification of cellular DNA leading to an abnormal growth of tissues. Of the many known types of cancer, only a few are successfully treated with chemotherapy. In fact, most cancers are best treated by surgical removal of the tumor. Unfortunately, many of the more lethal cancers do not involve a compact growth; rather, they affect the formed elements of the blood, especially leukocytes. Treating these widely dispersed cancers with surgery is not possible, as there is nothing for the surgeon to remove.

Chemotherapy is not nearly as safe or devoid of side effects as antibiotic therapy; however, scientists have yet to identify any unique characteristics of cancer cells that would allow them to develop drugs specific to those cells. Because cancer is the abnormal growth of normal cells, drugs that kill cancerous cells therefore also kill noncancerous cells. Chemotherapy is thus largely a balancing act aimed at maximizing the kill rate of cancer cells while minimizing the death of normal tissue. The one characteristic that most cancer cells share is rapid cell division and replication. Consequently, most antineoplastic agents have their greatest effect on cancer cells during miosis and on young, small cancers that are undergoing rapid growth.

The agents used to kill cancer cells are grouped according to their mechanism of action. Antimetabolite drugs mimic some of the enzymes and proteins needed for DNA replication but do not have the same effects; therefore, they prevent cells from reproducing. Their prototype is fluorouracil (Adrucil). Alkylating agents that interfere with DNA splitting include cyclophosphamide (Cytoxan) and mechlorethamine (Mustargen). Mitotic inhibitors also interfere with cell division; they include vinblastine (Velban) and vincristine (Oncovin).

Chemotherapy's primary side effects include nausea, vomiting, and other gastrointestinal disturbances, as well as hair loss and weakness. Almost all antineoplastic agents cause severe side effects and are given in conjunction with antiemetics.

DRUGS USED TO TREAT INFECTIOUS DISEASES AND INFLAMMATION

Infectious diseases are typically caused by bacteria, viruses, or funguses and may be treated with antimicrobial drugs developed to fight those particular invaders. We will discuss each broad class.

Antibiotics An **antibiotic** agent may either kill the offending bacteria (bactericidal agents) or so decrease the bacteria's growth that the patient's immune system can effectively fight the infection (bacteriostatic agents). In general, all of these agents share one of several mechanisms. Drugs in the penicillin and cephalosporin classes, as well as vancomycin (Vancocin), are bactericidal and act by inhibiting cell wall synthesis. Unlike animal cells, bacteria have hypertonic cell cytoplasm and depend on the rigid and relatively impermeable cell wall to maintain integrity. When cell wall synthesis is inhibited, osmotic pressure pulls water into the cell, and the cell ruptures, killing the bacteria. The macrolide, aminoglycoside, and tetracycline antibiotics inhibit protein synthesis, preventing the bacterial cell from replicating and thus spreading infection. These agents are usually bacteriostatic but can be bactericidal at high doses. Typical side effects from antibiotics include gastrointestinal dysfunction, which commonly results from a decrease in the natural gastrointestinal bacteria that inhabit the colon.

Antifungal and Antiviral Agents Fungi are parasitic microorganisms that cannot synthesize their own food. Fungal infections (mycoses) may be treated with several drugs. The azole antifungals inhibit fungal growth. Their prototype is

* **antibiotic** agent that kills or decreases the growth of bacteria.

ketoconazole (Nizoral). Drugs used to treat viruses work by a variety of mechanisms and include acyclovir (Zovirax) and zidovudine (Retrovir), which is commonly known as AZT. Protease inhibitors are one of the more promising classes of drugs for treating viruses such as HIV. Indinavir (Crixivan) is the prototype of this class.

Other Antimicrobial and Antiparasitic Agents While most diseases treated with the medications discussed in this section are uncommon in developed countries, they are leading causes of death in third-world countries. They include malaria, tuberculosis, leprosy, amebiasis, and helminthiasis. Tuberculosis is increasingly appearing in the United States in patients with compromised immune systems.

Malaria is a parasitic infection common in the tropics. It is transmitted by certain types of mosquitoes or, less commonly, by blood transfusion. Drugs used to treat malaria are called schizonticides. They include chloroquine (Aralen), mefloquine (Lariam), and quinine. Treatment is aimed at either preventing infestation (prophylactic treatment for individuals traveling to high risk areas) or killing the parasites in infected patients.

Tuberculosis is caused by bacteria that are transmitted through airborne droplets from the coughing and sneezing of infected patients. The bacteria can grow only in well-oxygenated areas. Because of the route of infection and the need for oxygen, most patients with tuberculosis have infestations in the lungs. Once in the lungs, the bacteria are typically "walled off," or enclosed in tubercules, and become dormant and noninfective. If the patient's immune system is compromised, the bacteria may become active again and begin to cause symptoms. Drugs commonly used to treat tuberculosis include isoniazid (Nydrazid, INH) and rifampin (Rifadin).

Amebiasis is a parasitic infection of the intestines common in tropical areas. Transmission most frequently occurs via the oral-fecal route from eating poorly cooked food contaminated by cooks who inadequately wash their hands. Drugs used to treat amebiasis include paromomycin (Humatin) and metronidazole (Flagyl).

Helminthiasis is caused by parasitic worms (helminths) including flatworms and roundworms. These worms usually invade the host's intestinal tract and attach themselves to the lumen wall with hooks or suckers. They cause symptoms by depriving the host of nutrients (especially in children); by obstructing the intestinal lumen, which leads to bowel obstruction; and by producing toxins. Treatment is aimed at either killing the organism outright or destroying its ability to latch onto the intestinal wall so it passes with the patient's feces. These drugs include mebendazole (Vermox) and niclosamide (Niclocide).

Leprosy, also known as Hansen's disease, is caused by bacteria. It leads to characteristic lesions, footdrop (plantar flexion), and plantar ulceration. Drugs used to treat it include dapsone (DDS, Avlosulfon), and clofazimine (Lamprene).

Nonsteroidal Anti-Inflammatory Drugs NSAIDs (nonsteroidal anti-inflammatory drugs) are commonly used as analgesics and antipyretics (fever reducers). Many are available over the counter, including acetaminophen and ibuprofen. As a group, these agents interfere with the production of prostaglandins, thereby interrupting the inflammatory process. NSAIDs are indicated for the relief of pain, fever, and inflammation associated with common headache, arthritis, dysmenorrhea, and orthopedic injuries. They are also commonly prescribed to relieve pain following trauma and surgery. Other NSAIDs include ketorolac (Toradol), piroxicam (Feldene), and naproxen (Naprosyn).

Uricosuric Drugs Uricosuric drugs are used to treat and prevent acute episodes of gout. Gout is an inflammatory disease caused by an altered metabolism of uric acid and marked by hyperuricemia (high levels of uric acid in the blood). It may present with acute episodes characterized by pain and swelling of joints. Left untreated, gout may lead to crystal deposits in various parts of the body that can cause kidney stones, nephritis, and atherosclerosis. Drugs used to treat gout include colchicine and allopurinol (Zyloprim).

Serums, Vaccines, and Other Immunizing Agents The human body has a complex series of systems that help prevent disease. The most important of these are the anatomical barriers such as the skin and mucous membranes that block the entrance of **pathogens** (disease causing organisms including viruses and bacteria). If pathogens get past these protective barriers, our immune system comes into play. This system consists of the spleen, lymph nodes, thymus, leukocytes, and proteins called antibodies in plasma. The ability to respond to pathogens is called **immunity.**

Immunity may be acquired passively or actively. It is passively acquired when antibodies pass directly into a person, either through artificial routes such as injection or through natural routes such as the placenta or breast milk. Immunity may also be actively acquired in response to the presence of a pathogen.

Actively acquired immunity occurs when T lymphocytes (a type of leukocyte that becomes specialized in the thymus gland) comes in contact with a new pathogen. The body produces an infinite variety of T-cell configurations. When the pathogen comes into contact with a T cell that is specific to it, that T cell begins to rapidly reproduce. Some of these cells become involved in the immune response to the pathogen, while others act as "memory" cells. The cells involved in the immune response either directly attack the pathogen (cell-mediated immunity) or activate the complement system, a complex cascade of events that leads to the immune response. The memory cells remain in the body in higher numbers so that the next time this specific pathogen enters the body, a much faster response is possible. At the same time, B cells (lymphocytes that differentiate or become more specialized in the body, as opposed to the thymus) that are specific for the invading pathogen begin to produce antibodies for that antigen. This process is called humoral immunity or antibody immunity. When an antibody contacts its specific antigen, it forms a complex that triggers the complement system, leading to the immune response.

Serums and vaccines may augment the immune system. A **serum** is a solution containing whole antibodies for a specific pathogen. The antibodies give the recipient temporary, passive immunity. A **vaccine** contains a modified pathogen that does not actually cause disease but still stimulates the development of antibodies specific to it. These pathogens may be either dead or attenuated (having a decreased disease-causing ability).

The best age for vaccination against disease is within the first two years of life, as the immune system is fairly immature.

Immune Suppressing and Enhancing Agents Available drugs can either suppress the immune system (immunosuppressants) or enhance it (immunomodulators). Suppressing the immune system is indicated to prevent the rejection of transplanted organs and grafted skin. Azathioprine (Imuran) is a commonly used immunosuppressant that acts by decreasing cell-mediated reactions and suppressing antibody production.

Immunomodulating agents enhance the natural immune reaction in immunosuppressed patients such as those with HIV. Zidovudine (Retrovir), commonly known as AZT, and several protease inhibitors such as ritonavir (Norvir) and saquinavir (Invirase) are examples of these agents.

✱ **pathogen** disease causing organism.

✱ **immunity** the body's ability to respond to the presence of a pathogen.

✱ **serum** solution containing whole antibodies for a specific pathogen.

✱ **vaccine** solution containing a modified pathogen that does not actually cause disease but still stimulates the development of antibodies specific to it.

DRUGS USED TO AFFECT THE SKIN

Dermatologic drugs are used to treat skin irritations. They are common over-the-counter medications. The many different general preparations include baths, soaps, solutions, cleansers, emollients (Lubriderm, Vaseline), skin protectants (Benzoin), wet dressings or soaks (Domeboro Powder), and rubs and liniments (Ben-Gay, Icy Hot). Prophylactic agents such as sunscreens are also available to help prevent skin disease and irritation.

DRUGS USED TO SUPPLEMENT THE DIET

Many disease processes affect the production, distribution, and utilization of essential dietary nutrients. Additionally, the body's intricate balance of fluid (including specific amounts of electrolytes) is a vital component of maintaining homeostasis. Dietary supplements can help to maintain needed levels of these essential nutrients and fluids.

VITAMINS AND MINERALS

Vitamins are organic compounds necessary for many different physiologic processes including metabolism, growth, development, and tissue repair. The body absorbs most vitamins through the gastrointestinal tract following dietary ingestion. Vitamins must be obtained from the diet, as the body cannot manufacture them. In developed countries, healthy adults usually receive adequate amounts of vitamins and do not need supplements. Vitamin supplements may, however, be indicated for special populations including pregnant and nursing women, patients with absorption disorders, the chronically ill, surgery patients, alcoholics, and the malnourished. Additionally, people on a strict vegetarian diet may need supplemental vitamins. Vitamins are either fat soluble or water soluble. The liver stores the fat soluble vitamins (A, D, E, and K), so the patient will become deficient only after long periods of inadequate vitamin intake. Vitamin D is unique in that the skin produces it with exposure to sunlight. The water soluble vitamins (C and those in the B complex), must be routinely ingested, as the body does not store them. After short periods of deprivation, patients may begin to experience vitamin deficiency. The B complex vitamins are grouped only because they occur together in foods; otherwise they share no significant characteristics. The individual B vitamins are named for the order in which they were discovered (B_1, B_2, B_3, and so forth). These vitamins also have specific names. For example, B_1 is also known as thiamine, a vitamin that plays a key role in carbohydrate metabolism. Table 6-9 details selected vitamins. Iron is an essential mineral necessary for oxygen transport and several metabolic processes. Iron supplements are the most common mineral supplement. They are indicated for iron deficiency.

FLUIDS AND ELECTROLYTES

Water comprises approximately 60 percent of a person's total body weight. The specific composition and amounts of this fluid are vital to a patient's well being. The specific amounts of electrolytes such as calcium, potassium, sodium, and chlorine are similarly important. This book's chapter on pathophysiology reviews the physiology of fluids and electrolytes and discusses acid-base balance. The indications and contraindications for administering fluids and electrolytes, as well as these medications' interactions are covered in Chapter 7 on medication administration and Chapter 19 on hemorrhage and shock.

Table 6-9 VITAMIN SOURCES AND DEFICIENCIES

Vitamin	Problems Resulting from Deficiency	Source
Fat Soluble		
A	Night blindness, skin lesions	Butter, yellow fruit, green leafy vegetables, milk
D	Bone and muscle pain, weakness, softening of bones	Fish, fortified milk, exposure to sunlight
E	Hyporeflexia, ataxia, anemia	Nuts, green leafy vegetables, wheat
K	Increased bleeding	Liver, green leafy vegetables
Water Soluble		
B_1 (thiamine)	Peripheral neuritis, depression, anorexia, poor memory	Whole grain, beef, pork, peas, beans, nuts
B_2 (riboflavin)	Sore throat, stomatitis, painful or swollen tongue, anemia	Milk, eggs, cheese, green leafy vegetables
B_2 (niacin)	Skin eruptions, diarrhea, enteritis, headache, dizziness, insomnia	Meat, eggs, milk
B_6 (pyridoxine)	Skin lesions, seizures, peripheral neuritis	Liver, meats, eggs, vegetables
B_9 (folic acid)	Megaloblastic anemia	Liver, fresh green vegetables, yeast
B_{12} (cyanocobalamin)	Irreversible nervous system damage, pernicious anemia	Fish, egg yolk, milk
C	Scurvy	Citrus fruits, tomatoes, strawberries

DRUGS USED TO TREAT POISONING AND OVERDOSES

The treatment for poisoning and overdose depends greatly on the substance involved. In general, therapy aims at eliminating the substance by emptying the gastric contents, by increasing gastric motility in order to decrease the time available for absorption, by alkalinizing the urine with sodium bicarbonate (for tricyclic antidepressant and salicylate overdose), or by filtering the substance from the blood with dialysis. When gastric emptying is indicated, syrup of ipecac is the drug of choice; otherwise, activated charcoal may be used as a gastric absorbent.

Actual antidotes are few; however, some medications are effective in treating certain overdoses or poisonings. General mechanisms for antidote action include receptor site antagonism, blocking enzyme actions involved with metabolism of the substance, and chelation (binding the substance with a stable compound such as iron so that it becomes inactive). Specific antidotes include acetylcysteine (Mucomyst) for acetaminophen overdose and deferoxamine for iron chelation. Organophosphates are a common ingredient in insecticides and herbicides as well as chemical weapons. They are aggressive acetylcholinesterase (AchE) inhibitors that prevent the breakdown of acetylcholine, leading to overstimulation of the parasympathetic nervous system as well as neuromuscular junctions. Signs and symptoms of this overstimulation may be remembered by the acronym SLUDGE (salivation, lacrimation, urination, defecation, gastric motility, and emesis). Other signs include bradycardia, hypotension, bronchospasm, muscle fasiculations, miosis (pupil constriction), and respiratory arrest. The antidotes for organophosphate poisoning are atropine and pralidoxamine (2-PAM, Protopam). Atropine antagonizes ACh, while pralidoxamine breaks the organophosphate-acetylcholinesterase bond, freeing AChE to break down the excess Ach.

SUMMARY

Pharmacology is a cornerstone of paramedic practice. Paramedics must have a solid understanding of its foundations (legal issues, terminology, drug forms, and routes), pharmacokinetics, and pharmacodynamics if they are to practice their profession safely. Additionally, paramedics must understand not only the medications they personally administer, but also the medications that their patients are taking on an ongoing basis. While you are not likely to remember everything in this chapter after your first reading, with diligent study and practice you can master this information. This chapter has barely broken the surface of pharmacology. To continue your education, you should take the time to understand the mechanisms and interactions of the medications your patients are taking. If you do not already know them (you will not in the majority of cases as you begin your career), look them up. Many very useful drug references are available today. Most are small and can be easily carried with you on your unit or in your station.

Finally, pharmacology is a dynamic field with new discoveries being made every day. If you take your responsibilities as a paramedic seriously and remain current on the latest changes in this field, you can be sure that you can give your patients the care they deserve.

CHAPTER 7

Medication Administration

Objectives

Part 1: Principles and Routes of Medication Administration (begins on p. 414)

After reading Part 1 of this chapter, you should be able to:

1. Review the specific anatomy and physiology pertinent to medication administration. (pp. 417–448)
2. Describe the indications, equipment needed, technique used, precautions, and general principles for the following:
   a. inhalation routes of medication administration. (pp. 421–425)
   b. parenteral routes of medication administration. (pp. 432–448)
   c. percutaneous routes of medication administration. (pp. 417–421)
   d. enteral routes of medication administration, including gastric tube administration and rectal administration. (pp. 425–432)
3. Describe the indications, contraindications, side effects, dosages, and routes of administration for medica-

tions commonly administered by paramedics. (pp. 417–448)
4. Discuss legal aspects affecting medication administration. (pp. 414–415, 417)
5. Discuss the "six rights" of drug administration and correlate them with the principles of medication administration. (p. 414)
6. Differentiate among the percutaneous routes of medication administration. (pp. 417–421)
7. Discuss medical asepsis and the differences between clean and sterile techniques. (pp. 415–416)
8. Describe uses of antiseptics and disinfectants. (pp. 415–416)
9. Describe the use of body substance isolation (BSI) procedures when administering a medication. (p. 415)

Continued

Objectives Continued

10. Describe disposal of contaminated items and sharps. (p. 416)
11. Synthesize a pharmacologic management plan including

medication administration. (pp. 414–448)

Part 2: Intravenous Access, Blood Sampling, and Intraosseous Infusion (begins on p. 448)

After reading Part 2 of this chapter, you should be able to:

1. Review the specific anatomy and physiology pertinent to medication administration. (pp. 448–487)
2. Describe the indications, equipment needed, technique used, precautions, and general principles for the following:

   a. peripheral venous or external jugular cannulation. (pp. 448–476)
   b. intraosseous needle placement and infusion. (pp. 480–487)
   c. obtaining a blood sample. (pp. 476–480)

Part 3: Medical Mathematics (begins on p. 487)

After reading Part 3 of this chapter, you should be able to:

1. Review mathematical equivalents. (pp. 487–490)
2. Differentiate temperature readings between the centigrade and Fahrenheit scales. (p. 489)

3. Discuss formulas as a basis for performing drug calculations. (pp. 490–495)
4. Describe how to perform mathematical conversions from the household system to the metric system. (pp. 488–489)

INTRODUCTION

Medications, or **drugs,** are foreign substances placed into the human body. They serve a variety of purposes such as controlling specific diseases like hypertension or helping the body cure diseases like cancer and infection.

Medication administration will be an important part of the medical care you provide as a paramedic. You may have to use medications to correct or prevent many life-threatening situations. You may also use them to stabilize or comfort a patient in distress. In addition to your knowledge of particular medications and their properties from the previous chapter on pharmacology, you must also be thoroughly skilled in drug administration. Specific drugs require specific routes and administration techniques. Their effectiveness depends directly upon their correct route of delivery. Incorrect or sloppy drug administration can have tremendous legal implications for the paramedic. More importantly, it equates to poor care that can harm or even kill the patient.

This chapter discusses the routes and techniques you will use to correctly deliver your patient's medications. It is divided into three parts:

Part 1: Principles and Routes of Medication Administration

Part 2: Intravenous Access, Blood Sampling, and Intraosseous Infusion

Part 3: Medical Mathematics

* **medications/drugs** foreign substances placed into the human body.

Part 1: Principles and Routes of Medication Administration

As a paramedic, you are responsible for ensuring that all emergency drugs are in place and ready for immediate use. Therefore, you must know your local drug distribution system. You will have to know where to obtain and replace each drug as it expires or is used, as another patient may require it at any time. You also will have to thoroughly document the administration and restocking of narcotics, as many local, state, and federal agencies mandate such record keeping.

Always be certain that you correctly give all drugs in the right dose. Medication errors may prove disastrous in terms of patient care and legal responsibility. Your knowledge of drug indications, contraindications, side effects, dosages, and routes of administration is crucial to effective patient care.

You can attain effective pharmacologic therapy and eliminate medication errors by following the six rights of drug administration:

Your knowledge of drug indications, dosages, and routes of administration is of paramount importance.

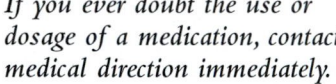

- *Right person*
- *Right drug*
- *Right dose*
- *Right time*
- *Right route*
- *Right documentation*

If you ever doubt the use or dosage of a medication, contact medical direction immediately.

In the field, you will be responsible for the safe and appropriate delivery of medications. If you ever doubt the use or dosage of a medication, contact medical direction immediately. You must repeat back, or echo, all drug orders issued by direct medical command. For example, if medical direction ordered you to administer 25 mg of diphenhydramine (Benadryl), you would echo, "Medic 101 copies the medication order for 25 mg of diphenhydramine to be administered slow IV push." By echoing, you confirm your reception and understanding of the order. If medical direction has issued an inappropriate medication or dosage, echoing may bring it to light and elicit an immediate correction. If you still find the order questionable after echoing, diplomatically request clarification or ask about the intent.

Pharmacologic therapy permits you to function as an extension of the physician. No room exists for medication errors, as once a drug is given it is difficult if not impossible to retrieve. In addition, withholding a needed medication can have catastrophic consequences. Concentration and knowledge are the keys to this component of paramedical care.

MEDICAL DIRECTION

Paramedics do not practice autonomously. You will operate under the license of a medical director who is responsible for all of your actions. This responsibility extends to the administration of medications.

The medical director determines which medications you will use and the routes by which you will deliver them. Some states have a "state drug list" whereby the medications a service carries are dictated by law or a legislative or regulatory agency. While some medications can be administered via off-line medical direction (written standing orders), you will need specific authorization for others after consulting on-line or direct medical direction. You must strictly abide by all of your medical director's guidelines.

Knowing all drug administration protocols is essential, especially which drugs to administer under standing orders and which to deliver only after getting authorization from medical direction. You can ill afford to waste valuable time looking up procedures and directives for the critical patient who requires immediate drug therapy. Furthermore, because inappropriate drug delivery can have serious consequences, you may face severe legal ramifications even if your patient suffers no harm.

BODY SUBSTANCE ISOLATION

Establishing routes for drug delivery presents the constant potential for exposure to blood and other body fluids. Always take appropriate **body substance isolation** (BSI) measures to decrease your risk of exposure. The type of BSI you use will vary according to the delivery route and your patient's condition. At a minimum, you should wear gloves. Optimally, you will also wear goggles and a mask. Remarkably, the simplest form of BSI is often the most neglected: hand washing. Washing your hands before and after patient contact is one of the most effective ways to decrease your exposure to infectious material. Chapter 1 includes a thorough discussion of BSI measures.

✱ **body substance isolation** (BSI) measures to decrease your risk of exposure to blood and body fluids.

MEDICAL ASEPSIS

Medical **asepsis** (*a-*, without; *sepsis,* infection) describes a medical environment free of pathogens. Many paramedical procedures, especially those related to drug administration, place the patient at increased risk for infection. The external environment is full of microorganisms, many of them pathogenic. Techniques such as intravenous access or endotracheal intubation can allow pathogens to enter the patient's body, where they may cause **local** or **systemic** complications.

✱ **asepsis** a condition free of pathogens.

✱ **local** limited to one area of the body.

✱ **systemic** throughout the body.

✱ **sterile** free of all forms of life.

STERILIZATION

The most aseptic environment is a sterile one. A **sterile** environment is free of all forms of life. Generally, environments are sterilized with extensive heat or chemicals. A sterile environment is difficult to attain in the prehospital setting. Consequently, you must practice medically clean techniques to minimize your patient's risk of infection. **Medically clean** techniques involve the careful handling of sterile equipment to prevent contamination. For example, much of the equipment used for drug administration is packaged sterilely. Once you open the package, you must use a medically clean technique to keep the equipment clean and uncontaminated until you use it. If you drop a piece of equipment on a dirty surface, you should discard it and obtain a new piece. Other medically clean techniques, including handwashing, glove changing, and discarding equipment in opened packages, help to prevent equipment and patient contamination. Remember, too, that many patients have lowered immunity levels or carry infectious diseases. Thus, keeping the ambulance and equipment clean is another essential medically clean procedure.

✱ **medically clean** careful handling to prevent contamination.

DISINFECTANTS AND ANTISEPTICS

When administering medications, you must use disinfectants and antiseptics to assure local cleanliness. Do not confuse disinfectants and antiseptics; the distinction is important. **Disinfectants** are toxic to living tissue. You will therefore

✱ **disinfectant** cleansing agent that is toxic to living tissue.

use them only on nonliving surfaces or objects such as the inside of an ambulance or laryngoscope blades after use. Never use disinfectants on living tissue. **Antiseptics** are not toxic to living tissue. They destroy or inhibit pathogenic microorganisms already on living surfaces and are generally used to cleanse the local area before needle puncture. Common antiseptics include alcohol and iodine preparations used either alone or together. Frequently, antiseptics are diluted disinfectants.

DISPOSAL OF CONTAMINATED EQUIPMENT AND SHARPS

Treat all blood and body fluids as potentially infectious.

Blood and body fluid can harbor infectious material that endangers the health care provider, family, bystanders, or the patient himself. Many times, the patient is infected with pathogenic organisms long before signs and symptoms appear. Therefore, you must treat all blood and body fluids as potentially infectious.

Drug administration commonly involves needles in direct contact with the patient's blood and body fluid. Once used, a needle presents a significant risk. Inadvertent needle sticks, the most common accident in health care as a whole, can transmit diseases between the patient and paramedic. Properly handling needles and other sharps before and after patient use can prevent many of these accidental needle sticks. To minimize or eliminate the risk of an accidental needle stick, take these precautions:

- *Minimize the tasks you perform in a moving ambulance.* Use needles as sparingly as possible in the back of a moving ambulance. When appropriate, perform all interventions involving needles on scene. If en route, it may be occasionally necessary to have the driver pull the ambulance to the side of the road and stop briefly. Most paramedics become quite proficient at completing these procedures in a moving ambulance.

- *Immediately dispose of used sharps in a sharps container.* A **sharps container** is a rigid, puncture-resistant container clearly marked as biohazardous. You can deposit whole needles and prefilled syringes in it, thus eliminating the need for bending or cutting. Some sharps containers have adapters that permit the easy removal of needles from blood draw equipment and syringes. You should also dispose of items such as used ampules in the sharps container. Avoid dropping sharps onto the floor for later disposal. In the heat of the moment, you may forget the sharp or mentally misplace it.

- *Recap needles only as a last resort.* If you absolutely must recap a needle, never use two hands to do so. Place the sharp on a stationary surface and replace the cap with one hand. While the one-hand method is still hazardous, it at least reduces the chance for an accidental needle stick.

By law, every medical organization must have a biological hazard exposure plan. Be familiar with yours. If you are exposed to blood or other body substances, follow the plan and immediately notify the appropriate resources. Remember that prevention is the best medicine.

MEDICATION ADMINISTRATION AND DOCUMENTATION

When administering medications, proper and thorough documentation is extremely important. You must record all information concerning the patient and the medication including:

- Indication for drug administration
- Dosage and route delivered
- Patient response to the medication—both positive and negative

You must also document the patient's condition and vital signs before medication administration as well as after. In addition to communicating all information to those to whom you transfer care, you must record it on a copy of the patient care report.

In emergent and nonemergent situations alike, you will administer a variety of medications through a variety of delivery routes. The routes of drug administration fall into four basic categories: percutaneous, pulmonary, enteral, and parenteral. Technically, drug deliveries through the rectum and pulmonary system are **topical** applications; however, accepted practice classifies these routes separately. Which route you use will depend on the drug you are administering and your patient's status.

PERCUTANEOUS DRUG ADMINISTRATION

Percutaneous medications are applied to and absorbed through the skin or mucous membranes. They are easy to administer and bypass the digestive tract, making their absorption more predictable.

TRANSDERMAL ADMINISTRATION

Medications given by the **transdermal** (*trans-*, across; *dermal,* skin) route promote slow, steady absorption. Nitroglycerin, hormones, and analgesics are commonly administered transdermally. Transdermal delivery can also produce localized effects, as with anti-inflammatories and other bacteriostatic and softening agents. Applying medication locally avoids passing larger quantities of the medication through the entire body, where it is not needed. Transdermal medications include lotions, ointments, creams, foams, wet dressings, adhesive backed applications, and suppositories.

To administer a transdermal medication, use the following technique:

1. Use BSI. Gloves avoid contaminating the medication and inadvertently getting it on your skin.
2. Clean and dry your patient's skin at the administration site.
3. Apply medication to the site as specified by the manufacturer. Avoid overdosing or underdosing when using lotion, ointment, cream, or foam.
4. Leave the medication in place for the required time. Monitor the patient for desirable or adverse effects.

You may need to place a dressing over the medication to protect the site and quantity of drug. Carefully follow all recommendations. Administration may

Content Review

ROUTES OF DRUG ADMINISTRATION
Percutaneous
Pulmonary
Enteral
Parenteral

✱ **topical medications** material applied to and absorbed through the skin or mucous membranes.

Content Review

PERCUTANEOUS ROUTES
Transdermal
Mucous Membrane

✱ **transdermal** absorbed through the skin.

vary subtly, depending upon the form of medication and the specific manufacturer's instructions.

Several factors can affect how quickly the skin absorbs transdermal medications. Thin skin, overdose, or penetrating solvents can increase the absorption rate. Conversely, thick skin, scar tissue, or peripheral vascular disease can decrease the rate. If these factors are present, consider alternative sites or dosage adjustments.

MUCOUS MEMBRANES

The mucous membranes absorb medications at a moderate to rapid rate. Similar to transdermal administration, drug delivery through the mucous membranes avoids the digestive tract and complications associated with that route. You can deliver drugs through the mucous membranes at several sites. However, specific drugs are made for specific sites and generally are not interchangeable.

Sublingual

✱ **sublingual** beneath the tongue.

Sublingual drugs are absorbed through the mucous membranes beneath the tongue (*sub-*, below; *lingual,* tongue). The sublingual region is extremely vascular and permits rapid absorption with systemic delivery. These medications are generally dissolvable tablets or sprays. One commonly administered sublingual medication is nitroglycerin.

To administer a medication via the sublingual route, follow these steps:

1. Use appropriate BSI.
2. Confirm the indication, medication, dose, sublingual route, and expiration date.
3. Have your patient lift his tongue toward the top and back of his oral cavity.
4. Place the pill or direct spray between the underside of the tongue and the floor of the oral cavity. Have your patient relax his tongue and mouth. If administering a pill, instruct the patient to let the pill dissolve and not to swallow.
5. Monitor the patient for desirable or adverse effects.

Buccal

✱ **buccal** between the cheek and gums.

The **buccal** region lies in the oral cavity between the cheek and gums. Buccal medications are generally tablets. Hormonal and enzyme preparations are typically given buccally.

To administer a medication buccally, follow these steps:

1. Use appropriate BSI.
2. Confirm the indication, medication, dose, buccal route, and expiration date.
3. Place the medication between the patient's cheek and gum. Instruct the patient to allow the pill or other preparation to dissolve. Ensure that the patient does not swallow the medication.
4. Monitor the patient for desirable or adverse effects.

FIGURE 7-1 Eye drop administration. Use a medicine dropper to place the prescribed dosage on the conjunctival sac.

Ocular

Ocular medications are topical medications that are administered through the mucous membranes of the eye. These are typically local medications for alleviating eye pain, treating infection, decreasing intraocular pressure, or lubricating the eyelid. Medications delivered by way of the eye are labeled for ophthalmic use and packaged as drops or ointments.

If medication is to be administered only to one eye, be sure to medicate the correct eye. The following abbreviations designate right, left, or both eyes:

o.d.	right eye *(oculus dexter)*
o.s.	left eye *(oculus sinister)*
o.u.	both right and left eyes *(oculus uterque)*

To administer a medication via eye drops, use the following technique (Figure 7-1):

1. Use gloves and appropriate BSI.
2. Have your patient lie supine or lay his head back and look toward the ceiling.
3. Pull the lower eyelid downward to expose the conjunctival sac. Never touch the eye.
4. Use a medicine dropper to place the prescribed dosage on the conjunctival sac. Never administer medications directly on the eye unless specifically instructed.
5. Instruct the patient to hold his eye(s) shut for one to two minutes.

Ocular medications may also be packaged as ointments. To apply an ointment, follow the same procedure as above, but carefully squeeze the ointment onto the conjunctival sac. If you administer too much medication, carefully blot away the excess drops or ointment with sterile gauze. The ointment will melt as it warms to body temperature and will spread smoothly across the surface of the eye.

* **ocular medication** drug administered through the mucous membranes of the eye.

FIGURE 7-2 Nasal medication administration.

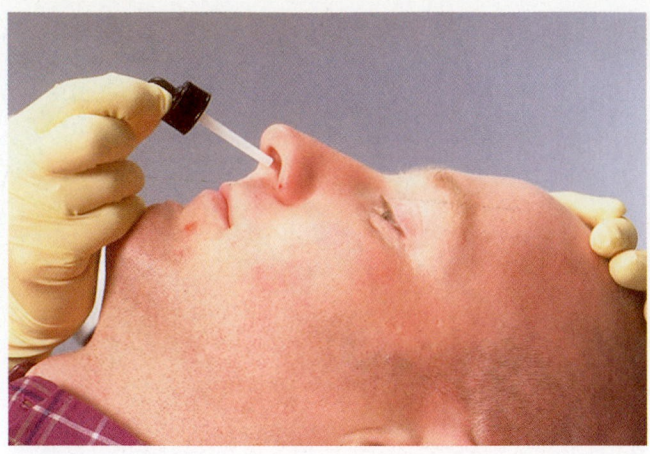

Nasal

✱ **nasal medication** drug administered through the mucous membranes of the nose.

The mucous membranes of the nose are another port for topical medication delivery. Given through the nares (nostrils), these **nasal medications** are usually drops or sprays intended for local effect. They commonly treat nasal congestion, hemorrhage, and infection.

To administer a medication via the nose, use the following technique (Figure 7-2):

1. Use gloves and appropriate BSI.
2. Have the patient blow his nose and tilt his head backwards.
3. Use a medicine dropper or squeezable nebulizer to administer the medication into the appropriate nare(s) according to the manufacturer's instructions.
4. Hold the nare(s) shut and/or tilt the head forward to distribute the medication.
5. Monitor the patient for desirable and undesirable effects.

Aural

Some medications are delivered to the mucous membranes of the ear and ear canal through drops or medicated gauze. These drugs primarily treat local infections and ear pain. Use the following technique to administer medicated drops (Figure 7-3):

1. Use gloves and appropriate BSI.
2. Confirm the indication, medication, dose, and expiration date.
3. Determine the correct ear for administration.
4. Have the patient lie in the lateral recumbent position with the affected ear upward.
5. Manually open the ear canal: for adult patients, pull the ear up and back; for pediatric patients, pull it down and back.
6. Administer the appropriate dose of medication with a medicine dropper.

FIGURE 7-3 Aural medication administration. Manually open the ear canal and administer the appropriate dose.

7. Have the patient continue to lie with his ear up for ten minutes.
8. Monitor the patient for desirable and undesirable effects.

Using medicated gauze or cotton is generally reserved for the hospital setting. If your local protocols permit you to administer these medications, follow the procedure outlined above, gently inserting the gauze into the ear instead of instilling medicated drops. Avoid tightly packing the ear canal.

PULMONARY DRUG ADMINISTRATION

Special medications can be administered into the pulmonary system via **inhalation** or **injection.** Generally gases, fine mists, or liquids, these drugs include those that promote bronchodilation for respiratory emergencies. Other inhaled drugs are mucolytics, antibiotics, and topical steroids. Inhalation can also be used for humidification and pulmonary decongestion.

NEBULIZER

Typically, drugs administered by inhalation are delivered with the aid of a **small volume nebulizer.** A nebulizer uses pressurized oxygen to disperse a liquid into a fine aerosol spray or mist. Inhalation carries the aerosol into the lungs. Figure 7-4 illustrates a typical nebulizer. The specific design depends upon the manufacturer, but they all work on the same principle and typically have the same parts:

- Mouthpiece
- Medication reservoir
- Oxygen port
- Relief valve
- Oxygen tubing
- Oxygen source

Content Review

PULMONARY MEDICATION MECHANISMS
Nebulizer
Metered dose inhaler
Endotracheal tube

* **inhalation** drawing of medication into the lungs along with air during breathing.

* **injection** placement of medication in or under the skin with a needle and syringe.

* **nebulizer** inhalation aid that disperses liquid into aerosol spray or mist.

FIGURE 7-4 Small volume nebulizer.

To administer a drug with a nebulizer, follow these steps:

1. Put the medication in the medication reservoir. If the medication is not diluted, combine it with 3–5 cc sterile saline solution. This will allow adequate aerosolization. Screw the reservoir in place.

2. Assemble the nebulizer.

3. Attach oxygen tubing to the oxygen port and oxygen source.

4. Set the oxygen source regulator for 5–8 liters per minute. Note: Never set the oxygen pressure outside of this range. Less than 5 liters per minute will not create enough pressure to aerosolize the medication. More than 8 liters per minute will create too much pressure and destroy the oxygen tubing or nebulizer at its weakest point. Furthermore, because of pressure restrictions, do not attach the nebulizer to an oxygen humidifier.

5. Place the nebulizer in the patient's mouth. Instruct him to exhale and then seal his lips around the mouthpiece. Now have him hold the nebulizer and slowly inhale as deeply as possible. Upon maximum inhalation, instruct the patient to hold in the medication for one to two seconds before exhaling. This permits maximum deposition and absorption. Continue this process until the medication is completely gone. Typically, this takes three to five minutes.

Nebulizers also come preattached to an oxygen facemask in both pediatric and adult sizes (Figure 7-5). Use nebulization facemasks for pediatric or adult patients who cannot hold the nebulizer. Nebulizers for those who require long-term therapy may be powered by a battery or other energy source.

For a nebulizer to be effective, the patient must have an adequate tidal volume and respiratory rate. If the tidal volume is shallow or respiratory rate low, the medication will not move from the nebulizer into the lungs. For patients with a poor tidal and/or respiratory rate who can not pull the medication into their lungs, you can connect nebulizers to a bag-valve mask and/or endotracheal tube.

(a) Nebulizer with attached face mask

Plastic face mask

Nebulizer

O₂

O₂

Valve

90° elbow

ET tube

Reservoir

Bag-valve unit

Nebulizer

(c) Nebulizer with bag-valve unit

"T" bar

ET tube

Nebulizer

O₂

(b) Nebulizer with endotracheal tube

FIGURE 7-5 Nebulizer with attached face mask, bag-valve mask, and endotracheal tube.

METERED DOSE INHALER

Inhaled medications are also delivered through **metered dose inhalers** (MDI). These small, handheld devices produce a medicated spray for inhalation. Patients with conditions such as asthma or COPD use metered dose inhalers to deliver a specific, or metered, dose of medication. A metered dose inhaler consists of two parts, a medication canister and a plastic shell and mouthpiece (Figure 7–6). Some metered dose inhalers come equipped with a spacer. The spacer is a cylindrical canister between the inhaler and the mouthpiece. Prior to self-administration, the patient will depress the inhaler sending a measured dose of drug into the spacer. The patient will then breathe in and out of the spacer through the mouthpiece, thus inhaling the drug into the lungs. This system is particularly useful for patients who have a hard time operating and inhaling the metered dose inhaler. This is common in the elderly and in young children. The spacer, when used in conjunction with a metered dose inhaler, is very effective.

✱ **metered dose inhaler** handheld device that produces a medicated spray for inhalation.

FIGURE 7-6   Metered dose inhaler.

Metered dose inhalers are usually self-administered. However, if your patient is incapacitated, you may have to physically assist with the administration or educate the patient or his caregivers in its use. To assist a patient in the use of a metered dose inhaler, follow this technique:

1. Insert the medication canister into the plastic shell.
2. Remove the cap from the mouthpiece.
3. Gently shake the MDI for 2–5 seconds.
4. Instruct the patient to maximally exhale.
5. Place the mouthpiece in the patient's mouth and have him form a seal with his lips.
6. As the patient inhales, press the canister's top downward to release the medication.
7. Have the patient hold his breath for several seconds.
8. Remove the inhaler from the patient's mouth and instruct him to breathe slowly.
9. If a second dose is necessary, wait according to the manufacturer's instructions. Then repeat.
10. In an acute respiratory emergency involving a patient with a metered dose inhaler, always use a nebulizer instead of the MDI. While the metered dose inhaler delivers a small amount of medication, the nebulizer delivers larger quantities of medication mixed with water and oxygen.

Nebulizers and metered dose inhalers offer several advantages. In respiratory emergencies, less medication is needed because it reaches its exact site of action. The lower dosage is less likely to promote side effects, and if the patient has an adverse reaction, implementing or discontinuing drug delivery is easy. Furthermore, because the patient can hold the nebulizer, he will benefit from feeling more in control of his overall therapy. Most importantly, if your patient is hypoxic you can administer inhaled medications with supplemental oxygen.

The nebulizer and metered dose inhaler also have disadvantages. Moving the aerosolized medication into the lungs depends on adequate ventilation. For the patient with a poor tidal and minute volume, nebulized medications are ineffective, as the drug cannot reach its site of action. In these cases, you should use the nebulizer in conjunction with a bag-valve mask and/or endotracheal tube. Additionally, the patient must exhibit an adequate level of consciousness and manual dexterity to hold the nebulizer and follow instructions correctly.

ENDOTRACHEAL TUBE

When you have not yet established an IV, you can administer certain medications such as lidocaine (Xylocaine), epinephrine, atropine, and naloxone (Narcan) through an endotracheal tube. Delivering liquid medications into the lungs permits rapid absorption through the pulmonary capillaries. In fact, some authorities believe pulmonary absorption is as fast as intravenous absorption.

When using an endotracheal tube, you must increase conventional IV dosages from two to two and one-half times. You also should dilute the medication in normal saline to create 10 ml of solution and then quickly inject it down the endotracheal tube. Several ventilations must follow to aerosolize the medication and enhance its absorption. Ideally, you can pass a commercially manufactured catheter through the endotracheal tube and inject the medication through it. If CPR is underway, stop compressions while you administer the medication and ventilate for aerosolization.

ENTERAL DRUG ADMINISTRATION

Enteral drug administration is the delivery of any medication that is absorbed through the gastrointestinal tract. The gastrointestinal tract, or alimentary canal, travels from the mouth to the stomach and on through the intestines to the rectum (Figure 7-7). You can administer enteral medications orally, through a gastric tube, or rectally.

Several advantages make the gastrointestinal tract the most common route for medication delivery. Aside from sheer convenience, it is the least expensive route, and its use requires little equipment and minimal training. In some instances, after you have delivered a drug you may be able to retrieve it by inducing vomiting, by removing it from the rectum, or simply by having the patient spit it out.

Conversely, enteral drug administration poses several disadvantages. Physical activity, emotions, or food can significantly alter the gastrointestinal tract's chemical and physical environment, making absorption unreliable. In addition, as all blood from the stomach and small intestine must pass through the hepatic circulatory system (portal circulation), the liver's condition can reduce the medication's effectiveness. A dysfunctional liver can significantly alter drug distribution and, in extreme cases, metabolize therapeutic medications into inert or harmful substances. Furthermore, a patient resistant to or *noncompliant* in taking medications makes administration via the enteral route very difficult.

* **enteral drug administration** the delivery of any medication that is absorbed through the gastrointestinal tract.

Mouth

Esophagus

Stomach

Large intestine

Small intestine

Rectum

Anus

FIGURE 7-7 Gastrointestinal tract.

ORAL ADMINISTRATION

* **oral drug administration** the delivery of any medication that is taken by mouth and swallowed into the lower gastrointestinal tract.

Oral drug administration denotes any medication taken by mouth (oral) and swallowed into the gastrointestinal (GI) tract. From the GI tract, the medication is absorbed and distributed throughout the body. When administering a medication by the oral route, you must be sure that the patient has an adequate level of consciousness to support his airway. Administering an oral medication to a patient who cannot support his airway may result in an airway occlusion or aspiration into the lungs. If aspiration into the lungs occurs, aspiration pneumonia and its deadly consequences may occur.

Medications for oral delivery come in a variety of forms, either solid or liquid.

- *Capsules.* Capsules contain liquid, dry, or beaded medication in a soluble casing. For maximum effectiveness, the patient must swallow them whole.
- *Tablets.* Tablets comprise medicated powder compressed into a small, solid disk. Typically, tablets may be scored to permit breaking in half or quarters when lesser dosages are required.

- *Pills.* Pills, comprised of medicated powder compressed into a small disk, are the same as tablets. In the past, the term pill was used to denote a solid medication taken by mouth. Over time, tablet has become the accepted term.
- *Enteric coated/time release capsules and tablets.* These forms of medication release the drug gradually as layers of the capsule or tablet slowly erode. Time release capsules or tablets must be swallowed whole.
- *Elixirs.* Elixirs are liquid medications combined with alcohol or placed in a sweetened fluid.
- *Emulsions.* Emulsions are medications combined with a fat or oil emulsifier.
- *Lozenges.* Lozenges are solid forms of medication that slowly dissolve in the mouth, thus permitting gradual swallowing.
- *Suspensions.* A suspension is a liquid that contains small particles of solid medication.
- *Syrups.* A syrup is a concentrated solution of sugar in water or another liquid to which a medication is added.

Equipment for Oral Administration

Administering oral medications is simple and easy. The basic equipment that you may need depends upon the medication and the patient's status:

- *Soufflé cup.* A soufflé cup is a paper or plastic cup. Placing a solid medication in a soufflé cup makes it easy to see and minimizes contact with the provider's hands.
- *Medicine cup.* A medicine cup is a plastic or glass cup with volumetric measurements on the side. It facilitates giving specific amounts of liquid medication. When you pour medication into the cup, the liquid does not form a flat surface but clings to the sides at a higher level, forming a *meniscus.* To compensate for the meniscus, measure the medication toward the center, at its lowest level.
- *Medicine dropper.* A medicine dropper has markings for measuring liquid volumes. You will use it for special medications and to administer medications to children or patients who cannot tolerate other forms of oral medication.
- *Teaspoon.* You will use these accurately sized measuring spoons to administer liquid medications. A teaspoon normally holds 5 milliliters of fluid; however, the volume of household teaspoons varies significantly. To ensure accurate medication administration, use a measured teaspoon or syringe.
- *Oral syringe.* Oral syringes are calibrated plastic syringes without a hypodermic needle. They are considered the most accurate oral means of administering liquid-based medications. When administering a medication with the oral syringe, place the end of the syringe in the patient's mouth and deliver only as much medication as the patient can safely swallow. Several administrations may be necessary to deliver a complete dose.
- *Nipple.* For the neonate or infant, liquid medication can be delivered with a plastic nipple.

Never use household teaspoons to measure medications, as they vary significantly in volume.

General Principles of Oral Administration

To administer medications orally, use the following technique:

1. Use appropriate BSI measures.
2. Note whether to administer the medication with food or on an empty stomach.
3. Gather any necessary equipment such as a soufflé cup or teaspoon; mix liquids or suspensions, or otherwise prepare medications as needed.
4. Have your patient sit upright (when not contraindicated).
5. Place the medication into your patient's mouth. Allow self-administration when possible; assist when needed.
6. Follow administration with 4–8 ounces of water or other liquid. Swallowing a liquid pushes the medication into the stomach.
7. Ensure that the patient has swallowed the medication and it is not hidden in his mouth. For some pediatric and psychiatric patients, you may have to visually confirm that the patient has swallowed the medication by inspecting the oral cavity.

GASTRIC TUBE ADMINISTRATION

For patients who have difficulty swallowing or whose nutritional status is poor, you may place a *gastric tube* to support or completely supplement nutritional requirements. Gastric tubes are also used in instances of drug overdose, trauma, and upper gastrointestinal bleeding. They may be surgically inserted directly into the stomach through the abdomen or indirectly through the nose (nasogastric tube) or mouth (orogastric tube). Placing a gastric tube through the abdominal wall is reserved for the hospital setting. In some EMS systems, paramedics insert orogastric or nasogastric tubes in the field for emergencies. A properly placed gastric tube allows enteral medication delivery. Activated charcoal for toxic ingestion is commonly administered through a nasogastric or orogastric tube. Other medications, many used in the nonacute setting, also are administered via the gastric tube. With modification, most oral medications can be administered this way. However, you should avoid administering time-release capsules and enteric-coated tablets through a gastric tube, as crushing them for delivery destroys their slow-release mechanism. Also, ensure that the medication has been sufficiently crushed so not to become trapped and occlude the gastric tube.

To administer a medication via a gastric tube, use the following technique (Procedure 7-1):

1. Confirm proper tube placement. Disconnect the tube from the drainage or suction unit or clamping device. Clamp the tube from the drainage or suction unit to avoid gastric contents spilling from either device. Attach a cone-tipped syringe to the proximal end of the gastric tube. Gently inject air while auscultating over the stomach. Following this, withdraw the plunger while observing for the presence of gastric fluid or contents, which indicates appropriate placement. Leave the tube disconnected from the drainage or suction unit.
2. Irrigate the gastric tube. To irrigate the gastric tube, draw up 50–100 ml of normal saline into a cone-tipped syringe. Insert the syringe into the open end of the gastric tube. With the syringe tip pointed at the

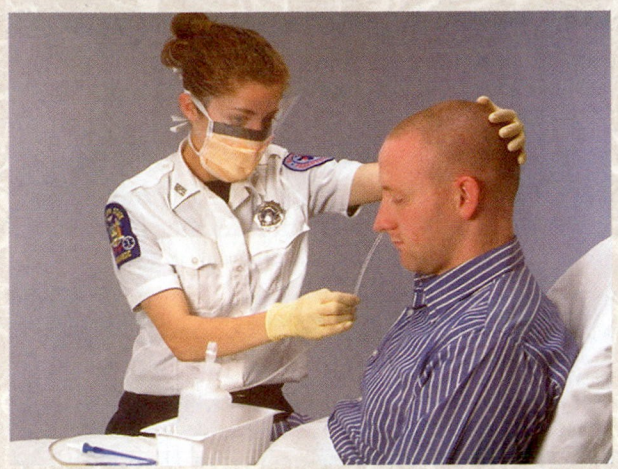

7-1a Confirm proper tube placement.

7-1b Withdraw the plunger while observing for the presence of gastric fluid or contents.

7-1c Instill medication into the gastric tube.

7-1d Gently inject the saline.

7-1e Clamp off the distal tube.

floor, gently inject the saline into the tube. If the saline encounters resistance, look for problems such as tube kinking. Also, have the patient lie on his left side and reattempt injection. If the saline still meets resistance, reattach the tube to the drainage or suction unit and contact medical direction for further directives.

3. Prepare the medication(s) for delivery. Crush tablets or empty capsules into 30 cc of warm water. Ensure that all particles are small so that they will not occlude the tube. You may administer liquid medications without further preparation.

4. Draw the medication into a 30–50 ml cone-tipped syringe and place the tip into open gastric tube. Gently administer the medication into the gastric tube. Forceful application may create considerable distention and patient discomfort.

5. Draw 50–100 ml of warm normal saline into a cone-tipped syringe and attach it to the open end of the gastric tube. Gently inject the saline. This facilitates the medication's passage into the stomach and rinses the tube, ensuring that the patient receives the entire dose. Repeated administrations may be necessary.

6. Clamp off the distal tube. Use a commercially manufactured device or hemostat to clamp shut the distal portion of the gastric tube for approximately 30 minutes after you administer the medication. Do not reattach to the drainage or suction unit. This will prevent the medication's inadvertent removal from the stomach.

If you must refill the syringe in order to administer the full dosage of medication, do not allow the syringe to empty completely before you detach it from the gastric tube. This prevents drawing air into the syringe and then introducing it into the stomach, which causes discomfort.

RECTAL ADMINISTRATION

The rectum's extreme vascularity promotes rapid drug absorption. Additionally, because medications given rectally do not pass through the liver, they are not subject to **hepatic alteration;** thus, their absorption is more predictable.

In the emergency setting, you may give certain drugs rectally if you cannot establish an intravenous line or use the oral route. These include diazepam (Valium) for protracted seizures or aspirin for cardiac or neurologic emergencies. In the nonacute setting, you may administer sedatives, antiemetics, or other specially prepared medications rectally.

Rectal administration may prove advantageous with the unconscious or pediatric patient, or when administering drugs with an objectionable taste or odor. Unfortunately, drug absorption may be erratic if gross fecal matter exists. In addition, some drugs may cause considerable anal or rectal irritation.

Rectal medications come in a variety of forms. In the emergency setting, they are typically liquid, thus permitting easy administration and rapid absorption. To administer a rectal medication in the emergent setting follow this technique:

1. Confirm the indication for administration and dose, and draw the correct quantity of medication into a syringe.

2. Place the hub of a 14-gauge Teflon catheter (removed from the angiocatheter) on the end of a needleless syringe (Figure 7-8).

3. Insert the Teflon catheter into the patient's rectum and inject the medication. Try to keep the medication in the lower part of the rectum. Administration higher in the rectum may result in the

* **hepatic alteration** change in a medication's chemical composition that occurs in the liver.

FIGURE 7-8 Catheter placement on needleless syringe.

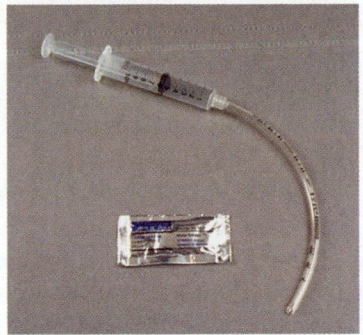

FIGURE 7-9 Syringe attached to endotracheal tube.

FIGURE 7-10 Prepackaged enema container.

medication's being absorbed by veins that deliver drug to the portal circulation.

4. Withdraw the catheter and hold the patient's buttocks together, thus permitting retention and absorption.

An alternative technique utilizes a small endotracheal tube instead of the Teflon angiocatheter. Remove the 15/22 mm BVM adapter and connect a syringe to the proximal end of the tube (Figure 7-9). Lubricate the tube and insert it into the rectum. Inject the medication, remove the tube, and hold the buttocks together.

In the nonemergent setting, suppositories or enemas are common methods for rectal administration. Because your responsibilities as a paramedic may include nonemergent clinical settings, you should master these techniques. Additionally, the rectal route may prove beneficial for a pediatric patient who resists oral administration or for whom IV access proves impractical.

Suppositories are medications packaged in a soft, pliable form. Generally refrigerated until they are used, they begin to melt at body temperature in the rectum. Some are lubricated to ease insertion. Suppositories can be lubricated by running a small amount of luke-warm tap water over the suppository prior to insertion. To administer a suppository, manually insert it into the rectum. Hold the buttocks shut for 5–10 minutes to allow for retention and absorption.

An **enema** is typically a liquid **bolus** of medication that is injected into the rectum. Medications given via this route are typically referred to as small volume enemas. They are typically prepackaged in a squeezable container with a rectal tip (Figure 7-10).

To administer a medicated small volume enema, use the following technique:

1. Apply appropriate BSI and confirm the need for administration via a small volume enema.
2. Place the patient on his left side. Flex his right leg to expose the anus.
3. Insert the prelubricated rectal tip into the anus and advance 3 to 4 inches.
4. Gently squeeze the medicated solution of the bottle into the rectum and colon.
5. Hold the buttocks together to enhance absorption into the rectal and intestinal tissue.

* **suppository** medication packaged in a soft, pliable form, for insertion into the rectum.

* **enema** a liquid bolus of medication that is injected into the rectum.

* **bolus** concentrated mass of medication.

✱ **parenteral** drug administration outside of the gastrointestinal tract.

✱ **syringe** plastic tube with which liquid medications can be drawn up, stored, and injected.

Only those medications with specific guidelines for rectal administration should be delivered through this route. Do not administer rectal medications in the presence of diarrhea, rectal bleeding, hemorrhoids, or any other situation involving severe anal irritation.

PARENTERAL DRUG ADMINISTRATION

Parenteral denotes any drug administration outside of the gastrointestinal tract. Broadly, this encompasses pulmonary and some topical forms of medication delivery; however, additional, specific criteria apply to parenteral administration. Typically, the parenteral route involves the use of needles as medications are injected into the circulatory system or tissues. Consequently, some forms of parenteral drug delivery afford the most rapid drug delivery and absorption.

SYRINGES AND NEEDLES

Frequently, giving medications via the parenteral route requires a syringe and hypodermic needle.

Syringe

A **syringe** is a plastic tube with which liquid medications can be drawn up, stored, and injected. Syringes range in size from 1 cc to 100 cc and greater. Remember that while medication dosages are generally given by weight (g/mg/mcg), syringes represent volume. Therefore, you must be prepared to mathematically convert these measurements.

A syringe's two major components are a barrel and a plunger (Figure 7-11). The tube-like barrel, or body, functions as a reservoir for medication. Markings on its side calibrate its overall volume. Smaller syringes are calibrated in 0.10 ml intervals, larger syringes in 1.0 ml intervals.

The plunger is a device that fits into the barrel. At one end it has a handle for pulling or pushing. At the opposite end, a rubber stopper fits snugly into the barrel. Pulling on the plunger draws material into the barrel; pushing on it expels material from the barrel. The rubber end forms a tight seal from which the fluid medication cannot escape.

The junction of the fluid and rubber stopper measures the total volume of liquid in the syringe. The barrel's maximum volume should correspond closely to the volume of medication needed. For example, to administer 2 ml of medication, a 3 ml syringe would prove most appropriate.

An adapter at the syringe's distal end is compatible with the hub of an IV catheter or, as many cases will require, a hypodermic needle.

FIGURE 7-11 Syringe.

FIGURE 7-12 Hypodermic
needle.

Hypodermic Needle

The **hypodermic needle** is a hollow metal tube used with the syringe to administer medications. It is sharp enough to easily puncture tissues, blood vessels, or IV medication ports.

The hypodermic needle's primary components include a hilt and shaft. The hilt is a threaded plastic tube that screws securely onto the syringe's distal adapter. The shaft is a thin metal tube through which medications can flow from the syringe into the delivery site. A bevel at the shaft's distal end accounts for its sharpness (Figure 7-12).

Hypodermic needles come in a variety of gauges and lengths. A needle's **gauge** describes its diameter. Generally, hypodermic needle gauges range from 18 to 27. The gauge and actual diameter are inversely related: the higher the gauge, the smaller the diameter. Thus, a 25-gauge needle's diameter is smaller than an 18-gauge needle's. Conversely, a 20-gauge needle's diameter is larger than a 22-gauge needle's. Hypodermic needle lengths generally range from 3/8″ to 1 1/2″. The package label lists the size of the syringe and the gauge and length of the hypodermic needle.

Because syringes and hypodermic needles frequently involve invasive procedures, they are packaged sterile. Never use either a syringe or a hypodermic needle from a package that has been opened or tampered with. Used hypodermic needles are sharp and present a biohazard. Dispose of them immediately after you complete any task involving their use.

MEDICATION PACKAGING

All medications delivered by the parenteral route are liquids. They are packaged in a variety of containers with which you must be familiar, as obtaining medication from each type requires a different procedure. The kinds of parenteral drug containers include:

- Glass ampules
- Single and multidose vials
- Nonconstituted drug vials
- Prefilled syringes
- Intravenous medication fluids

You must also be thoroughly familiar with the information included on the labels of all medication containers:

- *Name of medication.* The label lists both the generic and trade name of the medication. Always ensure that you have selected the right medication.

* **hypodermic needle** hollow metal tube used with the syringe to administer medications.

* **gauge** the size of a needle's diameter.

- *Expiration date.* All medications have an expiration date after which they cannot be used. Never use an expired medication.
- *Total dose and concentration.* The total dose of drug is the total weight (g/mg/mcg) of medication in the container. The concentration represents the weight of the drug per volume of fluid. For example, if 10 mg of a drug were packaged in 10 ml of fluid, the total dose would be 10 mg, and the concentration would be 10 mg/10 ml or 1 mg/ml. Beware, identical drugs can be packaged in different dosages and concentrations.

Always use the label printed directly on the container to confirm the correct medication.

These labels are printed directly on the vial, ampule, prefilled syringe, or IV medication bag. Always use them to confirm the correct medication.

Glass Ampules

* ampule breakable glass vessel containing liquid medication.

An **ampule,** or amp, is a breakable glass vessel containing liquid medication. It has a cone shaped top, thin neck, and circular tubular base for storing the medication (Figure 7-13). The thin neck is a vulnerable point where you intentionally break the ampule to retrieve its contents. Ampules usually range in volume from 1 to 5 ml. The least expensive form of drug packaging, they contain single doses of medication.

To obtain medication from a glass ampule you will need a syringe and needle. Use the following technique (Procedure 7-2):

FIGURE 7-13   Ampules.

1. Confirm medication indications and patient allergies.
2. Confirm the ampule label (medication name, dose, and expiration).
3. Hold the ampule upright and tap its top to dislodge any trapped solution.
4. Place gauze around the thin neck and snap it off with your thumb.
5. Place the tip of the hypodermic needle inside the ampule and withdraw the medication into the syringe.
6. Reconfirm the indication, drug, dose, and route of administration.
7. Administer the medication appropriately via the indicated route.
8. Properly dispose of the needle, syringe, and broken glass ampule.

Single and Multidose Vials

* vial plastic or glass container with a self-healing rubber top.

Vials are plastic or glass containers with a self-sealing rubber top (Figure 7-14). Vials may contain single or multiple doses of medication; the self-sealing rubber top prevents leakage from punctures and permits multiple access with a syringe and hypodermic needle. The medication inside the vial is packaged in a vacuum.

To obtain medication from a vial, follow these steps (Procedure 7-3):

FIGURE 7-14   Vials.

1. Confirm medication indications and patient allergies.
2. Confirm the vial label (name, dose, and expiration).
3. Determine the volume of medication to be administered.
4. Prepare the syringe and hypodermic needle. Because the vial is vacuum packed, you will have to replace the volume of medication removed with air in order to maintain equilibrium in the vial. Withdraw the plunger, to draw a volume of air into the syringe equal to the volume of medication to be administered. This technique permits easy medication retrieval from the vial.

7-2a   Hold the ampule upright and tap its top to dislodge any trapped solution.

7-2b   Place gauze around the thin neck . . .

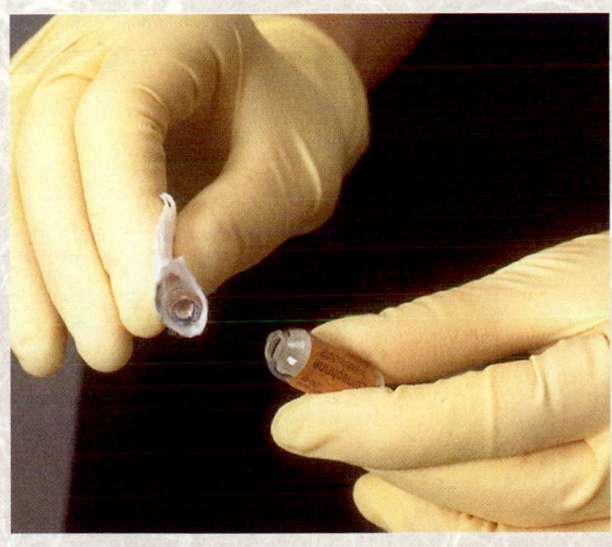

7-2c   . . . and snap it off with your thumb.

7-2d   Draw up the medication.

7-3a   Confirm the vial label.

7-3b   Prepare the syringe and hypodermic needle.

7-3c   Cleanse the vial's rubber top.

7-3d   Insert the hypodermic needle into the rubber top and inject the air from the syringe into the vial.

5. Cleanse the vial's rubber top with an antiseptic alcohol preparation.

6. Insert the hypodermic needle into the rubber top and inject the air from the syringe into the vial. Then withdraw the appropriate volume of medication.

7. Reconfirm the indication, drug, dose, and route of administration.

8. Administer appropriately via the indicated route.

9. Properly dispose of the needle, syringe, and vial.

Nonconstituted Drug Vial

The **nonconstituted drug vial,** extends the viability and storage time of drugs that have a short shelf life or are unstable in liquid form. The nonconstituted drug vial actually consists of two vials, one containing a powdered medication and one containing a liquid mixing solution (Figure 7-15). To prepare the drug you must mix it, or reconstitute it, by withdrawing the liquid solution from its vial and placing it in the powdered medication's vial. In a **Mix-o-Vial** system, the two vials are joined and you must squeeze them together to break the seal and mix.

To prepare a medication from a nonconstituted drug vial, use the following technique (Procedure 7-4):

1. Confirm medication indications and patient allergies.

2. Confirm the vial's label (name, dose, expiration date).

3. Remove all solution from the vial containing the mixing solution, using the same procedure as you would to withdraw medication from a single or multidose vial.

4. With an alcohol preparation, cleanse the top of the vial containing the powdered drug and inject the mixing solution.

5. Gently agitate or shake the vial to ensure complete mixture.

6. Determine the volume of newly constituted medication to be administered.

7. Prepare the syringe and hypodermic needle. Because the vial is vacuum packed, you will have to replace the volume of medication removed with air in order to retain equilibrium in the vial. By withdrawing the plunger, place into the syringe a volume of air equal to the volume of medication that will be removed. This technique permits easy medication retrieval from the vial.

8. Cleanse the medication vial's rubber top with an antiseptic alcohol preparation.

9. Insert the hypodermic needle into the rubber top and withdraw the appropriate volume of medication.

✳ **nonconstituted drug vial/Mix-o-Vial** vial with two containers, one holding a powdered medication and the other holding a liquid mixing solution.

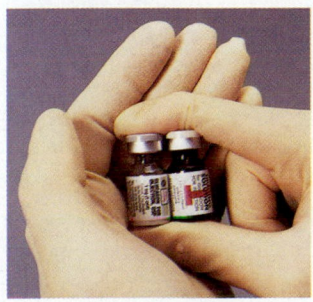

FIGURE 7-15 The nonconstituted drug vial actually consists of two vials, one containing a powdered medication and one containing a liquid mixing solution.

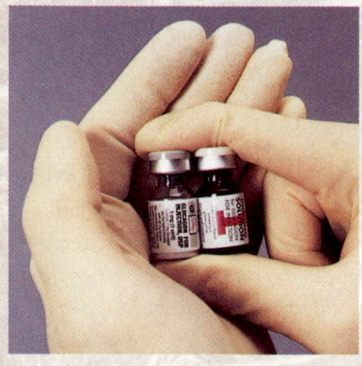

7-4a Nonconsituted drugs come in separate vials. Confirm the labels.

7-4b Remove all solution from the vial containing the mixing solution.

7-4c Cleanse the top of the vial containing the powdered drug and inject the solution.

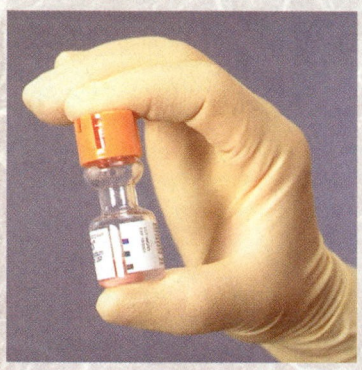

7-4d Agitate or shake the vial to ensure complete mixture.

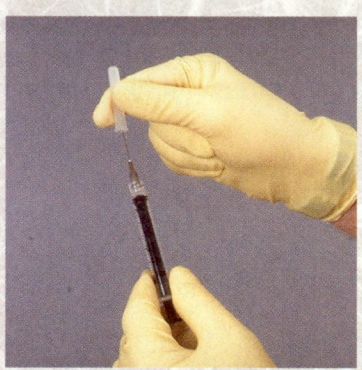

7-4e Prepare a new syringe and hypodermic needle.

7-4f Withdraw the appropriate volume of medication.

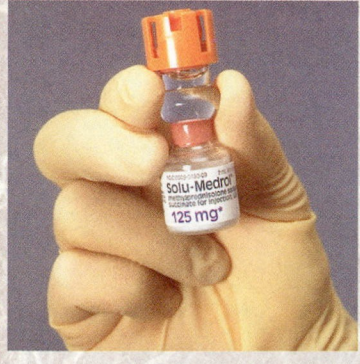

7-4g In the Mix-o-Vial system, the vials are joined at the neck. Confirm the labels.

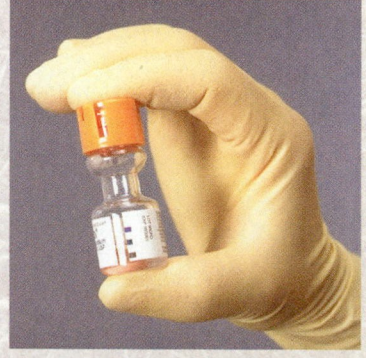

7-4h Squeeze the vials together to break the seal. Agitate or shake to mix completely.

7-4i Withdraw the appropriate volume of medication.

10. Reconfirm the indication, drug, dose, and route of administration.
11. Administer appropriately via the indicated route.
12. Monitor the patient for the desired effects.
13. Properly dispose of the needle and syringe.

In some instances you may have to place multiple medications into one syringe for a single delivery. For example, meperidine (Demerol) and promethazine (Phenergan) may be delivered in this manner. Meperidine, an analgesic, can cause nausea and vomiting when administered. To decrease the incidence of nausea and vomiting, you can simultaneously administer promethazine, an antiemetic. To perform this task, draw all medications in the appropriate order according to the procedures discussed. Always anticipate total volume and select an appropriate syringe size. To avoid complications, you must always be aware of drug incompatibilities.

Prefilled or Preloaded Syringes

Prefilled or **preloaded syringes** are packaged in tamper-proof containers with the medication already in the syringe. Because the syringe is prefilled, you do not need to draw the medication from another source. Generally, prefilled syringes contain standard dosages, thus decreasing the chance of dosage error.

The prefilled syringe consists of two parts, a syringe and a glass tube prefilled with liquid medication. The plastic syringe is similar to those described earlier; however, it does not have a plunger. Rather, you screw the prefilled glass tube into the syringe barrel and secure it (Figure 7-16). Pushing the glass container into the syringe barrel expels the medication through the attached hypodermic needle.

Follow these steps to administer a medication from a prefilled syringe:

1. Confirm medication indications and patient allergies.
2. Confirm the prefilled syringe label (name, dose, and expiration date).
3. Assemble the prefilled syringe. Remove the pop-off caps and screw together.
4. Reconfirm the indication, drug, dose, and route of administration.
5. Administer appropriately via the indicated route.
6. Properly dispose of the needle and syringe.

Intravenous Medication Solutions

Medicated solutions are another form of parenteral medication. They are packaged in an IV bag and administered as an IV **infusion**. IV medication solutions may be premixed or you may have to mix them. The section on intravenous drug infusions later in this chapter discusses their actual preparation and administration.

* **prefilled/preloaded syringe** syringe packaged in a tamper-proof container with the medication already in the barrel.

* **medicated solution** parenteral medication packaged in an IV bag and administered as an IV infusion.

* **infusion** liquid medication delivered through a vein.

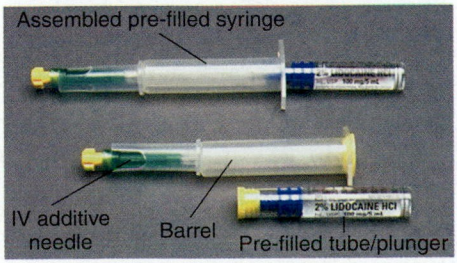

FIGURE 7-16 Prefilled syringes.

PARENTERAL ROUTES

Parenterally administered drugs can be absorbed locally or systemically. Additionally, depending on the route of administration, their absorption rate may be slow, sustained, or rapid. Parenteral delivery bypasses the digestive tract, thus making the drug's absorption, action, and onset more predictable. Because parenteral routes use hypodermic needles that contact body fluids, the risk of disease transmission is ever present.

Parenteral drug delivery employs the following routes:

- Intradermal injection
- Subcutaneous injection
- Intramuscular injection
- Intravenous access
- Intraosseous infusion

Specific medications require specific routes of parenteral delivery; therefore, you must be competent with every route. In this section we will discuss the specialized equipment, medications, and routes for intradermal, subcutaneous, and intramuscular injections. Because of their complexity, we will discuss intravenous access and intraosseous infusions separately in the following sections.

Whether you are administering a parenteral injection or an IV bolus or infusion, you should explain the entire procedure to the patient to help alleviate his anxiety. Finally, remember that hypoperfusion (hypovolemia or peripheral vascular disease, for instance), may significantly reduce parenteral absorption.

Intradermal Injection

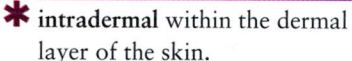 **intradermal** within the dermal layer of the skin.

Using a syringe and hypodermic needle, **intradermal** injections deposit medication into the dermal layer of the skin (*intra-*, within; *derma*, skin). The amount of medication placed in the dermal layer is quite small, typically less than 1 ml (Figure 7-17).

Capillaries in the dermis afford a very slow rate of absorption, with little or no systemic distribution. Rather, the bulk of medication remains localized in the area of administration. Intradermal delivery proves useful for allergy testing and tuberculin skin testing and for administering local anesthetics during suturing, wound debridement, and IV establishment.

The forearm and upper back are preferred sites for intradermal injections. They have little hair and are highly visible. Additionally, you should look for sites free of superficial blood vessels, which increase the chance for systemic absorption.

Capillaries in the dermis afford a very slow rate of absorption, with little or no systemic distribution.

FIGURE 7-17 Intradermal injection.

To administer an intradermal injection, you will need the following equipment:

- BSI protection
- Alcohol or betadine antiseptic preparations
- Packaged medication
- Tuberculin syringe (1 cc)
- 25–27-gauge needle, 3/8″–1″ long
- Sterile gauze and adhesive bandage

To administer an intradermal injection, follow these steps:

1. Assemble and prepare the needed equipment.
2. Apply BSI and confirm the drug, indication, dosage, and need for intradermal injection.
3. Draw up medication as appropriate.
4. Prepare the site with alcohol or betadine. The intended site must be cleansed of pathogens, therein decreasing the likelihood of infection. Generally, you will use alcohol or betadine antiseptics. To appropriately cleanse the site, start at the site itself and work outward with an expanding circular motion. This motion will push pathogens away from the intended site of puncture.
5. Pull the patient's skin taut with your nondominant hand.
6. Insert the needle, bevel up, just under the skin, at a 10°–15° angle.
7. Slowly inject the medication, look for a small bump, or wheal to form as medication is deposited and collects in the intradermal tissue.
8. Remove the needle and dispose of it in the sharps container.
9. Place the adhesive bandage over the site; use the gauze for hemorrhage control if needed.

Do not rub or massage the injection site. This promotes systemic absorption and nullifies the advantage of localized effect.

Subcutaneous Injection

Subcutaneous injections place medication into the subcutaneous tissue (*sub-*, below; *cutaneous*, skin). The subcutaneous layer consists of loose connective tissue between the skin and muscle (Figure 7-18). The subcutaneous tissue has few blood vessels and thus promotes slow, sustained absorption, which prolongs a

subcutaneous the layer of loose connective tissue between the skin and muscle.

The subcutaneous tissue has few blood vessels and thus promotes slow, sustained absorption, which prolongs a drug's effect on the body.

FIGURE 7-18 Subcutaneous injection.

FIGURE 7-19 Subcutaneous injection sites (injection sites shown in red).

drug's effect on the body. Like intradermal injections, no more than 1.0 ml of medication is administered subcutaneously. Administering more than 1.0 ml of medication can cause irritation and, possibly, an abscess.

Administer subcutaneous injections where you can easily pinch the skin on the upper arms, thighs, or occasionally, the abdomen (Figure 7-19). Easily pinched skin contains more subcutaneous tissue and readily separates from the muscle. All sites should be free of superficial blood vessels, nerves, and tendons. Additionally, avoid areas with tattoos or bruising.

To perform a subcutaneous injection, you will need the following equipment:

- BSI protection
- Alcohol or betadine antiseptic preparations
- Packaged medication
- Syringe (1–3 cc)
- 24–26-gauge hypodermic needle, 3/8″–1″ long
- Sterile gauze and adhesive bandage

To administer a subcutaneous injection, use the following technique (Procedure 7-5):

1. Assemble and prepare equipment.
2. Apply BSI and confirm the drug, indication, dosage, and need for subcutaneous injection.
3. Draw up the medication as appropriate.
4. Prepare the site with alcohol or betadine as described for an intradermal injection.
5. Gently pinch a 1″ fold of skin.
6. Insert the needle just into skin at a 45° angle with the bevel up.

7-5a   Prepare the equipment.

7-5b   Check the medication.

7-5c   Draw up the medication.

7-5d   Prep the site.

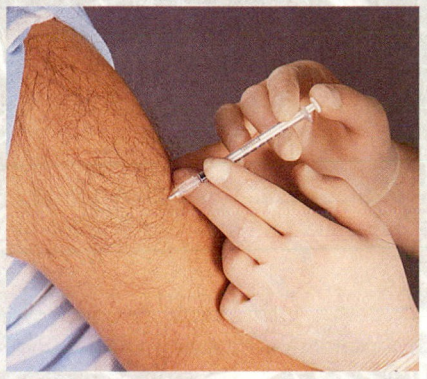

7-5e   Insert the needle at a 45° angle.

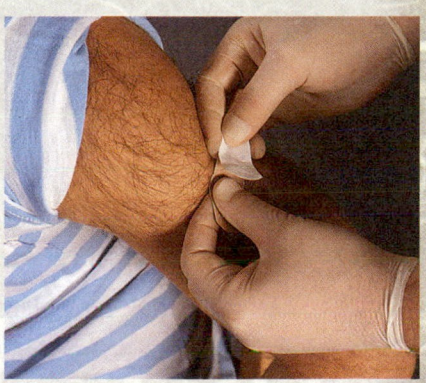

7-5f   Remove the needle and cover the puncture site.

7-5g   Monitor the patient.

7. Pull the plunger back to aspirate tissue fluid.

8. If blood appears, the hypodermic needle is in a blood vessel and absorption will be too rapid. Start the procedure over with a new syringe.

9. If no blood appears, proceed with step 10.

10. Slowly inject the medication.

11. Remove the needle and dispose of it in a sharps container.

12. Place an adhesive bandage over the site; use the gauze for hemorrhage control if needed.

13. Monitor the patient.

After you give the injection, gently rubbing or massaging the site will help initiate systemic absorption.

Some authorities recommend using an air plug in the syringe. This is approximately 0.1 ml of air that follows the injection and pushes the medication further into the subcutaneous tissue, thus preventing leakage or medication loss. To place an air plug in the syringe, aspirate approximately 0.1 ml of air into the barrel after you have drawn up the medication. Pointing the needle downward and perpendicular to the ground, tap the syringe with your finger to dislodge the air pocket. It will float to the top of the plunger, and from there it will follow the medication into the subcutaneous tissue.

You can also deliver a subcutaneous injection into the sublingual region, or fleshy tissue below the tongue. To administer a subcutaneous injection, you place the hypodermic needle of a small, medication-filled syringe into the sublingual tissue and then inject the medication as appropriate. Epinephrine in severe cases of asthma or anaphylaxis can be administered in this manner.

Intramuscular Injection

Intramuscular injections deposit medication into muscle (*intra-*, within; *muscular*, muscle). Muscle is extremely vascular and permits systemic delivery at a moderate absorption rate. Drug absorption through muscle is also relatively predictable. To reach the muscle, a needle must penetrate the dermal and subcutaneous tissue (Figure 7-20).

Several sites are used for intramuscular injections (Figure 7-21). Depending upon the site, varying quantities of medication can be delivered. These sites and their correlating volumes of medication include:

- *Deltoid*. The deltoid muscle is 3–4 finger breadths below the acromial process (the bony bump on the shoulder). It is highly vascular and permits easy access. You can deliver up to 2.0 ml into this muscle.

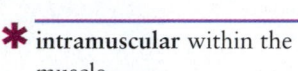
intramuscular within the muscle.

Content Review

INTRAMUSCULAR INJECTION SITES

Deltoid
Dorsal gluteal
Vastus lateralis
Rectus femoris

Muscle is extremely vascular and permits systemic delivery at a moderate absorption rate.

FIGURE 7-20 Intramuscular injection.

Vertical line

Preferred
site

Horizontal line

Hip

Preferred
site

Gluteal artery

Fold separating
the buttocks

Sciatic nerve

Deltoid
muscle

Preferred
site

Rectus
femoris

Vastus
lateralis

Preferred
site

FIGURE 7-21   Intramuscular
injection sites.

- *Dorsal Gluteal.* The dorsal gluteal muscle, or buttock, is a common administration point for intramuscular injections. Injections here can deliver 5.0 ml of medication or more. They cause little discomfort, but you must avoid the large sciatic nerve, which is the leg's major motor nerve. Damage to the sciatic nerve can decrease mobility or totally paralyze the leg. To help prevent neurological complication, envision an imaginary quadrant over the buttock; administer all injections in the upper and outer quadrant.

- *Vastus Lateralis.* The vastus lateralis muscle of the thigh is another common site for intramuscular injection, especially for pediatric patients. As at the dorsal gluteal muscle, injections here can deliver 5 ml of medication or more. To deliver medication at this site, imagine a grid of nine boxes. Administer injections in the middle, outer box, or anterolateral part of the muscle.

- *Rectus Femoris.* The rectus femoris lies over the femur and is closely associated with the vastus lateralis muscle. When utilizing the rectus femoris for intramuscular injection, place the medication into the center of the muscle at approximately mid-shaft of the femur. Up to 5 ml of drug volume can be administered into the rectus femoris.

When choosing a site, avoid bruised or scarred areas. Areas free of superficial blood vessels are most desirable.

To perform an intramuscular injection, you will need the following equipment:

- BSI protection
- Alcohol or betadine antiseptic preparation
- Packaged medication
- Syringe (1 ml to 5 ml, depending on dosage)
- 21–23-gauge hypodermic needle, 3/8″−1″ long
- Sterile gauze and adhesive bandage

Follow these steps to administer an intramuscular injection (Procedure 7-6):

1. Assemble and prepare the needed equipment.
2. Apply BSI and confirm the drug, indication, dosage, and need for intramuscular injection.
3. Draw up medication as appropriate.
4. Prepare the site with alcohol or betadine as described for an intradermal injection.
5. Stretch the skin taut over the injection site with your nondominant hand.
6. Insert the needle just into skin at a 90° angle with the bevel up.
7. Pull back the plunger to aspirate tissue fluid.
   - If blood appears, the hypodermic needle is in a blood vessel, and absorption of the medication will be too rapid. Start the procedure over with a new syringe.
   - If no blood appears proceed with step 8.
8. Slowly inject the medication.
9. Remove the needle and dispose of it in the sharps container.
10. Place an adhesive bandage over site; use gauze for hemorrhage control if needed.
11. Monitor the patient.

7-6a   Prepare the equipment.

7-6b   Check the medication.

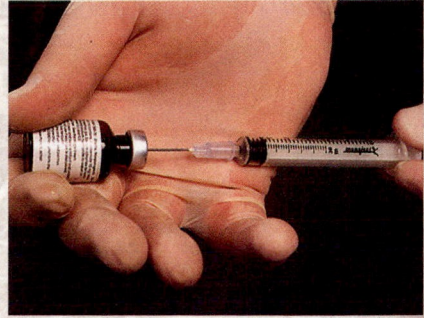

7-6c   Draw up the medication.

7-6d   Prepare the site.

7-6e   Insert the needle at a 90° angle.

7-6f   Remove the needle and cover the puncture site.

7-6g   Monitor the patient.

After administration, gently rubbing or massaging the site helps to initiate systemic absorption. Do not massage the site, however, if you have administered heparin or another anticoagulant. Again, some authorities recommend a 0.1 ml air plug as described under subcutaneous injection.

Intravenous and Intraosseous Routes

Two important parenteral drug administration routes—intravenous access and intraosseous infusion—are discussed in detail in Part 2.

Part 2: Intravenous Access, Blood Sampling, and Intraosseous Infusion

Objectives

In this part, we will discuss intravenous access, including types of venous access and the variety of equipment required, where and how to establish intravenous access, flow rates, and possible complications. We will also detail intravenous administration of medications (bolus and infusion). Venous blood sampling techniques will also be covered.

Additionally, this part of the chapter provides information on intraosseous medication administration, including techniques, possible complications, and contraindications. Intraosseous administration is a route most often used in pediatric patients under five years of age.

INTRAVENOUS ACCESS

✱ **intravenous access (cannulation)** surgical puncture of a vein to deliver medication or withdraw blood.

Intravenous *(IV)* access (*intra-*, within; *venous*, vein) or *cannulation,* is a routine paramedic procedure. Circulating blood transports chemicals, proteins, and fluids throughout the body. Venous circulation can likewise deliver medications and fluids into the body and provides an invaluable tool for treating the sick and injured.

The following situations indicate intravenous access:

- Fluid and blood replacement
- Drug administration
- Obtaining venous blood specimens for laboratory analysis

Since veins are easier to locate and penetrate, venous access is preferable to arterial access. Additionally, venous circulation pressure is lower than arterial and presents fewer hemorrhage control complications.

TYPES OF INTRAVENOUS ACCESS

Medical care providers use two types of intravenous access, peripheral and central. As a paramedic, you will most often perform peripheral intravenous access. Central venous access is rarely, if ever, performed in the prehospital setting.

Ulcer vein

Radial vein

Dorsal veins

External jugular vein

Dorsal venous arch

FIGURE 7-22   Peripheral IV access sites: veins of the arm, hand, neck, and foot.

Peripheral Venous Access

Although challenging, **peripheral venous access** is relatively easy to master. As its name implies, it uses peripheral veins. Common sites include the arms and legs and, when necessary, the neck. Figure 7-22 illustrates the specific veins commonly accessed on the hand, forearm, and leg.

As some patients' veins may not be readily visible, you must know venous topography. In these cases, you will have to locate veins based on anatomical layout and palpation. Exhaust all possibilities on the arms before trying to locate the veins of the legs. Leg veins are more difficult to access and present complications more frequently. For neonates and infants, you may access veins in the scalp. Chapter 42 on pediatrics explains that technique.

When establishing a peripheral IV, start at the distal end of the extremity and work proximally. Once you have attempted cannulation, the disruption in blood flow hinders using veins distal to that site. However, the purpose of access also determines site selection. For example, rapid fluid administration requires larger veins like the antecubital fossa, as opposed to the smaller veins of the hand. The external jugular vein is considered a peripheral vein and can be accessed when other peripheral sites are not available.

The major advantage of peripheral venous access is that it is relatively simple to perform because visualizing and accessing the veins is usually easy. Additionally, you can access peripheral veins while simultaneously doing other life sustaining procedures such as CPR or endotracheal intubation. Conversely, peripheral veins collapse in hypovolemia or circulatory failure, thus

✳ **peripheral venous access** surgical puncture of a vein in the arm, leg, or neck.

becoming difficult to locate and access. Furthermore, the peripheral veins of geriatric patients, pediatric patients, or those with peripheral vascular disease may be fragile and difficult to cannulate. Finally, peripheral veins may roll and elude IV placement.

Central Venous Access

* **central venous access** surgical puncture of the internal jugular, subclavian, or femoral vein.

Central venous access utilizes veins located deep within the body. These include the internal jugular, subclavian, and femoral veins. They are larger than peripheral veins and will not collapse in shock. Central IV lines are placed near the heart for long-term use. Typically, they are used when medical conditions require repeated access for medication and/or fluid delivery. They also are used for transvenous pacing or for monitoring central venous pressure.

* **peripherally inserted central catheter (PICC)** line threaded into the central circulation via a peripheral site.

A special type of central line is the **peripherally inserted central catheter,** or **PICC,** line. PICC lines are smaller than those routinely used for central access and are threaded into the central circulation via a peripheral site. PICC lines are most often used in infants and children requiring long term care.

Central venous access is typically restricted to the hospital setting because of its invasive nature and high risk of complications such as arterial puncture, pneumothorax, and air embolism. Central veins cannot be accessed during procedures such as CPR, and they often require a chest X-ray for placement confirmation. You may nonetheless encounter a central line during interfacility transports or in a chronically ill homebound patient. Protocols in some EMS systems allow paramedics to access existing central lines during emergency care. Still other systems allow their paramedics to place certain central lines. Always follow local protocols regarding central line access and insertion. For more information about central venous access, consult a text on advanced venipuncture techniques.

EQUIPMENT AND SUPPLIES FOR VENOUS ACCESS

To establish intravenous access, you will need the following specialized equipment and supplies.

Intravenous Fluids

* **intravenous fluid** chemically prepared solution tailored to the body's specific needs.

Intravenous fluids are chemically prepared solutions tailored to the body's specific needs. They replace the body's lost fluids and/or aid the delivery of IV medications. They also can keep a vein patent when no fluid or drug therapy is required.

Intravenous fluids come in four different forms: colloids, crystalloids, blood, and oxygen carrying fluids.

* **colloid** intravenous solutions containing large proteins that cannot pass through capillary membranes.

Colloids **Colloidal solutions** contain large proteins that cannot pass through the capillary membrane. Consequently, they remain in the circulatory system for a long time. In addition, colloids have osmotic properties that attract water into the circulatory system. A small quantity of colloid can significantly increase intravascular volume (volume of blood and fluid contained within the blood vessels). Common colloids include:

- *Plasma protein fraction (plasmanate).* Plasmanate is a protein-containing colloid. Its principle protein, albumin, is suspended with other proteins in a saline solvent.
- *Salt poor albumin.* Salt poor albumin contains only human albumin. Each gram of albumin will retain approximately 18 milliliters of water in the blood stream.

- *Dextran.* Dextran is not a protein but a large sugar molecule with osmotic properties similar to albumin's. It comes in two molecular weights: 40 000 and 70 000 daltons. Dextran 40 has from two to two and a half times the colloidal osmotic pressure of albumin. Anaphylactic reaction is a possible side effect.
- *Hetastarch (Hespan).* Like Dextran, hetastarch is a sugar molecule with osmotic properties similar to protein's. Hetastarch does not appear to share Dextran's side effects.

Although colloids help maintain vascular volume, using them in the field is not practical. Their high cost, short shelf life, and specific storage requirements suit them better to the hospital setting. However, the paramedic who works in an emergency department, aeromedical service, or at a mass casualty incident may have to administer colloidal solutions.

Crystalloids Crystalloids are the primary out-of-hospital IV solution. Crystalloids contain electrolytes and water but lack colloids' larger proteins and larger molecules. The many preparations of crystalloid solutions are classified by their tonicity (number of particles per unit volume) relative to that of body plasma:

* **crystalloid** intravenous solutions that contain electrolytes but lack the larger proteins associated with colloids.

- *Isotonic Solutions.* **Isotonic** solutions have a tonicity equal to blood plasma's. In a normally hydrated patient, they will not cause a significant fluid or electrolyte shift.
- *Hypertonic Solutions.* **Hypertonic** solutions have a higher solute concentration than do the cells. When administered to the normally hydrated patient, they cause fluid to shift out of the intracellular compartment and into the extracellular compartment. Later, solute will diffuse in the opposite direction.
- *Hypotonic Solutions.* **Hypotonic** solutions have a lower solute concentration than do the cells. When administered to a normally hydrated patient, they cause fluid to move from the extracellular compartment and into the intracellular compartment. Later, the solutes will move in the opposite direction.

* **isotonic** state in which solutions on opposite sides of a semi-permeable membrane are in equal concentration.

* **hypertonic** state in which a solution has a higher solute concentration on one side of a semi-permeable membrane than on the other side.

* **hypotonic** state in which a solution has a lower solute concentration on one side of a semi-permeable membrane than on the other side.

The particular type of IV solution you select depends on your patient's needs. The three most commonly used IV fluids in prehospital care are:

- *Lactated Ringer's.* Lactated Ringer's solution is an isotonic electrolyte solution. It contains sodium chloride, potassium chloride, calcium chloride, and sodium lactate in water.
- *Normal saline solution.* Normal saline is an isotonic electrolyte solution containing 0.90% sodium chloride in water.
- *5% dextrose in water* (D_5W). D_5W is a hypotonic glucose solution used to keep a vein patent and to supply calories needed for cellular metabolism. While D_5W initially increases circulatory volume, glucose molecules rapidly diffuse across the vascular membrane and increase the free water.

Both lactated Ringer's and normal saline solution are used for fluid replacement because of their immediate ability to expand the circulating volume. However, due to the movement of electrolytes and water, two thirds of either solution will be lost to the extravascular space within one hour. Crystalloids such as normal saline mixed with D_5W or half-strength normal saline (0.45 percent) are combinations or modifications of the above solutions.

Occasionally, you will have to warm or cool the IV fluid. A hypothermic patient may benefit from having a crystalloid warmed before and during fluid administration. Warm fluids assist in elevating the patient's core temperature. Conversely, cool fluids may benefit the patient with an increased core temperature. You can cool or warm fluids by storing them in a special temperature controlled compartment or by using the heater or air conditioner in the ambulance, helicopter, or mobile intensive care unit. Commercial fluid heaters are available. Their use is detailed later in this chapter. Some fluids, such as blood and some colloids, require constant storage in a cool environment.

Blood The most desirable fluid for replacement is whole blood. Unlike colloids and crystalloids, the hemoglobin in blood carries oxygen. Blood, however, is a precious commodity and must be conserved so that it can be of benefit to the most people. Its use in the field is generally limited to aeromedical services or mass casualty incidents. O-negative blood's universal compatibility makes it ideal for administration in the field. Chapter 35 on hematology discusses blood in detail.

Oxygen Carrying Solutions In development are fluids that can carry oxygen and off-load it for cellular use. These fluids, which remain experimental at present, show promise for treating hypovolemia in the field.

Packaging of Intravenous Fluids Most intravenous fluids and blood are packaged in soft plastic or vinyl bags of various sizes (50, 100, 250, 500, 1000, 2000, and 3000 ml) (Figure 7-23). Some contain medication that is incompatible with plastic or vinyl and must be packaged in glass bottles.

The IV-fluid container provides important information.

- *Label.* A label on every IV bottle or bag lists the fluid type and expiration date. Like any other medication, intravenous solutions have a shelf life; do not use them after their expiration date. Discard any fluid that appears cloudy, discolored, or laced with particulate. Additionally, avoid using any fluid whose sealed packaging has been opened or tampered with.
- *Medication Administration Port.* A medication port on IV-solution bags or bottles permits you to inject medication into the fluid for infusion.
- *Administration Set Port.* The administration set port is where you place the spike from the IV administration tubing.

Administration Tubing

Intravenous **administration tubing** connects the solution bag to the IV **cannula** that is inserted into the patient's vein. Administration tubing is made of very flexible clear plastic. You must select from several types of administration tubing according to your patient's need. All tubing is packaged in a sterile container. If the container is opened or appears damaged, select another administration set. Any pathogens on the tubing will enter the patient, possibly causing long-term complications.

Microdrip and Macrodrip Tubing Microdrip administration tubing delivers relatively small amounts of fluid to the patient. It is more appropriate when you need to restrict the overall fluid volume a patient will receive. **Macrodrip** administration tubing delivers relatively large amounts of fluid. It is more appropriate when volume replacement is necessary, as in shock, fluid replacement, or hypotension.

Expiration date
Normal saline fluid type
Medication administration port
Administration set port

FIGURE 7-23 IV solution containers.

Do not use any IV fluids after their expiration date; any fluids that appear cloudy, discolored, or laced with particulate; or any fluid whose sealed packaging has been opened or tampered with.

* **administration tubing** flexible, clear plastic tubing that connects the solution bag to the IV cannula.

* **cannula** hollow needle used to puncture a vein.

* **microdrip tubing** administration tubing that delivers a relatively small amount of fluid.

* **macrodrip tubing** administration tubing that delivers a relatively large amount of fluid.

FIGURE 7-24 Macrodrip and microdrip administration sets.

Flow regulator

Port for drug infusion

Drip chamber spike

Macrodrip

Microdrip

Drug infusion port

To effectively deliver intravenous fluids, you must be thoroughly familiar with the microdrip and macrodrip administration sets, their components, and their subtle differences (Figure 7-24).

- *Spike.* The **spike** is a sharp-pointed plastic device that you insert into the administration set port on the IV solution bag. A plastic sheath covering the spike keeps it sterile. When the sheath is removed, you must use a medically clean technique to avoid contaminating the spike. If the spike becomes contaminated, discard the administration set and start over with new tubing.

- *Drip Chamber.* The **drip chamber** is a clear plastic chamber that allows you to view the **drip rate.** The drip chamber is squeezable; when compressed, it collects fluid from the IV solution bag and acts as a reservoir for administration. For optimal fluid delivery, the drip chamber should be about one-third full; a line on the chamber marks the correct fluid level.

- *Drop Former.* Inside the drip chamber is a **drop former.** In microdrip administration tubing, the drop former is a hollow metal stylet. In macrodrip tubing, it is a large circular opening at the top of the drip

* **spike** sharp-pointed device inserted into the IV solution bag's administration set port.

* **drip chamber** clear plastic chamber that allows visualization of the drip rate.

* **drip rate** pace at which the fluid moves from the bag into the patient.

* **drop former** device that regulates the size of drops.

Intravenous Access **453**

chamber. The drop former regulates each drop's size. The narrow metal stylet in the microdrip tubing creates smaller drops; the wider opening in the macrodrip tubing creates larger drops. In either case, the drop former's precise calibration allows you to calculate fluid volumes by counting drops, or **gtts:**

- Microdrip   60 gtts = 1 ml
- Macrodrip   10 gtts = 1 ml

Depending upon the manufacturer, macrodrip sets may equate 15 or 20 gtts to 1 ml. You must know drops per milliliter to calculate flow rates or medicated infusion dosages.

- *Tubing.* Intravenous administration tubing is clear and very flexible. Thus, you can watch the solution flow through the administration set, and you can manipulate the tubing in tight situations. Some medications such as intravenous nitroglycerin are chemically incompatible with regular tubing and require special tubing.

- *Clamp.* IV administration tubing has a simple plastic clamp. When slid over the tubing, the clamp completely stops the flow of solution from the IV bag to the patient. It prevents both the entrainment of air into the tubing when changing IV bags and the backflow of medication when administering medications. You can also use it to stop infusion without disturbing the flow-regulator setting.

- *Flow Regulator.* The flow regulator is a dial enclosed in a triangular plastic casing. It allows infinite control of flow rates ranging from a continuous stream to completely stopped. Rolling the dial towards the IV solution bag increases the drip frequency; rolling the dial towards the patient decreases the drip frequency.

medication injection port self-healing membrane into which a hypodermic needle is inserted for drug administration.

- *Medication Injection Ports.* The **medication injection ports** have a self-sealing membrane into which you can insert a hypodermic needle for drug administration. Their design varies, depending upon the manufacturer. When possible, use the medication port nearest the patient.

needle adapter rigid plastic device specifically constructed to fit into the hub of an intravenous cannula.

- *Needle Adapter.* The **needle adapter** is a rigid plastic device at the administration tubing's distal end. It is specifically constructed to fit into the hub of an intravenous cannula. Similar to the spike, the needle adapter is sterile and covered by a protective cap. If it becomes contaminated at any time, start over with a new administration set.

extension tubing IV tubing used to extend a macrodrip or microdrip setup.

IV Extension Tubing Extension tubing is IV tubing used to extend the original macrodrip or microdrip setup. Its packaging clearly marks it as such. Like administration sets, extension tubing is sterile and must be handled accordingly.

Extension tubing also permits the paramedic to change the original administration tubing or the IV solution bag with little difficulty. For example, if you have to switch from a macrodrip set to a microdrip set, you can close the clamp on the extension and detach the primary tubing. Once you have flushed the new tubing with fluid, you place the needle adapter into the receiving port on the extension tubing and release the clamp. You can now resume fluid therapy without risking complications or having to painfully reinitiate a second IV line.

Electromechanical Pump Tubing Mechanical infusion devices may require specially manufactured pump tubing. Typically, pump tubing has special components that attach directly to the pump. Additionally, bladders and relief points permit you to void possible air bubbles. Many specific models of electromechanical infusion pumps require specific pump tubing. When using a mechanical infusion pump, be sure to have the appropriate tubing on hand.

Measured Volume Administration Set The **measured volume administration set** can deliver specific volumes of fluid with or without medication. It is especially advantageous for pediatrics, renal failure, or other patients who cannot tolerate fluid overload.

The measured volume administration set consists of either micro- or macrodrip tubing, with the addition of a large **burette chamber** marked in 1.0 ml increments. The burette chamber holds between 120 ml and 150 ml of fluid. Its components include:

- Flanged spike
- Clamp
- Airway handle
- Medication injection port
- Burette chamber
- Float valve
- Drip chamber
- Flow regulator
- Medication injection port
- Needle adapter

When opened, the airway handle on top of the burette chamber permits air to be displaced or replaced as fluid enters or exits the chamber. If a medication must be mixed in a specific amount of IV solution, you can add it through the medication administration port after correctly filling the chamber.

Blood Tubing Administering whole blood or blood components requires **blood tubing,** which contains a filter that prevents clots and other debris from entering the patient. Without exception, all blood must be filtered. Blood that is stored or delivered over an extended period is prone to form fibrin clots or to accumulate other debris. If these clots or debris enter the circulatory system, they can travel in the form of an embolus.

Many aeromedical and facility-based paramedics administer blood and must be familiar with blood tubing. Although most ambulances do not carry blood, paramedics may initiate normal saline with blood tubing in anticipation that whole blood or blood products will be required immediately in the emergency department.

Blood tubing comes in two configurations, straight and Y. Y tubing has two administration ports, one for blood and one for IV normal saline solution. Typically, blood is administered with normal saline. Fluids like lactated Ringer's increase the potential for blood coagulation. The two-port design permits immediate access to normal saline if the blood supply is exhausted or must be shut down, as for a transfusion reaction. When you use Y blood tubing, establish a traditional IV by connecting a bag of normal saline to the tubing. Attach the blood to the second port when needed, while maintaining strict medical asepsis. Using the flow regulator, discontinue the normal saline while opening the clamp regulating the flow of blood. Straight blood tubing has only one reservoir. Therefore, only blood is attached to the tubing. A medication administration port close to the needle adapter allows you to piggyback a secondary line of normal saline into the tubing.

Miscellaneous Administration Sets Some tubing now has a manual dial that can set drops per minute or specific flow rates. Some manufacturers have created a single drip chamber that can create either microdrips or macrodrips.

✳ **measured volume administration set** IV setup that delivers specific volumes of fluid.

✳ **burette chamber** calibrated chamber of Berutrol IV administration tubing that enables precise measurement and delivery of fluids and medicated solutions.

✳ **blood tubing** administration tubing that contains a filter to prevent clots or other debris from entering the patient.

FIGURE 7-25 Over-the-needle catheter.

Intravenous Cannulas

The intravenous cannula permits actual puncture and access into a patient's vein. The distal portion of the administration tubing connects to the IV cannula. The three basic types of IV cannulas are:

- Over-the-needle catheter
- Hollow-needle catheter
- Plastic catheter inserted through a hollow needle

✱ over-the-needle catheter/ angiocatheter semi-flexible catheter enclosing a sharp metal stylet.

Over-the-Needle Catheter Often called an **angiocatheter,** the semi-flexible **over-the-needle catheter** encloses a sharp metal stylet (needle) (Figure 7-25).

- *Metal stylet (needle).* The metal stylet punctures the skin and blood vessel. Blood flows through the hollow stylet to the flashback chamber.
- *Flashback chamber.* Blood in the clear plastic flashback chamber confirms placement of the stylet in the vein.
- *Teflon catheter.* The Teflon catheter slides over the metal stylet into a successfully punctured vein.
- *Hub.* Located on the back of the Teflon catheter, the hub receives the needle adapter of the administration tubing once removed from the metal stylet.

For peripheral venous access, the over-the-needle catheter is preferred since it is easy to place and anchor and permits freer movement of the patient.

✱ hollow-needle catheter stylet that does not have a Teflon tube but is itself inserted into the vein and secured there.

Hollow-needle Catheter For pediatrics or other patients with tiny, delicate veins, use **hollow-needle catheters** (Figure 7-26). These catheters do not have a Teflon tube; rather, the metal stylet itself is inserted into the vein and secured

FIGURE 7-26 Hollow-needle catheter.

FIGURE 7-27   Catheter inserted through the needle.

there. Because the sharp metal stylet can easily damage the vein, you must insert it very carefully. Some hollow-needle catheters have wings for guidance and securing into a vein. These hollow-needle catheters are referred to as winged catheters or butterfly catheters.

Catheter Inserted through the Needle The **catheter inserted through the needle** is also called an **intracatheter**. It consists of a Teflon catheter inserted through a large metal stylet (Figure 7-27). Used in the hospital setting to implement central lines, its proper placement requires great skill, as discussed previously.

The size of an intravenous cannula is expressed as its gauge. The *larger* the gauge, the *smaller* the diameter of the stylet and catheter. For example, a 22-gauge cannula is smaller than a 14-gauge cannula. The larger diameter, 14-gauge catheter allows greater flow rates than the smaller diameter 22-gauge cannula. When establishing venous access, choose the cannula size most appropriate for the patient condition. Typical uses for the various sizes of cannulas are:

* *22-gauge* Small gauges are used for *fragile* veins such as those of the elderly or children.
* *20-gauge* Moderate gauges are used for the average adult who does not need fluid replacement.
* *18-gauge, 16-gauge, or 14-gauge* Larger gauge cannulas are used to increase volume or to administer viscous medications such as dextrose. Blood can be administered only through a cannula that is 16 gauge or larger.

The largest gauge cannula that will fit into a vein is not always appropriate. A cardiac patient with large veins should not receive a 14-gauge cannula for medication administration, just as a multi-systems trauma patient with good veins should not receive a 22-gauge cannula for fluid administration. Remember that intravenous access is painful and causes discomfort not only to those receiving it but also to family members watching a loved one in distress.

Miscellaneous Equipment

The **venous constricting band** is a flat rubber band applied proximal to the intended puncture site. It impedes venous return, thereby engorging veins and making them easier to see. This helps you to select the best site and makes venipuncture easier. Never restrict arterial blood flow with the constricting band, and never leave it in place longer than two minutes.

Intravenous access is an invasive procedure; therefore you must use medically clean techniques, including antiseptic preparations, to prevent infection. Applying alcohol and betadine before and after venipuncture decreases the chance of infection.

Once you have established an IV, you must secure it to avoid losing the access. Medical tape and an adhesive bandage are inexpensive and easy to apply. You can

* **catheter inserted through the needle (intracatheter)** Teflon catheter inserted through a large metal stylet.

Intravenous access is painful and causes discomfort not only to those receiving it but also to family members watching a loved one in distress.

* **venous constricting band** flat rubber band used to impede venous return and make veins easier to see.

Never leave the constricting band in place more than two minutes.

also apply clear membranes over the site. Commercial devices manufactured specifically for this task are also available. Have gauze on hand for hemorrhage control if IV cannulation is unsuccessful or if blood leaks from around the site.

Obtaining a venous blood specimen at the time of venipuncture will save the patient from being stuck with a needle again later. This chapter's section on venous blood sampling discusses this technique in detail.

INTRAVENOUS ACCESS IN THE HAND, ARM, AND LEG

As a paramedic you will most often establish peripheral IVs in the hand, arm, or leg. The veins in these places are relatively easy to locate and accessing them causes the patient less pain. In addition, the likelihood of complications is less with these veins than with the external jugular vein (discussed later) or central IV initiation. Therefore, the veins of the hand, arm, and leg are the primary sites for IV initiation.

To establish a peripheral IV in the hand, arm, or leg, use the following technique (Procedure 7-7):

1. Confirm indication and type of IV setup needed. Gather and arrange all supplies and equipment beforehand to make the process easy and accessible.
   - IV fluid
   - Administration set
   - Intravenous cannula
   - Tape or commercial securing device
   - Venous blood drawing equipment
   - Venous constricting band
   - Antiseptic swab (betadine/alcohol)

   When appropriate, explain the entire process to the patient. Apply the proper BSI—gloves and goggles, as IV access is invasive and presents the potential for blood exposure.

2. Prepare all needed equipment. Examine the IV fluid for clarity and expiration date. Insert the administration tubing spike in the IV solution bag's administration set port. Squeeze fluid from the IV fluid container into the drip chamber until it reaches the fill line. Open the clamp and/or flow regulator to flush the solution through the administration tubing and expel trapped air bubbles. Shut down the flow regulator and replace the cap over the needle adapter. Remember that the IV administration set is sterile; if any contamination occurs you must replace the set with a new one.

3. Select the venipuncture site. Acceptable sites have clearly visible veins and are free of bruising or scarring. Straight veins are easier to cannulate than crooked ones.

4. Place the constricting band proximal to the intended site of puncture. Tighten it enough to impede venous blood flow without restricting arterial blood passage. Never leave the constricting band in place more than two minutes, as intrinsic changes will occur in the slowed venous blood.

5. Cleanse the venipuncture site. You must cleanse the intended site of pathogens to decrease the likelihood of infection. Alcohol and betadine are the most commonly used antiseptics. Start at the site itself and work outward in an expanding circle. This pushes pathogens away from the puncture site.

6. Insert the intravenous cannula into the vein. With your nondominant hand, pull all local skin taut to stabilize the vein and

7-7a Place the constricting band.

7-7b Cleanse the venipuncture site.

7-7c Insert the intravenous cannula into the vein.

7-7d Withdraw any blood samples needed.

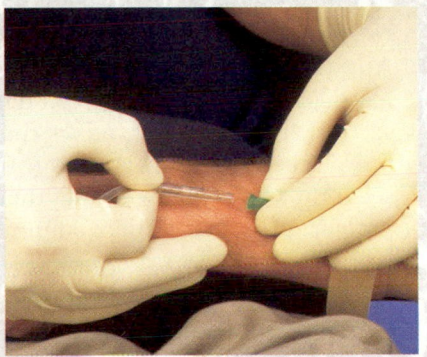

7-7e Connect the IV tubing.

7-7f Turn on the IV and check the flow.

7-7g Secure the site.

7-7h Label the intravenous solution bag.

prevent it from rolling. With the distal bevel of the metal stylet up, insert the cannula into the vein at a 10°–30° angle. Continue until you feel the cannula "pop" into the vein or see blood in the flashback chamber. The metal stylet is now in the vein; however, the Teflon catheter is not. To place the catheter into the vein, carefully advance the cannula approximately 0.5 cm further. (If you are using a butterfly cannula, it has no Teflon catheter, and you must carefully advance the needle itself.)

7. Holding the metal stylet stationary, slide the Teflon catheter over the needle into the vein. Place a finger over the vein at the catheter tip and tamponade (press gently downward to occlude the vein), thus preventing blood from flowing from the catheter and/or air from entraining into the circulatory system. Carefully remove the metal stylet and promptly dispose of it in the sharps container. Remove the venous constricting band.

8. Obtain venous blood samples as discussed in the section on venous blood sampling.

9. Attach the administration tubing to the cannula. Remove the protective cap from the needle adapter and tightly secure the needle adapter into the cannula hub. Open the flow regulator and allow the fluid to run freely for several seconds. Adjust the flow rate. Do not let go of the cannula and administration tubing until you have secured them as explained in step 10.

10. Apply antibiotic ointment to the site and cover it with an adhesive bandage or other commercial device. Loop the distal tubing and secure with tape. This makes the medication administration port more accessible and attaches the device to the patient more securely. Continue by taping the administration tubing to the patient, proximal to the venipuncture site.

11. Label the intravenous solution bag with the following information:
    • Date and time initiated
    • Person initiating the intravenous access

12. Continually monitor the patient and flow rate.

INTRAVENOUS ACCESS IN THE EXTERNAL JUGULAR VEIN

The external jugular vein is a large peripheral blood vessel in the neck, between the angle of the jaw and the middle third of the clavicle. It connects into the central circulation's subclavian vein. Since it lies so close to the central circulation, cannulation here offers many of the same benefits afforded by central venous access. Fluids and medications rapidly reach the core of the body from this site.

Consider accessing the external jugular only after you have exhausted other means of peripheral access or when a patient requires immediate fluid administration.

Consider accessing the external jugular only after you have exhausted other means of peripheral access or when a patient requires immediate fluid administration. This is an extremely painful site to access, so you typically will reserve its use for patients with a decreased or total loss of consciousness.

Cannulating the external jugular vein requires essentially the same equipment as other forms of peripheral IV access, plus a 10 ml syringe. You will not need a constricting band. To access the external jugular, use the following technique (Procedure 7-8):

1. Prepare all equipment as for peripheral IV access in an arm, hand, or leg. In addition, fill the 10 ml syringe with 3–5 ml of sterile

Peripheral Intravenous Access in an External Jugular Vein

7-8a Place the patient supine or in the Trendelenburg position.

7-8b Turn the patient's head to the side opposite of access and cleanse the site.

7-8c Occlude venous return by placing a finger on the external jugular just above the clavicle.

7-8d Point the catheter at the medial third of the clavicle and insert it, bevel up, at a 10°–30° angle.

7-8e Enter the external jugular while withdrawing on the plunger of the attached syringe.

saline. Attach the distal part of the syringe to the flashback chamber of a large bore, over-the-needle catheter. Apply the proper BSI protection.

2. Place the patient supine and/or in the Trendelenburg position. This position will increase blood flow to the chest and neck, thus distending the vein and making it easier to see. In addition, the supine-Trendelenburg position decreases the chance of air entering the circulatory system during cannulation.

3. Turn the patient's head to the side opposite of access. This maneuver makes the site easier to see and reach; do not perform it if the patient has traumatic head and/or neck injuries.

4. Cleanse the site with antiseptics. Start at the site of intended puncture and work outward one to two inches in ever increasing circles.

5. Occlude venous return by placing a finger on the external jugular just above the clavicle. This should distend the vein, again allowing greater visualization and ease of puncture. Never apply a venous constricting band around the patient's neck.

6. Position the intravenous cannula parallel with the vein, midway between the angle of the jaw clavicle. Point the catheter at the medial third of the clavicle and insert it, bevel up, at a 10°–30° angle.

7. Enter the external jugular while withdrawing on the plunger of the attached syringe. You will see blood in the syringe or feel a pop as the cannula enters the vein. Once inside the vein, advance the entire angiocatheter another 0.5 cm so the tip of the Teflon catheter lies within the lumen of the vein. Then slide the Teflon catheter into the vein and remove the metal stylet as previously described. Immediately dispose of the metal stylet.

8. Obtain venous blood samples as discussed in the section on venous blood sampling.

9. Attach the administration tubing to the IV catheter. Allow the intravenous solution to run freely for several seconds. Set the flow rate and secure as appropriate.

10. Monitor the patient for complications.

While using the external jugular vein has advantages, it also has distinct drawbacks. You may inadvertently puncture the airway or damage the nearby arterial vessels. Additionally, this is a painful entry site for the conscious patient. To minimize risks, perform the procedure very carefully.

INTRAVENOUS ACCESS WITH A MEASURED VOLUME ADMINISTRATION SET

When using a measured volume administration set, follow this procedure (Procedure 7-9):

1. Prepare the tubing by closing all clamps, and insert the flanged spike into the IV solution bag's spike port.

2. Open the airway handle. Open the uppermost clamp and fill the burette chamber with approximately 20 ml of fluid. Squeeze the drip chamber until the fluid reaches the fill line. Open the bottom flow regulator to purge air through the tubing. When all air is purged, close the bottom flow regulator.

Intravenous Access with a Measured Volume Administration Set

7-9a   Spike the solution bag.

7-9b   Open the uppermost clamp and fill the burette chamber with the desired volume of fluid.

7-9c   Close the uppermost clamp and open the flow regulator.

3. Continue to fill the burette chamber with the designated amount of solution.

4. Close the uppermost clamp and open the flow regulator until you reach the desired drip rate. Leave the airway handle open, so that air replaces the displaced fluid.

To refill the burette chamber, open the uppermost clamp until you have delivered the desired volume; then repeat step 4.

You can also use measured volume administration sets for continuous fluid administration. Fill the burette chamber with at least 30 ml of solution and close the airway handle. Leave the uppermost clamp open and adjust the rate with the lower flow regulator.

INTRAVENOUS ACCESS WITH BLOOD TUBING

To establish an IV with blood tubing, use the following procedure:

1. Prepare the tubing by closing all clamps, and insert the flanged spike into the spike port of the blood and/or normal saline solution (Y-configured tubing).

2. Squeeze the drip chamber until it is one-third full and blood covers the filter. Repeat for the normal saline if you are using Y tubing.

3. If you are using straight tubing, piggyback a secondary line of normal saline into the blood tubing, unless you plan to piggyback the straight blood tubing into a large bore primary line.

4. Flush all tubing with normal saline and blood as appropriate.

5. Attach blood tubing to the intravenous cannula or into a previously established IV line.

6. Ensure patency by infusing a small amount of normal saline. Shut down when you have confirmed patency.

7. Open the clamp(s) and/or flow regulator(s) that allows blood to move from the bag to the patient. Adjust the flow rate accordingly.

8. When blood therapy is complete or must be discontinued, shut down the flow regulator from the blood supply and open the regulator(s) for the normal saline solution.

FACTORS AFFECTING INTRAVENOUS FLOW RATES

If an IV does not flow properly, check for the following problems and correct them as appropriate.

- *Constricting band.* Has the venous constricting band been removed? This is probably the most common mistake both in and out of the hospital. Additionally, ensure that the patient is not wearing restrictive clothing that interferes with venous blood flow.

- *Edema at the puncture site.* Swelling at the IV site indicates fluid collection caused by infiltration. This **extravasation** occurs if you accidentally puncture the vein more than once, thus allowing IV solution and blood to escape from the second puncture and accumulate in the surrounding tissue. An infiltrated IV site is not usable.

Content Review

IV TROUBLESHOOTING

Constricting band still
  in place?
Edema at puncture site?
Cannula abutting vein
  wall or valve?
Administration set control
  valves closed?
IV bag too low?
Completely filled drip
  chamber?

＊ extravasation leakage of fluid or medication from the blood vessel that is commonly found with infiltration.

- *Cannula abutting the vein wall or valve.* If the distal tip of the cannula butts against a wall or valve, carefully reposition it. You may have to untape and retape the cannula once you have achieved an adequate flow rate. Additionally, you may need to use an arm board to keep the patient's extremity straight, as flexion may kink the vein at the site and impede the solution's flow.

- *Administration set control valves.* Ensure that the flow regulator is open. Be sure to check the flow regulator and clamps of both the primary and any secondary or extension tubing.

- *IV bag height.* When you move the patient, you may raise the cannulation site above the IV solution bag. This interrupts the solution's gravitational flow from the bag into the patient.

- *Completely filled drip chamber.* Is the drip chamber completely filled? You can easily correct this by inverting the bag and squeezing the fluid from the drip chamber back into the bag.

- *Catheter patency.* A blood clot at the end of the Teflon catheter or needle may obstruct the flow of solution from the IV solution bag into the body. If the flow slows, increase the IV drip rate to keep the catheter or needle clear. If the flow stops completely, cleanse the medication administration port closest to the IV entry site with alcohol preparations and insert a syringe and hypodermic needle. Gently aspirate back on the syringe until the blood clot is pulled into the syringe. Never flush an IV that has stopped running because of a clot. Flushing will force the clot into the circulatory system and can cause occlusions in the heart or lungs.

If flow remains inadequate after you have eliminated all of these possible causes, lower the IV bag below the insertion site. If blood flows into the IV administration tubing, the site is patent and the problem lies elsewhere. If the problem persists, remove the IV and reestablish it on another extremity, using all new equipment. If you do not observe blood return, the site is inoperable.

COMPLICATIONS OF PERIPHERAL INTRAVENOUS ACCESS

Even though it is a routine procedure, intravenous access is not trouble free. It can cause a number of complications.

Pain Pain at the puncture site occurs during needle penetration or with extravasation. To minimize pain, use a smaller gauge catheter or use a 1% lidocaine solution (without epinephrine) to anesthetize the overlying skin before insertion.

Local Infection Local infection occurs if you do not properly cleanse the site and thus introduce pathogens through the puncture. This complication does not become apparent until after the IV has been established for several hours.

Pyrogenic Reaction Pyrogens (foreign proteins capable of producing fever) in the administration tubing or IV solution can cause a pyrogenic reaction. The abrupt onset of fever (100°F–106°F), chills, backache, headache, nausea, and vomiting characterize these reactions. Cardiovascular collapse may also result.

Typically, a pyrogenic reaction will occur within one-half to one hour after you initiate an IV. If you suspect a pyrogenic reaction, immediately terminate the IV and reestablish access in the opposite side with new equipment and fluid.

Typically, pyrogenic reactions occur secondary to the use of intravenous solutions that have been contaminated with a microorganism or other foreign

Content Review

IV ACCESS COMPLICATIONS

Pain
Local infection
Pyrogenic reaction
Catheter shear
Inadvertent arterial
  puncture
Circulatory overload
Thrombophlebitis
Thrombus formation
Air embolism
Necrosis
Anticoagulants

* **pyrogen** foreign protein capable of producing fever.

matter. Pyrogenic reactions underscore the need to discard any fluid that is cloudy or any equipment that has been opened.

Allergic Reaction A patient receiving IV therapy may develop an allergic reaction. Most often allergic reactions accompany the administration of blood or colloidal (protein containing) solutions. In addition, some patients may react to the latex in some types of IV administration tubing.

The sudden onset of hives (urticaria), itching (pruritis), localized or systemic edema, or shortness of breath may signify an allergic reaction. If you suspect an allergic reaction, stop the IV infusion and remove the IV catheter. Treat the patient as discussed in Chapter 31 on allergies and anaphylaxis.

Catheter Shear A catheter shear can occur if you pull the Teflon catheter through or over the needle after you have advanced it into the vein. The soft plastic catheter will easily snag on the metal stylet's sharp point and shear off, thus forming a plastic **embolus**. Therefore, never draw the Teflon catheter over the metal stylet after you have advanced it.

* **embolus** foreign particle in the blood.

Inadvertent Arterial Puncture Because arteries may lie close to veins, accidental arterial puncture may occur. Arterial blood is bright red and characteristically spurts with each contraction of the heart. When an arterial puncture occurs, immediately remove the catheter and apply direct pressure to the site for at least five minutes. Do not release the pressure until the hemorrhage has stopped.

* **circulatory overload** an excess in intravascular fluid volume.

Circulatory Overload **Circulatory overload** occurs if you administer too much fluid for the patient's condition. You must monitor flow rates carefully, especially for patients with medical conditions such as kidney failure or heart failure who are intolerant of excessive fluid. Continually examine the patient for signs of circulatory overload (rales, tachypnea, dyspnea, and jugular venous distention, as discussed in Chapter 11 on physical exam techniques. If you encounter circulatory overload, adjust the flow rate.

* **thrombophlebitis** inflammation of the vein.

Thrombophlebitis **Thrombophlebitis,** or inflammation of the vein, is particularly common in long-term intravenous therapy. Redness and edema at the puncture site are typical signs of thrombophlebitis. This complication may also present as pain along the course of the vein, sometimes accompanied by inflammation and tenderness. Typically, thrombophlebitis does not occur until several hours after IV initiation. When you suspect thrombophlebitis, terminate the IV and apply a warm compress to the site.

* **thrombus** blood clot.

Thrombus Formation A **thrombus,** or blood clot, can form if IV access injures the vessel wall. A thrombus may form around the catheter and occlude the movement of fluid between the IV and the blood vessel. If you suspect a thrombus, restart the IV using new equipment. Do not attempt to dislodge the clot with a fluid bolus, as this may create an embolus that causes neurological or pulmonary complications.

* **air embolism** air in the vein.

Air Embolism **Air embolism** occurs when air enters the vein. Air embolus is most likely to occur during central venous access or when administration tubing has not been properly flushed. Failure to tamponade larger veins during cannulation may allow air into the vein.

* **necrosis** the sloughing off of dead tissue.

Necrosis **Necrosis,** or the sloughing off of dead tissue, occurs later in IV therapy as medication has extravasated into the interstitial space.

* **anticoagulant** drug that inhibits blood clotting.

Anticoagulants **Anticoagulant** drugs such as aspirin, Coumadin, or heparin increase the chance of bleeding and impede hemorrhage control during IV establishment. They drastically increase the complications of hematoma or infiltration.

CHANGING AN IV BAG OR BOTTLE

You may sometimes have to change an IV bag or bottle. This generally occurs when only 50 ml of solution remain and you must continue therapy after those 50 ml are depleted. Changing the solution bag or bottle is a sterile process. If the equipment becomes contaminated you should dispose of it.

To change the IV solution bag or bottle, use the following technique:

1. Prepare the new IV solution bag or bottle by removing the protective cover from the IV tubing port.
2. Occlude the flow of solution from the depleted bag or bottle by moving the roller clamp on the IV administration tubing.
3. Remove the spike from the depleted IV bag or bottle. Be careful not to drop or contaminate the spike in any way.
4. Insert the spike into the new IV bag of bottle. Ensure that the drip chamber is filled appropriately.
5. Open the roller clamp to the appropriate flow rate.

If air becomes entrained within the administration tubing during this process, cleanse the medication administration port below the trapped air and insert a hypodermic needle and syringe. Pull the plunger back to aspirate the trapped air into the syringe. After you have removed the air, adjust the IV flow rate as needed.

INTRAVENOUS DRUG ADMINISTRATION

Medications can be delivered through an existing IV line. As the IV line is seated directly into a vein, the blood rapidly absorbs these medications and distributes them throughout the body. Intravenous administration avoids many of the barriers to drug absorption in other routes. For example, drugs given via the gastrointestinal tract face enzymes and other chemicals that may deactivate, exacerbate, or in some other way alter the medication being administered. Likewise, local tissues can absorb drugs administered via the subcutaneous or intramuscular routes, thus preventing the total dosage from reaching the blood stream for delivery. The two methods for administering drugs through an IV line are intravenous bolus and intravenous infusion.

Intravenous Bolus

An intravenous bolus involves injecting the circulatory system with a concentrated dose of drug through the medication administration port of an established IV. This procedure requires the following equipment:

- BSI protection
- Alcohol antiseptic preparation
- Packaged medication
- Syringe (size depends upon the volume of drug you will administer)
- 18–20-gauge hypodermic needle, 1″–1 1/2″ long
- Existing intravenous line with medication port

To administer an intravenous medication bolus, use the following technique (Procedure 7-10):

1. Assure that the primary IV line is patent.
2. Confirm the drug, indication, dosage, and need for an IV bolus.
3. Draw up the medication or prepare a prefilled syringe as appropriate.

7-10a Prepare the equipment.

7-10b Prepare the medication.

7-10c Check the label.

7-10d Select and clean an administration port.

7-10e Pinch the line.

7-10f Administer the medication.

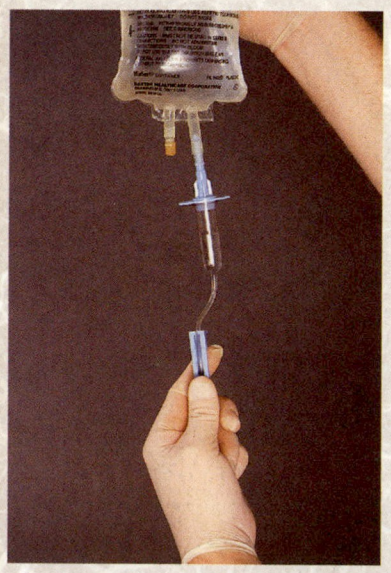

7-10g Adjust the IV flow rate.

7-10h Monitor the patient.

4. Cleanse the medication port nearest the IV site with an alcohol antiseptic preparation.

5. Insert a hypodermic needle through the port membrane.

6. Pinch the IV line above the medication port. This prevents the medication from traveling toward the fluids bag, forcing it instead toward the patient.

7. Inject the medication as appropriate.

8. Remove the hypodermic needle and syringe and release the tubing.

9. Open the flow regulator to allow a 20 cc fluid flush. The fluid will push the medication into the patient's circulatory system.

10. Dispose of the hypodermic needle and syringe as appropriate. Monitor the patient for desired or undesired effects.

Intravenous Drug Infusion

Many cardiac drugs and antibiotics are given as intravenous infusions (IV piggybacks). Intravenous drug infusions deliver a steady, continual dose of medication through an existing IV line. You may give them either as an initial dosage or to maintain drug levels after delivering an initial bolus.

Piggybacking IV infusions through an existing intravenous line gives you greater control over medication delivery and allows you easily to discontinue the infusion when therapy is complete or must be stopped. Never administer intravenous infusions as a primary IV line.

IV infusions are contained in bags or bottles of intravenous solution. If the IV infusion is premixed, read the label on the bag for the following information:

Never administer intravenous infusions as a primary IV line.

- Name of medication
- Total dosage in weight mixed in bag
- Concentration (weight per single cc)
- Expiration date

If the infusion is not premixed, make a label listing this information and attach it to the bag (Figure 7-28). Additionally, note the date and time you mixed the infusion, and initial it.

Use the following technique to administer a medication as an IV infusion (Procedure 7-11):

FIGURE 7-28 If an IV solution is not premixed, you will have to mix and label it yourself.

7-11a Select the drug.

7-11b Draw up the drug.

7-11c Select IV fluid for dilution.

7-11d Clean the medication addition port.

7-11e Inject the drug into the fluid.

7-11f Mix the solution.

7-11g Insert an administration set and connect to main IV line with needle.

1. Establish a primary IV line and assure patency.
2. Confirm administration indications and patient allergies.
3. Prepare the infusion bag or bottle. (If the infusion is premixed, continue to step 4.)
   a. Draw up the appropriate quantity of medication from its source with a syringe.
   b. Cleanse the IV bag or bottle's medication port with an alcohol antiseptic wipe.
   c. Insert the hypodermic needle into the medication port and inject the medication.
   d. Gently agitate the bag or bottle to mix its contents.
   e. Label the bag or bottle.
4. Connect administration tubing to the medication bag or bottle and fill the drip chamber to fluid line. Most infusions require microdrip tubing. If you use a mechanical infusion pump, you may need to use special tubing.
5. Place the hypodermic needle on the administration tubing's needle adapter and flush the tubing with solution. (The needle adapter typically accepts a 20-gauge needle.)
6. Cleanse the medication administration port on the primary line with alcohol and insert the secondary line's hypodermic needle. Secure the hypodermic needle and the secondary administration line with tape or another securing device.
7. Reconfirm the indication, drug, dose, and route of administration.
8. Shut down the primary line so that no fluid will flow from the primary solution bag.
9. Adjust the secondary line to the desired drip rate. If you are using a mechanical infusion pump set it accordingly.
10. Properly dispose of the needle and syringe.

When the infusion is complete, shut down the secondary line with the flow regulator or a clamp. Open the primary line and adjust it to the indicated drip rate. Remove the hypodermic needle from the medication administration port and properly dispose of all contents. If required by your local protocols, retain the medication bag to verify administration and for quality assurance.

You can also use measured volume administration tubing to administer medicated infusions. First, fill the burette chamber of a measured volume administration device with a specific volume of fluid. Then you can inject the drug through the medication injection site on top of the burette chamber. You must adjust the flow rate to deliver the precise amount of medication required. In addition, you can mix the medication within the IV bag or bottle as previously described and use the measured volume administration tubing solely for administering the infusion rather than for mixing it.

Heparin Lock and Saline Lock

When a patient requires occasional IV medication drips or boluses but does not need continuous fluid, heparin locks are used. A **heparin lock** is a peripheral IV port that does not use a bag of fluid. Like a typical IV start, it places an IV cannula into a peripheral vein; however, instead of IV administration tubing, it has attached short tubing with a clamp and a distal medication port (Figure 7-29). A heparin lock decreases the risk of accidental fluid overload and electrolyte derangement. You also may withdraw blood samples from the lock if it is in a suitable vein. For short-term

＊ **heparin lock** peripheral IV port that does not use a bag of fluid.

FIGURE 7-29 Heparin lock.

use, saline locks may be used. Sterile saline is injected following the drug. Saline remains in the lock to keep it open. For long-term use, a heparin lock is preferred. Although it functions the same as a saline lock, a heparin lock is filled with a low concentration solution of heparin, which aids in keeping any blood that gets into the device from clotting. Typically, a drug will be administered through the heparin lock. This is followed by a saline flush to assure that no drug remains in the lock or hub. Then, the lock and hub are filled with a heparin solution. This aids in keeping the IV site open for a long period of time.

Initiating a heparin lock requires the following equipment:

- IV cannula
- Heparin lock
- Syringe with 3 cc–5 cc sterile saline or commercial saline injection device
- Tape or commercial securing device
- Venous blood drawing equipment
- Venous constricting band
- Antiseptic swab (betadine/alcohol)

To place a heparin lock, follow these steps:

1. Select the venipuncture site.
2. Place the constricting band proximal to the puncture site.
3. Cleanse the venipuncture site with alcohol or betadine antiseptics.
4. Insert the intravenous cannula into the vein.
5. Slide the Teflon catheter into the vein.
6. Carefully remove the metal stylet and promptly dispose of it into the sharps container. Remove the venous constricting band.
7. Obtain venous blood samples, as explained under Venous Blood Sampling.
8. Attach the heparin lock tubing to the angiocatheter hub.
9. Cleanse the medication port and inject 3 ml–5 ml of sterile saline into the lock. Easy flow of the saline without edema at the puncture site indicates patency. If you encounter resistance or if edema forms, restart the procedure with new equipment.
10. Apply antibiotic ointment to the site and cover with an adhesive bandage or other commercial device. Secure the tubing to the patient.

To administer an IV medication bolus through a heparin lock, assemble the following equipment and supplies:

- BSI protection
- Alcohol antiseptic preparation
- Packaged medication
- Syringe (the size depends on the volume being administered)
- 18–20-gauge hypodermic needle 1–1 1/2″ long

After you have gathered all equipment and supplies, use the following technique to administer an IV medication bolus with a heparin lock:

1. Confirm the drug, indication, dosage, and need for an IV bolus.
2. Draw up the medication or prepare a prefilled syringe as appropriate.
3. Cleanse the medication port nearest the IV site with alcohol antiseptic preparation.
4. Ensure that the plastic clamp is open.
5. Insert the hypodermic needle through the port membrane.
6. Inject the medication as appropriate.
7. Remove the hypodermic needle and dispose of it in the sharps container.
8. Follow the medication administration with a 10–20 ml saline flush from another syringe.
9. Properly dispose of the hypodermic needle and syringe. Monitor the patient for desired or undesired effects.

If fluid administration becomes necessary, you can unscrew the medication port and insert IV administration tubing. Periodically flush with sterile saline or heparin to prevent clot formation and occlusion at the Teflon catheter's distal end.

Venous Access Device

A **venous access device** is a surgically implanted port that permits repeated access to the central venous circulation. Implanted just under the skin, venous access devices are constructed of a plastic or stainless steel injection port and flexible catheter. The injection port, which lies just beneath the skin, contains a self-sealing septum that allows repeated penetration and access into the venous circulation. The self-sealing septum is connected to a flexible catheter that is placed within the lumen of a central vein, most often the superior vena cava.

Typically, patients with venous access devices have chronic illnesses that require repeated intravenous access for medication administration, long-term intravenous therapy, or blood sampling. Generally, venous access devices are placed on the anterior chest near the third or fourth rib lateral to the sternum. A venous access device is apparent as a raised circle just beneath the skin.

Use of an indwelling central venous access device requires special training. Delivering a medication through the venous access device requires a special needle specific for the venous access device in question. A common needle, the **Huber needle,** has an opening on the side of its shaft instead of at the tip. When placed into the injection port, this configuration allows easy administration of medication

* **venous access device** surgically implanted port that permits repeated access to central venous circulation.

* **Huber needle** needle that has an opening on the side of the shaft instead of the tip.

into the venous access device. Never access a venous access device unless you have the specific needle unique for the particular device. Always ask the patient, family, or nursing staff about the type of venous access device. Often, they will have a supply of needles for the device.

To administer fluids, medication, or blood through a venous access device, you must first prepare the site using the following technique:

1. Take BSI measures.
2. Fill a 10 ml syringe with approximately 7 ml of normal saline.
3. Place a 21- or 22-gauge Huber needle (or other specialized needle) on the end of the syringe.
4. Cleanse the skin over the injection port with povidone-iodine or alcohol preparations.
5. Stabilize the site with one hand while inserting the Huber needle at a 90° angle. Gently advance it until it meets resistance. This signals that the needle has contacted the floor of the injection port.
6. Pull back on the plunger and observe for blood return. The presence of blood confirms placement.
7. Slowly inject the normal saline to assure patency.

To administer the medication by intravenous bolus, use the following technique:

1. Prepare the medication, fluid, or blood for administration.
2. Attach a 21- or 22-gauge Huber needle (or other specialized needle) to the end of the syringe.
3. Cleanse the skin over the injection port with povidone-iodine or alcohol preparations.
4. Insert the needle into the injection port at a 90° angle until the needle cannot be further advanced. Pull back on the plunger of the syringe and observe for the return of blood. The presence of blood confirms proper placement.
5. Inject the medication as appropriate.
6. Remove and dispose of the syringe appropriately.
7. With another syringe and attached specialized needle, administer a bolus of heparinized saline to clear the catheter of any blood clots or other obstruction.

If the venous access device is not patent or access proves difficult, contact medical direction for further directives.

To administer IV fluids, use the following technique:

1. Prepare a primary IV line. Be sure to prime or flush the air from the administration tubing.
2. Attach a 21- or 22-gauge Huber needle (or other specialized needle) to the primary IV administration tubing. Insert a 10 ml syringe and hypodermic needle filled with 7 ml of normal saline solution into the tubing medication delivery port nearest the venous access device.

3. Cleanse the skin over the injection port with povidone-iodine or alcohol preparations.

4. Insert the needle into the injection port at a 90° angle until it encounters resistance.

5. Pinch the administration tubing above the medication administration port and pull back on the syringe plunger. Observe for the return of blood. The presence of blood confirms proper placement.

6. Gently inject the 7 ml of normal saline solution.

7. Set the primary line to the appropriate flow rate.

If administering a secondary medicated infusion, continue as follows:

1. Prepare a secondary line containing the fluid, blood, or medicated solution for infusion.

2. Attach a hypodermic needle to the needle adapter of the secondary line. Insert the secondary line into a medication administration port on the primary tubing.

3. Shut down the primary line and infuse the medicated solution as appropriate. Look for ease of administration as a sign of patency.

4. When infusion is complete, administer a bolus of heparinized saline to clear the catheter of any blood clots or other obstruction.

Using a venous access device is a very sterile procedure. You must take care to clean the site before delivering medications. Other complications of using a venous access device include infection, thrombus formation, and dislodgment of the catheter tip from the vein.

Electromechanical Infusion Devices

Electromechanical infusion devices permit the precise delivery of fluid and/or medications through electronic regulation. Anytime that intravenous infusion occurs, electromechanical infusion pumps provide optimal delivery. Infusion devices are classified as either infusion controllers or infusion pumps.

Infusion Controllers Infusion controllers are gravity-flow devices that regulate the fluid's passage through the pump. Because infusion controllers do not use positive pressure, they will not force fluids into the **extravascular** space if you infiltrate the vein.

Infusion Pumps Infusion pumps deliver fluids and medications under positive pressure (Figure 7-30). This pressure can cause complications such as hematoma or extravasation if you infiltrate the vein. Some infusion pumps contain a pressure monitor and will warn you if they encounter the increased resistance that occurs with infiltration.

Syringe-type infusion pumps are gaining popularity for medical transport. Syringe pumps deliver their medications from a medical syringe without a hypodermic needle instead of from IV solution bags, fluids, or liquid medications (Figure 7-31). You place the syringe containing the medications in the pump, which uses computerized mechanics to gradually depress the plunger at the correct rate. These compact pumps prove advantageous during transport.

Manufacturers make many different electromechanical infusion pumps. Depending on the maker, pump compatibility may require specialized administration

✱ **infusion controller** gravity-flow device that regulates fluid's passage through an electromechanical pump.

✱ **extravascular** outside the vein.

✱ **infusion pump** device that delivers fluids and medications under positive pressure.

FIGURE 7-30 Infusion pump.

FIGURE 7-31 Syringe-type infusion pump.

tubing. With some computerized pumps, you can enter the basic information and then the pump will perform all medical calculations internally and automatically set the drip rate. Most infusion pumps contain internal monitoring devices that sound an alarm for problems such as infiltration, occlusion, or fluid source depletion. Electronic devices are prone to malfunction, so you must be prepared to perform all calculations and set the drip rate manually.

VENOUS BLOOD SAMPLING

The laboratory analysis of blood can provide valuable information about the sick and/or injured patient. The concentrations of electrolytes, gases, hormones, or other chemicals in blood can often shed light on the underlying causes of vague complaints such as dizziness or generalized weakness. Additionally, blood evaluation can confirm suspected conditions. For example, elevated cardiac enzymes in a patient's blood can confirm a suspected myocardial infarction.

In the field, you often will be the first to assess and treat an ill or injured patient. Many of your interventions can alter the blood's composition and erase important information. If you obtain venous blood samples before performing those interventions, they will enable the physician to evaluate the patient's original status.

Venous blood is commonly obtained via venipuncture. Thus, paramedics, who routinely initiate intravenous access, can simultaneously obtain blood samples. Doing so saves considerable hospital time and avoids multiple needle sticks.

You should obtain venous blood in the following situations:

- During peripheral access
- Before drug administration
- When drug administration may be needed

Never stop to draw blood if it will delay critical measures such as drug administration in cardiac arrest or transport in a multi-systems trauma.

Never stop to draw blood if it will delay critical measures.

Equipment for Drawing Blood

You will need the following equipment to obtain venous blood.

Blood tubes Blood tubes are made of glass and have color-coded, self-sealing rubber tops. Blood tube sizes for adults generally range from 5 ml to 7 ml; for pediatrics, from 2 ml to 3 ml (Figure 7-32). They are vacuum packed, and some contain a chemical anticoagulant. The different colored tops correspond to specific anticoagulants. A label on every blood tube identifies the type of additive and its expiration date. Do not use a blood tube after its expiration date, as both the anticoagulant and the vacuum lose their effectiveness.

Using blood tubes in their correct order is essential. If you do not follow the proper sequence, the various anticoagulants will cause cross contamination, skewing the results and rendering the blood useless. Table 7-1 lists anticoagulants, the order in which you should use them, and the colors of their tops.

FIGURE 7-32 Blood tubes.

Table 7-1	BLOOD TUBE SEQUENCE	
	Anticoagulant	**Color of Top**
1.	none	red
2.	citrate	blue
3.	heparin	green
4.	EDTA	purple
5.	Fluoride	gray

Miscellaneous Equipment Depending upon the technique you use to obtain venous blood, you will also need syringes, hypodermic needles, and commercially manufactured plastic sleeves called vacutainers.

Obtaining Venous Blood

Obtaining venous blood is a simple process; however, if the blood is to remain useable, you must pay strict attention to detail. You can obtain blood either from an angiocath or directly from the vein. Which technique you use will depend on the situation. In either case, venous blood samples are best obtained from sturdy veins such as the cephalic, basilic, or median. Smaller veins such as those on the back of the hand are more likely to collapse during retrieval, making the procedure difficult to complete.

Obtaining Venous Blood from an IV Angiocath The most convenient way to obtain venous blood is through an angiocath at the time of peripheral vascular access. In addition to blood tubes, you will need a tube holder (Figure 7-33). The tube holder is commonly referred to as a **vacutainer**. A special adapter called a leur lock fits into the tube holder. The **leur lock** has a rubber-covered needle used to puncture the self-sealing top of the blood tube. The remaining portion of the leur lock protrudes from the tube holder and fits snugly into the hub of the angiocath.

* **vacutainer** device that holds blood tubes.

* **leur lock** adapter with a rubber-covered needle used to puncture a blood tube's self-sealing top.

To obtain blood directly from the angiocath, use the following procedure:

1. Assemble and prepare all equipment. Inspect the blood tubes for expiration or damage and insert the leur lock into the vacutainer.
   Note: Never place blood tubes into the assembled vacutainer and leur lock until you are ready to draw blood. This will destroy the vacuum and render the blood tube useless.
2. Establish IV access with the angiocatheter. Do not connect IV administration tubing.
3. Attach the end of the leur adapter to the hub of the cannula.
4. In correct order, insert the blood tubes so that the rubber covered needle punctures the self-sealing rubber top. Blood should be pulled into the blood tube.
5. Fill all blood tubes completely, as the amount of anticoagulant is proportional to the tube's volume. Gently agitate the tubes to mix the anticoagulant evenly with the blood.
6. Tamponade the vein and remove the vacutainer and leur lock. Attach the IV and assure patency.
7. Properly dispose of all sharps.
8. Label all blood tubes with the following information:
   * Patient's first and last name
   * Patient's age and gender
   * Date and time drawn
   * Name of the person drawing the blood

Blood tube   Vacutainer

FIGURE 7-33 Vacutainer with leur sampling needle.

FIGURE 7-34   Obtaining a blood sample with a 20 ml syringe.

If commercial equipment is not available, use a 20 ml syringe (Figure 7-34). Attach the syringe's needle adapter to the angiocath hub and gently pull back the plunger. Blood will fill the syringe. When the syringe is full, remove it from the angiocath and place the IV line into the angiocath. Carefully attach a hypodermic needle to the syringe to puncture the tops of the blood tubes. In the appropriate order, place the collected blood into the blood tubes and gently agitate. When finished, properly dispose of all sharps and label the blood tubes.

Obtaining Blood Directly from a Vein When IV access is difficult or unobtainable, you may draw blood directly from the vein with a hypodermic needle. This technique is useful for routine sampling that will not require further IV access. To draw blood directly from a vein, you will need the same equipment as for obtaining blood from an angiocath. Instead of a leur lock, however, you will use a **leur-sampling needle** (Figure 7-35). A leur-sampling needle is similar to the leur lock, but instead of an angiocath adapter it has a long, exposed needle. The leur sampling needle screws into the vacutainer, and you insert the exposed needle directly into the vein. You will also need a constricting band and antiseptic wipes.

To obtain blood directly from a vein, use the following procedure:

1. Assemble and prepare all equipment. Inspect the blood tubes for expiration or damage, and insert the leur lock into the vacutainer.
2. Apply the constricting band and select an appropriate puncture site.
3. Cleanse the site with alcohol or betadine.
4. Insert the end of the leur sampling needle into the vein and remove the constricting band.
5. In the correct order, insert each blood tube so that the rubber-covered needle punctures the self-sealing rubber top. Blood should be pulled into the tube.

* leur-sampling needle long, exposed needle that screws into the vacutainer and is inserted directly into the vein.

FIGURE 7-35   Leur sampling needle.

6. Gently agitate the tube to evenly mix the anticoagulant with the blood. Completely fill all blood tubes, as the anticoagulant is proportional to the volume of the tube.
7. Place sterile gauze over the site and remove the sampling needle. Properly dispose of all sharps.
8. Cover the puncture site with gauze and tape or an adhesive bandage.
9. Label all blood tubes with the following information:
   - Patient's first and last name
   - Patient's age and gender
   - Date and time drawn
   - Person drawing the blood

Again, if commercial equipment is not available, you may use a 20-ml syringe. When using a syringe, attach an 18-gauge hypodermic needle to the end of the syringe and insert it into the vein. Gently pull back the plunger to fill the syringe with blood. When the syringe is full, remove the syringe and dress the puncture site. In the appropriate order, inject the collected blood into the blood tubes and gently agitate. When you have finished, properly dispose of all sharps and label the blood tubes.

Complications from drawing blood include damage to the vein wall, inadvertant removal of the IV angiocath and hemoconcentration and hemolysis of the blood sample. **Hemoconcentration** occurs when the constricting band is left in place too long, elevating the numbers of red and white blood cells in the sample. **Hemolysis** is the destruction of red blood cells. When red blood cells are destroyed, they release hemoglobin and potassium, thus rendering the blood unusable. Causes of hemolysis include vigorously shaking the blood tubes after they are filled, using too small a needle for retrieval, or too forcefully aspirating blood into or out of a syringe.

REMOVING A PERIPHERAL IV

You should remove any IV that will not flow or has fulfilled its need. To do so, completely occlude the tubing with the flow regulator and/or clamp. Remove all tape or other securing devices from the tubing and patient. Place a sterile gauze pad over the puncture site. Apply pressure to the gauze with the fingers or thumb of your nondominant hand. With your dominant hand, grasp the cannula at its hub and swiftly remove it, pulling straight back. The site may bleed, so apply direct pressure with the gauze for five minutes. Immediately dispose of all materials in the appropriate biohazard container. Apply an adhesive bandage or tape clean gauze over the site to protect against infection.

INTRAOSSEOUS INFUSION

Intraosseous infusions involve inserting a rigid needle into the cavity of a long bone (*intra-*, within; *os*, bone). The bone marrow contains a network of venous sinusoids that drain into the nutrient and emissary veins. These sinusoids accept fluids and drugs during intraosseous infusion and transport them to the venous system. Any solution or drug that can be administered intravenously, either bolus or infusion, can be administered by the intraosseous route.

Generally, you will use intraosseous infusions for the critical patient less than five years old when you cannot establish peripheral IV access. Less commonly, you may apply intraosseous infusions to adult patients. These patients have different access sites than pediatric patients, and rapid volume administration is not nearly as effective. Situations that might require an intraosseous route include shock, status epilepticus, trauma, and cardiac arrest, and critical pediatric patients where rapid IV access cannot be obtained. Initiate intraosseous lines only after 90 seconds or three unsuccessful attempts to establish peripheral IV access.

✱ **hemoconcentration** elevated numbers of red and white blood cells.

✱ **hemolysis** the destruction of red blood cells.

Remove any IV that will not flow or has fulfilled its need.

✱ **intraosseous** within the bone.

Initiate intraosseous lines only after 90 seconds or three unsuccessful attempts to establish peripheral IV access.

ACCESS SITE

The bone most commonly used for intraosseous access is the tibia. Pediatric access uses the proximal tibia. Adult and geriatric access uses the distal tibia. To properly locate appropriate sites and avoid complications, you must understand the anatomy and physiology of the tibia (Figure 7-36). The tibia is a long bone that transfers weight from the femur to the foot. In conjunction with the fibula, it permits walking. Its three main sections are the diaphysis, which comprises the middle, and the two epiphyses, one at either end. Epipheseal disks, or growth plates, between the diaphysis and the epiphyses, allow the tibia to grow and develop and are present in children. Damage to these disks during intraosseous access can cause long-term growth complications or abnormalities.

Within the diaphysis, the medullary canal holds the vascular bone marrow. When placed correctly, the distal part of the intraosseous needle will lie in the

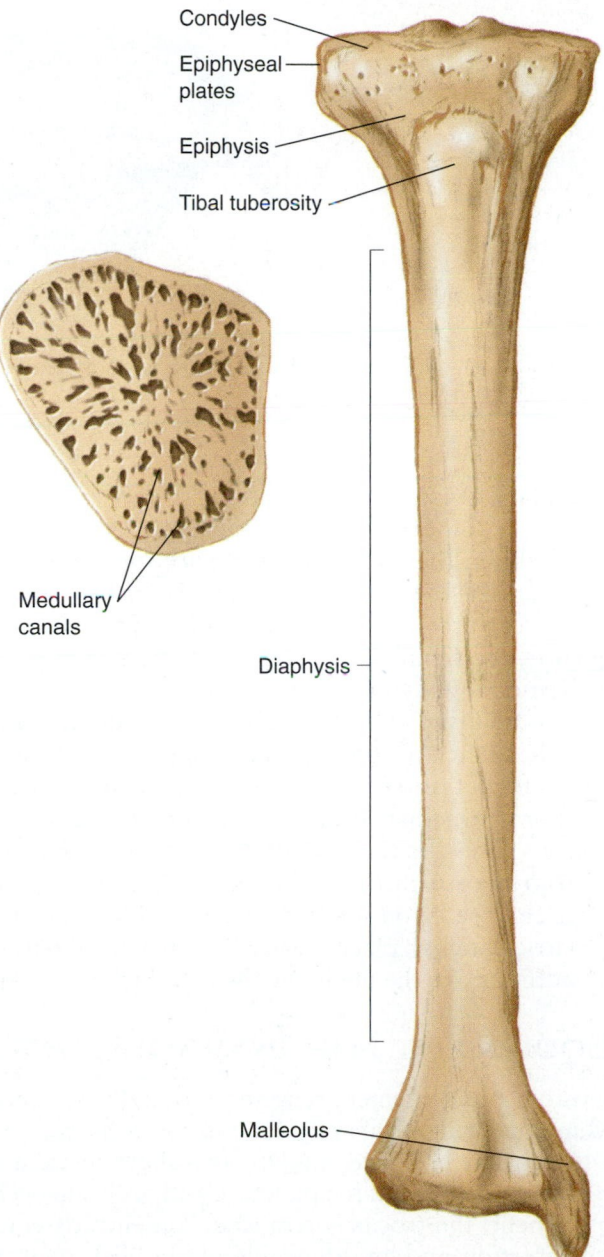

Condyles

Epiphyseal plates

Epiphysis

Tibal tuberosity

Medullary canals

Diaphysis

Malleolus

FIGURE 7-36 Tibia.

(a) pediatric

(b) adult

FIGURE 7-37   Pediatric and adult intraosseous needle placement sites.

medullary canal. On either side of the proximal tibia are the medial and lateral condyles. You can identify the proximal epiphysis by palpating the condyles.

Between the condyles, on the top of the anterior tibial crest, is a palpable bump called the tibial tuberosity. The tibial tuberosity lies at the level of the epipheseal growth plate, for which it provides an excellent reference. Consequently, the tibial tuberosity is extremely important in locating the appropriate pediatric intraosseous access site.

At the distal end of the tibia lie the lateral malleolus and the medial malleolus. They mark the distal epipheseal portion of the tibia and are important landmarks for intraosseous placement in the adult or geriatric patient.

For the pediatric patient (under five years old), you will establish intraosseous access on the medial aspect of the proximal tibia (Figure 7-37a). This site is from two to three finger-breadths below the tibial tuberosity. At this level, place the needle on the flat area medial to the anterior tibial crest. For adult or geriatric patients, place the needle at the distal part of the tibia, one to two finger-breadths above the medial malleolus (Figure 7-37b).

EQUIPMENT FOR INTRAOSSEOUS ACCESS

Intraosseous placement requires a specially designed needle and a 10 ml syringe. Manufactured specifically for intraosseous access, an intraosseous needle is a 14–18 gauge hollow cannula with a sharp metal **trocar** inside (Figure 7-38). The trocar gives strength for puncture and prevents occlusion during insertion. Upon placement, the trocar is removed. The intraosseous needle has a plastic handle for insertion and an adjustable plastic disk to stabilize the needle once it is in

✱ **trocar** a sharp, pointed instrument.

Adjustable
plastic disk

Cannula

Trocar

Handle

FIGURE 7-38   Intraosseous needle.

place. You will attach a 10 ml syringe with 3 to 5 ml of sterile saline to the intraosseous needle. The syringe and saline are used similarly to IV access of the external jugular vein. A large-bore spinal needle with a trocar in place is an acceptable substitute for an intraosseous needle.

Other equipment for intraosseous placement is similar to that for a peripheral intravenous access line (fluid, administration tubing, tape, antiseptics, and gauze). However, you will not use a constricting band or traditional cannula. Depending upon the specific intraosseous needle, you may need an adapter to connect the administration tubing and the needle.

PLACING AN INTRAOSSEOUS INFUSION

To place an intraosseous line use the following technique (Procedure 7-12):

1. Determine the indication for intraosseous access.
2. Assemble and check all equipment.
3. Position the patient. Rotate the leg toward the outside to expose the medial, proximal aspect of the tibia.
4. Locate the access site. Palpate the tibia and use all landmarks.
   - *Pediatric.* Locate the tibial tuberosity. Move from one to two finger breaths below the tibial tuberosity and find the flat expanse medial to the anterior tibial crest.
   - *Adult or geriatric.* Find the medial malleolus. Move from one to two finger breadths below the medial malleolus and locate the flat expanse medial to the anterior tibial crest.
5. Cleanse the site with alcohol or betadine. Start at the puncture site and work outward in an expanding circular motion.
6. Perform the puncture. Holding the needle perpendicular to the puncture site, insert it with a twisting motion until you feel a decrease in resistance or a "pop." When this occurs, the needle is in the medullary canal. Do not advance it any further. Generally, you will need to insert the needle only 2 to 4 mm for entry.
7. Remove the trocar and attach the saline-filled syringe. Slowly pull back the plunger to attempt aspiration into the syringe. Easy aspiration of bone marrow and blood confirms correct medullary placement.

7-12a Select the medication and prepare equipment.

7-12b Palpate the puncture site and prep with an antiseptic solution.

7-12c Make the puncture.

7-12d Aspirate to confirm proper placement.

7-12e Connect the IV fluid tubing.

7-12f Secure the needle appropriately.

7-12g Administer the medication. Monitor the patient for effects.

8. Once you have confirmed placement, rotate the plastic disk toward the skin to secure the needle.

9. Remove the syringe and attach the prepared administration tubing and solution. Set the appropriate flow rate.

10. Secure the needle as if securing an impaled object by surrounding it with bulky dressings and taping them securely in place. Commercial devices are available.

11. Periodically flush the needle to keep it patent.

Any solution or drug that can be administered by IV bolus or continuous infusion can also be delivered by the intraosseous route. Use the medicinal administration port on the primary administration tubing with the techniques as described under Intravenous Drug Administration.

When an intraosseous infusion is complete, shut down the secondary line with the flow regulator or a clamp. Open the primary line and adjust it to the indicated drip rate. Remove the hypodermic needle from the medication administration port and properly dispose of all contents if the infusion has been exhausted.

INTRAOSSEOUS ACCESS COMPLICATIONS AND PRECAUTIONS

Intraosseous access poses serious potential complications similiar to those of peripheral access: local infection, thrombophlebitis, air embolism, circulatory overload, and allergic reactions, plus the following:

- *Fracture.* Too large a needle or too forceful an insertion can fracture the tibia, particulary in very young children.

- *Infiltration.* Infiltration occurs when IV solution collects in the local tissues instead of in the intramedullary canal. Infiltration may occur if you run fluids through an incorrectly placed needle or if a fracture has occurred. An infusion that does not run freely or the formation of an edema at the puncture site indicates infiltration. If infiltration occurs, immediately discontinue infusion and restart on the other leg.

- *Growth plate damage.* An improperly located puncture may damage the growth plate and result in long-term growth complications.

- *Complete insertion.* To avoid complete puncture (needle passing through both sides of the tibia), stop advancing the needle once you feel the pop. If complete puncture occurs, remove the needle with a reverse twisting motion and start again on the other leg. Apply direct pressure and a sterile dressing over the site(s) for at least five minutes.

- *Pulmonary embolism.* If bone, fat, or marrow particles make their way into the circulatory system, pulmonary embolism may result. Use proper technique and watch for signs associated with pulmonary embolism (sudden onset of chest pain or shortness of breath).

Content Review

INTRAOSSEOUS ACCESS COMPLICATIONS

Fracture
Infiltration
Growth plate damage
Complete insertion
Pulmonary embolism
Infection

CONTRAINDICATIONS TO INTRAOSSEOUS PLACEMENT

Do not attempt intraosseous placement in the following situations:

- Fracture to the tibia or femur on the side of access
- Osteogenesis imperfecta—a congenital disease causing fragile bones
- Osteoporosis
- Establishment of a peripheral IV line

You must continually refresh your intraosseous access skills so that you can perform this technique properly when needed.

Part 3: Medical Mathematics

Proper drug administration requires basic mathematical proficiency. Because drug dosages are not always standardized, you may have to calculate amounts according to your patient's age, weight, or other medically related criteria. To properly prepare and administer medications, you must understand roman numerals and be proficient in multiplication, division, fractions, decimal fractions, proportions, and percentages. If you are deficient in one or more of these areas, refer to any text on basic and intermediate math.

METRIC SYSTEM

The metric system's three fundamental units are grams, meters, and liters. Prefixes denote values greater or less than the basic unit. Table 7-2 lists metric prefixes.

The most commonly used prefixes in pharmacology are *kilo-, centi-, milli-,* and *micro-*. The prefix *milli-* (*m*) refers to 1/1000. Thus, a *milliliter* equals 1/1000 of a liter. Similarly, a milligram is 1/1000 of a gram. The prefix *micro-* expresses 1/1 000 000. A *microgram* is 1/1 000 000 of a gram.

> **Content Review**
>
> ### FUNDAMENTAL METRIC UNITS
> Grams—mass
> Meters—distance
> Liters—volume

CONVERSION BETWEEN PREFIXES

If you know the prefixes and their numeric equivalents, you can easily convert measurements to smaller or larger units. To convert a measurement to a smaller

Table 7-2	METRIC PREFIXES	
Prefix	**Multiplier**	**Abbreviation**
kilo	1000	(k)
hecto	100	(h)
deka	10	(D)
deci	1/10 or 0.1	(d)
centi	1/100 or 0.01	(c)
milli	1/1000 or 0.001	(m)
micro	1/1 000 000 or 0.000001	(mcg or μg)

unit, multiply the original measurement by the numerical equivalent of the smaller measurement's prefix.

Example 1: Convert 3 grams to milligrams.

Milligrams (1/1 000) are smaller than grams; therefore, multiply 3 by 1000:

$$3 \text{ (grams)} \times 1000 \text{ (milli)} = 3000$$

$$3 \text{ grams} = 3000 \text{ milligrams}$$

Example 2: Convert 2.67 liters to milliliters.

Milliliters (1/1 000) are smaller than a liter; therefore multiply 2.67 by 1000:

$$2.67 \text{ liters} \times 1000 \text{ (milli)} = 2670$$

$$2.67 \text{ liters} = 2670 \text{ milliliters}$$

To convert a measurement to a larger unit, divide the original measurement by the numerical equivalent of the smaller measurement's prefix.

Example 3: Convert 1600 micrograms to grams.

A microgram is 1/1 000 000 the size of a gram; therefore, divide 1600 by 1 000 000:

$$1600/1 \ 000 \ 000 = 0.0016 \text{ grams}$$

$$1600 \text{ micrograms} = 0.0016 \text{ grams}$$

When converting a measurement to or from a prefix that is not the fundamental unit, first convert the *existing* measurement to the *fundamental* measurement. Then convert the fundamental measurement to the desired unit.

Example 4: Convert 5.6 milligrams to micrograms.

First, convert the 5.6 milligrams to grams:

$$5.6 \text{ milligrams}/1 \ 000 = 0.0056 \text{ grams (g)}$$

$$5.6 \text{ milligrams} = 0.0056 \text{ grams}$$

Now, convert 0.0056 grams to micrograms as previously described:

$$0.0056 \text{ (grams)} \times 1 \ 000 \ 000 = 5600 \text{ micrograms}$$

$$5.6 \text{ milligrams} = 5600 \text{ micrograms}$$

For the beginner, this technique avoids confusion. The more experienced provider will be able to make a direct conversion from milligrams to micrograms.

HOUSEHOLD AND APOTHECARY SYSTEMS OF MEASURE

In the past, pharmacology traditionally used the household and apothecary systems to measure drug dosages. Gradually, the metric system has replaced those systems, but you may occasionally encounter their remnants. Table 7-3 gives the metric equivalents of the household and apothecary units you will most likely confront.

Table 7-3	METRIC EQUIVALENTS	
Household	**Apothecary**	**Metric**
1 gallon	4 quarts	3.785 liters
1 quart	1 quart	0.946 liters
16 ounces	approximately 1 pint	473 milliliters
1 cup	approximately ½ pint	approximately 250 milliliters
1 tablespoon		approximately 16 milliliters
1 teaspoon		approximately 4–5 milliliters

WEIGHT CONVERSION

Some medications' dosages are calculated according to kilograms of body weight. To convert pounds to kilograms use the following formula:

$$\text{kilograms} = \text{pounds}/2.2$$

Example 5. How many kilograms does a 182 lb. person weigh?

$$\text{kilograms} = 182 \text{ lbs.}/2.2$$
$$\text{kilograms} = 82.7$$

TEMPERATURE

The international thermometric scale measures temperature in degrees Celsius. While degrees Celsius is often cited interchangeably with degrees centigrade, the two scales are slightly different. For practical purposes, however, you can think of them both as dividing the interval between the freezing and boiling points of water into 100 equal parts, with 0° being the freezing point and 100° being the boiling point. The household measurement system, on the other hand, divides the interval between the freezing and boiling points of water into 180 equal parts, with 32° being the freezing point and 212° being the boiling point. When taking a body temperature, use the following formulas to convert between degrees Fahrenheit and degrees Celsius:

$$°F = 9/5 \ °C + 32$$
$$°C = 5/9 \ (°F - 32)$$

Example 6: Convert 98.2 °F to °C

$$°C = 5/9 \ (98.2 - 32)$$
$$°C = 5/9 \ (66.2)$$
$$°C = 36.8$$
$$36.8°C = 98.2°F$$

Example 7: Convert 28.4 °C to °F

$$°F = 9/5 \ (28.4) + 32$$
$$°F = 51.12 + 32$$
$$°F = 83.1$$
$$83.1°F = 28.4°C$$

* unit predetermined amount of medication or fluid.

Converting between the different prefixes and between different systems of measurement is crucial in calculating drug dosages. You should continually practice all conversions, not only during your formal education but throughout your career in the emergency medical services.

UNITS

Some medications are measured in **units.** Penicillin, heparin, and insulin are administered in units. Units do not convert between the metric, household, and apothecary systems.

MEDICAL CALCULATIONS

Frequently you will have to apply basic mathematical principles to calculate specific quantities before administering medications and fluids. In prehospital care, the following forms of medications often require calculation:

- Oral medications
- Liquid parenteral medications
- Intravenous fluid administration
- Intravenous medication infusions

* stock solution standard concentration of routinely used medications.

Most medications are provided in **stock solution.** Therefore, you must calculate the exact amount of medication to remove from the stock for administration. To calculate basic drug dosage, you will need three facts:

- Desired dose
- Dosage on hand
- Volume on hand

* desired dose specific quantity of medication needed.

Desired Dose The **desired dose** is the specific quantity of medication needed. Most dosages are expressed as a weight (grams, milligrams, or micrograms). Dosages may be standard or calculated according to body weight or age.

* concentration weight per volume.

Dosage and Volume on Hand All liquid medications are packaged as concentrations. *Concentration* refers to weight per volume. A liquid medication's concentration is the drug's weight (grams, milligrams, or micrograms) per volume of liquid (ml) in which it is dissolved. For example, 50% Dextrose (D_{50}) is packaged as a concentration of 25 grams (weight) dextrose in 50 ml (volume) of water. From the concentration, you can determine the **dosage on hand** (weight) and the **volume on hand.** For 50% Dextrose, the dosage on hand is 25 grams and the volume on hand is 50 ml. Concentrations are identified on all drug packaging and labels.

* dosage on hand the amount of drug available in a solution.

* volume on hand the available amount of solution containing a medication.

Because you cannot see the desired dose dissolved in liquid, you must convert its weight to volume, a readily visible measurement, using the following formula:

$$\text{volume to be administered} = \frac{\text{volume on hand (desired dose)}}{\text{dosage on hand}}$$

To use this formula, you must express all weight and volume measurements with the same metric prefix. For example, if the desired dose is expressed in *milli*grams, the dosage on hand must also be expressed in *milli*grams, volume on hand in *milli*liters.

CALCULATING DOSAGES FOR ORAL MEDICATIONS

The following example illustrates how to calculate the volume of a specific drug dosage:

Example 1. A physician orders you to administer 90 mg of acetaminophen to a pediatric patient. The liquid acetaminophen is packaged as a concentration of 500 mg in 8 ml of solution. How much of the medication will you administer?

Because you cannot see the 90 mg of acetaminophen, you must convert this weight to a volume. To do so you need these facts:

desired dose = 90 mg

dosage on hand = 500 mg

volume on hand = 8 ml

Use the formula to calculate the dosage's volume:

$$\text{volume to be administered} = \frac{\text{volume on hand (8 ml)} \times \text{desired dose (90 mg)}}{\text{dosage on hand (500 mg)}}$$

volume to be administered = $(8 \times 90)/500$

volume to be administered = 720/500

volume to be administered = 1.44

Administer 1.44 ml of solution to deliver 90 mg of acetaminophen.

Another way to calculate drug dosages is the ratio (fraction) and proportion method. A ratio (fraction) illustrates a relationship between two numbers. A proportion is the comparison of two numerically equivalent ratios. Using the variable x, the above problem can be stated:

8 ml/500 mg = x ml/90 mg

To solve the problem, cross multiply the numerals:

8/500 = x/90

720/500 = x

1.44 = x

x = 1.44 ml

CONVERTING PREFIXES

The following example shows how to calculate the volume to be administered when the desired dose, the dosage on hand, and the volume on hand are not all expressed in metric units with the same prefix.

Example 2. A physician orders you to give 250 mg of a drug via IV bolus. The multidose vial contains 2 grams of the drug in 10 ml of solution. How much of the medication should you administer?

Because the desired dose is expressed as *milli*grams, the dosage on hand must be converted from grams to milligrams. In the metric system, 2 grams equal 2000 milligrams. You now know:

desired dose = 250 mg

dosage on hand = 2000 mg

volume on hand = 10 ml

Math Summary 1

$$x \text{ ml} = \frac{8 \text{ ml} \times 90 \text{ mg}}{500 \text{ mg}}$$

$$x \text{ ml} = \frac{720}{500}$$

$$x \text{ ml} = 1.44$$

Math Summary 2

$$\frac{500 \text{ mg}}{8 \text{ ml}} = \frac{90 \text{ mg}}{x \text{ ml}}$$

$$x \text{ ml} = \frac{720}{500}$$

$$x = 1.44 \text{ ml}$$

Now you can use the formula to calculate the volume to be administered:

$$\text{volume to be administered} = \frac{\text{volume on hand (10 ml)} \times \text{desired dose (250 mg)}}{\text{dosage on hand (2000 mg)}}$$

$$\text{volume to be administered} = (10 \times 250)/2000$$

$$\text{volume to be administered} = 2500/2000$$

$$\text{volume to be administered} = 1.25$$

Administer 1.25 ml of solution to deliver 250 mg medication.

You can also solve this problem using the ratio proportion as follows:

$$10 \text{ ml}/2000 \text{ mg} = x \text{ ml}/250 \text{ mg}$$

$$2500 = 2000 \, x$$

$$2500/2000 = x$$

$$1.25 = x$$

$$x = 1.25 \text{ ml}$$

Tablets also come in stock doses. If the dosage of one tablet or pill is more than needed, divide the tablet or pill to make the correct dose. Do not divide enteric or time-release capsules.

CALCULATING DOSAGES FOR PARENTERAL MEDICATIONS

You can use the same formula to calculate specific doses and volume for parenteral medication delivery.

> Example 3. A physician wants you to administer 5 milligrams of medication subcutaneously. The ampule contains 10 mg of the drug in 2 ml of solvent. How much medication should you use?

$$\text{desired dose} = 5 \text{ mg}$$
$$\text{dosage on hand} = 10 \text{ mg}$$
$$\text{volume on hand} = 2 \text{ ml}$$

$$\text{volume to be administered} = \frac{\text{volume on hand (2 ml)} \times \text{desired dose (5 mg)}}{\text{dosage on hand (10 mg)}}$$

$$\text{volume to be administered} = (2 \times 5)/10$$

$$\text{volume to be administered} = 10/10$$

$$\text{volume to be administered} = 1 \text{ ml}$$

Administer 1 ml of solution to deliver 5 mg of the medication.
Using the ratio and proportion method, the problem is solved as follows:

$$2 \text{ ml}/10 \text{ mg} = x \text{ ml}/5 \text{ mg}$$

$$10/10 = x$$

$$1 = x$$

$$x = 1.0 \text{ ml}$$

CALCULATING WEIGHT-DEPENDENT DOSAGES

Occasionally, you will have to calculate the desired dose according to the patient's weight.

Example 4. You must administer 1.5 mg/kg of lidocaine via IV bolus to a patient in stable ventricular tachycardia. The concentration of lidocaine is 100 mg in a prefilled syringe containing 10 ml of solution. The patient weighs 158 lbs.

Start by converting the patient's weight to kilograms:

$$\text{Kilograms} = \text{pounds}/2.2$$

$$\text{Kilograms} = 158 \text{ lbs.}/2.2$$

$$\text{Kilograms} = 71.82$$

The patient weighs approximately 72 kg.

Calculate the desired dose:

$$1.5 \text{ mg} \times 72 \text{ kg} = 108 \text{ mg}$$

You now know these three facts:

desired dose = 108 mg

dosage on hand = 100 mg

volume on hand = 10 ml

Use the same formula as before to calculate the volume to be administered:

$$\text{volume to be administered} = \frac{\text{volume on hand (10 ml)} \times \text{desired dose (108 mg)}}{\text{dosage on hand (100 mg)}}$$

$$\text{volume to be administered} = (10 \times 108)/100$$

$$\text{volume to be administered} = 1080/100$$

$$\text{volume to be administered} = 10.8$$

Administer 10.8 ml of solution to deliver 108 mg of lidocaine.

After you have calculated the desired dose, you can solve this problem using the ratio and proportion method as previously illustrated.

CALCULATING INFUSION RATES

To deliver fluid or medication through an IV infusion, you must calculate the correct infusion rate in drops per minute. To do so you must know the administration tubing's drip factor, as well as the volume on hand, desired dose, and dosage on hand.

Medicated Infusions

To calculate the correct IV infusion rate, use the following formula:

$$\text{drops/minute} = \frac{\text{volume on hand} \times \text{drip factor} \times \text{desired dose}}{\text{dosage on hand}}$$

Math Summary 6

$$x \text{ ml} = \frac{10 \text{ ml} \times 108 \text{ mg}}{100 \text{ mg}}$$

$$x \text{ ml} = \frac{1080}{700}$$

$$x = 10.8 \text{ ml}$$

Math Summary 7

$$\frac{100 \text{ mg}}{10 \text{ ml}} = \frac{108 \text{ mg}}{x \text{ ml}}$$

$$x \text{ ml} = \frac{1080}{100}$$

$$x = 10.8 \text{ ml}$$

Example 5. A physician wants you to administer 2 mg per minute of lidocaine to a patient. To prepare the infusion, you mix 2 grams of lidocaine in an IV bag containing 500 milliliters of 5 percent dextrose in water (D_5W). You will use a microdrip administration set (60 gtts/ml). Calculate the infusion rate.

$$\text{desired dose} = 2 \text{ mg}$$
$$\text{dosage on hand} = 2000 \text{ mg (2 grams)}$$
$$\text{volume on hand} = 500 \text{ ml}$$
$$\text{drip factor} = 60 \text{ gtts/ml}$$

Math Summary 8

$$\text{x drops/min} = \frac{500 \text{ ml} \times 60 \text{ gtts/ml} \times 2 \text{ mg}}{500 \text{ mg}}$$

$$\text{x drops/min} = \frac{60{,}000}{2{,}000}$$

$$\text{x drops/min} = 30$$

$$\text{drops/minute} = \frac{\text{volume on hand (500 ml)} \times \text{drip factor (60 gtts/ml)} \times \text{desired dose (2 mg)}}{\text{dosage on hand (2000 mg)}}$$

$$\text{drops/minute} = (500 \times 60 \times 2)/2000$$

$$\text{drops/minute} = 60\,000/2000$$

$$\text{drops/minute} = 30$$

Run the infusion at 30 drops/minute to infuse 2 mg lidocaine per minute.

Fluid Volume Over Time

Fluids with or without medications may require administration over a specific period of time. To deliver the fluid correctly you must calculate volume/time. This calculation, requires the following information:

- volume to be administered
- drip factor of the administration set (gtts/ml)
- total time of infusion (minutes)

infusion rate speed at which a medication is delivered intravenously.

To calculate the **infusion rate,** use this formula:

$$\text{drops/minute} = \frac{\text{volume to be administered (drip factor)}}{\text{time in minutes}}$$

Example 6. A physician tells you to administer 500 milliliters of normal saline solution to a patient over one hour (60 minutes). The administration tubing is a macrodrip set with a drip factor of 10 gtts/ml. At what drip rate would you run this infusion?

$$\text{volume to be administered} = 500 \text{ ml}$$
$$\text{administration set drip factor (gtts/ml)} = 10 \text{ gtts/ml}$$
$$\text{total time of infusion (minutes)} = 60 \text{ minutes}$$

Calculate the infusion rate:

Math Summary 9

$$\text{x drops/min} = \frac{500 \text{ ml} \times 10 \text{ gtts/ml}}{60 \text{ minutes}}$$

$$\text{x drops/min} = \frac{5{,}000}{60}$$

$$\text{x drops/min} = 83.3$$

$$\text{drops/minute} = \frac{(500 \text{ ml}) (10 \text{ gtts/ml})}{60 \text{ minutes}}$$

$$\text{drops/minute} = (500 \times 10)/60$$

$$\text{drops/minute} = 5000/60$$

$$\text{drops/minute} = 83.3$$

Set the flow rate at approximately 83 drops per minute to infuse 500 milliliters of normal saline in almost exactly 60 minutes.

You can use the same formula to determine how long it will take to use all the fluid in a container.

Example 7: You are transporting a patient with an IV antibiotic. The infusion rate is 45 gtts/minute and the administration tubing is a microdrip set (60 gtts/ml). 150 milliliters remain in the 500 milliliter bag of D_5W. How long until the antibiotic will complete infusion?

Use the same formula as in example 6; however, in this instance you will find time in minutes.

$$45 \text{ drops/minute} = \frac{(150 \text{ ml}) (60 \text{ gtts/ml})}{\text{time}}$$

$$45 = (150 \times 60)/\text{time}$$

$$45 = 9000/\text{time}$$

$$\text{time} = 9000/45$$

$$\text{time} = 200$$

$$45 \text{ drops/minute} = 200 \text{ minutes}$$

The antibiotic will complete infusion in 200 minutes, or 3 hours and 20 minutes.

Math Summary 10

$$45 \text{ gtts/min} = \frac{150 \text{ ml} \times 60 \text{ gtts/ml}}{\text{time}}$$

$$45 = \frac{9{,}000}{x}$$

$$x = \frac{9{,}000}{45}$$

$$x = 200 \text{ minutes}$$

Calculating Dosages and Infusion Rates for Infants and Children

Infants and children cannot tolerate under- or overdoses of medication and fluids. When you administer infusions to pediatric patients, you must calculate exact flow rates. Because infants and children differ drastically from adults in size and internal development, their dosages often depend on weight. Most weight dependent dosages express the patient's weight in kilograms, so you must make the appropriate conversion from pounds as discussed earlier. Occasionally, you may encounter a medication that is based on body surface area (BSA). Chemotherapeutic agents for children are often based on body surface area. While you will not initiate such drugs, you may encounter them on critical care transports either by ground or air. Many aids for calculating pediatric drug doses and infusion rates are available, including charts, forms, and length-based resuscitation tapes. While these devices are helpful, you should not rely on them exclusively. They are no substitute for knowledge.

SUMMARY

Drug administration is a fundamental skill used in the treatment of the sick and injured. For medications to be effective, they must be *safely* delivered into the body by the *appropriate* route. Many different routes for drug delivery are available to the paramedic; however, specific drugs require specific routes for administration.

It is your responsibility to be familiar with all routes of drug delivery and the techniques for establishing and utilizing them. You will use some routes of medication administration infrequently, and they will quickly fade from memory. Nonetheless, someone's well being may depend on your ability to utilize such a route in an emergency. Therefore, periodic review of all routes used in medication administration is highly recommended. In addition, you must accurately calculate many drug dosages. Dosage errors and inappropriate medication administration harm patient care and cast serious doubt on your ability.

CHAPTER 8

Airway Management and Ventilation

Objectives

After reading this chapter, you should be able to:

1. Describe the anatomy of the airway and the physiology of respiration. (See Chapter 3)
2. Explain the primary objective of airway maintenance. (p. 498)
3. Identify commonly neglected pre-hospital skills related to the airway. (p. 508)
4. Describe assessment of the airway and the respiratory system. (pp. 500–508)
5. Describe the modified forms of respiration and list the factors that affect respiratory rate and depth. (pp. 502–503)
6. Discuss the methods for measuring oxygen and carbon dioxide in the blood and their prehospital use. (pp. 505–508)
7. Define and explain the implications of partial airway obstruction with good and poor air exchange and complete airway obstruction. (p. 498)
8. Describe the common causes of upper airway obstruction, including:
   - the tongue (p. 499)
   - foreign body aspiration (p. 500)
   - laryngeal spasm (p. 499)
   - laryngeal edema (p. 499)
   - trauma (p. 499)

Continued

9. Describe complete airway obstruction maneuvers, including:
   - Heimlich maneuver (pp. 552–553)
   - removal with Magill forceps (pp. 552–553)
10. Describe causes of respiratory distress, including:
    - upper and lower airway obstruction (pp. 498–500)
    - inadequate ventilation (p. 500)
    - impairment of respiratory muscles (p. 500)
    - impairment of nervous system (p. 500)
11. Explain the risk of infection to EMS providers associated with airway management and ventilation. (pp. 508, 568)
12. Describe manual airway maneuvers, including:
    - head-tilt/chin-lift maneuver (pp. 508, 510)
    - jaw-thrust maneuver (p. 510)
    - modified jaw-thrust maneuver (p. 510)
13. Discuss the indications, contraindications, advantages, disadvantages, complications, special considerations, equipment, and techniques of the following:
    - upper airway and tracheobronchial suctioning (pp. 563–565)
    - nasogastric and orogastric tube insertion (pp. 565–566)
    - oropharyngeal and nasopharyngeal airway (pp. 511–515)
    - ventilating a patient by mouth-to-mouth, mouth-to-nose, mouth-to-mask, one/two/three person bag-valve mask, flow-restricted oxygen-powered ventilation device, automatic transport ventilator (pp. 568–572)
14. Compare the ventilation techniques used for an adult patient to those used for pediatric patients, and describe special considerations in airway management and ventilation for the pediatric patient. (pp. 540–544, 570)
15. Identify types of oxygen cylinders and pressure regulators, and explain safety considerations of oxygen storage and delivery, including steps for delivering oxygen from a cylinder and regulator. (p. 566)
16. Describe the indications, contraindications, advantages, disadvantages, complications, liter flow range, and concentration of delivered oxygen for the following supplemental oxygen delivery devices (p. 567):
    - nasal cannula
    - simple face mask
    - partial rebreather mask
    - nonrebreather mask
    - Venturi mask
17. Describe the use, advantages, and disadvantages of an oxygen humidifier. (p. 567)
18. Describe the indications, contraindications, advantages, disadvantages, complications, equipment, and technique for the following:
    - endotracheal intubation by direct laryngoscopy (pp. 524–528)
    - digital endotracheal intubation (pp. 532–535)
    - dual lumen airway (pp. 547–552)
    - nasotracheal intubation (pp. 544–546)
    - rapid sequence intubation (pp. 535, 537–540)
    - endotracheal intubation using sedation (pp. 535, 537–540)
    - open cricothyrotomy (pp. 558–562)
    - needle cricothyrotomy (translaryngeal catheter ventilation) (pp. 554–558)
    - extubation (p. 546)
19. Describe the use of cricoid pressure during intubation. (pp. 510–511, 525, 526)
20. Discuss the precautions that should be taken when intubating the trauma patient. (pp. 535, 536)
21. Discuss agents used for sedation and rapid sequence intubation. (pp. 537–540)
22. Discuss methods to confirm correct placement of the endotracheal tube. (pp. 527–531)

INTRODUCTION

Airway management and ventilation are the first and most critical steps in the initial assessment of every patient you will encounter. You must immediately establish and maintain an open airway while providing adequate oxygen delivery and carbon dioxide elimination for all patients. Without adequate airway maintenance and ventilation, the patient will succumb to brain injury or even death in as little as six to ten minutes. Early detection and intervention of airway and breathing problems, including bystander action, are vital to patient survival.

Your deliberate and precise use of simple, basic airway skills is the key to successful airway management and good patient outcome. Once you have applied the basic airway techniques to properly provide oxygenation and ventilation for your patient, you can use more sophisticated airway maneuvers and skills to further stabilize his airway. You must continually monitor and reassess the airway, being careful to watch for displacement of the endotracheal tube, mucus plugging, equipment failure, or the development of a **pneumothorax.**

This chapter will provide the information and skills you will need to manage even the most difficult airway. It begins with an overview of respiratory problems and then explores the initial assessment and management of the airway and ventilation. Finally it details enhanced airway management options for the more experienced paramedic.

RESPIRATORY PROBLEMS

Respiratory emergencies can pose an immediate life threat to the patient. You must calmly and quickly assess the severity of his illness or injury while considering the potential causes of and treatment for his respiratory distress. Often, he will give you little help, either because of anxiety or difficulty speaking. His respiratory difficulty may be due to airway obstruction, injury to upper or lower airway structures, inadequate ventilation caused by worsening of an underlying lung disease and fatigue, or central nervous system problems that threaten the airway or respiratory effort.

AIRWAY OBSTRUCTION

Blockage of the airway is an immediate threat to the patient's life and a true emergency. **Upper airway obstruction** may be defined as an interference with air movement through the upper airway. The tongue, foreign bodies, vomitus, blood, or teeth can all obstruct the upper airway.

Airway obstruction may be either partial or complete. Partial obstruction allows either adequate or poor air exchange. Patients with adequate air exchange can cough effectively; those with poor air exchange cannot. They often emit a high-pitched noise while inhaling (stridor), and their skin may have a bluish appearance (cyanosis). They also may have increased breathing difficulty, which can manifest as choking, gagging dyspnea, or (difficulty speaking) dysphonia. When you cannot feel or hear airflow from the nose and mouth, or when the patient cannot speak (aphonia), breathe, or cough, his airway is completely obstructed. He will quickly become unconscious and die if you do not relieve the obstruction. In the absence of breathing, difficulty ventilating the patient will indicate complete airway obstruction.

FIGURE 8-1   The tongue as airway obstruction.

The Tongue   The tongue is the most common cause of airway obstruction (Figure 8-1). Normally, the submandibular muscles directly support the tongue and indirectly support the epiglottis. Without sufficient muscle tone, though, the relaxed tongue falls back against the posterior pharynx, thus occluding the airway. This may produce snoring respiratory noises. At the same time, the epiglottis also may block the airway at the larynx. This at least diminishes airflow into the respiratory system, and the patient's breathing efforts may inadvertently suck the base of his tongue into an obstructing position. The patient's tongue can block his airway whether he is lateral, supine, or prone; however, the blockage depends on the position of the patient's head and jaw, so simple airway maneuvers such as the jaw-thrust can usually open his airway.

Foreign Bodies   Large, poorly chewed pieces of food can obstruct the upper airway by becoming lodged in the hypopharynx. These cases often involve alcohol consumption and denture dislodgement. Because they frequently occur in restaurants and are mistaken for heart attacks, they are commonly called "café coronaries." The patient may clutch his neck between the thumb and fingers, a universal distress signal. Children, especially toddlers, often aspirate foreign objects, as they have the tendency to put objects into their mouths.

Trauma   In trauma, particularly when the patient is unresponsive, loose teeth, facial bone fractures, and avulsed or swollen tissue may obstruct the airway. Secretions such as blood, saliva, and vomitus may compromise the airway and risk aspiration. Additionally, penetrating or blunt trauma may obstruct the airway by fracturing or displacing the larynx, allowing the vocal cords to collapse into the tracheal lumen.

Laryngeal Spasm and Edema   Since the glottis is the narrowest part of an adult's airway, edema (swelling) or spasm (spasmotic closure) of the vocal cords is potentially lethal. Even moderate edema can severely obstruct airflow and cause asphyxia (the inability to move air into and out of the respiratory system). Just beneath the mucous membrane that covers the vocal cords is a layer of loose tissue where blood or other fluids can accumulate. This tissue may swell following injury, and the swelling will be slow to subside. Causes of laryngeal spasm and edema include trauma, anaphylaxis, epiglottitis, and inhalation of superheated air, smoke, or toxic substances. The most common cause of spasm is overly aggressive intubation. It often occurs, too, immediately upon **extubation**, especially when the patient is semiconscious. Some authors propose that laryngeal spasm can sometimes be partially overcome by strengthening ventilatory effort, forceful upward pull of the jaw, or the use of muscle relaxants, although the success of these maneuvers is quite variable.

> The tongue is the most common airway obstruction.

> Since the glottis is the narrowest part of an adult's airway, edema or spasm of the vocal cords is potentially lethal.

* **extubation** removing a tube from a body opening.

Aspiration Vomitus is the most commonly aspirated material. Patients most at risk for this are those who are so obtunded (drowsy) that they cannot adequately protect their airways. This can occur with hypoxia, central nervous system toxins, or brain injury, among other causes. In addition to obstructing the airway, aspiration's other effects also significantly increase patient mortality. Vomitus consists of food particles, protein-dissolving enzymes, hydrochloric acid, and gastrointestinal bacteria that have been regurgitated from the stomach into the hypopharynx and oropharynx. If this mixture enters the lungs, it can result in increased interstitial fluid and pulmonary edema. The consequent marked increase in alveolar/capillary distance seriously impairs gas exchange, thus causing hypoxemia and hypercarbia. Aspirated materials can also severely damage the delicate bronchiolar tissue and alveoli. Gastrointestinal bacteria can produce overwhelming infections. These complications occur in 50%–80% of patients who aspirate foreign matter.

INADEQUATE VENTILATION

Insufficient minute volume respirations can compromise adequate oxygen intake and carbon dioxide removal. Additionally, oxygenation may be insufficient when conditions increase metabolic oxygen demand or decrease available oxygen. A reduction of either the rate or the volume of inhalation leads to a reduction in minute volume. In some cases, the respiratory rate may be rapid but so shallow that little air exchange takes place. Among the causes of such decreased ventilation are depressed respiratory function as from impairment of respiratory muscles or nervous systems, bronchospasm from intrinsic disease, fractured ribs, pneumothorax, hemothorax, drug overdose, renal failure, spinal or brain stem injury, or head injury. In some conditions, such as sepsis, the body's metabolic demand for oxygen can exceed the patient's ability to supply it. Additionally, the environment may contain a decreased amount of oxygen, as in high-altitude conditions or a house fire, which also produces toxic gases like cyanide and carbon monoxide. These situations of inadequate ventilation can lead to hypercarbia and hypoxia.

RESPIRATORY SYSTEM ASSESSMENT

Vigilance is the key to airway management in every patient.

Vigilance is the key to airway management in every patient. The trauma patient whose airway and breathing initially looked fine on exam may become symptomatic with the pneumothorax that was not initially evident. The asthma patient who initially responded to nebulizer treatment may have a sudden bronchospasm and worsen acutely. Minute-by-minute reassessment of the adequacy of every patient's airway and breathing is essential. The changes may be subtle increases in rate, worsening or onset of irregularity, or increased difficulty speaking.

INITIAL ASSESSMENT

* **ABCs** airway, breathing, and circulation.

The initial assessment's purpose is to identify any immediate threats to the patient's life, specifically airway, breathing, and circulation problems (**ABCs**). First, assess the airway to assure that it is patent. Snoring or gurgling may indicate potential airway problems. Next determine the adequacy of breathing. If the patient is comfortable, with a normal respiratory rate, alert, and speaking without difficulty, you may generally assume that breathing is adequate.

Patients with altered mental status warrant further evaluation. Feel for air movement with your hand or cheek. Look for the chest to rise and fall normally with each respiratory cycle. Listen for air movement and equal bilateral breath sounds. The absence of breath sounds on one side may indicate a pneumothorax

FIGURE 8-2   Bag-valve mask ventilation.

or hemothorax in the trauma patient. In an adult patient, the respiratory rate generally ranges between 12 and 20 breaths per minute. Breathing should be spontaneous, effortless, and regular. Irregular breathing suggests a significant problem and usually requires ventilatory support. Observe the chest wall for any asymmetrical movement. This condition, known as **paradoxical breathing,** may suggest a **flail chest.** Patients who show increased respiratory effort, insisting on upright, sniffing, or semi-Fowler's positioning, or those refusing to lie supine, should be considered to be in significant respiratory distress.

    If the patient is not breathing, or if you suspect airway problems, open the airway using the head-tilt/chin-lift or jaw-thrust maneuver, as described later in this chapter. If trauma is possible, use the jaw-thrust maneuver while stabilizing the cervical spine in neutral position. Once the airway is open, reevaluate the breathing status. If breathing is adequate, provide supplemental oxygen and assess circulation. Consider the use of airway adjuncts, as discussed later. If breathing is inadequate or absent, begin artificial ventilation (Figure 8-2). When assisting a patient's breathing with a ventilatory device (bag-valve mask or other positive-pressure device), or after placing an airway adjunct, (nasopharyngeal airway or oropharyngeal airway), or endotracheally intubating, monitor the chest's rise and fall to determine correct usage and placement. (We will discuss these ventilatory devices and mechanical airways in detail later in this chapter.)

* **paradoxical breathing** assymetrical chest wall movement that lessens respiratory efficiency.

* **flail chest** defect in the chest wall that allows a segment to move freely, causing paradoxical chest wall motion.

FOCUSED HISTORY AND PHYSICAL EXAMINATION

After you complete the initial assessment and correct any immediate life threats, conduct a focused history and physical exam while continuously monitoring the patient's airway, breathing, and circulation.

Focused History

The time when the patient and his family noted the onset of symptoms is important information, as is whether the acute event occurred suddenly or gradually. Identifying possible triggers such as allergens or heat also can help the patient avoid them in the future. Additionally, the symptoms' course of development since onset will help direct diagnosis and treatment. Have they been progressively worsening, recurrent, or continuous? Associated symptoms will further help to assess the cause of the patient's problem. Has he had fever or chills, productive cough, chest pain, nausea or vomiting, or diaphoresis? Does he think his voice sounds normal?

    The patient's past medical history will put his present complaints into perspective and help to identify the risk factors for a variety of likely diagnoses.

Determine whether the present episode is similar to any past episodes of shortness of breath, what medical evaluations have been done, and what they have found. Has the patient ever been admitted to the hospital for his complaints? Has he ever been intubated?

The recent history leading to the onset of symptoms is also important. Did the patient run out of medication? Has he been noncompliant with (not taken) his medications? Did he drink too much fluid or alcohol? Did he seize or vomit? Did he eat something that might induce an allergy? Did he receive any trauma? If an injury is involved, evaluate the mechanism of injury. Keep in mind that blunt trauma to the neck may have injured the larynx. Anything that makes the patient's condition better (ameliorates) or worse (exacerbates, aggravates) is also significant.

Physical Examination

Your physical examination of a patient with respiratory problems should continue the evaluation of his airway, breathing, and circulation begun during your initial assessment. Now you will use the physical examination techniques of inspection, auscultation, and palpation to evaluate his injury or illness in more detail and determine your plan of action. (Chapter 11 explains these techniques in detail.)

Inspection Begin the physical assessment by inspecting the patient. Evaluate the adequacy of his breathing. Note any obvious signs of trauma. Always remember to assess the skin color as an indicator of oxygenation status. Early in respiratory compromise, the sympathetic nervous system will be stimulated to help offset the lack of oxygen. When this happens, the skin will often appear pale and diaphoretic. **Cyanosis** (bluish discoloration) is another sign of respiratory distress. When oxygen binds with the hemoglobin, the blood appears bright red. Deoxygenated hemoglobin, on the other hand, is blue and gives the skin a bluish tint. This is not a reliable indicator, however, since severe tissue hypoxia is possible without cyanosis. In fact, cyanosis is considered a late sign of respiratory compromise. When it does appear, it usually affects the lips, fingernails, and skin. A red skin rash, especially if accompanied by hives, may indicate an allergic reaction. A cherry-red skin discoloration may on rare occasions be associated with carbon monoxide poisoning, as can bullae (large blisters).

Observe the patient's position. Tripod positioning (seated, leaning forward, with one arm forward to stabilize the body) may indicate COPD or asthma exacerbation; orthopnea (increased difficulty breathing while lying down) may indicate congestive heart failure, or asthma.

Next, inspecting for **dyspnea**—an abnormality of breathing rate, pattern, or effort—is essential. Dyspnea may cause or be caused by **hypoxia.** Prolonged dyspnea without successful intervention can lead to **anoxia** (the absence or near-absence of oxygen), which without intervention is a premorbid (occurring just before death) event, as the brain can survive only four to six minutes in this state. Remember that all interventions are useless if you do not establish a patent airway.

Also observe for the following modified forms of respiration:

- *Coughing*—forceful exhalation of a large volume of air from the lungs. This performs a protective function in expelling foreign material from the lungs.

- *Sneezing*—sudden, forceful exhalation from the nose. It is usually caused by nasal irritation.

- *Hiccoughing* (hiccups)—sudden inspiration caused by spasmodic contraction of the diaphragm with spastic closure of the glottis. It

* **cyanosis** bluish discoloration.

* **dyspnea** an abnormality of breathing rate, pattern, or effort.

* **hypoxia** oxygen deficiency.

* **anoxia** the absence or near-absence of oxygen.

serves no known physiologic purpose. It has, occasionally, been associated with acute myocardial infarctions on the inferior (diaphragmatic) surface of the heart.

- *Sighing*—slow, deep, involuntary inspiration followed by a prolonged expiration. It hyperinflates the lungs and reexpands atelectatic alveoli. This normally occurs about once a minute.
- *Grunting*—a forceful expiration that occurs against a partially closed epiglottis. It is usually an indication of respiratory distress.

Note any decrease or increase in the respiratory rate, one of the earliest indicators of respiratory distress. Also, look for use of the accessory respiratory muscles—intercostal, suprasternal, supraclavicular, and subcostal retractions—and the abdominal muscles to assist breathing. This indicates increased respiratory effort secondary to respiratory distress. In infants and children, nasal flaring and grunting indicate respiratory distress. COPD patients having difficulty breathing will purse their lips during exhalation. Monitor the patient's blood pressure, including any differences noted during expiration versus inspiration. Patients with severe chronic obstructive pulmonary disease may sustain a drop in blood pressure during inspiration. This drop is due to increased pressure within the thoracic cavity that impairs the ability of the ventricles to fill. Thus, decreased ventricular filling leads to decreased blood pressure. A drop in blood pressure of greater than 10 torr is termed **pulsus paradoxus** and may be indicative of severe obstructive lung disease.

Determine if the pattern of respirations is abnormal—deep or shallow in combination with a fast or slow rate. Some common abnormal respiratory patterns include:

* **pulsus paradoxus** drop in blood pressure of greater than 10 torr during inspiration.

- *Kussmaul's respirations*—deep, slow or rapid, gasping breathing, commonly found in diabetic ketoacidosis
- *Cheyne-Stokes respirations*—progressively deeper, faster breathing alternating gradually with shallow, slower breathing, indicating brain stem injury
- *Biot's respirations*—irregular pattern of rate and depth with sudden, periodic episodes of apnea, indicating increased intracranial pressure
- *Central neurogenic hyperventilation*—deep, rapid respirations, indicating increased intracranial pressure
- *Agonal respirations*—shallow, slow or infrequent breathing, indicating brain anoxia

Finally, observing altered mentation may be key in determining if breathing is adequate or if significant hypoxia may be present. If the patient's mental status is not normal, you must determine his usual baseline mental status before you can make this assessment.

Auscultation Following inspection, listen at the mouth and nose for adequate air movement. Then listen to the chest with a stethoscope (auscultate) (Figure 8-3). In a prehospital setting, you should auscultate the right and left apex (just beneath the clavicle), the right and left base (eighth or ninth intercostal space, midclavicular line), and the right and left lower thoracic back or right and left midaxillary line (fourth or fifth intercostal space, on the lateral aspect of the chest). When the patient's condition permits, you can monitor six locations on the posterior chest, three right, and three left. The posterior surface is preferable because heart sounds do not interfere with auscultation at this location.

FIGURE 8-3 Positions for auscultating breath sounds.

However, since patients are usually supine during airway management, the anterior and lateral positions usually prove more accessible. Breath sounds should be equal bilaterally. Sounds that point to airflow compromise include:

- *Snoring*—results from partial obstruction of the upper airway by the tongue
- *Gurgling*—results from the accumulation of blood, vomitus, or other secretions in the upper airway
- *Stridor*—a harsh, high-pitched sound heard on inhalation, associated with laryngeal edema or constriction
- *Wheezing*—a musical, squeaking, or whistling sound heard in inspiration and/or expiration, associated with bronchiolar constriction
- *Quiet*—diminished or absent breath sounds are an ominous finding and indicate a serious problem with the airway, breathing, or both

Beware of the quiet chest!

Sounds that may indicate compromise of gas exchange include:

- *Crackles* (rales)—a fine, bubbling sound heard on inspiration, associated with fluid in the smaller bronchioles
- *Rhonchi*—a coarse, rattling noise heard on inspiration, associated with inflammation, mucus, or fluid in the bronchioles

When you assess the effectiveness of ventilatory support or the correct placement of an airway adjunct, remember that air movement into the epigastrium may sometimes mimic breath sounds. Thus, listening to the chest should be only one of several means that you use to assess air movement. Another method of checking correct placement of an airway adjunct is to auscultate over the epigastrium; it should be silent during ventilation. When you provide ventilatory support, watch for signs of gastric distention. They suggest inadequate hyperextension of the neck, undue pressure generated by the ventilatory device, or improper placement of airway adjuncts.

Palpation Finally, palpate. First, using the back of your hand or your cheek, feel for air movement at the mouth and nose. (If an endotracheal tube is in place, you can check for air movement at the tube's adapter.) Next, palpate the chest for rise and fall. In addition, palpate the chest wall for tenderness, symmetry, abnormal motion, crepitus, and subcutaneous emphysema.

When ventilating with a bag-valve device, gauge airflow into the lungs by noting compliance. **Compliance** refers to the stiffness or flexibility of the lung tissue, and it is indicated by how easily air flows into the lungs. When compliance is good, airflow meets minimal resistance. When compliance is poor, ventilation is harder to achieve. Compliance is often poor in diseased lungs and in patients suffering from chest wall injuries or tension pneumothorax. If a patient shows poor compliance during ventilatory support, look for potential causes. Upper airway obstructions, which cause difficulty with mechanical ventilation, can mimic poor compliance. If ventilating the patient is initially easy but then becomes progressively more difficult, repeat the initial assessment and look for the development of a new problem, possibly related to the mechanical airway maneuvers. The following questions will aid this assessment:

* Is the airway open?
* Is the head properly positioned in extension (nontrauma patients)?
* Is the patient developing tension pneumothorax?
* Is the endotracheal tube occluded (a mucous plug or aspirated material)?
* Has the endotracheal tube been inadvertently pushed into the right or left mainstem bronchus?
* Has the endotracheal tube been displaced into the esophagus?
* Is the mechanical ventilatory equipment functioning properly?

Pulse rate abnormalities may also suggest respiratory compromise. Tachycardia (an abnormally fast pulse) usually accompanies hypoxemia in an adult, while bradycardia (an abnormally slow pulse) hints at anoxia with imminent cardiac arrest.

Noninvasive Respiratory Monitoring

Several available devices will help you measure the effectiveness of oxygenation and ventilation. Those measurements used most commonly in prehospital care are pulse oximetry, capnography, and esophageal detection devices. Peak expiratory flow testing can also be useful in the prehospital setting for some respiratory diseases.

Pulse Oximetry **Pulse oximetry** is widely used in prehospital emergency care. A pulse oximeter measures hemoglobin oxygen saturation in peripheral tissues (Figure 8-4). It is non-invasive (does not require entering the body), rapidly applied, and easy to operate. Pulse oximetry readings are accurate and continually reflect any changes in peripheral oxygen delivery. In fact, oximetry often detects problems with oxygenation faster than assessments of blood pressure, pulse, and respirations.

To determine peripheral oxygen saturation, you place a sensor probe over a peripheral capillary bed such as a fingertip, toe, or earlobe. In infants, you can wrap the sensor around the heel and secure it with tape. The sensor contains two light-emitting diodes and two sensors. One diode emits near-red light, a wavelength specific for oxygenated hemoglobin; the other emits infrared light,

* **compliance** the stiffness or flexibility of the lung tissue.

A fall in the pulse rate in a patient with airway compromise is an ominous finding.

* **pulse oximetry** a measurement of hemoglobin oxygen saturation in the peripheral tissues.

FIGURE 8-4   Pulse oximeter.

a wavelength specific for deoxygenated hemoglobin. Each hemoglobin state absorbs a certain amount of the emitted light, preventing it from reaching the corresponding sensor. Less light reaching the sensor means more of its type of hemoglobin is in the blood. The oximeter then calculates the ratio of the near-red and infrared light it has received to determine the **oxygen saturation percentage** (SaO_2).

Pulse oximeters display the SaO_2 and the pulse rate as detected by the sensors. They show the SaO_2 either as a number or as a visual display that also shows the pulse's waveform. The relationship between SaO_2 and the partial pressure of oxygen in the blood (PaO_2) is very complex. However, the SaO_2 does correlate with the PaO_2. The greater the PaO_2, the greater will be the oxygen saturation. Since hemoglobin carries 98% of oxygen in the blood while plasma carries only 2%, pulse oximetry accurately analyzes peripheral oxygen delivery.

Pulse oximetry is often called the "fifth vital sign." When available, you should use it in virtually any situation to determine the patient's baseline value, to guide patient care, and to monitor the patient's responses to your interventions. As a guide, normal SaO_2 varies between 95% and 99%. Readings between 91% and 94% indicate mild hypoxia and warrant further evaluation and supplemental oxygen administration. Readings between 86% and 91% indicate moderate hypoxia. You should generally give these patients 100% supplemental oxygen, exercising caution in those with COPD. Readings of 85% or lower indicate severe hypoxia and warrant immediate intervention, including the administration of 100% oxygen, ventilatory assistance, or both. Your goal is to maintain the SaO_2 in the normal (95–99%) range.

False readings with pulse oximetry are infrequent. When they do occur, the oximeter often generates an error signal or a blank screen. Causes of false readings include carbon monoxide poisoning, high-intensity lighting, and certain hemoglobin abnormalities. The absence of a pulse in an extremity also will cause a false reading. In hypovolemia and in severely anemic patients, the pulse oximetry reading may be misleading. While the SaO_2 reading may be normal, the total amount of hemoglobin available to carry oxygen may be so markedly decreased that the patient will remain hypoxic at the cellular level.

Pulse oximetry provides key information about the patient and is an important part of emergency care, including prehospital care. However, it is only one more assessment tool and does not replace other physical assessment or monitoring skills. Do not depend solely on pulse oximetry readings to guide care. Always consider and treat the whole patient.

Capnography **Capnography** is the measurement of exhaled carbon dioxide concentrations. The devices that make such measurements are called end-tidal carbon dioxide ($ETCO_2$) detectors. Their use in prehospital care is increasing, most commonly to assess proper placement of an endotracheal tube. Carbon dioxide's absence from the exhaled air strongly indicates that the tube is in the esophagus; its presence indicates proper tracheal placement.

End-tidal CO_2 detectors are available either as disposable colorimetric devices or as electronic monitors (Figures 8-5 and 8-6). They are attached either in-line or alongside the endotracheal tube and the ventilation device. A color change in the colorimetric device or a light on the electronic monitor confirms proper tube placement. On the colorimetric device, the low CO_2 content of inspired air makes the device purple, while the higher CO_2 content of expired air makes it yellow. Some electronic devices now combine pulse oximetry, $ETCO_2$ detection, blood pressure, pulse rate, respiratory rate, and temperature monitors in one unit (Figure 8-7).

Although the $ETCO_2$ detector is accurate, the $ETCO_2$ level falls precipitously during cardiac arrest. Therefore, these patients may not cause a color change on the $ETCO_2$ detector despite proper placement of the endotracheal tube.

* **capnography** the measurement of exhaled carbon dioxide concentrations.

FIGURE 8-5   Colorimetric end-tidal CO_2 detector.

FIGURE 8-6   Electronic end-tidal CO_2 detector.

FIGURE 8-7   Combined devices check pulse oximetry, $ETCO_2$, blood pressure, pulse, respiratory rate, and temperature.

As with pulse oximetry, you should use an ETCO$_2$ detector only in conjunction with other methods of assessing endotracheal placement. It does not replace actually visualizing the endotracheal tube's passage through the vocal cords.

Esophageal Detector Device The esophageal detector device (EDD) is a simple and inexpensive tool to help determine whether an endotracheal tube is in the trachea or the esophagus. It uses the anatomic principle that the trachea is a rigid tube and will not collapse with negative pressure, while the esophagus is a collapsible tube that flattens with negative pressure and does not allow air to enter the syringe. The EDD may be either a rigid syringe or a bulb syringe (Figure 8-8). Once you have intubated the patient, you attach the EDD to the proximal end of the endotracheal tube (ETT). Then you quickly pull back the syringe, aspirating air from the endotracheal tube. Easily withdrawn air confirms ETT placement in the trachea. If air is difficult or impossible to withdraw, the ETT is in the esophagus.

Peak Expiratory Flow Testing Peak expiratory flow testing utilizes a disposable plastic chamber into which the patient exhales forcefully after maximal inhalation. It can be used as a crude measure of respiratory efficacy. Improving measurements can indicate good response to treatment.

BASIC AIRWAY MANAGEMENT

Deciding if a patient has a patent airway is the most important step in the initial assessment. Airway management is one of the few prehospital interventions that is known to improve patient survival rates. Once you have determined that intervention is needed, you must use simple manual airway maneuvers and equipment before proceeding with more advanced techniques such as endotracheal intubation or placement of the CombiTube. Always provide supplemental oxygen to all patients for whom it is indicated; never withhold it even from the COPD patient. Be sure to always wear protective eyewear and gloves to avoid contact with the patient's body fluids. If you suspect cervical spine injury, perform modified airway techniques in conjunction with appropriate cervical spine stabilization. Once you have secured the airway, frequently reassess for an adequate airway and ventilation.

MANUAL AIRWAY MANEUVERS

Manual maneuvers are the simplest airway management techniques and are highly effective but often neglected in prehospital care. The head-tilt/chin-lift and the jaw-thrust are safe and dependable maneuvers for relieving obstruction by the tongue. Perform one of these techniques on all unconscious patients but not on responsive patients. If you suspect cervical spine injury, perform the modified jaw-thrust with in-line stabilization of the cervical spine.

Head–Tilt/Chin–Lift

In the absence of cervical spinal trauma, the head-tilt/chin-lift is the best technique for opening the airway in an unresponsive patient who is not protecting his own airway.

In the absence of cervical spine trauma, the head-tilt/chin-lift is the best technique for opening the airway in an unresponsive patient who is not protecting his own airway. The head-tilt is hazardous to patients with cervical spine injuries; do not use it for those patients. To perform the head-tilt/chin-lift:

1. Place the patient supine and position yourself at the side of the patient's head.

(a)

FIGURE 8-8 An esophageal intubation detector—bulb style. **a.** Squeeze the device and then attach it to the endotracheal tube. **b.** If the bulb refills easily upon release, it indicates correct placement. **c.** If the bulb does not refill, the tube is improperly placed.

(b)

(c)

Basic Airway Management **509**

2. Place one hand on the patient's forehead and, using firm downward pressure with your palm, tilt the head back.
3. Put two fingers of the other hand under the bony part of the chin and lift the jaw anteriorly to open the airway.

Caution: Avoid compressing the soft tissues of the neck and chin.

Jaw–Thrust Maneuver

A jaw-thrust is also acceptable for an unresponsive patient without the risk of cervical spine injury who cannot protect his airway.

1. Place the patient supine and kneel behind his head.
2. Apply fingers on each side of the jaw at the mandibular angles.
3. Lift the jaw forward (anterior) with a gentle tilting of the patient's head to open the airway.

For trauma patients, maintain the cervical spine in neutral position and use either the jaw-thrust without head-tilt or the modified jaw-thrust. You can perform both of these maneuvers with a cervical collar in place:

1. Jaw-thrust without head-tilt: lift the jaw by grasping under the chin and behind the teeth, without tilting the head. Use extreme caution with this technique, as even unresponsive patients can clench their teeth shut; do not use this method if the patient's mouth resists opening.
2. Modified jaw-thrust: lift the jaw using fingers behind the mandibular angles; do not tilt the head. Use this method if the patient's mouth resists opening.

Although they are simple and effective, none of these manual airway maneuvers protects the airway from aspiration. Additionally, the jaw-thrust and modified jaw-thrust are difficult to maintain for an extended time. The jaw-thrust is impossible to maintain if the patient becomes responsive or combative. Using them in conjunction with a bag-valve mask is often difficult and typically requires a second rescuer. Finally, maintaining the jaw-thrust requires you to keep your thumb in the patient's mouth.

Sellick's Maneuver

To help prevent regurgitation and reduce gastric distention, Sellick's maneuver applies gentle pressure posteriorly on the anterior cricoid cartilage (Figures 8-9 and 8-10). Since the esophagus lies just behind the cricoid cartilage, this maneuver will effectively close the esophagus to pressures as high as 100 cm/H$_2$O. It also facilitates intubation by moving the larynx posterior, bringing it into view.

To locate the cricoid cartilage, palpate the thyroid cartilage (Adam's apple) and feel the depression just below it (cricothyroid membrane). The prominence just inferior to this depression is the ring of cricoid cartilage. Using the thumb and index finger of one hand, apply pressure to the anterior and lateral aspects of the cricoid cartilage just next to the midline. In infants, use one fingertip and apply gentle downward pressure, taking care to avoid excessive pressure.

When you use this technique during bag-valve-mask ventilation and endotracheal intubation, a second rescuer is required, and you must remember that the patient will likely regurgitate when you release cricoid pressure. Ideally, therefore, once you have applied Sellick's maneuver, you must maintain it until endotracheal

FIGURE 8-9 Sellick's maneuver (cricoid pressure).

FIGURE 8-10a   Airway before applying Sellick's.

intubation is confirmed and personnel are ready to suction the oropharynx or place a nasogastric tube to decompress the stomach. Additionally, use caution in any patient with a suspected cervical spine injury, as movement of the neck in these patients could cause further spinal cord injury. Complications of Sellick's maneuver include esophageal rupture from unrelieved gastric pressure and obstruction of the trachea or laryngeal trauma from excessive manual pressure.

BASIC MECHANICAL AIRWAYS

In the absence of trauma, secretions, foreign bodies, and edema, basic manual airway maneuvers should clear the tongue from the air passages. However, the tongue often falls back to block the airway again. Two available airway adjuncts, the nasopharyngeal airway and the oropharyngeal airway correct this. These adjuncts cannot replace good head positioning, but they do help to lift the base of the tongue forward and away from the posterior oropharynx, establishing a patent airway. Always attempt any appropriate manual maneuvers before placing a mechanical airway.

Nasopharyngeal Airway

The **nasopharyngeal airway** is an uncuffed tube made of soft rubber or plastic. The nasopharyngeal airway follows the natural curvature of the nasopharynx, passing through the nose and extending from the nostril to the posterior pharynx just below the base of the tongue. It varies from 17 to 20 cm long, and its diameter ranges from 20 F to 36 F (**French**). A funnel-shaped projection at its proximal end helps prevent the tube from slipping inside a patient's nose and becoming lost or aspirated. The distal end is beveled to facilitate passage. You will use the nasopharyngeal airway to relieve soft tissue upper airway obstruction in cases where an oropharyngeal airway is not advised. Specific indications for the use of the nasopharyngeal airway include obtunded patients (with or without a suppressed gag reflex) and unconscious patients. If the patient does not tolerate the nasopharyngeal airway, you should remove it.

The nasopharyngeal airway's advantages are:

- It can be rapidly inserted and safely placed blindly.
- It bypasses the tongue, providing a patent airway.
- You may use it in the presence of a gag reflex.
- You may use it when the patient has suffered injury to his oral cavity (anything from trauma to the mandible to significant soft tissue damage to the tongue or pharynx).
- You may suction through it.
- You may use it when the patient's teeth are clenched.

Disadvantages of the nasopharyngeal airway are:

- It is smaller than the oropharyngeal airway.
- It does not isolate the trachea.
- It is difficult to suction through.
- It may cause severe nosebleeds if inserted too forcefully.
- It may cause pressure necrosis of the nasal mucosa.
- It may kink and clog, obstructing the airway.
- Inserting it is difficult if nasal damage (old or new) is present.
- You may not use it if the patient has or is suspected to have a basilar skull fracture.

Do not use the nasopharyngeal airway in patients who are predisposed to nosebleeds or who have a nasal obstruction. Also never use it when you suspect a basilar skull fracture, as the tube can inadvertently pass into the craninum.

The properly sized nasopharyngeal tube is slightly smaller in diameter than the patient's nostril, and in adults it is equal to or slightly longer than the distance from the patient's nose to his earlobe. Selecting the appropriate size is important. Too small a tube will not extend past the tongue; too long a tube may pass into the esophagus and result in hypoventilation and gastric distention with artificial ventilation (Figures 8-11 and 8-12). To insert the nasopharyngeal airway:

FIGURE 8-11 Nasopharyngeal airway.

FIGURE 8-12 Nasopharyngeal airway, inserted.

1. If the patient has no history of trauma, hyperextend his head and neck.

2. Assure or maintain effective ventilation. If indicated, hyperventilate the patient with 100% oxygen.

3. Lubricate the exterior of the tube with a water-soluble gel to prevent trauma during insertion. If possible, use a lidocaine gel in the alert or responsive patient; its anesthetic effect on the mucosa will make insertion more comfortable.

4. Push gently up on the tip of the nose and pass the tube into the right nostril. If the septum is deviated and you cannot easily insert the tube into the right nostril, use the left nostril. With the bevel oriented toward the septum, insert the tube gently along the nasal floor, parallel to the mouth. Avoid pushing against any resistance, as this may cause tissue trauma and airway kinking.

5. Verify appropriate position of the airway. Clear breath sounds and chest rise indicate correct placement. Also, feel at the airway's proximal end for airflow on expiration.

6. Hyperventilate the patient with 100% oxygen, if indicated.

While semiconscious patients tolerate a nasopharyngeal airway better than an oropharyngeal airway, it too may cause vomiting and laryngospasm. Insertion of the nasopharyngeal airway may injure the nasal mucosa, leading to bleeding, aspiration of clots, and the need for suctioning. Forceful insertion of the airway may lacerate the adenoids, causing considerable bleeding.

Oropharyngeal Airway

The **oropharyngeal airway** is a noninvasive semicircular plastic or rubber device designed to follow the palate's curvature. It holds the base of the tongue away from the posterior oropharynx, thus preventing it from obstructing the glottis. Its use is indicated in patients with no gag reflex.

When properly positioned, this device has several advantages:

- It is easy to place using proper technique.
- Air can pass around and through the device.
- It helps prevent obstruction by the teeth and lips.
- It helps manage unconscious patients who are breathing spontaneously or need mechanical ventilation.
- It makes suction of the pharynx easier, as a large suction catheter can pass on either side of the device.
- It serves as an effective bite block in case of seizures or to protect the endotracheal tube.

Disadvantages of the oropharyngeal airway are:

- It does not isolate the trachea or prevent aspiration.
- It cannot be inserted when the teeth are clenched. It may obstruct the airway if not inserted properly.
- It is easily dislodged.
- Return of the gag reflex may produce vomiting.

Do not use an oropharyngeal airway in conscious or in semiconscious patients who have a gag reflex, as it may cause vomiting or laryngospasm.

Do not use an oropharyngeal airway in conscious or in semiconscious patients who have a gag reflex, as it may cause vomiting (by stimulating the posterior tongue gag reflexes) or laryngospasm.

Oropharyngeal airways are available in sizes ranging from #0 (for neonates) to #6 (for large adults). Selecting the proper size is important. If the airway is too long, it can press the epiglottis against the entrance of the larynx, resulting in airway obstruction. If it is too small, it will not adequately hold the tongue forward. To measure for the appropriate oropharyngeal airway, place the flange beside the patient's cheek, parallel to the front of the teeth. A properly sized airway will extend from the patient's mouth to the angle of his jaw (Figure 8-13). To place the oropharyngeal airway:

1. If the patient has no history of trauma, hyperextend his head and neck. Open the mouth and remove any visible obstructions.
2. Assure or maintain effective ventilation; if indicated, hyperventilate the patient with 100% oxygen.
3. Grasp the patient's jaw and lift anteriorly.
4. With your other hand, hold the airway device at its proximal end and insert it into the patient's mouth. Make sure the curve is reversed, with the tip pointing toward the roof of the mouth.
5. Once the tip reaches the level of the soft palate, gently rotate the airway 180° until it comes to rest over the tongue.

FIGURE 8-13a Insert the Oropharyngeal airway with the tip facing the palate.

FIGURE 8-13b Rotate the airway 180° into position.

FIGURE 8-14 Improper placement of oropharyngeal airway.

6. Verify appropriate position of the airway. Clear breath sounds and chest rise indicate correct placement.

7. Hyperventilate the patient with 100% oxygen, if indicated.

Make sure the airway is correctly positioned. Improper placement can obstruct the airway by pushing the tongue back against the posterior oropharynx (Figure 8-14). The device's advancing out of the mouth during ventilatory efforts indicates improper placement. Improper technique can also cause dental or pharyngeal trauma. An alternative insertion method useful in both pediatric and adult patients is to press the tongue upward and forward with a tongue blade. Then, the airway can be advanced until the flange is seated at the teeth. This is the preferred method of airway insertion in infants and children.

ADVANCED AIRWAY MANAGEMENT

Inserting advanced mechanical airways requires special training. The preferred method of airway management is endotracheal intubation, as it is the only procedure that effectively isolates the trachea. In some EMS systems, endotracheal intubation is not available. These systems use other airway devices such as the Esophageal Tracheal CombiTube (ETC), Laryngeal Mask Airway (LMA), or Pharyngeo-tracheal Lumen (PtL), the esophageal gastric tube airway (EGTA), or the esophageal obturator airway (EOA).

ENDOTRACHEAL INTUBATION

Endotracheal intubation involves inserting an endotracheal tube into the trachea in order to provide the patient with a definitive, protected airway. It is clearly the preferred method of advanced airway management in prehospital emergency care, as it allows the greatest control of the airway in conjunction with a bag-valve mask unit or ventilator. Under most circumstances, it requires direct visualization of the larynx with a laryngoscope, though alternative methods are available. Successfully accomplishing endotracheal intubation requires more training than other techniques, and you must maintain ongoing proficiency to ensure patient safety. To assure the quality of your judgement and skill, you must continuously review field intubations and the criteria for performing them. You must also remember that, although endotracheal intubation affords the most effective airway control, you are bypassing important physiologic functions of the upper airway—warming, filtering, and humidifying the air before it enters the lower airway.

Endotracheal intubation is clearly the preferred method of advanced airway management in prehospital emergency care, as it allows the greatest control of the airway.

Content Review

ENDOTRACHEAL INTUBATION EQUIPMENT

- Laryngoscope (handle and blade)
- Endotracheal tube
- 10 ml syringe
- Stylet
- Bag-valve mask
- Suction device
- Bite block
- Magill forceps
- Tape or tube-holding device

 laryngoscope instrument for lifting the tongue and epiglottis in order to see the vocal cords.

Equipment

The equipment needed for endotracheal intubation includes: a laryngoscope (handle and blade), an appropriate-size endotracheal tube, a 10 ml syringe, a stylet, a bag-valve-mask, a suction device, a bite block, Magill forceps, and tape or a commercial tube-holding device.

Laryngoscope The **laryngoscope** is an instrument for lifting the tongue and epiglottis out of the way so that you can see the vocal cords. You will typically use it to place an endotracheal tube, but you may also use it in conjunction with Magill forceps to retrieve a foreign body obstructing the upper airway.

A laryngoscope consists of a handle and a blade. The handle may be either reusable or disposable. It houses batteries that power a light in the blade's distal tip. This light illuminates the airway, making it easier to see upper airway structures. The point attaching the handle and the blade is called the fitting. It locks the blade in place and provides electrical contact between the batteries and the bulb (Figure 8-15).

To prepare for intubation, attach the indentation on the proximal end of the laryngoscope's blade to the bar of the handle. It will click into place when properly seated. To determine if the laryngoscope is functional, raise the blade to a right angle with the handle until it clicks into place (Figure 8-16). The light should turn on and be bright and steady. A yellow, flickering light will not sufficiently illuminate the anatomic structures. If the light fails to go on, the problem may be either dead batteries or a loose bulb. Every airway kit should include spare parts. Infrequently, the contact points or the wire that runs through the blade to the bulb will fail.

Like the handle, the blade may be reusable or disposable. Two common types of blades are the curved blade (Macintosh blade) and the straight blade (often re-

Align identificaton with bar, press-forward to lock

Press to lock

FIGURE 8-15 Engaging the laryngoscope blade and handle.

Elevate blade to a right angle

FIGURE 8-16 Activating the laryngoscope light source.

ferred to as the Miller, Miller-Abbott, Wisconsin, or Flagg blade). Laryngoscope blades range in size from 0 for infants to 4 for large adults (Figure 8-17).

The curved blade is designed to fit into the vallecula (Figure 8-18). When you lift its handle anteriorly, the blade elevates the tongue and, indirectly, the epiglottis, allowing you to see the glottic opening. Because the curved blade does not touch the larynx itself, it should not traumatize or stimulate the very sensitive gag receptors on the posterior surface of the epiglottis. The curved blade also permits more room for viewing and ETT insertion. The straight blade, on the other hand, is designed to fit under the epiglottis (Figure 8-19). When you lift its handle anteriorly, the blade directly lifts the epiglottis out of the way.

Which blade you use is largely a matter of individual preference, but you should be skilled with both in order to accommodate patients' anatomic differences. A straight blade is better for endotracheal intubation in infants, because it stabilizes their floppier epiglottises and provides greater displacement of their relatively larger tongues. It also is better for the occasional adult patient with a floppy epiglottis or large tongue.

FIGURE 8-17 Laryngoscope blades.

FIGURE 8-18 Placement of
Mcintosh blade into vallecula.

FIGURE 8-19 Placement of
Miller blade under epiglottis.

* ETT endotracheal tube.

Endotracheal Tubes The endotracheal tube (**ETT**) is a flexible, translucent tube open at both ends and available in lengths ranging from 12 cm to 32 cm, with centimeter markings along its length (Figure 8-20). The proximal end has a standard 15-mm inside diameter/22-mm outside diameter connector that attaches to the ventilatory device, usually a BVM. The ETT is available with internal tube diameters ranging from 2.5 mm to 4.5 mm (uncuffed) and from 5.0 mm to 9.0 mm (cuffed). The distal end has a beveled tip to facilitate smooth movement through airway passages. When present, an inflatable 5 ml–10 ml cuff at the distal end of ETT sizes from 5.0 mm to 9.0 mm provides a seal between the ETT and the trachea. A thin inflation tube runs the length of the main tube from the distal cuff to a syringe. A one-way valve at the proximal end of the inflation tube permits the syringe to push air into the distal cuff or pull it out, but prevents air from escaping the cuff when the syringe is removed. A pilot balloon at the infla-

FIGURE 8-20   ETT and syringe.

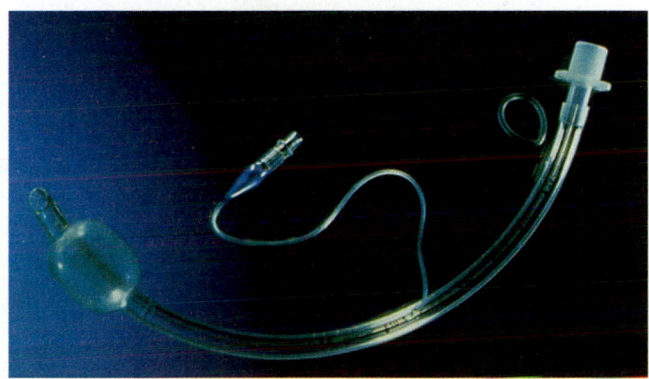

FIGURE 8-21   Endotrol ETT.

tion tube's proximal end, indicates whether the distal cuff is properly inflated. The pilot balloon should be partially inflated but soft, to avoid overinflating the distal cuff and inadvertently pressuring the tracheal mucosa. This could cause ischemia of the tracheal wall. Always check the distal cuff for leaks before insertion.

Suppliers typically prewrap an ETT in a curved shape. This is because the trachea lies anteriorly in the neck, and the tube must be directed upward to enter the glottic opening. On the Endotrol ETT, an O-shaped ring attaches to a plastic wire that runs the length of the tube and terminates distally (Figure 8-21). Pulling the ring bends the distal end of the tube upward and directs it into the glottic opening. This can facilitate placement of the tube without the need for a stylet.

Endotracheal tubes come in a variety of sizes. Markings on the tubes indicate their internal diameter in millimeters. The typical tube sizes for average-sized adult patients are 7.0–9.0 mm (females, 7.0–8.0 mm; males, 7.5–8.5 mm). A generally acceptable size for both male and female adults is 7.5 mm. (We discuss endotracheal intubation of children in detail later in this chapter.)

FIGURE 8-22 ETT, stylet, and syringe, unassembled.

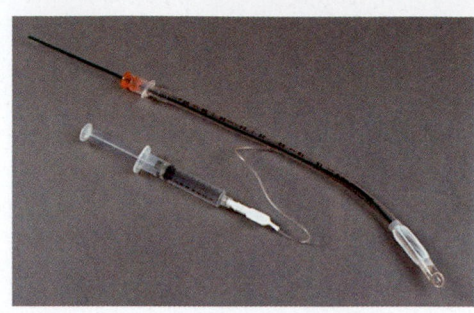

FIGURE 8-23 ETT, stylet, and syringe, assembled for intubation.

Stylet The malleable **stylet** is a plastic-covered metal wire used to direct the ETT anteriorly by bending its distal end into a J or hockey-stick shape (Figures 8-22 and 8-23). It is particularly useful in patients with extremely anterior laryngeal anatomy or those with short, fat necks with which head positioning can be difficult. Although using stylets is not mandatory, many paramedics prefer to use them in the prehospital setting because they afford greater control of the ETT. The wire stylet may damage tissues during intubation if it extends past the distal end of the ETT; therefore, you should keep it recessed at least 2 cm from the tip of the tube.

10 ml Syringe The syringe allows you to inflate the distal cuff just enough to avoid air leaks around the ETT without causing tracheal ischemia.

Tube–Holding Devices Tie-downs or tape secure the endotracheal tube once it is in the trachea. The reasons for securing the ETT are twofold. First, moving the patient about during resuscitation or transportation can easily dislodge the tube. Even if the ETT is not actually dislodged, its movement can still cause cardiovascular stimulation, an elevation in intracranial pressure, or injury to the tracheal mucosa. Second, the person providing ventilatory support may inadvertently push down on the ETT, forcing it into the right or left mainstem bronchus. Using tape requires extra care, as it can loosen when either the patient's face or the tube is moist. A number of commercial tube-holding devices are available.

FIGURE 8-24 Magill forceps.

Magill Forceps The **Magill forceps** are scissor-style clamps with circular tips. You will use them to remove foreign bodies or to redirect the endotracheal tube during nasotracheal intubation (Figure 8-24).

Lubricant Water-soluble lubricants facilitate inserting the ETT. Do not use petroleum-based lubricants; they may damage the ETT and cause tracheal inflammation.

Suction Unit A suction unit helps to remove secretions and foreign materials from the oropharynx during intubation attempts. It is a vital element that you must never forget. (We discuss suction units in more detail later in this chapter.)

End-Tidal CO$_2$ Detector or Other Confirmation Device These adjuncts to intubation are becoming the standard of care in most areas. You must be familiar with the devices, their role in intubation, and your local protocols' requirements for their use.

Additional Airways You should also have an oropharyngeal airway available during endotracheal intubation. You will occasionally use it as a block to prevent the patient from biting down on and collapsing the ETT.

Protective Equipment Endotracheal intubation, like many airway procedures, carries the risk of exposure to body substances. Because of this, it is essential to employ body substance isolation procedures. These include, but are not limited to, gloves, mask, protective eyewear, and possibly a gown. Remember, personal safety comes first!

Endotracheal Intubation Indications

Monitoring success rates for particular skills is not hard with an appropriate quality assurance program. Evaluating your ability to judge which patients you should intubate is considerably more difficult. Often the patient's condition may warrant trying nebulizer treatments or supplemental oxygen before deciding to intubate. A patient's continued distress and failure to respond to treatment clearly indicate intubation. In conjunction with the medical director, you are responsible for continually improving your judgement regarding the use of advanced airway management techniques. This includes recognizing subtle indicators that the patient's condition is worsening, before the onset of respiratory arrest.

Endotracheal intubation provides a definitive, secure, open airway for patients who are experiencing, or are likely to experience, upper airway compromise. Some of the indications for endotracheal intubation in these patients include respiratory or cardiac arrest; unresponsiveness without a gag reflex; inability to protect the airway, resulting in an increased risk of aspiration; obstruction due to foreign bodies, trauma, burns, or anaphylaxis. Endotracheal intubation also improves oxygenation and ventilation in patients with extreme lower airway difficulty. Some lower airway indications include severe respiratory distress due to diseases such as asthma, COPD, CHF, or pneumonia, as well as pneumothorax, hemothorax, or hemopneumothorax with respiratory difficulty. Clearly, then, endotracheal intubation may be indicated in breathing and apneic patients, though caution must be used in any patient with an intact gag reflex.

Do not attempt endotracheal intubation in the prehospital setting if epiglottitis is present, unless airway failure is imminent. Attempts to manipulate the airway in epiglottitis are very likely to result in vigorous laryngospasm. The most prudent management of epiglottitis is oxygenation of the patient without agitation. The preferred treatment for epiglottitis is rapid transport to the operating room for endotracheal intubation under more controlled conditions. This is carried out with the necessary equipment for emergency tracheostomy opened and ready for immediate use. Sometimes, these patients steadily worsen and loss of their airway is imminent and inevitable. In this case, the benefits from endotracheal intubation outweigh the risks. Regardless, the most experienced member of the crew should perform the procedure. Also, it is important to remember that there may be significant laryngeal edema and it may be necessary to insert a smaller than normal endotracheal tube. This should be kept in mind before undertaking this procedure. Always follow local protocols and contact medical direction regarding endotracheal intubation in cases where epiglottitis is present or suspected.

You are responsible for continually improving your judgement regarding airway management.

Content Review

ENDOTRACHEAL INTUBATION INDICATORS
- Respiratory or cardiac arrest
- Unconsciousness or obtusion without gag reflex
- Risk of aspiration
- Obstruction due to foreign bodies, trauma, burns, or anaphylaxis
- Respiratory *extremis* due to disease
- Pneumothorax, hemothorax, or hemopneumothorax with respiratory difficulty

Advantages of Endotracheal Intubation

- It isolates the trachea and permits complete control of the airway.
- It impedes gastric distention by channeling air directly into the trachea.
- It eliminates the need to maintain a mask seal.
- It offers a direct route for suctioning of the respiratory passages.
- It permits administration of the medications lidocaine, epinephrine, atropine, and naloxone via the endotracheal tube. (Use the mnemonic LEAN to remember these medications.)

Disadvantages of Endotracheal Intubation

- The technique requires considerable training and experience.
- It requires specialized equipment.
- It requires direct visualization of the vocal cords.
- It bypasses the upper airway's function of warming, filtering, and humidifying the inhaled air.

Complications of Endotracheal Intubation

Intubation presents a number of potential complications. Properly attending to detail and taking appropriate precautions will help you to avoid these problems.

Equipment Malfunction Equipment malfunctions consume valuable time when you are establishing a definitive airway and effective oxygenation and ventilation. Having a preassembled airway kit that is checked regularly will lessen the chances of this occurring. Ideally someone should check the airway kit daily to be sure that all needed supplies are present and that the bulb, batteries, and blade are in good working condition.

Teeth Breakage and Soft Tissue Lacerations Endotracheal intubation can injure the lips and teeth, but you can eliminate this hazard by carefully using the laryngoscope as an instrument, not a tool. When inserting the blade into the mouth and pharynx, guide it gently into place, avoiding pressure on the teeth. When manipulating the jaw anteriorly, use gentle traction upward and toward the feet rather than rotating and flexing your wrist, which will make the laryngoscope function as a lever. All levers require a fulcrum—and the only fulcrums available in your patient's mouth will be his upper incisors. A rotating/flexing action may thus break teeth. To avoid this hazard, lift the laryngoscope's handle (exposing the epiglottis) after you have applied the blade to the base of the tongue. After this, keep your wrist straight and do any lifting with your shoulder and arm.

If you use the laryngoscope too roughly, you can lacerate the patient's lips, tongue, or pharyngeal structures, producing profuse bleeding that is hard to control. This can also happen if you direct the tube away from midline into the pyriform sinuses or allow the stylet to protrude from the distal end of the ETT. In the larynx and lower airway, you might damage the vocal cords, cause laryngeal edema, or tear the trachea if you are not careful. A gentle technique and attention to detail are the keys to avoiding these complications.

Hypoxia Delays in oxygenation, either from interruption of basic airway techniques and BVM ventilation with 100% oxygen or from prolonged intubation attempts, can produce profound, life threatening hypoxia. Each patient's unique anatomy and unusual clinical situations can challenge even the most experienced

Content Review

COMPLICATIONS OF ENDOTRACHEAL INTUBATION

- Equipment malfunction
- Teeth breakage and soft tissue lacerations
- Hypoxia
- Esophageal intubation
- Endobronchial intubation
- Tension pneumothorax

paramedic. One basic rule that helps to avoid hypoxia during intubation is to limit each intubation attempt to no more than 30 seconds before reoxygenating the patient. To gauge this interval, some paramedics hold their breath from the time they stop ventilating the patient until they start again.

If you cannot pass the tube through the vocal cords on the first attempt, at least identify your landmarks and note any unique or difficult features that you may need to address. For example, too much edema might indicate a smaller ETT. Or the patient's larynx might be more anterior than you realized from his external anatomy, and you will need to use a different blade or change the ETT angle. You can then pass the tube on a subsequent attempt, after hyperventilating the patient with basic airway techniques and 100% oxygen using a BVM device.

Esophageal Intubation Misplacement of the ETT into the esophagus deprives the patient of oxygenation and ventilation. It is potentially lethal, resulting in severe hypoxia and brain death if you do not recognize it immediately. It also directs air into the stomach, encouraging regurgitation, which can lead to aspiration. Indicators of esophageal intubation include:

- An absence of chest rise and absence of breath sounds with mechanical ventilation
- Gurgling sounds over the epigastrium with each breath delivered
- Distention of the abdomen
- An absence of breath condensation in the endotracheal tube
- A persistent air leak, despite inflation of the tube's distal cuff
- Cyanosis and progressive worsening of the patient's condition
- Phonation (noise made by the vocal cords)
- No color change with colorimetric $ETCO_2$ detector
- A falling pulse oximetry reading

If you have any suspicion that the tube is in the esophagus, remove it immediately. Hyperventilate the patient with 100% oxygen and attempt endotracheal intubation with another tube.

Endobronchial Intubation If you pass the endotracheal tube successfully through the vocal cords and advance it too far, it likely will enter either the right or left mainstem bronchus. As discussed earlier, the ETT may be misplaced to either side, but it is more likely to pass into the right mainstem, which angles away from the trachea less acutely than does the left. In either case, the ETT ventilates only one lung and the result is hypoventilation and hypoxia from inadequate gas exchange. Also, when the bag-valve device **insufflates** enough air for two lungs into the smaller area of only one lung, it can create enough pressure to cause barotrauma such as a pneumothorax, worsening the patient's condition.

❋ **insufflate** to blow into.

You can avoid inserting the ETT too far by following these guidelines:

1. Advance the distal cuff no more than 1–2 cm past the vocal cords.
2. Once the tube is positioned, hold it in place with one hand to prevent it from being pushed any farther.
3. Inflate the cuff and firmly secure the tube in place with tape or a commercial tube-holding device.
4. Note the number marking on the side of the ETT where it emerges from the patient's mouth at the teeth, gums, or lips. This will allow you to quickly recognize any changes in tube placement.

Approximate ETT depth for the average adult is 21 cm at the teeth for women and 23 cm at the teeth for men, though this will vary.

Findings in endobronchial intubation include:

- Breath sounds present on one side of the chest but diminished or absent on the other
- Poor compliance (resistance to ventilations with the bag-valve device)
- Cyanosis, cardiac dysrhythmias, or other evidence of hypoxia

To resolve the problem, loosen or remove any securing devices and withdraw the ETT until breath sounds are present and equal bilaterally. Be certain to deflate the cuff when pulling back on the ETT.

Tension Pneumothorax Any tear in the lung parenchyma can cause a pneumothorax. If this is allowed to progress untreated, a tension pneumothorax, an accumulation of air or gas in the pleural cavity, may develop. A tension pneumothorax is a large pneumothorax that affects other structures in the chest. The expanding tension pneumothorax will adversely affect the other lung, the heart, and the structures of the mediastinum. It will eventually displace these structures away from the side of the chest with the tension pneumothorax. In addition to mainstem bronchus intubation, tension pneumothorax can result if you use too much of the bag-valve device's volume on a small adult or child or use the full bag-valve-device volume against diseased lungs with poor compliance. Tension pneumothorax is marked by progressively worsening compliance (more difficulty in ventilating), diminished unilateral breath sounds, hypoxia with hypotension, and distended neck veins. Often the trachea will deviate away from the side of the chest with the pneumothorax. Also, the marked increase in intrathoracic pressure resulting from the tension pneumothorax can prevent the ventricles from adequately filling. This can cause a decrease in cardiac output and will worsen the patient's overall condition. If you suspect tension pneumothorax, needle decompression of the chest is indicated, as described in Chapter 25 on thoracic trauma.

Orotracheal Intubation

The most widely preferred and, therefore, the most commonly used path for endotracheal intubation is the orotracheal route. Many medical personnel favor this route because it involves direct visualization of the vocal cords and a clear view of the ETT's passage through them. It is thus the most accurate method of intubation and the least likely to induce trauma to the airway. To perform orotracheal intubation in the absence of suspected trauma (Procedure 8-1):

1. Place the patient supine.
2. After using basic manual and adjunctive airway maneuvers to open the airway and ventilate, hyperventilate the patient with 100% oxygen.
3. While your partner ventilates the patient, prepare your intubation equipment, including suction, and be certain that all needed equipment is present and in good working order. Assemble and check the laryngoscope blade and handle to be certain you have a steady, bright light—then close the handle. Insert the stylet into the ETT, making sure to keep the distal end of the stylet at least 2 cm proximal to the distal tip of the ETT. You may choose to bend the

8-1a   Hyperventilate the patient.

8-1b   Prepare the equipment.

8-1c   Apply Sellick's maneuver and insert laryngoscope.

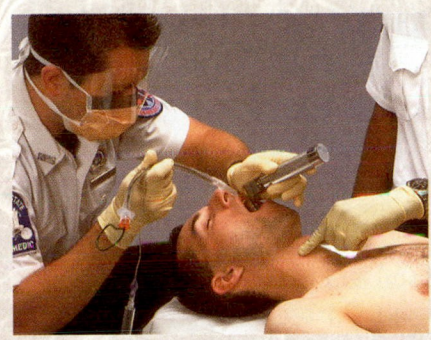

8-1d   Visualize the larynx and insert the ETT.

8-1e   Inflate the cuff, ventilate, and ausculatate.

8-1f   Confirm placement with an ETCO$_2$ detector.

8-1g   Secure the tube.

8-1h   Reconfirm ETT placement.

distal end of the ETT into a "hockey stick" shape just proximal to the distal cuff to help direct the ETT anteriorly. Apply water-soluble lubricant to the distal end of the ETT and reinsert. Leaving the ETT partially in its packaging until you are ready to insert it helps to keep it as clean as possible. Fill the 10 ml syringe with 5 ml to 10 ml of air and attach it to the valve at the proximal end of the ETT, using a twisting motion to lock it in place. Check the cuff for air leaks.

4. Turn on the suction and attach an appropriate tip.

5. Position the patient's head and neck. Remove any dentures or partial dental plates. To visualize the larynx, you must align the three axes of the mouth, the pharynx, and the trachea. To do this, place the patient's head in a "sniffing position" by flexing the neck forward and the head backward. Inserting a rolled towel or sheet under the patient's shoulders or the back of the head may help. Establishing this position is extremely difficult in patients with short, fat necks or whose motion is limited by such conditions as arthritis.

6. Hold the laryngoscope in your left hand whether you are right- or left-handed. Most laryngoscopes are designed for right-handed people; that is, the right-handed person must hold the laryngoscope in his left hand in order to manipulate the endotracheal tube with his right.

7. If you have not already done so, have your partner apply Sellick's maneuver (cricoid pressure) and maintain it until you confirm ETT placement in the trachea.

8. Insert the laryngoscope blade gently into the right side of the patient's mouth. With a gentle sweeping action, displace the tongue to the left. This pushes the tongue out of your line of vision and allows more room to manipulate the endotracheal tube.

9. Move the blade slightly toward the midline. Advance the Macintosh (curved) blade until the distal end is at the base of the tongue in the vallecula; advance the Miller (straight) blade until the distal end is under the epiglottis. As you advance the blade, move the patient's lower lip away from the blade using the index finger of your right hand.

10. Lift the laryngoscope handle slightly upward and toward the feet to displace the jaw. Be careful not to put pressure on the teeth. At this point, you can see any vomitus, blood, or secretions in the posterior pharynx. You likely will have to suction the airway clear. If the secretions are thick or copious, you may need to remove the suction tip and use the suction hose.

11. Upon lifting the jaw, determine if the laryngoscope blade is in proper position. You may need to adjust it before you can visualize the vocal cords. If you cannot see landmarks clearly, gently withdraw the blade, slowly and slightly. This may bring the vocal cords into view. If it does not, you might need to gently advance the blade farther into the hypopharynx.

12. Keeping your left wrist straight, use your left shoulder and arm to continue lifting the mandible and tongue to a 45° angle to the ground (up and toward the feet) until the glottis is exposed (Figure 8-25). Often you may not see the entire glottis, but you should see at least its posterior third or half. If the larynx lies anteriorly, a slight increase in your partner's pressure on the Sellick's maneuver should improve your view of the vocal cords.

FIGURE 8-25 Glottis visualized through laryngoscopy.

Occasionally, your partner will need to lessen the cricoid pressure slightly to allow you to visualize the vocal cords. Be ready to instruct him to apply more or less cricoid pressure.

13. Hold the ETT in your right hand with your fingertips as you would a dart or a pencil; this gives you control to gently maneuver the ETT. Advance the tube through the right corner of the patient's mouth, and direct it toward the midline.

14. Directly visualizing the vocal cords, pass the ETT gently through the glottic opening until its distal cuff disappears beyond the vocal cords; then advance it another 1–2 cm.

15. Hold the tube in place with your hand to prevent its displacement; do not let go under any circumstance until it is taped or tied securely in place. Attach a bag-valve device to the 15/22-mm connector on the tube; have the ETCO$_2$ detector attached to the bag-valve device as your local protocols require.

16. Inflate the distal cuff with 5–10 ml of air. To avoid tracheal trauma or ischemia from excessive cuff pressure, apply only enough pressure to prevent air leakage around the ETT during ventilation. Listen for any air leak and adjust the cuff's pressure as needed. When cuff pressure is correct, remove the syringe, using a twisting motion to prevent any air leak.

17. Check for proper tube placement. While listening for equal bilateral breath sounds over the chest, watch to see that the chest rises and falls symmetrically. Listen over the epigastrium to be certain you hear no gastric sounds. Look for moisture condensation in the exhaled breath; it should appear in the ETT during each exhalation.

18. Hyperventilate the patient with 100% oxygen. Gently insert an oropharyngeal airway to serve as a bite block.

19. Secure the ETT with umbilical tape, while maintaining ventilatory support. Loop the tape around the tube at the level of the patient's teeth, attaching it tightly to the tube without kinking or pinching it. Then wrap the tape around the patient's head, and tie it at the side of his neck. Alternatively, use a commercial tube-holding device.

20. Repeat step 17 periodically to confirm proper ETT placement. Also repeat step 17 after any major patient movement or movement of his head or neck. (Neck manipulation can displace the tube up to 5 cm.) Continue to support the tube manually while maintaining ventilatory support.

Verification of Proper Endotracheal Tube Placement Continuously checking and rechecking tube placement is an important responsibility during endotracheal intubation. The hypervigilance with which you must monitor the patient's clinical condition cannot be overemphasized. You can employ a number of methods in the field to confirm correct ETT placement. You should put them to maximum use, but do not become overly reliant on technology. The patient's clinical condition should be the deciding factor in your patient management decisions.

The most reliable method of confirming proper ETT placement is direct visualization of its passage through the vocal cords. This requires the proper use of a laryngoscope and continued visualization of the vocal cords throughout intubation. If you do this, you have little chance of inadvertently intubating the esophagus.

The hypervigilance with which you must monitor the patient's clinical condition cannot be overemphasized.

Following ETT placement, watch to be sure that the patient's chest rises with ventilations. If the ETT is misplaced in the esophagus, the chest will not rise. You also should auscultate for breath sounds. Their equal presence over both sides (apices and bases) of the chest and their absence over the epigastrium helps to confirm proper ETT placement. Conversely, their absence over the chest and their presence over the epigastrium indicates an esophageal intubation. Breath sounds present on one side but absent or diminished on the other indicate that the ETT may be advanced too deeply into one of the mainstem bronchi, that bronchial obstruction may be present, or that a pneumothorax is present. Absent breath sounds bilaterally may indicate esophageal intubation.

End-tidal CO_2 detectors and esophageal detector devices can be helpful. Adequate levels of exhaled carbon dioxide, as detected by an end-tidal CO_2 detector, confirm proper endotracheal tube placement. The ability to withdraw air readily from an esophageal detector device's syringe further confirms placement of the ETT in the trachea. Resistance to air withdrawal, or the creation of a vacuum, denotes esophageal intubation.

Also observe the endotracheal tube's contents. Exhaled air approaches 100% humidity. Usually, the ambient relative humidity is less than 100%. Thus, condensation inside the ETT suggests its proper placement. Because the gastric sphincter relaxes in critically ill patients and the high pressures of a bag-valve mask create gastric distention, patients frequently vomit and aspirate during resuscitation. If you misplace the ETT into the esophagus, you may observe an efflux of gastric contents through the ETT, particularly with subsequent ventilation attempts. Because aspiration into the trachea also may have occurred, you might see vomitus in the ETT even with proper endotracheal intubation; nonetheless, this finding always should raise suspicion of esophageal intubation and prompt further investigation.

It is important to assure proper endotracheal tube placement. Allegations of improperly placed endotracheal tubes are a major reason for paramedic malpractice suits. Because of this, it is important to verify *and document* proper endotracheal tube placement. In fact, it is ideal to verify and document at least three different indicators of proper placement. These may include:

- Visualization of the tube passing between the cords
- Presence of bilateral breath sounds
- Absence of breath sounds over the epigastrium
- Positive end-tidal CO_2 change on an $ETCO_2$ device
- Verification of endotracheal placement by an esophageal detector device
- Presence of condensation inside the endotracheal tube
- Absence of vomitus inside the endotracheal tube
- Absence of phonation, or vocal sounds, once the tube is placed

In addition, an increase in the oxygen saturation will help support proper placement of the endotracheal tube. Likewise, a rise and fall of the chest indicates endotracheal intubation. Worsening gastric distention may indicate possible esophageal placement. Any gastric distention should be investigated. Remember, though, it is not uncommon for gastric distention to develop prior to endotracheal intubation due to mechanical ventilation. Even in experienced hands, it is very difficult to avoid gastric distention with mechanical ventilation until an endotracheal tube is placed.

Transillumination Intubation Since a bright light in the trachea is visible (transilluminates) through the soft tissue of the anterior neck, an ETT with a lighted

FIGURE 8-26 Lighted stylet for endotracheal intubation.

stylet can facilitate correct intubation (Figure 8-26). The stylet is a plastic cable with a malleable, retractable wire running through its center and a small, high-intensity bulb at its distal end. An on-off switch and power supply at the stylet's proximal end control the bulb, which begins to blink about 30 seconds after it is turned on. This blinking makes detecting the light's transilluminations easier.

You can confirm correct ETT placement by observing the stylet's light through the anterior neck's soft tissue; esophageal intubation results in little or no light being visible. Because you can place the ETT safely and correctly without directly visualizing the glottic opening, you can perform endotracheal intubation without manipulating a trauma patient's head and neck. Several studies have shown the transillumination technique to be fast, dependable, and atraumatic.

This technique's biggest limitation is that bright ambient light can make the transillumination difficult to see. Therefore, it works best in a darkened room and with thin patients. When attempting this procedure, reduce ambient light; in direct or bright daylight, shade the patient's neck.

To perform transillumination intubation:

1. While maintaining ventilatory support, hyperventilate the patient with 100% oxygen.

2. Prepare and check your equipment. The endotracheal tube's diameter should be 7.5–8.5 mm. You will need to cut the ETT to a length of 25–27 cm to accommodate the stylet. Place the stylet in the ETT and lock the ETT in place at its proximal end. Using the sliding mechanism on the handle, adjust the stylet and bend it into a hockey-stick shape just proximal to the distal cuff.

3. With the patient supine and his head in neutral position, kneel along either his right or left side, facing his head.

4. Turn on the stylet light.

5. With your index and middle fingers inserted deeply into the patient's mouth and your thumb under his chin, lift his tongue and jaw forward (Figure 8-27).

6. With the proximal end of the ETT directed toward the patient's feet, insert the tube/stylet into the mouth and advance it gently through the oropharynx into the hypopharynx.

FIGURE 8-27 Insertion of
lighted stylet/ETT.

FIGURE 8-28 Lighted stylet/ETT in position.

7. Use a "hooking" action with the tube/stylet to lift the epiglottis
   out of the way (Figure 8-28).
8. When you see a circle of light at the patient's Adam's apple, the
   stylet is placed correctly (Figure 8-29). A diffuse, dim, hard-to-see,
   or absent light indicates that the ETT/stylet combination is in the

Tube stat

FIGURE 8-29   Transillumination of a lighted stylet.

esophagus. A bright light lateral and superior to the Adam's apple indicates that it has moved into the right or left pyriform fossa. To correct either of these placements, withdraw the tube and reattempt intubation after ventilating the patient with 100% oxygen for several minutes, using proper basic manual and adjunct airway maneuvers.

9. After the ETT is properly placed, hold the stylet stationary. Advance the tube off the stylet into the larynx approximately 1–2 cm, while simultaneously retracting the internal wire from the stylet using the O-ring at its proximal end.

10. Once the light is in the correct position and you have partially advanced the ETT while partially retracting the stylet wire, hold the tube firmly in place with one hand and remove the stylet.

11. Attach the bag-valve device to the endotracheal tube's 15/22 mm connector and deliver several breaths, inflating the distal ETT cuff and checking for proper placement as usual.

12. Secure the ETT, recheck placement, and maintain ventilatory support. Continue periodic assessment of the airway.

FIGURE 8-30   Blind orotracheal intubation by digital method.

Digital Intubation Some situations may require you to perform digital intubation. This technique dates to the eighteenth century, when people performed intubations without the benefit of a laryngoscope. Instead, they used digital (finger), or tactile (touch), intubation (Figure 8-30).

Digital intubation is still useful for a number of situations in the prehospital setting. It is suggested when a patient is deeply comatose or in cardiac arrest and when proper positioning is difficult. The classic example is an unresponsive trauma patient with a suspected cervical spine injury. Since the digital technique does not require manipulation of the head and neck, it is of great value here. It may also be useful in extrication situations where the confined space prevents properly positioning the patient. Also, because digital intubation does not require visualization, it may be helpful when facial injuries distort the patient's anatomy or when you cannot suction copious amounts of blood, vomitus, or other secretions for a proper view of the airway.

Digital intubation is risky for the paramedic; it may stimulate even a deeply comatose patient to clamp down and bite your finger. Do not use it with conscious patients or with unconscious patients who have a gag reflex. To perform digital intubation:

1. Use blood and body fluid precautions.
2. While maintaining ventilatory support with basic manual and adjunctive airway maneuvers, hyperventilate the patient with 100% oxygen.
3. Prepare and check your equipment. You will need the following items: an appropriately sized ETT, a malleable stylet, water-soluble lubricant, a 5–10 ml syringe, a bite block, and umbilical tape or a commercial anchoring device. Insert the stylet into the endotracheal tube and bend the ETT/stylet into a J shape.

FIGURE 8-31   Digital intubation. Insert your middle and index fingers into the patient's mouth.

4. While another team member stabilizes the patient's head and neck in an in-line (neutral) position, kneel at the patient's left shoulder, facing his head. Place a bite block device between the patient's molars to help protect your fingers.

5. Insert your left middle and index fingers into the patient's mouth (Figure 8-31). By alternating fingers, "walk" your hand down the midline while simultaneously tugging gently forward on the tongue. You may also use gauze to hold and extend the tongue more effectively, which may facilitate palpation of the glottis. This lifts the epiglottis up and away from the glottic opening, within reach of your probing fingers.

6. Palpate the arytenoid cartilage posterior to the glottis and the epiglottis anteriorly with your middle finger (Figure 8-32). Press the epiglottis forward, and insert the endotracheal tube into the mouth, anterior to your fingers (Figure 8-33).

7. Advance the tube, pushing it gently with your right hand. Use your left index finger to keep the tip of the ETT against your middle finger. This will direct the tip to the epiglottis.

8. Use your middle and index fingers to direct the tip of the ETT between the epiglottis (in front) and your fingers (behind). Then with your right hand advance the ETT through the cords while simultaneously maneuvering it forward with your left index and middle fingers. This will prevent it from slipping posteriorly into the esophagus.

9. Hold the tube in place with your hand to prevent its displacement. Attach a bag-valve device with an $ETCO_2$ detector to the 15/22-mm connector on the ETT; inflate the distal cuff with 5–10 ml of air; check for proper tube placement.

FIGURE 8-32 Digital intubation. Walk your fingers and palpate the patient's epiglottis.

FIGURE 8-33 Digital intubation—insertion of the ETT.

534

10. Hyperventilate the patient with 100% oxygen. Gently insert an oropharyngeal airway to serve as a bite block. Secure the ETT with umbilical tape. Repeat steps to confirm proper ETT placement and maintain ventilatory support. Continue your airway assessment periodically.

Trauma Patient Intubation Airway management and ventilatory support in the trauma patient are essential for a successful outcome. Appropriate treatment of all other injuries is meaningless if you do not assure a patent airway and adequate oxygenation and ventilation.

The trauma patient presents a number of obstacles to effective airway management and ventilation. Some of them may be the need for extrication, blood in the oropharynx, distorted anatomy due to injury, and the need to protect the cervical spine. Getting an adequate seal on a mask is very difficult when the patient is being extricated or has significant facial trauma. You must keep the cervical spine in a neutral, in-line position throughout your management of all patients with known or suspected cervical spine trauma. Digital intubation, transillumination intubation, and nasotracheal intubation (described later in this chapter) provide potential solutions for some patients when trauma complicates airway management, but visualizing the vocal cords is still preferable. You can do this effectively using direct laryngoscopy-assisted orotracheal intubation with manual in-line stabilization of the cervical spine (Procedure 8-2).

To perform orotracheal intubation with in-line stabilization:

1. After basic manual and adjunctive airway maneuvers, have your partner maintain in-line stabilization while kneeling at the patient's side, facing his head. This is done by placing both hands over the patient's ears with the little, ring, and middle fingers under the occiput, the index fingers anterior to the ears, and the thumbs on the face over the maxillary sinuses.

2. Apply slight pressure in a caudal direction (toward the feet) to support and immobilize the head.

3. Proceed gently with orotracheal intubation, remembering the need to minimize movement of the cervical spine.

Rapid Sequence Intubation Your most immediate concern with every patient you treat is to maintain a patent airway and adequate oxygenation and ventilation. Clearly, if a patient is in cardiac or respiratory arrest, or is unconscious or obtunded and not protecting his airway, endotracheal intubation is indicated. Quite commonly, however, you may have an awake patient, perhaps with significantly altered mental status, who is hypoxic even on 100% oxygen because of respiratory distress or a worsening airway disorder. This patient is working his hardest to breathe but does not have adequate gas exchange to support life. His altered mental status indicates that some level of significant hypoxia is putting essential brain functions at risk.

You cannot perform orotracheal intubation on this patient until he fatigues enough to have respiratory failure, with resultant unconsciousness and decreased muscle tone. By then, however, he will have suffered prolonged hypoxia, possibly accompanied by a myocardial infarction, brain damage, or vomiting with aspiration. If a patient clearly is precipitously failing maximal aggressive medical management, or if the history of his problem clearly indicates that he will not be able to or already cannot protect his airway, then active intervention is appropriate to control the airway and provide adequate ventilation. The safest way to do this is an advanced airway procedure called rapid sequence intubation or **rapid sequence intubation** (RSI). Classic rapid sequence induction is an anesthetic procedure

Appropriate treatment of a trauma patient's other injuries is meaningless if you do not assure a patent airway and adequate oxygenation and ventilation.

* **rapid sequence intubation** giving medications to sedate (induce) and temporarily paralyze a patient and then performing orotracheal intubation.

8-2a Hyperventilate the patient and apply manual C-spine stabilization.

8-2b Apply Sellick's maneuver and intubate.

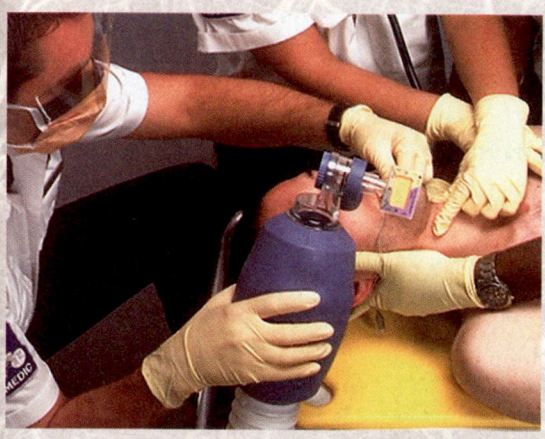

8-2c Ventilate the patient and confirm placement.

8-2d Secure the ETT and place a cervical collar.

8-2e Reconfirm placement.

whereby patients rapidly receive induction of general anesthesia followed by endotracheal intubation. In emergency medicine, we do not administer general anesthesia, but we have borrowed other elements of this technique in order to rapidly obtain an airway in a patient who has altered mental status. While the term *rapid sequence induction (RSI)* describes the classic procedure, it has been modified in the emergency medicine setting *to rapid sequence intubation (RSI)*. Again, the difference is that the latter does not utilize a general anesthetic agent.

Rapid sequence intubation involves preoxygenating the patient to the best level possible given his condition, carefully monitoring him, and giving medications to induce (sedate) and temporarily paralyze him. You then proceed with orotracheal intubation in a controlled manner. Patients who are candidates for RSI are either awake, responsive, agitated, or combative, or have a significant gag reflex, clenched teeth, or too much airway muscle tone to allow intubation. Indications for RSI intubation include:

- Impending respiratory failure due to intrinsic pulmonary disease such as COPD, CHF, asthma, or pneumonia
- Acute airway disorder that threatens airway patency such as facial burns, laryngeal or upper airway trauma, and epiglottitis
- Altered mental status with significant risk of vomiting and aspiration, as in head trauma (a Glasgow Coma Score of 8 or less), drug or alcohol intoxication, status epilepticus

The basic physiology involved in rapid sequence induction centers around the neuromuscular junction—the connection between peripheral nerves and skeletal muscle. Nerve impulses travel down the nerve and release a chemical (neurotransmitter) which stimulates (depolarizes) skeletal muscle, resulting in contraction. Acetylcholine is the primary neurotransmitter, and blocking its action results in relaxation of skeletal (voluntary) muscle. There are two ways to block the neuromuscular junction. Depolarizing agents substitute themselves into the neuromuscular junction in place of acetylcholine. They have a stimulating effect as they work, which produces fasciculations (generalized involuntary muscle twitching). Succinylcholine is a depolarizing agent, and is the most commonly used paralytic agent for RSI. Nondepolarizing agents block the uptake of acetylcholine and do not allow stimulation of the muscle. Thus they do not cause fasciculations. Vecuronium, atracurium, and pancuronium are typical examples of nondepolarizing neuromuscular blocking agents.

Paralyzing the patient causes complete muscular relaxation and allows you to take control of his precarious clinical condition. In addition to paralyzing the airway muscles, these agents also immobilize the respiratory muscles, so the patient becomes apneic and requires mechanical ventilation. Esophageal and stomach muscles, and therefore sphincter tone, also relax, posing the risk of vomiting and aspiration. Succinylcholine (Anectine), the agent preferred for neuromuscular blockade in emergency medical care, is a depolarizing drug. As mentioned, it causes fasciculations just before initiating paralysis. These fasciculations may increase the tendency to vomit and may increase intracranial pressure. Conditions that elevate serum potassium preclude the use of succinylcholine, which transiently increases serum potassium, and thus can lead to life-threatening hyperkalemia. Side effects, which are dose related, include bradycardia and other dysrhythmias, as well as hypertension. The guidelines for using succinylcholine include:

- Dose: 1.5 mg/kg, IV bolus in adults; 2.0 mg/kg, IV bolus in children less than 10 years old
- Onset of action: 60–90 seconds

Succinylcholine is the preferred neuromuscular blocking agent for emergency RSI.

Content Review

COMMON PARALYTIC AGENTS

- Succinycholine
- Vecuronium
- Atracurium
- Pancuronium

- Duration: 3–5 minutes
- Contraindications: penetrating eye injuries, patients with burns greater than eight hours' duration, massive crush injuries, and neurologic injuries greater than one week out

Vecuronium (Norcuron) is a nondepolarizing agent; thus, it does not cause fasciculations. It is generally the second-line paralytic when succinylcholine is contraindicated, because it has fewer cardiac and hypotensive side effects than other nondepolarizing agents. In much smaller doses as a premedication, or priming dose, to succinylcholine or to a paralyzing dose of vecuronium it effectively lessens or prevents fasciculations. It also blunts succinylcholine's bradycardic effect. This priming (or premedication) dose is given two minutes before the paralytic agent. Guidelines for using vecuronium include:

- Dose: 0.15 mg/kg IV bolus (paralyzing)
        0.01 mg/kg IV bolus (priming)
- Onset: 2–3 minutes
- Duration: 45 minutes

Atracurium (Tracrium) is a nondepolarizing paralytic useful for patients with kidney or liver disease because these conditions do not prolong its duration. Some patients experience hypotension from the histamine release that this drug causes. The usual dosage of 0.5 mg/kg IV has a duration of 20–30 minutes.

Pancuronium (Pavulon) is a nondepolarizing paralytic that has been used frequently in the past. The advantage of its relatively rapid onset (3–5 minutes), is offset by its major disadvantage, a long (60-minute) duration. It also produces tachycardia due to its effects on the heart. Better agents are currently available.

If you cannot intubate a paralyzed patient he has no definitive airway. You must ventilate him mechanically for the duration of the paralysis (assuming you can mechanically maintain a patent airway). If the airway is lost during the procedure, you must be prepared to initiate a surgical airway (cricothyrotomy). Nothing works as fast as succinylcholine or is of as short a duration; therefore, it is the preferred neuromuscular blocking agent for emergency RSI.

Neuromuscular blocking agents do not affect mental status or pain sensation; therefore, you must use sedating and amnestic drugs to ease the awake, aware patient's anxiety and discomfort and to decrease his gag reflex, thereby increasing patient compliance and enhancing the ease of intubation. If the patient is already obtunded (from a drug overdose or head injury, for example), sedating him is pointless; omit that step. If the patient's injuries are causing significant pain and his clinical condition does not contraindicate their use, give small doses of pain medications as indicated.

When hypovolemia is present or when significant trauma is present with hypotension or a strong likelihood for hypotension, avoid induction agents that cause hypotension. Agents that blunt ICP response are good choices for the patient with head injury. Table 8-1 details general guidelines for common sedative (induction) agents. If you are able to identify that the patient has an allergy or sensitivity to a particular agent, you should not administer that agent.

Two other agents, atropine and lidocaine are appropriate for use as premedication agents in RSI, if indicated. Table 8-2 outlines their use.

Most patients with emergent airway conditions have eaten or drunk something within a few hours before the onset of their emergency conditions. Thus, you should consider every emergency patient to have a full stomach and be at risk

Table 8-1   GUIDELINES FOR SEDATIVE (INDUCTION) AGENTS

Induction Agent	Dose	Onset	Duration (min)	Advantages	Disadvantages
Midazolam (Versed)	0.1–0.3 mg/kg	1–3 min.	20–30 min.	Amnesia effects, good sedative	Hypotension
Diazepam (Valium)	0.2–0.5 mg/kg	2–3 min.	30–40 min.	Amnesia effects	Hypotension, respiratory depression
Etomidate (Amidate)	0.3 mg/kg	1–2 min.	5 min.	Little affect on blood pressure, decreases intracranial pressure (ICP)	Suppresses cortisol → not good for head injured patients
Ketamine (Ketalar)	1–2 mg/kg	≤ 1 min.	10–20 min.	Decreases bronchospasm, little hypotension, amnesia	Increases ICP
Sodium Thiopental	3–5 mg/kg	≤ 1 min.	5 min.	Blunts ICP changes	Significant hypotension, bronchospasm
Propofol (Diprivan)	1–1.5 mg/kg	≤ 1 min.	3–5 min.	Rapid onset, good sedative effects	Significant hypotension
Fentanyl	3–5 mcg/kg	1–2 min.	30–40 min.	Little affect on blood pressure; blunts ICP changes	Can cause muscle rigidity in chest wall

Table 8-2   ALTERNATIVE SEDATIVE (INDUCTION) AGENTS

Agent	Dose	Indication	Contraindication Precaution
Atropine	0.01-0.02 mg/kg (min.–max./0.1–0.4)	Pediatric patients, bradycardia	Cannot give less than 0.1 mg
Lidocaine	1 mg/kg	Head injury	Allergy

of vomiting and aspiration. This is another reason why you should expediently intubate the patient after the onset of paralytic effect and **apnea**. Remember to always have a working suction device at the patient's side during airway maneuvers. Likewise, application of Sellick's maneuver will help prevent aspiration.

    To perform rapid sequence intubation:

1. Preoxygenate the patient with 100% oxygen using basic manual and adjunctive maneuvers, and using a bag-valve mask if indicated.

2. Prepare your equipment, supplies, and patient. In addition to the usual intubation equipment, be certain you have at least one, and preferably two, secure and working IV lines. Place the patient on a cardiac monitor and pulse oximeter. Draw the appropriate doses of medications into syringes and label them.

3. If the patient is alert, administer a sedative (induction) agent, such as midazolam (Versed) prior to administering any neuromuscular blocking agents.

4. Apply Sellick's maneuver (cricoid pressure) and maintain until you confirm proper ETT placement.

✳ **apnea** temporary stop in breathing

5. Per local protocols, consider premedicating the patient with a priming dose of vecuronium. This is especially important in children, where fasiculations from succinylcholine can cause musculoskeletal trauma. Also, if indicated in local protocols, consider premedicating with lidocaine and atropine.

6. Paralyze the patient, administering succinylcholine 1.5 mg/kg IV bolus and continue oxygenation. Alternatively, vecuronium (Norcuron) can be used as a blocking agent. It has a slower onset of action.

7. Once adequate relaxation is obtained, insert the ETT through the patient's vocal cords at the onset of apnea and jaw relaxation, using the orotracheal intubation procedure previously explained. Because you have preoxygenated the patient, BVM ventilation is generally not indicated before the first intubation attempt, unless prolonged. Not ventilating the patient at this juncture will help prevent gastric distention and regurgitation. If you are unable to pass the tube after 20–30 seconds, stop, hyperventilate the patient with 100% oxygen for two minutes, and then try again. Remember that the patient's lower esophageal sphincter tone is decreased, so ventilating during paralysis makes gastric distention and vomiting more likely, even with cricoid pressure. Your goal is to rapidly place the ETT properly in the trachea to minimize these complications, but do not avoid BVM hyperventilation with 100% oxygen in the hypoxic patient.

8. Confirm proper placement of the ETT into the trachea. Inflate the distal cuff, ventilate with a bag-valve device with a CO_2 detector attached, and look for the appropriate color change. Watch for the chest to rise and fall with ventilations. Auscultate with each ventilation for bilateral breath sounds over the chest and no gastric sounds over the stomach.

9. Release Sellick's maneuver.

10. Insert a bite block device, secure the ETT in place, reconfirm placement, and continue ventilating the patient. Continually assess the patient's condition and recheck ETT placement.

11. Check with medical direction or follow your local protocol for indications for continuing paralysis with vecuronium during transport. This will depend largely on your patient's medical condition and combativeness after the paralytic and induction agent wear off, as well as on your anticipated transport time to the hospital.

Pediatric Intubation

Pediatric airway emergencies generally produce more anxiety than adult emergencies among both medical care providers and family. It is important to take appropriate steps to separate the parent from the pediatric patient with significant respiratory distress or apnea in order to effectively manage the airway. While the indications, procedures, and precautions for airway management in children are fundamentally the same as in adults, you must take additional precautions and remember several significant differences. These concerns revolve around variances in anatomy, as discussed in Chapter 3. To review the anatomical features of the pediatric airway:

- The structures are proportionally smaller and more flexible than an adult's.
- The tongue is larger in relation to the oropharynx.
- The epiglottis is floppy and round ("omega" shaped).

- The glottic opening is higher and more anterior in the neck.
- The vocal cords slant upward, toward the back of the head, and are closer to the base of the tongue.
- The narrowest part of the airway is the cricoid cartilage, not the glottic opening as in adults.

A straight laryngoscope blade is preferred for most pediatric patients, although straight or curved may be useful for adolescents. Also, selecting the appropriate tube diameter for children is critical. Too large a tube can cause tracheal edema and/or damage to the vocal cords, while too small a tube may not allow exchange of adequate ventilatory volumes. Table 8-3 lists general guidelines for selecting ETT size according to the child's age. Another guide for children's sizes is:

$$\text{ETT size (mm)} = (\text{Age in years} + 16) \div 4$$

Correct tube size for an eight-year-old, for instance, would be $(8 + 16) \div 4$, or 6 mm. You can also measure tube size by matching it to the diameter of the child's smallest finger. Usually you will use noncuffed endotracheal tubes with infants and children under the age of eight years, because the round narrowing of these patients' cricoid cartilage forms a suitable cuff.

The depth of insertion of the distal tip for pediatric endotracheal tubes should be 2–3 cm below the vocal cords, as deeper insertion may result in mainstem intubation or injury to the carina. The uncuffed ETT has a black glottic marker at its distal end that should be placed at the level of the vocal cords. The cuffed ETT should be placed so that the cuff is just below the vocal cords. For detailed guidelines regarding depth of insertion for different age groups, refer to Table 8-3. Alternately, you can use the formula $(3 \times \text{ETT inside diameter}) - 1$.

Also remember that infants and small children have greater vagal tone than adults. Therefore, laryngoscopy and passage of an endotracheal tube are more likely to precipitate a vagal response, dramatically slowing the child's heart rate and decreasing cardiac output and blood pressure. To guard against this complication, you must monitor heart rate throughout the procedure, and you may give atropine (0.02 mg/kg, 0.1 mg minimum) IV bolus. If heart rate falls below 60 beats per minute (or below 80 beats per minute in an infant), stop the procedure and reinitiate ventilations with 100% oxygen.

The indications for endotracheal intubation in a pediatric patient are the same as those for adults:

- Ventilatory support with a bag-valve mask is inadequate.
- Cardiac or respiratory arrest.

Table 8-3 APPROXIMATE SIZE OF ETT FOR PEDIATRICS

Patient's Age	ETT Size	Type	Depth of ETT Insertion	Laryngoscope Blade Size
Premature infant	2.5–3.0	Uncuffed	8 cm	0 straight
Full-term infant	3.0–3.5	Uncuffed	8–9.5 cm	1 straight
Infant to one year	3.5–4.0	Uncuffed	9.5–11 cm	1 straight
Toddler	4.0–5.0	Uncuffed	11–12.5 cm	1–2 straight
Preschool	5.0–5.5	Uncuffed	12.5–14 cm	2 straight
School age	5.5–6.5	Uncuffed	14–20 cm	2 straight
Adolescent	7.0–8.0	Cuffed	20–23 cm	3 straight or curved

8-3a   Hyperventilate the child.

8-3b   Position the head.

8-3c   Insert the laryngoscope.

8-3d   Insert the ETT and ventilate the child.

8-3e   Confirm placement and secure the ETT.

- It is necessary to provide a route for drug administration (LEAN) or ready access to the airway for suctioning.
- Prolonged artificial ventilation is needed.

Additionally, if local protocols allow, you may use endotracheal intubation in a child with epiglottitis if his condition is rapidly deteriorating.

To perform endotracheal intubation on a pediatric patient (Procedure 8-3):

1. After initiating basic manual and adjunctive maneuvers, hyperventilate the patient with 100% oxygen, using the appropriately-sized BVM.

2. Prepare and check your equipment. As stated earlier, a straight blade laryngoscope is usually preferred in infants and small children, since it provides greater displacement of the tongue and better visualization of the relatively cephalad and anterior epiglottis. Also, with children younger than eight years old, use an uncuffed endotracheal tube. Due to the short distance between the mouth and the trachea, you rarely need a stylet to position the tube properly. Remember to lubricate the ETT with water-soluble gel.

3. Place the patient's head and neck in an appropriate position. You should maintain a pediatric patient's head in a sniffing position (perhaps by placing a towel under his head), unless you know of or suspect trauma. In case of trauma, proceed with manual in-line stabilization of the cervical spine.

4. Have your partner apply gentle cricoid pressure (Sellick's maneuver).

5. Hold the laryngoscope in your left hand and insert it gently into the right side of the patient's mouth. With a sweeping action, displace the tongue to the left.

6. Move the blade slightly toward the midline, and then advance it until the distal end reaches the base of the tongue.

7. Look for the tip of the epiglottis, and position the laryngoscope properly. Keep in mind that a child—particularly an infant—has a shorter airway and a higher glottis than an adult. Because of this, you may see the cords much sooner than you expect.

8. If you cannot see the glottis, bring the blade gently and slowly out until the vocal cords fall into view. Lift the epiglottis gently with the tip of the laryngoscope. Be certain not to use the teeth or gums as a fulcrum.

9. Grasp the endotracheal tube in your right hand and, under direct visualization of the vocal cords, insert it through the right corner of the patient's mouth into the glottic opening. Pass it through until the distal 10 mm or distal cuff of the ETT disappears 2 cm–3 cm beyond the vocal cords. In some cases, advancing an endotracheal tube will be difficult at the level of the cricoid. Do not force the ETT through this region, as it may cause laryngeal edema and bleeding.

10. Hold the tube in place with your left hand, and attach an infant- or child-size bag-valve device to the 15/22 mm connector and deliver several breaths, checking for proper tube placement. Watch for the chest to rise and fall symmetrically with each ventilation. Auscultate for equal, bilateral breath sounds at the lateral chest wall, high in the axilla. Breath sounds over the epigastrium should be absent with ventilations. The patient should improve clinically,

with pinker color and increased heart rate. Additionally, use the end-tidal CO_2 detector as previously discussed.

11. If the tube has a distal cuff, inflate it with just enough air to prevent any air leaks.

12. Secure the ETT with tape or a commercial device as with an adult patient, note placement of distance marker at teeth/gums, recheck for proper placement, and continue ventilatory support. Periodically reassess ETT placement, and watch the patient carefully for any clinical signs of difficulty. As with the adult patient, allow no more than 30 seconds to pass without ventilating your patient.

NASOTRACHEAL INTUBATION

* **nasotracheal route** through the nose and into the trachea.

The orotracheal route is usually preferred for intubation as it affords more control over the airway. In a few circumstances, however, the **nasotracheal route** (through the nose and into the trachea) may be useful. As a rule this is a "blind" procedure without direct visualization of the vocal cords. To perform nasotracheal intubations, you can often visualize the vocal cords with a laryngoscope and guide the ETT with Magill forceps. But if this is possible, orotracheal intubation is generally feasible and preferred. Potential indications for blind nasotracheal intubation include:

- Possible spinal injury
- Clenched teeth, preventing opening the patient's mouth
- Fractured jaw, oral injuries, or recent oral surgery
- Significant angioedema (facial and airway swelling)
- Obesity
- Arthritis, preventing placement in the sniffing position

Nasotracheal intubation is not recommended in the following situations:

- Suspected nasal fractures
- Suspected basilar skull fractures
- Significantly deviated nasal septum or other nasal obstruction
- Cardiac or respiratory arrest
- Unresponsive patient

Advantages of Nasotracheal Intubation When the patient's condition indicates its use, nasotracheal intubation offers the following advantages:

- The head and neck can remain in neutral position.
- It does not produce as much gag response and is better tolerated by the awake patient.
- It can be secured more easily than an orotracheal tube.
- The patient cannot bite the ETT.

Disadvantages of Nasotracheal Intubation The following disadvantages of nasotracheal intubation discourage its use unless clearly indicated by the patient's condition:

- It is more difficult and time-consuming to perform than orotracheal intubation.
- It is potentially more traumatic for patients. Passage of the tube may lacerate the pharyngeal mucosa or larynx during insertion.

FIGURE 8-34 Blind nasotracheal intubation.

- The tube may kink or clog more easily than an orally placed endotracheal tube.
- It poses a greater risk of infection, because the ETT introduces nasal bacteria into the trachea.
- Improper placement is more likely when performing blind nasotracheal intubation, as the tube's passage through the glottic opening cannot be visualized.
- Blind nasotracheal intubation requires that the patient be breathing.

Nasotracheal Intubation Technique To perform blind nasotracheal intubation (Figure 8-34):

1. Using basic manual and adjunctive maneuvers, open the airway and ventilate the patient with 100% oxygen.
2. Prepare your equipment and place the patient supine. If you suspect cervical spine injury, maintain the head and neck in neutral position with manual in-line stabilization.
3. Inspect the nose and select the larger nostril as your passageway.
4. Apply topical anesthesia with Hurricaine spray or topical lidocaine.
5. Insert the ETT into the nostril, with the bevel along the floor of the nostril or facing the nasal septum. This will help avoid damage to the turbinates. Next, gently guide the ETT from anterior to posterior.
6. As you feel the tube drop into the posterior pharynx, listen closely at its proximal end for the patient's respiratory sounds. These sounds are loudest when the ETT is proximal to the epiglottis. When the ETT's tip reaches the posterior pharyngeal wall, you must take care to direct it toward the glottic opening. At this

point, the tip of the ETT may catch in the pyriform sinus. If it does, you will feel resistance, and the skin on either side of the Adam's apple will tent. To resolve pyriform sinus placement, slightly withdraw the ETT and rotate it to the midline.

7. With the patient's next inhaled breath, advance the ETT gently but quickly into the glottic opening. Continue passing the ETT until the distal cuff is just past the vocal cords. At this point, the patient may cough, buck, or strain. Gagging or vocal sounds are signs of esophageal placement, while slight bulging and anterior displacement of the larynx usually indicate correct tracheal placement. When you place the ETT correctly in the trachea, you will see the patient's exhaled air as condensation in the ETT and feel it coming from the proximal end of the ETT.

8. Holding the ETT with one hand to prevent displacement, inflate the distal cuff with 5–10 ml of air, connect a bag-valve device with an $ETCO_2$ detector attached, hyperventilate the patient with 100% oxygen, and confirm proper placement of the ETT. Observe the chest rise and fall with ventilations, auscultate breath sounds over the chest bilaterally, and verify no gastric sounds with each ventilation.

9. Secure the ETT and reconfirm proper placement. Continue to observe the patient's condition, maintain ventilatory support, and frequently recheck ETT placement.

Field Extubation

Infrequently, an intubated patient will awaken and be intolerant of the ETT. This happens most often with respiratory distress patients who undergo rapid sequence intubation. When the paralytic medications wear off and they awaken from the induction medications, they may struggle against the intubation and ventilation. This usually indicates sedation and, perhaps, repeat paralysis, as extubation will cause continued respiratory distress with loss of a definitive airway. If the patient is clearly able to maintain and protect his airway and accomplish adequate spontaneous respirations and is not under the influence of any sedating agents, and if reassessment indicates the problem that led to endotracheal intubation is resolved, extubation may be indicated. However, you must consider the high risk of laryngospasm, involuntary closure of the glottis, upon extubation, especially in the awake patient. Laryngospasm may prohibit successful reintubation attempts. Additionally, in repeat attempts at rapid sequence intubation the medications will produce variable responses and do not ensure relaxation of the laryngospasm. The need for field extubation is extremely rare.

To perform field extubation:

1. Continue blood and body fluid precautions. Ensure patient's oxygenation. A crude method for accomplishing this in the field is to be certain that the patient's mental status, skin color, and pulse oximetry are optimal on room air with the ETT in place.

2. Prepare intubation equipment and suction.

3. Confirm patient responsiveness.

4. Suction the patient's oropharynx.

5. Deflate the ETT cuff.

6. Remove the ETT upon cough or expiration.

7. Provide supplemental oxygen as indicated.

8. Reassess the adequacy of the patient's ventilation and oxygenation.

FIGURE 8-35 ETC airway—
tracheal placement.

ESOPHAGEAL TRACHEAL COMBITUBE

The **Esophageal Tracheal CombiTube** (ETC) is a dual-lumen airway with a ventilation port for each **lumen.** The longer, blue port is the distal port; the shorter, clear port is the proximal port, which terminates in the hypopharynx. The ETC has two inflatable cuffs—a 15-ml cuff just proximal to the distal port and a 100-ml cuff just distal to the proximal port.

It is inserted blindly through the mouth into the posterior oropharynx and then gently advanced. Upon insertion one port enters the trachea and the other enters the esophagus (Figures 8-35 and 8-36). To determine which port has entered the trachea and is to be ventilated, first ventilate the longer external port, since esophageal insertion is highly likely. Now auscultate the chest. If you hear breath sounds over the chest and none over the stomach, continue ventilating through the longer external port. If you hear ventilation sounds over the stomach without breath sounds over the chest, stop ventilating through the longer port and attach the bag-valve device to the shorter port. The distal cuff isolates the distal port, and the larger proximal cuff isolates the proximal port, encouraging air that is insufflated into the hypopharynx to enter the trachea.

Advantages of the Esophageal Tracheal CombiTube

- It provides alternate airway control when conventional intubation techniques are unsuccessful or unavailable.

✳ **Esophageal Tracheal CombiTube** dual-lumen airway with a ventilation port for each lumen.

✳ **lumen** the tunnel through a tube.

Content Review

INTUBATION DEVICES

- Endotracheal tube (ETT)
- Esophageal CombiTube (ETC)
- Laryngeal mask airway (LMA)
- Phyrngo-tracheal lumen airway (PtL)
- Esophageal gastric tube (EGTA)
- Esophageal obturator airway (EOA)

FIGURE 8-36 ETC airway—esophageal placment.

- Insertion is rapid and easy.
- Insertion does not require visualization of the larynx or special equipment.
- The pharyngeal balloon anchors the airway behind the hard palate.
- The patient may be ventilated regardless of tube placement (esophageal or tracheal).
- It significantly diminishes gastric distention and regurgitation.
- It can be used on trauma patients, since the neck can remain in neutral position during insertion and use.
- If the tube is placed in the esophagus, gastric contents can be suctioned for decompression through the distal port.

Disadvantages of the Esophageal Tracheal CombiTube

- Suctioning tracheal secretions is impossible when the airway is in the esophagus.
- Placing an endotracheal tube is very difficult with the ETC in place.
- It cannot be used in conscious patients or in those with a gag reflex.

- The cuffs can cause esophageal, tracheal, and hypopharyngeal ischemia.
- It does not isolate and completely protect the trachea.
- It cannot be used in patients with esophageal disease or caustic ingestions.
- It cannot be used with pediatric patients.
- Placement of the CombiTube is not foolproof—errors can be made if assessment skills are not adequate.

Inserting the Esophageal Tracheal CombiTube

To insert the Esophageal Tracheal CombiTube:

1. Complete basic manual and adjunctive maneuvers and provide supplemental oxygen and ventilatory support with a bag-valve mask and hyperventilation.
2. Place the patient supine and kneel at the top of his head.
3. Prepare and check the equipment.
4. Place the patient's head in neutral position. Stabilize the cervical spine if cervical injury is possible.
5. Insert the ETC gently at midline through the oropharynx, using a tongue-jaw-lift maneuver, and advance it past the hypopharynx to the depth indicated by the markings on the tube. The black rings on the tube should be between the patient's teeth.
6. Inflate the pharyngeal cuff with 100 ml of air and the distal cuff with 10–15 ml of air.
7. Ventilate through the longer blue proximal port with a bag-valve device connected to 100% oxygen, while auscultating over the chest and stomach. If you hear bilateral breath sounds over the chest and none over the stomach, secure the tube and continue ventilating.
8. If you hear gastric sounds over the chest instead of breath sounds, change ports and ventilate through the clear connector. Confirm breath sounds over the chest with no gastric sounds. Use multiple confirmation techniques as previously discussed (visualize, auscultate, use $ETCO_2$ detector, monitor clinical improvement).
9. Secure the tube and continue ventilating with 100% oxygen.
10. Frequently reassess the airway and adequacy of ventilation.

LARYNGEAL MASK AIRWAY

The **laryngeal mask airway** (LMA) may assist with ventilations in the unconscious patient without laryngeal reflexes when tracheal intubation is unsuccessful. It has an inflatable distal end (similar to a face mask) which is placed in the hypopharynx and then inflated (Figure 8-37). A bag-valve device at the proximal end assists respirations (similar to an endotracheal tube). The laryngeal mask airway can be disposable and comes in various sizes. Its blind insertion requires less skill and training than endotracheal intubation. The laryngeal mask airway's disadvantage is that it does not isolate the trachea; therefore, it does not protect the airway from regurgitation and aspiration. Also, it cannot be used in a patient who has a gag reflex or is semiconscious. You must weigh these disadvantages against the benefits of establishing a patent airway.

FIGURE 8-37 Laryngeal Mask Airway.

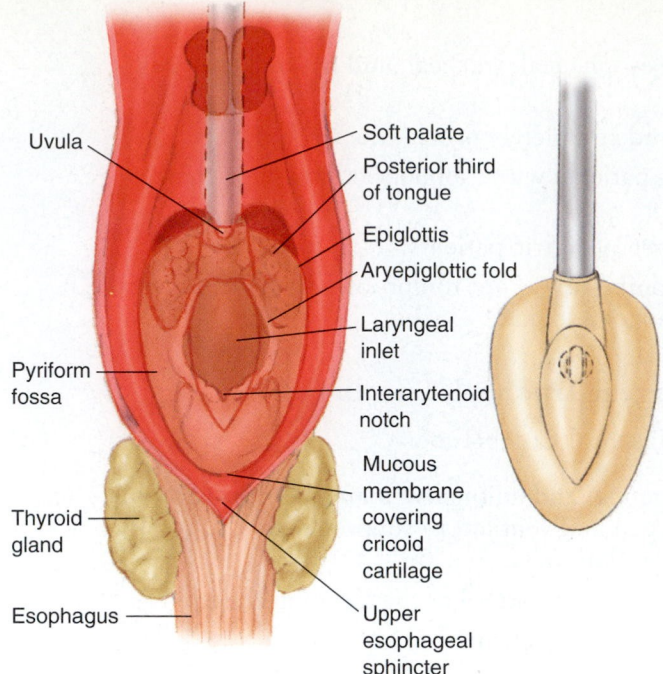

FIGURE 8-38 Pharyngo-tracheal lumen airway.

PHARYNGO-TRACHEAL LUMEN AIRWAY

* pharyngo-tracheal lumen airway (PtL) is a two tube system.

The **pharyngo-tracheal lumen airway** (PtL) is a two-tube system (Figure 8-38). The first tube is short, with a large diameter; its proximal end is green. A large cuff encircles the tube's lower third. When inflated, the cuff seals the entire oropharynx. Air introduced at this tube's proximal end will enter the hypo-pharynx. The second tube is long, with a small diameter, and clear. It passes through and extends approximately 10 cm beyond the first tube. This second tube may be inserted blindly into either the trachea or the esophagus. A distal cuff, when inflated, seals off whichever anatomical structure the tube has entered. When the second tube enters the trachea, you will ventilate the patient through it.

Each of the PtL's tubes has a 15/22 mm connector at its proximal end, allowing the attachment of a standard ventilatory device. A semi-rigid plastic stylet in the clear plastic tube allows redirection of the oropharyngeal cuff while the other cuff remains inflated. An adjustable, cloth neck strap holds the tube in place. When the long, clear tube is in the esophagus, deflating the cuff in the oropharynx allows you to move the device to the left side of the patient's mouth. This may permit endotracheal intubation while continuing esophageal occlusion. However, placement of an endotracheal tube with a PtL already in place is difficult at best.

Advantages of the Pharyngo-Tracheal Lumen Airway

- It can function in either the tracheal or esophageal position.
- It has no face mask to seal.
- It does not require direct visualization of the larynx and, thus, does not require the use of a laryngoscope or additional specialized equipment.
- It can be used in trauma patients, since the neck can remain in neutral position during insertion and use.
- It helps protect the trachea from upper airway bleeding and secretions.

Disdvantages of the Pharyngo-Tracheal Lumen Airway

- It does not isolate and completely protect the trachea from aspiration.
- The oropharyngeal balloon can migrate out of the mouth anteriorly, partially dislodging the airway.
- Intubation around the PtL is extremely difficult, even with the oropharyngeal balloon deflated.
- It cannot be used in conscious patients or those with a gag reflex.
- It cannot be used in pediatric patients.
- It can only be passed orally.

Inserting the Pharyngo-Tracheal Lumen Airway

To insert the pharyngo-tracheal lumen airway:

1. Complete basic manual and adjunctive maneuvers and provide supplemental oxygen and ventilatory support with a BVM and hyperventilation.
2. Place the patient supine and kneel at the top of his head.
3. Prepare and check the equipment.
4. Place the patient's head in the appropriate position. Hyperextend the neck if there is no risk of cervical spine injury. Maintain neutral position with stabilization of the cervical spine if cervical spine injury is possible.
5. Insert the PtL gently, using the tongue-jaw-lift maneuver.
6. Inflate the distal cuffs on both PtL tubes simultaneously with a sustained breath into the inflation valve.
7. Deliver a breath into the green oropharyngeal tube. If the patient's chest rises and you auscultate bilateral breath sounds, the long

clear tube is in the esophagus. Inflate the pharyngeal balloon and continue ventilations via the green tube.

8. If the chest does not rise and you auscultate no breath sounds, the long clear tube is in the trachea. Remove the stylet from the clear tube and ventilate the patient through that tube.

9. Attach the bag-valve device to the 15 mm connector, secure the tube, and continue ventilatory support with 100% oxygen.

10. Multiple placement confirmation techniques are again essential, as are good assessment skills. Misidentification of placement has been reported. Frequently reassess the airway and adequacy of ventilation.

If the patient regains consciousness or if the protective airway reflexes return, remove the PtL. It is best to remove the PtL before endotracheal intubation.

Complications of PtL placement include:

- Pharyngeal or esophageal trauma from poor technique
- Unrecognized displacement of the long tube from the trachea into the esophagus
- Displacement of the pharyngeal balloon

ESOPHAGEAL GASTRIC TUBE AIRWAY AND ESOPHAGEAL OBTURATOR AIRWAY

Although clearly better devices have made them obsolete, the esophageal gastric tube airway and esophageal obturator airway are still available in some areas. Our discussion is intended solely to familiarize you with these devices. They both stimulate the gag reflex, so you must use them only for patients with no gag reflex. Both can cause esophageal rupture. They can be inserted with the head in neutral position.

The esophageal gastric tube airway (EGTA) is a hollow tube. A cuff just proximal to the distal, open port blocks air to the esophagus. The EGTA is inserted into the esophagus, with ventilation via the attached, inflatable mask through air holes at the level of the hypopharynx. A second port on the face mask allows you to extend a gastric tube through the distal port into the stomach for decompression of contents. If the gastric tube enters the trachea, the airway and gastric suction ports on the mask are not interchangeable.

The esophageal obturator airway (EOA) is a hollow tube with a closed end and a distal cuff intended to block air from the esophagus. It is inserted into the esophagus, with ventilation via an attached face mask through air holes at the level of the hypopharynx. The EOA does not allow gastric suctioning, and improper placement in the trachea introduces a closed tube into the airway.

Contraindications to EOA insertion are:

- Age less than 16 years
- Height less than 5 feet or more than 6 feet, 7 inches
- Possible ingestion of caustic poisons
- History of esophageal disease or alcoholism.

FOREIGN BODY REMOVAL UNDER DIRECT LARYNGOSCOPY

Direct visualization of the larynx with a laryngoscope may enable you to remove an obstructing foreign body using Magill forceps or a suction device (Figure 8-39). Initially, you should carry out basic life support maneuvers for airway obstruction, in-

FIGURE 8-39   Foreign body removal with direct visualization and Magill forceps.

cluding the Heimlich maneuver, finger sweep, and chest thrust. As you recall from your basic training, the Heimlich maneuver involves initiating a forceful upward thrust with your fist on the choking patient's abdomen, halfway between the umbilicus and the xiphoid process. Use suction as indicated. If these fail to alleviate the obstruction, direct visualization of the airway for foreign body removal is indicated. The procedure for visualizing the airway is identical to that used for orotracheal intubation.

SURGICAL AIRWAYS

With proper training and frequent practice, including the use of rapid sequence intubation procedures, you will be able to secure most airways in the field by endotracheal intubation. Occasionally, however, extreme circumstances prohibit successful endotracheal intubation. In these situations, performing a surgical airway technique may be the only way to ensure your patient's survival. Two different techniques, **needle cricothyrotomy** (also called translaryngeal cannula ventilation) and **open cricothyrotomy,** both provide access to the airway through the cricothyroid membrane. A needle cricothyrotomy, is generally the easier procedure but makes providing adequate ventilation more difficult; an open cricothyrotomy is the more difficult procedure but allows for more effective oxygenation and ventilation.

You should use surgical airway procedures only after you have exhausted your other airway skills and have decided that no other means will establish

✳ **needle cricothyrotomy** surgical airway technique that inserts a 14-gauge needle into the trachea at the cricothyroid membrane.

✳ **open cricothyrotomy** surgical airway technique that places an endotracheal or tracheostomy tube directly into the trachea through a surgical incision at the cricothyroid membrane.

an airway. Even when performed correctly, these procedures are highly invasive and prone to complications which you must recognize and treat immediately. The major long-term complication, tracheal **stenosis,** can cause difficulty if the patient requires intubation at some point in the future. You must
master the skills for performing surgical airways and continually practice
them under the direct supervision of the physician medical director, who
should determine that you can perform the technique and that you understand
and can treat its possible complications.

Indications that warrant a surgical cricothyrotomy include problems that
prevent intubating or ventilating a patient by the nasal or oral routes. Massive
facial or neck trauma is the most common cause. Some cases involve so much
facial or airway distortion that you cannot identify normal landmarks. Other
indications of a surgical cricothyrotomy include total upper airway obstruction
due to epiglottitis, severe anaphylaxis, burns to the face and respiratory tract,
posterior laceration of the tongue, or the inability to open the mouth. You can
perform surgical airways with the patient's head and neck in neutral position.
Contraindications to performing surgical airways in the field include inability to
identify anatomical landmarks (including trauma and short, fat necks), crush
injury to the larynx, tracheal transection, and underlying anatomical abnormalities such as trauma, tumor, or subglottic stenosis.

Needle Cricothyrotomy

*The only indication for a
surgical airway is the inability
to establish an airway by any
other method.*

Though it is an invasive surgical procedure that you must master before performing it in the field, a needle cricothyrotomy is technically easier to accomplish
than an open cricothyrotomy and has a lower complication rate. It can be rapidly performed, does not manipulate the cervical spine, and provides adequate
ventilation when performed properly. It is a temporary airway, used until a larger
diameter, definitive airway is provided. It does not interfere with subsequent
intubation attempts because it uses a 14-gauge needle, which has a relatively
small diameter so that an ETT can pass beside it. However, because the catheter
does not fill the tracheal diameter, needle cricothyrotomy cannot protect the
patient against aspiration.

This procedure requires different oxygenation and ventilation techniques
than other airway maneuvers. Transtracheal jet insufflation (ventilation) uses
a high-pressure jet ventilator to force oxygen through the small-diameter
catheter and provide adequate oxygenation and ventilation. Because very high
pressures insufflate large volumes of oxygen, **barotrauma,** including pneumothorax, is a potential complication. This procedure is not indicated if
exhalation is not possible or if adequate high-pressure ventilation equipment
is not available.

Needle Cricothyrotomy Complications The potential complications of needle
cricothyrotomy with jet ventilation include:

- Barotrauma from overinflation
- Excessive bleeding due to improper catheter placement
- Subcutaneous emphysema from improper placement into the
  subcutaneous tissue, excessive air leak around the catheter, or
  laryngeal trauma
- Airway obstruction from compression of the trachea secondary to
  excessive bleeding or subcutaneous air
- Hypoventilation from use of improper equipment, incorrect use of
  the jet ventilator, or misplacement of the catheter

FIGURE 8-40 Anatomical landmarks for cricothyrotomy.

Hyoid bone

Epiglottis

Thyroid gland

Thyroid cartilage

Cricothyroid membrane

Cricoid cartilage

Trachea

FIGURE 8-41 Locate/palpate the cricothyroid membrane.

Needle Cricothyrotomy Technique To perform needle cricothyrotomy with jet ventilation:

1. Place the patient supine and hyperextend the head and neck (maintain neutral position if you suspect cervical spine injury). Position yourself at the patient's side. Manage the patient's airway with basic maneuvers and supplemental oxygen, and prepare your equipment.

2. Gently palpate the inferior portion of the thyroid cartilage and the cricoid cartilage. The indention between the two is the cricothyroid membrane (Figures 8-40 and 8-41).

3. Prepare the anterior neck with povidone-iodine swabs. Firmly grasp the laryngeal cartilages and reconfirm the site of the cricothyroid membrane.

4. Attach a large-bore IV needle, with a catheter (adults: 14- or 16-gauge; pediatrics: 18- or 20-gauge) to a 10 or 20 ml syringe. Carefully insert the needle into the cricothyroid membrane at midline, directed 45° caudally (towards the feet) (Figure 8-42). Often you will feel a pop as the needle penetrates the membrane.

FIGURE 8-42   Proper positioning for cricothyroid puncture.

FIGURE 8-43   Advance the catheter with the needle.

5. Advance the needle no more than 1 cm, then aspirate with the syringe. If air returns easily, the catheter is in the trachea. If blood returns or you feel resistance to return, reevaluate needle placement. After you confirm proper placement, hold the needle steady and advance the catheter. Then withdraw the needle (Figure 8-43).

6. Reconfirm placement by again withdrawing air from the catheter with the syringe. Secure the catheter in place (Figure 8-44).

FIGURE 8-44 Cannula properly placed in the trachea.

FIGURE 8-45 Jet ventilation with needle cricothryrotomy.

7. Check for adequacy of ventilations. Look for chest rise with each ventilation, and listen for bilateral breath sounds in the chest. If spontaneous ventilations are absent or inadequate, begin transtracheal jet ventilation.

8. Connect one end of the oxygen tubing to the catheter and the other end to the jet ventilator.

9. Open the release valve to introduce an oxygen jet into the trachea (Figure 8-45). Then adjust the pressure to allow adequate lung expansion (usually about 50 psi, compared with about 1 psi through a regulator).

10. Watch the chest carefully, turning off the release valve as soon as the chest rises. Exhalation then occurs passively through the

glottis, due to elastic recoil of the lungs and chest wall. Deliver at least 20 breaths per minute to insure adequate oxygenation and ventilation. The inflation-to-deflation time ratio should be approximately 1:2, as with normal respirations. Keep in mind that you may need to adjust this to the patient's needs, particularly in COPD and asthma patients, who often require a longer expiration time.

11. Continue ventilatory support, assessing for adequacy of ventilations and looking for the development of any potential complications.

Open Cricothyrotomy

An open cricothyrotomy is preferred to needle cricothyrotomy when a complete obstruction prevents a glottic route for expiration. Indications are the same as for needle cricothyrotomy. It involves obtaining an airway by placing an endotracheal or tracheostomy tube directly into the trachea through a surgical incision at the cricothyroid membrane. It can be rapidly performed and does not manipulate the cervical spine. Its greater potential complications mandate even more training and skills monitoring than with the needle method.

Contraindications are the same as for needle cricothyrotomy. Additionally, open cricothyrotomy is contraindicated in children under the age of 12 because the cricothyroid membrane is small and underdeveloped.

Cricothyrotomy Complications Complications that can occur with this invasive procedure include:

- Incorrect tube placement into a false passage
- Cricoid and/or thyroid cartilage damage
- Thyroid gland damage
- Severe bleeding
- Laryngeal nerve damage
- Subcutaneous emphysema
- Vocal cord damage
- Infection

Open Cricothyrotomy Technique To perform an open cricothyrotomy (Procedure 8-4):

1. Locate the thyroid cartilage and the cricoid cartilage. Find the cricothyroid membrane between the two cartilages.
2. Clean the area with iodine-containing solution if time permits, while your partner sets up suction, pulse oximetry, and cardiac monitor.
3. Stabilize the cartilages with one hand, while using a scalpel in the other hand to make a 1 to 2 cm vertical skin incision over the membrane.
4. Find the cricothyroid membrane again and make a 1 cm incision in the horizontal plane through the membrane, avoiding nearby veins and arteries, as well as the recurrent laryngeal nerve.
5. Insert curved hemostats into the membrane incision and spread it open.

8-4a Locate the cricothyroid membrane.

8-4b Stabilize the larynx and make a 1–2 cm skin incision over cricothyroid membrane.

(continued)

8-4c   Make a 1 cm horizontal incision through the cricothyroid membrane.

8-4d   Using a curved hemostat, spread the membrane incision open.

8-4e   Insert an ETT (6.0) or Shiley (6.0).

8-4f   Inflate the cuff.

8-4g   Confirm placement.

8-4h   Ventilate.

8-4i   Secure the tube, reconfirm placement, and evaluate the patient.

6. Insert either a cuffed endotracheal tube (6.0-mm or 7.0-mm) or tracheostomy tube (6 or 8 Shiley), directing the tube into the trachea.

7. Inflate the cuff and ventilate.

8. Confirm placement with auscultation, end-tidal CO_2 detector, and chest rise.

9. Secure the tube in place.

We cannot stress enough that you must continuously practice this skill with the medical director's involvement before you are allowed to perform it.

MANAGING PATIENTS WITH STOMA SITES

Often patients who have had a laryngectomy (removal of the larynx) or tracheostomy (surgical opening into the trachea) breathe through a **stoma,** an opening in the anterior neck that connects the trachea with the ambient air. These patients frequently have tracheostomy tubes, which consist of an inner and outer cannula, in place to keep the soft tissue stoma open (Figure 8-46).

✳ **stoma** opening in the anterior neck that connects the trachea with ambient air.

FIGURE 8-46 Tracheostomy cannulae.

A patient with a stoma often has problems with excessive secretions. A laryngectomy produces a less effective cough, making it more difficult to clear secretions. If these secretions organize, they form a mucous plug that can occlude the stoma and, thus, the airway. A stoma apparatus generally has a fixed outer portion and an inner cannula. The inner cannula can be easily removed and cleaned, then replaced. Timely replacement of the outer cannula is important if it must also be removed, because the stoma can constrict within just a few hours to prohibit its replacement without dilation.

As the external stoma site narrows, so can the inner tracheal diameter; either can produce potentially life-threatening stenosis. Any acute inflammation that leads to soft tissue swelling can worsen this by further reducing the stoma and tracheal diameter. Further, this stenosis may make the cannula very difficult or impossible to replace. In this case, choose the largest diameter ETT that will pass through the stoma to maintain the airway before complete obstruction occurs. Lubricate the ETT, instruct the patient to exhale, and gently insert the ETT to about 1–2 cm beyond the distal cuff. Inflate the cuff, then confirm comfort, patency, and proper placement. Be certain to suspect and check for improper placement into the surrounding subcutaneous tissue, which will produce a false lumen. Subcutaneous emphysema as well as the lack of clinical improvement in the patient, indicates a false lumen.

You must use extreme caution with any suctioning, as this process can itself cause soft tissue swelling. In order to suction, begin by preoxygenating the patient with 100% oxygen. Inject 3 ml sterile saline down the trachea through the stoma. Instruct the patient to exhale, then gently insert the catheter until resistance is met. While the patient coughs or exhales, suction the airway during withdrawal of the catheter.

When the patient with a stoma requires ventilatory assistance, the bystander may use the mouth-to-stoma technique, while rescue personnel will generally use a BVM device. If you use the mouth-to-stoma technique, it is preferable to use a pocket mask to cover the stoma for protection from communicable disease. For either technique, locate the stoma site and expose it. Obtain a tight seal around the stoma site, and check for adequate ventilation. Be sure to seal the mouth and nose if you note air leaking from these sites.

Timely replacement of a stoma device's outer cannula is important because the stoma can constrict within just a few hours to prohibit its replacement without dilation.

SUCTIONING

Anticipating complications when managing airways is the key for successful outcomes. You must be prepared to **suction** all airways in order to remove blood or other secretions and for the patient to vomit. Suctioning equipment must be readily available for all patients, to prevent a simple vomiting episode from becoming a complicated aspiration episode that increases the patient's risk for greater morbidity or mortality.

* suction to remove with a vacuum-type device.

SUCTIONING EQUIPMENT

Many different suctioning devices are available. They may be handheld, oxygen-powered, battery-operated, or mounted (nonportable). To suit the prehospital environment, your equipment should be lightweight, portable, durable, generate a vacuum level of at least 300 mmHg when the distal end is occluded, and allow a flow rate of at least 30 liters per minute when the tube is open. In addition to a portable device, the ambulance should have a mounted, vacuum-powered suction device that can generate stronger suction and can be a backup device in case of equipment failure. The most commonly used suction catheters are either

Table 8-4 TYPES OF SUCTIONING CATHETERS

Hard/rigid catheter	Soft catheters
A large tube with multiple holes at the distal end	Long, flexible tube; smaller diameter than hard-tip catheters
Suctions larger volumes of fluid rapidly	Cannot remove large volumes of fluid rapidly
Standard size	Various sizes
Used in oropharyngeal airway only	Can be placed in the oropharynx, nasopharynx, or down the endotracheal tube
Removes larger particles	Suction tubing without catheter (facilitates suctioning of large debris)

hard/rigid catheters ("Yankauer" or "tonsil tip") or soft catheters ("whistle tip"). Table 8-4 summarizes their differences.

Because suctioning reduces a patient's access to oxygen, you should limit each attempt to 10 seconds. If possible, hyperventilate the patient with 100% oxygen before and after each effort. Clear any fluids from the upper airway first, as assisted breathing may cause aspiration. Do not apply suction while inserting the catheter. Apply suction only as you withdraw the catheter after properly positioning it.

Complications of suctioning are related to hypoxia from prolonged suctioning attempts without proper ventilation. The decrease in myocardial oxygen supply can cause cardiac dysrhythmias. Suctioning can also stimulate the vagus nerve, causing bradycardia and hypotension, or the anxiety of being suctioned can cause hypertension and tachycardia. Stimulation of the cough reflex will cause a patient to cough, causing an increase in intracranial pressure and reducing cerebral blood flow.

SUCTIONING TECHNIQUES

You must have suction equipment by any patient who has airway compromise and will need airway management. To suction a patient:

1. Wear protective eyewear, gloves, and face mask.
2. Preoxygenate the patient; this may require hyperventilating him.
3. Determine the depth of catheter insertion by measuring from the patient's earlobe to his lips.
4. With the suction turned off, insert the catheter into your patient's pharynx to the predetermined depth.
5. Turn on the suction unit and place your thumb over the suction control orifice; limit suction to 10 seconds.
6. Continue to suction while withdrawing the catheter. When using a whistle-tip catheter, rotate it between your fingertips.
7. Hyperventilate the patient with 100% oxygen.

In many cases you will suction extremely viscous, or thick, secretions, that can obstruct the flow of fluid through the tubing. To reduce this problem, suction water through the tubing between suctioning attempts. This dilutes the secretions and facilitates flow to the suction canister. Most suction units have small water canisters for this purpose.

Tracheobronchial Suctioning

You may have to suction some patients through an endotracheal tube or a tracheostomy tube to remove secretions or mucous plugs that can cause respiratory distress. Suctioning these patients risks hypoxia, so oxygenating them before and after the procedure is essential. If possible, use sterile technique to avoid contaminating the pulmonary system. Use only the soft-tip catheter to avoid damaging any structures, and be certain to prelubricate it. Once you have preoxygentated the patient with 100% oxygen, lubricate the catheter tip with a water soluble gel and gently insert it until you feel resistance. Then apply suction for only 10–15 seconds while extracting the catheter. Ventilation and oxygenation are mandatory immediately after each suctioning attempt. You may have to inject 3–5 centimeters of sterile water down the endotracheal tube to help loosen thick secretions.

GASTRIC DECOMPRESSION

A common problem with ventilating a nonintubated patient is gastric distention, which occurs when the procedure's high pressures trap air in the stomach. As the stomach expands with this trapped air, the risk of vomiting rises. The enlarged stomach also pushes against the diaphragm, inhibiting the lungs' expansion and increasing their resistance to ventilation. Once the patient has gastric distention, you should place a tube in his stomach for gastric decompression, using either the nasogastric or orogastric approach.

Nasogastric tube placement is generally preferred in awake patients as it allows them to talk, while orogastric tube placement is recommended in patients with facial fractures to avoid placing the tube through a skull fracture into the brain. Indications for gastric tube placement include the need for decompression because of the risk of aspiration or difficulty ventilating. In addition, large-bore gastric tubes are occasionally placed for gastric lavage in hypothermia and some overdose emergencies. The possibility of esophageal bleeding dictates extreme caution in patients with esophageal disease or trauma. Avoid placing gastric tubes in the presence of an esophageal obstruction because of the increased risk of esophageal perforation. Both routes effectively accomplish gastric decompression; the orogastric route adds the advantage of allowing the use of a larger bore tube for lavage. Disadvantages of both routes include discomfort to patients and minor interference with orotracheal intubation. In patients with facial fractures, use orogastric routes to avoid placing the tube through a skull fracture into the brain. When no contraindication exists, nasogastric tube placement for gastric decompression is generally preferred. Both routes put the patient at risk for vomiting, misplacement into the trachea, or trauma and bleeding from poor technique.

As for any other invasive procedure, you should always wear protective eyewear, gloves, and face shield whenever you place a nasogastric or orogastric tube. To place a nasogastric or orogastric tube:

1. Prepare the patient's head in a neutral position while preoxygenating.
2. Determine the length of tube insertion by measuring from the epigastrium to the angle of jaw, then to the tip of the nares.
3. If the patient is awake, use a topical anesthetic to the nares or oropharynx. Suppress the gag reflex with a topical anesthetic applied into the posterior oropharynx or with IV lidocaine.
4. Lubricate the distal tip of the gastric tube and gently insert the tube into the nares and along the nasal floor or, alternately, into the oral cavity at midline. Advance the tube gently. If the patient is awake, encourage swallowing to facilitate the tube's passage.

5. Advance to the predetermined mark on the tube.

6. Confirm placement by injecting 30–50 ml of air while listening to the epigastric region for air sounds. Inability to speak that develops after gastric tube placement indicates malposition of the tube through the vocal cords and into the trachea. If this occurs, you must remove the tube.

7. Apply suction. Note gastric contents that pass through the tube.

8. Secure the tube in place.

OXYGENATION

Oxygen is an important drug, and you must thoroughly understand its indications and precautions. Providing supplemental oxygen to patients who are frankly hypoxic will diminish the hypoxia's secondary effects on organs such as the brain and the heart. You should provide supplemental oxygen to patients who are in shock or at risk of shock, regardless of their oxygen saturation. Although the patient may be oxygenating his arterial blood well, the oxygen may not be reaching his cells effectively. The increased oxygen levels may help improve perfusion.

Never withhold oxygen from any patient for whom it is indicated. However, use caution with COPD patients. These patients lose the impulse to breathe at normal or supranormal oxygen levels. Their normal respiratory regulatory mechanism (elevated $PaCO_2$) has failed, and their impulse to breathe is triggered by a low PaO_2, or hypoxia. This is termed hypoxic drive. As a general approach, slowly increase these patients' oxygen until their breathing is less labored and they are more comfortable, though not necessarily back to their baseline. Watch your patient closely to be sure his decreased breathing effort does not signal impending respiratory failure. If this occurs, be ready to support the patient's ventilations, using basic maneuvers, adjuncts, and BVM.

OXYGEN SUPPLY AND REGULATORS

Oxygen is supplied either as a compressed gas or a liquid. Compressed gaseous oxygen is stored in an aluminum or steel tank in 400 liter (D), 660 liter (E), or 3,450 liter (M) volumes. To calculate how long the oxygen will last:

tank life in minutes = (tank pressure in psi × 0.28) ÷ liters per minute

Liquid oxygen is cooled to aqueous form and warmed back to its gaseous state for delivery. Although liquid oxygen requires less storage space than an equal amount of compressed oxygen, you must keep it upright and accommodate other special requirements for its storage and transfer.

Regulators for oxygen tanks are either **high-pressure regulators,** which are used to transfer oxygen at high pressures from tank to tank, or **therapy regulators,** which are used for delivering oxygen to patients. The default pressure for therapy regulators is 50 psi, which is controlled within the regulator to allow for adjustable low-flow oxygen delivery.

OXYGEN DELIVERY DEVICES

Oxygen delivery to patients is measured in liters of flow per minute (L/min). A number of delivery devices are available; the patient's condition will dictate which method you use. You must continually reassess the patient who requires oxygen therapy to be certain that the method of delivery and flow rate are adequate. You

---

Never withhold oxygen from any patient for whom it is indicated.

* **high-pressure regulator** regulator used to transfer oxygen at high pressures from tank to tank.

* **therapy regulator** pressure regulator used for delivering oxygen to patients.

You must continually reassess the patient who requires oxygen therapy to be certain that the method of delivery and flow rate are adequate.

should not use these devices for patients with poor respiratory effort, severe hypoxia, or apnea or for patients who exhibit mouth breathing.

Nasal Cannula The **nasal cannula** is a catheter placed at the nares. It provides an optimal oxygen supplementation of up to 40% when set at 6 L/min flow. At flow rates above 6 L/min, the nasal mucous membranes become very dry and easily break down. Patients generally tolerate the nasal cannula well. It is indicated for low to moderate oxygen requirements and long-term oxygen therapy.

Venturi Mask The **venturi mask** is a high-flow face mask that uses a venturi system to deliver relatively precise oxygen concentrations, regardless of the patient's rate and depth of breathing. As oxygen passes into the mask through a jet orifice in the base of the mask, it entrains room air. The device then delivers the resulting mixture to the patient. Some venturi masks have dial selectors to control the amount of ambient air taken in; others have interchangeable caps. Either type can deliver concentrations of 24%, 28%, 35%, or 40% oxygen. The liter flow depends on the oxygen concentration desired. The venturi mask is particularly useful for COPD patients, who benefit from careful control of inspired oxygen concentration.

Simple Face Mask The simple face mask is indicated for patients requiring moderate to high oxygen concentrations. Side ports allow room air to enter the mask and dilute the oxygen concentration during inspiration. Flow rates generally range from about 6 L/min to 10 L/min, providing 40%–60% oxygen at the maximum rate, depending on the patient's respiratory rate and depth. Delivery of volumes beyond 10 L/min does not enhance oxygen concentration.

Partial Rebreather Mask The partial rebreather mask is indicated for patients requiring moderate to high oxygen concentrations when satisfactory clinical results are not obtained with the simple face mask. One-way discs that cover the partial rebreather mask's side ports prevent the inspiration of room air. Minimal dilution occurs with inspiration of residual expired air along with the supplemental oxygen. Maximal flow rate is 10L/min.

Nonrebreather Mask The nonrebreather mask has one-way side ports as well, but also has an attached reservoir bag to hold oxygen ready to inhale. It provides the highest oxygen concentration of all oxygen delivery devices available, 80%–95% at 15 L/min. It is not indicated as continuing support for poor respiratory effort and severe hypoxia; however, you should place it initially to attempt to preoxygenate these patients while you prepare to intubate them, unless initial ventilatory support with BVM and 100% oxygen is indicated.

Small–Volume Nebulizer Nebulizer chambers containing 3–5 cc of fluid are attached to a face mask that allows for delivery of medications in aerosol form (nebulization). Pressurized oxygen or air enters the chamber to create a mist, which the patient then inspires. Oxygen is the usual carrier, but in many COPD cases, supplemental oxygen by nasal cannula with nebulization using air is preferred.

Oxygen Humidifier You can provide humidified oxygen to the patient by attaching a sterile water reservoir to the oxygen outlet. Humidified oxygen benefits patients with croup, epiglottitis, or bronchiolitis, as well as those patients receiving long-term oxygen therapy.

VENTILATION

Many of your cases in the field will call for ventilatory support. These situations will range from apneic patients to less obvious instances when patients are experiencing depressed respiratory function. Remember that an unconscious

* **nasal cannula** catheter placed at the nares.

* **venturi mask** high-flow face mask that uses a venturi system to deliver relatively precise oxygen concentrations.

The venturi mask is particularly useful for COPD patients, who benefit from careful control of inspired oxygen concentration.

Content Review

OXYGEN DELIVERY DEVICES

- Nasal cannula
- Venturi mask
- Simple face mask
- Partial rebreather mask
- Nonrebreather mask
- Small-volume nebulizer
- Oxygen humidifier

If you do not correct any significant decrease in the patient's rate or depth of breathing, respiratory or cardiac arrest may occur.

patient's respiratory center may not function adequately. A significant decrease in the patient's rate or depth of breathing will lead to decreased respiratory minute volume, hypercarbia, hypoxia, and a lowered pH. If you do not correct this, respiratory or cardiac arrest may occur. Effective ventilatory support requires a tidal volume of at least 800 ml of oxygen at 12–20 breaths per minute.

When providing ventilatory support, you must generate enough force to overcome the elastic resistance of the lungs and chest wall, as well as the frictional resistance in the respiratory passageways, without overinflating the lungs. This is similar to blowing up a balloon; you must overcome the balloon's resistance in order to inflate it. Keep in mind that air will travel the path of least resistance. If you do not maintain a tight seal between the ventilation mask and your patient's face, air will flow out of the gaps rather than through the respiratory passageways.

Effective artificial ventilation requires: a patent airway, an effective seal between the mask and the patient's face, and delivery of adequate ventilatory volumes. Exercise care when you attempt to generate enough pressure to ventilate the lungs. Too much pressure may lead to gastric distention and regurgitation. Also, be certain that you allow the patient to exhale between delivered breaths.

Exercise care when you attempt to generate enough pressure to ventilate the lungs.

MOUTH-TO-MOUTH/MOUTH-TO-NOSE VENTILATION

Mouth-to-mouth and mouth-to-nose ventilation are the most basic methods of rescue ventilation. Both are indicated in the presence of apnea when no other ventilation devices are available. They require no special equipment, yet both allow an adequate seal between the rescuer and the patient and can provide effective ventilatory support, with adequate tidal volumes and oxygenation; however, the capacity of the person delivering the ventilations limits both methods. Also, both methods provide only limited oxygen—the rescuer's expired air will contain only 17% oxygen. This procedure's major drawback is its potential for exposing either the rescuer or the patient to communicable diseases through contact with blood and other body fluids. Take care not to hyperinflate the patient's lungs or to hyperventilate yourself.

MOUTH-TO-MASK VENTILATION

The pocket mask is a clear plastic device that you place over an apneic patient's mouth and nose. It prevents direct contact between you and your patient's mouth, thus reducing the risk of contamination and subsequent infection. It may be easier to obtain a good seal on the patient's face using a mask. However, the mask is only useful if it is readily available. Do not use it in awake patients.

A variety of pocket masks are available. Some are reusable, others are disposable. Most are small and compact enough to fit in a pocket or purse, and you should always carry one. Because of the increasing risks of infectious diseases, you should use a disposable mask whenever you ventilate a patient. These devices usually have a one-way valve that prevents you from contacting the patient's expired air. The valve may also provide an inlet for supplemental oxygen; mouth-to-mask ventilation combined with an oxygen flow rate of 10 L/min can deliver an inspired oxygen concentration of approximately 50%. To apply the mouth-to-mask technique, position the head to open the airway by one of the previously discussed methods, position the mask to obtain a good seal, and provide adequate ventilatory volumes. As with mouth-to-mouth and mouth-to-nose methods, hyperinflation of the patient's lungs, gastric distention in the patient, and hyperventilation in the rescuer are potential complications.

BAG-VALVE DEVICES

For patients with apnea or an unsatisfactory respiratory effort, prehospital and emergency department personnel most commonly use the bag-valve device. Used correctly the bag-valve device assists in ventilating patients by expanding the lungs and improving alveolar ventilation, thus preventing hypoxia. When using the bag-valve device with the mask (BVM), the paramedic must still open the airway with either the jaw-thrust or head-tilt/chin-lift maneuver. Nor should you use the BVM in awake patients who do not tolerate the procedure.

The **bag-valve mask** consists of an oblong, self-inflating, silicone or rubber bag with two one-way valves (an air/oxygen-inlet valve and a patient valve) and a transparent plastic face mask, which is available in three sizes: neonatal, child, or adult. Some bag-valve masks have a built-in colorimetric end-tidal CO_2 detector (Figure 8-47). With the increasing risks of transmitting infectious diseases, bag-valve masks should be disposable. Do not reuse them.

You can use bag-valve masks with or without oxygen. Without oxygen they deliver only room air (21% oxygen) to the patient; with oxygen attached, the deliverable amount of oxygen increases to 60%–70%. The bag-valve device also has an adjunct oxygen reservoir or corrugated tubing that can deliver 90%–95% oxygen when coupled with an oxygen source. If possible, connect all patients who require a bag-valve device to an oxygen reservoir with oxygen at 15 L/min.

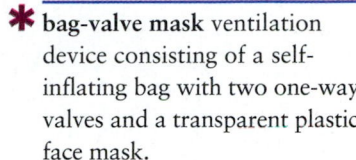

* **bag-valve mask** ventilation device consisting of a self-inflating bag with two one-way valves and a transparent plastic face mask.

Do not reuse bag-valve masks.

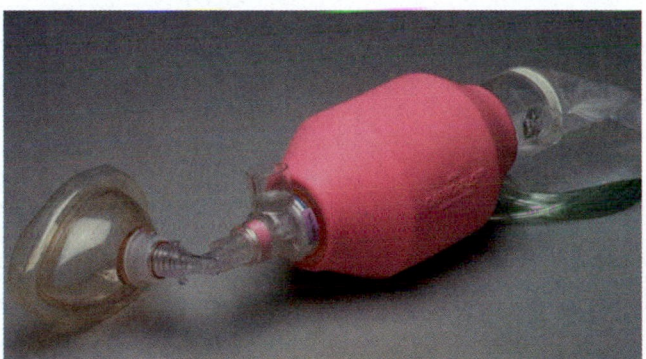

FIGURE 8-47 Bag-valve-mask with built-in colorimetric ETCO$_2$ detector.

Bag-valve masks for pediatric cases may have a pop-off valve. Bag-valve masks for adults should not have pop-off valves, because patients with high airway resistance and poor lung compliance will activate the pop-off valve, thus preventing effective ventilation.

One, two, or three rescuers may perform bag-valve-mask ventilation. One-person BVM ventilation is the most difficult method to master because obtaining and maintaining the mask seal can be challenging. You must not only keep the airway open with a jaw-thrust or chin-lift but at the same time keep the mask sealed well and squeeze the BVM to deliver an adequate tidal volume. Two-person BVM ventilation is the most efficient method, providing superior mask seal and tidal volumes when applied correctly. It requires the availability of an adequate number of trained medical personnel. Three-person BVM ventilation also provides excellent mask seal and volume delivery, but it requires more personnel, and it crowds access to the patient's airway.

To perform the two-person BVM method, the first rescuer maintains the mask seal while the second squeezes the bag. With the three-person BVM method, the first rescuer applies manual airway maneuvers, the second maintains the mask seal, and the third squeezes the bag. Observe the patient for chest rise, development of gastric distention, and changes in compliance of the bag with ventilation. Complications of BVM ventilation include inadequate volume delivery if there is a poor mask seal or improper technique, barotrauma from overinflation of the lungs, and gastric distention.

Ventilation of Pediatric Patients The differences in the pediatric patient's anatomy require some variation in ventilation technique. First, his relatively flat nasal bridge makes achieving mask seal more difficult. Pressing the mask against the child's face to improve the seal can obstruct his airway, which is more compressible than an adult's. You can best achieve the mask seal with the two-person BVM technique, using jaw thrust to maintain an open airway.

For BVM ventilation, the bag size depends on the child's age. Full-term neonates and infants will require a pediatric BVM with a capacity of at least 450 ml. For children up to eight years of age, the pediatric BVM is preferred, though for patients in the upper age range you can use an adult BVM with a capacity of 1500ml if you do not maximally inflate it. Children older than eight years require an adult BVM to achieve adequate tidal volumes. Additionally, be certain that the mask fits properly, from the bridge of the nose to the cleft of the chin. If a length-based resuscitation tape (Broselow Tape) is available, you can use it to help determine the proper size.

To achieve a proper mask seal, place the mask over the patient's mouth and nose; avoid compressing the eyes. Using one hand, place your thumb on the mask at the apex and your index finger on the mask at the chin (C-grip). Apply gentle pressure downward on the mask to establish an adequate seal. Maintain the airway by lifting the bony prominence of the chin with the remaining fingers forming an *E* under the jaw; avoid placing pressure on the soft area under the chin. You may use the one-rescuer technique, although the two-rescuer technique will be more effective.

Ventilate according to current standards, obtaining chest rise with each breath. Begin the ventilation and say "squeeze," providing just enough volume to initiate chest rise—be very careful not to overinflate the child's lungs. Allow adequate time for exhalation, saying "release, release." Continue ventilations, saying "squeeze, release, release." To assess adequacy of ventilations, look for adequate chest rise, listen for lung sounds at the third intercostal space, midaxillary line, and assess for clinical improvement (skin color and heart rate).

DEMAND VALVE DEVICE

The **demand valve device**, also called the manually-triggered oxygen-powered ventilation device or flow-restricted, oxygen-powered ventilation device, will deliver 100% oxygen to a patient at its highest flow rates (40 liters per minute maximum). Flow is restricted to 30 cm H_2O or less to diminish gastric distention that can occur with its use. The device is rugged, compact, and easy to handle. It also includes an easy-to-locate manual control button. In addition, the entire device can be attached to a face mask or a mechanical airway (Figure 8-48).

The complete system consists of high-pressure tubing that connects to an oxygen supply, and a valve that is activated by a push button or lever. When the valve is opened, oxygen flows to the patient. Most of these units also contain an inspiratory release valve that makes them useful in treating spontaneously breathing patients who need high oxygen concentrations. The slight negative pressure created by inhalation opens the valve. The greater the inspiratory effort, the higher the flow. When inhalation ceases, so does oxygen flow. This helps to decrease the likelihood of overinflation during ventilation of a patient with respiratory effort. The indications for use of oxygen-powered ventilation devices include the need for high-volume, high-oxygen-concentration delivery in awake, compliant patients. You may use it in unconscious patients, but must be extremely cautious, as you cannot measure delivered volumes or feel lung compliance. The demand valve device is easy to use and provides high oxygen concentrations. However, the demand valve device has several drawbacks. During ventilation, it does not give the rescuer a sense of chest compliance; thus, you must take care not to overinflate the lungs. The high pressures that the device generates may injure the lungs, which can lead to pneumothorax and subcutaneous emphysema. Also, the demand valve resuscitator may open the esophagus, causing gastric distention in patients who have not been intubated. Finally, the demand valve resuscitator's high flow rate will quickly

* **demand valve device** a ventilation device that is manually operated by a push button or lever.

FIGURE 8-48   Demand valve and mask.

FIGURE 8-49 Portable
mechanical ventilator.

drain a portable oxygen cylinder. You will have to use another means of ventilatory support if the cylinder requires changing during patient management.

The demand valve resuscitator is not recommended for use with patients under the age of 16. Because of the sudden high pressures that this device can produce, you should use it with extreme caution in intubated patients or those with chest trauma.

AUTOMATIC TRANSPORT VENTILATOR

Several compact mechanical ventilators are available for prehospital care. Designed for convenience and easy use during patient care and transport, these lightweight and durable portable devices offer a number of advantages. They maintain minute volume better than bag-valve devices, and they tolerate temperatures ranging from −30°F to 125°F with great dependability. In cardiac arrest, the automatic ventilator allows you to interpose chest compressions between mechanical breaths. They are mechanically simple and adapt to a portable oxygen supply.

The compact ventilator typically comes with two or three controls: one for the ventilatory rate, the other for tidal volume (Figure 8-49). It also has a standard 15/22 mm adapter, so that you can attach it to a variety of airway devices. Some of these automatic units deliver controlled ventilation only. Others function as intermittent mandatory ventilators, reverting to controlled mechanical ventilation in patients who are not breathing. Tidal volume in most is adjustable, while the ventilatory rate may be either fixed or adjustable. The inspired oxygen concentration is usually fixed at 100%, but it may be adjustable.

Many of these ventilators have a pop-off valve that prevents pressure-related injury. When airway pressure exceeds a preset level (typically 60 cmH$_2$O), the valve opens, venting some of the tidal volume. This feature can hinder ventilating patients with cardiogenic pulmonary edema, adult respiratory distress syndrome (ARDS), pulmonary contusion, bronchospasm, or other disorders in which high airway pressures must be overcome. Consider using a bag-valve device if this problem occurs. Also, these devices generally have no alarms to warn of possible tube displacement or barotrauma.

As a rule, you should not use mechanical ventilators in children less than five years old, awake patients, or patients with obstructed airways or increased airway resistance, as described above. Otherwise, when indicated, the device can prove a valuable tool. In intubated patients, the mechanical ventilator allows you to perform other vital tasks. Its disadvantages are that it can be difficult to secure and proper functioning depends on oxygen tank pressure.

SUMMARY

Airway assessment and maintenance is the most critical step in managing any patient. If you do not promptly establish a definitive airway and provide proper ventilation, the patient's outcome will be poor. Frequently reassessing the airway is mandatory to ensure that the patient has not decompensated, requiring additional airway procedures. Successful management of all airways requires the paramedic to follow the proper management sequence.

Basic airway and management skills can make the difference between a successful outcome and a poor patient prognosis. Once you have mastered these basic skills and made them a part of airway management in every patient, you should learn and utilize advanced skills such as intubation, RSI, and cricothyrotomy. You must maintain proficiency in all airway skills, especially the more advanced techniques, through ongoing continuing education, physician medical direction, and testing with each EMS service. If you cannot do this, it is in the patient's best interest to focus on less sophisticated airway skills. If you anticipate that every airway will be complicated, apply basic airway skills before using advanced procedures, and perform frequent reassessments, you will give the patient his best chance for meaningful survival.

CHAPTER 9

Therapeutic Communications

Objectives

After reading this chapter, you should be able to:

1. Define communication. (p. 575)
2. Identify internal and external factors that affect an interview. (pp. 575–577, 582–583)
3. Identify strategies for developing rapport with the patient. (p. 576)
4. Discuss open-ended and closed, questions. (pp. 580–581)
5. Discuss common errors made when interviewing patients. (pp. 582–583)
6. Identify the nonverbal skills used in patient interviewing. (pp. 578–579)
7. Identify interview methods used to assess mental status. (p. 581)
8. Discuss strategies for interviewing a patient who is not motivated to talk. (pp. 581, 583–584)
9. Describe the use of, and differentiate between, facilitation, reflec-

tion, clarification, empathetic responses, confrontation, and interpretation. (p. 582)
10. Differentiate strategies used for interviewing hostile and cooperative patients. (pp. 581, 587)
11. Summarize developmental considerations that influence patient interviewing. (pp. 578, 581, 584–585)
12. Define the unique interviewing techniques for patients with special needs. (pp. 583–587)
13. Discuss cross-cultural interviewing considerations. (pp. 586–587)
14. Given several preprogrammed simulated patients, provide a patient interview using therapeutic communication. (pp. 575–587)

INTRODUCTION

Communication should be easy. After all, **communication** is only a matter of exchanging common symbols—written, spoken, or other kinds such as signing and body language. However, as you know, even in the best circumstances, communication can be a challenge. EMS providers have a particularly difficult job of it, because they must communicate with strangers who are in crisis.

As a paramedic, you must learn how to use every available strategy to make sure that you understand your patients and they, in turn, understand you. You also must be able to communicate well with the patient's relatives, bystanders, and other EMS providers. Strategies you will use include persistently paying attention to word choices, tones of voice, facial expressions, and body language. You will learn to minimize external and internal distractions and to adjust your personal communication style to fit each new situation, especially when dealing with children, elderly people, people of different cultures, and hostile people.

Helpful core traits for effective communication in EMS include a genuine liking for people, a sincere desire to be part of a helping profession, an understanding of human strengths and weaknesses, and **empathy,** or the ability to view the world through another's eyes while remaining true to yourself.

* **communication** the exchange of common symbols—written, spoken, or other kinds such as signing and body language.

Helpful core traits for effective communication in EMS include a genuine liking for people, a sincere desire to be part of a helping profession, an understanding of human strengths and weaknesses.

* **empathy** identification with and understanding of another's situation, feelings, and motives.

* **encode** to create a message.

* **decode** to interpret a message.

* **feedback** a response to a message.

BASIC ELEMENTS OF COMMUNICATION

Communication consists of a sender, a message, a receiver, and feedback. First, the sender has to **encode,** or create a message; that is, he must write, speak, or otherwise place symbols common to both parties in an understandable format. This may mean translating the message into another language, using words a child can understand, or writing the words on paper. The receiver then must **decode,** or interpret, the message, ideally with the same meaning the sender intended to convey. Finally, the receiver gives the sender **feedback** (a response to the message). If by way of this response, the sender believes the message was received accurately, both parties can congratulate themselves on communicating successfully.

Unfortunately, partial or complete failure to communicate occurs often. There are abundant reasons for this. In EMS those reasons include:

- Prejudice, or lack of empathy, particularly by the paramedic toward the patient or situation
- Lack of privacy, which inhibits a patient's responses to questions
- External distractions, such as traffic, crowds, loud music, EMS radios, or TVs
- Internal distractions, or thinking about things other than the situation at hand

One way to minimize failure is to keep in mind that patience and flexibility are hallmarks of a good communicator.

Content Review

REASONS FOR FAILING TO COMMUNICATE
- Prejudice
- Lack of privacy
- External distractions
- Internal distractions

Patience and flexibility are hallmarks of a good communicator.

* **patient interview** interaction with a patient for the purpose of obtaining in-depth information about the emergency and the patient's pertinent medical history.

Content Review

WAYS TO BUILD TRUST AND RAPPORT

- Use the patient's name.
- Address the patient properly.
- Modulate your voice.
- Use a professional but compassionate tone.
- Explain what you are doing and why.
- Keep a kind, calm expression.
- Use an appropriate style of communication.

Content Review

HOW TO REMEMBER A NAME

- Say the name out loud three times.
- "See" the name in bold capital letters.
- "Feel" yourself write the name.

TRUST AND RAPPORT

As a representative of EMS, you are granted a certain amount of the public's trust at each new emergency scene. You have to earn the rest by putting the patient and others at ease and by letting them know you are on their side, you respect their comments, and you want to help. Little courtesies such as asking the patient his name and thereafter pronouncing it correctly can help to accomplish this goal. So can recognizing and responding with compassion to signs of discomfort or suffering. Once trust is established, rapport follows.

With good rapport, the people you are serving will follow your lead, even if that means some pain (such as with a needle stick) and inconvenience (such as canceling a trip to have a medical evaluation at the hospital). The people with whom you work also will be more motivated to do difficult and sometimes dangerous tasks. Remember that effective communication begins and ends with trust and rapport. Without them, your safety could be at risk.

PROFESSIONAL BEHAVIORS

First impressions are crucial. What others see in you during the first few seconds of an encounter can lay the foundation for success or failure. The patient relies almost exclusively on visual input, so your physical presentation—from facial expression to the appearance of your clothing—matters. Even though encounters with patients are typically brief, patients usually remember them for a very long time. Make sure your first impression is a positive one. The elements of a good first impression involve all conventional professional standards, including:

- Clean, neat uniform that allows you to be easily identifiable as a paramedic
- Good personal hygiene, including clean, cut fingernails and inoffensive breath. Also avoiding use of colognes and perfumes.
- Physical fitness
- Overall professional demeanor that is calm, capable, and trustworthy
- Facial expression that is open, interested, caring. Avoiding expressions of disdain or disgust.
- Confident (not arrogant) stance
- Appropriate gait. Avoiding running or strolling.
- Consideration for the patient, such as wiping your feet on the doormat before entering the residence

The next period of interaction with your patient is the time for obtaining in-depth information about the emergency and the patient's medical history. This may be called the **patient interview**. A good starting point is always to assure the patient's privacy, which also minimizes inhibitions and distractions. It helps to be sure that lighting is adequate and noise is minimized. Equipment that might be alarming (such as needles) should be placed out of the patient's sight.

Other ways to help build the trust and rapport you need to conduct a patient interview include the following:

- *Use your patient's name.* It is a powerful tool for forming a quick bond. A technique for remembering a name involves three steps: First, say the patient's name out loud three times in the first minute. Then "see" the patient's name in your mind in bold capital letters.

Finally, "feel" yourself writing the name in your imagination. Some people actually write the name on their paperwork, but this does not work as well as the mental imagery.

- *Address your patient properly.* Use formal forms of address, such as "Mr." and "Mrs." or "Ms.," as appropriate. Never call patients "honey," "dude," or any name other than their own. Also, be careful about shortening children's names. If a child is introduced to you as "Matthew," use that name, or ask the child if he goes by a nickname such as "Matt."

- *Modulate your voice.* Pay attention to your volume. Speak quietly and in low tones. If the patient is hard of hearing or difficult to control, speak up. Check your pitch; some people find it hard to hear high voices. Also, check your rate of speaking. Be especially aware that people in crisis may have difficulty taking in information at a normal rate, so slow down.

- *Use a professional but compassionate tone of voice.* Avoid tones that portray sarcasm, irritation, anger, or other emotions that fail to serve the patient.

- *Explain what you are doing and why.* This helps to ease your patient's anxiety, especially if he is in pain. For example, if you must immobilize a broken bone, explain that a splint will help to prevent movement and more pain. Also tell the patient that applying a splint may be painful but once applied, the broken limb should be more comfortable. (Note: Never make false promises or false assurances. They violate your patient's trust.)

- *Keep a kind, calm facial expression.* Remember that facial expressions can reflect a wide variety of emotions and conditions, including relaxation, relief, pain, fear, anger, sorrow, and so on. No matter what the emergency, maintain a kind-looking poker face. It will convince others that you can handle things.

- *Use the appropriate style of communication.* There is a wide range to choose from. In general, patients will respond well to a calm, re-assuring demeanor, but be prepared to use a tough, authoritative approach when needed. Also, if a situation requires you to be firm, be completely firm. Do not let your facial expression, for example, kill the effect (such as one that says, "Gosh, I hope they believe me!").

At the end of a call, a final word or two can be very helpful, particularly after emotional calls. A "goodbye and good luck" can help bring the event to a close for the patient and family.

COMMUNICATION TECHNIQUES

GENERAL GUIDELINES

Patients generally respond to questioning in one of three ways: They may pour out information easily, they may reveal some things and conceal others that might be embarrassing or shameful, or they may resist, hiding information from themselves and, therefore, from you. The patient who conceals information or resists giving it may be trying to maintain a certain image or may be fearful about how others will respond (perhaps with ridicule or rejection). To get the information you need, you must be consistently professional, nonjudgmental, and willing to talk about any concern the patient may have.

To get the information you need, you must be consistently professional, nonjudgmental, and willing to talk about any concern the patient may have.

Nonverbal Communication

* **nonverbal communication**
gestures, mannerisms, and
postures by which a person
communicates with others;
also called *body language*.

Nonverbal communication, or body language, consists of gestures, mannerisms, and postures by which a person communicates with others. Your position within the environment and in relation to your patient is part of that language. Examples include the following:

Content Review

ELEMENTS OF NONVERBAL COMMUNICATION
- Distance
- Relative level
- Stance

- *Distance* (Table 9-1). In the U.S., the socially acceptable distance between strangers is 4 to 12 feet. A "comfortable" distance may be described as twice the length of a patient's arm. In most cases, paramedics are able to break social convention and quickly enter a patient's "intimate space" (1.5 feet or less) because people intuitively understand the need for medical personnel to get "hands on" with them. However, if the patient stiffens or backs away from you, the best strategy may be to linger at a less threatening distance until you have built more trust and rapport.

- *Relative level.* A different message is sent to the patient each time you stand at his eye level, above it, or below it. Remaining at eye level indicates equality. Standing above or over the patient imparts an air of authority, but it also can be intimidating. Dropping below eye level indicates a willingness to let the patient have some control of the situation, a strategy that can be especially helpful when your patient is an elderly adult or a child.

* **open stance** a posture or body
position that is relaxed and
suggests confidence, ease,
warmth, and attentiveness.

- *Stance* (Figure 9-1). Arms extended, open hands, relaxed large muscles, and a nodding head characterize an **open stance.** A paramedic who has an open stance sends the message that he is confident and at ease. When it is safe to do so, use this stance to communicate warmth and attentiveness.

* **closed stance** a posture or
body position that is tense and
suggests negativity, discomfort, fear, disgust, or anger.

A **closed stance** is just the opposite. In this position, arms are flexed, or arms are crossed tightly over the chest. The fists are clenched or a finger may be pointing. The head may be shaking negatively. The body is square to the patient or, in some cases, may turn slightly away. This posture suggests disinterest, discomfort, disgust, fear, or anger and sends negative signals to the patient.

Table 9-1 INTERPERSONAL ZONES

Zone	Distance	Characteristics
Intimate zone	0 to 1.5 feet	Visual distortion occurs.
		Best for assessing breath and other body odors.
Personal distance, or "personal space"	1.5 to 4 feet	Perceived as extension of self.
		No visual distortion.
		Body odors are not apparent.
		Voice is moderate.
		Much of patient assessment, and sometimes patient interviewing, may occur at this distance.
Social distance	4 to 12 feet	Used for impersonal business transactions.
		Perceptual information is much less detailed than at personal distance.
		Patient interview may occur at this distance.
Public distance	12 feet or more	Allows impersonal interaction with others.
		Voices must be projected.

FIGURE 9-1a   An open stance.

FIGURE 9-1b   A closed stance.

Watch your patient's body language, too. It can tell you how well communication with him is going. If the patient has a closed stance, you may need to change your approach.

Eye Contact

A powerful source of effective communication comes with eye contact. While you are interviewing the patient, use it as much as possible. (Always remove sunglasses while working with patients.) Even when you are taking notes, look at the patient frequently. Eye contact is one way to send a message to your patient, whether it is a compassionate "I care about you" or a stern "settle down now." You name it. With eye contact, you can hold the attention of a patient so powerfully that your patient can feel you are helping him hang on in desperate circumstances.

Of course, using eye contact means that the other person is looking at you, too, which can be unnerving, especially if you are unfamiliar with this technique. If you feel uncomfortable, look at the bridge of the other person's nose for a bit of relief. Then try direct eye contact again. Build this skill over time, and it will serve you well.

Compassionate Touch

Another communication skill is touching (Figure 9-2). The ability to hold a hand, or even hug, in the right circumstances can yield information that would otherwise not be given. Some paramedics need to learn this skill the way they learn how to use an IV. That is, it can be awkward at first, but it is worth the effort. Nothing builds trust and rapport, or calms patients, faster than the power of touch. How effective it is depends on the patient's age, gender, cultural background, past experience, and current setting. Be careful to touch appropriately. There is a line between compassion and improper intimacy. Remember that as a paramedic, you must always carefully guard the integrity of the public's trust in you.

> *Nothing builds trust and rapport, or calms patients, faster than the power of touch.*
>
>

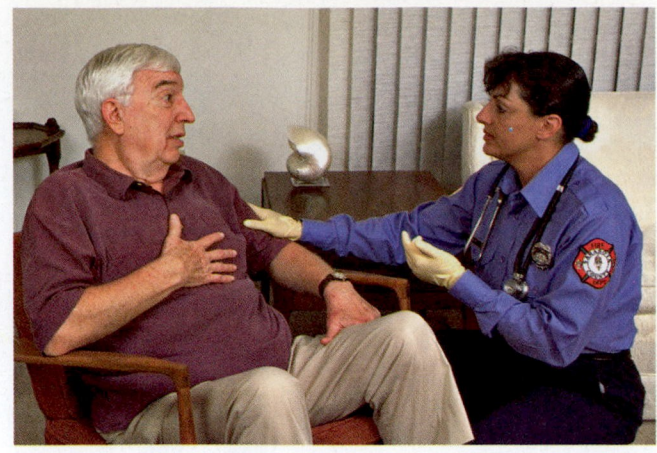

INTERVIEW TECHNIQUES

From the moment of your first contact with the patient, your job is to find out all information relevant to the present emergency. You need to identify the patient's chief complaint (the reason why 911 was called), find out the circumstances that caused the emergency, and determine the patient's condition. Much of this is accomplished by asking questions, observing the patient, and listening effectively.

Questioning Techniques

An important part of patient assessment is gathering information that is accurate, complete, and relevant to the present emergency. To begin, you must identify the patient's chief complaint. Although dispatch probably will have given you an idea of what the emergency is about, it is important for you to let the patient state the chief complaint in his own words. If you were to ask **leading questions** (ones that guide the patient's replies), such as: "Are you having chest pain?" or "I see you've injured your arm. How does it feel?", you could easily miss a serious problem. So, instead, ask **open-ended questions,** such as: "What happened that led you to call 911?" or "What seems to be the problem?" They will allow your patient to respond in an unguided, spontaneous way. They also encourage patients who are reluctant to speak to describe their complaint in a way that might not be possible otherwise.

The patient's chief complaint should then drive the evolution of all other questions to be asked. For example, if your patient's chief complaint is chest pain, you are required to obtain answers to a specific set of questions. But instead of asking them as if you were reading a shopping list, individualize the process. For example, you would have to find out if a patient with chest pain takes any medications. If your patient tells you that his chief complaint is "chest pain so bad even the nitroglycerin tablets aren't helping," your question about medications might be worded: "What medications do you take in addition to nitroglycerin?" This tells the patient you have been listening, which can yield a greater rapport. Other questioning techniques include the following:

- *Continue to ask open-ended questions.* They do not limit the patient's responses, which can help to reveal unexpected but important facts. For example, instead of asking a patient with abdominal pain "Did you have breakfast today?" which can be answered with either a "yes" or a "no," ask: "What have you eaten today?"
- *Use direct questions,* when necessary. Direct questions, or **closed questions,** ask for specific information. ("Did you eat lunch?" or

> ✱ **leading questions** questions framed to guide the direction of a patient's answers.
>
> ✱ **open-ended questions** questions that permit unguided, spontaneous answers.

> ✱ **closed questions** questions that ask for specific information and require only very short or yes-or-no answers. Also called *direct questions.*

"Does the abdominal pain come and go like a cramp, or is it constant?") These questions are good for three reasons: They fill in information generated by open-ended questions. They help to answer crucial questions when time is limited. And they can help to control overly talkative patients, who might want to tell you about their gall-bladder surgery in 1949 when the chief complaint is a sprained ankle.

- *Do not ask leading questions.* Avoiding them means avoiding being taken down a path unrelated to the current emergency.

- *Ask only one question at a time, and allow complete answers.* If you ask more than one question, the patient may not know which one to answer and may leave out portions of information or become confused.

- *Listen to the patient's complete response before asking the next question.* By doing so, you might find that you need to ask a question that is different from the one you were expecting to ask.

- *Use language the patient can understand.* In general, people do not understand medical terms. For example, you may need to use "pee" instead of "urine," or "breaths" instead of "respirations." However, be careful to avoid jargon and slang. Also keep in mind that children are very literal and concrete minded. Never tell a child, for example, that you are going to "take" her blood pressure. Say instead that you are going to "measure" it.

- *Do not allow interruptions, if possible,* unless your partner or other EMS personnel need to give you patient care information of a critical nature. Interruptions will interfere with your patient's and your trains of thought. Interruptions also can cause you to miss information important to the patient's medical care.

Observing the Patient

Observe the patient during the interview. External signs such as overall appearance, including clothing, jewelry, and other physical signs, may give you some indication of the patient's condition. Other clues you pick up may offer you a way to explore the patient's internal experiences, or mental status.

So, while you are interacting with the patient, observe his level of consciousness and body movements. Assess his rate and clarity of speech, his thinking, and his ability to pay attention, concentrate, and comprehend. You may be able to check the patient's orientation to person, place, and time, and his remote, recent, and immediate memory. Explore his mood and energy level, too. Watch for evidence of autonomic responses (sweating, trembling, and so on) and for unusual facial movements such as a tic around the mouth, nose, or eyes. Note that lack of eye contact can suggest that the patient is shy, withdrawn, confused, bored, intimidated, apathetic, or depressed.

Many people do not cope well with being the center of attention. Be aware of various defense mechanisms people may use, so you can be prepared to deal with them if necessary. For example, if your patient is self-grooming (fixing hair or straightening clothes), it may be that he needs some reassurance. If the patient keeps shifting focus away from your questions, back off for a bit and then return to the topic from a different angle.

If the patient is acting out and hostile, point out the behavior in a professional manner, ask if the behavior is intentional, let him know that such behavior defeats the purpose of calling for help, and then name behaviors you would rather see. If there is any indication that the patient's hostility may threaten your safety or that of your crew, maintain distance and an exit path. (Additional information about hostile patients appears later in this chapter.)

Effective Listening and Feedback

Few people practice the art of listening well. Usually, they think about what they are going to say next while others are still talking to them. There may be less than a one-half second gap between speakers, and many people cannot even wait that long and instead finish others' sentences for them.

Listening is an active skill, not a passive one. It requires your complete attention, and it requires constant practice. In order to listen well, you must focus on the messenger. Stop doing other things. Discipline yourself to cease any internal dialogue that can distract or interrupt you mentally. Never finish the other person's sentences, and do not consider your response until the speaker has finished speaking. Allow some silence when the speaker has stopped.

Once the speaker has stopped talking, provide feedback to confirm that you have understood his message correctly. Feedback techniques include:

- *Silence.* Give the patient time to gather his thoughts and add to what has been said.

- *Reflection.* To check your understanding and to reassure the speaker, echo his message back to him using your own words.

- *Facilitation.* Encourage the speaker to provide more information.

- *Empathy.* Let your body language show that you understand, so that the patient feels accepted and more open to talking.

- *Clarification.* Ask the speaker to help you understand, when you need to eliminate confusion about what has been said.

- *Confrontation.* Focus the patient on one particular factor of the interview.

- *Interpretation.* State your interpretation of the information; that is, link events, make associations, identify an implied cause, or draw conclusions.

- *Explanation.* Share factual or objective information related to the message.

- *Summarization.* Briefly review the interview and your interpretation of the situation. Ask open-ended questions, if needed, to allow the patient to clarify details.

Traps of interviewing, or common errors made when listening and providing feedback to patients, include the following:

- *Providing false assurances.* Never make any promises you cannot keep. For example, saying "everything will be all right" is a terrible false reassurance.

- *Giving advice.* People call 911 because they are seeking advice, but the paramedic must be careful how it is conveyed. Saying "my opinion is that your chest pain should be evaluated at the hospital" is acceptable advice. Saying "I think you would be crazy not to get seen by a doctor" is not.

- *Authority.* Remember that EMS is not a power trip. Although paramedics are imbued with the power to do a difficult job, that power must never be used inappropriately. A paramedic provides a vital public service. Doing so correctly requires constant attention to protecting the public's trust and avoiding behaviors that might be interpreted as abuse of power.

- *Using avoidance language.* Avoidance language is "an unproductive conflict strategy in which a person takes mental or physical flight from the actual conflict," according to communication expert Joseph DeVito.[1] For example, a person who chooses to change the conversation rather than get into a discussion about something difficult may use avoidance language. If a paramedic does this, the patient's whole story may not be revealed.

- *Distancing.* When the paramedic is insensitive to distancing, he or she may stand too close or too far from patient to attain optimal rapport. Noticing the effects of distancing and adjusting accordingly is a hallmark of a good communicator.

- *Professional jargon.* Although it is necessary to make sure the patient knows what you are doing and why, it is unnerving for him to hear that you are going to "slip a line and jam a tube." So, watch your language and make sure you are speaking at your patient's comprehension level.

- *Talking too much.* Remember that listening is also a part of communication.

- *Interrupting.* As already discussed, good listening skills require you to wait until your patient answers you fully.

- *Using "why" questions.* The question "why" often steers a conversation toward blame, such as: "Why did you put your hand in the lawnmower while it was running?" or "Why didn't you call for help three hours ago?" This type of question is counterproductive.

Demonstrating good listening and feedback skills on an emergency call is challenging. So many things are happening, it can seem like a whirlwind. It may be necessary to apply monitoring equipment to the patient while you ask questions, for example. If this happens, reassure the patient by saying something like: "I know it seems overwhelming to you, but please understand that I am listening to your answers while I work."

PATIENTS WITH SPECIAL NEEDS

Patients generally are more than willing to answer your questions, though some will require more time and a variety of techniques. Note that difficult interviews stem from several sources. The patient's condition, including a developing cognitive impairment, may impact his ability to talk. The patient may be afraid to talk to you because of a psychological disorder, language or cultural difference, or even the difference between your ages. Or the patient intentionally may want to deceive you (to hide illegal drug abuse, for example).

Use the same techniques on a patient who is reluctant to talk to you as you would on any other patient, but use them in a slightly different way. For example, start your interview in the usual manner. If the patient does not respond to your questions, take time to develop rapport by reviewing the reason dispatch gave for the call. Attempt to ask open-ended questions. If unsuccessful, try direct questions including ones that require only a yes-or-no response. Accept that you may not be able to obtain any elaboration or details about the facts. Provide positive feedback to any response the patient provides.

If the patient continues to be reluctant, be sure the patient understands your questions. Rule out language barriers and hearing difficulties. Once you know the patient can understand you, continue to ask questions about the critical

Content Review

SOURCES OF DIFFICULT INTERVIEWS
- Patient's physical condition
- Patient's fear of talking
- Patient's intentions to deceive

[1]J. DeVito, *Essentials of Human Communication,* Third Edition (New York City: Longman, 1999).

information you need to know to progress with treatment. If you cannot get even this much, attempt to rule out pathology (disease) by asking family members or others at the scene how long the patient has been uncommunicative.

If you determine that pathology is not the cause, you may need to continue to build trust and rapport with the patient. One way to do this is to encourage him to ask you questions about your equipment, profession, medical care, or any topic that might start conversation. Model how you would like the patient to respond to your questions by answering his fully.

Further information on communicating with patients who require a special effort on your part follows. These patients include children and their parents, elderly people, people who are blind or deaf, people of other cultures, and people who are hostile or uncooperative.

Children

Effective communication with pediatric patients (infants, children, and adolescents) depends on their age. Have a good idea of what to expect at each stage of development so that your efforts to communicate can be appropriate. (See Chapter 5.)

In general, you can start by talking to the caregivers, then gradually approach the patient. Remember your body language. When dealing with younger children especially, it will help to get down to their eye level (Figure 9-3). Children pick up on anxiety easily and often take cues from what they observe, so it is very important to stay calm. Then introduce yourself, and use the child's name often. Be careful not to clam up and work silently.

Even if your own anxieties and the pressure of the medical requirements of the call are taxing your limits, talk! Tell the child everything: what you are looking at ("Now let's look at this arm . . .") and why it is important (". . . so we can be sure it's okay, too."). Explain your equipment, and if there is time, let the child see how the equipment works. Above all, explain what you intend to do, even to very young children. (For example, you might say, "Alexander, I am going to make your leg hurt less by putting on this splint. I will need to make the leg move first, which might hurt some. But after that, it should be a lot better. Okay?") Never tell a child that something will not hurt when, in actuality, it will. Once you have lost the trust of a child, it is very difficult to regain it.

Most important, you must build trust. Once you have that, a child will put up with a lot. Giving a child a stuffed toy may be helpful. Also, be sure to move

Never tell a child that something will not hurt when it will. Once you have lost the trust of a child, it is very difficult to regain it.

FIGURE 9-3 Getting down to patient's level can help improve communications on a pediatric call.

slowly, talk gently, explain everything, and be honest. To engage children, ask questions, and when you answer their questions, be sure not to talk down. Use straightforward language. Never try to hide the fact that something is wrong. When something will hurt or will be at all uncomfortable, tell them. The more matter-of-fact and informative you can be, the better. If you are fair about the difficult parts and avoid springing nasty surprises, you will find greater overall cooperation. The need to be gentle whenever possible should be obvious.

If a child is especially fearful, let him play with a toy or other object and then gradually increase contact. Do not be in a hurry to touch a child unless the situation is critical. Use lots of eye contact and compassionate touch, too. Keep in mind that even if the child cannot understand you, your tone of voice is reassuring and your words and actions will be meaningful to the family and bystanders. Ask the child for feedback frequently, wait for an answer, and acknowledge that answer. Involve the child in decision making whenever possible. If he is crying, do not take it personally and do not tell him to stop. Instead, try saying, "Go ahead and cry until you don't want to cry any more." Lending control in this way can work wonders.

Be aware that young children are very literal. Word choice is important. As noted earlier, do not "take" a pulse, "measure" it. A blood-pressure cuff does not "squeeze," it "hugs." When one child was told that she would fly to the hospital, she started to cry. "I don't know how to fly," she wailed. Think about what you say.

With pediatric patients, it is important to understand that caregivers, especially parents, may be very concerned and upset. Remember that you must manage them as well as your patient. Common responses include crying, emotional outbursts, anger, guilt, and confusion, which may be directed at you. Do not take it personally. You must build trust and rapport with the parents as well as with the child.

Sometimes parents interfere with emergency care and must be separated from the child. Usually, however, it is most effective to let the parents stay and, if appropriate, even hold the child. No matter how parents behave, always treat them with courtesy, respect, and understanding. Avoid raising your voice. Tell them that you know they want help for their child. They need your support and understanding, too.

When possible, allow parents to remain with the pediatric patient.

Note that for younger children (ages 1 to 6), most of your conversation will be with caregivers. Be aware that you are collecting information about the child's history from an adult's point of view, but do not put the caregiver on the defensive. Be careful to be nonjudgmental, especially if it appears that the child has not been provided with proper care or safety before your arrival. Be observant but not confrontational.

Elderly Patients

Be careful of your own prejudices with all special populations, but particular with the elderly. Be respectful of them. Always use a formal means of address, such as "Mr." and "Mrs." or "Ms." Speak slowly and clearly. Interviews might take longer, because many elders cannot process a lot of information quickly due to interfering physical disabilities and the fact that they can fatigue easily. Remember that the use of compassionate touch can be a welcome and important means of nonverbal support.

Always treat the elderly with the respect that our elders deserve.

Give the elderly patient choices whenever possible. Take along their "living assists," such as walkers, hearing aids, and eyeglasses, and their book of phone numbers to facilitate reaching family or friends. Many elderly people are set in their ways and can be stubborn, but if you respect their dignity and do not rush them, you usually can build enough rapport to work with them effectively.

Patients with Sensory Impairment

Blind people, including the sighted patients whose injuries may require covering the eyes, benefit from verbal communication. Tell them everything you are going to do before doing it. If you need to have them walk, lead them by letting them hold onto your bended arm. Use touch as a form of contact for reassurance.

Ask hearing-impaired and deaf patients their preferred method of communication: lip reading, signing, or writing. Writing often is necessary—and the best method of communication—in the out-of-hospital environment. Always be sure your face is illuminated when you speak to them. At night, also be sure that the deaf person who is trying to lip-read is not blinded by a flashlight. If the patient has some hearing, speak normally and do not exaggerate your enunciation of words or use too much volume, which can distort sound. Be aware that many hearing-impaired patients will nod "yes," even if they do not understand what was said or asked, possibly in a misguided effort to be agreeable.

Language and Cultural Considerations

An emergency situation in which people of different cultures and languages must interact requires you to be especially compassionate. To accomplish this, you must understand that cultures vary and **ethnocentrism,** or viewing your own life as the most desirable, acceptable, or best, and acting in a superior manner, will only hinder communication. Then, you must imagine the additional fear and frustration a patient in crisis feels when he tries to explain the emergency to a paramedic who cannot speak his language or understand his attitudes. To really empathize with him, you must be able to avoid **cultural imposition;** that is, avoid imposing on him your own beliefs, values, and patterns of behavior.

In a transcultural situation in which your patient also does not speak your language, you have the opportunity to make the experience less stressful by being caring and calm—and finding an interpreter. Some important principles when using an interpreter are:

* Children of immigrants may act as interpreters. If this occurs, remember to keep what you have to say at the appropriate age level.
* Recognize that the emergency may cause distressing emotions in the interpreter, especially if the interpreter is a child.
* Speak slowly.
* Phrase questions carefully and clearly.
* Address both the patient and the interpreter.
* Ask only one question at a time, and wait for a complete response.
* Understand that the information you receive may not be reliable.
* Have patience.

Cultural differences include more than just language differences. People of some cultures are more comfortable at a variety of distances when communicating; some expect health-care workers to have all the answers to their illnesses; some treat ill or injured family members in different ways. Asian, Native American, Indochinese, and Arab people may consider direct eye contact impolite or aggressive and may thus demonstrate respect to you by averting their eyes. The welts on a feverish Southeast Asian child may not be from abuse, but rather from a folk practice known as "coin rubbing" or "coining," which many believe will draw out fever.

Understand that both you and the patient may bring cultural stereotypes to the situation. If either of you acts as if one culture is superior to the other, the situation could be ripe for problems. As with any call, create an appropriate professional relationship, but keep in mind that the rules about interpersonal space, eye contact, and touching may all be very different from those you know. As you can see, it is a good idea to study the various cultures typical to your area. Be open to the different ways of people, and do not act as if your way is the only correct way to manage things. There is no reason to impose your beliefs, values, and patterns of behavior on others.

* **ethnocentrism** viewing one's own life as the most desirable, acceptable, or best, and acting in a superior manner to another culture's way of life.

* **cultural imposition** the imposition of one's beliefs, values, and patterns of behavior on people of another culture.

Many cultures have established and accepted folk-medicine beliefs. While these may seem strange, they are very important to those who believe and practice them. If you work in an area with a concentration of a particular ethnic group, try to learn about the folk-medicine beliefs and practices of that group.

Hostile or Uncooperative Patients

There are times when you will need to build rapport with someone who cannot or does not want you to. If this is the case, be sure you are not threatening. Avoid confrontation, but keep trying until you are successful. Use the same questioning techniques you usually use. Sometimes patients open up if you clearly explain the benefits and advantages of cooperation. You also may be able to obtain the information you need from observing the scene and from questioning the patient's family, bystanders, or even law enforcement officers.

Set limits and establish boundaries with an uncooperative patient, if necessary. If the patient is sexually aggressive, for example, clarify your professional role for the patient. Tell him in a way that you are certain he understands that you are there to provide emergency medical care. Be sure to document unusual situations, and ask witnesses to document their observations as well. In extreme cases, consider having a same-sex witness ride in the back of your ambulance or tape record all interactions.

If a patient is blatantly hostile, or there is any hint that your safety is jeopardized, be sure to stay far enough away from the patient. Monitor him closely, and never leave the patient alone without adequate assistance. Also, to prevent a hostile situation from getting worse, be sure to have an appropriate show of force (enough personnel to overpower the patient), if necessary. Remember, your personal safety is paramount. Always be sure you have a clear path to the nearest exit, and always position yourself so you can observe others entering or exiting the area. Know local protocols regarding the use of restraints and psychological medications. Don't hesitate to call for law enforcement back-up if necessary.

TRANSFERRING PATIENT CARE

When you arrive at the scene of an emergency, EMS-trained First Responders may already be there. Before they transfer patient care to you, be sure to listen to their report carefully. Integrate the information they give you into the questions you ask your patient; he will trust you more if he sees you have listened to your colleagues. Say something like: "The First Responder said you felt dizzy before you fell today. Were there any other sensations you can remember?"

If the emergency department is busy, the receiving nurse or doctor may appear to be distracted. If this is true, important medical information could get lost. In non-critical circumstances, therefore, respectfully stand your ground until the nurse or doctor looks at you. Then say, "Are you the person who will be listening to my hand-off report?" If so, follow up with, "Are you ready to listen, or would you rather wait a moment?" Also, be sure to introduce the patient by name and to say goodbye to the patient before you leave.

SUMMARY

The skills required to manage medical situations are obviously an important part of emergency care. Remember, much of the information you will gather from all your patients is extremely personal. You will need an enormous degree of sensitivity to recognize and respond to the signs of suffering in order to create an ideal, individualized process of communication.

DIVISION 2

PATIENT ASSESSMENT

CHAPTER 10

History Taking

Objectives

After reading this chapter, you should be able to:

1. Describe the techniques of history taking. (pp. 591–594)

2. Describe the structure, purpose, and how to obtain a comprehensive health history. (pp. 591–607)

3. List the components of a comprehensive history of an adult patient. (pp. 594–602)

INTRODUCTION

In the majority of medical cases, you will base your field diagnosis on the patient history. Clearly, how you conduct the patient interview and the questions you ask will determine how much relevant medical information your patient reveals. In medical cases, obtaining an adequate history of your patient's **chief complaint**, recent illnesses, and significant past medical history is as important as, if not more important than, the physical exam. The information you gather will direct the physical exam and reveal clues to your patient's problem. Although we present the history by itself in this chapter, you will most likely conduct it simultaneously with parts of the physical exam.

The ability to elicit a good history is the foundation for providing good care to patients you have never met before. To conduct a good interview you must gain your patient's trust in just a very short time. Then you must ask the right questions, listen intently to your patient's answers, and respond accordingly. In this chapter we will discuss both the verbal and nonverbal components of taking a comprehensive medical history.

We present the medical history in its entirety, as a well-structured, yet flexible, tool having several component procedures that are conducted in order. In reality, your patient's answers will alter the sequence of your questioning, and some of the information in this chapter will not readily adapt itself to prehospital emergency medicine. As you gain clinical experience, you will learn which components of the history are appropriate to the particular situations you encounter. Whether your patient is critical or stable, the situation determines the length and completeness of the interview. For example, complicated medical cases require a close investigation of your patient's chief complaint and past history. Trauma cases, on the other hand, are generally sudden events not precipitated by medical conditions and require only a modified approach to history taking.

The interview is the focal point of your relationship with your patients. It establishes the bonding necessary for effective and efficient patient care. By asking a series of well-designed questions you begin to build a profile of your patients. You also should have a good understanding of their problems and a list of causes (**differential field diagnosis**) to explain their signs and symptoms. Often, learning about your patient's history, medications, and even their lifestyle will reveal clues to your final field diagnosis.

* chief complaint the reason the ambulance was called.

The ability to elicit a good history lays the foundation for good patient care.

* differential field diagnosis the list of possible causes for your patient's symptoms.

ESTABLISHING PATIENT RAPPORT

Your patients will form an opinion about you within the first few minutes, so you must establish a positive rapport quickly. This is not always easy. The situation, the patient, and the conditions will determine your ability to establish rapport. You can do several things, however, to facilitate this task. By asking them the right questions you will discover their chief complaint and their symptoms. By responding to them with empathy, you will win their trust and encourage them to discuss freely their problems with you. Their answers will also help you decide which areas require in-depth investigation and on which body systems to focus.

SETTING THE STAGE

Sometimes you will assess a patient from a long-term care facility. If your patient's chart is available, as in a nursing home or extended care facility, review it before conducting the interview. Quickly note his age, sex, race, marital status, address, and occupation. The insight into your patient's life experiences that you begin developing with this information may provide subtle clues to help steer your questioning. Determine any past medical problems or previous referrals for the same condition. Note any treatments rendered and their effects. On emergency scenes, review the first responder's run sheet. Look for the chief complaint, a brief history including a current medication list, and vital signs. Be careful not to let your patient's chart, his past medical history, or someone else's first impression bias your possible field diagnoses. Always accept such information gratefully, but briefly reconfirm it with the patient and conduct your interview with an open mind.

If possible, conduct the interview in a quiet room, alone, with no distractions. Since you are asking your patient to divulge very intimate information, privacy encourages open communication. It should be a place where you and your patient can sit down and comfortably talk about his current problem and past experiences. Unfortunately, on emergency runs, you conduct the patient interview in a variety of settings beyond your control from the kitchen floor to a busy street corner or a crowded bus. Often the back of your ambulance is where your patient will disclose important personal information to you. Some patients, however, will still be reluctant to reveal intimate information to a nonphysician in the emergency setting. Paramedics are often surprised at the hospital when their patients tell a different story to the physician in the emergency department, but this is common. To maximize your chances of obtaining a good history, practice the following techniques for developing better patient rapport.

LANGUAGE AND COMMUNICATION

Use appropriate language. Nothing distances you from your patient more quickly than sophisticated medical terminology. "Have you ever had a heart attack?" is better than "Have you ever had an MI?" Effective communication means connecting with your patient. Most of your patients will not understand medical terms. Use an appropriate level of questions, but do not appear condescending. Other barriers to communication include cultural differences, language differences, deafness, speech impediments, and even blindness. When you encounter such obstacles, try to enlist someone who can communicate with your patient and act as an interpreter. An alternative is to adopt a conservative approach toward assessment, field diagnosis, and treatment.

Listening is an important part of the interview. The old saying, "Listen to your patient; he will tell you what is wrong," explains why it is crucial for a skilled clinician to be a good listener. Listen closely to what your patients tell you. Be careful not to develop tunnel vision from dispatch information. Begin your assessment without any preconceived notions about your patient's injuries or illnesses. Also watch for subtle clues that your patient may not be telling the truth. For example, your patient tells you that his chest pain went away, but his facial expressions and body language suggest otherwise. Developing good communication skills takes time and practice.

Avoid working your way in strict order down any prearranged list of questions (such as those in this chapter). Use these lists as a guide only. Listen to your patients and watch for clues to important signs, symptoms, emotions, or other factors. Then modify your questions to follow those clues. The following practices promote **active listening**.

Facilitation Maintain sincere eye contact, use concerned facial gestures, and lean forward while you listen. Cues such as "Mm-hmm," "Go on," or "I'm listening" all help your patient open up. Sometimes strategic silence is also helpful.

* **active listening** the process of responding to your patient's statements with words or gestures that demonstrate your understanding.

Content Review

ACTIVE LISTENING SKILLS
Facilitation
Reflection
Clarification

Reflection Repeat your patient's words. This encourages him to provide more details. Just make sure not to disturb his train of thought. For example:

> *Patient:* I can't breathe.
> *You:* You can't breathe?
> *Patient:* No, it feels like I can't take in a full breath because my chest hurts.
> *You:* Your chest hurts, too?
> *Patient:* Yes, it started this morning when I was working in the yard. I usually take a Nitro but I'm all out.

This simple reflection encouraged the patient to reveal facts about his history of heart disease. If the paramedic had merely investigated the chief complaint of dyspnea, discovering its true cause may have taken longer. Since the primary problem is not always the chief complaint, allowing your patient to take the lead is sometimes advantageous.

Clarification In crisis, patients often cannot clearly describe what they feel. They will use vague, general words. Do not hesitate to ask for clarification. For example:

> *You:* Do you have any allergies?
> *Patient:* Yes, the last time I took penicillin I had a bad reaction.
> *You:* Can you describe the reaction?
> *Patient:* Well, I got itchy all over with a rash.
> *You:* Did you have any difficulty breathing or feel like you were choking?
> *Patient:* Oh, no, just the itching and rash.

By asking for clarification you distinguish between a simple allergic reaction and life threatening anaphylaxis.

TAKING A HISTORY ON SENSITIVE TOPICS

Paramedic students normally have difficulty questioning their patients about embarrassing, sensitive, or very personal topics such as sexual activities, death and dying, physical deformities, bodily functions, and domestic violence. Even though you may feel uneasy discussing these matters, you may learn important information about your patient's illness. To become more comfortable dealing with these subjects, watch experienced clinicians discuss them with their patients. Familiarize yourself with and practice some opening questions on sensitive topics that both put your patient at ease and encourage him to talk about it. If a particular area makes you most uncomfortable, attend a lecture or seminar and learn how professionals deal with this subject daily. Make the unfamiliar familiar and it will seem less imposing.

Let's look at two sensitive topics—physical violence and the sexual history. Your patient may not want to reveal a history of physical abuse. You should consider it when any of the following conditions are present:

- Injuries that are inconsistent with the story given
- Injuries that embarrass your patient
- A delay between the time of the injury and seeking help
- A past history of "accidents"
- Suspicious behavior of the supposed abuser

To earn your patient's trust, try to make him or her feel that the problem is not uncommon and that you understand the reasons. For example, you can ask your female patient, "Sometimes when husbands and wives argue a lot, it leads to physical fighting. I noticed you have some bruises. Can you tell me what happened? Did someone hit you?" With active listening techniques, such questioning will help establish a rapport that encourages open communication.

Taking a sexual history can be the most embarrassing and uncomfortable topic for an inexperienced health care provider. The sexual history is normally taken later during the history but can be a part of the present illness or past history, depending on your patient's chief complaint. For example, if your patient complains of a genitourinary problem, the sexual history becomes important during the present illness questioning. If your patient has a history of sexually transmitted disease, then the sexual history is relevant to the past history. Whenever you begin the sexual history, it is helpful to prepare your patient with introductory statements and questions like, "Now I need to ask you some questions about your sexual health and activity. It may help me determine the cause of your problem and provide better care for you. This information will be strictly confidential. May I begin?" If your patient consents, proceed as follows: "Are you sexually active? Have you had sex with anyone in the last six months? Do you have more than one partner? Do you have sex with men, women, or both? Do you take precautions to avoid infection or unwanted pregnancy? Do you have any problems or concerns about your sexual function?" This may seem very uncomfortable for the beginning paramedic but with time and clinical experience you will develop a sense of where and when these questions are appropriate. It is critical that you remain calm, objective, and nonjudgmental regardless of how your patient answers.

THE COMPREHENSIVE PATIENT HISTORY

This section presents the components of a comprehensive patient history in a systematic order. In practice, you will ultimately select only those components that apply to your patient's situation and status. For example, if you conduct preemployment physical exams for a company, you may use the entire form. On the other hand, if you respond to a gasping patient in acute pulmonary edema, you will focus on the present illness. Common sense and clinical experience will determine how much of the following history to use.

Common sense and clinical experience will determine how much of the history to use.

Content Review

ELEMENTS OF THE PATIENT HISTORY

Preliminary data
Chief complaint
Present illness/injury
Past history
Current health status
Review of systems

PRELIMINARY DATA

For documentation, always record the date and time of the physical exam. Determine your patient's age, sex, race, birthplace, and occupation. This provides a starting point for the interview and establishes you as the interviewer. Who is the source of the information you receive about your patient? Is it the competent patient himself, his spouse, a friend, or a bystander? Are you receiving a report from a first responder, the police, or another health care worker? Do you have the medical record from a transferring facility? After you have gathered the information, you should establish its reliability, which will vary according to the source's knowledge, memory, trust, and motivation. Again, reconfirm the information with the patient, if possible. This is a judgment call based on your experience. For example, if the patient information you received from a particular EMT first responder has been accurate in the past, you probably will trust it again. On the other hand, if the nurse at a physician's office has repeatedly provided you with erroneous information, you probably will doubt her accuracy.

THE CHIEF COMPLAINT

The history begins with an open-ended question about your patient's chief complaint. The chief complaint is the pain, discomfort, or dysfunction that caused your patient to request help. In a medical case, it may be a woman's call for help because she has chest pain. In a trauma case, it may be a bystander's call for assistance to a "man down" or a police officer's reporting an injury in an auto collision. Your patient may have called for more than one symptom. It is important to begin with a general question that allows your patient to respond freely. For example, "Why did you call us today?" or "What seems to be the problem?" Avoid the tunnel vision that often biases paramedics who focus on dispatch information that may or may not accurately describe the situation. As you interview and assess your patient, the chief complaint becomes more specific.

The chief complaint differs from the **primary problem.** While the chief complaint is a sign or symptom noticed by the patient or a bystander, the primary problem is the principal medical cause of the complaint. For example, your patient's chief complaint may be leg pain, while the primary problem is a tibia fracture. When possible, report and record the chief complaint in your patient's own words. For example, "I am having a hard time breathing" is better than "the patient has dyspnea." For the unconscious patient, the chief complaint becomes what someone else identifies or what you observe as the primary problem. In some trauma situations, for instance, the chief complaint might be the mechanism of injury such as "a gunshot to the chest," or "a fall from 25 feet."

* **primary problem** the underlying cause for your patient's symptoms.

THE PRESENT ILLNESS

Once you have determined the chief complaint, explore each of your patient's complaints in greater detail. Be naturally inquisitive when exploring the events surrounding these complaints. A practical template for exploring each complaint follows the mnemonic OPQRST—ASPN, an acronym for *Onset, Provocation, Quality, Region/Radiation, Severity, Time, Associated Symptoms,* and *Pertinent Negatives.* This line of questioning provides a full, clear, chronological account of your patient's symptoms.

Onset Did the problem develop suddenly or gradually? What was your patient doing when the symptoms started? In medical emergencies, investigate your patient's activities at the time of, or shortly before, the signs or symptoms developed. In some cases, especially trauma, you may have to gather information from a few weeks before the onset of symptoms. For example, the signs and symptoms of a subdural hematoma may not appear until weeks following an injury. Was the patient exercising or exerting himself, or at rest or sleeping? Was he eating or drinking? If so, what? In trauma cases, assure that a medical problem did not cause the accident. For example, the sudden onset of an illness such as a seizure or syncope may have caused a fall.

Provocation/Palliation What provokes the symptom (makes it worse)? Does anything palliate the symptom (make it better)? In many illnesses, certain factors such as motion, pressure, and jarring may increase or decrease pain, discomfort, or dysfunction. Does eating, movement, exertion, stress, or anything else provoke the current problem. Positioning also may be a factor. Your patient may wish to curl up and lie on his side to reduce abdominal pain. Your congestive heart failure patients will sit bolt upright to ease respiration. They also may sleep with several pillows raising their upper body to relieve paroxysmal nocturnal dyspnea (PND), a sleep-disturbing breathing difficulty caused by fluid that accumulates in the lungs when they are supine. Ask your patient how breathing affects the discomfort. Deep breathing may increase the acute abdomen patient's pain. A patient with pleuritic or rib-fracture pain will not breathe deeply, whereas breathing may not affect the pain of angina. Any patient with respiratory pain will breathe with shallower but more frequent breaths.

If your patient took a medication shortly before you arrived, its effect or lack of effect may help determine the problem. Drugs such as bronchodilators, hypoglycemic agents, antihypertensives, and anticonvulsants are commonly prescribed and taken at home. Investigate any medication used to relieve a problem

Content Review

PRESENT ILLNESS— OPQRST–ASPN

Onset of problem
Provocative/**P**alliative factors
Quality
Region/radiation
Severity
Time
Associated **S**ymptoms
Pertinent **N**egatives

and note its effectiveness. Ask about any activity, medication, or other circumstance that either alleviates or aggravates the chief complaint.

Quality How does your patient perceive the pain or discomfort? Ask him to explain how the symptom feels, and listen carefully to his answer. Does your patient call his pain crushing, tearing, oppressive, gnawing, crampy, sharp, dull, or otherwise? Quote his descriptors in your report.

Region/Radiation Where is the symptom? Does it move anywhere else? Identify the exact location and area of pain, discomfort, or dysfunction. Does your patient complain of pain "here," while holding a clenched fist over the sternum, or does he grasp the entire abdomen with both hands and moan? If your patient has not done so, ask him to point to the painful area. Identify the specific location, or the boundary of the pain if it is regional.

Determine if the pain is truly pain (occurring independently) or **tenderness** (pain on palpation). Also determine if the pain moves or radiates. Localized pain occurs in one specific area, while radiating pain travels away from the source, in one, many, or all directions. Evaluate moving pain's initial location and progression and any factors that affect its movement.

Note any pain that may be referred from other parts of the body. **Referred pain** is felt in a part of the body away from the source of the disease or problem. The heart and diaphragm are two areas that most commonly produce referred pain. Cardiac problems such as myocardial infarction or anginal pain are usually referred to the left arm, with occasional referral to the neck, jaw, and back. Pain associated with irritation of the diaphragm (most commonly blood in the abdomen of the supine patient) generally is referred to the clavicular region.

Severity How bad is the symptom? Severity is the intensity of pain or discomfort felt by your patient. Ask him how bad the pain feels, and then have him compare it to other painful problems he has experienced. Sometimes a patient can describe the severity of the pain on a scale from one to ten, with ten being the worst pain he has ever felt. Also notice the amount of discomfort your patient's condition causes. How easy is it to distract your patient from his concern over the pain? Is your patient very still and resistive to your touch? Is he writhing about? The answers should give you a good idea of the intensity of your patient's pain.

Time When did the symptoms begin? Is a symptom constant or intermittent? How long does it last? How long has this symptom affected your patient? For several days, hours, or just a few minutes or seconds? When did any previous episodes occur? How does this episode's length vary from earlier ones?

Associated Symptoms What other symptoms commonly associated with the chief complaint in certain diseases can help rule in your field diagnosis. For example, if the chief complaint is chest pain, ask, "Are you short of breath? Are you nauseous? Have you vomited? Are you dizzy or light-headed?" The presence of these symptoms would help support a field diagnosis of cardiac chest pain.

Pertinent Negatives Are any likely associated symptoms absent? Their absence is as important to the field diagnosis as their presence, because they help rule out a particular disease or injury. Note any element of the history or physical exam that does not support a suspected or possible field diagnosis. For example, it is significant if your patient who complains of chest pain denies shortness of breath, nausea, and lightheadedness.

THE PAST HISTORY

The past medical history may provide significant insights into your patient's chief complaint and your field diagnosis. Look in-depth at your patient's general state of health, childhood and adult diseases, psychiatric illnesses, accidents or

---

✱tenderness pain that is elicited through palpation.

✱referred pain pain that is felt at a location away from its source.

The past medical history may provide significant insights into your patient's chief complaint and your field diagnosis.

injuries, surgeries, and hospitalizations. They may reveal general or specific clues that will help you to correctly assess his current problem. Your patient's condition, the situation, and time constraints will determine how much information you can and should gather on the scene. For example, asking about childhood diseases may not be relevant for your acute cardiac or trauma patient.

General State of Health How does your patient perceive his general state of health?

Childhood Diseases What childhood diseases did your patient have? Did he have mumps, measles, rubella, whooping cough, chickenpox, rheumatic fever, scarlet fever, or polio? Again, this line of questioning's relevance depends on the patient and the situation.

Adult Diseases Is your patient a diabetic? Does he have a history of heart disease, breathing problems, high blood pressure, or similar conditions? A preexisting medical problem may contribute to your patient's current problem or influence his care during the next few hours. To discover significant preexisting medical problems, ask if your patient has recently seen a physician or been hospitalized. If so, for what conditions? If you discover a preexisting problem, investigate its effects on your patient. When did the problem last affect him? Is your patient on any special diets or prescribed medications or restricted in activity? Even with the trauma patient, do not forget that a medical problem may have led to an accident or may complicate the effects of trauma. Also, obtain the name of your patient's physician since it may be helpful to the emergency department staff.

Psychiatric Illnesses Does your patient have a history of mental illness? Has he ever been diagnosed with depression, mania, schizophrenia, or other problems? Is he being treated for a mental illness? If so, what medications is he taking? Has he ever had thoughts of suicide? Has he ever attempted suicide? Tailor these questions for patients you suspect of having a mental illness.

Accidents or Injuries Has your patient ever had a serious accident or injury requiring hospitalization? Has he had a previous injury that could be a factor in his current problem? For example, a seemingly minor head injury one week ago may present now as a subdural hematoma in your unconscious elderly patient. Keep this line of questioning to relevant information only. An old football injury or childhood laceration is probably not influencing your patient's chest pain and respiratory distress today. But his pneumonectomy (surgical removal of a lung) probably is the reason for the absence of lung sounds on his right side.

Surgeries or Hospitalizations Has your patient had any other hospitalizations or surgeries not already mentioned. Again, these may offer some insight into your suspected field diagnosis. For example, your patient is an 85-year-old man with a long history of congestive heart failure and no history of chronic lung disease. He suddenly presents with severe difficulty in breathing and audible wheezing. You should suspect the obvious—a cardiac problem. Don't look for the five-legged cat.

CURRENT HEALTH STATUS

The current health status assembles all the factors in your patient's present medical condition. Here, you try to gather information that completes the puzzle surrounding your patient's primary problem. Look for clues and correlations among the various sections of this part of the history. For example, your patient is a heavy smoker, has many allergies to inhaled particles, works in a coal mine, and frequently uses bronchodilating medications. He now complains of shortness of breath and expiratory wheezing. He is probably having an exacerbation of his chronic lung disease.

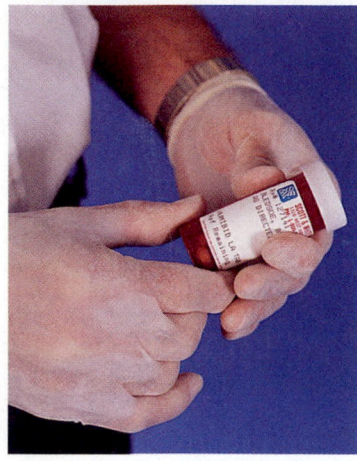

FIGURE 10-1 You should take your patient's medications with you to the hospital, when practical.

Current Medications Is your patient taking any medications? These include over-the-counter drugs, prescriptions, home remedies, vitamins, and minerals. If so, why? Your patient's explanation may not be medically accurate, but it may help to determine underlying conditions. For example, your 65-year-old patient tells you she takes a "water pill." You can safely assume she takes a **diuretic,** and has a history of renal or cardiac problems. A medication not taken as prescribed may be responsible for the current medical problem—possibly by under- or over-medication. A recently prescribed medication may cause an allergic or untoward (severe and unexpected) reaction. It also may be out of date and no longer effective. Even for trauma, emergency department personnel will need to know what medications your patient is taking. For example, if your patient takes warfarin, an anticoagulant, it would interfere with the normal clotting process and actually promote bleeding. If practical, bring your patient's medications to the hospital (Figure 10-1).

Allergies Does your patient have any known allergies, especially to penicillin, the "caine" family (local anesthetics), tetanus toxoid, and narcotics? These agents are occasionally given in emergency situations. What type of reaction did your patient have to the medication? For example, was it just a mild allergic reaction with a rash and itching or localized swelling or anaphylactic shock? Knowledge of your patient's allergies may prevent additional complications during the emergency department visit, especially if he becomes disoriented or unconscious during transport. If your patient is short of breath with wheezing, ask about environmental allergies. In cases of possible anaphylaxis, ask about allergies to drugs, to foods such as shellfish, nuts, and dairy products, and to insect bites and stings.

Tobacco Does your patient use tobacco? If so, how (cigarettes, cigars, pipe, smokeless, or other), how much, and for how long? To quantify his smoking history, multiply the number of packs smoked per day by the number of years he has smoked. The result is his pack/year history. For example, if your patient smoked two packs of cigarettes per day for 25 years, he is a 50 pack/year smoker. Anything over 30 pack/years is considered significant.

Alcohol, Drugs, and Related Substances Alcohol and drugs are often contributing factors in, if not the primary cause of, your patient's medical problems. Your job is not to pass judgment, but to gather data that will help direct your patient's medical treatment. Remaining nonjudgmental will aid you in your questioning. Start with a general question such as "How much alcohol do you drink?" If you suspect a drinking problem may be a factor, you can use the CAGE questionnaire (an alcoholism screening instrument) to determine the presence of alcoholism. Reserve this line of questioning for the chronic patient in a controlled setting. It would be inappropriate in a bar with an unruly, intoxicated patient.

The CAGE Questionnaire

Have you ever felt the need to **C**ut down on your drinking?

Have you ever felt **A**nnoyed by criticism of your drinking?

Have you ever had **G**uilty feelings about drinking?

Have you ever taken a drink first thing in the morning as an **E**ye-opener?

Two or more "yes" answers suggest alcoholism and further lines of inquiry.

Ask about blackouts, accidents, or injuries that happened while drinking. Also ask about alcohol-related job losses, marital problems, and arrests while under the influence of alcohol. Similarly, ask about drug use. For example, "Do you use marijuana, cocaine, heroin, sleeping pills, or painkillers? How much do you take? How do these drugs make you feel? Have you had any bad reactions?" As your patients realize you are not judging their substance abuse, they may feel more comfortable telling you about their patterns of use.

Diet Ask about your patient's normal daily intake of food and drink. Perhaps your 78-year-old retiree just moved to the Arizona desert and underestimated the increased fluid loss due to sweating. He does not realize he needs to increase his daily fluid intake, and now he presents weak and dizzy from dehydration. Are there any dietary restrictions or supplements? Ask specifically about his use of foods with stimulating effects such as coffee, tea, cola drinks, and other beverages containing caffeine. For example, your 23-year-old patient with a rapid heart beat (200 beats per minute) drinks continuous cups of coffee each morning at her highly stressful job.

Screening Tests Ask about certain screening tests that may have been done for your patient. Some examples include a purified protein derivative (PPD) test for suspected tuberculosis, Pap smears and mammograms for female problems, stool testing for occult blood, and cholesterol tests. Record the dates of the tests and their results.

Immunizations Ask your patient about his immunizations for diseases such as tetanus, pertussis, diphtheria, polio, measles, rubella, mumps, influenza, hepatitis B, and pneumococcal vaccine. For example, ask the parent of a child suspected of epiglottitis if he had the hemophilus influenza B vaccine. The H-flu is a common cause for epiglottitis in children.

Sleep Patterns Ask your patient what time he normally goes to bed and arises. Does he take daytime naps? Does he have problems falling asleep or staying asleep?

Exercise and Leisure Activities Does your patient exercise regularly or lead a sedentary existence? Sometimes your patient's lifestyle will support your field diagnosis.

Environmental Hazards Ask about possible hazards in the home, in school, and at the workplace. For example, your patient may live or work in an area with high levels of toxic substances. Many health problems can be traced to these environmental causes.

Use of Safety Measures In an auto accident, did your patient use a seat restraint system? Were all passengers belted in? Did the air bag deploy? Such information aids you and the emergency department staff in determining the extent of damage caused by a particular mechanism of injury. For bicycle, in-line skate, and skateboard injuries, ask about the use of helmets and knee and elbow pads.

Family History Since many disease processes are hereditary, the medical history of immediate family members is important. In the nonemergency setting you may explore deep into the family tree and chart the medical history of grandparents, parents, aunts, and uncles. In the emergency setting, learning that your 45-year-old patient with chest pain had a father and brother who both died of heart attacks in their late forties is important information. Look for a family history of diabetes, heart disease, hypercholesterolemia, high blood pressure, stroke, kidney disease, tuberculosis, cancer, arthritis, anemia, allergies, asthma, headaches, epilepsy, mental illness, alcoholism, drug addiction, and any symptoms like your patient's.

Since many disease processes are hereditary, it is important to learn the medical history of immediate family members.

Home Situation and Significant Others Who lives at home with your patient? Ask him about his home life—or lack of one. Ask about friends, family, support groups, loved ones. Find out if he has a support network and whom it includes. Who takes care of him when he needs help? Loneliness and isolation may complicate your patient's physical symptoms.

Daily Life Ask your patient to describe his typical day. When does he get up? What does he do first? Then what? Such questions reveal a lot about your patient's state of mind and general wellness. Is he busy, active, and motivated to get up in the morning? Does he merely exist from the time he awakens and go through life with no purpose or direction? Is he under high levels of stress from morning to night in a job that requires him to take his problems home with him? Find out what kind of life your patient leads. It may reveal a lot about his illness.

Important Experiences Ask about your patient's upbringing and home life growing up. How much schooling does he have? Was he in the military? What kinds of jobs has he held? What is his financial situation? Is he married, single, divorced, or widowed? What does he do for fun and relaxation? Is he retired or looking forward to retirement? Again, the answers give you a broader picture of your patient.

Religious Beliefs Some religions forbid certain treatments and have guidelines regarding the management of illness and injury. For example, some forbid whole blood transfusions. Knowing if your patient is guided by these beliefs can help you understand and care for him better. These questions require some expression of sensitivity, or it might be best to ask broadly if he has any limitations in medical care.

The Patient's Outlook Find out what your patient thinks and how he feels about the present and future.

REVIEW OF SYSTEMS

The **review of systems** is a series of questions designed to identify problems your patient has not already mentioned. It is a system-by-system list of questions that are more specific than those asked during the basic history. Again, the patient's chief complaint, condition, and clinical status determine how much, if any, of the review of systems you will use. For example, if your patient complains of chest pain, you may want to review the respiratory, cardiac, gastrointestinal, and hematological systems. If your patient complains of a headache, you may want to review the **HEENT** (head, eyes, ears, nose, and throat), neurologic, peripheral vascular, and psychiatric systems. Let your patient lead you through the history. The following sampling includes a few of the many questions that you might ask.

General What is your patient's usual weight, and have there been any recent weight changes? Has he had weakness, fatigue, or fever?

Skin Has your patient noticed any new rashes, lumps, sores, itching, dryness, color change, or changes in nails or hair? Could cosmetics or jewelry have caused these problems?

Head, Eyes, Ears, Nose, and Throat (HEENT) Has your patient had headaches or recent head trauma? How is his vision? Does he wear glasses or contact lenses? When was his last eye exam? Has he experienced any of the following: pain, redness, excessive tearing, double vision, blurred vision, spots, specks, flashing lights? Has he ever had glaucoma or cataracts? How is his hearing? Does he use hearing aids? Has he ever experienced ringing in the ears (**tinnitus**), vertigo, earaches, infection, or discharge? Does he have frequent colds, nasal stuffiness, nasal discharge, hay fever, nosebleeds, sinus problems? Does he wear dentures? When was his last dental exam? Describe the condition of his teeth and gums. Do his gums bleed? Does he get a sore tongue, dry mouth, frequent sore throats, or hoarseness? Does he have lumps or swollen glands? Has he ever had a goiter, neck pain, difficulty swallowing, or stiffness?

Respiratory Has your patient ever had wheezing, coughing up blood (**hemoptysis**), asthma, bronchitis, emphysema, pneumonia, TB, or pleurisy? When was his last chest X-ray? Is he coughing now? If so, can you describe the sputum?

✳ **hemoptysis** coughing up blood.

Cardiac Has your patient ever had heart trouble, high blood pressure, rheumatic fever, heart murmurs, chest pain or discomfort, palpitations, shortness of breath (**dyspnea**), shortness of breath while lying flat (**orthopnea**), or peripheral edema? Has he ever been awakened from sleep with shortness of breath (**paroxysmal nocturnal dyspnea**)? Has he ever had an ECG or other heart tests?

✳ **dyspnea** the sensation of having difficulty in breathing.

✳ **orthopnea** difficulty in breathing while lying supine.

✳ **paroxysmal nocturnal dyspnea** sudden onset of shortness of breath at night.

Gastrointestinal Has your patient ever had trouble swallowing, heartburn, loss of appetite, nausea/vomiting, regurgitation, vomiting blood (**hematemesis**), indigestion? How often does he move his bowels? Describe the color and size of his stools. Have there been any changes in his bowel habits? Has he had rectal bleeding or black, tarry stools, hemorrhoids, constipation, diarrhea? Has he had abdominal pain, food intolerance, or excessive belching or passing of gas? Has he had jaundice, liver or gallbladder problems, or hepatitis?

✳ **hematemesis** vomiting blood.

Urinary How often does your patient urinate? Has he ever had excessive urination (**polyuria**), excessive urination at night (**nocturia**), burning or pain while urinating, blood in the urine (**hematuria**), urgency, reduced caliber or force of urine flow, hesitancy, dribbling, or incontinence? Has he ever had a urinary tract infection or stones?

✳ **polyuria** excessive urination.

✳ **nocturia** excessive urination at night.

✳ **hematuria** blood in the urine.

Male Genital Has your patient ever had a hernia, discharge from or sores on the penis, testicular pain or masses? Has he ever had a sexually transmitted disease? If so, how was it treated?

Female Genital At what age did your patient have her first menstrual period? Describe the regularity, frequency, duration, and amount of bleeding of her periods. When was her last menstrual period? Does she bleed between periods or after intercourse? Has she ever had difficulty with her period (**dysmenorrhea**) or premenstrual tension? At what age did she become menopausal? Were there symptoms or bleeding? Has she ever had any vaginal discharge, lumps, sores, or itching? Has she ever had a sexually transmitted disease? If so, how was it treated? How many times has she been pregnant? How many deliveries? Any abortions (spontaneous or induced)? Some health care personnel use the G-P-A-L system to document a patient's history of pregnancy:

✳ **dysmenorrhea** menstrual difficulties.

Gravida	How many times pregnant?
Para	How many viable births?
Abortions	How many abortions?
Living	How many living children?

Has she ever had complications of pregnancy? Does she use birth control? If so, what type? If postmenopausal, is she on hormone replacement therapy?

Peripheral Vascular Has your patient ever had intermittent calf pain while walking (**intermittent claudication**), leg cramps, varicose veins, or blood clots?

✳ **intermittent claudication** intermittent calf pain while walking that subsides with rest.

Musculoskeletal Has your patient ever experienced muscle or joint pain, stiffness, arthritis, gout, or backache? Describe the location or symptoms.

Neurologic Has your patient ever experienced any of the following: fainting, blackouts, seizures, speech difficulty, vertigo, weakness, paralysis, numbness or loss of sensation, tingling, "pins and needles," tremors, or other involuntary movements?

Hematologic Has your patient ever been anemic? Has he ever had a blood transfusion? If so did he have a reaction to it? Does he bruise or bleed easily?

Endocrine Has your patient ever had thyroid trouble? Did he ever experience heat or cold intolerance, or excessive sweating? Does he have diabetes? Has he ever had excessive thirst, hunger, or urge to urinate?

Psychiatric Is he nervous? Is he under much stress and tension? Has he ever been depressed? Has he ever thought of committing suicide?

SPECIAL CHALLENGES

No matter how long you practice as a paramedic, some patients will present with special circumstances that challenge your skills. Your ability to deal with them will improve with time and practice.

SILENCE

Silence can become very uncomfortable if you are impatient. Why has your patient suddenly become silent? This question has no single answer. His silence can have many meanings and many uses. It may result from an organic brain condition that prevents him from forming thoughts. Or it may be due to dysarthria (difficulty in speaking due to muscular impairment). Maybe he is just collecting his thoughts or trying to remember details. Or maybe he is deciding whether he trusts you. He might be clinically depressed, or perhaps, he simply deals with situations by being quiet.

What do you do during the silence? Stay calm and observe your patient's nonverbal clues. Is he in pain? Is he scared? Is he on the verge of becoming hysterical or combative, or is he about to cry? You can encourage him to continue speaking by confronting him with your perceptions. For example, "I see you are obviously very upset about this. Do you want to talk about it?" If you sense your patient is not responsive to your questions, perform a brief orientation exam. Speak to him in a loud voice and call him by name. Shake him gently if he does not respond. If this does not elicit a response, assume a neurological problem and proceed accordingly.

Sometimes your behavior might have caused the silence. Are you asking too many questions too quickly? Have you offended your patient? Have you frightened him? Have you been insensitive? Have you failed to respond to your patient's needs? If your patient suddenly becomes silent, try to determine why, what is happening, and what you should do about it.

OVERLY TALKATIVE PATIENTS

The patient who rambles on can be just as frustrating to deal with as the one who will not talk at all. Why is your patient talking so fast and so much? Some patients react to stress this way. Maybe he has a lot to say. Maybe he needs someone to talk to; some lonely patients will take any opportunity to communicate with another human being. What can you do in the emergency setting when time is scarce? This problem has no perfect solution. You can lower your goals and accept a less comprehensive history. You can briefly give your patient free rein.

You can focus on the important areas and ask closed-ended questions about them. You can interrupt him frequently and summarize what he says. Above all, try not to become impatient.

PATIENTS WITH MULTIPLE SYMPTOMS

Patients often present with multiple complaints. For example, your elderly patient may present you with a barrage of symptoms from an extensive medical history. Your challenge is to discover the chief complaint and why she called you today. If she complains of symptoms that suggest multiple disease states, the challenge is compounded. In these types of cases, you must sort through a multitude of information quickly and recognize patterns that lead you to a correct field diagnosis.

Some patients will answer "Yes" to every question you ask. They have every symptom you mention; although possible, this phenomenon is not probable. Your patient might simply misunderstand or be trying hard to cooperate; more than likely he has an emotional problem and requires a psychosocial assessment. Document your findings on your prehospital care report and request a psychological referral. Asking the patient what single complaint led him to call for help today often helps.

ANXIOUS PATIENTS

Anxiety is a natural reaction to stress. People who face serious illness or injury can be expected to exhibit some degree of anxiety. Sometimes this manifests itself as simple nervousness, tenseness, sweating, or trembling. Some patients will fall silent, while others will ramble. Still others may exhibit anxiety attacks marked by a rapid heart rate, nausea and vomiting, chest pain, and shortness of breath. When you detect signs of anxiety, encourage your patient to speak freely about it. For example, you can say, "I see you are concerned about this. Do you want to talk about it?"

PATIENTS NEEDING REASSURANCE

Appropriate reassurance is a cornerstone of patient care. You must be careful, however, not to be overly reassuring or to prematurely reassure your anxious patient. It is natural to say, "Relax, everything is going to be all right. We are going to take care of you and get you to the hospital. Just relax and you will be all right." But your patient may have anxiety about something of which you are not aware. For instance, if your chest pain patient is anxious, you might naturally assume he is apprehensive about dying. In reality he may be anxious about something entirely different. He may be embarrassed about his anxieties, and instead of helping him deal with them, you have helped him cover them up. Now he may decide you are not interested in what is really bothering him and block further communication. Listen carefully to your patient before offering reassurance.

ANGER AND HOSTILITY

You will often encounter angry patients or their families. They might be angry for many reasons. Your patient is sick, perhaps dying. The family is anticipating their future loss. Often they will lash out at the easiest target—you. Sometimes you cannot do anything quickly enough or well enough for them. Understand that their anger is a natural part of the grieving process and they may be merely venting their frustration. Unfortunately you find yourself at the receiving end of their outbursts. Try to accept their feelings without getting defensive or angry in return.

INTOXICATION

Dealing with belligerent, intoxicated patients challenges even the most experienced paramedic. These patients are irrational, they disrupt your control of the scene, and they rarely allow you to examine them. First and foremost, make sure your environment is safe. If your patient acts violently, call for the police before attempting any interaction. As you approach your patient, introduce yourself and offer a handshake. Avoid any challenging body language or remarks. Appear friendly and nonjudgmental, but always stay alert for a potential violent outburst. If your patient is shouting or cursing, do not try to get him to stop or to lower his voice. Listen to what he says, not how he says it, and try to understand his situation before making a clinical judgment. Sometimes a genuine offer of a place to sit will help calm an agitated, intoxicated person. Then you can begin your assessment.

CRYING

Sometimes your patients will cry. This can make any paramedic uncomfortable. Crying is just another form of venting, an important clue to your patient's emotions. Accept it as a natural release and do not try to suppress it. Be patient, allow your patient to cry, and then offer a supportive remark. Quiet acceptance and supportive remarks will open the lines of communication once your patient composes himself.

DEPRESSION

* **depression** a mood disorder characterized by hopelessness and malaise.

Depression is a common problem in medicine. It is also commonly misdiagnosed or ignored. It often presents with symptoms such as insomnia, fatigue, weight loss, or mysterious aches and pains. Depression is potentially lethal, so you must recognize its signs and evaluate its severity just as you would chest pain or shortness of breath. Ask your patient if he has ever thought about committing suicide; if he is currently thinking about suicide; if he has the means to commit suicide; and if he has ever attempted it. The more exact and precise his suicide plan, the more apt he is to carry it out.

SEXUALLY ATTRACTIVE OR SEDUCTIVE PATIENTS

Occasionally you will encounter a patient who is attracted to you or to whom you are attracted. These feelings are natural. The key is not to allow these feelings to affect your behavior. Always keep your relationship professional. If necessary, clearly tell any patient who behaves seductively that you are there on a professional basis, not a personal one. Afterward, determine if how you dressed, what you did, or what you said helped your patient get the wrong impression about your relationship. Did you send the wrong signals? Whenever possible, always have a partner with you to avoid any accusations of improper behavior or touching.

CONFUSING BEHAVIORS OR HISTORIES

* **dementia** a deterioration of mental status that is usually associated with structural neurological disease.

* **delirium** an acute alteration in mental functioning that is often reversible.

You may encounter a patient whose story you just cannot follow. No matter what you ask, the answers leave you confused and frustrated. You cannot seem to develop a clear picture about your patient's problems. In fact, his answers don't even seem to make any sense. For example, you ask, "When did your headache begin?" and he answers, "My head feels like a squirrel." In these cases, the problem is most likely psychotic (mental illness) or organic (**dementia** or **delirium**). Also consider head injury or other physiological conditions such as stroke.

Many psychotic patients live and function in their communities, with varying degrees of success. Some will provide an accurate past history, others will not. If your patient's behavior seems distant, aloof, inappropriate, or even bizarre, suspect a mental illness such as schizophrenia. It may be helpful to focus your assessment on this patient's mental status, with special emphasis on thought, perceptions, and mood.

Delirium and dementia are disorders relating to cognitive function. Delirium is common in the acutely ill or intoxicated patient; dementia occurs more frequently in the elderly. These patients often cannot provide clear, accurate histories. Their descriptions of their symptoms and their accounts of how things happened will be vague and inconsistent. They may appear inattentive to your questions and hesitant in their answers. They may even make up stories to fill in the gaps in their memories. In these cases, do not spend too much time trying to get a detailed history, because you will only become more frustrated. Focus on the mental status exam, with special emphasis on level of response, orientation, and memory. For a more detailed discussion of these problems, see Chapter 38 on psychiatric and behavioral emergencies.

LIMITED INTELLIGENCE

You can usually obtain an adequate history from a patient with limited intelligence. Do not assume that he will not be able to provide accurate information concerning his current or past medical status. Also, do not overlook obvious omissions because your patient appears to be giving you a good story. Try to evaluate your patient's education and mental abilities. If you suspect severe mental retardation, obtain the patient's history from family or friends. Above all, show a genuine interest in your patient and try to establish a positive relationship. Then, communication can still happen.

LANGUAGE BARRIERS

Few things are more frustrating than responding to an automobile accident with several patients who speak a language you do not understand. It is almost impossible to get an accurate history of the event. In these cases, try to locate an interpreter. Sometimes a family member speaks both languages and is willing to translate for you. Often, however, family members cause more confusion by paraphrasing what the patient and you are saying. Instead of hearing your patient's exact words, you hear the translator's version, and the true meanings become vague. Do not waste time using your broken foreign language from high school, because you will invariably confuse everyone involved.

HEARING PROBLEMS

The challenge of communicating with a hearing-impaired person is much like that of overcoming a language barrier. Some options, however, afford a degree of flexibility. You can try handwritten questions, but they can be time consuming. Sign language is effective if the patient practices it and you find a proficient interpreter. If your patient reads lips, you must modify your communication techniques accordingly. Always face him directly in a well-lit setting, and speak slowly in a low-pitched voice. Avoid covering your mouth and trailing off the end of your sentences. If your patient has one good ear, use that to your advantage. If he wears a hearing aid, make sure it is working. If he has eyeglasses, make sure he wears them. Augment your speech with hand gestures and facial expressions.

BLINDNESS

Blind patients present special problems. They need you to identify yourself immediately, since they cannot see your uniform. Always announce yourself and explain who you are and why you are there. If possible, take your patient's hand to establish a personal contact and to show him where you are. Remember that nonverbal communications such as hand gestures, facial expressions, and body language are useless in these cases. Your voice is your only tool for effective communication.

TALKING WITH FAMILIES OR FRIENDS

You will often encounter patients who cannot give you any useful information. In these cases, find a third party who can augment the patient history and offer a useful adjunct to the patient's answers (Figure 10-2). The typical case is the postictal patient who cannot describe his seizure activity to you. Another example is learning from his friend that your patient's wife died in an automobile accident just three weeks ago. Now you better understand why your patient appears depressed and suicidal. Make sure that patient confidentiality is a priority when you accept personal information from a family member, friend, or bystander. Patient assessment is a comprehensive history and physical exam process.

SUMMARY

This chapter dealt with taking a good history. While it presented the patient history in its entirety, common sense will determine which parts are appropriate for a given situation. Most of a paramedic's work is patient contact. It is making a connection with people in crisis. Patients most often comment on the attitudes of their paramedics. How well did they relate to them? Did they make them feel at ease? Did they care for them? Patients rarely comment on a paramedic's technical skills. Top-notch paramedics are technically skillful and treat all their patients with dignity and compassion. This begins with the history.

Good patient interaction can lead to good patient outcomes, improved patient satisfaction, and better adherence to treatment. As a paramedic you have the first opportunity to treat your patient when he enters the health care world. Let his first impression of the health care industry be your caring, compassionate, professional demeanor. Conducting effective and efficient interviews and communicating with your patient are essential to good medical practice. Medical interviewing is a basic clinical skill that must be learned and practiced, much like airway management.

CHAPTER 11

Physical Exam Techniques

Objectives

After reading this chapter, you should be able to:

1. Define and describe the techniques of inspection, palpation, percussion, auscultation. (pp. 610–614)
2. Describe the evaluation of mental status. (pp. 676–678)
3. Evaluate the importance of a general survey. (pp. 622–629)
4. Describe the examination of the following body regions, differentiate between normal and abnormal findings, and define the significance of abnormal findings:
   - skin, hair, and nails (pp. 630–635)
   - head, scalp, and skull (pp. 636, 638)
   - eyes, ears, nose, mouth, and pharynx (pp. 636–645)
   - neck (pp. 645–647)
   - thorax (anterior and posterior) (pp. 647–652)
   - arterial pulse including rate, rhythm, and amplitude (pp. 652–656)
   - jugular venous pressure and pulsations (pp. 652–656)
   - heart and blood vessels (pp. 652–656)
   - abdomen (pp. 656–657, 658–659)
   - male and female genitalia (pp. 657, 660)
   - anus and rectum (pp. 660–661)

Continued

Objectives Continued

- peripheral vascular system (pp. 671, 673–675, 661–671)
- musculoskeletal system (pp. 661–671)
- nervous system (pp. 675–681)
- cranial nerves (pp. 678–681)

5. Describe the assessment of visual acuity. (pp. 636, 638)
6. Explain the rationale for the use of an ophthalmoscope and otoscope. (pp. 620, 639–642)
7. Describe the survey of respiration. (pp. 615–617; 648–652)
8. Describe percussion of the chest. (pp. 649, 650, 652)
9. Differentiate the percussion notes and their characteristics. (pp. 612–613)
10. Describe special examination techniques related to the assessment of the chest. (pp. 647–652)

11. Describe the auscultation of the chest, heart, and abdomen. (pp. 649–655, 656–658)
12. Distinguish between normal and abnormal auscultation findings of the chest, heart, and abdomen and explain their significance. (pp. 649–655, 656–658)
13. Describe special techniques of the cardiovascular examination. (pp. 652–656)
14. Describe the general guidelines of recording examination information. (pp. 695–696)
15. Discuss the examination considerations for an infant or child. (pp. 690–695)

PHYSICAL EXAMINATION APPROACH AND OVERVIEW

Although assessment of a medical patient formally starts with the history, the physical examination actually begins when you first set eyes on your patient. Upon meeting him you immediately assess his general appearance, level of consciousness, breathing effort, and skin color. If you initially use touch as a reassuring gesture, you can also assess skin condition and peripheral pulses. Your physical assessment continues throughout the history as you ask questions and observe your patient's body language, facial expressions, and general demeanor. Thus, you cannot draw an exact dividing line between the history and the physical exam. In emergency street medicine, the two usually occur simultaneously.

The purpose of the physical exam is to investigate areas that you suspect are involved in your patient's primary problem. As we covered the entire history in the previous chapter, we present the entire physical exam in this one. Again, if you practice in a setting other than the prehospital, such as conducting pre-employment physicals for a company, you might perform the entire physical examination outlined here. On an emergency run, you limit the exam to only those aspects that you decide are appropriate. Practice and clinical experience will dictate your ability to apply the skills you learn in this section to real situations.

EXAMINATION TECHNIQUES

Four techniques—inspection, palpation, auscultation, and percussion—are the foundation of the formal physical exam. Each can reveal information essential to a comprehensive patient assessment.

Inspection

* **inspection** the process of informed observation.

Inspection is the process of informed observation (Figure 11-1). A simple, noninvasive technique that clinicians often take for granted, it is also one of their most valuable tools in appraising patient condition. With a keen eye, you can evaluate your patient's condition in great detail.

Inspection begins when you first meet your patient and continues while you take his history. Often, this first impression forms the basis for your history because you

FIGURE 11-1 Inspect your patient's body for signs of injury or illness.

will judge your patient's clinical status immediately. Notice how he presents himself. Is he conscious and alert or unconscious and flaccid? Is he lying on the floor, sitting upright, or limping badly on one foot? Is he breathing normally or gasping for each breath? You can learn a great deal about your patient's neurological, musculoskeletal, and respiratory systems just by careful observation. Watch for changes in his emotional and mental status throughout the history and physical exam.

During the formal physical exam, consciously evaluate each body area, looking for discoloration, unusual motion, or deformity. Pay special attention to areas where you most expect to find signs and where the patient complains of symptoms. For example, if your patient struck his chest against a bent steering wheel, you would expect to see chest wall abnormalities. Remember that you may not notice the skin color changes that follow a significant contusion until after your patient arrives at the emergency department.

Effective inspection depends on good lighting, adequate time, and a curiosity for looking beyond the obvious. During your inspection, draw on your past clinical experiences to identify the signs of illness and injury. Knowing what you are looking for is essential. Do not hurry. Give yourself enough time to inspect and then to process what you see. Inspection is an ongoing process that should not end until you transfer your patient to emergency department staff. Finally, while respecting your patient's modesty and dignity, never allow clothing to obstruct your examination.

Palpation

Palpation is usually the next step in assessing your patient, although sometimes you will inspect and palpate your patient simultaneously. **Palpation** involves using your sense of touch to gather information. With your hands and fingers you can determine a structure's size, shape, and position. You also can evaluate its temperature, moisture, texture, and movement. You can check for growths, swelling, tenderness, spasms, rigidity, pain, and crepitus. When you become skilled at this procedure, you can detect a distended bladder, an enlarged liver, a laterally pulsating abdominal aorta, or the position of a fetus.

Certain parts of your hands and fingers are better than others for specific types of palpation. For example, the pads of your fingers are more sensitive than the tips for detecting position, size, consistency, masses, fluid, and crepitus; therefore, you would use them to palpate lymph nodes or rib fractures (Figure 11-2). The palm

✱ **palpation** using your sense of touch to gather information.

FIGURE 11-2 Palpate with the pads of your fingers to detect masses, fluids, and crepitus.

of your hand is better for sensing vibrations such as fremitus. Because its skin is thinner and more sensitive, the back of your hand or fingers is better for evaluating temperature.

Palpation may be either deep or light. You control its depth by applying pressure with your hand and fingers. Since deep palpation may elicit tenderness or disrupt tissue or fluid, you should always perform light palpation first. Use light palpation to assess the skin and superficial structures. Press in approximately one centimeter. Apply the same gentle pressure you use to feel a pulse. Too much pressure dulls your sensitivity and can injure your patient.

To assess visceral organs such as those in the abdomen, use deep palpation. Apply pressure by placing the fingers of the opposite hand over the sensing fingers and gently pressing in about four centimeters. This will increase your sensitivity to any masses, guarding, or other abdominal pathology. Feel for areas of warmth that might reflect injury before significant edema or discoloration occur. Observe how your patient responds with facial expressions while you palpate tender areas. Even if he is unconscious, he may respond to pain with facial expressions or purposeful or purposeless motion.

Palpation begins your physical invasion of your patient. Three common sense tips will help make it therapeutic and respectful. Keep your hands warm, keep your fingernails short, and be gentle to avoid discomfort or injury to your patient.

To make palpation therapeutic and respectful, keep your hands warm, keep your fingernails short, and be gentle.

* percussion the production of sound waves by striking one object against another.

Percussion

Percussion is the production of sound waves by striking one object against another. In this technique, you strike a knuckle on one hand with the tip of a finger on the opposite hand. The impact causes vibrations that produce sound waves from four to six centimeters deep in the underlying body tissue. We hear these sound waves as percussion tones. The density of the tissue through which the sound must travel determines the degree of percussion. The denser the medium, the quieter the tone. The tone's resonance or lack of resonance indicates whether the underlying region is filled with air, air under pressure, fluid, or normal tissue. Listen to each sound and evaluate its meaning (Table 11-1).

Move across the area that you are percussing and compare sounds with what you know to be normal there. For example, in the chest you expect to hear the resonant sound of a healthy lung filled with air and tissue. In a pneumothorax or emphysema, however, you may hear the hyperressonant sound of air trapped in the chest. In a hemothorax, you may hear the dull sound of blood in the same area.

Percussion is simple. Place one hand on the area of the body you wish to percuss. Use a finger of that hand (usually the middle finger) as the striking surface. Sharply tap the distal knuckle of that finger with the tip of your other middle finger (Figure 11-3). The tap should come from snapping the wrist, not the forearm or shoulder. Snap the finger back quickly to avoid dampening the sound. When

Table 11-1	PERCUSSION SOUNDS				
Sound	**Description**	**Intensity**	**Pitch**	**Duration**	**Location**
Tympany	Drumlike	Loud	High	Medium	Stomach
Hyperresonance	Booming	Loud	Low	Long	Hyperinflated lung
Resonance	Hollow	Loud	Low	Long	Normal lung
Dull	Thud	Medium	Medium	Medium	Solid organs—liver
Flat	Extremely dull	Soft	High	Short	Muscle, atelectasis

FIGURE 11-3 Percuss your patient to evaluate vibrations and sounds.

percussing the chest, make sure the finger lies between the ribs and parallel to them. In this way you will percuss the tissue underneath the ribs, not the ribs themselves.

A wall in your home is a good place to practice your percussion skills. As you percuss the air-filled area between studs, you will hear a hollow, resonant sound. Wall spaces filled with insulation will sound less resonant. When you percuss over a wall stud, you will notice a flatter, dull sound. You can apply this principle to the percussion of body cavities. Compare the sounds on the affected side with those on the unaffected side. The key is knowing what is normal, so above all you must practice percussion on healthy people in order to recognize abnormalities in sick or injured patients.

Unfortunately at most emergency scenes, especially those in the street, noise prevents percussing your patient effectively. Your clinical experience and common sense will tell you when to use this valuable assessment technique.

Auscultation

Auscultation involves listening for sounds produced by the body, primarily the lungs, the heart, the intestines, and major blood vessels. It is difficult to master. You may hear some sounds clearly, such as stridor, the high-pitched squeal of a partially obstructed upper airway. Most, however, require a stethoscope. You should perform auscultation in a quiet environment. Unfortunately, this is not always practical in emergency services. Hearing the low amplitude heart and lung sounds against on-scene noise or in-transit background noise may be especially difficult.

For your patient's comfort, warm the end piece of your stethoscope with your hands before auscultating. To auscultate, hold the end piece of your stethoscope between your second and third fingers and press the diaphragm firmly against your patient's skin (Figure 11-4). If you are using the bell side, place it evenly and lightly on the skin. Avoid touching the tubing with your hands or allowing it to rub any surfaces. Make sure the earpieces point anteriorly before you put them in your ears.

Listen for the presence of sound and its intensity, pitch, duration, and quality. When reporting and recording lung sounds, always note abnormal sounds (crackles, wheezes), their locations (bilateral, right lower lobe, bases), and their timing during the respiratory cycle (inspiratory, end-expiratory). Sometimes, closing your eyes helps you concentrate on the sounds by eliminating visual stimuli. Try to isolate and concentrate on one sound at a time. Generally, auscultate after you have used other assessment techniques. The only exception is the abdomen, which you should auscultate before palpation and percussion. A paramedic should be

You must practice percussion on healthy people in order to recognize abnormalities in sick or injured patients.

✳ **auscultation** listening with a stethoscope for sounds produced by the body.

FIGURE 11-4 Auscultate body sounds with the stethoscope.

proficient in auscultating blood pressure, lung sounds, heart sounds, bowel sounds, and arterial bruits. As with any other physical assessment tool, you cannot detect abnormalities unless you know what is normal. Take every opportunity to auscultate lung, heart, and bowel sounds regularly.

Measurement of Vital Signs

Measure vital signs early in the physical examination and, in emergency situations, repeat them often and look for trends.

The four basic vital signs in medicine are pulse, respiration, blood pressure, and body temperature. While any complete physical examination should include all four, the first three are most important in prehospital care. They are the primary indicators of your patient's health. Measure them early in the physical examination and, in emergency situations, repeat them often and look for trends. For example, in a serious head injury, watch for your patient's systolic blood pressure to rise, his pulse pressure to widen, and his pulse rate to fall. These trends suggest an increase in intracranial pressure, a serious medical emergency. Conversely, a falling blood pressure with an increasing pulse rate may indicate shock. As a paramedic you should become an expert at taking vital signs on patients of every age.

Pulse As the heart ejects blood through the arteries, a pulse wave results. Each pulse beat corresponds to a cardiac contraction and results from the ejected blood's impact on the arterial walls. The pulse is a valuable indicator of circulatory function. Your patient's pulse rate, rhythm, and quality indicate his hemodynamic (circulatory) status and the critical nature of his condition. *Rate* refers to the number of pulsations felt in one minute. It can be slow (bradycardic), normal, or fast (tachycardic). *Rhythm* refers to the pulse's pattern and the equality of intervals between beats. It can be regular, regularly irregular, or irregularly irregular. *Quality* refers to the pulse's strength. Terms such as bounding or thready are used to describe the pulse's quality.

✱ **pulse rate** number of pulses felt in one minute.

✱ **pulse rhythm** pattern and equality of intervals between beats.

✱ **pulse quality** strength, which can be weak, thready, strong, or bounding.

✱ **bradycardia** pulse rate lower than 60.

✱ **tachycardia** pulse rate higher than 100.

The normal pulse rate for an adult is 60–100 beats per minute. Rates below 60 are bradycardic; rates above 100 are tachycardic. **Bradycardia** may indicate an increase in parasympathetic nervous system stimulation. It might also be the result of a head injury, hypothermia, severe hypoxia, or drug overdose. Bradycardia is sometimes a normal finding in the well-conditioned athlete. Treat bradycardia only if it compromises your patient's cardiac output and general circulatory status. **Tachycardia** usually indicates an increase in sympathetic nervous system stimulation with which the body is compensating for another problem such as blood loss, fear, pain, fever, or hypoxia. It is an early indicator of shock and may indicate ventricular tachycardia, a life-threatening cardiac dysrhythmia.

The pulse's rhythm, when present, may be regular, regularly irregular, irregularly irregular, or grossly chaotic. Irregular pulse rates may be due to extra beats, skipped beats, or pacemaker problems and usually indicate a cardiac abnormality. The rhythm's effect on cardiac output determines if intervention is necessary.

The pulse's quality can be weak, strong, or bounding. Weak, thready pulses indicate a decreased circulatory status such as shock. Strong, bounding pulses may indicate high blood pressure, heat stroke, or increasing intracranial pressure. The pulse location may be another indicator of your patient's clinical status. The presence of a carotid pulse generally means that his systolic blood pressure is at least 60 mmHg. The presence of peripheral pulses indicates a higher blood pressure; their absence suggests circulatory collapse. Practice locating each of the pulse locations (Figure 11-5). As with other vital signs, take your patient's pulse frequently in the emergency setting and note any trends.

Respiration Since oxygen and carbon dioxide exchange is essential to sustain life, **respiration** must occur continuously and must be effective. The lungs supply the arteries with oxygen and maintain the blood's pH by eliminating or retaining carbon dioxide. These two functions occur during respiration. Continuously observe your patient's respiratory rate, effort, and quality. Look for subtle signs of distress. Recognize when your patient requires rapid intervention such as aggressive airway management, positive pressure ventilation, and oxygenation. These interventions, some invasive, often will make the difference between life and death.

* **respiration** exchange of oxygen and carbon dioxide in the lungs and at the cellular level.

Recognizing when your patient's respiration requires rapid intervention often will make the difference between life and death.

Peripheral Pulse Sites

Temporal – lateral to eye orbit

Carotid – medial to and below angle of jaw

Brachial – just medial to biceps tendon

Radial – thumb side of wrist

Ulnar – little finger side of wrist

Femoral – just below inguinal ligament

Popliteal – just behind knee

Dorsalis pedis – top of foot

Posterior tibial – behind medial malleolus

FIGURE 11-5   Know each pulse location.

✳ **respiratory rate** number of times patient breathes in one minute.

✳ **tachypnea** rapid breathing.

✳ **bradypnea** slow breathing.

> *Very rapid or very slow breathing rates require rapid intervention to ensure that the adequate exchange of gases continues.*
>
>

✳ **respiratory effort** how hard patient works to breathe.

✳ **quality of respiration** depth and pattern of breathing.

✳ **tidal volume** amount of air one breath moves in and out of lungs.

✳ **blood pressure** force of blood against arteries' walls as the heart contracts and relaxes.

✳ **systolic blood pressure** force of blood against arteries when ventricles contract.

✳ **diastolic blood pressure** force of blood against arteries when ventricles relax.

✳ **Korotkoff sounds** sounds of blood hitting arterial walls.

Your patient's **respiratory rate** is the number of times he breathes in one minute. In general the normal respiratory rate for a healthy adult at rest is 12 to 20 breaths per minute. Rapid breathing (**tachypnea**) can be the result of hypoxia, shock, head injury, or anxiety. Slow breathing (**bradypnea**) can be caused by drug overdose, severe hypoxia, or central nervous system insult. Very rapid or very slow breathing rates require rapid intervention to ensure that the adequate exchange of gases continues.

Your patient's **respiratory effort** is how hard he works to breathe. Normal inhalation involves using the respiratory muscles (diaphragm and intercostals) to increase the chest's inner diameter. It is an active process that requires energy. The increasing space creates negative pressure, like a vacuum, that draws air into the lungs. Exhalation is the passive process of the respiratory muscles' elastic recoil. This normally effortless process can become difficult with some respiratory conditions. For example, an airway obstruction may compromise inhalation. The resultant increased breathing effort is evident in accessory muscle use, retractions, and possibly abnormal breath sounds.

Diseases such as asthma and emphysema, where the smaller airways collapse and trap air in the distal airways, may obstruct exhalation. Exhalation then becomes an active process that leads to respiratory distress and failure. Some injuries can decrease the respiratory effort. Rib fractures, for example, will cause a decrease in chest wall expansion because it hurts to breathe. A pneumothorax decreases effective gas exchange because the air enters the pleural space instead of the alveoli. Children become tired and decrease their respiratory effort, making their condition even worse. Evaluating your patient's respiratory effort will provide invaluable information about his respiratory status.

The **quality of respiration** refers to its depth and pattern. The depth, or **tidal volume,** of respiration is the amount of air your patient moves in and out of his lungs in one breath. The normal depth for a healthy adult at rest should be approximately 500 ml, just enough to cause the chest to rise. The tidal volume may increase during exercise or anxiety. It may decrease in the presence of a rib injury when every breath hurts.

Assess your patient's respiratory depth by inspecting and palpating the chest wall for symmetrical chest expansion, by feeling and listening for air movement and noise from the nose and mouth, and by auscultating for lung sounds. The depth may be shallow, normal, or deep. Once again, to recognize inadequate respiratory depth, you must know what is normal. The respiratory pattern should be regular. Variations in respiratory pattern can be associated with specific diseases (Table 11-2). Some irregular patterns such as Cheyne-Stokes may indicate serious brain or brain stem problems.

Blood Pressure Blood pressure is the force of blood against the arteries' walls as the heart contracts and relaxes. It is equal to cardiac output times the systemic vascular resistance. Any alteration in the cardiac output or the vascular resistance will alter the blood pressure. An important indicator of your patient's condition, blood pressure is measured during both systole and diastole. **Systolic blood pressure** (the higher numeric value) measures the maximum force of blood against the arteries when the ventricles contract. **Diastolic blood pressure** (the lower numeric value) measures the pressure against the arteries when the ventricles relax and are filling with blood. The diastolic blood pressure is a measure of systemic vascular resistance and correlates well with changes in vessel size. The sounds of the blood hitting the arterial walls are called the **Korotkoff sounds.**

Many factors may influence your patient's blood pressure. Anxiety, for example, may cause it to rise. His position (sitting, lying, standing) also may affect the measurement. If your patient has recently been smoking, exercising, or eating, you must wait at least five to ten minutes to allow his blood pressure to return to

Table 11-2 BREATHING PATTERNS

	Condition	Description	Causes
∿∿∿∿	Eupnea	Normal breathing rate and pattern	
∿∿∿∿∿	Tachypnea	Increased respiratory rate	Fever, anxiety, exercise, shock
∿∿∿	Bradypnea	Decreased respiratory rate	Sleep, drugs, metabolic disorder, head injury, stroke
———	Apnea	Absence of breathing	Deceased patient, head injury, stroke
∿∿∿	Hyperpnea	Normal rate, but deep respirations	Emotional stress, diabetic ketoacidosis
⋀⋀⋀⋀	Cheyne-Stokes	Gradual increases and decreases in respirations with periods of apnea	Increasing intracranial pressure, brain stem injury
⋀⋀⋀	Biot's	Rapid, deep respirations (gasps) with short pauses between sets	Spinal meningitis, many CNS causes, head injury
⋀⋀⋀⋀⋀	Kussmaul's	Tachypnea and hyperpnea	Renal failure, metabolic acidosis, diabetic ketoacidosis
⋀⋀⋀⋀⋀	Apneustic	Prolonged inspiratory phase with shortened expiratory phase	Lesion in brain stem

a resting level before you measure it. Because of these many intangibles, you should never use blood pressure as the single indicator of your patient's condition. Always correlate it with his other clinical signs of end-organ **perfusion** such as level of response, skin color, temperature, and condition, and peripheral pulses.

The average blood pressure in the healthy adult is 120/80. Females usually will have a lower blood pressure until menopause. **Pulse pressure** is the difference between the systolic and diastolic pressures. For example, a blood pressure of 120/80 represents a pulse pressure of 40 mmHg. A normal pulse pressure is generally 30–40 mmHg. In certain conditions, such as pericardial tamponade or tension pneumothorax, the pulse pressure will narrow. In others, such as increasing intracranial pressure or fever, the pulse pressure will widen. Again, take your physiologically unstable patient's blood pressure as often as every five minutes to chart trends.

What is normal? This question has no easy answer. Generally, systolic blood pressure in adults ranges from 100 to 135 mmHg, diastolic from 60 to 80 mmHg. **Hypertension** in adults is defined as a pressure higher than 140/90. A blood pressure of 130/70, however, may represent hypertension if a patient's usual pressure is 90/60 or **hypotension** if his usual pressure is 170/90. The numbers are not as important as detecting trends and assessing end-organ perfusion. Do not define hypotension by numbers but by whether perfusion is adequate to sustain life.

Hypertension can result from cardiovascular disease, kidney disease, stroke, or head injury, where it is a classic sign of increasing intracranial pressure. It may be a predisposing factor to, and preexist in, stroke or cardiovascular disease. Did the hypertension occur before or after the condition? Hypotension usually indicates shock due to cardiac insufficiency (cardiogenic shock), low blood volume (hypovolemic shock), or massive vasodilation (vasogenic shock). Orthostatic hypotension is a decrease in your patient's blood pressure when he stands or sits up.

If you suspect shock due to blood or fluid volume loss and you do not suspect a spinal injury, perform a tilt test. Take your patient's pulse and blood pressure while he is supine. Then have him sit up and dangle his feet, then stand. In 30–60 seconds retake his vital signs. The healthy patient's vital signs should not change. The tilt test is positive either if his pulse rate increases 10–20 beats per minute or if his systolic blood pressure drops 10–20 mmHg. (Research has found

Never use blood pressure as the single indicator of your patient's condition; always correlate it with his other clinical signs of end-organ perfusion.

✱ **perfusion** passage of blood through an organ or tissue.

✱ **pulse pressure** difference between systolic and diastolic pressures.

✱ **hypertension** blood pressure higher than normal.

✱ **hypotension** blood pressure lower than normal.

that an increase in heart rate is a more sensitive indicator of hypovolemia than a decrease in systolic blood pressure.) This finding is common in patients suspected of hypovolemia.

Body Temperature The body works hard to maintain a temperature of approximately 98.6°F (37°C). This temperature reflects the balance between heat production and heat loss through the skin and respiratory system. Even a slight variance can mean that significant events are happening within the body or on the body from environmental factors. Assess your patient's temperature to approximate his internal core temperature.

An increase in body temperature (**hyperthermia**) can result from environmental extremes, infections, drugs, or metabolic processes. Ordinarily the body's cooling mechanisms maintain a steady core temperature. In an extremely hot and humid environment or in cases like heat stroke, the cooling mechanisms can fail and the core temperature will rise despite an internal thermostat that wants to maintain a normal temperature. Fever, on the other hand, results when the body tries to make its internal environment inhospitable to invading organisms. It often presents with a history of illness. The skin is somewhat dry until the fever breaks and the body's cooling mechanisms begin to take effect. As the body temperature rises, it begins to threaten body processes, specifically those of the brain. A temperature of up to 102°F (38°C) increases metabolism markedly. As body temperature rises above 103°F (39°C), the neurons of the brain may denature. At temperatures above 105°F (41°C), brain cells die and seizures may occur.

Extreme cold also affects body temperature. When peripheral vasoconstriction and shivering mechanisms can no longer balance heat production and loss, core temperature drops (**hypothermia**). At a body temperature of 93°F (34°C), normal body warming mechanisms begin to fail. As the core temperature drops below 90°F (31°C), shivering stops, heart sounds diminish and cardiac irritability increases. If the temperature drops much below 70°F (22°C), your patient will present with a deathlike appearance and, possibly, irreversible asystole (absence of heartbeat).

A variety of methods can provide accurate temperature readings. You can use glass thermometers to take oral, rectal, or axillary temperatures. A rectal thermometer is the preferred device for children younger than six years old and for patients with an altered level of consciousness. An axillary temperature reading is the least accurate of the three methods.

EQUIPMENT

To conduct a comprehensive physical examination you will need a stethoscope, a sphygmomanometer, an ophthalmoscope, an otoscope, a scale, and other equipment. The ophthalmoscope, otoscope, and scale are not considered prehospital assessment tools.

Stethoscope The **stethoscope** is a basic paramedic tool used to auscultate most sounds (Figure 11-6). It transmits sound waves from the source through an end piece and along rubber tubes to the ear. One side of the end piece is a rigid diaphragm that best transmits high-pitched sounds such as heart sounds and blood pressure sounds. The diaphragm also screens out low-pitched sounds such as lung sounds and bowel sounds. The other side of the end piece is a bell that uses the skin as a diaphragm. The sounds that the bell transmits vary with the amount of pressure exerted. For example, with light pressure the bell picks up low-pitched sounds; with firm pressure it acts like the diaphragm and transmits high-pitched sounds. Whether you use the bell or the diaphragm depends on which sounds you are auscultating. To hear blood pressure or heart sounds, for instance, use the diaphragm; to hear lung or bowel sounds, use the bell side.

Even a slight variance in body temperature can mean that significant events are happening within the body.

✳ **hyperthermia** increase in body's core temperature.

✳ **hypothermia** decrease in body's core temperature.

Content Review

PHYSICAL EXAMINATION EQUIPMENT
• Stethoscope
• Sphygmomanometer
• Ophthalmoscope
• Otoscope
• Scale
• Tongue blades
• Thermometer
• Penlight
• Visual acuity chart/card
• Reflex hammer

✳ **stethoscope** tool used to auscultate most sounds.

Accurate auscultation depends in part on the quality of your instrument. Your stethoscope should have the following important characteristics:

- A rigid diaphragm cover
- Thick, heavy tubing that conducts sound better than thin, flexible tubing
- Short tubing (30–40 cm) to minimize distortion
- Earpieces that fit snugly—large enough to occlude the ear canal—and are angled toward the nose to project sound toward the eardrum
- A bell with a rubber-ring edge to ensure good contact with the skin

Sphygmomanometer The circumstances and the patient care setting determine what type of equipment you use to measure blood pressure (Figure 11-7). Intensive care unit staff commonly use intra-arterial pressure devices for critically ill patients who need continuous monitoring. When a noisy environment makes auscultation difficult or when the sounds are especially weak, a doppler device that amplifies the sounds is useful. You will see these devices in the emergency department, newborn nursery, emergency vehicles, and labor and delivery suites. The most familiar blood-pressure measuring device is the aneroid **sphygmomanometer.** You will use it with your stethoscope to auscultate the sounds of the blood moving through an artery, usually the brachial artery. Because your patient's blood pressure is important in evaluating his condition, you must be able to measure it accurately.

A sphygmomanometer includes a bulb, a cuff, and a manometer. The cuff has an airtight, flat, rubber bladder enclosed within a fabric cover. Cuffs are available

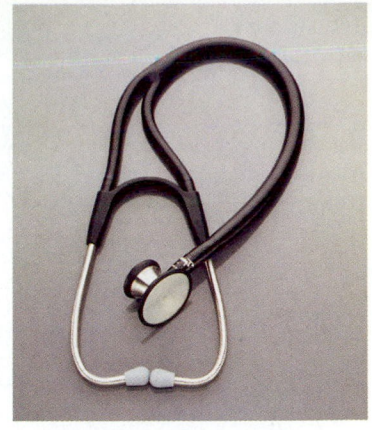

FIGURE 11-6 Use a stethoscope to auscultate most sounds.

 sphygmomanometer blood pressure measuring device comprising a bulb, a cuff, and a manometer.

Because your patient's blood pressure is important in evaluating his condition, you must be able to measure it accurately.

FIGURE 11-7 Use a blood pressure device suited to the circumstances. Clockwise from upper left: aneroid sphygmomanometer, mercury sphygmomanometer, digital electronic, and doppler device.

in various sizes and designs. Flexible tubing attaches the rubber bulb to the cuff. Squeezing the bulb pumps air into the cuff's bladder. A control valve allows you to inflate and deflate the cuff. To inflate the cuff, close the valve by turning it clockwise; to deflate the cuff, open the valve by turning it counterclockwise.

The **manometer** is a pressure gauge with a scale calibrated in millimeters of mercury (mmHg). Each line represents 2 mmHg. The heavy lines are 10 mmHg of mercury apart. The aneroid manometer displays the scale on a circular dial. As the pressure in the bladder changes, the needle moves and indicates the pressure reading at a given moment. When you use an aneroid sphygmomanometer, keep the dial in plain sight. The aneroid types lose their calibration, so you will need to calibrate them periodically against a mercury-type device.

The mercury sphygmomanometer displays the scale along a glass tube connected to a reservoir of mercury. As pressure in the cuff increases, the mercury in the tube rises. When using a mercury sphygmomanometer, keep the scale at eye level and vertical. Available as portable, wall-mounted, or floor units, mercury sphygmomanometers are more accurate than aneroid, but they are impractical for prehospital use.

Ophthalmoscope An **ophthalmoscope** allows you to examine the interior of your patient's eyes. It is a handheld device comprised of a light source and a series of lenses and mirrors (Figure 11-8).

Otoscope To visualize the ear canal and tympanic membrane you will need an **otoscope**. The otoscope provides illumination for inspecting the ear canal and tympanic membrane (eardrum) and the internal nose. It has a light source, a speculum you insert into the ear canal, and a magnifying glass through which you visualize the inner structures of the ear (Figure 11-9).

Scale The standing platform scale measures weight and height (Figure 11-10). To measure weight it uses a system of counterbalanced weights that you calibrate before each use. Your patient simply stands on the scale, and you add or

FIGURE 11-8 Visualize the interior of your patient's eyes with an ophthalmoscope.

FIGURE 11-9 An otoscope enables you to inspect the ear canal and tympanic membrane.

FIGURE 11-10 Use a platform scale to measure your patient's weight and height.

FIGURE 11-11 Essential assessment tools.

subtract weight in small increments until it balances. To measure your patient's height, pull up the height adjustment and position the head piece at his crown. Electronic scales are becoming more popular. They calculate your patient's weight electronically and display it as a digital readout. You also calibrate them before each use.

Additional Equipment Besides the above items, you will need sterile tongue blades to inspect inside the mouth and to initiate a gag reflex; a penlight to test your patient's pupillary responses; a visual acuity chart or card to measure visual acuity; a reflex hammer to test deep tendon reflexes; and a thermometer to measure body temperature (Figure 11-11). The danger of breakage limits glass thermometers' usefulness in the prehospital setting, and their inability to record temperatures below 96°F (36°C) prevents them from helping you evaluate the hypothermic patient. Available battery-operated devices measure temperature orally, rectally, and in the ear canal. If your service operates in areas of low environmental temperatures, equip your ambulance with a low-reading thermometer. Some of these items, such as the ophthalmoscope, otoscope, and scale, will be more suited to a medical clinic setting than to a typical prehospital scene.

THE GENERAL APPROACH

How you approach your patient, both in the emergency setting and elsewhere, will set the stage for an efficient and effective patient assessment. Most patients are apprehensive about a physical examination. They feel exposed and vulnerable, and they fear painful procedures. This anxiety is multiplied in an emergency. You must recognize your patient's apprehension and take steps to alleviate it. Display confidence and skill while you complete your history and physical exam.

If you systematically assess your patient's complaints and efficiently perform your duties, he should feel safe. Then add the personal touches of active listening, a reassuring voice, and gestures that convey your sincere compassion and interest. Most patients will respond favorably. Let your patient know that you are not just checking off items on a diagnostic list; you are conducting a personal examination of *his* problems.

How you approach your patient, both in the emergency setting and elsewhere, will set the stage for an efficient and effective patient assessment.

Proficiency will come only with clinical practice. In time, you will become adept at focusing the exam on your patient's chief complaint and present illness. In the emergency setting, no matter how nervous and apprehensive you may be, never let your patient see anything but a calm, professional, confident demeanor. This will help alleviate his anxiety about disclosing personal information to, and being examined by, a nonphysician. Try to remain objective, even when confronted by alarming or disgusting information. A bad bedsore, a perverted sexual story, or black tarry stools (melena) can test even the most experienced clinician's composure. Simply thinking about how embarrassed your patient must be may help you keep your own poise.

OVERVIEW OF A COMPREHENSIVE EXAMINATION

The key to an effective comprehensive exam is integrating each individual section into a unified patient assessment.

This section gives an overview of the comprehensive physical exam. Later in the chapter we will discuss each component in detail. The key to an effective comprehensive exam is to integrate each individual section into a unified patient assessment. Chapter 12 provides a template for conducting a problem-oriented patient assessment on both medical and trauma patients.

As a paramedic, you will determine which elements of the comprehensive exam to use. You will base your decision on your patient's presenting problem and clinical status. For example, if you are conducting comprehensive physicals for your fire department, you may choose to use the entire examination. If you are assessing a child just struck by an automobile and lying unconscious in the street, you will narrow your focus to the child's injuries. A comprehensive examination should include a general survey and a detailed assessment of anatomical regions.

THE GENERAL SURVEY

A general survey is the first part of a comprehensive examination. It begins with noting your patient's appearance and goes on to include vital signs and other assessments.

Appearance

A thorough evaluation of your patient's appearance can provide a great deal of valuable information about his health. Note his level of consciousness, posture, and any obvious signs of distress, such as sitting upright gasping for each breath or slumped to one side. Is his motor activity normal or does he have noticeable tremors or paralysis? Observe his general state of health, his dress, grooming, and personal hygiene. Obvious odors can also furnish significant information.

Level of Consciousness Is your patient awake? Is he alert? Does he speak to you in a normal voice? Are his eyes open, and does he respond to you and others in the environment? If he is not apparently awake, speak to him in a loud voice. If he does not respond to your verbal cues, shake him gently. If he still does not respond, apply a painful stimulus such as pinching a tendon, rubbing his sternum, or rolling a pencil across a nail bed. Note his response.

Signs of Distress Is your patient in distress? For example, does he have a cardiac or respiratory problem, as evidenced by labored breathing, wheezing, or a cough? Is he in pain, as evidenced by wincing, sweating, or protecting the painful area? Is he anxious, as evidenced by his facial expression, cold moist palms, or nervous fidgeting?

Apparent State of Health Is your patient healthy, robust, and vigorous? Or is he frail, ill-looking, or feeble? Does he have an obvious abnormality? Base your evaluation of his general state of health on your observations throughout the interview and physical examination.

Vital Statistics Vital statistics, weight and height, are used widely in clinical medicine. Accurately measuring your patient's weight and height with a scale, however, is not a practical prehospital assessment procedure. You will occasionally estimate your patient's weight to administer medications of which the dose is weight dependent. You also may use a **Broselow Tape** to measure your infant patient's length. The Broselow tape provides information concerning drug dosages, airway management adjuncts, and intravenous calculations based on your patient's height.

Note your patient's general stature. Is he lanky and slender, short and stocky, muscular and symmetrical? Does he have any obvious deformities or disproportionate areas? Is he extremely thin or obese? If obese, is the fat evenly distributed or is it concentrated in his trunk? Has he gained or lost weight recently?

Sexual Development Is your patient's sexual maturity appropriate for his or her age and gender? Consider such indicators as voice, facial and body hair, and breast size.

Skin Color and Obvious Lesions Is your patient's skin pale, suggesting decreased blood flow or anemia? Does he have central (lips, oral mucosa) or peripheral (nail beds, hands) cyanosis, the bluish color resulting from decreased oxygenation of the tissues? Does he have the yellow color of jaundice or high carotene levels? Note any rashes, bruises, scars, or discoloration.

Posture, Gait, and Motor Activity Observe your patient's posture and presentation. Is he sitting straight up and forward, bracing his arms (tripodding)? This suggests a serious breathing problem such as acute pulmonary edema or airway obstruction. Does one side of his body droop and seem immobile, suggesting a stroke? Does he sit quietly or does he seem restless? Does he have tremors or other involuntary movements?

Dress, Grooming, and Personal Hygiene Does your patient dress appropriately for the climate and situation? Are his clothes clean and properly fastened? Are they conventional for his age and social group? Abnormalities in dress might suggest the cold intolerance of hypothyroidism or the hiding of a skin rash or needle marks, or they might simply reflect personal preference. Look at his shoes. Are they clean? Do they have holes, slits, open laces, or other alterations to accommodate painful foot conditions such as gout, bunions, or edema? Does he wear a slipper, or slippers, instead of shoes? Is he wearing unusual jewelry such as a copper bracelet for arthritis or a medical information tag? Do his grooming and hygiene seem appropriate for his age, lifestyle, occupation, and social status? Does his lack of concern over appearance (overgrown nails and hair, for instance) suggest a long illness or depression?

Odors of Breath or Body Does your patient have any unusual or striking body or breath odors? The acetone breath of a diabetic, the bitter-almond breath of a cyanide poisoning, the putrid smell of bacterial infection, or the obvious smell of alcohol may give important clues to the underlying problem. Avoid tunnel-vision when you smell alcohol, which often masks other serious illnesses such as liver failure or injuries such as a subdural hematoma.

Facial Expression Watch your patient's facial expressions throughout your interaction. His face should reflect his emotions during the interview and physical exam. The patient with hyperthyroidism may stare intently. The Parkinson's patient's face may appear immobile.

* **vital statistics** height and weight.

* **Broselow Tape** a measuring tape for infants that provides important information regarding airway equipment and medication doses based on your patient's length.

Vital Signs

Take a complete set of vital signs to include pulse, respiration, blood pressure, and temperature.

Pulse To take the pulse of a conscious adult or large child, the most accessible and commonly used location is the radial artery. With the pads of your first two or three fingers, compress the radial artery onto the radius, just below the wrist on the thumb side (Procedure 11-1a). In the unconscious patient, begin by checking his carotid pulse. To locate the carotid pulse, palpate medial to and just below the angle of the jaw. Locate the thyroid cartilage (Adam's apple) and slide your fingers laterally until they are between the thyroid cartilage and the large muscle in the neck (sternocleidomastoid). In infants and small children, use the brachial artery or auscultate for an apical pulse. Remember that auscultating an apical pulse does not provide information about your patient's hemodynamic status. To locate the brachial artery, feel just medial to the biceps tendon. Auscultate the apical pulse just below the left nipple. First, note your patient's pulse rate by counting the number of beats in one minute. If his pulse is regular, you can count the beats in fifteen seconds and multiply that number by four. If his pulse is irregular, you must count it for a full minute to obtain an accurate total. Note also the pulse's rhythm and quality.

Respiration To measure your patient's respiratory rate, place one hand on your patient's chest and count the breaths he takes in thirty seconds (Procedure 11-1b). Multiply that number by two. Because your patient may consciously or subconsciously control his breathing, try to evaluate it without his knowing. Also assess his respiratory effort and quality of respiration.

Blood pressure To measure your patient's blood pressure, first choose the arm you will use. Remove any clothing that covers the upper arm; do not take the blood pressure over clothing, if possible. Look for a dialysis shunt in patients with renal failure. Do not take a blood pressure in that arm. Place the arm in a slightly flexed position, palm up and fingers relaxed. Support the upper arm at the level of your patient's heart.

Use the correct size cuff to obtain an accurate measurement. Its width should be one half to one third the circumference of your patient's arm. For most adults, unless they are obese or extremely slim, the large size cuff (15 cm wide) will suffice. If your patient has an obese arm, use a larger cuff. If the larger cuff is still too small, use your patient's forearm and place your stethoscope over the radial artery. For all patients, use a cuff that covers approximately two thirds of his upper arm or thigh. Using a cuff that is too wide, too narrow, too long, or too short will result in an inaccurate measurement.

Turn the control valve counterclockwise to open it; squeeze all the air out of the bladder before applying the cuff. Locate the brachial artery by palpating on the medial side of the antecubital space until you feel a pulse. Place the lower edge of the cuff one inch above the antecubital space. Find the center of the bladder (usually marked on the cuff with an arrow), and place it directly over the artery. Fasten the cuff so it is smooth and fits tightly enough to obtain an accurate reading. If you have difficulty inserting a finger between the cuff and your patient's arm, it is snug enough. Also make sure the rubber tubing is clear of the cuff. Check the placement of the manometer so you can see it easily.

Now palpate the radial artery. With your other hand, turn the control valve completely clockwise and squeeze the bulb rapidly to inflate the cuff to approximately 30 mmHg over the point where the radial pulse disappears. Place your stethoscope directly over the brachial artery and hold it firmly in place without pressing on the artery (Procedure 11-1c). Turn the control valve counterclockwise slowly and steadily to deflate the cuff at a rate of 2–3 mmHg per heart beat. Deflating too slowly or too rapidly will cause an inaccurate reading.

As you slowly deflate the cuff, watch the manometer and listen for the Korotkoff sounds. When you hear the first pulse beat, note the reading on the manometer dial or mercury column. This is the systolic pressure. Continue deflating the cuff until the pulsations diminish or become muffled. This is the diastolic pressure.

If you do not obtain a reading, wait 30 seconds to allow the blood pressure to normalize before inflating the cuff again. Sometimes you can palpate the artery during the deflation. The point at which you feel the pulse return marks the systolic reading. You cannot evaluate the diastolic pressure with the palpation method. To take your patient's blood pressure with a Doppler, follow the same procedure as for the palpation method, but instead of palpating for the return of the pulse, place the Doppler device over the palpated artery and listen for the "whooosh" of flowing blood indicating the systolic measurement (Procedure 11-1d). Record the blood pressure on your patient's chart. Include the systolic and diastolic pressures (for instance, 134/78), the arm used (right/left), and your patient's position (lying, sitting, standing).

Temperature The type of glass thermometer you use determines how long you must leave it in place to get an accurate reading. To take your patient's temperature orally with a glass thermometer, place the thermometer under his tongue for at least 3–4 minutes. It may provide a false reading if your patient has swallowed liquid or smoked within 15–30 minutes. To use a rectal thermometer, lubricate it well and then insert it 1.5 inches into the rectum; leave it in place for at least 2-3 minutes. If you use an axillary thermometer, it must remain under your patient's armpit at least 10 minutes. If your service uses battery operated devices, become familiar with them and follow the manufacturer's instructions for their use (Procedure 11-1e). For example, when using the tympanic membrane device, place the speculum into the ear canal, push the button and hold it for two to three seconds, then remove the device (Procedure 11-1f). The temperature is then displayed on a digital readout.

Additional Assessment Techniques

Additional assessment techniques include pulse oximetry, cardiac monitoring, and blood glucose determination.

Pulse Oximetry The **pulse oximeter** is a noninvasive device that measures the oxygen saturation of your patient's blood. It can reliably indicate your patient's cardiorespiratory status because it may tell you how well he is oxygenating the most peripheral vessels of his circulatory system. It also quantifies the effectiveness of your interventions such as oxygen therapy, medications, suctioning, and ventilatory assistance. For example, on room air, your patient's reading is 92%; after two minutes of high-flow oxygen therapy, it is 99%, showing a definite improvement.

The pulse oximeter has a probe-sensor and a monitoring unit with digital readouts. Attach the probe-sensor clip to your patient's finger, toe, or earlobe (Figure 11-12). The probe directs two lights (one red and one infrared) through a small area of tissue. The lights penetrate the tissue and are absorbed. Since saturated and desaturated hemoglobin absorb the lights differently, the sensors can determine their individual concentrations. The result is a measurement of your patient's oxygen saturation, or SaO_2.

Normal oxygen saturation at sea level should be between 96% and 100%. Generally, if the reading is below 95%, suspect shock, hypoxia, or respiratory compromise. Provide your patient with the appropriate airway management and supplemental oxygen and watch him carefully for further changes. Any reading below 90% requires aggressive airway management, positive pressure ventilation, or oxygen administration. The unresponsive patient may require invasive airway management and positive pressure ventilation.

* **pulse oximeter** noninvasive device that measures the oxygen saturation of blood.

11-1a Assess the pulse as an indicator of circulatory function.

11-1b Count your patient's respirations.

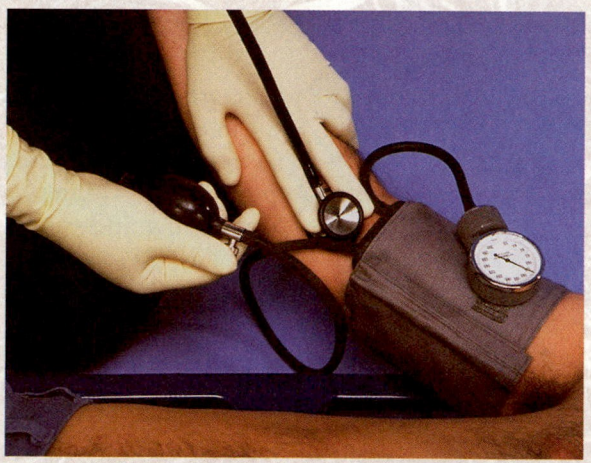

11-1c Assess blood pressure with a sphygmomanometer and stethoscope.

11-1d If you cannot hear blood pressure with a stethoscope, use an ultrasonic Doppler.

11-1e Use a battery-operated oral thermometer to take your patient's temperature.

11-1f Use a specially designed, battery-operated thermometer to measure temperature inside the ear.

FIGURE 11-12 Pulse oximetry allows you quickly and accurately to determine your patient's oxygenation status.

FIGURE 11-13 The cardiac monitor is essential to managing advanced cardiac life support.

Several factors affect the accuracy of a pulse oximetry reading. The sensors can accurately measure the oxygen saturation only if blood flow through the tissue is adequate. Most pulse oximeters display a digital readout of the pulse rate; others display a pulsation wave. In either case, if the display does not match your patient's actual pulse, the SaO_2 reading will be erratic. If your patient has decreased blood flow through the tissue, as in hypovolemia or hypothermia, you will obtain a false reading.

In cases of carbon monoxide (CO) poisoning, your saturation readings will be high while your patient's tissues are severely ischemic. This is because the CO molecule saturates the hemoglobin molecule 200 times more easily than does oxygen and the pulse oximetry probe cannot distinguish between hemoglobin that is bound to carbon monoxide and hemoglobin that is bound to oxygen. Your patient's hemoglobin is in fact saturated, but with carbon monoxide, not oxygen. Other than these limitations, the pulse oximeter, when teamed with other patient assessment techniques, can be a useful tool in the prehospital setting.

Cardiac Monitoring The **cardiac monitor** is essential in assessing and managing the patient who requires advanced cardiac life support (ACLS) (Figure 11-13). The most simple prehospital machines monitor the electrical activity of the heart in three "leads" or positions. These "limb leads" adequately identify life-threatening cardiac rhythms. Also available for prehospital use are 12-lead ECGs. They are essential in gathering data to confirm a myocardial infarction.

Other features of cardiac monitors include pacing capabilities and the "quick-look" paddles and the "hands-off" defibrillation pads used in cardiac arrest. The paddles, which you place on your patient's chest, allow you to check

* **cardiac monitor** machine that displays and records the electrical activity of the heart.

the cardiac rhythm and deliver a rapid electrical countershock. The hands-off defibrillation pads have two large electrodes that you attach to the chest wall. These replace the paddles and allow you to deliver a countershock without fear of injuring yourself.

All monitor-defibrillators can deliver a synchronized countershock in the presence of an unstable tachycardia. Most have a transcutaneous pacemaker that is placed externally on the chest and provides an electrical impulse to stimulate cardiac contraction in cases of bradycardia and heart blocks. This is a temporary measure until a permanent pacemaker can be implanted. Finally, some ECG machines have a "code summary" feature that prints out the electrical record of events and their times. This helps you document your patient's progress while in your care.

The cardiac monitor is a useful tool for measuring electrical activity, but it has one major disadvantage. It cannot tell you if the heart is pumping efficiently, effectively, or at all. The ECG reading does not necessarily correlate with the mechanical function of the heart. Electrical activity can exist with no mechanical contraction. Always assess your patient and compare what you see on the monitor with the rate and quality of the pulse.

Always compare what you see on a cardiac monitor with what you feel for a pulse.

Blood Glucose Determination In cases of altered mental status due to diabetic emergencies, seizures, and strokes, you will want to measure your patient's blood glucose level. The arrival of inexpensive, handheld **glucometers** makes this test easy to perform in the field. Most diabetic patients do it several times each day at home by themselves.

✱ glucometer tool used to measure blood glucose level.

To perform this procedure you will need a glucometer with test strips, a finger stick device with sterile lancets, alcohol wipe, and tissue or gauze pads. Simply place a drop of your patient's capillary blood from a finger stick onto a chemical reagent strip (Figure 11-14). Following the manufacturer's instructions, place the test strip in the glucometer and wait for the reading to appear. This procedure takes less than one minute to perform.

Since all glucometers work differently, you must read the manufacturer's instructions carefully. The slightest mistake can alter the measurement's accuracy. For example, make sure the code numbers on the test strips match those on the digital reading. Also make sure you do not allow alcohol to contaminate the blood. Glucometers are moderately accurate when used properly and calibrated daily.

FIGURE 11-14 Use a glucometer to determine your patient's blood glucose.

Content Review

ANATOMICAL REGIONS

- Skin
- Head, eyes, ears, nose, throat
- Neck
- Chest
- Abdomen
- Extremities
- Posterior body
- Neurological

ANATOMICAL REGIONS

After you complete the general survey, you will examine the body regions and systems in more detail. Again, the specific situation and your experience and common sense will determine whether you conduct a thorough examination, as you would when performing physicals for an insurance company, or narrow the focus of your examination, as you might in an emergency setting.

THE SKIN

Although you will observe your patient's skin throughout your assessment, a comprehensive physical exam must also include a concentrated inspection of all areas of the skin. The skin provides data on a variety of systemic problems in addition to skin-related disorders. Examining the skin requires good light and a keen eye. The characteristics of normal skin vary with your patients' racial, ethnic, and familial backgrounds. Evaluate its color, moisture, temperature, texture, mobility and turgor, and any lesions. Always wear protective gloves if your patient has any areas of open skin, exudative lesions, or rashes.

Content Review

SKIN CHARACTERISTICS TO ASSESS

- Color
- Moisture
- Temperature
- Texture
- Mobility and turgor
- Lesions

Color Normal skin color in light-skinned people is pink, indicating adequate cardiorespiratory function and vascular integrity. This means that the capillaries in the skin are well-oxygenated. The bright red oxyhemoglobin in the oxygen-rich blood circulating through the capillary beds gives the epidermis its pink appearance. A pale color suggests decreased blood flow through the skin. This is typical in hypothermia, hypovolemia, and compensatory shock, where blood flow through the distal capillary beds is severely diminished. It also is common in anemia, in which your patient's red blood cell count is low. As the hemoglobin loses its oxygen to the tissues, it changes to the darker, blue deoxyhemoglobin. Increased deoxyhemoglobin causes cyanosis, a bluish skin color. Cyanosis means that less oxygen is available at the tissue level.

Evaluate skin color where the epidermis is thinnest. This includes the fingernails and lips and the mucous membranes of the mouth and conjunctiva. In dark-skinned people, evaluate the sclera, conjunctiva, lips, nail beds, soles, and palms. Note any discoloration caused by vascular changes underneath the skin. Petechiae are small, round, flat, purplish spots caused by capillary bleeding from a variety of etiologies. Ecchymosis is a blue-black bruise resulting from trauma or bleeding disorders. Jaundice first appears in the sclera and then, in the late stages of liver disease, all over the skin. If only your patient's palms, soles, and face are yellow, he may have carotanemia, a harmless nutritional condition caused by eating a diet high in carrots and yellow vegetables or fruits.

Moisture Inspect and palpate the skin for dryness, increased sweating, and excessive oiliness. Dry skin, common during the cold winter months and in the elderly, may be the result of other conditions. Excessive oiliness, especially where the sebaceous glands are concentrated in the face, neck, back, chest, and buttocks, may suggest acne or hyperthyroidism. Increased sweating may indicate a sympathetic nervous system response to anxiety, fear, or exertion.

Temperature Use the backs of your fingers to feel the skin temperature in several different locations. Compare symmetrical body areas. Generalized warming or cooling suggests an environmental, infectious, or thyroid problem. Localized warmth may indicate bleeding or swelling.

Texture Feel your patient's skin. Is it rough or smooth? Are there large patches or small areas of scaling? Observe the skin's thickness. Thin and fragile skin is a sign of debilitating disease in the elderly. Thick skin often occurs with eczema and psoriasis. Inspect the palms and soles for calluses.

Mobility and Turgor Test the skin's **turgor** and elasticity by picking up a fold of skin over a bony prominence and then releasing it. Normal skin immediately returns to its original state. Poor turgor (tenting) results from dehydration. Test the skin's mobility by moving it over the bony prominence. Decreased mobility suggests edema or scleroderma, a progressive skin disease.

✳ **turgor** normal tension in the skin.

Lesions A skin **lesion** is any disruption in normal tissue. Skin lesions are classified as vascular, involving a blood vessel (Figure 11-15); primary, arising from previously

✳ **lesion** any disruption in normal tissue.

Purpura – Reddish-purple blotches, diameter more than 0.5 cm

Spider angioma – Reddish legs radiate from red spot

Petechiae – Reddish-purple spots, diameter less than 0.5 cm

Venous star – Bluish legs radiate from blue center

Ecchymoses – Reddish-purple blotch, size varies

Capillary hemangioma – Irregular red spots

FIGURE 11-15 Vascular skin lesions.

normal skin (Figure 11-16); or secondary, resulting from changes in primary lesions (Figure 11-17). Skin lesions can take any shape, color, or arrangement. Note their anatomical location and distribution. Are they generalized or localized? Do they involve exposed surfaces or areas that fold over? Do they relate to possible irritants such as wristbands, bracelets, necklaces? Are they linear, clustered, circular, or dermatomal (following a sensory nerve pathway)? What type are they? Inspect and feel all skin lesions carefully. Skin tumors are another variety of skin lesion. These include basal cell and squamous cell carcinomas, malignant melanomas, Kaposi's sarcoma in AIDS, actinic keratosis, and seborrheic keratosis.

When you detect a skin lesion, use anatomical landmarks to describe its exact location on the skin's surface. Describe its shape in terms such as oval, spherical, irregular, or tubular. Sometimes sketching an outline of the lesion is helpful. Record the size of the mass in centimeters, carefully measuring its length, width, and depth.

Macule – Flat spot, color varies from white to brown or from red to purple, diameter less than 1 cm

Plaque – Superficial papule, diameter more than 1 cm, rough texture

Patch – Irregular flat macule, diameter greater than 1 cm

Wheal – Pink, irregular spot varying in size and shape

Papule – Elevated firm spot, color varies from brown to red or from pink to purplish red, diameter less than 1 cm

Nodule – Elevated firm spot, diameter 1–2 cm

FIGURE 11-16   Primary skin lesions.

Describe the consistency of the mass exactly as it feels to you (for instance, soft, firm, edematous, cystic, or nodular). Of particular concern is its mobility. If the mass is affixed to a specific structure, suspect a malignancy. Note any pain or tenderness surrounding the mass upon palpation. Pulsation in the mass is another significant finding. For example, a mass that pulsates in all directions suggests an aneurysm.

THE HAIR

Inspect and palpate the hair, noting its color, quality, distribution, quantity, and texture. Is there hair loss? Is there a pattern to the loss? Patients undergoing chemotherapy for cancer may experience generalized hair loss. Failure to develop normal hair growth during puberty may indicate a pituitary or hormonal problem. Abnormal facial hair growth in women (hirsutism) also may indicate

Tumor – Elevated solid, diameter more than 2 cm, may be same color as skin

Pustule – Elevated area, diameter less than 1 cm, contains purulent fluid

Vesicle – Elevated area, diameter less than 1 cm, contains serous fluid

Cyst – Elevated, palpable area containing liquid or viscous matter

Bulla – Vesicle with diameter more than 1 cm

Telangiectasia – Red, threadlike line

FIGURE 11-16 (CONTINUED) Primary skin lesions.

Fissure – Linear red crack ranging into dermis

Scar – Fibrous, depth varies, color ranges from white to red

Erosion – Depression in epidermis, caused by tissue loss

Keloid – Elevated scar, irregular shape, larger than original wound

Ulcer – Red or purplish depression ranging into dermis, caused by tissue loss

Excoriation – Linear, may be hollow or crusted, caused by loss of epidermis leaving dermis exposed

FIGURE 11-17 Secondary skin lesions.

a hormonal imbalance. Part the hair in several places and palpate the scalp (Figure 11-18). A normal scalp is clean with no scaling, lesions, redness, lumps, or tenderness. Dandruff is characterized by mild flaking, psoriasis by heavy scaling, and seborrheic dermatitis by a greasy scaling. Try to differentiate the flaking of dandruff from the nits (eggs) of lice. andruff flakes off the hair easily, while nits firmly attach themselves to the hair shaft.

Feel the hair texture. In white people a soft hair texture is normal; in black people a coarser texture is normal. Very dry, brittle, or fragile hair is abnormal. Inspect and palpate the eyebrows. Note the quality and distribution of the hair and any scaling of the underlying skin. When assessing hair remember that the normal quantity and distribution of hair is related to gender and racial group. For instance, men have more trunk and body hair than women. Native American men have less facial and body hair than white men. In addition, Caucasians have more abundant and coarser body hair than Asians.

Scale – Elevated area of excessive exfoliation, varies in thickness, shape, and dryness, and ranges in color from white to silver or tan

Lichenification – Thickening and hardening of epidermis with emphasized lines in skin, resembles lichen

Crust – Reddish, brown, black, tan, or yellowish dried blood, serum, or pus

Atrophy – Skin surface thins and markings disappear, semitransparent parchment-like appearance

FIGURE 11-17 (CONTINUED)   Secondary skin lesions.

THE NAILS

Inspect and palpate the fingernails and toenails. Observe the color beneath the transparent nail. Normally it is pink in Caucasians and black or brown in blacks. Note if the nails appear blue-black or purple, brown, or yellow-gray. Look for lesions, ridging, grooves, depressions, and pitting. Depressions that appear in all nails are usually caused by a systemic disease. Gently squeeze the nail between your thumb and forefinger to test for adherence to the nail bed. A boggy nail suggests the clubbing seen in systemic cardiorespiratory diseases. The condition of the fingernails also can provide important insight into your patient's self care and hygiene. Check the toenails for any deformity or injury such as being ingrown.

FIGURE 11-18   Inspect and palpate your patient's hair and scalp.

THE HEAD

You can also examine the skull when you inspect and palpate the scalp and hair. Look for any wounds or active bleeding. Observe the general size and contour of the skull. Palpate the cranium from front to back (Procedure 11-2a). It should be symmetrical and smooth. Note any tenderness or deformities (depressions or protrusions). An indentation in the skull may suggest a depressed skull fracture. Note any areas of unusual warmth.

Inspect the face. Is it symmetrical? Are there any involuntary movements? Note any masses or edema. Observe the bony orbits of the eye for periorbital ecchymosis, a bluish discoloration also known as "raccoon eyes." Also check the mastoid process for discoloration (Procedure 11-2b). These are classic signs of a basilar skull fracture. They normally will not appear on the scene but will present hours after the injury occurs. Palpate the facial bones for stability and note any crepitus or loose fragments (Procedure 11-2c). Note whether your patient's facial expressions change appropriately with his mood.

Evaluate the TMJ. Place the tip of your index finger into the depression in front of the tragus (the cartilaginous projection just in front of the ear's outer opening) and ask your patient to open his mouth (Procedure 11-2d). The tips of your fingers should drop into the joint space. Palpate the joint for tenderness, swelling, and range of motion. Sometimes, you may hear a clicking or snapping. This is neither unusual nor problematic unless it is accompanied by pain, swelling, and crepitus. Test for range of motion by asking your patient to open and close his mouth, jut and retract his jaw, and move it from side to side. Finally, assess the skin of the face for color, pigmentation, texture, thickness, hair distribution, and lesions.

THE EYES

The ideal environment for an eye exam is a quiet room, free from distractions, in which you can control the lighting and make your patient comfortable. First, test for visual acuity. Place your patient 20 feet from a **visual acuity wall chart** or have him hold a **visual acuity card** 14 inches from his face. Ask him to cover one eye with a card and begin reading the lines (Procedure 11-3a). Record the visual acuity grade next to the smallest line in which he can read at least one half of the letters. The result is written as a fraction. The first number represents the distance away from the chart. The second number is the distance from which a normal eye could read the line. Normal is 20/20. A result of 20/70 means that a normal eye could read the line from 70 feet away but your patient could only read it from 20 feet. If no chart is available, you can have your patient count your raised fingers, read from a distance something you have printed, or distinguish light from dark. This type of exam is routinely conducted as part of a comprehensive physical exam in a clinic setting.

Test the visual fields by confrontation. Sit directly in front of your patient. Have him cover his left eye while you cover your right eye. Ask him to look at your nose. Extend your left arm to the side and slowly bring it toward you. Ask your patient to say when he first sees your finger. Use your own peripheral vision as a guide. If he sees your finger when you do, his visual field is grossly normal in that direction. Do this test in all four quadrants (left and right, up and down). Then perform the same test with the other eye (Procedure 11-3b). Any abnormalities suggest a defect in peripheral vision. Some common abnormalities include a horizontal defect (loss of vision in the upper or lower half of an eye), a blind eye, bitemporal hemianopsia (loss of vision in the outside half of each eye), left or right homonymous hemianopsia (loss of vision in the right half of both eyes or the left half of both eyes), or homonymous quadrantic defect (loss of vision in the same quadrant of both eyes). Record the area of defect as illustrated in Figure 11-19.

* **visual acuity wall chart/card** wall chart or handheld card with lines of letters used to test vision.

VISUAL FIELD ABNORMALITIES

Horizontal defect

Blind eye

Bitemporal hemianopsia

Homonymous hemianopsia

Homonymous quadrantic defect

Left Right

FIGURE 11-19 Visual field abnormalities.

Now examine the external eyes. Place yourself directly in front of your patient. Inspect his eyes for symmetry in size, shape, and contour. Do they look alike? Do they protrude (proptosis)? Are they properly aligned? Note the eyelids' position relative to the eyeballs. They should cover the upper quarter of the iris. Are the eyes totally exposed or do the eyelids droop (ptosis)? Have your patient close his eyes. Do they close completely? Do you see any edema, inflammation, or mass? Note the eyelid's color. It should be pink, indicating good central oxygenation. If the lid is pale, your patient could be in shock or anemic. If cyanotic, he could have central hypoxemia. Are there any lesions?

Carefully observe the lids' shape and inspect their contours for any growths. If you see any drainage, note its color and consistency. Do the eyelashes turn inward to scrape against the eyeball or outward to prevent the complete closure of the eye? Are they clean and free from debris? Is there a stye (reddened swelling of the inner eyelid)? Quickly assess the regions of the lacrimal sacs and glands for swelling, excessive tearing, or dryness of the eyes.

Now ask your patient to look up while you pull down both lower eyelids to inspect the sclera and conjunctiva (Procedure 11-3c). Be careful not to put pressure on the eyeball. Ask your patient to look left and right, up and down. The conjunctiva should be clear and transparent, with no redness or cloudiness. Redness or a cobblestone appearance suggests an allergic or infectious conjunctivitis. Bright red blood in a sharply defined area surrounded by normal tissue, not extending into the iris, indicates a hemorrhage under the conjunctiva. Look for any nodules, swelling, or discharge. The normal sclera is white. A yellow sclera suggests the jaundice of liver disease.

With an oblique light source, inspect each cornea for opacities. Also check the lens for opacities that you may see through the pupil. Inspect the iris when you inspect the cornea. Shine the light directly from the lateral side and look for a crescent-shaped shadow on the medial side of the iris. Since the iris is flat, the light should cast no shadow. A shadow could suggest glaucoma, caused by a blockage that restricts aqueous humor from leaving the anterior chamber. This increases intraocular pressure and threatens your patient's eyesight.

Inspect the size, shape, and symmetry of the pupils. Are they unusually large (excessive dilation) or unusually small (excessive constriction)? Are they equal? Some patients (20%) have unequal pupils, a condition known as anisocoria; if the difference in the pupil's size is less than two millimeters and they react normally to light, anisocoria is benign. To test the pupils, first shine a light into one eye and observe that eye's reaction (Procedure 11-3d). This tests the eye's direct response. The pupil should constrict. Repeat this test for the other eye. Now shine a light into one eye and observe the other eye's reaction. This tests the eye's

11–2a Palpate the cranium from front to back.

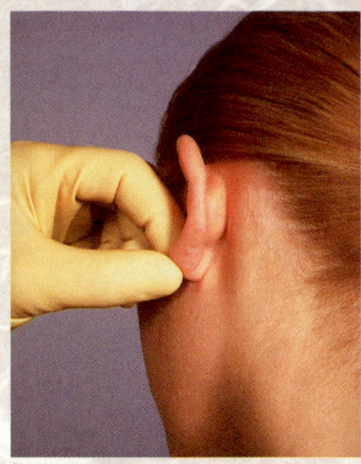

11–2b Inspect the mastoid process.

11–2c Palpate the facial bones.

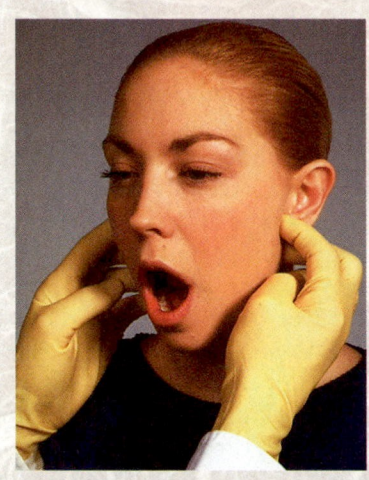

11–2d Palpate the TMJ.

Procedure 11-3   Examining the Eyes

11-3a Use a visual acuity chart to test visual acuity.

11-3b Test peripheral vision.

11-3c   Inspect the external eye.

11-3d   Test the pupil's reaction to light.

11-3e   Test for accommodation.

11-3f   Move your finger in an *H* pattern to test your patient's extraocular muscles.

11-3g   Check the corneal reflex.

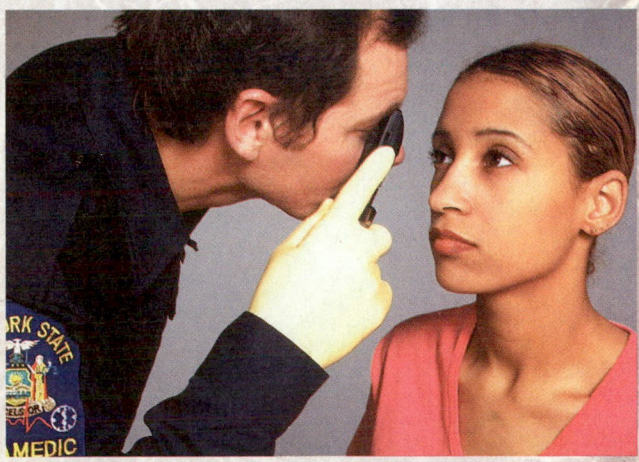

11-3h   Visualize the interior eye with an ophthalmoscope.

consensual response. Both eyes should react simultaneously to the light. Repeat this test for the other eye.

Normal pupils react to light briskly. A sluggish pupil suggests pressure on the oculomotor nerve (CN-III) from increased intracranial pressure. Bilateral sluggishness may indicate global hypoxia to the brain tissue or an adverse drug reaction. Constricted pupils suggest an opiate overdose, whereas fixed and dilated pupils usually mean brain death.

Now have your patient focus on an object in the distance. Then, ask him to focus on an object right in front of him. As he focuses on the near object, his pupils should constrict (near response). Now have your patient follow your finger or a pen, pencil, or similar object as you move it from a distance to the bridge of his nose (Procedure 11-3e). His eyes should converge on the object as the pupils constrict (accommodation). Finally, have your patient follow your finger as you move it in an *H* pattern in front of him (Procedure 11-3f). This tests the integrity of the extraocular muscles. Normal eye movements to follow your finger will be conjugate (together). Nystagmus is a fine jerking of the eyes; it may be normal if noted at the far extremes of the test. Check the corneal reflex by touching the eye gently with a strand of cotton and watch for your patient to blink (Procedure 11-3g).

Using an ophthalmoscope, visualize the eye's anterior chamber for cells, blood (hyphema), and pus (hypopyon) (Procedure 11-3h). Also visualize the retina, blood vessels, and optic nerve. Look for foreign bodies under the eyelid or in the cornea, check the cornea for lacerations, abrasions, and infection, and examine the vitreous humor. Look also for cataracts, papilledema caused by increased intracranial pressure, arterial and venous occlusions, and retinal hemorrhages, common clinical conditions you can visualize with an ophthalmoscope. Examining the eye's interior with an ophthalmoscope is a detailed process that is very difficult to master; it requires skill and practice.

Examining the eye's interior with an ophthalmoscope is a detailed process that is very difficult to master and requires skill and practice.

THE EARS

Begin examining the external ears from in front of your patient. Are they symmetrical? Then examine each ear separately. Inspect the auricles for size, shape, symmetry, landmarks, color, and position on the head. Observe the surrounding area for deformities, lumps, skin lesions, tenderness, and erythema (redness). Pull the helix upward and outward and note any tenderness or discomfort (Procedure 11-4a). Press on the tragus and on the mastoid process (Procedure 11-4b). Pain or tenderness in any of these areas suggests infection such as otitis or mastoiditis. Discoloration in this area is known as Battle's sign, a common, but late, finding in a basilar skull fracture. An earache may arise from the ear itself or be referred from another place through adjoining and shared sensory nerve pathways. Sources of referred pain may include sinus problems, a bad tooth, temporomandibular joint pain, the common cold, a sore throat, and the cervical spine.

Inspect for discharge (otorrhea) from the ear canal (Procedure 11-4c). The discharge may contain mucus, pus, blood, or cerebrospinal fluid that may have leaked from the skull through a fracture in its base. Injuries to the ear itself can result from blunt trauma to the side of the head, causing temporary or permanent damage to the outer or middle ear. A ruptured eardrum can result from sticking a sharp object into the ear canal or from a pressure wave caused by an explosion.

Check hearing acuity by having your patient close one ear. Test the open ear by whispering, then speaking, in its direction (Procedure 11-4d). Repeat this test for the other ear. Hearing loss can result from many causes. These include trauma, accumulation of debris (particularly cerumen, or "wax") in the ear canal, tympanic membrane rupture, certain drugs, previous surgery, or even prolonged exposure to loud noise. Tinnitus is the perception of abnormal noise in the ear. It usually presents as a buzzing or ringing and is associated with some degree of hearing loss.

11-4a   Examine the external ear.

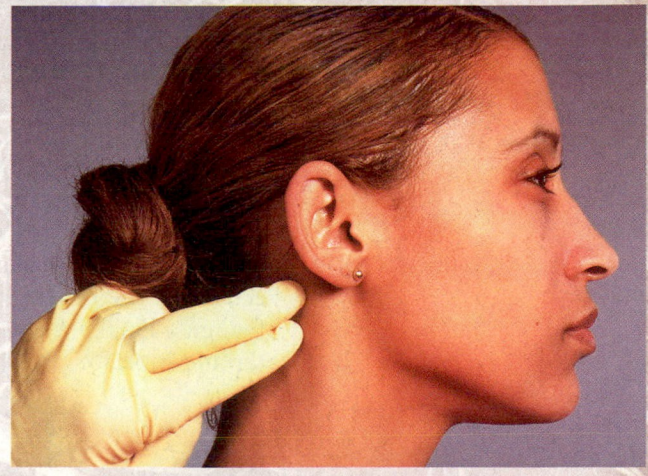

11-4b   Press on the mastoid process.

11-4c   Inspect the ear canal for drainage.

11-4d   Whisper in your patient's ear.

11-4e   Visualize the inner ear canal and tympanic membrane.

Visualize the inner ear canal and tympanic membrane using an otoscope. Attach to the otoscope the largest speculum that will fit into your patient's ear canal. Hold the otoscope either upward or downward. To enter the canal, first tilt your patient's head slightly away from you. Grasp the auricle gently and pull slightly up and backward to straighten the external canal (Procedure 11-4e). Insert the speculum gently and examine the ear canal for cerumen, discharge, redness, lesions, perforations, and foreign bodies.

Now focus farther back on the eardrum itself and note its color. The tympanic membrane should be a pearly, translucent gray. A change in color suggests a middle ear or tympanic membrane abnormality such as fluid or infection behind the eardrum. Observe the landmarks of the drum. You will need to move the scope around to visualize the drum's entirety. Begin with the light reflection in the anterior inferior quadrant. It should be sharp and bright. Then, check the center of the drum for bulging or protractions. Note the long process of the malleus. Finally move to the rim of the drum. Follow along the drum's perimeter and look for perforations from a ruptured tympanic membrane.

THE NOSE

Check your patient's nose from the front and from the side and note any deviation in shape or color. Also note any nasal flaring, an indication of respiratory distress. Palpate the external nose for depressions, deformities, and tenderness (Procedure 11-5a).

To inspect the nose's internal structures, tilt your patient's head back slightly. Insert the speculum of your otoscope and check the nasal septum for deviation and perforations (Procedure 11-5b). Erosions suggest intranasal cocaine abuse. Examine the nasal mucosa for evidence of drainage and note the color, quantity, and consistency of the discharge. Rhinitis (a runny nose) may produce a watery, clear fluid, as seen in seasonal allergies. If the discharge appears thick and yellow, suspect an infection. Epistaxis (a nosebleed) may be caused by trauma or a septal defect.

Test for nasal obstruction by occluding one side of the nose and having your patient breathe through the other side (Procedure 11-5c). It is normal for one side to be more patent than the other. A deviated septum, foreign body, excessive secretions, or mucosal edema may cause abnormal obstructions.

Inspect and palpate the frontal and maxillary sinuses for swelling and tenderness. To palpate the frontal sinus, press your thumbs upward, deep under the orbital ridges (Procedure 11-5d); to palpate the maxillary sinuses, press up under the zygomatic arches (cheeks) (Procedure 11-5e). You also can tap on each area for similar symptoms. Swelling or tenderness suggests a sinus infection or obstruction.

THE MOUTH

Assess the mouth from anterior to posterior, starting with the lips. Note their condition and color. They should be pink, smooth, and symmetrical and devoid of lesions, swelling, lumps, cracks, or scaliness. Gently palpate the lips with the jaw closed and note any lesions, nodules, or fissures, especially at the corners (Procedure 11-6a). Observe the undersurfaces of the upper and lower lips (Procedure 11-6b). They should be wet and smooth. Look for any of the lip abnormalities in Table 11-3.

To examine the mouth you will need a bright light and a tongue blade. Holding the tongue blade like a chopstick will give you good downward leverage. Examine the oral mucosa for color, ulcers, white patches, and nodules. The oral mucosa should appear pinkish-red, smooth, and moist. Note the color of the gums and teeth. The gums should be pink with a clearly defined margin surrounding each tooth. Inspect the teeth for color, shape, and position. Are any missing or

11-5a Palpate the external nose.

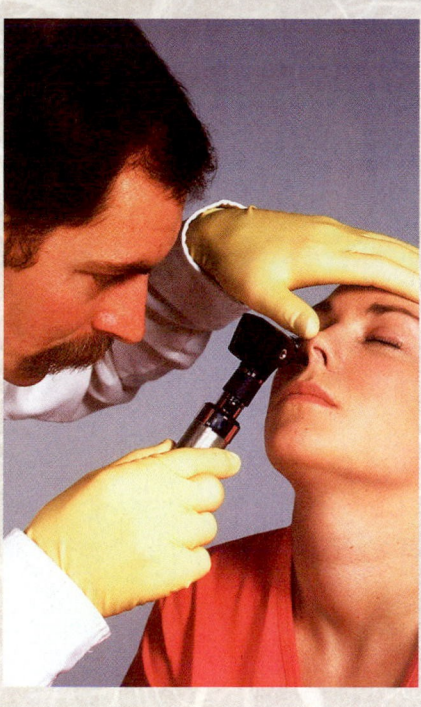

11-5b Inspect the internal nose with an otoscope.

11-5c Inspect the nose for nasal obstruction.

11-5d Palpate the frontal sinus.

11-5e Palpate the maxillary sinus.

11-6a   Palpate the lips.

11-6b   Inspect the lips' undersurfaces.

11-6c   Examine the buccal mucosa.

11-6d   Inspect the tongue using a gauze pad and a gloved hand.

11-6e   Inspect under the tongue.

11-6f   Have your patient say "aaahhh" while you examine the soft palate and uvula.

Table 11-3 LIP ABNORMALITIES

Lips	Cause
Dry, cracked lips	Dehydration, wind damage
Swelling/edema	Infection, allergic reaction, burns
Lesions	Infection, irritation, skin cancer
Pallor	Anemia, shock
Cyanosis	Respiratory or cardiac insufficiency

loose? Suspect periodontal disease if the gums are swollen, bleed easily, and are separated from the teeth by large crevices that trap food. Use a tongue blade to move the lateral lip to one side while you examine the buccal mucosa and parotid glands (Procedure 11-6c). Note the buccal mucosa's color and texture.

Ask your patient to stick his tongue straight out and then to move it from side to side. Coating of the tongue indicates dehydration. Note its color and normally velvety surface. Hold the tongue with a 2″ × 2″ gauze pad and a gloved hand to manipulate it for inspection (Procedure 11-6d). Make sure to inspect the sides and bottom of the tongue because malignancies are more likely to develop there, especially in patients over age 50 who smoke, chew tobacco, or drink alcohol (Procedure 11-6e). The undersurface should be smooth and pink; often you can see the bluish discoloration of dilated veins or the yellowish tint of early jaundice. Inspect the floor of the mouth, the submandibular ducts, and the fold over the sublingual gland.

Now examine the normally white hard palate and the normally pink soft palate (Procedure 11-6f). Check them for texture and lesions. Observe the posterior pharyngeal wall. Press the blade down on the middle third of the tongue and have your patient say "aaaaahhhh." Examine the posterior pharynx, the palatine tonsils, and the movement of the uvula. Inspect the tonsils for color and symmetry. Look for exudate (pus), swelling, ulcers, or drainage. The uvula should move straight up with no deviation.

Note any odors from your patient's mouth. The smell of alcohol, feces (bowel obstruction), acetone (diabetic ketoacidosis), gastric contents, or the bitter-almond smell of cyanide poisoning may all provide important clues to your patient's problem. Also look for any fluids or unusual matter in your patient's mouth. For example, coffee-grounds-like material suggests an upper gastrointestinal (GI) bleed. Pink-tinged sputum indicates acute pulmonary edema, whereas a green or yellow phlegm suggests a respiratory infection. Pay special attention to anything in your patient's mouth that can eventually obstruct his upper airway, including dentures or missing teeth.

Pay special attention to anything in your patient's mouth that can eventually obstruct his upper airway.

THE NECK

Briefly inspect your patient's neck for general symmetry and visible masses. Note any obvious deformity, deviation, tugging, masses, surgical scars, gland enlargement, or visible lymph nodes. Examine any penetrating injuries to the neck closely for damage to the trachea or major blood vessels; handle gently to avoid dislodging a clot that has halted bleeding. Immediately cover any open wounds with an occlusive dressing to prevent air from entering a lacerated jugular vein during inspiration. Look for jugular vein distention while your patient is sitting upright and at a 45° degree incline.

Palpate the trachea for midline position (Procedure 11-7a). Then gently palpate the carotid arteries and note their rate and quality of their pulses (Procedure 11-7b). Now palpate the butterfly-shaped thyroid gland from behind your patient. Rest your thumbs on his trapezius muscles and place two fingers of each

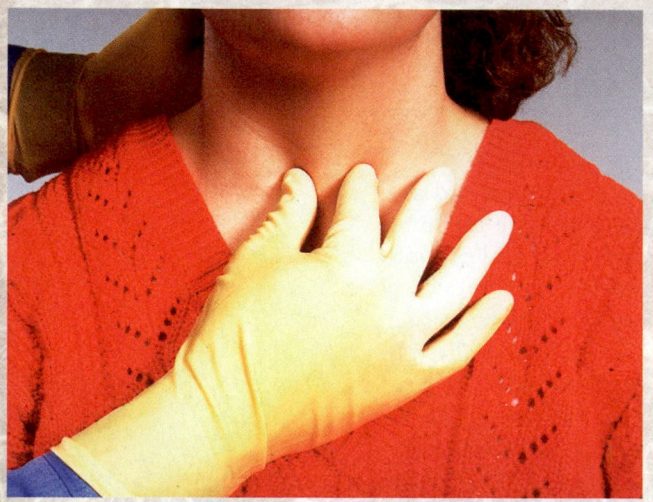

11-7a Assess the trachea for midline position.

11-7b Palpate the carotid arteries.

11-7c Palpate the thyroid gland.

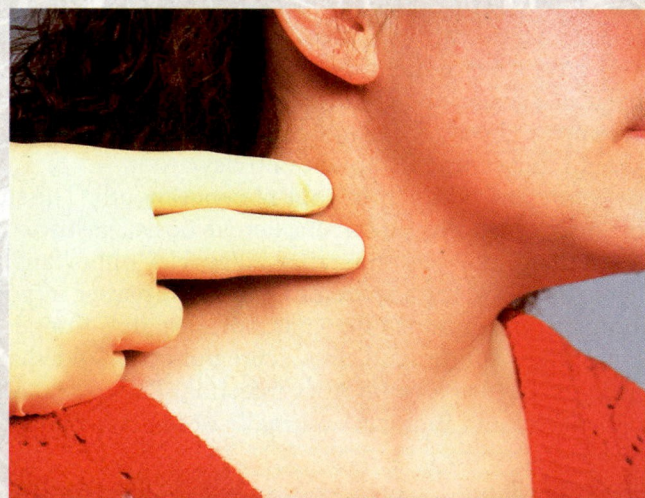

11-7d Palpate the lymph nodes.

Table 11-4 LYMPH NODE EXAM

Node	Exam
Preauricular	Press on the tragus and "milk" anteriorly
Postauricular	Palpate on or under the mastoid process
Occipital	Palpate at the base of the skull lateral to the thick bands of muscle
Submental	Palpate at the base of the mandible under the chin
Submaxillary	Palpate along the underside of the jawline
Anterior cervical	Palpate anterior to the sternocleidomastoid muscle
Posterior cervical	Palpate posterior to the sternocleidomastoid muscle
Deep cervical	Encircle and palpate the sternocleidomastoid muscle
Supraclavicular	Palpate just above the clavicle in the deep groove

hand on the sides of the trachea just beneath the cricoid cartilage (Procedure 11-7c). Have your patient swallow and feel for the movement of the gland. If you can feel it, it should be small, smooth, and free of nodules. Examining the lymph nodes requires a systematic approach (Table 11-4). Using the pads of your fingers palpate the nodes by moving the skin over the underlying tissues in each area (Procedure 11-7d). When swollen, the nodes are palpable, sometimes even visible. Note their size, shape, mobility, consistency, and tenderness. Tender, swollen, and mobile nodes suggest inflammation, usually from infection. Hard or fixed nodes suggest a malignancy. Inspect and palpate for subcutaneous emphysema, the presence of air just below the skin. This generally suggests a tear in the tracheo-bronchial tree or a pneumothorax.

THE CHEST AND LUNGS

To assess the chest and thorax you will need a stethoscope with a bell and diaphragm, a marking pen, and a centimeter ruler. Have your patient sit upright, if possible, and expose his entire chest. At the same time, try to maintain your female patient's dignity when assessing her thorax and lungs by keeping her breasts covered. Perform your exam in the standard sequence—inspect, palpate, percuss, auscultate—and compare the findings from side to side. Always try to visualize the underlying lobes of the lungs during your exam.

Observe your patient's breathing. Look for signs of acute respiratory distress. Now count the respiratory rate and note his breathing pattern. Obviously-prolonged inhalation or exhalation indicates difficulty moving air in or out of the lungs. Do you hear sounds of an upper airway obstruction (inspiratory stridor) or a lower airway obstruction (expiratory wheezing, rhonchi)? Any gross abnormalities in the respiratory rate or pattern require rapid emergency intervention.

Inspect the anterior chest wall and assess its symmetry. Funnel chest (pectus excavatum) is a condition in which the lower portion of the sternum is depressed (Figure 11-20). With a pigeon chest (pectus carinatum), the sternum curves outward. Do both sides of your patient's chest wall rise in unison? Note whether he is using neck muscles during inhalation or abdominal muscles during exhalation. If his skin retracts in the area above his clavicles (supraclavicular), at the notch above his sternum (suprasternal), and between his ribs (intercostal), suspect a ventilation problem. If multiple ribs are fractured, creating a "floating segment" or "traumatic flail chest," you may find paradoxical (opposite) movement of that part of the chest wall during breathing.

Any gross abnormalities in the respiratory rate or pattern require rapid emergency intervention.

Funnel chest   Pigeon chest   Barrel chest

FIGURE 11-20   Chest wall abnormalities.

Now look at his chest from the side. Normally an adult's thorax is twice as wide as it is deep. That is, the transverse diameter of the chest wall is usually twice the antero-posterior diameter. In infants, the elderly, or patients with chronic pulmonary disease, however, the antero-posterior diameter is increased, giving them a barrel chest appearance.

Posterior Chest Examination

Next examine the posterior chest. Ask your patient to fold his arms across his chest and breathe normally during the exam. This moves his scapulae out of the way and allows you more access to his posterior lung fields. Inspect his posterior chest for deformities and symmetrical movement as he breathes. Some patients may exhibit thoracic kyphoscoliosis, an abnormal spinal curvature that deforms the chest and makes your lung exam more challenging. Inspect the intercostal spaces for retractions or bulging; both are abnormal. Retractions may appear when airflow is impeded during inspiration. Bulging may appear when airflow is impeded during exhalation. Respiratory movement should be smooth and effortless. When it is not, suspect underlying respiratory disease or structural impairment.

Palpate the rib cage for rigidity. Feel for tenderness, deformities, depressions, loose segments, asymmetry, and crepitus. Then evaluate for equal expansion. First, locate the level of the posterior 10th rib. To do this, find the lowest rib and simply move up two more ribs. An alternate method for locating the posterior 10th rib is to palpate the spinous processes. Ask your patient to touch his chin to his chest. The most prominent spinous process is the 7th cervical vertebra. Locate it and count down to T-10 in the midline. Now place your hands parallel to the 10th rib on your patient's back with your fingers spread. Lightly grasp his lateral rib cage with your spread hands (Procedure 11-8a). Ask him to inhale deeply. Normally the distance between your thumbs will increase symmetrically by three to five centimeters during deep inspiration. If you detect decreased thoracic expansion or feel unilateral delay, suspect a disorder of the underlying lung, pleura, or diaphragm.

When your patient speaks, you can feel vibrations on his chest wall. This is known as tactile fremitus. Place the palm of your hand on your patient's chest wall and have him say "ninety-nine or one-on-one." As he does, palpate the posterior chest; feel the vibrations in different areas of the chest wall and compare symmetrical areas of the lungs (Procedure 11-8b). Identify and note any

11-8a Palpate the posterior chest for excursion.

11-8b Palpate the posterior chest for tactile fremitus.

11-8c Percuss the posterior chest.

11-8d Auscultate the posterior chest.

11-8e Palpate the anterior chest for excursion.

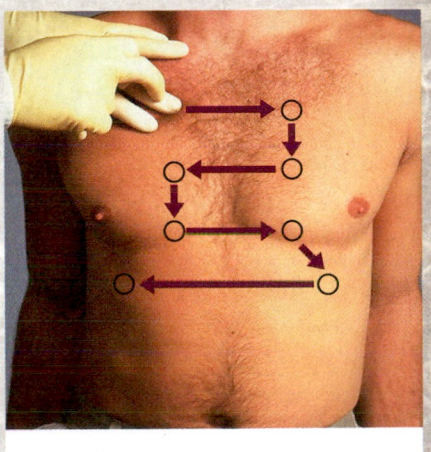

11-8f Percuss the anterior chest.

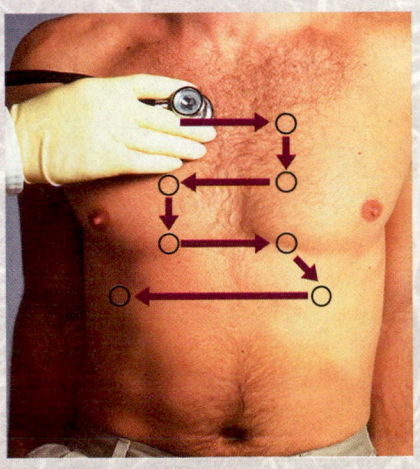

11-8g Auscultate the anterior chest.

areas of increased, decreased, or absent vibrations. You will feel increased fremitus when sound transmission is enhanced through areas of consolidated lung tissue such as in a tumor, pneumonia, or pulmonary fibrosis. You will feel decreased or absent fremitus when sound transmission is diminished in a certain area, as may occur with a pleural effusion, emphysema, or pneumothorax.

Percuss your patient's posterior chest to determine whether the underlying tissues are air-filled, fluid-filled, or solid. Also percuss to determine the position and boundaries of the diaphragm and underlying organs. Percuss both sides of the chest symmetrically from the apex to the base at five-centimeter intervals, avoiding bony areas such as the scapulae (Procedure 11-8c). Percuss at least twice in each area and compare both sides of the thorax. Identify and note any area of abnormal percussion. For example, a hyperresonant sound in the right chest may indicate a pneumothorax, whereas a dull sound in the same area may indicate a hemothorax. Assess the percussion sounds according to their quality, intensity, pitch, and duration. Practice percussing the chest so that you will become familiar with the normal resonance of the lungs and be able to identify abnormal sounds.

Next assess for diaphragmatic excursion. Identify the level of the diaphragm during quiet breathing by percussing for dullness as the diaphragm moves during the respiratory cycle. Percuss at the lower rib margin on one side and note when dullness (muscle) replaces resonance (air). With a pen mark the location of the diaphragm at the end of inhalation and at the end of exhalation. The distance between the marks is the diaphragmatic excursion. In the normal healthy adult at rest, the diaphragmatic excursion should be approximately six centimeters. Now measure diaphragmatic excursion on the opposite side and compare the marks. If you find asymmetrical diaphragmatic levels, a paralyzed phrenic nerve may be the problem. Here, reevaluate your patient's respiratory depth for adequacy and provide the appropriate intervention as needed.

Auscultate your patient's chest for normal breath sounds, adventitious breath sounds, and voice sounds. Auscultate all lung fields and compare side-to-side. Evaluate the normal breath sounds produced by airflow through the upper and lower airways. These include tracheal, bronchial, bronchovesicular, and vesicular breath sounds (Table 11-5).

Besides the normal breath sounds already mentioned you also may hear adventitious sounds. These include crackles, wheezes, rhonchi, stridor, and pleural rubs.

Also known as "rales," **crackles** are light crackling, popping, nonmusical sounds heard usually during inspiration. They are produced by air passing through moisture in the broncho-alveolar system or from the abrupt opening of closed alveoli. Early inspiratory crackles, associated with chronic bronchitis and heart failure, begin shortly after inspiration starts, and they stop soon thereafter. These are coarse crackles—loud, low pitched, and long, similar to the sound of water boiling. They are often audible at the mouth.

Content Review

ADVENTITIOUS BREATH SOUNDS

- Crackles
- Wheezes
- Rhonchi
- Stridor
- Pleural rubs

✳ crackles light crackling, popping, nonmusical sounds heard usually during inspiration.

Table 11-5	NORMAL BREATH SOUNDS		
Sound	**Description**	**Location**	**Duration**
Tracheal	Very loud, harsh	Over the trachea	Nearly equal inspiratory and expiratory phases
Bronchial	Loud, high pitch, hollow	Over the manubrium	Prolonged expiratory phase
Bronchovesicular	Soft, breezy, lower pitch	Between the scapulae / 2nd—3rd ICS lateral to the sternum	Approximately equal inspiratory and expiratory phases
Vesicular	Soft, swishy, lowest pitch	Lung periphery	Prolonged inspiratory phase

Late inspiratory crackles, associated with congestive heart failure and interstitial lung diseases, begin in the first half of the inspiratory phase and continue into late inspiration. They are fine crackles—soft, high pitched, and very brief, similar to the sound of Rice Krispies crackling. They commonly appear first at the base of the lungs and move upward as your patient's condition worsens. Usually, you can expect them to shift to dependent regions with changes in your patient's position. For example, if your heart failure patient is sitting up, expect to hear crackles first in the bases. If he is bedridden, expect to hear crackles first in the back.

Wheezes are continuous, high-pitched musical sounds similar to a whistle. They result when air moves through partially obstructed smaller airways. Their causes include asthma, bronchospasm, and foreign bodies. You may hear them without a stethoscope or by auscultating the chest during any or all phases of the respiratory cycle. They often originate in the small bronchioles and first appear at the end of exhalation. The closer to inspiration they appear, the worse your patient's condition.

Rhonchi are continuous sounds with a lower pitch and a snoring quality. They are caused by secretions in the larger airways, a common finding in bronchitis (diffuse) and pneumonia (localized). Rhonchi usually appear in early exhalation but may occur in early inspiration as well.

Stridor is a predominantly high pitched inspiratory sound. It indicates a partial obstruction of the larynx or trachea.

Pleural friction rubs are the squeaking or grating sounds of the pleural linings rubbing together. They occur where the pleural layers are inflamed and have lost their lubrication. Pleural rubs are common in pneumonia and pleurisy (inflammation of the pleura). Because these sounds occur whenever your patient's chest wall moves, they appear during the entire respiratory cycle.

You may hear no breath sounds in some areas. This may result from effusion (fluid in the pleural space causing a decrease in functional lung tissue) or consolidation (infectious pus causing collapsed alveoli). In either case, note the area's size and intervene appropriately to ensure adequate ventilation and oxygenation of your patient.

Auscultate the posterior chest systematically. Have your patient fold his arms across his chest and breathe through his mouth more deeply and slowly than usual. Auscultate the same areas you percussed and compare the bilateral findings (Procedure 11-8d). Listen for at least one full breath at each location. Be alert for patient discomfort or hyperventilation. Note the pitch, intensity, and duration of each inspiratory and expiratory sound. If the sounds are decreased, suspect impaired airflow or poor sound transmission. If the sounds are absent, suspect no airflow. Note whether you hear sounds where you normally should. For example, when you auscultate over the peripheral lung fields, you should not hear tracheal, bronchial, or bronchovesicular breath sounds. Listen carefully and note what you hear, where you hear it, and when you hear it during the respiratory cycle. Also note whether the sounds change when your patient coughs or changes position.

If you hear abnormally located tracheal, bronchial, or bronchovesicular breath sounds, assess your patient's transmitted voice sounds. Ask him to repeat the words "ninety-nine" as you auscultate his chest wall. Normally you should hear muffled, indistinct sounds. Hearing the words clearly is an abnormal finding known as **bronchophony**. Bronchophony occurs when fluid (water, blood) or consolidated tissue (pus, tumor) replaces the normally air-filled lung. After you check your patient for bronchophony, assess him for **whispered pectoriloquy** and **egophony**. For pectoriloquy, ask your patient to whisper "ninety-nine" while you auscultate. As with bronchophony, the words will be clear and distinct if sound transmission through an area is abnormally enhanced. For egophony, ask him to repeat the long *e* sound while you auscultate. You should hear a muffled, long *e*. If vocal resonance is abnormally increased, you will hear an *a* sound instead. This is known as "*e* to *a* egophony."

* **wheezes** continuous, high-pitched musical sounds similar to a whistle.

* **rhonchi** continuous sounds with a lower pitch and a snoring quality.

* **stridor** predominantly inspiratory wheeze associated with laryngeal obstruction.

* **pleural friction rub** the squeaking or grating sound of the pleural linings rubbing together.

* **bronchophony** abnormal clarity of patient's transmitted voice sounds.

* **whispered pectoriloquy** abnormal clarity of patient's transmitted whispers.

* **egophony** abnormal change in tone of patient's transmitted voice sounds.

Anterior Chest Examination

Your examination of the anterior chest will be similar to your examination of the posterior chest. Begin by having your patient lie supine with his arms relaxed but slightly abducted at his sides. Look for any gross deformities or asymmetrical movements. Does the chest wall rise symmetrically? Is there accessory muscle use? Look for abnormal retractions in the suprasternal, supraclavicular, and intercostal areas. Also check for callused elbows from tripodding (leaning with elbows on a table or chair arms), and finger clubbing—both common signs of chronic lung disease. Is the trachea midline or deviated; does it tug during inhalation? In cases of tension pneumothorax the trachea will deviate away from the affected side. In cases of pulmonary fibrosis and atelectasis it will tug toward the affected side during inhalation.

Palpate the anterior chest for deformities and areas of tenderness. Check for chest expansion by placing your thumbs along the costal margins on both sides and gently grasping the lateral rib cage (Procedure 11-8e). Ask your patient to inhale deeply. Normally your thumbs will separate symmetrically and the distance between them will increase from three to five centimeters. If you detect decreased thoracic expansion or feel unilateral delay, suspect a disorder of the underlying lung, pleura, or diaphragm.

As with the posterior chest, test for tactile fremitus, bronchophony, whispered pectoriloquy, and egophony if you detect abnormal breath sounds.

Percuss your patient's anterior chest to help determine whether the underlying tissues are air-filled, fluid-filled, or solid and to determine the position and boundaries of the diaphragm and underlying organs. Percuss each side of your patient's anterior chest from its apex to its base at five centimeter intervals at the mid-clavicular lines (Procedure 11-8f). Percuss at least twice in each area and compare both sides of the thorax. Identify and note any area of abnormal percussion. Remember that when percussing the right chest, you will hear dullness at the upper border of the liver. On the left side, you will hear the normal resonance of the lung change to tympany when you reach the stomach. You also will percuss an area of cardiac dullness from the 3rd to the 5th intercostal spaces.

Finally, auscultate the anterior and lateral thorax systematically. Have your patient breathe through his mouth more deeply and slowly than usual. Auscultate the same areas you percussed and compare symmetrical areas (Procedure 11-8g). Listen for at least one full breath at each location. Be alert for patient discomfort or hyperventilation. As with posterior chest auscultation, note the pitch, intensity, and duration of each inspiratory and expiratory sound and whether you heard sounds where you should normally expect them. Listen for adventitious sounds. If you hear abnormally located tracheal, bronchial, or bronchovesicular breath sounds, assess for bronchophony, whispered pectoriloquy, and egophony.

THE CARDIOVASCULAR SYSTEM

* **diastole** phase of cardiac cycle when ventricles relax.

* **systole** phase of cardiac cycle when the ventricles contract.

To assess cardiac function, you must understand the cardiac cycle. During **diastole,** the heart's resting period, the ventricles relax. The pressure in the atria is greater than the pressure in the ventricles. This opens the tricuspid valve on the right side and the mitral valve on the left, allowing blood from the atria to fill the ventricles. During **systole** the ventricles contract and the tricuspid and mitral valves close, preventing backflow into the atria. The vibrations of these valves' closings generate the first heart sound—S_1, or the "lub." The increased pressure in the right ventricle opens the pulmonic semilunar valve, sending deoxygenated blood to the lungs. The increased pressure in the left ventricle opens the aortic semilunar valve, sending freshly oxygenated blood to the body. At the end of systole, as pressure in the ventricles falls, the pulmonic and aortic semilunar valves

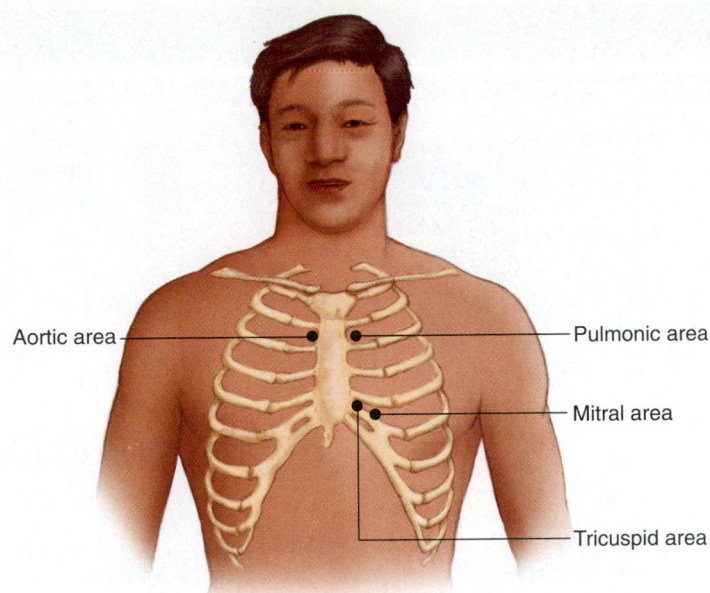

Aortic area

Pulmonic area

Mitral area

Tricuspid area

FIGURE 11-21 Sites for cardiac auscultation.

close tightly to prevent backflow. These vibrations generate the second heart sound—S_2, or the "dub." This cycle repeats approximately 60–100 times per minute in the healthy adult at rest. Extra sounds known as heart murmurs result when valves do not fully open or close, causing turbulent flow that an experienced clinician can detect.

You must auscultate for heart sounds at the proper places on the chest wall (Figure 11-21). Always listen downstream. For example, since the tricuspid and mitral valves direct blood flow to the ventricles, which are toward your patient's feet, listen for S_1 at the apex of the heart. This is found near the lower left sternal border. Since the aortic and pulmonic valves direct blood flow to the lungs and aorta, which are toward your patient's head, listen for S_2 at the base of the heart. This is found at the 2nd intercostal space near the sternum.

Begin your cardiovascular assessment by inspecting for signs of arterial insufficiency or occlusion in your patient's trunk and extremities. Look for skin pallor and other signs of decreased perfusion. Now assess the arterial pulses. Inspect the carotid arteries for visible pulsations just medial to the sternocleidomastoid muscles. Palpate the carotid arteries at the level of the cricoid cartilage to avoid pressing on the carotid sinus (Procedure 11-9a). Never palpate both carotids simultaneously; doing so may decrease cerebral blood flow. Assess the carotid pulse for rate, rhythm, and quality. Does its quality vary? Do the variations correspond to respiration? For example, in pulsus paradoxus, the amplitude of the pulse diminishes with inspiration and increases with exhalation. Do you feel a vibration or humming (**thrills**) when you palpate the carotid artery? If so, auscultate the area with your stethoscope for **bruits,** the sounds of turbulent blood flow around a partial obstruction (Procedure 11-9b).

If you have not already taken your patient's blood pressure, do so now. Also check for jugular venous pressure, which approximates your patient's right atrial pressure. Position your patient supine, with his head elevated to about 30°. Turning your patient's head away from the side you are assessing, identify the external jugular veins on both sides and locate the pulsations of the internal jugular veins. Look for the pulsation in the area around the suprasternal notch and where the sternocleidomastoid muscle inserts on the clavicle and manubrium.

Content Review

HEART SOUNDS
- S_1—"lub"
- S_2—"dub"
- Split S_1—"la-lub"
- Split S_2—"da-dub"
- S_3—"lub-dub-dee" (Kentucky)
- S_4—"dee-lub-dub" (Tennessee)
- Click
- Snap
- Pericardial friction rub
- Murmur

✶ **thrill** vibration or humming felt when palpating the pulse.

✶ **bruit** sound of turbulent blood flow around a partial obstruction.

11-9a   Assess the carotid pulse.

11-9b   Auscultate for bruits.

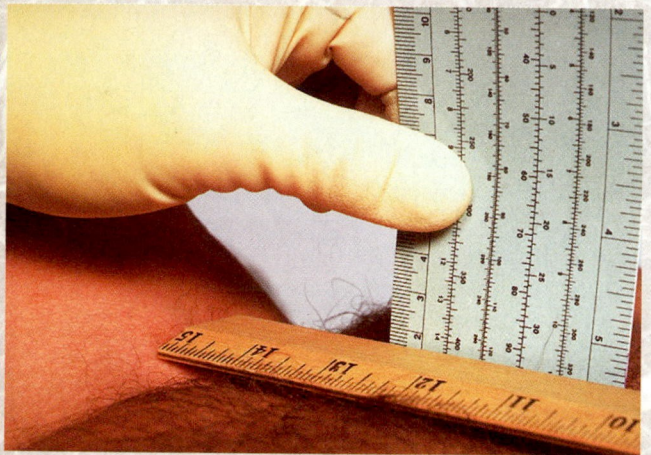

11-9c   Measure jugular venous pressure.

11-9d   Palpate for the apical impulse (PMI).

11-9e   Percuss for the PMI.

11-9f   Auscultate for heart sounds.

Now identify the internal jugular vein's highest point of pulsation (the point where the pulse diminishes) and measure its vertical distance from the sternal angle (midline at the 2nd costal cartilage). To do this, place a ruler perpendicular to the chest at the sternal angle and position a straightedge at a right angle to the ruler (Procedure 11-9c). Lower the straightedge until it rests atop the jugular vein pulsation. The corresponding ruler mark is your measurement. Normal venous pressure is 1–2 cm. If you cannot visualize the pulsations, observe the point where the external jugular veins collapse and use the same measuring parameters.

Examine the external jugular veins for equality of distention. Abnormal bilateral distention indicates fluid volume overload or that something such as congestive heart failure or cardiac tamponade is blocking venous return to the heart. Unilateral distention suggests a localized problem.

With your patient's head still raised to about 30°, inspect and palpate the chest for the apical impulse, or PMI (Procedure 11-9d). When examining a woman with large breasts, gently displace the left breast upward and laterally, if needed, or ask her to do this for you. First, look for a pulsation at the cardiac apex, normally at the 5th intercostal space just medial to the mid-clavicular line. This pulsation represents the PMI. It helps you locate the left ventricle's apex.

If you cannot see the pulsation, ask your patient to exhale and stop breathing for a few seconds. Lateral displacement of the PMI indicates an enlarged right ventricle. The PMI may be displaced upward and to the left in pregnant women. If your patient is obese or has a very muscular chest wall or a barrel chest you may not detect the PMI. Percussion may help if you have difficulty palpating the PMI. Start lateral and work your way toward the midline (Procedure 11-9e). When you hear a change from resonance (lung) to dull (heart), you have located the PMI.

Using the diaphragm of your stethoscope, auscultate your patient's anterior chest for normal heart sounds and for abnormal or extra heart sounds (Procedure 11-9f). Listen for the high-pitched sounds of S_1 at the 5th intercostal space at the left sternal border (tricuspid valve) and at the PMI (mitral valve) using the diaphragm of your stethoscope. Listen for the high-pitched sounds of S_2 at the 2nd intercostal space at the right sternal border (aortic valve) and 2nd intercostal space at the left sternal border (pulmonic valve). For a comprehensive auscultation of heart sounds, you should also listen at the 3rd and 4th intercostal spaces. Although nothing is specifically behind those spaces, you may hear something there that you will not hear in the other places if the heart is not anatomically perfect.

Because the mitral and aortic valves (left side) close slightly before the tricuspid and pulmonic valves (right side), you may hear two sets of sounds instead of one. This is known as splitting. A split S_1 sounds like "la-lub," a split S_2 like "da-dub." Instead of "lub-dub" you will hear "la-lub—da-dub." Splitting of S_2 during inspiration is normal in healthy children and young adults. Expiratory or persistent splitting suggests an abnormality.

You also may hear extra or abnormal heart sounds, depending on your patient's age and condition. A third heart sound, S_3, is sometimes called the ventricular gallop. It is the "dee" of "lub-dub-dee" and has the same cadence as the word "Kentucky." This extra heart sound develops from vibrations that result when blood fills a dilated ventricle. Commonly heard in children and young adults, an S_3 is usually considered pathologic in patients over age 30. It generally develops with ventricular failure and ventricular volume overload and disappears when the problem is resolved. S_3 is a low-pitched sound heard in early to mid-diastole. Listen for S_3 at the apex using the bell of your stethoscope with your patient lying on his left side.

Atrial gallop is the fourth heart sound, S_4. It is the "dee" of "dee-lub-dub" and has the same cadence as the word "Tennessee." An S_4 develops from vibrations produced in late diastole when atrial contraction forces blood into a ventricle that has decreased compliance or that resists filling and causes volume overload. It usually disappears when the problem is resolved. Listen for the low-pitched S_4 at the apex using the bell of your stethoscope with your patient lying on his left side.

Experienced cardiologists can also detect clicks, snaps, friction rubs, and murmurs. An ejection click results from a stiff or stuck valve. An opening snap results when a stenotic mitral or tricuspid valve's leaflets recoil abruptly after ventricular diastole. A pericardial friction rub occurs when inflammation causes the heart's visceral and parietal surfaces to rub together at each heartbeat. A murmur is a rumbling or vibrating noise that results from turbulent blood flow through the heart valves, a large artery, or a septal defect.

THE ABDOMEN

To examine the abdomen, you need good lighting, a relaxed patient, and exposure from above the xiphoid process to the symphysis pubis. Make sure your patient does not have a full bladder. Make him comfortable in the supine position with one pillow under the head and another under the knees. Have him place his hands at his sides. This helps relax his abdominal muscles, making the examination easier for you and more comfortable for him.

Ask your patient to point out any areas of pain or tenderness. Examine these areas last. Use warm hands and a warm stethoscope and keep your fingernails short. If your hands are cold, palpate your patient through his clothes until your hands warm up. Begin your exam slowly and avoid any quick, unexpected movements. Monitor your patient's facial expressions for pain and discomfort. During the exam, distract him with conversation or questions. Use inspection, auscultation, percussion, and palpation to perform the exam. Always auscultate before percussing or palpating, because these manipulations may alter your patient's bowel motility and resulting bowel sounds.

When you examine the abdomen you will assess the gastrointestinal organs and other nearby organs and structures. Inspect the skin of the abdomen and flanks for scars, dilated veins, stretch marks, rashes, lesions, and pigmentation changes. Look for discoloration over the umbilicus (**Cullen's sign**) or over the flanks (**Grey-Turner's sign**); these are late signs suggesting intra-abdominal bleeding. Assess the size and shape of your patient's abdomen to determine whether it is scaphoid (concave), flat, round, or distended. Ask the patient if it is its usual size and shape. Note its symmetry. Check for bulges, hernias, or distended flanks. **Ascites** appears as bulges in the flanks and across the abdomen and indicates edema caused by congestive heart failure. A distended bladder or pregnant uterus can cause a suprapubic bulge. Bulges in the inguinal or femoral areas suggest a hernia.

Now look at your patient's umbilicus. Note its location and contour and observe for any signs of herniation or inflammation. Check for any visible pulsation, peristalsis (the wavelike motion of organs moving their contents through the digestive tract), or masses. You may see the normal pulsation of the aorta just lateral to the umbilicus. If you notice a bounding or exaggerated pulsation, suspect an aortic aneurysm. Visible peristalsis may indicate a bowel obstruction.

Next auscultate for bowel sounds and other sounds such as bruits throughout the abdomen. To auscultate for bowel sounds, first warm your diaphragm in your hand, because a cold diaphragm might cause abdominal tension. Gently place the diaphragm on your patient's abdomen and proceed systematically, listening for bowel sounds in each quadrant. Note their location, frequency, and character.

Normal bowel sounds consist of a variety of high-pitched gurgles and clicks that occur every 5–15 seconds. More frequent sounds indicate increased bowel motility in conditions such as diarrhea or an early intestinal obstruction. Occasionally you may hear loud, prolonged, gurgling sounds known as **borborygmi**. These indicate

Cullen's sign discoloration around the umbilicus (occasionally the flanks) suggestive of intra-abdominal hemorrhage.

Grey-Turner's sign discoloration over the flanks suggesting intra-abdominal bleeding.

ascites bulges in the flanks and across the abdomen, indicating edema caused by congestive heart failure.

borborygmi loud, prolonged, gurgling bowel sounds indicating hyperperistalsis.

hyperperistalsis. Decreased or absent sounds suggest a paralytic ileus or peritonitis. Listen at least two minutes for bowel sounds if the abdomen is silent. Bruits are swishing sounds that indicate turbulent blood flow. To confirm bruits use the bell of your stethoscope and listen in areas over abdominal blood vessels such as the aorta and renal arteries (Procedure 11-10a). If you hear a bruit, suspect an arterial disorder such as an abdominal aortic aneurysm or renal artery stenosis.

Percussing the abdomen produces different sounds based on the underlying tissues. These sounds help you detect excessive gas and solid or fluid-filled masses. They also help you determine the size and position of solid organs such as the liver and spleen. Percuss the abdomen in the same sequence you used for auscultation. Note the distribution of tympany and dullness. Expect to hear tympany in most of the abdomen; expect dullness over the solid abdominal organs such as the liver and spleen.

Palpate the abdomen last to detect tenderness, muscular rigidity, and superficial organs and masses. Before you begin palpation, ask your patient if he has any pain or tenderness. If he does, ask him to point to the area with one finger. Palpate that area last, using gentle pressure with a single finger. Ask him to cough and tell you if and where he experiences any pain. If coughing causes pain, suspect peritoneal inflammation.

Now ask your patient to take slow, deep breaths with his mouth open, and have him flex his knees to relax his abdominal muscles. Perform light palpation by moving your hand slowly and just lifting it off the skin (Procedure 11-10b). Palpate all areas in the same sequence you used for auscultation and percussion. Watch your patient's face for signs of discomfort. Identify any masses and note their size, location, contour, tenderness, pulsations, and mobility. Abdominal pain upon light palpation suggests peritoneal irritation or inflammation. If you feel rigidity or guarding while palpating, determine whether it is voluntary (patient anticipates the pain or is not relaxed) or involuntary (peritoneal inflammation).

Next palpate the abdomen deeply to detect large masses or tenderness. Use one hand on top of another and push down slowly (Procedure 11-10c). Assess for rebound tenderness by pushing down slowly and then releasing your hand quickly off the tender area. If the peritoneum is inflamed, your patient will experience pain when you let go. Alternatively, hold your hand one centimeter above your patient's abdomen at rest. Then ask him to push his abdomen out to touch your hand. Limitation by pain suggests peritoneal irritation.

If you note a protruding abdomen with bulging flanks and dull percussion sounds in dependent areas, you might perform two tests for ascites. First assess for areas of tympany and dullness while your patient is supine. Then ask him to lie on one side. Percuss again, noting once more any areas of tympany and dullness. If your patient has ascites, the area of dullness will shift down to the dependent side and the area of tympany will shift up. To test for fluid wave, ask an assistant to press the edge of his hand firmly down the midline of your patient's abdomen (Procedure 11-10d). With your fingertips, tap one flank and feel for the impulse's transmission to the other flank through excess fluid. If you detect the impulse easily, suspect ascites.

THE FEMALE GENITALIA

Except in cases of trauma or abuse, you rarely would be expected to examine the female genitalia. Before examining the external female genitalia, make sure that the room is warm and quiet and that your patient's bladder is empty. Be sure to maintain privacy during this examination. To reduce any anxiety or embarrassment your patient may feel, explain what you are doing during the exam. Expose her body areas only as necessary, be sensitive to her feelings, and project a professional demeanor. Place a pillow under her head and shoulders to help relax her abdominal muscles.

11-10a   Auscultate for renal bruits.

11-10b   Light abdominal palpation.

11-10c   Deep abdominal palpation.

11-10d   Test for ascites.

Begin your assessment by inspecting your patient's external genitalia. Look at the mons pubis, labia, and perineum for abnormalities such as inflammation, swelling, or lesions. These abnormalities may signal a sebaceous cyst or a sexually transmitted disease such as syphilis or herpes simplex virus infection. Check the bases of the pubic hair for signs of lice such as excoriation, or small, itchy, red maculopapules.

Now retract the outer labia and inspect the inner labia and urethral meatus (opening). Assess for vaginal discharge. The normal discharge is clear or cloudy and has little or no odor. A white, curd-like discharge with no odor or a yeasty, sweet odor may suggest a fungal infection (candidiasis). A yellow, green, or gray discharge with a foul or fishy odor may suggest a bacterial infection (gonorrhea or Gardnerella). Examining the external female genitalia can be an embarrassing, uncomfortable experience, especially for male clinicians. Remember it is probably twice as awkward for your patient. It is customary for male clinicians to have a female partner present during the examination.

THE MALE GENITALIA

Except for trauma, you rarely would be expected to inspect the male genitalia. Before examining the male genitalia make sure that the room is warm and quiet and that your patient's bladder is empty. Be sure to maintain privacy during this examination. To reduce any anxiety or embarrassment your patient may feel, explain what you are doing during the exam. Expose his body areas only as necessary, be sensitive to his feelings, and project a professional demeanor.

Begin your assessment by inspecting your patient's penis and scrotum. Note any inflammation, and inspect the skin around the base of the penis for abnormalities such as lesions that may be caused by sexually transmitted diseases. Also check the bases of the pubic hair for signs of lice such as excoriation or small, itchy, red maculopapules. Next inspect the glans for signs of degeneration or other abnormalities. If the foreskin is present, ask your patient to retract it. Note any abnormalities and the location of the urethral meatus. Inspect the anterior surface of the scrotum and note its contour. Then lift the scrotum to inspect its posterior surface and note any swelling or lumps. Expect acute epididymitis or testicular torsion if your patient has scrotal swelling and lower abdominal pain. Testicular torsion requires immediate intervention.

Assess any discharge from the urethral meatus. Normally no discharge is present. A profuse, yellow discharge may be a sign of gonorrhea. A scant, clear or white discharge may suggest a nongonococcal urethritis. Examining the male genitalia can be an embarrassing, uncomfortable experience, especially for female clinicians. Remember it is probably twice as awkward for your patient. It is customary for female clinicians to have a male partner present during the examination.

THE ANUS

Examining the anus is normally not a prehospital assessment practice. Unless your patient presents with rectal bleeding, there will be no reason for you to examine this area. Because routine internal rectal and prostate examinations are beyond the scope of this course, this section will focus on the external anal exam. As always, your aim is gentleness, a calm demeanor, and talking to your patient about what you are doing.

Before examining the anus make sure the room is warm and quiet. Be sure to maintain privacy during this examination. To reduce any anxiety or embarrassment your patient may feel, explain what you are doing during the exam. Drape your patient appropriately and expose his body areas only as necessary; be sensitive to his feelings and project a professional demeanor. Place your patient on his left side with his legs flexed and his buttocks near the edge of the examination table. Glove your hands and spread the buttocks apart. Inspect the sacrococcygeal and perianal areas for lumps, ulcers, inflammations, rashes, or excoriation. Palpate any abnormal areas carefully and note any tenderness or inflammation. If appropriate, obtain a fecal sample and test it for occult blood. Simply smear a small sample onto a special test slide and add a couple drops of developer onto the sample. If it turns blue, there is blood in the stool.

THE MUSCULOSKELETAL SYSTEM

An examination of the musculoskeletal system must include a detailed assessment of function and structure. Inspect and palpate your patient's joints, their structure, their range of motion, and the surrounding tissues. Begin your assessment with a general observation of posture, build, and muscular development. Watch how your patient's body parts move, and observe their resting positions. Begin the exam with your patient sitting to evaluate his head, neck, shoulders, and upper extremities. Then have him stand to assess his chest, back, and ilium; ask him to walk so that you can assess his gait. Finally, ask him to lie down to examine his hips, knees, ankles, and feet.

Inspect for swelling in or around joints, changes in the surrounding tissue, redness of the overlying skin, deformities, and symmetry of impairment. Swelling may be caused by trauma to the area or by excess synovial fluid in the joint space or tissues surrounding the joint. Tissue changes may include muscle atrophy, skin changes, and subcutaneous nodules resulting from rheumatoid arthritis or rheumatic fever. Skin redness may suggest inflammation or arthritis. Deformities may be produced by restricted range of motion, misalignment of the articulating bones, dislocation (complete separation of bone ends), or subluxation (partial dislocation). Symmetrical impairment is usually associated with a disorder such as rheumatoid arthritis.

Inspect and palpate each body part, then test its range of motion and muscle strength as explained in the Motor System section later in this chapter. Examine each joint and compare joints on opposite sides for equal size, shape, color, and strength. Swelling in a joint usually involves the synovial membrane or a bursa, which will feel spongy on deep palpation within the joint space. It also may involve the surrounding structures such as ligaments, cartilage, tendons, or the bones themselves. Redness of the overlying skin suggests a non-traumatic joint inflammation such as arthritis, gout, or rheumatic fever. Palpate for tenderness in and around the joint. Try to identify the specific structure that is tender, such as a ligament or tendon. Some common causes of a tender joint include arthritis, tendinitis, bursitis, or osteomyelitis. With the back of your hand, feel over the tender area for increased heat, which suggests arthritis.

After you have inspected and palpated each body part with your patient at rest, assess range of motion. Test each joint for passive range of motion, range of motion against gravity, and range of motion against resistance. First test the joint's passive range of motion by moving it in the directions that it normally allows. For example, test the elbow, a hinge joint, for flexion and extension. Note any resistance and whether the range of motion is within normal limits. Now test range of motion against gravity by asking your patient to perform the same movements by himself. Again, note the range of motion and any difficulties. Finally, test range of motion against resistance. Have your patient perform the same movements while you apply resistance.

An examination of the musculoskeletal system must include a detailed assessment of function and structure.

Content Review

STEPS IN EVALUATING JOINTS

1 Inspection
2 Palpation
3 Passive range of motion
4 Range of motion against gravity
5 Range of motion against resistance

Passive and active range should be equal. A discrepancy indicates either a muscle weakness or a joint problem. If your patient has difficulty with passive and active tests, suspect a joint problem. If he has difficulty only with active tests, suspect a weakened muscle or nerve disorder. A decreased range of motion could indicate arthritis or injury, while an increased range of motion suggests a loosening of the structures that support the joint.

Listen for **crepitation** (or **crepitus**), the crunching sounds of unlubricated parts rubbing against each other, while you manipulate the joint. Crepitus may indicate an inflamed joint or osteoarthritis. An obvious traumatic deformity could indicate a sprained ligament, a bone fracture, or a dislocation. In these cases, modify your manipulation and range of motion exam accordingly. Non-traumatic deformities are caused by arthritis or the misalignment of bones. Avoid manipulating a painful joint.

* crepitation (or **crepitus**) crunching sounds of unlubricated parts in joints rubbing against each other.

The Extremities

Wrists and Hands Begin by inspecting your patient's hands and wrists. Next palpate them by feeling the medial and lateral aspects of the DIP joints and then the PIP joints with your thumb and forefinger (Procedure 11-11a). Note any swelling, sponginess, bony enlargement, or tenderness. Then palpate the tops and bottoms of these joints in the same manner. Now ask your patient to flex his hand slightly so you can examine each MCP. Compress the MCP joints by squeezing the hand from side-to-side between your thumbs and fingers and note any swelling, tenderness, or sponginess (Procedure 11-11b). Finally, palpate each wrist joint with your thumbs and note any swelling, sponginess, or tenderness (Procedure 11-11c). If your patient has had swelling of both his wrists or finger joints for several weeks, suspect an inflammatory condition such as rheumatoid arthritis.

To assess range of motion, ask your patient to make a fist with each hand and then open his fist and extend and spread his fingers. He should be able to make a tight fist and spread his fingers smoothly and easily. Next ask him to flex and then extend his wrist. Normal flexion is 90°, extension 70° (Procedure 11-11d). Check for radial and ulnar deviation by asking your patient to flex his wrist and move his hands medially and laterally. Normal radial movement is 20°, ulnar movement 45° (Procedure 11-11e).

If your patient complains of hand pain and numbness, especially at night, suspect carpal tunnel syndrome, the painful inflammation of the median nerve. To detect additional signs of this disorder, hold your patient's wrists in acute flexion for 60 seconds (Procedure 11-11f). In carpal tunnel syndrome, he will develop numbness or tingling in the areas innervated by the median nerve—the palmar surface of his thumb, index, and middle fingers, and part of his ring finger. Throughout these maneuvers watch for deformities, redness, swelling, nodules, or muscular atrophy.

Elbows To examine the elbow, support your patient's forearm with your hand so that his elbow is flexed about 70° (Procedure 11-12a). Inspect the elbow joint and note any deformities, swelling, or nodules. Palpate the joint structures for tenderness, swelling, or thickening. Press on the medial and lateral epicondyles (Procedure 11-12b). Inflammation of either the medial epicondyle (tennis elbow) or of the lateral epicondyle (golfer's elbow) suggests tendinitis at those muscle insertion sites. To assess range of motion, ask your patient to flex and extend his elbow (Procedure 11-12c). Normally he will flex his elbow up to 160° and return it back to the neutral position. Then ask him to keep his elbows flexed and

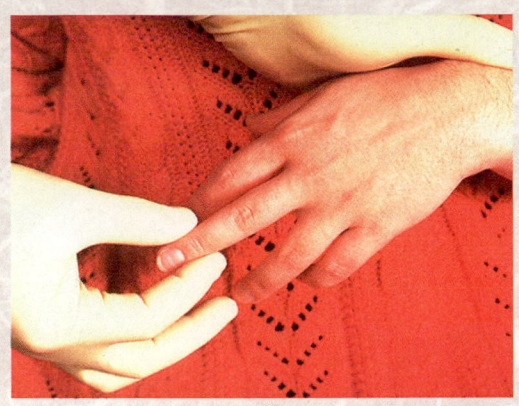

11–11a   Palpate the DIP and PIP joints.

11–11b   Palpate the MCP joint.

11–11c   Palpate the wrist.

Extension

Neutral

Flexion

11–11d   Assess wrist flexion and extension.

Ulna Deviation

Radial Deviaton

Neutral

11–11e   Assess radial and ulnar deviation.

11–11f   Test for carpal tunnel syndrome.

11-12a   Inspect the elbow.

11-12b   Palpate the lateral and medial epicondyles.

Flexion

Extension

11-12c   Assess elbow flexion and extension.

Supination   Pronation

11-12d   Assess supination and pronation of the wrist.

his arms at his sides. Now have him turn his palms up and then down. Normally both supination and pronation are 90° (Procedure 11-12d).

Shoulders To assess your patient's shoulders look at them from the front and then look at his scapulae from the back. Inspect the entire shoulder girdle for swelling, deformities, or muscular atrophy. Before you palpate, ask your patient if he has any pain in his shoulders. If so, have him point to it with one finger; palpate this area last. Palpate the shoulders with your fingertips, moving along the clavicles out toward the humerus (Procedure 11-13a). Palpate the sternoclavicular joint, acromioclavicular joint, subacromial region, and the bicipital groove for tenderness (biceps tendinitis) or swelling (bursitis). Now palpate over the greater tubercle of the humerus as you abduct the arm at the shoulder. Then palpate the scapulae.

To assess range of motion ask your patient to raise both arms forward and then straight overhead (flexion) (Procedure 11-13b). Expect to see forward flexion of 180°. Next ask him to extend both arms behind his back (extension). Normal extension is 50°. Now have him raise both arms overhead from the side (abduction) (Procedure 11-13c). Normal abduction is 180°. Then ask him to lower his arms and swing them as far as he can across his body (adduction). Normal shoulder adduction is 75°. Finally have him adduct his shoulders to 90°, pronate, and flex his elbows 90° to the front of his body. Now ask him to rotate his shoulders to the "goal post" position (external rotation) (Procedure 11-13d). Normal external rotation is 90°. Finally, ask him to place both hands behind the small of his back (internal rotation). Normal internal rotation is 90°. During these motions, cup your hands over your patient's shoulders and note any crepitus.

Ankles and Feet Inspect the foot and ankle for obvious deformities, nodules, swelling, calluses, or corns. Palpate the anterior aspect of each ankle joint with your thumbs and note any sponginess, swelling, or tenderness (Procedure 11-14a). Feel along the Achilles tendon for tenderness or nodules. Exert pressure between your thumbs and fingers on each metatarsophalangeal joint (Procedure 11-14b). Acute inflammation of these joints suggests gout. Tenderness is an early sign of rheumatoid arthritis.

To test range of motion, ask your patient to bring his foot upward (dorsiflexion) (Procedure 11-14c). Normal dorsiflexion is 20°. Then have him point it downward (plantar flexion). Normal plantar flexion is 45°. Next, while stabilizing the ankle with one hand, grasp the heel with the other hand and invert the foot, then evert it (Procedure 11-14d). Normal inversion is 30°, normal eversion 20°. These four movements test the ankle joint's stability. A sprained ankle will cause your patient pain when the injured ligament is stretched or torn. Since the lateral ligaments are smaller and weaker than the medial ligaments, lateral sprains are more common, causing severe pain upon inversion and plantar flexion. In arthritis, pain and tenderness will accompany movement in any direction. Finally, flex and extend the toes (Procedure 11-14e). Expect a great range of motion in these joints, especially the big toes.

Knees Inspect your patient's knees for alignment and deformities. Look for the concave areas that usually appear on each side of the patella and just above it. The absence of these concavities indicates swelling in the knee or the surrounding structures. If swelling is present, milk the medial aspect of the knee firmly upward two or three times to displace the fluid. Then press the knee just behind the lateral margin of the patella and watch for a return of

11-13a   Palpate the shoulder with your fingertips.

11-13b   Assess shoulder flexion and extension.

11-13c   Assess shoulder abduction and adduction.

11-13d   Assess internal and external shoulder rotation.

11-14a   Palpate the ankle and foot.

11-14b   Palpate the metatarsal-phalangeal joints.

11-14c   Assess dorsiflexion and plantar flexion.

11-14d   Assess inversion and eversion of the foot.

11-14e   Test flexion and extension of the toes.

fluid (a positive sign for effusion) (Procedure 11-15a). Feel for any thickening or swelling around the patella; these suggest synovial thickening or effusion. Compress the patella and move it against the femur (Procedure 11-15b). Note any pain or tenderness.

To test for range of motion, have your patient flex his knee to 90°. Press your thumbs into the joint and palpate along the tibial margins from the patellar tendon laterally. Palpate along the course of each ligament and note any points of tenderness. If your patient has tenderness, expect damage to the meniscus or to lateral ligaments. If you feel irregular bony ridges, suspect osteoarthritis. Now test for stability of the medial and collateral ligaments by moving the knee joint from side to side with the knee flexed to 30° (Procedure 11-15c). There should be little movement if the joint is stable. Evaluate the anterior and posterior cruciate ligaments by using the "drawer" test. Try to move the knee joint anterior and posterior, much like opening and closing a drawer (Procedure 11-15d). Again, if the ligaments are strong, there should be little movement.

Now have your patient sit at the edge of the exam table with his lower legs dangling. Ask him to extend his leg. Normal extension is 90° (Procedure 11-15e). Ask him to roll over and try to touch his foot to his back. Normal flexion is 135°. With your patient standing, inspect the posterior surface of his legs, especially the popliteal region behind his knees. Note any deformity or abnormalities such as bowlegs, knock-knee, or flexion contracture, the inability to fully extend the knee.

Hips Inspect the hips for deformities, symmetry, and swelling. Palpate for tenderness all around the joint, including the three bursa and greater trochanter of the femur (Procedure 11-16a). Test the hip's range of motion with your patient supine. Ask him to raise his knee to his chest and pull it firmly against his abdomen. Observe the degree of flexion at the knee and hip (normally 120°) (Procedure 11-16b). Now flex the hip at 90° and stabilize the thigh with one hand while you grasp the ankle with the other. Swing the lower leg medially to evaluate external rotation and laterally to evaluate internal rotation (Procedure 11-16c). Normal external rotation is 40°, normal internal rotation 45°. Arthritis restricts internal rotation. To test for hip abduction, have your patient extend his legs. Then while you stabilize the anterior superior iliac spine with one hand, abduct the other leg until you feel the iliac spine move. This marks the degree of hip abduction, which is normally 90° (Procedure 11-16d). If your patient complains of hip pain or if range of motion is limited, palpate the three bursa for swelling (bursitis) and tenderness.

The Spine

To assess your patient's spine, first inspect his head and neck for deformities, abnormal posture, and asymmetrical skin folds. The head should be erect and the spine straight. Ask your patient to bend forward slightly while you visually identify the spinous processes, the paravertebral muscles, the scapulae, the iliac crests, and the posterior iliac spines (usually marked by dimples). Draw imaginary horizontal lines across the shoulders and iliac crests. Now draw an imaginary vertical line from T1 to the space between the buttocks (gluteal cleft). Any deviations suggest a variety of pathologies.

Next observe your patient from the side. Evaluate the curves of the cervical, thoracic, and lumbar spine and note any irregularities. Common abnormalities

Examining the Knee

11-15a Palpate the knee.

11-15b Palpate the patella.

11-15c Test the collateral ligaments of the knee.

11-15d Test the cruciate ligaments of the knee.

Extension

Flexion

11-15e Assess knee flexion and extension.

11-16a Palpate the hip.

11-16b Assess hip flexion with the knee flexed.

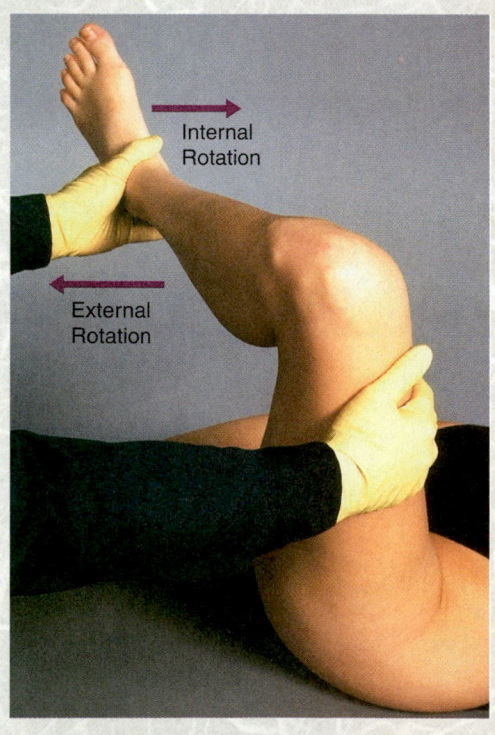

Internal Rotation

External Rotation

11-16c Assess external and internal rotation of the hip.

Adduction

Abduction

11-16d Assess hip abduction and adduction.

Table 11-6	SPINAL CURVATURES
Condition	**Description**
Normal	Concave in cervical and lumbar regions, convex in thorax
Lordosis	Exaggerated lumbar concavity (swayback)
Kyphosis	Exaggerated thoracic concavity (hunchback)
Scoliosis	Lateral curvature

of the spine include lordosis, scoliosis, and kyphosis (Table 11-6). Using the pads of your fingers, palpate the spinous processes for tenderness (Procedure 11-17a). Feel the supporting structures for muscle tone, symmetry, size, and tenderness or spasms. If your patient exhibits tenderness of the spinous processes and paravertebral muscles, suspect a herniated intervertebral disk, most commonly found between L4 and S1.

Now test range of motion. First test for flexion by asking your patient to touch his chin to his chest (Procedure 11-17b). Flexion is normally 45°. Next, ask him to bend his head backward. This tests extension, which normally is up to 55°. Now test for rotation by asking your patient to touch his chin to each shoulder (Procedure 11-17c). Normal rotation is 70° on each side. Finally ask him to touch his ears to his shoulders without raising his shoulders. This assesses lateral bending, which normally is 40° on each side (Procedure 11-17d). Now test for flexion of the lower spine with your patient standing. Ask him to bend and touch his toes (Procedure 11-17e). Note the smoothness and symmetry of movement, the range of motion, and the curves in the lumbar region. Normal flexion ranges from 75° to 90°. If the lumbar area remains concave or appears asymmetrical during this exam, your patient may have a muscle spasm. Next stabilize your patient's pelvis with your hands and have him bend sideways; normal lateral bending is 35° on each side (Procedure 11-17f). To assess hyperextension, ask him to bend backwards toward you; normal hyperextension is 30° (Procedure 11-17g). Finally test spinal rotation by asking your patient to twist his shoulders one way, then the other. Normally they will rotate 30° to each side (Procedure 11-17h).

If your patient complains of lower back pain radiating down the back of one leg, assess it by having him lie supine on the table. Ask him to raise his straightened leg until he feels pain. Note the angle of elevation at which the pain occurs, as well as the quality and distribution of the pain. Now dorsiflex your patient's foot. If this causes a sharp pain that radiates from your patient's back down his leg, suspect compression of the nerve roots of the lower lumbar region. Repeat this test with the other leg. Increased pain in the affected leg when the opposite leg is raised confirms the finding.

THE PERIPHERAL VASCULAR SYSTEM

To assess your patient's peripheral vascular system, inspect both arms from the fingertips to the shoulders. Note their size and symmetry. Observe swelling, venous congestion, the color of the skin and nail beds, and the skin texture. Yellow or brittle nails or poor color in the fingertips indicates chronic arterial insufficiency. Palpate the peripheral arteries to evaluate pulsation and capillary refill

Procedure 11-17 Assessing the Spine

11-17a Palpate the spine.

11-17b Test flexion and extension of the head and neck.

11-17c Test rotation of the head and neck.

11-17d Assess lateral bending of the head and neck.

11-17e Assess flexion of the lower spine.

11-17f Assess lateral bending of the lower spine.

11-17g Assess spinal extension.

11-17h Assess spinal rotation.

Table 11-7   ASSESSING A PERIPHERAL PULSE

Score	Description
0	Absent pulse
1+	Weak or thready
2+	Normal
3+	Bounding

and to assess skin temperature (Procedure 11-18a and 11-18b). To palpate a peripheral pulse, lightly place your fingerpads over the artery's pulse point. Slowly increase the pressure until you feel a maximum pulsation. Note the rate, regularity, equality, and quality of the pulses. Count the number of beats in one minute. Then determine whether the pulse is regular, regularly irregular, or irregularly irregular. Finally, assess the quality of the pulse by noting its amplitude and contour; rate its quality from 0 to 3+ as shown in Table 11-7. Determine if it is absent, normal, weak, or bounding, and note any thrills, humming vibrations that feel similar to the throat of a purring cat. Thrills suggest a cardiac murmur or vascular narrowing. Expect the pulse of a normal adult to range between 60 and 100 beats per minute with a regular rhythm and normal amplitude.

Compare peripheral pulses bilaterally. If you detect a weak or absent pulse in one extremity, suspect an arterial occlusion proximal to the pulse point. Also compare distal and proximal pulses for equality. If you cannot palpate a distal artery move proximally to another artery. For example, if you cannot palpate the radial artery, move to the the brachial artery in the antecubital area. While you are at the elbow, you can also assess the epitrochlear lymph nodes; they will be palpable only if inflamed.

Next assess the feet and legs. Have your patient lie down and ask him to remove his socks. Inspect the legs from the feet to the groin. Note their size and symmetry. Evaluate the presence of swelling, venous congestion, the color of the skin and nail beds, and the skin texture. Note any venous enlargement. Evaluate scars, pigmentation, rashes, and ulcers. Palpate and compare the femoral pulses (Procedure 11-18c). Note the rate, regularity, equality, and quality of the pulses. Palpate the popliteal pulse behind the knee, the dorsalis pedis pulse on top of the foot, and the posterior tibial pulse just behind the medial malleolus (Procedure 11-18d through 11-18f). Feel the temperature of the legs, feet, and toes with the back of your fingers and compare both sides. Unilateral coldness indicates an arterial occlusion. Bilateral coldness is due to an environmental problem, bilateral occlusion (saddle embolus) or to a general circulatory problem (shock). Palpate the superficial inguinal lymph nodes for enlargement and tenderness.

Observe the legs for edema, the presence of an abnormal amount of fluid in the tissues. Compare one leg and foot with the other. Note their relative size and symmetry. Are veins, tendons, and bones easily visible under the skin? Edema will usually obscure these structures. Palpate for pitting edema by pressing firmly with your thumb for five seconds over the top of the foot, behind each medial ankle, and over the shins (Procedure 11-18g). **Pitting** is a depression left by the pressure of your thumb. Normally there should be no depression. If edema is present evaluate the degree of pitting that can range from slight to marked (Figure 11-22). You can grade the depth of the pitting according to the appropriate scale in Table 11-8. Expect the pit to disappear within ten seconds after you release the pressure. Bilateral edema suggests a central circulatory problem such as congestive heart failure or renal failure; unilateral edema suggests a lower extremity circulation abnormality such as deep vein thrombosis or venous occlusion. Note the extent of the edema. How far up the leg does it spread? The higher the edema, the more severe the problem.

✻ **pitting** depression that results from pressure against skin when pitting edema is present.

11-18a   Palpate the radial artery.

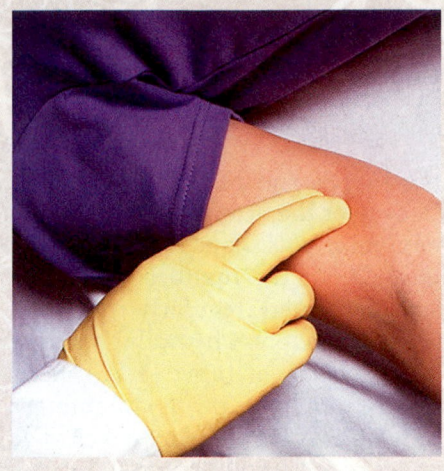

11-18b   Palpate the brachial artery.

11-18c   Palpate and compare the femoral arteries.

11-18d   Palpate the popliteal pulse.

11-18e   Palpate the dorsalis pedis pulse.

11-18f   Palpate the posterior tibial pulse.

11-18g   Palpate for edema.

+1 Slight pitting edema   +4 Deep pitting edema

FIGURE 11-22   Assessing for edema.

Table 11-8	PITTING EDEMA SCALE
Score	**Description**
1+	One quarter inch or less
2+	One quarter to one half inch
3+	One half to one inch
4+	One inch or more

During your assessment, look for visible venous distention. An associated swollen, painful leg suggests a deep vein thrombosis (DVT). Palpate the femoral vein just medial to the femoral artery. If you detect a tender femoral vein, flex the knee and palpate the calf for tenderness, another classic sign of DVT. Is there a local redness or warmth? Feel for a cordlike vessel. Evaluate the skin for discoloration, ulcers, and unusual thickness. Finally, ask your patient to stand. Evaluate his legs for varicose veins and, if present, palpate them for signs of thrombophlebitis (redness, swelling, pain, and tenderness).

THE NERVOUS SYSTEM

A comprehensive physical exam includes a thorough evaluation of your patient's mental status and thought processes. On the scene of an emergency, you would limit your mental exam to level of consciousness and basic orientation questions such as "What is your name?" "Where are you right now?" "What day is it today?" If you are conducting a full physical exam or evaluating someone with altered mentation, some or all of the following techniques will be useful.

When you conduct a neurological exam, you are attempting to answer two vital questions. First, are the findings symmetrical or unilateral? Second, if the signs are unilateral, is the site of origin in the central nervous system (brain and spinal cord) or in the peripheral nervous system (everything else). You will conduct many parts of the neuro exam while you assess other anatomical areas and systems. For example, you can examine the cranial nerves while evaluating the head and face. You can note any weaknesses or abnormal neurological findings while evaluating the arms and legs during the musculoskeletal exam.

A nervous system exam covers five areas: mental status and speech, the cranial nerves, the motor system, the reflexes, and the sensory system. This section presents the complete neuro exam. The chief complaint, clinical condition of your patient, and time constraints will determine which parts you actually use.

A neurological exam attempts to answer two vital questions: are the findings symmetrical or unilateral, and if unilateral, where do they originate?

Content Review

FIVE AREAS OF NEUROLOGICAL EXAM
- Mental status and speech
- Cranial nerves
- Motor system
- Sensory system
- Reflexes

Mental Status and Speech

Generally you will evaluate your patient's mental status and speech when you begin your interview. During this time you will assess his level of response, general appearance and behavior, and speech. If you detect abnormalities, continue your assessment with more specific questioning or testing as presented here.

Appearance and Behavior First, assess your patient's level of response. Is he alert and awake? Does he understand your questions? Are his responses appropriate and timely, or does he drift off the topic easily or lose interest? If you detect an abnormality, continue with more specific questions. Is he lethargic (drowsy, but answers questions appropriately before falling asleep again)? Is he obtunded (opens his eyes and looks at you but gives slow, confused responses)? Sometimes you must arouse your patient repeatedly by gently shaking him or shouting his name. If he does not respond to your verbal cues, assess him with painful stimuli for coma or stupor. The stuporous patient is arousable for short periods but is not aware of his surroundings. The comatose patient is in a state of profound unconsciousness and is totally unarousable.

If your patient is awake and alert, observe his posture and motor behavior. Does he lie in bed or prefer to walk around? His posture should be erect and he should look at you. A slumped posture and a lack of facial expression may indicate depression. Excessive energetic movements or constantly watchful eyes suggest tension, anxiety, or a metabolic disorder. Watch the pace, range, and character of his movements. Are they voluntary? Are any parts immobile? Do his posture and motor activity change with the environment? Some possible findings are listed in Table 11-9.

Observe your patient's grooming and personal hygiene. How is he dressed? Are his clothes clean, pressed, and properly fastened? Is his appearance appropriate for the season, climate, and occasion? A deterioration in grooming and personal hygiene in the previously well-groomed person may suggest an emotional problem, a psychiatric disorder, or an organic brain disease. Patients with obsessive-compulsive behavior may exhibit excessive attention to their appearance. Note your patient's hair, teeth, nails, skin, and beard. Are they well groomed? Compare one side to another. One-sided neglect may suggest a brain lesion.

Also observe your patient's facial expressions. Are they appropriate? Do they vary when he talks with others and when the topic changes or is his face immobile throughout the interaction? Can he express happiness, sadness, anger, or depression? Patients with Parkinson's disease have facial immobility, a mask-like appearance.

Speech and Language Note your patient's speech pattern. Normally a person's speech is inflected, clear and strong, fluent and articulate, and varies in volume. It should express thoughts clearly. Is your patient excessively talkative or silent? Does he speak spontaneously or only when you ask him a direct question? Is his speech slow and quiet, as in depression? Is it fast and loud, as in a manic episode? Does he speak clearly and distinctly? Does he have dysarthria

Table 11-9 POSTURE AND BEHAVIOR	
Motor Activity	**Meaning**
Tense posture, restlessness, fidgeting	Anxiety
Crying, hand wringing, pacing	Agitated, depression
Hopeless, slumped posture, slowed movements	Depression
Singing, dancing, expansive movements	Manic

(defective speech caused by motor deficits), dysphonia (voice changes caused by vocal cord problems), or aphasia (defective language caused by neurologic damage to the brain)? With expressive aphasia his words will be garbled; with receptive aphasia, his words will be clear but unrelated to your questions. Your patient with aphasia may have such difficulty talking that you mistakenly suspect a psychotic disorder.

Mood Observe your patient's verbal and nonverbal behavior for clues to his mood. Note any mood swings or behaviors that suggest anxiety or depression. Is he sad, elated, angry, enraged, anxious, worried, detached, or indifferent? Assess the intensity of your patient's mood. How long has he been this way? Is his behavior normal for the circumstances? For example, anxiety is normal for someone having a heart attack; if your heart attack patient did not act frightened and concerned, that would be abnormal. If your patient is depressed, is he suicidal? If you suspect the possibility of suicide, ask him directly, "Have you ever thought of committing suicide? Are you currently thinking of committing suicide?"

Thought and Perceptions Assess how well your patient organizes his thoughts when he speaks. Is he logical and coherent? Does he shift from one topic to an unrelated topic without realizing that the thoughts are not connected? These "loose associations" are typical in schizophrenia, manic episodes, and other psychiatric disorders. Does he speak constantly in related areas with no real conclusion or end-point? Such "flight of ideas" is most often associated with mania. Does he ramble with unrelated, illogical thoughts and disordered grammar? You may see this "incoherence" in severe psychosis. Does he make up facts or events in response to questions? You may see this "confabulation" in amnesia. Does he suddenly lose his train of thought and stop in mid-sentence before completing an idea? Such blocking occurs in normal people but is pronounced in schizophrenia.

Assess the thought content of your patient's responses as they occur during the interview. For example, "You said you thought you were allergic to your mother. Can you tell me why you think that way?" In this way you can ask about your patient's unpleasant or unusual comments. Allow him the freedom to explore these thoughts with you. Is your patient driven to try to prevent some unrealistic future result (compulsion)? Does he have a recurrent, uncontrollable feeling of dread and doom (obsession)? Does he sense that things in the environment are strange or unreal (feelings of unreality)? Does he have false personal beliefs that other members of his group don't share (delusions)? Compulsions and obsessions are neurotic disorders, while delusions and feelings of unreality are psychotic disorders.

Determine whether your patient perceives imaginary things. Does he see visions, hear voices, smell odors, or feel things that aren't there? Ask him about these false perceptions just as you would ask about anything else. For example, "When you see the pink elephants, what are they doing?" Decide whether your patient is misinterpreting what is real (illusions) or seeing things that are not real (hallucinations). Both illusions and hallucinations may occur in schizophrenia, post traumatic stress disorders, and organic brain syndrome. Auditory and visual hallucinations are common in psychedelic drug ingestion, while tactile hallucinations suggest alcohol withdrawal.

Insight and Judgment During the interview you will most likely evaluate your patient's insight and judgment. Does he understand what is happening to him? Does he realize that what he thinks and how he feels is part of the illness? Patients with psychotic disorders may not have insight into their illness. Judgment refers to your patient's ability to reason appropriately. Does your mature patient respond appropriately to questions concerning his family and personal life? Ask him what he would do if he cut himself shaving. Proper judgment means that your patient can evaluate the data and provide an adequate response. Impaired judgment is common in emotional problems, mental retardation, and organic brain syndrome.

Memory and Attention Assess your patient's orientation. Does he know his name? Person disorientation suggests trauma, seizures, or amnesia. Does he know the time of day, day of the week, month, season, and year? Time disorientation may suggest anxiety, depression, or organic brain syndrome. Does he know where he is, where he lives, the name of the city and state? Place disorientation suggests a psychiatric disorder or organic brain syndrome. Your patient should be oriented to person, time, and place and respond appropriately to your questions.

To assess your patient's ability to concentrate, use the following three exercises. First, have him repeat a series of numbers back to you (digit span). Normally, a person can repeat at least five numbers forward and backward. Then, ask him to start from 100 and subtract seven each time (serial sevens). A normal person can complete this in ninety seconds with fewer than four errors. Finally, ask your patient to spell a common five-letter word backward (spelling backward). Poor performance in these tests may suggest delirium, dementia, mental retardation, loss of calculating ability, anxiety, or depression.

Memory can be divided into three grades, immediate, recent, and remote. First, test your patient's immediate memory. Ask him to repeat three or four words that have no correlation such as "desk," "toothbrush," "six," and "blue." This tests immediate recall and is similar to digit span. Next, test your patient's recent memory by asking him what he had for lunch or to repeat something he told you earlier in the interview. Make sure the information you ask for is verifiable. Finally, test for remote memory by asking about facts such as his wife's name, son's birthday, or his social security number. Ask him to describe the house in which he grew up or the schools he attended. Long-term and short-term memory problems may be due to amnesia, anxiety, or organic causes. Finally, test your patient's ability to learn new things. Give him the names of three or four items such as "man, chair, grass, and hot dog." Ask him to repeat them. This tests registration and immediate recall. About five minutes later ask him to repeat them again. Normally, he will be able to name all four. Note his accuracy, his awareness of whether he is correct, or if he tries to confabulate by making up new words.

The Cranial Nerves

The 12 pairs of cranial nerves originate from the base of the brain and provide sensory and motor innervation, mostly to the head and face. Each pair bears the name of its function and carries either sensory fibers, motor fibers, or both. Table 11-10 lists the cranial nerves' names, their specific functions, and the areas they innervate.

Most likely you will conduct parts of the cranial nerve exam when you assess other areas such as the eyes, ears, throat, and musculoskeletal system. The following is the cranial nerve exam in its entirety.

CN-I Test your patient's olfactory nerve by having him close his eyes and compress one nostril while you present him with a variety of common, nonirritating odors (Procedure 11-19a). Repeat the test with each nostril. Ask him to identify the odor. Most people will do so easily. If your patient cannot, several causes are possible. Bilateral loss of smell suggests head trauma, nasal stuffiness, smoking, cocaine use, or a congenital defect. A unilateral loss of smell without nasal disease suggests a frontal lobe lesion.

Table 11-10 CRANIAL NERVES

CN	Name	Function	Innervation
I	Olfactory	Sensory	Smell
II	Optic	Sensory	Sight
III	Oculomotor	Motor	Pupil constriction; superior rectus, inferior rectus, inferior oblique muscles
IV	Trochlear	Motor	Superior oblique muscles
V	Trigeminal	Sensory	Opthalmic (forehead), maxillary (cheek), and mandibular (chin) regions
		Motor	Chewing muscles
VI	Abducens	Motor	Lateral rectus muscle
VII	Facial	Sensory	Tongue
		Motor	Face muscles
VIII	Acoustic	Sensory	Hearing balance
IX	Glossopharyngeal	Sensory	Posterior pharynx, taste to anterior tongue
		Motor	Posterior pharynx
X	Vagus	Sensory	Taste to posterior tongue
		Motor	Posterior palate and pharynx
XI	Accessory	Motor	Trapezius muscles Sternocleidomastoid muscles
XII	Hypoglossal	Motor	Tongue

CN-II Test the optic nerve with the visual acuity and visual field tests described earlier in this chapter in the anatomical regions section on the eyes.

CN-III Test the oculomotor nerve with the optic nerve when you perform pupil reaction tests. Inspect the size and shape of your patient's pupils and compare one side to the other. A slight inequality may be normal. Usually the pupil is mid-point. Constricted or dilated pupils may result from medications, drug abuse, glaucoma, and neurologic disease. Darken the room, if possible, to test for pupillary reaction. Ask your patient to look straight ahead. Shine a bright light obliquely into one of his pupils. Watch for direct reaction (pupillary constriction in the same eye) and for consensual reaction (pupillary constriction in the opposite eye). Repeat this test on the other side. Now assess for the near response, asking your patient to follow your finger as you move it in toward the bridge of his nose. Watch for his pupils to constrict and his eyes to converge.

CN-III, IV, VI Test the oculomotor, trochlear, and abducens nerves by evaluating your patient's extraocular movements (EOM). Ask him to follow your finger with only his eyes as you move it through the six cardinal positions of gaze (Procedure 11-19b). Make a wide "H" in the air with your finger. Observe for conjugate (together) movements of your patient's eyes in each direction. Normally your patient can follow your finger with no strabismus (deviation) or nystagmus (involuntary movements). Inability to move in any direction can be the result of a problem with a cranial nerve, an ocular muscle, or an eye orbit that may be fractured and impinging on the muscle or nerve. Finally, look for ptosis (a droopy eyelid) that may be the result of CN-III palsy or myasthenia gravis.

11-19a   Test the olfactory nerve by having your patient identify common odors.

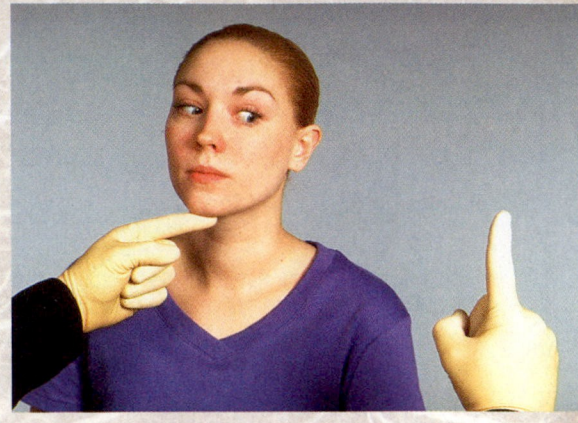

11-19b   Test the oculomotor, trochlear, and abducens nerves by evaluating your patient's extraocular movements.

11-19c   Test motor function of the trigeminal nerve by palpating the temporal and masseter muscles.

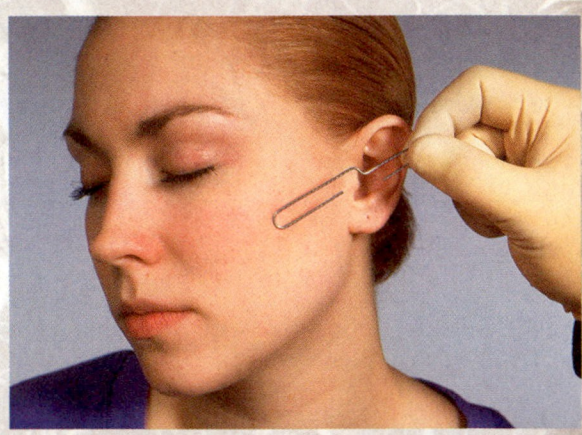

11-19d   Test sensory function of the trigeminal nerve with sharp and dull objects.

11-19e   Test the glossopharyngeal and vagus nerves with a tongue blade.

11-19f   Test the spinal accessory nerve by having your patient shrug her shoulders against resistance.

CN-V Test motor function by asking your patient to clench his teeth while you palpate the temporal and masseter muscles (Procedure 11-19c). Note the strength of the muscle contraction. Unilateral weakness or the inability to contract suggests a trigeminal nerve lesion. Bilateral dysfunction suggests motor neuron involvement.

To test for sensory function in the three main divisions of the trigeminal nerve, first ask your patient to close his eyes. Using something sharp and something dull, lightly scrape the objects across the forehead, cheek, and chin on both sides and ask your patient to distinguish the sensations (Procedure 11-19d). The two ends of a paper clip work well for this procedure; straighten one end and use its tip as the sharp object. Unilateral loss of sensation suggests a trigeminal nerve lesion. Finally, test the corneal reflex. Ask your patient to look up and away as you touch his cornea lightly with some fine cotton fibers. He should blink. Repeat this test on the other eye.

CN-VII First assess your patient's face at rest and during conversation. Note any asymmetry, eyelid drooping, or abnormal movements such as tics. Test the facial nerve by having your patient assume a variety of facial expressions. Ask him to raise his eyebrows, frown, show his upper and lower teeth or smile, and puff out his cheeks. Also ask him to close his eyes tightly so that you cannot open them; then to test muscle strength, try to open them. Bell's palsy is an inflammation of CN-VII. Your patient will present with unilateral facial drooping from paralysis of this nerve.

CN-VIII Ask your patient to occlude one ear with a finger. Then whisper something softly into the other ear. Ask him to repeat what you said. Any loss of hearing warrants further testing to detect air and bone conduction problems. Test the acoustic nerve for the senses of hearing and balance. Ask your patient to stand erect and close his eyes. Now evaluate his balance and then ask him to open his eyes. If he doesn't become dizzy and opens his eyes to your command, the eighth nerve is functioning appropriately.

CN-IX, X Test the glossopharyngeal and vagus nerves together. Listen to your patient's voice. Hoarseness suggests a vocal cord problem; a nasal quality suggests a palate problem. Ask your patient to swallow; note any difficulties. Ask him to open his mouth and say "aaahhh"; watch for the soft palate and uvula to rise symmetrically. The posterior pharynx should move medially. If the vagus nerve is paralyzed, the soft palate and uvula will deviate toward the side of the lesion. Test the gag reflex with a tongue blade on the posterior tongue (Procedure 11-19e). Absence of a gag reflex suggests a lesion in one of these nerves.

CN-XI Inspect the upper portions of your patient's trapezius muscles and sternocleidomastoid muscles for symmetry at rest. To test his trapezius muscles, place your hands on his shoulders and ask him to raise his shoulders against resistance (Procedure 11-19f). Now test his sternocleidomastoid muscles. Place your hands along his face and ask him to turn his head to each side as you apply resistance. Note any bilateral or unilateral weaknesses. A supine patient with bilateral weakness of the sternocleidomastoids will have trouble lifting his head.

CN-XII First evaluate your patient's speech articulation. Then ask him to stick out his tongue; watch for a midline projection. A CN-XII lesion will make the tongue deviate away from the affected side. Have your patient move his tongue from side to side as you watch for symmetry.

You may conduct a cranial nerve exam according to this sequence. More likely, you will develop your own efficient system of testing these nerves.

The Motor System

Inspect your patient's general body structure, muscle development, positioning, and coordination. What is his position at rest? Is he erect or does he slump to one side, suggesting unilateral paralysis or weakness? Note any obvious asymmetries, deformities, or involuntary movements. Are there tremors, tics, or fasciculations (twitches)? If so, note their location, rate, quality, rhythm, amplitude, and relation to your patient's posture, activity, fatigue, emotion, and other factors. For example, if your patient's hand begins to shake only when you ask him to perform a task with it such as writing his name or lifting a spoon, this suggests a postural tremor. Conversely, a tremor at rest that may disappear with voluntary movement suggests Parkinson's disease. To assess involuntary movement, observe your patient throughout the exam.

To determine your patient's muscle bulk, observe the size and contour of his muscles. Look for atrophy, a decrease in bulk and strength; hypertrophy, an increase in bulk and strength; or pseudohypertrophy, an increase in bulk and decrease in strength, as in muscular dystrophy. Flattened or concave contours, especially with fasciculations, may result from lower motor neuron disease. Some degree of muscle atrophy may be a normal part of the aging process or may result from the effects of diabetes on the peripheral nervous system. Look for signs of general muscle atrophy by checking for flattening of the thenar (thumb) muscle and for furrowing between the metacarpals. Unilateral muscle atrophy in the hands suggests median or ulnar nerve paralysis.

To assess muscle tone, feel the muscle's resistance to passive stretching in the extremities. Ask your patient to relax one of his arms. Then put the arm, wrists, and hands through a moderate range-of-motion exam (Procedure 11-20a). Repeat the exam in the lower extremities. If you detect decreased resistance, shake the hand loosely back and forth. It should move freely, but it should not be floppy (flaccid). Increased resistance may be caused by tension. Does the resistance persist throughout the motion (lead-pipe rigidity), or does it vary? If the resistance increases at the extreme limits of the movement, it is called spasticity. A ratchet-like jerkiness in the resistance is known as "cog-wheel rigidity," a common finding in a patient faking his symptoms or trying to resist your examination. Table 11-11 describes some common muscle tone findings.

Now focus on your patient's muscle strength. First, assess the strength of his grip. Test both grips simultaneously and compare them. Cross your middle finger over the top of your index finger to prevent your fingers from being hurt; then ask your patient to squeeze them as hard as possible (Procedure 11-20b). Normally you will have difficulty removing your fingers from your patient's grip. Continue testing all of the muscle groups listed in Table 11-12. While assessing muscle strength remember that each patient's age, gender, size, and muscular training will affect your exam results. When comparing sides, your patient's dominant side will be stronger. Test for muscle strength by having your patient move actively against your

Table 11-11	MUSCLE TONE
Finding	**Description**
Spasticity	Increased tone when passive movement applied, especially at the end of range. Common in stroke.
Rigidity	Increased rigidity throughout movement (lead-pipe). Common in Parkinson's disease and extra pyramidal reactions. Cog-wheel motion is a patient-applied resistance.
Flaccidity	Loss of muscle tone causing limb to be loose. Common in stroke, spinal cord lesion, and Guillain-Barré syndrome.
Paratonia	Sudden changes in tone with passive movement. Can be increased or decreased resistance. Common in dementia.

Table 11-12 MUSCLE STRENGTH TESTS

Muscles	Nerves	Test
Biceps	C5, C6	Flexion of the elbow
Triceps	C6, C7, C8	Extension of the elbow
Wrist extensors	C6, C7, C8, radial nerve	Extension of the wrist
Fingers	C8, T1, ulnar nerve	Finger abduction
Thumb	C8, T1, median nerve	Thumb opposition
Iliopsoas	L2, L3, L4	Hip flexion
Hip extensor	S1	Hip extension
Hip abductors	L4, L5, S1	Hip abduction
Hip adductors	L2, L3, L4	Hip adduction
Quadriceps	L2, L3, L4	Knee extension
Hamstrings	L4, L5, S1, S2	Knee flexion
Feet	L4, L5	Dorsiflexion
Calf muscles	S1	Plantar flexion

resistance (Procedure 11-20c). If the muscle is too weak to perform against resistance, have him try the movement against gravity or with gravity eliminated (you support the limb). Grade muscle strength on a scale from 1 to 5 (Table 11-13).

To assess your patient's position sense and coordination, first observe his gait. Ask him to walk across the room, turn, and come back. Normally he will be able to maintain his balance, swing his arms at his side, and turn easily. If his gait is ataxic—uncoordinated, reeling, or unstable—suspect cerebellar disease, loss of position sense, or intoxication. Next ask him to walk heel-to-toe in a straight line. This "tandem walking" may reveal an ataxia not previously seen. Now ask your patient to walk first on his toes, then on his heels. This will assess plantar flexion and dorsiflexion of the ankle as well as balance. Next, ask him to hop in place on each foot in turn. Difficulty hopping may result from leg muscle weakness, lack of position sense, or cerebellar dysfunction. Now ask him to do a shallow knee bend on each leg in turn. Difficulty doing this suggests muscle weakness in the pelvic girdle and legs. If your patient is old and unable to hop or do knee bends, have him rise from a sitting position without arm support, or step up onto a stool.

Next perform the Romberg test. Ask him to stand with his feet together and his eyes open. Now have him close his eyes for 20 to 30 seconds. Observe his ability to remain upright with minimal swaying and no support. Losing his balance indicates a positive Romberg test caused by ataxia from a loss of position

Table 11-13 MUSCLE STRENGTH SCALE

Score	Description
5	Active movement against full resistance with no fatigue
4	Active movement against some resistance and gravity
3	Active movement against gravity
2	Active movement with gravity eliminated
1	Barely palpable muscle contraction with no movement
0	No visible or palpable muscle contraction

11-20a   Assess the elbow's range of motion.

11-20b   Test your patient's grip.

11-20c   Test arm strength.

11-20d   Test for pronator drift.

11-20e   Test for coordination with rapid alternating movements.

11-20f   Test coordination with point-to-point testing.

11-20g   Assess coordination with heel-to-shin testing.

sense. An inability to maintain his balance with his eyes open and feet together represents a cerebellar ataxia. Now check your patient for pronator drift. Ask him to stand with his arms straight out in front of him with his palms up and his eyes closed (Procedure 11-20d). Ask him to maintain this position for 20 to 30 seconds. Normally your patient can do this easily. If one forearm pronates, suspect a mild hemiparesis. If it drifts sideways or upward, suspect a loss of position sense.

To assess your patient's coordination, test for rapid alternating movements. These maneuvers can be difficult to describe, so you should always demonstrate them to your patient. Ask him to repeat them as rapidly as possible while you observe for speed, rhythm, and smoothness. He should repeat all movements with both sides of the body. Keep in mind that his dominant hand usually will perform better than his nondominant hand. If his movements are slow, irregular and clumsy, suspect cerebellar or extrapyramidal tract disease or upper motor neuron weakness.

First, have your patient tap the distal joint of his thumb with the tip of his index finger as rapidly as possible. Then ask him to place his hand, palm up, on his thigh, quickly turn it over palm down, and return it palm up (Procedure 11-20e). Have him repeat this movement as quickly as possible for 15 seconds; evaluate both hands. Next have him perform point-to-point testing. Ask him to alternate touching your index finger and his nose several times while you observe for accuracy and smoothness (Procedure 11-20f). Note any tremors or difficulty performing this task, indicating cerebellar disease; evaluate both hands. Now assess for point-to-point testing in his legs. Ask him to touch his heel to the opposite knee, then run it down his shin to his big toe (Procedure 11-20g). Note the smoothness and accuracy of his actions. Repeat the test with the other leg. To test your patient's position sense, have him close his eyes and repeat this test for both legs. Abnormalities suggest cerebellar disease.

The Sensory System

To assess the sensory system, test for pain, light touch, temperature, position, vibration, and discriminative sensations. Remember to compare distal areas to proximal areas, to compare symmetrical areas bilaterally, and to scatter the stimuli to assess most of the dermatomes. Ask your patient to close his eyes for each of these tests. To test for pain sensation, touch your patient's skin with a sharp object and ask him to tell you whether it is sharp or dull. Compare areas as you move along the different regions, intermittently substituting a dull object for the sharp one. To test for light touch, softly touch him with a fine piece of cotton. Ask him to tell you whenever he feels the cotton. An abnormality suggests a peripheral neuropathy. Test for temperature sensation by touching his skin with a vial filled with either hot or cold liquid. Then test for position sense by pulling one of his toe's upward and asking him to tell you whether it is up or down. Test for vibration sense by placing the stem of a vibrating tuning fork against a bony prominence (Figure 11-23). Finally, test for discriminative sensation by putting a familiar object such as a key in your patient's hand and asking him to identify it.

Reflexes

The sensory pathways manage conscious sensation and participate in the reflex arc. The reflex arc connects some sensory impulses directly to motor neurons, triggering immediate responses to noxious stimuli such as touching your hand to a flame. Deep tendon reflexes are a similar involuntary response to direct muscular stretch. Striking a slightly flexed tendon with a reflex hammer sends

FIGURE 11-23   Test vibration sense with a tuning fork.

an impulse to the spinal cord, where a reflex arc occurs (Figure 11-24). This immediately sends a motor response back to the tendon, which begins the muscle contraction.

When you perform a nervous system exam, also test your patient's superficial and deep tendon reflexes. Always compare one side to the other. Grade the reflexes on a scale of 0 to 4+ (Table 11-14) and record your findings on a stick figure. A hyperactive response suggests upper motor neuron disease. A diminished response or no response suggests damage to the lower motor neurons or spinal cord.

FIGURE 11-24   A reflex arc depicts muscle tension over time.

Table 11-14 REFLEX SCALE

Grade	Description
0	No response
+	Diminished, below normal
++	Average, normal
+++	Brisker than normal
++++	Hyperactive, associated with clonus

Deep tendon reflexes can be tested at several places on the body. Use the pointed end of a reflex hammer for striking small areas, the flat end for striking larger areas. First ask your patient to relax. Then properly position the limb you are testing. Quickly strike the tendon using wrist motion only.

Biceps Support your patient's arm in the slightly flexed position with your thumb directly over the distal biceps tendon in the antecubital space (Procedure 11-21a). Strike your thumbnail with the point of the reflex hammer and watch for contraction of the biceps muscle and the resulting flexion of the elbow. This tests for spinal nerves C5 and C6.

Triceps Flex your patient's arm at a right angle. With the point of your reflex hammer, strike the triceps tendon along the posterior aspect of the distal humerus (Procedure 11-21b). Watch for triceps contraction and the resulting elbow extension. This tests spinal nerves C6, C7, and C8.

Brachioradialis Support your patient's arm with the forearm slightly pronated (Procedure 11-21c). Now strike his radius about two inches above his wrist. Watch for contraction of the brachioradialis and the resulting flexion and supination of the forearm. This tests cervical nerves C5 and C6.

Quadriceps Have your patient sit with his leg hanging off the end of the exam table. Tap the tendon just below the patella and watch for the quadriceps to contract and extend the knee (Procedure 11-21d). This tests lumbar nerves L2, L3, and L4.

Achilles With your patient sitting, dorsiflex the foot at the ankle and strike the Achilles tendon (Procedure 11-21e). Watch for the calf muscles to contract and cause plantar flexion of the foot. This tests sacral nerves S1 and S2.

Abdominal/Plantar Now test the superficial abdominal reflexes and plantar response. These are initiated by stimulating the skin instead of muscle. Assess the plantar reflex by stroking the lateral aspect of the sole from the heel to the ball of your patient's foot, curving medially across the ball (Procedure 11-21f). Begin with the lightest stimulus that will elicit a response. If you detect no response, be more firm. Watch for plantar flexion of the toes. Note if the big toe dorsiflexes while the other toes fan out. Known as a positive **Babinski response**, this indicates a central nervous system lesion.

✱ **Babinski response** big toe dorsiflexes and the other toes fan out when sole is stimulated.

Test the abdominal reflex by lightly stroking each side of the abdomen above and below the umbilicus with an irregular object such as a reflex hammer, a broken cotton swab or a split tongue blade (Procedure 11-21g). Note the contraction of the abdominal muscles and how the umbilicus deviates to the stimulus. The area above the umbilicus is innervated by thoracic nerves T8, T9, and T10. The area below the umbilicus is innervated by thoracic nerves T10, T11, and T12. The absence of abdominal reflexes can suggest either a central or peripheral nervous system disorder.

11-21a   Test the biceps reflex (cervical nerves C5 and C6).

11-21b   Test the triceps reflex (cervical nerves C6, C7, and C8).

11-21c   Test the brachioradialis reflex (cervical nerves C5 and C6).

11-21d   Test the quadriceps reflex (lumbar nerves L2, L3, and L4).

11-21e   Test the Achilles reflex (sacral nerves S1 and S2).

11-21f   Test the plantar reflex (central nervous system).

11-21g   Test abdominal reflexes (thoracic nerves T8, T9, T10, T11, and T12).

PHYSICAL EXAMINATION OF INFANTS AND CHILDREN

Conducting a physical examination of a sick or injured child can challenge any clinician. Your success will depend on several factors. First, you must be familiar with the anatomical differences between children and adults. Second, you must understand the physical and psychological developmental stages of the different age groups. Most importantly, you must practice these skills daily.

BUILDING PATIENT AND FAMILY RAPPORT

Children are not just small adults, and you cannot treat them as if they were.

Children are not just small adults, and you cannot treat them as if they were. Children are naturally apprehensive of strangers and new things. A sick or injured child is a frightened child. He fears pain, separation from his family, and unfamiliar surroundings. Dealing with these fears paves the way for a successful encounter with the child and his parents. You are a stranger. In uniform, you become even more ominous. Gaining your pediatric patient's trust becomes a vital part of your assessment. Unless he requires emergency critical care, take time to establish a rapport with him. This will help to ensure continuous cooperation.

The more invasive the procedure, the later in the exam you should perform it.

While different age groups have specific fears and characteristics, the following general rules apply to pediatrics as a whole. Remain calm and confident. Be direct and honest about what you are doing, especially if you are performing a painful procedure. If possible, do not separate the child from his parents. Instead, elicit their help in obtaining the history and allow them to help hold the child while you conduct your exam. The more invasive the procedure, the later in the exam you should perform it—unless, of course, your patient is critically ill or injured. (Never delay important procedures or techniques on the critically ill or injured child.) Once your patient begins crying and carrying on, the more difficult the rest of your exam will be, if not impossible. Finally, provide continuous reassurance and feedback to your patient and his family members. This helps reduce everyone's anxiety over what is wrong, what you are doing, and what comes next.

Position yourself at the child's eye level, use a soft voice, and smile a lot. Often a small toy, such as a teddy bear, can distract your patient while you examine him. If you are using diagnostic equipment, allow the child to handle it while you explain how it works. Make sure your movements are slow and deliberate, and explain everything you are doing.

ANATOMY AND THE PHYSICAL EXAM

To assess a child properly, you must understand his unique anatomy (Figure 11-25). The anatomical differences among age groups will alter your interpretation of physical findings. For example, since an infant's skin is thinner and contains less subcutaneous fat, you can expect environmental temperature extremes to affect him more severely.

This section deals with examining infants and children in the clinical situation. The pediatric chapter, Chapter 42, discusses a more detailed pediatric assessment.

General Appearance

Especially in the emergency setting, note whether your patient looks toxic, or sick. A toxic child appears not to recognize or respond to his parents. He may look tired and have a decreased respiratory effort and may have mottled skin or a generalized rash. He may be gray or cyanotic and just look very sick, usually from

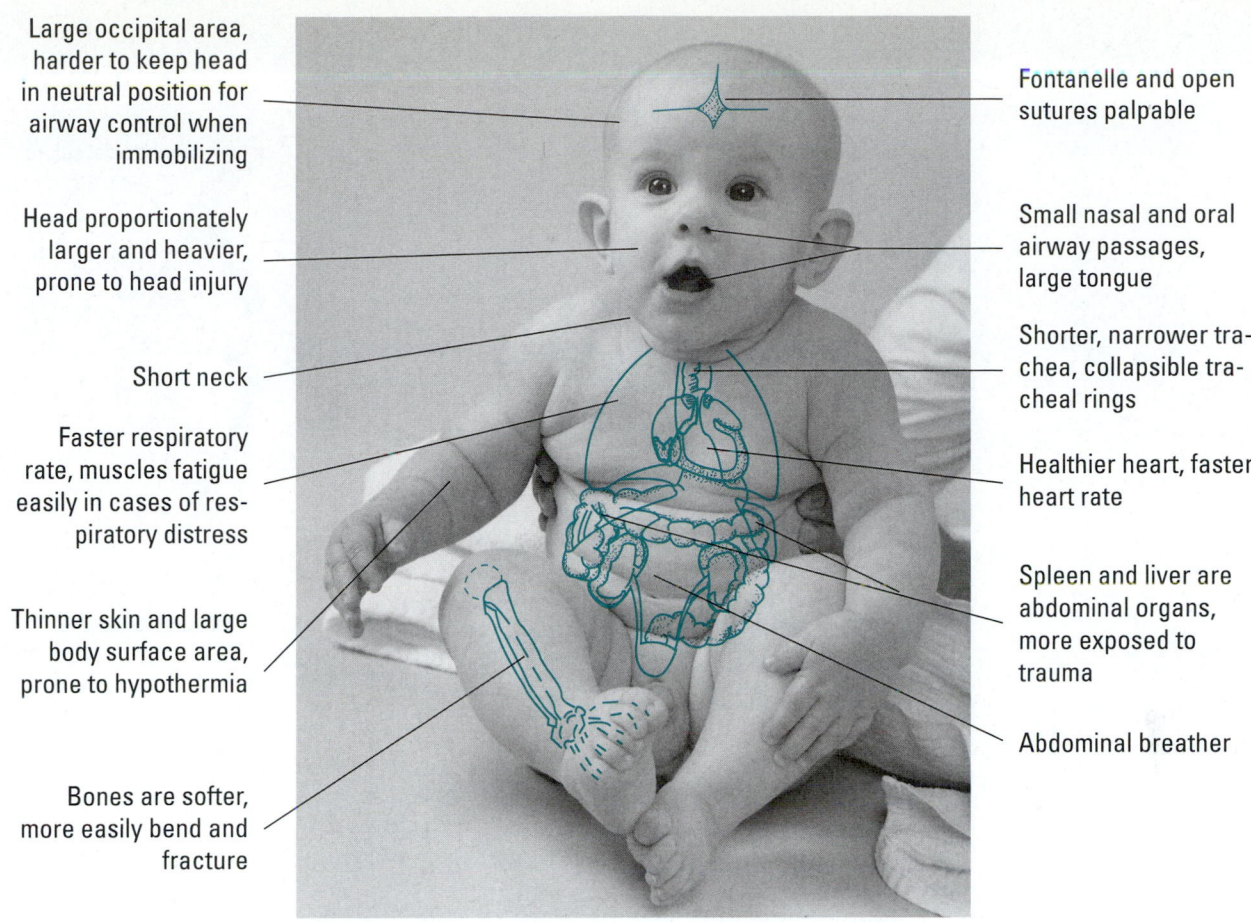

Large occipital area, harder to keep head in neutral position for airway control when immobilizing

Head proportionately larger and heavier, prone to head injury

Short neck

Faster respiratory rate, muscles fatigue easily in cases of respiratory distress

Thinner skin and large body surface area, prone to hypothermia

Bones are softer, more easily bend and fracture

Fontanelle and open sutures palpable

Small nasal and oral airway passages, large tongue

Shorter, narrower trachea, collapsible tracheal rings

Healthier heart, faster heart rate

Spleen and liver are abdominal organs, more exposed to trauma

Abdominal breather

FIGURE 11-25 Pediatric anatomy and physiology. You must understand a child's unique anatomy to assess him properly.

some type of bacterial process. These children, who present with the signs and symptoms of respiratory failure or shock, usually require rapid transport while you provide aggressive resuscitation procedures (advanced airway management, oxygenation and ventilation, intravenous access, and rapid fluid administration).

Head and Neck

The bones of the skull are soft and the fontanelles ("soft spots," spaces between a child's cranial bones) stay opened until about 18 months (Figure 11-26). From this time until about age five, cartilage connects the sutures. This allows the skull to expand as the brain grows. Check the sutures for bulging (increased intracranial pressure) or sunkenness (dehydration). In infants, a soft bulging spot following a history of trauma suggests a head injury with increasing intracranial pressure. The same finding associated with a fever suggests meningitis.

Because a child's airways are so much smaller than an adult's, a minor obstruction can create an acute respiratory problem. Watch the child's face for signs of distress and increased respiratory effort, such as nasal flaring. Children in acute respiratory distress will appear anxious and not interested in their surroundings. Also watch for retractions and head bobbing. Listen for stridor, wheezing, and grunting as further signs of severe breathing problems. As the child speaks, listen for hoarseness (upper airway obstruction) or moaning

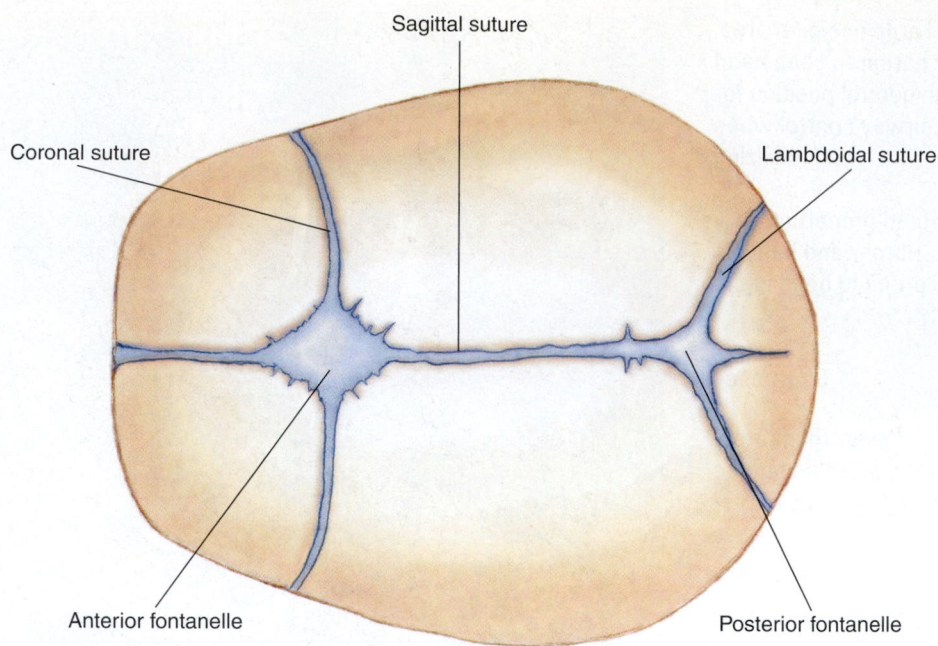

Sagittal suture

Coronal suture

Lambdoidal suture

Anterior fontanelle

Posterior fontanelle

FIGURE 11-26 Fontanelle of the infant skull.

(decreasing level of consciousness). These findings always require appropriate intervention and rapid transport. Remember, a crying or screaming child has a patent airway.

Observe the child's face for signs of pain and discomfort as you continue your examination. Inspect his eyes as you would an adult's. Assess the outer ear for position. The top of the ear should be on a horizontal line with the outer corner of the eye. As a child grows, the anatomy of the external ear canal changes. In infancy the canal curves downward, so you should pull down the auricle to see the tympanic membrane at the distal end of the canal. As the child grows, the canal starts to move up and backward, and the ear is relatively higher and farther back on the head. Remember to pull the auricle upward and backward to afford the best view with the otoscope. Brace your hand against the child's skull to prevent injury from sudden movement.

Choose the largest speculum that will fit comfortably into the child's ear. Tilt the child's head away from you. Hold the otoscope firmly in one hand and, with your free hand, pull the ear appropriately to straighten the ear canal. Slowly insert the speculum one-fourth to one-half inch into the canal. Observe the amount, texture, and color of wax and the presence of foreign bodies. Inspect the tympanic membrane for color, light reflex, and bony landmarks. Repeat the same steps for the other ear.

Inspect the child's mouth much the same as you would for the adult. A young child's mouth is small, while the tongue is relatively large, so examining his oral cavity will be a challenge. Examine the nose using the nasal speculum and penlight or the appropriate attachment to the otoscope. To examine the mucous membrane, tip the child's head back and use the otoscope to inspect for color or swelling.

Evaluate the child's neck for stiffness, which—when associated with a fever—suggests meningitis. Evaluate for lymphadenopathy (enlarged lymph nodes) in the neck by assessing the nodes' size, warmth, tenderness, and mobility. Certain infectious diseases like mononucleosis, rubella, and mumps are associated with lymphadenopathy. Nodes commonly feel enlarged due to recurrent upper respiratory infection.

Hoarseness, suggesting an upper airway obstruction, or moaning, suggesting decreased consciousness, requires intervention and rapid transport.

Table 11-15	NORMAL PEDIATRIC VITAL SIGNS		
Age Group	**Respiratory Rate**	**Heart Rate**	**Systolic BP**
Newborn	30–60	100–180	60–90
Infant	30–60	100–160	87–105
Toddler	24–40	80–110	95–105
Preschooler	22–34	70–110	95–110
School Age	18–30	65–110	97–112
Adolescent	12–26	60–90	112–128

Chest and Lungs

The rib cage in infants and small children is elastic and flexible. Because it comprises more cartilage than bone at this age, rib fractures are rare. On the other hand, lung contusions are common, because the lung tissue is very fragile. Small children also have a mobile mediastinum with a greater tendency to develop a tension pneumothorax. The chest muscles are not well developed, so children are mostly diaphragm breathers until about age seven.

The chest muscles are considered accessory muscles in the young child; to evaluate his breathing, observe both the chest and abdomen for movement. A child in severe respiratory distress may exhibit a "see-saw" pattern in which his sternum and abdomen rise and fall in opposition to each other. Count the respiratory rate without touching your patient, if possible. Assess the rate, quality, and depth of his respirations. Normal respiratory rates vary with age, but generally they decrease as the child grows older. Table 11-15 gives normal vital signs for the various pediatric age groups. Auscultate for breath sounds with the bell of your stethoscope at the mid-axillary lines (Figure 11-27). Use this location to avoid hearing transmitted breath sounds from the opposite lung fields.

Cardiovascular

Unless the child has a congenital defect, his heart will be strong and healthy. His heart rate will vary with age, but generally it will decrease as he gets older. If the child is alert and uncooperative, measure his pulse rate by listening to the heart. Place your stethoscope between the sternum and nipple on your patient's left side. Children have thin chest walls, so you will usually be able to observe the apical impulse of the heart.

FIGURE 11-27 Place your stethoscope along your young patient's mid-axillary line.

FIGURE 11-28 Gradually increase the pressure when palpating a young patient's abdomen.

Remember that tachycardia or bradycardia can both be a response to hypoxia in infants and young children. Bradycardia is the initial response to this condition in the newborn; without aggressive intervention, cardiopulmonary arrest will soon follow. Blood pressure will vary in children, but generally it will rise as they grow older. Children respond to hypovolemia by increasing cardiac function.

Abdomen

A child's liver and spleen are proportionally larger and more vascular than an adult's. Thus they extend beyond the rib cage and are more exposed. Likewise, the child's immature abdominal muscles provide less protection than an adult's. Inspect the abdomen first for movement. Normally only respiratory movements should be visible; peristalsis is not normally observable. Next, assess contour. The abdomen normally bulges by the end of inspiration. Note any asymmetry. Inspect the groin area for inguinal hernias, common in male children. Finally, look at the umbilicus for any hernias, common in children under three years. Percuss and auscultate the abdomen as in the adult.

Before you begin palpating the abdomen, make sure the child is comfortable. Bend his knees to relax the abdominal muscles and make palpation easier. Your hands should be warm. If the child is ticklish, cover his hands with yours as you palpate. Begin with light palpation and gradually increase the pressure (Figure 11-28). Palpate all four quadrants. Deep palpation is performed next. You are feeling for masses and tenderness. The child's facial expression is a better guide to pain than his words, since he may interpret your pressure as pain.

Musculoskeletal

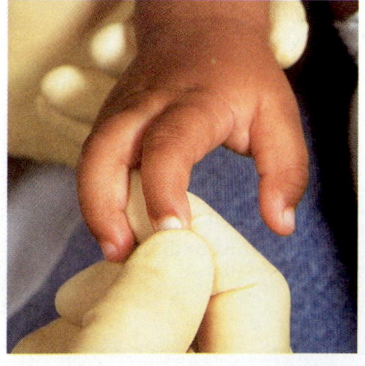

FIGURE 11-29 Pressing a child's fingernail is one of several ways to assess capillary refill. The child's capillary refill time is a good indicator of the child's peripheral perfusion status.

Evaluate pulses, sensation, movement, and warmth in all four extremities. Check for capillary refill and feel for peripheral pulses (Figure 11-29). Evaluate the skin, which reveals important clues in children. Its color, turgor, moisture, and temperature are key indicators of his cardiovascular system's condition. Unlike the adult's, the child's capillary refill time accurately reflects his peripheral perfusion status. When examining the musculoskeletal system, remember the growth and posture at different stages of the child's development. For example, a toddler walks with a broad base for support and is likely to appear bowlegged. A teenager with poor posture may suffer from a skeletal problem such as scoliosis.

Palpate the upper and lower extremities for swelling, tenderness, and contractions. Next have the child demonstrate the range of motion of his joints while you feel for smoothness of movement. Examine all joints. Check muscle strength in all muscle groups by asking the child to prevent you from moving a part of his body. A child's bones are more likely to break at the ends, where growth takes place. Until the child reaches adolescence, when these areas become as strong as the rest of the bone, injuries that occur near the joints are more likely to damage the bone than the ligaments or tendons. Assess the child's muscle coordination by having him stand and then hop on one foot. Repeat this for the other foot. Children usually enjoy this aspect of the physical examination. You can also have the child skip or jump.

Nervous System

The child's general behavior, level of consciousness, and orientation are signs of cerebral function. You have asked the parents to comment on their child's behavior during the history taking. You have observed the child's behavior throughout the examination and already have learned much about his cerebral function by interacting with him. Now test specific functions such as language and recall. You will have checked most of the 12 cranial nerves during your head and neck exam.

You can test for cerebellar function with several games that children usually enjoy. First, as you move your finger, ask the child to touch his nose and then your finger. Consistent past-pointing should arouse your suspicion. An alternate test is to have the child pat his knees alternately with the palms and backs of his hands. Check for sensation over the child's face, trunk, arms, and leg. Check for hot and cold sensation by alternately touching the skin with warm and cold test tubes. Ask the child to close his eyes and tell you which he feels. Be sure to test for reflexes on both sides of the body, just as with an adult. If the child has difficulty relaxing, test the parent's reflexes to show that it does not hurt.

Remember, the most important characteristic of a physical assessment is thoroughness. Be systematic in your approach and, with practice, you will be able to do a complete and accurate physical assessment.

The most important characteristic of a physical assessment is thoroughness.

RECORDING EXAMINATION FINDINGS

After you perform the history and physical examination, it is time to record the findings on your patient's chart, or permanent medical record. The information you enter enables you and other members of the health care team to identify health problems, make a diagnosis, plan the appropriate care, and monitor your patient's response to treatment. The patient record is only as good as the accuracy, depth, and detail you provide.

All health care clinicians follow a standard format when charting patient information. Using it and appropriate medical terminology will allow everyone to easily read and understand your assessment findings. While your first attempts at writing a complete history and physical exam will be lengthy and possibly disorganized, clinical experience will eventually lead to a more efficient and organized record.

Your patient's chart is a legal document, and any information you enter may be used in court. Proper documentation is vital to your protection. Present the data legibly, accurately, and truthfully. They should represent the findings of your history and physical examination—no more, no less. State your assessment, your analysis of the problem, and your management plan clearly and exactly. No question should ever arise about your assessment or care of your patient if you document it properly.

Be sure to include all data about your assessment. You cannot formulate an impression unless you have clearly spelled out the positive and negative details upon which it was made. Remember that the absence of a sign or symptom (pertinent negative) may be just as important as its presence. Record everything in writing. If you do not document a neuro exam, you will never convince anyone that you performed it, especially not a plaintiff's lawyer or a jury. Be complete but avoid unnecessary words. For example, say "pale," not "pale in color." Also avoid lengthy repetitive

The patient record is only as good as the accuracy, depth, and detail you provide.

Record everything in writing.

phrases such as "patient states." Use accepted abbreviations and symbols whenever possible. Avoid using vague adjectives such as *good, normal,* and *poor,* because they are open to interpretation by other providers. Document what your patient tells you, not what you infer or interpret. Use direct quotes whenever possible.

The universally accepted organization for patient charts follows the SOAP format. SOAP stands for <u>S</u>ubjective, <u>O</u>bjective, <u>A</u>ssessment, and <u>P</u>lan. Use this format when writing your patient's chart. Subjective information is what your patient tells you. It comprises the chief complaint, the history of present illness, the past history, the current health status, and the review of systems. Objective information includes the data collected from the general survey, vital signs, head-to-toe anatomical exam, systems-oriented exam, and neurological exam, including the mental status. These are the data you gathered by inspection, palpation, percussion, auscultation, and other techniques of physical examination. Objective information also includes the results of any laboratory tests. The assessment summarizes the relevant data for each problem identified in the history and physical exam. The plan outlines your management strategy in three categories: diagnostic (how you will assess progress), therapeutic (any treatments), and educational (what you need to teach your patient). Chapter 15, "Documentation," deals with prehospital documentation in detail.

Content Review

SOAP
- Subjective
- Objective
- Assessment
- Plan

SUMMARY

This chapter has presented both a regional and a systems approach to physical examination. The setting, chief complaint, and clinical status of your patient will dictate how much of the physical exam you actually use. For example, if you are hired to conduct preemployment physicals, you may decide to conduct a complete examination. If you are at the scene of a critically ill or injured patient, you will assess only those areas relevant to the situation. If your patient presents with a minor, isolated musculoskeletal injury, you may focus your exam on that area and system. As you become more experienced, making these decisions will become easier.

CHAPTER 12

Patient Assessment in the Field

Objectives

After reading this chapter, you should be able to:

1. Recognize hazards/potential hazards associated with the medical and trauma scene. (pp. 701–708)
2. Identify unsafe scenes and describe methods for making them safe. (pp. 701–708)
3. Discuss common mechanisms of injury/nature of illness. (pp. 710–712)
4. Predict patterns of injury based on mechanism of injury. (pp. 710–711, 722–724)
5. Discuss the reason for identifying the total number of patients at the scene. (pp. 708–709)
6. Organize the management of a scene following size-up. (pp. 701–708)
7. Explain the reasons for identifying the need for additional help or assistance during the scene size-up. (pp. 701, 704–708)
8. Summarize the reasons for forming a general impression of the patient. (pp. 712–714)
9. Discuss methods of assessing mental status/levels of consciousness in the adult, infant, and child patient. (pp. 714–715)

Continued

Objectives Continued

10. Discuss methods of assessing and securing the airway in the adult, child, and infant patient. (pp. 715–716)
11. State reasons for cervical spine management for the trauma patient. (pp. 713–714)
12. Analyze a scene to determine if spinal precautions are required. (pp. 714–715, 722–724)
13. Describe methods for assessing respiration in the adult, child, and infant patient. (pp. 716–717)
14. Describe the methods used to locate and assess a pulse in an adult, child, and infant patient. (pp. 717–720)
15. Discuss the need for assessing the patient for external bleeding. (p. 720)
16. Describe normal and abnormal findings when assessing skin color, temperature, and condition. (p. 720)
17. Explain the reason and process for prioritizing a patient for care and transport. (pp. 720–722)
18. Use the findings of the initial assessment to determine the patient's perfusion status. (pp. 717–720, 721)
19. Describe orthostatic vital signs and evaluate their usefulness in assessing a patient in shock. (p. 740)
20. Describe the medical patient physical examination. (pp. 736–740)
21. Differentiate between the assessment for an unresponsive, altered mental status, and alert medical patients. (pp. 735–743)
22. Discuss the reasons for reconsidering the mechanism of injury. (pp. 724–725)
23. Recite examples and explain why patients should receive a rapid trauma assessment. (p. 724)
24. Describe the trauma patient physical examination. (pp. 724–733)
25. Describe the elements of the rapid trauma assessment and discuss their evaluation. (pp. 724–734)
26. Identify cases when the rapid assessment is suspended to provide patient care. (pp. 724–725)
27. Discuss the reason for performing a focused history and physical exam. (pp. 722, 735, 743)
28. Describe when and why a detailed physical examination is necessary. (p. 744)
29. Discuss the components of the detailed physical examination. (pp. 744–750)
30. Explain what additional care is provided while performing the detailed physical exam. (pp. 744–750)
31. Distinguish between the detailed physical exam that is performed on a trauma patient and that of the medical patient. (pp. 744–750)
32. Differentiate between patients requiring a detailed physical exam and those who do not. (p. 744)
33. Discuss the rationale for repeating the initial assessment as part of the ongoing assessment. (pp. 751–753)
34. Describe the components of the ongoing assessment. (pp. 751–754)
35. Describe trending of assessment components. (pp. 751–754)
36. Discuss medical identification devices/systems. (p. 730)
37. Given several preprogrammed and moulaged medical and trauma patients, provide the appropriate scene survey, initial assessment, focused assessment, detailed assessment, and ongoing assessments. (pp. 700–754)

INTRODUCTION

Patient assessment means conducting a problem-oriented evaluation of your patient and establishing priorities of care based on existing and potential threats to human life. In the previous two chapters you studied the techniques of performing a comprehensive history and physical exam. Such all-inclusive evaluations are best suited for patients without a chief complaint. They also establish a baseline health evaluation for patients admitted to the hospital. As a paramedic, however, you will certainly never perform a comprehensive exam in the acute setting. It is too time consuming and yields too much irrelevant information. Instead you will use your foundation of knowledge, skills, and tools to assess the acutely ill or injured patient. With time and clinical experience you will learn which components of the comprehensive exam apply to your particular patient.

Now you can use the pertinent components of the comprehensive history and physical exam to perform patient assessments—problem-oriented assessments based on your patient's chief complaint. The basic components of patient assessment include the initial assessment; the focused history and physical exam, including vital signs; an ongoing assessment; and in some cases, a detailed physical exam.

Your patient's condition will determine which components you use and how you use them. For example, for trauma patients with a significant mechanism of injury, you will perform an initial assessment followed by a rapid trauma assessment (a head-to-toe exam aimed at traumatic signs and symptoms) and, if time allows, a detailed physical exam en route to the hospital. For patients with minor, isolated trauma, an initial assessment followed by a focused physical exam is warranted. For the responsive medical patient, you will conduct an initial assessment followed by a focused history and physical exam. Finally, for the unresponsive medical patient, you will perform an initial assessment followed by a rapid medical assessment (a head-to-toe exam aimed at medical signs and symptoms). In all cases, you will perform an ongoing assessment en route to the hospital to detect changes in patient condition.

The initial assessment's goal is to identify and correct immediately life-threatening conditions. These include airway compromise, inadequate ventilation, and major hemorrhage. During this rapid evaluation you use a variety of maneuvers and special equipment to manage any life threats as you find them. Immediately following the initial assessment you will establish the priorities of care. People such as the trauma patient with unstable vital signs and the unresponsive medical patient require a rapid head-to-toe exam and immediate transport to the hospital. Patients with minor, isolated trauma and most medical emergencies allow time to perform further assessments and provide care before transport.

Your proficiency in performing a systematic patient assessment will determine your ability to deliver the highest quality of prehospital advanced life support (**ALS**) to sick and injured people. Paramedic patient assessment is a straightforward skill, similar to the assessment you might have performed as an EMT-Basic. It differs, however, in depth and in the kind of care you will provide as a result. Your assessment must be thorough, because many advanced life support procedures are potentially dangerous. Safely and appropriately performing advanced procedures such as administration of drugs, defibrillation, synchronized cardioversion, needle decompression of the chest, or endotracheal intubation will depend upon your assessment and correct field diagnosis. If your assessment does not reveal your patient's true problem, the consequences can be devastating.

As always, common sense dictates how you proceed in the field. When you assess the responsive medical patient, the history reveals the most important diagnostic information and takes priority over the physical exam. For the trauma patient and the unresponsive medical patient, the reverse is true. Yet trauma may cause a medical emergency, and conversely, a medical emergency may cause trauma. Only by performing a thorough patient assessment can you discover the true cause of your patient's problems. This chapter provides problem-oriented patient assessment templates based on the information and techniques presented in the previous two chapters. You will need to refer to those chapters for the details of taking a history and conducting a physical exam.

SCENE SIZE-UP

Scene size-up is the essential first step at any emergency. Before you enter a scene, take the necessary time to judge the situation. Fire officers drive just past a burning house so they can see three of its sides before they make strategic decisions. Follow their lead. Never rush into any situation; first stop and look around (Figure 12-1).

Never rush into any situation; first stop and look around.

Upon arrival, determine whether the scene is safe. Does the situation require special body substance isolation precautions? Is the mechanism of injury or the nature of illness obvious? Are there multiple patients? Do you need immediate additional resources? After an initial scene assessment, if necessary, report to your dispatcher what you have, what you need, and what you are doing. This way, you keep everyone informed and your dispatcher can send any necessary additional support.

While size-up is your initial responsibility, remember that it is also an ongoing process. Emergency scenes are dynamic and can change suddenly. An injury to a child call can erupt into a violent domestic dispute if one parent blames the other. A hazardous material spill can ignite. An improperly stabilized car can shift. Always be alert for subtle signs of danger, and avoid becoming a patient yourself.

Always be alert for subtle signs of danger.

Sizing up the scene gives you important information that will guide your actions. In trauma, a brief size-up of the accident scene reveals the mechanism of injury. From this, you can estimate the degree of energy transfer and possible

Sizing up the scene gives you important information that will guide your actions.

FIGURE 12-1   Always stop to size up the scene before going in.

seriousness of injuries. In a medical emergency, you can sometimes determine the nature of your patient's illness from clues at the scene. The smell of a lower gastrointestinal bleed, the sound of a hissing oxygen tank, or the sight of drug paraphernalia provides clues and an initial insight into your patient's situation. Learn to use all your senses when sizing up the scene.

The components of a scene size-up include:

- Body substance isolation
- Scene safety
- Location of all patients
- Mechanism of injury
- Nature of the illness

Content Review

COMPONENTS OF SCENE SIZE-UP

Body substance isolation
Scene safety
Location of all patients
Mechanism of injury
Nature of the illness

BODY SUBSTANCE ISOLATION

Body fluids frequently contain health-threatening pathogens. The best defense against bloodborne, body-fluid-borne, and airborne agents is to take appropriate body substance isolation precautions. Your goal is to prevent infectious disease from spreading to yourself or to others. Make sure that personal protective equipment such as gloves, masks, gowns, and eye protection is available on every emergency vehicle, and take the appropriate precautions on every emergency call (Figure 12-2). Your patient's clinical condition and the procedures you perform will determine the required precautions.

Most body isolation procedures are simply common sense. Wash your hands thoroughly before and after treating each patient whenever possible (Figure 12-3). This simple technique is the most effective method of preventing disease transmission between patients and their health care workers. Wear latex or vinyl gloves anytime you expect to contact blood or other body fluids. This includes the mucous membranes, any areas with broken skin, or items soiled with blood or body fluids. Since you often cannot wash your hands before examining your patient, you should wear gloves also to avoid exposing your patient to your germs. If you are managing multiple patients, you should attempt to change gloves between patients in order to prevent cross-contamination. Discard all contaminated gloves in the appropriate biohazard bag (Figure 12-4).

Always use all the equipment recommended for a particular procedure or patient to maximize your protection against communicable diseases. If blood, vomit, or secretions might splash near your eyes, nose, or mouth, wear a face mask and protective eyewear. Such situations may include arterial bleeding, childbirth, invasive procedures such as endotracheal intubation, and oral suctioning, as well as

The best defense against bloodborne, body-fluid-borne, and airborne pathogens is to take body substance isolation precautions.

Washing your hands is the most effective method of preventing disease transmission between you and your patients.

Always use all the equipment recommended for a particular procedure or patient to maximize your protection against communicable diseases.

FIGURE 12-2   Always wear the appropriate personal protective equipment (PPE) to prevent exposure to contagious diseases.

FIGURE 12-3 Careful, methodical hand washing helps reduce exposure to contagious disease.

FIGURE 12-4 Place all contaminated items in the appropriate biohazard bag.

FIGURE 12-5 With a suspected tuberculosis patient, you may place a surgical-type mask on the patient while you wear a NIOSH-approved respirator. Monitor the patient's airway and breathing carefully.

during clean-up when heavy scrubbing is necessary. If you expect large blood splashes, such as in emergency childbirth, wear a gown to protect your clothing.

Consider masking both yourself and your patient whenever the potential for airborne transmission of disease exists (Figure 12-5). The National Institute of Occupational Safety and Health has designed high-efficiency particulate air (**HEPA**) respirators to filter out the tuberculosis bacillus (TB). Always wear a

FIGURE 12-6 Look for potential hazards during scene size-up.

properly fitted HEPA mask if you are managing a patient with suspected TB, especially when performing procedures like endotracheal intubation, oral suctioning, and administering nebulized medications. These procedures present a high risk for the transmission of airborne particles.

SCENE SAFETY

Scene safety simply means doing everything possible to ensure a safe environment for yourself, your crew, other responding personnel, your patient, and any bystanders—in that order. Your personal safety is the top priority at any emergency scene. Make sure you are not injured while providing care. If you become a patient yourself, you will do your own patient little good. You must determine that no hazards may endanger the lives of people on the scene. If your scene is unsafe, either make it safe or wait until someone else does (Figure 12-6).

As the first unit on the scene, you may overestimate your capability to manage a rescue situation. Do not attempt a hazardous rescue unless you are properly clothed, equipped, and trained. Individual acts of courage are sometimes necessary, but modern rescue operations emphasize safety first, not heroics. Foolish heroics often end in tragedy. If in doubt, it is better to err on the side of caution than to risk personal harm.

Many factors can make an emergency scene unsafe. Through experience you will learn to identify them quickly. Do not become complacent. Sometimes even the most nonthreatening, harmless-looking scene can turn into a disaster (Figure 12-7). If you are not sure the scene is safe, do not enter. As you approach a scene, immediately evaluate the surrounding area. Is it as your dispatcher's information has led you to expect, or does something just not look right? What do the bystanders' faces tell you? Are they angry, scared, or panicked? Be alert for situations that look or feel suspicious. If necessary, wait until law enforcement personnel secure the scene. Use all your senses to evaluate a scene and learn to trust your intu-

FIGURE 12-7 Even the most peaceful-looking scene can pose potential dangers.

ition. If your instincts tell you not to enter or to get out, follow them. They are the subconscious sum of your experiences. Listen to them; they are probably correct.

Carefully look for and identify on-scene hazards before even attempting to reach your patient. To do otherwise places you, other rescuers, and your patient at risk. Remember that you may find such dangers at either medical or trauma scenes. Potential hazards include fire, structural collapse, traffic, unstable surfaces, and broken glass or jagged metal. Other risks involve hazardous materials—chemical spills, radiation, or gas leaks that might ignite or explode. A simple spark can set off a gas leak or oil spill. Electric wires threaten both fire and electric shock. Look around to determine the possibility of lightning, avalanche, rock slides, cave-ins, or similar dangers. Other potential hazards include poisonous or caustic substances; biological agents; germ-infested materials; confined spaces such as vessels, trenches, mines, silos, or caves; and extreme heights. In every case, let common sense dictate scene management.

Crime scenes pose a special threat. When responding to a call in which the initial dispatch includes words such as *shooting, stabbing,* or *domestic dispute,* wait for law enforcement personnel to secure the scene before entering (Figure 12-8). In fact, do not even enter the neighborhood, as sitting in your ambulance on the scene may undermine an already unstable environment. If possible, turn off your lights and siren and stage your vehicle a few blocks away, where it cannot be seen from the scene. Refer to the crime scene awareness section of Chapter 48 for more information on this topic.

In every case, let common sense dictate scene management.

FIGURE 12-8 Wait for the police before entering a potentially hazardous scene.

Do not even consider entering hazardous scenes unless you have the proper clothing, equipment, and training to work in them.

A prompt call for backup can save critical minutes in a life-threatening situation.

Content Review

MINIMUM RESCUE-OPERATION EQUIPMENT

Four-point suspension helmets
Eye goggles and industrial safety glasses
High-quality hearing protection
Leather work gloves
High-top steel-toed boots
Insulated coveralls
Turnout gear

Crash scenes requiring heavy-duty rescue procedures, scenes where toxic substances are present, crime scenes with a potential for violence, or scenes with unstable surfaces like slippery slopes, ice, or rushing water all call for specialized crews, additional medical supplies, and sophisticated equipment (Figure 12-9). Do not even consider entering such situations unless you have the proper clothing, equipment, and training to work in them. Because getting backup requires extra time, this phase is critical. A prompt call to your dispatch center can save critical minutes in a life-threatening situation.

Without the appropriate protective gear, you will jeopardize your safety and your patient's. To participate in a rescue operation, you should have at least the following equipment immediately available: four-point suspension helmets, eye goggles or industrial safety glasses, high-quality hearing protection, leather

FIGURE 12-9 Never enter a specialized rescue situation without proper training and equipment.

FIGURE 12-10 Full protective gear, including eye protection, helmet, turnout gear, and gloves.

FIGURE 12-11 Self-contained breathing apparatus (SCBA).

work gloves, high-top steel-toed boots, insulated coveralls, and turnout gear (Figure 12-10). Only personnel thoroughly trained in hazardous material (haz-mat) suits or self-contained breathing apparatus (SCBA) should use them (Figure 12-11). These items are often supplied on specialty support vehicles such as haz-mat response units and heavy-rescue trucks (Figure 12-12).

After you ensure that responding personnel have adequate safety equipment to manage the rescue scene, consider patient safety. Many considerations for rescuer safety also apply to patients. Additionally, patient safety equipment should at least include construction-type hard hats, eye goggles, hearing and respiratory protection, protective blankets, and protective shielding. You will need these to protect your patient during rescue operations (Figure 12-13). Patient safety also includes simple measures such as removing them from unstable environments such as temperature extremes, smoky rooms, or hostile crowds. For example, the simplest way to begin managing a patient suffering from hypothermia is to move him into a warm environment.

Safe, orderly, and controlled incident management is essential for everyone's safety. Call for specialty personnel to stabilize wreckage or turn off electrical power. Make sure someone routes traffic safely around a vehicle collision. Control bystanders and spot potential human hazards. Be certain that a hostile crowd or someone who assaulted your patient is not ready to attack you. Scenes involving toxic exposures, environmental hazards, and violent patients are

Content Review

MINIMUM PATIENT-SAFETY EQUIPMENT
Construction-type hard hats
Eye goggles
Hearing and respiratory protection
Protective blankets
Protective shielding

Safe, orderly, and controlled incident management is essential for everyone's safety.

FIGURE 12-12   Hazardous materials responses require special training and equipment.

FIGURE 12-13   Protect the patient from hazards at the scene.

especially worrisome. When possible, have law enforcement personnel establish a tape line to cordon off the hazard zone to protect bystanders who do not realize the potential dangers of watching operations (Figure 12-14).

LOCATION OF ALL PATIENTS

Scene size-up also includes a search of the area to locate all of the patients. Ask yourself if other persons could be involved in the accident or affected by the medical problem. Determine where you are most likely to find the most seriously affected patients and how many patients will need transport. The mechanism of injury or the nature of the illness can help you determine the number of patients. For example, a two-car accident must include at least two drivers. Clues such as diaper bags, child auto seats, toys, coloring books, clothing, or twin spider-web impact marks in the windshield should lead you to search for more patients, especially children, than

Searching the area to locate all patients.

FIGURE 12-14   Tape lines help to keep bystanders out of hazardous scenes.

those who may be readily apparent. Some medical situations such as carbon monoxide poisoning can affect an entire household. A hazardous liquid spill in the chemistry lab can affect students and staff in an entire wing of a school.

If you find more patients than you can safely and effectively manage, call for assistance early. If possible, you should do this before you make contact with any patients, because you are less likely to call for help once you become involved with patient care. Often, as you proceed into a scene, more patients become apparent. It is wise to overestimate when asking for help at the scene.

Initiate the mass casualty plan according to your local protocols (Figure 12-15). Again, try not to become involved in patient care, for two important functions must occur in the initial stages of any mass casualty incident—command and triage. If you and your partner find yourselves in a situation that overwhelms your resources, one of you should establish command while the other begins triaging patients. The command person performs a scene size-up, determines the needs of the incident, makes a radio report requesting the necessary additional help, and directs on-coming crews to their duties (Figure 12-16). The triage person performs a triage exam on every patient and prioritizes them for immediate or delayed transport (Figure 12-17). He may perform simple life-saving procedures such as opening the airway or controlling bleeding, but as a rule he should not stop to provide intensive care for any one patient.

Call for assistance early; it is wise to overestimate when asking for help.

FIGURE 12-15   Follow local protocols when you respond to a mass-casualty incident.

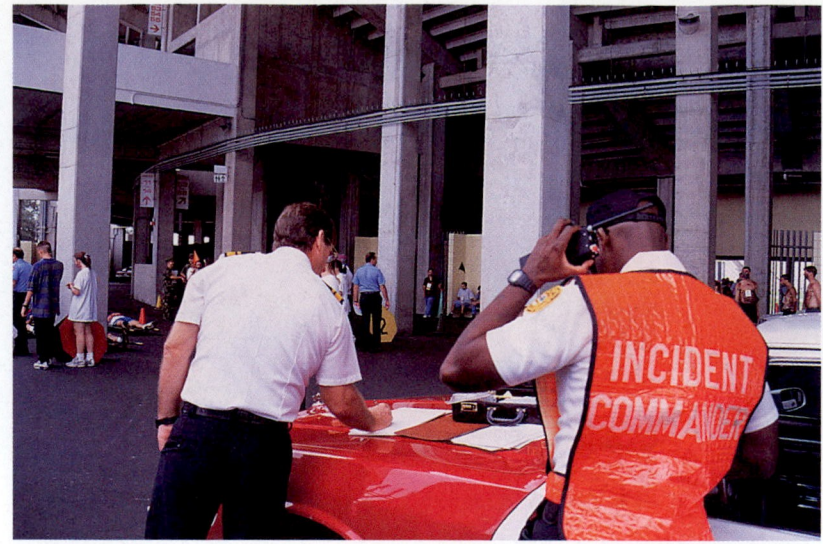

FIGURE 12-16 The incident commander directs the response and coordinates resources at a multiple-casualty incident.

FIGURE 12-17 The triage person examines and prioritizes patients.

MECHANISM OF INJURY

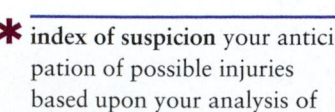 **mechanism of injury** combined strength, direction, and nature of forces that injured your patient.

The **mechanism of injury** is the combined strength, direction, and nature of forces that injured your patient. It is usually apparent through careful evaluation of the trauma scene and can help you anticipate both the location and the seriousness of injuries. Identify the forces involved, the direction from which they came, and the bodily locations affected (Figure 12-18). For example, in a fall injury, how high was the patient, what did he land on, and what part of his body hit first? If your patient jumped from a height and landed on his feet, expect lower extremity, pelvic, and lumbar spine injuries.

In an automobile accident, the mechanism of injury is the process by which forces are exchanged between the automobile and what it struck, between your patient and the automobile's interior, and among the various tissues and organs as they collide with one another within the patient. Close inspection of the automobile and the forces, or various collisions, can lead to an **index of suspicion** (a prediction of injuries based on the mechanism of injury) for possible injuries. What does the car look like? If the windshield is cracked, expect head and neck

index of suspicion your anticipation of possible injuries based upon your analysis of the event.

FIGURE 12-18   With trauma, try to determine the mechanism of injury during scene size-up.

injuries. If the steering wheel is bent, expect chest and abdominal injuries. With a major intrusion into the passenger compartment, expect major trauma.

Expect a pedestrian struck by a car to have fractures of the lower extremities. If the auto was moving at 20 miles per hour, expect less severe fractures than if it were moving at 55 miles per hour. Also, internal injuries are less likely at lower speeds than at higher speeds. By evaluating the strength and nature of impact, you can anticipate which organs are injured and the degree of their damage.

For a gunshot patient, determine the type of gun used, the range of the shot, and if an exit wound exists. This information will enable you to estimate the damage along the bullet's path and to formulate an index of suspicion for your patient's possible injuries. Expect the internal injuries from serious blunt trauma to be more extensive and severe than those you see externally. Often the mechanism of injury is the only clue to the possibility of serious internal injury. Chapters 17 and 18 on blunt and penetrating trauma describe the mechanisms of these injuries in depth.

Often the mechanism of injury is the only clue to the possibility of serious internal injury.

NATURE OF THE ILLNESS

Determine the nature of the illness from bystanders, family members, or your patient himself. If he is alert and oriented, he is usually the best source of information about his problem. If he is unresponsive, disoriented, or otherwise unable to provide information, rely on family members, bystanders, or visual cues for this information.

The scene can give additional clues to your patient's condition. How is he positioned? Does he sit bolt upright gasping to breathe? Are pill bottles or drug paraphernalia nearby? Is medical-care equipment such as an oxygen tank, a nebulizer, or a glucometer in the room? For example, if you respond to a "difficulty breathing" call and your patient is using his nebulizer when you arrive, suspect a history of pulmonary disease such as asthma, emphysema, or chronic bronchitis. If your patient is an agitated 17-year-old with a rapid pulse and you notice crack cocaine ampules on the floor, suspect a substance abuse problem.

* **initial assessment** prehospital process designed to identify and correct life-threatening airway, breathing, and circulation problems.

* **general impression** your initial, intuitive evaluation of your patient.

Sometimes the nature of the illness is not readily apparent. Your patient with severe difficulty breathing, for instance, may be suffering from respiratory disease, a cardiac problem, an allergic reaction, or a toxic exposure. Remember that the nature of your patient's illness may be very different from his chief complaint.

THE INITIAL ASSESSMENT

The **initial assessment** exemplifies the basis of all prehospital emergency medical care. Its goal is to identify and correct immediately life-threatening patient conditions of the <u>A</u>irway, <u>B</u>reathing, or <u>C</u>irculation (**ABCs**). If you find these conditions during this part of your assessment, treat them at once. For example, open a closed airway, provide ventilation, or control hemorrhage before moving on. Immediately following the initial assessment, decide priority regarding immediate transport or further on-scene assessment and care. The initial assessment consists of the following steps:

- Forming a general impression
- Stabilizing the cervical spine as needed
- Assessing a baseline mental status
- Assessing the airway
- Assessing breathing
- Assessing circulation
- Determining priority

The initial assessment should take less than one minute, unless you have to intervene with life-saving measures. Perform the initial assessment as part of your ongoing assessment throughout the patient contact, especially after any major intervention or whenever your patient's condition changes.

FORMING A GENERAL IMPRESSION

The **general impression** is your initial, intuitive evaluation of your patient. It will help you determine his general clinical status (stable vs. unstable) and priority for immediate transport. Base your first impression on the information you gather from the environment, the mechanism of injury, the nature of the illness, the chief complaint, and your instincts.

Your patient's age, gender, and race often influence your index of suspicion. Very old and very young patients are more apt to have severe complications from injury or illness. For example, age is a factor in burn mortality, along with degree and body percentage. A 25-year-old patient with third degree burns over 50% of his body will have a 75% chance of mortality. A 45-year-old patient with the same burns will have a 95% chance of mortality. Suspect a female of child-bearing age with lower abdominal pain and vaginal bleeding to have a life-threatening gynecological emergency known as ruptured ectopic pregnancy. Black Americans have a higher incidence of hypertension and cardiovascular disease than members of other races.

Determine whether your patient's problem results from trauma or from a medical problem. Sometimes this will not be readily apparent. For example, did your patient slip and fall or get dizzy and fall? Note your patient's face and his posture and decide whether rapid intervention or a more deliberate approach is warranted. With experience you will be able to recognize even the most subtle clues of a patient in critical condition. Generally, the more serious the condition, the quieter your patient will be. Look at, listen to, and smell the environment. Gather as many clues as possible as you enter the scene.

Take the necessary body substance isolation precautions with every patient. Then, if your patient is alert, identify yourself and begin to establish a rapport. For example, "Hello, I'm Jen Stevens, a paramedic with ALS Ambulance Service. I'm here to help you." This establishes your level of training, authority, and reason for being at your patient's side. It also allows your patient to refuse care. As discussed in Chapter 2 on medical/legal aspects of advanced prehospital care, you cannot provide care without either implied or informed consent.

Reassure your patient. Listen to him and do not trivialize his complaints. Frequently we forget how significant an injury or illness, even a minor one, seems to a patient. With your experience, his problem may seem small, but for your patient it is a real concern. The ill or injured patient may worry about the long-term consequences for work, child care, and finances. Understand these fears and support your patient psychologically as well as physiologically.

Listen to your patient and do not trivialize his complaints.

If the mechanism of injury is significant or if your patient is unresponsive, have your partner manually stabilize your patient's head and neck (Figure 12-19a). Do this before establishing his mental status and continue manual stabilization until you fully immobilize him to a long spine board. If your patient is awake, explain what you are doing and ask him not to move his neck. You do not want him to turn his head when you try to assess mental status. Ask your partner to maintain

FIGURE 12-19a Manually stabilize the head and neck on first patient contact.

FIGURE 12-19b Place a folded towel under your young patient's shoulders to keep the airway aligned.

your patient's head in a neutral position as you begin your assessment. If your patient is a small child, place a small towel or pad beneath the shoulders to maintain proper alignment of the cervical spine (Figure 12-19b). This will compensate for the large occiput of the child's head, which normally would flex his neck when he was placed on a flat surface.

MENTAL STATUS

Your assessment of baseline mental status is crucial for all patients with serious head trauma.

Your assessment of baseline mental status is crucial for all patients. For example, when you deliver your head injury patient to the emergency department, the neurosurgeon will want a chronological report of your patient's mental status from the time you arrived on the scene. This vital information helps the surgical team diagnose a deteriorating brain injury. If the patient was alert and oriented when you arrived, then became sleepy en route, and within 30 minutes was responsive only to deep pain stimuli, the suspicion for epidural hematoma is high. Rapid surgical intervention can save lives in most cases if the diagnosis is made quickly. Your baseline mental status documentation is critical to these patients' emergency care. Establishing a baseline mental status is also crucial in assessing the variety of medical situations that cause altered levels of response. Drug overdoses, poisonings, diabetic emergencies, sepsis, hypoxia, and hypovolemia are just a few of the many conditions that result in altered mentation. For the stroke patient, identifying the time of the symptoms' onset is critical for the emergency physician to consider administering clot-dissolving drugs within the three-hour window of opportunity. This is possible only with your accurate assessment of your patient's change in mental status.

To record your patient's mental status, use the acronym *AVPU*. Your patient either is <u>A</u>lert, responds to <u>V</u>erbal stimuli, responds only to <u>P</u>ainful stimuli, or is <u>U</u>nresponsive. Perform this exam by starting with verbal, then moving to painful stimuli only if he fails to respond to your verbal cues.

Alert An alert patient is awake, as evidenced by open eyes. He may be oriented to person (who he is), place (where he is), and time (day, month, and year) and give organized, coherent answers to your quetions. He also may be disoriented and confused. For example, the patient with a suspected concussion will often present as dazed and confused. The hypoxic or hypoglycemic patient may present as combative. The shock patient may be restless and anxious. If his eyes are open and he appears awake, he is categorized as alert. Children's responses to your questions will vary with their age-related physical and emotional development. Infants and young children usually will be curious but cautious when a stranger approaches. Their level of response may not indicate the gravity of their condition. In fact, the quiet child is usually the seriously injured or ill child.

Verbal If your patient appears to be sleeping but responds when you talk to him, he is responsive to verbal stimuli. He can respond by speaking, opening his eyes, moaning, or just moving. Note the level of his verbal response. Does he speak clearly, mumble inappropriate words or make incomprehensible sounds? Children may respond to your verbal commands by turning their heads or stopping activity. For infants you may have to shout to elicit a response.

Pain If your child or adult patient does not respond to verbal stimuli, try to elicit a response with painful stimuli. Pinch his fingernails or rub your knuckles on his sternum and watch for a response. Again, he may respond by waking up, speaking, moaning, opening his eyes, or moving. Note the type of his motor response to the painful stimuli. Is his response purposeful or nonpurposeful? If he tries to move your hand away or to move himself away from the pain, it is purposeful. **Decorticate** (arms flexed, legs extended) or **decerebrate** (arms and legs extended) posturing is nonpurposeful and suggests a serious brain injury. For the infant, flick the soles of the feet and expect crying as the appropriate response.

* **decorticate** arms flexed, legs extended.

* **decerebrate** arms and legs extended.

Unresponsive The unresponsive patient is comatose and fails to respond to any noxious stimulus. The AVPU scale describes your patient's general mental status. Avoid using terms such as *semi-conscious, lethargic,* or *stuporous* since they are broadly interpreted and you have not had a chance to conduct a comprehensive neurological exam at this point. Your patient's response to stimulation will tell you a great deal about his condition. Any alteration or deterioration in mental status may indicate an emergent or already serious problem. A patient with an impaired mental status may have lost, or be in danger of losing, the ability to protect his airway. Take immediate steps to protect your patient's airway by proper positioning, use of airway adjuncts, or intubation, as appropriate. Provide oxygen to any patient with diminished mental status and seek out its cause.

Any alteration in mental status may indicate an emergent or already serious problem.

AIRWAY ASSESSMENT

If your patient is responsive and can speak clearly, you can assume that his airway is patent. If your patient is unconscious, however, his airway may be obstructed. The supine unconscious patient's tongue often obstructs his upper airway. Because the mandible, tongue, and epiglottis are all connected, gravity allows these structures to block your patient's upper airway as his facial muscles relax.

You can open your patient's airway with one of two simple manual maneuvers, the jaw thrust and the head-tilt/chin-lift. For the trauma patient with a suspected cervical spine injury, use the jaw thrust, to avoid movement of the cervical spine. Place your thumbs on your patient's cheeks and lift up on the angle of the jaw with your fingers. For all other patients, use the head-tilt/chin-lift. Place one hand on your patient's forehead and lift up under the chin with the fingers of your other hand. To open the airways of infants and young children, apply a gentle and conservative extension of the head and neck. These patients' upper airway structures are very flexible and are easily kinked when their necks are flexed or hyperextended. You must constantly readjust their airways to maximize patency.

To assess your patient's airway, look for chest rise while you listen and feel for air movement. If the airway is clear, you should hear quiet air flow and feel free air movement. A noisy airway is a partially obstructed airway. Snoring occurs when the tongue partially blocks the upper airway. In this case, reposition the head and neck and reevaluate. Gurgling indicates that fluid such as blood, secretions, or gastric contents is blocking the upper airway. Gently open and examine the mouth for foreign bodies you can remove easily and quickly. Use aggressive suctioning to remove blood, vomitus, secretions, and other fluids (Figure 12-20).

You must constantly adjust infants' and young children's airways to maximize patency.

The high-pitched inspiratory screech of stridor is caused by a life-threatening upper airway obstruction that may be due to a foreign body, severe swelling, allergic reaction, or infection. If you suspect a foreign body obstruction and your patient exhibits poor air movement, a weak cough, or a diminishing mental status, immediately deliver abdominal thrusts (Heimlich maneuver) to dislodge the object. If your patient is less than one year old, use back blows and chest thrusts instead of abdominal thrusts. If these maneuvers are ineffective, remove the object under direct laryngoscopy with Magill forceps.

Stridor signals a potentially life-threatening airway obstruction.

Other causes of stridor require vastly differently approaches. Upper respiratory infections such as croup or epiglottitis call for blow-by oxygen and a quiet ride to the hospital; respiratory burns demand rapid endotracheal intubation; and anaphylaxis necessitates vasoconstrictor medications. Since these vastly different management techniques are potentially life-threatening when applied inappropriately, your correct field diagnosis is critical. If your patient presents with stridor, take time to evaluate the history and clinical signs and symptoms for foreign body obstruction (sudden onset while eating), epiglottitis (fever, illness, drooling, inability to swallow), respiratory burns (history of facial burns, hoarseness), and anaphylaxis (hives, history of allergies).

FIGURE 12-20 Suction fluids from your patient's airway.

The softer, expiratory whistle of wheezing is caused by constricted bronchioles, the smaller, lower airways. You will hear it in cases such as asthma, bronchitis, emphysema, or other causes of bronchospasm. Bronchiolitis, a lower respiratory infection, often causes these sounds in infants and young children. Wheezing patients require a bronchodilator medication to dilate the bronchioles and reduce airway resistance.

If your patient is not moving air, he is in respiratory arrest. Immediately provide ventilation with a bag-valve mask. Ventilate adult patients at a minimum of 12 breaths per minute and all children at a minimum of 20 breaths per minute. If you cannot ventilate the lungs, reposition the head and neck and try again. If there is still no air movement, assume a complete obstruction and begin measures to correct it.

Once you have cleared the airway, keeping it open may require constant attention. In these cases, insert a basic airway adjunct to help keep the tongue from blocking the upper airway. If your patient is unconscious and lacks a gag reflex, insert an oropharyngeal airway. If he has a gag reflex or significant oro-facial trauma, insert a nasopharyngeal airway. Be cautious using a nasopharyngeal airway if you suspect a basilar skull fracture. If he has no gag reflex and cannot protect his airway, you will need to use advanced techniques to maintain airway patency. These include endotracheal intubation, multi-lumen airways such as the Pharyngotracheal Lumen (PL) airway and the Esophageal Tracheal CombiTube (ETC), and transtracheal techniques such as needle or surgical cricothyroidotomy. The multi-lumen airways are not appropriate for use in children. All of these devices for maintaining upper airway patency are described in detail in Chapter 8 on airway management and ventilation. If your patient has an airway problem or an altered mental status, administer high concentration oxygen by nonrebreather mask.

BREATHING ASSESSMENT

Assess your patient for adequate breathing. Immediately note any signs of inadequate breathing. These include:

- Altered mental status, confusion, apprehension, or agitation
- Shortness of breath while speaking

Once you have cleared the airway, keeping it open may require constant attention.

Content Review

SIGNS OF INADEQUATE BREATHING

Altered mental status
Shortness of breath
Retractions
Asymmetric chest wall movement
Accessory muscle use
Cyanosis
Audible sounds
Abnormal rate or pattern
Nasal flaring

Table 12-1	**RESPIRATORY RATES**	
Age	**Low Rate**	**High Rate**
Newborn	30	60
Infant (<1 year)	30	60
Toddler (1–2 years)	24	40
Preschooler (3–5 years)	22	34
School age (6–12 years)	18	30
Adolescent (13–18 years)	12	26
Adult (>18 years)	12	20

- Retractions (supraclavicular, suprasternal, intercostal)
- Asymmetric chest wall movement
- Accessory muscle use (neck, abdominal)
- Cyanosis
- Audible sounds
- Abnormally rapid, slow, or shallow breathing
- Nasal flaring

Assess the respiratory rate and quality. Normal respiratory rates vary according to your patient's age. Abnormally fast or slow rates (Table 12-1) actually decrease the amount of air that reaches the alveoli for gas exchange. For patients with abnormally fast or slow respiratory rates and decreased tidal volumes, provide positive pressure ventilation with, for example, a bag-valve mask and supplemental oxygen, to ensure full lung expansion and maximum oxygenation. Note the respiratory pattern. Rapid (tachypneic), deep (hyperpneic) respirations are a compensatory mechanism and suggest the body is attempting to rid itself of excess acids. They may indicate a diabetic problem, severe acidosis, or head injury. They also may result from hyperventilation syndrome or from simple exertion. Kussmaul's respirations (deep, rapid breathing) accompanied by a fruity breath odor are a classic sign of a patient in a diabetic coma. In either case, always ensure an adequate inspiratory volume and administer high-flow oxygen. Cheyne-Stokes respirations, a series of increasing and decreasing breaths followed by a period of apnea, most likely result from a brain stem injury or increasing intracranial pressure. Biot's respirations, identified by short, gasping, irregular breaths, may signify severe brain injury. Again, ensure adequate inspiratory volume and provide ventilation with supplemental oxygen as needed.

If your trauma patient's breathing is inadequate, immediately conduct a rapid trauma assessment of the neck and chest before moving on to circulation. Identify and correct any life-threatening conditions such as a sucking chest wound, a flail chest, or a tension pneumothorax. If your patient exhibits adequate breathing, move directly to circulation.

CIRCULATION ASSESSMENT

The **circulation assessment** consists of evaluating the pulse and skin and controlling hemorrhage. Go directly to the wrist and feel for a radial pulse (Procedure 12-1a). Its presence suggests a systolic blood pressure of at least 80 mmHg. If the radial pulse is absent, check for a carotid pulse (Procedure 12-1b). The carotid pulse's presence suggests a systolic blood pressure of at least 60 mmHg. In the infant, palpate the brachial pulse (Procedure 12-1c) or, if necessary, auscultate the apical pulse.

If your patient's breathing is inadequate, immediately conduct a rapid trauma assessment of the neck and chest and provide positive pressure ventilation with supplemental oxygen.

circulation assessment evaluating the pulse and skin and controlling hemorrhage.

12-1a   To assess an adult's circulation feel for a radial pulse.

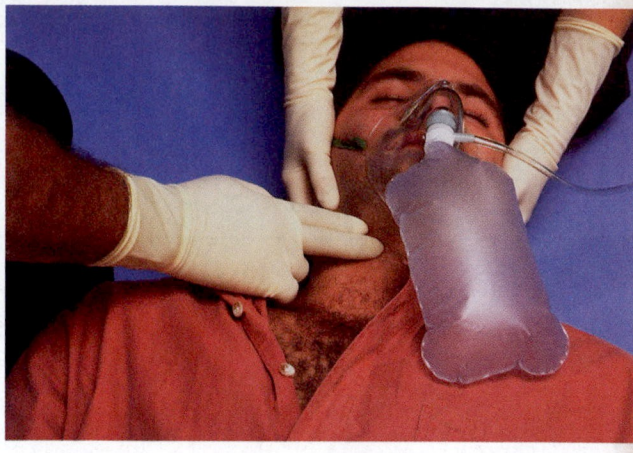

12-1b   If you cannot feel a radial pulse, palpate for a carotid pulse.

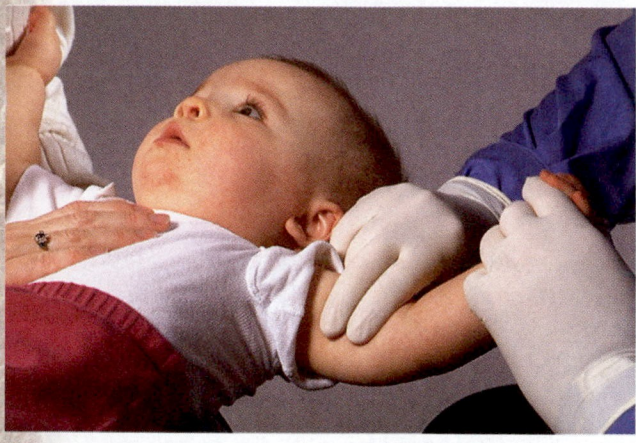

12-1c   To assess an infant's circulation, palpate the brachial pulse.

12-1d   Control major bleeding.

12-1e   Assess the skin.

12-1f   Capillary refill time provides important information about the circulatory status of infants and young children.

12-1g   Elevate your patient's feet if you suspect circulatory compromise.

12-1h   Apply a pneumatic antishock garment according to your local protocol.

12-1i   En route to the hospital, establish an IV.

Table 12-2	NORMAL PULSE RATE RANGES		
Age		**Low Rate**	**High Rate**
Newborn		100	180
Infant (<1 year)		100	160
Toddler (1–2 years)		80	110
Preschooler (3–5 years)		70	110
School age (6–12 years)		65	110
Adolescent (13–18 years)		60	90
Adult (>18 years)		60	100

If the pulse is absent in the adult patient, begin chest compressions immediately, evaluate the cardiac rhythm, and provide prompt defibrillation as needed. In the child, immediately begin cardiopulmonary resuscitation (CPR).

Assess your patient's pulse for rate and quality as detailed in Chapter 11. The normal heart rate varies with your patient's age (Table 12-2). Very fast rates (tachycardia) and very slow rates (bradycardia) may indicate a life-threatening cardiac dysrhythmia. Note the quality of the pulse. The normal pulse should be regular and strong. An irregular pulse may indicate a cardiac dysrhythmia requiring advanced cardiac life support procedures. In head injury, heat stroke, or hypertension, you will often find a strong, bounding pulse. A weak, thready pulse usually indicates poor perfusion due to fluid loss, pump failure, or massive vasodilation.

Stop your patient's bleeding if you haven't already done so (Procedure 12-1d). Major bleeding usually originates with trauma, but it also can result from a medical emergency. For example, vaginal bleeding, rectal bleeding, and even a nosebleed associated with hypertension can result in life-threatening blood loss. For external bleeding, employ any appropriate measures for hemorrhage control, including direct pressure and elevation, pressure dressings, pressure points, and the last-resort tourniquet. Internal bleeding is not easily controlled in the prehospital setting and demands initiating transport as soon as possible.

Assess the skin for temperature, moisture, and color (Procedure 12-1e). Peripheral vasoconstriction decreases peripheral perfusion to the skin early in shock. The skin may appear mottled (blotchy), cyanotic (bluish), pale, or ashen. It may also feel cool and moist (clammy). This often indicates that warm, circulating blood has been shunted away from the skin to the core of the body to maintain perfusion of vital organs. If you find any of these signs, suspect conditions related to or caused by poor perfusion. In infants and young children capillary refill is a reliable indicator of circulatory function (Procedure 12-1f). In adults, smoking, medications, cold weather, or chronic conditions of the elderly may affect capillary refill, so you should always also consider the other indicators of circulatory function.

If your patient shows signs of circulatory compromise, consider elevating his legs to support venous return to the vital organs (Procedure 12-1g). Keep him warm, and on adult patients only, apply and inflate the pneumatic antishock garment as indicated by your local protocol (Procedure 12-1h). Chapter 19 on hemorrhage and shock explains this procedure fully. Consider starting large-bore intravenous lines en route to the hospital and infusing fluids to augment your patient's circulating blood volume (Procedure 12-1i). Also consider using vasoconstricting drugs and antidysrhythmic medications for other specific causes of poor perfusion.

PRIORITY DETERMINATION

Once you have conducted an initial assessment, determine your patient's priority. If his initial assessment suggests a serious illness or injury, conduct a rapid head-to-toe

Internal bleeding is not easily controlled in the prehospital setting and demands initiating transport as soon as possible.

Do not delay transport for detailed assessments and procedures that you can provide en route to the hospital.

FIGURE 12-21   Expedite transport for a high priority patient and continue assessment and care en route.

assessment to identify other life threats and transport him immediately to the nearest appropriate facility that can deliver definitive care (Figure 12-21). Do not delay transport for detailed assessments and procedures that you can provide en route to the hospital. Consider top priority and rapid transport for the following patients:

- Patients with a poor general impression
  - Apnea
  - Pulselessness
  - Obvious severe distress
- Patients with altered mental status
- Patients with airway compromise
  - Obstructive sounds such as gurgling, snoring, or stridor
  - Vomitus, secretions, blood, or foreign bodies obstructing the airway
  - Inability to protect the airway (absence of a gag reflex)
- Patients with abnormal breathing
  - Rates less or greater than normal for age
  - Absent or diminished air movement and breath sounds
  - Retractions
  - Accessory muscle use
- Patients with poor circulation
  - Weak or absent peripheral pulses
  - Pulse rates less or greater than normal for age
  - Irregular pulse
  - Pale, cool, diaphoretic skin
  - Uncontrolled bleeding
- Obvious serious or multiple injuries

In these cases, decide whether to stabilize your patient on the scene or expedite transport and initiate advanced life support procedures en route. On the way to

Content Review

TOP PRIORITY PATIENTS
Poor general impression
Unresponsive
Responsive but cannot
  follow commands
Difficult breathing
Signs and symptoms of
  hypoperfusion
Complicated childbirth
Chest pain and blood
  pressure below 100 systolic
Uncontrolled bleeding
Severe pain
Multiple injuries

Content Review

TYPES OF PATIENTS
Trauma patient with
  significant mechanism
  of injury
Trauma patient with
  isolated injury
Responsive medical patient
Unresponsive medical patient

the hospital you can conduct a detailed history and physical exam and provide additional care as time allows. If your patient is stable, before transport you can conduct a focused history and physical exam—a problem-oriented patient assessment—followed by a detailed physical exam either at the scene or during transport as the situation requires, if time allows.

The initial assessment is the crucial first-step in providing life-saving measures to seriously ill or injured patients. It should take you less than one minute to perform, yet it will provide you with enough vital information to confirm your priority determination.

✳ **focused history and physical exam** problem-oriented assessment process based on initial assessment and chief complaint.

✳ **major trauma patient** person who has suffered significant mechanism of injury.

Content Review

ORDER OF FOCUSED HISTORY AND PHYSICAL EXAM FOR MAJOR TRAUMA PATIENTS
Initial assessment
Rapid trauma assessment
Packaging
Rapid transport and
  ongoing assessment

Content Review

PREDICTORS OF SERIOUS INTERNAL INJURY
Ejection from vehicle
Death in same passenger
  compartment
Fall from higher than 20 feet
Rollover of vehicle
High-speed vehicle collision
Vehicle-pedestrian collision
Motorcycle crash
Penetration of head, chest,
  or abdomen

Your assessment of trauma patients must look beyond obvious injuries to the mechanism of injury.

THE FOCUSED HISTORY AND PHYSICAL EXAM

The **focused history and physical exam** is the second stage of patient assessment. It is a problem-oriented process based on your initial assessment and your patient's chief complaint. How you conduct the focused history and physical exam will depend on which of four general categories your patient's initial presentation falls under:

- Trauma patient with a significant mechanism of injury or altered mental status
- Trauma patient with an isolated injury
- Responsive medical patient
- Unresponsive medical patient

Each type of patient requires a vastly different approach.

THE MAJOR TRAUMA PATIENT

The **major trauma patient** is one who has sustained a significant mechanism of injury or has an altered mental status from the incident. For serious trauma patients, you will conduct an initial assessment followed by a rapid trauma assessment, package your patient, provide rapid transport to the emergency department, and perform an ongoing assessment en route, in that order. If time allows, you can also perform a detailed assessment.

Mechanism of Injury

Begin the focused history and physical exam for major trauma patients by reconsidering the mechanism of injury (Figure 12-22). Although trauma poses a serious threat to life, its appearance often masks your patient's true condition. Extremity injuries, for example, are frequently obvious and grotesque, yet they rarely cause death. Conversely, life-threatening problems such as internal bleeding and rising intracranial pressure often occur with only subtle signs and symptoms. Your assessment of trauma patients must look beyond obvious injuries to the mechanism of injury for evidence that suggests life-threatening situations. Certain mechanisms predictably cause serious internal injury:

- Ejection from a vehicle
- Fall from higher than 20 feet
- Rollover of vehicle

- High-speed vehicle collision with resulting severe vehicle deformity
- Vehicle-pedestrian collision
- Motorcycle crash
- Penetration of the head, chest, or abdomen

Additional considerations for infants and children include:

- Fall from higher than ten feet
- Bicycle collision
- Medium-speed vehicle collision with resulting severe vehicle deformity

These mechanisms' presence suggests a high index of suspicion for serious injury. Quickly transport patients to a trauma center when either the mechanism of injury or your patient's clinical presentation indicates a likelihood of internal injury.

Other significant mechanisms of injury can result from seat belts, airbags, and child safety seats. Do not rule out serious injury just because your patient wore a seat belt. Seat belts can actually cause injuries, even when worn properly. Always ask your patient if he wore a seat belt and look for bruises across the chest or around the waist. If present, expect hidden internal injuries.

In general, airbags have been effective devices in preventing serious injury by protecting passengers from hitting the windshield, steering wheel, and dashboard. They deploy only when the front of the car hits another object. But they are not without complication. For example, they are designed to cushion the chests of large adults. If the passenger is a child or a short adult, the airbag will hit him in the face, causing injury. Also, airbags are designed to deflate automatically within seconds after inflation, which may allow passengers to be propelled into the steering wheel or dashboard. For this reason, they may not be effective without the seat belt. Always lift the deployed bag and inspect the steering wheel for deformity. If you discover a bent steering wheel, suspect serious internal injury (Figure 12-23).

A child safety seat, when used appropriately, also can save a life. But if the safety seat is not securely fastened to the car seat, it can come loose and be thrown when the collision occurs, causing severe head, neck, and body cavity

> ### Content Review
>
> **ADDITIONAL PREDICTORS OF SERIOUS INTERNAL INJURY FOR INFANTS AND CHILDREN**
>
> Fall from higher than ten feet
> Bicycle collision
> Medium-speed vehicle collision

Quickly transport patients with a high likelihood of internal injury to an appropriate medical facility.

Do not rule out serious injury just because your patient wore a seat belt.

Always lift a deployed airbag and inspect the steering wheel for deformity.

FIGURE 12-23 A bent steering wheel signals potentially serious injuries. (*Courtesy of Edward T. Dickinson, MD*)

trauma to its occupant. If the safety seat is used in the car's front seat, the child can suffer a serious injury when the airbag deploys.

If your initial assessment rules out any immediate life threat, examine the suspected area of trauma. Physical signs of trauma such as abrasions or contusions confirm your index of suspicion. If you do not identify any physical evidence, reexamine the mechanism of injury and evaluate your patient's vital signs. You will miss many serious injuries if your index of suspicion is too low.

Usually you will distinguish between those patients who need on-the-scene stabilization and those who need rapid transport after your initial assessment and rapid trauma assessment. Whether to transport your patient immediately or to attempt more extensive on-the-scene assessment and care is among your most difficult decisions, but the care you provide will be more effective if you decide quickly. As a rule, patients who experience the mechanisms of injury listed earlier or who display serious clinical findings should be transported quickly with intravenous access and other procedures attempted en route. Remember, you often arrive at the patient's side only minutes after the accident. He may not yet have lost enough blood internally to demonstrate signs of shock or progressive head injury. If in doubt, transport to an appropriate medical facility without delay. It is always best to err on the side of precaution.

Rapid Trauma Assessment

After you finish your initial assessment, conduct a rapid trauma assessment to identify all other life-threatening conditions. Every trauma patient with a significant mechanism of injury, altered mental status, or multiple body-system trauma should receive a rapid trauma assessment. If your patient is responsive, ask him about symptoms as you proceed with your exam. Do not, however, focus totally on the areas your patient identifies as his chief problem. A patient with multiple injuries usually complains about his most painful injury. Sometimes, this may not be his most serious problem. Assess your patient systematically and avoid the tunnel-vision invited by dispatch information, first responders' reports, and your patient's chief complaint.

Assume that any trauma patient has a spinal injury if he has injuries above the shoulders, has a significant mechanism of injury, or complains of weakness, numbness, or spinal pain. Maintain spinal immobilization throughout your rapid trauma exam.

As you proceed through the exam and discover additional information about your patient, reconsider your decision to transport. Things can change unexpectedly, especially with children. For example, your child patient who appeared stable

It is always best to err on the side of precaution.

Avoid the tunnel vision invited by dispatch information, first responder's reports, and your patient's chief complaint.

suddenly deteriorates, requiring you to expedite transport to the closest appropriate facility. The hallmark of an experienced paramedic is the ability to improvise, adapt to new situations, and overcome obstacles that hinder good patient care.

The **rapid trauma assessment** is not a detailed physical exam but a fast, systematic assessment for other life-threatening injuries. Since you perform it before packaging your patient for transport, you must conduct it quickly. First, reassess your patient's mental status using the AVPU mnemonic and compare your findings with the baseline mental status from your initial assessment. Pay special attention to the head, neck, chest, abdomen, and pelvis. Injuries in these areas can occur with limited signs and symptoms, yet they may rapidly lead to patient deterioration and death. When inspecting an area for injury, keep in mind that the discoloration of contusions will develop over time and may not be apparent at first. Remember, your major concern may not be the injury you see but the internal injuries beneath the superficial wounds. Palpate to identify other signs such as tenderness, deformity, crepitation, symmetry, subcutaneous emphysema, or paradoxical movement. Compare muscle tone and tissue compliance from one side of the body or from one limb to another.

The mnemonic DCAP-BTLS may be helpful. The letters represent eight common signs of injury for which you are looking during most of this assessment: <u>D</u>eformities, <u>C</u>ontusions, <u>A</u>brasions, <u>P</u>enetrations, <u>B</u>urns, <u>T</u>enderness, <u>L</u>acerations, and <u>S</u>welling.

Head Assess the head for DCAP-BTLS and crepitation (Procedure 12-2a). The scalp is extremely vascular and lacks the protective vasospasm mechanism that helps control bleeding. Thus even the most minor lacerations tend to bleed profusely. Inspect the scalp for lacerations that are hidden under hair matted with clotted blood. Look for blood flowing into the hair, and examine your gloved fingers periodically for blood or other body fluids (Procedure 12-2b). If you detect uncontrolled bleeding from the scalp, apply a direct pressure dressing immediately. A simple scalp laceration can cause a life-threatening hemorrhage.

Palpate the skull for open wounds, depressions, protrusions, lack of symmetry, and any unusual warmth. Use cupped hands and do not probe with your fingers. If you feel a depression, stop palpating it, as this risks pushing a broken piece of bone into the brain. If you find an impaled object, stabilize it in place with bulky dressings. If your patient presents with an altered mental status and any abnormality in the structure of the skull, consider this a serious emergency and expedite transport while you continue your assessment and treatment.

Neck Inspect and palpate the neck for DCAP-BTLS and crepitation (Procedure 12-2c). Immediately cover any lacerations that may involve the major blood vessels such as the carotid arteries and jugular veins with an occlusive dressing. This is a high pressure area and your patient can suffer significant blood loss quickly. Because inspiration generates negative pressures in the chest, the jugular veins may draw in air. This can result in a massive air embolus that prevents the heart from pumping blood.

Examine the jugular veins for abnormal distention. In a patient lying supine without circulatory compromise, these veins should distend slightly. If they do not, your patient may be hypovolemic. In the **semi-Fowler's position** (sitting up at 45°), the veins should not distend. Distention beyond 45° is significant because something is inhibiting blood return to the chest. In the trauma patient, this may be the result of cardiac tamponade or tension pneumothorax.

Inspect and palpate the position of the trachea. It should lie midline and remain fixed during the breathing cycle. Tugging to one side during inspiration suggests a pneumothorax on that side. Displacement to one side may indicate a tension pneumothorax on the opposite side as the entire mediastinum is pushed away from the injury.

* **rapid trauma assessment** quick check for signs of serious injury.

Content Review

DCAP-BTLS
Deformities
Contusion
Abrasions
Penetration
Burns
Tenderness
Lacerations
Swelling

Immediately cover any neck lacerations that may involve the major blood vessels.

* **semi-Fowler's position** sitting up at 45°.

Finally, inspect and palpate the neck for **subcutaneous emphysema,** the crackling sensation caused by air just underneath the skin. This condition is the result of air leaking from the respiratory tree into the tissues of the neck. It strongly indicates a serious neck or chest injury.

Now palpate the posterior neck for evidence of spinal trauma (Procedure 12-2d). Gently feel the spinous processes and note any deformities, swelling, and tenderness. If you feel a muscle spasm, consider it a reflex sign following injury somewhere along the spinal column. When a corroborating mechanism of injury is present, suspect a significant spinal injury requiring immobilization. At this point you can apply a cervical spinal immobilization collar (CSIC). Have someone maintain head and neck stabilization even after applying the collar until your patient is fully fastened to the long board.

Chest Look for signs of acute respiratory distress. If your patient has an upper airway obstruction, he may need to create tremendous negative pressures within his chest just to draw in air. To do so he will use accessory muscles in his neck and chest to help lift the chest wall. These negative pressures may cause suprasternal, supraclavicular, and intercostal retractions. A patient with a lower airway obstruction may have difficulty moving air out. To do so, he may use his abdominal muscles to force the diaphragm upward and inward. He also may purse his lips during exhalation in an attempt to maintain a back pressure to keep the airways open. Infants and small children grunt to maintain this back pressure. Accessory muscle use always indicates a patient in respiratory distress due to a difficulty in moving air. Assist these patients with positive pressure ventilation and supplemental oxygen as needed.

Quickly inspect and then palpate the chest. Begin palpating at the clavicles and work down and around the rib cage, checking for stability. Palpate the clavicles over their entire length, bilaterally (Procedure 12-3a). These bones, which fracture more frequently than any other bone in the human body, are located directly over the subclavian artery and vein and the superior-most aspect of the lung. Their fracture and displacement may lacerate the vessels or puncture lung tissue, leading to hemothorax, pneumothorax, hypovolemia, or all three.

Be especially careful when palpating the ribs. Beneath each rib lie an artery, a vein, and a nerve that overaggressive palpation can easily damage. Classical soft-tissue injury signs may not be present because the ecchymotic coloration of bruising likely will not have had time to develop. Look for erythema caused by impact to the ribs. The first three ribs are well supported by muscles, ligaments, and tendons. Because of the energy required to fracture them, you should suspect major damage to the underlying organs, especially vascular structures, when they are broken.

If you notice the crackling of subcutaneous emphysema during chest palpation, suspect pneumothorax or a tracheo-bronchial tear. This condition results when air collects in the soft tissues. Subcutaneous air will normally flow from the upper chest to the neck and head. In some cases, it will drastically change your patient's facial features before your eyes.

Observe for equal, symmetrical, effortless chest rise. The chest should rise with inhalation and fall with exhalation. An abnormality in the chest wall may inhibit this process. For example, a patient with a rib fracture hesitates to expand his chest because it hurts. The fracture of two or more adjacent ribs in two or more places causes an unstable flail (floating) segment which may be evidenced by paradoxical chest wall movement. Paradoxical movement may not appear early in a flail segment because the muscles surrounding the fractured ribs may contract spasmodically, securing the ribs in place. As the muscles fatigue and relax, the flail segment becomes obvious in the paradoxical movement. A flail chest greatly reduces air movement. The underlying lung contusion and subsequent decreased tidal volume limit the air available for gas exchange. To ensure enough air movement for adequate gas exchange, assist ventilation with a bag-valve mask and supplemental oxygen. If the flail segment is loose, stabilize it to the chest wall with a large pad and tape (Procedure 12-3b).

Inspect your patient's chest front and back for open wounds. The lungs expand because they adhere to the inner chest wall. This adherence is made possible by the presence of two thin membranes, the visceral pleura, which covers the lungs, and the parietal pleura, which covers the inner chest wall. A film of liquid between these two layers creates a negative-pressure bond that forces the lungs to expand with the chest wall. Any opening in this system can disrupt adherence and cause the lung to collapse. Since air follows the path of least resistance, it may enter the chest cavity through the hole instead of through the respiratory tract. Thus, you should seal any open wounds with an occlusive dressing such as Vaseline gauze at the end of exhalation. Tape the dressing on three sides only to create a "one-way valve" effect, allowing air to escape but not be drawn in (Procedure 12-3c). Remember to check carefully under the armpits and back for knife and small-caliber gunshot wounds. You can easily miss these because the elastic skin closes quickly over the wound and limits external bleeding.

Auscultate both lungs quickly at each mid-axillary line for equal and adequate air movement. Unequal air movement may indicate the presence of a collapsed lung from a pneumothorax or hemothorax. Absent sounds on one side and diminished sounds on the other may suggest a life-threatening condition known as tension pneumothorax. This condition also presents with severe respiratory distress, accessory muscle use, retractions, tachycardia, hypotension, narrowing pulse pressure, and distended neck veins. Tracheal deviation may be a late sign of tension pneumothorax. If authorized, perform needle decompression immediately. Insert a large-bore IV catheter into the pleural space at the second intercostal space over the tip of the rib, midclavicular line, allowing the trapped air to escape and release the tension (Procedure 12-3d). Only through practice and repetition will you gain the confidence to recognize the difference between adequate and diminished lung sounds. Again, for patients with inadequate lung sounds, administer 100% oxygen and assist ventilation with a bag-valve mask as needed.

Abdomen Inspect and palpate the abdomen for DCAP-BTLS and crepitation. Note any areas of bruising and guarding. Exaggerated abdominal-wall motion to assist respiration may result from spinal injury, airway obstruction, or respiratory muscle failure. Solid organs such as the kidneys, liver, and spleen can bleed enough blood into the abdominal cavity to cause profound shock.

Two characteristic areas for bruising are over the umbilicus (**Cullen's sign**) and over the flanks (**Grey-Turner's sign**). Both signs indicate intra-abdominal hemorrhage but usually will not occur until hours after the injury. Perform deep palpation over each quadrant and note any tenderness, rigidity, and guarding. Be careful, because deep palpation sometimes can aggravate the problem. Avoid spending time needlessly trying to make a specific diagnosis. You need only to recognize the possibility that an intra-abdominal hemorrhage exists and that your patient requires immediate transport to an appropriate medical facility for surgery.

Hollow organs such as the stomach and intestines, when injured, spill their toxic contents into the abdomen, irritating the peritoneum, the inner-abdominal lining. Testing for rebound tenderness will help you determine if your patient's peritoneum is irritated. Gently palpate an area and let your hand up quickly. If your patient experiences pain with this release, it is likely due to peritoneal irritation. If you suspect intra-abdominal hemorrhage, provide oxygen and expedite transport. En route to the hospital, provide IV fluid resuscitation as needed.

✱ **Cullen's sign** bruising over the umbilicus.

✱ **Grey-Turner's sign** bruising over the flanks.

Avoid spending time needlessly trying to make a specific diagnosis during rapid trauma assessment of the abdomen.

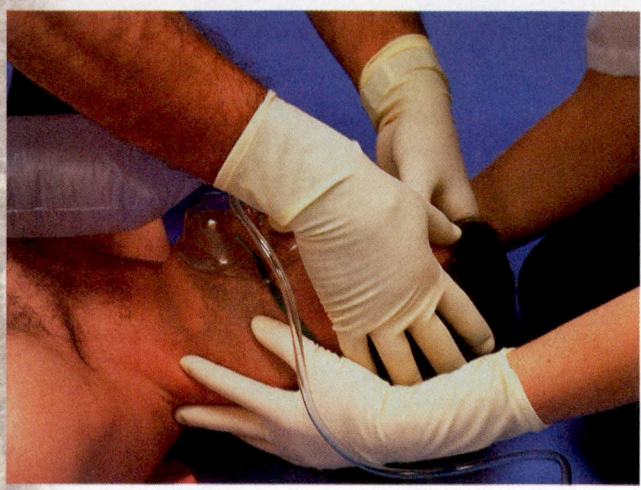

12-2a The first step in the rapid trauma assessment is to palpate the head.

12-2b Periodically examine your gloves for blood.

12-2c Inspect and palpate the anterior neck. Pay particular attention to tracheal deviation and subcutaneous emphysema.

12-2d Inspect and palpate the posterior neck. Note any tenderness, irregularity, or edema.

12-3a   Palpate the clavicles.

12-3b   Stabilize flail chest.

12-3c   Seal any sucking chest wound with tape on three sides.

12-3d   Perform needle decompression to relieve tension pneumothorax if authorized.

Pelvis Examine the pelvis for DCAP-BTLS and crepitation. The importance of a stable pelvic ring cannot be overemphasized. A patient with a pelvic fracture or dislocation risks lacerating the iliac arteries and veins, major blood vessels running through that area. He can easily lose a significant amount of blood into the pelvic cavity.

Evaluate the pelvic ring at the iliac crests and symphysis pubis. With the palms of your hands, direct pressure medially and posteriorly (Procedure 12-4a and 12-4b). Then press posteriorly on the symphysis pubis, being careful not to entrap the penis or cause injury to the urinary bladder. Any pain, instability, or crepitus suggests a pelvic fracture. Always immobilize the pelvis before transport to prevent movement and a possible circulatory catastrophe. The pneumatic antishock garment may be used as a splint to immobilize an unstable pelvic fracture.

Do not spend time splinting an unstable patient's fractures on the scene.

Extremities Inspect and palpate all four extremities for DCAP-BTLS and crepitation (Procedure 12-4c and 12-4d). Splint fractures en route to the hospital if your patient is unstable. Do not spend time splinting fractures on the scene.

Before placing your patient on a backboard and immobilizing his spine, evaluate distal neurovascular function by checking for pulses, sensation, and the ability to move (Procedure 12-4e and 12-4f). If you cannot locate a pulse, determine the adequacy of perfusion by assessing the temperature, color, and condition of the skin of the extremity. Assume vascular compromise if pulse is absent, the extremity is cool, or the skin is ashen or cyanotic. The inability to feel and move both legs indicates complete spinal cord disruption. Diminished sensation or diminished motor ability may indicate a partial disruption. Weakness or disability on only one side of the body suggests brain injury due to a stroke or head injury. Evaluate these functions again after spinal immobilization to make certain they have not changed. Report and record all extremity function tests. Check for Medic Alert tags, which will identify a medical condition that may complicate the injury (Figure 12-24).

FIGURE 12-24 Medic alert tags can give important information about the patient's condition and medical history.

12-4a Assess the integrity of the pelvis by gently pressing medially on the pelvic ring.

12-4b Compress pelvis posteriorly.

12-4c Palpate the legs.

12-4d Palpate the arms.

12-4e Palpate the dorsalis pedis pulse to evaluate distal circulation in the leg.

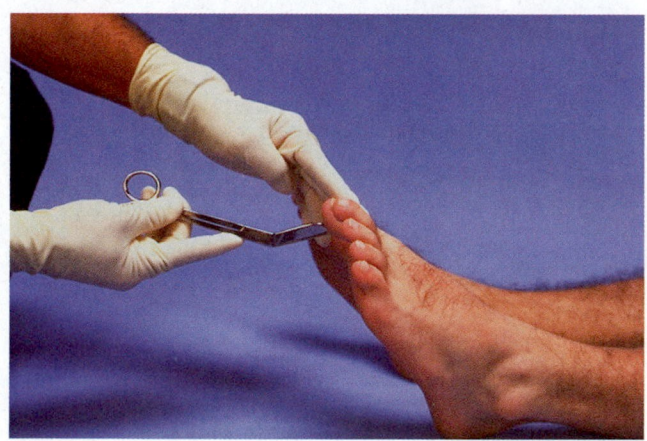

12-4f Assess distal sensation and motor function.

FIGURE 12-25   Inspect and palpate the posterior body.

Posterior Body If you suspect a spinal injury, carefully maintain manual stabilization of the head and spine as you log-roll the patient onto his side. Then inspect and palpate the posterior trunk for DCAP-BTLS and crepitation (Figure 12-25). Particularly note any tenderness in the spinal area. Palpate the buttocks to rule out hemorrhage, contusion, or other injury. Though predominantly soft tissue, this area is a large mass and can conceal considerable internal blood loss. Next place the long spine board snugly against your patient's body and maintain alignment of the head and spine as you log-roll him into a supine position on the spine board. He is now ready to be secured to the spine board and transported.

Vital Signs

Take a baseline set of vital signs, either at the scene or during transport, as your patient's condition and circumstances allow. These vital signs include pulse rate and quality, blood pressure, respiration rate and quality, and skin temperature and condition. During your EMT-B training, you may have learned to include pupils as part of your vital sign check. Including a basic pupil response check (direct response to light) as part of your baseline and serial vital sign assessment is acceptable; however, during the detailed physical exam you may perform an expanded assessment of the pupils (consensual response, near-far response, and accommodation) as outlined in Chapter 11.

History

The history consists of four elements: the chief complaint, the history of present illness, the past history, and the current health status. (Refer to Chapter 10 for a detailed description of taking a history.) For major trauma cases when time is critical, use an abbreviated format that forms the acronym SAMPLE: **S**ymptoms, **A**llergies, **M**edications, **P**ast medical history, **L**ast oral intake, and **E**vents preceding the incident. This handy mnemonic is especially useful for eliciting a quick history from your trauma patient. If your patient cannot provide this information, elicit it from family, friends, and bystanders.

Content Review

BASELINE VITAL SIGNS

Pulse rate and quality
Blood pressure
Respiration rate and quality
Skin condition

Content Review

SAMPLE HISTORY

Symptoms
Allergies
Medications
Past medical history
Last oral intake
Events preceding the incident

The Focused History and Physical Exam   **733**

THE ISOLATED-INJURY TRAUMA PATIENT

Focus your minor-trauma assessment on the specific injury and conduct a DCAP-BTLS exam in that area.

Some trauma patients sustain an isolated injury such as a cut finger or sprained ankle. These patients have no significant mechanism of injury and show no signs of systemic involvement such as poor peripheral perfusion, altered mental status, tachycardia, or breathing problems. They do not require an extensive history or comprehensive physical exam. To treat the trauma patient with an isolated injury, first ensure his hemodynamic status via the initial assessment. Then conduct your focused history and physical exam on the specific isolated injury. Use the mnemonic DCAP-BTLS to evaluate the injured area and take a full set of vital signs. Then, if time allows, this is an excellent opportunity to use some of the advanced assessment techniques you learned in Chapter 11. After your exam of the isolated injury, take a SAMPLE history. Remember that some trauma patients may complain of an isolated problem but actually have more significant injuries. Avoid tunnel vision and develop a low threshhold for suspecting other injuries based on the mechanism of injury and your patient's story.

IN THE FIELD

1. Your patient is a young football player who twisted his knee and lies on the ground, complaining loudly of knee pain. After a quick initial assessment and DCAP-BTLS assessment, you conclude that your patient is in stable condition with no signs or symptoms of systemic involvement and good distal neurovascular function. Before splinting your patient's leg, you decide to elicit more information through a detailed exam of the knee. You inspect the normal concavities for evidence of excessive fluid in the joint by "milking the knee joint" on one side and looking for a fluid wave on the opposite side. Next you palpate the medial and lateral collateral ligaments for tenderness. Then, if doing so does not cause your patient undue pain, you examine the stability of the collateral ligaments with the "side-to-side" test and the cruciate ligaments with the "drawer test." Finally, you assess the knee's passive range of motion (flexion and extension) and note any limitations.

2. Your patient sustains a laceration to the palm of his hand from a breadknife. After you have controlled the bleeding and ensured no systemic involvement or major loss of blood, you decide to examine the hand further before bandaging it. You conduct a DCAP-BTLS exam and note that distal neurovascular function is intact. Knowing that the flexor tendons all run through the palm of the hand, you examine each tendon's function through a full range of motion exam. You ask your patient to make a fist, then open his hand and extend all of his fingers. You note any abnormalities, pain, or limitations in the range of motion.

3. Your patient is a teenager who was punched in the eye during a minor altercation with a classmate. After determining that he had no loss of consciousness and that he is alert and oriented with stable vital signs, equal and reactive pupils, and no signs or symptoms of serious head injury, you may conduct a more detailed exam of the injured eye. First you inspect the external structures for discoloration, deformity, or swelling and find all three. You palpate the orbit of the eye for tenderness and deformity. You look for evidence of hyphema (blood in the anterior chamber), indicating severe blunt trauma. You then examine your patient's visual acuity with a visual acuity card. With a penlight, you check for direct and consensual response to light and for the near-far reflex and accommodation. Finally, you assess the integrity of the extraocular muscles with the H test.

FIGURE 12-26 Begin treatment while you assess your responsive medical patient.

THE RESPONSIVE MEDICAL PATIENT

Assessing the responsive patient with a medical emergency is entirely different from assessing the trauma patient for two reasons. First, the history takes precedence over the physical exam. This is because, in the majority of cases, you will formulate your field diagnosis from your patient's story. The physical exam serves mostly to support your diagnostic impression. Second, your physical exam is aimed at identifying signs of medical complications such as inflammation, infection, and edema rather than signs of injury. The focused physical exam evaluates pertinent areas suggested by the history. Remember that you will begin treatment as you conduct your assessment. For example, while interviewing your patient who complains of chest pain, simultaneously take vital signs, administer oxygen, provide cardiac monitoring, and start an IV if appropriate (Figure 12-26). The following focused history and physical exam pertains to the responsive medical patient. For a more detailed description of the information and techniques outlined here, refer to Chapters 10 and 11.

Listen to your patient; he will tell you what is wrong.

The History

Conscious, alert patients can usually tell you a great deal about their illness. Remember the old medical adage, "Listen to your patient; he will tell you what is wrong." Ask questions and then listen intently to your patient's answers. Since children may not be able to describe their illness and medical history clearly, look to their parents for this information. Elderly patients may pose several obstacles to the clear communication of medical information. They are more likely to be confused, to have poor short-term and long-term memory, and to have hearing, speech, or sight difficulties. Obtaining an accurate history from such patients requires patience, empathy, and outstanding communication skills.

The history consists of four elements: the chief complaint, the history of the present illness, the past history, and the current health status.

The Chief Complaint
The **chief complaint** is the pain, discomfort, or dysfunction that caused your patient to request help. Ask your patient, "What seems to be the problem?"

> **Content Review**
>
> **ELEMENTS OF THE HISTORY FOR RESPONSIVE MEDICAL PATIENTS**
> Chief complaint
> History of present illness
> Past history
> Current health status

* **chief complaint** the pain, discomfort, or dysfunction that caused your patient to request help.

Content Review

OPQRST—ASPN

Onset
Provocation/Palliation
Quality
Region, radiation
Severity
Time
Associated symptoms
Pertinent negatives

Content Review

ELEMENTS OF THE PAST MEDICAL HISTORY

General state of health
Childhood and adult
  diseases
Psychiatric illnesses
Accidents and injuries
Surgeries and
  hospitalizations

Content Review

ELEMENTS OF THE CURRENT HEALTH STATUS

Current medications
Allergies
Tobacco use
Alcohol and substance abuse
Diet
Screening exams
Immunizations
Sleep patterns
Exercise and leisure activities
Environmental hazards
Use of safety measures
Family history
Social history

Let the diagnostic impression you formed during the history guide your examination of a responsive medical patient.

The History of Present Illness Discover the circumstances surrounding the chief complaint, following the acronym OPQRST—ASPN:

Onset	What was your patient doing when the problem/pain began? Did emotional or environmental factors contribute to the problem?
Provocation/**P**alliation	What makes the problem/pain worse or better?
Quality	Can your patient describe the problem/pain?
Region/**R**adiation	Where is the problem/pain and does it radiate anywhere?
Severity	How bad is the problem/pain? Can your patient rate it on a scale of 10?
Time	When did the problem/pain begin? How long does the pain last?
Associated **S**ymptoms	Is your patient having any other problems?
Pertinent **N**egatives	Are any likely associated symptoms absent?

Past Medical History The past medical history may provide significant insights into your patient's chief complaint and your field diagnosis. It includes your patient's general state of health, childhood and adult diseases, psychiatric illnesses, accidents and injuries, surgeries and hospitalizations. If your history taking reveals significant medical problems, investigate in more detail. Note when your patient first recognized the problem and how it affected him. How frequently did it happen and what medical care did he seek? Was the treatment effective or did the problem recur?

Current Health Status The current health status assembles all of the factors regarding your patient's medical condition. It tries to gather information that will complete the puzzle surrounding your patient's primary problem. The elements of the current health status include current medications, allergies, tobacco use, alcohol and substance abuse, diet, screening exams, immunizations, sleep patterns, exercise and leisure activities, environmental hazards, the use of safety measures, and any pertinent family or social history. Look for clues and correlations among the various sections of this part of the history. If your patient is critical and your time is limited, use the abbreviated SAMPLE format to elicit the history.

Focused Physical Exam

Once you have obtained the history, begin a focused physical exam based on the information you elicited from your patient. Let the diagnostic impression you formed during the history guide your examination. For example, if you suspect a myocardial infarction, examine areas pertinent to a patient having a heart attack—cardiac and respiratory systems, chest, neck, and peripheral perfusion. It would be pointless and impractical to test deep tendon reflexes, extraocular movements, or the elbow's range of motion. Use those exam techniques presented in Chapter 11 that pertain to your patient's special situation and clinical status.

Three common presentations among your responsive medical patients will be cardiac chest pain/respiratory distress, altered mental status, and acute abdomen. The following sections outline problem-oriented physical exams for those complaints. Note that for each of these cases, the focused physical exam is different. As you gain clinical experience you will be able to quickly assess your patient's pertinent areas according to your suspected field diagnosis. Likewise, clinical judgment and the seriousness of your patient's condition will determine which exam techniques you use on the scene and which you use en route to the hospital.

Chest Pain/Respiratory Distress For a patient complaining of chest pain or respiratory distress, assess the following:

HEENT (head, eyes, ears, nose, and throat) Note the color of the lips. Lip cyanosis is an ominous sign of central circulatory hypoxia. For a patient complaining of chest pain or respiratory distress, assess the following: Examine the oral mucosa for pallor suggesting decreased circulation as in shock. Inspect any fluids in the mouth. Pink, frothy sputum (the result of plasma proteins' mixing with air and red blood cells in the alveoli) is a classic sign of acute pulmonary edema. Always keep the mouth clear of any fluids that may block the upper airway by aggressive suctioning. Note any swelling, redness, or hives, suggesting an allergic reaction.

Neck Observe the neck for accessory muscle use and retractions, signs of acute respiratory distress. Retractions in the supraclavicular (above the clavicles) and suprasternal (above the sternum) notches indicate your patient is having difficulty inhaling. Palpate the carotid arteries for rate, quality, and equality; if you detect weak or unequal pulses, auscultate for bruits. Examine the jugular veins for abnormal distention. In a patient lying supine without circulatory compromise, these veins should distend slightly. This is normal. If the jugular veins do not distend in the supine position, your patient may be hypovolemic. In the semi-Fowler's position (sitting up at 45°), the veins should disappear. Distention beyond 45° is significant because something is inhibiting blood return to the chest. This may be the result of cardiac tamponade, tension pneumothorax, or right heart failure. Inspect and palpate the position of the trachea. It should lie midline and remain fixed during the breathing cycle. Tugging to one side during inspiration suggests a pneumothorax on that side. Displacement to one side may indicate a tension pneumothorax on the opposite side as the entire mediastinum is displaced.

Chest Assess the respiratory rate and pattern again and administer oxygen or ventilation as needed. Note the length of the inspiratory and expiratory phases. A prolonged inspiratory phase suggests an upper airway obstruction. A prolonged expiratory phase suggests a lower airway obstruction such as in asthma and emphysema. Inspect and palpate the chest wall for symmetry of movement and intercostal retractions. A barrel chest suggests a history of emphysema. Look for the classic midline scar from open heart surgery or the typical bulge of an implanted pacemaker or defibrillator.

Auscultate all lung fields (anterior to posterior, apices to bases) and compare side-to-side. Report and record the sounds you hear (crackles, wheezes), where you hear them (in the bases, apices, diffuse), and when they occur during the respiratory cycle (inspiratory, expiratory). For example, if your patient has bilateral inspiratory rales, you might suspect congestive heart failure or pulmonary edema. If he has diffuse expiratory wheezing, you might suspect the bronchospasm associated with asthma or chronic obstructive pulmonary disease. The presence of both would suggest acute pulmonary edema. A localized wheeze might indicate a pulmonary embolism, a foreign body aspiration, or an infection. Patients with unilateral (one-sided) decreased breath sounds require further testing such as tactile fremitus, bronchophony, egophony, or whispered pectoriloquoy. Percuss the chest and back for hyperresonance (asthma, emphysema, pneumothorax) and dullness (pulmonary edema, pleural effusion, pneumonia).

Cardiovascular Inspect for signs of arterial insufficiency or occlusion in your patient's trunk and extremities. Look for skin pallor and other signs of decreased perfusion. Inspect and palpate the chest for the PMI. Assess central and peripheral pulses for equality, rate, regularity, and quality. Auscultate for heart sounds, identifying S1, S2, and any additional sounds.

> *Always keep the mouth clear of any fluids that may block the upper airway by aggressive suctioning.*
>
>

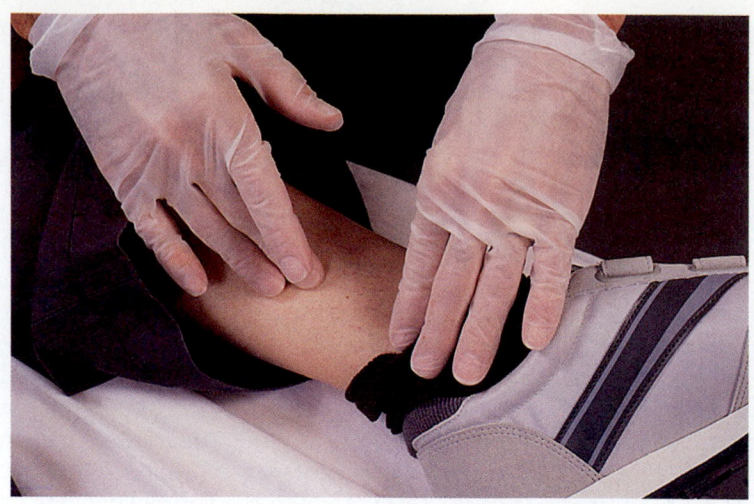

Figure 12-27   Check for peripheral edema.

Abdomen   Look for exaggerated abdominal muscle use during exhalation, a sign of lower airway obstruction as seen in asthma and emphysema. Inspect and palpate the abdomen for distention due to air or fluid. Ascites is an accumulation of fluid within the abdominal cavity caused by increased pressure in the systemic circulation as seen in patients with right heart failure. It is also common in patients with cirrhosis of the liver, where portal circulation (to and from the liver) is increased. This is often seen in patients with right heart failure or cirrhosis of the liver. Inspect and palpate the flanks and presacral area for edema in bedridden patients suspected of having congestive heart failure. Check for unusual pulsation of the descending aorta, just left of the umbilicus. Palpate for liver enlargement or upper quadrant tenderness suggesting ulcer disease, gall bladder disease, or pancreas problems, all of which can be confused as chest pain.

Extremities   Perform neurovascular checks on both hands and feet. These consist of checking for pulses, sensation, and the ability to move. Pay special attention to the equality of pulses in all extremities. Unequal pulses in the upper extremities suggest a thoracic aneurysm; unequal pulses in the lower extremities suggest an abdominal aneurysm. Assume vascular compromise if the pulse is absent, the limb is cool, or the skin is cyanotic or ashen. In cardiac and respiratory emergencies, evaluate the lower extremities for pitting edema. Depress the skin on the tibial plateau (Figure 12-27). If the depression remains after you remove your finger, pitting edema exists. This is a sign of chronic fluid retention as seen in heart and renal failure. Examine the fingernails for pitting. Check the wrists for Medic Alert identification.

Altered Mental Status   For a patient with an altered mental status, assess the following:

HEENT   Inspect and palpate the head to rule out any evidence of trauma. For example, your stroke patient may have suffered a skull fracture from falling on the floor. Palpate the fontanels of the infant for sunkenness (dehydration) and bulging (increasing intracranial pressure). Examine the face for symmetry. Unilateral facial drooping may indicate a stroke or inflammation of the facial nerve (Bell's Palsy). Examine the pupils for direct and consensual response to light. One pupil's getting larger or reacting more slowly to light could indicate a deteriorating brain pathology such as a stroke. A small portion of the population, however, has unequal pupils, a benign condition known as anisocoria. Bilaterally sluggish pupils usually suggest decreased blood flow to the brain and hypoxia. Fixed and dilated pupils indicate severe brain anoxia. Your patient's pupils also may dilate from sympathomimetic or anticholinergic drug use. Pinpoint pupils suggest a narcotic drug overdose or pontine hemmorhage (bleeding within the pons). Next, test for near response and accommodation. Test the integrity of the extraocular muscles with the "H" test. Normally your patient will move his eyes conjugately (together) to follow your finger. He may exhibit a nystagmus, a fine jerking of the eyes. At the far extremes of the test, nystagmus may be normal, but if you observe it during all extraocular movements it suggests a pathology. Examine the conjunctiva for redness (irritation), pallor (hypoperfusion), or cyanosis (hypoxia). Inspect the sclera for jaundice.

Chest   Inspect, palpate, and auscultate the chest for any signs of cardiorespiratory involvement.

Abdomen   Look for evidence of trauma or internal bleeding. Listen for bowel sounds that are absent in anticholinergic drug ingestions.

Pelvis   Look for evidence of incontinence.

Extremities   Perform neurovascular checks on both hands and feet. These consist of checking for pulses, sensation, and the ability to move. Assume vascular compromise if the pulse is absent, the limb is cool, or the skin is cyanotic or ashen. Since the motor and sensory nerves run along different pathways in the spinal cord, you must check your patient's extremities both for mobility and for sensation of light touch and pain. As with trauma patients, the inability to feel and move both legs indicates complete spinal cord disruption. Diminished sensation or diminished motor ability indicates a partial disruption. Weakness or disability on only one side suggests brain dysfunction such as a stroke. Report and record all extremity function tests.

Posterior Body   Inspect the posterior body for deformities of the spine. Also check for evidence of incontinence. In the supine patient, inspect the flanks for presacral edema.

Neuro   Reassess your patient's level of consciousness and compare his response to your earlier findings. Note his speech pattern and any deficits in speech or language. Observe mood swings or behaviors that suggest anxiety or depression. Determine your patient's person, time, and place orientation. Does he know his name, the day of the week, and where he is? Perform the one-minute cranial nerve exam outlined in Table 12-3. Inspect general body structure, muscle development, positioning, and coordination. Note any obvious asymmetries, deformities, or involuntary movements. Assess muscle tone by feeling the muscle's resistance to passive stretching in the extremities. Note the degree of resistance. Test for muscle strength by applying resistance during the range of motion evaluation. Check for pronator drift and watch for any drifting sideways or upward. Assess for coordination and cerebellar function, using rapid alternating movements and point-to-point testing. Note seizure activity tremors.

Table 12-3   ONE-MINUTE CRANIAL NERVE EXAM

Cranial Nerves	Test
I	Normally not done.
II, III	Direct response to light.
III, IV, VI	"H" test for extraocular movements.
V	Clench teeth; palpate massiter and temporal muscles. Test sensory to forehead, cheek, and chin.
VII	Show teeth.
IX, X	Say "aaaahhhh"; watch uvula movement. Test gag reflex.
XII	Stick out tongue.
VIII	Test balance (Romberg test) and hearing.
XI	Shrug shoulders, turn head.

Acute Abdomen For a patient complaining of abdominal pain, assess the following:

HEENT Notice any unusual odors coming from your patient's mouth. The smell of alcohol does not rule out a serious medical condition. The sweet smell of ketones suggests diabetes. A fecal odor may indicate a lower-bowel obstruction. The acidic smell of gastric contents means that your patient has vomited and may again. Inspect any fluids in the mouth. Coffee-ground emesis (vomiting) results from blood's mixing with stomach acids and suggests an upper GI bleed. Fresh blood usually means recent hemorrhage from the upper gastrointestinal tract.

Chest Listen to breath sounds. Crackles may indicate pneumonia, a cause of upper abdomen pain.

Abdomen Look for discoloration over the umbilicus (Cullen's sign) or over the flanks (Grey-Turner's sign) suggesting intra-abdominal bleeding. Check for any visible pulsation, peristalsis, or masses. If you notice a bounding or exaggerated pulsation, suspect an aortic aneurysm. Visible peristalsis may indicate a bowel obstruction. Auscultate for bowel sounds and renal bruits. Percussing the abdomen produces different sounds based on the underlying tissues. Percuss the abdomen in the same sequence you used for auscultation. Note the distribution of tympany and dullness. Expect tympany in most of the abdomen; expect dullness over the solid abdominal organs such as the liver and spleen.

Palpate the abdomen last to detect tenderness, muscular rigidity, and superficial organs and masses. The normal abdomen is soft and non-tender. Abdominal pain upon light palpation suggests peritoneal irritation or inflammation. If you feel rigidity or guarding while palpating, determine whether it is voluntary (patient anticipates the pain or is not relaxed) or involuntary (peritoneal inflammation). Then palpate the abdomen deeply to detect large masses or tenderness. If the peritoneum is inflamed, your patient will experience pain when you let go.

Posterior Body Inspect the posterior body for evidence of rectal bleeding.

Baseline Vital Signs

Prehospital medicine employs four basic vital signs: blood pressure, pulse, respiration, and temperature. As mentioned earlier, you may add a basic pupil assessment to this list. Your patient's vital signs are your windows to what is happening inside his body. They provide a unique, objective capsule assessment of his clinical status. Vital signs indicate severe illness and the urgency to intervene. Subtle alterations in these vital signs are often the only indication that your patient's condition is changing. They can warn you that your patient is deteriorating, or they can reassure you that he is responding to therapy.

Of the physical assessment techniques, taking accurate sets of vital signs reveals the most important information. As a paramedic you must assess these signs on every patient you evaluate. If your patient is with you for an extended time, measure and record his vital signs at intervals as his clinical condition dictates. Always reevaluate the vital signs after invasive procedures such as endotracheal intubation or fluid resuscitation and after any sudden change in your patient's condition. Accurate records of these numbers are invaluable when documenting your patient assessment.

If you suspect your patient of being hypovolemic, consider performing an orthostatic vital sign exam, commonly known as the tilt test. Take your patient's pulse and blood pressure while he is supine. Then have him sit up and dangle his feet. Finally, tell him to stand. Then in 30–60 seconds retake the vital signs. They should not change in the healthy patient. An increase in the pulse rate of 10–20 beats per minute or a drop in blood pressure of 10–20 mmHg, is a positive tilt test. This is a common finding in patients suspected of hypovolemia. Chapter 11 describes vital sign evaluation in detail.

Always reevaluate vital signs after invasive procedures and after any sudden change in your patient's condition.

Additional Assessment Techniques

Additional techniques include pulse oximetry, cardiac monitoring, and blood glucose determination. Refer to Chapter 11 for detailed descriptions of these techniques.

Pulse Oximetry The pulse oximeter is a noninvasive device that measures the oxygen saturation of your patient's blood. It is usually a good indicator of cardiorespiratory status because it tells you how well your patient is oxygenating the most distal ends of his circulatory system. It also quantifies the effectiveness of your interventions such as oxygen therapy, medications, suctioning, and ventilatory assistance. Normal oxygen saturation at sea level should be between 96% and 100%. Generally, if the reading is below 95%, suspect shock, hypoxia, or respiratory compromise. Provide your patient with the appropriate airway management, supplemental oxygen, and watch him carefully for further changes. Any reading below 90% requires aggressive airway management, positive pressure ventilation, or oxygen administration.

Cardiac Monitoring The cardiac monitor, which measures electrical activity, is essential in assessing and managing the patient who requires advanced cardiac life support (**ACLS**) measures. You should apply it to any patient you suspect of having a serious illness or injury. Its one major disadvantage, however, is that it cannot tell you if the heart is pumping efficiently, effectively, or at all. Always assess your patient and compare what you see on the monitor with what you feel for a pulse. If available, perform 12-lead ECG monitoring to identify the presence and location of a possible myocardial infarction.

Blood Glucose Determination In cases of altered mental status, such as diabetic emergencies, seizures, and strokes, measure your patient's blood sugar level. The arrival of inexpensive, hand-held glucometers makes this test simple and easy to perform in the field.

Emergency Medical Care

After conducting your physical exam, provide the necessary emergency medical care authorized by your medical director via standing orders. Then contact the on-line medical direction physician to request further orders. For example, you may administer 50 percent dextrose to an adult patient (25 percent dextrose to a pediatric patient) with documented hypoglycemia (Figure 12-28), intubate a patient in severe respiratory distress, or apply external cardiac pacing to a patient with third degree heart block. Always base your emergency care on your patient's signs and symptoms as obtained through a thorough focused history and physical exam. Finally, en route to the hospital conduct an ongoing assessment as described later in this chapter.

Apply the cardiac monitor to any patient you suspect of having a serious illness or injury.

Always base care of responsive medical patients on your patient's signs and symptoms as obtained through a thorough focused history and physical exam.

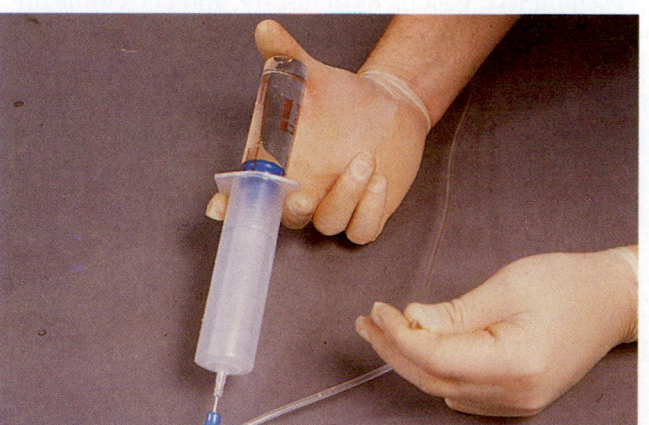

FIGURE 12-28 Administer 50 percent dextrose to a patient in insulin shock.

Again, if time allows, in certain situations you may wish to selectively use some of the advanced assessments described in Chapter 11. For example, en route to the hospital you might conduct a complete neurological exam for your patient who complains of stroke-like symptoms. This would comprise a full mental status assessment including orientation, appearance and behavior, speech and language, mood, thoughts and perceptions, insight and judgment, and memory and attention; a cranial nerve exam; a motor system assessment including muscle bulk, tone, and strength; a sensory exam including sharp and dull identification, temperature discrimination, position and vibration sense, and discriminative sensation; and deep tendon, as well as superficial, reflex tests. For your patient with upper respiratory distress and flu symptoms you may decide to examine the posterior pharynx and tonsils for redness and exudate; palpate the cervical lymph nodes for presence and tenderness; and thoroughly assess the lungs for tactile fremitus, egophony, bronchophony, and whispered pectoriloquoy. For your patient suspected of having acute appendicitis, you may wish to use the psoas test. Ask your patient to bring his right knee to his chest, contracting the iliopsoas muscle group. This motion usually causes pain as the muscles rub against the inflamed appendix. Your clinical experience and judgment will guide these types of decisions. The scope of paramedic practice is changing, not in procedures but in assessment capabilities. You will learn much more than your predecessors about anatomy and physiology, pathophysiology, and patient assessment. In time, you will learn which exam techniques yield the most relevant information and use them in your daily practice.

THE UNRESPONSIVE MEDICAL PATIENT

Since he cannot tell you what is wrong, the unresponsive medical patient requires an entirely different approach than the responsive patient. Assess the unresponsive medical patient much as you would a trauma patient. Begin with the initial assessment; then conduct a rapid head-to-toe exam known as the rapid medical assessment; and finally take a brief history from family or friends. This approach to the unresponsive medical patient also will help you to detect whether trauma may be involved.

After conducting the initial assessment, position your patient so that his airway is protected. If the cervical spine is not involved, place your patient in the recovery position—laterally recumbent. This will prevent secretions from obstructing his airway. Now begin the rapid medical assessment. The rapid medical assessment is similar to the rapid trauma assessment, except that you will look for signs of illness, not injury. Assess the head, neck, chest, abdomen, pelvis, extremities, and posterior aspect of the body. Perform the entire exam with the unresponsive patient. Then, assess baseline vital signs: pulse, blood pressure, respiration, and temperature. Finally, obtain a history from bystanders, family members, friends, or medical identification devices or services. If possible it should include the chief complaint, history of the present illness, past medical history, and current health status.

Evaluate your data and provide emergency medical care while performing additional tests such as cardiac monitoring, blood glucose determination, and pulse oximetry as needed. Consider your unresponsive patient unstable and expedite transport to the hospital, performing an ongoing assessment every five minutes en route.

Expedite transfer of unresponsive medical patients to the hospital and perform an ongoing assessment every five minutes en route.

IN THE FIELD

The rapid assessment is not a comprehensive history and physical exam, but a practical, systematic assessment aimed at quickly identifying the cause of your patient's unresponsive condition. Your care for a patient with a coma of unknown origin, for example, might go something like this:

You are dispatched to an "unresponsive person" in a residential neighborhood. Your patient is an elderly man who presents laterally recumbent on the floor of his bathroom. You conduct an initial assessment while your partner elicits information from the patient's wife:

General: Your patient appears pale and diaphoretic, moaning unintelligibly. You find no apparent signs of trauma, and he appears to have slumped to the floor from the toilet.

Mental Status: You establish your patient's mental status with the AVPU mnemonic. He responds to your voice but cannot answer your questions.

Airway: You open your patient's airway with a head-tilt/chin-lift maneuver and observe his breathing. His airway is clear. His breathing is rapid and shallow, but not labored. You ask another rescuer to administer positive pressure ventilation with supplemental oxygen while you continue with your assessment.

Circulation: You palpate his radial pulse, and note its absence. His carotid pulse is slow, irregular, and weak. His skin is pale, cool, and clammy, indicating poor peripheral perfusion.

You prioritize this patient high because of his altered mental status; his rapid, shallow breathing; and his poor peripheral perfusion. You suspect shock and begin a rapid medical assessment.

HEENT: You note lip cyanosis, a sign of central hypoxia. You see no lip pursing, nasal flaring, or other signs of increased breathing effort such as retractions or accessory muscle use. You smell no unusual odors or fluids from the mouth. The face is symmetrical; the pupils are equal and round, but react to light sluggishly. The trachea is midline, there is no JVD.

Chest: You note symmetrical chest wall movement and an equal and adequate rise and fall of the chest with each ventilation. You note some crackles in the lung bases. Your patient has no surgical scars.

ABD: You see no ascites or abdominal distention, no rigidity or guarding, no rebound tenderness, no renal or carotid bruits, no needle marks, no surgical scars or pulsating masses.

Pelvis: You see no evidence of bladder or bowel incontinence or of rectal bleeding.

Extremities: No finger clubbing, no medical identification, no needle marks. Peripheral circulation is poor with no radial or pedal pulses. You note no needle marks, but some pitting edema in lower extremities.

Posterior: You note some edema in your patient's flanks.

Vitals: Heart rate, 46 and regular; BP, 78/38; respirations, 36 and shallow.

Additional: ECG monitor shows third-degree AV block; pulse oximetry, 92% on room air, 99% with oxygen; blood glucose, 110.

Your patient's wife reveals his long history of heart disease and a long list of cardiac medications. Your field diagnosis is cardiogenic shock due to the bradycardic rate of the third-degree block. While your partner initiates an IV, you set up for immediate external cardiac pacing.

THE DETAILED PHYSICAL EXAM

The **detailed physical exam** uses many components of the comprehensive evaluation presented in the previous two chapters. It is a careful, thorough process of eliciting the history and conducting a physical exam. The detailed physical exam is a luxury, designed for use en route to the hospital, if time allows, for patients with significant trauma or serious medical illnesses. Ironically, with critical patients you usually will not have time to perform this in-depth exam because you will be preoccupied with performing ongoing assessments and providing emergency care. So you will seldom, if ever, perform a complete exam in the field. In fact, physicians in the emergency department rarely perform a detailed exam on their critical patients. It is too comprehensive and time-consuming and yields little relevant information.

In the emergency setting, individualize the exam to your patient's particular situation.

In the emergency setting, use a modified approach. You can individualize the exam to your patient's particular situation in many ways. For example, for the multi-trauma patient, perform a head-to-toe survey that is more detailed and slower than the rapid trauma assessment yet focuses on injury. For the 17-year-old football player who presents with shoulder pain, you may perform the entire portion of the shoulder exam. Palpating the abdomen and auscultating heart sounds would yield little useful information. For your stable patient who complains of abdominal pain, you may conduct an extensive history as detailed in Chapter 10, instead of the abbreviated SAMPLE history. Often you will elicit vital information from a seemingly obscure question during the review of systems. Again, clinical experience and your patient's condition will determine how you proceed with the detailed exam.

When you conduct the detailed exam you will use components of the comprehensive exam presented in Chapters 10 and 11. Refer to those chapters for a complete description of the components outlined in this section. Interview your patient to ascertain the history, then conduct a systematic head-to-toe physical exam. Place special emphasis on those areas suggested by your patient's chief complaint and present problem. Remember that the physical exam can be an anxiety-provoking experience for both the patient and the examiner. Using a professional, calm demeanor will minimize this anxiety. The following example illustrates how you might conduct a detailed physical exam for a multi-trauma patient en route to the hospital.

Aggressively suction patients with facial fractures to keep the upper airway clear.

Head Palpate the cranium from front to back for symmetry and smoothness (Procedure 12-5a). Note any tenderness, deformities, and areas of unusual warmth. Inspect and palpate the facial bones for stability and note any crepitus or loose fragments (Procedure 12-5b). Any instability or asymmetry of the eye orbits, nasal bones, maxilla, or mandible suggests a facial bone fracture. In these cases, pay careful attention to the upper airway for obstruction from blood, bone chips, and teeth. Suction these patients aggressively to keep the upper airway clear.

When the base of the skull is fractured, blood and fluid from the brain can seep into the soft tissues around the eyes and ears and can drain from the ears or nose. Observe the bony orbits of the eye and the mastoid process behind the ears for discoloration. **Periorbital ecchymosis** (raccoon's eyes) is a black and blue discoloration surrounding the eye sockets. **Battle's sign** is a similar discoloration over the mastoid process just behind the ears (Procedure 12-5c). They are both late signs and usually are not visible on the scene unless a previous injury exists. Evaluate the temporomandibular joint for tenderness, swelling, and range of motion.

Eyes Examine the external structure of the eyes for symmetry in size, shape, and contour. Inspect the sclera and conjunctiva for discoloration, swelling, and exudate. Inspect the eyes for discoloration, foreign bodies, or blood in the anterior chamber (hyphema). Hyphema suggests that a tremendous blunt trauma to the anterior part of the eye has occurred. Check the pupils for equality in size and reaction to light (Procedure 12-5d). Bilaterally sluggish pupils usually suggest decreased cerebral perfusion and hypoxia. Fixed and dilated pupils indicate severe cerebral anoxia. Unequal pupils may indicate a variety of pathologies, including brain lesions, meningitis, drug poisoning, third-nerve paralysis, and increasing intracranial pressure.

Examine the eyes for conjugate movement, their ability to move together. Muscle or nerve damage to the eyes and certain drugs can cause dysconjugate gaze, in which the eyes seem to look in different directions. Check for extraocular movements. Note any inability of the eyes to follow your finger as you draw a large imaginary "H" in front of them; this indicates either nerve damage or an orbital fracture impinging on the extraocular muscles (Procedure 12-5e). Test for visual acuity and peripheral vision, if appropriate.

Ears Examine the external ears and observe the surrounding area for deformities, lumps, skin lesions, tenderness, and erythema. Examine the ear canal for drainage (Procedure 12-5f). A basilar skull fracture can cause blood and clear cerebrospinal fluid to leak into the auditory canals and flow to the outside. Do not try to block this flow; just cover it with sterile gauze to prevent an easy route for infection. Check for hearing acuity as appropriate.

Nose and Sinuses Check your patient's nose from the front and from the side and note any deviation in shape or color. Palpate the external nose for depressions, deformities, and tenderness. Examine the nares for flaring, a sign of respiratory distress, especially in small children. Pay special attention to infants less than three months old. They are mainly nose breathers and need a clear, unobstructed nasal cavity for respiration. Examine the nasal mucosa for evidence of drainage and note the color, quantity, and consistency of the discharge (Procedure 12-5g). A clear, runny discharge may indicate leaking cerebral spinal fluid (CSF) from a basilar skull fracture. Test for nasal obstruction.

The nasal cavity has a rich blood supply to warm the inspired air. Unfortunately, this can make bleeding in the nasal cavity severe and very difficult to control. If unconscious, these patients require aggressive suctioning. The patient who swallows this blood may complain later of nausea and vomiting.

Mouth and Pharynx Note the condition and color of the lips. Lip cyanosis is an ominous sign of central circulatory hypoxia. Examine the oral mucosa for pallor suggesting poor perfusion as in shock (Procedure 12-5h). Ask your patient to extend his tongue straight out and then move it from side to side. Press a tongue blade down on the middle third of the tongue and have your patient say "aaaahhhh." Examine the movement of the uvula. Asymmetrical movement of the uvula suggests a cranial nerve lesion. Note any odors or fluids coming from your patient's mouth; they can provide clues to infection, poisoning, and metabolic processes such as diabetic ketoacidosis.

Lip cyanosis is an ominous sign of central circulatory hypoxia.

Neck Briefly inspect the neck for general symmetry. Note any obvious deformity, deviation, tugging, masses, surgical scars, gland enlargement, or visible lymph nodes. Examine any penetrating injuries to the neck closely for injury to the trachea or major blood vessels. Look for jugular vein distention while your patient is sitting up and at a 45° incline. Palpate the trachea for midline position (Procedure 12-5i). Then, palpate the carotid arteries and note their rate and quality.

Chest and Lungs Observe your patient's breathing. Look for signs of acute respiratory distress. Count his respiratory rate and note his breathing pattern. Inspect the anterior and posterior chest walls for symmetrical movement. Note the use of neck muscles (sternocleidomastoids, scalene muscles) during inhalation or abdominal muscles during exhalation. Accessory muscle use suggests partial

12-5a Inspect and palpate the cranium from front to back.

12-5b Inspect and palpate the facial bones.

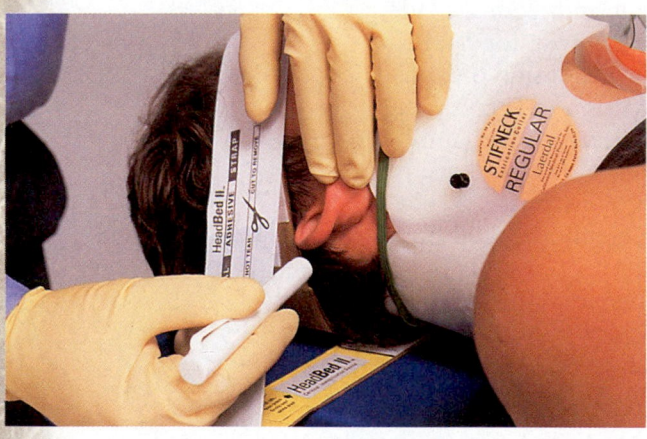

12-5c Inspect the mastoid process for Battle's sign.

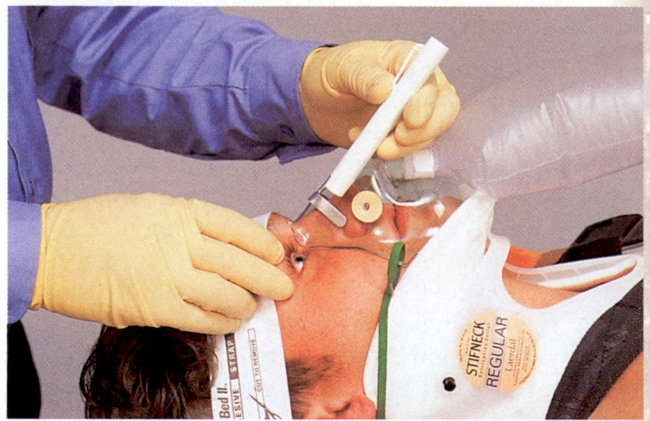

12-5d Check the pupils for reaction to light.

12-5e Check for extraocular movement.

12-5f Inspect the ear canal for drainage.

12-5g Examine the nasal mucosa for drainage.

12-5h Examine the oral mucosa for pallor.

12-5i Palpate the trachea for midline position.

airway obstruction and difficulty moving air. Inspect the intercostal spaces for retractions or bulging.

Palpate the rib cage for rigidity (Procedure 12-6a). Feel for tenderness, deformities, depressions, loose segments, asymmetry, and crepitus. Evaluate for equal expansion. Percuss the chest symmetrically from the apices to the bases. Identify and note any area of abnormal percussion. Auscultate all lung fields and compare side-to-side (Procedure 12-6b).

Percussion can also provide evidence regarding chest pathology. If the region is hyperresonant, the thorax may contain air under pressure (tension pneumothorax). If the region is dull to percussion, it may be filled with blood (hemothorax) or other fluid (pleural effusion). Be sure to compare the sounds left-to-right and, during examination of the posterior body, front-to-back to confirm your evaluation.

Cardiovascular System Look for skin pallor and other signs of decreased perfusion. Inspect and palpate the carotid arteries for rate, rhythm, and quality or amplitude. Inspect and palpate the chest for the PMI. Auscultate for normal, abnormal, and extra heart sounds.

Abdomen Inspect the skin of the abdomen and flanks for scars, dilated veins, stretch marks, rashes, lesions, and pigmentation changes. Look for Cullen's sign or Grey-Turner's sign suggesting intra-abdominal bleeding. Assess the size and shape of your patient's abdomen and note its symmetry. Palpate the abdomen last to detect tenderness, muscular rigidity, and superficial organs and masses (Procedure 12-6c). Assess for rebound tenderness, a classic sign of peritoneal irritation, by pushing down slowly and then releasing your hand quickly off the tender area.

Pelvis Reevaluate the pelvic ring at the iliac crests and symphysis pubis (Procedure 12-6d). With the palms of your hands, direct pressure medially and posteriorly. Then press posteriorly on the symphysis pubis, being careful not to entrap the penis or cause injury to the urinary bladder. Any pain, instability, or crepitus suggests a pelvic fracture. Always immobilize the pelvis before transport to prevent movement and a possible circulatory catastrophe. If your patient presents in shock with an unstable pelvis, apply and inflate the pneumatic antishock garment.

Genitalia The external genitalia are extremely vascular and can bleed profusely when lacerated. Control hemorrhage in this area with direct pressure. Examine the male organ for priapism, a painful, prolonged erection usually caused by spinal cord injury or blood disturbances. Suspect a major spinal cord injury in any patient with a priapism. The female genitalia are somewhat well-protected from all but penetrating injury.

If you suspect your patient may have been raped or sexually abused, limit your assessment and management to only those techniques that are essential to patient stabilization. If possible, have a member of the same sex treat these patients. This may relieve any hostilities and anxiety that might be directed toward a caregiver of the opposite sex. Encourage the patient not to bathe. One of your most important tasks is to provide emotional support and reassurance. (For more on this subject, see Chapter 44 on abuse and assault.)

Anus and Rectum Examining the anus is normally not a prehospital assessment practice. If your patient presents with severe rectal bleeding apply direct pressure to the area with sterile pads and be prepared to treat him for shock. You will have no other reason to examine this area.

One of your most important tasks for possible victims of rape or sexual abuse is to provide emotional support and reassurance.

Peripheral Vascular System Inspect all four extremities, noting their size and symmetry. Palpate the peripheral arteries for pulse rate and quality. Assess the skin for temperature, moisture, color, and capillary refill.

12-6a   Palpate the ribcage.

12-6b   Auscultate the lungs.

12-6c   Palpate the abdomen.

12-6d   Evaluate the pelvis.

Musculoskeletal System Reinspect and palpate all four extremities. Inspect and palpate your patient's joints, their structure, their range of motion, and the surrounding tissues. Inspect for swelling in or around joints, changes in the surrounding tissue, redness of the overlying skin, deformities, and symmetry of impairment. Compare both sides for equal size, shape, color, and strength. Palpate for tenderness in and around the joint. Try to identify the specific structure that is tender, such as a ligament, or tendon.

Test for range of motion passively and against gravity and resistance. Difficulty during passive range of motion tests suggests a joint problem. Difficulty with gravity or against resistance suggests a muscular weakness or nerve problem. Listen for crepitation, the crunching sounds of unlubricated parts rubbing against each other, while you manipulate the joint. Perform distal neurovascular checks.

Nervous System A nervous system exam covers five areas: mental status and speech; the cranial nerves; the motor system; the reflexes; and the sensory system.

Mental Status and Speech First, assess your patient's level of consciousness and compare his response to your earlier findings. Observe his posture and motor behavior and his grooming and personal hygiene. Note his speech pattern and use of language. Observe your patient's mood from his verbal and nonverbal behavior. Assess his thought content, perceptions, insight and judgment, memory, attention, and learning ability.

Cranial Nerves Test any cranial nerves that you have not already checked. (Review Table 3-3 for a quick, reliable, practical, cranial nerve exam that should take no longer than one minute to perform.)

Motor System Inspect your patient's general body structure, muscle development, positioning, and coordination. Note any obvious asymmetries, deformities, or involuntary movements. Assess muscle tone by feeling the muscle's resistance to passive stretching in the extremities. Test for muscle strength by applying resistance during the range of motion evaluation. Check for pronator drift and watch for any drifting sideways (laterally) or upward (superiorly). Assess for coordination and cerebellar function, using rapid alternating movements and point-to-point testing.

Reflexes Test your patient's deep tendon reflexes with a reflex hammer and note any hyperactive or diminished response. Check the biceps, triceps, brachioradialis, quadriceps, and Achilles reflexes. Test the superficial abdominal reflexes and plantar response.

Sensory System Test for pain, light touch, temperature, position, vibration, and discriminative sensations. Compare distal areas to proximal areas, symmetrical areas bilaterally, and scatter the stimuli to assess most of the dermatomes. Assess your patient's ability to distinguish sharp from dull sensations.

VITAL SIGNS

Take another set of vital signs and compare them to earlier sets to detect any trends, patterns that indicate either an improvement or deterioration in your patient's condition. These trends include a rising or falling pulse rate and blood pressure; an increasing or decreasing respiratory rate and effort; changing skin temperature, color, and condition; and changing pupillary equality and response to light. Such trends may suggest specific pathologies that you will learn in Chapters 16 to 26 on trauma emergencies and Chapters 27 to 40 on medical emergencies.

RECORDING EXAM FINDINGS

Record all exam findings on the appropriate run sheet or chart. Remain objective and nonjudgmental when recording the data. Chapter 15, "Documentation," gives detailed instructions on writing patient care reports.

Content Review

AREAS OF NERVOUS SYSTEM EXAM

Mental status and speech
Cranial nerves
Motor system
Reflexes
Sensory system

Content Review

REFLEX TESTS

Biceps
Triceps
Brachioradialis
Quadriceps
Achilles
Abdominal plantar

Content Review

SENSORY SYSTEM TESTS

Pain
Light touch
Temperature
Position
Vibration
Discriminative

ONGOING ASSESSMENT

En route to the hospital, conduct an ongoing series of assessments to detect trends, determine changes in your patient's condition, and assess the effectiveness of your interventions. Patient condition can change suddenly. You must steadfastly reassess mental status, airway patency, breathing adequacy, circulation, and any deterioration in areas already compromised (Procedure 12-7a). Conduct your ongoing assessment every fifteen minutes for stable patients, every five minutes for unstable patients. Compare your findings to the baseline findings and note any trends.

MENTAL STATUS

Recheck your patient's mental status by performing the AVPU exam frequently during transport. Any deterioration in mental status is cause for great concern. The brain demands a constant supply of oxygen and glucose and a constant elimination of waste products. When it is deprived of either, even briefly, expect rapid mental status changes. A falling level of response indicates either a direct or indirect brain pathology. For example, following a head injury, your patient who was alert and oriented at the scene gradually becomes sleepy and eventually unarousable. You should suspect a life-threatening increase in intracranial pressure (pressure inside the enclosed skull) and expedite transport to the appropriate medical facility. Or your patient with an intra-abdominal hemorrhage becomes increasingly less arousable due to the decreased oxygenated blood flow to the brain (indirect pathology). Or sometimes patients improve following your interventions. After you administer 50% dextrose to your hypoglycemic diabetic patient, for instance, he becomes alert and begins talking.

You must steadfastly reassess mental status, ABCs, and any areas already compromised.

Any deterioration in mental status is cause for great concern.

AIRWAY PATENCY

The patency of your patient's airway can change instantly. Bleeding, vomiting, and even secretions can suddenly obstruct the upper airway. Be prepared to suction your patient quickly. Respiratory burns and anaphylaxis can cause life-threatening swelling in a matter of minutes. Croup and epiglottitis also can quickly deteriorate into total upper airway occlusion.

Endotracheal intubation is the best way to secure the airway in patients with no gag reflex. But endotracheal tubes can become dislodged easily during transport. Recheck for tube placement frequently during transport and every time you move your patient onto a back board, onto the stretcher, or onto the hospital gurney.

The price of proper airway management is eternal vigilance and a pessimistic outlook— anything that can go wrong will go wrong. Be prepared for the worst.

BREATHING RATE AND QUALITY

A change in respiratory rate or quality might indicate improvement or deterioration. A sudden increase in rate or respiratory effort suggests deterioration. For example, if your patient suddenly begins to gasp for air, has retractions, and uses his accessory neck muscles, he has a serious problem. Sometimes the signs are not so obvious. Subtle increases in respiratory rate can suggest a developing problem. A decrease in rate and effort could mean that your treatments are effective and your patient is improving. For example, after you administer an albuterol treatment, your patient breathes easier and his lung sounds improve. In infants and young children, however, a decrease in rate and effort may mean that your patient is exhausted and requires aggressive intervention. If, while assisting ventilation with a bag-valve mask, your partner suddenly complains that squeezing the bag is becoming more difficult, consider the possibility that a tension pneumothorax is developing or that bronchospasm or laryngospasm may be occurring. Airway and breathing management require constant reevaluation.

12-7a   Reevaluate the ABCs.

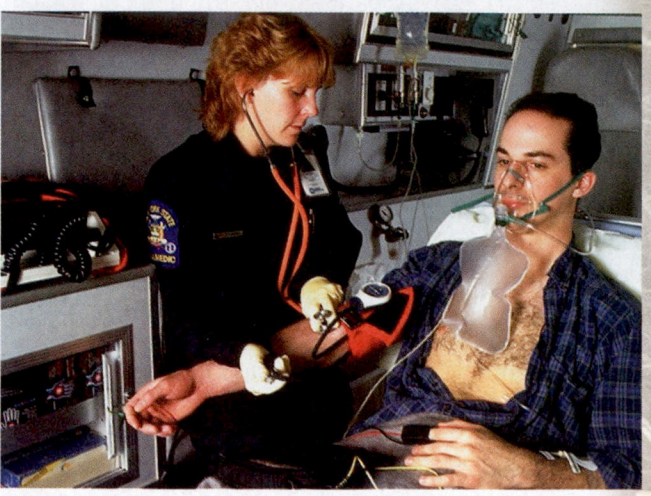

12-7b   Take all vital signs again.

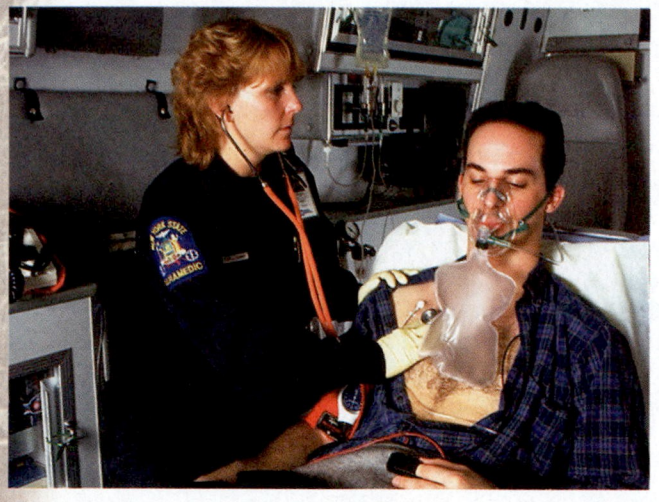

12-7c   Perform your focused assessment again.

12-7d   Evaluate your interventions' effects.

PULSE RATE AND QUALITY

Check central and peripheral pulses and compare the findings to earlier measurements. A rising pulse rate could indicate shock, hypoxia, or cardiac dysrhythmia. A falling rate could mean the terminal stage of shock or a rise in intracranial pressure. A sudden change in rate or regularity may suggest a cardiac dysrhythmia. The loss of peripheral pulses could mean decompensating shock.

SKIN CONDITION

Similar to mental status, the skin quickly reflects the body's hemodynamic status. Reevaluate your patient's skin color, temperature, and condition. Cyanosis suggests decreased oxygenation. Lip cyanosis indicates central hypoxia (overall oxygen status), while peripheral cyanosis indicates decreased oxygen to the tissues. Pallor and coolness suggest decreased circulation to the skin, as seen in shock. If your patient suddenly develops hives after you administer a medication, suspect an allergic reaction. A localized redness and warmth could indicate bleeding under the skin or vasodilation. Cyanosis and coolness in a lower extremity suggest a peripheral vascular problem such as an arterial occlusion. A deep vein thrombosis will result in redness, swelling, and warmth in the lower leg.

TRANSPORT PRIORITIES

Sometimes stable patients suddenly deteriorate en route to the hospital. For example, the formerly conscious and alert head-injury patient now responds only to pain. Or your stable cardiac patient suddenly develops a life-threatening dysrhythmia. Or your patient suddenly cannot breathe because his simple pneumothorax has developed into a tension pneumothorax. In these cases, while you provide life-saving treatments, change your transport decision to a higher priority. By the same token, if your unstable patient becomes stable, you may wish to downgrade your priority transport decision and decrease the danger and liability of driving with lights and siren on.

VITAL SIGNS

Reassessing vital signs reveals trends clearly (Procedure 12-7b). A rising pulse rate combined with a falling blood pressure indicates shock. A decreasing pulse rate combined with a rising blood pressure, associated with an irregular respiratory pattern, suggests a rise in intracranial pressure. Any change in heart rate could indicate a cardiac dysrhythmia. A narrowing pulse pressure with a weakening pulse indicates cardiac tamponade, a tension pneumothorax, or hypovolemic shock. Reevaluate your critical patient's vital signs every five minutes and look for changes.

Reevaluate your critical patient's vital signs every five minutes.

FOCUSED ASSESSMENT

Elicit your patient's chief complaint again to determine if the problem still exists or if other problems have arisen. Often following trauma your patient will develop more complaints en route to the hospital as the excitement of the incident begins to wear off. Patients often focus on their major injuries and might not even be aware of other problems. Repeat your focused assessment as your patient's chief complaint dictates (Procedure 12-7c).

EFFECTS OF INTERVENTIONS

Evaluate the effects of any interventions (Procedure 12-7d). Did the albuterol treatment help open the lower airways? Did the oxygen and nitroglycerin relieve the chest pain? What are the affects of the fluid challenge? Is the pneumatic anti-shock garment inhibiting your patient's breathing? Did your intervention help or harm your patient? Is he getting better or worse? Know the expected therapeutic benefits of your interventions, and then evaluate whether they worked. For example, you administer lidocaine to convert ventricular tachycardia. Following administration, observe your patient's electrocardiogram for changes while noting any harmful side effects such as nausea, vomiting, or seizures.

MANAGEMENT PLANS

Have the courage to admit it if your plan is not working and the flexibility to change it.

Evaluate whether your care is working. If it is not, consider another management plan. Develop the courage to admit when your plan is not working and the flexibility to change your course of action. For example, your patient, an elderly man with a history of congestive heart failure (CHF) and chronic obstructive pulmonary disease (COPD), presents with severe difficulty breathing and audible wheezing. You suspect he is having an exacerbation of his COPD and administer two nebulizer treatments and begin transporting. En route, however, he is not improving, and now you also can hear crackles bilaterally. At this point, you suspect he is in CHF and change your management to administering nitroglycerin, furosemide, and morphine.

Patients often present with multiple complaints, symptoms, and histories. Formulating a definitive diagnosis is difficult without the hospital's labs, X-rays, and other assessment tools. Your ability to reassess your patient, reevaluate your field diagnosis, and alter your management plan will optimize patient care.

Your ability to reassess your patient, reevaluate your field diagnosis, and alter your management plan will optimize patient care.

SUMMARY

Patient assessment is the key to providing effective prehospital emergency medical care. Its components include the initial assessment, the focused history and physical exam, vital signs, ongoing assessment, and the detailed physical exam. The initial assessment is designed to identify life-threatening airway, breathing, and circulation problems. The focused history and physical exam is designed to identify the signs and symptoms surrounding your patient's chief complaint. It is a problem-oriented approach that is easily modified to match your patient's clinical situation. The ongoing assessment is designed to reevaluate your patient for changes in status en route to the hospital. The detailed physical exam is a comprehensive head-to-toe evaluation designed to identify any conditions not already found. Although more suited to a clinical setting, it is intended to be done en route to the hospital if time allows.

The four general types of patients require distinctly different assessment approaches. The trauma patient with a significant mechanism of injury should receive an initial assessment, a rapid trauma assessment, and rapid transport. The patient with isolated, minor trauma, such as a cut finger or sprained ankle, should receive a physical exam focused on his particular problem or area. The responsive medical patient requires an initial assessment, a history and physical exam that focuses on his chief complaint, and vital signs. The unresponsive medical patient requires an initial assessment, followed by a rapid head-to-toe medical assessment and rapid transport. You will perform detailed history and physical exam techniques en route to the hospital if time and your patient's condition allow.

The assessment templates in this chapter are only guidelines. They do not dictate an exact procedure for assessing every patient. Instead, they provide general chronological guides to help you make critical transport and management decisions. As a paramedic you will be expected to use clinical judgment when deciding which assessment tools to use for your particular patient and situation. With time and experience, you will become adept at assessing real patients in crisis. The more effective and efficient you become with this process, the better your patient care will be.

CHAPTER 13

Clinical Decision Making

Objectives

After reading this chapter, you should be able to:

1. Compare the factors influencing medical care in the out-of-hospital environment to other medical settings. (p. 758)

2. Differentiate between critical life-threatening, potentially life-threatening, and non-life-threatening patient presentations. (pp. 758–759)

3. Evaluate the benefits and shortfalls of protocols, standing orders, and patient care algorithms. (pp. 759, 760)

4. Define the components, stages, and sequences of the critical thinking process for paramedics. (pp. 759–767)

5. Apply the fundamental elements of critical thinking for paramedics. (pp. 765–767)

6. Describe the effects of the "fight or flight" response and its positive and negative effects on a paramedic's decision making. (p. 764)

7. Summarize the "six *R*s" of putting it all together: *R*ead the patient, *R*ead the scene, *R*eact, *R*eevaluate, *R*evise the management plan, *R*eview performance. (p. 767)

8. Given several preprogrammed and moulaged trauma and medical patients, demonstrate clinical decision making. (pp. 757–767)

INTRODUCTION TO CRITICAL THINKING

As a paramedic you eventually will face your "moment of truth." You will confront a situation that requires you to make a critical decision. Often, you will have several options, but choosing the best one may mean the difference between life and death. And you will be all alone. Others may be at the scene, but as the paramedic, you will be responsible for that decision. That you someday will have to make a decision on which your patient's life hinges is a sobering thought.

In the 1970s, with rare exceptions the first paramedics made few critical decisions. They usually worked under rigidly-written protocols developed by their medical director. Mostly, they were required to contact the medical direction physician who, after hearing their report, would diagnose the patient's problem and order treatment. They were no more than technicians who needed only good psychomotor skills to conduct patient assessments and follow orders. As prehospital care has evolved, paramedics now do much more than collect data for the physician to evaluate. You not only will have to gather information, but analyze it, form a field diagnosis, and devise a management plan. In most cases you will do these things before contacting your medical direction physician.

Twenty-first-century paramedics are prehospital practitioners of emergency medicine—not field technicians. To fill this role, you will need to develop your critical decision making skills—to be able to think rationally about what you are doing. Because patients seldom present with the classic textbook signs and symptoms, you will encounter situations that appear totally unfamiliar. These cases will call for you to use sound judgment in devising a management plan that meets your patient's needs. Making such decisions requires **clinical judgment**, using your knowledge and experience to make critical decisions regarding patient care. No one can teach you clinical judgment; you must develop it from experience. Unfortunately, experience often includes making bad decisions. We learn from our mistakes, if someone points them out and explains them to us. Your hospital and field preceptors will do this for you during this program.

During this program, your instructors also will place you in as many problem-solving situations as possible to begin developing your clinical judgment. The number and type of supervised patient contacts you make during this program will determine how much clinical judgment you develop as a student. The more types of cases you see during your clinical rotations, the more clinically competent you will be when you complete your education.

PARAMEDIC PRACTICE

As a paramedic, you must gather, evaluate, and synthesize much information in very little time. You will obtain this information using your senses (sight, smell, hearing, and touch) during the history and physical exam. Analyzing these data will involve the total of your education, training, and clinical experience. For example, as you enter a patient's home, the sound of his gasping for breath with audible wheezes startles you. Having heard wheezing before and having learned in class that it results from a variety of problems will help you to make what is called a differential diagnosis. The differential diagnosis is a preliminary list of possible causes for your patient's problem. For example, a differential diagnosis for diffuse wheezing might include asthma, emphysema, bronchitis, and acute pulmonary edema. Now you conduct a history and physical exam and arrive at a **field diagnosis,** or impression.

Your next step will involve applying your clinical experience and exercising independent decision making as you develop and implement a management plan.

As a paramedic you inevitably will face your moment of truth—a critical decision that can mean the difference between life and death.

Twenty-first-century paramedics are prehospital practitioners of emergency medicine—not field technicians.

✳ clinical judgment the use of knowledge and experience to diagnose patients and plan their treatment.

✳ field diagnosis prehospital evaluation of the patient's condition and its causes.

For example, your gasping and wheezing patient is an elderly male who presents with severe difficulty breathing. He has a history of cardiac and pulmonary disease, and you are not sure which problem precipitates this episode. You gather information and make an initial field diagnosis of congestive heart failure. You immediately administer medications (nitroglycerin, furosemide, morphine) to reduce cardiac preload, ease the workload of the heart, and increase urine production. You also decide to intubate and ventilate your patient to ease his respiratory effort. This decision to administer potentially life-threatening drugs requires you to think clearly and work effectively under pressure. Few prehospital situations create more pressure than a patient struggling to breathe.

The prehospital emergency medical setting is unlike any other medical care environment. Paramedics carry out the same tasks as other clinicians. They assess patients, obtain vital signs, start IVs, manage airways, and perform many other invasive procedures. The difference is that paramedics perform these procedures in various uncontrolled and unpredictable environments under circumstances that do not exist in other clinical settings and without information gathered from laboratory results and X-ray. For example, starting an IV line in a well lit, quiet hospital room is not a major challenge. Starting one while balancing yourself in the back of a rapidly moving ambulance is. Often you will use your skills in seemingly unmanageable circumstances. The key is to block out the distractions and focus on the task. Experienced paramedics do this better than anyone.

PATIENT ACUITY

* **acuity** the severity or acuteness of your patient's condition.

Not everyone who calls 911 has a life-threatening emergency. Just the opposite is true. The vast majority of our patients are people who want transportation to the hospital for non-life-threatening problems. For others, the emergency department is their only health care option, even for a sore throat. The spectrum of care in the prehospital setting includes three general classes of patient **acuity**: those with obvious critical life threats, those with potential life threats, and those with non-life-threatening presentations. Patients with obvious life-threatening conditions include major multisystem trauma; devastating single system trauma; end stage disease presentations such as liver or renal failure when the patient is in the last days of his terminal illness and is close to death; and acute presentations of chronic diseases such as asthma or emphysema. These patients present with serious airway, breathing, circulation, or neurological problems and often require aggressive resuscitation. Potential life-threatening conditions include serious multisystem trauma and multiple disease etiologies such as a diabetic with cardiac complications. Non-life-threatening presentations include isolated minor illnesses and injuries. You will be expected to manage cases in all three categories. In a typical twelve-hour shift you may manage a patient in cardiac arrest; deliver a baby; control a lacerated, spurting artery; and transfer an elderly woman back to her nursing home. The wide range of patient types, degrees of severity, and complicating environmental factors makes out of hospital care a unique form of emergency medicine.

Arriving at a management plan for patients with minor medical and traumatic events requires little critical thinking or clinical judgment. For example, if your patient has a fractured tibia, you will splint the leg and transport him to the emergency department for X-rays and casting. You have no real life-saving decisions to make. On the opposite end of the acuity spectrum, patients with obvious life-threats such as cardiac arrest and major trauma also require few critical decisions because caring for them is largely rote and standardized. For cardiac arrest, you perform CPR and work through the protocol associated with your patient's cardiac rhythm. For major trauma, you manage the ABCs while providing rapid transport to a trauma center.

acuity the severity or acuteness of your patient's condition.

Content Review

CLASSES OF PATIENT ACUITY
- Critically life-threatening
- Potentially life-threatening
- Non-life-threatening

Patients who fall between minor medical and life-threatening on the acuity spectrum pose the greatest challenge to your critical thinking abilities. These patients might become unstable at any moment. For example, if your patient is an infant with signs of respiratory distress, you must recognize the signs of early respiratory failure and take precautionary measures to keep him from deteriorating to respiratory arrest. In these cases, you use your knowledge of pediatric respiratory assessment, your skills in airway and breathing management, and your clinical judgment to determine how and when to intervene. You will constantly reassess and revise your interventions as needed.

PROTOCOLS AND ALGORITHMS

Paramedics function in an emergency medical services system under the license of a medical director. Every state has enacted legislation allowing paramedics to practice medicine in the field and describing the scope of their practice. Within these laws, state and local EMS medical directors devise **protocols** that detail exactly what paramedics can do. Protocols are standards that include general and specific procedures for managing certain patient conditions. For example, every system will develop standards for managing asthma, congestive heart failure, and tension pneumothorax. Each will also develop protocols for special situations such as physician-on-scene, radio failure, and termination of resuscitation. **Standing orders** authorize you to perform certain procedures before contacting your medical direction physician. For example, you may administer oxygen, start an IV, and administer aspirin and nitroglycerin to a patient with cardiac chest pain. For repeat nitro orders, you may have to consult the physician. Patient care **algorithms** are flow-charts with arrows, lines, and boxes arranged schematically (Figure 13-1). To use them, you simply start at the top and follow wherever your patient's signs and symptoms lead.

Protocols, standing orders, and patient care algorithms provide a standardized approach to emergency patient care. However, they address only "classic patients." Unfortunately, many patients present with atypical signs and symptoms, often requiring you to use clinical judgment and instinct to develop a management plan. Patients frequently present with nonspecific complaints that do not match any specific algorithm. Sometimes your patients just do not clearly describe what is bothering them. Another limitation of protocols is that they cannot adequately cover multiple disease etiologies such as the patient with chronic obstructive pulmonary disease and congestive heart failure. When your patient with this multiple history presents with severe difficulty breathing, you must quickly identify the underlying condition that is causing the present problem and follow the appropriate protocol. Nor do protocols deal with managing more than one patient problem at a time in possible multiple treatment situations. For example, your stroke patient also presents with shock and with bilateral Colles' fractures and a fractured hip from the fall. Protocols are standards designed to promote consistent patient care in common situations. They are written also to allow you, in consultation with the medical direction physician, to use clinical judgment to provide optimum care in unusual situations. The linear thinking, or "cookbook medicine," that protocols promote should not restrict you from consulting with your medical direction physician in difficult or unusual cases.

CRITICAL THINKING SKILLS

The ability to think under pressure and make decisions cannot be taught; it must be developed. As a paramedic, you will be a team leader on emergency scenes. In

* **protocol** standard that includes general and specific principles for managing certain patient conditions.

* **standing orders** treatments you can perform before contacting the medical control physician for permission.

* **algorithm** schematic flow chart that outlines appropriate care for specific signs and symptoms.

RESUSCITATION OF A NEWBORN

Newborn is delivered.

Suction, dry, wrap in newborn blanket, and resuction.

Evaluate breathing.

Nonbreathing or gasping   Spontaneous

Evaluate heart rate.

Provide positive pressure ventilation with high concentration oxygen for 15 to 30 seconds.

Below 100 beats/minute

Evaluate heart rate.

Above 100 beats/minute

Below 60 beats/minute
• Continue ventilations.
• Provide chest compressions.

Above 100 beats/minute
• Assess for spontaneous respirations.
• Stop positive pressure ventilations when spontaneous respirations are effective.

Evaluate color.

60 to 100 beats/minute	
Heart rate not increasing • Continue ventilations. • Provide chest compressions if heart rate is below 80 beats/minute	Heart rate increasing • Continue ventilations.

Pink or peripheral cyanosis
• Observe and monitor.

Blue
• Provide oxygen.

FIGURE 13-1   To use a patient care algorithm, follow the arrows to your patient's symptoms and provide care as indicated.

that role you must make sound, reasonable decisions regarding your patient's care. Several aspects of this program will help you to develop this essential skill. In the classroom you will work on case histories. In the labs you will practice patient scenarios on moulaged victims. In the hospital you will assess and help manage real patients in the emergency department and critical care units. In the field internship, you will assess and manage patients in the streets. In all of these settings you will begin developing clinical judgment.

FUNDAMENTAL KNOWLEDGE AND ABILITIES

First, you must have an excellent working knowledge of anatomy and physiology and of the pathophysiology of your patient's disease or injury. To assess and manage a patient with difficulty breathing, for instance, you must know which organs and body systems are involved in breathing. You must understand the process of normal breathing and each body system's role in that effort. You must recall the factors that inhibit normal breathing and recognize the signs and symptoms of respiratory distress. For example, a patient might wheeze because of lower airway obstruction from secretions, bronchoconstriction, edema, or any combination of these conditions. All reduce the inner diameter of the airways, restricting airflow and making moving air in and out of the lungs difficult. Managing this patient would require a knowledge of the respiratory and cardiovascular causes of wheezing, because their treatments are vastly different. Respiratory causes for generalized wheezing include asthma and bronchitis, which you would manage with bronchodilators. Cardiac causes for wheezing include congestive heart failure, which you would manage with vasodilators and diuretics. Without a good working knowledge of these diseases, you might make a mistaken and potentially devastating field diagnosis.

You also must be able to focus on many specific data. When you conduct a patient assessment, you will evaluate all relevant information while focusing on specific important findings. You will be inundated with information requiring you to establish relationships and form conclusions. Your patient who presents with difficulty breathing and wheezing in the previous example would require an in-depth history and focused examination of his cardiac and respiratory systems. You also would assess other systems relative to his chief complaint (HEENT, musculoskeletal, neurological, and lymphatic), while remaining focused on the primary problem (cardiorespiratory). Although his chief complaint is difficulty breathing, his primary problem might be cardiac, muscular, infectious, allergic, or neurologic.

You must be able to organize the information you obtain and form concepts from it. Initially you elicit your patient's chief complaint and begin to formulate a **differential field diagnosis.** As you conduct the history and a clearer picture of your patient's problem emerges, you narrow your differential field diagnosis to the most probable disease. For example, your patient has severe difficulty breathing and inspiratory stridor. Your differential field diagnosis might include foreign body obstruction, epiglottitis, respiratory burns, anaphylaxis, laryngeal trauma, and throat cancer. Then you learn that he is hoarse and febrile, has had a sore throat for two days, and in the past six hours has had increasing difficulty swallowing. You now suspect epiglottitis. This ability to formulate a working field diagnosis is essential for paramedics.

You must be able to identify and deal with medical ambiguity. Many patients present with vague signs and symptoms. It is not unusual for a patient to complain of "just not feeling right." He will provide you with an imprecise story and you will be unable to arrive at a specific field diagnosis. In these cases, your field diagnosis will have to be generalized: "abdominal pain" or "general illness." Often it will be almost impossible to definitively diagnose your patient without laboratory results, X-rays, and other tests.

You must be able to differentiate between relevant and irrelevant data. You will have to sift the important data from the many bits of information you receive during your patient assessment. A positive family history for sudden cardiac death is relevant for your patient with chest pain; for your patient with a fractured arm it is not. Pupil and extraocular movement exams are relevant for trauma and for patients with an altered mental status; for a patient with asthma or arthritis they are not. When you radio the medical direction physician, you

Content Review

DECISION-MAKING REQUIREMENTS

- Knowing anatomy, physiology, and pathophysiology
- Focusing on large amounts of data
- Organizing information
- Identifying and dealing with medical ambiguity
- Differentiating between relevant and irrelevant data
- Analyzing and comparing similar situations
- Explaining decisions and constructing logical arguments

* **differential field diagnosis** the list of possible causes of your patient's symptoms.

will report critical information only. Likewise, in your written documentation you will record relevant information and omit the rest.

You must be able to analyze and compare similar and contrasting situations. What were the similarities between your last three stroke patients? Did all three have facial drooping, slurred speech, and unilateral paralysis? Did they all have a history of hypertension? Can you depend on any patterns of presentation for future calls like this? Have some patient presentations been unusual? Have any patients presented with signs of stroke but had a different diagnosis? For example, your patient is a 45-year-old woman who presents with right-sided facial drooping. Your initial impression may be stroke, but further investigation reveals no other neurological deficits. You now change your impression to Bell's Palsy, caused by inflammation of the facial nerve (CN-VII). You must be able to recall the factors that help rule in or rule out a particular disease or injury.

You must be able to explain your decisions and construct logical arguments. Often, the emergency physician will want to know what you were thinking when you made your field diagnosis. You must be able to express yourself rationally while you make your case. These are the times when you demonstrate your professionalism to other health care providers. Observe the following conversation:

Physician: Why did you think your patient had Bell's Palsy and not a stroke? How can you rule out a stroke in the field?

Paramedic: Well, she had paralysis on the entire right side of her face, indicating a lesion of the seventh cranial nerve, rather than the lower facial paralysis of a stroke. All other neuro tests were negative.

Physician: OK, I agree, good job!

Through interactions such as this, you establish credibility with the emergency physician. The next time you contact him regarding a patient, he is more apt to trust your assessment and judgment.

USEFUL THINKING STYLES

As a paramedic, you will face confusing emergencies that would challenge even the most knowledgeable, analytical care provider. You must be able to stay calm and not panic. Your self-control in the face of extreme chaos will set the example for other team members to follow. Even when you are struggling to maintain your composure—especially then—never let others know. The key is focusing on the task and blocking out the distractions. Be like the duck—cool and calm on the water's surface, while paddling feverishly underneath.

Assume and plan for the worst, and always err on the side of benefiting your patient. For example, if you are deliberating whether to immobilize your patient, initiate advanced life support procedures, or administer oxygen, just do it! It is better to err by providing care than by withholding it. Be pessimistic! Anticipate all potential bad side effects of your treatments and prepare "plan B." For example, as you deliver a bronchodilating drug to your severe asthmatic patient, anticipate that it will not work and mentally prepare to intubate him and perform positive pressure ventilation. Or while you are administering atropine to your patient with symptomatic bradycardia, plan ahead for external cardiac pacing and dopamine, if atropine therapy fails to restore adequate circulation.

Establish and maintain a systematic assessment pattern. Practice your assessments until they become second nature, and you will avoid skipping and missing steps. Be disciplined and stay focused, especially when you are confronted with a complex emergency scene. For example, your patient lies moaning

---

Content Review

FACILITATING BEHAVIORS
- Stay calm
- Plan for the worst
- Work systematically
- Remain adaptable

Be like the duck—cool and calm on the water's surface, while paddling feverishly underneath.

Except for safety concerns, never allow anything to distract you from your most important job—assessing and caring for your patient.

on the ground in a pool of blood. Bystanders are screaming at you to help him; others are trying to tell you what happened. The police are gathering the story and trying unsuccessfully to talk with your patient. You must gain control of this scene. You do so by focusing on your patient and performing a systematic assessment. Use common acronyms (MS-ABC, OPQRST, SAMPLE) or make up your own to help you remember the key elements of your assessment. Except for safety concerns, never allow anything to distract you from your most important job—assessing and caring for your patient.

The different situations you encounter will require a variety of management styles. Adapting your styles of situation analysis (reflective vs. impulsive), data processing (convergent vs. divergent), and decision making (anticipatory vs. reactive) to each situation will enable you to provide the best possible care in every case.

Reflective vs. Impulsive Some situations call for you to be **reflective,** take your time, and figure out what is wrong with your patient. You have a patient who complains of "not feeling well." She has a long history of cardiac, renal, respiratory, and diabetic problems. Since she is in no real distress and is hemodynamically stable, you can take your time to determine her primary problem. Other situations call for immediate action. They require you to make an instinctive, **impulsive** decision and manage your patient's life-threatening condition. For example, if your patient presents apneic and pulseless, you will immediately begin CPR and prepare for rapid defibrillation. If he presents with a spurting artery, you will at once take measures to control the hemorrhage. If he is choking and has a weak, ineffective cough, you will quickly perform the Heimlich maneuver. You have to think fast in these situations.

Divergent vs. Convergent To process the data you receive from your patient and the scene, you can use either a divergent approach or a convergent approach. The **divergent** approach considers all aspects of a situation before arriving at a solution. It is insightful and works well when you are confronted with complex scenarios. For example, your emotionally distraught, stable patient presents with multiple problems and a long, complicated medical history. You need to consider the physical, emotional, and psychological aspects of his condition before making a field diagnosis and management plan. Likewise, extricating a victim from a wooded scene requires you to weigh a variety of environmental and medical factors before selecting a mode of transport.

On the other hand, the **convergent** approach focuses narrowly on a situation's most significant aspects. This technically oriented approach relies heavily on step-by-step problem solving and is best suited for simple, uncomplicated situations that require little thought or reflection. For example, you have an unresponsive, apneic, pulseless patient who presents in ventricular fibrillation. Your immediate concern is simple and straightforward—you manage the ABCs and defibrillate him as quickly as possible. Experienced paramedics employ both approaches effectively in the appropriate situations.

Anticipatory vs. Reactive Your decision-making process can be either anticipatory or reactive. You either anticipate the possible ramifications of your actions in a proactive way or you react to events as you encounter them. For example, your patient presents with a severe laceration and severe blood loss. The bleeding is controlled. Now you can either anticipate his going into shock and begin measures before it happens, or you can wait until he shows signs of shock and then act. Unfortunately, by then it is often too late to do anything about it. Whenever possible, it is best to anticipate problems and act before they occur.

* **reflective** acting thoughtfully, deliberately, and analytically.

* **impulsive** acting instinctively without stopping to think.

* **divergent** taking into account all aspects of a complex situation.

* **convergent** focusing on only the most important aspect of a critical situation.

Whenever possible, anticipate problems and act before they occur.

THINKING UNDER PRESSURE

autonomic nervous system part of the nervous system that controls involuntary actions.

When you must make a critical decision, physical influences may help or hinder your ability to think clearly. Your **autonomic nervous system,** which controls your involuntary actions, may respond by secreting "fight or flight" hormones. These hormones will enhance your visual and auditory acuity and will improve your reflexes and muscle strength. However, they may also impair your ability to think critically and diminish your ability to assess and concentrate. In these instances you will revert to your most basic instincts. Many an inexperienced paramedic has been "mentally paralyzed" by a complicated, critical call. With experience, you will learn to manage your nervousness and maintain a steadfast, controlled demeanor.

pseudo-instinctive learned actions that are practiced until they can be done without thinking.

One way to enhance your ability to remain in control is to raise your technical skills to a **pseudo-instinctive** level. This means that you do not have to concentrate on them to perform them. For example, you do not think about tying your shoes, you just tie them. Such "muscle memory" is essential when performing emergency medical skills. When you set up for an Albuterol nebulizer treatment, for instance, you automatically fit together the pieces of the device and administer the treatment without hesitation. This way you can concentrate on your patient's condition, controlling the scene, and managing the multitude of items that usually complicate any emergency call. Concentrating on more than one thing simultaneously is difficult, if not impossible.

Maintaining your composure, especially during a chaotic, complicated call is key to developing a management plan for the best patient outcome.

MENTAL CHECKLIST

Thinking under pressure is not easy. Maintaining your composure, especially during a chaotic, complicated call is key to developing a management plan for the best patient outcome. Developing a routine mental checklist is a good way to stay focused and systematic. Pilots work through their preflight checklists routinely before ever turning over their engines. Medical clinicians develop acronyms and mnemonics to remember critical elements during stressful incidents. For example, when conducting an initial assessment, use the acronym MS-ABC. Use OPQRST to elicit your patient's present history, or use SAMPLE when time is critical. You can adopt the following checklist any time you must make a critical decision.

Scan the Situation Stand back and scan the situation. Sometimes you can miss subtle signs if you focus too narrowly on one aspect of your patient's problem. Look for environmental factors and other not-so-obvious clues. For example, your patient lies unconscious and cyanotic on the floor. You rule out any airway, breathing, or circulation problems. No medical history is available and no medication bottles are present. When you detect a fruity odor on your patient's breath, you suspect diabetic ketoacidosis.

Stop and Think Do not do anything without stopping and weighing your actions. Consider all of your options before you act. Remember that for every action there is a reaction. Know what reactions to expect and anticipate their possible harmful effects. For example, after administering lidocaine, monitor your patient closely for the expected benefits (eradication of ventricular tachycardia) and early signs of toxicity (numbness and tingling to the lips, drowsiness, nausea).

Decide and Act Once you have assessed the situation, make your decision and act confidently. Announce your management plan to your crew with a combination of authority, confidence, and respect. Convey the feeling that you know your actions are correct and will work. This confidence helps reassure

Content Review

MENTAL CHECKLIST
- Scan the situation
- Stop and think
- Decide and act
- Maintain control
- Reevaluate

your patient, his family, your crew, and other responders even in the most stressful situations.

Maintain Control To maintain clear, efficient control of the scene and everyone involved, you must first control yourself. Many situations will challenge your inner strength and self-control. You will eventually be in charge of a scene where everyone seems out of control. These chaotic incidents can occur anywhere and anytime. Your job is to remain steadfast under fire.

Reevaluate Regularly reevaluate your plan's effects and revise it accordingly. Never assume that your plan is working to perfection. Anticipate ways your patient might deteriorate and devise alternate plans. Conduct an ongoing assessment en route to the hospital and be prepared to revise your management plan. For example, if you note increased lung congestion after administering fluids, stop the infusion.

THE CRITICAL DECISION PROCESS

Understanding the **critical-thinking** process is essential for a paramedic. Your ability to analyze data effectively and devise a practical management plan optimizes patient care. You can conduct the most comprehensive history and physical exam, but if you cannot analyze the data and devise the proper management plan, your efforts will be fruitless. The critical-thinking process has five steps: forming a concept, interpreting the data, applying the principles, evaluating the results, and reflecting on the incident. To explain the critical decision-making process, we will consider a nineteen-year-old female patient with a sudden onset of sharp pain to her right lower quadrant with some vaginal bleeding.

✱ **critical thinking** thought process used to analyze and evaluate.

FORM A CONCEPT

The first step in critical decision making is to gather information and form a concept of your patient and the scene. You will get this information by assessing the general environment and the immediate surroundings. Note the mechanism of injury, if applicable. Then observe your patient's mental status, skin color, positioning, and note any deformities or asymmetry. In our sample case, your patient presents at home, sitting on a sofa. At first glance, she appears pale, diaphoretic, and anxious. Next you conduct an initial assessment, focusing on the MS-ABCs. Your initial goal is to identify and manage critical life-threats. In this case, your general impression is of an alert and oriented but anxious young woman in moderate distress who presents with a clear airway; good air movement, as evidenced by her ability to converse in complete sentences; a strong, rapid, regular pulse; and cool, moist skin.

Now you ascertain your patient's chief complaint, history of present illness, past history, and current health status, while observing her affect (her general demeanor and attitude) and her degree of distress. You determine that her chief complaint is lower right quadrant pain that began suddenly 30 minutes ago. She also states she began bleeding at around the same time. She denies any nausea, vomiting, or diarrhea. You learn she has a past history of pelvic inflammatory disease and an active, unprotected sex life with multiple partners. Her last menstrual period was six weeks ago. She has had four pregnancies but no viable births. She appears in moderate distress.

> **Content Review**
>
> **STEPS IN CRITICAL DECISION MAKING**
> - Form a concept
> - Interpret the data
> - Apply the principles
> - Evaluate
> - Reflect

Finally, you conduct a focused physical exam of the appropriate areas. This includes any diagnostic testing, such as an electrocardiogram, pulse oximetry, and blood glucose testing. You take a full set of vital signs, which can help you identify most life-threatening conditions. Remember that your patient's age, underlying physical and medical condition, and current medications can influence her vital signs. For example, the use of beta blockers could cause a general decrease in her pulse and blood pressure. Your patient has some deep palpation tenderness in the lower right quadrant but no rebound tenderness, and the rest of her abdomen is soft and nontender. She has minor bleeding at this time and has used only one sanitary pad since the bleeding began. Her vital signs are: HR—110 and regular; respirations 20, not labored; BP—120/86.

INTERPRET THE DATA

After you assess the patient you will interpret all of your data in light of your knowledge and experience. In this case, your knowledge base includes female reproductive anatomy, the physiology of a normal pregnancy, and the pathophysiology of pregnancy complications along with their classic signs and symptoms. It also involves the anatomy, physiology, and pathophysiology of the cardiovascular system and the signs and symptoms of shock. Your experience base includes every patient you have assessed and managed with a similar presentation. Your attitude toward managing patients with these symptoms also becomes a factor, because your experience may prejudice you. Consider all of the data and determine the most common and statistically probable conditions that fit your patient's initial presentation. This is your differential field diagnosis. Then, consider the most serious condition that fits your patient's situation. In our example, a field diagnosis of a ruptured ectopic pregnancy is obvious. When a clear medical diagnosis is elusive, base your treatment on the presenting signs and symptoms.

APPLY THE PRINCIPLES

With your field diagnosis in mind, you devise a management plan that covers all contingencies. You will use written protocols, standing orders, and all the interventions at your disposal to manage your patient's particular problem. Sometimes patients present with atypical signs and symptoms. For example, a patient who presents with a sore throat and cough may actually be having a heart attack and congestive heart failure. Other times a protocol for your patient's problem simply may not exist. For example, your system may not have a protocol for facilitated intubation in head injuries. In these cases, consult with your medical direction physician for guidance in providing optimum care to your patient. The physician's emergency medical expertise and experience can be invaluable to you and your patient in unusual and difficult cases.

In our example, although your patient presents with relatively normal vital signs and is fully alert and oriented, you are very concerned. A basic principle of medicine is that all females of child-bearing age with lower abdominal pain are pregnant until proven otherwise. You initiate advanced life support precautions en route to the hospital, including high-flow oxygen and two large-bore intravenous lines. Her presentation, has led you to expect the worst. If her fallopian tube ruptures and begins to hemorrhage, she will need rapid fluid resuscitation and general shock management. Your experience includes similar patients who suddenly suffered a life-threatening hemorrhage from a ruptured fallopian tube. Again, your attitude becomes a factor in that you will not allow her stable presentation to undermine your initial instinct—that she is potentially in serious trouble.

EVALUATE

During the ongoing assessment you reassess your patient's condition and the effects of your standing order/protocol interventions. In other words, you determine if your treatment is improving your patient's condition and status. For example, has the Albuterol helped your patient's breathing? Did the nitro and oxygen relieve the chest pain? Is the hemorrhage under control? Reflect on your actions and either continue your original plan, discontinue treatment, or take a completely different approach. You may alter your initial impression if your patient's condition worsens or if you discover new information. If time and circumstances allow a detailed exam, you may discover less obvious problems.

In our sample case, your patient remains in potentially unstable condition. Your repeat assessment shows her vital signs are holding with the infusion of IV fluids. She is alert and not as anxious as before, and her skin is becoming warm and normal in color. You deliver her to the emergency department in stable, but guarded, condition.

REFLECT

After the call, discuss your field diagnosis and care with the emergency physician. Compare your field diagnosis with his diagnosis. Conduct a run critique with your crew and discuss ways to improve your assessment and management of this case and future cases. Add this data to your information and experience base for future calls. Make every patient contact a learning experience. In this case, the emergency physician confirms your field diagnosis with lab tests and an ultrasound.

Make every patient contact a learning experience.

PUTTING IT ALL TOGETHER

A helpful mnemonic for the critical decision making process is the "six Rs":

1. **R**ead the scene—Observe the general environmental conditions, the immediate surroundings, and any mechanism of injury.

2. **R**ead the patient—Observe his level of consciousness, skin color, position, location, and any obvious deformity or asymmetry. Talk to him to determine the chief complaint and whether it is a new problem or a worsening of a preexisting condition. Touch him to evaluate skin temperature and condition, pulse rate and quality. Auscultate for problems with the upper and lower airways. Identify any life threats with the ABCs and take a full set of vital signs.

3. **R**eact—Address any life-threats as found, determine the most common and serious existing conditions, and treat him accordingly.

4. **R**eevaluate—Conduct a focused and detailed physical assessment, note any response to your initial management interventions, and discover other less obvious problems.

5. **R**evise the management plan—Change or stop interventions that are not working or are causing your patient's condition to worsen, or try something new.

6. **R**eview your performance at run critique—Be honest and critically evaluate your performance, always looking for better ways to manage a particular case presentation.

> **Content Review**
>
> ### THE SIX RS
>
> 1. **R**ead the scene
> 2. **R**ead the patient
> 3. **R**eact
> 4. **R**eevaluate
> 5. **R**evise the management plan
> 6. **R**eview your performance

SUMMARY

Clinical decision making is an essential paramedic skill that you will develop with time and experience. The prehospital environment is unlike any other medical care setting and you will have to make decisions in less-than-optimal and sometimes dangerous conditions. Most times you will have the benefit of consulting with your medical direction physician in difficult and unusual situations; other times you may not. Your ability to gather information, analyze it, and make a critical decision may someday be the difference between your patient's life and death. This is inevitable. How well you prepare for that challenge will determine your ultimate success. The process begins in your paramedic training program. You must develop a good working knowledge of anatomy, physiology, pathophysiology, and the principles of emergency medicine. In time, through repeated patient contacts, you will develop the clinical judgment you need to make effective patient care decisions.

The critical-decision-making process involves a series of steps that experienced clinicians do almost unconsciously. First you gather information (history and physical exam) to form an initial impression and then interpret it against your knowledge and experience to develop a working field diagnosis. You next apply the principles of emergency medicine to devise and implement a management plan and evaluate the effects of your treatments. Then you reevaluate and revise your plan as necessary. Finally you compare your findings with the emergency physician's diagnosis and discuss alternate ways to manage similar patients. With every patient contact, your experience grows and your clinical judgment improves. This is the essence of paramedic practice.

CHAPTER 14

Communications

Objectives

After reading this chapter, you should be able to:

1. Identify the role and importance of verbal, written, and electronic communications in the provision of EMS. (pp. 773–778)

2. Describe the phases of communications necessary to complete a typical EMS response. (pp. 775–778)

3. List factors that impede and enhance effective verbal and written communications. (pp. 773–775)

4. Explain the value of data collection during an EMS response. (pp. 774, 783)

5. Recognize the legal status of verbal, written and electronic communications related to an EMS response. (pp. 773–774, 786–787)

6. Identify current technology used to collect and exchange patient and/or scene information electronically. (pp. 779–783)

7. Identify the various components of the EMS communications system and describe their function and use. (pp. 772, 775–778)

Continued

Objectives Continued

8. Identify and differentiate among the following communications systems:

   - Simplex (p. 779)
   - Multiplex (p. 780)
   - Duplex (p. 780)
   - Trunked (pp. 780–781)
   - Digital communications (p. 781)
   - Cellular telephone (p. 781)
   - Facsimile (p. 782)
   - Computer (pp. 782)

9. Describe the functions and responsibilities of the Federal Communications Commission. (pp. 786–787)

10. Describe the role of emergency medical dispatch and the importance of prearrival instructions in a typical EMS response. (pp. 775–778)

11. List appropriate caller information gathered by the emergency medical dispatcher. (pp. 776–777)

12. Describe the structure and importance of verbal patient information communication to the hospital and medical direction. (pp. 783–786)

13. Diagram a basic communications system. (pp. 773–774)

14. Given several narrative patient scenarios, organize a verbal radio report for electronic transmission to medical direction. (pp. 783–786)

INTRODUCTION TO COMMUNICATION

Knowledge of communications plays an important role in your paramedic training. All aspects of prehospital care require effective, efficient communications. During a routine transfer or a life-threatening emergency run, you will communicate with a wide variety of people. They will include:

- The emergency medical dispatcher (EMD) whose job it is to manage an entire system of EMS response and readiness, not just your call. You will transmit administrative information such as "responding," "arrived," "transporting," and "back-in-service." The EMD must know the location of all his resources to manage the system effectively. On a serious emergency call, the EMD can be your best ally by securing for you the resources you need to manage your incident.

- Your patient, his family, bystanders, and others who may, at times, not understand what you are doing and become obstructive. Quite often, people misconstrue your actions and words. You must try to keep them well-informed.

- Personnel from other responding agencies, such as the police department, fire department, or mutual aid ambulances who may not share your priorities at the scene. You must communicate effectively with other responders to coordinate and implement your treatment plan. You will accomplish this face-to-face and via the radio. These communications require you to exhibit confidence and authority.

- Health care staff from physicians' offices, health care facilities, and nursing homes who usually do not understand the extent of your training or abilities. Often, uninformed staff will call you "ambulance drivers." In these cases, you must exhibit professionalism and a calm demeanor while you ask pertinent questions and discuss the case intelligently.

- The medical direction physician who has extended his license to you in the field. The physician's expertise and advice can be a tremendous resource for you during the call. You will need to communicate patient information and scene assessment effectively to him. He can prepare for your arrival if you have communicated to him the needs of your patient. For example, you are transporting a patient with a serious head injury who exhibits a decreasing level of consciousness. By reporting this information, the emergency department can arrange for the trauma team, including a neurosurgeon, to meet you in the ED upon arrival. In such cases, good communication results in good patient care.

You must interact effectively with everyone involved in the call to coordinate a unified effort resulting in top-quality patient care. EMS is the ultimate team endeavor. Your performance as a paramedic is just one component in a series of interactions that ensure continuous first-rate care. From the call taker to the rehabilitation specialist, every player in this continuum is equally important—only their roles differ. Communication is not merely one aspect of an EMS response; it is the key link in the chain that results in the best possible patient outcome. Effective communication optimizes patient care during every phase of the EMS response.

Communication is the key link in the chain that results in the best possible patient outcome.

VERBAL COMMUNICATION

Factors that can enhance or impede effective communication may be either **semantic** (the meaning of words) or technical (communications hardware). Communication requires a mutual language. For example, a city unit and a county unit that use different **10-code** systems will find it difficult to communicate effectively. A 10-10 may mean a working fire in one system and a cardiac emergency in another. Thus, many EMS systems have changed from using 10-codes to plain English.

When reporting your patient's condition to the medical direction physician, you should use terminology that is widely accepted by both the medical and emergency services communities. Using a 10-code system with which the ED staff is unfamiliar would be inappropriate. Telling the medical direction physician that you have a victim of a 10-21-Golf (assault with a gun) may be meaningless. Conversely, if the medical direction physician asks you for your pregnant patient's EDC (due date) or her LMP (last menstrual period) and you do not know those acronyms, you have failed to communicate. The receiver must be able to decode the sender's message.

Your communication network must consist of reliable equipment designed to afford clear communication among all agencies within the system. This becomes a challenge in systems that cover large geographical areas or where terrain interferes with transmission and reception. If you want to communicate with a unit clear across the county but your radio is not powerful enough to transmit that far, communication will be difficult, if not impossible. A system that covers a large geographical expanse can place repeaters strategically throughout its service area. These devices receive transmissions from a low-powered source and rebroadcast them at a higher power (Figure 14-1).

* **semantic** related to the meaning of words.

* **10-code** radio communications system using codes that begin with the word *ten*.

Your communication network must consist of reliable equipment designed to afford clear communication among all agencies within the system.

FIGURE 14-1   Example of an EMS system using repeaters.

Your regional EMS system may consist of many agencies that have conducted business for decades on different **radio bands** and **frequencies.** City units may transmit on **ultrahigh frequency** (UHF) radio waves because they penetrate concrete and steel well and are less susceptible to interference. County units may use a low band frequency because those waves travel farther and better over varied terrain. In any event, communicating between agencies will be difficult unless all units share a common frequency. This is rarely the case. The spectrum of communications equipment currently ranges from antiquated radios to mobile data terminals mounted inside emergency vehicles. Geographically integrating communications networks would enable routine and reliable communication among EMS, fire, law enforcement, and other public safety agencies. This would in turn facilitate coordinated responses during both routine and large-scale operations. Developing the necessary hardware (equipment and network) and software (language) will be essential to improving emergency communications.

WRITTEN COMMUNICATION

Written records are another important aspect of EMS communications. Your **prehospital care report** (PCR) is a written record of events that includes administrative information such as times, location, agency, and crew, as well as medical information. It will be used by hospital staff, agency administrators, system quality-assurance/improvement committees, insurance and billing departments, researchers, educators, and lawyers. The data collected from your PCR can help to monitor and improve patient care through medical audits, research, education, and system policy changes. Furthermore, your written documentation becomes a legal record of the incident and may become part of your patient's permanent medical record. All legal rules regarding confidentiality and disclosure pertain to your PCR.

The same factors that influence verbal communication also affect written communication. Be objective, write legibly, thoroughly document your patient's assessment and care, and use terminology that is widely accepted in the medical community (Figure 14-2). Finally, your PCR illustrates your professionalism. A sloppy, incomplete PCR suggests sloppy, inefficient care. The chapter on documentation deals with PCRs and other written communications in much greater detail.

FIGURE 14-2 The prehospital care report is as important as the run itself. Complete it promptly, accurately, and legibly.

Using industry terminology appropriately provides a common means of communicating with other emergency care professionals.

TERMINOLOGY

Every industry develops its own terminology. Doing so makes communication within the industry more clear, concise, and unambiguous. The airline industry, for example, uses the term *payload* to describe the total weight of everything (passengers, fuel, luggage, and other items) on an airplane. Musical composers and arrangers use words like *fortissimo, allegro,* and *a cappella* to describe a specific tempo or style.

The medical field also uses an extensive list of terms, acronyms, and abbreviations that allow quick, accurate communication of complex information. (The documentation chapter includes an extensive table of standard charting abbreviations.) An emergency physician may request a CBC (complete blood count), ABGs (arterial blood gases), or a CIP (cardiac injury profile)—common terms describing diagnostic tests run on acutely ill patients. The emergency services industry has further developed its own terms for radio communication (Table 14-1). These words or phrases shorten air time and transmit thoughts and ideas quickly. For example, *copy, 10-4,* and *roger* mean "I heard you and I understand what you said." Using industry terminology appropriately is an important part of effective communication. It provides a common means of communicating with other emergency care professionals.

Table 14-1 COMMON RADIO TERMINOLOGY

Term	Meaning
Copy, 10-4, roger	I understand
Affirmative	Yes
Negative	No
Stand by	Please wait
Repeat	Please repeat what you said
Land-line	Telephone communications
Rendezvous	Meet with
LZ	Landing zone (helicopter)
ETA	Estimated time of arrival
Over	I am finished with my transmission
Mobile status	On the air, driving around
Stage	Wait before entering a scene
Clear	End of transmission
Unfounded	We cannot find the incident/patient
Be advised	Listen carefully to this

THE EMS RESPONSE

Your ability to communicate effectively during a stressful EMS response will determine the success or failure of your efforts. A brilliant assessment and management plan will be futile if you cannot communicate it to others. Dealing effectively with your patient and bystanders requires a variety of communication skills such as empathy, confidence, self-control, authority, and patience. Your clinical experience will suggest which skills to use in any particular situation. For example, you might use confidence and an authoritative posture when dealing with unruly bystanders. On the other hand, you would need to be gentle and empathetic with a child or an elderly grandmother. If you were in charge of an incident, you would have to communicate your authority within the structure of the emergency scene to providers from other responding agencies. Delegating tasks, listening to initial reports, and coordinating the scene require effective communication and interpersonal skills.

The sequence of an EMS response illustrates the importance of communications in prehospital care. A typical EMS response includes the following chain of events.

Detection and Citizen Access To begin the response to any emergency once it has occurred, someone must detect the problem and summon EMS (Figure 14-3). Any citizen with an urgent medical need should have a simple and reliable mechanism for accessing the EMS system. In the United States, most people access EMS by telephone; thus, a well-publicized universal telephone number such as 911 provides direct citizen access to the communications center. At enhanced 911 (E-911) communication centers, a computer displays the caller's telephone number and location. The centers also have instant call-back capabilities, should the caller hang up too soon. The 911 system has been available since the late 1960s. Currently, 96 percent of the population in the United States enjoy a 911 system. Highway call boxes, citizens band (CB) radio, and amateur radio all provide alternate means of accessing emergency help in some regions.

Calls to 911 usually connect the caller to a public safety answering point (**PSAP**), which then directs the caller to the appropriate agency for dispatch and response. In some systems, the PSAP call taker will elicit the information and

> *A brilliant assessment and management plan will be futile if you cannot communicate it to others.*
>

Content Review

EMS RESPONSE COMMUNICATIONS

- Detection and citizen access
- Call taking and emergency response
- Prearrival instructions
- Call coordination and incident recording
- Discussion with medical direction physician
- Transfer communications
- Back in service, ready for next call

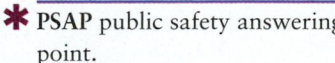 **PSAP** public safety answering point.

determine the nature of the response. In others, he will simply answer with the question, "Is this a police, fire, or medical emergency?" and transfer the caller to the appropriate dispatcher, who will then elicit the information. Many systems use computerized technology at the PSAP to connect the caller automatically with the appropriate agency. Some even provide language translation. Future global positioning systems will allow the dispatcher to pinpoint a cellular-phone caller's location. Additionally, automakers are installing communications computers in some automobiles. When involved in an accident, these "black boxes" automatically will provide the dispatcher with the location, speed, type of collision, projected damage, and suspected severity of injury.

In some systems, all public safety agencies are located within the same facility. In others, they are connected electronically. No one way is best. If the public receives timely, appropriate responses to all emergency calls, the system is effective.

Call Taking and Emergency Response The emergency medical dispatcher (**EMD**) is the public's first contact with the EMS system and plays a crucial role in every EMS response. The most important information the call taker must obtain is the address of the incident, the caller's name, the call-back number, and other pertinent factors. Ideally, he also will ascertain the nature of the emergency and other pertinent factors.

In a coordinated system known as **priority dispatching,** medical dispatchers interrogate a distressed caller using a set of medically-approved questions to elicit essential information about the chief complaint (Figure 14-4). Then, the dispatcher follows established guidelines to determine the appropriate level of response (Figure 14-5). These predetermined guidelines are based on criteria approved by the medical director. For example, an elderly man with a history of heart problems who is complaining of chest pain radiating to his left arm may indicate a priority-one response (life-threatening emergency, lights and siren). In some systems, the appropriate response may include a fire-department basic-life-support first responding unit, a paramedic engine company, and a transporting ambulance. Other systems may require only a paramedic ambulance. This form of call-screening, when done appropriately, saves time and money because only the necessary re-

✱ **EMD** emergency medical dispatcher.

✱ **priority dispatching** system using medically-approved questions and predetermined guidelines to determine the appropriate level of response.

FIGURE 14-4 Priority dispatching and pre-arrival medical instruction have enhanced the efficiency of the EMS system.

FIGURE 14-5 The dispatcher determines the appropriate level of response according to established guidelines.

sources are sent. It also limits the liability associated with lights and siren response to possible life-threatening incidents. Many private and public EMS systems throughout the United States use the priority dispatching system.

Prearrival Instructions Many EMS systems provide **prearrival instructions,** a service that is considered the standard of care. Prearrival instructions complement the call screening process in a priority dispatch system. As the dispatcher sends the appropriate response, the caller remains on the line and receives prearrival instructions for suitable emergency measures such as cardiopulmonary resuscitation or hemorrhage control. During prearrivals, the dispatcher also can obtain further information for the responding units. In the case of cardiac arrest, the dispatcher can relay information concerning the presence of a living will, a "Do Not Resuscitate" (DNR) form, or other advanced directives. In another case, a unit en route to a baby who had stopped breathing could reduce their response speed if they learned that the child had started breathing and was conscious. Prearrival instructions have saved many lives since 1974. They also are useful for comforting a distressed caller or providing emotional support to bystanders, family members, or the patient himself.

 prearrival instructions dispatcher's instructions to caller for appropriate emergency measures.

Call Coordination and Incident Recording After sending the appropriate response and providing prearrival instructions, the emergency medical dispatcher's main duties are support and coordination. He will provide the responding units with any additional resources needed and record information about the call such as times, locations, and units involved. Your dispatcher can be your best friend. He can assign the resources you need to manage an incident—additional medical personnel to help with a cardiac arrest, for instance, or the fire department to provide specialized rescue. He also may facilitate communication with other agencies, hospitals, communication centers, and support services.

Discussion with Medical Direction Physician After conducting your assessment and initiating care as outlined by your local protocols, you will contact the medical direction physician to discuss the case. Following consultation, he may give you further orders for interventions such as medications or other medical procedures. The many ways to conduct this communication include the radio, telephone, and cellular phone. Taping these communications for use later is advisable. For example, if a discrepancy arose as to your orders, you could always refer to the tape, which never lies. At this point, you continue treatment and prepare your patient for transport. You will contact your dispatcher, who will record when you leave the scene and when you arrive at your destination.

Transmitting clear, concise, controlled reports will encourage your medical direction physicians to trust your assessments and on-scene treatment plans.

Your professional relationship with your medical direction physicians must be based on trust. Transmitting clear, concise, controlled reports will encourage your medical direction physicians to accept your assessments and on-scene treatment plans. Your ability to communicate effectively on the radio will cast a large part of your professional reputation. The general radio procedures and standard format sections later in this chapter offer guidelines for communicating with your medical direction physician and transmitting patient information (Figure 14-6).

Never leave your patient until you formally transfer responsibility for his care.

Transfer Communications As you transfer care of your patient to the receiving facility staff, you must give the receiving nurse or physician a formal verbal briefing (Figure 14-7). This report should include your patient's vital information, chief complaint and history, physical exam findings, and any treatments rendered. Do not assume that the receiving nurse heard your radio report and knows of your patient. Some systems require the receiving nurse to sign the prehospital care report (PCR) to verify and document the transfer of care. In any case, never leave your patient until you have completed some type of formal transfer of care, because you may be charged with abandonment. Many systems likewise require the medical direction physician to sign the PCR for any medications administered by paramedics, especially if they included controlled substances such as morphine or diazepam. In all cases, end your documentation with transfer of care information on your PCR.

FIGURE 14-6 You will discuss each case with the medical direction physician and follow his instructions for patient care.

COMMUNICATION TECHNOLOGY

EMS systems can use all of today's various communication technologies. These include the more traditional forms of radio communication as well as innovations in radio technology and other media.

RADIO COMMUNICATION

Many types of radio transmission are possible, with new technologies being developed every day. Usage may vary from system to system. This section discusses some of the more common technologies in use today.

Simplex The most basic communications systems use **simplex** transmissions. These systems transmit and receive on the same frequency and thus cannot do both simultaneously (Figure 14-8). After you transmit a message, you must release the transmit button and wait for a response. This slows communication because you have to wait for all traffic to stop before you can speak. It also makes the system more formal and prevents open discussion. Simplex communication systems are most effective on the scene, when the incident commander or EMS dispatcher must transmit orders or directions without interruption. Most dispatch systems and on-scene communications use simplex transmissions.

✱ **simplex** communication system that transmits and receives on the same frequency.

FIGURE 14-8 Simplex communications systems transmit and receive on the same frequency.

FIGURE 14-9 Duplex communications systems use two frequencies for each channel.

Portable unit

Voice and ECG
(not at same time)

Frequency 1

Voice

Frequency 2

Base station

✱ **duplex** communication system that allows simultaneous two-way communications by using two frequencies for each channel.

Duplex Duplex transmissions allow simultaneous two-way communications by using two frequencies for each channel (Figure 14-9). Each radio must be able to transmit and receive on each channel. For example, on channel one, a hospital base station might transmit on 468.000 megahertz (MHz) and receive on 478.000 MHz. Field radios would then transmit on 478.000 MHz and receive on 468.000 MHz—just the opposite. Either party could then transmit and receive on the same channel simultaneously.

Duplex systems work like telephone communications. Many areas use them for communications between the field paramedic and the medical direction physician. The duplex system's major advantage is that one party does not have to wait to speak until the other party finishes his transmission. This allows a much freer discussion and consultation between physician and paramedic. For example, the medical direction physician can interrupt your report with an important question or concern. On the other hand, this ability to interrupt can be a disadvantage when abused.

Duplex systems all allow you to transmit either voice messages or data such as ECG strips.

✱ **multiplex** duplex system that can transmit voice and data simultaneously.

Multiplex Multiplex systems are duplex systems with the additional capability of transmitting voice and data simultaneously (Figure 14-10). This enables you to carry on a conversation with the medical direction physician while you are transmitting an ECG strip. Speaking while you are transmitting the ECG strip, however, causes much interference on the ECG strip.

✱ **trunking** communication system that pools all frequencies and routes transmissions to the next available frequency.

Trunking Many communications systems operating in the 800 MHz range use **trunking** to hasten communications. Trunked systems pool all frequencies. When a radio transmission comes in, a computer routes it to the first available frequency. The computer routes the next transmission to the next available frequency, and so on. When a transmission terminates, that fre-

FIGURE 14-10 Multiplex systems can transmit voice and data at the same time.

quency becomes available and reenters the pool of unused frequencies. Trunking thus frees the dispatcher or field unit from having to search for an available frequency.

Digital Communications Voice transmission can be time-consuming and difficult to understand. The trend toward combining radio technology with computer technology has encouraged a shift from voice (analog) to **digital communications.** Digital radio equipment is becoming increasingly popular in emergency services communication systems. This technology translates, or encodes, sounds into digital code for broadcast. Digital transmission is much faster and much more accurate than analog transmission. Since the messages are transmitted in condensed form, they help to ease the overcrowding of radio frequencies. Also, because you need a decoder to translate digital transmissions back into voice, scanners cannot monitor them. Your communications, therefore, are considerably more secure than over the radio. Many cellular phone companies now use digital transmissions. Future technology will link patient-monitoring devices to a small computer equipped with a radio for transmission.

The **mobile data terminals** in many emergency vehicles are a basic form of digital communications. They are mounted in the vehicle cab and wired to the radio. When a data transmission such as the address of the incident comes in, the terminal displays the message on a screen or prints it in hard copy. Responders can reply by punching a button to send a message such as "en route," "arrived," or "transporting to the hospital." Though somewhat restrictive and primitive, these terminals have reduced on-air time to a minimum even in the busiest systems. It is important to remember, however, that voice communications will always have a place in emergency services. Crews will always need to speak to one another, to physicians and nurses, or to dispatchers.

ALTERNATIVE TECHNOLOGIES

Among the more common alternatives to radio communications are the cellular telephone, the facsimile machine, and the computer.

Cellular Telephone Many EMS systems have found that **cellular telephones** are a cost-effective way to transmit essential patient information to the hospital (Figure 14-11). Cellular technology is available in even the most remote areas of the country. A cellular telephone service is divided into regions called cells. These cells are radio base stations, with which the mobile telephone communicates. When the transmission leaves one cell's range, another cell picks it up immediately, without interruption.

Like duplex radio transmissions, cellular phones make communication less formal, promote discussion, and reduce on-line times. They further allow the medical direction physician to speak directly with the patient and offer the further advantages of being widely available and highly reliable. Because the ECG signal is digitized, the hospital receives a better signal than if it were transmitted over radio waves. The telephones themselves are inexpensive, but cellular telephone systems charge a monthly fee for their use. Their major disadvantage is that each cell can handle only a limited number of calls. Geography can interfere with the cellular telephone's signals, and in large metropolitan areas the cells often fill up and become unavailable, especially during peak hours. Other disadvantages are that anyone with a scanner can monitor conversations on analog cellular phones; cellular phones require an external antenna; and the cellular phone system will deny access to a cell if you do not know or forget the personal identification number (PIN). Despite their limitations, cellular telephones have become a popular medium for dispatching, on-scene, and medical direction communications.

* **digital communications** data or sounds are translated into a digital code for transmission.

* **mobile data terminal** vehicle-mounted computer keyboard and display.

* **cellular telephone system** telephone system divided into regions, or cells, that are served by radio base stations.

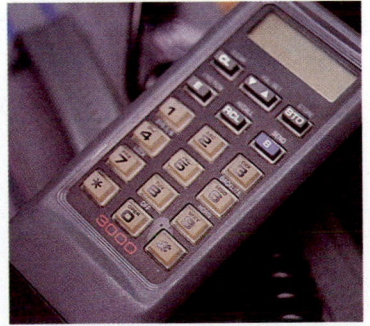

FIGURE 14-11   Cellular telephones have made it possible to transmit high quality facsimiles, computer data, and 12-lead ECGs.

Facsimile A **facsimile machine** (fax) provides a quick way to send printed information. This machine "reads" the printed information, digitizes it line-by-line, and transmits it to another machine, which then decodes it and prints a facsimile of the original. A fax machine enables health care agencies to exchange medical information immediately. Future systems will allow EMS responders to access a patient's medical record from a general data base; responders or database operators will be able to send the same information to the receiving facility. With some electronic run sheet systems, you will be able to transmit your patient information to the receiving hospital long before you arrive. This technology's one obvious limitation is that both the sending and the receiving agency must have access to a fax machine and a telephone line.

Computer Computers have entered every aspect of our daily lives. In emergency services communications, they have revolutionized system management and incident data collection. Most dispatchers no longer enter data via pen and pencil, time stamping machines, or typewriters. They can make a permanent record of any incident's events in real time. Computers also make research faster and easier. For example, if you wanted to determine the day of the week when most cardiac calls happen, or what time of day is busiest, or which area of a city needs more coverage, you could retrieve the pertinent data from your computerized records immediately. You can program your system to provide whatever type of data you want, in whatever format you desire. It also eliminates the need to enter retrospective data when conducting research. For example, the times, locations, and particulars of a call already will be in the computer files for immediate retrieval during a research project. A computer's limitations include its own power, speed, and capacity, as well as its operator's ability. Also, rigidly programmed machines that function only in certain restrictive ways can limit your flexibility.

NEW TECHNOLOGY

New technology is being developed every day. The National Aeronautics and Space Administration (NASA) has pioneered communications that allow television viewers to hear and see astronauts in space. Ground crews can monitor each astronaut's biological function and maintain a permanent record throughout the trip. And they have been doing this for decades.

In comparison to other industries, public safety communication systems are nearly archaic. Most EMS agencies still document patient assessment and care with hand-written run sheets, and some use radio equipment so old that replacement tubes are no longer available. But times are changing rapidly. Time constraints, storage space, and congested radio traffic necessitate developing new systems that will allow paramedics to transmit, receive, and store vital patient information quickly and reliably. Someday computer-based technology, digital satellite transmission, and electronic storage and retrieval of patient information will replace radio communications, written documentation, and file cabinets filled with EMS run sheets. These technologies are costly, but they already exist.

Current documentation systems already allow you to record all aspects of your EMS response electronically, by use of a **touch pad**. With pen-based reporting systems you can record patient information on a handheld computer. These systems do away with written documentation and capture information in real time, eliminating your need to estimate times after the call. Some systems integrate diagnostic technology and enable you to transmit ECG and pulse oximetry readings to the hospital before arrival. Such advanced knowledge of diagnostic test results from the field may radically change a medical direction physician's decisions and reduce the time needed to make an in-hospital diagnosis and begin therapy. Transmitting a 12-lead ECG, for example, will reduce the time before paramedics in transit or receiving emergency department personnel can begin cardiac muscle-saving thrombolytic therapy for the patient with a suspected myocardial infarction. In some cases paramedics will be able to start therapy en route. Other systems allow you to receive important medical information from your patient's permanent record while on the scene or in transit. For instance, at the home of a patient with an altered mental status and no family to relate his history, you might access his medical records and attain his history via a computerized data base. In this type of system, the transferring facility, the receiving hospital, and you can all access this information simultaneously.

A disadvantage of electronic recording systems is the absence of a "paper record" of the incident, should the information be accidentally erased or destroyed. The legal guidelines that apply to written and spoken communication also apply to electronic reporting. You must maintain patient confidentiality, you must be objective, and you must not **slander** or **libel** another person.

REPORTING PROCEDURES

As a paramedic, you must effectively relay all relevant medical information to the receiving hospital staff. Initially, you might do this over the radio or by cellular telephone. Later, when you deliver your patient to the emergency department, you can give additional information in-person to the appropriate receiving hospital personnel.

One of your most important skills will be gathering essential patient information, organizing it, and relaying it to the medical direction physician. The medical direction physician will then issue appropriate orders for patient care. The amount and type of information you relay to the medical direction physician will depend on the type of technology you use, your patient's priority, and your local communication **protocols**. For example, if communications in your region are not secured (private) you must limit the type of information you can communicate without breaching patient confidentiality. The acuteness of your patient's clinical status and the amount of local radio traffic also may determine the length of your report. For a critical patient you may give a brief report while you tend to your patient's medical needs. For a complicated medical emergency, you may wish to communicate a greater share of the results of your history and physical exam to the medical direction physician.

STANDARD FORMAT

Communicating patient information to the hospital or to the medical direction physician is a crucial function within the EMS system. Verbal communications, which may occur via radio or land-line, give the hospital enough information on your patient's condition to prepare for his care. These communications also should initiate the medical orders you need to treat your patient in the field. A standard format for transmitting patient assessment information helps to achieve those goals in several ways. First, it adds to the medical communications system's efficiency. Second, it helps the physician to assimilate information about the patient's condition quickly. Third, it assures that medical information is complete. In general, your verbal reports to medical direction should include the following information:

- Identification of unit and provider
- Description of scene
- Patient's age, sex, and approximate weight (for drug orders)
- Patient's chief complaint and severity

---

* **slander** to orally defame another person.

* **libel** to defame another person in writing.

One of your most important skills will be gathering essential patient information, organizing it, and relaying it to the medical direction physician.

* **protocol** predetermined, written guidelines for patient care.

- Brief, pertinent history of the present illness or injury (OPQRST)
- Pertinent past medical history, medications, and allergies (SAMPLE)
- Pertinent physical exam findings
- Treatment given so far/request for orders
- Estimated time of arrival at the hospital
- Other pertinent information

The formats and contents of reports for medical and trauma patients differ to include only the information relevant to either type of emergency. Reports for medical patients emphasize the history in the beginning of the report; reports for trauma patients emphasize the injuries and the physical exam.

After transmitting your report, you will await further questions and orders from the medical direction physician. Upon arrival, your spoken report will give essential patient information to the provider assuming care. It should include a brief history, pertinent physical findings, treatment, and responses to that treatment.

GENERAL RADIO PROCEDURES

Using the radio properly will make your communications skillful and efficient. All of your transmissions must be clear and crisp, with concise, professional content (Figure 14-12). Always follow these guidelines for effective radio use:

1. Listen to the channel before transmitting to assure that it is not in use.
2. Press the transmit button for one second before speaking.
3. Speak at close range, approximately two–three inches, directly into, or across the face of, the microphone.
4. Speak slowly and clearly. Pronounce each word distinctly, avoiding words that are difficult to understand.
5. Speak in a normal pitch, keeping your voice free of emotion.
6. Be brief. Know what you are going to say before you press the transmit button.
7. Avoid codes unless they are part of your EMS system.
8. Do not waste air time with unnecessary information.

FIGURE 14-12 The professionalism of your communications reflects on the professionalism of your patient care.

9. Protect your patient's privacy. When appropriate:
   - Use telephone rather than radio.
   - Turn off external speaker.
   - Do not use your patient's name; doing so violates FCC regulations.
10. Use proper unit or hospital numbers, and correct names or titles.
11. Do not use slang or profanity.
12. Use standard formats for transmission.
13. Be concise in order to hold the attention of the person receiving your radio report.
14. Use the **echo procedure** when receiving directions from the dispatcher or orders from the physician. Immediately repeating each statement will confirm accurate reception and understanding.
15. Always write down addresses, important dispatch communications, and physician orders.
16. When completing a transmission, obtain confirmation that your message was received and understood.

Occasionally, communications equipment will not function properly. Even a weak battery can disrupt clear communication. If you are far from the base station, particularly if you have a portable radio, try to broadcast from higher terrain. Structures that contain steel and concrete can interfere with radio transmission. Simply moving outside the building or near a window may improve communications. If that does not work, try to telephone.

> **✱ echo procedure** immediately repeating each transmission received during radio communications.

MODEL VERBAL REPORTS

The following examples demonstrate professional verbal reports for a medical patient and for a trauma patient. Neither report takes more than forty-five seconds, and each gives the medical direction physician enough information to make an initial diagnosis and prepare for arrival. As you read them, consider how they follow the principles of effective communication discussed throughout this chapter, and note their differences in format and information.

Medical Patient

Paramedic Identification:	This is NAVAC ambulance 4, Paramedic Smith.
Patient Identification:	We have a 63-year-old, 70-kg alert male, patient of Dr. Welby.
Subjective Data:	He complains of sudden onset of substernal chest pain radiating to the neck for the past half hour. He also complains of shortness of breath and nausea. He has a past history of cardiac problems and takes nitroglycerin, Isordil, and Procardia XL.
Objective Data:	He appears in moderate distress at this time, clutching his chest, but able to speak in full sentences. Vitals: BP—138/80; pulse—88 and regular; respirations 24 and slightly labored; skin warm and dry. He has clear lung sounds bilaterally, no JVD, peripheral edema or ascites. ECG shows

> **Content Review**
>
> **ELEMENTS OF MEDICAL PATIENT REPORT**
> - Paramedic identification
> - Patient identification
> - Subjective data
> - Objective data
> - Plan

sinus rhythm with an occasional unifocal PVC. Pulse oximetry is 92% on room air.

Plan: We have him on oxygen at 15 liters-per-minute via nonrebreather mask, we have a saline lock in place, and have given him 2 baby aspirin and 3 nitros with no relief. Request permission to administer 1–3 milligrams of morphine IV until relief of pain. Our ETA is 20 minutes.

Trauma Patient

Paramedic Identification: This is DeWitt Rescue 7, Paramedic Jones.

Patient Identification: We have a 23-year-old unresponsive female.

Mechanism of Injury: She was the unbelted driver in a high-speed, head-on one-car versus telephone pole accident with severe damage to the car and intrusion into the passenger compartment.

Injuries: She has a major head and chest trauma and shows signs of decompensated shock. Vitals are BP—76 by palpation; pulse—120 weak and regular, carotid only; respirations 40 and shallow; skin cool, pale, and clammy. She has a depressed skull fracture in the left parietal region, and a right-sided flail chest. Her pupils are unequal and slow to react, no drainage from the ears or nose, no Battle's sign or raccoon's eyes. Trachea is midline, no JVD. She shows paradoxical chest wall movement and is cyanotic with diminished lung sounds on the right side. Pulse oximetry is 88% on room air.

Plan: We have the patient fully immobilized, have stabilized the flail segment and are assisting ventilation with a bag-valve mask and supplemental oxygen. We have an IV of normal saline running wide open and are starting a second line. Our ETA is 20 minutes.

REGULATION

The **Federal Communications Commission** (FCC) controls and regulates all nongovernmental communications in the United States. This includes AM and FM radio, television, aircraft, marine, and mobile land frequency ranges. The FCC has designated frequencies within each radio band for special use. They include public safety frequencies in both the **very high frequency** band (VHF) and the ultrahigh frequency band (UHF). The FCC's primary functions include:

* Licensing and allocating radio frequencies.
* Establishing technical standards for radio equipment.
* Licensing and regulating the technical personnel who repair and operate radio equipment.

✳ **Federal Communications Commission** agency that controls all nongovernmental communications in the United States.

✳ **very high frequency** radio frequency band from 30 to 300 megahertz

- Monitoring frequencies to assure appropriate usage.
- Spot-checking base stations and dispatch centers for appropriate licenses and records.

The FCC requires all EMS communications systems to follow appropriate governmental regulations and laws. You must stay abreast of and obey any FCC regulations that apply to your communications.

SUMMARY

As one of the fundamental aspects of prehospital care, accurate communications help ensure an EMS system's efficiency. Communications begin when the citizen accesses the EMS system and end when you complete your patient report. Your spoken messages must be understandable, and your written messages must be legible. All of your communications must be concise and complete and conform to national and local protocols. The more sophisticated and advanced your EMS system grows, the more sophisticated and advanced its communications—and, accordingly, your communications skills—must become.

CHAPTER 15

Documentation

Objectives

After reading this chapter, you should be able to:

1. Identify the general principles regarding the importance of EMS documentation and ways in which documents are used. (pp. 789–791)
2. Identify and properly use medical terminology, medical abbreviations, and acronyms. (pp. 792, 794–797)
3. Explain the role of documentation in agency reimbursement. (p. 790)
4. Identify and eliminate extraneous or nonprofessional information. (p. 802)
5. Describe the differences between subjective and objective elements of documentation. (pp. 802–804)
6. Evaluate a finished document for errors and omissions and proper use and spelling of abbreviations and acronyms. (pp. 799, 801–802)
7. Evaluate the confidential nature of an EMS report. (p. 812)
8. Describe the potential consequences of illegible, incomplete, or inaccurate documentation. (pp. 799, 801–802)

Continued

INTRODUCTION

In this age of litigation, treating your patient and documenting his care are separate but equally important duties. Your written **prehospital care report** (**PCR**) is the only truly factual record of events. When written correctly it accurately describes your assessment and care throughout the emergency call. It documents exactly what you did, when you did it, and the effects of your interventions. It can be your best friend or your worst enemy in a court proceeding.

Your PCR is your sole permanent, complete written record of events during the ambulance call. The dispatch center may have a record of the call times and audio tapes of radio transmissions, and your patient will have his memory of the call. You and other responders also may have some recollections about the call. Your PCR, however, will always be considered the most comprehensive and reliable record of the event. In addition, it reflects your professionalism. A well-written, thorough PCR suggests a thorough, efficient assessment and quality care. A sloppy, incomplete PCR suggests sloppy, inefficient care.

Document exactly what you did, when you did it, and the effects of your interventions.

* **Prehospital Care Report PCR** the written record of an EMS response.

Your PCR reflects your professionalism.

USES FOR DOCUMENTATION

Your PCR will be a valuable resource for a variety of people. They include medical professionals, EMS administrators, researchers, and occasionally, lawyers.

MEDICAL

Hospital staff (nurses and physicians) may need more information from you than they can get before you have to take another call. For example, they may want a chronological account of your patient's mental status from the time you arrived on the scene. Your PCR can tell the emergency department staff of your patient's condition before he arrived at the hospital. It serves as a baseline for comparing assessment findings and detecting trends that indicate improvement or deterioration. The surgical staff will want to know the mechanism of injury and other pertinent findings during your initial assessment of your patient and the scene.

If your patient is admitted to the hospital, the floor or intensive care unit staff may need more information about his original condition than he can remember. In addition, your PCR provides them with information from people at the scene to whom they might not have access—family, bystanders, first responders, or other witnesses. Knowing about the circumstances that led to the event or the mechanism of injury may also help rehabilitation specialists to provide better therapy. Your PCR becomes an important document that helps ensure your patient's continuous effective care (Figure 15-1).

ADMINISTRATIVE

EMS administrators must gather information for quality improvement and system management. Information regarding **response times,** call location, the use of lights and siren, and date and time is vital to evaluating your system's readiness to respond to life threatening emergencies. It also is essential to providing information of community needs. The quality improvement or quality assurance committee will use PCRs to identify problems with individual paramedics or with the EMS system. In some agencies, the billing department will need to determine which services are billable. Insurance carriers may need to know more about the illness or injury to process the claim. Some states will use your PCR data to allocate funding for regional systems.

Your PCR is an important document that helps ensure your patient's continuity of care.

* **response time** time elapsed from when a unit is alerted until it arrives on the scene.

Prehospital Care Report

Agency Name	ARLINGTON RESCUE

MILEAGE					
END	2 4 4 9 6
BEGIN	2 4 4 7 6
TOTAL	0 0 0 2 0

USE MILITARY TIMES	
CALL REC'D	0 7 0 5
ENROUTE	0 7 0 7
ARRIVED AT SCENE	0 7 1 9
FROM SCENE	0 7 3 8
AT DESTIN	0 7 5 4
IN SERVICE	0 8 1 0
IN QUARTERS	0 8 3 2

Dispatch Information: CARDIAC

Call Location: 124 CYPRUS ST 2nd FLOOR

CHECK ONE: ☑ Residence ☐ Health Facility ☐ Farm ☐ Indus. Facility ☐ Other Work Loc. ☐ Roadway ☐ Recreational ☐ Other

LOCATION CODE: 0 1 2 4

CALL TYPE AS REC'D
☑ Emergency
☐ Non-Emergency
☐ Stand-by

MECHANISM OF INJURY
☐ MVA (✓ seat belt used → N/A)
☐ Fall of _____ feet N/A
☐ Unarmed assault
☐ GSW
☐ Knife
☐ Machinery
☐ _____

FIGURE 15-1 The run data in a prehospital care report is vital to your agency's efforts to improve patient care.

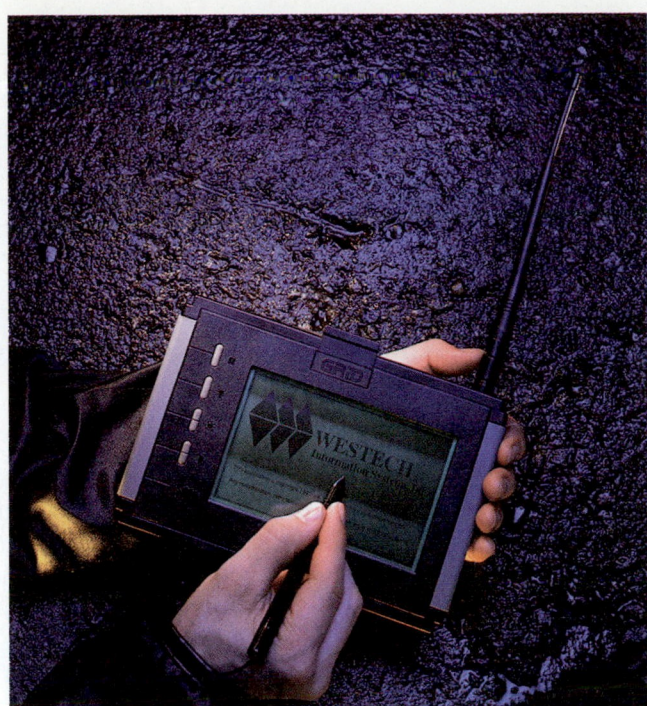

RESEARCH

Your PCR may give researchers useful data about many aspects of the EMS call. For example, they may analyze your recorded data to determine the efficacy of certain medical devices or interventions such as drugs and invasive procedures. They also may use the data to cut costs, alter staffing, and shorten response times. Some systems use computerized or electronic PCRs and a computerized database to analyze the data (Figure 15-2). Regardless of the method you use, your written documentation provides the basis for continuously improving patient care in your EMS system.

LEGAL

Your PCR becomes a permanent part of your patient's medical record. Lawyers may refer to it when preparing court actions, and in a legal proceeding it might be your sole source of information about the case. You may be called upon to testify in a case where your PCR becomes the central piece of evidence in your testimony. Or your PCR may serve as evidence in a criminal case and help determine the accused's innocence or guilt. Each state has its own laws regarding the length of time the hospital must keep its records.

Always write your PCR as if you knew you would have to refer to it someday in a court proceeding. Describe your patient's condition when you arrived and during your care, and note his status upon arrival at the hospital. Always document his condition before and after any interventions, and avoid writing any subjective opinions such as "the patient is intoxicated, obnoxious, and looks like a crack-addict." After your PCR is written, ask your partner to review it for completeness and accuracy. A complete, accurate, and objective account of the emergency call may be your best and only defense against a plaintiff's attorney who will try to find inconsistencies and ambiguities in your account.

Your PCR provides the basis for continuously improving patient care in your EMS system.

A complete, accurate, and objective account of the emergency call may be your best and only defense in court.

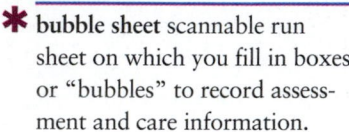
* **bubble sheet** scannable run sheet on which you fill in boxes or "bubbles" to record assessment and care information.

If you do not know how to spell a word, look it up or use another word.

You must be familiar with your local EMS system's acronyms and abbreviations.

Every EMS system has its own specific requirements for documentation. The type of call record used also varies from system to system. Some systems use reports with check boxes, some **bubble-sheets,** computer scannable reports on which you record patient information by filling in boxes or "bubbles" (Figure 15-3). Still others may use computerized documentation. The particular type of operational data collected, such as time intervals, will also differ among systems. For example, proprietary EMS agencies may require more billing information than community-based volunteer agencies. The general characteristics of a well-written PCR, though, remain constant among all agencies and systems.

MEDICAL TERMINOLOGY

An essential component of good documentation is the appropriate use of medical terminology. Medical terms, though sometimes difficult to spell, transform your report into a universally accepted medical document. Learning the meanings and correct spellings of the medical terms that you will use in your PCRs is essential. Misused or misspelled words reflect poorly on your professionalism and may confuse the report's readers.

If you do not know how to spell a word, look it up or use another word. Many paramedics carry pocket-size medical dictionaries in their ambulances for this purpose. Using "plain English" is acceptable when you do not know the appropriate medical term or its correct spelling. "Chest" is just as accurate as "thorax" and better than "thoracks." "Belly" is not as professional as "abdomen," but it is still better than "abodemin."

ABBREVIATIONS AND ACRONYMS

Medical abbreviations and acronyms allow you to increase the amount of information you can write quickly on your report (Table 15-1 on pages that follow). They also pose problems, however, because they can have multiple meanings. For instance, their meanings can vary in different areas of medicine. Is "CP" chest pain, cardiovascular perfusion, or cerebral palsy? Is "CO" cardiac output or carbon monoxide? Is "BLS" basic life support or burns, lacerations, and swelling? These are all common abbreviations with more than one accepted meaning. Furthermore, many abbreviations are specific to one community. You must be familiar with those used in your local EMS system.

Abbreviations and acronyms can cause considerable confusion when someone unfamiliar with the call reads your report. Health care professionals who are not familiar with local customs or with emergency medicine might not understand them. One way to clarify the meaning of a new abbreviation or acronym is to write it out the first time you use it, followed by the abbreviation or acronym in parenthesis. After that, you can use the abbreviation alone throughout the report. The following examples illustrate how abbreviations and acronyms can shorten your narratives. In standard English the report might be written:

> The patient is a 54-year-old conscious and alert male who complains of sudden onset of chest pain and shortness of breath which started 20 minutes ago. He has taken 2 nitroglycerin with no relief. He denies any nausea, vomiting, or dizziness. He has a past history of coronary artery disease, a heart attack 3 years ago, and high blood pressure. He takes nitroglycerin as needed, Procardia XL, hydrochlorothiazide, and potassium. He has no known drug allergies.

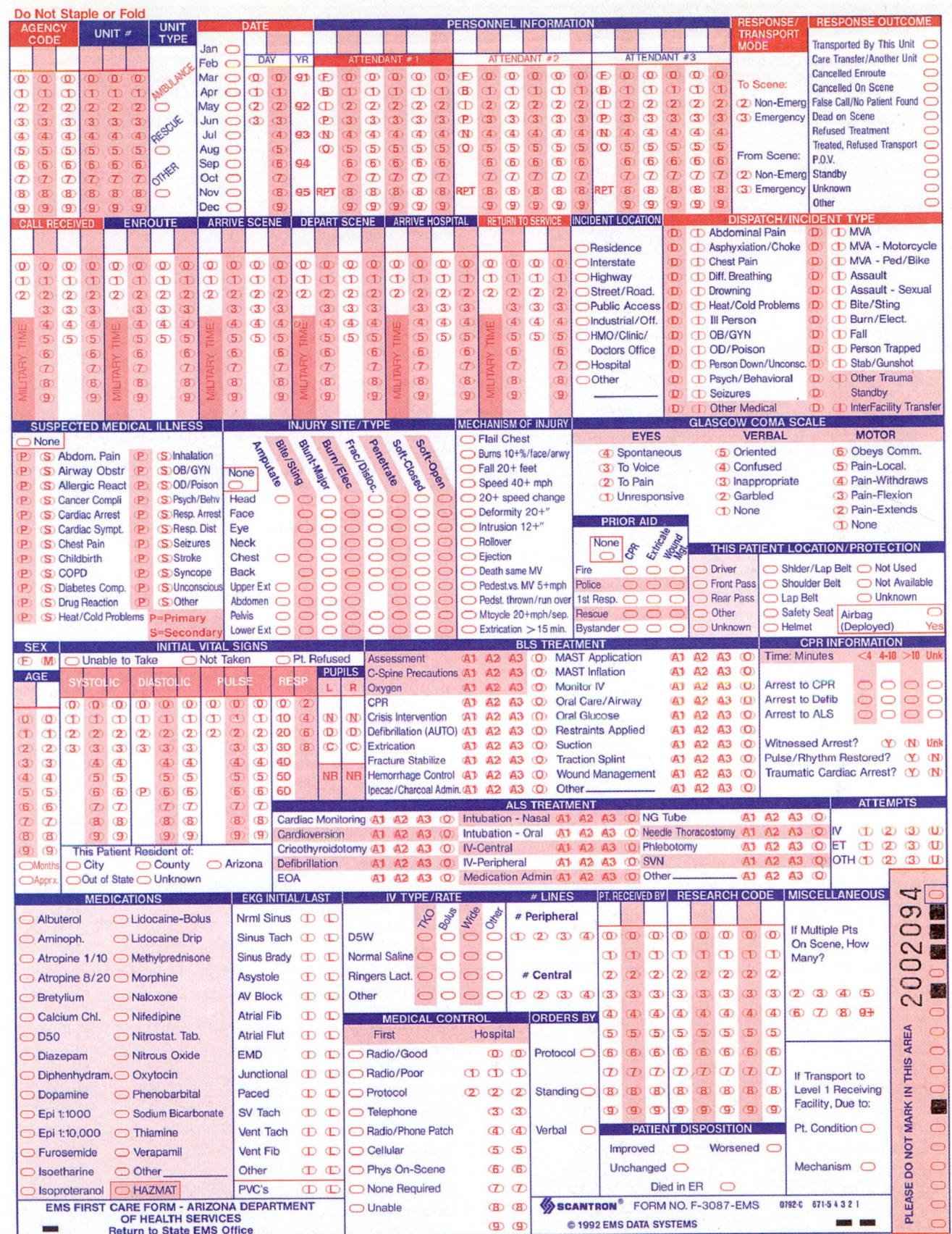

FIGURE 15-3 This prehospital care report's format allows a computer to scan its information.

Table 15-1 STANDARD CHARTING ABBREVIATIONS

Patient Information/Categories

Asian	A	Medications	Med
Black	B	Newborn	NB
Chief complaint	CC	Occupational history	OH
Complains of	c/o	Past history	PH
Current health status	CHS	Patient	Pt
Date of birth	DOB	Physical exam	PE
Differential diagnosis	DD	Private medical doctor	PMD
Estimated date of confinement	EDC	Review of systems	ROS
Family history	FH	Signs and symptoms	S/S
Female	♀	Social history	SH
Hispanic	H	Visual acuity	VA
History	Hx	Vital signs	VS
History and physical	H&P	Weight	Wt
History of present illness	HPI	White	W
Impression	IMP	Year-old	y/o
Male	♂		

Body Systems

Abdomen	Abd	Gynecological	GYN
Cardiovascular	CV	Head, eyes, ears, nose, and throat	HEENT
Central nervous system	CNS	Musculoskeletal	M/S
Ear, nose, and throat	ENT	Obstetrical	OB
Gastrointestinal	GI	Peripheral nervous system	PNS
Genitourinary	GU	Respiratory	Resp

Common Complaints

Abdominal pain	abd pn	Lower back pain	LBP
Chest pain	CP	Nausea/vomiting	n/v
Dyspnea on exertion	DOE	No apparent distress	NAD
Fever of unknown origin	FUO	Pain	pn
Gunshot wound	GSW	Shortness of breath	SOB
Headache	H/A	Substernal chest pain	sscp

Diagnoses

Abdominal aortic aneurysm	AAA	Insulin-dependent diabetes mellitus	IDDM
Abortion	Ab	Intracranial pressure	ICP
Acute myocardial infarction	AMI	Mass casualty incident	MCI
Adult respiratory distress syndrome	ARDS	Mitral valve prolapse	MVP
Alcohol	ETOH	Motor vehicle crash	MVC
Atherosclerotic heart disease	ASHD	Multiple sclerosis	MS
Chronic obstructive pulmonary disease	COPD	Non-insulin-dependent diabetes mellitus	NIDDM
Chronic renal failure	CRF	Organic brain syndrome	OBS
Congestive heart failure	CHF	Otitis media	OM
Coronary artery bypass graft	CABG	Overdose	OD
Coronary artery disease	CAD	Paroxysmal nocturnal dyspnea	PND
Cystic fibrosis	CF	Pelvic inflammatory disease	PID
Dead on arrival	DOA	Peptic ulcer disease	PUD
Delirium tremens	DTs	Pregnancies/Births (gravida/para)	G/P
Deep vein thrombosis	DVT	Pregnancy-induced hypertension	PIH
Diabetes mellitus	DM	Pulmonary embolism	PE
Dilation and Curettage	D&C	Rheumatic heart disease	RHD
Duodenal ulcer	DU	Sexually transmitted disease	STD
End-stage renal failure	ESRF	Transient ischemic attack	TIA
Epstein-Barr virus	EBV	Tuberculosis	TB
Foreign body obstruction	FBO	Upper respiratory infection	URI
Hepatitis B virus	HBV	Urinary tract infection	UTI
Hiatal hernia	HH	Venereal disease	VD
Hypertension	HTN	Wolff-Parkinson-White syndrome (disease)	WPW
Infectious disease	ID		
Inferior wall myocardial infarction	IWMI		

| Table 15-1 | STANDARD CHARTING ABBREVIATIONS (continued) |

Medications

Angiotensin-converting enzyme	ACE	Lactated Ringer's, Ringer's Lactate	LR, RL
Aspirin	ASA	Magnesium sulfate	Mg^{++}
Bicarbonate	HCO_3^-	Morphine sulfate	MS
Birth control pills	BCP	Nitroglycerin	NTG
Calcium	Ca^{++}	Nonsteroidal antiflammatory agent	NSAID
Calcium channel blocker	CCB	Normal saline	NS
Calcium chloride	$CaCl_2$	Penicillin	PCN
Chloride	Cl^-	Phenobarbital	PB
Digoxin	Dig	Potassium	K^+
Dilantin (phenytoin sodium)	DPH	Sodium bicarbonate	$NaHCO_3$
Diphendydramine	DPHM	Sodium chloride	NaCl
Diphtheria-Pertussis-Tetanus	DPT	Tylenol	APAP
Hydrochlorothiazide	HCTZ		

Anatomy/Landmarks

Abdomen	Abd	Lymph node	LN
Antecubital	AC	Medial collateral ligament	MCL
Anterior axillary line	AAL	Metacarpalphalangeal (joint)	MCP
Anterior cruciate ligament	ACL	Metatarsalphalangeal (joint)	MTP
Anterior-posterior	A/P	Midaxillary line	MAL
Distal interphalangeal (joint)	DIP	Posterior axillary line	PAL
Dorsalis pedis (pulse)	DP	Posterior cruciate ligament	PCL
Gallbladder	GB	Proximal interphalangeal (joint)	PIP
Intercostal space	ICS	Right lower lobe	RLL
Lateral collateral ligament	LCL	Right lower quadrant	RLQ
Left lower lobe	LLL	Right middle lobe	RML
Left lower quadrant	LLQ	Right upper lobe	RUL
Left upper lobe	LUL	Right upper quadrant	RUQ
Left upper quadrant	LUQ	Temporomandibular joint	TMJ
Left ventricle	LV	Tympanic membrane	TM
Liver, spleen, and kidneys	LSK		

Physical Exam/Findings

Arterial blood gas	ABG	Hemoglobin	Hgb
Bilateral breath sounds	BBS	Inspiratory	Insp
Blood sugar	BS	Jugular venous distention	JVD
Breath sounds	BS	Laceration	lac
Cardiac injury profile	CIP	Level of consciousness	LOC
Central venous pressure	CVP	Moves all extremities (well)	MAEW
Cerebrospinal fluid	CSF	Nontender	NT
Chest X-ray	CXR	Normal range of motion	NROM
Complete blood count	CBC	Palpation	Palp
Computerized tomography	CT	Passive range of motion	PROM
Conscious, alert, and oriented	CAO	Point of maximal impulse	PMI
Costovertebral angle	CVA	Posterior tibial (pulse)	PT
Deep tendon reflexes	DTR	Pulse	P
Dorsalis pedis (pulse)	DP	Pupils equal and reactive to light	PEARL
Electrocardiogram	EKG, ECG	Pupils equal, round, reactive to light	
Electroencephalogram	EEG	and accomodation	PERRLA
Expiratory	Exp	Range of motion	ROM
Extraocular movements (intact)	EOMI	Respirations	R
Fetal heart tones	FHT	Tactile vocal fremitus	TVF
Full range of motion	FROM	Temperature	T
Full term normal delivery	FTND	Unconscious	unc
Heart rate	HR	Urinary incontinence	UI
Heart sounds	HS		
Heel-to-shin (cerebellar test)	H→S		

Table 15-1   STANDARD CHARTING ABBREVIATIONS (continued)

Miscellaneous Descriptors

After (post-)	p̄	Not applicable	n/a
After eating	pc	Number	No or #
Alert and oriented	A/O	Occasional	occ
Anterior	ant.	Pack years	pk/yrs, p/y
Approximate	≈	Per	/
As needed	prn	Positive	+
Before (ante-)	ā	Posterior	post.
Before eating (*ante cibum,* before meal)	a.c.	Postoperative	PO
Body surface area (%)	BSA	Prior to arrival	PTA
Celsius	C°	Radiates to	→
Change	Δ	Right	Ⓡ
Decreased	↓	Rule out	R/O
Equal	=	Secondary to	2°
Fahrenheit	F°	Superior	sup.
Immediately	stat	Times (for 3 hours)	× (×3h)
Increased	↑	Unequal	≠
Inferior	inf.	Warm and dry	W/D
Left	Ⓛ	While awake	WA
Less than	<	With (*cum*)	c̄
Moderate	mod.	Within normal limits (*or* we never looked)	WNL
More than	>	Without (*sine*)	s̄
Negative	−	Zero	0
No, not, none	Ø		

Treatments/Dispositions

Advanced cardiac life support	ACLS	Nasogastric	NG
Advanced life support	ALS	Nasopharyngeal airway	NPA
Against medical advice	AMA	No transport—refusal	NTR
Automated external defibrillator	AED	Nonrebreather mask	NRM
Bag-valve mask	BVM	Nothing by mouth	NPO
Basic life support	BLS	Occupational therapy	OT
Cardiopulmonary resuscitation	CPR	Oropharyngeal airway	OPA
Carotid sinus massage	CSM	Oxygen	O₂
Continuous positive airway pressure	CPAP	Per square inch	psi
Do not resuscitate	DNR	Physical therapy	PT
Endotracheal tube	ETT	Positive end-expiratory pressure	PEEP
Estimated time of arrival	ETA	Short spine board	SSB
External cardiac pacing	ECP	Therapy	Rx
Intermittent positive-pressure ventilation	IPPV	Treatment	Tx
Long spine board	LSB	Turned over to	TOT
Nasal cannula	NC	Verbal order	VO

Medication Administration/Metrics

Centimeter	cm	Kilogram	kg
Cubic centimeter	cc	Liter	L
Deciliter	dL	Liters per minute	LPM, L/min
Drop(s)	gtt(s)	Microgram	mcg
Drops per minute	gtts/min	Milliequivalent	mEq
Every	q	Milligram	mg
Grain	gr	Milliliter	ml
Gram	g, gm	Millimeter	mm
Hour	h, hr, or °	Millimeters of mercury	mmHg
Hydrogen-ion concentration	pH	Minute	min
Intracardiac	IC	Orally	po
Intramuscular	IM	Subcutaneous	SC, SQ
Intraosseous	IO	Sublingual	SL
Intravenous	IV	To keep open	TKO
Intravenous push	IVP		
Joules	j		
Keep vein open	KVO		

Table 15-1   STANDARD CHARTING ABBREVIATIONS (continued)

Cardiology

Atrial fibrillation	AF	Paroxysmal atrial tachycardia	PAT
Atrial tachycardia	AT	Paroxysmal supraventricular tachycardia	PSVT
Atrioventricular	AV	Premature atrial contraction	PAC
Bundle branch block	BBB	Premature junctional contraction	PJC
Complete heart block	CHB	Premature ventricular contraction	PVC
Electromechanical dissociation	EMD	Pulseless electrical activity	PEA
Idioventricular rhythm	IVR	Supraventricular tachycardia	SVT
Junctional rhythm	JR	Ventricular fibrillation	VF
Modified chest lead	MCL	Ventricular tachycardia	VT
Normal sinus rhythm	NSR	Wandering atrial pacemaker	WAP

Using abbreviations and acronyms, the same report might be written:

Pt. is 54 y/o CAO male c/o sudden onset CP/SOB × 20 min. Pt took NTG × 2 s̄ relief. ∅ n/v, dizziness. PH: CAD, AMI × 3y, HTN. Meds: NTG prn, Procardia XL, HCTZ and K$^+$; NKDA.

TIMES

Incident times are another important but perilous part of the PCR. The times you record on your PCR are considered the official times of the incident. For medical and legal purposes, you must ensure their accuracy.

The PCR typically has spaces for the time the call was received, the dispatch time, the time of arrival at the scene, time of departure from the scene, time of arrival at the hospital, and time back in service. Other time intervals are important, as well. The time you and your crew arrived at the patient's side is often very different from the time the ambulance arrived at the scene—when your patient is on the fourth floor of a building without an elevator, for example, or in a field several hundred yards from the road. Whatever the reason, document in your report any significant discrepancies between your arrival at the scene and your arrival at the patient. The times of vital signs assessment, medication administration, certain medical procedures as local protocols require, and changes in patient condition are also important and require accurate documentation.

One common problem with documenting times is inconsistencies among the dispatch center clock, the ambulance clock, and your watch. Imagine a report that documents that the ambulance arrived on scene at 20:32 according to the dispatch time, that CPR was started at 20:29 according to your watch, and the first defibrillation was administered at 20:43 according to the defibrillator's internal clock. While we may recognize this phenomenon and tend to discount the accuracy of the recorded times, they are nonetheless the official, legal times. Whenever possible, therefore, record all times from the same clock. When that is not possible, be sure that all the clocks and watches you use are synchronized. If they cannot be synchronized and the documented times seem to conflict with each other, explain this in your narrative. A simple statement such as "All time intervals on the scene were documented using my watch, all other times are those reported by the dispatch center" will suffice.

Whenever possible, record all times from the same clock.

COMMUNICATIONS

Your communications with the hospital are another important item to document. Though your system may make voice recordings of those communications, the recordings are usually not kept indefinitely. Again, the PCR will likely be the only permanent record of your discussion with the medical direction physician. Specifically, you should document any medical advice or orders you receive and the results of implementing that advice and those orders. In some situations you might need to document what you reported to the physician and/or discussed with him, so the reader will be able to understand the decision-making process. Finally, always document the physician's name on your PCR and, if possible, have him sign it to verify your treatments.

Document any medical advice or orders you receive and the results of implementing that advice and those orders.

PERTINENT NEGATIVES

The patient assessment and medical interventions are the essence of the EMS event and become the core of your PCR. We will discuss specific approaches to documenting assessment and interventions later in this chapter, but some general rules apply regardless of the method.

Document all findings of your assessment, even those that are normal.

Document all findings of your assessment, even those that are normal. Although the positive findings are usually of most interest, some negative findings—known as pertinent negatives—are also important. For example, if your respiratory distress patient does not have swollen ankles or crackles, that helps rule out a field diagnosis of congestive heart failure. Or if your patient with a broken leg does not have loss of sensory or motor function, it suggests he has no serious neurologic injury. You should include such information in your report.

The pertinent negatives vary for each chief complaint. In general, if a positive assessment finding for any given chief complaint would be important, a negative finding probably is pertinent. Even though these findings do not warrant medical care or intervention, your seeking them demonstrates the thoroughness of your examination and history of the event.

ORAL STATEMENTS

Also essential to every PCR, regardless of approach, are the statements of witnesses, bystanders, and your patient. They help to document the mechanism of injury, your patient's behavior, the events leading up to the emergency, and any first aid or medical care others rendered before you arrived. They also may include information regarding the disposition of personal items such as wallets or purses. At crime scenes, document safety-related information such as weapons disposition. Your PCR may be the only written report of what happened to a murder weapon. Other details such as where you first saw a victim, what position he was in, and the time you arrived on the scene may be crucial evidence someday in a criminal proceeding.

Whenever possible, quote the patient—or other source of information—directly. Clearly identify the quotation with quotation marks, and identify its source. For example:

> Bystanders state the patient was "acting bizarre and threatening to jump in front of the next passing car."

ADDITIONAL RESOURCES

Document all of the resources involved in the event. If an air-medical service transported your patient, your documentation should include your assessment and all interventions up to the point when you transferred care. Identify the air-medical service and your patient's ultimate destination, if you know it. If other EMS, fire, rescue/extrication, or law enforcement agencies were involved in the call, document their roles. This can be particularly important in mutual aid calls, when many different agencies cooperate in your patient's care. Also include personnel from the coroner's or medical examiner's office for dead-on-arrival (DOA) scenes.

If a physician stops to help, identify him by name and document his qualifying credentials. If one of your medical direction physicians is on the scene and directs care, document his activities. Likewise document the names, credentials, and activities of any other medically qualified personnel present who offer to help. Your clinical experience and local protocols will determine how you integrate qualified health care workers into your emergency scene. Document that integration carefully.

ELEMENTS OF GOOD DOCUMENTATION

A well-written PCR is accurate, legible, timely, unaltered, and professional. Each of these traits is essential.

COMPLETENESS AND ACCURACY

The accurate PCR should be precise but comprehensive. Include all of the relevant information that anyone might be expected to want later, and exclude superfluous information. For example, if your patient's foot was run over by a lawn mower, reporting that his great toe on that foot had been amputated six years ago would be important; documenting that he had his tonsils removed when he was three years old probably would not. That you applied direct pressure to the bleeding foot is pertinent; that the lawn mower was a John Deere model 6354 is not.

Many PCRs provide check boxes and a space for written narratives (Figure 15-4). You should complete both the narrative and check-box sections of every PCR. All check-box sections of a document must show that you attended to them, even if you did not use a given section on a call. The check boxes can help to ensure that routine, common information is recorded for every call, but no PCR has a check box for every possible chief complaint, assessment finding, or intervention.

The narrative is the core of the documentation. Even if you document something in a check-box, repeating that information in the narrative might be worthwhile. By doing so, you can expand on the yes-or-no limitations of the check box to explain the timing, the assessment findings, the circumstances, or the changes in patient condition associated with the indicated action.

Remember that proper spelling, approved abbreviations, and proper acronyms also affect your PCR's accuracy. Misspelled words lose their meaning; many abbreviations are not universally recognized; and several acronyms have more than one meaning. Make sure that the meaning of any abbreviation or acronym is clear.

LEGIBILITY

Poor penmanship and illegible reports lead to poor documentation. Some EMS providers say, "I wrote it, and I can read it. That's all that matters." This is simply not true. The PCR does not exist solely for its author's reference. It is a permanent record that many different people use. Your handwriting must be neat enough that other people can read and understand the report—especially the narrative. It must also be neat enough that you can read and understand it yourself many years from now, long after the event has faded from your memory. Your writing must be heavy enough to transfer to any carbon copies. Using a ball-point pen whenever possible makes carbon copies more legible and makes it difficult for someone to tamper with the document. Clearly mark the check boxes to eliminate any doubt that a check mark is not just a meaningless scratch. Always remember that other members of the health care team may use the report for medical information, research, or quality improvement.

Your handwriting must be neat enough that other people can read and understand the report.

Prehospital Care Report
FOR BLS FR USE ONLY

Recycled Paper

M	D	Y		RUN NO.		AGENCY CODE	VEH. ID.

DATE OF CALL

Name

Address

Ph #

AGE | DOB M D Y | SEX M F

Physician

CARE IN PROGRESS ON ARRIVAL:
☐ None ☐ Citizen ☐ PD/FD/Other First Responder ☐ Other EMS

MECHANISM OF INJURY
☐ MVA (✓ seat belt used →) ☐ Fall of ____ feet ☐ GSW ☐ Machinery
☐ Struck by vehicle ☐ Unarmed assault ☐ Knife ☐ _____

Agency Name

Dispatch Information

Call Location

CHECK ONE ☐ Residence ☐ Health Facility ☐ Farm ☐ Indus. Facility
☐ Other Work Loc. ☐ Roadway ☐ Recreational ☐ Other

CALL TYPE AS REC'D.
☐ Emergency
☐ Non-Emergency
☐ Stand-by

COMPLETE FOR TRANSFERS ONLY
Transferred from ☐☐☐
☐ No Previous PCR
☐ Unknown if Previous PCR
Previous PCR Number ☐ - ☐☐☐☐☐

☐ Extrication required _____ minutes

Seat belt used? ☐ Yes ☐ No ☐ Unknown

Seat Belt Use Reported By ☐ Crew ☐ Patient ☐ Police ☐ Other

MILEAGE
END
BEGIN
TOTAL

LOCATION CODE

USE MILITARY TIMES
CALL REC'D
ENROUTE
ARRIVED AT SCENE
FROM SCENE
AT DESTIN
IN SERVICE
IN QUARTERS

CHIEF COMPLAINT

SUBJECTIVE ASSESSMENT

PRESENTING PROBLEM
If more than one checked, circle primary

☐ Airway Obstruction
☐ Respiratory Arrest
☐ Respiratory Distress
☐ Cardiac Related (Potential)
☐ Cardiac Arrest

☐ Allergic Reaction
☐ Syncope
☐ Stroke/CVA
☐ General Illness/Malaise
☐ Gastro-Intestinal Distress
☐ Diabetic Related (Potential)
☐ Pain _____

☐ Unconscious/Unresp.
☐ Seizure
☐ Behavioral Disorder
☐ Substance Abuse (Potential)
☐ Poisoning (Accidental)

☐ Other _____

☐ Shock
☐ Head Injury
☐ Spinal Injury
☐ Fracture/Dislocation
☐ Amputation

☐ Major Trauma
☐ Trauma-Blunt
☐ Trauma-Penetrating
☐ Soft Tissue Injury
☐ Bleeding/Hemorrhage

☐ OB/GYN
☐ Burns
Environmental
☐ Heat
☐ Cold
☐ Hazardous Materials
☐ Obvious Death

PAST MEDICAL HISTORY	V I T A L S I G N S	TIME	RESP	PULSE	B.P.	LEVEL OF CONSCIOUSNESS	GCS	R PUPILS L	SKIN	STATUS
☐ None ☐ Allergy to ___ ☐ Hypertension ☐ Stroke ☐ Seizures ☐ Diabetes ☐ COPD ☐ Cardiac ☐ Other (List) ☐ Asthma			Rate: ☐ Regular ☐ Shallow ☐ Labored	Rate: ☐ Regular ☐ Irregular		☐ Alert ☐ Voice ☐ Pain ☐ Unresp.		Normal Dilated Constricted Sluggish No-Reaction	☐ Unremarkable ☐ Cool ☐ Pale ☐ Warm ☐ Cyanotic ☐ Moist ☐ Flushed ☐ Dry ☐ Jaundiced	C U P S
			Rate: ☐ Regular ☐ Shallow ☐ Labored	Rate: ☐ Regular ☐ Irregular		☐ Alert ☐ Voice ☐ Pain ☐ Unresp.		Normal Dilated Constricted Sluggish No-Reaction	☐ Unremarkable ☐ Cool ☐ Pale ☐ Warm ☐ Cyanotic ☐ Moist ☐ Flushed ☐ Dry ☐ Jaundiced	C U P S
Current Medications (List)			Rate: ☐ Regular ☐ Shallow ☐ Labored	Rate: ☐ Regular ☐ Irregular		☐ Alert ☐ Voice ☐ Pain ☐ Unresp.		Normal Dilated Constricted Sluggish No-Reaction	☐ Unremarkable ☐ Cool ☐ Pale ☐ Warm ☐ Cyanotic ☐ Moist ☐ Flushed ☐ Dry ☐ Jaundiced	C U P S

OBJECTIVE PHYSICAL ASSESSMENT

COMMENTS

TREATMENT GIVEN

☐ Moved to ambulance on stretcher/backboard
☐ Moved to ambulance on stair chair
☐ Walked to ambulance
☐ Airway Cleared
☐ Oral/Nasal Airway
☐ Esophageal Obturator Airway/Esophageal Gastric Tube Airway (EOA/EGTA)
☐ EndoTracheal Tube (E/T)
☐ Oxygen Administered @ ___ L.P.M., Method _____
☐ Suction Used
☐ Artificial Ventilation Method _____
☐ C.P.R. in progress on arrival by: ☐ Citizen ☐ PD/FD/Other First Responder ☐ Other

☐ C.P.R. Started @ Time ▶ ☐☐☐☐   Time from Arrest Until C.P.R. ▶ ☐☐☐ Minutes
☐ EKG Monitored (Attach Tracing) [Rhythm(s) _____]

☐ Defibrillation/Cardioversion No. Times ☐ ☐ Manual ☐ Semi-automatic

☐ Medication Administered (Use Continuation Form)
☐ IV Established Fluid _____ Cath. Gauge ☐☐
☐ Mast Inflated @ Time _____)
☐ Bleeding/Hemorrhage Controlled (Method Used: _____)
☐ Spinal Immobilization Neck and Back
☐ Limb Immobilized by ☐ Fixation ☐ Traction
☐ (Heat) or (Cold) Applied
☐ Vomiting Induced @ Time ___ Method _____
☐ Restraints Applied, Type _____
☐ Baby Delivered @ Time ___ In County _____
   ☐ Alive ☐ Stillborn ☐ Male ☐ Female
☐ Transported in Trendelenburg position
☐ Transported in left lateral recumbent position
☐ Transported with head elevated
☐ Other _____

DISPOSITION (See list)

DISP. CODE ☐☐☐

CONTINUATION FORM USED YES ←

CREW	IN CHARGE	DRIVER'S NAME	NAME	NAME
	☐ EMT ☐ AEMT #	☐ CFR ☐ EMT ☐ AEMT #	☐ CFR ☐ EMT ☐ AEMT #	☐ CFR ☐ EMT ☐ AEMT #

© COPYRIGHT 1986 NEW YORK STATE DEPARTMENT OF HEALTH

AGENCY COPY/WHITE

EMS 100 (11/86) provided by NYS-EMS PROGRAM
DOH 3822 (6/94)

FIGURE 15-4 Complete both the narrative and check-box sections of every PCR.

The ~~left~~ *right pupil was fixed and dilated*

FIGURE 15-5 The proper way to correct a prehospital care report is to draw a single line through the error, write the correct information beside it, and initial the change.

TIMELINESS

As a rule, you should avoid writing your report in the ambulance during transport of your patient for two reasons. First, the bumpy ride makes it difficult to write neatly. More importantly, your time is better spent communicating with your patient and conducting ongoing assessments. Most hospitals have an area where you can sit and complete your paperwork.

Ideally, you should complete your report immediately after you complete the emergency call, when the information is fresh in your mind and you can check with your partner or patient if you have any questions about the events. At times you may be too busy to complete the entire documentation immediately following a call. If so, make notes on scratch paper and write enough of the report that you will be able to finish it completely and accurately later. The sooner you finish it, the more details you are likely to recall and the better the report will be.

Ideally, you should complete your report immediately after you complete the emergency call.

ABSENCE OF ALTERATIONS

Mistakes happen. During a busy shift or in the middle of the night you will check the wrong box, misspell a word, or omit important information. You will be thinking of one medication and write another's name on your report. If you make a mistake writing your report, simply cross through the error with one line and initial it (Figure 15-5). Some systems may expect you to date the correction, as well. Do not scribble over or blacken out any area of the call report. Never try to hide an error. Such foolish tactics only raise the reader's curiosity about what you wrote originally. After crossing out the error, continue with the correct information. If you find the error after you've already written several more sentences, submit an **addendum.**

Whenever possible, have everyone involved in the call read or reread the PCR before you submit it. Make all corrections before you submit the report to the hospital or to the EMS administrative offices. Do not make changes on the original report after you have submitted it. If for any reason you need to make corrections after you have submitted the report, or some portion of it, place an addendum. Simply note on the original report, "See addendum," and attach the addendum to the original report. Write the addendum on a separate sheet of paper or on an official form if one exists. Likewise, if more information comes to your attention after you have submitted the report, write a supplemental narrative on a separate report form.

Write any addendum to your report as soon as you realize that you made an error or that additional information is needed. Note the purpose of the revision and why the information did not appear on your original report. The addendum should document the date and time that it was written, the reason it was written, and the pertinent information. Only the original author of a report should attach an addendum, as it is part of the official call record. Agencies should have separate forms for other EMS personnel, supervisors, or citizens who, for some reason, want to contribute to the documentation.

Never try to hide an error.

* addendum addition or supplement to the original report.

PROFESSIONALISM

Write your report in a professional manner. Remember that someday it may be scrutinized by hospital staff, quality improvement committees, supervisors, lawyers, and the news media. Your patient's family may request, and is entitled to, a copy of your report from your agency. Write cautiously and avoid any remarks that might be construed as derogatory. **Jargon** can be confusing and does little to enhance your image. Do not describe a patient well known to EMS providers as a "frequent flyer." Never include slang, biased statements, or irrelevant opinions. Include only objective information. "The patient smelled of beer and had slurred speech and difficulty walking" are factual statements. "The patient was very drunk" is an inference; even if accurate, it is still just your opinion. **Libel** and **slander** are, respectively, writing or speaking false and malicious words intended to damage a person's character. Always write and speak carefully. A seemingly innocent phrase or comment can come back to haunt you.

NARRATIVE WRITING

The narrative is the part of the written report in which you depict the call at length. Less structured than the check-box or fill-in sections of your report, the narrative allows you the freedom to describe your assessment findings in detail. When other people read your report, they usually will rely on your written narrative for the most relevant information. For example, as you transfer care to the emergency department nurse, she will usually scan your PCR for information concerning your patient's history, vital signs, and physical exam.

NARRATIVE SECTIONS

Any patient documentation includes three sections of importance—the subjective narrative, the objective narrative, and the assessment/management plan.

Subjective Narrative

The subjective part of your narrative typically comprises any information that you elicit during your patient's history. This includes the chief complaint (CC), the history of present illness (HPI), the past history (PH), the current health status (CHS), and the review of systems (ROS). In trauma, this also includes the mechanism of injury, as told to you by your patient or bystanders. The following is a typical subjective narrative on a patient complaining of shortness of breath:

CC: The patient is a 74-year-old conscious black female who complains, "I can't catch my breath."

HPI: Gradual onset of severe shortness of breath for the past 3 hours; began while sitting in living room watching television; nothing provokes or relieves the dyspnea; her son states this is worse than usual for her. She has had a 3-day history of some vague chest discomfort. She denies any chest pressure, nausea, or dizziness.

PH: She has a 5-year history of heart problems and congestive heart failure; hospitalized for this problem 3 times in the past 5 years; no surgeries.

CHS: Meds: Isosorbide, nitroglycerin, furosemide, digoxin, potassium; No known drug allergies; 50 pack/year smoker; non-drinker; non-drug abuser.

ROS: Resp: Unproductive cough for 1 day; audible wheezing; no hx of COPD or asthma; last chest X-ray 1 year ago. Card: no palpitations, pressure, or pain; + orthopnea; + paroxysmal nocturnal dyspnea; + edema for past few days; past ECG 1 year ago. GU: No changes in urinary patterns. Per. Vasc: + pitting edema for few days; cold feet.

Objective Narrative

The objective part of your narrative usually includes your general impression and any data that you derive through inspection, palpation, auscultation, percussion, and diagnostic testing. This includes vital signs, physical exam, and tests such as cardiac monitoring, pulse oximetry, and blood glucose determination.

To document your physical exam you can use either of two approaches—head-to-toe or body systems. While the medical community accepts both extensively, emergency medical services more often uses the head-to-toe approach.

Content Review

APPROACHES TO THE PHYSICAL EXAM
- Head-to-toe
- Body systems

Head-to-Toe The head-to-toe approach is well suited for any call when you perform an entire physical exam, because you document your findings in the same order that you conducted the exam—from head-to-toe. Remember that even though you may have conducted your pediatric assessment from toe-to-head, you should document it in head-to-toe order. This style encourages you to be systematic and thorough. It is appropriate for major trauma and serious medical emergencies, when you examine every body area and system. Include all circulatory and neurological findings within the body area you are documenting. For example, when recording findings in the extremities, include distal neurovascular function. When documenting the head, include the results of cranial nerve testing. The following illustrates the head-to-toe approach for a patient from an automobile accident:

General:	The patient presents in the front seat of the car, in moderate distress with bruises to his forehead and some facial lacerations. Pt. is alert and oriented to self, time, and place.
Vital signs:	Pulse—100 strong, regular radial, BP—110/88; Resp—24 non-labored; skin pale and cool.
HEENT:	Depression to right frontal bone, minor bleeding controlled prior to arrival; no drainage from ears, nose. No periorbital ecchymosis or Battle's sign; pupils equal and reactive to light; extraocular movements intact, cranial nerves II—XII intact.
Neck:	Trachea midline; no jugular vein distention; + cervical spine tenderness.
Chest:	Equal expansion; bruises across the chest wall; no deformities; equal bilateral breath sounds.
Abdomen:	Soft, non-tender.
Pelvis:	Unstable pelvic ring; pain upon palpation.
Extremities:	+ Circulation, sensory, and motor function in all four extremities; no deformities noted.
Posterior:	No injuries noted.
Labs:	Sinus tachycardia no ectopy, pulse oximetry 97% on supplemental oxygen.

Body Systems The body systems approach focuses on body systems instead of body areas. It is best suited to screening and preadmission exams in which you conduct a comprehensive exam involving all body systems. Each body system has different key components that you should assess and document.

When you use the body systems approach in emergency medicine, you usually will focus only on the system, or systems, involved in the current illness or injury. For example, a patient having an asthma attack would require an in-depth evaluation of the respiratory system. Another patient with lower abdominal pain would need a close examination of the gastrointestinal system. Neither patient would require a full head-to-toe physical exam but, instead, intensive documentation of the affected body system or systems. The body systems approach can be one of the most comprehensive approaches to documentation.

The following illustrates a body systems approach for a patient with chest pain and shortness of breath:

General:	Patient is a healthy-looking female who presents sitting upright in her chair, able to speak in phrases only.
Vital Signs:	Pulse—90; BP—170/80; Resp—28 labored; skin—warm and diaphoretic
HEENT:	+ Lip cyanosis and pursing; some nasal flaring; pink, frothy sputum; jugular veins distended.
Respiratory:	Good respiratory effort; accessory neck muscle use; trachea midline; + intercostal, supraclavicular, suprasternal retractions; = chest expansion; diffuse crackles and wheezing in all lung fields, decreased breath sounds.
Per. Vasc.:	+ Ascites fluid wave; + 2 pitting edema in lower extremities; strong peripheral pulses.
Labs:	Sinus tachycardia with occasional unifocal premature ventricular contractions. Pulse oximetry—92% room air; 97% on supplemental oxygen.

Assessment/Management

In the assessment/management section, you document what you believe to be your patient's problem. This is also known as your **field diagnosis,** or impression. For example, your field diagnosis for a patient with chest pain may be "possible angina or rule/out myocardial infarction." You do not have to make an exact diagnosis. When you are not sure, simply document what you suspect is the general problem. Sometimes, for instance, your field impression might be "rule out acute abdomen, or seizures." *Rule out* identifies possible diagnoses that you believe the emergency physician should evaluate.

Record your complete management plan from start to finish. This includes how you packaged and moved your patient to the ambulance. Did you carry him on a stair-chair or on a backboard fully immobilized or did he walk? List any interventions you completed before contacting your medical control physician. For example, did you control bleeding with direct pressure? Did you start an IV? Then describe any orders from the medical control physician, and always include his name. Describe how you transported your patient and the effects of any interventions such as drug administration or other invasive procedures. Include the results of ongoing assessments and any changes in your patient's condition. Finally, describe your patient's condition when you transferred care to the emergency department staff. The following example is a management plan for a trauma patient with a pelvic fracture whose condition deteriorates en route to the hospital.

* **field diagnosis** what you believe to be your patient's problem, based on your history and physical exam.

Record your complete management plan from start to finish.

On-Scene

Extrication:	Rapid extrication from vehicle, placed supine on backboard
Airway:	Airway cleared with suctioning, nasopharyngeal airway inserted
Breathing:	Oxygen @ 15 liters/min via non rebreather mask
Circulation:	Foot of stretcher raised 30°; bleeding from arm laceration controlled with dry sterile dressing and direct pressure; PASG applied; IV—16 ga. left antecubital area—normal saline run KVO per Dr. Johnson.

Transport

Transported by ground ambulance to University Hospital with full body immobilization supine on long spine board; ETA 10 minutes.

Ongoing:	Patient becomes restless and anxious; VS: pulse—120 weak carotid only, BP—50 palpated, Resp—28, skin: cool, pale, clammy with some mottling; PASG inflated; initial IV run wide open; second IV 16 ga. right antecubital normal saline—run wide open.

Arrival

Patient transferred to ED staff restless; VS: pulse 120, BP—80 palpated, Resp—26, skin—mottled and cool.

GENERAL FORMATS

The mnemonics SOAP and CHART identify two common patterns for organizing a narrative report. These acronyms provide templates for most medical and trauma reports. They help you to arrange your history, physical exam, and management plan into a logical, readable structure. They are widely used because they group information in categories that differentiate between subjective and objective information. For example, someone wanting only to determine your patient's medications can find that list easily in either the SOAP or CHART format. Either pattern is acceptable and effective when used consistently.

SOAP

SOAP stands for *S*ubjective, *O*bjective, *A*ssessment, and *P*lan. The detailed SOAP format includes:

Subjective:	• Chief complaint
	• History of present illness
	• Past History
	• Current health status
	• Family History
	• Psychosocial History
	• Review of systems
Objective:	• Vital Signs
	• General impression
	• Physical exam
	• Diagnostic tests

Assessment:	• Field diagnosis
Plan:	• Standing orders
	• Physician orders
	• Effects of interventions
	• Mode of transportation
	• Ongoing assessment

CHART

CHART stands for *C*hief complaint, *H*istory, *A*ssessment, *R*x (treatment), and *T*ransport. The detailed CHART format includes:

Chief Complaint

History:	• History of present illness
	• Past History
	• Current health status
	• Review of systems

Assessment:	• Vital signs
	• General impression
	• Physical exam
	• Diagnostic tests
	• Field diagnosis

| Rx: | • Standing orders |
| | • Physician orders |

Transport:	• Effects of interventions
	• Mode of transportation
	• Ongoing assessment

Other Formats

Like patient assessment itself, documentation is not "one-size-fits-all." No one narrative format is ideal for all situations. Two additional formats—patient management and call incident—are appropriate in certain circumstances.

Patient Management The patient management format is preferred for some critical patients, such as those in cardiac arrest, when you focus on immediately managing a variety of patient problems and not on conducting a thorough history and physical exam. This format is a chronological account from the time you arrived on the scene until you transferred care to someone else. It emphasizes your assessment and management of the conditions you found. Simply begin your chart with a description of the event and any other pertinent information and then document your management, starting with your airway, breathing, and circulation (ABCs) assessment. Record everything in real time and in absolute chronological order, and always include the results of your interventions. A patient management chart would look like this:

> Patient is an 89-year-old Hispanic male who was found by his wife unconscious on the floor immediately after collapsing. He presents pulseless and apneic.

No single narrative format is ideal for all situations.

Use the patient management format for critical patients when you focus on immediately managing a variety of patient problems.

Time	Intervention
1320	Airway cleared with suctioning; quick look—ventricular fibrillation.
1321	Defibrillation @ 200, 300, 360 joules—no change.
1322	CPR begun; oropharyngeal airway inserted, ventilation with BVM @ 12/min with supplemental oxygen.
1324	IV 18-gauge left antecubital area—normal saline KVO; epinephrine 1:10,000 1 mg IVP.
1325	Defibrillation @ 360 joules—no change; lidocaine 100 mg IVP.
1327	Defibrillation @ 360 joules—patient converts to normal sinus rhythm rate of 72 with strong peripheral pulses, BP—110/76, no spontaneous respirations. ET tube inserted. + lung sounds bilaterally with BVM.
1328	Ventilation continued @ 12/min via BVM; lidocaine infusion 2 mg/min.
1332	Patient transferred to ambulance on stretcher—transported to University Hospital.
1335	Patient has spontaneous respirations @ 20/min, + bilateral breath sounds; becoming more awake; HR—72, BP—120/76.
1340	Arrived at UH—Patient is conscious, alert and oriented with retrograde amnesia.

Call Incident The call incident approach simply emphasizes the mechanism of injury, the surrounding circumstances, and how the incident occurred. Use this approach to begin documenting a trauma call with a significant mechanism of injury. It is most suitable when the events surrounding the call might be significant. It would be inappropriate for a man sitting in his living room with chest pain or for someone who simply cut his finger with a carving knife. You may use this style in both the subjective and objective sections of your PCR. The following example shows call incident documentation for a motor vehicle crash:

Use the call incident approach to begin documenting a trauma call with a significant mechanism of injury.

Subjective: The patient is a 46-year-old conscious and alert white male who was an unrestrained driver in a low-speed, head-on, two-car motor vehicle crash, moderate front-end damage, no passenger compartment intrusion, deformity to windshield, dashboard, and steering wheel. Patient states he "reached for cigarette on floor and when he looked up, there was another vehicle in front of him." He denies any loss of consciousness and can recall all details prior to and immediately following the crash. Patient complains of pain to the head, neck, chest, and hip from being thrown against the dashboard and windshield.

Objective: The patient presents in the front seat of the car, appears in moderate distress with bruises to his forehead, facial lacerations, and a deformed left leg. His left leg is pinned underneath the dashboard with his left foot hooked around the brake pedal. Upon arrival, fire department rescue personnel were holding manual stabilization of his head and neck and stabilizing the vehicle.

These are not the only systems of documentation. Indeed, you may use some combination of these systems or develop a unique format for your regional system. The important thing is for your documentation to be complete, accurate, and consistent. By using the same system to document every call, you will be less likely to accidentally overlook or omit something.

SPECIAL CONSIDERATIONS

Some circumstances create special problems for EMS documentation. Patient refusals, calls where transport is unnecessary, multiple patients, and mass casualties are among the more common examples. In these and other unusual circumstances, take extra care to document everything that happened during the call.

PATIENT REFUSALS

Two types of patients might refuse care. The first type is the person who is not seriously ill or injured and simply does not want to go to the hospital. For example, the belted driver of a minor automobile crash has an abrasion on his knee from striking the dashboard. He is alert and oriented, has no other injuries, and claims he will seek medical attention if it bothers him later. This type of patient usually signs your PCR in a special place marked "Refusal of Care," and you return to service.

The second type of patient is more worrisome. This patient refuses care even though you feel he needs it. This is known as **against medical advice**, or **AMA.** Some legal experts regard AMA as your failure to convince your patient to accept necessary treatment and transport. Such patient refusals are particularly troublesome because they have the most potential to end badly. Still, patients retain the right to refuse treatment or transportation if they are competent to make that decision and are not actively suicidal. While you cannot make a legal determination of competence (sometimes it takes a court decision), document that you believe your patient was competent to refuse care. Though specific laws vary from state to state, your patient will demonstrate competence by his understanding of the circumstances and the risks associated with refusing care and by accepting those risks and the responsibility for refusing care. Assess your patient as thoroughly as possible, with special emphasis on his mental status and behavior. Pay extra attention to any patient suspected of being under the influence of drugs or alcohol. Clearly document that your patient has an adequate mental status and understands your field diagnosis, alternative treatments, and the consequences of refusing care. Also record his reason for refusing care (Table 15-2).

Even after you document your patient's competence, most patient refusals require more thorough documentation than the typical EMS run because the opportunity for and consequences of abandonment charges are tremendous. Simply having your patient sign your PCR is not sufficient. Again, document that you described your patient's injuries to him and that he understood the risks of refusing treatment and trans-

* against medical advice (AMA) your patient refuses care even though you feel he needs it.

Patients retain the right to refuse treatment or transportation if they are competent to make that decision.

Table 15-2	REFUSAL OF CARE DOCUMENTATION CHECKLIST

❏ Thorough patient assessment
❏ Competency of patient
❏ Your recommendation for care and transport
❏ Explanation to the patient about possible consequences of refusing care, including possibility of death, if appropriate
❏ Other suggestions for accessing care
❏ Willingness to return if patient changes mind
❏ Patient's understanding of statements and suggestions and apparent competence to refuse care based on that understanding

port. Inform him of potential complications from injuries that might not be obvious. Discuss those associated risks also, and document this discussion. Also document any involvement of your patient's family or friends. Since ruling out serious injury is all but impossible in the field, you may need to make clear the possibility of your patient's dying. Although this might seem extreme, it plainly conveys that the risks are serious. A patient who was informed that he was at risk of dying, refused care, and subsequently had his leg amputated because of an infection would have a hard time convincing a jury that he did not think the risks were serious.

In many systems, you must contact the medical direction physician before allowing a patient to refuse transport. If you confer with a physician, document any information, advice, or orders that the physician gives you. If your patient speaks directly to the physician, document that as well. Once more, document that your patient understands the circumstances and the risks and still chooses to refuse transport. Note that you instructed him to call an ambulance or go to the emergency department if his condition worsens, or if he just changes his mind. You can ask a bystander or law enforcement officer to witness the patient refusal, although this is not always required.

Your documentation also should include a complete narrative with quotations and statements from others on the scene. For example, if your patient's wife and son plead with him to go to the hospital, include their comments in your report. If your system uses a specific form for patient refusals, complete that paperwork as well (Figure 15-6). The additional form, however, is not a substitute for a complete documentation of the circumstances.

RELEASE FROM RESPONSIBILITY

DATE _____ 19 _____ TIME _____ a.m. / p.m.

This is to certify that _____

is refusing ☐ TREATMENT ☐ TRANSPORTATION

against the advice of the attending Emergency Medical Technician and of the Phoenix Fire Department, and when applicable, the base hospital and the base hospital physician.

I acknowledge that I have been informed of the following:

1. The nature and potential of the illness or injuries.
2. The potential risks of delaying treatment and transportation, up to and including death.
3. The availability of ambulance transportation to a hospital for treatment.

Nevertheless, I assume all risks and consequences of my decision, including further physical deterioration, loss of limb, paralysis, and even death, and hereby release the attending Emergency Medical Technician and the Phoenix Fire Department, and when applicable, the base hospital and the base hospital physician from any ill effects which may result from my refusal.

Witness _____   Signed: **X** _____

Witness _____   Relationship to Patient _____

Refusal must be signed by the patient; or by the nearest relative or legal guardian in the case of a minor, or when patient is physically or mentally incompetent.

☐ Patient refuses to sign release despite efforts of attending Emergency Medical Technician to obtain such signature after informing patient of concerns listed in numbers 1, 2, and 3 above.

GUIDELINES — Patient Refusal Documentation

In addition to those items normally documented (chief complaint, history of present illness, mechanism of injury, physical assessment, etc.) the following items should be recorded, regardless of patient's cooperation:

- Mental Status (orientation, speech, etc.)
- Suspected presence of alcohol or drugs
- Patient's exact words (as much as possible) in the refusal of care OR the signing of the release form
- Circumstances or reasons (including exact words of patient, if possible) for INCOMPLETE ADVISEMENT (risk of injury, abusiveness, unruliness, risk of injury other than from patient, etc.)
- Advice given to patients' guardian(s)

FIGURE 15-6   One example of a refusal of care form.

SERVICES NOT NEEDED

Some systems allow you to determine that your patient does not need ambulance transport. Although such policies help to reduce ambulance utilization rates, the risks of denying transport are even greater than those of patient refusals. In these cases, the documentation must clearly demonstrate that transport was unnecessary. As with patient refusals, document any discussion you have with the emergency department physician and any advice you give to your patient.

Transportation may not be needed for other reasons, as well. Ambulances are often called to minor accidents where no injuries have occurred. When this happens, first responders such as the fire department rescue unit or a police agency might cancel the ambulance. If the ambulance is canceled en route, document the canceling authority and the time of notification. If you arrive on the scene and find no patients, document that. If, when you arrive, you are canceled by on-scene personnel, document that you made no patient contact and record the person and agency who canceled you. The difference is considerable between "no patients found" and "only minor injuries, patients refusing transport." Although they might refuse transport, evaluate people with even the most minor injuries. Consider them patients and document them accurately.

MASS CASUALTY INCIDENTS

Multiple patients, mass casualties, and disasters all present special documentation problems. The number of patients needing care and transport during such situations may overwhelm you. Often, more than one ambulance crew cares for the many patients. Some EMS personnel may fill only support roles and never actually provide patient care. Obtaining complete patient information might be impossible, and completing documentation for one patient before going on to care for others might be impractical.

In these situations, you must weigh your patients' needs against the demand for complete documentation. Document as much as possible—as quickly as possible—on your PCR. You can complete the documentation later as an addendum. If you cannot remember the particulars of a specific patient or transport, do not guess. Document only what you know to be factual and accurate. A simple note at the end of the documentation explaining the circumstances will account for any missing information.

Some EMS agencies use special forms for multiple patient events, and most provide a general incident report form or record that anyone connected with the call may complete. You should become familiar with local policies and procedures for documenting these situations. Many systems use **triage tags** to record vital information on each patient quickly. A triage tag has just enough room for your patient's vital information—name, major injuries, vital signs, treatment, and priority (urgent, non-urgent). You affix it to your patient, and it remains there throughout the event; you can transfer its information to your PCR later. Whatever your local policies, document as completely and accurately as possible without detracting from patient care.

CONSEQUENCES OF INAPPROPRIATE DOCUMENTATION

Inappropriate documentation can have both medical and legal consequences. The medical consequences of inadequate documentation are potentially the most serious. Health care providers across several disciplines may refer to your PCR in planning their care for a patient. Do not guess about your patient's medical prob-

---

The risks of denying transport are even greater than those of patient refusals.

* triage tags tags containing vital information, affixed to your patient during a multi-patient incident.

Whatever your local policies regarding multiple patients and mass casualties, document as completely and accurately as possible without detracting from patient care.

lems if you are not certain. An inaccurate or incomplete report can affect patient care for many hours, even days, after the ambulance call ends. Failing to document a medication allergy or documenting an incorrect medical history could have grave effects. If no one can read your sloppy report, it is useless despite the importance of its information. Good documentation now enables good care later.

The potential legal consequences of inadequate documentation are enormous. If poor documentation results in inappropriate care, you may be held responsible. Or if the documentation does not make it clear that you informed a patient of the risks when he refused transport, you may be legally accountable for any harmful consequences. If the documentation does not explicitly say the patient in ventricular fibrillation was defibrillated immediately, you might be accused of providing inadequate care. Even though you did everything appropriately, poor, incomplete, or inaccurate documentation will encourage anyone who is pursuing a frivolous lawsuit. Good documentation discourages such actions. Always remember that if it is not documented, you did not do it.

Inaccurate, incomplete, illegible documentation also reflects poorly on the EMS provider writing the report. Missing information, misspelled words, and poor penmanship give the impression of a sloppy, incompetent provider. Good documentation, on the other hand, enhances the EMS provider's professional stature.

Good documentation now enables good care later.

Poor, incomplete, or inaccurate documentation encourages frivolous lawsuits; good documentation discourages them.

CLOSING

As a paramedic you will assume responsibility for your documentation. Although documentation is often a begrudged task, it is one of the most important parts of an EMS call. Ensuring that your documentation is complete, accurate, legible, and appropriate is one of your professional responsibilities. As a professional, you should recognize this responsibility and set a positive example for others as you fulfill it.

Your report's confidentiality cannot be overemphasized. Confidentiality is your patient's legal right. Do not discuss your report with anyone not medically connected directly with the case. Generally, you are allowed to share patient information with another health care provider who will continue care, with third-party billing companies, with the police if it is relevant to a criminal investigation, and with the court if it issues a subpoena. Your report also may be used for quality assurance or research. In these cases, block out the patient's name.

Computer charting will certainly become common in the future. Several systems now on the market allow you to enter data electronically, transmit that information to the receiving facility, and immediately receive a printed report. When you use such systems, remember that the principles of effective documentation still apply.

Ƨ UMMARY

Regardless of the system you use for documentation, all EMS records should possess the same basic attributes. Appropriate terminology, proper spelling, accepted abbreviations and acronyms, and accurate times are essential. A description of the patient assessment and interventions, including pertinent negatives and communications with on-line physicians, is equally important. Finally, all of the personnel and resources involved in a call must be documented. The record must be accurate and precise, free of jargon, and neatly written. Corrections should be made properly, including the use of an addendum when appropriate.

Prehospital care providers may use many systems of documentation, including the CHART and SOAP formats. Whatever system you use, it is best if you use the same one consistently. This results in more reliable, complete documentation and reduces the chances of omitting important information. Any of the existing documentation systems can incorporate a head-to-toe assessment of the patient. Special situations such as multiple patients and refusals of transportation require extra attention. They are often the most difficult calls to document, yet they are also the calls for which good documentation can be most valuable. A complete narrative—in addition to any check boxes or filled-in "bubbles"—is the best way to ensure that all the necessary information is documented.

Although EMS providers frequently dislike documentation, it is one of the most important parts of the EMS call. Ensuring that the documentation is complete, accurate, legible, and appropriate is one of an EMS provider's professional responsibilities. Your PCR is the only permanent record of the ambulance call and the only permanent reflection of your professionalism.

DIVISION 3

TRAUMA EMERGENCIES

CHAPTER 16

Trauma and Trauma Systems

Objectives

After reading this chapter, you should be able to:

1. Describe the prevalence and significance of trauma. (pp. 815–816)
2. List the components of a comprehensive trauma system. (pp. 816–818)
3. Identify the characteristics of community, area, and regional trauma centers. (p. 817)
4. Identify the trauma triage criteria and apply them to narrative descriptions of trauma patients. (pp. 819–822)
5. Describe how trauma emergencies differ from medical emergencies in the scene size-up, assessment, prehospital emergency care, and transport. (pp. 819–822)
6. Explain the "Golden Hour" concept, and describe how it applies to prehospital emergency medical service. (pp. 820–821)
7. Explain the value of air medical service in trauma patient care and transport. (pp. 820–821)

INTRODUCTION TO TRAUMA AND TRAUMA CARE

Trauma is a physical injury or wound caused by external force or violence. It is the number four killer in the United States today behind cardiovascular disease, stroke, and cancer. It is, however, the leading killer of persons under age 44. As such, trauma steals the greatest number of productive years from its victims. It also may be the most expensive medical problem because of the productivity losses it causes in its victims and the high cost of initial care, rehabilitation, and often lifelong maintenance of those victims.

Trauma accounts for about 150,000 deaths per year, with auto crashes responsible for about 44,000 and gunshot wounds another 38,000. Other deaths are attributed to falls, blasts, stabbings, crush injuries, and sports injuries. In addition to the great death toll from trauma, many more of its victims are injured and carry lifelong physical reminders of their experiences with it.

Your role in trauma care, as a member of the Emergency Medical Services team, is to understand the structure and objectives of the trauma care system, to promote injury prevention, and to provide the seriously injured trauma patient with proper assessment, aggressive care, and rapid transport to the most appropriate facility. The remainder of this chapter will help you with these responsibilities as it further defines trauma, explains the components of trauma care systems, identifies the capabilities of different levels of trauma centers, and more fully defines your role as a care provider in the trauma system.

TRAUMA

The types of trauma can range from slight abrasions or scratches to the fatal, multiple-system injuries that might result from a high-speed automobile-versus-pedestrian collision. Trauma is broken down into two major categories, blunt and penetrating. **Penetrating trauma** occurs when an arrow, bullet, knife, or other object enters the body and exchanges energy with human tissue, thereby causing injury. **Blunt trauma** is injury that occurs as the energy and forces of collision with an object—not the object itself—enter the body and damage tissue. These two categories of trauma are discussed in greater detail in the next two chapters of this book.

Although trauma poses a serious threat to life, its presentation often masks the patient's true condition. Extremity injuries, for example, infrequently cause death. Yet they are often obvious and grotesque (Figure 16-1). On the other hand, life-threatening problems, such as internal bleeding and shock, may occur with only subtle signs and symptoms. When assessing a trauma patient, you must look beyond obvious injuries for evidence that suggests a life-threatening condition. When such a condition is found, you must assure rapid access to the trauma system for your patient.

Serious and life-threatening injury occurs in fewer than 10 percent of trauma patients. In most patients with life-threatening injury, however, the injury is internal and is likely to involve the head or body cavity hemorrhage. Prehospital care can neither properly nor definitively stabilize these patients and their injuries in the field. The best care you as a paramedic can offer is to secure the airway, assure adequate respirations, control any significant external hemorrhage, and rapidly transport the patient to definitive trauma care. That care is only available at a specialized treatment facility with rapid access to surgery—a trauma center.

Some 90 percent of trauma patients do not have serious, life-threatening injuries. You can best care for these patients by providing thorough on-scene

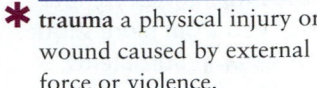 **trauma** a physical injury or wound caused by external force or violence.

Trauma is the leading killer of persons under age 44 in the United States.

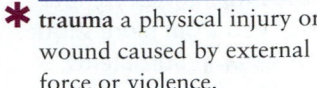 **penetrating trauma** injury caused by an object breaking the skin and entering the body.

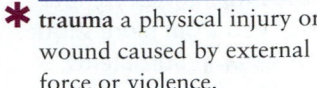 **blunt trauma** injury caused by the collision of an object with the body in which the object does not enter the body.

Life-threatening problems, such as internal bleeding and shock, may occur with only subtle signs and symptoms.

When assessing a trauma patient, look beyond obvious injuries for evidence that suggests a life-threatening condition.

FIGURE 16-1 In prehospital care, it is essential that gruesome, non-life-threatening injuries do not distract you from more subtle, life-threatening problems. *(Courtesy of Edward T. Dickinson, MD)*

assessment and stabilization followed by conservative transport to the nearest general hospital or other appropriate health care facility.

It is essential that you determine the difference between trauma patients with serious, life-threatening conditions and those less seriously injured patients during your assessment. You will be aided in making this determination by using guidelines known as trauma triage criteria. These criteria involve consideration of the mechanisms by which patients are injured and of the physical or clinical findings indicating internal injury. Using these criteria, which will be discussed in detail later in this chapter, will help you properly direct patients as they enter the trauma care system.

THE TRAUMA CARE SYSTEM

In the mid-to-late 1960s, several medically oriented groups investigated the death toll on U.S. highways. Their studies revealed that victims of vehicle crashes suffered not only from the injuries received in the crashes but also from the lack of an organized approach to bringing these victims into the health care system. The studies also demonstrated that most hospitals were inadequately equipped and staffed to care for the victims of these crashes. These investigations led to passage of the Highway Safety Act of 1966 and to the development of today's Emergency Medical Services system.

More than two decades later, the American College of Surgeons, recognizing that the system of caring for severely injured trauma victims was still inadequate, successfully worked to achieve passage of the Trauma Care Systems Planning and Development Act of 1990. This act helped establish guidelines, funding, and state-level leadership and support for the development of trauma systems.

The trauma system is predicated on the principle that serious trauma is a *surgical disease*. This means that the proper care for serious internal trauma is often immediate surgical intervention to repair internal hemorrhage sites. While patients with life-threatening injuries account for less than 10 percent of all trauma patients, immediate surgical care of these patients can drastically reduce trauma mortality and morbidity.

Care for seriously injured trauma patients is expensive and complicated. A well-designed EMS system will allocate limited resources in a way that provides the most efficient and effective care for these patients. Such a system utilizes hospitals with special resources and commitment to trauma patient care. These hospitals are designated as trauma centers.

Serious trauma is a **surgical disease**; *its proper care is immediate surgical intervention to repair internal hemorrhage sites.*

TRAUMA CENTER DESIGNATION

The current model for a trauma system includes three levels of **trauma center,** with an increased ability and commitment to provide trauma care at each level (Table 16-1).

The Level I, or regional, trauma center is a hospital, usually a university teaching center, that is prepared and committed to handle all types of specialty trauma (Figure 16-2). These centers provide neurosurgery, microsurgery (limb reattachment), pediatric care, burn care, and care for multi-system trauma. They also provide leadership and resource support to other levels of the regional trauma system through system coordination and continuing medical and public education programs. When population density does not permit a commitment to the requirements of a Level I trauma center, a Level II trauma center may act as the regional trauma center.

The Level II, or area, trauma center, has an increased commitment to trauma care, but not as great as a Level I facility. It has surgical care capability available at all times for incoming trauma patients. Level II centers can handle all but the most seriously injured specialty and multi-system trauma patients. Staff at these facilities can stabilize those patients in preparation for transport to a Level I trauma center.

The Level III, or community, trauma center is a general hospital with a commitment to special staff training and resource allocation for trauma patients. These centers are located in smaller cities situated in generally rural areas. They are well prepared to care for most trauma victims and to stabilize and triage more seriously injured ones for transport to higher level trauma centers.

In some remote areas, there is provision for an additional level of trauma center. In these areas, seriously injured trauma patients may be taken to a Level IV trauma facility for stabilization and care before transport, often by helicopter, to a more distant, higher-level trauma center. In these areas, the incidence of trauma does not support the resource allocation necessary to meet the requirements of a trauma center; by default, some other type of health care facility is identified as a trauma transport destination.

> *The modern trauma system includes three levels of trauma center, each with an increased ability and commitment to providing trauma care.*
>
>

✱ **trauma center** a hospital that has the capability of caring for acutely injured patients; trauma centers must meet strict criteria to use this designation.

Table 16-1   CRITERIA FOR TRAUMA CENTER DESIGNATION

Level I—Regional Trauma Center

Commits resources to address all types of specialty trauma 24 hours a day, 7 days a week.

Level II—Area Trauma Center

Commits the resources to address the most common trauma emergencies with surgical capability available 24 hours a day, 7 days a week; will stabilize and transport specialty cases to the regional trauma center.

Level III—Community Trauma Center

Commits to special emergency department training and has some surgical capability, but will usually stabilize and transfer seriously injured trauma patients to a higher level trauma center as needed.

Level IV—Trauma Facility

In remote areas, a small community hospital or medical care facility may be designated a trauma receiving facility, meaning that it will stabilize and prepare trauma patients with moderate to serious injuries for transport to a higher level facility.

FIGURE 16-2 The R. Adams Cowley Shock Trauma Center in Baltimore, Maryland, is an example of a Level I trauma facility.

The design of a trauma system should be flexible in order to meet the needs of the region it serves. In urban and suburban areas, there are just a few trauma centers to assure that each receives adequate patient volume to maintain staff proficiency and to assure that resources are being effectively used. In rural regions, a Level III center may act as the regional trauma center because the incidence of serious trauma does not support any greater commitment. In some areas, a Level IV facility may be all that is available and thus becomes the default destination for seriously injured trauma patients. Consult your Emergency Medical Services system plan to determine the intended patient flow patterns in your region.

SPECIALTY CENTERS

Beyond classification as trauma centers, certain medical facilities may be designated as specialty centers. Such facilities may include neurocenters, burn centers, pediatric trauma centers, and centers specializing in hand and limb reattachment by microsurgery. One other specialty service is hyperbaric oxygenation, which is important in the treatment of carbon monoxide poisoning and problems related to SCUBA diving.

Specialty centers have made a commitment of trained personnel, equipment, and other resources to provide services not usually available at a general or trauma hospital. These centers are also more likely to provide a higher level of intensive care and state-of-the-art injury management than other facilities are able to. Be aware of the specialty services available in your system as well as the protocols defining when patients should be directed to them.

YOUR ROLE AS AN EMT-PARAMEDIC

As an EMT-Paramedic, your tasks in the trauma system are likely to include triage of trauma patients against standards established by your medical direction authority (trauma triage criteria) and assurance of the rapid assessment, care, and transport of patients to the closest appropriate medical facility (Figure 16-3). For those patients that meet trauma triage criteria, the appropriate facility is the nearest trauma center.

Trauma triage criteria are guidelines established to help you determine which patients require the services of a trauma center and which do not. The presence of certain mechanisms of injury and clinical findings have been proven, by research, to accurately reflect the potential for serious injury and the need for the intensive services available only at a trauma center. Compare your patient's mechanism of injury and any physical assessment findings to these pre-established criteria. These criteria are listed in detail later in this chapter. If your patient meets any of the criteria, rapid transport is required.

*❋ **trauma triage criteria** guidelines to aid prehospital personnel in determining which trauma patients require urgent transportation to a trauma center.*

MECHANISM OF INJURY ANALYSIS

To help determine the **mechanism of injury,** mentally recreate the accident from evidence available at the scene. You should identify the forces involved in the incident, the direction from which they came, and the areas of the patient's body affected by these forces. In an automobile collision, for example, the mechanism of injury includes the energy exchange process between the auto and what it struck, between the patient and the auto's interior, and among the various tissues and organs as they collide, one with another, within the patient. Close inspection of the mangled auto reveals evidence about the collision and the forces at work in it. (See Chapter 17, "Blunt Trauma," and Chapter 18, "Penetrating Trauma.")

*❋ **mechanism of injury** the processes and forces that cause trauma.*

FIGURE 16-3 Your role as a paramedic attending a trauma patient is to assure the ABCs and prepare the patient for rapid transport.

You will begin your consideration of the mechanism of injury during the scene size-up. Later, you should reconsider the mechanism of injury as the first step of the focused history and physical exam for the trauma patient.

INDEX OF SUSPICION

The information you gather during your consideration and reconsideration of the mechanism of injury suggests an **index of suspicion** for possible injuries. This index is an anticipation of possible injuries based upon analysis of the event. For example, a pedestrian struck by a car can be expected to have lower extremity fractures. Further, if the auto were moving at 20 miles per hour, fracture severity would be less than if it were moving at 55 miles per hour. Also, the probability of internal injury at lower speeds is less than it would be at higher speeds. By evaluating the strength of the impact and its nature, you can anticipate the structures and organs damaged and the degree to which they have been damaged.

In addition to developing an index of suspicion for specific injuries, you will also examine the trauma patient for physical signs of injury, both during the initial assessment and during the rapid trauma assessment or the focused history and physical exam. The physical signs suggesting serious trauma include the signs and symptoms of shock and those of internal head injury. Since shock and head injury are the great killers in trauma, be watchful for the earliest evidence of their existence. Remember, the body compensates well for the internal loss of blood and hides serious signs of injury until late in the shock process. If you have any reason to suspect that a patient has sustained serious internal injury, move to enter that patient rapidly into the trauma system. Otherwise, provide frequent ongoing assessment to assure that progressive signs of shock and internal head injury are discovered as early as possible.

THE GOLDEN HOUR

Time is a very important consideration in the survival of seriously injured trauma patients. Research has demonstrated that patient survival rates increase dramatically as time from the trauma incident to the beginning of surgery decreases. The current goal for incident-to-surgery time is 1 hour, often referred to as the **Golden Hour.**

Factors such as the location of the incident and time needed to extricate a patient all consume a portion of the Golden Hour. Many of these factors will be beyond your control; for that reason, it is vital to keep time spent on factors over which you do have control to the minimum. Ideally, you should provide the initial and rapid trauma assessments, emergency stabilization, patient packaging and initiation of transport in under 10 minutes. When distances or traffic conditions present prolonged ground transport times, reduce transport times by using an air medical service if possible.

Air medical service, usually provided by helicopter, has added a weapon in the fight against time for the seriously injured trauma patient (Figure 16-4). The helicopter travels much faster than ground transport and in a straight line from the crash scene to the trauma center.

Be aware, however, that air medical transport is not appropriate in all cases. Trauma patients must be in relatively stable condition for it to be utilized. Additionally, the limited space within the aircraft and its associated engine noise make in-flight care difficult. Further, combative patients may endanger the

---

Consideration of the mechanism of injury begins during the scene size-up. The mechanism of injury should be reconsidered as the first step of the focused history and physical exam for trauma patients.

* index of suspicion the anticipation of injury to a body region, organ or structure based on analysis of the mechanism of injury.

If you have any reason to suspect that the patient has sustained serious internal injury, move to enter him or her rapidly into the trauma system.

* Golden Hour the 60 minute period after a severe injury; it is the maximum acceptable time between the injury and initiation of surgery for the seriously injured trauma patient.

Initial patient assessment, emergency stabilization, patient packaging, and initiation of transport should ideally take less than 10 minutes.

FIGURE 16-4   An air medical services helicopter can significantly reduce transport time from the accident scene to the trauma center.

safety of the flight crew and the aircraft. Adverse weather conditions can also limit the use of air medical transport. Finally, air medical transport services are very expensive and can be used most effectively only as part of a comprehensive EMS trauma system. Follow local protocols about when and how to request air medical transport.

THE DECISION TO TRANSPORT

The decision either to transport a patient immediately or to attempt more extensive on-scene care is among the most difficult you must make. The trauma triage criteria are designed to help you with this decision. As a rule, transport patients who experience certain mechanisms of injury or display key clinical findings quickly, with intravenous access and other time-consuming procedures attempted en route. Indicators for immediate transport are given in Table 16-2.

In applying trauma triage criteria, it is best to err on the side of precaution. If a patient does not fit the stated criteria, be suspicious. Remember, you often arrive at the patient's side only minutes after the accident. The patient may not yet have lost enough blood internally to exhibit signs of shock or progressive head injury. If in doubt, transport to a trauma center without delay.

These criteria are designed for the "over-triage" of trauma patients. They assure that patients with very subtle signs and symptoms, yet with significant and serious injuries, are not missed during assessment. Use of these criteria means that you will transport some patients to trauma centers unnecessarily. However, transporting a patient who may not need the resources of a trauma center is far better than not transporting a patient who truly needs the care available only there.

In applying trauma triage criteria, it is best to err on the side of precaution.

Table 16-2	TRAUMA TRIAGE CRITERIA INDICATING NEED FOR IMMEDIATE TRANSPORT

Mechanism of Injury

- Falls greater than 20 feet (3 times the victim's height)
- Pedestrian/bicyclist versus auto collisions
  —Struck by a vehicle traveling over 5 MPH
  —Thrown or run over by vehicle
- Motorcycle impact at greater than 20 MPH
- Ejection from a vehicle
- Severe vehicle impact
  —Speed at impact greater than 40 MPH
  —Intrusion of more than 12 inches into occupant compartment
  —Vehicle deformity greater than 20 inches
- Rollover with signs of serious impact
- Death of another occupant in the vehicle
- Extrication time greater than 20 minutes

Significant mechanism of injury considerations with infants and children include the following:

- A fall of greater than 10 feet (3 times the victim's height)
- A bicycle/vehicle collision
- A vehicle collision at medium speed
- Any vehicle collision where the infant or child was unrestrained

Physical Findings

- Revised Trauma Score less than 11
- Glasgow Coma Scale less than 14
- Systolic blood pressure less than 90
- Respiratory rate less than 10 or greater than 29
- Pulse less than 50 or greater than 120
- Penetrating trauma (except distal extremities)
- Two or more proximal long-bone fractures
- Flail chest
- Pelvic fractures
- Limb paralysis
- Burns to more than 15 percent of body surface area
- Burns to face or airway

One of the best and most cost-effective ways of reducing mortality and morbidity is to prevent trauma in the first place.

INJURY PREVENTION

One of the best, most cost-effective ways of reducing mortality and morbidity is to prevent trauma in the first place. Several programs in this vein have been very effective. Programs promoting seat belt use and awareness of the dangers of drinking and driving have encouraged teenagers and adults to drive more safely and responsibly. Other programs, like "let's not meet by accident," increase society's awareness of trauma systems as well as an appreciation for safety-oriented behaviors. Safety programs for users of boats and firearms also raise safety awareness and assist in injury prevention. The Emergency Medical Services system has a responsibility to support such programs and to promote their development where they do not exist. As an EMS provider, you should participate and encourage your peers to participate.

Technical developments such as better highway design, airbag restraint systems, and vehicles constructed to absorb the energy of crashes have also played major parts in greatly reducing the yearly highway death toll. Paramedics have a responsibility to support the development and use of these new designs and technologies as a way of further reducing trauma deaths and injuries.

DATA AND THE TRAUMA REGISTRY

As with all emergency medical services, research is the only way to recognize those trauma care practices and procedures that benefit patients and those that do not. In the trauma system, the **trauma registry** is a uniform and standard set of data collected by regional trauma centers. This data is analyzed to determine how well the system is performing and to identify factors that may contribute to or lessen chances of patient survival.

It is important that you do all that you can to support this research effort by assuring that your prehospital care reports accurately and completely describe the findings of your assessments, the care you provide to patients, the results of ongoing assessments, and the times associated with calls. You should also consider taking part in and supporting prehospital research projects if the opportunity presents itself.

* **trauma registry** a data retrieval system for trauma patient information, used to evaluate and improve the trauma system.

QUALITY IMPROVEMENT

Trauma system Quality Improvement (QI), or Quality Management (QM) is another way of examining system performance with the aim of providing better patient care. In the QI process, committees look at selected care modalities (called indicators) to determine if designated standards of care are being met. For trauma system QI, the committees would study the application of trauma triage criteria, performance of field skills, and amounts of time spent in various aspects of response, care, and transport of patients. QI committees may also look at select calls to determine if their documentation accurately reflects the results of assessment and the care given. If the system standards are not being met, the committees may suggest such steps as continuing education programs or modification of protocols. As a member of the trauma system, you should become actively involved in such programs and encourage the participation of your peers.

SUMMARY

Trauma remains one of the greatest tragedies of our modern society. It accounts for large numbers of deaths and disabling injuries and often affects individuals who are in their most productive years of life. A well-designed and well-implemented trauma system offers a way of lessening the impact of these traumas.

As a paramedic, you are a part of the trauma system. You are charged with evaluating trauma patients by comparing their mechanisms of injury and the physical signs of their injuries to pre-established trauma triage criteria in order to determine which patients should enter the trauma system and which could be best cared for at a general hospital. In the presence of severe, life-threatening trauma, you must assure rapid assessment, on-scene care, and appropriate transport to provide your patients with the best chances for survival.

CHAPTER 17

Blunt Trauma

Objectives

After reading this chapter, you should be able to:

1. Identify, and explain by example, the laws of inertia and conservation of energy. (p. 826)

2. Define kinetic energy and force as they relate to trauma. (pp. 826–827)

3. Compare and contrast the types of vehicle impacts and their expected injuries. (pp. 829–832, 834–848)

4. Discuss the benefits of auto restraint and motorcycle helmet use. (pp. 832–834, 845)

5. Describe the mechanisms of injury associated with falls, crush injuries, and sports injuries. (pp. 854–857)

6. Identify the common blast injuries and any special considerations

regarding their assessment and proper care. (pp. 848–854)

7. Identify and explain any special assessment and care considerations for patients with blunt trauma. (pp. 834–857)

8. Given several preprogrammed and moulaged blunt trauma patients, provide the appropriate scene size-up, initial assessment, rapid trauma or focused physical exam and history, detailed exam, and ongoing assessment and provide appropriate patient care and transportation. (pp. 834–857)

INTRODUCTION TO BLUNT TRAUMA

Blunt trauma is the most common cause of trauma death and disability. It results from an energy exchange between an object and the human body, without intrusion of the object through the skin (Figure 17-1). The energy exchange causes a chain reaction among various body tissues that crushes and stretches their structures, resulting in injury beneath the surface. Blunt trauma is especially confounding because the true nature of the injury is often hidden, and evidence of the serious injury is very subtle or even absent.

To properly care for victims of blunt trauma, you should understand the injury process and its results. This study, called kinetics of trauma, gives insight into the events that produce injury, known as the mechanism of injury. This insight then helps you develop an index of suspicion, an anticipation of the nature and severity of likely injuries. Armed with an index of suspicion, you then better focus your trauma patient assessment, triage, and care because you know what happened and the injuries the event is likely to have produced.

Let us look at the kinetics of blunt trauma, vehicular collisions, blast injuries, and other types of blunt trauma to better understand these prevalent mechanisms of injury and their physiologic results.

Blunt trauma is the most common cause of trauma death and disability.

Blunt trauma can be deceptive because the true nature of the injury is often hidden and evidence of the serious injury is very subtle or even absent.

FIGURE 17-1 Blunt trauma is the most common cause of injury and trauma-related death. It is a physical exchange of energy from an object or surface transmitted through the skin into the body's interior.

KINETICS OF BLUNT TRAUMA

* **kinetics** the branch of physics that deals with motion, taking into consideration mass and force.

Kinetics is a branch of physics dealing with forces affecting objects in motion and the energy exchanges that occur as objects collide. These collisions, or impacts, are the events that induce injury in patients. An understanding of kinetics helps you appreciate and anticipate the results of auto and other impacts. The two basic principles of kinetics are the law of inertia and the law of energy conservation. Further, the kinetic energy and force formulas quantify the energy exchange process between the moving object and the human body. These laws and formulas best describe what happens during impact and help in our understanding of blunt trauma.

INERTIA

* **inertia** tendency of an object to remain at rest or remain in motion unless acted upon by an external force.

* **motion** the process of changing place; movement.

The law of **inertia,** as described by Sir Isaac Newton and also known as Newton's first law, helps explain what happens during blunt trauma. The first part of his first law states: "A body in **motion** will remain in motion unless acted upon by an outside force." As an example, think of identical autos moving at 55 miles per hour. One car brakes for a red light; the other rams into a bridge abutment. An "outside force" stops the motion of both vehicles, but with very different results. In the first case, the car's brakes absorb the energy of motion. In the second, the front bumper and grill, the frame, and eventually the occupants of the car absorb the energy as the car stops.

The second part of the law states: "A body at rest will remain at rest unless acted upon by an outside force." Examples of this include an auto accelerating from a stop sign or a stopped vehicle propelled forward by a rear-end collision. In the first case, the auto engine provides the force to initiate movement. In the second, the energy of the moving vehicle provides the force as the stopped car absorbs the energy and jolts ahead.

CONSERVATION OF ENERGY

* **energy** the capacity to do work in the strict physical sense.

The law of conservation of energy states: "**Energy** can neither be created nor destroyed. It only changes from one form to another." In an auto crash, as in other trauma, identifying probable energy changes helps you assess the impacts of various collisions. Kinetic energy, possessed by a moving car and its passengers, transforms into other energy forms whenever a car stops.

If an auto slows down gradually for a stop sign, the brakes develop friction against the turning wheels, producing heat. During an auto crash, however, the energy of motion is converted at a much faster rate into different forms. This conversion of energy is manifest in the sound of impact, the deformation of the auto's structural components, the heat in the twisted steel, and the injuries to passengers as they collide with the vehicle interior. When all the kinetic energy converts to other energy forms, the auto and its passengers come to a stop.

KINETIC ENERGY

* **kinetic energy** the energy an object has while it is in motion. It is related to the object's mass and velocity.

* **mass** a measure of the matter that an object contains; the property of a physical body that gives the body inertia.

* **velocity** the rate of motion in a particular direction in relation to time.

Kinetic energy is the energy of motion. It is a function of an object's **mass** and its **velocity** (Figure 17-2). (While mass and weight, and velocity and speed, are not identical, we will consider them as such for these discussions.) Kinetic energy of an object while in motion is measured by the following formula:

$$\text{Kinetic Energy} = \frac{\text{Mass (or weight)} \times \text{Velocity (or speed)}^2}{2}$$

This formula illustrates that if you double an object's weight, you double its kinetic energy. It is twice as damaging to be hit by a 2-pound baseball as to be hit by a 1-pound ball. It is three times as damaging to be hit by a 3-pound ball, and so on.

FIGURE 17-2 Increasing mass directly increases kinetic energy, while increasing velocity exponentially increases kinetic energy.

As speed (velocity) increases, there is a larger (squared) increase in kinetic energy. Being hit with a 1-pound baseball traveling at 20 miles per hour is four times as injurious as being hit with the same ball moving at 10 miles per hour. If speed increases to 30 miles per hour, trauma is nine times worse. This concept plays a key role in understanding the devastating effects of a gunshot wound in which a small bullet can do great damage (as discussed in Chapter 18, "Penetrating Trauma").

Kinetic energy is the measure of how much energy an object in motion has, not necessarily how much injury occurs. Two autos traveling at 55 miles per hour have about the same kinetic energy. The same two autos would have the same kinetic energy once they have stopped, even if one came to rest by hitting a bridge. The difference between these two events is the rate of slowing. This rate is proportional to the crash force.

FORCE

Newton's second law of motion explains the forces at work during a collision. It is summarized by the formula below:

Force = Mass (Weight) × Acceleration (or Deceleration)

The formula emphasizes the importance of the rate at which an object changes speed, either increasing (**acceleration**) or decreasing (**deceleration**). Slow changes in speed are usually uneventful. Normal deceleration, such as slowing for a stop sign, covers about 120 feet (from 55 miles per hour to 0 miles per hour at a braking rate of 22 feet/10 miles per hour). It therefore rarely results in injury. On the other hand, colliding with a bridge abutment and slowing from 55 miles per hour to 0 miles per hour in a matter of inches produces tremendous force and devastating injuries.

✱ **acceleration** the rate at which speed or velocity increases.

✱ **deceleration** the rate at which speed or velocity decreases.

TYPES OF TRAUMA

When significant kinetic energy is applied to human anatomy, we call it trauma. Trauma is defined as a wound or injury that is externally and violently produced by some outside force. The injury may be either blunt (closed) or penetrating (open) (Figure 17-3).

Trauma can be categorized as either blunt or penetrating.

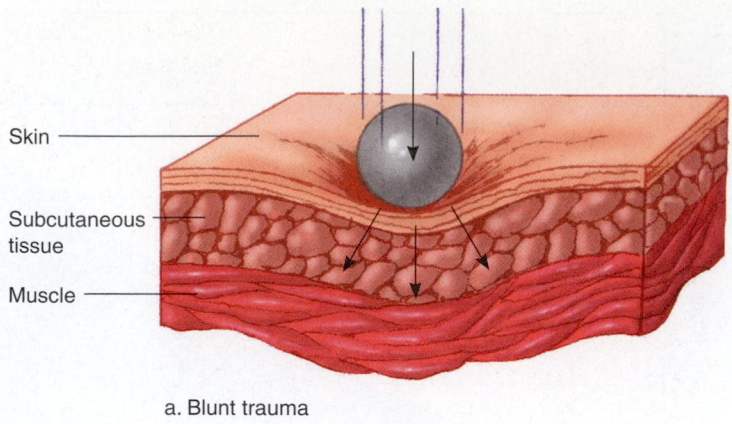

Skin

Subcutaneous tissue

Muscle

a. Blunt trauma

Skin

Subcutaneous tissue

Muscle

b. Penetrating trauma

FIGURE 17-3 Blunt trauma results when an object or force impacts the body and kinetic energy is transferred to the involved body tissues. Penetrating injury is produced when an object enters the body resulting in direct injury.

Blunt trauma occurs when a body area is struck by, or strikes, an object. The transmission of energy, rather than the object, damages the tissues and organs beneath the skin as they collide with one another. An example of this is hitting your thumb with a hammer. The thumb is compressed between the hammer (which pushes the tissue) and the board (which resists the motion). Tissue injury results as flesh and bone are trapped between these two forces (acceleration and deceleration). Skin and muscle cells stretch and crush, blood vessels tear, and bone may fracture.

Blunt trauma can also induce injury deep within the body cavity. Forces of compression cause hollow organs like the bladder or bowel to rupture, spilling their contents and hemorrhaging. In the thorax, alveoli or small airways may burst, permitting air to enter the pleural space. Solid organs, such as the spleen, liver, pancreas, and kidneys, may contuse or lacerate, leading to swelling, blood loss, or both.

Other blunt trauma may result from the effects of rapid speed change on organ attachment. An example is the liver, which is suspended in the abdomen by the *ligamentum teres*. During severe deceleration, the liver may be sliced by the ligament in a way similar to cheese when cut by a wire cheese cutter. Similarly, the aorta may be injured as the chest slows and the heart, which is suspended from the great vessels, twists upon impact. Layers of the vessel are torn apart, and blood enters the injury with the force of the systolic blood pressure. The aorta balloons like a defective tire, leading to a tearing chest pain, circulatory compromise, and immediate or delayed **exsanguination** (severe blood loss).

Wounds that break the skin are classified as penetrating trauma. Penetrating trauma occurs when the energy source (such as a knife or bullet) progresses into the body. Energy may also be transmitted to surrounding body tissue, thus extending the trauma beyond the pathway of the object. This frequently happens with high velocity gunshot wounds.

As a paramedic, you will encounter both blunt and penetrating trauma. The balance of this chapter deals with examples of blunt trauma. Examples of penetrating trauma are discussed in Chapter 18.

* **exsanguination** the draining of blood to the point at which life cannot be sustained.

BLUNT TRAUMA

Blunt trauma most commonly results from motor vehicle crashes involving automobiles, motorcycles, pedestrians, or recreational vehicles (all-terrain vehicles, watercraft, snowmobiles). It can also result from explosions, falls, crush injuries, and sports injuries.

AUTOMOBILE CRASHES

Vehicular crashes (sometimes called motor vehicle crashes or MVCs) account for a large proportion of paramedic responses. Each year over 100,000 serious collisions occur on U.S. highways. Some 44,000 people lose their lives in these crashes, while many more are seriously injured or permanently disabled. As a paramedic, you must be prepared to offer rapid assessment and appropriate care to victims of these crashes. To this end, you must recognize the various types of vehicular impacts, identify possible mechanisms of injury, and form a reasonable index of suspicion for specific injuries. Analysis of the types of impacts and the events associated with them help you form this index of suspicion.

Events of Impact

There are basically five types of vehicle impacts—frontal, lateral, rotational, rear-end, and rollover. Each type progresses through a series of five events (Figure 17-4). These events are:

1. *Vehicle Collision.* Vehicle collision begins when the auto strikes an object. Kinetic energy converts to vehicle damage or is transferred to the object hit by the auto. The force developed in the crash depends upon the stopping distance. If the auto slides into a snow bank, damage is limited. If the auto strikes a concrete retaining wall, the damage is much greater. The degree of auto deformity is a good indicator of strength and direction of forces experienced by its occupants. The auto collision slows or stops the vehicle.

2. *Body Collision.* Body collision occurs when a vehicle occupant strikes the vehicle's interior. The vehicle and its interior have slowed dramatically during the crash, but an unrestrained occupant remains at or close to the initial speed. As the occupant contacts the interior, energy is transferred to the vehicle or is transformed into the initial tissue deformity, compression, stretching, and trauma. If the vehicle collision causes intrusion

Vehicle collision

Auto hits tree

Impact points
Head vs. windshield

Body Collisions

Chest/abdomen
vs. steering wheel

Knee vs. dash

FIGURE 17-4 An automobile crash generates four major collisions: the vehicle collision, the body collision, the organ collision, and secondary collisions.

into the passenger compartment, this displacement may further injure occupants or otherwise worsen the injury process.

3. *Organ Collisions.* Organ collision results as the occupant contacts the vehicle's interior and slows or stops. Tissues behind the contacting surface collide, one into another, as the occupant's body comes to a halt. This causes compression and stretching as tissues and organs violently press into each other. In the process, organs may also twist or decelerate, and tear at their attachments or at blood vessels. The result is blunt trauma.

Organ collision

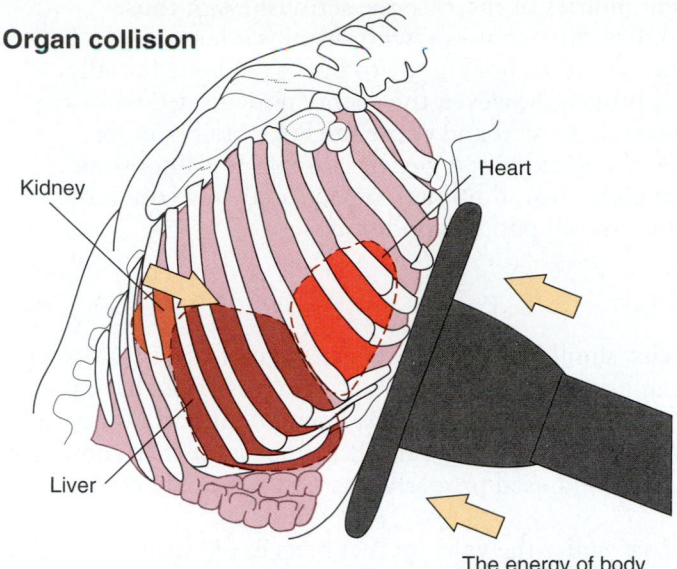

Kidney

Heart

Liver

The energy of body collision is transmitted to the interior.

Secondary collisions

FIGURE 17-4 (CONTINUED)

4. *Secondary Collisions.* Secondary collisions occur when a vehicle occupant is impacted by objects traveling within the auto. During the crash, objects—such as those in the back seat, on the back window ledge, or in the back of a van—or other unrestrained passengers may continue to travel at the auto's initial speed. They then impact an occupant who has come to rest within the auto. It is important to consider the possibility of any secondary collisions and their effects on occupants when developing an index of suspicion for injuries.

5. *Additional Impacts.* Additional impacts occur when a vehicle receives a second impact—for example, when it hits a vehicle, is deflected, then hits a parked car. This second impact may induce

Secondary collisions may cause a patient's injuries or increase their severity.

additional patient injuries or increase the seriousness of those already received. Consider someone who sustains a femur fracture. It takes a great deal of energy to break the bone initially. Once the bone is broken, however, the energy now needed to move those bone ends around and cause further, possibly more severe, injury to nerves and blood vessels is small. It is important to consider what effect any additional impacts may have upon the initial injuries and overall patient condition.

Restraints

Restraints have had a profound effect in reducing crash-related deaths.

Restraints such as seat belts, shoulder straps, airbags, and child safety seats have a profound effect on the injuries associated with auto crashes. They have played a substantial role in reducing crash-related deaths from about 55,000 a year in the early 1970s to about 44,000 in recent years. It is important that you determine if restraints were used—and used properly—as you anticipate the possible results of an auto crash.

EMS workers should recognize the value of seat belts in reducing auto crash mortality and morbidity. Hence, all ambulance personnel must employ seat belts when in the patient care area of the vehicle and especially while driving. Securing the lap belt firmly provides positive positioning so drivers and other crew members are not as adversely affected by the gravitational forces (G forces) sometimes associated with emergency driving.

Seat belt use should be mandatory for all EMS personnel.

Seat Belts Use of seat belts and shoulder straps prevents the wearer's continuing and independent movement during a vehicle crash. The occupant slows with the auto rather than moving rapidly forward and impacting the interior suddenly. The occupant's ultimate deceleration rate is thus reduced, lessening the likelihood of serious injury from collisions within the vehicle. Seat belts and shoulder straps also lessen the chances that the wearer will be ejected from the vehicle.

Although seat belts and shoulder straps significantly reduce injury severity, they may cause some, usually much less serious, injuries. A lap belt worn alone does not restrain the torso, neck, or head from continuing forward. These body regions may impact the dash or steering wheel, resulting in chest, neck, and head injuries. The sudden folding of the body at the waist during extreme impacts when only a lap belt is worn may result in intra-abdominal or lower spine injuries. If the lap belt is worn alone and too high, abdominal compression and spinal (T12 to L2) fractures may result. If worn too low, it may cause hip dislocations. If the shoulder strap is worn alone, it may cause severe neck contusions, lacerations, possible spinal injury, and even decapitation in more violent crashes. In very strong impacts, the shoulder strap may induce chest contusions and, in some cases, rib fractures. Further, the seat belt and/or shoulder strap do not protect against intrusions into the passenger compartment. In severe crashes, the dashboard may displace into the front seat, trapping or crushing the lower extremities of occupants.

Airbags Airbags, also called supplemental restraint systems (SRS), work much differently than seat belts and are extremely effective for frontal crashes. They inflate explosively upon auto impact, producing a cushion to absorb the energy exchange. Their ignition is dependent on several detectors sensing a very strong frontal deceleration, as can only occur with serious vehicle impact. Only after these detectors all agree does the explosive agent ignite. The ignition instantaneously fills the bag, slightly before or just as the occupant collides with it. The explosive gases escape quickly as the occupant compresses the bag, cushioning the impact much as the inflated bags used by pole-vaulters and movie stuntmen do. Like seat belts, airbags are credited with dramatically reducing vehicular death and trauma (Figure 17-5).

FIGURE 17-5 Airbags cushion the driver from the forces of impact and significantly reduce mortality and morbidity in frontal impact crashes.

Airbags are positioned in the steering wheel, and their presence is indicated by an "SRS" (Supplemental Restraint System) sticker on the windshield and/or on the steering wheel itself. They may also be located in the dash for the front seat passenger. Steering wheel and dash-mounted airbags offer significant protection only in frontal impact collisions. This protection is only for the first impact and not subsequent ones.

Airbags may induce injury during their ignition and rapid inflation. As the bag inflates, especially from the steering wheel, it may impact the driver's fingers, hands, and forearms, possibly causing dislocations and fractures. In persons of small stature seated very close to the steering wheel, airbag inflation may also cause nasal fractures, minor facial lacerations, and contusions. The residue from airbag inflation may cause some irritation of the eyes; this can be relieved with gentle irrigation. Whenever an airbag has deployed, check beneath it for steering wheel deformity, which is indicative of injury to the driver.

Passenger airbags have inflated in minor impacts and pushed infant and child safety seats into seats with tremendous force. In some cases, infants and children have been severely injured or killed by inflation of the bags. For this reason, it is recommended that parents secure child carriers in the back seat when a passenger airbag system is in place.

Auto manufacturers are starting to install airbags in the seat sides, adjacent to the doors in some cars, for protection in lateral impact crashes. Some manufacturers also install airbags in the headliners above doors to provide protection for the head in such crashes. Since little experience has been gained with these types of restraints, their benefits and potential drawbacks are not well known. However, lateral impacts do account for a very high mortality rate that may be mediated with lateral-impact and head-protection airbags.

Child Safety Seats The child's anatomy makes protection in vehicle crashes difficult. Because a child's size changes so quickly with increasing age, normal restraint

While airbags can cause injury, they have, overall, greatly reduced injury and death in vehicular crashes.

Properly used child safety seats provide the best protection for infants and small children riding in vehicles.

systems are designed for adults only. Small children should be placed in appropriate child safety seats to assure their relative safety during an auto impact. With infants and very small children, the child safety seat is positioned facing to the rear and held firmly to the seat with the seat belt. This positioning best distributes frontal impact forces and prevents unrestrained infant movement. As the child grows in size, the child carrier is turned facing forward and used as a small seat. The seat belt then crosses the child at the waistline.

Children held in an adult's lap or arms are not well protected during a crash. The holder may grasp them too tightly during impact or, more likely, will not (or cannot) hold on tightly enough. If the child is not held, he becomes an unrestrained moving object and will impact the vehicle interior suffering serious, possibly fatal, injury.

When evaluating the results of an auto impact, always be sure to examine for and ask questions about the use of restraints. Determine if seat belts and shoulder straps were used and used properly, if airbags deployed during the crash, and if child carriers were properly positioned and secured. If these restraints were properly employed, the severity of injuries to the vehicle occupants will very likely be reduced.

Types of Impact

As you have read, there are five general types of auto impacts. They are:

- Frontal
- Lateral
- Rotational
- Rear-end
- Rollover

The following is a breakdown of the frequency of different types of motor-vehicle impacts (Figure 17-6). Figures reflect an urban setting. In a more rural area, anticipate a greater percentage of frontal impacts with corresponding reductions in other categories.

Frontal: 32 percent

Lateral: 15 percent

Rotational: 38 percent

Rear End: 9 percent

Rollover: 6 percent

Note that rotational impact includes four sub-categories: left front, right front, left rear, and right rear.

Content Review

TYPES OF VEHICLE IMPACT
Frontal
Lateral
Rotational
Rear-end
Rollover

FIGURE 17-6 Incidence of motor vehicle impacts.

FIGURE 17-7 Frontal impact often results in a significant exchange of energy and serious injuries.

Frontal Impact Frontal impact is the most common type of impact (Figure 17-7) and produces three pathways of patient travel. They are:

1. *Down-and-Under Pathway.* In the down-and-under pathway, the occupant slides downward as the vehicle comes to a stop. The knees contact the fire wall, under the dash, and absorb the initial impact. Knee, femur, and hip dislocations or fractures are common. Once the lower body slows, the upper body rotates forward, pivoting at the hip, and crashing against the steering wheel or dash. Chest injuries like flail chest, myocardial contusion, and aortic tears result. If the neck contacts the steering wheel, tracheal and vascular injury may occur. An injury process frequently associated with steering wheel impact is the "paper bag" syndrome (Figure 17-8). The driver takes a deep breath in anticipation of the collision. Lung tissue (alveoli, bronchioles, and larger airways) ruptures when the chest impacts the steering wheel, much like an inflated paper bag caught between clapping hands. Pneumothorax and pulmonary contusion may result.

2. *Up-and-Over Pathway.* In the up-and-over pathway, the occupant tenses the legs in preparation for impact (Figure 17-9). With vehicle slowing, the unrestrained body's upper half pivots forward and upward. The steering wheel impinges the femurs, causing possible bilateral fractures. In addition, it compresses and decelerates the abdominal contents, causing hollow-organ rupture and liver laceration. Traumatic compression may also force abdominal contents against the diaphragm, causing it to rupture and allowing organs to enter the thoracic cavity. As the body continues forward, the lower chest impacts the steering wheel and

Frontal impact is the most common type of vehicle crash.

Content Review

MECHANISMS ASSOCIATED WITH FRONTAL IMPACTS
Down-and-under pathway
Up-and-over pathway
Ejection

The up-and-over pathway accounts for over half of the deaths in vehicular crashes.

Deceleration

Compression

Precrash

Impact

FIGURE 17-8 The "paper bag" syndrome results from compression of the chest against the steering column.

Forces of impact to head and neck

Forces of impact to chest

FIGURE 17-9 The up-and-over pathway is associated with frontal impact crashes.

may account for the same thoracic injuries seen with the down-and-under pathway.

The same forward motion propels the head into the windshield, leading to soft tissue injury, skull or facial fractures, and internal head injury. Neck injury may result from hyperextension, hyperflexion, or the compressional forces of windshield impact. As the body is thrown upward and forward, the head contacts the windshield. The rest of the body tries to push the head through the windshield. The result is a compressional force on the cervical spine called **axial loading.** This loading may result in collapse of support elements of the vertebral column. Over half of vehicular deaths are attributed to the up-and-over pathway.

3. *Ejection.* The up-and-over pathway may lead to ejection of an unrestrained occupant. Such a victim experiences two impacts: (1) contact with the vehicle interior and windshield and (2) impact with the ground, tree, or other object. This mechanism of injury is responsible for about 27 percent of vehicular fatalities. While ejection may occur with other types of impact, it is most commonly associated with frontal impact.

Recognize that a frontal impact crash interposes more vehicle between the point of impact and the vehicle occupants. Modern vehicle design techniques use this area of the vehicle (called the **crumple zone**) to absorb the impact forces and limit occupant injury (Figure 17-10). Patients in vehicle collisions such as those involving vans and lateral impacts do not benefit from these energy absorbing crumple zones. In these circumstances, the apparent vehicle damage may be less than in a frontal impact crash, even though the forces delivered to the occupants are greater.

✱ **axial loading** application of the forces of trauma along the axis of the spine; this often results in compression fractures of the spine.

✱ **crumple zone** the region of a vehicle designed to absorb the energy of impact.

Occupants of a vehicle without a crumple zone may experience greater forces in a collision even though damage to the vehicle itself may not appear as severe as damage to a vehicle with a crumple zone involved in a similar crash.

FIGURE 17-10 Crumple zones provide significant protection with both frontal and rear-end impacts but much less in cases of lateral impacts.

FIGURE 17-11 A lateral impact collision presents the least amount of crumple zone between the vehicle's exterior and its passenger compartment.

Lateral Impact The kinetics of lateral impact are the same as for frontal impact with two exceptions. First, occupants present a different profile (turned 90 degrees) to collision forces. Second, the amount of structural steel between the impact site and the vehicle interior is greatly reduced (Figure 17-11). Lateral impacts account for 15 percent of all auto accidents, yet they are responsible for 22 percent of vehicular fatalities. When a lateral impact occurs, the index of suspicion for serious and life-threatening internal injuries must be higher than vehicle damage alone suggests.

With lateral impacts, there is an increase in upper extremity injuries (Figure 17-12). The ribs fracture laterally on the side of impact instead of anteriorly. The clavicle, humerus, pelvis, and femur may fracture on the impact side. Cervical spine injury occurs as the body moves laterally while the head remains stationary. Vertebrae may fracture with the rapid lateral motion as may the skull as it smashes into the window. Lateral compression, affecting the body cavity, may give rise to diaphragm rupture, pulmonary contusion, splenic injury (to the driver), and much more. Aortic aneurysm may occur with this in-

Maintain a higher index of suspicion of serious injury when assessing lateral impact crashes because the degree of injury may be greater than the damage alone would indicate.

FIGURE 17-12 In a lateral impact collision, an occupant may experience lateral impact to the head, lateral bending of the neck, twisting of the heart and the aorta, and humerus, clavicular, pelvic, and femur fractures.

jury mechanism. The heart, which is not firmly attached in the central thorax, moves violently toward the impact as the body accelerates. This twists the aorta, tearing its inner layer, the intima. Blood seeps between the connective tissue layers and the vessel begins to delaminate. The aorta may rupture immediately or over the next few hours.

Evaluation of lateral impact collisions should take into consideration any unrestrained passenger opposite the impact site. If the driver's side is struck and such a passenger is not belted, the passenger becomes an object that will strike and injure the driver shortly after initial impact.

FIGURE 17-13 In rotational impacts, the energy exchange is more gradual and there may be less injury than vehicle damage suggests. There may, however, be multiple impacts.

Rotational Impact In rotational impact, the auto is struck at an **oblique** angle and rotates as the collision forces are expended (Figure 17-13). The ensuing rotation causes injuries similar to those from frontal and lateral impacts. Acceleration (or deceleration) is greatest farther from the center of the auto and closest to impact. Autos involved are deflected from their paths rather than being stopped abruptly. While rotational impact injuries can be serious, they are often less than vehicle damage might suggest. With the deflection of the impact, the occupant's stopping distance is much greater, deceleration is more gradual, and injuries are generally less serious.

Rear-end Impact In rear-end impact, the collision force pushes the auto forward (Figure 17-14). Within the vehicle, the seat propels the occupant forward. If the headrest is not up, the head is unsupported and remains stationary. The

FIGURE 17-14 In rear-end impacts there is generally good protection for the body, except for the head and neck. *(Courtesy of Edward T. Dickinson, MD)*

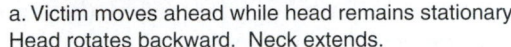

a. Victim moves ahead while head remains stationary. Head rotates backward. Neck extends.

b. Head snaps forward. Head rotates forward. Neck flexes.

FIGURE 17-15   The effects of a rear-end collision on the occupant of a vehicle.

neck extends severely, stretching the neck muscles and ligaments while the head rotates backward. Once acceleration ceases, the head snaps forward and the neck flexes. This rapid and extreme hyperextension followed by hyperflexion may result in severe connective tissue and cervical vertebra injuries (Figure 17-15). There is also risk of injury when the auto finally ends its acceleration and an unrestrained occupant is thrown forward.

Rollover Auto rollover is normally caused by a change in elevation and/or a vehicle with a high center of gravity (Figure 17-16). As the vehicle rolls, it impacts the ground at various points. The occupant experiences an impact with each

FIGURE 17-16   Rollover crashes result in multiple impacts and, possible, multiple injury mechansims.

impact of the vehicle. These impacts can be especially violent due to the absence of crumple zones and internal padding at the multiple points of impact (vehicle sides and roof). The type of injuries expected with a rollover relate to the specific vehicle impacts involved. Remember, any injury occurring with the first collision is likely to be compounded with subsequent impacts. A common result of rollover is ejection or partial ejection with a limb or head trapped between the rolling vehicle and the ground. Restraints are especially effective in reducing ejection and injury during rollover.

Vehicle Crash Analysis

Vehicle crashes often produce hazards not only to the vehicle occupants but also to bystanders and care providers. Be alert for these hazards during the scene size-up. Such hazards may include hot engine and transmission parts, hot fluids such as radiator coolant or engine oil, caustic substances such as battery acid and automatic transmission or steering fluids, and the sharp, jagged edges of torn metal or broken glass. Also remain aware of the potential for danger from traffic moving near the crash site or from electrical power lines that may have been downed by the crash.

The visual examination of the crash scene can tell you a great deal about what happened to the patient(s) and what injuries should be suspected.

During the scene size-up, evaluate the vehicle to determine the direction of impact and the amount of vehicle damage. From the angle of impact, visualize the direction of forces expressed on the crash victims and the strength of those forces. Realize that the front and rear structures of the modern cars are designed to crumple during impact to absorb kinetic forces. While moderate-speed impacts may destroy the vehicle, the passengers may escape with little injury. Occupants in lateral and rollover impacts do not benefit from such crumple zones and frequently suffer injuries more directly related to the kinetic forces.

As you evaluate the collision, consider the relative sizes of the impacting vehicles or objects. A large, heavy vehicle impacting a smaller, lighter one will experience lesser acceleration or deceleration forces than the smaller vehicle. In this case, there is likely to be more severe vehicle damage to the smaller vehicle and more serious injuries to its occupants as well. Similar considerations apply with objects impacted by vehicles. For example, a large, well-rooted tree that does not move will cause much more damage during an impact than will a telephone pole that shears off.

When evaluation of the outside of the vehicle is complete, look at the passenger compartment (Figure 17-17). Determine if there is any intrusion, which indicates the presence of forces greater than those that could be absorbed by the crumple zones. Quickly look for signs of occupant/interior impacts. A spider-webbed windshield suggests a severe impact between the occupant's head and the glass. A deformed steering wheel suggests injury to the driver's chest or upper abdomen. A dented dash suggests injury to the knees or injuries transmitted to the femur or hip. Deformities of the gas, brake, or clutch pedals suggest foot injury. Deployed and deflated airbags may indicate chest, forearm, or hand injury.

In very severe impacts, collision forces may push the dashboard and firewall into the passenger compartment, entrapping and crushing the lower extremities of occupants against the seat. In such cases, parts of the vehicle, like the foot pedals, turn indicator arms, shift levers, and instrument panel knobs or switches may be physically imbedded in crash victims. This complicates extrication because the seat and the dash must be separated carefully to free the trapped victim. In these cases, the area should be carefully examined before and while any extrication equipment is used. Ongoing examinations should be provided frequently during extrication in order to ensure that the process does not result in further, unnecessary harm to the patient.

Assess whether restraints have been used or airbags deployed. Use of these devices may limit the severity of injuries in frontal impacts. Conversely, their non-use

FIGURE 17-17 Study the interior of a crashed vehicle carefully to identify the strength and direction of forces expressed to the patient.

may suggest more severe injuries. Check the positions of headrests in rear-impact collisions. Their proper positioning may limit neck hyperextension and injury.

Intoxication Whenever you evaluate motor vehicle trauma, consider the possibility of alcohol intoxication. Figures from states requiring mandatory alcohol-level testing after fatal auto collisions reveal that more than 50 percent of the drivers were legally intoxicated. Alcohol also contributes to many recreational-vehicle accidents, boating accidents, and accidental drownings.

Whenever you suspect alcohol intoxication, your assessment must be more diligent. Remember, alcohol interferes with the patient's level of consciousness and masks signs and symptoms of injury. Intoxication may be hard to differentiate from the signs of head injury. It also anesthetizes the patient somewhat to trauma pain. These factors make the mechanism of injury analysis and the resultant index of suspicion even more important. Otherwise, significant injuries may be overlooked or brushed off as symptoms of alcohol intoxication.

Alcohol intoxication is associated with most serious crashes.

Vehicular Mortality Examination of the effects of motor vehicle trauma on the human anatomy reveals certain areas to be especially prone to life-threatening injury. A study of the incidence of mortality and the associated location of trauma provides the findings in Table 17-1.

Trauma to the head and body cavity accounts for 85 percent of vehicular mortality. For this reason, the rapid trauma assessment should be directed at the head, neck, thorax, abdomen, and pelvis. Once you assure the airway, breathing,

Head and body cavity trauma account for 85 percent of deaths in vehicular crashes.

Table 17-1	MOTOR VEHICLE FATALITIES
(Incidence by Body Area)	
Head	47.7 %
Internal (chest/abdominal/pelvic)	37.3 %
Spinal and chest fracture	8.3 %
Fractures to the extremities	2.0 %
All other	4.7 %

and circulation, proceed to the rapid trauma assessment, looking at areas where your index of suspicion suggests injury. Examine the head, chest, and abdomen first to identify any evidence of life-threatening injuries.

Crash Evaluation As a paramedic, you must be thoroughly practiced in the assessment of trauma patients, especially because of the high incidence of serious injury associated with auto crashes. Whenever you respond to an accident, analyze the five types of collisions associated with vehicle impact. In each case, ask yourself these questions:

- How did the objects collide?
- From what direction did they come?
- At what speed were they traveling?
- Were the objects similarly sized or grossly different? (For example, did a car and a semi-truck collide?)
- Were any secondary collisions or additional transfers of energy involved?

In analyzing the mechanisms of injury, also consider the cause of the crash.

- Did wet pavement or poor visibility contribute to the accident?
- Was alcohol involved?
- Is there an absence of skid marks? If so, what happened to the driver to prevent him from braking?

Examine the auto interior, which is the mass struck by the moving occupant.

- Does the windshield show evidence of impact by the victim's head?
  – Is it bloody or broken in the characteristic spider web or star shape?
  – Has it been penetrated by the patient's head or body?
- Is the steering wheel deformed or collapsed?
- Is the dash indented where the knees or head hit it?
- Has the impact damage extended into the passenger compartment (intrusion)?

Answers to such questions complement your mechanism of injury analysis and help you to develop accurate indices of suspicion.

MOTORCYCLE CRASHES

In addition to auto crashes, as a paramedic you will respond to many motorcycle crashes. Because of the lack of protective vehicle structure, motorcycle crashes often result in serious trauma, even at low speeds. The rider, rather than the structural steel, absorbs much of the crash energy (Figure 17-18). Injuries can be severe, with an especially high incidence of head trauma. The motorcycle crash impacts differ somewhat from those of an auto crash. The four types of motorcycle impacts include the following: frontal, angular, sliding, and ejection.

In a frontal, or head-on impact, the bike dips downward, propelling the rider upward and forward. The handlebars catch the rider's lower abdomen or pelvis, causing abdominal and/or pelvic injury. Occasionally, the rider travels through a higher trajectory. In such cases, the handlebars can trap the femurs, often resulting in bilateral fractures.

An angular impact occurs when the bike strikes an object at an oblique angle. The rider's lower extremity is trapped between the object struck and the bike. This may fracture or crush the foot, ankle, knee, and femur. Open wounds often result.

Serious trauma is likely with even low-speed motorcycle crashes because of the lack of protective vehicle structure.

FIGURE 17-18 Motorcycle crashes result in serious trauma because the cycle provides little protection for its rider.

Sliding impact occurs when an experienced rider, facing an imminent crash, "lays the bike down." The rider slides the bike sideways into the object, so that the bike hits the object first, absorbing much of the energy. Laying the bike down also reduces the chances of ejection. The result is an increase in lacerations, abrasions, and minor fractures, with a decrease in more serious injuries.

Ejection during a motorcycle crash is common and usually results in serious injury. It may occur with any of the mechanisms previously described and result in the following impacts:

- Initial bike/object collision
- Rider/object impact
- Rider/ground impact

Likely injuries include skull fracture and/or head injury, spinal fractures and paralysis, internal thoracic or abdominal injury, and extremity fractures.

In assessing a motorcycle crash, remember that protective equipment affects injury patterns. A helmet can reduce the incidence and severity of head injury by 50 to 66 percent. Use of a helmet, however, neither increases nor decreases the incidence of spinal trauma. Leather clothing and boots protect the rider against open soft-tissue injury, but they can also hide underlying contusions and fractures.

Helmets reduce the incidence and severity of head injuries in motorcycle crashes, but they have no effect on the incidence of spinal trauma.

PEDESTRIAN ACCIDENTS

Some vehicular accidents involve pedestrians, who are often severely injured because of the mass and speed of the object hitting them and because of their lack of protection. Adults and children suffer different types of injuries because of differing

FIGURE 17-19   An adult frequently turns away from a collision with an automobile and thus impacts the vehicle first with a leg. Because of a higher center of gravity, such patients are often thrown onto the hood and into the windshield.

anatomical size and differing responses to the impending accident. Recognition of these differences helps you anticipate injuries and provide the necessary treatment.

Adult pedestrians generally turn away from oncoming vehicles and present a lateral surface to impact. Anatomically, impact is low. The bumper strikes the lower leg first, fracturing the tibia and fibula. Energy transmitted to the opposing knee can lead to ligament injury. As the lower extremities are propelled forward with the car, the upper and lateral body crashes into the hood causing femur, lateral chest, or upper extremity fractures. The victim then slides into the windshield, leading to head, neck, and shoulder trauma. The adult may be further injured when thrown to the ground. This secondary collision may cause additional injury or compound those already received (Figure 17-19).

In contrast to adults, children usually turn toward an oncoming vehicle. Because of their smaller anatomy, injuries are located higher on children's bodies. The bumper impacts the femurs or pelvis, causing fracture. Children are frequently thrown in front of the vehicle because of their smaller size and lower center of gravity. They may then be run over or pushed to the side by the vehicle. If a child is thrown upward, injuries are similar to those of an adult (Figure 17-20).

When evaluating the injuries associated with auto-vs.-pedestrian accidents, look carefully at the scene. Try to determine the speed of the vehicle at time of impact and the distance the pedestrian was thrown. This information may be useful to the emergency department personnel in their determination of suspected injuries.

RECREATIONAL VEHICLE CRASHES

Over the past years, recreational vehicle usage has increased, and with it, the incidence of related trauma. Recreational vehicle crashes often cause injuries similar to those associated with auto crashes. Drivers and passengers of recreational vehicles, however, do not have the structural protections and restraint systems found in autos. Complicating injuries is the fact that recreational vehicles travel off road, which means there is often difficulty in reaching and retrieving victims once collisions are detected. The major types of vehicles most often involved in recreational vehicle crashes are snowmobiles, watercraft, and all-terrain vehicles (ATVs).

In pedestrian-vs.-automobile crashes, adults tend to turn away from the oncoming vehicle before impact, while children turn toward it.

Recreational vehicles usually lack the structure and the restraint systems that offer significant protection to automobile drivers and passengers.

FIGURE 17-20   In collisions with autos, children often turn toward the impact and, because of their lower body heights, are frequently thrown in front of the vehicle.

Snowmobile crashes can be very violent because the speeds at which snowmobiles travel can approach those of cars and snowmobiles offer no crumple zones for impact absorption. These accidents commonly result in ejections, crush injuries secondary to rollover, and glancing blows against obstructions in the snow. Riders also experience severe head and neck injuries from collisions with other vehicles, including autos, other snowmobiles, or with stationary objects such as trees. Snowmobile trauma may include severe neck injury when the rider runs into an unseen wire fence. The anterior neck is deeply lacerated, causing airway compromise, severe bleeding, and, in some cases, complete decapitation. Injuries to snowmobilers may be compounded by the effects of cold exposure and hypothermia.

Watercraft accidents commonly result from impact with other boats or obstructions, submerged or otherwise (Figure 17-21). These vehicles are not designed to absorb the energy of impacts nor are the occupants provided with restraint systems. As a result, watercraft crashes can cause serious injuries, even though the speeds of typical watercraft are substantially lower than those of autos. Trauma in these crashes is further complicated by the potential for drowning if the occupants are thrown into the water or the boat sinks. In northern areas, water temperatures can also rapidly induce hypothermia. Alcohol is frequently associated with watercraft accidents.

The use of personal watercraft, commonly called jet skis, for water recreation has increased greatly in recent years, as has the incidence of watercraft accidents. Jet skis are especially dangerous in the hands of inexperienced riders. The high speeds

FIGURE 17-21   Watercraft accidents are common, may involve either objects on the surface or submerged, and present the risks of drowning or hypothermia.

Blunt Trauma   **847**

attained by these watercraft contribute to the incidence and severity of injury associated with crashes. Although the craft's propulsion unit is protected and unlikely to cause trauma, collision with other watercraft, as well as objects and people in the water, lead to blunt trauma, again complicated by the potential for drowning.

There are two types of ATVs: the three- and four-wheeled versions (Figure 17-22). The three-wheeled ATV is notoriously unstable, especially when ridden by children, young adults, persons of lower body weight, or those with limited vehicle experience. The ATV's center of gravity is relatively high, contributing to the likelihood of rollover during quick turns. As with snowmobiles, a significant incidence of frontal collision is common with both types of ATVs. The injuries expected might include upper and lower extremity fracture and head and spine injury.

BLAST INJURIES

*oxidizer an agent that enhances combustion of a fuel.

Explosions can be caused by dust, as in a grain elevator, by fumes, such as gasoline or natural gas, or by explosive compounds (combustible and **oxidizer** mixes) such as dynamite, gun powder, and TNT. The explosion may be the result of an accident or intentional act of terrorism or warfare. The blast magnitude may range from that of a small firecracker in the hands of a teenager to a nuclear detonation.

Explosion

An explosion occurs when an agent or environment combusts. During a conventional (non-nuclear) explosion, the fuel and oxidizing agent combine instantaneously. Chemical bonds are broken down and reestablished, releasing tremendous energy in the form of rapidly moving molecules, known to us as heat. This heat creates a great pressure differential between the exploding agent and the surrounding air. This heat and the pressure differential produce several mechanisms of injury including a pressure wave, blast wind, projectiles, heat, and displacement of persons near the blast (Figure 17-23).

Pressure Wave

As the combustible agent ignites and burns explosively, it immediately heats the surrounding air. The molecules of heated air move very fast, increasing the pressure of the exploding cloud. The rapid increase in pressure compresses adjacent

FIGURE 17-23 An explosion releases tremendous amounts of heat energy, generating a pressure wave, blast wind, and projection of debris.

air. Adjacent air, in turn, pushes against air farther out from the point of ignition, and a **pressure wave** begins to move away from the blast epicenter. This is not a gross air movement but rather a narrow compression wave moving rapidly outward, similar to a wave through water (where the wave and not the water moves). This narrow wave, called **overpressure**, results in a drastic but brief increase, then decrease, in air pressure as it passes. The blast overpressure wave moves outward slightly faster than the speed of sound through the air or water, and its strength decreases quickly.

When the explosion involves a dust, aerosol, or gas cloud, the result is an area, not a single point, of detonation. The exploding cloud's pressure is extremely lethal, and the area it involves can be extensive. A bomb's casing or confined spaces, such as a building interior, contain the pressure of an explosion until the structure ruptures. The ensuing rapid release of the pressure enhances the peak overpressure and the potential for injury and death.

Underwater detonation also greatly enhances the potential for injury and death associated with the pressure wave. Water is a non-compressible medium that transmits the overpressure efficiently. Any submerged portion of the victim is subject to the rapid compression and then decompression. The lethal range for an explosive charge increases threefold with an underwater detonation.

Upon striking the body, the overpressure wave instantly compresses, then decompresses, the body's air-filled spaces, causing trauma. This rapid compression/decompression may produce injury to the middle ear, sinuses, bowel, or lungs. Because overpressure intensity diminishes rapidly as the wave travels outward, most life-threatening compression injuries are usually limited to people in close proximity to the detonation, with the exceptions of gas-cloud ignitions and underwater detonations.

A victim's orientation to the blast wave is also an important factor in the production of injuries. The greater the surface a victim presents to the blast wave, the greater the impact and damage. People standing and facing directly toward or away from the blast experience the greatest pressure effect. People lying on the ground, with their heads away from or toward the blast, experience the least pressure effects. In water, the same is true, although the more deeply submerged a victim is, the greater the damaging effects of the overpressure.

✱ **pressure wave** area of overpressure that radiates outward from an explosion.

Content Review

MECHANISMS ASSOCIATED WITH BLASTS

Pressure wave
Blast wind
Projectiles
Personnel displacement
Confined spaces and
  structural collapses
Burns

✱ **overpressure** a rapid increase then decrease in atmospheric pressure created by an explosion.

Underwater detonation increases the lethal range of an explosion threefold.

Blast Wind

Following the pressure wave and traveling just behind it, is the **blast wind.** This is the actual outward movement of heated and expanding combustion gases from the explosion epicenter. The blast wind has less strength but greater duration than the pressure wave. It causes much less direct injury, although in powerful blasts it may propel debris or displace victims, which will, in turn, produce injuries.

Projectiles

If the exploding material is contained by a casing, as with military **ordnance** or a pipe bomb, or by a structure, as with a garage filled with gas fumes, the container holds the explosive force until the container breaks apart. The parts of the container then become high-speed projectiles, behaving much like bullets and bound by the same laws of physics. Although they are not as fast as bullets and they lack good aerodynamic properties, they can cause serious injury beyond the injury zone of the blast's pressure wave itself. Some military ordnance contains special arrow-shaped missiles called **flechettes.** Their design gives the flechettes a greater following surface and aligns the missiles in flight, reducing their wind resistance and increasing their range and penetrating ability.

If the victim is in very close proximity to a strong blast, the casing and debris may move forcefully enough to tear off limbs or cause serious open wounds. The blast debris—glass fragments, building materials, or casing elements—may also impale itself in the skin and soft tissue. While the wounds caused by blast debris are normally small, large and heavy fragments may penetrate deeply into victims and cause serious tissue damage and hemorrhage.

Personnel Displacement

The pressure wave and blast wind may be strong enough to physically propel victims away from the center of the blast. Those victims then become projectiles and impact the ground, objects, debris, or other personnel, resulting in blunt or, in some cases, penetrating trauma. While the effects of this mechanism of injury are limited when compared to those produced by the pressure wave, blast wind, or projectiles, significant injuries can occur.

Confined Space Explosions and Structural Collapses

The effects of explosive devices are usually limited in range because the pressure wave and debris radiate outward in all directions from a central point. This rapidly reduces the overpressure and the concentration and, to a lesser degree, the velocity of projectiles. When an explosion occurs in a confined space, however, the pressure wave maintains its energy longer. There is also danger of structural collapse, and debris from the confining structure can increase the blast's projectile content. The blast overpressure also bounces off walls and, where pressure waves meet, the pressure greatly increases. The result can be extremely deadly overpressures. The most lethal blasts are those causing structural collapses followed by those involving confined spaces.

Structural collapses may cause severe crush-type injuries. The collapses may also make victims difficult to locate and, once found, difficult to extricate because of the weight of the material entrapping them. Damage to structures may present further hazards to rescuers and victims, including the possibility of additional collapses, electrocution, fire, or secondary explosion due to gas or fuel leaks.

Burns

An explosion can create tremendous heat. This heat may cause flash burns to those very close to the detonation. These injuries are generally superficial or partial thickness burns and may occur in conjunction with other trauma. However, victims may also be burned as the heat of the blast ignites combustibles such as clothing, debris, other munitions, or fuel. These secondary burns may be full thickness and extensive.

Some military and terrorist devices are designed to induce damage and injury through combustion. Napalm, for an example, is a highly **incendiary,** jelly-like substance that clings to people or structures when spread by a blast. It can produce severe or fatal full-thickness burns. Other ordnance uses materials, such as phosphorus, that spontaneously combust when exposed to air.

Blast Injury Phases

The injuries produced by explosions are usually classified into three types depending on the phases of the blast that caused them: primary, secondary, and tertiary (Figure 17-24).

Primary Blast Injuries Primary blast injuries are caused by the heat of the explosion and the overpressure wave. The pressure injuries are the most serious and life-threatening injuries associated with the explosion. Burn injuries are generally limited unless caused by secondary combustion.

Secondary Blast Injuries Secondary blast injuries include trauma caused by projectiles. These injuries may be as or more severe than the primary blast injuries. Projectiles from an explosive blast do have the ability to extend the range of injury beyond that caused by the blast wave and wind. High concentrations of projectiles may also create multiple body penetrations and impalements over large areas of a victim's body. The resulting injuries may produce severe bleeding.

Tertiary Blast Injuries Tertiary blast injuries include those injuries resulting from personnel displacement and structural collapse. Blast victims may be thrown against walls, the ground, or other obstructions and suffer blunt and/or penetrating trauma. When the blast results in a structural collapse, crush injuries may also result. These injuries can be extensive and result in soft skeletal, nervous, and vascular tissue and organ destruction.

Blast Injury Assessment

Blast injuries produce extreme trauma in those who are close to the blast epicenter. Blasts in densely populated areas may also involve large numbers of victims. Your role as an EMT-Paramedic is to survey and size up the scene and do what you can to secure it for further EMS operations. This normally involves implementing the incident command system and assuring overall scene management. Once command is established and operational, you will likely begin caring for patients by applying the normal assessment priorities (the ABCs of the initial assessment) and then focusing on the seriously injured but salvageable blast victims. If the number of victims exceeds the immediate capabilities of your EMS system, employ disaster triage.

Determine, if possible, whether the blast was the result of terrorist action. If you suspect that it was, be alert to the possibility that other explosive devices may be set or the area booby-trapped to endanger rescuers. Assure that police and bomb squad personnel sweep the area before you and your team enter it.

Carefully evaluate the scene for secondary hazards. Look for such things as gas leaks, disrupted electrical wiring, sharp debris, and the possibility of further structural collapse. During the scene size-up, determine the location of the

* incendiary an agent that combusts easily or creates combustion.

Content Review

BLAST INJURY PHASES

Primary—caused by heat of explosion and overpressure wave

Secondary—caused by blast projectiles

Tertiary—caused by personnel displacement and structural collapse

Employ disaster triage and activate the jurisdiction's disaster plan if the number of blast victims exceeds EMS system capacities.

Secondary Injuries:
missiles and debris
being propelled

Tertiary Injuries:
impacts with hard
surfaces or structural
collapses

Primary Injuries:
burns and pressure
injuries

FIGURE 17-24 Blasts can cause injury with the initial blast, when the victim is struck by debris, or when the victim is thrown by the blast or injured by structural collapse.

Pulmonary injuries are the most common and serious trauma associated with explosions.

epicenter of the blast. Note the presence of greater destruction and injury as you progress toward the epicenter. As you get closer, your index of suspicion for serious injury increases.

The most common and serious trauma associated with explosions is lung injury. Pulmonary injury may not manifest itself immediately, so anticipate it in anyone with any other significant signs or symptoms of blast trauma. Evaluate breathing and breath sounds frequently, carefully watching and listening for any dyspnea and crackles or other signs of respiratory congestion. At the first sign of breathing problems, consider high-flow oxygen and rapid transport.

Some blast victims may experience hearing loss due to the pressure wave. After experiencing the emotional impact of the blast itself, this injury can be extremely anxiety-producing for victims. Do your best to calm and reassure these patients. Remember that they will find it difficult to understand what others are saying and will not be able to follow spoken commands.

Blast Injury Care

The effects of a serious explosion can produce injuries to the lungs, abdomen, and ears that involve special care considerations. Otherwise, care for blunt trauma, punctures/penetrations, and burns as you would for these injuries if they were produced by other mechanisms.

Lungs Pulmonary blast trauma is the most frequent and life-threatening pressure injury associated with an explosion. The blast-induced pressure wave rapidly and forcefully compresses and distorts the chest cavity, individual air passages, and the alveoli. During compression/decompression, the air pressures in these areas do not have time to equalize, as they do with normal respiration. The extreme pressure damages or ruptures the thin and delicate alveolar walls, resulting in fluid accumulation, hemorrhage, and possibly even the entry of air directly into the blood-stream from the alveoli. Fluid accumulation (pulmonary edema) makes the lungs less elastic and air movement more difficult. The victim finds it more laborious and energy-consuming to breathe. Alveolar wall rupture releases blood into the alveoli and may allow air to enter the capillaries. The victim may spit or cough up blood or a frothy mixture of blood and air. If the air enters the bloodstream, it may then travel through the pulmonary circulation to the heart and then to other critical organs causing small obstructions to circulation called **emboli**. These emboli may cause stroke-like signs, myocardial infarction, or even death.

A patient history of exposure to a detonation should leave you suspicious of the possibility of lung injury. Since lung injury occurs more frequently with blasts than other pressure injuries and is usually more serious, assess carefully for signs and symptoms of lung injury in patients with abdominal and ear injuries. Lung injury patients may have progressively worsening crackles, difficulty breathing (**dyspnea**) and, in extreme cases, may cough up blood or blood-tinged sputum (**hemoptysis**). Patients occasionally experience a reduced level of consciousness or small, stroke-like episodes. If there is any reason to suspect lung injury from a blast, transport the victim immediately to the closest trauma center or other appropriate facility.

If it becomes necessary to ventilate a blast injury patient, do so with caution. The mechanism of injury may have damaged the alveolar-capillary walls and opened small blood vessels to the alveolar space. Positive pressure ventilations may push small air bubbles into the vascular system and create emboli. These emboli may quickly travel to the heart and brain, where they can cause further injury or death. The pressure of the ventilations may also induce **pneumothorax** by pushing air past blast-induced lung defects and into the pleural space. If possible, place a victim in the left lateral recumbent position with the head somewhat down. This positioning will discourage emboli from traveling up the carotid arteries and toward the brain.

Despite the risks associated with ventilating blast injury patients, always provide positive pressure ventilations to any casualty with serious dyspnea. Use only the pressure needed to obtain moderate chest rise and respiratory volumes. High concentration oxygen, as supplied with a reservoir, is also helpful because the bloodstream absorbs small oxygen bubbles more easily than the nitrogen of room air.

Abdomen The blast wave's sudden compression/decompression may also damage the air-filled bowel. Violent movements of the bowel wall cause hemorrhage and possible wall rupture. Rupture releases bowel contents into the abdominal cavity leading, over time, to severe infection and irritation (peritonitis).

Blast injuries to the abdomen require no special attention in the early stages of care. The impact of associated injuries—the bowel hemorrhage and spillage of bowel contents—on the patient's overall condition takes time to develop and is not usually apparent at the emergency scene. The only exceptions are when the blast is extremely powerful or the patient was very close to the detonation. In

* **emboli** undissolved solid, liquid, or gaseous matter in the bloodstream that may cause blockage of blood vessels.

* **dyspnea** labored or difficult breathing.

* **hemoptysis** expectoration of blood from the respiratory tract.

* **pneumothorax** collection of air or gas in the pleural cavity between the chest wall and lung.

Provide careful positive pressure ventilations to any blast injury patient with serious dyspnea.

these cases, be alert for signs and symptoms of developing shock and provide rapid transport and fluid resuscitation as needed.

Ears The ears suffer greatly from blast wave forces associated with ordnance explosion, artillery fire, and even repeated small-arms fire at close range. The structure of the ears explains this. The middle ear is an air-filled cavity containing the organs of hearing (cochlea and stapes) and of positional sense (semicircular canals). The pina (the external portion of the ear) focuses and directs pressure waves (normally, sound waves) through the external auditory canal to the eardrum. The eardrum (tympanic membrane) permits the passage of sound waves but excludes the movement of air into the middle ear. The eustachian tube provides a mechanism for equalizing small and gradual changes in atmospheric pressure between the middle ear and the outside atmosphere. During blast overpressure, however, the eustachian tube cannot equalize the rapid pressure changes. The pressure on the tympanic membrane becomes so great that the membrane stretches or ruptures, resulting in acute hearing loss. The pressure change may be so great as to fracture the delicate bones of hearing, also resulting in acute hearing loss. Hearing losses associated with blasts may be temporary or permanent.

Often ear injuries, even with as much as a third of the eardrum torn, will improve over time without much attention. Direct your care to supporting the victim and assuring that the ear canal remains uncontaminated.

Penetrating Wounds Care for penetrating wounds as you would for any serious open wound. Remove as much of the contaminating material as is practical, and cover the site with a sterile dressing. If you encounter a large embedded or impaled object, stabilize the object by securing gauze pads around it or cover it with a non-Styrofoam paper cup to prevent movement during transport. Large areas of damaged tissue are prone to infection, so keep the wound as clean as possible. Care of penetrating trauma will be discussed at greater length in Chapter 18.

Burns Blasts can also cause extensive burn injuries either from the explosions themselves or from the ignition of other munitions or fuels or of debris or clothing. Care for burn injuries is discussed in detail in Chapter 21.

OTHER TYPES OF BLUNT TRAUMA

Blunt trauma can be caused by still other mechanisms. These include falls, crush injuries, and sports injuries.

Falls

The potential for injury from a fall depends on the height and stopping distance.

In terms of physics, falls are a release of stored gravitational energy. The greater the distance a person falls, the greater the impact velocity, the greater the exchange of energy, and the greater the resultant trauma. As with auto impacts, stopping distance may be more important than the height of the fall. A person may dive pleasurably from a 12-foot platform into deep water, but a fall from a second story window to a concrete sidewalk results in serious injury. Newton's Second Law—

$$\text{Force} = \text{Mass} \times \text{Acceleration (or Deceleration)}$$

—illustrates that the more rapid the deceleration (the shorter the stopping distance), the greater the force and resultant injury. The nature of the impact surface contour may also affect the nature of the injury. An irregular surface, like building rubble or a stairway, may focus the force of impact, increasing the seriousness of the injury.

Trauma resulting from a fall is dependent upon the area of contact and the pathway of energy transmission. If the victim lands feet first, energy is transmitted up

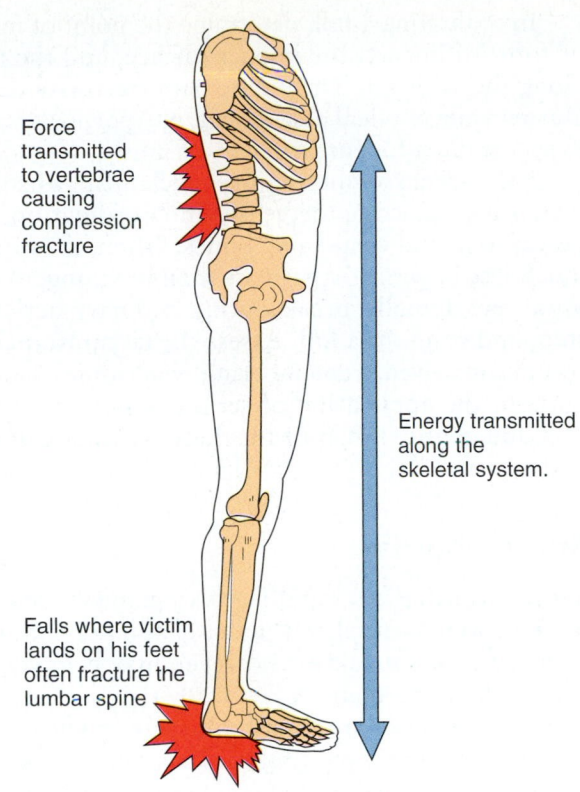

Force transmitted to vertebrae causing compression fracture

Energy transmitted along the skeletal system.

Falls where victim lands on his feet often fracture the lumbar spine

the skeletal structure through the calcaneus, tibia, femur, pelvis, and lumbar spine (Figure 17-25). Fractures along this skeletal pathway are common. The lumbar spine is especially prone to compression injury because it is the only skeletal component supporting the entire upper body. As the victim continues the collision, he may fall forward or backward. In forward falls, an outstretched arm may attempt to break the impact, resulting in shoulder, clavicle, and wrist fractures. Pelvic, thoracic, and head injury may result from a backward fall. In some cases, the fall will progress with the patient continuing a straight impact. The tongue may be bitten deeply as the weight of the cranium pushes the maxilla against the mandible as it impacts the sternum.

The initial impact may involve other body surfaces with kinetic energy transmitted from the contact point toward the body's center of mass. In diving injuries, the patient's head meets with the lake or pool bottom, while the rest of the body compresses the cervical spine between the head and shoulders. Axial loading crushes the vertebrae, disrupts the spinal cord, and paralyzes the patient. This may result from even a very shallow dive, as from poolside or from within the water.

If the victim falls on outstretched arms, the impact energy is transmitted along the skeletal system from the hand and wrist, to the forearm, elbow, arm, and shoulder. In these cases, the clavicle often fractures because it is the smallest weight-bearing bone along the pathway of impact transmission. With collapse of the upper extremities, the head and neck may experience energy exchange and injury as may the shoulders upon collision with the impact surface.

In severe falls, with a person dropping more than three times his own height (20 feet for the adult, 10 feet for the small child), focus your attention on potential internal injuries. Rapid deceleration causes many organs to be compressed, displaced, and twisted. The heart, for example, is held in the center of the thorax by the aorta, the vena cavae, and the *ligamentum arteriosum*. When the victim contacts the ground, the heart is pulled downward with such force that it may tear from its aortic attachments, thus leading to immediate exsanguination.

In evaluating a fall, determine the point of impact, the fall height or velocity or force of impact, the impact surface, and the transmission pathway of forces along the skeleton. Then anticipate fracture sites and possible internal injuries. During your physical assessment, pay particular attention to the areas where you expect trauma for further signs of injury.

Falls are a common injury mechanism for older or geriatric patients. With increasing age come decreases in coordination, deficits in eyesight and depth perception, and weakening bones. Often, the forces required to break bones are much less in geriatric patients than in younger ones. A brittle bone, like the femur, may actually break during ordinary activities, such as walking down a step, and result in a fall. Assess the circumstances surrounding the fall and the trauma involved, remembering that some fractures in the elderly can occur without the application of serious kinetic forces. Provide careful immobilization and gentle transport for these patients and assure that they are comforted and reassured.

Sports Injuries

Sports medicine is a rapidly growing and extensive field, one that certainly cannot be covered completely in this chapter or text. Understanding some basic principles of sports medicine, however, may help you to better understand and care for the injured athlete.

Sports injuries are most commonly produced by extreme exertion, fatigue, or by direct trauma forces. Injuries can be secondary to acceleration, deceleration, compression, rotation, hyperextension, or hyperflexion. These forces leave behind soft-tissue damage to muscle, connective tissue injury to tendons and ligaments, skeletal trauma to long bones or the spinal column, as well as internal damage to either hollow or solid organs.

When a debilitating sports-related injury occurs, transport the athlete to an emergency department for a complete examination before further participation in the sport is allowed. Injuries that present with minimal pain may be significantly worsened by the stress of further competition. Such stress may cause complete ligament rupture or other soft-tissue injury and increase the potential for permanent disability.

In some contact sports, athletes may experience severe impacts (Figure 17-26). If collision leads to any period of unconsciousness, neurologic deficit, or lowered level of orientation, assure that the individual is evaluated by emergency department personnel. There is often a strong desire by coaches and players alike for the athlete's return to the game. Until head and cervical spine injury can be ruled out, however, discourage such action.

Protective gear reduces the chance for and significance of injuries. Gear, however, can sometimes be a contributing factor in sports injuries. In major contact sports, for example, shoes are designed to give maximum traction, using cleats to lock the foot firmly in position. In football, a player might be struck, forcing the body to turn on an immobile foot. Ligaments in the knee may tear, resulting in severe and disabling leg injury. In other cases, protective gear may hinder your complete assessment and patient stabilization.

A newer helmet design for high-school contact sports uses an air-filled bladder to immobilize the head within the device. This fixation may be adequate to immobilize the head within the helmet in cases of suspected spinal injuries. While it is difficult to immobilize a spherical helmet to the flat surface of a spine board, it may be preferable to attempting helmet removal. If your protocols require, attempt to immobilize the head and helmet to the long spine board, leaving the shoulder pads in place to help maintain the head and neck in a neutral position.

If a collision leads to any loss of consciousness, neurological deficit, or altered level of consciousness, the athlete should be evaluated by emergency department personnel.

FIGURE 17-26   Contact sports may result in the exchange of great kinetic forces and produce serious injuries. (Allsport NY)

Crush Injuries

Crush injuries are common types of trauma. They may result from mechanisms such as structural collapse as in an explosion, an industrial or agricultural accident where a limb is caught in machinery, or when a limb is caught under a vehicle. These mechanisms direct great force to soft tissues and bones, compressing surfaces together while stretching semifluid soft tissues laterally. The result may be severe tissue disruption and serious associated hemorrhage.

The injury may be further compounded if the crushing pressure remains in place for an extended period of time. The pressure can disrupt blood flow to and through the limb, causing anaerobic metabolism and some tissue death. This causes a build-up of toxins in the blood stream. If blood flow returns to the limb, the blood may carry these toxins back to the central circulation. This acidic and toxic blood may then induce cardiac dysrhythmias or seriously damage the kidneys. Another consequence of the release of the crushing pressure is severe and difficult-to-control hemorrhage. The blood vessels within the limb are severely damaged, and bleeding results from many difficult-to-identify locations. With severe and prolonged crush injury entrapment, prehospital care may include sodium bicarbonate and other medications to combat the effects of acidosis, limit damage, and improve kidney function.

SUMMARY

Blunt trauma accounts for most injury deaths and disabilities. While vehicle crashes are the most frequent cause of blunt trauma, blast injuries, sports injuries, crush injuries, and falls also account for significant mortality and morbidity. Blunt trauma is difficult to assess accurately so you, as the care provider, must look carefully at the mechanism of injury and subtle physical signs to help anticipate serious internal injury. Careful analysis of the mechanism of injury, followed by development of indices of suspicion for injury can help guide you to recognize those patients needing rapid entry into the trauma system and those best served by on-scene care and transport to the nearest appropriate care facility.

CHAPTER 18

Penetrating Trauma

Objectives

After reading this chapter, you should be able to:

1. Explain the energy exchange process between a penetrating object or projectile and the object it strikes. (pp. 859–863)

2. Determine the effects that profile, yaw, tumble, expansion, and fragmentation have on projectile energy transfer. (pp. 860–863)

3. Describe elements of the ballistic injury process including direct injury, cavitation, temporary cavity, permanent cavity, and zone of injury. (pp. 860–863, 866–869)

4. Identify the relative effects a penetrating object or projectile has when striking various body regions and tissues. (pp. 869–873)

5. Anticipate the injury types and the extent of damage associated with high-velocity/high-energy projectiles, such as rifle bullets; with medium-energy/medium-velocity projectiles such as handgun and shotgun bullets, slugs, or pellets; and with low-energy/low-velocity penetrating objects, such as knives and arrows. (pp. 863–866)

Continued

INTRODUCTION TO PENETRATING TRAUMA

Modern society is experiencing a great increase in the number and severity of penetrating traumas, especially gunshot wounds. About 38,000 deaths occur each year as a result of shootings, and the number is growing. Many additional mechanisms, including knives, arrows, nails, and pieces of glass or wire, can also cause penetrating trauma. As is the case with auto crashes, physical laws govern the energy exchange process associated with penetrating trauma. Therefore, the types of weapons and projectiles involved and the characteristics of the tissue they impact all affect the severity of injury with penetrating trauma. Understanding the principles of energy exchange and projectile travel will help you to anticipate the potential for injuries, to recognize the injuries that have occurred, and, ultimately, to adequately assess and care for victims of penetrating trauma.

PHYSICS OF PENETRATING TRAUMA

The basic principles of physics that you read about in association with blunt trauma in the last chapter also apply to instances of penetrating trauma. When a projectile strikes a target, it exchanges its energy of motion, more properly called kinetic energy, with the object struck. As you recall, an object's kinetic energy is equal to its mass times the square of its velocity:

$$\text{Kinetic Energy} = \frac{\text{Mass (weight)} \times \text{Velocity (speed)}^2}{2}$$

Thus, the greater the mass of an object, the greater the energy. If you double the mass of an object, it will have twice the kinetic energy if the speed of the object remains the same. However, the speed (or velocity) of an object has a squared relationship to its kinetic energy. If you double the speed of an object, its kinetic energy increases by fourfold. If the speed triples, the energy increases by ninefold, and so on (Figure 18-1).

This relationship between mass and velocity explains why very small and relatively light bullets traveling very fast have the potential to do great harm. It also makes clear why different weights of bullets traveling at different velocities cause different amounts of damage. For example, handguns, shotguns, and low-powered rifles are considered to be medium-energy/medium-velocity weapons. They deliver their bullets, slugs, and pellets much faster than low-energy/low-velocity objects like

FIGURE 18-1 The extreme velocity of firearm projectiles gives them great kinetic energy and the potential to do great damage.

knives and arrows travel but still are slower than bullets delivered by high-energy/high-velocity weapons like assault rifles. Thus, a handgun bullet is generally smaller and much slower (250 to 400 meters per second) than a rifle bullet. A hunting rifle, on the other hand, commonly expels a slightly heavier bullet at speeds of 600 to 1,000 meters per second. Hence, the high-energy rifle bullet's kinetic energy is three to nine times greater than the medium-energy handgun bullet's and can be expected to do significantly more damage. Experience in Northern Ireland suggests that rifle bullets are between two and four times as lethal as handgun bullets.

The Law of Conservation of Energy (energy can be neither created nor destroyed) explains why the projectile kinetic energy is transformed into damage as it slows. If a projectile like a bullet remains within the object struck, then all its energy is transferred to the object. If the projectile passes completely through the object, then the energy transferred to the object is equal to the kinetic energy just prior to entry minus the energy remaining in the projectile as it exits.

Studies suggest that wounds from rifle bullets are from two to four times more lethal than wounds from handgun bullets.

BALLISTICS

The study of the characteristics of projectiles in motion and their effects upon objects they impact is called **ballistics.** The basic physics described above is the starting point for this study. One aspect of ballistics is **trajectory,** or the curved path that a bullet follows once fired from a gun. As it travels through the air, the bullet is constantly pulled downward by gravity. The faster the bullet, the flatter its curve of travel and the straighter its trajectory.

A second, more significant, aspect of projectile travel is energy dissipation. Factors that affect energy dissipation include drag, cavitation, profile, stability, expansion, and shape. As a bullet travels through the air, it experiences wind resistance, or **drag.** The faster it travels, the more drag it experiences and the greater the slowing effect. Since this represents a reduction in bullet speed, it also means, if all else is equal, that the damage caused by a bullet fired at close range will be more severe than from one fired at a distance.

Objects traveling relatively slowly, and without much kinetic energy, like knives or arrows, will affect only the tissue they contact. High- or medium-velocity projectiles, like rifle or handgun bullets, however, set a portion of the semi-fluid body tissue in motion, creating a shock wave and a temporary cavity in the tissue. This stage of the destruction process is known as **cavitation** and is related to the bullet's velocity and how quickly it gives up its energy. The energy exchange rate is related to the size of the projectile's contacting surface, called its profile, and to its shape.

* **ballistics** the study of projectile motion and its interactions with the gun, the air, and the object it contacts.

* **trajectory** the path a projectile follows.

* **drag** the forces acting on a projectile in motion to slow its progress.

* **cavitation** the outward motion of tissue due to a projectile's passage, resulting in a temporary cavity and vacuum.

Profile

The **profile** is the portion of the bullet you would see if you looked at it as it traveled toward you. The larger this surface profile, the greater the energy exchange rate, the more quickly the bullet slows, and the more extensive the damage to surrounding tissue. For bullets that remain stable during their travel and do not deform, the profile is the bullet's diameter, or **caliber.** To increase the energy exchange rate, bullets are designed to become unstable as they pass from one medium to another or to deform through expansion or fragmentation.

Stability

The location of a bullet's center of mass affects its stability both during its flight and when it impacts a solid or semi-solid object. The longer the bullet, the farther the center of mass is from its leading edge. If the bullet is deflected from straight flight—for example, by the barrel exhaust or by a gust of wind—the lift created by the projectile's tip passing through air at an angle will cause the bullet to tumble. If it continues to tumble, the bullet will slow and the accuracy of the shot will be diminished. To prevent tumbling, bullets are sent spinning through the air by the gun barrel's rifling. This rotation gives a bullet gyroscopic stability like a spinning top. If the spinning bullet is slightly deflected, it will wobble, or **yaw,** then slowly return to straight flight.

When a bullet impacts a dense substance, several things happen. If there is already a yaw, the yaw greatly increases as the bullet begins its penetration. This occurs as the bullet's mass tries to overrun the leading edge. Secondly, the gyroscopic spin designed for stability in air becomes insufficient. A bullet would need to spin at a rate 30 times greater in body tissue than in air to maintain the same stability. The result may be tumbling and a great increase in the bullet's presenting profile. Since a rifle bullet is generally longer than a handgun bullet and has its center of mass farther back from the leading edge, it is more likely to tumble once it hits body tissue (Figure 18-2). With increased tumbling and a larger presenting profile, a rifle bullet's kinetic energy exchange rate increases, as does its potential for causing damage. In human tissue, a rifle bullet generally rotates 180 degrees and then continues its travel base first.

* **profile** the size and shape of a projectile as it contacts a target; it is the energy exchange surface of the contact.

* **caliber** the diameter of a bullet expressed in hundredths of an inch. (.22 caliber = 0.22 inches); the inside diameter of the barrel of a handgun, shotgun, or rifle.

* **yaw** swing or wobble around the axis of a projectile's travel.

FIGURE 18-2 The presenting surface, or profile, of a bullet changes as it tumbles when it contacts human tissue.

FIGURE 18-3 Some bullets are designed to mushroom on impact, thus increasing their profile, energy exchange rate, and damage potential.

Expansion and Fragmentation

Projectiles also may increase their profile and their energy exchange rate by deforming when they strike a medium denser than air. As the bullet's nose contacts the target, it is compressed by the weight of the rest of the bullet behind it. The nose of the bullet mushrooms outward as the rear of the bullet pushes into it, increasing the projectile's diameter (Figure 18-3). In some cases, the initial impact forces are so great that the bullet separates into several pieces or fragments. This fragmentation increases the energy exchange rate of impact because the total surface area of the fragments is much greater than that of the original bullet profile (Figure 18-4). While handgun bullets are made of relatively soft lead, their velocity, and hence their kinetic energy, is generally not sufficient to cause significant deformity. However, some bullets (dum-dums or wad-cutters) are specifically designed to mushroom and/or fragment upon impact and thereby increase the damage they cause. Rifle bullets have much greater velocities than handgun bullets and much more kinetic energy. They are more prone to deform when contacting human tissue, especially bullets used for big-game hunting. Most military ammunition is fully jacketed with impact-resistant metal and seldom deforms solely with soft tissue collision.

FIGURE 18-4 Some firearm projectiles may break apart, or fragment, on contact, greatly increasing their profile and damage potential.

Secondary Impacts

The energy exchange between a projectile and body tissue can also be affected by any object the projectile strikes during its travel. Branches, window glass, or articles of clothing may all deflect a bullet and induce yaw and tumble. They may also cause bullet deformity, and thereby increase the energy exchange rate once the bullet impacts the victim.

A special type of secondary impact occurs when the bullet collides with body armor. Kevlar™ and other synthetic fabrics can effectively resist the kinetic energy generated by medium-energy projectiles. This energy is absorbed by the armor and distributed to the victim in much the same way that the recoil of a gun is distributed to the shooter. The impact of the bullet may produce blunt trauma in the person hit (for example, myocardial contusion), but such injuries are generally less damaging than penetration by the bullet would have been. High-energy projectiles may pass through body armor, but in doing so they dissipate some of their energy as blunt trauma, thereby reducing the penetrating kinetic energy as the bullet strikes body tissue. Bullet deformity may increase the rate of energy exchange, but the reduction in kinetic energy reduces the overall injury potential. Ceramic inserts for body armor will stop penetration of most rifle bullets but not without causing significant, but less lethal blunt trauma.

Shape

In addition to profile, other aspects of the shape of the bullet affect the energy exchange rate and the resulting damage. Handgun ammunition is rather blunt, is more resistant to travel through human tissue, and releases kinetic energy more quickly. Rifle bullets are more pointed and cut through the tissue more efficiently. However, if the rifle bullet tumbles, it will present a different shape and may exchange energy more rapidly both because of the shape and the increase in profile. If a bullet fragments, the irregular shape of the fragments mean that the projectile will give up its energy more rapidly and through more erratic pathways than either an intact handgun or rifle bullet.

SPECIFIC WEAPON CHARACTERISTICS

Weapons that commonly cause wounds encountered by paramedics include handguns, domestic rifles, assault rifles, shotguns, and knives and arrows. Each type of weapon has certain characteristics associated with the injuries it produces (Figure 18-5).

While body armor protects against penetration, impact may result in less lethal but still serious blunt injury.

Content Review

FACTORS AFFECTING ENERGY EXCHANGE BETWEEN A PROJECTILE AND BODY TISSUE
Velocity
Profile
Stability
Expansion and
 fragmentation
Secondary Impacts
Shape

FIGURE 18-5 Firearms include (top to bottom) handguns, assault rifles, domestic rifles, and shotguns.

FIGURE 18-6 The energy of
the handgun projectile is
limited by low projectile
weight and its relatively slow
velocity.

Handgun

The handgun is often a small-caliber, short-barreled, medium-velocity weapon with limited accuracy that is most effective at close range. Because a handgun does not fire a high-velocity, high-energy projectile as a rifle does, its potential for causing damage is limited. The blunter shape of the bullet and, less frequently, its softer composition and associated mushrooming and fragmentation, may release the bullet's energy more rapidly. The damage is still, however, less than that of the higher energy rifle bullet. The severity of injury is usually related to the organs directly damaged by the bullet's passage (Figure 18-6).

Some handguns fire automatically (machine pistols). They continue to discharge bullets until the trigger is released or the magazine empties. While the energy for each projectile remains the same, the damage potential associated with automatic weapons is increased because of the likelihood of multiple impacts or multiple victims.

Rifle

The domestic hunting rifle fires a heavier projectile than the handgun, through a much longer barrel, and with much greater muzzle velocity. It is either a manually loaded, single-shot weapon with some mechanical loading action to advance the next shell, or a semi-automatic weapon, in which the next shell is fed into the chamber by recoil or exhaust gases. However, no more than one bullet is expelled by each squeeze of the domestic hunting rifle's trigger. The high-energy rifle bullet travels much farther, with greater accuracy, and retains much more of its kinetic energy than does the handgun projectile. Due to the rifle bullet's high speed and energy, it transfers great damaging energy to the target (Figure 18-7). This results in extensive wounds with injuries that extend beyond the projectile's immediate track. Domestic hunting ammunition is especially lethal. It is often designed to expand dramatically on impact, greatly increasing the energy delivery rate and the size of both the temporary cavity and the wound pathway.

The damage caused by high-energy rifle bullets can extend well beyond the actual track of the projectile.

Assault Rifle

The assault rifle differs from the domestic hunting rifle in that it generally has a larger magazine capacity and will fire in both the semi-automatic and automatic mode. Examples of these weapons include the M16 and the AK47. The resulting injuries are similar to injuries produced by domestic hunting rifles, although multiple wounds and casualties can be expected. Military ammunition is fully jack-

FIGURE 18-7 The energy carried by a rifle bullet is very damaging because of its heavier weight and very high velocity.

eted and not designed for expansion and, while still very deadly, the energy delivery is not as severe as with domestic hunting ammunition. Assault weapons in terrorist hands, however, may be loaded with domestic hunting-type ammunition. This greatly increases their injury potential.

Shotgun

The shotgun expels a single projectile (a slug) or numerous spheres (pellets or shot) at medium velocity. The shell is loaded with a particular size of lead shot, varying from 00 (about 1/3 inch in diameter) to #9 shot (about the size of a pin head). The size of the projectile compartment is approximately the same with various types of loads. This means that the larger the shot, the smaller the number of projectiles. Each projectile shares a portion of the total muzzle energy and adds to the resistance as it moves through air. The shotgun is limited in range and accuracy; however, injuries sustained at close range can be very severe or lethal (Figure 18-8).

Knives and Arrows

In contrast to high- or medium-velocity projectiles such as rifle or handgun bullets, knives, arrows, and other slow-moving, penetrating objects cause low-velocity, low-energy wounds. Because low-velocity objects do not produce either a pressure shock wave or cavitation, damage is usually limited to physical injury caused by

FIGURE 18-8 A shotgun propels small projectiles with limited velocity. However, because of the large number of projectiles, the weapon can be extremely damaging at close range.

FIGURE 18-9 As a bullet passes through a gel designed to simulate human tissue, it demonstrates the wounding process.

The extent of damage is often difficult to assess with wounds caused by low-velocity, low-energy projectiles such as knives and arrows. Suspect internal hemorrhage and/or injury to body organs.

direct contact between the blade or object and the victim's tissue. The severity of a low-velocity penetrating wound, however, can often be difficult to assess because the depth and angle of the object's insertion cannot be determined from the visible wound. In addition, an attacker may move the penetrating object about inside the victim, then leave it in place or withdraw it. The penetration can result in serious internal hemorrhage or injury to individual or multiple body organs.

The hunting tips designed for arrows can be especially damaging. These feature three razor-tipped, pointed barbs that are intended to smoothly cut tissue. These tips produce severe internal hemorrhage. Also, any movement of an arrow while it is impaled in the victim increases both the tissue damage and hemorrhage rate.

DAMAGE PATHWAY

The damage pathway that a high-velocity projectile inflicts results from three specific factors. They are the direct injury, the pressure shock wave, and cavitation, or the creation of a temporary cavity. These three factors can also create a permanent cavity and a zone of injury (Figure 18-9).

THE PROJECTILE INJURY PROCESS

The spinning bullet smashes into a semi-fluid target (such as human tissue) with great speed and kinetic energy. The tip of the bullet impacts tissue, pushing the tissue forward and to the side along the pathway of its travel. This tissue collides with adjacent tissue, ultimately creating a shock wave of pressure moving forward and lateral to the projectile. This shock wave continues to move perpendicular to the bullet's path as it passes. The rapid compression of tissue laterally and the stretching of the tissue as it moves outward from the bullet path crushes and tears the tissue structure. The motion creates a pocket, or cavity, behind the bullet. The pressure within this cavity is reduced, creating suction. This suction draws air and debris into the cavity from the entrance wound and from the exit wound, if one is present. The body tissue's elasticity then draws the sides of the cavity back together, causing the entrance wound, exit wound, and wound pathway to close completely or remain only partially open.

The bullet's exchange of energy with the body leaves various tissues disrupted and injured. Tissue in the direct pathway of the bullet suffers most. It is severely contused and likely to have been torn from its attachments. In addition to the directly injured tissue, other debris, blood, and air are found along the bullet's pathway. The cavitational wave stretches and tears adjacent tissue, damag-

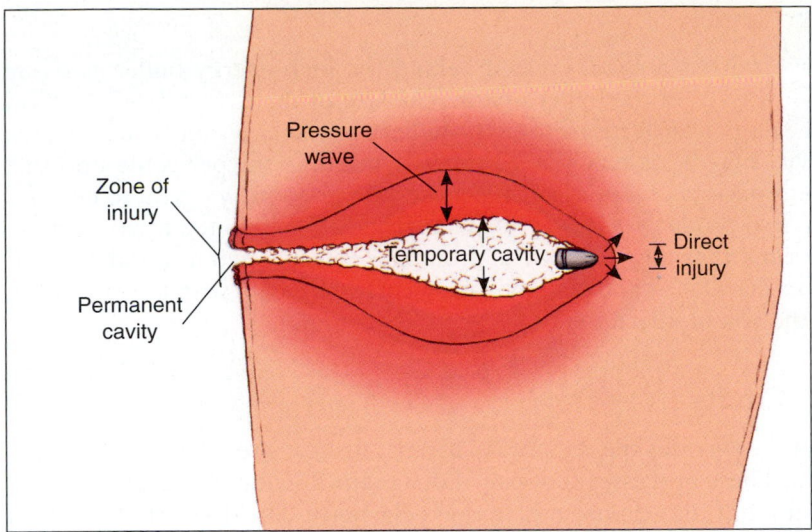

FIGURE 18-10 As a projectile passes through tissue it creates a pressure wave and temporary cavity, with results that include direct injury, a permanent cavity, and a zone of injury.

ing cell walls and small blood vessels. The adjacent tissue is injured, but will likely regain its normal function slowly. Larger blood vessels torn by the bullet and the cavitational wave release their precious fluid in large quantities into the damage pathway. Over time, this pathway, because of the disruption in circulation and the introduction of infectious material with the drawing-in of debris, may experience severe infection, which will prolong the healing process.

Direct Injury

Direct injury is the damage done as the projectile strikes tissue, contuses and tears that tissue, and pushes the tissue out of its way. The direct injury pathway is limited to the profile of the bullet as it moves through the body or the profiles of resulting fragments as the bullet breaks apart. Except for magnum rounds (generating particularly high velocities), handgun bullet damage is usually limited to direct injury.

Pressure Shock Wave

When a high-velocity, high-energy projectile strikes human flesh, it creates a pressure shock wave (Figure 18-10). Since most human tissue is semi-fluid and elastic, the impact of the projectile transmits energy outward very quickly. The tissue cells in front of the bullet are pushed forward and to the side at great speed. They push adjacent cells forward and outward, creating a moving wave of pressure and tissue. The faster and blunter the bullet, the greater the effect. With high-velocity rifle bullets, pressures are extreme, approaching 100 times normal atmospheric pressure.

The pressure wave travels very well through fluid, such as blood, and may injure blood vessels distant from the projectile pathway. Air-filled cavities, such as the small air sacs (alveoli) of the lung, compress very easily and absorb the pressure, quickly limiting the shock wave and the resulting temporary cavity. Solid and dense organs, like the liver and spleen, suffer greatly as the pressure wave moves through them, causing internal hemorrhage and, in extreme cases, fracture.

The severity of injury in cases of bullet wounds usually depends on the organs damaged by the bullet's passage.

Temporary Cavity

The temporary cavity is a space created behind the high-energy bullet as tissue moves rapidly away from the bullet's path. The size of the cavity depends upon the amount of energy transferred during the bullet's passage. With rifle bullets, the temporary cavity may be as much as 12 times larger than the projectile's profile. After the bullet's passage, tissue elasticity causes the temporary cavity to close.

Cavitation also produces a sub-atmospheric pressure within the cavity as it expands. This means that air is drawn in from the entrance wound and the exit wound, if one exists. Debris and contamination enter the cavity with the in-flowing air, adding to the risk of infection.

Permanent Cavity

The movement that creates the temporary cavity crushes, stretches, and tears the affected tissues. These processes seriously damage the area in and adjacent to the bullet's path and may also damage the tissue's elasticity. The tissue thus may not return to its normal orientation, resulting in a permanent cavity that in some cases may be larger than the bullet's diameter. This cavity is not a void but is filled with disrupted tissues, some air, fluid, and debris.

Zone of Injury

Associated with most projectile wounds is a zone of injury that extends beyond the permanent cavity. This zone contains contused tissue that does not function normally and may be slow to heal because of cell and tissue damage, disrupted blood flow, and infection.

LOW-VELOCITY WOUNDS

Weapons such as knives, ice picks, arrows, or flying objects such as blast debris or wires thrown by a lawn mower can cause low-velocity penetrating trauma. In these cases, the relatively slow speed of the object limits the kinetic energy exchange rate as it enters the victim's body. Consider, for example, the stabbing of a victim by a 150-pound attacker who strikes with a knife moving at about 3 meters per second. Although the mass behind the penetration of the knife blade is significantly greater than a rifle bullet's, the velocity of the knife is vastly lower. This means that injury in such cases is usually restricted to the tissue actually contacted by the penetrating object (Figure 18-11).

FIGURE 18-11 Damage caused by a low-velocity wounding process, such as that caused by a wire thrown by a lawnmower, is limited to the object's path of travel.

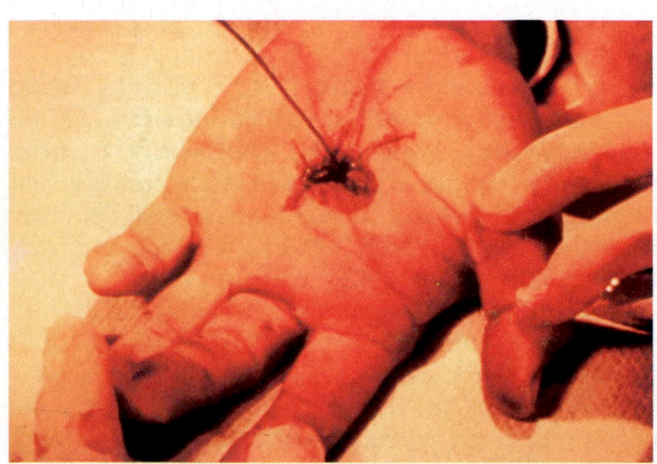

While the injury is limited to the penetrating object's pathway, that object may be twisted, moved about, or inserted at an oblique angle. As a result, the entrance wound may not reflect the depth of the object's penetration, the extent of its motion within the body, or the actual organs and tissues it contacts and injures.

Characteristics of the attacker and victim are important to keep in mind when assessing cases of low-velocity penetrating trauma. Knife-wielding males, for example, most often strike with a forward, outward, or crosswise stroke. Females usually strike with an overhand and downward stroke. Victims of these attacks initially attempt to protect themselves by using their arms. This means they often receive deep upper-extremity lacerations (commonly called defense wounds). If an attack continues, injuries are often directed to the chest, abdomen, face, neck, or back.

SPECIFIC TISSUE/ORGAN INJURIES

The extent of damage that a penetrating projectile causes within the body varies with the particular type of tissue it encounters. The density of an organ affects how efficiently the projectile's energy is transmitted to surrounding tissues. The tissue's connective strength and elasticity, called **resiliency**, also influence how much tissue damage occurs with the kinetic energy transfer. Structures and tissues within the body that behave differently during projectile passage include connective tissue, solid organs, hollow organs, lungs, and bone.

* resiliency the connective strength and elasticity of an object or fabric.

CONNECTIVE TISSUE

Muscles, the skin, and other connective tissues are dense, elastic, and held together very well. When exposed to the pressure and stretching of the cavitational wave, these types of tissue characteristically absorb energy while limiting tissue damage. The wound track closes due to the resiliency of the tissue, and serious injury is frequently limited to the projectile's pathway.

ORGANS

Another factor that has profound effects on the victim's potential for survival is the particular organ involved in a penetrating injury. Some organs, like the heart and brain, are immediately necessary for life functions, and serious injury may cause immediate death. When large blood vessels are involved, the hemorrhage can be rapid and severe. A penetrating injury to the urinary bladder, on the other hand, may not receive surgical intervention for several hours without threatening the patient's life. When evaluating a wound's seriousness, anticipate the organs injured and the effect their injury is likely to have on the patient's condition and survivability.

Solid Organs

Solid organs such as the liver, spleen, kidneys, pancreas, and brain have the density but not the resiliency of muscle and other connective tissues. When struck by the forces of bullet impact, these tissues compress and stretch, resulting in greater damage more closely associated with the size of the temporary cavity than with the bullet's profile. The tissue returns to its original location, not because of its own elasticity but because of the resiliency of surrounding tissues or the organ capsule. Hemorrhage associated with solid organ projectile damage is often severe.

Be alert to the possibility of severe hemorrhage if you suspect that a projectile has damaged a solid organ.

Hollow Organs

Hollow organs such as the bowel, stomach, urinary bladder, and heart are muscular containers holding fluid. The fluid within is non-compressible and rapidly transmits the impact energy outward. If the container is filled and distended with fluid at the time of impact, the energy released can tear the organ apart explosively (Figure 18-12). Slower and smaller projectiles may produce small holes in an organ and permit slow leakage of its contents. If this occurs with the heart, it may produce **pericardial tamponade** (blood filling the pericardial sac, thus limiting heart function) or moderate and slowly life-threatening hemorrhage. If the container is not distended, it is more tolerant of cavitational forces. If a hollow organ, such as the bowel or stomach holds air, the air compresses with the passage of the pressure wave and somewhat limits the extent of injury. (Large blood vessels respond to projectile passage much like hollow, fluid-filled, organs.)

✱ pericardial tamponade filling of the pericardial sac with fluid, which in turn limits the filling and function of the heart.

LUNGS

The lungs consist of millions of small, elastic, air-filled sacs. As the bullet and its associated pressure wave pass, the air is compressed, thereby slowing and limiting the transmission of the cavitational wave. Injury to lung tissue in cases of penetrating trauma is generally less extensive than can be expected with any other body tissue.

A bullet may, however, open the chest wall or disrupt larger airways, thus permitting air to escape into the thorax (pneumothorax) or creating a valve-like defect that results in accumulating pressure within the chest (tension pneumothorax). Bullet wounds only infrequently induce an open pneumothorax (sucking chest wound) because the entrance wound diameter is usually limited to the bullet caliber. Explosive exit wounds of high-powered rifles or close-range shotgun blasts, however, may be large and cause significant disruption of the chest wall integrity. In these cases, a pneumothorax is a more likely outcome.

Injury to lung tissue in cases of penetrating trauma is generally less extensive than can be expected with any other body tissue.

Suspect the possibility of pneumothorax when there has been a significant disruption of chest wall integrity.

BONE

In contrast to lung tissue, bone is the densest, most rigid, and non-elastic body tissue of all. When struck by a projectile or its associated pressure wave, bone resists displacement until it fractures, often into numerous pieces. These bone fragments then may distribute the impact energy to surrounding tissue. The projectile's contact with bone may also significantly alter the projectile's path through the body.

GENERAL BODY REGIONS

Several body regions deserve special attention regarding projectile wounds. They include the extremities, abdomen, thorax, neck, and head (Figure 18-13). A projectile's passage also has a special effect on the first and last tissue contacted, the sites of the entrance and the exit wounds.

Extremities

The extremities consist of skin covering muscles and surrounding large long bones. An extremity injury may be debilitating but does not immediately threaten life unless there is severe hemorrhage associated with it. The severity of injury is limited by the resiliency of the skin and muscle, although if the bone is involved, the degree of soft tissue damage may be increased. In recent military experience, extremity injuries account for between 60 and 80 percent of injuries yet result in less than 10 percent of fatalities. The remaining 20 to 40 percent of penetrating injuries are divided among wounds of the abdomen, thorax, and head and account for more than 90 percent of mortality.

Abdomen

The abdomen (including the pelvic cavity) is the largest body cavity and contains most of the human organs. The area is not well protected by skeletal structures other than the upper pelvic ring, the lower rib cage border, and the lumbar vertebral column. The passage of a projectile through the abdominal cavity can produce a significant cavitational wave. The major occupant of the cavity, the bowel, is very tolerant of compression and stretching, but the liver, spleen, kidneys, and

> **Content Review**
>
> **BODY REGIONS DESERVING SPECIAL ATTENTION WITH PENETRATING TRAUMA**
> Extremities
> Abdomen
> Thorax
> Neck
> Head

Some 90 percent of penetrating trauma mortality involves the head, thorax, and abdomen.

pancreas are highly susceptible to injury and hemorrhage. Since these organs occupy the upper abdominal quadrants, you should consider any penetrating projectile injury to this area to be serious and to have the potential to cause severe internal hemorrhage. Serious consequences should also be anticipated with injuries to the abdominal aorta and inferior vena cava, which are located along the spinal column in the posterior and central abdomen.

If a projectile perforates the small or large bowel, those organs may spill their contents into the abdominal cavity. This spillage results in serious peritoneal irritation due to chemical action or infection, although the signs and symptoms take some time to develop. If the injury process disrupts the blood vessels, the free blood will not result in abdominal irritation.

Thorax

Within the chest is a cavity formed by the ribs, spine, sternum, clavicles, and the diaphragm's strong muscle. This thoracic cavity houses the lungs, heart, and major blood vessels as well as the esophagus and part of the trachea. The impact of a bullet with the ribs may induce an explosive energy exchange that injures the surrounding tissue with numerous bony fragments. Lung tissue can absorb much of the cavitational energy while sustaining limited injury itself. However, the heart and great vessels, as fluid-filled containers, may suffer greatly from the energy of the bullet's passage. The damage to these structures and the associated massive hemorrhage may cause almost instant death. Because of the pressure-driven dynamics of respiration, any large chest wound may compromise breathing. Air may pass through a wound instead of the normal airway (pneumothorax) or may build up under pressure within the chest wall (tension pneumothorax).

Neck

The neck is an anatomical area traversed by several critical structures. These include the larynx, the trachea, the esophagus, several major blood vessels (the carotid and vertebral arteries and the jugular veins), and the spinal cord. Penetrating trauma in this area is very likely to damage vital structures and lead to airway compromise, severe bleeding, and/or neurological dysfunction. Associated swelling and hematoma formation may compromise circulation and the airway. Additionally, any large penetrating wound may permit air to be drawn into an open external jugular vein and immediately threaten life due to the resulting pulmonary emboli.

Head

The skull is a hollow, strong, and rigid container, housing the brain's delicate semi-solid tissue. It is highly susceptible to projectile injury. If a bullet penetrates the skull, its cavitational energy is trapped within the cavity and subjects the brain to extreme pressures. If the released kinetic energy is great enough, the skull may explode outward. In some cases, a bullet may enter the skull and not have enough energy to exit; in such a case, the bullet may continue to travel along the interior of the skull, disrupting more and more brain matter. Bullet wounds to the head, particularly those that penetrate the skull, are especially lethal.

The destructive forces released by a projectile wound to the head may also disrupt the airway and/or the victim's ability to control his own airway. The head and face are also areas with an extensive supply of blood vessels. Penetrating trauma may damage these vessels and result in serious and difficult-to-control hemorrhage.

A frequent occurrence associated with suicide attempts is severe damage to the facial region. As the individual places a shotgun or rifle under the chin and pulls the trigger, the head tilts up and back. This directs the blast entirely to the facial region, but the projectile(s) may not enter the cranium or strike any immediately life-threatening structures. There is, however, serious bleeding. The bleeding and the associated damage can make the airway very hard to control. In these cases, use of an endotracheal tube to secure the airway can be difficult because many airway structures and landmarks are often obliterated by the blast.

Entrance Wound

Entrance wounds are usually the size of the bullet's profile. At this point, cavitational wave energy has not had time to develop and contribute to the wounding process (Figure 18-14). The situation is different, however, with bullets that deform or tumble during flight. With these projectiles, the initial impact can be especially violent, producing a much larger and more disrupted entry wound than the caliber of the bullet alone would suggest.

Bullet entry wounds sustained at close range, a few feet or less, display special characteristics. Such wounds may be marked by elements of the barrel exhaust and bullet passage. Tattooing from the propellant residue may form a darkened circle or an oval (if the gun is held at an angle) around the entry wound and contaminate the wound itself. At the wound site, you may notice a small (usually 1 to 2 mm) ridge of discoloration around the entrance caused by the spinning bullet. If the gun barrel is held very close or against the skin as the weapon is fired, it may push the barrel exhaust into the wound producing subcutaneous emphysema (air within the skin's tissue) and crepitus to the touch. If the barrel is held a few inches from the skin, you may notice some burns caused by the hot gases of the barrel exhaust.

Exit Wound

The exit wound is caused by the physical damage from both the passage of the bullet itself and from the cavitational wave. Since the pressure wave is moving forward and outward, the wound may have a "blown outward" appearance. The exit wound may appear as stellate, referring to the tears radiating outward in a star-like fashion (Figure 18-15). Because the cavitational wave has had time to develop, the exit wound may more accurately reflect the potential for damage caused by the bullet's passage than the entrance wound. If the bullet expends all its kinetic energy before it can exit the body, there is no exit wound and the bullet remains within the body. If the bullet does exit, the kinetic energy expended within the body is equal to the kinetic energy before impact minus the energy that remains in the bullet as it leaves the body.

An exit wound may more accurately reflect the potential damage caused by a bullet's passage through the body than an entrance wound.

FIGURE 18-15 A bullet's exit wound often has a "blown outward" appearance, with stellate tears.

SPECIAL CONCERNS WITH PENETRATING TRAUMA

SCENE SIZE-UP

The scene size-up for a shooting or stabbing raises special concerns not associated with most other emergency care situations. The very nature of these injuries should suggest the possibility of danger from further violence and potential injury to you and your crew. Do not approach a shooting or stabbing scene unless and until law-enforcement personnel arrive and secure it and direct you to enter and provide care. If law-enforcement personnel are not yet on the scene when you arrive, stage your vehicle at least a block away and out of sight of the scene. Once police or other law-enforcement personnel arrive, bring your vehicle closer to the scene but keep the police and their vehicles between you and the shooting or stabbing site. Wait there for the police to indicate that it is safe to approach the patient (Figure 18-16).

Once you reach the patient, survey carefully to determine that there are no weapons within the patient's reach. Consider the possibility that the victim may be carrying a knife or other weapon. If you have any doubts, request that the police search the victim for weapons before you begin to provide care.

As you carefully survey the scene of a shooting, try to reconstruct the event. Attempt to determine the victim's original position and his or her angle to and distance from the shooter. This helps you determine the angle at which the bullet entered the patient (which may not otherwise be revealed by the entrance wound) and whether the wound was received at point blank range or from a distance. Also try to determine the caliber of weapon and its type—handgun, rifle, or shotgun.

If the call involves a knifing injury, attempt to determine the gender and approximate weight of the attacker and the length of the blade. (You probably will

In cases involving shootings or stabbings, always be sure that police have secured the scene before you enter it.

Consider the possibility that the patient may be carrying a weapon and have the police search him if necessary.

FIGURE 18-16 Assure that any potentially violent scene is safe and secured by police before entering.

not be able to determine the wound depth.) This information will help the emergency department determine the potential severity of the wound.

As you move on to your assessment of the patient, do all that you can to preserve the crime scene while providing any needed patient care. Disturb only those materials around the patient that you must move in order to render care. Cut around any bullet or knife holes in clothing and give the clothing to police for use as evidence. If there is ever any doubt about what to do, however, err on the side of providing patient care. (See Chapter 48, the section on "Crime Scene Awareness.") If the victim is obviously dead, employ your jurisdiction's protocols for handling the body, but try to do so without disturbing evidence that may be crucial in determining what happened.

PENETRATING WOUND ASSESSMENT

When assessing the victim of penetrating trauma, try to determine the pathway of the penetrating object and the organs that may have been affected by the wound. Anticipate the impact of potential organ injury and use this determination in setting priorities for on-scene care or rapid transport of the victim. Remember, however, that a bullet may not travel in a straight line between entrance and exit wounds. Often, a very small shift in a bullet's pathway may mean the difference between tearing open a large blood vessel or missing critical organs completely. The human body is also a dynamic place. The diaphragm moves the kidneys, pancreas, liver, spleen, and heart during respirations, so whether or not these organs are injured may be somewhat dependent on the phase of respiration in which the injury occurs.

It is often hard to anticipate the severity of a projectile wound. Injuries to the large blood vessels, heart, and brain may be immediately or rapidly fatal, while injuries to solid organs (liver, pancreas, kidneys, or spleen) may also be deadly but take more time in working their effects. Consequently, always suspect the worst with bullet wounds that involve the head, chest, or abdomen. Provide rapid transport in these cases, and treat shock aggressively.

Make every effort to preserve evidence at a crime scene, but remember that care of the patient takes priority.

Provide rapid transport for patients with bullet wounds to the head, chest, or abdomen and treat aggressively for shock.

PENETRATING WOUND CARE

Certain penetrating wounds need special attention. These include wounds of the face and chest and those involving impaled objects. Their care is described below; care for other penetrating injuries and shock is discussed in later chapters.

Facial Wounds

Some facial gunshot wounds destroy many airway landmarks (Figure 18-17). With wounds like these, endotracheal intubation is extremely difficult. You might find it helpful to visualize the larynx with the laryngoscope while another

FIGURE 18-17 Facial wounds may distort or destroy airway landmarks.

If endotracheal intubation cannot be accomplished in a patient whose airway landmarks have been destroyed by a gunshot wound, emergency cricothyrotomy or cricothyrostomy may be necessary to create a route for ventilations.

✳ **cricothyrotomy** a surgical incision into the cricothyroid membrane, usually to provide an emergency airway.

✳ **cricothyrostomy** the introduction of a needle or other tube into the cricothyroid membrane, usually to provide an emergency airway.

Anticipate a developing tension pneumothorax if your assessment reveals frothy blood in a patient with a bullet wound to the chest.

✳ **prognosis** the anticipated outcome of a disease or injury.

rescuer gently presses on the chest. Look for any bubbling during the chest compression, and try to pass the endotracheal tube through the bubbling tissue. Then, very carefully assure that the endotracheal tube is properly placed in the trachea and that lung ventilation is adequate.

If this approach is not effective, two related techniques may restore the airway, at least for long enough to reach more definitive care. These techniques are the **cricothyrotomy** and the **cricothyrostomy.** These emergency surgical or needle airway procedures perforate the membrane between the thyroid and cricoid cartilages, providing a route for ventilation directly into the lower airway. (These techniques are discussed in detail in Chapter 23, "Head, Facial, and Neck Trauma.")

Chest Wounds

The chest wall is rather thick and resilient. It requires a large wound to create an opening big enough to permit free air movement through the chest wall, an open pheumothorax. Wounds caused by small-caliber handguns usually result in no air movement, while wounds caused by shotgun blasts and exiting high-velocity bullets more commonly cause such injuries. If frothy blood is associated with a chest wound, anticipate a developing tension pneumothorax, in which air builds up under pressure within the thorax. Remember, it takes pressure to push air through the wound and froth the blood. If you completely seal the chest wound, you may stop any outward air flow. This can increase both the speed of development of the tension pneumothorax and its severity. Cover any open chest wound with an occlusive dressing sealed on three sides (Figure 18-18). If dyspnea is significant, assess for tension pneumothorax and perform needle decompression as indicated (see Chapter 25, "Thoracic Trauma").

Always consider the possibility of heart and great vessel damage with a penetrating chest wound. These injuries may lead rapidly to severe internal hemorrhage and death. Another serious complication of penetrating chest trauma is pericardial tamponade. This condition occurs when an object or projectile perforates the heart and permits blood to leak into the pericardial sac. As blood accumulates in the sac, the heart no longer fully fills with blood and circulation slows. If pericardial tamponade is uncorrected, the **prognosis** for the patient is very poor. However, a needle introduced into the pericardial space, a procedure available at the emergency department, can quickly alleviate the life threat. Therefore, if you suspect this condition, arrange for rapid transport. The assessment of pericardial tamponade is discussed in Chapter 25, "Thoracic Trauma."

FIGURE 18-18 Seal open chest wounds and assure adequate respirations.

Impaled Objects

If an object that causes a low-velocity wound lodges in the body, removal of the object may be dangerous for the patient. If the object bent as it hit a bone upon entry, attempts at removal may cause further injury. If the object is held firmly by soft tissue, it may obstruct blood vessels, thereby restricting blood loss; removal of the object may then increase hemorrhage.

Immobilize impaled objects in place where and as they are found and transport the patient. The only impaled objects that you should remove are those lodged in the cheek or trachea that interfere with the airway or those that you must remove to provide CPR.

Immobilize impaled objects in place. Only remove those that have lodged in the cheek or those that interfere with the airway or that prevent CPR.

SUMMARY

Penetrating injuries, especially those associated with gunshot wounds are responsible for a high incidence of prehospital trauma and death. Your understanding of the mechanisms of injury that produce these wounds and an understanding of the types of injuries caused by these mechanisms (index of suspicion) can help you rapidly identify serious life threats and assure these patients receive rapid transport to a trauma center. Special prehospital care techniques such as sealing an open pneumothorax and managing a difficult airway can also help you stabilize the patient in the field and help assure that he safely reaches definitive care.

CHAPTER 19

Hemorrhage and Shock

Objectives

After reading this chapter, you should be able to:

1. Describe the epidemiology, including the morbidity/mortality and prevention strategies, for shock and hemorrhage. (pp. 886–888, 896–898)

2. Discuss the anatomy, physiology, and pathophysiology of the cardiovascular system. (see Chapters 3 and 4)

3. Define shock based on aerobic and anaerobic metabolism. (see Chapter 4)

4. Describe the body's physiological response to changes in blood volume, blood pressure, and perfusion. (pp. 896–900)

5. Describe the effects of decreased perfusion at the capillary level. (pp. 897–898)

6. Discuss the cellular ischemic, capillary stagnation, and capillary washout phases related to hemorrhagic shock. (pp. 897–898)

7. Discuss the various types and degrees of shock and hemorrhage. (pp. 886–888, 898–900)

8. Predict shock and hemorrhage based on mechanism of injury. (pp. 890, 900–901)

9. Identify the need for intervention and transport of the patient with hemorrhage or shock. (pp. 889–893, 900–903)

Continued

INTRODUCTION TO HEMORRHAGE AND SHOCK

The loss of the body's most important and dynamic medium, blood, is called **hemorrhage.** Acute and continuing loss of blood robs the body of its ability to provide oxygen and nutrients to, and remove carbon dioxide and waste products from, the body's elemental building blocks, the cells. In the absence of an adequate volume of circulating blood, the cells and the organs dysfunction and, ultimately, the organism itself dies. The transition between normal function (**homeostasis**) and death is called **shock.** The ability to recognize hemorrhage and shock and to care for them are critical skills for the EMT-Paramedic and are essential to reducing mortality and morbidity in trauma patients. This chapter provides you with an understanding of the cardiovascular system as it relates to hemorrhage and shock and then describes how to recognize and care for these life-threatening assaults on the human body.

✳ **hemorrhage** an abnormal internal or external discharge of blood.

✳ **homeostasis** the natural tendency of the body to maintain a steady and normal internal environment.

✳ **shock** a state of inadequate tissue perfusion.

The EMT-Paramedic must be able to recognize hemorrhage and shock in trauma patients in order to reduce mortality and morbidity.

HEMORRHAGE

As noted previously, hemorrhage is loss of blood from the closed vascular system because of injury to the blood vessels. Hemorrhage is usually classified based on the injured vessel from which it flows: capillary, venous, or arterial.

Capillary hemorrhage generally oozes from the wound, normally an abrasion, and clots quickly on its own. The blood is usually bright red because it is well oxygenated.

Venous hemorrhage flows more quickly, though it, too, generally stops in a few minutes. Bleeding associated with venous hemorrhage is generally dark red because the blood has already given up its oxygen as it passed though the capillary beds.

Bleeding associated with arterial hemorrhage flows very rapidly, often spurting from the wound. This blood is well oxygenated and appears bright red as it escapes from the wound. The blood volume lost can be extreme because of the pressure behind arterial bleeding. The spurting nature of arterial hemorrhage results from the variations in the blood pressure driving the blood loss.

While it is convenient to determine the type of hemorrhage, the nature and depth of a wound may make it hard to differentiate between heavy venous and arterial bleeding. Internal hemorrhage cannot be classified by type with the diagnostic techniques available to paramedics providing prehospital care.

It may be hard to differentiate between heavy venous and arterial bleeding in the field; likewise, paramedics cannot classify internal hemorrhage by type when providing prehospital care.

* clotting the body's three-step response to stop the loss of blood.

* vascular phase step in the clotting process in which smooth blood vessel muscle contracts, reducing the vessel lumen and the flow of blood through it.

CLOTTING

The body's response to local hemorrhage is a complex three-step process called **clotting** (Figure 19-1). As a blood vessel is torn and begins to lose blood, its smooth muscle contracts. This reduces its lumen and the volume and strength of blood flow through it. This is called the **vascular phase.**

At the same time, the vessel's smooth interior lining (the tunica intima) is disrupted, causing a turbulent blood flow. The disturbed blood flow causes frictional damage to the surfaces of the platelets, making them adherent. Platelets then stick to collagen, a protein fiber found in connective tissue, on the vessel's injured inner surface, and to other injured tissue in the area. The blood vessel walls also become adherent. If they are small enough, like capillaries, they may stick together, further occluding blood flow. As platelets adhere to the vessel walls, they **aggregate,** or collect, other platelets. This is the **platelet phase,** the second step of the clotting process. These events occur almost immediately after injury and effectively halt hemorrhage from capillaries and small venous and arterial vessels. While this is a rapid method of hemorrhage control, the resulting clot is unstable.

As time passes, the wound initiates the third and final step of the process, **coagulation.** In this phase, enzymes are released into the bloodstream, initiating a complex sequence of events. These enzymes come from the damaged blood vessel and surrounding tissue (the extrinsic pathway), from the damaged platelets (the intrinsic pathway), or from both. The release of the enzymes triggers a series of chemical reactions that result in the formation of strong protein fibers, or **fibrin.** These fibers entrap red blood cells and form a stronger, more durable clot. This further collection of cells halts all but the most severe hemorrhage. Coagulation normally takes from 7 to 10 minutes. Over time, the cells trapped in the clot protein matrix slowly contract, drawing the wound and the injured vessel together.

The nature of the wound also affects how rapidly and well the clotting mechanisms respond to hemorrhage (Figure 19-2). If the wound lacerates the vessel cleanly in a transverse fashion, the muscles of the vessel wall contract. This retracts the vessel into the tissue, thickening the now shortened tunica media. This thickening further reduces the vessel's lumen, reduces blood flow, and assists the clotting mechanism. If the blood vessel is lacerated longitudinally rather than transversely,

* aggregate to cluster or come together.

* platelet phase second step in the clotting process in which platelets adhere to blood vessel walls and to each other.

* coagulation the third step in the clotting process, which involves the formation of a protein called fibrin that forms a network around a wound to stop bleeding, ward off infection, and lay a foundation for healing and repair of the wound.

* fibrin protein fibers that trap red blood cells as part of the clotting process.

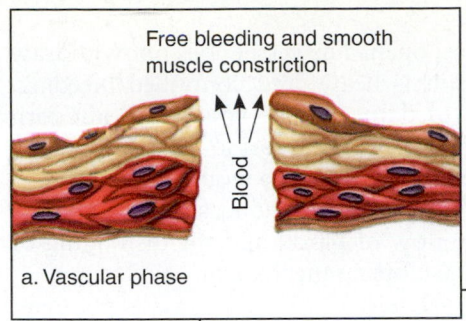

Free bleeding and smooth
muscle constriction

a. Vascular phase

Platelet agglutination

b. Platelet phase

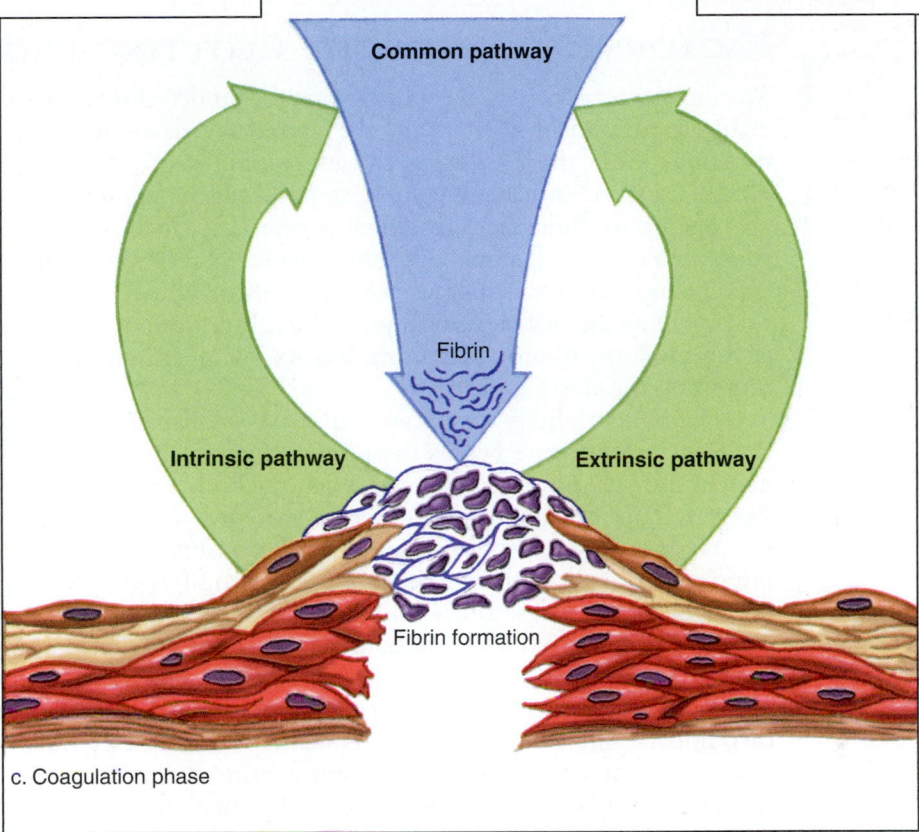

Common pathway

Fibrin

Intrinsic pathway

Extrinsic pathway

Fibrin formation

c. Coagulation phase

FIGURE 19-1   The three steps of the clotting process are the vascular phase, the platelet phase, and coagulation.

FIGURE 19-2   The type of
blood vessel injury often
affects the nature of the
hemorrhage.

a. A clean lateral cut permits the vessel
to retract and thicken its wall.

b. A longitudinal cut to the vessel
causes the wound to open.

the smooth muscle contraction pulls the vessel open. The vessel does not withdraw and the lumen does not constrict. The result is heavy and continued bleeding. Crushing trauma often produces this type of damage. The vessels are not torn cleanly and do not withdraw. The actual hemorrhage site is lost in the disrupted tissue, resulting in severe, hard-to-control bleeding from a large wound area.

If a severe hemorrhage continues, frank hypotension reduces the blood pressure at the hemorrhage site. This limits the flow of blood and the dislodging of clots, thus improving the effectiveness of the clotting mechanism.

FACTORS AFFECTING THE CLOTTING PROCESS

The clotting process can be either helped or hindered by a variety of factors. For example, movement at or around the wound site, as in the manipulation of a fracture, may break the developing clot loose and disrupt the forming fibrin strands. For this reason, immediate wound immobilization (splinting) is beneficial.

Aggressive fluid therapy, which is often provided in cases of severe hemorrhage, may adversely impact the effectiveness of clotting mechanisms. Aggressive fluid resuscitation may increase blood pressure, which in turn increases the pressure pushing against the developing clots. In addition, the water and salts used in fluid therapy dilute the clotting factors, platelets, and red blood cells, further inhibiting the clotting process.

The patient's body temperature also has an effect on the clotting process. As the body temperature begins to fall, as it may in shock states, clot formation is neither as rapid nor as effective as when the body temperature is 98.6° F (37° C) degrees. Thus it is important to keep a patient with severe hemorrhage warm.

Medications may interfere with the body's ability to form a clot and halt both internal and external hemorrhage. Aspirin modifies the enzymes on the surface of platelets that cause them to aggregate after an injury. Ibuprofen and other NSAIDs (non-steroidal anti-inflammatory drugs) may have a similar but temporary effect. Heparin and warfarin (Coumadin®) interfere with the normal generation of protein fibers that produce a stable clot. While these drugs may prevent thrombosis and emboli in patients with heart disease, they may prolong or worsen hemorrhage when that patient is injured. Try to gather information on whether the patient uses such medications when taking the patient history.

HEMORRHAGE CONTROL

Hemorrhage is either internal or external. While there are a number of steps you can take to control external hemorrhage in the field, prehospital care of internal hemorrhage is more limited.

External Hemorrhage

External hemorrhage is easy to identify and care for. It presents with blood oozing, flowing, or spurting from the wound. Bleeding from capillary and venous wounds is easy to halt because the pressure driving it is limited (Figure 19-3). Usually **direct pressure** on the wound or a combination of direct pressure and elevation work quite well in stopping the bleeding. Bleeding from an arterial wound, however, is powered by the arterial blood pressure and escapes from the blood vessel with significant force. The normal control and clotting mechanisms help reduce blood loss but do not stop it if the injured vessel is large. To stop bleeding from such a wound, pressure on the bleeding site must exceed the arterial pressure. Direct digital pressure on the site of blood loss, maintained by a dressing and pressure bandage, is most effective. Elevation of the wound area and use of pressure points may also be necessary if the bandage cannot apply enough pressure directly to the hemorrhage site.

Content Review

FACTORS HINDERING THE CLOTTING PROCESS

Movement of the wound site
Aggressive fluid therapy
Low body temperature
Medications such as aspirin, heparin, or Coumadin

Immediate immobilization (splinting) of the wound site aids the clotting process.

⚷

✱ **direct pressure** method of hemorrhage control that relies on the application of pressure to the actual site of the bleeding.

FIGURE 19-3a Hemorrhage control: apply direct pressure.

FIGURE 19-3b Hemorrhage control: elevate the extremity above the level of the heart.

FIGURE 19-3c Hemorrhage control: if bleeding does not stop, apply direct fingertip pressure.

FIGURE 19-3d Hemorrhage control: if bleeding continues, apply pressure to a pressure point.

Be extremely cautious if you consider using a **tourniquet.** Employ the device *only* to halt persistent, life-threatening hemorrhage. If you apply the tourniquet at a pressure less than the arterial pressure, blood continues to flow into the limb, while the tourniquet restricts venous flow out. The limb's arterial and venous pressures then rise, as does the rate of hemorrhage. If the tourniquet meets its objective and halts all blood flow to the limb, blood loss stops, but so does circulation to the distal extremity. During this absence of perfusion, **lactic acid,** potassium, and other **anaerobic** metabolites accumulate in the stagnant blood. When the tourniquet is released, the resumption of blood flow may transport these toxins into the central circulation with devastating results (Figure 19-4). Once you apply the tourniquet, therefore, leave it in place until the patient is in the emergency department or some other facility where the negative effects of re-perfusion can be addressed. If you must apply a tourniquet, use a wide cravat or belt or a blood pressure cuff. A thin or narrow constricting device may damage tissue beneath the tourniquet. Despite these hazards, the tourniquet may be essential in halting life-threatening arterial hemorrhage.

* **tourniquet** a constrictor used on an extremity to apply circumferential pressure on all arteries to control bleeding.

Use a tourniquet only as a last resort to halt persistent, life-threatening hemorrhage.

* **lactic acid** compound produced from pyruvic acid during anaerobic glycolyis.

* **anaerobic** able to live without oxygen.

Internal Hemorrhage

Internal hemorrhage is associated with almost all serious blunt and penetrating trauma. As with external hemorrhage, internal hemorrhage can involve capillary, venous, or arterial blood loss. The blood can accumulate in the tissue itself, forming a

a. Blood pressure cuff positioned but not inflated. Normal blood flow.

Arteriole

Body cells

Capillary

Venule

b. Inflation of B/P cuff as a tourniquet cuts off circulation. Blood flow stagnates and metabolic byproducts accumulate.

CO_2

Waste products

c. Release of cuff restores circulation. Returning blood flow pushes acidic byproducts back into the central circulation.

CO_2

Waste products

FIGURE 19-4 Release of a tourniquet may send accumulated toxins into the central circulation with devastating results for the patient.

visible or hidden contusion, or it can be forced between **fascia** and form a pocket of blood called a **hematoma**. In most of these cases, the hemorrhage is self-limiting because the pressure within the tissue or fascia controls the blood loss. However, large contusions, massive soft tissue injuries, and large hematomas, especially those affecting large muscle masses like the thighs or buttocks, can account for moderate blood and body fluid loss. Fractures of the humerus and tibia/fibula may account for 500 to 750 mL of loss, while femur fractures may account for up to 1,500 mL of loss.

In body cavities such as the chest and the abdominal, pelvic, and retroperitoneal spaces, the resistance to continuing blood loss does not develop. With bleeding in these areas, loss continues unabated until the normal clotting process is effective, the blood pressure drops significantly, or surgical intervention is provided. The best indicators of significant internal hemorrhage are the mechanism of injury (MOI), local signs and symptoms of injury, and the early signs and symptoms of blood loss and shock. If a patient has sustained significant trauma to the chest, abdomen, or pelvis, anticipate significant, continuing, and uncontrolled blood loss. Such a patient requires rapid transport to a trauma center or hospital for surgical repair of any damaged vessels.

You can assist the natural internal hemorrhage control mechanisms in the extremities by providing a patient with immobilization and elevation. Continued movement of the injury site, especially if it is associated with a long bone fracture, disrupts the clotting process, causing further soft tissue, nervous, and vascular damage, and continuing the blood loss. If the patient is a victim of serious or multisystem trauma, however, do not spend time on the scene with aggressive skeletal immobilization. Instead, quickly splint the patient to a long spine board and begin transport. Provide splinting of individual limbs if time permits during transport.

Internal hemorrhage is often associated with injuries to specific organs and can be related either to trauma or to pre-existing medical problems. Internal hemorrhage can also present with external signs of injury or disease in addition to the signs and symptoms of blood loss. These signs can help you identify the nature and location of the blood loss.

The nasal cavity is lined with a rich supply of capillaries to warm and help humidify incoming air. Hypertension, a strong sneeze, or direct trauma may rupture the vessels supplying these capillary beds and produce the moderate to severe hemorrhage called **epistaxis**. Prolonged epistaxsis can result in hypovolemia, while blood flowing down the posterior nasal cavity, down the esophagus, and into the stomach may result in nausea, followed by vomiting (Figure 19-5). Trauma to the

* **fascia** a fibrous membrane that covers, supports, and separates muscles and may also unite the skin with underlying tissue.

* **hematoma** collection of blood beneath the skin or trapped within a body compartment.

Provide a patient with suspected internal bleeding with immobilization and elevation (of extremities) to aid the body's hemorrhage control mechanisms.

* **epistaxis** bleeding from the nose resulting from injury, disease, or environmental factors; a nosebleed.

FIGURE 19-5a To control nosebleed, have the patient sit leaning forward.

FIGURE 19-5b Pinch the fleshy part of the patient's nostrils firmly together.

Content Review

STAGES OF HEMORRHAGE

Stage 1—blood loss of up to 15%; patient may display some nervousness and marginally cool skin with slight pallor

Stage 2—blood loss of 15 to 25%; patient displays thirst, anxiety, restlessness, cool, clammy skin, increased respiratory rate

Stage 3—blood loss between 25 and 35%; patient experiences air hunger, dyspnea, severe thirst, anxiety, restlessness; survival unlikely without rapid intervention

Stage 4—blood loss greater than 35%; pulse barely palpable, respirations ineffective; patient lethargic, confused, moving toward unresponsiveness; survival unlikely

With hemorrhage patients, determine the relative severity of blood loss, the need for aggressive intervention, the length of time since the incident that caused the trauma, the current stage of hemorrhage, and how quickly the patient is moving from one stage to another.

oral cavity may likewise result in serious hemorrhage, followed by ingestion of blood, nausea, and then emesis.

There are also outward signs that indicate hemorrhage in the lungs and respiratory system. For example, degenerative diseases, such as tuberculosis or cancer, or chest trauma may rupture pulmonary vessels. This leads to the release of blood into the lower airways or alveolar space. The patient may then cough up bright red blood, a sign called hemoptysis.

Trauma, caustic ingestion, degenerative disease (for example, cancer), and rupturing **esophageal varicies** may lead to hemorrhage along the esophagus. In these pathologies, blood is likely to travel, via peristalsis, into the stomach, where it collects. Gastric hemorrhage due to ulceration or trauma may also result in the accumulation of blood in the stomach. A significant collection of blood acts as a gastric irritant, inducing vomiting. If the blood is evacuated early, it is bright red in color. If blood remains in the stomach for some time, emesis resembles coffee grounds in both color and consistency.

Hemorrhage in the small or large bowel can be associated with trauma, degenerative disease, or diverticulitis (small pouches in the walls of the bowel that collect material, become infected, and may burst). Bowel hemorrhage may present as bleeding from the rectum, or the blood may be digested before release, producing a black and tarry stool called **melena.**

Rectal injury may be caused by pelvic fracture or direct trauma. This presents with bleeding, which may be severe.

Vaginal hemorrhage may be associated with trauma, degenerative disease, menstruation, ectopic pregnancy, placenta previa, and potential or actual miscarriage. Urethral hemorrhage is generally minor and may reflect damage to the prostate or urethra. Blood in the urine reflects bladder injury.

Non-traumatic forms of hemorrhage may be either acute or chronic. Acute hemorrhage moves the victim rapidly toward shock and is quickly recognizable. Chronic hemorrhage is likely to be rather limited in volume, but it does continue over time. The resulting loss depletes the body of red blood cells and leads to **anemia.** This condition reduces the blood's oxygen-carrying capacity, and the patient experiences fatigue and lethargy. Clotting factors may likewise be depleted, which increases the rate of fluid loss and makes any secondary hemorrhage more difficult to control.

STAGES OF HEMORRHAGE

Fluid accounts for about 60 percent of the body's weight and is distributed among the cellular, interstitial, and vascular spaces. The cells contain about 62 percent of the total fluid volume, while the interstitial (non-vascular) space holds 26 percent. Four to five percent of body fluid is found in other spaces such as the ventricles of the brain and meninges (cerebrospinal fluid). The remaining 7 percent of fluid volume resides in the vascular space. This fluid, called plasma, and the blood cells account for 7 percent of the average adult male's body weight (about 6.5 percent in the female). Fluid in the vascular space is distributed among the heart, arteries, veins, and capillaries and accounts for 5 liters (10 units) of blood volume in the healthy 70-kg adult male.

The effects of hemorrhage can be categorized into four progressive stages as blood volume is lost. These stages relate to the volume of blood lost in acute hemorrhage and that result in "classic" signs and symptoms. Remember, however, that each individual's response to blood loss may vary as may the rate and progress of the loss. Use these categories to help determine the relative severity of the loss and the need for aggressive intervention. It is also important to identify the following: the length of time elapsed since the incident that caused the trauma; the stage of hemorrhage the victim is in when you arrive at his side; and how quickly the patient is moving from one stage to another (Table 19-1).

Table 19-1 — PATIENT SIGNS ASSOCIATED WITH STAGES OF HEMORRHAGE

Stage	Blood Loss	Vasoconstriction	Pulse Rate	Pulse (Pressure) Strength	Blood Pressure	Respiratory Rate	Respiratory Volume
1	<15%	↑	↑	→	→	→	→
2	15–25%	↑↑	↑↑	↓	→	↑	↑
3	25–35%	↑↑↑	↑↑↑	↓↓	↓	↑↑	↓
4	>35%	↓↓	Variable	↓↓↓	↓↓↓	↓	↓↓

Stage 1 Hemorrhage

Stage 1 hemorrhage is a blood loss of up to 15 percent of the circulating blood volume. In the 70-kg male that is approximately 500 to 750 mL of blood, about the amount you might give during a blood drive. The healthy human system can easily compensate for such a blood loss volume by constricting the vascular beds, especially on the venous side. In this stage, the blood pressure remains constant as do the **pulse pressure**, respiratory rate, and renal output. The central venous pressure may drop slightly, but it returns to normal quickly. The pulse rate elevates slightly, and the patient may display some signs of **catecholamine** (epinephrine and norepinephrine) release, notably nervousness and marginally cool skin with a slight pallor.

Stage 2 Hemorrhage

Stage 2 hemorrhage occurs as 15 to 25 percent (750 to 1,250 mL) of the blood volume is lost. The body's first-line compensatory responses can no longer maintain blood pressure, and secondary mechanisms are now employed. Tachycardia becomes very evident, and the pulse strength begins to diminish (the pulse pressure is noticeably narrowed). A strong release of catecholamines increases peripheral vascular resistance. This maintains systolic blood pressure but results in peripheral vasoconstriction and cool, clammy skin. Anxiety increases, and the patient may begin to display restlessness and thirst. Thirst is present as fluid leaves the intracellular and interstitial spaces and the osmotic pressure of the blood changes. Renal output remains normal, but the respiratory rate increases.

Stage 3 Hemorrhage

Stage 3 hemorrhage occurs when blood loss reaches between 25 to 35 percent of blood volume (1,250 to 1,750 mL). The body's compensatory mechanisms are unable to cope with the loss, and the classic signs of shock appear. Rapid tachycardia is present as the blood pressure begins to fall. The pulse is barely palpable as the pulse pressure remains very narrow. The patient experiences air hunger and tachypnea. Anxiety, restlessness, and thirst become more severe. The level of responsiveness decreases, and the patient becomes very pale, cool, and diaphoretic. Urinary output declines. Without rapid intervention, this patient's survival is unlikely.

Stage 4 Hemorrhage

Stage 4 hemorrhage occurs with a blood loss of greater than 35 percent of the body's total blood supply. The patient's pulse is barely palpable in the central arteries, if one can be found at all. Respirations are very rapid, shallow, and ineffective. The patient is very lethargic and confused, moving rapidly toward unresponsiveness.

* **pulse pressure** difference between the systolic and diastolic blood pressures.

* **catecholamine** a hormone, such as epinephrine or norepinephrine, that strongly affects the nervous and cardiovascular systems, metabolic rate, temperature, and smooth muscle.

Without rapid intervention, survival of a Stage 3 hemorrhage patient is unlikely.

The skin is very cool, clammy, and extremely pale. Urinary output ceases. Even with aggressive fluid resuscitation and blood transfusions, patient survival is unlikely.

These descriptions of the stages of hemorrhage presume that the patient is a normally healthy adult. Any pre-existing condition may affect the volume of blood loss required for movement from one stage to another as well as the speed at which the patient moves through the stages. The patient's state of hydration, from dehydrated to fluid-rich, may also affect how quickly and to what degree compensation takes place.

The rate of the blood loss also has a profound effect on how quickly a patient moves from stage 1 to stage 4. If the blood loss is very rapid, the compensatory mechanisms may not work as effectively. On the other hand, a small wound bleeding uncontrollably but very slowly for days may not move the patient from stage 1 to stage 2, even with a loss much greater than 750 mL.

Certain categories of patients—pregnant women, athletes, obese patients, children, and the elderly—react differently to blood loss. The blood volume of a woman in late pregnancy is 50 percent greater than normal. This patient may lose rather large volumes of blood before progressing through the various stages of hemorrhage. Although the mother in this circumstance appears to be somewhat protected from the effects of serious hemorrhage, the fetus is deprived of good circulation early in the blood loss and is more susceptible to harm.

A well-conditioned athlete often has greater fluid and cardiac reserves than a typical patient. This means he or she may move more slowly through the early stages with greater percentages of loss needed to advance from one stage to another.

The obese patient, on the other hand, has a blood volume close to 7 percent of ideal body weight, but not actual body weight. Thus, the blood volume as a percentage of actual body weight is lower than 7 percent. This means that what appears to be only a small blood loss may have a more serious effect in such a patient.

In infants and young children, blood volumes approximate 8 to 9 percent of body weight, volumes that are proportionally about 20 percent greater than those of adults. However, compensatory mechanisms in infants and children are neither as well developed nor as effective as those in adults. These young patients may not show early signs and symptoms of compensation as clearly as adults. They may instead move quickly into the later stages of shock. Suspect hemorrhage early with child and infant trauma and treat it aggressively.

The elderly are likewise more adversely affected by blood loss. They have lower volumes of fluid reserves, and their compensatory systems are less responsive to fluid losses. These patients may also be on medications, such as beta-blockers, that further reduce the body's ability to respond to blood loss and varying blood pressures or on medications, such as aspirin, Coumadin®, and heparin, that interfere with the body's natural hemorrhage control system. Often, elderly patients do not experience the tachycardia associated with blood loss, and their blood pressures drop before those of healthy adults. Signs of blood loss and shock may be masked by reduced perceptions of pain in the elderly and by lowered levels of mental acuity due to disease. The elderly also do not tolerate periods of inadequate tissue perfusion well because of chronic cardiovascular inefficiency.

Suspect hemorrhage early in cases of child and infant trauma and treat it aggressively.

Be aware that signs and symptoms of blood loss in elderly patients may be masked by use of medications, bodily changes, reduced perception of pain, and the effects of disease.

HEMORRHAGE ASSESSMENT

The assessment of various types of trauma patients will be the subject of the next few chapters. In these chapters, only the aspects of assessment that are pertinent to those pathologies will be addressed. Please refer to the patient assessment chapters (Chapter 10, "History Taking"; Chapter 11; "Physical Exam Techniques"; Chapter 12, "Patient Assessement in the Field"; Chapter 13, "Clinical Decision Making) for a more complete discussion of trauma assessment.

The assessment of the hemorrhage patient is directed at identifying the source of the hemorrhage and halting any serious and controllable loss. During assessment, you should also examine the circumstances of injury to approximate the volume of blood lost and the rate of past and continuing hemorrhage. This process begins with the scene size-up and continues throughout transport and care.

The assessment of the hemorrhage patient is directed at identifying the source of the hemorrhage and halting any serious and controllable loss.

Scene Size–up

Remember that body substance isolation precautions are essential during the assessment of trauma patients. A patient's blood and other body fluids may contain pathogens capable of transmitting HIV, hepatitis, and other diseases to you. Conversely, you may transmit infectious agents to the wounds of the patients you assess and care for. In fact, the risk of your transmitting disease or infection to a patient with open wounds or burns is probably much greater than the risk that he or she will transmit disease or infection to you. For these reasons, always observe body substance isolation precautions with all trauma patients. These precautions include the use of gloves and a mask when you inspect or palpate any injured area, especially one with open wounds (Figure 19-6). If there is spurting blood, as with arterial hemorrhage, if a patient is combative, or if there is airway trauma with or without bleeding, also wear eye protection and a disposable gown to protect your uniform. Be sure to wash your hands before each ambulance call and do so immediately afterwards as well. Scrub vigorously when washing to remove as much of the bacterial load as possible.

Body substance isolation procedures protect the patient as well as the care giver.

If your gloves become contaminated with earth, debris, blood, or body fluids while caring for a patient, change them immediately. If you will be assessing or treating multiple patients, consider double gloving. This means that you put on two or more sets of gloves and remove a set each time you complete assessment of one patient and move on to the next. Place any contaminated gloves, clothing, dressings, or other materials in a bio-hazard bag and assure proper disposal.

The handling of needles presents special problems for prehospital personnel. Once a needle is used, it carries the potential of introducing a patient's blood directly

FIGURE 19-6   When caring for a hemorrhaging patient, employ appropriate body substance isolation procedures.

into a care giver's or bystander's tissues. This greatly increases the likelihood of disease transmission. When dealing with needles, always assure that they are not recapped, but rather placed in a properly marked and secure, puncture-resistant sharps container. Should you be stuck with a needle, continue your care, but document the incident immediately upon arrival at the emergency department. Wash and cover the wound, then report the incident to your service's infection control officer or other designated officer. There are several prophylactic regimes available that may protect against the transmission of some infectious diseases. Even more important, you can guard against some diseases, such as hepatitis, by obtaining immunizations before you begin your career as a care provider.

Patients may see your gloves and then feel uncomfortable about being treated by someone who is "afraid to touch them." Assure those patients that the gloves and other precautions are for their protection as well as yours.

When appropriate BSI precautions have been taken, continue with the scene size-up. Evaluate the mechanism of injury to anticipate sites of both external and internal hemorrhage. Anticipating external hemorrhage sites focuses your subsequent assessment and care, while anticipating internal hemorrhage affects your decision on whether to provide rapid transport.

When evaluating the mechanism of injury (MOI), also attempt to determine the amount of time that has elapsed between the injury and your evaluation of it. Knowing the length of this time period is very important in determining the amount and rate of blood loss. For example, if you arrive on a scene 3 minutes after an accident and find a patient losing 150 mL of blood per minute, you can estimate that 450 mL of blood have been lost. You would not expect the patient to display the signs and symptoms of stage 1 hemorrhage. If, however, you arrive 10 minutes after the incident, the same patient, losing blood at the same rate, will have lost 1,500 mL of blood and is likely to have reached stage 3. In both these cases, the patient is suffering serious, life-threatening hemorrhage. Good assessment and recognition assures provision of a proper course of care. However, the earlier you arrive at the patient's side, the harder it is to identify serious hemorrhage. For this reason, you must be aware of and appreciate the progressive effects of blood loss and use both the MOI analysis and the time since an incident to increase your suspicions of a problem. Remember, the sooner the signs of later stages of hemorrhage appear, the greater the rate and volume of blood loss.

The sooner the signs of the later stages of hemorrhage appear, the greater the rate and volume of blood loss.

Initial Assessment

As you begin the initial assessment, form a general impression of the patient. Be especially alert for any signs and symptoms of internal hemorrhage. These early signs are very subtle and may go unnoticed unless you deliberately look for them. Correct any immediate life threats and provide in-line stabilization if you suspect spinal injury. Assess the patient's initial mental status to determine alertness, orientation, and responsiveness. Be alert for any signs of anxiety, confusion, or combativeness. Any central nervous system deficit may be secondary to hemorrhage, so be suspicious.

Assess both airway and breathing carefully, noting any tachypnea or air hunger. Administer oxygen via nonrebreather mask at a rate of 15 L/minute. When assessing circulation, pay special attention to the pulse strength (the pulse pressure) and rate. Remember that the pulse pressure narrows well before the systolic pressure begins to drop. The pulse rate, too, may suggest developing shock. A fast—and especially a fast, weak (thready)—pulse may be the first noticeable sign of serious internal blood loss. Note also skin color and condition. Pale or mottled skin is an early sign of shock, while cool and clammy skin is also an indicator of potential blood loss and shock.

Complete the initial assessment by establishing patient priorities. Decide, based on your findings to this point, whether the patient is to receive a rapid trauma assessment or a focused history and exam. If any indication, mechanism of injury, sign or symptom suggests serious internal hemorrhage or uncontrolled external hemorrhage, consider the rapid trauma assessment and then immediate transport for the patient.

Focused History and Physical Exam

Your initial assessment findings and the evaluation of the mechanism of injury determine how you will proceed with the focused history and physical exam. For trauma patients who have a significant MOI, continue spinal immobilization, and perform a rapid trauma assessment crest. Then obtain baseline vital signs and a patient history.

For trauma patients who have no significant mechanism of injury and who have revealed no critical findings during initial assessment, perform an assessment focused on the area of injury, then obtain baseline vital signs and gather a patient history. Finally, provide care as appropriate and transport.

With both these types of trauma patients, perform ongoing assessments during transport. If time and the patient's condition permit, you may also perform a detailed physical exam. However, you should never delay transport to perform the detailed examination.

Rapid Trauma Assessment For trauma patients with a significant MOI, you perform a rapid trauma assessment, inspecting and palpating the patient in an orderly fashion from head to toe. Pay particular attention to areas where critical trauma has occurred and areas where the MOI suggests forces were focused.

Carefully and quickly observe the head for serious bleeding. Internal head injury rarely accounts for the classic signs of shock. However, the scalp bleeds profusely because the vessels there are large and lack the ability to constrict as well as other peripheral vessels. If any external bleeding appears serious, halt it immediately.

Next, examine the neck. The carotid arteries and jugular veins are located close to the skin's surface. Injury to them can produce rapid and fatal exsanguination. An added danger is the aspiration of air directly into an open jugular vein. At times, venous pressure, due to deep inspiration, can be less than atmospheric pressure. Air may then be drawn into the vein, traveling to the heart and forming emboli, which then lodge in the pulmonary circulation. Quickly control any serious hemorrhage from neck wounds with sterile occlusive dressings. If spinal injury is suspected, apply a rigid cervical collar when assessment of the neck is complete, but maintain in-line manual immobilization until the patient is immobilized to a spine board.

Visually sweep the chest and abdomen for any serious external hemorrhage, though such bleeding is infrequent there. You are more likely to note signs of blunt or penetrating trauma, suggesting internal injury and hemorrhage within. Look to the abdomen for signs of soft tissue injury, contusions, abrasions, rigidity, and guarding and tenderness that suggest internal injury.

Quickly examine the pelvic and groin region. Test the integrity of the pelvic ring by pressing gently on the iliac crest. Remember that pelvic fracture can account for blood loss of more than 2,000 mL. Lacerations to the male genitalia may also account for serious external hemorrhage.

Assess the extremities and rule out fractures of the femur, tibia/fibula, or humerus. Keep in mind that femur fracture can account for up to 1,500 mL of blood loss, while each tibia/fibula or humerus fracture may contribute an additional 500 to 750 mL of blood loss. Hematomas and large contusions may account for up to 500 mL of blood loss in the larger muscle masses. Quickly check

> **Content Review**
>
> ### INJURIES THAT CAN CAUSE SIGNIFICANT BLOOD LOSS
>
> Fractured pelvis (2,000 mL)
> Fractured femur (1,500 mL)
> Fractured tibia (750 mL)
> Fractured humerus (750 mL)
> Large contusion (500 mL)

Early

Pain, tenderness, swelling, or discoloration of suspected injury site

Bleeding from mouth, rectum, vagina, or other orifice

Vomiting of bright red blood

Tender, rigid and/or distended abdomen

Late

Anxiety, restlessness, combativeness, or altered mental status

Weakness, faintness, or dizziness

Vomiting of blood the color of dark coffee grounds

Thirst

Melena

Shallow, rapid breathing

Rapid, weak pulse

Pale, cool, clammy skin

Capillary refill greater than 2 seconds (most reliable in infants and children under 6)

Dropping blood pressure

Dilated pupils sluggish in responding to light

Nausea and vomiting

✳ **hematochezia** passage of stools containing red blood.

✳ **orthostatic hypotension** a decrease in blood pressure that occurs when a person moves from a supine or sitting to an upright position.

✳ **tilt test** drop in the systolic blood pressure of 20 mmHg or an increase in the pulse rate of 20 beats per minute when a patient is moved from a supine to a sitting position; a finding suggestive of a relative hypovolemia.

---

distal pulse strength and muscle tone in the extremities, comparing findings in the opposing extremities.

Finally, visually sweep the body, including the posterior, for any external hemorrhage that may have gone unnoticed in your examination to this point.

At the end of the rapid trauma assessment, assess the patient's vital signs, obtain a patient history if possible, and inventory the injuries that may contribute to shock. Provide rapid transport for any patient with a MOI or physical findings that meet trauma triage criteria (see Chapter 16, "Trauma and Trauma Systems"). Any patient with injuries likely to induce hemorrhage at the level of stage 2 or greater should likewise receive immediate transport. If travel time to the trauma center will exceed 20 minutes, consider requesting air medical transport. Be sure to record the results of your assessment carefully. Compare this information with signs and symptoms you discover during the ongoing assessment to identify trends in the patient's condition.

Perform a detailed physical exam only when all immediate life threats have been addressed. Normally, this would be when you are en route to the hospital or trauma center or when transport has been delayed for some reason.

Focused Physical Exam Employ the focused trauma assessment for patients without a significant MOI, for example, a patient who has lacerated his or her finger with a knife. In such cases, the hemorrhage can be controlled on the scene and the MOI does not suggest additional problems. With such patients, focus your exam on the area injured, inspecting and palpating the area thoroughly, looking for additional injuries beyond the one that prompted the call. Control the hemorrhage, if you have not already done so. Obtain baseline vital signs and a patient history, and prepare and transport the patient.

In some cases, you may wish to perform a rapid trauma assessment, even though the patient does not have a significant MOI. This would be the case, for example, if you suspect the patient has more injuries than he or she has complained of or if his or her condition suddenly begins to deteriorate. With such patients, it may be necessary to perform a rapid head-to-toe examination, inspecting and palpating all body regions.

Additional Assessment Considerations In the trauma patient with a significant MOI or the medical patient showing signs and symptoms of blood loss and shock, it is important to search for evidence of internal hemorrhage. This evidence may be in the form of blood, or material suggestive of blood, flowing from the body orifices. Bright red blood from the mouth, nose, rectum, or other orifice suggests direct bleeding. The vomiting of material that looks like coffee grounds is associated with partially digested blood in the stomach, suggestive of a long-term and slow hemorrhage. A black, tarry stool called melena suggests blood has remained in the bowel for some time. **Hematochezia** is stool with frank blood in it and reflects active bleeding in the colon or rectum.

In the patient with non-specific complaints—general ill feeling, anxiousness, restlessness—or a lowered level of responsiveness, suspect and look for other signs of internal hemorrhage. Watch for an increasing pulse rate, rising diastolic blood pressure (narrowing blood pressure), and cool and clammy skin.

Also observe for dizziness or syncope when the patient moves from a supine to a sitting or standing position. This condition is called **orthostatic hypotension** and is suggestive of a volume loss, possibly attributable to internal hemorrhage. This phenomenon is the basis of the **tilt test,** which can be employed to determine blood or fluid loss and the body's reduced ability to compensate for normal positional change. Perform this test only on patients who do not already display signs and symptoms of shock. Prepare for the test by obtaining blood pressure and pulse rates from the patient in a supine or seated position. Then have the supine patient move to a seated position or the seated patient stand up and obtain another set of blood pressure and pulse rates. If the systolic blood pressure drops more than 20 mmHg or the pulse rate rises more than 20 beats per minute, the test is considered positive, indicating hypovolemia.

Ongoing Assessment

Once you have rendered all appropriate life-saving care, perform ongoing assessments frequently—at least every 5 minutes with unstable patients and every 15 minutes with stable ones. Reevaluate your general impression, and reassess the patient's mental status, airway, breathing, and circulation, and obtain additional sets of vital signs. Compare each set of findings with earlier ones to determine if the patient's condition is stable, deteriorating, or improving. Pay special attention to the pulse pressure because it is a clear indicator of the body's efforts to compensate for hypovolemia. Also pay particular attention to changes in mental status, noting any increasing anxiety or restlessness.

HEMORRHAGE MANAGEMENT

The management of hemorrhage is an integral part of care for the trauma patient, one that begins during the initial assessment and is shaped by findings of the rapid trauma assessment or the focused physical exam.

First, assure that the airway is patent, that the patient is breathing adequately, and that you have administered high flow oxygen. If you have not, establish and maintain the airway and provide the necessary ventilatory support. Be prepared to provide endotracheal intubation if necessary to secure the airway.

Assure that the patient has a pulse. If not, initiate CPR, attach a monitor-defibrillator, and employ advanced cardiac life support measures. Rule out pericardial tamponade and tension pneumothorax as possible causes of cardiac dysfunction. Understand that cardiac arrest in trauma cases due to hypovolemia carries an extremely poor prognosis. When resources are scarce, your efforts may be better utilized caring for other salvageable patients.

During the initial assessment, care for serious (arterial and heavy venous) hemorrhage only after any airway and breathing problems are corrected. Quickly apply a pressure dressing held in place by self-adherent bandage material or a firmly tied cravat. Return to provide better hemorrhage control after you complete the initial and rapid trauma assessments and set priorities for care of the hemorrhages and other trauma you discover. If the patient displays early signs of shock, consider applying a PASG and initiating fluid therapy; do not, however, delay transport in order to carry out these measures.

During the initial assessment, care for serious hemorrhage only after any airway and breathing problems are corrected.

Once you have completed the focused history and physical exam stage of assessment, begin caring for injuries, including hemorrhage, as you have prioritized them. As you work down your injury priority list and come to a wound, inspect the site to identify the type and exact location of bleeding. This helps you apply pressure—either digitally or with dressings and bandages—most effectively to halt the blood flow. With cases of external hemorrhage, it is important to identify the exact source and type of bleeding and to be sure to look at the wound site.

Document your findings on the prehospital care report. If you document and convey this information clearly to the emergency department staff, you will reduce the need for others to open the wound (thus disrupting the clotting process) to determine and describe its nature.

Direct pressure controls all but the most persistent hemorrhage (Figure 19-7). Although systolic blood pressure drives arterial hemorrhage, you can stop such a hemorrhage with simple finger pressure properly applied to the source of the bleeding. If a wound looks as though it may pose a problem, insert a wad of dressing material over the site of the heaviest bleeding and apply a bandage over the

Direct pressure usually controls all but the most persistent hemorrhage.

FIGURE 19-7 In most cases of moderate to severe external hemorrhage, direct pressure, maintained by a bandage and dressing, will control bleeding.

dressing. This focuses pressure on the site and away from the surrounding area. If bleeding saturates the dressing, cover it with another dressing and apply another bandage to keep pressure on the wound. Removing the soaked bandage and dressing disrupts the clotting process and prolongs the hemorrhage. If, however, the wound continues to bleed through your layers of dressings and bandages, consider removing the dressing materials you have applied, directly visualizing the exact site of bleeding, and then re-applying a wad of dressing and firm direct pressure to the precise hemorrhage site.

If direct pressure alone does not halt the blood flow to an extremity, consider elevation. Elevation reduces the systolic blood pressure because the heart has to push the blood against gravity and up the limb. Employ elevation only when there is an isolated bleeding wound on a limb and movement will not aggravate any other injuries.

If bleeding still persists, find an arterial pulse point proximal to the wound and apply firm pressure there (Figure 19-8). This further reduces the blood pressure within the limb and should reduce the hemorrhaging.

Other techniques that can aid in hemorrhage control include limb splinting and the use of pneumatic splints. Splinting helps maintain the stability of the wound site, thus assisting the mechanisms by which clots develop. Splinting may also protect the site from injuries that might occur if the patient is jostled during extrication and transport or as you assess and care for other wounds. Pneumatic splints can also prevent movement of an injured limb. They may also be helpful in holding dressings in place and in applying direct pressure to a limb circumferentially.

Consider using a tourniquet only as a last resort when hemorrhage is prolonged and persistent. As mentioned earlier, there are hazards associated with tourniquet use. Apply a blood pressure cuff just proximal to the hemorrhage site and inflate it to apply a pressure about 30 mmHg greater than the systolic blood pressure. Assure there is no continued bleeding after you apply the tourniquet, and mark the patient's forehead with the letters "TQ" and the time of application.

Specific Wound Considerations

There are several types of wounds that require special attention for hemorrhage control. They include head wounds, neck wounds, large gaping wounds, and crush injuries.

Head injuries raise some special concerns regarding hemorrhage control. Head wounds may be associated with both severe hemorrhage and the loss of

a. Radial artery for hand.

b. Brachial artery for forearm.

c. Femoral artery for thigh.

d. Popliteal artery for leg and foot.

FIGURE 19-8   Common pressure points for hemorrhage control.

skull integrity (fracture). Control bleeding with such wounds very carefully, using gentle direct pressure around the wound site and against the stable skull. Fluid drainage from the ears and nose may be secondary to skull fracture. Cerebrospinal fluid, as it escapes the cranial vault, relieves building intracranial pressure. Halting the flow of fluid would end this relief mechanism and compound the increase in pressure. In addition, stopping the flow may provide a pathway for pathogens to enter the meninges and cause serious infection (meningitis). Cerebrospinal fluid quickly regenerates as the injury heals. Thus, if there is hemorrhage from either the nose or ear canal, simply cover the area with a soft, porous dressing and bandage it loosely.

Neck wounds carry the risk of air being drawn into the venous circulation with life-threatening results. Cover any open neck wound with an occlusive dressing held firmly in place. Do not employ circumferential bandages to create direct pressure with neck wounds. Digital pressure controls most, if not all, neck bleeding. It may, however, be necessary to apply and maintain this manual pressure continuously during the patient's prehospital care.

With head injury patients, do not attempt to stop the flow of blood or fluid from the nose or ear canal, but cover the area with porous dressing to collect the material and bandage loosely.

Cover any open neck wound with an occlusive dressing held firmly in place.

Gaping wounds often present hemorrhage control problems. With such wounds, bleeding originates from many sites and their open nature prevents application of uniform direct pressure. To manage bleeding from such a wound, create a mass of dressing material approximating the volume and shape of the wound. Place the material with the sterile, non-adherent side down on the wound and bandage it firmly in place.

Controlling hemorrhage associated with crush injuries can be particularly challenging. The source of hemorrhage in such cases is frequently difficult to determine, and the vessels are damaged in such a way that the normal hemorrhage control mechanisms may be ineffective. Place a dressing around and over the crushed tissue and a pneumatic splint over that and inflate to apply pressure and hold the dressing in place. If bleeding is heavy and persistent, consider using a tourniquet but keep in mind the precautions discussed previously.

Transport Considerations

Consider rapid transport for any patient who experiences serious external hemorrhage that you cannot control and for any patient with suspected serious internal hemorrhage.

Consider rapid transport for any patient who experiences serious external hemorrhage that you cannot control and for any patient with suspected serious internal hemorrhage. Be vigilant for any signs of compensation for blood loss and for the early signs of shock. Monitor your patient's mental status, pulse rate, and blood pressure (for narrowing pulse pressure). When in doubt, transport.

Understand that serious hemorrhage can have a significant psychological impact on patients. Stress triggers the "fight-or-flight" response, increases heart rate and blood pressure, increases the body's metabolic demands, works against the body's hemorrhage control mechanisms, and contributes to the development of shock. Do what you can to ease the anxieties of such patients. Communicate freely with them, and explain what care measures you are taking and why. Be especially alert to their comfort needs and address them as appropriate. If possible, keep these patients from seeing their injuries or the serious injuries affecting friends and other accident victims.

SHOCK

Shock is the underlying killer of all trauma patients and often presents with only subtle signs and symptoms.

A simple medical definition of shock is "a state of inadequate tissue perfusion." Beyond that simple definition, however, shock is the transitional stage between normal life, called homeostasis, and death. It is the underlying killer of all trauma patients and often presents with only subtle signs and symptoms until the body can no longer compensate. Then the victim moves quickly, and often irreversibly, toward death. Because of this, you, as a paramedic, must understand the process of shock and recognize its earliest signs and symptoms.

Cells are the microscopic building blocks of the human body. When cells cease to function—and if the process is not reversed—the result is cell death, which leads to tissue death, then to organ failure, and ultimately to the death of the organism. In order for cells to function, they must be continually perfused by blood, as carried through the capillaries, in order to receive a constant supply of oxygen and other nutrients and to eliminate waste products.

Shock is a tissue perfusion problem affecting the individual body cells. There are many causes of shock, though all are commonly manifested by signs and symptoms of cardiovascular system compensation followed by decompensation and, ultimately, collapse. The best way to understand shock and how body systems compensate for it is to look at the cell and its functions and then to examine how the body provides for the cells' metabolic needs and how this process can fail. Normal cell **metabolism** is discussed in Chapter 3, while the pathophysiology of shock is discussed in Chapter 4.

* **metabolism** the total changes that take place in an organism during physiological processes.

THE BODY'S RESPONSE TO BLOOD LOSS

The sympathetic nervous system and the hormones it releases begin progressive responses as hemorrhage causes blood to leave the cardiovascular system. As the draw down of the vascular volume reaches the heart, the right atrium does not completely fill. This means the atrium's output does not engorge the ventricle. Cardiac contractility therefore suffers as the ventricular myocardium does not stretch. The stroke volume drops, and there is an immediate drop in the systolic blood pressure. This reduced pressure reduces the cardiovascular system's ability to drive blood through the capillary beds. The baroreceptors in the neck recognize this decrease in blood pressure and signal to the medulla oblongata. The vasomotor center increases the peripheral vascular resistance and increases venous tone, while the cardioacceleratory center increases heart rate and contractile strength. With the reduced venous capacitance and a slight increase in heart rate and peripheral vascular resistance, the blood pressure returns to normal, as does tissue perfusion. These actions normally compensate for small blood losses. If the blood loss stops, the body reconstitutes the blood from the interstitial fluid and replaces the lost red blood cells gradually, without noticeable or ill effects.

Cellular Ischemia

If blood loss continues, the venous system constricts to its limits in order to maintain cardiac preload. However, it becomes more and more difficult for the venous system to compensate because its limited musculature begins to tire. Peripheral vascular resistance also continues to increase to maintain the systolic blood pressure. As it does, the diastolic blood pressure rises, the pulse pressure narrows, and the pulse weakens. The constriction of arterioles means that less and less blood is directed to the non-critical organs, and those organs' supply of oxygen is reduced. The skin, the largest of the non-critical organs, receives reduced circulation and becomes cool, pale, and moist. If the hemorrhage continues, some non-critical organ cells begin to starve for oxygen. Anaerobic metabolism is their only energy source, and carbon dioxide and lactic and other acids begin to accumulate. Cellular hypoxia begins, followed by **ischemia**. The heart rate increases, but slowly, because the other compensatory mechanisms are still effectively maintaining preload.

* **ischemia** a blockage in the delivery of oxygenated blood to the cells.

As the blood loss increases, more and more body cells are deprived of their oxygen and nutrient supplies, and more and more waste products accumulate. The bloodstream becomes acidic, and the body's chemoreceptors stimulate an increase in depth and rate of respirations. Circulating catecholamines and increasing acidosis cause alterations in the level of orientation, and the patient becomes anxious, restless, and possibly combative. Ischemia now affects not only non-critical organs but also the arterioles. These vessels, which also require oxygen, become hypoxic and begin to fatigue. Meanwhile, the coronary arteries are providing a decreasing amount of oxygenated blood to the laboring heart.

If the blood loss stops, the blood draws fluid from within the interstitial space, at a rate of up to 1 L per hour, to restore its volume, and erythropoietin accelerates the production of red blood cells. The kidneys reduce urine output to conserve water and electrolytes, and a period of thirst provides the stimulus for the patient to drink liquids and replace the lost volume on a more permanent basis. Transfusion with whole blood may be required at this point. While some signs of circulatory compromise and fatigue are present, the patient's recovery is probable with a period of rest.

Capillary Microcirculation

If blood loss continues, sympathetic stimulation and reduced perfusion to the kidneys, pancreas, and liver cause release of hormones. Angiotensin II further increases peripheral vascular resistance and reduces the blood flow to more of the body's tissues. If the blood loss continues, circulation is further limited to only those organs most critical to life. This further decrease in circulation leads to an increase in cellular hypoxia in non-critical tissues, and more cells begin to use anaerobic metabolism for energy in a desperate attempt to survive. The build-up of lactic acid and carbon dioxide relaxes the pre-capillary sphincters. The circulating blood volume is diminished both by the continued hemorrhage and by fluid loss as the capillary beds engorge. Post-capillary sphincters remain closed, forcing fluids into the interstitial spaces by **hydrostatic pressure.** The circulatory crisis worsens as the compensatory mechanisms begin to fail. Interstitial edema reduces the ability of the capillaries to provide oxygen and nutrients to and remove carbon dioxide and other waste products from the cells. The capillary and cell membranes also begin to break down. Red blood cells begin to clump together, or agglutinate, in the hypoxic and stagnant capillaries forming columns of coagulated cells called **rouleaux.**

Capillary Washout

The building acidosis from the accumulating lactic acid and carbon dioxide (carbonic acid) finally causes relaxation of the post-capillary sphincters. With relaxation, those byproducts along with potassium (released by the cells to maintain a neutral environment in the presence of building acidosis) and the columns of coagulated red blood cells are dumped into the venous circulation. This **washout** causes profound metabolic acidosis and releases microscopic emboli. Cardiac output drops toward zero; peripheral vascular resistance drops toward zero; blood pressure drops toward zero; cellular perfusion, even to the most critical organs, drops toward zero. The body moves quickly and then irreversibly toward death.

STAGES OF SHOCK

The shock process, as described above, can be divided into three stages based on presenting signs and symptoms. The stages are progressively more serious and include compensated, decompensated, and irreversible shock (Table 19-2).

Compensated Shock

Compensated shock is the initial shock state. In this stage, the body is still capable of meeting its critical metabolic needs through a series of progressive compensating actions (Figure 19-9). These progressive compensations create a series of signs and symptoms that range from the subtle to the obvious. The compensated shock stage ends with the precipitous drop in blood pressure. Compensated shock is the shock stage in which prehospital interventions and rapid transport are most likely to meet with success.

The body's first recognizable response to serious blood loss is probably an increase in pulse rate. However, a rate increase due to blood loss may be difficult to differentiate from tachycardia due to excitement and the "fight-or-flight" response. The first sign usually attributable to shock is a narrowing pulse pressure and weakening pulse strength (weak and rapid pulse). As the condition becomes more serious, vasoconstriction causes the victim's skin to become pale, cyanotic, or ashen as blood is directed away from the skin and toward the more critical organs. The skin becomes cool and moist (clammy), and capillary refill times begin to exceed 3 sec-

---

* **hydrostatic pressure** the pressure of liquids in equilibrium; the pressure exerted by or within liquids.

* **rouleaux** group of red blood cells that are stuck together.

* **washout** release of accumulated lactic acid, carbon dioxide (carbonic acid), potassium, and rouleaux into the venous circulation.

* **compensated shock** hemodynamic insult to the body in which the body responds effectively. Signs and symptoms are limited, and the human system functions normally.

Compensated shock is the shock stage in which prehospital interventions and rapid transport are most likely to meet with success.

Content Review

STAGES OF SHOCK
Compensated
Decompensated
Irreversible

Table 19-2 THE STAGES OF SHOCK

Compensated Shock

Initial stage of shock in which the body progressively compensates for continuing blood loss.

- Pulse rate increases
- Pulse strength decreases
- Skin becomes cool and clammy
- Progressing anxiety, restlessness, combativeness
- Thirst, weakness, eventual air hunger

Decompensated Shock

Begins when the body's compensatory mechanisms can no longer maintain preload.

- Pulse becomes unpalpable
- Blood pressure drops precipitously
- Patient becomes unconscious
- Respirations slow or cease

Irreversible Shock

Shortly after the patient enters decompensated shock, the lack of circulation begins to have profound effects on body cells. As they are irreversibly damaged, the cells die, tissues dysfunction, organs dysfunction, and the patient dies.

---

onds. As compensation becomes more acute, the victim becomes anxious, restless, or combative and complains of thirst and weakness. Near the end of the compensated shock stage, the patient may experience air hunger and tachypnea.

Decompensated Shock

Decompensated shock begins as the body's compensatory mechanisms can no longer respond to a continuing blood loss. Mechanisms that initially compensated for blood loss now fail, and the body moves quickly toward complete

✱ **decompensated shock** continuing hemodynamic insult to the body in which the compensatory mechanisms break down. The signs and symptoms become very pronounced, and the patient moves rapidly toward death.

FIGURE 19-9 In compensated shock, the body reduces venous capacitance in response to blood loss.

a. Normal hydration   b. Hypovolemia and venous compensation collapse. Entry into decompensated shock is indicated by a precipitous drop in systolic blood pressure. Despite all compensatory mechanisms, venous return is inadequate, and the heart no longer has enough blood volume to pump. Even extreme tachycardia produces little cardiac output. No amount of vascular resistance can maintain blood pressure and circulation. Even the most critical organs of the body are hypoperfused. The heart, already hypoxic because of poor perfusion and the increased oxygen demands created by tachycardia, begins to fail. This state may be indicated by the presence of a bradycardia. In this stage, the brain is extremely hypoxic. This means that the patient displays a rapidly dropping level of responsiveness. The brain's control over bodily functions, including respiration, ceases, and the body takes on a death-like appearance.

Irreversible Shock

Irreversible shock exists when the body's cells are badly injured and die in such quantities that the organs cannot carry out their normal functions. While aggressive resuscitation may restore blood pressure and pulse, organ failure ultimately results in organism failure. The transition to irreversible shock is very difficult to identify in the field. Clearly, the longer a patient is in decompensated shock, the more likely it is that he or she has moved to irreversible shock.

Shock Assessment

You must be able to recognize shock as early as possible in your patient assessment and begin to provide care just as promptly. You must search out the signs and symptoms of shock in each phase of the assessment process: the scene size-up, the initial assessment, the rapid trauma assessment or focused history and physical exam, and—when appropriate—the detailed physical exam. Further, you must carefully monitor for the development or progression of shock with frequent ongoing assessments during care and transport of the trauma patient.

Scene Size-up

Anticipate shock during the scene size-up. Analyze the forces that caused the trauma and their impacts on your patient for the possibility of both external and internal injury and hemorrhage. Look especially for injury mechanisms that might result in internal chest, abdominal, or pelvic injuries or in external hemorrhage from the head, neck, and extremities. Apply trauma triage criteria as early as practical to identify the patients who are most likely to require immediate transport to the trauma center and access to air medical transport, if appropriate.

Initial Assessment

The initial assessment directs your attention to the body systems/patient priorities that present the early signs of shock. Determine the patient's level of consciousness, responsiveness, and orientation. Any mental deficit or restlessness, anxiety, or combativeness may be due to blood loss and hypovolemia. As you assess the airway and breathing, apply high flow oxygen. Watch for tachypnea and air hunger, which are late signs of shock. When assessing circulation, recall that tachycardia suggests hypovolemia. Baseline rates suggestive of tachycardia are about 160 in the infant, 140 in the preschooler, 120 in the school-age child and 100 in the adult. An increase of 20 beats per minute above any of these rates suggests a significant blood loss. The weaker the pulse, the more the patient is compensating for blood loss.

Carefully observe the patient's body surface and be quick to anticipate potential shock, either as a cause of or a contributing factor to the patient's condition. Look also to the general condition of the skin. It should be warm, pink, and dry. If it is cyanotic, gray, ashen, pale, and cool and moist (clammy), suspect peripheral vasoconstriction, an early sign of shock.

Watch the pulse oximeter for the saturation value and keep it above 95 percent, if possible. As compensation increases and the pulse strength diminishes, the pulse oximeter readings will become more and more unreliable. If you note erratic or intermittent readings with the device, suspect increasing cardiovascular compensation and progressing shock as the reason.

Conclude the initial assessment by establishing patient priorities. If any indication, MOI, sign or symptom suggests serious internal hemorrhage or uncontrolled external hemorrhage, consider rapid trauma assessment. If the patient has minor and isolated injuries, move to the focused history and physical exam.

Focused History and Physical Exam

As noted earlier, the order in which the steps of the focused history and physical exam are performed vary with the patient's MOI. For trauma patients who have no significant mechanism, perform an assessment focused on the area of injury, then obtain baseline vital signs and gather a patient history. For trauma patients who have a significant MOI, continue spinal immobilization and perform a rapid trauma assessment and then obtain baseline vital signs and a patient history. Remember that trauma patients with significant mechanisms of injury are the most likely to suffer from shock.

The rapid trauma assessment is performed on a patient with a significant MOI or signs of shock or serious injury.

Rapid Trauma Assessment   When you have a trauma patient with a significant MOI, perform a rapid trauma assessment, inspecting and palpating the patient from head to toe (Figure 19-10). Immediately control any significant hemorrhage. Put a dressing and bandage over the wound and apply direct pressure. Provide more complete hemorrhage control once you attend to the other priorities.

Be sure to examine areas of the body where you expect to find serious injury, as suggested by your scene size-up. Pay special attention to the areas most likely to produce serious, life-threatening injury: the head, neck, chest, abdomen, and pelvis. Minor reddening may be the only sign of a developing contusion and serious internal injury. Also examine the neck veins. In the supine, normovolemic patient, they should be full. If they are flat, suspect hypovolemia.

During your rapid trauma assessment, rule out the possibility of obstructive shock. Assess the chest to identify any tension pneumothorax. Look for dyspnea,

The focused physical exam is performed on a trauma patient with an expected, isolated, non-serious injury.

a hyperinflated chest, distended jugular veins, resonant percussion, and diminished or absent breath sounds on the affected side, lower tracheal shift to the opposite side, and any subcutaneous emphysema. Consider pleural decompression if the signs suggest tension pneumothorax (see Chapter 25, "Thoracic Trauma"). Also suspect and search for pericardial tamponade. Look for penetrating injury, distended jugular veins, muffled or distant heart tones, tachycardia, and progressive and extreme hypotension. Pericardial tamponade requires immediate and rapid transport to a trauma center. If the patient received significant anterior chest trauma, suspect myocardial contusion. Apply an ECG monitor and analyze the cardiac rhythm.

During assessment, be alert to the possibility that hemorrhagic shock is not the problem or is not the only problem affecting your patient.

During the assessment, be alert to the possibility that hemorrhagic shock is not the problem or is not the only problem affecting your patient. Conditions such as stroke, epilepsy, or heart attack can lead to auto crashes and other traumatic events. Be careful to rule out cardiogenic shock by questioning the patient about crushing substernal chest pain and looking for pulmonary edema, jugular vein distention, and cardiac dysrhythmias (see Chapter 28, "Cardiology"). Also suspect and check for neurogenic shock (see Chapter 24, "Spinal Trauma"). Look for the presence of pink and warm skin below the point of nervous system injury, while the skin above the injury is pale, cool, and clammy. Other shock states such as anaphylactic, septic, and diabetic shock are not likely unless the patient history suggests them.

Take a quick set of vital signs, keying in on both the pulse rate and pulse pressure. If the pulse is weak, its rate is elevated, or the pulse pressure is diminished, suspect serious hemorrhage. Gauge your findings against the MOI and the time from the injury to your assessment. The shorter the time and the more pronounced the signs and symptoms, the more rapidly the patient is moving toward decompensation and then irreversible shock.

Complete this step of the assessment process by gathering a patient history. Listen to any patient complaints of weakness, thirst, or nausea, which may be further signs of shock. Be especially alert for patient complaints suggestive of a myocardial infarction. Be prepared to monitor the heart for dysrhythmias.

At the end of the rapid trauma assessment or the focused history and physical exam, inventory your findings. Set the patient's priority for transport, and set priorities for the order in which you will care for injuries. Again, if any indication, MOI, sign or symptom suggests serious internal hemorrhage or uncontrolled external hemorrhage, consider rapid transport for the patient. Approximate the probable volume of blood lost to fractures, large contusions, and hematomas. Also note the probable locations of internal hemorrhage and attempt to approximate blood loss from them. Identify all significant injuries and assign each a priority for care. While you may not complete care for all the injuries, setting priorities assures that you quickly address those injuries most likely to contribute to the patient's hypovolemia and shock.

Detailed Physical Exam

Consider performing a detailed physical exam on a potential shock patient only after all priorities have been addressed and the patient is either en route to the trauma center or circumstances such as a prolonged extrication prevent immediate transport. If you have the time, assess the patient from head to toe and look for any additional signs of injury. Remember that your early arrival at the patient's side may mean that the ecchymosis (black-and-blue discoloration) associated with injuries has not had time to develop. So be very careful to look for reddening (erythema) and areas of local warmth, suggestive of trauma.

Ongoing Assessment

After completing the initial assessment and the rapid trauma assessment or focused history and physical exam, perform serial ongoing assessments. Reassess mental status, airway, breathing, and circulation. Reestablish patient priorities and reassess and record the vital signs. This ongoing assessment allows you to identify any trends in the patient's condition. Pay particular attention to the pulse rate and pulse pressure. If the pulse rate is increasing and the difference between the diastolic and systolic pressures is decreasing, suspect increasing compensation and worsening shock. Perform a focused assessment for any changes in symptoms the patient reports. Also, check the adequacy and effectiveness of any interventions you have performed. Provide this ongoing assessment every 5 minutes for the seriously injured patient or for any patient who displays any of the signs or symptoms of shock.

SHOCK MANAGEMENT

Airway and Breathing Management

Management of the shock patient begins with corrective actions taken during the initial assessment. One of the primary principles of shock care is to assure the best possible chance for tissue oxygenation and carbon dioxide offload. Accomplish this by assuring or providing good ventilations with supplemental high flow oxygen (15 L/min via nonrebreather mask). If the patient is moving air ineffectively (at a breathing rate less than 12/min or with inadequate respiratory volume), provide positive pressure ventilations.

Positive pressure ventilation to the breathing patient, called **overdrive respiration,** is coordinated with the patient's breathing attempts if possible (Figure 19-11). However, assure that the ventilations provide both a good respiratory volume (at least 800 mL) and an adequate respiratory rate (at least 12 to 16 per minute). Overdrive respiration may be indicated in patients with rib fractures, flail chest, spinal injury with diaphragmatic respirations, head injury, or any condition in which the patient, because of bellows system or respiratory control failure, is not breathing adequately on his own.

If necessary, guard the airway with endotracheal intubation. If the patient is unconscious or semiconscious and unable to protect his airway, be aggressive in your care. Rapid sequence intubation may be required. Shock patients frequently vomit, and gastric aspiration presents a serious, possibly fatal, consequence.

If there is any sign of tension pneumothorax, confirm it and provide pleural decompression either at the 2nd intercostal space, mid-clavicular line or at the 5th intercostal space, mid-axillary line (see Chapter 25, "Thoracic Trauma"). Continue to monitor the patient because it is common for the catheter to clog and the tension pneumothorax to reappear. Insert another needle close to the first to relieve any subsequent build-up of pressure.

Hemorrhage Control

Provide rapid control of any significant external hemorrhage. Use direct pressure, direct pressure and elevation where practical, and pressure points as needed. Apply a tourniquet to control serious and continuing hemorrhage only if it is absolutely necessary. Remember, there are serious consequences with both proper and improper use of a tourniquet.

Fluid Resuscitation

The field treatment of choice for fluid resuscitation in trauma cases is blood. Blood, however, must be refrigerated, typed, and cross-matched. (O-negative blood may be given in emergency circumstances.) Blood also has a short shelf life and is costly

A primary principle of shock care is to assure the best possible chance for tissue oxygenation and carbon dioxide offload; do this by providing supplemental high-flow oxygen or positive pressure ventilation.

* **overdrive respiration** positive pressure ventilation supplied to a breathing patient.

FIGURE 19-11 Assure that the potential shock patient receives adequate ventilation, using overdrive respiration, if necessary.

The most practical choice for prehospital fluid resuscitation is lactated Ringer's solution.

for field use. The most practical fluid for prehospital administration, then, is lactated Ringer's solution. Lactated Ringer's best matches the electrolyte concentration of plasma and does not produce the hyperchloremic acidosis associated with the infusion of large volumes of normal saline. However, normal saline is an acceptable second choice and has few drug and fluid incompatability problems.

Some hypertonic and synthetic solutions show promise for fluid resuscitation. None of these, however, has been identified as superior to isotonic electrolyte solutions for prehospital use. Hypertonic solutions can mobilize the interstitial and cellular fluid volumes to replace lost blood volume, but they are not able to carry either the oxygen or the clotting factors essential for hemorrhage control. Synthetic agents are now available that can carry oxygen and may, in the future, assist the clotting process. These agents, however, are expensive, have short shelf lives, and pose some patient compatibility problems.

When administering fluids to a trauma patient or to any patient who may need large fluid volumes, consider the internal lumen size of both the catheter and administration set. Fluid flow is proportional to the fourth power of the internal diameter. This means that if you double the lumen's diameter, the same fluid under the same pressure will flow 16 times more quickly. Hence, use the largest catheter you can introduce into the patient's vein and use a large-bore trauma or blood administration set (Figure 19-12).

Catheter length and fluid pressure also influence fluid flow. The longer the catheter, the greater the resistance to flow. The ideal catheter for the shock patient is relatively short, 1½″ or shorter. An increase in pressure increases fluid flow. This means that the higher you position the bag or the greater the pressure differential between the solution and the venous system, the faster the fluid flow. If you cannot elevate the fluid bag, position it under the patient or place it in a pressure infuser or a blood-pressure cuff inflated to 100 or 200 mmHg.

Electrolyte administration is indicated for patients with the classic signs and symptoms of shock. When you have controlled external hemorrhage and there is no reason to suspect serious internal hemorrhage, employ aggressive fluid resuscitation. Moderate fluid resuscitation is also prudent for patients with blunt trauma to the chest or abdomen. Administer 1 L of lactated Ringer's solution rapidly via IV (Figure 19-13). Use trauma or blood tubing to assure unimpeded flow, and initiate the IV with a large-bore (14- or 16-gauge) catheter. In children, infuse 20 mL/kg of body weight rapidly when you see any signs and symptoms of shock. Administer a second fluid bolus if the vital signs do not improve after the first bolus or if, at some later time, the patient again begins to deteriorate. The objective of fluid resuscitation in the field is not the return of normal vital signs but the stabilization of vital signs until the patient reaches the trauma center.

The objective of prehospital fluid resuscitation is not the return of normal vital signs but the stabilization of vital signs until the patient reaches the trauma center.

FIGURE 19-13   Supplies for initiating IV therapy.

If penetrating trauma to the chest exists and/or you cannot control other hemorrhage, be more conservative with fluid administration. Cautiously control fluid volume, remembering that your goal is maintaining vital signs, not improving them. Increases in blood pressure can dislodge developing clots and disrupt the normal clotting processes. The result may be further hemorrhage with further dilution of the clotting factors and hemoglobin. Closely monitor your patient's vital signs, and administer lactated Ringer's solution to keep the patient's mental status and pulse pressure at a steady level. Maintain the blood pressure at a steady level even if it has dropped below 100 mmHg, and studies suggest that a blood pressure of 88 mmHg may be optimal for the patient with continuing internal hemorrhage. Do not, however, let the pressure drop below 50 mmHg.

Temperature Control

Trauma and blood loss deal serious blows to the mechanisms that normally adjust the body's core temperature. Reduced body activity reduces heat production to subnormal levels. Cutaneous vasoconstriction decreases the skin's ability to act as part of the body's temperature control system. The result is a patient highly susceptible to fluctuations in body temperature. In cases of trauma, patients commonly lose heat more rapidly than normal. At the same time, the heat-generating reflexes, like shivering, are ineffective and, in fact, are counterproductive to the shock care process.

In all except the warmest environments, help conserve body temperature by covering the patient with a blanket and keeping the patient compartment of the ambulance very warm. If you infuse fluids, assure that they are well above room temperature—ideally at body temperature or slightly above (no more than 104°F). Use fluid warmers or keep IV solutions in a compartment that is warmer than the rest of the ambulance. Be very sensitive to any patient complaints about being cold, and provide whatever assistance you can to assure that heat loss is limited.

In all but the warmest environments, cover the hemorrhage or shock patient with a blanket and keep the patient compartment of the ambulance very warm.

Pneumatic Anti-Shock Garment

The pneumatic anti-shock garment (PASG), sometimes referred to as the medical anti-shock trouser (MAST), is a device designed to apply firm circumferential pressure around the lower extremities, pelvis, and lower abdomen. The device is intended to compress the vascular space, thereby accomplishing four objectives:

* To increase peripheral vascular resistance by pressurizing the arteries of the lower abdomen and extremities.
* To reduce the vascular volume by compressing venous vessels.

* **pneumatic anti-shock garment (PASG)** garment designed to produce uniform pressure on the lower extremities and abdomen; used with shock and hemorrhage patients in some EMS systems.

- To increase the central circulating blood volume with blood returned from areas under the garment.
- To immobilize the lower extremities and the pelvic region.

Research has determined that the garment is responsible for a return of about 250 mL of blood to the central circulation and probably reduces the venous capacitance by the same volume. The PASG also does seem to increase the peripheral vascular resistance, although this may be detrimental to patients with uncontrolled internal hemorrhage.

Research has further revealed potential problems with PASG use. The abdominal component of the PASG pressurizes the abdominal cavity, increasing the work associated with breathing and, in some cases, reducing chest excursion. Application of the garment also increases mortality when used in cases of penetrating chest trauma. In light of this information, it is imperative that you understand the limitations of the device and comply with your local protocols and medical direction when considering use of the PASG.

The PASG is a puncture-resistant, easy to clean, three-compartment trouser attached to the patient circumferentially around the lower abdomen and extremities with Velcro® closures. The compartments can be inflated either independently or all together with a foot- or electric-powered pump. However, the abdominal segment should be inflated with the leg segments or after them, never before. A PASG may or may not come with pressure gauges, although all models should be equipped with pop-off valves to prevent inflation above 110 mmHg.

Indications for PASG use include shock patients with controlled hemorrhage, patients with pelvic fracture and instability with hypotension, patients with possible neurogenic shock, and any shock patients with uncontrolled hemorrhage below the mid-abdomen. Pulmonary edema and cardiogenic shock are contraindications to PASG application and inflation. Use the PASG with caution for patients in late pregnancy, patients with suspected diaphragmatic ruptures, and patients with objects impaled in the abdomen or with abdominal eviscerations. In these cases, do not inflate the abdominal section because doing so increases intra-abdominal pressure.

Begin application of the PASG by removing the patient's clothing, although you may leave on the undergarments for patient modesty if they are not bulky (Procedure 19-1). Assess areas of the patient's body that will lie beneath the garment, as these regions will be hidden from view and inaccessible once the PASG is applied. Then move the patient onto a spine board or other patient-carrying device with an opened garment positioned for application. One application technique calls for securing the garment's Velcro® attachments at the ends of their travel and having a caregiver at the patient's feet put one arm through each of the garment's leg sections from the foot ends. That caregiver then grasps the patient's toes while another caregiver then pulls the garment off the first caregiver's arms, onto the patient's legs, and up to the small of the patient's back. Alternatively, you may slide the device under the patient from the feet with the extra garment and the anterior abdominal segment folded between the legs. Position the PASG so that the upper portion of the abdominal segment is just below the rib margin. Secure the abdominal and leg segments with the Velcro® strips, assuring that they hold the segments firmly around the limbs and abdomen. This reduces the air volume necessary to inflate the PASG.

Quickly take baseline vital signs, and then inflate the PASG slowly. Watch for any change (improvement) in your patient's mental status, skin color, or pulse rate. If you notice such a change, stop the inflation and re-assess vital signs and level of responsiveness. The intent of PASG use is to stabilize the patient's condition, not to return the blood pressure and circulation to normal levels. As with too-aggressive fluid resuscitation, inflation of PASG to a point where blood pressure increases can interfere with the clotting process or even increase internal hemorrhage, thus moving the patient more quickly toward decompensation and death. If vital signs

Penetrating chest trauma, pulmonary edema, and cardiogenic shock are contraindications to PASG application and inflation.

19-1a Monitor the patient before PASG application.

19-1b Prepare the PASG.

19-1c Position the patient.

19-1d Wrap the legs, following the manufacturer's recommendations.

19-1e Wrap the abdomen last.

19-1f Connect the tubing.

19-1g Inflate the PASG, both legs first.

19-1h Monitor the patient.

19-1i Close the stopcock valve

and the level of responsiveness deteriorate, continue PASG inflation until you regain the level of your baseline findings. Once the pop-off valves release, stop inflation. Then inflate the garment every few minutes until the pop-off valves release to assure that the PASG maintains its maximum pressure.

Carefully monitor respirations during PASG inflation. The device may put pressure on the diaphragm, thus increasing the work of respiration as well as reducing respiratory excursion. Also listen carefully for breath sounds. The PASG may increase blood pressure and respiratory congestion as well. If you hear any crackles in the chest or if the patient complains of difficulty breathing, halt the PASG inflation.

The PASG should not be deflated in the prehospital setting. The release of circumferential pressure reduces peripheral vascular resistance, expands the size of the vascular space, and removes about 250 mL of blood from the active circulation. This could seriously harm the healthy patient and have devastating effects on one who is compensating for shock.

The PASG should not be deflated in the prehospital setting.

Pharmacological Intervention

In shock, pharmacological interventions are generally limited, especially in hypovolemic patients. The sympathetic nervous system efficiently compensates for low volume, and no agent has been shown effective in the prehospital setting, other than intravenous fluid and, in some cases, blood and blood products. For cardiogenic shock, fluid challenge, vasopressors like dopamine, and the other cardiac drugs are indicated (see Chapter 28, "Cardiology"). For spinal and obstructive shock, consider intravenous fluids like normal saline and lactated Ringer's solution. For distributive shock, consider IV fluids, dopamine, and use of the PASG.

The patient who has experienced trauma sufficient to induce hemorrhage and hypovolemia will be anxious and bewildered. As the care provider at the patient's side, it is your responsibility to be calm and reassuring, thus counteracting the natural "fight-or-flight" response (Figure 19-14). By acting in this manner, you not only help your patient deal with the event's emotional trauma but also combat some of the negative effects of sympathetic stimulation.

FIGURE 19-14 Emotional support for the seriously injured trauma patient is an important part of shock patient care.

Summary

Significant hemorrhage and its serious consequence, shock, are genuine threats to the trauma patient's life. The signs of these threats are often subtle or hidden, especially if bleeding is internal. Only through careful analysis of the mechanism of injury during the scene size-up and careful evaluation of the patient during the assessment process can you recognize and then treat these life-threatening problems. Treatment often involves rapidly bringing the patient to the services of a trauma center and, while doing so, providing aggressive care—supplemental oxygen, positive pressure ventilations, fluid resuscitation, and use of a PASG as necessary—aimed at maintaining vital signs, not necessarily improving them. With this approach, you afford your patient the best chance for survival.

CHAPTER 20

Soft-Tissue Trauma

Objectives

After reading this chapter, you should be able to:

1. Describe the incidence, morbidity, and mortality of soft-tissue injuries. (p. 912)
2. Describe the anatomy and physiology of the integumentary system, including epidermis, dermis, and subcutaneous tissue. (see Chapter 3)
3. Identify the skin tension lines of the body. (pp. 916–917)
4. Predict soft-tissue injuries based on mechanism of injury. (pp. 932–935)
5. Discuss blunt and penetrating trauma. (pp. 912–919)
6. Discuss the pathophysiology of soft-tissue injuries. (pp. 912–929)
7. Differentiate among the following types of soft-tissue injuries:

a. Closed (pp. 913–915)
   i. Contusion
   ii. Hematoma
   iii. Crush injuries
b. Open (pp. 915–919)
   i. Abrasions
   ii. Lacerations
   iii. Incisions
   iv. Avulsions
   v. Impaled objects
   vi. Amputations
   vii. Punctures

8. Discuss the assessment and management of open and closed soft-tissue injuries. (pp. 932–951)
9. Discuss the incidence, morbidity, and mortality of crush injuries. (pp. 914–915, 946–948)

Continued

10. Define the following conditions:
   a. Crush injury (pp. 914–915, 927–928, 946–947)
   b. Crush syndrome (pp. 915, 928, 947–948)
   c. Compartment syndrome (pp. 948–949)
11. Discuss the mechanisms of injury, assessment findings, and management of crush injuries. (pp. 914–915, 927–928, 946–947)
12. Discuss the effects of reperfusion and rhabdomyolysis on the body. (pp. 928, 946–948)
13. Discuss the pathophysiology, assessment, and care of hemorrhage associated with soft-tissue injuries, including:
   a. Capillary bleeding (pp. 920, 937)
   b. Venous bleeding (pp. 920, 937)
   c. Arterial bleeding (pp. 920, 937–940)
14. Describe and identify the indications for and application of the following dressings and bandages: (pp. 929–931)
   a. Sterile/nonsterile dressing
   b. Occlusive/nonocclusive dressing
   c. Adherent/nonadherent dressing
   d. Absorbent/nonabsorbent dressing
   e. Wet/dry dressing
   f. Self-adherent roller bandage
   g. Gauze bandage
   h. Adhesive bandage
   i. Elastic bandage

15. Predict the possible complications of an improperly applied dressing or bandage. (pp. 929–931, 943)
16. Discuss the process of wound healing, including:
   a. Hemostasis (pp. 921–922)
   b. Inflammation (p. 922)
   c. Epithelialization (p. 922)
   d. Neovascularization (p. 923)
   e. Collagen synthesis (p. 923)
17. Discuss the assessment and management of wound healing. (pp. 920–929)
18. Discuss the pathophysiology, assessment, and management of wound infection. (pp. 923–925)
19. Formulate treatment priorities for patients with soft-tissue injuries in conjunction with:
   a. Airway/face/neck trauma (pp. 949–950)
   b. Thoracic trauma (open/closed) (p. 950)
   c. Abdominal trauma (pp. 950–951)
20. Given several preprogrammed and moulaged soft tissue trauma patients, provide the appropriate scene size-up, initial assessment, rapid trauma or focused physical exam and history, detailed exam, and ongoing assessment and provide appropriate patient care and transportation. (pp. 932–951)

INTRODUCTION TO SOFT-TISSUE INJURIES

The skin is one of the largest, most important organs of the human body, comprising 16 percent of total body weight. It provides a protective envelope that keeps invading pathogens out while containing body substances and fluids. It is also a key organ of sensation as well as a radiator of excess body heat in warm weather and a conservator of heat in cold conditions. Even as it accomplishes these various functions, the skin remains a durable, pliable, and accommodating tissue, and one that is very able to repair itself.

Known collectively as the **integumentary system,** the skin is the first tissue of the human body to experience the effects of trauma. Because skin covers the entire body surface, any penetrating injury or the kinetic forces of blunt injury must pass through it before impacting on other vital organs. Often, the signs of this energy transmission can only be observed with very careful examination of the skin. Therefore, the skin is of great significance at all stages of the patient assessment process.

Trauma to the skin may present as open injuries—abrasions, lacerations, incisions, punctures, avulsions, and amputations—or as closed injuries—contusions, hematomas, and crush injuries. Such injuries infrequently threaten life but may endanger blood vessels, nerves, connective tissue, and other important internal structures. Uncontrolled blood loss may lead to hypovolemia and shock, while the wound may provide a pathway for infection.

*** integumentary system** skin, consisting of the epidermis, dermis, and subcutaneous layers.

EPIDEMIOLOGY

Soft tissue injuries are the most common type of trauma.

Soft-tissue injuries are by far the most common form of trauma. Over 10 million patients present to emergency departments annually with soft-tissue wounds, many of which require closure. Most, but not all, open wounds require only simple care and limited suturing. A significant minority, however, damage arteries, nerves, or tendons and can lead to permanent disability. Uncontrolled external hemorrhage of an otherwise uncomplicated open wound is a very rare but completely preventable situation that sometimes occurs with this type of injury and can result in death. Of the open wounds presenting to emergency departments, up to 6.5 percent will eventually become infected, resulting in significant morbidity.

Closed wounds share a similar epidemiology, except that they are probably even more common than open injuries. Most minor "bumps and bruises" never reach the paramedic, as most patients elect to self-treat all but the most serious cases. Despite their frequency and usually minor nature, closed injuries *can* result in significant pain, suffering, and morbidity. Infection, however, is not usually a complication with closed wounds. Risk factors for soft-tissue wounds include age (especially school-age children and the elderly), alcohol or drug abuse, and occupation. Laborers, machine operators, and others whose hands and body parts are exposed to heavy objects, machines, or tools are at great risk.

Simple measures can reduce risks and prevent soft-tissue injuries. For example, locating playgrounds on grass, sand, gravel or other forgiving surfaces and padding of equipment in them can cut injury rates among children. In factories, machine guards, fail-safe switches, and similar engineering controls can reduce injuries. Protective clothing such as steel-toed boots and leather gloves also provide simple methods of reducing the incidence and severity of soft-tissue injuries.

PATHOPHYSIOLOGY OF SOFT-TISSUE INJURY

Although we often take the skin's functions for granted, soft-tissue injury can seriously affect health, causing severe blood and fluid loss, infection, hypothermia, and other problems.

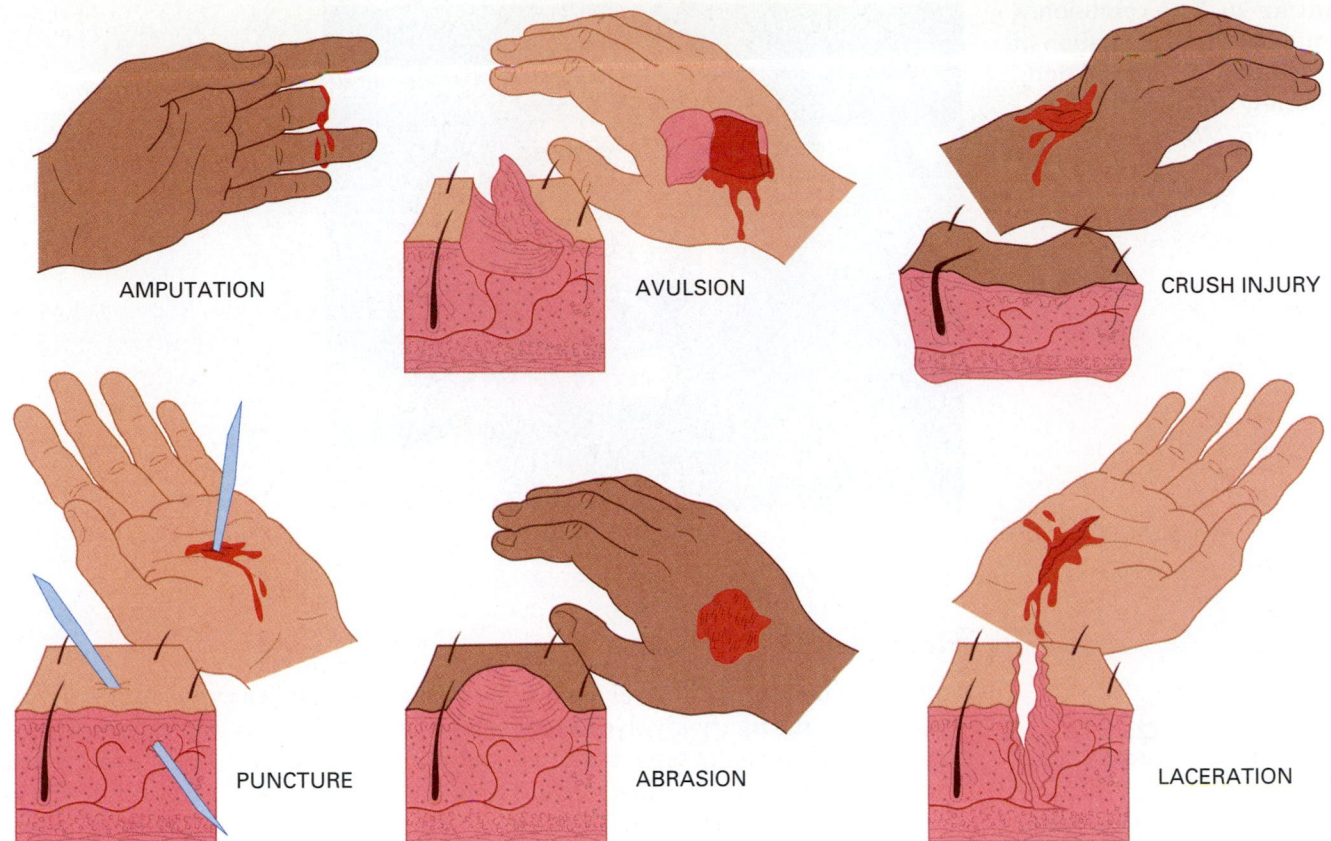

FIGURE 20-1 Types of open soft-tissue injuries.

Trauma is a violent transfer of energy that produces an open or closed wound to the skin and possible injury to the structures underneath. Wounds can be either blunt or penetrating (Figure 20-1). While all penetrating wounds are open, blunt trauma can, on occasion, create open wounds. Common soft-tissue injuries include closed wounds—contusions, hematomas, and crush injuries—and open wounds—abrasions, lacerations, incisions, punctures, avulsions, and amputations. Each type of wound is different and deserves special consideration.

CLOSED WOUNDS

Contusions

Contusions are blunt, non-penetrating injuries that crush and damage small blood vessels (Figure 20-2). Blood is drawn to the inflamed tissue, causing a reddening called **erythema.** Blood also leaks into the surrounding interstitial spaces through damaged vessels. As the hemoglobin within the free blood loses its oxygen, it becomes dark red and then blue, resulting in the black-and-blue discoloration called **ecchymosis.** Because the development of ecchymosis is a progressive process, the discoloration may not be evident during prehospital care.

Contusions are more pronounced in areas where the mechanism causing the injury (for example, a steering wheel) and skeletal structures (such as the ribs or skull) trap the skin. Occasionally, a chest injury displays an erythematous or ecchymotic outline of the ribs and sternum, reflecting an impact with the auto dashboard or some other blunt object. Early signs of such an injury may be difficult to identify, but they will become more evident as time passes and discoloration increases.

* **contusion** closed wound in which the skin is unbroken, although damage has occurred to the tissue immediately beneath.

Content Review

TYPES OF CLOSED WOUNDS
Contusions
Hematomas
Crush injuries

* **erythema** general reddening of the skin due to dilation of the superficial capillaries.

* **ecchymosis** blue-black discoloration of the skin due to leakage of blood into the tissues.

FIGURE 20-2 A contusion. Note that the discoloration of a contusion is a delayed sign. *(Courtesy of Edward T. Dickinson, MD)*

Hematomas

Soft-tissue bleeding can occur within the tissue and at times can be quite significant. When the injury involves a larger blood vessel, most commonly an artery, the blood can actually separate tissue and pool in a pocket called a **hematoma**. These injuries are very visible in cases of head trauma because of the unyielding skull underneath. Hematomas tend to be less pronounced in other body areas, even though they can contain significant hemorrhage. Severe hematomas to the thigh, leg, or arm may contribute significantly to hypovolemia. A hematoma in the thigh, for example, can contain over a liter of blood before swelling becomes noticeable.

✱ **hematoma** collection of blood beneath the skin or trapped within a body compartment.

Crush Injury

The term **crush injury** describes a collection of traumatic insults that include crush injury and crush syndrome. A body part that is crushed, possibly by a heavy object, sustains deep injury to the muscles, blood vessels, bones, and other internal structures (Figure 20-3). Damage can be massive, despite minimal signs displayed

✱ **crush injury** mechanism of injury in which tissue is locally compressed by high pressure forces.

FIGURE 20-3 A crush injury.

FIGURE 20-4 Abrasions.

on the skin itself. **Crush syndrome** is the term used to describe the systemic effects of a crush injury. If the pressure that causes a crush injury remains in place for several hours, the resulting destruction of skeletal muscle cells leads to the accumulation of large quantities of myoglobin (a cell protein), potassium, lactic acid, uric acid, and other toxins. When the pressure is released, these products enter the bloodstream. They circulate, causing a severe metabolic acidosis. These materials are also toxic to the kidneys and heart. Crush syndrome is thus a potentially life-threatening trauma event. It will be discussed in more detail later in this chapter.

OPEN WOUNDS

Abrasions

Abrasions are typically the most minor of injuries that violate the protective envelope of the skin. They involve a scraping or abrasive action that removes layers of the epidermis and the upper reaches of the dermis (Figure 20-4). Bleeding can be persistent but is usually limited because the injury involves only superficial capillaries. If the injury compromises a large area of the epidermis, it carries the danger of serious infection.

Lacerations

A **laceration** is an open wound that penetrates more deeply into the dermis than an abrasion (Figure 20-5). A laceration tends to involve a smaller surface area,

✳ **crush syndrome** systemic disorder of severe metabolic disturbances resulting from the crush of a limb or other body part.

> **Content Review**
>
> **TYPES OF OPEN WOUNDS**
> Abrasions
> Lacerations
> Incisions
> Punctures
> Avulsions
> Amputations

✳ **abrasion** scraping or abrading away of the superficial layers of the skin; an open soft-tissue injury.

✳ **laceration** an open wound, normally a tear with jagged borders.

FIGURE 20-5 Lacerations (secondary to animal bite).

being limited to the tissue immediately surrounding the penetration. It endangers the deeper and more significant vasculature—arteries, arterioles, venules, and veins—as well as nerves, muscles, tendons, ligaments, and perhaps some underlying organs. As with an abrasion, the injury breaks the skin's protective barrier and provides a pathway for infection.

Note that the skin does not merely hang on the flesh, but rather is spread over the body and attached to fit the contours of the underlying structures. This creates natural stretch or tension in the skin. The orientation of tension in the skin is revealed in characteristic patterns called **tension lines** (Figure 20-6). The effects of tension on the skin become evident when the skin is transected, as with a laceration. Lacerations cutting across the tension lines have a tendency to be pulled apart and thus spread widely or gape. Lacerations parallel to the tension lines tend to gape very little. Wounds that spread widely tend to bleed more than those with minimal gaping. Large gaping wounds heal more slowly and are more likely to leave noticeable scars than wounds that spread less.

The tension represented by skin tension lines can be either static or dynamic. Static tension is noted in areas with limited movement of the tissue and structures beneath, as in the anterior abdomen or between joints in the extremities. Dy-

* **tension lines** natural patterns in the surface of the skin revealing tensions within.

FIGURE 20-6 Tension lines of the skin.

namic tension lines occur in areas subject to great movement, as in the skin over joints like the elbow, wrist, or knee. The increased motion in areas with dynamic skin tension lines means that the clotting and tissue mending processes in these areas are more frequently interrupted, disrupting and complicating skin repair.

You should note the laceration's orientation to the skin tension lines during your assessment of the patient. Remember that if the orientation parallels those lines, the wound may remain closed. If it is perpendicular to them, the wound may gape open.

Incisions

An **incision** is a surgically smooth laceration, often caused by a sharp instrument such as a knife, straight razor, or piece of glass. Such a wound tends to bleed freely. In all other ways, it is a laceration.

* **incision** very smooth or surgical laceration, frequently caused by a knife, scalpel, razor blade, or piece of glass.

Punctures

Another special type of laceration is the **puncture**. It involves a small entrance wound with damage that extends into the body's interior (Figure 20-7). The wound normally seals itself and presents in a way that does not reflect the actual extent of injury. If the puncture penetrates deeply, it may involve not just the skin but underlying muscles, nerves, bones, and organs. A puncture additionally carries an increased danger of infection. A penetrating object introduces bacteria and other pathogens deep into a wound. There, the disrupted tissue and blood vessels, along with a reduced oxygen level, create a warm and moist environment that is ideal for the colonization of bacteria.

* **puncture** specific soft-tissue injury involving a deep, narrow wound to the skin and underlying organs that carries an increased danger of infection.

Impaled Objects

An **impaled object** is not a wound itself, but rather a wound complication often associated with a puncture or laceration. Impaled objects are important for the damage they may cause if withdrawn. Frequently, embedded objects are irregular in shape and become entangled in important structures such as arteries,

* **impaled object** foreign body embedded in a wound.

FIGURE 20-7 A puncture wound.

FIGURE 20-8   An impaled object.

nerves, or tendons (Figure 20-8). Their removal in the field can result in further damage. Perhaps more critically, the embedded object may have lacerated a large blood vessel and the object's presence temporarily blocks, or tamponades, blood loss. Removal of the object may cause an uncheckable flow of blood. This situation is particularly dangerous when the object is impaled in the neck or trunk, where the application of effective direct pressure is difficult or impossible.

Avulsions

* **avulsion** forceful tearing away or separation of body tissue; an avulsion may be partial or complete.

Avulsion occurs when a flap of skin, although torn or cut, is not torn completely loose from the body (Figure 20-9). Avulsion is frequently seen with blunt trauma to the skull, where the scalp is torn and folds back. It may also occur with animal bites and machinery accidents. The seriousness of the avulsion depends upon the area involved, the condition of the circulation to (and distal to) the injury site, and the degree of contamination.

* **degloving injury** avulsion in which the mechanism of injury tears the skin off the underlying muscle, tissue, blood vessels, and bone.

A special type of avulsion is the **degloving injury.** In this wound, the mechanism of injury tears the skin off the underlying muscle, connective tissue, blood vessels, and bone. It is a particularly gruesome injury, occurring occasionally with farm and industrial machinery. The device pulls the skin off with great force as the skeletal tissue underneath is held stationary. The wound exposes a large area of tissue and is often severely contaminated. The injury carries with it a poor prognosis. If, however, the vasculature and innervation remain intact, there may be some hope for future use of the digit or extremity.

FIGURE 20-9   An avulsion.

FIGURE 20-10   A ring-type degloving injury.

A variation of the degloving process is the ring injury (Figure 20-10). As a person jumps or falls, the ring is caught, pulling the skin of the finger against the weight of the victim. The force may tear the upper layers of tissue away from the phalanges, exposing the tendons, nerves, and blood vessels. Although the ring injury involves a smaller area, it is otherwise a degloving injury.

Amputations

The partial or complete severance of a digit or limb is an **amputation** (Figure 20-11). It often results in the complete loss of the limb at the site of severance. The hemorrhage associated with the amputation may be limited if the limb or digit is cut cleanly or may be severe and continuing if the wound is a jagged or crushing one. The surgeon may attempt to reattach the amputated part or use its skin for grafting as he repairs the remaining limb. If this skin is unavailable, the surgeon may have to cut the bone and musculature back further to close the wound. This reduces the length of the limb as well as its future usefulness.

✳ **amputation** severance, removal, or detachment, either partial or complete, of a body part.

FIGURE 20-11   An amputation of the first two fingers.

ARTERIAL	**VENOUS**	**CAPILLARY**
• Pulsating flow • Bright red color	• Steady, slow flow • Dark red color	• Slow, even flow • Bright red color

FIGURE 20-12 Hemorrhage. Arterial hemorrhage is bright red and flows rapidly from a wound. Venous hemorrhage is darker red and flows slowly. Capillary hemorrhage is also bright red and flows slowly.

HEMORRHAGE

Soft-tissue injuries frequently cause blood loss, ranging from inconsequential to life threatening. The loss can be arterial, venous, or capillary (Figure 20-12). Bleeding can be easy or almost impossible to control. Hemorrhage is usually dark red with venous injury, red with capillary injury, and bright red with arterial injury. The rate of hemorrhage also varies from oozing capillary, to flowing venous, to pulsing arterial bleeding. In practice, it may be hard to differentiate among the types and origins of hemorrhage. It is important, however, to determine the rate and quantity of blood loss. This information helps you to decide upon the most effective means of stopping the blood flow and to prioritize the patient for care and transport.

Often the nature of the soft-tissue wound may be more important than the size or type of vessel involved in determining the severity of the blood vessel injury. If a moderately sized vein or artery is cut cleanly, the muscles in its wall contract. This constricts the vessel's lumen and retracts the severed vessel into the tissue. As the muscle is drawn back from the wound, it thickens and further restricts the lumen. This restricts blood flow, reduces the rate of loss, and assists the clotting mechanisms. Therefore, clean lacerations and amputations generally do not bleed profusely. If, on the other hand, the vessel is not severed cleanly but is laid open instead, muscle contraction opens the wound, thereby increasing and prolonging blood loss.

WOUND HEALING

Wound healing is a complex process that begins immediately following injury and can take many months to complete. Wound healing is an essential component of homeostasis, the process whereby the body maintains a uniform environment for itself. Although it is useful to divide the wound healing process into stages or parts, it is important to note that these phases overlap considerably and are intertwined physiologically (Figure 20-13).

During assessment, it is important to determine the rate and quantity of hemorrhage.

Content Review

STAGES OF WOUND HEALING
Hemostasis
Inflammation
Epithelialization
Neovascularization
Collagen synthesis

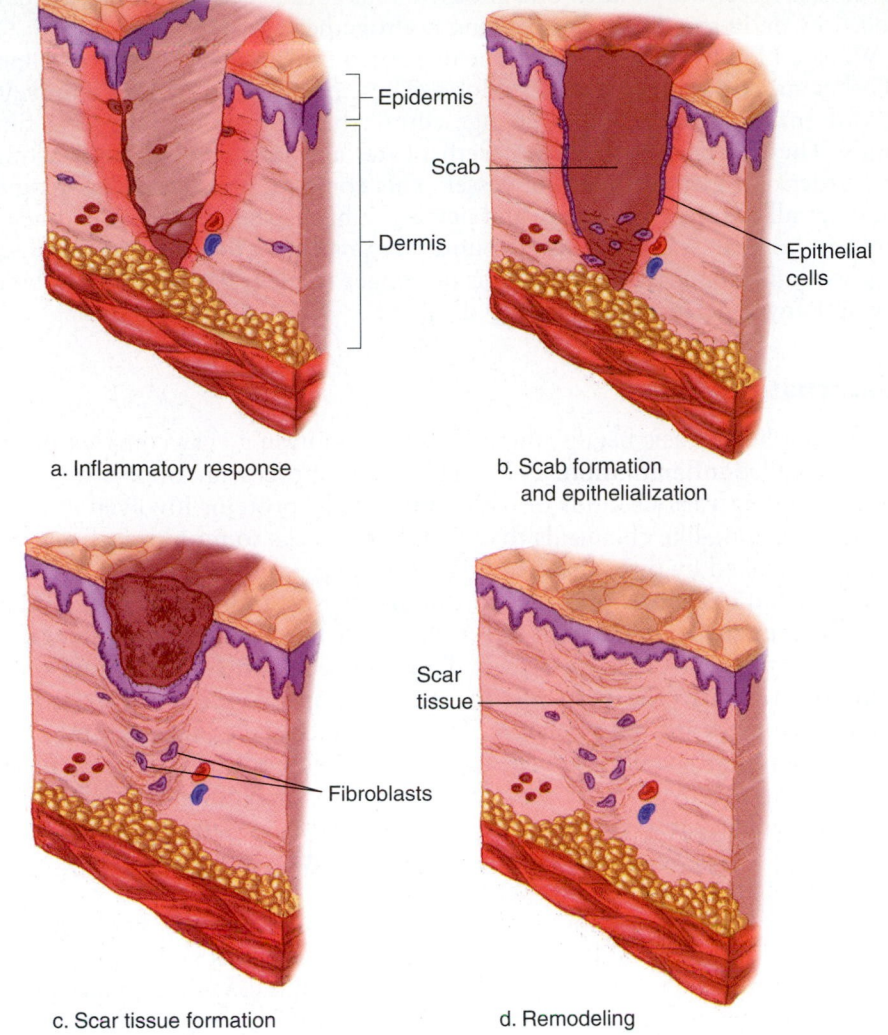

a. Inflammatory response

b. Scab formation and epithelialization

Epidermis

Scab

Epithelial cells

Dermis

c. Scar tissue formation

Fibroblasts

d. Remodeling

Scar tissue

FIGURE 20-13   The wound healing process.

Hemostasis

Arguably the most important aspect of wound healing is the body's ability to stop most bleeding on its own. This process is called **hemostasis.** Without hemostasis, even the most trivial nicks and scratches would continue to bleed, leading to life-threatening hemorrhage. Hemostasis has three major components related to the vasculature, the platelets, and the clotting cascade.

Hemostasis begins almost immediately following injury. Arteries, arterioles, and some veins are endowed with a muscular layer that reflexively constricts the vessel in response to local injury. The longitudinal muscles, too, play a role by retracting the cut ends of larger vessels back into the contracted muscle, thus reducing flow. This immediate response usually reduces but does not entirely stop bleeding. Capillaries, which do not have a muscle layer, cannot contract and thus continue to bleed. This explains the continuing but minor bleeding associated with capillary wounds such as paper cuts and minor abrasions.

Platelets begin the clotting process. The damaged vessel wall becomes "sticky," as do the platelets in the turbulent flow of the disrupted vessel. Platelets

* **hemostasis** the body's natural ability to stop bleeding, the ability to clot blood.

stick to the vessel wall and to one another. This forms a platelet plug, reducing blood flow or, in small vessels, stopping it altogether.

When a blood vessel is injured, the disrupted tunica intima exposes collagen and other structural proteins to the blood. These proteins activate a complicated series of enzyme reactions that change certain blood proteins into long fibrin strands. These strands then entrap erythrocytes and produce a gelatinous mass that further occludes the bleeding vessel. This complex process, called coagulation, stops all but the most severe and persistent hemorrhage. With time, the clot shrinks or contracts, bringing the wound margins closer together, further facilitating wound healing. When the clot is no longer needed, it is reabsorbed by the body and any superficial scab merely drops off.

Inflammation

Shortly after hemostasis begins, the body sets in motion a very complex process of healing called **inflammation**. The inflammatory process involves a host of elements including various kinds of white blood cells, proteins involved in immunity, and hormone-like chemicals that signal other cells to mobilize.

Cells damaged by direct trauma or by invading pathogens release a number of proteins and chemicals into the surrounding tissue and blood. These agents, called **chemotactic factors,** recruit cells responsible for consuming cellular debris, invading bacteria, or other foreign or damaged cells and for beginning the inflammatory process. The first cells to arrive are specialized white blood cells called **granulocytes** and **macrophages.** These cells (also called phagocytes) are capable of engulfing bacteria, debris, and foreign material, digesting them, and then releasing the byproducts in a process called **phagocytosis.** Other white blood cells called lymphocytes, in combination with immunoglobulins or immune proteins, are also mobilized. Lymphocytes attack invading pathogens directly or through an antibody response.

The injury process, the material released from injured cells, and the debris released as the phagocytes destroy invading cells cause mast cells to release histamine. Histamine dilates pre-capillary blood vessels, increases capillary permeability, and increases blood flow into and through the injured or infected tissue. This brings much-needed oxygen and more phagocytes to the injured area and draws away the byproducts of cell destruction and repair. The increasing blood flow and local tissue metabolism also increase tissue temperature, which may in turn denature pathogen membranes. This response produces a swollen (edematous), reddened (erythematous), and warm region, characteristic of inflammation in response to local infection or injury. The result of the inflammation stage is the clearing away of dead and dying tissue, removal of bacteria and other foreign substances, and the preparation of the damaged area for rebuilding.

Epithelialization

Epithelialization is an early stage in wound healing in which epithelial cells migrate over the surface of the wound. The stratum germinativum cells rapidly divide and regenerate, thus restoring a uniform layer of skin cells along the edges of the healing wound. In clean, surgically prepared wounds, complete epithelialization may take place in as little as 48 hours. Except in minor, superficial wounds, the new epithelial layer is not a perfect facsimile of the original, undamaged skin. Instead, the new skin layer may be thinner, pigmented differently, and devoid of normal hair follicles. However, the new skin is usually quite functional and cosmetically similar to the original. If the wound is very large, epithelialization may be incomplete, and collagen will show through as a shiny, pinkish line of tissue called a scar.

✳ **inflammation** complex process of local cellular and biochemical changes as a consequence of injury or infection; an early stage of healing.

✳ **chemotactic factors** chemicals released by white blood cells that attract more white blood cells to an area of inflammation.

✳ **granulocytes** white blood cells charged with the primary purpose of neutralizing foreign bacteria.

✳ **macrophage** immune system cell that has the ability to recognize and ingest foreign pathogens.

✳ **phagocytosis** process in which a cell surrounds and absorbs a bacterium or other particle.

✳ **epithelialization** early stage of wound healing in which epithelial cells migrate over the surface of the wound.

Neovascularization

In order for healing to take place, new tissue must grow and regenerate. That requires blood rich in oxygen and nutrients. The body responds to this increased demand by generating new blood vessels in a process called **neovascularization.** These vessels bud from undamaged capillaries in the wound margins and then grow into the healing tissue. Neovascularized tissue is very fragile and has a tendency to bleed easily. It takes weeks to months for the newly formed blood vessels to become fully resistant to injury and for the surrounding tissue to strengthen enough to protect the new and delicate circulation.

* **neovascularization** new growth of capillaries in response to healing.

Collagen Synthesis

Collagen is the body's main structural protein. It is a strong, tough fiber forming part of hair, bones, and connective tissue. Scar tissue, cartilage, and tendons are almost entirely collagen. Specialized cells called **fibroblasts** are brought to the wound area and synthesize collagen as an important step in rebuilding damaged tissues. Collagen binds the wound margins together and strengthens the healing wound. It is important to note that as the wound heals, it is not "as good as new." Regenerated skin has only about 60 percent of the tensile strength of undamaged skin at 4 months, when the scar is fully mature. This accounts for the occasional re-injury and reopening of wounds weeks or months after healing. The fibroblasts continue to reshape the scar tissue and shrink the wound for months after the scab falls off. This **remodeling** involves reorganizing collagen fibers into neat, parallel bands, strengthening the healing tissue still more. Remodeling can continue for up to 6 to 12 months after the initial injury, so the final cosmetic outcome of the healing process may not be evident until then.

* **collagen** tough, strong protein that comprises most of the body's connective tissue.

* **fibroblasts** specialized cells that form collagen.

* **remodeling** stage in the wound healing process in which collagen is broken down and relaid in an orderly fashion.

INFECTION

Infection is the most common and, next to hemorrhage, the most serious complication of open wounds. Approximately 1 in 15 wounds seen at the emergency department results in a wound infection. These infections delay healing. They may also spread to adjacent tissues and endanger cosmetic appearances. Occasionally, they cause widespread or systemic infection, called sepsis.

The most common causes of skin and soft-tissue infections are the Staphylococcus and Streptococcus bacterial families. These bacteria are gram positive (gram staining is a procedure to differentiate between types of bacteria), aerobic, and very common in the environment. Staphylococcus bacteria frequently colonize on the surface of normal skin, so it is not surprising to find them driven into wounds by the forces of trauma. Less commonly, wound infections are caused by other bacteria such as gram-negative rods, including pseudomonas aeruginosa (diabetics and foot puncture wounds) and pasteurella multocida (cat and dog bites).

It takes bacteria a few days to grow into numbers sufficient to cause noticeable signs or symptoms of infection. Infections appear at least 2 to 3 days following the initial wound and commonly present with pain, tenderness, erythema, and warmth. Infection earlier than that is very unusual. Pus, a collection of white blood cells, cellular debris, and dead bacteria, may be visible draining from the wound. The pus is usually thick, pale yellowish-to-greenish in color, and has a foul smell. Visible red streaks, or **lymphangitis,** may extend from the wound margins up the affected extremity proximally. These streaks represent inflammation of the lymph channels as a result of the infection. The patient may also complain of fever and malaise, especially if the infection has begun to spread systemically.

Infection is the most common complication of open wounds.

* **lymphangitis** inflammation of the lymph channels, usually as a result of a distal infection.

Infection Risk Factors

Risk factors for wound infections are related to the host's health, the type and location of the wound, any associated contamination, and the treatment provided. Diabetics, the infirm, the elderly, and individuals with serious chronic diseases such as COPD are at greater risk for infection and heal more slowly and less efficiently than healthy individuals. Patients with any significant disease or pre-existing medical problem such as cancer, anemia, hepatic failure, or cardiovascular disease have difficulty mobilizing the immune and tissue-repair response necessary for good wound healing. HIV and AIDS attack the body's immune system and seriously impair its ability to ward off infection, increasing risk significantly. Smoking constricts blood vessels and robs healing tissues of needed oxygen and nutrients, also increasing infection risk.

Several drugs detract from the body's ability to fight infection. Persons on immunosuppressant medications such as prednisone or cortisone (corticosteroids) and non-steroidal anti-inflammatory drugs (NSAIDs) such as ibuprofen are also at increased risk for serious infection. Colchicine, a drug used to treat gout, also reduces the body's inflammation response. Neoplastic agents, which are used to combat rapidly reproducing cells in cancer patients, also disrupt cell regeneration at an injury site.

The type of wound—for example, a puncture or an extensive crush injury—may influence the likelihood of infection.

The wound type strongly affects the likelihood of a wound infection. A puncture wound traps contamination deep within tissue where there is a perfect environment for bacterial growth. Avulsion tears away blood vessels and supporting structures, robbing the damaged tissue of its blood supply, a critical factor in preventing or reducing infection. Crush injuries and other wounds that produce large areas of injured or dead (devitalized) tissue provide an excellent environment for bacterial growth and are at great risk for wound infection.

In a similar fashion, wound location influences infection risk. Well-vascularized areas such as the face and scalp are very resistant to infection. Distal extremities, the feet in particular, are at greater risk.

Clean objects, such as uncontaminated sheet metal or a clean knife, usually leave only small amounts of bacteria in a wound and, consequently, do not often cause infections. On the other hand, objects contaminated with organic matter and bacteria, such as a nail on a barnyard floor, a knife used to clean raw meat, or a piece of wood, pose much greater risks of infection. The infection risk associated with bites caused by mammals, and carnivores in particular, is very great. Bites by humans, cats, and dogs are among the most common and most serious types of bites.

The type of treatment provided for a wound affects the risk of infection. Use of sterile dressings and clean examination gloves minimizes wound contamination during prehospital treatment. Gloves protect not only the rescuer but also the patient from contaminants on the rescuer's hands. Irrigation of wounds with sterile saline using a pressurized stream device has been shown to reduce bacterial loads and reduce infection rates. Closing wounds (with sutures or staples, for example) increases infection risks as compared to leaving wounds open. However, the risks associated with wound closure are frequently accepted in order to achieve the best possible cosmetic outcome and more rapid healing.

In most cases, routine use of antibiotics with wounds does not help reduce infection rates and, in fact, may increase the likelihood of infection with antibiotic-resistant microorganisms. Antibiotics may be helpful if given within the first hour or so after deep major wounds, such as those from gunshots or stabbings, puncture wounds to the feet, and wounds where retention of a foreign body is suspected.

Infection Management

Despite the potential problems noted above, the mainstay in treatment for infections is the use of chemical bactericidals, also know as antibiotics. Antibiotics for the treatment of gram-positive infections include the antistaphylococcal penicillin, cephalosporin, and erythromycin in patients allergic to penicillin. The pharmalogical approach against pseudomonas often requires the use of two drugs, while pasteurella is adequately treated with penicillin.

On occasion, a wound forms a collection of pus called an abscess and requires a minor incision and drainage to correct. Surgical removal of this material helps the body return to normal more quickly.

Gangrene One of the rarest and most feared wound complications is **gangrene.** Gangrene is a deep space infection usually caused by the anaerobic bacterium *Clostridium perfringens*. These bacteria characteristically produce a gas deep within a wound, causing subcutaneous emphysema and a foul smell whenever the gas escapes. Once they have become established, the bacteria are particularly prolific and can rapidly involve an entire extremity. Left unchecked, gangrene frequently leads to sepsis and death. In the days before antibiotics, amputation was frequently necessary to stop the spread of the disease. Modern treatment with a combination of antibiotics, surgery, and hyperbaric oxygenation effectively arrests most cases of gangrene early in their course.

> ✱ **gangrene** deep space infection usually caused by the anaerobic bacterium *Clostridium perfringens*.

Tetanus Another highly feared but, fortunately, rare complication of wound infections is tetanus, or lockjaw. Tetanus is caused by the bacterium *Clostridium tetani,* and like its cousin *Clostridium perfringens,* it is anaerobic. Tetanus presents with few signs or symptoms at the local wound site, but the bacteria produce a potent toxin that causes widespread, painful, involuntary muscle contractions. Early observers noted mandibular trismus, or jaw-clenching ("lockjaw"). There is an antidote for the tetanus toxin, but it only neutralizes circulating toxin molecules, not those already bound to the motor endplates. Thus, treatment is slow and recovery prolonged.

Fortunately, tetanus is preventable through immunization. Widespread immunization has reduced incidence to a very few cases. The standard immunization is a series of three shots in childhood, with boosters every 10 years thereafter. It is common practice in emergency departments to provide boosters to wound patients if they have not been immunized in the past 5 years.

OTHER WOUND COMPLICATIONS

Several circumstances or conditions can interfere with normal wound healing processes. These conditions include impaired hemostasis, re-bleeding, and delayed healing.

Impaired Hemostasis

Several medications can interfere with hemostasis and the clotting process. Aspirin is a powerful inhibitor of platelet aggregation, and it is used clinically to help prevent clot formation in the coronary and cerebral arteries of patients at risk for myocardial infarction or cerebrovascular accident (stroke). Thus, a side effect of aspirin use is a prolongation of clotting time, an important consideration in a patient who has sustained significant trauma or is undergoing major surgery. Likewise, anticoagulants, such as Coumadin® (warfarin) and heparin, and thrombolitics, such as TPA and streptokinase, interfere with or break down the protein fibers that form clots and are used to prevent or destroy obstructions at critical locations. They also adversely affect clot development in soft-tissue wounds. Penicillins may increase clotting times and interfere with blood cell production. Additionally, abnormalities in proteins involved in the fibrin formation cascade may result in delayed clotting, as is the case in hemophiliacs.

> *Some medications, like aspirin, warfarin, and heparin, can interfere with the clotting process.*
>
>

Re-bleeding

Despite treatment that provides adequate initial control of bleeding, re-bleeding is possible from any wound. Movement of underlying structures, such as muscles or bones, or of the bandage or dressing material may dislodge clots and re-institute hemorrhage.

Also, hemorrhage that appears to have been stopped may actually be bleeding into an oversized dressing until it saturates the dressing and pushes through it. Monitor your dressings and bandages frequently to assure that blood loss is not continuing.

Partially healed wounds are also at risk for re-bleeding. Postoperative wounds in particular can start bleeding again with life-threatening results. Because patients are discharged from hospitals more quickly today than in the past and return home sooner after surgery, be wary of this potential complication.

Delayed Healing

* **serous fluid** a cellular component of blood, similar to plasma.

In some patients, the wound repair process may be delayed or even arrested, resulting in incomplete wound healing. Persons at greatest risk for this complication are diabetics, the elderly, the chronically ill, and the malnourished. Seriously or chronically infected wounds and wounds in locations with limited blood flow (distal extremities) are also at risk for incomplete healing. Incompletely healed wounds remain tender and are easily re-injured. A pale yellow or blood-tinged **serous fluid** may drain from them. Out-of-hospital treatment of incompletely healed wounds includes frequent changes of sterile, non-adherent dressings and protection of the wound.

Compartment Syndrome

* **compartment syndrome** muscle ischemia that is caused by rising pressures within an anatomical fascial space.

Compartment syndrome is a complication of closed and, occasionally, open wounds. In compartment syndrome, an extremity injury causes significant edema and swelling in the deep tissues. Because the extremity muscles are encapsulated in tough, inflexible fasciae, the swollen tissue has "nowhere to go," and the pressure in the compartment rises (Figure 20-14). When the pressure rises above 45 to 60 mmHg, the blood flow to that muscle group or compartment is compromised and ischemia ensues. If the condition continues for more than a few hours, irreversible damage and permanent disability may result. The muscle mass may die and its contribution to limb function may be lost. Frequently, the resulting scar tissue shortens the length of the muscle strand and produces what is called Volkmann's contracture, thus further reducing the usefulness of the limb after compartment syndrome. All extremities may experience compartment syndrome, but the lower extremities, especially the calf, are at greatest risk because of their bulk and fascial anatomy.

Abnormal Scar Formation

* **keloid** a formation resulting from overproduction of scar tissue.

During the healing process, scar tissue sometimes develops abnormally. A **keloid** is excessive scar tissue that extends beyond the boundaries of a wound. It develops most commonly in darkly pigmented individuals and develops on the sternum, lower abdomen, upper extremities, and ears. Another healing abnormality is hypertrophic scar formation. This is an excessive accumulation of scar tissue, usually within the injury border, that is often associated with dynamic skin tension lines, like those at flexion joints.

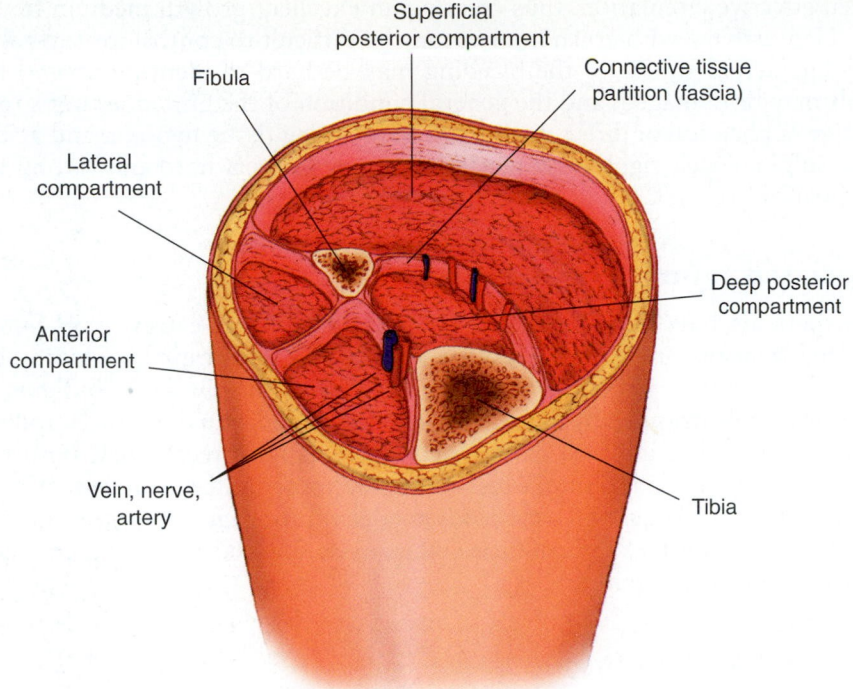

FIGURE 20-14 Musculoskeletal compartments segregated by fascia.

Labels on figure:
- Superficial posterior compartment
- Fibula
- Connective tissue partition (fascia)
- Lateral compartment
- Deep posterior compartment
- Anterior compartment
- Vein, nerve, artery
- Tibia

Pressure Injuries

A special type of soft-tissue injury is the pressure injury, which is caused by prolonged compression of the skin and tissues beneath. This may occur in the chronically ill (bed-ridden) patient, the patient who falls and remains unconscious for hours (due to alcohol intoxication, stroke, or drug overdose), or the patient who is entrapped with no crushing mechanism. The patient's weight against the ground or other surface compresses tissue and induces hypoxic injury. The injury is similar to a crush injury, although the mechanism is more passive and more likely to go unnoticed. Pressure injury may also occur when a long spine board, PASG, air splint, or rigid splint remains on a patient for an extended period of time.

Pressure injuries may occur if a long spine board, splint, or PASG is left on a patient for an extended period.

CRUSH INJURY

Crush injury involves a trauma pattern in which body tissues are subjected to severe compressive forces. A crush injury can be relatively minor—for example, one that involves only a finger or part of an extremity—or it can be massive—one that affects much or all of the body. The mechanisms of injury can be varied. A packing machine might compress a worker's finger or extremity; a collapsed jack might trap a mechanic's leg under a car wheel; the seat and steering column might compress a driver's chest between them in an auto crash; or debris from a building collapse or trench cave-in might bury a construction worker.

A crush injury disrupts the body's tissues—muscles, blood vessels, bone, and, in some cases, internal organs. With such injuries, the skin may remain intact and the limb may appear normal in shape, or the skin may be severely cut and bruised and the extremity mangled and deformed. In both cases, however, the damage within is extensive. The injury often results in a large area of destruction with limited effective circulation, thus creating an excellent growth medium for bacteria. Hemorrhage with crush injuries may be difficult to control for several reasons: The actual source of the bleeding may be hard to identify; several large vessels may be damaged; and the general condition of the limb does not support effective application of direct pressure. The resulting tissue hypoxia and acidosis may result in muscle rigor, with muscles that may feel very hard and "wood-like" on palpation.

Associated Injury

When patients have been subjected to mechanisms that cause crush injuries, those mechanisms or others associated with them often result in additional injuries. For example, patients who have received crush injuries in building collapses or when entrapped by machinery may suffer additional fractures and open or closed soft-tissue injuries. Falling debris can cause direct injury, both blunt and penetrating. Dust and smoke can cause respiratory and eye injuries. Also, entrapment for any length of time leads to dehydration and hypothermia. You should consider all these possibilities when assessing and providing emergency care to victims of crush injury.

CRUSH SYNDROME

Crush syndrome occurs when body parts are entrapped for 4 hours or longer. Shorter periods of entrapment may result in direct body part damage, but they usually do not cause the broad, systemic complications of crush syndrome. The crushed skeletal muscle tissue undergoes **necrosis** and cellular changes with resultant release of metabolic byproducts. This degenerative process, called traumatic **rhabdomyolysis** (skeletal muscle disintegration), releases many toxins. Chief among these byproducts of cellular destruction are myoglobin (a muscle protein), phosphate and potassium (from cellular death), lactic acid (from anaerobic metabolism), and uric acid (from protein breakdown). These byproducts accumulate in the crushed body part but, because of the entrapment and the resulting minimal circulation through the injured tissue, do not reach the systemic circulation. Once the limb or victim is extricated and the pressure is released, however, the accumulated byproducts and toxins flood the central circulation.

High levels of myoglobin can lodge in the filtering tubules of the kidney, especially with patients who are in hypovolemic (shock) states, leading to renal failure, a leading cause of delayed death in crush syndrome. More immediate problems include hypovolemia and shock from the flow of sodium, chloride, and water into the damaged tissue. Increased blood potassium (hyperkalemia) can reduce the cardiac muscle's response to electrical stimuli, induce cardiac dysrhythmias, and lead to sudden death. Rising phosphate levels (hyperphosphatemia) can lead to abnormal calcifications in the vasculature and nervous system, compounding problems for the patient. In addition, as oxygenated circulation returns to the cells the aerobic process by which uric acid is produced can operate again, thus increasing cellular acidity and injury.

INJECTION INJURY

A unique type of soft-tissue injury is the injection injury. A bursting high-pressure line, most commonly a hydraulic line, may inject fluid through a patient's skin and into the subcutaneous tissues. If the pressure is strong enough, the fluid may push between tissue layers and travel along the limb (Figure 20-15). The fluid thus injected—for example, a petroleum-based hydraulic fluid—may then chemically damage the surrounding tissue. The body's repair mechanisms are unprepared to

* **necrosis** tissue death, usually from ischemia.

* **rhabdomyolysis** accute disease that involves the destruction of skeletal muscle.

remove the great quantities of injected material, and the resulting damage is severe. A limb may be lost due to the direct physical damage from the injection process, from the chemical damage done by the injected material, or from infection that develops after the injection.

DRESSING AND BANDAGE MATERIALS

There are several types of dressings and bandages that are effective in prehospital care. A dressing is the material placed directly on the wound to control bleeding and maintain wound cleanliness (Figure 20-16). A bandage is the material used to hold a dressing in place and to apply direct pressure to control hemorrhage (Figure 20-17). Dressings and bandages have various designs and are used for a variety of purposes in emergency care.

Sterile/Nonsterile Dressings

Sterile dressings are cotton or other fiber pads that have been specially prepared to be without microorganisms. They are usually packaged individually and remain sterile for as long as the package is intact. Once the packaging is opened,

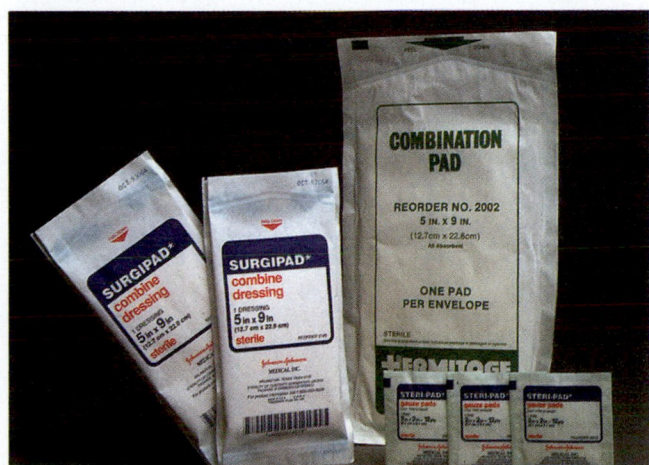

a. A variety of sterile dressings.

b. Occlusive dressings.

FIGURE 20-16 Assorted dressings used in the care of soft-tissue injuries.

FIGURE 20-17 Kerlix®, a type of self-adherent roller bandage.

sterile dressings become contaminated by airborne dust and particles that harbor bacteria and other microorganisms. Sterile dressings are designed to be used in direct contact with wounds.

Nonsterile dressings are clean—that is, free of gross contamination—but are not free of microscopic contamination and microorganisms. Nonsterile dressings are not intended to be applied directly to a wound, but rather to be placed over a sterile dressing to add bulk or absorptive power.

Occlusive/Nonocclusive Dressings

Some dressings, such as sterilized plastic wrap and petroleum-impregnated gauze, are designed to prevent the movement of fluid and air through them. These dressings are called occlusive and are helpful in preventing air aspiration into chest wounds (open pneumothorax) and open neck wounds (air emboli into the jugular vein). Most dressing material is nonocclusive.

Adherent/Nonadherent Dressings

Adherent dressings are untreated cotton or other fiber pads that will stick to drying blood and fluid that has leaked from open wounds. Adherent dressings have the advantage of promoting clot formation and thus reducing hemorrhage, but their removal from wounds can be quite painful. Removal or disturbance of an adherent dressing is also likely to break the clot and cause re-bleeding. Nonadherent dressings are specially treated with chemicals such as polymers to prevent the wound fluids and clotting materials from adhering to the dressing. Nonadherent dressings are preferred for most uncomplicated wounds.

Absorbent/Nonabsorbent Dressings

Absorbent dressings readily soak up blood and other fluids, much as a sponge soaks up water. This property is helpful in many bleeding situations. Nonabsorbent dressings absorb little or no fluid and are used when a barrier to leaking is desired. The clear membrane dressings frequently placed over intravenous puncture sites are good examples of nonabsorbent dressings. Most other dressings used in prehospital care are absorbent dressings.

Wet/Dry Dressings

Wet dressings are sometimes applied to special types of wounds such as burns. They are also used in the hospital to effect healing in some complicated post-operative wounds. Sterile normal saline is the usual fluid used to wet dressings. Wet dressings provide a medium for the movement of infectious material into wounds, however, and are not commonly used in prehospital care, except with injuries such as abdominal eviscerations or burns involving only a limited body surface area. Dry dressings are the type most often employed for wounds in prehospital care.

Self-adherent Roller Bandages

The most common and convenient bandage material is the soft, self-adherent, roller bandage (Kling or Kerlix). It has limited stretch and resists unraveling as it is rolled over itself. It conforms well to body contours and is quick and easy to use. This bandage is most appropriate for injuries located where it can be wrapped circumferentially. It comes in rolls from 1 to 6 inches wide.

Gauze Bandages

Like soft, self-adherent bandages, gauze bandages are a convenient material for securing dressings. They do not stretch, however, and thus do not conform as well to body contours as the self-adherent material, but they are otherwise functional for bandaging. Since gauze bandages do not stretch, they may increase the pressure associated with tissue swelling at injury sites. Gauze usually comes in rolls from 1/2 to 2 inches wide.

Adhesive Bandages

An adhesive bandage (or adhesive tape) is a strong plastic, paper, or fabric material with adhesive applied to one side. It can effectively secure a small dressing to a location where circumferential wrapping is impractical. When used circumferentially, an adhesive bandage does not allow for any swelling and permits pressure to accumulate in the tissues beneath it. Adhesive bandages usually come in widths that range from 1/4 to 3 inches.

Elastic (or Ace) Bandages

Elastic bandages stretch easily and conform to the body contours. Elastic bandages provide stability and support for minor musculoskeletal injuries, but they are not commonly used in prehospital care. When you do use these bandages, however, remember that it is very easy to apply too much pressure with them. Each consecutive wrap applied will contain and add to pressure on the wound site. Swelling associated with the wound may increase the pressure until blood flow through and out of the affected limb is reduced or stopped.

Triangular Bandages

Triangular bandages, or cravats, are large triangles of cotton fabric. They are strong, non-elastic bandages commonly used to make slings and swathes and, in some cases, to affix splints. They can also be used to hold dressings in place, but they do not conform as well to body contours as soft, self-adherent bandages and do not maintain pressure or immobilize wound dressings very well.

ASSESSMENT OF SOFT-TISSUE INJURIES

Proper evaluation of the skin can tell you more about the body's condition after trauma than any other aspect of patient assessment. Not only is the skin the first body organ to experience the effects of trauma, it is the first and often the only organ to display them. Therefore, assessment of the skin and its injury must be deliberate, careful, and complete. While the processes that cause soft-tissue injuries and the manifestations of those injuries vary, prehospital assessment is a simple, well-structured process. Follow the assessment process carefully and completely to ensure that you establish the nature and extent of each injury. Doing so enables you to assign soft-tissue injuries, and other injuries associated with them, the appropriate priorities for care.

Assessment of patients with soft-tissue wounds follows the same general progression as the assessment of other trauma patients. First, size up the scene, ruling out potential hazards, identifying the mechanism of injury, and determining the need for additional medical and rescue resources. Next, perform a quick initial assessment and identify and care for any immediately life-threatening injuries. For the patient with a mechanism of injury or signs and symptoms that suggest serious trauma, you will perform a rapid trauma assessment and use trauma triage criteria to determine the need for rapid transport. For a patient with no significant mechanism of injury and no indication from the initial assessment of a serious injury or life threat, perform a focused trauma assessment and gather vital signs and patient history at the scene. Perform a detailed physical exam only if conditions warrant and time permits. Provide serial ongoing assessments to track your patient's response to his injuries and your care.

SCENE SIZE-UP

During the scene size-up, look for evidence that will help you determine the mechanism of injury and anticipate the likely injuries and their severity. While soft-tissue injuries are not usually life threatening, they can suggest other, serious life threats. Remember: No injury mechanism can impact the human body without first traveling through the skin. Identify where injury is likely and be prepared to carefully examine the skin for evidence that suggests internal injury. Consider mechanisms of injury that could cause entrapment and either crush injury or crush syndrome.

Be alert to the fact that the mechanisms that injured the patient may still be present and pose threats to you and other rescuers. Rule out or eliminate any threats to yourself or fellow care providers before entering the scene (Figure 20-18).

FIGURE 20-18 During the scene size-up, rule out hazards, don gloves, and analyze the mechanism of injury.

Because trauma and injuries that penetrate the skin are likely to expose you to the hazards of contact with a patient's body fluids, don sterile gloves and observe other body substance isolation procedures as you approach the patient. Recognize that arterial bleeding and hemorrhage associated with the airway can cause blood to splatter at the scene. If you suspect these injuries, don splash protection for your eyes and clothing.

INITIAL ASSESSMENT

Begin your initial assessment by establishing manual cervical in-line immobilization if you suspect significant head or spine injury and forming a general impression of the patient. Determine the patient's level of consciousness and assess the airway, breathing, and circulation. Assess perfusion by noting skin color, temperature, and condition and by assessing capillary refill.

During this assessment, pay particular attention to the location and types of visible wounds to gain further understanding of the mechanism of injury and whether it produced blunt or penetrating trauma. If responsive, the patient may be able to give you critical information about how the wound occurred. If the patient is unable to speak, First Responders or bystanders may be able to provide this information. Correct any immediate threats to the patient's life as you discover them.

FOCUSED HISTORY AND PHYSICAL EXAM

Use the information you have gathered through the initial assessment to determine how to proceed in the assessment process. Patients with serious trauma, suggested by a significant mechanism of injury or the findings of the initial assessment, will receive a rapid trauma assessment. All other patients will receive a focused trauma assessment.

Significant Mechanism of Injury—Rapid Trauma Assessment

In the rapid trauma assessment, you will perform a swift evaluation of the patient's head, neck, chest, abdomen, pelvis, extremities, and posterior body. Examine these areas for signs of internal or life-endangering injuries. Quickly investigate any discolorations, deformities, temperature variations, abnormal muscle tone, or open wounds.

Assure that any wounds you discover, or the injuries suggested beneath them, do not involve or endanger the airway or breathing or contribute significantly to blood loss. Focus your immediate care during the rapid trauma assessment on continuing to assure the patient's airway and breathing and then on controlling severe blood loss.

Inspect and palpate areas where the mechanism of injury suggests serious injuries may exist. Again, look for discoloration, temperature variation, abnormal muscle tone, and deformity suggestive of trauma (Figure 20-19). If the mechanism of injury suggests open wounds, sweep body areas hidden from sight with gloved hands; this will rule out the possibility of unseen blood loss and pooling. Control moderate to severe hemorrhage immediately. Hemorrhage control need not be definitive, but should stop continuing significant blood loss. Once more serious injuries are cared for, you can return and dress and bandage wounds more carefully.

Survey bleeding wounds to determine the type of hemorrhage—arterial, venous, or capillary. Attempt to approximate the volume of blood lost since the time of the accident, which suggests the rate of blood loss.

Carry out your exam using the methods described in "Assessment Techniques" later in this chapter. Apply a cervical spinal immobilization collar once you have

FIGURE 20-19 Often the only signs of serious internal injury are external soft-tissue injuries. *(Courtesy of Edward T. Dickinson, MD)*

completed the rapid assessment of the head and neck. Continue to provide manual immobilization, however, until the patient is fully immobilized to a backboard.

When the rapid trauma assessment is complete, obtain a set of baseline vital signs and a patient history. Be sure to maintain manual in-line immobilization while the signs and history are being gathered. If you have enough personnel, the vital signs and history may be obtained simultaneously as the rapid trauma assessment is performed.

When obtaining the history, be sure to question the patient about medications, especially those that may have some direct relevance to soft-tissue injuries. For example, the patient's tetanus history is important with any penetrating trauma. Determine if the patient has had a tetanus booster and how long ago it was given. Note that a patient's routine use of aspirin or blood thinners—for example, heparin or warfarin for stroke or MI risk—may impact the body's ability to halt even minimal hemorrhage. Ask about use of anti-inflammatory medications, such as prednisone, because those medications reduce the inflammatory response and slow the normal healing process. Question the patient about any pre-existing diseases. Note that certain diseases, especially HIV, AIDS, or anemia, increase the risks of infection and the problems of hemorrhage control.

At the conclusion of the rapid trauma assessment, confirm the decision either to transport the patient immediately with further care provided en route to the hospital or to remain at the scene and complete treatment of non-life-threatening injuries. Consider the rate and volume of any blood loss and any uncontrollable bleeding in this decision.

If your patient's condition merits care at the scene, prioritize the soft-tissue wounds you have identified to establish an order of care to follow. The few moments taken to sort out injuries and to plan the management process saves valuable time in the field. This also ensures that you provide early care for injuries with the highest priority.

No Significant Mechanism of Injury— Focused Trauma Assessment

When a patient has a soft-tissue injury but neither a significant mechanism of injury nor an indication of a serious problem from the initial assessment—for example, a cut finger or a knee abrasion from a fall—the sequence of assessment steps is different than for a patient with a significant injury mechanism. Begin this phase of the assessment with a focused trauma assessment, which is an exam directed at the injury site—the finger or the knee in the examples noted above. A full head-to-toe rapid trauma assessment is not necessary in most such cases.

Direct the focused assessment at the chief complaint and any area of injury suggested by the mechanism of injury. Use the examination techniques of inquiry, inspection, and palpation (described below) to evaluate the injury and the surrounding area. In the case of a wound to an extremity, be sure to check the distal extremity for pulses, capillary refill, color, and temperature. Then, obtain a set of baseline vital signs and a history from the patient. If any of your findings suggest the patient has more serious injuries, perform a rapid trauma assessment and consider rapid transport.

Depending on the nature of the patient's injury, you may decide to provide transport or to refer/release the patient. If you are treating an isolated injury such as a cut finger, your system's protocols may prescribe whether you may release/refer the patient or transport the patient. More and more often, EMS systems are employing release/referral protocols to increase system efficiency. If you do transport, provide ongoing assessment.

DETAILED PHYSICAL EXAM

Once the rapid or focused trauma assessment has been completed, vital signs and history gathered, and necessary emergency care steps have been taken, you may perform a detailed physical exam. Like the rapid trauma assessment, this head-to-toe evaluation of the skin (and the rest of the body) involves the techniques of inquiry, observation, and palpation. The detailed exam should follow a planned and comprehensive process, ideally progressing from head to toe although the order is not critical. The main purpose of the detailed assessment is to pick up any additional information regarding the patient's condition and to search for any unsuspected or subtle injuries. Manage any additional injuries you discover during the examination. The detailed physical exam is usually performed during transport or on scene if transport has been delayed. Never delay transport to perform it, and only perform it if the patient's condition permits.

The detailed head-to-toe examination should be performed at the scene only if significant and life-threatening bleeding can be ruled out.

ASSESSMENT TECHNIQUES

The assessment techniques described below can be used during both the rapid trauma assessment and the detailed physical exam.

Inquiry

Question the patient about the mechanism of injury, any pain, pain on touch or movement, and any loss of function or sensation specific to an area. Additionally, attempt to determine the exact nature of the pain or sensory or motor loss by using elements of the OPQRST mnemonic (see Chapter 12, "Patient Assessment in the Field"). Question the patient about signs and symptoms before touching an area.

Inspection

Continue the exam by carefully observing a particular body region. Identify any discolorations, deformities, or open wounds in those regions.

Determine if any discoloration is local, distal, or systemic, reflecting local injury, circulation compromise, or systemic complications such as shock. Contusions, blood vessel injuries, dislocations, and fractures may cause local discoloration, including erythema or ecchymosis. Distal discoloration may present as a pale, cyanotic, or ashen-colored limb distal to the point of circulation loss. You may also notice systemic discoloration, such as pale, ashen, or grayish skin in all limbs, suggestive of hypovolemia and shock.

Examine any deformities you find to determine their cause. Is the deformity due to a developing hematoma, to the normal swelling associated with the inflammatory process, or to underlying injuries?

Inspect any wounds you discover in detail. Study the wound to determine its depth and evaluate its potential for damage to underlying muscles, nerves, blood vessels, organs, or bones. If possible, identify the object that caused the wound and determine the amount of force transmitted by it to the body's interior. Ascertain if there are any foreign bodies, contamination, or impaled objects in the wound. Finally, identify the nature and location of any hemorrhage.

Observe each wound carefully so you can describe it to the attending physician after you dress and bandage the injury. This information will help the emergency department staff prioritize the patient's injuries. Careful observation will also aid you in preparation of your prehospital care report. Adequate lighting is crucial for evaluating wounds. If necessary, defer this portion of the detailed physical exam until better lighting is available, as in the back of the ambulance.

If a patient's limb or digit has been amputated, have other rescuers conduct a brief but thorough search for the amputated part. If the part cannot be located immediately or remains entrapped, do not delay transport. Instead, leave someone at the scene to continue the search. Ensure that once the body part is retrieved, it is properly handled, packaged, and brought to the same hospital as the patient.

The wound should be observed in such a way that it can later be described to the attending physician.

Palpation

In addition to questioning the patient and inspecting the body regions, you should palpate the body's entire surface. Be alert for any deformity, asymmetry, temperature variation, unexpected mass, or localized loss of skin or muscle tone. Gently palpate all apparent closed wounds for evidence of tenderness, swelling, crepitus, and subcutaneous emphysema. Avoid palpating the interior of open wounds, which may introduce contamination and disturb the clotting process. Ascertain the presence or absence of distal pulses and capillary refill time with any extremity injury. Also, check motor and sensory function distal to any extremity wound and compare findings with those from the opposite limb.

ONGOING ASSESSMENT

During transport, provide an ongoing assessment, reassessing the patient's mental status, airway, breathing, and circulation, gathering additional sets of vital signs, and evaluating the sites of the patient's injuries. Also inspect any interventions you have performed. Provide an ongoing assessment at least every 5 minutes with unstable patients and every 15 minutes with stable patients. If you note any change in the patient's condition, modify your priorities for transport and care accordingly.

MANAGEMENT OF SOFT-TISSUE INJURY

Once you complete your patient assessment, take steps to manage the soft-tissue injury, either in the field or en route to the hospital. Control of blood loss, prevention of shock, and decontamination of affected areas take priority. The following sections describe some of the most important of these care steps.

Unless you note extensive bleeding, wound management by dressing and bandaging is a late priority in the care of trauma patients. Dress and bandage wounds whose bleeding does not represent a life threat only after you stabilize your patient by caring for higher-priority injuries.

The management of minor wounds is a late priority in the care of the trauma patient, unless extensive bleeding is noted.

OBJECTIVES OF WOUND DRESSING AND BANDAGING

The dressing and bandaging of a wound has three basic objectives. These are to control all hemorrhaging, to keep the wound as clean as possible, and to immobilize the wound (Procedure 20-1). The appearance of the final dressing and bandage is not as critical as achievement of these three objectives.

Hemorrhage Control

The primary method—and the most effective one—of controlling hemorrhage associated with soft-tissue injury is direct pressure. In cases of serious hemorrhage flowing from a wound with some force, place a small dressing directly over the site of the bleeding and apply pressure directly to it with a finger. When the bleeding is the more commonly encountered slow-to-moderate type, use a dressing that has been sized to cover and pad the wound. Then simply wrap the dressing with a soft, self-adherent bandage using moderate pressure to halt the blood loss. Monitor the wound frequently to assure bleeding has stopped.

Elevation can assist in the control of hemorrhage, although it is generally not as effective as direct pressure. Elevation reduces arterial pressure in the extremity and increases venous return. Elevation can thus reduce edema and increase blood flow through the wound and injured extremity. This promotes good oxygenation and wound healing. Do not elevate a limb, however, if doing so will cause any further harm as would be the case if the patient has a suspected spinal or associated musculoskeletal injury or if there is an object impaled in the limb.

Use pressure points to assist with bleeding control and the clotting process when direct pressure and elevation together do not control it. Locate a pulse point immediately proximal to the wound and above a bony prominence. Apply firm pressure and maintain it for at least 10 minutes. Assure that the hemorrhage does not continue.

Occasionally, bleeding from a soft-tissue injury can be difficult to control. If the bleeding continues despite the use of direct pressure, elevation, and pressure points, reassess the wound to be sure you have determined the exact site of blood loss. Then reapply direct digital pressure to that precise point. Too often, hemorrhage continues because the bandaging technique distributes pressure over the entire wound site rather than focusing it directly on the source of the bleeding. The force driving the hemorrhage is no greater than the patient's systolic blood pressure, and properly applied digital pressure can thus easily provide a pressure greater than this to compress the vessel and halt any blood loss.

In certain circumstances, the use of direct pressure, elevation, and a pressure point may not control hemorrhage. Crush injuries and amputations are situations in which normal bleeding control measures are often ineffective. With these traumatic injuries, several blood vessels are jaggedly torn, confounding the body's normal hemorrhage control mechanisms and making it difficult to pinpoint the source of bleeding. Even if the source of bleeding can be found, applying firm direct pressure to it may be difficult. In such cases, the application of a tourniquet may be useful. The tourniquet should be considered the last option for controlling hemorrhage. If properly applied, the tourniquet will stop the flow of blood; however, its use has serious associated risks. Keep the following precautions in mind whenever you consider using a tourniquet.

1. If the pressure applied is insufficient, the tourniquet may halt venous return while permitting continued arterial blood flow into the extremity, increasing the rate and volume of blood loss.

The three objectives of bandaging are to control hemorrhage, to keep the wound clean, and to immobilize the wound site.

A combination of techniques for hemorrhage control may be effective when bleeding is resistant to direct pressure.

To halt hemorrhage, apply firm pressure to the site for at least 10 minutes.

20-1a   Apply direct pressure with a dressing to the site of hemorrhage.

20-1b   Elevate the hemorrhage site if there is no serious musculoskeletal injury.

20-1c   Apply additional dressings as needed.

20-1d   If serious hemorrhage persists, expose the wound and place digital pressure with a gloved hand on the site of bleeding.

20-1e   Bandage the dressing in place, maintaining pressure on the wound.

20-1f   Apply digital pressure to a proximal artery if the hemorrhage persists.

a. Place a bulky dressing over the distal artery.

b. Apply a pressure exceeding the systolic pressure.

FIGURE 20-20   The steps of tourniquet application.

c. Secure the tourniquet and monitor the wound site for continuing hemorrhage.

2. When the tourniquet is applied properly, the entire limb distal to the device is without circulation. Hypoxia, ischemia, and necrosis may permanently damage the tissue distal to the tourniquet.

3. When circulation is restored, the blood flows and pools in the extremity, adding to any hypovolemia. In addition, any blood that returns to the central circulation is highly hypoxic, acidic, and toxic. This blood can cause shock, lethal dysrhythmias, renal failure, and death. The return of circulation may also restart hemorrhage and introduce emboli into the central circulation.

Do not use a tourniquet unless you cannot control severe bleeding by any other means. Place it just proximal to the wound site, but stay away from the elbow or knee joints (Figure 20-20). Apply the tourniquet in a way that will not injure the tissue beneath. For example, do not use very narrow material, like rope or wire, for a tourniquet; applying great pressure to a limb with such material may cause serious injury in the compressed tissue. Instead, select a 2-inch or wider band for compression.

A readily available, effective, and easily controllable tourniquet is the sphygmomanometer (regular for the upper extremity and thigh for the lower). It is wide, simple to apply, rapid to inflate, and easy to monitor. Inflate it to a pressure 30 mmHg above the patient's systolic blood pressure and beyond the pressure at which the patient's hemorrhage ceases.

Once you apply a tourniquet, leave it in place until the patient arrives at the emergency department. Monitor the tourniquet during transport to assure that it does not lose pressure, and watch for signs of renewed bleeding. If bleeding starts again, increase the tourniquet pressure. Alert the hospital staff to your use of the tourniquet during transport as well as upon arrival. Mark the patient's forehead clearly with the letters "TQ," and note the time the tourniquet was applied.

Do not release a tourniquet in the field except under exceptional circumstances and then only during consultation with medical direction. Be prepared to provide vigorous fluid resuscitation, ECG monitoring, dysrhythmia treatment, and rapid transport if a tourniquet release is attempted.

Do not use a tourniquet unless you cannot control bleeding by any other means.

Once applied, a tourniquet should be left in place until the patient arrives at the emergency department.

Management of Soft-Tissue Injury   **939**

Sterility

Once you halt severe bleeding, keep the wound as sterile as possible. Under field conditions, this may simply mean keeping the wound as clean as reasonably possible. With very small open wounds, like an IV start or a small laceration, you may consider the application of an antibacterial ointment to help with infection control. However, the effectiveness of such ointments on larger wounds is limited, and ointments are not generally applied to these wounds.

Under normal conditions, you need not cleanse the wound. If a wound is grossly contaminated, however, irrigate it with normal saline or lactated Ringer's solution. A 1,000 mL bag of saline, connected to a macrodrip administration set and pressurized by squeezing the bag under your arm, may allow rapid and gentle wound cleansing. Try to move any contamination from the center of the wound outward. You may also carefully remove larger particles—glass, gravel, debris, and so forth—if you can do this swiftly and without inducing further injury.

Apply a bandage to make the dressing appear as neat as time and the conditions under which you are working will allow. Often, this is as easy as covering the entire dressing with wraps of soft, self-adherent roller bandage. The neat appearance calms and reassures the patient, while the bandaging reduces contamination and the chances of post-trauma infection.

Immobilization

Immobilization is an important, but frequently overlooked, component of hemorrhage control.

The last objective of bandaging is immobilization. The stability of the wound site helps the natural clotting mechanisms operate and reduces the patient's discomfort. Maintaining gentle pressure with the bandage may reduce pain and local swelling. Immobilize the limb with bandaging material to the patient's body or to a rigid surface such as a padded board or ladder splint.

When immobilizing a limb, do not use elastic bandaging material or apply the bandage too tightly. The edema that develops rapidly with an injury puts increasing pressure on underlying tissue. This pressure may quickly reduce or halt circulation.

Frequently monitor any limb that you bandage circumferentially to assure that the distal pulse remains strong and that the distal extremity maintains good color and does not swell. If you cannot locate the distal pulse, monitor capillary refill, skin color, and temperature. If signs or symptoms suggest that the distal circulation is compromised, elevate the extremity, if possible, and check and consider loosening the bandage.

Pain and Edema Control

Treat painful soft-tissue injuries or those likely to cause large debilitating edema with the application of cold packs and moderate-pressure bandages. Cold reduces inflammatory response and local edema. It also dulls the pain associated with serious soft-tissue trauma. Use a commercial cold pack or ice in a plastic bag wrapped in a dry towel and apply it to the wound. Do not use a cold pack directly against the skin as it cools beyond any therapeutic value. Direct application of a cold pack may also cause tissue freezing, especially in areas with reduced circulation.

Some moderate pressure over the wound area may also help reduce pain and wound edema. In cases where the patient reports severe pain, consider use of morphine sulfate or other analgesics for patient comfort. Administer morphine in 2 mg increments titrated to pain relief every 5 minutes (up to a total of 10 mg).

ANATOMICAL CONSIDERATIONS FOR BANDAGING

Each area of the body has specific anatomical characteristics. Your application of bandages and dressings should take these characteristics into account to provide effective prehospital wound care (Figure 20-21).

a. Head and/or ear bandage.

b. Cheek and ear bandage
(be sure mouth will open).

c. Hand bandage.

d. Shoulder bandage.

e. Foot and/or ankle bandage.

FIGURE 20-21   Good bandaging uses the natural body curves and the self-adherent characteristics of bandages to hold dressings firmly in place.

Scalp

The scalp has a rich supply of vessels that can bleed heavily when injured. It's commonly said that head wounds rarely account for shock, but scalp hemorrhage can be severe and difficult to control and can lead to the loss of moderate to large volumes of blood.

In scalp hemorrhage uncomplicated by skull fracture, direct pressure against the skull is effective in the control of bleeding. To hold a dressing in place and maintain pressure, wrap a bandage around the head, capturing the occiput or brow or, in some cases, passing the bandage under the chin (while still allowing for jaw movement).

If a head wound is complicated by fracture, be very careful in your application of pressure. Apply gentle digital pressure around the wound and attempt to locate the small scalp arteries that feed it to use as pressure points. Then simply hold a dressing on the wound without much pressure.

Face

Facial wounds are frequently gruesome and bleed heavily. Gentle direct pressure to these wounds can effectively control hemorrhage. You can maintain this pressure by wrapping a bandage around the head. Be careful to assure a clear airway and use your bandaging to splint any facial instability.

Remember, blood is a gastric irritant and swallowed blood may induce emesis. Be ready to provide suctioning in patients with oral or nasal hemorrhage because unexpected emesis may compromise the airway.

Ear or Mastoid

Wounds to the ear region can be easily bandaged by wrapping the head circumferentially. Use open gauze to collect, not stop, any bleeding or fluids flowing from the ear canal. These materials may contain cerebrospinal fluid and halting their flow may add to any increasing intracranial pressure.

Neck

Minor neck wounds may be lightly wrapped circumferentially with bandages or taped to hold dressings in place. If bleeding is moderate to severe, however, direct manual pressure may be necessary because the amount of pressure applied by circumferential wrapping may compromise both the airway and circulation to and from the head. In cases of large wounds or moderate to severe bleeding, also consider using an occlusive dressing to prevent aspiration of air into a jugular vein.

Shoulder

The shoulder is an easy area to bandage as soft, self-adherent roller bandages readily conform to body contours. Use the axilla, arm, and neck as points of fixation, but be careful not to put pressure on the anterior neck and trachea.

Trunk

For minor trunk wounds, adhesive tape may be sufficient to hold dressings in place. With larger wounds, bandaging can be more difficult because you must wrap the patient's body circumferentially to apply direct pressure to a wound. Applying a bandage in this way may require moving the patient unnecessarily and risk causing or worsening an injury. Consider instead using a ladder splint that is negotiated beneath the patient's torso, folded to the curve of the back, and then folded outward sharply at each end to serve as a bandaging fixation point. You then wrap the bandage between the ends of the ladder splint to hold the dressing in place.

Groin and Hip

The groin and the hip are easy places to affix a dressing. Bandage by following the contours of the upper thighs and waist, similar to the technique of bandaging a shoulder. Be careful here, though. Any movement of the patient is likely to affect the tightness of the bandage and the amount of pressure over the dressing. With these injuries, therefore, bandage after the patient is in final position for transport.

Elbow and Knee

Joints, especially the elbow and knee, are difficult to bandage. Bandage using circumferential wraps and then splint the area to assure that the bandage does not loosen with movement. If possible, place the joint in a position halfway between flexion and extension. This position, called the position of function, relaxes the muscles controlling the joint and the skin tension lines, and is most comfortable for the patient during long transports or periods of immobilization.

Hand and Finger

Hand and finger injuries are easy to bandage by simple circumferential wrapping. Again, consider placing the hand or digit in the position of function, halfway between flexion and extension. Accomplish this by placing a large, bulky dressing in the palm of the patient's hand and then wrapping around it. You may use a malleable finger splint to obtain the position of function and then wrap circumferentially to splint the finger.

Ankle and Foot

Ankle and foot wounds are also easy to bandage by wrapping circumferentially and by using the natural body contours. If strong direct pressure is needed to maintain hemorrhage control, start your wrapping from the toes and work proximally. This assures that the pressure of bandaging does not form a venous tourniquet and compromise circulation to this very distal injury.

COMPLICATIONS OF BANDAGING

Bandaging can lead to some complications, although such occurrences are infrequent. If a bandage—particularly a circumferential bandage—is too tight, the area beneath it may continue to swell, increasing pressure in the area of the wound. This can lead to decreased blood flow and ischemia distal to the bandage. Pressure can build to such an extreme that the bandage acts like a tourniquet. Pain, pallor, tingling, a loss of pulses, and prolonged capillary refill time are typical signs of developing pressure and ischemia. Avoid this complication by making bandages snug but not too tight. A useful technique is to wrap a bandage only so tight that one finger can still be easily slipped beneath it.

Bandages and dressings left on too long can become soaked with blood and body fluids and then serve as incubators for infection. This problem usually takes at least 2 to 3 days to develop and is not a common concern in most prehospital settings.

The size of the dressing is an important consideration in bandaging. An unnecessarily large and bulky dressing can prevent proper inspection of a wound and hide contamination and continued serious bleeding. Too small a dressing can become lost in a wound and become, in effect, a foreign body. This is most frequently a problem with large, gaping wounds and deep wounds that penetrate the thoracic or abdominal body cavities. When dressing a wound, choose a dressing just larger than the wound yet not so small as to become lost in it.

Frequently check the pressure beneath a bandage to assure good distal circulation.

CARE OF SPECIFIC WOUNDS

Some circumstances—amputations, impaled objects, and crush syndrome cases—deserve special attention during the patient management process. These injuries can challenge even the seasoned paramedic to provide the most appropriate care.

Amputations

Amputations may bleed either heavily or minimally. Attempt to control hemorrhage with direct pressure by applying a large, bulky dressing to the wound. If this fails to control hemorrhage, consider using a tourniquet just above the point of severance. If there is a crushing wound associated with the limb loss, apply the

FIGURE 20-22 Amputated parts should be put in a dry bag, sealed, and placed in cool water that contains a few ice cubes.

Current recommendations for managing amputated body parts includes dry cooling and rapid transport.

tourniquet just above the crushed area. Do not delay patient transport while locating or extricating the amputated body part. Transport the patient immediately, and then have other personnel transport the part once it is located or released from entrapment.

Current recommendations for managing separated body parts include dry cooling and rapid transport. Place the amputated part in a plastic bag and immerse the bag in cold water (Figure 20-22). The water may have a few ice cubes in it, but avoid direct contact between the ice and the injured part. Even if the amputated part cannot be totally reattached, skin from it may be used to cover the limb end (Figure 20-23).

a. An amputated hand.

b. A successfully reimplanted hand.

FIGURE 20-23 Amputated parts should be located and transported with the patient to the hospital for possible reimplantation.

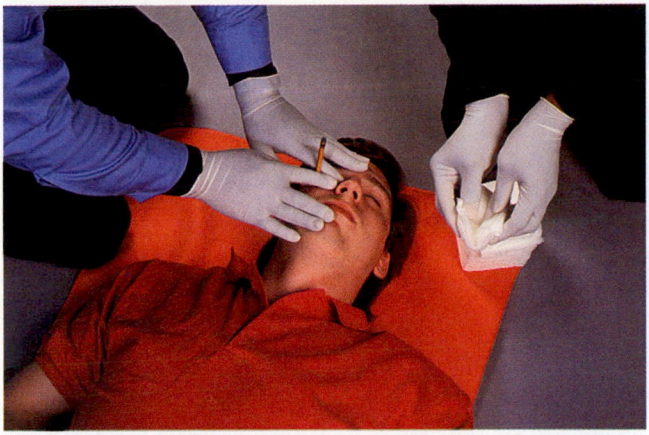

a. Manually stabilize any impaled object.

b. Use bulky padding or dressing to immobilize the object.

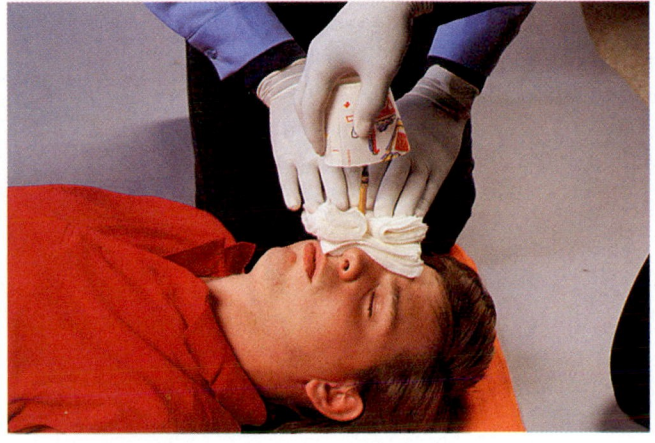

c. If the object protrudes, cover it with a paper cup.

d. Bandage the cup and padding securely in place.

FIGURE 20-24   Stabilization of an impaled object.

Impaled Objects

When possible, immobilize all impaled objects in place (Figure 20-24). Position bulky dressings around the object to stabilize it, and tape over the dressings to hold them in place. Try to make movement of the patient to the ambulance and transport to the emergency department as smooth and nonjarring as possible. Remember that any movement of the impaled object is likely to cause continued internal bleeding and additional tissue damage.

Do not remove impaled objects because of the risk of serious, uncontrollable bleeding.

If the impaled object is too large to transport or is affixed to something that cannot be moved, such as a reinforcing rod set in concrete, consider cutting it. Use appropriate techniques and tools depending on the circumstances of the impalement. A hand or power saw, an acetylene torch, or bolt cutters might be employed. Whatever tools and techniques are used, be sure to take steps to limit the heat, vibration, or jolting transmitted to the patient. Provide the best possible support for both the object and the patient during the cutting procedure.

There are some special circumstances in which you *should* remove an impaled object. For example, you may remove an object impaled in the cheek if the removal is necessary to maintain a patent airway (Figure 20-25). In this case, be prepared to apply direct pressure to the wound both from inside the cheek (intraorally) and externally.

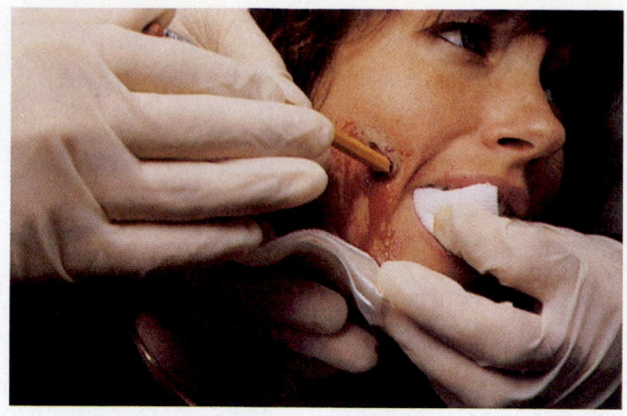

FIGURE 20-25 Objects impaled in the cheek may be removed because the sites of hemorrhage can be controlled and the object may interfere with airway control.

Only remove impaled objects that obstruct the airway or prevent CPR.

Another object that would require removal is one impaled in the central chest of a patient who needs CPR. In such a circumstance, the risk associated with not performing resuscitation outweighs the risk of removing the object. Be aware, however, that a trauma patient who needs CPR has a very poor prognosis.

Another complication associated with an impaled object occurs when a patient is impaled on an object that cannot be cut or moved. In such a case, contact medical direction for advice and guidance. If the object is impaled in a limb, bleeding may be controllable. If it has entered the head, neck, chest, or abdomen, it may not be.

Crush Syndrome

The key to successful prehospital management of a crush syndrome patient is anticipation of the problem and prevention of its effects. Since, by definition, all crush syndrome patients are victims of prolonged entrapment, cases can be identified before extrication is complete. The focus of prehospital crush injury care is on rapid transport, adequate fluid resuscitation, diuresis, and—possibly—systemic alkalinization.

The prehospital approach to crush syndrome is similar to that with other trauma patients. Assuring scene safety is particularly important in these cases. Crush syndrome victims are often buried in heavy rubble or other large debris, and access may be difficult (Figure 20-26). You may need to request the assistance of specialized personnel and their equipment—urban search and rescue teams, or trench, heavy, or confined space rescue teams. Never place yourself or other rescuers in unreasonable danger when providing care or attempting a rescue.

Once the scene is safe and you can reach the patient, conduct an initial assessment. Remove debris from around the head, neck, and thorax to minimize airway

FIGURE 20-26 Explosion and structural collapse frequently produce crush injury and crush syndrome.

obstruction and restriction of ventilation. Control any reachable and obvious bleeding. Perform as much of the initial and rapid trauma assessment as possible, keeping in mind that portions of the patient's body will be inaccessible as a result of the entrapment. The dark, dusty, and cramped conditions of many confined space rescues may force you to improvise. Be alert for signs and symptoms of associated injuries such as dust inhalation, dehydration, and hypothermia.

Remember that the greater the body area compressed and the longer the time of entrapment, the greater the risk of crush syndrome. Initially, a trapped patient will usually complain only of entrapment symptoms: pain, lack of motor function, tingling, or loss of sensation in the affected limb. The patient may also experience flaccid paralysis and sensory loss in the limb unrelated to the normal distribution of peripheral nerve control and sensation.

As long as the body part is still trapped and the metabolic byproducts of the crush injury are confined to the entrapped part, the patient will not experience the full effects of crush syndrome. With extrication, however, toxic byproducts are released into the circulation, and the patient may rapidly develop shock and die. If the patient survives the initial release of the byproducts, he remains at great risk of developing renal failure with serious morbidity or delayed death. Note, too, that a crush injury may also induce compartment syndrome (explained below), especially with prolonged entrapment.

Once you have assured the patient's ABCs, turn your attention to obtaining IV access. Intravenous fluids and selected medications are important in treating crush syndrome. Initiate two large-bore IVs if possible. Because of the entrapment, it may be necessary to consider alternative IV sites such as the external jugular vein or the veins of a lower extremity. Avoid any site distal to a crush injury.

When you encounter crush syndrome, it is unlikely that your protocols will address it. Contact the trauma center for medical direction and communicate, on-line, with the emergency physician. Expect to provide frequent vital sign and patient updates, and be prepared to administer large fluid volumes and, possibly, alkalizing agents.

Infuse 1,000 to 1,500 mL (20-30 mL/kg) of normal saline or, more ideally, 5 percent dextrose in 1/2 normal saline, even in a patient not yet showing signs of shock. Avoid lactated Ringer's or other solutions containing potassium. Then, infuse solution at a rate of 1,000 mL/hr (20 mL/Kg/hr) for as long as the patient remains trapped (up to 12 L in 24 hours). Continue this infusion rate until the patient reaches the hospital. As with all patients receiving large volumes of crystalloids, periodically query the patient for symptoms of shortness of breath and auscultate the lungs for evidence of pulmonary edema (e.g., crackles). Stop or reduce the fluid flow rate if you suspect pulmonary edema. In young, healthy adults and children, this rarely occurs at the fluid flow rates described here.

Alkalinization of the blood and urine is a consideration for preventing and treating crush syndrome. In combination with fluid resuscitation, alkalinization can correct acidosis, help prevent renal failure, and help correct hyperkalemia. Administer sodium bicarbonate 1 mEq/kg initially, followed by 0.25 mEq/kg/hr thereafter. It is preferable to add the bicarbonate to the normal saline bag rather than administering it as a bolus or IV push.

Note: The milliequivalent (mEq) is a means of measuring electrolytes in a standard solution and is based upon the molecular weight of the electrolyte in question.

Diuretics may help keep the kidneys well perfused and more resistant to failure during crush syndrome. Mannitol, an osmotic diuretic, is the drug of choice as it draws interstitial fluid into the vascular space and eliminates it as mannitol is excreted by the kidneys. Furosemide, a loop diuretic, inhibits the reabsorption of both sodium and chloride. Its use is not advisable in hypovolemic states because it may add to the electrolyte imbalance.

Consider applying a tourniquet before the entrapping pressure is released if you have been unable to medicate the patient and provide fluid resuscitation. The tourniquet will sequester the toxins and prevent reperfusion injury. Tourniquet use, however, will continue the development of crush syndrome and worsen its effects.

In cases where the entrapping object may not be moved for many hours or days, medical direction may consider field amputation. This operation will likely be performed by a physician responding to the scene but, in dire circumstances, may be performed by a paramedic under the on-line direction of the emergency physician.

Cardiac (ECG) monitoring is important with all crush syndrome patients. Dysrhythmias may develop at any time but are most likely to occur immediately following the release of pressure upon extrication. Sudden cardiac arrest should be treated in the usual fashion with defibrillation and cardiac drugs as appropriate. Consider 500 mg calcium chloride IV push (in addition to the sodium bicarbonate) to counteract life-threatening dysrhythmias induced by hyperkalemia. Watch for the tenting, or peaking, of the T-wave, a prolonged P-R interval, and S-T segment depression. Be sure to flush the IV line between infusions or to use different lines because calcium chloride and sodium bicarbonate precipitate.

Once the patient is freed from entrapment, be prepared to treat rapidly progressing shock. Continue the normal saline infusions at 30 mL/kg/hr and provide additional boluses of sodium bicarbonate as needed. Rapidly transport the patient to an appropriate hospital (usually a trauma center) for all cases of suspected crush syndrome.

Prehospital care of the crushed limb or body parts requires no special techniques. Cover open wounds and splint fractures, keeping in mind that progressive swelling will necessitate ongoing reassessment, with monitoring of distal circulation and the tightness of bandages, straps, and splints. Handle all crushed limbs gently because the ischemic tissue is prone to injury. Elevation of severely crushed extremities is not indicated in the prehospital setting.

Care at the hospital for crush injury is aggressive and may use techniques such as debridement and hyperbaric oxygenation. During hyperbaric oxygenation, the patient is placed in a chamber with artificially high concentrations of oxygen under several atmospheres of pressure. This drives oxygen into poorly oxygenated tissue to help with the destruction of anaerobic bacteria and to increase tissue oxygenation for repair and regeneration, ultimately reducing tissue necrosis and edema. Hyperbaric oxygenation is most effective when provided early in the course of care.

Hospital care for crush injuries also includes administration of several medications as well as hemodialysis to help salvage the kidneys from the ravages of myoglobin and other toxic agents. Allopurinol, a xanthine oxidase inhibitor, interferes with the production of uric acid, a byproduct of skeletal muscle destruction, and may help reperfusion of both the kidneys and the skeletal muscles. It is most effective if administered immediately before release of the compression. Amiloride hydrochloride is a potassium-sparing diuretic that inhibits the sodium/calcium exchange. Mannitol, tetanus toxoid, and prophylactic antibiotics may also be administered in the hospital to treat crush syndrome.

Compartment Syndrome

The most prominent symptom of compartment syndrome is severe pain, often out of proportion to the physical findings. Other signs are often subtle or absent, or they may be overshadowed by the original injury such as a fracture or contusion. Some people suggest using the six Ps—pain, paresthesia, paresis, pressure, passive stretching pain, pulselessness—to identify compartment syndrome, but many of these signs are not dependable or they appear very late in the course of the injury. (Passive stretching pain is pain or an increase in pain noted by a patient as a muscle is extended by a care provider.) Motor and sensory functions are usually normal with compartment syndrome, as are distal pulses. Even capillary refill shows little change. It is important to note that compartment syndrome rarely occurs within the first 4 hours after an acute injury. It is more likely to appear 6 to 8 hours (or as much as a day or more) after the initial injury. Recognition of compartment syndrome can be challenging and requires a healthy suspicion for the problem.

The first step in prehospital treatment for compartment syndrome is care of the underlying injury. Splint and immobilize all suspected fractures, and use traction as appropriate for femur fractures. Apply cold packs to severe contusions. Elevation of the affected extremity is the single most effective prehospital treatment for compartment syndrome. This reduces edema, increases venous return, lowers compartment pressure, and helps prevent ischemia. In the hospital, compartment syndrome is treated surgically, through a procedure that incises the restrictive fascia, a fasciectomy.

SPECIAL ANATOMICAL SITES

Several anatomic sites provide challenges to care of soft-tissue injuries. These include the face and neck, the thorax, and the abdomen.

Face and Neck

Soft-tissue injuries to the face and neck present potential challenges owing to the anatomical relationships of the airway and great vessels. Injuries to the face may result in blood and tissue debris in the airway, posing risks of airway obstruction, asphyxia, and aspiration (Figure 20-27). Pooled secretions and tissue edema may add to airway problems. Trauma to the face or neck may also distort the anatomical structures of the upper airway, leading to airway compromise, and complicating attempts at endotracheal intubation.

Emergency treatment of face and neck injuries can be challenging and may tax your skills. First, gain control of the airway. Open the airway using manual maneuvers. If you suspect the possibility of spinal injury, use the jaw-thrust maneuver in conjunction with in-line manual immobilization. Aggressively suction blood, saliva, and debris from the pharynx, but avoid stimulating the gag reflex in the patient or inducing emesis. Insert an oro- or nasopharyngeal airway as needed.

Visualized endotracheal intubation is the gold standard for securing the airway, but achieving it is fraught with complications in cases of face and neck trauma. Secretions and blood may prevent adequate visualization even with aggressive suctioning. Airway edema can distort the anatomy beyond recognition, and even prevent passage of the ET tube. In all cases, meticulous and absolute confirmation of tube placement is mandatory to avoid fatal hypoxia.

In desperate circumstances, needle or surgical cricothyrotomy may be lifesaving. Avoid placing the needle or making the incision through neck hematomas to avoid life-threatening bleeding.

FIGURE 20-27 Severe facial soft-tissue injuries may interfere with airway control and distort landmarks used for intubation.

Once you have secured the airway, focus your attention on any serious facial or neck bleeding. Direct pressure is usually successful for bleeding control, but be certain to avoid compressing or occluding the airway. Pressure points and tourniquets should not be used because of the risks they present of cerebral ischemia and strangulation. Open neck wounds also carry the danger of air aspiration and emboli. Cover any open neck wound with an occlusive dressing, which should then be held or bandaged firmly in place. Because of the neck's anatomy, you may have to maintain digital pressure throughout the course of prehospital care to assure effective bleeding control.

Thorax

Superficial soft-tissue injury to the thorax may suggest more serious intrathoracic injuries. The pleural space extends superiorly to the supraclavicular fossa and inferiorly to include the entire rib cage both anteriorly and posteriorly. Trauma to this area is likely to injure both the pleura and lungs. Small "lacerations" may actually be deep, penetrating stab or gunshot wounds with resultant hemothorax, pneumothorax, pericardial tamponade, penetrating heart trauma, or injury to the great vessels, esophagus, bronchi, or diaphragm. A seemingly minor "rib bruise" may be the only visible sign of serious lung or cardiac contusions beneath.

Never explore a thoracic open wound beyond its edges. Probing may create a pneumothorax or induce serious bleeding.

Perform a thorough physical examination to detect any signs of internal bleeding, pulmonary edema, dysrhythmias, or shock. However, never explore a thoracic wound beyond the skin edges. Probing deeper can convert a minor wound to a pneumothorax or a bleeding disaster. Consider all thoracic wounds to be potentially life threatening until evidence proves otherwise. See Chapter 25, "Thoracic Trauma," for detailed care procedures.

Dress all open thoracic wounds with sterile dressings in the usual fashion. Be alert, however, for the presence of air bubbling, subcutaneous emphysema, crepitus, or other hints of open pneumothorax. Be extremely cautious about making an airtight seal on any thoracic wound because doing so can rapidly lead to tension pneumothorax and death. Instead, use an occlusive dressing sealed on three sides and be prepared to assist ventilations. Auscultate the chest and monitor respirations frequently. Watch the occlusive dressing so that it does not seal with blood against the chest wall and convert a simple pneumothorax into a tension pneumothorax.

Watch any open chest wound for the development of a pneumothorax or tension pneumothorax.

Abdomen

The peritoneal cavity extends approximately from the symphysis pubis inferiorly to the diaphragm superiorly. Since the diaphragm rises and falls with respiration, so too does the border between the abdominal and thoracic cavities. You cannot know the exact position of the diaphragm at the time the injury occurred, so suspect associated injuries to both abdominal and thoracic organs if the soft-tissue injury involves the region between the rib margin and the 5th rib anteriorly, the 7th rib laterally, and the 9th rib posteriorly.

Blunt or penetrating trauma to the abdomen can injure both hollow and solid organs, penetrate or rupture the diaphragm, and cause serious internal bleeding. Anteriorly and just underlying the rib margin are the liver on the right and the spleen on the left. Posteriorly, the kidneys (not true abdominal organs since they lie retroperitoneally) are located in the costovertebral angle region. Hollow organs—the bowel, stomach and urinary bladder—may rupture. In addition to bleeding copiously, these organs may release their contents and inflame the peritoneum.

Consider any soft-tissue wound in the abdominal region as potentially damaging to the underlying organs. Signs and symptoms of internal damage can be subtle, particularly early on. Eviscerations and other massive injuries are obvious, but other internal injuries that are just as serious may not be apparent. Prehospital treatment is primarily supportive and includes assuring adequate oxygenation, preventing shock, and dressing open wounds (see Chapter 26, "Abdominal Trauma").

WOUNDS REQUIRING TRANSPORT

Transport any patient with a wound that involves a structure beneath the integument for emergency department evaluation. This includes wounds involving, or possibly involving, nerves, blood vessels, ligaments, tendons, or muscles. Also transport any patient with a significantly contaminated wound, a wound involving an impaled object, or a wound that was received in a particularly unclean environment. Also transport any patient with a wound with likely cosmetic implications, such as facial wounds or large gaping wounds.

SOFT-TISSUE TREATMENT AND REFER/RELEASE

In some EMS systems, paramedics are permitted to treat and release patients with minor and superficial soft-tissue injuries or treat and refer them to their personal physicians. This generally occurs under on-line medical direction or according to strict protocols.

In such circumstances, you must evaluate and dress the wound. Then explain to the patient the steps to follow for continuing care of the injury. Tell the patient of the need to change the dressing and to monitor the injury site for further hemorrhage or developing infection. Provide the patient with simple written instructions (approved and/or published by medical direction) explaining wound care, monitoring, protection, dressing change, cleansing, and the signs of problems such as infection or hemorrhage.

Instruct the patient to contact a physician if certain signs and symptoms appear and describe those signs and symptoms thoroughly. Assure that the patient has the means to obtain physician or health care provider follow-up and again stress the circumstances in which such follow-up care should be sought. During any referral or release, if the patient's tetanus immunization history is unclear or it has been longer than 5 years since the last immunization, instruct the patient to obtain a tetanus booster.

Document all refer/release incidents carefully in the prehospital care report. The report should include a description of the nature and extent of the wound and of the care provided for it. Note in the report all instructions and materials provided to the patient and any medical direction you received.

SUMMARY

Soft-tissue injury may compromise the skin—the envelope that protects and contains the human body. Any trauma must penetrate the skin before it can harm the interior organs and threaten life. Any damage to the skin may interfere with its ability to contain water and blood and to prevent damaging agents from entering. For these reasons, the assessment and care of soft-tissue injuries are important parts of prehospital care.

Assess wounds carefully since they may provide the only overt signs of serious internal injury. Realize that discoloration and swelling take time to develop and may not be as apparent in the field as when you present the patient at the emergency department. Look carefully for the early signs of wounds, and use the mechanism of injury to locate potential trauma sites. When caring for soft-tissue injuries, keep in mind the basic goals: controlling hemorrhage, keeping the wound as clean as possible, and immobilizing the injury site.

CHAPTER 21

Burns

Objectives

After reading this chapter, you should be able to:

1. Describe the anatomy and physiology of the skin and remaining human anatomy as they pertain to thermal burn injuries. (see Chapter 3)

2. Describe the epidemiology, including incidence, mortality, morbidity, and risk factors for thermal burn injuries as well as strategies to prevent such injuries. (p. 954)

3. Describe the local and systemic complications of a thermal burn injury. (pp. 954–956, 966–969)

4. Identify and describe the depth classifications of burn injuries, including superficial burns, partial-thickness burns, and full-thickness burns. (pp. 964–965)

5. Describe and apply the "rule of nines," and the "rule of palms" methods for determining body surface area percentage of a burn injury. (pp. 965–966)

6. Identify and describe the severity of a burn including a minor burn, a moderate burn, and a critical burn. (pp. 972–974)

7. Describe the effects age and pre-existing conditions have on burn severity and a patient's prognosis. (pp. 968, 973)

Continued

Objectives Continued

8. Discuss complications of burn injuries caused by trauma, blast injuries, airway compromise, respiratory compromise, and child abuse. (pp. 962–964, 969–971, 977–978)

9. Describe thermal burn management including considerations for airway and ventilation, circulation, pharmacological and non-pharmacological measures, transport decisions, and psychological support/communication strategies. (pp. 969–978)

10. Describe special considerations for a pediatric patient with a burn injury and describe the criteria for determining pediatric burn severity. (pp. 965–966, 968, 973)

11. Describe the specific epidemiologies, mechanisms of injury, pathophysiologies, and severity assessments for inhalation, chemical, and electrical burn injuries and for radiation exposure. (pp. 977–985)

12. Discuss special considerations that impact the assessment, management, and prognosis of patients with inhalation, chemical, and electrical burn injuries and with exposure to radiation. (pp. 977–985)

13. Differentiate between supraglottic and subglottic inhalation burn injuries. (pp. 962–963)

14. Describe the special considerations for a chemical burn injury to the eye. (p. 982)

15. Given several preprogrammed, simulated thermal, inhalation, electrical, and chemical burn injury and radiation exposure patients, provide the appropriate scene size-up, initial assessment, rapid trauma or focused physical exam and history, detailed exam, and ongoing assessment and provide appropriate patient care and transportation. (pp. 969–985)

INTRODUCTION TO BURN INJURIES

The incidence of burn injuries in the United States and other developed countries has been declining for several decades. Despite the decline, an estimated 1.25 to 2 million Americans are treated for burns annually and 50,000 are hospitalized. Some 3 to 5 percent of these burns are considered life threatening. Persons at greatest risk for serious burns include the very young and old, the infirm, and workers, such as firefighters, metal smelters, and chemical workers. Burn injuries remain the second leading cause of death in children under 12 years of age and the fourth overall cause of trauma death.

Much of the national decline in burn mortality is attributed to improved building codes, safer construction techniques, and the use of smoke detectors. Smaller but still important effects are attributed to educational campaigns aimed primarily at school children. Other simple and inexpensive measures that have helped prevent burns include keeping cigarette lighters and matches away from children and reducing household hot-water temperatures to below scalding levels.

Burns are a specific subset of soft-tissue injuries with a specific pathologic process. While the term "burn" suggests combustion, the actual process that produces burn injuries is much different. The human body is predominantly water and does not support combustion. Instead, body tissues change chemically, evaporating water and denaturing the proteins that make up cell membranes. The result can be widespread damage to the skin, or integumentary system.

Although the skin and its functions are often taken for granted, burn injury to this organ can subject a patient to severe fluid loss, infection, hypothermia, and other injuries.

PATHOPHYSIOLOGY OF BURNS

Burns result from the disruption of proteins in the cell membranes. Burns can be caused by several different mechanisms including thermal, electrical, chemical and radiation energies. Being able to understand the mechanism of a burn and to determine the degree and area of burn helps you assess the seriousness of the burn and thus guide your care.

Content Review

BASIC TYPES OF BURNS
Thermal
Electrical
Chemical
Radiation

TYPES OF BURNS

Soft-tissue burns occur secondary to thermal (heat), electrical, chemical, or radiation insults to the body. While the resulting burns are much the same, the damage process differs with the various mechanisms. The following sections describe each of these four types of burns.

Thermal Burns

A thermal burn causes damage by increasing the rate at which the molecules within an object move and collide with each other. We measure the energy of this molecular motion as temperature. At a temperature greater than absolute zero, the molecules of any object move about. As the object's temperature increases, so does the speed of the molecules and the incidences of their collisions with other molecules. These changes in internal energy cause many substances—for example, steel—to expand with increasing temperature. Heat energy may also cause chemical changes. As temperature increases, substances such as gasoline may combine with oxygen. The nature of matter may change as well. Water, for example, may change into ice (with decreasing heat energy) or steam (with increasing heat energy). An egg changes its nature as the proteins break down, or **denature**, in a hot frying pan. This is why cooked eggs have a rubbery consistency.

Similar changes also take place in burned tissue. As molecular speed increases, the cell components, especially membranes and proteins, begin to break down just like the egg in a frying pan. The result of exposure to extreme heat is progressive injury and cell death.

The extent of burn injury relates to the amount of heat energy transferred to the patient's skin. The amount of that heat energy in turn depends upon three components of the burning agent: its temperature, the concentration of heat energy it possesses, and the length of its contact time with the patient's skin.

Obviously, the greater the temperature of an agent, the greater the potential for damage. However, it is also important to consider the amount of heat energy possessed by the object or substance. Receiving a blast of heated air from an oven at 350°F is much less damaging than contact with hot cooking oil at the same temperature. In general, water, oils, and other liquids have a fairly high heat energy content. This content is roughly related to the density of the material. In a similar fashion, solids also usually have a high heat content. Gases, on the other hand, usually have less capacity to hold heat owing to their less dense nature.

Duration of exposure to the heat source is also obviously important in determining the severity of a burn. A patient's momentary contact with hot oil would result in less damage than if the oil were poured into his or her shoe.

A burn is a progressive process, and the greater the heat energy transmitted to the body, the deeper the wound. Initially, the burn damages the epidermis by the increase in temperature. As contact with the substance continues, heat energy penetrates further and deeper into the body tissue. Thus, a burn may involve the epidermis, dermis, and subcutaneous tissue as well as muscles, bone, and other internal tissue.

At the level of local tissues, thermal burns cause a number of effects collectively termed **Jackson's theory of thermal wounds.** This theory helps us understand the physical effects of high heat and helps explain a number of clinical effects (Figure 21-1).

With a burn, the skin nearest the heat source suffers the most profound changes. Cell membranes rupture and are destroyed, blood coagulates, and structural proteins denature. This most damaged area is the **zone of coagulation.** If the zone of coagulation penetrates the dermis, the resulting injury is termed a full-thickness or third degree burn. Adjacent to this area is a less damaged yet still inflamed region where blood flow decreases that is called the **zone of stasis.** More distant from the burn source is a broader area where inflammation and changes in blood flow are limited. This is the **zone of hyperemia;** this zone accounts for the erythema (redness) associated with some burns.

Large burns have profound pathological effects on the body as a whole. In general, these effects are important in any burn that covers more than 15 to 20 percent of the patient's body surface area. To understand these effects and the resulting burn shock, you must first learn a little about the progression of burns.

The body's response to burns occurs over time and can usefully be classified into four stages. The first stage occurs immediately following the burn and is called the **emergent phase.** This is the body's initial reaction to the burn. This phase includes a pain response as well as the outpouring of catecholamines in response to the pain and the physical and emotional stress. During this stage, the patient displays tachycardia, tachypnea, mild hypertension, and mild anxiety.

✳ **denature** alter the usual substance of something.

✳ **Jackson's theory of thermal wounds** explanation of the physical effects of thermal burns.

Content Review

EFFECTS OF HEAT ACCORDING TO JACKSON'S THEORY OF THERMAL WOUNDS

Zone of coagulation—most damaged area nearest heat source; cell membranes rupture and are destroyed, blood coagulates, structural proteins denature

Zone of stasis—adjacent to most-damaged region; inflammation present, blood flow decreased

Zone of hyperemia—area farthest from heat source; limited inflammation and changes in blood flow

✳ **zone of coagulation** area in a burn nearest the heat source that suffers the most damage and is characterized by clotted blood and thrombosed blood vessels.

✳ **zone of stasis** area in a burn surrounding the zone of coagulation and that is characterized by decreased blood flow.

✳ **zone of hyperemia** area peripheral to a burn that is characterized by increased blood flow.

✳ **emergent phase** first stage of the burn process that is characterized by a catecholamine release and pain mediated reaction.

Zone of hyperemia

Zone of stasis

Zone of coagulation

Epidermis

Dermis

Subcutaneous tissue

FIGURE 21-1 The zones of injury commonly caused by a thermal burn.

The **fluid shift phase** follows the initial phase and can last for up to 18 to 24 hours. The fluid shift phase begins shortly after the burn and reaches its peak in 6 to 8 hours. You are therefore likely to see it in the prehospital setting. In this phase, damaged cells release agents that initiate an inflammatory response in the body. This increases blood flow to the capillaries surrounding the burn and increases the permeability of the capillaries to fluid. The response results in a large shift of fluid away from the **intravascular space** into the **extravascular space** (massive edema). Note that the capillaries leak fluid (water, electrolytes, and some dissolved proteins) and not blood cells. Blood loss from burns uncomplicated by other trauma is usually minimal.

After the fluid shift phase comes the **hypermetabolic phase,** which may last for many days or weeks depending on the burn severity. This phase is characterized by a large increase in the body's demands for nutrients as it begins the long process of repairing damaged tissue. Gradually this phase evolves into the **resolution phase,** in which scar tissue is laid down and remodeled, and the burn patient begins to rehabilitate and return to normal function.

Electrical Burns

Electricity's power is the result of an electron flow from a point of high concentration to one of low concentration. The difference between the two concentrations is called the **voltage.** It is helpful to envision voltage as the "pressure" of the electric flow. The rate or the amount of flow in a given time is termed the **current** and is measured in **amperes.**

Another factor that affects the flow of electricity is **resistance.** Resistance is measured in **ohms.** Copper electrical wire has very little resistance and allows a free flow of electrons. Tungsten (the filament in a light bulb) is moderately resistant and heats, glows, and emits light as more and more current is applied to it.

The relationship between current (I), resistance (R), and voltage (V) is well known as **Ohm's law:**

$$V = IR \text{ or } I = V/R$$

Like tungsten, the internal parts of the human body are moderately resistant to the flow of electricity. The skin, on the other hand, is highly resistant to electrical flow. Moisture or sweat on the skin lowers this resistance. If the human body is subjected to voltage, the body initially resists the flow. If the voltage is strong enough, the current begins to pass into and through the body. As it does, heat energy is created. The heat produced is proportional to the square of the current flow and is related to power, P, as expressed in **Joule's law:**

$$P = I^2R$$

The highest heat occurs at the points of greatest resistance, often at the skin. This accounts for the severe "entry" and "exit" wounds sometimes seen in electrical injuries. Dry, callused skin can have enormous resistance values, ranging from 500,000 to 1,000,000 ohms/cm. Wet skin, particularly the thin skin on the palm side of the arm or on the inner thigh can have values as low as 300 to 10,000 ohms/cm. Mucous membranes have very low resistance (100 ohms/cm) and allow even small currents to pass. This accounts for the relative ease with which household current can cause lip and oral burns in children who accidentally bite electrical cords (Figure 21-2).

With small currents, the heat energy produced is of little consequence. But if the voltage or current is high, profound body damage can occur. The longer the duration of contact, the greater the potential for injury. Electrical burns can be particularly damaging because the burn heats the victim from the inside out, causing great damage to internal organs and structures while possibly leaving little visible damage on the surface, save for the entry and exit wounds (Figure 21-3).

Thermal injury due to electrical current occurs as energy travels from the point of contact to the point of exit. At both these points, the concentration of electricity is great, as is the degree of damage you might expect. The smaller the area of contact, the greater the concentration of current flow and the greater the injury. Between the entrance and exit points, the energy spreads out over a larger cross-sectional area and generally causes less injury. Electrical current may follow blood vessels and nerves because they offer less resistance than muscle and

* **Ohm's law** the physical law identifying that the current in an electrical circuit is directly proportional to the voltage and inversely proportional to the resistance.

* **Joule's law** the physical law that the rate of heat production is directly proportional to the resistance of the circuit and to the square of the current.

Electrical burns can be particularly damaging because the current burns the victim from the inside out.

a. Entrance wound.

b. Exit wound.

FIGURE 21-3   Injuries due to electrical shock.

bone. This may lead to serious vascular and nervous injury deep within the involved limbs or body cavity.

Electrical contact also interferes with control of muscle tissue. The passage of current, especially alternating current, severely disrupts the complicated electrochemical reactions that control muscles. If contact with a current as small as 20 to 50 milliamperes (mA) is maintained for a period of time, the muscles of respiration may be immobilized. The result is prolonged respiratory arrest, anoxia, hypoxemia, and—eventually—death. Electrical currents greater than 50 mA may also disrupt the heart's electrical system, causing ventricular fibrillation accompanied by ineffective pumping action. Alternating electrical current such as that found in household current can also cause tetanic convulsions or uncontrolled contractions of muscles. If the victim is holding a wire at such a time, the victim may be unable to let go, thereby prolonging the exposure and increasing the severity of injury. This can occur with as little as 9 mA of current.

Electrical injury may also disrupt muscular and other tissue, leading to its degeneration. As the tissue dies, it releases materials toxic to the human body. These materials may damage the liver and kidneys, leading to failure.

At times, electrical energy may cause flash burns secondary to the heat of current passing through adjacent air. Air is very resistant to the passage of electrical current. If the current is strong enough and the space through which it passes is small, the electricity arcs, producing tremendous heat. If the patient's skin is close by, the heat may severely burn or vaporize tissue. In addition, the heat may ignite articles of clothing or other combustibles and produce thermal burns.

Chemical Burns

Chemical burns denature the biochemical makeup of cell membranes and destroy the cells. Such injuries are not transmitted through the tissue as are thermal injuries. Instead, a chemical burn must destroy the tissue before it can chemically burn any deeper. This fact generally limits the "burn" process unless very strong chemicals are involved (Figure 21-4). Agents that can cause chemical burns are too numerous to mention. However, the most common causes of these burns are either strong acids or bases (alkalis).

Both acids and alkalis burn by disrupting cell membranes and damaging tissues on contact. As they cause damage, acids usually form a thick, insoluble mass, or coagulum, at the point of contact. This process is called **coagulation necrosis** and helps to limit the depth of acid burns. Alkalis, however, do not form a protective coagulum. Instead, the alkali continues to destroy cell membranes,

FIGURE 21-4 A chemical burn to the ear.

releasing the intercellular and interstitial fluid, destroying tissue in a process called **liquefaction necrosis**. This process allows the alkali to rapidly penetrate the underlying tissue, causing progressively deeper burns. For this reason, alkali burns can be quite serious.

Radiation Injury

Nuclear radiation has bombarded Earth since long before recorded time. It is a daily, natural phenomenon. Radiation becomes a danger when people are exposed to synthetic sources that greatly increase the intensity of radiation. Medicine and industry use radioactive materials for diagnostic testing and treatment and for energy production. Deaths from exposure to radiation are extremely rare as are serious injuries because of the safety measures commonly used with the handling of nuclear materials. The risk of injury comes from accidents associated with improper handling, either in the on-site environment or during transport. In addition, the possibility of large-scale exposure to radiation from terrorist acts is considered to be increasing.

Nuclear radiation causes damage through a process known as **ionization**. A radioactive energy particle travels into a substance and changes an internal atom (Figure 21-5). In the human body, the affected cell either repairs the damage, dies, or goes on to produce damaged cells (cancer). The cells most sensitive to radiation injury are the cells that reproduce most quickly, like those responsible for erythrocyte, leukocyte, and platelet production (bone marrow), cells lining the intestinal tract, and cells involved in human reproduction.

We commonly encounter four types of radiation. These are:

- *Alpha Radiation* The nucleus of an atom releases **alpha radiation** in the form of a small helium nucleus. Alpha radiation is a very weak energy source and can travel only inches through the air. Paper or clothing can easily stop alpha radiation. This radiation also cannot penetrate the epidermis. On the subatomic scale, however, alpha particles are massive and can cause great damage over the short distance they travel. Alpha radiation is only a significant hazard if the patient inhales or ingests contaminated material, thus bringing the source in close proximity to sensitive respiratory and digestive tract tissue.

✱ **liquefaction necrosis** the process in which an alkali dissolves and liquefies tissue.

✱ **ionization** the process of changing a substance into separate charged particles (ions).

✱ **alpha radiation** low level form of nuclear radiation; a weak source of energy that is stopped by clothing or the first layers of skin.

Content Review

TYPES OF RADIATION

Alpha—very weak, stopped by paper, clothing, or the epidermis

Beta—more powerful than alpha; can travel 6-10 feet through air; can penetrate some clothing and the first few millimeters of skin

Gamma—most powerful ionizing radiation; great penetrating power; protection requires thick concrete or lead shielding

Neutron—great penetrating power, but uncommon outside nuclear reactors and bombs

TYPES OF RADIATION

Alpha
Beta
Gamma

DISTANCE

An object at twice
the distance from the source
receives one-fourth the amount of exposure

TIME (EXAMPLE SHOWS 300 r/hr)

FIGURE 21-5   The injury considerations associated with nuclear radiation.

* **beta radiation** medium-strength radiation that is stopped with light clothing or the uppermost layers of skin.

• *Beta Radiation* A second type of radiological particle produces **beta radiation.** Its energy is greater than that of alpha radiation. However, the beta particle is relatively lightweight, with the mass of an electron. Beta radiation can travel 6 to 10 feet through air and can penetrate a few layers of clothing. Beta particles can invade the first few millimeters of skin and thus have the potential for causing external as well as internal injury.

- *Gamma Radiation* **Gamma radiation,** also known as x-rays, is the most powerful type of ionizing radiation. It has the ability to travel through the entire body or ionize any atom within. Its lack of mass or charge (it is pure electromagnetic energy) helps give it great penetrating power. Gamma radiation evokes the greatest concern for external exposure. It is the most dangerous and most feared type of radiation because it is difficult to protect against. Many feet of concrete or many inches of lead are needed to protect against the highest-energy gamma rays. Fortunately, exposure to high-energy gamma rays occurs only in individuals who are exposed to nuclear blasts, are near the cores of nuclear reactors, or are very close to highly radioactive materials. More modest amounts of concrete, steel, or lead can provide shielding from the more common and lower-energy x-rays and gamma rays.

- *Neutron Radiation* Neutrons are small, yet moderately massive subatomic particles with no charge. Their small size and lack of charge account for their great penetrating power. Fortunately, strong **neutron radiation** is uncommon outside of nuclear reactors and bombs.

Exposure to radiation and the effects of ionization can occur through two mechanisms. In the first, an unshielded person is directly exposed to a strong radioactive source, for example, an unstable material such as uranium. The second mechanism of exposure is contamination by dust, debris, or fluids that contain very small particles of radioactive material. These contaminants give off weaker radiation than a direct radioactive source like uranium. However, the close proximity of these contaminants to the body and their longer contact times with it may result in greater exposure and contamination. Note that most substances, including human tissue, do not give off radiation. The patient himself is not the danger in a radiological exposure incident. Any danger comes from the radioactive source such as the contaminated material on the patient.

Three factors are important to keep in mind whenever you are called to incidents of radiation exposure. They include the duration of exposure, the distance from the radioactive source; and the shielding between you, the patient, and the source. Knowledge of these three factors can limit your exposure and potential for injury.

- *Duration.* Radiation exposure is an accumulative danger. The longer you or the patient remain exposed to the source, the greater the potential for injury.

- *Distance.* Radiation strength diminishes quickly as you travel farther from the source. The effect is similar to that of a light bulb's intensity. At a few feet, you can easily read by it, while at a few hundred feet the light barely casts a shadow. Mathematically, the relationship is inverse and squared. As you double your distance from the radioactive source, its strength drops to one fourth. As you triple the distance, its strength diminishes to one ninth, and so on.

- *Shielding.* The more material between you and the source, the less radioactive exposure you experience. With alpha and beta radiation, shielding is very easy to provide and reasonably effective. With gamma and neutron sources, dense objects such as earth, concrete, metal, and lead are needed to provide any real protection.

Radiation exposure is measured with a Geiger counter, while cumulative exposure is recorded by a device called a dosimeter. They record units of radiation expressed as either the **rad** or the **Gray** (Gy), with 1 Gray equal to 100 rads.

✱ **gamma radiation** powerful electromagnetic radiation emitted by radioactive substances with powerful penetrating properties; it is stronger than alpha and beta radiation.

✱ **neutron radiation** powerful radiation with penetrating properties between that of beta and gamma radiation.

Content Review

FACTORS AFFECTING EXPOSURE TO RADIATION
Duration of exposure
Distance from the source
Shielding from the source

✱ **rad** basic unit of absorbed radiation dose.

✱ **Gray** a unit of absorbed radiation dose equal to 100 rads.

Different tissues are sensitive to different levels of absorbed radiation. As little as 0.2 Gy can cause cataracts in exposed eyes and damage the blood-cell-producing bone marrow (also called hematopoietic) tissue. The radiation dose that is lethal to about 50 percent of exposed individuals is approximately 4.5 Gy.

With whole body exposure, and as the radiation dose increases, the signs and symptoms of exposure appear earlier and become more severe. The first signs of serious exposure are slight nausea and fatigue, occurring between 4 and 24 hours after exposure. As the radiation dose moves into the lethal range, the severity of the nausea increases and is joined by anorexia, vomiting, diarrhea, and malaise. Erythema of the skin may be present, and fatigue becomes more intense. These signs appear within 2 to 6 hours. With exposure to even higher, fatal doses, the patient displays all the signs of radiation exposure almost immediately and soon thereafter experiences confusion, watery diarrhea, and physical collapse. Note that the signs and symptoms of radiation exposure and the injuries associated with it vary because individual sensitivity to radiation exposure varies greatly.

Prolonged exposure to even small amounts of radiation may produce long-term and delayed problems. Infertility is a potential injury, because the cells producing eggs and sperm are very susceptible to ionization damage. Cancer is another delayed and severe side effect. It may occur years or even decades after a radiation exposure.

Inhalation Injury

Inhalation injury may be associated with burns, especially if the injury occurred in an enclosed space.

The burn environment frequently produces inhalation injury. This is especially true if the patient is in a closed space or is unconscious. A patient who is unconscious or trapped in a smoke-filled area eventually inhales gases, heated air, flames, or steam. The inhalation results in airway and respiratory injury.

You can expect to find the following inhalation conditions in a burn environment (Figure 21-6). Keep them in mind as you survey the scene and take the necessary protective measures.

Toxic Inhalation Modern residential and commercial construction uses synthetic resins and plastics that release toxic gases as they burn. Combustion of these materials can form such toxic agents as compounds of cyanide and hydrogen sulfide. If a patient inhales these gases, the gases react with the lung tissue, causing internal chemical burns, or they diffuse across the alveolar-capillary membrane and enter the bloodstream, causing systemic poisoning. The signs and symptoms of these injuries may present immediately following exposure or their onset may be delayed for an hour or two after inhalation. Toxic inhalation injury occurs more frequently than thermal inhalation burns.

Suspect carbon monoxide poisoning in any patient who was in an enclosed space during combustion.

Carbon Monoxide Poisoning An additional concern associated with the burn environment is carbon monoxide (CO) poisoning. Suspect it in any patient who has been within an enclosed space during combustion. Carbon monoxide is created during incomplete combustion, like that which may occur with a faulty heating unit or when someone tries to heat a room with an unvented device like a barbecue grill. Poisoning occurs because carbon monoxide has an affinity for hemoglobin more than 200 times greater than oxygen. If your patient inhales carbon monoxide, even in the smallest quantities, the carbon monoxide displaces oxygen in the hemoglobin and remains there for hours. The result is hypoxemia. Hypoxemia, which is difficult to detect, subtly compromises the delivery of oxygen to the patient's vital organs. If carbon monoxide inhalation is associated with airway burns, the respiratory compromise will be further compounded.

Airway Thermal Burn Another, though less frequent, injury is the airway thermal burn. Very moist mucosa lines the airway and helps insulate it against heat damage. Because of this mucosa, **supraglottic,** or upper airway, structures may absorb the

* **supraglottic** referring to the upper airway.

Extreme heat
Carbon monoxide
Toxic gases

Airway burns from thermal injuries, toxic gases.
Systemic poisoning from CO, cyanide, other toxic gases.

FIGURE 21-6   Hazards of fire in an enclosed environment.

heat and prevent lower airway burns. High levels of thermal energy are required to evaporate the fluid and injure the cells. Inspiration of hot air or flame rarely produces enough heat to cause significant thermal burns to the lower airway.

Superheated steam has greater heat content than hot, dry air and can cause **subglottic,** or lower airway, burns. Superheated steam is created under great pressure and can have a temperature well above 212°F. A common hazard to firefighters, superheated steam develops when a stream of water strikes a hot spot and vaporizes explosively. The blast can dislodge the mask of a firefighter's self-contained breathing apparatus, exposing him or her to superheated steam inhalation. The steam contains enough heat energy to severely burn the upper airway. It also may damage the lower respiratory tract, although this happens less frequently.

Risk factors for inhalation injuries associated with burns include standing in the burn environment (hot gases rise), screaming or yelling there (the open glottis allows toxic gases to enter the lower airway), and being trapped in a closed burn environment.

* subglottic referring to the lower airway.

Superheated steam is a common cause of airway burns.

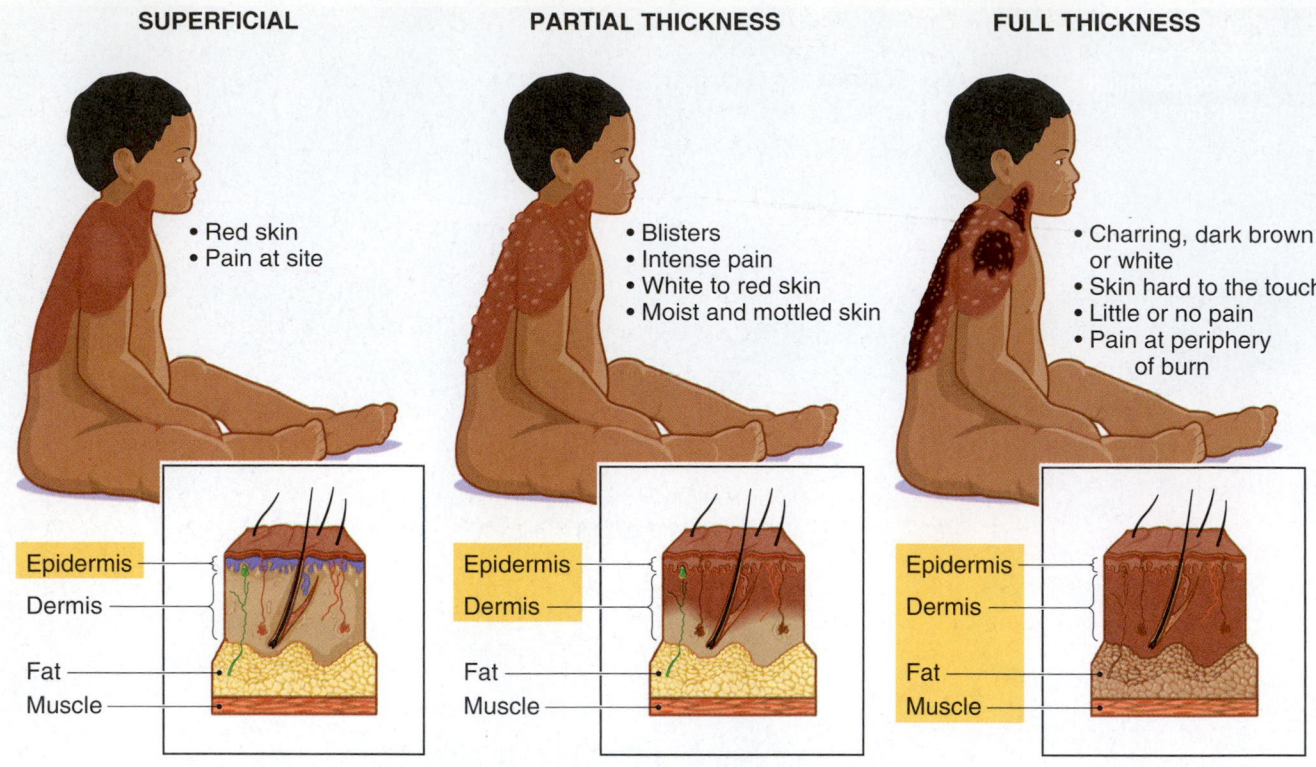

SUPERFICIAL
- Red skin
- Pain at site

PARTIAL THICKNESS
- Blisters
- Intense pain
- White to red skin
- Moist and mottled skin

FULL THICKNESS
- Charring, dark brown or white
- Skin hard to the touch
- Little or no pain
- Pain at periphery of burn

Epidermis
Dermis
Fat
Muscle

FIGURE 21-7 Classification of burns by depth.

With any thermal or smoke-related chemical burn injury to the respiratory tract, there is the danger of airway restriction, severe dyspnea, and possible respiratory arrest. The airway is a narrow tube, lined with extremely vascular tissue. If damaged, this tissue swells rapidly, seriously reducing the size of the airway lumen. The patient presents with minor hoarseness, followed precipitously by dyspnea. Stridor or high-pitched "crowing" sounds on inspiration are ominous signs of impending airway obstruction. Other clues leading you to suspect potential airway burns include singed facial and nasal hair, black-tinged (carbonaceous) sputum, and facial burns. The airway injury may be so extensive as to induce complete respiratory obstruction and arrest. Accurate assessment is important because 20 to 35 percent of patients admitted to burn centers and some 60 to 70 percent of burn patients who die have an associated inhalation injury.

DEPTH OF BURN

After you determine the burn source and assess the possibility of associated inhalation injury, you need to assess the burn's severity. One element in determining the severity of a burn is the depth of damage it causes. Depth of burn damage is normally classified into three categories (Figure 21-7).

Superficial Burn

* **superficial burn** a burn that involves only the epidermis; characterized by reddening of the skin; also called a first-degree burn.

The **superficial burn,** also termed a first-degree burn, involves only the epidermis. It is an irritation of the living cells in this region and results in some pain, minor edema, and erythema. It normally heals without complication.

Partial Thickness Burn

The **partial thickness burn,** also termed a second-degree burn, penetrates slightly deeper than a superficial burn and produces blisters. Heat energy travels into the dermis, involving more of the tissue and resulting in greater destruction. The partial thickness burn is similar to a superficial burn in that it is reddened, painful, and edematous. You can differentiate it from the superficial burn only after blisters form. Because there are many nerve endings in the dermis, both superficial and partial thickness burns are often very painful. With both superficial and partial thickness burns, the dermis is still intact and complete skin regeneration is very likely.

The sunburn is a common, but specialized type of burn. Ultraviolet radiation causes the burn rather than normal thermal processes. The radiation penetrates superficially and damages the uppermost layers of the dermis. Sunburn can present as either a superficial or partial thickness burn.

Another similar type of burn occurs as someone watches an arc welder without proper protection. The lens of the eye focuses the high-intensity ultraviolet light on the retina, where it burns the tissue. This results in delayed eye pain and, possibly, transient blindness.

Full Thickness Burn

The **full thickness,** or third-degree, **burn,** penetrates both the epidermis and the dermis and extends into the subcutaneous layers or even deeper, into muscles, bones, and internal organs. These burns destroy the tissue's regenerative properties and the peripheral nerve endings. The injury is painless because of the nerve destruction, but the margins of the full thickness burn are frequently partial thickness burns, which can be quite painful. The full thickness burn takes on various colorations depending on the nature of the burning agent and the damaged, dying, or dead tissue. They can be white, brown, or a charred color and typically have a dry, leather-like appearance. Because the burn destroys the entire dermis, healing is difficult unless the wound is small or skin grafting is possible.

BODY SURFACE AREA

Another factor affecting burn severity is how much of a person's **body surface area** (BSA) the burn involves. There are two approaches to estimating the BSA involved in a burn. The first, the rule of nines, is useful in estimating large burn areas. The second method, the rule of palms, is helpful in assessing smaller wounds more accurately.

Rule of Nines

The **rule of nines** identifies 11 topographical adult body regions, each of which approximates 9 percent of the patient's BSA (Figure 21-8). These regions include the entire head and neck; the anterior chest; the anterior abdomen; the posterior chest; the lower back (the posterior abdomen); the anterior surface of each lower extremity; the posterior surface of each lower extremity; and each upper extremity. The genitalia make up the remaining 1 percent of BSA.

Because infant and child anatomy differs significantly from that of adults, you modify the rule of nines to maintain an accurate approximation of BSA. Divide the head and neck area into the anterior and posterior surface and award 9 percent for each. Reduce the surface area of each lower extremity by 4 1/2 percent to ensure the total body surface area remains at 100 percent. The rule of nines is at best an approximation of the area burned. It is, however, an expedient and useful tool to help measure the burn's extent.

* **partial thickness burn** burn in which the epidermis is burned through and the dermis is damaged; characterized by redness and blistering; also called a second-degree burn.

Content Review

DEPTH OF BURN

Superficial (1st degree)—
involves only the
epidermis; produces pain,
minor edema, and
erythema (redness)
Partial thickness
(2nd degree)—involves
epidermis and dermis;
produces pain, edema,
erythema, blisters
Full thickness (3rd degree)—
involves all skin layers and
possibly structures
beneath; painless, but
tissue is destroyed; white,
brown, or charred,
leather-like appearance

* **full thickness burn** burn that damages all layers of the skin; characterized by areas that are white and dry; also called third-degree burn.

* **body surface area** (BSA) amount of a patient's body affected by a burn.

* **rule of nines** method of estimating amount of body surface area burned by a division of the body into regions, each of which represents approximately 9 percent of total BSA (plus 1 percent for the genital region).

THE RULE OF NINES

Head and neck 9%

Upper back 9%

Anterior chest 9%

Each upper extremity 9%

Anterior abdomen 9%

Lower back 9%

External genitalia 1%

Each anterior lower extremity 9%

Each posterior lower extremity 9%

Genitalia   9%

13.5%

1%

13.5%   9%/9%

9%/9%

9%

Posterior trunk 9%/9%

FIGURE 21-8   The rule of nines.

FIGURE 21-9   Using the rule of palms, the surface of the patient's palm represents approximately 1% of BSA and is helpful in estimating the area of small burns.

Rule of Palms

The **rule of palms,** an alternative system for approximating the extent of a burn, uses the palmar surface as a point of comparison in gauging the size of the affected body area (Figure 21-9). The patient's palm (the hand less the fingers) represents about 1 percent of the BSA, whether the patient is an adult, a child, or an infant. If you can visualize the palmar surface area and apply it to the burn area mentally, you can then obtain an estimate of the total BSA affected.

The rule of palms is easier to use for local burns of up to about 10 percent BSA, while the rule of nines is simpler and more appropriate for larger burns. Many other burn approximation techniques exist that are both more specific to age and, in general, more accurate. However, these techniques are more complicated and time consuming to use. Both the rule of nines and the rule of palms provide reasonable approximations of BSA when used properly in the field.

SYSTEMIC COMPLICATIONS

Burns cause several systemic complications. These can affect the overall severity of a burn. Typical complications include hypothermia, hypovolemia, eschar formation, and infection.

Hypothermia

A burn may disrupt the body's ability to regulate its core temperature. Tissue destruction reduces or eliminates the skin's ability to contain the fluid within. The burn process releases plasma and other fluids, which seep into the wound. There they evaporate and rapidly remove heat energy. If the burn is extensive, uncontrolled body heat loss induces rapid and severe hypothermia.

Hypovolemia

Hypovolemia also may complicate the severe burn. The inability of damaged blood vessels to contain plasma causes a shift of proteins, fluid, and electrolytes into the burned tissue. Additionally, the loss of plasma protein reduces the blood's ability, via osmosis, to draw fluids from the uninjured tissues. This in turn compromises the body's natural response to fluid loss and may produce a profound hypovolemia. Although this is a serious complication of the extensive burn, it takes hours to develop. Modern aggressive fluid resuscitation can effectively counteract this aspect of the burn process.

A related complication is electrolyte imbalance. With the massive shift of fluid to the interstitial space, the body's ability to regulate sodium, potassium, and other electrolytes becomes overwhelmed. In addition, large thermal and electrical burns can lead to massive tissue destruction with a resultant release of breakdown products into the bloodstream. Potassium is one such breakdown product and its oversupply, or hyperkalemia, can lead to life-threatening cardiac dysrhythmias. Careful ECG monitoring and appropriate fluid resuscitation can help prevent hyperkalemic complications.

Eschar

Skin denaturing further complicates full thickness thermal burns. As the burn destroys the dermal cells, they become hard and leathery, producing what is known as an **eschar**. The skin as a whole constricts over the wound site, increasing the pressure of any edema beneath and restricting the flow of blood (See Figure 21-10). If the extremity burn is circumferential, the constriction may be severe enough to occlude all blood flow into the distal extremity. In the case of a thoracic burn, eschar may drastically reduce chest excursion and respiratory tidal volume.

✱ **eschar** hard, leathery product of a deep full thickness burn; it consists of dead and denatured skin.

Infection

Although infection is the most persistent killer of burn victims, its effects do not appear for several days following the acute injury. Pathogens invade the wound shortly after the burn occurs and continue to do so until the wound heals. These pathogens pose a hazard to life when they grow to massive numbers, a process that takes days or weeks. To reduce the patient's exposure to infectious pathogens, carefully employ body substance isolation, use sterile dressings and clean equipment, and avoid gross contamination of the burn.

FIGURE 21-10 The constriction created by an eschar can limit chest excursion or cut off blood flow to and from a limb.

Organ Failure

As noted above, the burn process releases material from damaged or dying body cells into the bloodstream. Myoglobin from the muscles clogs the tubules of the kidneys and, with hypovolemia, may cause kidney failure. Hypovolemia and the circulating by-products of cellular destruction may also induce liver failure. In addition, the release of cellular potassium into the blood stream affects the heart's electrical system, causing dysrhythmias and possible death.

Special Factors

Consider any patient with a pre-existing illness or disease or any pediatric or geriatric patient as having a more serious burn injury.

Certain factors involving the burn patient's overall health and age will also affect the patient's response to a burn and should influence your field decisions regarding treatment and transport. Geriatric and pediatric patients and patients who are already ill or otherwise injured have greater difficulty coping with burn injuries than do healthy individuals. The pediatric patient has a high body surface area to body weight ratio, which means the fluid reserves needed for dealing with the effects of a burn are low. Geriatric patients have reduced mechanisms for fluid retention and lower fluid reserves. They are also less able to combat infection and more apt to have underlying diseases. Ill patients are already using the energy of their bodies to fight their diseases; with burns, these patients have additional medical stresses to combat. The fluid loss that accompanies a burn also compounds the effects of blood loss in a trauma patient. This patient now must recover from two injuries.

Physical Abuse

When assessing any burn, particularly in a child or an elderly and infirm adult, be alert for any signs of potential physical abuse. Look for mechanisms of injury that don't make sense, such as stove burns on an infant who cannot yet stand or walk. Certain burn patterns should also give rise to suspicion. Multiple circular burns each about a centimeter in diameter may reflect intentional cigarette burns. Infants who have been dipped in scalding hot water will have characteristic circumferential burns to their buttocks as they raise their feet and legs in an attempt to avoid the burning water (Figure 21-11). Branding is an unusual form of abuse

FIGURE 21-11 Burn injury from placing a child's buttocks in hot water as punishment.

and is sometimes seen in ritualistic or hazing ceremonies in some organizations. In all cases of suspected abuse, document your findings objectively and accurately, report them to the person assuming patient care in the emergency department, and notify the proper authorities as state and local laws require.

ASSESSMENT OF THERMAL BURNS

Skin evaluation tells more about the body's condition than any other aspect of patient assessment. Not only is the skin the first body organ to experience the effects of burns, it is the first and often the only organ to display them. Therefore, assessment of the skin and the associated burns must be deliberate, careful, and complete.

While the burn process varies, assessment is simple and well structured. Assess burn patients carefully and completely to assure that you establish the nature and extent of each injury. This helps you to assign burns the appropriate priority for care.

The assessment of thermal burns follows established procedures for performing the scene size-up, the initial assessment, the rapid trauma assessment or focused history and physical exam, the detailed physical exam, and the ongoing assessment.

SCENE SIZE-UP

The safety of your patients, fellow rescuers, and yourself depends upon a complete and thorough scene size-up. Look around carefully as you arrive at the scene to assure there is no continuing danger to you or your patient. Examine the scene to assure it is safe for you to enter. If there is any doubt, do not enter until the scene is made safe by appropriate emergency personnel (Figure 21-12).

On calls involving burn patients, be wary of entering enclosed spaces, such as a bedroom or a garage, if there is recent evidence of a fire. Even small fires can cause intense heat in small, enclosed spaces. This can rapidly lead to a near-explosive process (called flashover) in which the contents of a room rise in temperature to the point of rapid ignition. Flashover is frequently fatal to victims caught in the immediate area.

Another significant hazard at fire-ground scenes is the buildup of toxic gases. Carbon monoxide, cyanide, and hydrogen sulfide are common byproducts of

Be wary of entering any enclosed space associated with a fire because of the dangers of flashover and toxic gases.

FIGURE 21-12 Never enter a fire scene until it has been safely contained by appropriately trained personnel.

combustion and can be produced in large quantities in some fires. Cyanide, in particular, can kill after as little as 15 seconds of exposure, a time short enough to fell any would-be rescuer without proper protection.

Never enter any potentially hazardous scene. Instead, assure that the fire is thoroughly extinguished or that the patient is brought to you by persons skilled in working in hazardous environments who are using proper personal protective equipment. Assure that the area where you will be caring for the patient is free from dangers such as structural collapse, contamination, electricity, and any other hazards.

Once at the burn patient's side, stop the burning process so it no longer threatens you or the patient. Extinguish any overt flame using copious irrigation, as water is available. As an alternative, a heavy wool or cotton blanket (avoid most synthetics such as nylon or polyester) will smother flames.

Quickly survey the patient for other materials he or she is wearing that may continue the burn process. Remember that burn patients may be an actual hazard both to themselves and to you. Leather articles, such as shoes, belts, or watchbands, can smolder for hours and continue to induce thermal injury. Watches, rings, and other jewelry may also hold and transmit heat or may restrict swelling tissue and occlude distal circulation. Synthetics (such as a nylon windbreaker) produce great heat as they burn and leave a hot, smoldering residue once the overt flames are out. Remove materials like those described above as soon as possible. Be careful as you check for and remove these items. They may be hot enough to burn you.

Once the scene is safe and there are no further dangers to you or others, consider the burn mechanism. Ask yourself: "Is there any possibility that the patient was unconscious during the fire or trapped within the building?" If so, be ready to place a special emphasis upon your assessment and management of the patient's airway and breathing. Watch for any signs of airway restriction, and be alert to possible poisoning from carbon monoxide or other toxic gases.

Also consider and examine for other mechanisms of injury associated with the burn. Remember that the victim, in attempting to escape the flames, may have fallen down a flight of stairs or jumped from a second- or third-story window. Anticipate skeletal and internal injuries. In cases of electrical burns, consider the possibility that muscle spasms caused by contact with high voltage may also have caused skeletal fractures. Be aware that trauma injuries will increase the severity of the burn's impact on your patient.

Conclude the scene size-up by considering the need for other resources to manage the scene and treat the patient. Request additional EMS, police, and fire personnel and equipment as necessary. If you suspect serious airway involvement or carbon monoxide poisoning, consider requesting air medical service to reduce transport time to the hospital or burn/trauma center.

INITIAL ASSESSMENT

Start your initial assessment by forming a general impression of the patient. Rule out any danger of associated trauma or the possibility of head and spine injury. Evaluate the patient's level of consciousness, and, if the patient displays an altered state of consciousness, consider toxic inhalation as a cause. Protect the patient from further cervical injury if indicated by the suspected mechanism of injury or by the patient's symptoms.

Next, assure the airway is patent. If it is not, protect it. You must give the airway of a burn patient special consideration. Look for the signs of any thermal or inhalation injury during your initial airway exam (Figure 21-13). Look carefully at the facial and nasal hairs to see if they have been singed. Examine any sputum and the areas around the mouth and nose for carbonaceous residue or any other evidence of inhalation. Listen for airway sounds, such as stridor, hoarseness, or coughing, that indicate irritation or inflammation of the mucosa.

Look for and extinguish smoldering shoes, belts, or watchbands early in the assessment of burn patients.

Such sounds should alert you to the possibility that the airway has been injured and that progressive swelling of the airway is likely. Stridor, in particular, is a serious finding. Consider a patient with any signs of respiratory involvement as a potential acute emergency, and provide immediate care and transport.

With patients in whom respiratory involvement is suspected, provide high-flow, high-concentration oxygen, and prepare the equipment for endotracheal intubation. High-concentration oxygen (at levels approaching 100 percent) is especially important for burn patients because they may be suffering from carbon monoxide poisoning. Very high oxygen percentages more effectively provide oxygen to body cells and may reduce the half-life of the carbon monoxide by up to two thirds.

Burn patients may progress rapidly from mild dyspnea to total respiratory arrest. While the intubation of a respiratory burn patient may be difficult in the field, there are distinct advantages to performing it early. The edema is progressive and gradually reduces the airway lumen. If intubation is delayed until the patient becomes extremely dyspneic or goes into respiratory arrest, the airway may be so edematous that it will be difficult, if not impossible, to intubate.

If you elect field intubation for the burn patient (and medical direction approves), perform it quickly and carefully. The airway is already narrowing, and the normal trauma associated with intubation could make matters worse. Intubation can be more complicated if the patient is conscious and fights the process. Consider using rapid sequence intubation techniques and pharmacological adjuncts including sedatives and paralytics. Use succinylcholine (see Chapter 23, "Head, Facial, and Neck Trauma") cautiously, if at all, since it may worsen the hyperkalemia sometimes associated with severe burns. You may also find nasotracheal intubation useful. In any case, select the crew member with the most experience to assure that intubation is completed quickly and with the least amount of associated airway trauma.

As with all intubation, it is best to maintain an airway using the largest endotracheal tube possible. Be sure, however, to have several tubes smaller than you would normally use ready, because edema may have reduced the size of the airway. Select the largest tube that you think will easily pass through the cords. In extreme cases, creation of a surgical airway by either cricothyrotomy or needle cricothyrostomy may be a lifesaving necessity; in such cases follow local protocols or on-line medical direction.

Assure that the patient's breathing is adequate in both volume and rate. Carefully assess tidal volume if there are circumferential burns of the chest, because the developing eschar may restrict chest excursion. Ventilate as necessary via bag-valve mask using the reservoir and high-flow oxygen.

In cases of severe airway burns, intubate early. If intubation is delayed until the patient arrives at the emergency department, the airway may be so edematous that it may be difficult or impossible to intubate.

FIGURE 21-14   A partial thickness burn.

FIGURE 21-15   A deep full thickness burn.

FOCUSED AND RAPID TRAUMA ASSESSMENT

The focused history and physical exam for the burn patient are much the same as for any other trauma patient, beginning with a rapid trauma assessment or a focused physical exam and proceeding to the taking of baseline vital signs and a patient history. With a burn patient, however, you must also accurately approximate the area of the burn and its depth. This approximation guides your care and helps emergency department personnel prepare for patient arrival.

Except in cases of very localized burns, examine the patient's entire body surface, both anterior and posterior. Remove any clothing that was or could have been involved in the burn. If any of the clothing adheres to the burn or resists removal, cut around it as necessary.

Apply the rule of nines to determine the total body surface area (BSA) burned. Add 9 percent if the burn involves an entire "rule of nines" region. If it only involves a portion, add that proportion of 9 percent. For example, if 1/3 of the upper extremity is burned, the surface area approximation is 3 percent (1/3 of 9 percent = 3 percent). For small burns, use the rule of palms to approximate the affected BSA.

The depth of a burn injury is also an important consideration. Identify areas of painful sensation as partial thickness burns (Figure 21-14). Consider those that present with limited or absent pain as probable full thickness burns (Figure 21-15). This differentiation is difficult because partial thickness injury and its associated pain commonly surrounds the full thickness burn (Figure 21-16). See Table 21-1 for the characteristics of the different types of burns.

FIGURE 21-16   A hand wound displaying both partial and full thickness burns.

Table 21-1	CHARACTERISTICS OF VARIOUS DEPTHS OF BURNS		
	Superficial (1st Degree)	Partial Thickness (2nd Degree)	Full Thickness (3rd Degree)
Cause	Sun or minor flame	Hot liquids, flame	Chemicals, electricity, hot metals, flame
Skin color	Red	Mottled red	Pearly white and/or charred, translucent, and parchment-like
Skin	Dry with no blister	Blisters with weeping	Dry with thrombosed blood vessels
Sensation	Painful	Painful	Anesthetic
Healing	3–6 days	2–4 weeks	May require skin grafting

A third consideration in determining the severity of a burn is the area of the body affected. The face, hands, feet, joints, genitalia, and circumferential burns deserve particular consideration. Each presents with special problems to patients and their recovery.

You have already assessed the face for burns to eliminate respiratory involvement. But this area also needs special consideration for aesthetic reasons. Facial damage and scarring may be more socially debilitating than a joint or limb burn. Carefully assess and give a high priority to these injuries, even if you do rule out respiratory involvement.

Consider burns involving the feet or the hands as serious. These areas are critical for much of the patient's daily activities. Serious burns and the associated scar tissue make thermal hand or foot injuries very debilitating. Assess these areas and communicate the precise location of the injury and the degree of the burn to the receiving physician. Joint burns can likewise be debilitating for patients. Scar tissue replaces skin, leading to loss of joint flexibility and mobility. Give any burn assessed as full thickness that involves the hands, feet, or joints a higher priority than a burn of equal surface area and depth elsewhere.

Also pay particular attention to burns that completely ring an extremity, the thorax, the abdomen, or the neck. Due to the nature of a full thickness burn, the area underneath the burn may be drastically compressed as an eschar forms. The resulting constriction may hinder respirations, restrict distal blood flow, or cause hypoxia of the tissues beneath. Carefully assess any burn encircling a part of the body for distal circulation or other signs of vascular compromise. Once you note such an injury, perform ongoing assessments to monitor distal circulatory status.

Finally, assign a higher priority to any burns affecting pediatric or geriatric patients or patients who are ill or otherwise injured. Serious burns cause great stress for these patients. The massive fluid and heat loss as well as the infection often associated with burns challenge the ability of body systems to perform adequately. Consider a burn more serious whenever it is accompanied by any other serious patient problem.

Once you determine the depth, extent, and other factors that contribute to burn severity, categorize the patient as having either minor, moderate, or severe burns. Use the criteria in Table 21-2 as a guide.

The severity of a burn should be increased one level with pediatric and geriatric patients and patients suffering from other trauma or acute medical problems. Also consider burns as critical with a patient who shows any signs or symptoms of respiratory involvement. Such patients require immediate transport to a burn (or trauma) center, if possible (see Table 21-3).

The burn center is a hospital with a commitment to providing specialty treatment to burn patients. That commitment includes measures necessary to reduce the risk of infection presented by serious burns. The center must also have the resources to perform delicate skin grafts necessary to replace destroyed skin. Because serious burns leave scar tissue that covers joints and other important areas

Burns to the face, hands, feet, joints, genitalia, and circumferential burns are of special concern.

The head-to-toe examination should continue at the scene only if significant and life-threatening burns can be ruled out.

Table 21-2	BURN SEVERITY
Minor	
Superficial: BSA < 50 percent (sunburns, etc.)	
Partial thickness: BSA < 15 percent	
Full thickness: BSA < 2 percent	
Moderate	
Superficial: BSA > 50 percent	
Partial thickness: BSA < 30 percent	
Full thickness: BSA < 10 percent	
Critical	
Partial thickness: BSA > 30 percent	
Full thickness: BSA > 10 percent	
Inhalation injury	
Any partial or full thickness burns involving hands, feet, joints, face, or genitalia	

Source: American Burn Association.

and affects movement, the center can provide rehabilitation programs requiring prolonged patient stays and intensive nursing care. While immediate transport to a burn center is not as critically time dependant as transport for other seriously injured patients to a trauma center, the burn center's resources can optimize a patient's recovery prospects. Review your local protocols for criteria regarding patient transport to a burn center.

Conclude the focused history and physical exam by prioritizing the patient for transport. Rapidly transport any patient with full thickness burns over a large portion of the BSA. Patients with associated injuries to the face, joints, hands, feet, or genitalia are also candidates for immediate transport. Other cases needing rapid transport include patients who have experienced smoke, steam, or flame inhalation, or any geriatric, pediatric, otherwise ill, or trauma patient. Direct these patients to the nearest burn center as described by your local protocols or by on-line medical direction.

ONGOING ASSESSMENT

Conduct ongoing assessments for all burn patients, every 15 minutes for minor burns and every 5 minutes for moderate or critical burns. Although the burn injury mechanism has been halted, the nature of the burn will continue to affect

Table 21-3	INJURIES THAT BENEFIT FROM BURN CENTER CARE
Partial thickness (2nd-degree) burn greater than 15 percent of BSA	
Full thickness (3rd-degree) burn greater than 5 percent BSA	
Significant burns to the face, feet, hands, or perineal area	
High-voltage electrical injuries	
Inhalation injuries	
Chemical burns causing progressive tissue destruction	
Associated significant injuries	

Source: American Burn Association.

the patient. In addition to monitoring vital signs, watch for early signs of hypovolemia and airway problems. Also be cautious of aggressive fluid therapy. Monitor for lung sounds and respiratory effort suggestive of pulmonary edema, and slow the fluid resuscitation if any signs develop. Also carefully monitor distal circulation and sensation with any circumferential burn. Finally, monitor the ECG to identify any abnormalities, which may be caused by electrolyte imbalances secondary to fluid movement and tissue destruction.

MANAGEMENT OF THERMAL BURNS

Once you complete your burn patient assessment and correct or address any immediate life threats, you can begin certain burn management steps, either in the field or en route to the hospital. These include the prevention of shock, hypothermia, and any further wound contamination.

Thermal burn management can be divided into two categories: that for local and minor burns and that for moderate to severe burns.

LOCAL AND MINOR BURNS

Use local cooling to treat minor soft-tissue burns involving only a small proportion of the body surface area at a partial thickness. Provide this care only for partial thickness burns that involve less than 15 percent of the BSA or very small full thickness burns (less than 2 percent BSA). Cooling of larger surface areas may subject the patient to the risk of hypothermia. Cold or cool water immersion has some effect in reducing pain and may limit the depth of the burning process if applied immediately (within 1 or 2 minutes) after the burn.

Cool water immersion of minor localized burns may be effective if accomplished in the first few minutes after a burn.

If you have not already done so, remove any article of clothing or jewelry that might possibly act to constrain edema. As body fluids accumulate at the injury site, the site begins to swell. If the swelling encounters any constriction, it increases pressure on other tissue and may, in effect, serve as a tourniquet. This pressure may result in the loss of pulse and circulation distal to the injury. Evaluate distal circulation and sensation frequently during care and transport.

Also provide the burn patient with comfort and support. Even rather minor burns can be very painful. Calm and reassure the patient; in severe cases, consider diazepam or morphine sulfate analgesia.

Standard in-hospital treatment for minor burns includes the application of topical (not systemic) antibiotic ointments such as silver sulfadiazine and bulky sterile dressings. Encourage the patient, as much as possible, to keep the burn elevated. Provide analgesia in either oral or parenteral form as burns can be quite painful. Full thickness burns are open wounds, so any patient without an up-to-date tetanus immunization is given a booster of tetanus-diphtheria toxoid.

MODERATE TO SEVERE BURNS

Use dry, sterile dressings to cover partial thickness burns that involve more than 15 percent BSA or full thickness burns involving more than 5 percent of the BSA. Dressings keep air movement past the sensitive partial thickness burn to a minimum, and thereby reduce pain. Bulky sterile dressings also provide padding against minor bumping and other trauma. In full thickness burns, they provide a barrier to possible contamination.

Keep the patient warm. When burns involve large surface areas, the patient loses the ability to effectively control body temperature. If the burn begins to seep fluid, as in a full thickness burn, evaporative heat loss can be extreme. Cover such an area with dry sterile dressings, cover the patient with a blanket, and maintain a warm environment.

Cover extensive partial and full thickness burns with dry sterile dressing, keep the patient warm, and initiate fluid resuscitation.

FIGURE 21-17   Separate burned toes and fingers with dry sterile gauze.

When treating full thickness burns to the fingers, toes, or other locations where burned surfaces may contact each other, place soft, non-adherent bandages between the burned skin areas (Figure 21-17). Without this precaution, the disrupted and wet wounds would stick together and cause further damage when pulled apart for care at the emergency department.

If the surface area of the burn is great, medical direction may ask you to provide aggressive fluid therapy during prehospital care. While hypovolemia is not an early development after a burn, fluid migration into the wound later during the burn cycle eventually leads to serious fluid loss. Early and aggressive fluid therapy can effectively reduce the impact of this fluid loss.

If burns cover all the normal IV access sites, you may place the catheter through tissue with partial thickness burns, proximal to any more serious injury. (Full thickness burns usually damage the blood vessels or coagulate the blood, making intravenous cannulation difficult and possibly impeding effective fluid flow.) Be careful with insertion. The skin may be leathery, but the tissue underneath is very delicate.

Establish intravenous routes in any patient with moderate to severe burns. Introduce two large-bore catheters and hang 1,000 mL bags of either normal saline (preferred) or lactated Ringer's solution. Current fluid resuscitation formulas recommend 4 mL of fluid for every kilogram of patient weight multiplied by the percentage of body surface area burned:

$$4 \text{ mL} \times \text{Patient weight in kg} \times \text{BSA burned} = \text{Amount of fluid}$$

Thus for a 70-kg patient with 30 percent BSA burned, the calculation is

$$4 \times 70 \times 30 = 8,400 \text{ mL}$$

The patient needs half this amount of fluid in the first 8 hours after the burn. This particular fluid resuscitation protocol is known as the Parkland formula. Other variations exist and may be in use in your local area. In most prehospital situations where transport time is short (less than 1 hour), an initial fluid bolus of 0.5 mL of fluid for every kilogram of patient weight multiplied by the percentage of BSA burned is reasonable:

$$0.5 \text{ ml} \times \text{Patient weight in kg} \times \text{BSA burned} = \text{Amount of fluid}$$

Thus, for an 80-kg patient with 20 percent BSA burned, the calculation is

$$0.5 \times 80 \times 20 = 800 \text{ mL}$$

You may repeat this infusion once or twice during the first hour or so of care.

Be cautious and conservative when administering fluids to the burn patient if there is any possibility of airway or lung injury. Rapid fluid administration may worsen airway swelling or the edema that accompanies toxic inhalation. Carefully monitor the airway and auscultate for breath sounds frequently whenever you administer fluid to a burn patient.

Burns are quite painful, yet the pain is often paradoxical to the burn severity. Less severe superficial and partial thickness (first- and second-degree) burns are very uncomfortable, while extensive full thickness (third-degree) burns are often almost without pain. Provide patients in severe pain with narcotic analgesia. Consider morphine in 2 mg IV increments every 5 minutes until suffering is relieved. Use morphine with caution as it may depress the respiratory drive and increase any existing hypovolemia.

Infection is another classic and deadly problem associated with extensive soft-tissue burns. This life-threatening condition does not develop until well after pre-hospital care is concluded. However, proper field care can significantly reduce mortality and morbidity. Providing a clean environment and sterile dressings can lessen the bacterial load for the patient. Avoid prophylactic antibiotics because their early use has been shown to actually worsen outcomes for burn patients.

In dire circumstances medical direction may request you to perform an emergency escharotomy. To do this, you incise the burned tissue through the eschar, perpendicular to the constriction. Be certain to incise about 1 cm deeper than the developing eschar to assure the release of pressure. If adequate respirations or distal pulses do not return after the escharotomy, medical direction may request you to repeat the procedure a short distance from the first incision.

Emergency department personnel will continue fluid resuscitation for serious burn patients according to the Parkland or another suitable formula. They will perform arterial blood gas evaluation to determine oxygen tension, carbon monoxide concentration, and cyanide poisoning levels. Urine output and cardiac monitoring are instituted as well. The staff will assure adequate administration of parenteral narcotic analgesia and provide tetanus immunization if necessary. They will closely evaluate severe circumferential burns for eschar development. If the blood flow in an extremity or respirations are impaired, the physician may perform an escharotomy.

INHALATION INJURY

If you suspect thermal (or chemical) airway burns and airway compromise is imminent, intubation can be life saving. Once you assure the patient's airway, provide high-flow oxygen by nonrebreather mask at 15 lpm. Oxygen not only counters hypoxia but is also therapeutic in carbon monoxide and cyanide poisoning. Consider transport to a center capable of providing hyperbaric oxygen therapy for patients with suspected carbon monoxide poisoning. The hyperbaric chamber provides oxygen under the pressure of two or more atmospheres. This pushes oxygen into the patient's bloodstream, carrying it directly to the body's cells. Hyperbaric oxygenation also drives carbon monoxide from the hemoglobin, shortening the time to recovery. If hyperbaric oxygen therapy is available in your area, any smoke inhalation or suspected carbon monoxide poisoning patient should be considered for treatment at the facility.

Suspect cyanide toxicity in patients with severe symptoms such as dyspnea, chest pain, altered mental status, seizures, and unconsciousness. To be effective, antidotal treatment of serious cyanide poisoning must be started early. Vapor exposures are likely to result in severe respiratory distress or apnea in addition to unconsciousness. Rapid airway intervention with endotracheal intubation and ventilatory support with a bag-valve mask are initial priorities. However, a rapid shift to antidotal therapy is essential to save the patient.

Be cautious and conservative when administering fluids to the burn patient with inhalation injury.

Early intubation can be life saving for the inhalation injury patient.

FIGURE 21-18   A cyanide antidote kit.

Administration of the antidote for cyanide is a two-stage process, first using a nitrite compound, followed by a sulfur-containing compound (Figure 21-18). The nitrite acts by converting the hemoglobin (the primary oxygen-carrying protein in the blood) to methemoglobin. Methemoglobin then binds the cyanide, removing it from the cytochrome$_{a3}$ (an enzyme necessary for oxygen processing by cells). The sulfur-containing antidote then removes the cyanide by forming a nontoxic compound, excreted in the urine.

Ambulances serving industrial areas with high cyanide use may carry antidote kits containing amyl nitrite, sodium nitrite, and sodium thiosulfate. If an IV is already established, administer 300 mg sodium nitrite over 2 to 4 minutes for adults. If an IV is not yet established, crush one amyl nitrate ampule for the patient to inhale. If the patient has spontaneous respirations, place the ampule under an oxygen mask with high-flow oxygen running. In patients needing ventilatory support, place the ampule in the bag or oxygen reservoir of the bag-valve mask. Do not let the ampule fall into the patient's mouth or down the endotracheal tube. Always follow inhaled amyl nitrate with intravenous sodium nitrite, and do not use amyl nitrite if the patient has already received sodium nitrite.

Following administration of IV sodium nitrite, administer 12.5 gm of sodium thiosulfate for the adult. Avoid sodium thiosulfate unless the patient has received IV sodium nitrite, as it does not work well by itself. A highly effective and much safer antidote (related to vitamin B_{12}) is on the horizon, but is not yet available for general use in the United States.

ASSESSMENT AND MANAGEMENT OF ELECTRICAL, CHEMICAL, AND RADIATION BURNS

ELECTRICAL INJURIES

Be certain that the power has been shut off before you approach the scene of a suspected electrical injury. Until it is, do not allow anyone to approach the patient or the proximity of the electrical source. Remember that an energized power line need not spark or whip around to be deadly; a power line simply lying on the ground can still present a significant danger. Note also that some utility lines have breakers that will try to re-establish power periodically. Establish a safety

Until the power is off, no one should be allowed to approach the electrical burn patient.

zone if there is any question about the status of lines that are down. Keep vehicles and personnel at a distance from downed lines or the source pole that is greater than the distance between the power poles. Also be aware that downed power lines may energize metal structures such as buildings, vehicles, or fences.

Once the scene is secure, assess the patient and prepare him or her for transport. Search for both an entrance and an exit wound. Look specifically for possible contact points with both the ground and the electrical source. In some circumstances, multiple entrance and exit wounds are present. Remember that electrical current passes through the body and therefore may result in significant internal burns, especially to blood vessels and nerves, while the assessment reveals only minimal superficial findings. Rapidly progressive cardiovascular collapse can follow contact with an electrical source. Also, examine the patient for any fractures resulting from forceful muscle contractions caused by the current's passage.

As with thermal burns, look for smoldering shoes, belts, or other items of clothing. Such items may continue the burning process well after the current is shut off. Also remove rings, watches, and any other constrictive items from the fingers, limbs, and the neck.

Perform ECG monitoring for possible cardiac disturbances in victims of electrical burns. Electrical current may induce dysrhythmias including bradycardias, tachycardias, ventricular fibrillation, and asystole. Assure that emergency department personnel examine any patient who has sustained a significant electrical shock. The damage the current causes may be internal and not apparent to you or your patient during assessment. Consider any significant electrical burn or exposure patient as a high priority for immediate transport.

Lightning strikes to humans occur more than 300 times each year in the United States and result in over 100 deaths. Strikes to people riding tractors, on open water, on golf courses, and under trees are most common, and men are the victims of 75 percent of all strikes. A lightning strike is a high-voltage (up to 100,000 volts), high-current (10,000 amperes), and high-temperature (50,000°F) event that lasts only a fraction of a second. A direct strike will impart this energy to the patient (Figure 21-19). However, the lightning will often strike a nearby object with some voltage traveling sideways (sideflash) or the voltage may radiate outward in alternate pathways from the strike point, thus diminishing the voltage (step voltage).

By the time anyone reaches the victim of a lightning strike, the electricity has long since dissipated. (There will be, however, a continued risk of further strikes as long as the storm remains nearby.) There is no danger of electrical shock from touching the victim of a lightning strike. The victim's clothing, however, may continue to smolder, so remove it as necessary. Among other serious effects, lightning can produce a sudden cessation of breathing. Despite being apneic and perhaps pulseless, these patients frequently survive with prompt prehospital intervention.

Treat visible burns ("entrance" and "exit" wounds) just as any thermal burn with cooling, if necessary, followed by the application of dry sterile dressings. Do not focus too much on the visible burns, but instead recognize that the electricity has passed through the body, possibly causing widespread internal effects.

Treat cardiac or respiratory arrest in electrical burn patients with aggressive airway, ventilatory, and circulatory management. Patients in cardiac arrest because of contact with electrical current have a high survival rate if prehospital intervention is prompt. Check immediately for ventricular fibrillation and defibrillate if necessary. Secure the airway with an endotracheal tube and begin ventilations and chest compressions. The usual resuscitative procedures for cases of cardiac arrest apply equally when the cause of the arrest is electrical injury; they might include the use of vasopressors and antidysrhythmics.

For serious electrical burn injuries, initiate at least two large bore IVs and give an initial 20 mL/kg fluid bolus. If the electrical burn is severe, provide additional

Monitor the electrical burn patient for abnormalities in the ECG.

FIGURE 21-19 A typical lightning strike injury.

fluid using the Parkland or another formula. Consider use of sodium bicarbonate and mannitol, usually at the discretion of medical direction, to prevent the complications of rhabdomyolysis (discussed in Chapter 20, "Soft Tissue Trauma") and hyperkalemia. The usual starting dose is 1 mEq/kg for sodium bicarbonate and 10 g for mannitol.

CHEMICAL BURNS

As you perform the scene size-up, identify the nature of the chemical spill/contamination and, if possible, approach from upwind. Identify the location of the chemical and assure that it poses no hazard to you, other rescuers, or the public. Be wary of toxic fumes and cross-contamination from the patient and the surrounding environment. If necessary, have hazardous material team members evacuate and decontaminate the victim before you begin assessment and care. Seek out personnel on the scene who are familiar with the agent and consult with them regarding dangers posed by the agent and any specific medical care and patient handling procedures required with it.

During your assessment and care, always wear medical examination gloves, but never presume that they will protect you from the agent. Take appropriate protective action against airborne dust, toxic fumes, and splash exposure for both yourself and the patient (goggles and mask as needed). Wear a disposable gown if there is danger of the agent contacting your clothing. Make certain the agent is isolated and no longer a danger to the patient or others. Have any of the patient's clothing that you suspect may be contaminated removed, and isolate it from accidental contact. Save the clothing and assure that it is disposed of properly. Identify the type of agent, its exact chemical name, the length of the patient's contact time with it, and the precise areas of the patient's body affected by it.

As you begin your initial assessment, assure that the patient is alert and fully oriented and that airway and breathing are unaffected by the contact. If there is any airway restriction or respiratory involvement, consider early intubation. As airway tissue swells, the obstruction worsens and intubation becomes more

In dealing with a chemical burn, take all precautions to assure that no one else becomes contaminated.

difficult. Monitor the patient's heart rate and consider ECG monitoring, because many chemicals (for example, organophosphates) may affect the heart. If the patient is stable, begin the rapid trauma assessment.

Examine any chemical burn carefully to establish the depth, extent, and nature of the injury. If you suspect the involvement of phenol, dry lime, sodium or riot agents, treat as indicated below.

- *Phenol* A gelatinous caustic called phenol is used as a powerful industrial cleaner. Phenol is very difficult to remove because it is sticky and insoluble in water. Alcohol, which dissolves it, is frequently available in places where phenol is regularly used. You can use the alcohol to remove the phenol and follow removal with irrigation using large volumes of cool water.

- *Dry Lime* Dry lime is a strong corrosive that reacts with water. It produces heat and subsequent chemical and thermal injuries. Brush dry lime off the patient gently, but as completely as possible. Then rinse the contaminated area with large volumes of cool to cold water. While the water reacts with any remaining lime, it cools the contact area and removes the rest of the chemical. By rinsing with water, you assure the lime reacts with that water rather than with the water contained within the patient's soft tissues.

- *Sodium* Sodium is an unstable metal that reacts destructively with many substances, including human tissue. It reacts vigorously with water, creating extreme heat, explosive hydrogen gas, and possible ignition. Sodium is normally stored submerged in oil because the metal reacts with oxygen in the air. If a patient is contaminated with sodium, decontaminate him or her quickly by gentle brushing. Then cover the wound with oil used to store the substance.

- *Riot Control Agents* These agents, which include CS, CN (Mace), and oleoresin capsicum (OC, pepper spray), deserve special mention because people are the targets of their intended use and because that use is frequent. These agents cause intense irritation of the eyes, mucous membranes, and respiratory tract. In general, they do not cause permanent damage when properly deployed. Patients who have contacted them typically present with eye pain, tearing, and temporary "blindness." Coughing, gagging, and vomiting are not uncommon. Treatment is supportive and most patients recover spontaneously within 10 to 20 minutes of exposure to fresh air. If necessary, irrigate the patient's eyes with normal saline if you suspect that any riot agent particles remain in the eye.

If it has not been done earlier, decontaminate the patient who has come in contact with any other chemical capable of causing tissue damage. Stop the damage by irrigating the site with large volumes of water (see Figure 21-20). Water rinses away the offending material and dilutes any water-soluble agents. The water also reduces the heat and rate of the chemical reaction and, ultimately, the chemical's effects upon the patient's skin. If the contamination is widespread, douse the patient with large volumes of water. Use a garden hose or low-pressure water from a fire truck. Assure that the water is neither warm nor too cold.

When the patient has been thoroughly rinsed for a few minutes, remove any remaining clothing. Take care that the process does not contaminate rescuers. If the agent is dangerous, save all clothing and contain the rinse water for proper disposal at a later time. Next, gently wash the burn with a mild soap (such as ordinary dish detergent) and a gentle brush or sponge. Be careful not to cause further

Irrigation with copious amounts of cool water is indicated for burns from an unknown chemical agent.

FIGURE 21-20 Chemical burns should be flushed with large quantities of water. Dry lime should be first brushed away before applying cool water.

Chemical burn . . . flood area with water

Dry lime . . . brush from skin and clothing, then irrigate

soft-tissue damage. After washing, gently irrigate the wound with a constant flow of water. While the pain and the burning process may appear to subside, it is important to continue the irrigation until the patient arrives at the emergency department. If practical, transport the label from the corrosive's container or a sample of the agent (safely contained and marked) along with the patient. On arrival at the hospital, be sure to describe to emergency department personnel, and enter in your prehospital care report, any first aid given prior to your arrival.

Do not use any antidote or neutralizing agent. Neutralizing agents often react violently with the contaminants they neutralize. They may ultimately increase the heat of the reaction and induce thermal burns. In some cases, the antidote or neutralizing agent is more damaging to the skin than the contaminant.

With chemical burns, pay particular attention to the patient's eyes. Eyes are very sensitive to chemicals and can easily be damaged, even by weak agents. Prompt treatment of chemical eye injury is critical and can reduce damage and preserve eyesight. Ask the patient about chemical contact with the eyes, eye pain, vision changes, and contact lens use. Examine the eyes for eyelid spasm (**blepharospasm**), conjunctival erythema, discoloration, tearing, and other evidence of burns or irritation.

Irrigate chemical splashes that involve the eye with large volumes of water. Alkali burns are especially damaging and with them you should flush the eye for at least 15 minutes. Irrigate acid burns for at least 5 minutes. Flush splashes of an unknown agent for up to 20 minutes. Do not, however, delay transport while irrigating.

A useful technique for irrigation is to hang a bag of normal saline (lactated Ringer's is an acceptable substitute) and use the flow regulator to control the flow of fluid into the nasal corner of the eye. Turn the patient's head to the side to facilitate drainage and avoid cross-contaminating the other eye with the waste fluid. Be alert for contact lenses in cases where chemicals are splashed into the eyes. Chemicals may become trapped under the lenses, preventing adequate irrigation. Gently remove the lenses, continuing irrigation.

Do not use any antidote or any neutralizing agent on chemical burns.

blepharospasm twitching of the eyelids.

Irrigate all alkali burns to the eye for at least 15 minutes.

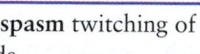

RADIATION BURNS

An incident involving potential radiation exposure or burns must be a concern during both dispatch and response phases of the emergency call. Because radiation can neither be seen nor felt, it can endanger EMS personnel unless the hazard has been anticipated and proper precautions taken. If you suspect radiation exposure, approach the scene very carefully (Figure 21-21). If the incident occurs at a power generation plant or in an industrial or a medical facility, seek out personnel knowledgeable about the radioactive substance being used. Such persons are always on staff, and frequently on site, at these facilities. Stay a good distance from the scene and assure that bystanders, rescuers, and patients remain remote from the source of the exposure. Remember that distance and the nature of the materials, like concrete or earth, between you and the radiation source reduce potential exposure. If the exposure may be from dust or fire, approach from and remain upwind of the radiation source.

In radiation exposure incidents, assure that personnel trained in radiation hazards isolate the source, contain it, and test the scene for safety. If this is impossible, move the patient to a site remote from the radioactivity source where you can give care without danger either to yourself or the patient. Plan the removal carefully. Use as much shielding as possible and keep exposure times to a minimum. Remember, the dose of radiation received is related to three primary factors: duration, distance, and shielding.

If you must carry out a patient removal, use the oldest rescuers for the evacuation team. This approach is prudent because many of the effects of radiation exposure become evident many years after the exposure. If you use older rescuers, they will more likely be past their reproductive years and have fewer years of life left if and when a problem does surface. This concern is especially important with pregnant females and young adults of both sexes. Remember that radiation damages the reproductive system very easily.

If there is a risk that patients are contaminated, assure that they are properly decontaminated before you begin assessment and care. If available for this task, use persons knowledgeable in decontamination and monitoring techniques who have the appropriate protective gear. If this is not possible, don goggles, a mask, gloves, and a disposable gown. Direct the evacuation team to place the patients in a decontamination area remote from your vehicle and other personnel and where any contamination can be contained. Have the patients disrobe or carefully disrobe them, rinse them with large volumes of water, then wash them with a soft brush and rinse again. Ordinary dish detergent is effective as a cleansing agent. Scrub, or

Because radiation can be neither seen nor felt, it can endanger EMS personnel unless proper precautions are taken.

Duration, distance, and shielding are important factors in determining radiation dose exposure.

FIGURE 21-21 Warning labels may indicate the presence of radioactive materials.

cut off and then scrub, any areas of body hair. As in incidents of chemical contamination, save all clothing and decontamination water and dispose of them safely. Perform decontamination before moving the patients to the ambulance.

Carefully document the circumstances of the radioactive exposure. If possible, identify the source and strength of the agent. Determine the patient's proximity to the source during the exposure as well as the length of exposure.

Once decontaminated, treat a radiation exposure patient as you would any other patient. Because the human body by itself cannot be a source of ionizing radiation, the decontaminated patient poses no threat to you or your crew. Remember, however, that any contaminated material remaining on the patient or any contamination transferred to you does provide a source of radiation exposure and may contaminate you and your vehicle.

The actual assessment of a patient exposed to radiation is quite simple and usually reveals minimal signs or symptoms of injury. Only extreme exposures result in the classical presentation of nausea, vomiting, and malaise. Burns are extremely rare, although they may occur if the exposure is extremely intense. Even though a patient seems well, the delayed consequences of high-dose radiation exposure can be devastating. If you note any early patient complaints, record the findings in the patient's own words and include the time the complaint first was made. This information is helpful in determining the patient's degree of radiation exposure (Table 21-4).

Treat the symptoms of the radiation injury patient, make the patient as comfortable as possible, and offer psychological support. Cover any burns with sterile dressing and, if general symptoms are noticeable, provide oxygen and initiate an IV. Maintain the patient's body temperature and provide transport to the emergency department.

Once properly decontaminated, the radiation injury patient presents no radiation danger to care givers.

Table 21-4 DOSE-EFFECT RELATIONSHIPS TO IONIZING RADIATION

Whole Body Exposure Dose (RAD)	Effect
5–25	Asymptomatic. Blood studies are normal.
50–75	Asymptomatic. Minor depressions of white blood cells and platelets in a few patients.
75–125	May produce anorexia, nausea, and vomiting, and fatigue in approximately 10–20% of patients within 2 days.
125–200	Possible nausea and vomiting. Diarrhea, anxiety, tachycardia. Fatal to less than 5% of patients.
200–600	Nausea and vomiting. Diarrhea in the first several hours. Weakness, fatigue. Fatal to approximately 50% of patients within 6 weeks without prompt medical attention.
600–1,000	"Burning sensation" within minutes. Nausea and vomiting within 10 minutes. Confusion, ataxia, and collapse within 1 hour. Watery diarrhea within 1 to 2 hours. Fatal to 100% within short time without prompt medical attention.

Localized Exposure Dose (RAD)	Effect
50	Asymptomatic
500	Asymptomatic (usually). May have risk of altered function of exposed area.
2,500	Atrophy, vascular lesion, and altered pigmentation.
5,000	Chronic ulcer, risk of carcinogenesis.
50,000	Permanent destruction of exposed tissue.

ONGOING ASSESSMENT

Monitor patients with inhalation, chemical, and electrical burns and radiation exposure patients for signs of increasing complications associated with their burn mechanisms. Also monitor blood pressure, pulse, and respirations and trend any changes. Perform these evaluations every 15 minutes in stable patients and every 5 minutes in unstable patients.

SUMMARY

Burn injuries may compromise the skin—the protective envelope that protects and contains the human body. Burn damage to the skin may interfere with its ability to contain water within the body and to prevent damaging agents from entering. For these reasons, assessment and care of these soft-tissue injuries are important.

Assess the burn to determine its depth and the extent of the body surface area it involves. Be sensitive to any respiratory, joint, hand, foot, or circumferential regions affected by the burn. Give special consideration to pediatric and geriatric burn patients and to burn patients who are also ill or otherwise injured. Consider all these factors in determining the overall severity of a burn. If the patient's condition warrants, institute aggressive care. Anticipate airway compromise and fluid loss. Secure the airway very early in prehospital care. Initiate IV access, and begin fluid administration.

Electrical, chemical, or radiation burns require special care and assessment. An electrical burn requires careful assessment to determine the area and depth of burn involvement and should be followed by wound site dressing and cardiac monitoring. Chemical burns need rapid and effective decontamination. Radiation burns call for extreme care in removing the patient from the radiation source and in providing decontamination and supportive care.

CHAPTER 22

Musculoskeletal Trauma

Objectives

After reading this chapter, you should be able to:

1. Describe the incidence, morbidity, and mortality of musculoskeletal injuries. (pp. 987–988)
2. Discuss the anatomy and physiology of the muscular and skeletal systems. (see Chapter 3)
3. Predict injuries based on the mechanism of injury, including: (pp. 988–994)
   - Direct
   - Indirect
   - Pathologic
4. Discuss the types of musculoskeletal injuries, including:
   - Fractures (open and closed) (pp. 991–993)
   - Dislocations/fractures (pp. 990–991)
   - Sprains (p. 990)
   - Strains (p. 990)
5. Describe the six "Ps" of musculoskeletal injury assessment. (p. 999)
6. List the primary signs and symptoms of extremity trauma. (pp. 996–1001)

Continued

INTRODUCTION TO MUSCULOSKELETAL TRAUMA

In trauma, incidences of musculoskeletal injury are second in frequency only to soft-tissue injuries. They usually result from application of significant direct or transmitted blunt kinetic forces. Skeletal or muscular injuries may also occasionally result from penetrating mechanisms of injury. Millions of Americans sustain musculoskeletal injuries each year from a variety of sources including sports injuries, motor vehicle crashes, falls, and acts of violence. These incidents can cause a variety of injuries to the body's bones, cartilage, ligaments, muscles,

Incidences of musculoskeletal injury are second in frequency only to soft-tissue injuries in trauma.

or tendons. While injuries to the upper extremities can be painful and sometimes debilitating, they rarely threaten life. Lower extremity injuries, on the other hand, are generally associated with a greater magnitude of force and greater secondary blood loss and, thus, more often constitute threats to life or limb. In addition, the same forces responsible for a musculoskeletal injury may damage internal organs, nerves, and blood vessels, causing serious problems throughout the body. In fact, most patients (up to 80 percent) who suffer multi-system trauma, experience significant musculoskeletal injuries.

PREVENTION STRATEGIES

Stopping injury before it occurs—injury prevention—is the optimal way of dealing with musculoskeletal injuries. Strategies for preventing musculoskeletal injuries include application of modern vehicle and highway designs and safe driving practices, including the use of restraint systems. Auto crashes are the greatest single cause of musculoskeletal injuries, and improved vehicle safety has done much to reduce injury incidence and severity. Workplace safety standards developed and enforced by the Occupational Safety and Health Administration (OSHA) have done much to reduce on-the-job injuries. These standards include criteria for proper footwear, scaffolding, fall protection devices, and the like. Sports injuries, which most commonly affect the musculature, joints, and long bones, account for a significant number of traumas. While protective gear, improved equipment design, and better conditioning of athletes has reduced injuries, the very nature of contact sports means that these activities remain a significant cause of injury. Household accidents and falls also account for many musculoskeletal injuries, and use of good safety practices—for example, proper footwear, well-designed railings, proper use of step ladders—can reduce injury incidence at home.

PATHOPHYSIOLOGY OF THE MUSCULOSKELETAL SYSTEM

The musculoskeletal injury process is a complicated one, resulting in much more damage than the disruption of an inert structural element of the body. Bone is alive and requires a continuous supply of oxygenated circulation. Bone lies deep within muscle tissue, and major nerves and blood vessels parallel it as they travel to the distal extremity. At points of articulation, there is a complex arrangement of ligaments, cartilage, and synovial fluid that holds the joint together while permitting a wide range of movement. Finally, the muscles attach and direct skeletal movement through the collections of fibers, fasciculi, and muscle bodies connected to the skeletal system by tendons. This complex arrangement of connective, skeletal, vascular, nervous, and muscular tissue is endangered whenever significant kinetic forces are applied to the extremities. If the forces are severe enough, they are likely to cause muscular, joint, or skeletal injury.

MUSCULAR INJURY

Muscular injuries may result from direct blunt or penetrating trauma, overexertion, or problems with oxygen supply during exertion. These injuries include contusions, penetrating injuries, fatigue, strains, sprains, cramps, and spasms. Muscular problems usually do not contribute significantly to hypovolemia and shock, with the exceptions of severe contusions with large associated hematomas and penetrating injuries with extensive hemorrhage.

Contusion

Severe trauma frequently crushes muscles between a blunt force and the skeletal structure beneath. This damages both the muscle cells and the blood vessels that supply them. Small blood vessels rupture, leaking blood into the interstitial spaces and causing pain, erythema, and then ecchymosis. Blood in the interstitial spaces and muscle cell damage set off the body's inflammatory response. Capillary beds engorge with blood, and fluid shifts to the interstitial space, leading to tissue edema. The injury may also cause blood to pool beneath tissue layers in a hematoma. In more massive body muscles, like those of the thigh, buttocks, calf, or arm, large volumes of blood may accumulate, contributing significantly to hypovolemia. A large hematoma or significant muscular edema will increase the diameter of the injured limb, especially as compared to the opposing uninjured limb. For the most part, however, signs of muscle injury remain hidden beneath the skin.

Compartment Syndrome

Contusion, crush injury, and fracture may damage the soft tissue of the extremity and cause both internal hemorrhage and swelling. As the swelling and pooling of blood increase, pressure may build within the fascial compartment that contains them. This pressure first restricts capillary blood flow and compresses and damages nerves. If the pressure continues to build, it restricts and then halts venous return through the limb and ultimately stops arterial circulation. The first signs of this developing injury are tension (a feeling like a contracted muscle) within the limb and some loss of distal sensation, especially in the webs of the fingers or toes. The patient may complain of pain and appear more seriously injured than the mechanism of injury or outward signs might suggest. In addition, your moving of the patient's limb (passive extension) may elicit increased pain. Pulse deficit is a late sign of compartment syndrome.

Penetrating Injury

Deep lacerations may penetrate skin and subcutaneous tissues, thus affecting muscle masses and tendons below. Massive wounds involving a large percentage of a muscle body or those injuring or severing a tendon may reduce the distal limb's strength or render muscular control ineffective. When a tendon or muscle is cut, contraction of the opposing muscle moves the limb while the injured muscle/tendon is unable to return the limb toward the neutral position. Such injuries call for surgical intervention to identify and rejoin the damaged tendon or muscle body. These wounds may also introduce infectious agents, damage muscle tissue, and affect the muscle's blood supply. The resulting infection, ischemia, or a combination of the two may result in further tissue injury and poor healing.

Fatigue

Muscle **fatigue** occurs as the muscles reach their limit of performance. Exercise draws down the muscle's oxygen and energy reserves and causes accumulation of metabolic by-products. The cell environment becomes hypoxic, toxic, and energy deprived. Fewer and fewer muscle fibers are able to contract. The strength of the muscle mass diminishes, and further exertion becomes painful. Until adequate circulation restores oxygen and the muscle cells can replenish energy sources, the muscle fibers and muscle body remain weakened.

✱ **fatigue** condition in which a muscle's ability to respond to stimulation is lost or reduced through overactivity.

Muscle Cramp

Cramping is not really an injury, but an "angina" of the muscle tissue. Muscle pain results when exercise consumes the available oxygen and energy sources and

✱ **cramping** muscle pain resulting from overactivity, lack of oxygen, and accumulation of waste products.

the circulatory system fails to remove metabolic waste products. The pain begins during or immediately after vigorous exercise or after the limb has been left in an unusual position for a period of time (obstructing circulatory flow). Cramping is usually associated with continuous muscle contraction (spasm). Changing the limb's position or massaging it may help return the circulation and reduce the pain. Once rest and adequate circulation restore the metabolic balance, the pain of muscle cramp usually subsides.

Muscle Spasm

✳ **spasm** intermittent or continuous contraction of a muscle.

In muscle **spasm,** the affected muscle goes into an intermittent (clonic) or continuous (tonic) contraction. The spasm may be firm enough to feel like the deformity associated with a fracture and can confound assessment. (The extreme of muscle spasm is rigor mortis, an anoxic, rigid, whole-body muscle spasm that occurs after death.) As with the cramp, the spasm usually subsides uneventfully with the restoration of circulation.

Strain

✳ **strain** injury resulting from overstretching of muscle fibers.

A **strain** occurs when muscle fibers are overstretched by forces that exceed the strength of the fibers. The muscle fibers then stretch and tear, causing pain that increases with any use of the muscle. The injury may occur with extreme muscle stress, as during heavy lifting or sprinting, or at times of fatigue, when only a limited number of fibers are in contraction. With a strain, the fibers are damaged without internal bleeding, edema, or discoloration. The site of injury is generally painful to palpation, and patients normally report pain that limits use of the affected muscle.

> **Content Review**
>
> #### TYPES OF JOINT INJURY
> Sprain
> Subluxation
> Dislocation

JOINT INJURY

Joint injuries include sprains, subluxations, and dislocations. The following sections detail the pathologies behind each of these injuries.

Sprain

✳ **sprain** tearing of a joint capsule's connective tissues.

✳ **subluxation** partial displacement of a bone end from its position in a joint capsule.

A **sprain** is a tearing of a joint capsule's connective tissues, specifically a ligament or ligaments. This injury causes acute pain at its site, followed shortly by inflammation and swelling. Ecchymotic discoloration occurs over time, but not usually during prehospital care. The tearing of ligaments weakens the joint. Continued use of the joint may lead to its complete failure. Sprains are classified, or graded, according to their severity, using the following criteria:

> **Content Review**
>
> #### TYPES OF SPRAINS
> Grade I—minor and incomplete capsule tear; painful, but minimal swelling; joint stable
> Grade II—significant but incomplete tear; moderate to severe pain, swelling; joint intact but unstable
> Grade III—complete tear; severe pain and spasm; joint unstable

- *Grade I* Minor and incomplete tear. The ligament is painful, and swelling is usually minimal. The joint is stable.
- *Grade II* Significant but incomplete tear. Swelling and pain range from moderate to severe. The joint is intact but unstable.
- *Grade III* Complete tear of the ligament. Due to severe pain and spasm, the sprain may present as a fracture. The joint is unstable.

Subluxation

A **subluxation** is a partial displacement of a bone end from its position within a joint capsule. It occurs as the joint separates under stress, stretching the ligaments. The subluxation differs from the sprain in that it more significantly reduces the joint's integrity. The injured joint is painful and swells quickly, its range

a. Presentation of a knee dislocation.

b. X-ray of the dislocation.

FIGURE 22-1   Knee dislocation. *(Courtesy of Edward T. Dickinson, MD)*

of motion is limited, and the joint is unstable. Hyperflexion, hyperextension, lateral rotation beyond the normal range of motion, or application of extreme axial force are common causes of subluxations.

Dislocation

A **dislocation** is a complete displacement of bone ends from their normal joint position (Figure 22-1). The joint then fixes in an abnormal position with noticeable deformity. The site is painful, swollen, and immobile. This type of injury carries with it the danger of entrapping, compressing, or tearing blood vessels and nerves. Dislocation occurs when the joint moves beyond its normal range of motion with great force. By its nature, a dislocation has serious associated ligament damage and may involve injury to the joint capsule and articular cartilage.

> ✳ **dislocation** complete displacement of a bone end from its position in a joint capsule.

BONE INJURY

The fracture is an involved process that ultimately disrupts the continuity of the bone. When extreme compressional forces or significant lateral forces exceed the tensile strength of a bone, the bone fractures.

A fracture may be caused by direct injury—for example, an auto bumper impacts a patient's femur or a high-powered rifle bullet slams into a patient's thigh and, then, femur. The cause of the fracture may also be indirect. This might occur when a bike rider is thrown over the handlebars and braces the fall with an outstretched upper extremity. In this case, the energy of impact is transmitted from the hand to the wrist, to the forearm, to the arm, to the shoulder, to the clavicle. The transmitted force fractures the clavicle and may cause internal injury to blood vessels and the upper reaches of the lung. For this reason, always analyze the mechanism of injury carefully, recognizing that kinetic forces may be transmitted and cause injury far from the point of impact. Remember, 80 percent of multi-system trauma cases have associated serious musculoskeletal injury.

As kinetic energy is transmitted to the bone and the bone fractures, the collagen, osteocytes, salt crystals, blood vessels, nerves, and medullary canal of the bone, as well as its periosteum and endosteum (the inner lining of the medullary canal) are disrupted. If the broken bone ends displace, they may further injure surrounding muscles, tendons, ligaments, veins, and arteries. The result is a serious insult to the limb structure.

> *Recognize that kinetic forces may be transmitted through the skeletal system and cause injury remote from the impact site.*
>
>

FIGURE 22-2 Open and closed fractures.

Open

Closed

Content Review

TYPES OF FRACTURES

Open
Closed
Hairline
Impacted
Transverse
Oblique
Comminuted
Spiral
Greenstick
Epiphyseal

✳ **closed fracture** a broken bone in which the bone ends or the forces that caused it do not penetrate the skin.

✳ **open fracture** a broken bone in which the bone ends or the forces that caused it penetrate the surrounding skin.

✳ **hairline fracture** small crack in a bone that does not disrupt its total structure.

✳ **impacted fracture** break in a bone in which the bone is compressed on itself.

Vascular damage may restrict blood flow to the distal limb, increasing capillary refill time, diminishing pulse strength and limb temperature, and causing discoloration and paresthesia (a "pins-and-needles" sensation). Nerve injury may result in distal paresthesia, anesthesia (loss of sensation), paresis (weakness), and paralysis (loss of muscle control). Muscle or tendon damage may interfere with the victim's ability to move the limb. If muscle tissue is badly damaged where fasciae firmly contain it, compartment syndrome may develop.

If the bone does not seriously displace and the forces causing fracture do not penetrate, the surrounding skin remains intact and the resulting injury is termed a **closed fracture**. If the sharp bone ends displaced by the forces causing the fracture or other subsequent motion of the limb lacerate through the muscle, subcutaneous tissue, and skin, the result is termed an **open fracture** (Figure 22-2). An open fracture may also occur when a bullet travels through the limb and fractures the bone. Open fractures carry the risk of associated infection within the disrupted soft, bone, and medullary tissues. Such an infection may seriously reduce the bone's ability to heal. Where bones are located very close to the skin, as with the tibia (the shin), an open fracture can occur with relatively minimal bone displacement.

Surprisingly, some fractures may be relatively stable (Figure 22-3). When the bone suffers a small crack that doesn't disrupt its total structure, the injury is termed a **hairline fracture**. This type of injury weakens the bone and is painful, but the bone remains in position, retaining some of its strength. Another type of relatively stable bone injury is the **impacted fracture**. In some cases of compression, the bone impacts upon itself resulting in a compressed but aligned bone. As in a hairline fracture, the bone in an impacted fracture remains in position and retains some of its original strength. The danger with both hairline and impacted fractures is that further stress and movement may fracture the remaining bone and displace the bone ends, increasing both the severity of the injury and its healing time.

Impacted

Oblique

Transverse

Comminuted

Greenstick

Spiral

FIGURE 22-3   Types of fractures.

There are several fracture types whose physical characteristics can be revealed only by x-rays. For example, the **transverse fracture** is a complete break in the bone that runs straight across it at about a 90-degree angle. A fracture that runs at an angle across the bone is considered an **oblique fracture**. A fracture in which the bone has splintered into several smaller fragments is a **comminuted fracture**; this type of fracture is often associated with crushing injuries or the impact of a high-velocity bullet. Fractures involving a twisting motion may result in a curved break around the bone shaft known as a **spiral fracture**. Spiral fractures can occur with twisting motions, as when a child's arm is rotated by an adult or when an adult's limb is pulled into machinery like an auger.

The **fatigue fracture** is associated with prolonged or repeated stress such as walking. The bone generally weakens and fractures without the application of great kinetic force. An example is the metatarsal fatigue fracture, also known as a march fracture.

A very infrequent but serious complication of fracture is fat embolism. The bone's disruption may damage adjacent blood vessels and the medullary canal. The injury may then release fat, stored in a semi-liquid form, into the wound site where it enters the venous system and travels to the heart. The heart distributes the fat to the pulmonary circulation where it becomes pulmonary emboli. Fat embolism is usually associated with severe or crush injuries or post-injury manipulation of larger long bone fractures.

✱ **transverse fracture** a break that runs across a bone perpendicular to the bone's orientation.

✱ **oblique fracture** break in a bone running across it at an angle other than 90 degrees.

✱ **comminuted fracture** fracture in which a bone is broken into several pieces.

✱ **spiral fracture** a curving break in a bone as may be caused by rotational forces.

✱ **fatigue fracture** break in a bone associated with prolonged or repeated stress.

Pediatric Considerations

The bones of infants, young children and, to a degree, older children contain a greater percentage of cartilage than those of adults and are still growing from the epiphyseal plate. Pediatric patients thus often sustain different types of fractures than adults do.

The flexible nature of pediatric bones is responsible for the **greenstick fracture,** a type of partial fracture. The injury disrupts only one side of the long bone and remains angulated, resisting alignment due to the disrupted bone fibers on the fracture side. During the bone repair process, the injured side experiences more rapid growth than the other side. This results in increasing angulation of the bone as it heals. Surgeons often complete a greenstick fracture by breaking the bone fully, thereby assuring proper healing.

A child's bone grows at the epiphyseal plate, which forms a weak spot in the diaphysis. In pediatric trauma, this is a common site of the long bone disruption called an **epiphyseal fracture.** If the growth plate is disrupted, the disruption may lead to a reduction or halt in bone growth, a condition most commonly involving the proximal tibia.

Geriatric Considerations

The aging process causes several changes to the musculoskeletal system. A gradual, progressive decrease in bone mass and collagen structure begins at about the age of 40 and results in bones that are less flexible, more brittle, and more easily fractured. The bones also heal more slowly. The aging adult also loses some muscle strength and coordination, increasing the likelihood of skeletal injury. Fractures of the lumbar spine and femoral neck occur because of stress, often without history of significant trauma.

Another age-related and more significant problem secondary to poor bone remodeling is called **osteoporosis.** Osteoporosis is an accelerated degeneration of bone tissue due to loss of bone minerals, principally calcium. It typically affects women more than men and becomes most serious after menopause. The condition leads to increases in bone structure degeneration, spinal curvature, and incidences of fractures.

Pathological Fractures

Pathological fractures result from disease pathologies that affect bone development or maintenance. Such problems may be caused by tumors of the bone, periosteum, or articular cartilage or by diseases that release agents that increase osteoclast activity and osteoporosis. Other diseases and infections can have the same impact on bone tissue and result in fracture, especially in older patients. Radiation treatment may also kill bone cells, resulting in localized bone degeneration, weakened bones, and fractures. These fractures are not likely to heal well, if they heal at all.

GENERAL CONSIDERATIONS WITH MUSCULOSKELETAL INJURIES

The potential effects of trauma can be better anticipated when the skeletal structure and the musculature are examined together. It is important to note that long bones are smallest through the diaphysis and largest at the epiphyseal area, or joint. On the other hand, the external extremity diameter is greatest surrounding the midshaft due to the placement of skeletal muscle. This anatomical relationship is significant when looking at the potential for nervous or vascular injury.

---

* greenstick fracture partial fracture of a child's bone.

* epiphyseal fracture disruption in the epiphyseal plate of a child's bone.

* osteoporosis weakening of bone tissue due to loss of essential minerals, especially calcium.

Since there is limited soft tissue surrounding joints, joint fractures, dislocations, and—to a lesser degree—subluxations and sprains may cause severe problems beyond the direct injury. Any swelling, deformity, or displacement may compromise the nerve and vascular supply to the distal extremity. Fractures near a joint are more likely to compress or sever blood vessels or nerves. With shaft fractures, neurovascular injury is less likely, although manipulation of the fracture site or gross deformity may still endanger vessels and nerves running along the bone.

Areas around the joints are further endangered because blood vessels supplying the epiphysis enter the long bone through the diaphysis. If a fracture close to the epiphysis displaces the bone ends, it may compromise this blood supply with devastating results. The distal bone tissue may die without adequate circulation, destroying the joint and its function.

Once injury occurs, the stability of the extremity is reduced. Any additional movement can increase pain, damage to soft tissues, and the possibility of vascular or nerve involvement. Even slight manipulation can cause internal trauma. For example, a fractured femur has bone ends that are about the size of a broken broom handle. If, during extrication, splinting, and patient transport, the bone ends move about within the soft tissue, the resulting damage may be much more severe than that which initially occurred with the fracture. Manipulation of the injury site may also increase the likelihood of introducing bone fragments or fat emboli into the venous system, causing pulmonary embolism.

Another complication associated with long bone fracture is muscle spasm induced by pain. In a long bone fracture, pain causes the surrounding muscles to contract. This contraction forces the broken bone ends to override the fracture site. The result, in the case of the femur, is two broom-handle-sized bones driven into the muscles of the thigh, causing a cycle of more pain, more spasm, and more damage.

Because there is limited soft tissue surrounding joints, injuries there may cause severe problems beyond the direct injury because blood vessels and nerves may be affected.

BONE REPAIR CYCLE

The bone repair cycle is a complex process that results in almost complete healing. When trauma fractures a bone, the periosteum tears, as do local blood vessels, soft tissues, and the endosteum. Blood fills the injured area and congeals, establishing a red blood cell and collagen clot. This hemorrhagic clot is not very stable, but does begin the bone repair process. Osteocytes from the bone ends begin to multiply rapidly and produce osteoblasts. These osteoblasts lay down salt crystals within the collagen clot fibers. This establishes lengthening and widening regions of skeletal tissue from each disrupted bone end. Over time, the two growing ends join and form a large knob of cancellous bone, called the **callus**, that encapsulates the fracture site.

✱ callus thickened area that forms at the site of a fracture as part of the repair process.

As the process continues, the deposition of salts and the increasing collagen fiber matrix strengthen the callus and stabilize the bone to near-normal strength. Then osteoclasts dissolve salt crystals and collagen in areas where stress is minimal, while osteoblasts lay down new collagen and salts in high-stress areas. Through this process, the bone is remodeled until it looks very much like it did before the injury. If a fracture occurs when a patient is young and the bone ends are well aligned, there may be little evidence to suggest an injury ever occurred. If the bone ends are misaligned or if the bone experiences stress, infection, or movement before it has a chance to heal properly, the injury site may never return to normal and may leave the person with some disability.

INFLAMMATORY AND DEGENERATIVE CONDITIONS

Patients suffering from inflammatory and degenerative conditions may complain of joint pain, tenderness, and fatigue. These patients may also have difficulty walking and moving, may require additional assistance with their normal daily activities, and be prone to musculoskeletal injuries. Common inflammatory diseases of the musculoskeletal system include bursitis, tendinitis, and arthritis.

Bursitis

* **bursitis** acute or chronic inflammation of the small synovial sacs.

Bursitis is an acute or chronic inflammation of the bursae, the small synovial sacs that reduce friction and cushion ligaments and tendons from trauma. Bursitis may result from repeated trauma, gout, infection, and, in some cases, unknown etiologies. A patient with bursitis experiences localized pain, swelling, and tenderness at or near a joint. Commonly affected locations include the olecranon (elbow), the area just above the patella, and the shoulder.

Tendinitis

* **tendinitis** inflammation of a tendon and/or its protective sheath.

Tendinitis is characterized by inflammation of a tendon and its protective sheath and has a presentation similar to that of bursitis. Repeated trauma to a particular muscle group is a common cause of the condition, which usually affects the major tendons of the upper and lower extremity.

Arthritis

* **arthritis** inflammation of a joint.

* **osteoarthritis** inflammation of a joint resulting from wearing of the articular cartilage.

Arthritis is literally an inflammation of a joint. Three of the most common types of arthritis are osteoarthritis, rheumatoid arthritis, and gout (more formally known as gouty arthritis).

Osteoarthritis, which is also known as degenerative joint disease, is the most common type of connective tissue disorder. It is characterized by a general degeneration, or "wear-and-tear," of articular cartilage that results in irregular bony overgrowths. Signs and symptoms include pain, stiffness, and diminished movement in the joints. Joint enlargement may be visible, especially in the fingers. Predisposing factors for osteoarthritis include trauma, obesity, and aging.

* **rheumatoid arthritis** chronic disease that causes deterioration of peripheral joint connective tissue.

Rheumatoid arthritis is a chronic, systemic, progressive, and debilitating disease resulting in deterioration of peripheral joint connective tissue. It is characterized by inflammation of the synovial joints, which causes immobility, pain, increased pain on movement, and fatigue. The disease occurs two to three times more frequently in women than in men. In extreme cases, flexion contractures may develop due to muscle spasms induced by inflammation.

* **gout** inflammation of joints and connective tissue due to build-up of uric acid crystals.

Gout is an inflammation in joints and connective tissue produced by an accumulation of uric acid crystals. It occurs most frequently in males who often have high concentrations of uric acid in the blood. Uric acid is a metabolism endproduct that is not easily dissolved. Signs and symptoms of gout include peripheral joint pain, swelling, and possible deformity.

MUSCULOSKELETAL INJURY ASSESSMENT

With the majority of patients, fractures, dislocations, or muscular injuries only infrequently threaten life or seriously contribute to the development of shock. In most circumstances, a patient with an isolated fracture, dislocation, or trauma to muscular or connective tissue will receive complete assessment and management at the scene.

On the other hand, serious musculoskeletal injury is common in a patient who presents with other serious injuries. As you read earlier, energy is often transmitted from the point of impact along the skeletal system to the internal organs. Thus, when you discover a skeletal injury, always look for indications of the severity of the trauma forces and the possibility that the forces also caused internal injuries.

When you discover a skeletal injury, always look for indications of the severity of the trauma forces and the possibility that the forces also caused internal injuries.

As with any trauma patient, the assessment process progresses through the scene size-up, the initial assessment, either the rapid trauma assessment or focused exam and history, the detailed physical examination when appropriate, and serial ongoing assessments. You will usually focus your attention on musculoskeletal injuries during the rapid trauma assessment or focused exam and history and then as part of the detailed physical exam.

SCENE SIZE-UP

Remember to assure scene safety and don the appropriate personal protective equipment before approaching any scene. Gloves are mandatory when dealing with open musculoskeletal wounds, but those wounds, by themselves, do not usually suggest the need for protective eyewear, mask, or gown. Since most musculoskeletal injuries result from trauma, analyze the mechanism of injury to anticipate the nature and severity of those injuries. Enhance your analysis of the mechanism of injury by talking with the patient, family members, and bystanders to identify what happened and how.

INITIAL ASSESSMENT

It is imperative that assessment of the trauma patient begin with an evaluation of the patient's mental status and ABCs. During this initial assessment, you must also identify the potential for spinal injury and the need for spinal precautions. Remember, any serious musculoskeletal injury suggests kinetic energy forces sufficient to cause spinal injury, so always take spinal precautions with such an injury. Proceed with the initial assessment and assure that any life-threatening injuries are addressed before moving on in the assessment process. Never let the gruesome nature of a musculoskeletal injury distract you from performing a proper initial assessment and identifying and caring for life-threatening injuries first (Figure 22-4).

Patients with musculoskeletal injuries are classified into four categories:

- Patients with life- and limb-threatening injuries
- Patients with life-threatening injuries and minor musculoskeletal injuries
- Patients with non-life-threatening injuries but serious limb-threatening musculoskeletal injuries
- Patients with non-life-threatening injuries and only isolated minor musculoskeletal injuries

Perform a rapid trauma assessment for those patients with possible life- or limb-threatening injuries. A patient without life threat but with serious musculoskeletal

Any serious musculoskeletal injury suggests kinetic energy forces sufficient to cause spinal injury, so always take spinal precautions.

Never let the gruesome nature of a musculoskeletal injury distract you from identifying and caring for more subtle, but life-threatening injuries first.

Content Review

CLASSIFICATION OF PATIENTS WITH MUSCULOSKELETAL INJURIES

Life- and limb-threatening injuries

Life-threatening injuries, minor musculoskeletal injuries

Non-life-threatening injuries, serious limb-threatening injuries

Non-life-threatening injuries, isolated minor musculoskeletal injuries

FIGURE 22-4   As you begin assessment, examine the patient quickly for musculoskeletal injuries, but remember that they are not often life threatening.

injury may receive the rapid trauma assessment or the focused exam and history, depending upon the mechanism of injury and the information you discover during the initial assessment. Provide patients with isolated and simple musculoskeletal injuries with a focused exam and history, though you must remain watchful for any sign or symptom of more serious injury and the need for both a rapid trauma assessment and rapid patient transport to a trauma center.

RAPID TRAUMA ASSESSMENT

The rapid trauma assessment is performed on any patient with any sign, symptom, or mechanism of injury that suggests serious injury. While musculoskeletal injuries do not often cause life-threatening hemorrhage, remember that 80 percent of patients with serious multi-system trauma have associated musculoskeletal injury. When you have evidence of serious musculoskeletal injury, maintain a high index of suspicion for serious internal injury.

Perform the rapid trauma assessment in a carefully ordered way, progressing through an evaluation of the head, neck, chest, and abdomen, and arriving at the pelvis. Pay particular attention to the possibility of pelvic fracture, because such an injury may account for hemorrhage of more than 2 liters. Check the stability of the pelvic ring by directing firm pressure downward, then inward on the iliac crests, and then directing gentle downward pressure on the symphysis pubis. If the pressure reveals any instability or crepitus or elicits a response of pain from the patient, suspect pelvic fracture. Crepitus is a grating sensation felt as bone ends rub against one another. If you feel crepitus once, presume that bone injury exists and do not attempt to recreate the sensation. Consider the patient a candidate for aggressive fluid resuscitation and rapid transport.

In assessing the thighs, look for signs of tissue swelling and femur fracture. Each femur fracture may account for as much as 1,500 mL of blood loss. Evidence of this loss may be hidden within the tissue and muscle mass of the thigh, so compare one thigh to the other to evaluate swelling. If you find evidence of either pelvic or bilateral femur fracture, apply the pneumatic anti-shock garment (PASG), and inflate all compartments to a pressure that immobilizes the pelvis and the lower extremities. Monitor for the signs that the patient is compensating for blood loss, and consider both aggressive fluid resuscitation and rapid transport.

While fractures and muscular injuries of the extremities may not by themselves produce shock, they may significantly contribute to hypovolemia. Consider the effects of these injuries in your decision on whether to provide rapid transport or on-scene care. Further, fractures and dislocations may entrap or damage blood vessels or nerves, thus seriously threatening the future use of a limb. Quickly survey each limb and check the distal pulses, temperature, sensation (if the patient is conscious), motor function, and muscle tone.

Complete the rapid trauma assessment by gathering a patient history and a baseline set of vital signs (which may be done at the same time the physical assessment is being performed). If the rapid trauma assessment reveals a serious threat to life or limb, rapidly transport the patient to the nearest appropriate facility.

FOCUSED HISTORY AND PHYSICAL EXAM

The focused history and physical exam directs your attention to the injuries found or suggested during the initial assessment by the mechanism of injury and the patient's signs and symptoms. This step of the assessment process is performed for patients without life-threatening injuries and permits both assessment and care focused on isolated injuries.

A pelvic fracture may account for hemorrhage of more than 2 liters.

A femur fracture may account for as much as 1,500 mL of blood loss.

a. A fracture will often present with deformity.

b. An x-ray of the fracture.

FIGURE 22-5   Presentation of a forearm fracture.

Begin the focused physical exam by observing and inquiring carefully for signs and symptoms of fracture, dislocation, or other musculoskeletal injury in each limb with suspected injury (Figure 22-5). Expose and visualize the entire limb by removing any restrictive clothing or cutting it away carefully. In doing so, avoid manipulation of any potential injury site. Inspect the injury site carefully to locate any deformities (angulation or swelling), discolorations (unlikely in the first minutes after the incident), and indications of soft-tissue wounds that suggest injury beneath. Any unusual limb placement, asymmetry, or inequality in limb length (when compared to the opposing limb) should also arouse suspicion of musculoskeletal injury. Consider the possibility that any open wounds communicate with an associated fracture or dislocation. Observe for any contamination or sign of the bone protruding. Question the patient about pain, pain with attempted movement, discomfort, or unusual feeling or sensation. Also inquire about weakness, paralysis, paresthesia, or anesthesia. It may be helpful to think of the "six Ps" as a way to remember the key elements to be alert for when evaluating an extremity:

- *Pain.* The patient may report this upon palpation (tenderness) or movement.
- *Pallor.* The patient's skin may be pale or flushed, and capillary refill may be delayed.
- *Paralysis.* The patient may have inability or difficulty in moving an extremity.
- *Paresthesia.* The patient may report numbness or tingling in the affected extremity.
- *Pressure.* The patient reports a feeling of tension within the extremity.
- *Pulses.* These may be diminished or absent in the extremity.

If you do not identify a specific injury, palpate the extremity for instability, deformity (swelling or angulation), crepitus, unusual motion (joint-like motion where a joint doesn't exist), muscle tone (normal, flaccid, or spasming), or any regions of unusual warmth or coolness. Palpate the entire anterior and posterior surfaces, then the lateral and medial surfaces. Your assessment must be gentle, yet complete. Record any abnormal signs. When assessing the feet, carefully evaluate the distal circulation. Assess pulses for presence and relative strength, and

Content Review

THE SIX PS IN EVALUATING LIMB INJURY
Pain
Pallor
Paralysis
Paresthesia
Pressure
Pulses

FIGURE 22-6 Evaluate the distal extremity for pulse, temperature, color, sensation, and capillary refill.

then compare bilaterally. Test the skin for humidity, and warmth. Suspect circulatory compromise if capillary refill time is prolonged compared to the uninjured limb. Observe the skin for discoloration, noting any erythema, ecchymosis, or any abnormal hue (pale, ashen, or cyanotic). Approximate the level at which any deficit begins, and note any relation to possible extremity injury.

In a conscious and responsive patient, evaluate sensation and muscle strength distal to the injury (Figure 22-6). Check tactile (touch) response by touching or stroking the bottom of the foot with the blunt end of a bandage scissors or other similar instrument. Ask the patient to describe the feeling. If the patient is responsive and if there is no indication that the limb is injured, ask the patient to push down with the balls of both feet (plantar flexion) against your hands. Then ask the patient to pull upward with the top of the feet (dorsiflexion), again against your hands. If you feel any unilateral or bilateral weakness or the patient reports any pain, document the finding on the prehospital care report and look for the cause. Check abnormal sensation and the patient's ability to wiggle the toes or fingers.

Assess for potential upper extremity injury in a manner similar to your assessment of the lower extremity. Expose, observe, question about, and then palpate the limb as described above. Determine tactile response by using the back of the patient's hand. Test muscular strength by having the patient squeeze two of your fingers. Compare strength and sensation bilaterally, identify any deficit, and attempt to locate the cause. Evaluate the upper extremity and assure it is uninjured before you use it for blood pressure determination.

When the assessment of an extremity suggests injury, treat the limb as though a fracture or dislocation exists.

When the assessment of an extremity suggests injury, treat the limb as though a fracture or dislocation exists because the only definitive way to rule out these injuries is x-ray examination. Also note that splinting protects strains, sprains, and subluxations as well as fractures and dislocations from further injury. Treating a soft-tissue or muscular injury as a fracture or dislocation produces nothing more harmful than slight discomfort for the patient. Failure to immobilize an injury properly, however, may lead to additional soft, skeletal, connective, vascular, or nervous tissue damage and possibly cause permanent harm.

Form a clear mental picture of the injury site and be able to describe it to the emergency physician.

If possible, find the exact site of injury and determine if it involves a joint area or a long bone shaft. Form a clear visual image of the injury site in your mind so that you can describe the injury in the patient care report and to the receiving physician. Remember that the splinting device (e.g., the PASG for a femur fracture) may hide the site from view, leaving the attending physician unable to determine what exists beneath it. A good description of the wound may delay the need to remove the splint to view the injury.

One complication of musculoskeletal injury to the extremities is compartment syndrome. This condition results from bleeding into, or edema within, a muscle mass surrounded by fasciae that do not stretch. The build-up of pressure then compresses capillaries and nerves, leading to local tissue ischemia and then necrosis, with some loss of distal sensation. A pulse deficit may be a very late finding in compartment syndrome. Suspect compartment syndrome in any patient who has any paraesthesia, especially in the webs between the medial toes or fingers, who has an extremity injury with a firm mass or increased skin tension at the injury site, or who has pain out of proportion to the nature of the injury or pain that increases when you move the limb (passive stretching). Also suspect compartment syndrome in any unconscious patient with a swollen limb. Compartment syndrome most often occurs in the forearm or leg.

During the physical exam, question the patient about the symptoms of injury. Assure that your verbal investigation is detailed and complete. Determine the nature and location of pain and tenderness or dysfunction. The patient's description of the fracture or dislocation event may also be helpful. The patient may state that he felt the bone "snap" or the joint "pop out." Determine if the bone snapped, thus causing the fall, or whether the fall caused the fracture. Evaluate for the amount of pain and discomfort the patient is experiencing with the injury. For example, an elderly patient may present with a fractured hip and limited pain, a presentation usually related to a degenerative disease and secondary fracture. These findings may suggest that you adopt a less aggressive approach to care for this patient, focusing upon the patient's comfort rather than upon traction splinting and shock care. Also identify the signs and symptoms of injury as well as pertinent patient allergies, medications, past medical history, last oral intake, and events leading up to the incident.

Compare the findings of your assessment to the index of suspicion for injury you developed during the scene size-up. If you have found less significant injury than you suspected, consider reevaluating the patient to assure that no injury has been overlooked. If you find a more significant injury, suspect other severe injury may have occurred elsewhere and expand your focused exam.

As you conclude the focused history and physical exam, identify all injuries found, prioritize them, and establish the order of care for them. Identify the extent to which each injury may contribute to hemorrhage and shock. Then prioritize the patient for transport. Taking these few moments to sort out what is wrong with the patient and to plan care steps will increase the efficiency of your patient care, reduce on-scene time, and ensure that the patient receives the proper care at the right time.

DETAILED PHYSICAL EXAM

After you have ruled out or addressed potential threats to the patient's life or limbs, attended to any serious problems, and assessed any suspected injuries, you may perform a detailed physical exam. You will most likely perform the detailed physical exam on the patient who is unconscious or has a lowered level of consciousness. The exam may be performed at the scene or, more likely, while en route to the hospital. The detailed physical exam is a search for the signs and symptoms of further injury. It is performed as a head-to-toe evaluation, looking specifically where you have not looked before and with enough care to identify any subtle indications of injury. Be alert for the signs and symptoms of internal or external injury or hemorrhage. Use the same assessment techniques for evaluating musculoskeletal injuries during the detailed physical exam that you employed during the rapid trauma assessment and focused history and physical exam.

At the conclusion of the rapid trauma assessment or the focused exam, identify all injuries and prioritize them for care.

ONGOING ASSESSMENT

The ongoing assessment focuses on serial measurement of the patient's vital signs, level of consciousness, and the signs and symptoms of the major trauma affecting the patient. For patients with musculoskeletal injuries, monitor distal sensation and pulses frequently. Remember to ask about the patient's complaints and description of the musculoskeletal injury, watching for any changes in the responses. As time passes and the effects of the "fight-or-flight" response wear off, the patient may display more significant and specific symptoms of injury. The patient may also begin to complain of other injuries masked earlier by the chief complaint and of other major pain or discomfort. If this occurs, provide a focused assessment on the area of complaint and modify your patient priorities as additional injuries are found.

SPORTS INJURY CONSIDERATIONS

Many of the musculoskeletal injuries you attend as an EMT-Paramedic are associated with sports activities. Activities such as football, basketball, soccer, baseball, in-line skating, skiing, snowboarding, bicycling, wrestling, hiking, and rock climbing often lead to injury for participants. When you are called to the scene of a sports injury, assess the mechanism of injury and determine whether there was a major kinetic force involved, a hyperextension or flexion injury, or a fatigue-type injury. Athletic injuries often affect major body joints like the shoulder, elbow, wrist, shoulder, knee, and ankle. Injuries in these areas are especially troubling for patients because serious ligament damage might preclude future participation in a sport and limit limb usefulness. It is imperative that any potentially significant sports injury be attended to by an emergency department physician. The competitive natures of players, teammates, coaches, and athletic trainers may lead them to downplay injuries in order to keep an injured athlete in competition. Allowing an injured athlete to keep playing, however, places additional stress on the injury and may result in further, and more debilitating, damage.

MUSCULOSKELETAL INJURY MANAGEMENT

Management of musculoskeletal injuries is not normally a high priority in trauma patient care. It usually does not occur until after you have completed the initial assessment, stabilized the airway, breathing, and circulation, and finished the rapid trauma assessment. While the focus of care for the serious trauma patient is the current life threats, some protection for serious musculoskeletal injuries is provided by moving the patient as a unit (with axial alignment) and by packaging the patient for transport using the long spine board (see Chapter 24, "Spinal Trauma"). These techniques help you reduce the risks of aggravating musculoskeletal injuries, increasing hemorrhage, and worsening shock and patient outcome. However, do not let gruesome musculoskeletal injury distract you from the priorities of trauma management.

Fractures of the pelvis and, to a lesser degree, the femur can significantly contribute to hypovolemia and shock. These injuries deserve a high priority in patient care. Other musculoskeletal injuries that merit a priority for care include those that threaten a limb, such as injuries with loss of distal circulation or sensation (most commonly joint injuries), and those that cause compartment syndrome (most likely leg or forearm injuries). You may prioritize other injuries by the relative size of the bone fractured or the body area involved and by the energy that was required to cause injury. Prioritize the patient's musculoskeletal injuries for care, then proceed with splinting and transport.

During the ongoing assessment, be sure to ask about the patient's complaints and description of the musculoskeletal injury, because over time, the patient may display more significant and specific symptoms of injury and complain of other injuries masked earlier by the chief complaint.

Any potentially significant sports injury should be attended to by an emergency department physician.

GENERAL PRINCIPLES OF MUSCULOSKELETAL INJURY MANAGEMENT

The objectives of musculoskeletal injury care are to reduce the possibility of any further injury during patient care and transport and to reduce the patient's discomfort. Accomplish these goals by protecting open wounds, positioning the extremity properly, immobilizing the injured extremity, and monitoring neurovascular function in the distal limb. In some cases, care involves manipulating the injury to reestablish distal circulation and sensation or simply to restore normal anatomic position for the patient expecting prolonged extrication or transport. In most cases, care for musculoskeletal injuries will also include application of a splinting device.

As you begin to care for a patient with musculoskeletal injuries, talk to him and explain what you are doing, why, and what impact it will have on the patient. Alignment and splinting will likely first cause an increase in pain followed by a significant reduction in it. By telling the patient of this in advance, you will increase confidence in both your intent to help and your ability to provide care.

Protecting Open Wounds

If there is any open wound in close proximity to the fracture or dislocation, consider the fracture or dislocation to be an open one. Carefully observe the wound and note any signs of muscle, tendon, ligament, or vascular injury and be prepared to describe the wound in your report and at the emergency department. Cover the wound with a sterile dressing held in place with bandaging or a splint. Frequently, the attempts to align a limb, the splinting process, or the application of traction will draw protruding bones back into the wound. This is an expected consequence of proper care but must be brought to the attention of the attending emergency department physician.

Positioning the Limb

Proper limb positioning is essential to assure patient comfort, to reduce the chances of further limb injury, and to encourage venous drainage. Proper positioning is different with fractures and dislocations, although splinting with the limb in a normal anatomical position, the position of function, is beneficial for both.

Limb alignment is appropriate for any fractures of the mid-shaft femur, tibia/fibula, humerus, or radius/ulna. Alignment can be maintained by using the air splint, padded rigid splint, PASG, or traction splint. Proper alignment of a fracture enhances circulation and reduces the potential for further injury to surrounding tissue. It is also very difficult to immobilize a limb with a fracture in an unaligned, angulated position because the fracture segments are short and buried in soft tissue. Perform any limb alignment with great care so as not to damage the tissue surrounding the fracture site. During the process, the proximal limb should remain in position while you bring the distal limb to the position of alignment using gentle axial traction. Stop the process when you detect any resistance to movement or when the patient reports any significant increase in pain.

Generally, you should not attempt alignment of dislocations and serious injuries within 3 inches of a joint. Only attempt to manipulate such injury sites if the distal circulation is compromised. In such a case, try to move the joint while another care provider palpates the distal pulse. If the pulse is restored, if you meet significant resistance to movement, or if the patient complains of greatly increased pain, stop the manipulation and splint the injured limb as it is. Be sure to transport the patient quickly, because a loss of circulation can endanger the future usefulness of the limb.

Content Review

BASICS OF MUSCULOSKELETAL INJURY CARE

Protecting open wounds
Proper positioning
Immobilizing the injury
Monitoring of neurovascular function

Stop realignment attempts when you detect any resistance to movement or when the patient reports any significant increase in pain.

Do not attempt alignment of dislocations and serious injuries within 3 inches of a joint.

If you suspect a limb will remain dislocated for an extended period, as during lengthy transports or prolonged patient entrapments, consider reducing the dislocation. Apply a firm and progressive traction to the limb, which draws the dislocated ends away from each other and moves the joint toward normal positioning. When (and if) the bone ends "pop" back into position, assure there is a distal pulse and immobilize the limb in the position of function.

Proper positioning of injured limbs is important for maintaining distal circulation and sensation and increasing patient comfort. Deformities and extremes of flexion or extension put pressure on the soft tissues and may compress nerves and blood vessels. These positions also fatigue the surrounding muscles and increase the pain associated with the injury. By placing the uninjured joints of the limb halfway between flexion and extension in what is called the position of function, you place the least stress on the joint ligaments and the muscles and tendons surrounding the injury. Place the limb in the position of function whenever possible (Figure 22-7). Note, however, that some injuries and some splinting devices commonly used for musculoskeletal injuries may preclude this positioning.

When possible, place injured limbs in the position of function or neutral position.

When practical, elevate the injured limb. This will assist with venous drainage and reduce the edema associated with musculoskeletal injury.

Immobilizing the Injury

The aim in immobilizing musculoskeletal injuries is to prevent further injury caused by the movement of broken bone ends and bone ends dislodged from a joint and by further stress placed on muscles, ligaments, or tendons already injured by a strain, sprain, subluxation, dislocation, or fracture. This immobilization is usually accomplished through the use of a splinting device.

Since most long bones lie buried deep within the musculature of the extremities, it is very difficult to immobilize them directly. Hence, we immobilize the joint above and the joint below the injury, regardless of whether the injury occurs at a joint or mid-shaft in a long bone. This assures that no motion is transmitted through the injury site as might occur, for example, with the rotation (supination/pronation) of the radius against the ulna at the elbow when the wrist turns.

Wrap any splinting device or associated bandage from a distal point to a proximal one. This assures that the pressure of bandaging moves any blood into the systemic circulation and does not trap it in the distal limb. This method of wrapping thus assists venous drainage and the healing process. Apply firm pressure when wrapping, but be sure you can easily push a finger beneath the wrapping.

Checking Neurovascular Function

It is imperative that you identify the status of the circulation, motor function, and sensation distal to the injury site before, during, and after splinting of all musculoskeletal injuries. The check before splinting identifies a baseline condition and establishes that the initial injury has not disrupted circulation. The check during splinting assures that inadvertent limb movement or circumferential pressure does not compromise distal circulation. The check after splinting identifies any restriction caused by progressive swelling of the injured area against the splinting device. Clearly identify and document these evaluations whenever you apply a splint.

To perform this evaluation, first palpate for a pulse and assure it is equal in strength to that of the opposing limb. If the pulse cannot be located or is weak, check capillary refill and skin temperature, color, and condition. Again compare your findings to the opposing limb. Ask the patient to describe the sensation when you rub or pinch the bottom of the foot or back of the hand and ask him to move the fingers or toes. The patient response establishes your baseline circulation, sensory, and motor findings. Reevaluate pulse, motor function, and sensation frequently during the remaining care and transport. If a care provider is holding the limb while you apply the splint, have him or her monitor both pulse and skin temperature. That care provider can then immediately note any compromise in circulation.

Always check pulses, motor function, and sensation in the distal extremity before, during, and after splinting.

SPLINTING DEVICES

An essential part of managing any musculoskeletal system injury is the use of devices to immobilize a limb and permit patient transport without causing further injury. These devices, called splints, are designed to help you reduce or eliminate any movement of the injured extremity. Splints come in several forms that can assist in immobilizing common fractures and dislocations associated with musculoskeletal trauma (Figure 22-8). They include rigid, formable, soft, traction, and other splints.

Rigid Splints

Rigid splints, as the name implies, are firm and durable supports for the injured limb. They can be constructed of cardboard, plastic, metal, synthetic products, or wood. Such devices very effectively immobilize injury sites but require adequate padding to lessen patient discomfort. This padding may be built into the splint or may simply be a bulky dressing affixed to the splint with soft bandaging. Several types of commercially available rigid splints are used in prehospital

FIGURE 22-8 A variety of splints are available for musculoskeletal injuries.

care. They are usually flat and rigid devices and are about 3 inches wide and from 16 to 48 inches long. The injured limb that is in alignment is immobilized to the splint by circumferential wrapping, while an angulated limb may be held in position by cross-wrapping at two locations.

A special form of rigid splint is the preformed splint. It is usually a stamped metal or preformed plastic or fiberglass device shaped to the contours of the distal limbs. These splints are usually available for the ankles and hands.

Formable Splints

Another type of rigid splint is the formable, or malleable, splint. It is made up of a material that you can easily shape to match the angulation of a limb. You then affix the formed splint to the limb with circumferential bandaging. Formable splints include both the ladder splint, which is a matrix of soft metal wires soldered together, and the metal sheet splint, which is made up of thin aluminum or another easily shaped metal.

Soft Splints

Soft splints use padding or air pressure to immobilize an injured limb in place. Among the varieties of soft splints are air splints, which include the PASG, and pillow splints.

The air splint provides immobilization as air pressure fills the splint and compresses the limb. Since the splint is a formed cylinder, and may include shaping for the foot, it immobilizes the limb in an aligned position. Air splints should not be used with long bone injuries at or above the knee or elbow because they cannot prevent movement of hip or shoulder joints and are thus unable to immobilize the proximal joints of the limb. Air splints also apply a pressure that may be helpful in controlling both external and internal hemorrhage. While these devices may limit assessment of the distal extremity, they do permit observation because they are transparent. (Note that the PASG is not transparent, so carefully assess the patient from the rib cage to the feet before applying and inflating it.)

Monitor pressure within the air splint or PASG, as it may change with changes in altitude or temperature.

Monitor air splints carefully with any changes in temperature or atmospheric pressure. Increases in ambient heat or decreases in pressure, as during an ascent in a helicopter, will increase the pressure within the splint. Conversely, decreases in temperature or a descent in a helicopter will decrease pressure in the splint. Constantly monitor the pressure in the air splint and PASG to assure it does not rise or fall during your care.

The pillow splint is a comfortable splint for ankle and foot injuries. The foot is simply placed on the pillow while the outer fabric is drawn around the foot and pillow. The outer fabric is pinned together or wrapped circumferentially with bandage material around the injury site. This device applies gentle and uniform pressure to effectively immobilize the distal extremity. Using a bulky blanket or two and wrapping them firmly may also provide the same type of immobilization.

Traction Splints

The traction splint was developed during World War I and used extensively during World War II. This splint dramatically reduced both mortality and limb loss from femur fractures caused by projectile wounds, blast injuries, and other traumas. Today, the traction splint is the mainstay of prehospital care for the isolated traumatic femur fracture.

The traction splint is a frame that applies a pull (traction) on the injured extremity and against the trunk. The application of traction is useful when splinting the femur, which is surrounded by very heavy musculature. Frequently, the

a. A bipolar frame traction splint.

b. A unipolar frame traction splint.

FIGURE 22-9   Traction splints.

pain of fracture initiates muscle spasm that causes the bone ends to override each other causing further pain and muscle spasm and aggravating the original injury. The traction splint prevents overriding of the bone ends, lessens patient pain, and may help relax any muscle spasm.

There are basically two styles of traction splint, the bipolar frame device and the unipolar device (Figure 22-9). The bipolar (Hare or Thomas) traction splint has a half ring that fits up and against the ischial tuberosity of the pelvis. A distal ratchet connects to a foot harness and pulls traction from the foot and against the pelvis. The frame lifts and supports the limb and a foot stand suspends the injured limb above the ground. This construction helps prevent motion of the limb during movement of the patient, while the elevation supplied by the stand enhances venous drainage. The unipolar (Sager) traction splint uses a single lengthening shaft to pull a foot harness against pressure applied to the pubic bone. The unipolar splint does not elevate or stabilize the extremity, so you must observe greater care whenever you move the patient. You can use the unipolar splint in conjunction with the PASG.

Other Splinting Aids

Vacuum splints can conform to the exact shape of a limb (Figure 22-10). An injured limb is placed on a bag of small plastic particles. The splint is shaped around the limb and then the air is withdrawn from the device. The suction locks the particles in position, immobilizing the splint to the contours of the limb. The

FIGURE 22-10 Suction the air out of a vacuum splint until the device is rigid. Reassess pulse, motor function, and sensation in the extremity after application.

only disadvantage to vacuum splinting is that during air evacuation there is a small amount of shrinkage and a reduction in the splinting effect.

Cravats or Velcro® straps can augment the effectiveness of rigid splints. You can secure the lower extremities, one to the other, to help the patient control the musculoskeletal injury site or you can use a sling and swathe to help immobilize a splinted upper extremity to the chest. Fractures of the humerus are difficult to immobilize because the shoulder is such a large and mobile part of the body. A sling may hold the elbow at a fixed angle, while a swathe secures the limb against the body to limit further shoulder motion. By holding a thumb in the fold of the elbow, the patient can easily reduce any motion of the limb and complement the splinting process.

In some cases of serious musculoskeletal injury, other injuries preclude the splinting of individual fractures and dislocations. In such cases, you may splint the limbs to the body with cravats or bandage material and immobilize the patient to the long spine board. Simply strap the body and limbs to the board and transport the patient as a unit. While this is not definitive splinting, it will provide reasonable protection for musculoskeletal injuries.

FRACTURE CARE

Consider any injury within 3 inches of a joint to be a joint injury.

For prehospital care purposes, consider a joint injury to be any muscular or connective tissue injury or dislocation or fracture within 3 inches of a joint. Fractures are then defined as shaft injuries at least 3 inches away from the joint. These definitions are essential because injury near the joint carries a higher incidence of blood vessel and nerve involvement and requires a different approach to positioning and splinting.

Begin fracture care by assuring distal pulses, sensation, and motor function. Then align the limb for splinting. Quickly recheck the circulation and motor and sensory function below the injury. If you identify any neurovascular deficit, attempt to correct the problem by gentle repositioning, even if the limb is relatively aligned. If the limb is angulated, proceed with realignment. Remember that most splinting devices are designed to immobilize aligned limbs and that alignment provides the best chance for assuring good neurovascular function distal to the injury.

To move an injured limb from an angulated position into alignment, use gentle distal traction applied manually. Have an assisting EMT immobilize the proximal limb in the position found. Grasp the distal limb firmly and apply traction along the limb's axis, gently moving it from the angulated to an aligned position. Should you feel any resistance to movement or notice a great increase in patient discomfort, stop the alignment attempt and splint the limb as it lies. Once you complete alignment, recheck the distal neurovascular function. If it is adequate, proceed with splinting. If function is inadequate, move the limb around slightly while another care provider monitors for a pulse. If one attempt at gentle manipulation does not reestablish a pulse, splint and transport the patient quickly.

Proceed with splinting by selecting an appropriate device and secure the limb to it in a way that assures you immobilize both the fracture site and the adjacent joints. Have the care provider who is holding the limb apply a gentle traction to stabilize the limb (and monitor the distal pulse) during splinting. If you apply your splint properly, the device may maintain this traction and provide greater stabilization of the limb and greater patient comfort. Secure the limb to the body (upper extremity) or to the opposite limb (lower extremity) to protect it and to give the patient some control over the limb.

JOINT CARE

Joint care, too, begins with assessment for distal neurovascular function. If you find pulse, sensation, and motor function to be adequate, immobilize the joint in the position found. Use a ladder or other malleable splint, shaped to the limb's angle, or cross-wrap with a padded rigid splint to immobilize the joint in place. Assure that your splinting immobilizes the injured joint and both the joint above and the joint below the injury. If not, secure the limb firmly to the body to immobilize these joints.

If circulation or motor or sensory function is lost below the joint injury, consider moving the limb to reestablish it. While you gently move the limb, have another care provider monitor the circulation and sensation. If you can reestablish neurovascular function quickly, splint the limb in the new position. If not, splint and provide quick transport.

With some joint injuries, you may attempt to return the displaced bone ends to their normal anatomic position. This process is called **reduction** and has both benefits and hazards. An early return to normal position reduces stress on the ligaments and basic joint structure and facilitates better distal circulation and sensation. On the other hand, the process creates the risk of trapping blood vessels or nerves as the bone ends return to their normal anatomic position. Attempt reduction of a dislocation only when you are sure the injury *is* a dislocation, when you expect the patient's arrival at the emergency department to be delayed (prolonged extrication or long transport time), or when there is a significant neurovascular deficit. Do not attempt a reduction if the dislocation is associated with other serious patient injuries. Consult your protocols and medical direction to determine the criteria for attempting dislocation reduction used in your system.

When performing a joint reduction, you attempt to protect the articular surface while directing the bones back to their normal anatomic position. Begin the process by providing the patient with analgesic therapy to reduce pain associated with the injury and the reduction itself. Then have an assisting care provider hold the proximal extremity in position and provide a counter-traction during the reduction. You then apply traction to pull the bone surfaces apart, reducing the pressure between the non-articular surfaces. Slowly increase traction and direct the displaced limb toward its normal anatomic position. Successful relocation is indicated when you feel the joint "pop" back into position, the patient experiences a lessening of pain, and the joint becomes mobile within at least a few minutes of the procedure. Carefully evaluate the distal circulation, sensation, and motor function after the reduction. If the procedure does not meet with success within a few minutes, splint the limb as it is and provide rapid transport for the patient. If the reduction is successful, splint the limb in the position of function and transport.

Unless you identify a neurovascular deficit, immobilize joint injuries as you find them.

---

* **reduction** returning of displaced bone ends to their proper anatomic orientation.

MUSCULAR AND CONNECTIVE TISSUE CARE

Injuries to the soft tissues of the musculoskeletal system deserve special care. While such injuries are not usually life threatening, they can be very painful, and in some cases, threaten limbs. For example, compartment syndrome can restrict capillary blood flow, venous blood return, and nerve function beyond the site of the injury. If such an injury is not discovered and relieved, it may produce severe disability. Deep contusions and especially large hematomas can also contribute to blood loss and hypovolemia. Once you care for life threats, fractures, joint injuries, and other limb threats, give injuries to muscular and connective tissues your attention.

To manage these muscle, tendon, and ligament injuries, immobilize the region surrounding them. Doing so will reduce the associated internal hemorrhage and pain. Provide gentle circumferential bandaging (loose enough to let you slide a finger underneath) to further reduce hemorrhage, edema, and pain, but be sure to monitor distal circulation and loosen the bandage further if there are any signs of neurovascular deficit. Application of local cooling will reduce both edema and patient discomfort. Be careful to wrap any cold or ice pack in a dressing to prevent too drastic a cooling and any consequent injury. You may apply heat to the wound after 48 hours to enhance both circulation and healing. If possible, place the limb in the position of function and elevate the extremity to assure good venous return, limit swelling, and reduce patient discomfort. Monitor distal neurovascular function to assure your actions do not compromise circulation, sensation, or motor function.

CARE FOR SPECIFIC FRACTURES

Pelvis

Always consider a pelvic fracture patient to be a candidate for rapid transport.

Pelvic fractures involve either the iliac crest or the pelvic ring. While iliac crest fractures may reflect serious trauma, they do not represent the patient life-threat suggested by ring fractures. Iliac crest fractures are often isolated and stable injuries that you can care for by simple patient immobilization.

Pelvic ring fractures, on the other hand, are often serious, life-threatening events. The ring shape of the pelvis provides strength to the structure, but when it breaks, two fracture sites usually result. The kinetic forces necessary to fracture the pelvic ring are significant and are likely to produce fractures and internal injuries elsewhere. In addition, the pelvis is actively involved in blood cell production, has a rich blood supply, and its interior surface is adjacent to major blood vessels serving the lower extremities. Injury to the pelvic ring, therefore, can result in heavy hemorrhage that is likely to empty into the pelvic and retroperitoneal spaces and account for blood loss in excess of 2 liters. Such injury may also result in circulation loss to one or both lower extremities. Pelvic fractures may also be associated with hip dislocations and injuries to the bladder, female reproductive organs, the urethra, the prostate in the male, and the end of the alimentary canal (anus and rectum). Clearly, pelvic ring fractures are very serious injuries.

The objectives of pelvic injury care are to stabilize the fractured pelvis, support the patient hemodynamically, and provide rapid transport to a trauma center. Because of the potential for severe blood loss and the difficulty of immobilizing the broken pelvic ring, application of the PASG is standard practice with pelvic fractures (Figure 22-11). Inflate the PASG until it stabilizes the pelvis and hip joint. Start two large-bore IVs, and hang two 1,000 mL bags of lactated Ringer's solution or normal saline. Set up using trauma tubing and pressure infusion sets for rapid infusion because aggressive fluid administration may be necessary. Be prepared to run 1,000 mL of solution immediately to maintain the blood pressure at between 90 and 100 mmHg. Once the initial bolus of fluid is administered, the IV lines need only run at a "to-keep-open" rate unless there are further signs of hy-

FIGURE 22-11 The PASG is an effective splint for traumatic pelvic fractures and helps control internal hemorrhage.

povolemic compensation or the blood pressure dips below 90 mmHg. Always consider a pelvic fracture patient to be a candidate for rapid transport.

Femur

Femur fractures may be traumatic, resulting from the application of very strong and violent forces, or atraumatic, resulting from degenerative diseases. Patients with disease-induced fractures usually are of advancing age and present with a history of a degenerative disease, a clouded or limited history of trauma, and only moderate discomfort. Care for such patients by immobilizing them as found and then providing gentle transport. Generally, you can provide effective splinting by placing the patient on a long spine board and padding with pillows and blankets for patient comfort. Use of a traction splint is not essential because pain is not inducing the spasms that cause broken bone ends to override.

A patient who has suffered a traumatic femur fracture usually experiences extreme discomfort, often writhing in pain. In such a case, providing distal traction immobilizes both bone ends, relieves muscle spasms, and reduces the associated pain. Traction splinting is the best avenue for care of the hemodynamically stable patient with an isolated femur fracture. However, the traction splint is not indicated if the patient has concurrent serious knee, tibia, or foot injuries.

Proximal fractures (surgical neck and intertrochanteric fractures) are frequently caused by hip injuries, transmitted forces, or the degenerative effects of aging. Midshaft fractures often result from high-energy, lateral traumas and are associated with significant blood loss. Injuries to the distal femur (condylar and epicondylar fractures) can be extensive and are likely to involve blood vessels, nerves, and connective tissue. The energy necessary to fracture the femur may be sufficient to dislocate the hip and cause serious internal injuries elsewhere in the body.

If the femur fracture is concurrent with a severe pelvic fracture, you may best achieve limb immobilization and hemodynamic stability by using the PASG alone. A traction splint may apply pressure to the fractured pelvis, thereby causing further bone displacement and hemorrhage. Also, if the early signs of shock are present or if the history suggests that the patient has sustained trauma severe enough to induce shock, the PASG may be a better choice because it effectively splints the entire region and contributes to hemodynamic stability.

You may find it difficult to differentiate between proximal fractures of the femur (hip fractures) and anterior hip dislocations. Generally, a femur fracture presents with the foot externally rotated (turned outward) and the injured limb shortened when compared to the other. This difference may be slight and may be unnoticeable if the patient's legs are not straight and parallel. An anterior dislocation presents similarly to the femur fracture, but with the head of the femur protruding in the inguinal region. When in doubt, treat as a dislocation.

If you suspect femur fracture, align the limb, determine the status of circulation and sensory and motor function, and apply the traction splint (Figure 22-12). (If you use manual traction to align the femur, maintain it until the splint is applied and continues the traction.) Adjust the length of the splint to the injured extremity, position the device against the pelvis, and secure it in position with the inguinal strap. With a bipolar splint, apply the ankle hitch, provide gentle traction, and elevate the distal limb to place the splint's ring against the ischial tuberosity. With a unipolar splint, position the T-shaped support against the pubic bone and simply apply the ankle hitch. Assure that hitch and splint hold the foot and limb in an anatomic position as you apply firm traction. Position and secure the limb to the splint with straps, then gently move the patient and splint to the long spine board. Firmly secure the patient and limb for transport.

Guide your application of traction by the patient's response. Ask the patient how the limb feels as you initiate and increase the amount of traction. Stop the

Atraumatic femur fractures may be splinted by gently placing the patient on a long spine board.

application of traction when the limb is immobilized and patient discomfort decreases. Remember, as the traction splint prevents the overriding of bone ends, the pain of injury decreases. This reduces the strength of muscle spasm and lets the limb return toward its initial length. This, in turn, reduces the traction provided by the splint, which means that the bone ends will no longer be as well immobilized. Check the amount of traction frequently to assure that it does not lessen during your care. If the patient reports increasing pain, consider increasing traction gradually until some reduction in pain is noted.

When the need for rapid transport or other patient injuries preclude the use of the traction splint, consider using the long spine board for immobilizing and transporting the femur fracture patient. Use long padded rigid splints, one medial and one lateral, to quickly splint the injured limb, and then tie that limb to the uninjured one. Use an orthopedic stretcher or another device or movement technique to transfer the patient to a long spine board and secure the patient firmly on it.

Tibia/Fibula

Fractures of the leg bones, the tibia and the fibula, can occur separately or together. The tibia is the most commonly fractured leg bone and may be broken by direct force, crushing injury, or twisting forces. Tibial fracture is likely to cause an open wound. Fibular fractures are often associated with damage to the knee or ankle. If the tibia is fractured and the fibula is intact, the extremity may not angulate, but it is not able to bear weight. If only the fibula is broken, the limb may be relatively stable. Injuries to either bone may result in compartment syndrome. Direct trauma suffered during an auto crash or athletic impact frequently causes these tibia and fibula injuries.

Fibular fractures are relatively stable, while tibial fractures are not.

Align the injured limb, assess circulation, sensation, and motor function, and then immobilize the limb with gentle traction. A full-leg air splint (one that accommodates the foot) or lateral and medial padded rigid splints will provide effective immobilization (Figure 22-13). You may also use a cardboard splint as long as it accommodates the full limb and is rigid enough to maintain immobilization. After you splint the injured limb, secure it to the uninjured leg. This affords some protection against uncontrolled movement and may reassure the patient that he still has some control over the extremity.

Clavicle

The clavicle is the most frequently fractured bone in the human body. Fractures to it usually result from transmitted forces directed along the upper extremity that cause relatively minor skeletal injury. The clavicle, however, is located adjacent to both the upper reaches of the lung and the vasculature that serves the up-

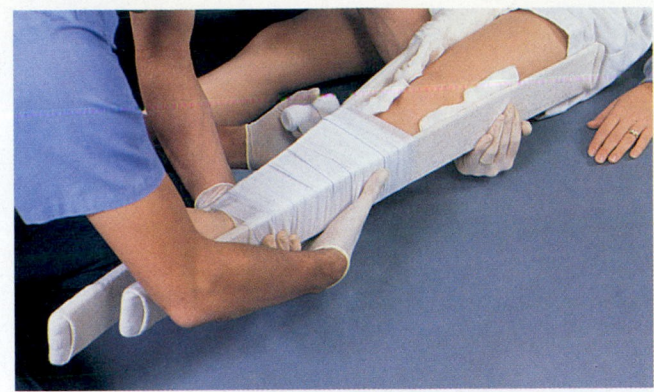

FIGURE 22-13 Placement of long padded board splints laterally and medially can effectively splint tibia/fibula fractures.

per extremity and head. Hence, an injury to the clavicle has the potential to cause serious internal injury, especially if very powerful mechanisms of injury are involved. The clavicular fracture patient often presents with pain and the shoulder shifted forward with palpable deformity along the clavicle. Accomplish splinting either by immobilizing the affected limb in a sling and swathe or by wrapping a figure-eight bandage around the shoulders, drawing the shoulders back, and then securing the bandage tension. Monitor the patient carefully for any sign of internal hemorrhage or respiratory compromise.

Humerus

A fractured humerus is very difficult to immobilize at its proximal end. The proximal humerus is buried within the shoulder muscles, and the shoulder joint is very mobile atop the thoracic cage. The axillary artery runs through the axilla, making it difficult to apply any mechanical traction to the limb without compromising circulation. Hence, the most effective techniques for splinting this fracture are to apply a sling and swathe to immobilize the bent limb against the chest or to tie the extended and splinted limb to the body.

The preferred technique is to use the sling and swathe. Apply a short padded rigid splint to the lateral surface of the arm to distribute the pressure of the swathing and better immobilize the arm. Sling the forearm with a cravat, catching just the wrist region and not the elbow. This permits some gravitational traction in the seated patient and prevents inadvertent application of pressure by the sling, which could push the limb together. Then use several cravats to gently swathe the arm and forearm to the chest. If the patient is conscious, have him place the thumb of the uninjured extremity in the fold of the elbow to help control the injured limb's motion. This gives the patient control over the limb, decreases limb movement, and increases patient comfort.

You may also immobilize the limb by using a long padded rigid splint affixed to the extended limb. Place the splint along the medial aspect of the upper extremity and assure that it does not apply pressure to the axilla. Such pressure disrupts axillary artery blood flow to the limb and is uncomfortable for the patient. Secure the splint firmly to the limb, wrapping from the distal end toward the proximal end. Then secure the splint to the supine patient's body, and move the patient and splint to a long spine board.

Radius/Ulna

The forearm may fracture anywhere along its length and the fracture may involve the radius, the ulna, or both. Most commonly, fracture occurs at the distal end of the radius, just above the articular surface. This is known as a Colles's fracture, and it presents with the wrist turned up at an unusual angle. Another term

FIGURE 22-14 A full-arm air splint can effectively splint fractures of the radius and/or ulna.

FIGURE 22-14 A full-arm air splint can effectively splint fractures of the radius and/or ulna.

for this injury is the "silver fork deformity" because it is contoured like a fork and the distal limb often becomes ashen. As with most joint fractures, the major concern here is for distal circulation and innervation. If you find a neurovascular injury, use only slight adjustments to restore nervous or circulatory function because movement in this area is likely to cause further injury.

Splint forearm fractures with a short, padded rigid splint affixed to the forearm and hand. Secure the hand in the position of function by placing a large wad of dressing material in the palm to maintain a position like that of holding a large ball. Place the rigid splint along the medial forearm surface and wrap circumferentially from the fingers to the elbow. Leave at least one digit exposed to permit checking for capillary refill. Bend the elbow across the chest and use a sling and swathe to hold the limb in position. This provides relative elevation and improved venous drainage in both seated and supine patients.

The air splint or long padded rigid splint, tied firmly to the body, may also adequately immobilize forearm fractures (Figure 22-14). When using these devices, remember to place the hand in the position of function to increase patient comfort.

When possible, leave a distal digit exposed to evaluate capillary refill and skin color and temperature.

CARE FOR SPECIFIC JOINT INJURIES

Hip

The hip may dislocate in two directions, anteriorly and posteriorly. The anterior dislocation presents with the foot turned outward and the head of the femur palpable in the inguinal area. The posterior dislocation is most common and presents with the knee flexed and the foot rotated internally. The displaced head of the femur is buried in the muscle of the buttocks. Immobilize a patient with either type of dislocation on a long spine board using pillows and blankets as padding to maintain the patient's position and provide comfort. If distal circulation, sensation, or motor function is severely compromised, consider one attempt at reduction of a posterior dislocation. (Consult local protocols and medical direction to identify criteria for reduction attempts.) However, do not attempt reduction if there are other serious injuries, like a pelvic fracture, associated with the hip dislocation. Anterior dislocations in general cannot be managed by reduction in the prehospital setting.

For reduction of a posterior hip dislocation, have a care provider hold the pelvis firmly against the long spine board or other firm surface by placing downward pressure on the iliac crests. Flex both the patient's hip and knee at 90 degrees and apply a firm, slowly increasing traction along the axis of the femur. Gently rotate the femur externally. It takes some time for the muscles to relax, but when they do the head of the femur will "pop" back into position. If you feel this "pop" or if the patient reports a sudden relief of pain and is able to extend the leg easily, the reduction has likely been a success. Immobilize the patient in a comfortable position, either in flexion (not to exceed 90 degrees) or fully supine with the hip and leg in full extension. Reevaluate sensation, motor function, and circulation. If the femur head does not move into the acetabulum after a few minutes of your attempted reduction, immobilize the patient as found and consider rapid transport.

Knee

Knee injuries may include fractures of the femur, the tibia, or both, patellar dislocations, or frank dislocations of the knee. Because the knee is such a large joint and bears such a great amount of weight, an injury to it is serious and threatens the patient's future ability to walk. Another concern with knee injury is possible injury to the major blood vessel traversing the area, the popliteal artery. This artery is less mobile than blood vessels in other joints, which leaves it more subject to injury and distal vascular compromise.

Immobilize knee joint fractures and patellar dislocations in the position found unless distal circulation, sensation, or motor function is disrupted. If the limb is flexed, splint it with two medium rigid splints, placing one medially and one laterally (Figure 22-15). Cross-wrap with bandage material to secure the limb in position. You may also use ladder or malleable splints, conformed to the angle of the limb and placed anteriorly and posteriorly, or a vacuum splint to immobilize the knee. If the limb is extended, simply apply two padded rigid splints or a full-leg air splint.

Dislocation of the patella is more common than dislocation of the knee joint and usually leaves the knee in a flexed position with a lateral displacement of the patella. The injured knee appears significantly deformed, though patellar dislocation has a lower incidence of associated vascular injury than does knee dislocation.

Anterior dislocations of the knee produce an extended limb contour that lifts at the knee (moving from proximal to distal) while posterior dislocations produce a limb that drops at the knee. (Assure that the injury is not a patellar dislocation.) If there is neurovascular compromise, have another care provider immobilize the femur. You should then grasp the limb just above the ankle and at the calf muscle and apply a firm and progressive traction, first along the axis of the tibia and then pulling the limb toward alignment with the femur. With posterior dislocations, a third care provider may provide moderate downward pressure on the distal femur and upward pressure on the proximal tibia to facilitate the reduction. As with most dislocations, success is measured by feeling the bone end "pop" back into place, hearing the patient report a dramatic reduction in pain, and noting a freer movement of the limb at the knee joint. Once you reduce the knee dislocation, immobilize the joint in the position of function and transport the patient. If you cannot

Immobilize knee injuries in the position found unless you discover significant distal circulation, sensation, or motor deficit.

FIGURE 22-15 Angulated knee dislocations can be immobilized with two padded rigid splints.

FIGURE 22-16 A pillow splint can be used with injuries to the ankles and feet.

reduce the dislocation with a few minutes of distal traction, immobilize the extremity in the position found and transport quickly. Perform a knee dislocation reduction even if the patient has good distal circulation and nervous function when the time to definitive care will exceed 2 hours.

Ankle

Ankle injuries often produce a distal lower limb that is grossly deformed, either due to malleolar fracture, dislocation, or both. Sprains are also injuries of concern, although with them the limb remains in anatomic position. Splint sprains or non-displaced fractures with an air splint (shaped to accommodate the foot) or with long rigid splints positioned on either side of the limb, padded liberally, and wrapped firmly. You may also use a pillow splint, especially if there is any ankle deformity (Figure 22-16). Apply local cooling to ease the pain and reduce swelling.

Ankle dislocation may occur in any of three directions: anteriorly, posteriorly, and laterally. The anterior dislocation presents with a dorsiflexed (upward pointing) foot that appears shortened. The posterior dislocation appears to lengthen the plantar flexed (downward pointing) foot. The lateral dislocation is most common and presents with a foot turned outward with respect to the ankle. If distal neurovascular compromise indicates the need for reduction, have a care provider grasp the calf, hold it in position, and pull against the traction you apply. You then grasp the heel with one hand and the metatarsal arch with the other. Pull a distal traction to disengage the bone ends and protect the articular cartilage during the relocation. For anterior dislocations, move the foot posteriorly with respect to the ankle; with lateral dislocations, rotate the foot medially; with posterior dislocations, pull the heel toward you and the foot toward you, then away. The joint should return to normal position with a "pop," a reduction in patient pain, and an increase in the mobility of the joint. Apply local cooling and immobilize the limb. If the procedure does not result in joint reduction within a few minutes, splint the joint as found and provide rapid transport.

Foot

Injuries to the foot include dislocations and fractures to the calcanei (heel bones), metatarsals, and phalanges. Injuries to the calcanei generally result from falls and can cause significant pain and swelling. Injuries to the metatarsals and phalanges can result from penetrating or blunt trauma or the typical "stubbing" of a toe. Fatigue fractures of the metatarsal bones, or "march fractures," are relatively common. These injuries are reasonably stable, even though the extremity cannot bear weight. When foot or ankle injury is suspected, anticipate both bilateral foot injuries and lumbar spinal injury.

Immobilize foot injuries in much the same way you do with ankle injuries. Use pillow, vacuum, ladder or air splints (with foot accommodation). If possible, leave some portion of the foot accessible so you can monitor distal capillary refill or, at least, skin temperature and color.

Shoulder

Fractures to the shoulder most commonly involve the proximal humerus, lateral scapula, and distal clavicle. Dislocations can include anterior, posterior, and inferior displacement of the humoral head. Anterior dislocations displace the humoral head forward, resulting in a shoulder that appears "hollow" or "squared-off," with the patient holding the arm close to the chest and forward of the mid-axillary line. Posterior dislocations rotate the arm internally, and the patient presents with the elbow and forearm held away from the chest. Inferior dislocations displace the humoral head downward, with the result that the patient's arm is often locked above the head.

You should immobilize shoulder injuries, like all joint injuries, as found, unless pulse, sensation, or motor function distal to the injury is absent. Immobilize anterior and posterior dislocations with a sling and swathe and, if needed, place a pillow under the arm and forearm. Immobilization of any inferior dislocation (with the upper extremity fixed above the head) will call for ingenuity on your part in splinting. In such cases, immobilize the extended arm in the position found. Using cravats, tie a long, padded splint to the torso, shoulder girdle, arm, and forearm to immobilize the arm above the head. Gently move the patient to the long spine board and secure both splint and patient to the spine board.

Begin reduction of anterior and posterior shoulder dislocations by placing a strap across the patient's chest, under the affected shoulder (through the axilla) and across the back. Have a care provider prepared to pull counter traction across the chest and superiorly using the strap. You, meanwhile, should flex the patient's elbow, drawing the arm somewhat away from the body (abduction) and pull firm traction along the axis of the humerus. Some slight internal and external rotation of the humerus may facilitate reduction. For reduction of inferior dislocations, have one care provider hold the thorax while you flex the elbow. Gradually apply firm traction along the axis of the humerus and gently rotate the arm externally. If the joint does not relocate in a few minutes, immobilize it as it lies and transport the patient. If reduction is successful, immobilize the upper extremity in the normal anatomic position with a sling and swathe.

Elbow

Elbow injuries display a high incidence of nervous and vascular involvement, especially in children. As in the knee, the blood vessels running through the elbow region are held firmly in place. The probability is good, therefore, that any fracture or dislocation will involve the brachial artery and the medial, ulnar, and radial nerves. Assess the distal neurovascular function and, if you detect a deficit, move the joint very carefully and minimally to restore distal circulation. Then splint the elbow with a single padded rigid splint, providing cross-strapping as necessary, or use a ladder splint bent to conform to the angle of the limb (Figure 22-17). Keeping the wrist slightly elevated above the elbow, secure the limb to the chest using a sling and swathe. This position increases venous return and reduces the swelling and pain associated with the injury.

Elbow dislocations should not be reduced in the prehospital setting.

Wrist/Hand

Fractures of the hand and wrist are commonly associated with direct trauma. They present with very noticeable deformity and significant pain reported by the

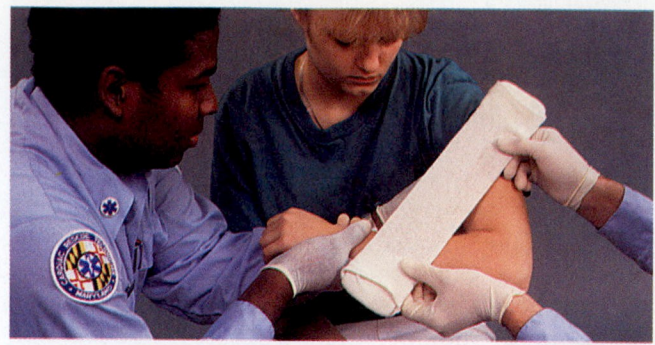

When splinting the distal upper extremity, place padding in the palm of the hand to maintain the position of function.

patient. These fractures are of serious concern to the patient. Since the hand and wrist bones are small, any fracture is in close proximity to a joint. Exercise concern when you care for these injuries because of the possibility of vascular and neural involvement.

You can effectively immobilize musculoskeletal injuries of the forearm, wrist, hand, or fingers with a padded rigid or air splint. Place a roll of bandaging, a wad of dressing material, or some similar object in the patient's hand to maintain the position of function. Then secure the extremity to the padded board or inflate the air splint. Be sure to leave some portion of the distal extremity accessible so that you can monitor the adequacy of perfusion and sensation. Place the wrist above the elbow to assist venous return and reduce distal swelling.

Hand and wrist injuries are very common, particularly among athletes and children. A particular type of wrist fracture is the Colles's fracture in which the wrist has a "silver fork" appearance. Fortunately, such injuries are seldom serious and can be managed in the prehospital setting quite easily.

Finger

Forces may displace the phalanges from their joints, resulting in deformity and pain. Displacement usually occurs between the phalanges or between the proximal phalanx and the metacarpal and causes the bone to be moved either anteriorly or posteriorly. (Amputations are multi-system injuries that severely damage the musculoskeletal system. They are addressed in depth in Chapter 20, "Soft-Tissue Trauma.")

Splint finger fractures using tongue blades or small, malleable splints designed for the purpose that you shape to the contour of the injured finger. The finger may also be taped to the adjoining fingers to limit additional motion. The hand is then placed in the position of function and further immobilized.

Finger dislocations usually involve the proximal joint (and sometimes the distal joint) with the digit commonly displacing posteriorly. If reduction is indicated, grasp the distal finger and apply a firm distal traction. Then direct the digit toward the normal anatomic position by moving its proximal end. You should feel the finger "pop" into place, and the digit should resume its normal alignment when compared to the uninjured finger on the other hand. Splint the finger with a slight bend (10 to 15 degrees) and immobilize the hand in the position of function.

SOFT AND CONNECTIVE TISSUE INJURIES

Tendon, ligament, and muscle injuries are rarely life-threatening.

Tendon, ligament, and muscle injuries are rarely, if ever, life threatening. Massive muscular contusions and hematomas can, however, contribute to hypovolemia, while ligament and tendon injuries can endanger the future function of a limb. Be careful about permitting the patient to put further stress on a limb, especially with higher grades of sprains. The weakened ligaments may fail completely, resulting in dislocation or complete joint instability. For the purpose of care, treat these injuries as you would dislocations and immobilize the adjacent joints. Monitor distal neurovascular function because tissue swelling within the circumferential wrapping of a splint may compress blood vessels and nerves. Care for muscular injuries with immobilization, gentle compression with snug (but not overly tight) dressings, and local cooling to suppress edema and pain using cold packs or ice wrapped in dressing material. Be watchful for signs of compartment syndrome, especially in the calf and forearm regions.

Open wounds involving the muscles, tendons, and ligaments can be severe and debilitating. Carefully evaluate such wounds for signs of connective tissue involvement. Be especially watchful with deep open injuries close to the joints. With such wounds, the likelihood of tendon and ligament disruption is great and may affect the use of the joint, the muscles controlling the joint, or the muscles controlling joint movement distal to the injury. Carefully evaluate for circulation, sensation, and motor function below these injuries.

Injury to a muscle or tendon may limit its ability to either extend or flex the limb. The opposing muscle moves the limb, while the injured muscle cannot return it to the normal position. With limb injuries, note any unusual limb position, especially if the patient is unable to return the limb to a neutral position. At any sign of pain or dysfunction, splint the limb.

Care for muscular injuries with immobilization, gentle compression with snug dressings, and local cooling to suppress edema and pain.

MEDICATIONS

Medications are frequently administered to the patient with musculoskeletal injury to relieve pain and to premedicate before the relocation of a dislocation. Medications used include nitrous oxide, diazepam, meperidine, nalbuphine, and morphine.

Sedatives/Analgesics

Nitrous Oxide Nitrous oxide (Nitronox®) is a nitrogen and oxygen compound in a gas state. It is administered in the prehospital setting for its anesthetic properties, specifically to reduce the perception of pain in cases of musculoskeletal injuries. For prehospital care, it is administered in a 50 percent nitrous oxide and 50 percent oxygen mixture via a special regulator and a self-administration mask. Self-administration of nitrous oxide prevents over-medication because the patient will drop the mask when too heavily sedated.

Nitrous oxide is non-explosive, and its analgesic effects dissipate within 2 to 5 minutes of discontinuing administration. High concentrations of nitrous oxide may lead to hypoxia and may cause respiratory depression and vomiting. These side effects are minimized, however, because the gas is pre-mixed with oxygen by the administration set during prehospital delivery.

The chief concern with the use of nitrous oxide is that is diffuses easily into air-filled spaces in the body, increasing the pressure within them. This diffusion is especially dangerous in patients with pneumothorax or tension pneumothorax, bowel obstruction, and middle ear obstruction. Rule out COPD and these pathologies before you administer nitrous oxide in the prehospital setting.

The nitrous oxide administration device consists of two cylinders of equal size, one holding oxygen (green) and the other, nitrous oxide (blue). The gases are mixed in a special blender/regulator and distributed to the patient when his inspiration generates a less-than-atmospheric pressure. (In other countries, both gases are pre-mixed in one cylinder, reducing the weight and size of the administration device.) The patient must hold the administration mask firmly to the face to trigger administration, thus preventing administration in a patient who is heavily sedated. Nitrous oxide is a controlled substance and its use is carefully monitored for provider abuse.

Diazepam Diazepam (Valium®) is a benzodiazepine with both anti-anxiety and skeletal muscle relaxant qualities. The drug reduces the patient's perception and memory of pain. It is used with musculoskeletal injuries and to premedicate patients before painful procedures such as cardioversion and dislocation reduction. It is administered in a slow IV bolus of 5 to 15 mg, not to exceed 5 mg/minute, into a large vein. Diazepam is rather fast acting, with IV effects occurring almost immediately and reaching peak effectiveness in 15 minutes. Its duration of effectiveness is from 15 to 60 minutes. Do not mix diazepam with any other drugs, and flush the IV line before and after administration. Administer diazepam as close to the IV catheter as possible, and do not inject it into a plastic IV bag. Diazepam is readily absorbed by plastic, which quickly reduces its concentration.

Diazepam is usually supplied in single-use vials or pre-loaded syringes containing 2 mL of a 5 mg/mL solution (10 mg). Administer 5 to 15 mg IV and repeat in 10 to 15 minutes if necessary.

The effects of diazepam may be reversed by the administration of flumazenil. Usually, 2 mL of a 0.1 mg/mL solution is given IV (over 15 seconds) with a second dose repeated at 60 seconds.

Morphine Morphine sulfate (Duramorph®, Astramorph®) is an opium alkaloid used to relieve pain (narcotic analgesic), to sedate, and to reduce anxiety. It is used with musculoskeletal injuries for its ability to reduce pain perception. Morphine may reduce vascular volume and cardiac preload by increasing venous capacitance and may thus decrease blood pressure in the hypovolemic patient. It should not be administered to a patient with hypovolemia or hypotension. Its major side effects are respiratory depression and possible nausea and vomiting.

Morphine is available in 10 mL single-use vials or Tubex® units of a 1 mg/mL solution or as 1 mL of a 10 mg/mL solution vial for dilution with 9 mL normal saline. Administer a 2 mg bolus slowly IV, repeating as necessary every few minutes to effect.

Naloxone hydrochloride (Narcan®) is a narcotic antagonist that can quickly reverse the effects of narcotics (morphine, meperidine, and nalbuphine) and should be available anytime you use morphine sulfate. Naloxone is administered as an IV bolus of 0.4 to 2 mg, repeated every 2 to 3 minutes until effective. Naloxone is a shorter-acting drug than morphine, so repeat doses may be necessary.

Meperidine Meperidine hydrochloride (Demerol®) is a narcotic analgesic with properties similar to those of morphine, although it may produce less smooth muscle relaxation, constipation, and cough reflex suppression. As with morphine, it is used with musculoskeletal injuries for its ability to reduce the patient's perception of pain. It also may produce respiratory depression and hypotension, especially in the patient who is volume depleted.

Meperidine is supplied in single-dose vials and preloaded syringes and in concentrations of from 10 to 100 mg/mL. It may be administered in doses of 50 to 100 mg IM. For IV administration use a concentration of 10 mg/mL diluted in normal saline or lactated Ringer's solution and inject slowly in doses of 50 to 100 mg. Narcan® will reverse its effects.

Nalbuphine Nalbuphine hydrochloride (Nubain®) is a synthetic narcotic analgesic with properties much like those of morphine. It is equivalent on a milligram-to-milligram basis to morphine, although it antagonizes some of the actions of that drug. Nalbuphine does not generally decrease blood pressure, although it may produce respiratory depression and bradycardia. Unlike morphine and meperidine, it is not a controlled substance. It is a rapid acting—within 2 to 3 minutes—drug with a long duration of effectiveness—3 to 6 hours.

Nalbuphine is supplied in ampules or preloaded syringes containing 1 mL of a 10 or 20 mg/mL solution. It is administered IV in a dose of 5 mg, then 2 mg repeated as needed up to 20 mg. Narcan® will reverse its effects.

OTHER MUSCULOSKELETAL INJURY CONSIDERATIONS

Other areas for special consideration with musculoskeletal injuries include pediatric injuries, athletic injuries, patient refusals and referrals, and the psychological support for the patient with musculoskeletal injury.

Pediatric Musculoskeletal Injury

Children are at higher risk than adults for musculoskeletal injuries due to their activity levels and incompletely developed coordination. Special injuries affecting them include greenstick fractures and epiphyseal fractures.

The incomplete nature of the greenstick fracture produces a stable but angulated limb in the young child. The injured limb is painful and will not bear weight. In these cases, do not attempt to realign the limb and understand that the orthopedic specialist will probably complete the fracture to permit proper healing.

Epiphyseal fractures disrupt the child's growth plate and endanger future bone growth. This injury is likely with fractures within a few inches of the joint because the epiphyseal plate is a point of skeletal weakness. Treat these fractures as you would for an adult, but recognize that they are potentially limb-threatening injuries.

Athletic Musculoskeletal Injuries

Athletes, especially those involved in contact sports like football, soccer, basketball, and wrestling, have a higher incidence of musculoskeletal injuries than the general public. Injuries to the joints, often serious knee and ankle sprains, are common reasons for calls to EMS. Such injuries are especially important because they occur in individuals who are at least moderately well conditioned and result from the application of significant kinetic forces. When you are called to the side of an injured athlete, be especially sensitive to the potential for residual disability caused by these injuries and be predisposed to transport instead of permitting the patient to remain at the scene.

Knowing the athletic trainers in your area may help your on-scene operations run more smoothly and efficiently. In many cases, the athletic trainer works under the supervision of a local physician much as you work under medical direction. It is important for trainers to understand that, once you are called to the scene, the injured athlete becomes a patient of the EMS system and will be treated under the system's medical direction and protocols. Also, as the representative of that system, you are likely to assume responsibility for decisions about care and transport of the patient. Assuring that trainers understand these facts may eliminate confrontations over care of injured athletes.

Athletic trainers use the acronym RICE to identify the recommended treatment for sprains, strains, and other soft tissue injuries. RICE stands for: *Rest* the extremity, *Ice* for the first 48 hours, *Compression* with an elastic bandage, and *Elevation* for venous drainage. This is consistent with standard emergency care for sprains and strains. (Note, however, that the application of the elastic bandage in this case is to strengthen the limb for further activity and is not recommended for prehospital care.)

Patient Refusals and Referral

In some situations, you may encounter a patient suffering from an isolated sprain or strain with no significant mechanism of injury and no other signs, symptoms, or complaints. This patient may refuse your assistance or be a

Knowing the athletic trainers in your area may help your on-scene operations run more smoothly and efficiently.

Content Review

RICE PROCEDURE FOR STRAINS, SPRAINS, SOFT TISSUE INJURIES
Rest the extremity.
Ice for first 48 hours.
Compress with elastic bandage.
Elevate extremity

candidate for on-scene treatment and referral for follow-up medical care. Evaluate the need for immobilization and x-rays and determine if the patient should seek immediate care in an emergency department or see a personal physician. Any referral to a personal physician must be done in conjunction with medical direction and following local protocol.

Psychological Support for the Musculoskeletal Injury Patient

Regardless of the specific type of injury sustained, patients need psychological as well as physiological support. Too often, we concentrate all efforts on the patient's injuries, forgetting the emotional impact that the incident and the emergency care measures employed have on the patient. Keep in mind that patients are not frequently exposed to injuries. They do not know what effects injuries will have on their lives or what to expect from medical care in the prehospital, emergency department, or in-hospital settings. Remember that you can have a significant impact on a patient's emotional response to trauma. Displaying a concerned attitude and a professional demeanor and communicating frequently and compassionately with patients will go far to calm and reassure them. Simple attention paid to the patient may make the experience with prehospital emergency medical service one that is remembered positively.

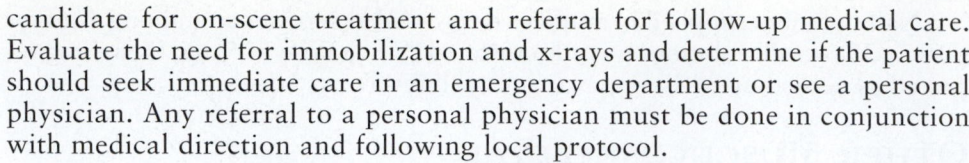

Summary

Injuries to the bones, ligaments, tendons, and muscles of the extremities rarely threaten your patient's life. Major exceptions to this statement are pelvic and serious or bilateral femur fractures, in which associated hemorrhage can contribute significantly to hypovolemia and shock. In addition, serious musculoskeletal trauma suggests the possibility of other, life-threatening trauma and, in fact, occurs in about 80 percent of cases of major multi-system trauma. The presence of serious musculoskeletal trauma should increase your index of suspicion for other serious internal injuries.

Care for isolated musculoskeletal trauma is usually delayed until the ABCs and other patient life-threats are stabilized. The goals of the care are to protect any open wounds, position affected limbs properly, immobilize the area of injury, and carefully monitor distal extremities to assure neurovascular function.

Pelvic and bilateral femur fractures are immobilized through application of the PASG. This device both provides splinting for the pelvis, hip joint, and upper portion of the lower extremity and helps control internal blood loss in the region. Manage other fractures by aligning the extremity with gentle traction and immobilizing it by splinting. In cases where you discover a loss of distal neurovascular function, move the extremity slightly to restore distal neurovascular function and then splint.

Joint injuries carry a greater risk of damage to distal circulation, sensation, and motor function. Splint these injuries as you find them unless there is distal neurovascular compromise. If that is the case, employ gentle manipulation to restore circulation, motor function, or sensation. If gentle manipulation is unsuccessful and transport is to be delayed, attempt reduction of dislocations for the hip, knee, ankle, shoulder, or finger as permitted by local protocol.

Care for injuries to connective and muscular tissues by immobilizing the area of injury in the position of function. Evaluate distal extremities for pulse, capillary refill, color, temperature, sensation, and motor function before, during, and after any immobilization or movement of a limb and provide frequent monitoring thereafter.

CHAPTER 23

Head, Facial, and Neck Trauma

Objectives

After reading this chapter, you should be able to:

1. Describe the incidence, morbidity, and mortality of head, facial, and neck injuries. (p. 1026)
2. Explain head and facial anatomy and physiology. (see Chapter 3)
3. Differentiate between the following types of facial injuries, highlighting the defining characteristics of each (see Chapter 3):
   a. Eye
   b. Ear
   c. Nose
   d. Throat
   e. Mouth
4. Predict head, facial, and other related injuries based on mechanism of injury. (pp. 1026–1027)
5. Differentiate between facial injuries based on the assessment and history. (pp. 1039–1044)
6. Explain the pathophysiology, assessment, and management for patients with eye, ear, nose, throat, and mouth injuries. (pp. 1039–1067)
7. Explain anatomy and relate physiology of the CNS to head injuries. (pp. 1031–1038)

Continued

Objectives Continued

8. Distinguish between facial, head, and brain injury. (pp. 1028–1044)
9. Explain the pathophysiology of head/ brain injuries. (pp. 1026–1039)
10. Explain the concept of increasing intracranial pressure (ICP). (pp. 1035–1037)
11. Explain the effect of increased and decreased carbon dioxide on ICP. (pp. 1035–1037)
12. Define and explain the process involved with each of the levels of increasing ICP. (pp. 1035–1037)
13. Relate assessment findings associated with head/brain injuries to the patho-physiologic process. (pp. 1028–1039)
14. Classify head injuries (mild, moderate, severe) according to assessment findings. (pp. 1031–1035)
15. Identify the need for rapid interven-tion and transport of the patient with a head/brain injury. (pp. 1045, 1052)
16. Describe and explain the general management of the head/brain injury patient, including pharmacological and non-pharmacological treatment. (pp. 1053–1065)
17. Analyze the relationship between carbon dioxide concentration in the blood and management of the airway in the head/brain injured patient. (pp. 1035–1036)
18. Explain the pathophysiology, assess-ment, and management of a patient with:
   a. scalp injury (pp. 1028–1029, 1048–1049, 1053–1065)
   b. skull fracture (pp. 1029–1031, 1046, 1048–1049, 1053–1065)
   c. cerebral contusion (pp. 1032, 1053–1065)
   d. intracranial hemorrhage (including epidural, subdural, subarachnoid, and intracerebral hemorrhage) (pp. 1032–1034, 1053–1065)
   e. axonal injury (including concussion and moderate and severe diffuse axonal injury) (pp. 1034–1035, 1053–1065)
   f. facial injury (pp. 1039–1044, 1053–1065)
   g. neck injury (pp. 1044–1045, 1046, 1047, 1050–1053, 1065)
19. Develop a management plan for the removal of a helmet for a head-injured patient. (p. 1047)
20. Differentiate between the types of head/brain injuries based on the assessment and history. (pp. 1026–1053)
21. Given several preprogrammed and moulaged head, face, and neck trauma patients, provide the appropriate scene size-up, initial assessment, rapid trauma or focused physical exam and history, detailed exam, and ongoing assessment and provide appropriate patient care and transportation. (pp. 1045–1067)

INTRODUCTION TO HEAD, FACIAL, AND NECK INJURIES

Head, facial, and neck injuries are common with major trauma. Approximately 4 million people experience significant head impact each year, with 1 in 10 requiring hospitalization. While most of these hospitalizations are due to relatively minor injuries, severe head injury is the most frequent cause of trauma death. It is especially lethal in auto crashes and frequently produces significant long-term disability in patients who survive them. Gunshot wounds that penetrate the cranium result in a mortality of about 75 to 80 percent. Injuries to the face and neck threaten critical airway structures as well as the significant vasculature found in these regions.

The populations most at risk for serious head injury are males between the years of 15 and 24, infants and young children, and the elderly. Education programs promoting safe practices in many different fields and the use of head protection, seat belts, and airbags have had major effects on reducing head injury mortality and morbidity. The use of helmets for bicycling, rollerblading, and motorcycling and in contact sports like football has also significantly reduced the incidence of serious head injury. In motorcycle crashes, for example, helmet use reduces serious head injury by more than 50 percent. Once a head injury occurs, however, time becomes a critical consideration. Intracranial hemorrhage and progressing edema can increase the intracranial pressure, hypoxia, and the internal and permanent damage done.

PATHOPHYSIOLOGY OF HEAD, FACIAL, AND NECK INJURY

Head, facial, and neck injuries are difficult to assess in the prehospital setting, yet they commonly threaten life or may expose victims to lifelong disability. A clearer appreciation of the anatomy of these regions, of the various mechanisms of injury affecting them, and of the specific pathologic processes related to head, facial, and neck injury can help you better anticipate, assess, and then manage these injuries and their effects on the human system.

MECHANISMS OF INJURY

Injuries to the head, neck, and face are divided by mechanisms of injury into blunt (closed) and penetrating (open).

Blunt Injury

The structures of the head, face, and neck protect very well against most blunt trauma. At times, however, the forces producing blunt trauma are of such magnitude as to compromise the body's well-designed protective mechanisms. For example, head injuries most frequently result from auto and motorcycle crashes and account for more than half of vehicle crash deaths. Sports-related impacts, falling objects, falls, and acts of violence, like assault with a club, are other less common, but still significant mechanisms of head injury (Figure 23-1).

The face is another area frequently subjected to blunt trauma. Significant facial injury occurs less frequently than head injury in auto impacts because the head's frontal or parietal regions are more likely to impact the windshield than the face. The same holds true for falls, as the arms, chest, or head absorb energy as the conscious victim tries to protect the facial area from injury. Intentional violence is less likely to spare the facial region. The face is often the target of blows from a fist or from impact-enhancing objects like sticks or clubs. The middle and inner ears and the eyes are very well protected against most blunt trauma, though ear injury may be caused by compressional forces associated with diving or explosions. The eyes may occasionally be injured by impacts from smaller blunt objects like a racquetball, baseball, or tennis ball.

The neck is anatomically well protected from most blunt trauma because the head and chest protrude more anteriorly. Laterally, the neck is protected as the shoulders protrude a significant distance from the neck. The neck is, however, a point of impact in special situations. For example, during an auto crash the neck may strike the steering wheel or be injured by a shoulder strap that is worn without a lap belt. The region may also be impacted by objects during fights or traumatically constricted or distracted during an attempted suicide by hanging.

Penetrating Injury

Penetrating injuries to the head, face, and neck are not as common as those resulting from blunt trauma, but they can be just as severe and potentially life threatening. In addition, a penetrating injury to the head suggests the meninges have been opened, producing a route for potentially serious infection.

Penetrating injuries to the head, face, and neck usually result from either gunshots or stabbings. Gunshot wounds are most common and especially hideous because bullets release tremendous energy as they slow during collision with skeletal and central nervous tissue. Similarly, explosions propel projectiles, either intrinsic to the explosive device or from debris produced by the blast, that may penetrate and damage this region. Knife wounds to the head and face tend to be superficial because of the region's extensive skeletal components. The anterior and lateral neck, however, are not as well protected, and wounds there may compromise both the airway and major blood vessels, quickly threatening the patient's life.

There are many other types of penetrating injuries that may involve the head, face, and neck. Some examples include the "clothesline" impact with a wire fence while a victim is riding an all-terrain vehicle or snowmobile; bites from humans, dogs, and other animals; or a tongue bitten when the victim traps it between the teeth during an impact. Infrequently, a fall may impale a person on a fixed object such as a concrete reinforcing bar, producing a penetrating injury.

Blunt and penetrating injury mechanisms have different impacts depending on the structures they involve. The following sections discuss the pathologic processes of injuries as they affect the head, face, and neck.

FIGURE 23-2 Scalp wounds can bleed heavily.

HEAD INJURY

Head injury is defined as a traumatic insult to the cranial region that may result in injury to soft tissues, bony structures, and the brain. Let us look at head injury as it progresses from the exterior to the interior, examining scalp, cranial, and brain injuries.

Scalp Injury

The most superficial head injuries involve the scalp (Figure 23-2). A scalp injury may also be the only overt indication of deeper, more serious injury beneath. The scalp overlies the firm cranium and is very vascular. Its blood vessels lack the ability to constrict as effectively as those elsewhere in the body; hence, scalp wounds tend to bleed heavily. Some people believe that head injuries do not result in shock; this, however, assumes that the hemorrhage they cause is easy to control. In fact, any serious blood loss from scalp wounds can contribute to shock and, if left uncontrolled, may itself cause hypovolemia and shock. Scalp wounds further provide a route for infection because emissary veins drain from the dural sinuses, through the cranium, and into the superficial venous circulation. Because of rich circulation to the area, scalp wounds tend to heal well.

Scalp wounds may present in a manner that confounds assessment. Usually, blunt trauma creates a contusion that, because of the firm skull underneath, expands outwardly in a very rapid and noticeable way. However, blunt trauma may also tear underlying fascia and areolar tissue, causing it to separate. This can leave an elevated border surrounding a depression, mimicking the contour of a de-

The presentation of scalp wounds may make them difficult to assess.

FIGURE 23-3   Various types of skull fractures.

pressed skull fracture. On the other hand, the scalp's blood vessels may bleed into a depressed skull fracture, fill any depression, and conceal the injury's true nature.

A common and special type of scalp wound is the avulsion. Areolar tissue is only loosely attached to the skull, and glancing blows can create a shearing force against the scalp's border. Such blows frequently tear a flap of scalp loose and fold it back against the uninjured scalp, exposing a portion of the cranium. The mechanism of injury may also seriously contaminate the wound and may cause moderate hemorrhage unless the avulsed tissue folds back sharply, compressing the blood vessels.

Cranial Injury

Because of its spherical shape and skeletal design, the skull does not fracture unless trauma is extreme. Such fractures may present as linear, depressed, comminuted, or basilar in nature (Figure 23-3). Linear fractures are small cracks in the cranium and represent about 80 percent of all skull fractures. The temporal bone is one of the thinnest and most frequently fractured cranial bones. If there are no associated intracranial injuries, a linear fracture poses very little danger to the patient. In contrast, a depressed fracture represents an inward displacement of the skull's surface and results in a greater likelihood of intracranial damage. Comminuted fractures involve multiple skull fragments that may penetrate the meninges and cause physical harm to the structures beneath.

A common type of skull fracture involves the base of the skull. This area is permeated with foramina (openings) for the spinal cord, cranial nerves, and various blood vessels. The basilar skull also has hollow or open structures such as

The temporal bone is one of the thinnest and most frequently fractured cranial bones.

Retroauricular ecchymosis (Battle's sign).

Bilateral periorbital ecchymosis (racoon eyes).

the sinuses, the orbits of the eye, the nasal cavities, the external auditory canals, and the middle and inner ears. These spaces weaken the skull and leave the basilar area prone to fracture.

The signs of basilar skull fracture vary with the injury's location (Figure 23-4). If the fracture involves the auditory canal and the lower lateral areas of the skull, hemorrhage may migrate to the mastoid region (just posterior and slightly inferior to the ear). This causes a characteristic discoloration called **retroauricular ecchymosis** or "Battle's sign." Another classic sign of basilar skull fracture is **bilateral periorbital ecchymosis,** sometimes referred to as "raccoon eyes." This is a dramatic discoloration around the eyes associated with orbital fractures and hemorrhage into the surrounding tissue. Both retroauricular ecchymosis and bilateral periorbital ecchymosis take time to develop; neither is likely to develop during the period after an injury when the patient is under paramedic care.

Basilar skull fracture can tear the dura mater, opening a wound between the brain and the body's exterior. Such a wound may permit cerebrospinal fluid to seep out through a nasal cavity or an external auditory canal and also provide a possible route for infection to enter the meninges.

This type of wound may also provide an escape for cerebrospinal fluid in the presence of increasing intracranial pressure. Escaping cerebrospinal fluid may mediate the rise in ICP and somewhat limit damage to the brain. (While cerebrospinal fluid is an important medium, the body can regenerate it quite rapidly.) Blood mixed with cerebrospinal fluid and flowing from the nose, mouth, or ears will demonstrate the target or "halo" sign (a dark red circle surrounded by a lighter yellowish one) when dropped on a pillow or towel (Figure 23-5). Normal blood demonstrates a narrow concentric ring of yellowish coloration surrounding the red circle produced by the less mobile erythrocytes. If cerebrospinal fluid is mixed with the blood, this outer ring is much larger. Be aware, however, other fluids, like lacrimal or nasal fluids or saliva, may cause a similar response. Hence, the halo sign is most reliable when associated with fluid leaking from the ear.

Bullet impacts induce specific types of cranial fracture. The entrance wound often produces a comminuted fracture and sends bone fragments into the brain. Often the bullet's kinetic energy is sufficient to permit the bullet to exit from the cranium and cause a second fracture. This exit wound site is blown outward and is often more severe in appearance than the entrance wound.

In many cases, the energy of the projectile's passage through the cranium causes a cavitational wave of extreme pressure, which is contained and enhanced by the rigid container of the skull. The result is extreme damage to the cranial

* **retroauricular ecchymosis** black-and-blue discoloration over the mastoid process (just behind the ear) that is characteristic of a basilar skull fracture. (Also called Battle's sign.)

* **bilateral periorbital ecchymosis** black-and-blue discoloration of the area surrounding the eyes. It is usually associated with basilar skull fracture. (Also called raccoon eyes.)

The "halo sign" is most reliable when associated with fluid leaking from the ear.

The glucose level of CSF is normally half that of the blood. If you are unsure whether a clear fluid is water or CSF, check the glucose level of the fluid and compare it to the patient's blood glucose level.

FIGURE 23–5 The "halo test" can detect the presence of cerebrospinal fluid. If CSF is present, it will diffuse faster across a paper towel or gauze because it is thinner than blood.

contents, and, if the transmitted kinetic energy is strong enough, the skull may fracture and "explode" outward.

Another type of wound occurs when a bullet enters the cranium at an angle, is deflected within, and continues to move along the cranium's interior until its energy is completely exhausted. This process does devastating damage to the cerebral cortex and is rarely survivable.

A special type of cranial injury involves an impaled object. As is the case with objects impaled in most other regions of the body, any further motion of the object may cause additional hemorrhage and tissue damage. When the object is impaled in the cranium, the situation is especially serious. Brain tissue is much more delicate than other body tissue, does not immobilize the object as well, and is easily injured by the object's motion. As with objects impaled elsewhere, removal of the impaled object from the cranium may cause further injury and increase blood accumulation.

Note that a cranial fracture, by itself, is a skeletal injury that will heal with time; it does not, by itself, threaten the brain. Rather, it is the possibility of injury beneath and suggested by the skull fracture that is of greatest concern. The forces necessary to fracture the cranium are extreme and likely to cause injury within.

> *A cranial fracture, by itself, is a skeletal injury that will heal with time. However, the forces necessary to fracture the skull are often sufficient to induce brain injury.*

Brain Injury

Brain injury is defined by the National Head Injury Foundation as "a traumatic insult to the brain capable of producing physical, intellectual, emotional, social, and vocational changes." It is classified as a direct or indirect injury to the tissue of the cerebrum, cerebellum, or brainstem.

Direct Injury Direct (or primary) injury is caused by the forces of trauma and can be associated with a variety of mechanisms. Rapid acceleration (or deceleration) or penetrating injury can cause mechanical injury to nervous system cells and impair their function. The forces causing direct injury can also disrupt blood vessels, both restricting blood flow through the injured area and causing irritation of nervous tissue as blood flows into it. Remember that the brain is specially protected from contact with some of the blood's content by the blood-brain barrier. Injury disrupts this barrier. Lastly, serious jarring may damage capillary walls, affect their permeability, and cause a fluid shift to the interstitial space, or tissue edema. Most frequently, there is a mixture of these mechanisms associated with direct brain injury.

FIGURE 23-6   Coup and contrecoup movement of the brain.

Two specific types of direct brain injury are coup and contrecoup injury (Figure 23-6). **Coup** injuries are tissue disruptions that occur directly at the point of impact. These injuries are inflicted as the brain displaces toward the impact surface and collides with the interior of the cranium. They are most common in the frontal region because its interior surface is rough and irregular. In contrast, the occipital areas are smooth and coup injuries occur there less frequently. Coup injury may also occur as the brain slides along the rough contours at the base of the skull.

Contrecoup injuries produce tissue damage away from the impact point as the brain, floating in cerebrospinal fluid inside the cranium, "sloshes" toward the impact, then away from it, again impacting the interior of the skull. For example, a blow to the forehead might result in injury to the occipital region (visual center) and produce visual disturbances (seeing stars). Contrecoup injury to the frontal region of the brain is most common (from an impact to the occipital region) again because the frontal bones have an irregular inner surface.

Direct brain injuries can be further assigned to one of two specific categories—focal or diffuse.

Focal Injuries   Focal injuries occur at a specific location in the brain and include contusions and intracranial hemorrhages.

Cerebral Contusion   A cerebral contusion is caused by blunt trauma to local brain tissue that produces capillary bleeding into the substance of the brain. The contusion is relatively common with blunt head injuries and often produces prolonged confusion or other types of neurologic deficit. This pathology may result from a coup or contrecoup mechanism and may occur at one or several sites in the brain. The localized form of the injury manifests with dysfunctions related to the site of the injury. For example, a patient who suffers a contusion of the frontal lobe after trauma to the forehead may experience personality changes. (Remember, the frontal lobe is the most commonly injured lobe.)

Intracranial Hemorrhage   Bleeding can occur at several locations within the brain, each presenting with a different pathologic process. These injuries—proceeding

Dura mater

Epidural
hematoma

FIGURE 23-7 Epidural hematoma.

Dura mater

Subdural
hematoma

FIGURE 23-8 Subdural hematoma.

from the most superficial to the deepest—are epidural, subdural, and intra-cerebral hemorrhages. In contrast to patients with concussions and contusions, expect the intracranial hemorrhage patient to deteriorate during your assessment and care because of associated indirect injury such as increasing intracranial pressure.

Bleeding between the dura mater and the skull's interior surface is called **epidural hematoma** (Figure 23-7). It usually involves arterial vessels, often the middle meningeal artery in the temporal region. Because the bleeding is from a relatively high-pressure vessel, intracranial pressure builds rapidly, compressing the cerebrum and increasing the pressure within the skull. As pressure builds, the patient moves quickly toward unresponsiveness. The hemorrhage-induced increase in intracranial pressure reduces oxygenated circulation to the nerve cells (indirect injury). Bleeding may be so extensive that it displaces the brain away from the injury site, pushing it toward the foramen magnum. Although the progression is both rapid and life threatening, immediate surgery can frequently reverse it.

Bleeding within the meninges, specifically beneath the dura mater and within the subarachnoid space, is called **subdural hematoma** (Figure 23-8). This type of bleeding occurs very slowly and may have a subtle presentation because blood loss is usually due to rupture of a small venous vessel, often one of those bridging to the dural sinuses. The vessel most commonly involved is the superior sagittal sinus. Because the subdural hemorrhage occurs above the pia mater, it does not cause the cerebral irritation associated with intracerebral hemorrhage. The free blood in the cerebrospinal fluid may clog the structures responsible for the fluid's reabsorption, which can result in an increasing intracranial pressure. The patient usually does not show overt signs and symptoms until hours or even days after the injury. Because of this delay, subdural hemorrhage is difficult to detect in the prehospital setting.

* **epidural hematoma** accumulation of blood between the dura mater and the cranium.

* **subdural hematoma** collection of blood directly beneath the dura mater.

* intracerebral hemorrhage bleeding directly into the tissue of the brain.

* diffuse axonal injury type of brain injury characterized by shearing, stretching, or tearing of nerve fibers with subsequent axonal damage.

* concussion a transient period of unconsciousness. In most cases, the unconsciousness will be followed by a complete return of function.

Suspect subdural hematoma in a medical (non-trauma) patient who demonstrates neurologic signs and symptoms. Careful history taking may uncover a recent mechanism of injury, such as a fall, that could cause this presentation. You occasionally encounter such pathologies with the elderly or with chronic alcoholics. Because both the aging process and chronic alcoholism reduce the size of the brain, head impact causes greater and less controlled motion of the brain within the cranium. This increases the likelihood of injury and, specifically, the subdural hematoma.

Intracerebral hemorrhage results from a ruptured blood vessel within the substance of the brain. Although blood loss is generally minimal, it is particularly damaging. Tissue edema results because free blood, outside the blood vessels, irritates the nervous tissue. Intracerebral hemorrhage often presents much like a stroke with the manifestations occurring very quickly. The particular presentation relates to the area of the brain involved. Normally, the signs and symptoms will progressively worsen with time.

Diffuse Injuries   Diffuse injuries involve a more general scenario of injury and include mild (concussions), moderate, and severe axonal disruptions. During head impact, a shearing, tearing, or stretching force is applied to the nerve fibers and causes damage to the axons, the long communication pathways of the nerve cells. This pathology is frequently distributed throughout the brain and thus is called **diffuse axonal injury (DAI)**. Diffuse axonal injuries are common among vehicle occupants involved in collisions and in pedestrians struck by vehicles because of the severe acceleration/deceleration mechanisms. DAIs can range from the mild (a concussion) to the severe and life threatening (a brainstem injury).

Concussion   A **concussion** is a mild to moderate form of DAI and is the most common outcome of blunt head trauma. It represents nerve dysfunction without substantial anatomic damage (i.e., a normal head CT scan). Concussion results in a transient episode of neuronal dysfunction (confusion, disorientation, event amnesia), followed by a rapid return to normal neurologic activity. Prehospital management of concussion consists of frequent neurologic assessments with attention to the airway, to respiratory effort, and to subtle changes in the level of consciousness. Most patients survive with no neurologic impairment.

A concussion, contusion, intracerebral hemorrhage, subdural hematoma and epidural hematoma may occur alone or in combination with one another. For example, an injury may cause a patient to sustain a concussion and an epidural hematoma concurrently. The concussion results in immediate unconsciousness, which resolves after only a few minutes. The patient becomes conscious and alert, but then later exhibits a deteriorating level of consciousness. This interim period of consciousness, called a lucid interval, occurs while the epidural hematoma expands.

Moderate Diffuse Axonal Injury   Here again, shearing, stretching, or tearing of the axons occurs, but now there is minute bruising of brain tissue. This type of injury is often referred to as the "classic concussion." If the cerebral cortex or reticular activating system of the brainstem is involved, the patient may be rendered unconscious. This type of injury is more severe than a mild concussion, occurs in 20 percent of all severe head injuries, and comprises 45 percent of all DAI cases. Moderate DAI is commonly associated with basilar skull fracture. Although most patients survive this injury, some degree of residual neurological impairment is common.

Short- and long-term signs and symptoms associated with moderate DAI include immediate unconsciousness, followed by persistent confusion, inability to concentrate, disorientation, and retrograde and anterograde amnesia. The victim may also complain of headache, focal neurological deficits, light sensitivity (photophobia), and disturbances in smell and other senses. Anxiety may be present, and the patient may experience significant mood swings.

Severe Diffuse Axonal Injury Severe DAI (previously known as brainstem injury) is a significant mechanical disruption of many axons in both cerebral hemispheres with extension into the brainstem. Approximately 16 percent of all severe head injuries and 36 percent of all cases of DAI are classified as severe. Many patients do not survive this type of injury; those that do, have some degree of permanent neurological impairment. The patient experiencing severe DAI is unconscious for a prolonged period of time and displays the signs of increased ICP (Cushing's reflex) and decerebrate or decorticate posturing.

Indirect Injury Indirect (or secondary) injuries are the result of factors that occur because of, though after, the initial (or primary) injury. These processes are progressive and cause the patient deterioration often associated with serious head injuries. The indirect injuries may be as or more damaging than the initial injury because of the unique design of the skull and the especially delicate nature of central nervous system tissue.

Indirect injuries are caused by two distinct pathologic processes. The first process is a diminishing circulation to brain tissue (intracranial perfusion) due to an increasing intracranial pressure and possibly exacerbated by hypoxia, hypercarbia, and systemic hypotension. The second process is progressive pressure against, or physical displacement of, brain tissue secondary to an expanding mass within the cranium. Both these pathologies continue and expand the nervous tissue injury and cause some of the specific and progressive signs and symptoms associated with head injury.

Intracranial Perfusion The brain is one of the body's most perfusion-sensitive organs. Any injury that affects perfusion has a rapid and devastating effect on the brain and its control of body systems. Cerebral, cerebellar, and brainstem perfusion may be disrupted both by increasing intracranial pressure and by low systemic blood pressure (hypotension).

As mentioned earlier, the cranial volume is fixed and does not vary. The cerebrum, cerebellum, and brainstem account for 80 percent (1,200 mL) of this volume. Venous, capillary, and arterial blood account for most of the remaining space, or about 12 percent (150 mL), while cerebrospinal fluid accounts for roughly the remaining 8 percent (90 mL). Any increase in the size of one internal component must be matched by a similar reduction in another component. If it is not, the intracranial pressure will rise.

As a mass expands within the cranium, the first means of compensating for the expansion is compression of the venous blood vessels. If the mass continues to expand, the next intracranial volume affected is the cerebrospinal fluid, which is pushed out of the cranium and into the spinal cord. These mechanisms respond very quickly and maintain an ICP very close to normal. However, once they reach their compensatory limits, the intracranial pressure rises quickly and begins to restrict arterial blood flow. The reduction in cerebral blood flow triggers a rise in the systemic blood pressure in an attempt to assure adequate cerebral perfusion, a process known as autoregulation. The greater the pressure of arterial blood flow, the greater the ICP. This increase in ICP further increases the resistance to cerebral blood flow, producing more hypoxia and hypercarbia. The resulting additional increase in systolic blood pressure and then ICP, leads to a worsening, eventually deadly, cycle (Figure 23-9). If the mass, injury (edema), or hemorrhage continues to expand, the ICP becomes so high that cerebral circulation all but stops.

Another factor affecting ICP and circulation through the brain is the level of carbon dioxide in the cerebrospinal fluid. As the carbon dioxide level rises, the cerebral arteries dilate to encourage greater blood flow and reduce the hypercarbia. In

Remember,
$$CPP = MAP - ICP$$
⚷

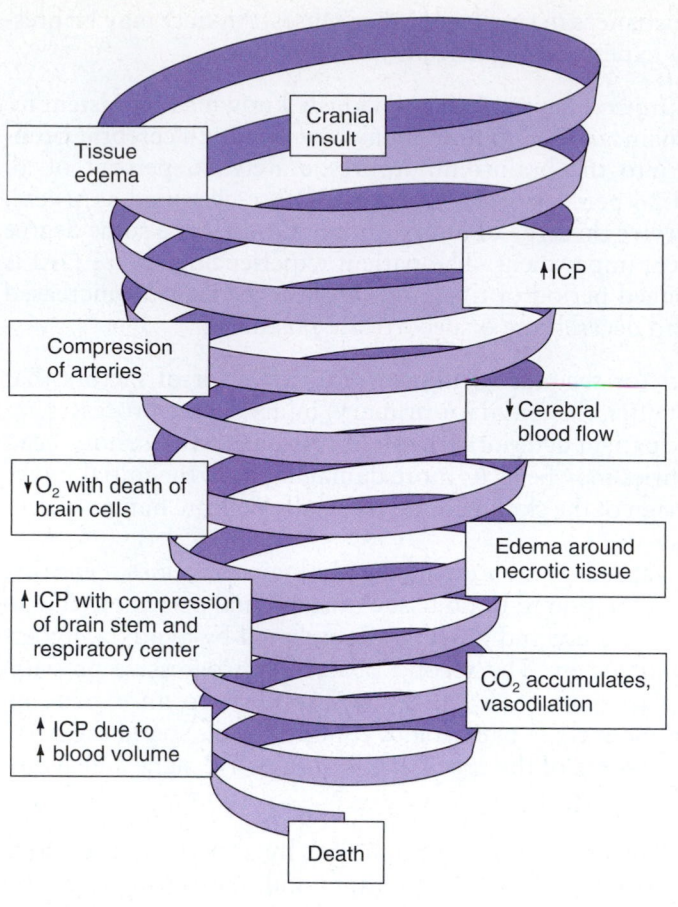

FIGURE 23-9 Pathway of deterioration following central nervous system insult.

Labels in figure:
- Cranial insult
- Tissue edema
- ↑ICP
- Compression of arteries
- ↓Cerebral blood flow
- ↓O₂ with death of brain cells
- Edema around necrotic tissue
- ↑ICP with compression of brain stem and respiratory center
- CO₂ accumulates, vasodilation
- ↑ ICP due to ↑ blood volume
- Death

the presence of an already high ICP, this process can have devastating results. The brain's response to high carbon dioxide concentrations and the increasing ICP causes the classical hyperventilation and hypertension associated with head injury. Low levels of carbon dioxide, on the other hand, can also have dire effects, triggering cerebral arterial constriction. In extreme cases, the resulting constriction can all but stop circulation through the brain.

Two systemic problems frequently associated with trauma and sometimes related to brain injury are low blood pressure and poor ventilation. These problems seriously compound any existing head injury through a tertiary injury mechanism.

Hypotension, especially in the brain-injured patient with increasing ICP, may contribute to poor cerebral perfusion pressure. In turn, diminished cerebral circulation causes increasing acidosis (retained carbon dioxide) and anaerobic metabolism. This induces further neural cell injury due to hypoxia and acidosis. At the same time, vasodilation (in response to increasing acidosis and carbon dioxide levels) elevates any existing intracranial pressure.

Hypoxia, secondary to shock or chest injury, increases the severity of any head injury. The reduced blood oxygen levels increase the cellular hypoxia at and around the injury site. Since central nervous tissue is extremely dependent upon good cellular oxygenation, neural cell damage becomes more severe.

Pressure and Structural Displacement As hemorrhage accumulates or edema increases in a region of the brain, this expansion pushes uninjured tissue away from the injury site. Even in the absence of increased ICP, such expansion puts pressure on adjacent brain cells, most commonly along the brainstem. As the mass continues to increase in size, it may physically compress brainstem components. With fur-

Low blood pressure and poor respiratory exchange seriously compound any existing head injury.

ther expansion, it may push the brain tissue against and around the falx cerebri and the tentorium cerebelli. Because these are basically immobile structures within the skull, the displacement results in a process called herniation. With herniation, a portion of a brain structure is pushed into and through an opening, physically disrupting the structure and compromising its blood supply. If the displacement affects the upper brainstem by pushing it through the tentorium incisura, it causes vomiting, changes in the level of consciousness, and pupillary dilation. If the displacement affects the medulla oblongata by pushing it into the foramen magnum, it results in disturbances in breathing, blood pressure, and heart rate.

Signs and Symptoms of Brain Injury

Direct injury, increasing intracranial pressure, and compression and displacement of brain tissue produce an altered level of orientation and of consciousness as well as specific signs and symptoms related to the central nervous system structure(s) affected. The actual process of brain injury can be mapped as the pressure increases and the injury moves from the cortical surface and down the brainstem.

As a portion of the cerebral cortex is disrupted by injury, the specific activity it controls is affected. For example, if the frontal lobe is injured, the patient will likely present with alterations in personality. If the occipital region is affected, visual disturbances are expected. A large region of cortical disruption may reduce the patient's level of awareness. The patient may become unaware of the circumstances leading up to the incident (**retrograde amnesia**) or following it (**anterograde amnesia**) or disoriented (to time, place, and person), confused, or combative. Focal deficits, like hemiplegia or weakness, or seizures may also result. When intracranial injury extends to components of the ascending reticular activating system in the brainstem, the patient may display an altered level of arousal, including lethargy, somnolence, or coma.

If the compression results from a building mass along the central region of the cerebrum, pressure is first directed to the midbrain, then the pons, and finally to the medulla oblongata. The signs and symptoms of this progressive pressure and structural displacement are somewhat predictable and are known as the central syndrome.

In this syndrome, upper brainstem compression produces an increasing blood pressure to maintain cerebral perfusion pressure and a reflex decreasing heart rate in response to vagus nerve (parasympathetic) stimulation of the SA node and AV junction. The patient may also exhibit a characteristic cyclic breathing pattern called **Cheyne-Stokes respirations**. This consists of increasing, then decreasing respiratory volumes, followed by a period of apnea. The combination of an increasing blood pressure, slowing pulse, and erratic respirations is a classical sign of brainstem pressure or injury called **Cushing's reflex** (Figure 23-10). If the brain injury involves the hypothalamus, the patient may experience vomiting, frequently without nausea, and body temperature changes. The pupils remain small and reactive. Decorticate posturing (body extension with arm flexion) in response to painful stimuli may occur as the neural pathways through the upper brainstem are disrupted.

As the middle brainstem becomes involved the pulse pressure widens and the heart rate becomes bradycardic. Respirations now may be deep and rapid (central neurologic hyperventilation). Increasing intracranial pressure may also induce pupil sluggishness or non-reactivity (bilaterally since the pathology involves compression from above) as the oculomotor nerve (CN-III) is compressed. The patient develops extension (decerebrate) posturing. Few patients ever function normally again once they have reached this ICP level.

Finally, as the pressure reaches the lower brainstem the pupils become fully dilated and unreactive. Respirations become ataxic (erratic with no characteristic

Content Review

SIGNS AND SYMPTOMS OF BRAIN INJURY

Altered level of consciousness
Altered level of orientation
Alterations in personality
Amnesia
   Retrograde
   Anterograde
Cushing's reflex
   Increasing blood pressure
   Slowing pulse rate
   Erratic respirations
Vomiting (often without nausea)
Body temperature changes
Changes in reactivity of pupils
Decorticate posturing

* **retrograde amnesia** inability to remember events that occurred before the trauma that caused the condition.

* **anterograde amnesia** inability to remember events that occurred after the trauma that caused the condition.

* **Cheyne-Stokes respirations** respiratory pattern of alternating periods of apnea and tachypnea.

* **Cushing's reflex** response due to cerebral ischemia that causes an increase in systemic blood pressure, which maintains cerebral perfusion during increased intracranial pressure.

FIGURE 23-10 How systolic blood pressure and pulse rate respond to increasing intracranial pressure.

rhythm) or may even cease altogether. The pulse rate is often very irregular with great swings in rate. ECG conduction disturbances become apparent, including QRS complex, S-T segment, and T-wave changes. As control over blood pressure is disrupted, the patient becomes hypotensive. The patient no longer responds to painful stimuli, and the skeletal muscles become flaccid. Patients rarely survive once the ICP rises to this level.

If the mass causing the compression is located more laterally than in the central syndrome described above, the signs and symptoms occur in a less predictable sequence. The pupillary responses, sluggishness, non-reactivity, and dilation, are usually ipsilateral (on the same side) as the expanding mass.

Pediatric Head Trauma

Pediatric head trauma has a very different pathology than that in the older patient. The skull is not fully formed at birth and is still rather cartilaginous. It will distort more easily with the force of an impact and transmit that force more directly to the delicate central nervous tissue. On the other hand, the incomplete formation of the skull with its "soft spots" (the anterior and posterior fontanelles) permits some intracranial expansion. The fontanelles bulge outward with increasing intracranial pressure. Generally, then, this softer skeletal structure increases the direct injury associated with head trauma in the very young pediatric patient but slows the progression of increasing intracranial pressure.

As noted earlier, the blood and cerebrospinal fluid represent about 20 percent of the total volume of the adult cranium (about 240 mL). A blood loss into the cranium cannot account for a significant component of hypovolemia in the adult. A pediatric patient, however, has a proportionally larger head, the ability to accommodate increased fluids because of the fontanelles, and a much smaller total body fluid volume and reserves. In the pediatric patient, therefore, intracranial hemorrhage may significantly contribute to hypovolemia.

When treating an infant with head, face, or neck injury, pay particular attention to the airway. Infants are obligate nasal breathers and must have a patent nasal passage and pharynx to assure a clear airway. Hyperextension of the head will obstruct the airway as the tongue pushes the soft pallet closed. Assure proper head positioning, and ventilate using both the mouth and nose.

In the pediatric patient, intracranial hemorrhage may significantly contribute to hypovolemia.

Glasgow Coma Scale

The **Glasgow Coma Scale** (GCS) is a standardized evaluation method used to measure a patient's level of consciousness. The scale assesses the best eye opening, verbal, and motor response and awards points for the various responses. Responses must be determined for both sides of the patient and any side-to-side differences noted. (A fuller discussion of the scale is found later in this chapter.)

✱ **Glasgow Coma Scale** scoring system for monitoring the neurological status of patients with head injuries.

Eye Signs

Pay close attention to the eyes when evaluating a patient with possible head trauma. The eyes are a very specialized body tissue (like central nervous system tissue) and a very visible special sense organ. The eyes can give indications of problems with cranial nerves CN-II, III, IV, and VI and with perfusion associated with cerebral blood flow. The surface of the eye is very dependent on good perfusion and lacrimal fluid flow. If perfusion is diminished, the eyes loose their luster quickly. The eyes also give quick, highly visible signs of the patient's demeanor—anxiety, fear, anger, etc.

Pupil size and reactivity also give clues to underlying conditions. Depressant drugs or cerebral hypoxia will reduce pupillary responsiveness, while extreme hypoxia causes them to dilate and fix. An expanding cranial lesion places progressive pressure on the oculomotor nerve (CN-III), causing the ipsilateral (same side) pupil to become sluggish, then dilated, then fixed. This occurs because the outer oculomotor nerve contains parasympathetic fibers. As increasing pressure interferes with these nerve fibers, the pupil dilates and is unable to constrict. If one pupil is fixed yet shows some response to consensual stimulation (light variations in the other eye), the problem most likely lies with the oculomotor nerve.

Evaluation of the eyes is very important in patients with suspected head injury.

FACIAL INJURY

Facial injury is a serious trauma complication, not only because of the cosmetic importance people place on facial appearance, but also because of the region's vasculature and the location of the initial airway and alimentary canal structures and the organs of sight, smell, taste, and hearing present there. Remember, too, that serious facial injuries suggest associated head and spinal injuries.

Facial Soft Tissue Injury

Facial soft tissue injury is common and can threaten both the patient's airway and physical appearance. Because of the ample supply of arterial and venous vessels, injuries in the region may bleed heavily, contributing to hypovolemia. Facial injuries are often the result of violence, like bullet or knife wounds. Superficial injuries and hemorrhage rarely affect the airway. With deep lacerations, however, blood may accumulate and endanger the airway or enter the digestive tract and induce vomiting. Serious blunt or penetrating injury to the soft tissues and skeletal structures supporting the pharynx may reduce the patient's ability to control the airway, increasing the likelihood of foreign body or fluid aspiration and airway compromise. Hypoxia caused by aspiration is more likely caused by blood than by other fluids or physical obstruction.

Remember, the process of inspiration creates a less-than-atmospheric pressure in the lungs to draw air in. This reduction in pressure may collapse damaged structures along the airway that are normally held open by bony or cartilaginous formations. Soft tissue swelling may also rapidly restrict the airway or close it completely. Swelling and deformity from trauma may distort the facial region so landmarks are hard to recognize, making airway control even more difficult. In serious facial soft tissue injury, always consider the likelihood of associated injury, especially basilar skull fracture and spine injury.

Patients with serious facial soft tissue injuries are likely to have associated injury, especially basilar skull fractures and spine injuries.

Content Review

LE FORT FACIAL FRACTURES

I—slight instability to maxilla; no displacement

II—fracture of both maxilla and nasal bones

III—fracture involving entire face below brow ridge (zygoma, nasal bone, maxilla)

✱ **Le Fort criteria** classification system for fractures involving the maxilla.

With a Le Fort II injury, the mid-face and zygoma move concurrently. This results in the "dish-face" description often given to this injury.

✱ **diplopia** double vision.

Facial Dislocations and Fractures

Trauma may result in open or closed facial fractures with significant associated pain, swelling, deformity, crepitus, and hemorrhage. Common injuries include mandibular, maxillary, nasal, and orbital fractures and dislocations.

Mandibular dislocation occurs as the condylar process displaces from the temporomandibular joint, just anterior to the ear. This dislocation may result in the malocclusion of the mouth, misalignment of teeth, deformity of the facial region at or around the joint, immobility of the jaw, and pain. The patient's ability to control the airway may be decreased, but dislocation is not usually a significant airway or breathing threat.

Fractures of the mandible are painful, present with deformity along the jaw's surface, and may result in the loosening of a few teeth. An open mandibular fracture may produce a blood-stained saliva. Mandibular fracture may represent a serious life threat if the patient is placed supine. With such a fracture, the tongue is no longer supported at its base and may displace posteriorly, blocking the airway even in a conscious patient. Always look for a second fracture site when you encounter a patient with a mandibular fracture.

Maxillary fractures are classified according to **Le Fort criteria** (Figure 23-11). A slight instability involving the maxilla alone usually presents with no associated displacement and is classified as a Le Fort I fracture. A Le Fort II fracture results in fractures of both the maxilla and nasal bones. Le Fort III fractures characteristically involve the entire facial region below the brow ridge, including the zygoma, nasal bone, and maxilla. The Le Fort II and III fractures usually result in cerebrospinal fluid leakage and may endanger the patency of the nasal and oral portions of the airway.

Dental injury is commonly associated with serious blunt facial trauma. Teeth may chip, break, loosen, or dislodge from the mandible or maxilla. They may then become foreign objects drawn (aspirated) into the airway. Note that a dislodged tooth may be re-implanted if fully intact and handled properly during prehospital care.

Orbital (blowout) fractures most commonly involve the zygoma or maxilla of the inferior shelf. Zygomatic arch fractures are painful and present with a unilateral depression over the prominence of one cheek. The fracture may entrap the extraocular muscles, reducing the eye's range of motion and can cause blurred or double vision (**diplopia**). Zygomatic fracture may also entrap the masseter muscle and limit jaw movement. With maxillary bone fracture, the patient often experiences significant swelling and pain in the maxillary sinus region. Although these injuries are not life threatening, they warrant evaluation by emergency department staff.

A special type of facial injury is that associated with a suicide attempt using a rifle or shotgun. The victim places the barrel under the chin but in an effort to push the trigger, stretches and tilts the head back. The gunshot blast is directed under the chin and at the facial region but may be deflected from entering the cranium. The result is a very disrupted facial region with most of the structures of, and supporting, the airway destroyed. The patient may still be conscious, there is usually heavy bleeding, and the remains of the airway are hard to locate. With such a patient, the airway is in serious danger of obstruction and attempts to secure it are very challenging.

Nasal Injury

Nasal injuries are painful and often create a grossly deformed appearance, but they are not usually life threatening. While dislocation or fracture of the cartilage and nasal bone may interfere with nasal air movement, the swelling and associated hemorrhage are more likely threats to the airway. However, the conscious and alert patient is usually very able to control the airway.

Le Fort I   **Le Fort II**   **Le Fort III**

FIGURE 23-11   Le Fort facial fracture classification.

Epistaxis (nosebleed) is a common nasal problem. Bleeding can be spontaneous as well as traumatic and can be further classified as either anterior or posterior. Anterior hemorrhage comes from the septum and is usually due to bleeding from a network of vessels called Kisselbach's plexus. Such hemorrhage bleeds slowly and is usually self limiting. Posterior hemorrhage may be severe and cause blood to drain down the back of the patient's throat. In epistaxis secondary to severe head trauma with likely basilar skull fracture, the integrity of the nasal cavity's posterior wall may be compromised. Attempts at nasal airway, nasogastric tube, or nasotracheal tube insertion may permit the tube to enter the cerebral cavity and directly damage the brain.

Ear Injury

The external ear, or pinna, which is exposed to the environment, is frequently subjected to trauma. It has a minimal blood supply and does not often bleed heavily when lacerated. In glancing blows, the pinna may be partially or completely avulsed. In a folding type of injury, the cartilage may separate. Due to the poor blood supply, external ear injuries do not heal as well as other facial wounds.

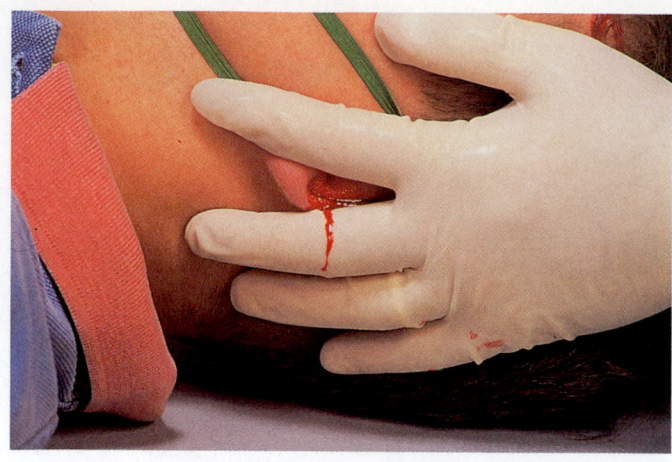

The internal portions of the ear—the external auditory canal and the middle and inner ear—are well protected from trauma by the structure of the skull. Injury only results from objects forced into the ear or from rapid changes in pressure as in diving accidents or explosions. With an explosion—even with repeated small arms fire—the pinna focuses the rapidly changing air pressure and directs it into the external auditory canal. This enhanced pressure irritates or ruptures the tympanum and, if strong enough, fractures the small bones of hearing (the ossicles). The result can be temporary or permanent hearing loss. In a diving injury, the changing pressure is not equalized by the eustachian tube (also called the pharyngotympanic passage) and eventually builds until the eardrum ruptures. Water floods the middle ear and interferes with the function of the semicircular canals. The patient experiences vertigo, an extremely dangerous sensation when near weightless under water.

Basilar skull fracture may also disrupt the external auditory canal and tear the tympanum. If the dura mater is torn, cerebrospinal fluid may flood the middle ear and seep outward through the torn tympanum (Figure 23-12). As with the other mechanisms described earlier, hearing loss may result.

Tympanic injuries are not life threatening and, in many cases, repair themselves, even with a rupture that tears as much as half the tympanum. However, a victim with an acute hearing loss can be quite apprehensive and anxious. The patient may be frustrated when unable to hear and understand questions or instructions. Such a patient may also be unable to hear sounds of approaching danger such as traffic noise.

Eye Injury

Although the orbit is a very effective protective housing for the eye, penetrating and some blunt trauma may cause serious injury. The anterior eye structures are extremely specialized and, like most specialized tissues, do not regenerate effectively. If significant penetrating injury occurs, especially if accompanied by loss of the eye's fluids—aqueous or vitreous humor—the patient's sight is threatened, possibly with permanent loss. A penetrating object is likely to disturb the integrity of the anterior and possibly the posterior chamber. In addition, removal of the object may allow fluids to leak from the chambers and further threaten the patient's vision. Penetrating injuries may be caused by foreign bodies so small that they are difficult to see with the naked eye. Suspect the presence of such bodies if the patient reports a history of sudden eye pain and the sensation of an impaled foreign body after using a power saw or grinder, especially when working with metal.

FIGURE 23-13   Laceration of the eyelid.

Similarly, small foreign particles that land on the eye's surface can also cause ocular injury. The object may embed in the surface of the eyelid and then drag across the cornea as the eye blinks. Corneal abrasions or lacerations result, often causing intense and continuing pain even after the object is cleared from the eye. These lacerations are usually superficial but can be deep (Figure 23-13).

Blunt trauma may result in several ocular presentations. Hemorrhage into the anterior chamber pools, displaying a collection of blood in front of the iris and pupil. This condition, called **hyphema,** is a potential threat to the patient's vision and requires evaluation by an ophthalmologist and may result in hospital admission.

A less serious, but equally dramatic, eye injury is a sub-conjunctival hemorrhage. This may occur after a strong sneeze, vomiting episode, or direct eye trauma, such as orbital fracture. It occurs when a small blood vessel in the sub-conjunctival space bursts, leaving a portion of the eye's surface blood red (Figure 23-14). Sub-conjunctival hemorrhage often clears without intervention and rarely causes any residual scars or impairment.

✱ **hyphema** blood in the anterior chamber of the eye, in front of the iris.

A hyphema is a sight-threatening injury.

Occasionally, blood will completely fill the anterior chamber resulting in what is called an "eight-ball" hyphema. This can easily be missed without close examination.

FIGURE 23-14   Sub-conjunctival hemorrhage.

*Most trauma surgeons feel that
any neck injury that penetrates
the most superficial muscle
(platysma) should be surgically
explored.*

Blunt trauma may fracture the orbital structures surrounding the eye and produce an injury called eye avulsion. In such a case, the eye is not really avulsed but appears to protrude from the wound as the structure of the orbit is crushed and depressed. If the eye as well as the nerves and vasculature remain intact, sight in the eye can usually be salvaged.

Two other, more serious ocular problems involve the retina. **Acute retinal artery occlusion** is not an injury but rather a vascular emergency caused when an embolus blocks the blood supply to one eye. The patient complains of sudden and painless loss of vision in the eye. In **retinal detachment,** which may be traumatic in origin, the retina separates from the eye's posterior wall. The patient complains of a dark curtain obstructing part of the field of view. Both of these conditions are true emergencies in which the patient's eyesight is at risk.

Soft tissue lacerations can occur around the eye and involve the eyelid. If not properly identified and repaired, such an injury may disrupt the function of the lacrimal duct and interrupt lubrication and oxygenation of the cornea. Another soft tissue problem may occur if a contact lens is left in the eye of an unconscious patient. The contact lens will then obstruct the normal lacrimal fluid flow across the eye. This loss of circulation may dry out the eye's surface and cause hypoxic injury. The result is usually severe eye pain and possible damage to the cornea.

NECK INJURY

The neck is protected from impact by the more anterior head and chest and by its own skeletal and muscular structures. The neck's major skeletal component is the cervical vertebral column, which is strengthened by interconnecting ligaments. The neck muscles provide additional protection to the vital structures in the neck. They include the muscles that support and move the head through a large range of motion as well as the shoulder muscles that help move the upper extremities and act as auxiliary breathing muscles. The skeletal structures and muscles of the neck protect the airway, carotid and jugular blood vessels, and the esophagus very well from all but anterior blunt trauma and deep penetrating trauma. Such trauma may result in serious injuries to the airway, cervical spine, blood vessels, and other structures in the region.

Blood Vessel Trauma

Blunt trauma to a blood vessel may produce a serious and rapidly expanding hematoma. This hematoma may be trapped within the fascia of the region and apply restrictive pressure to the jugular veins. Laceration of the external jugular vein, or deep laceration involving the internal jugular vein or the carotid arteries may result in severe hemorrhage due to the large size of the vessels and the volume of blood they carry (Figure 23-15). Their laceration and subsequent hemorrhage can rapidly lead to hypovolemia and shock. Arterial interruption may cause subsequent brain hypoxia and infarct, mimicking the signs and symptoms of a stroke. An open neck wound affecting the external jugular vein may permit formation of an air embolism as the venous pressure drops below atmospheric pressure with deep respirations.

Airway Trauma

Trauma may also injure the trachea. Severe blunt or penetrating trauma may separate the larynx from the trachea, fracture or crush either of these two structures, or open the trachea to the environment. These injuries may result in serious hemorrhage that threatens the airway, vocal cord contusion or swelling, destruction of the integrity of the airway and collapse on inspiration, disruption of normal airway landmarks, and restrictive soft tissue swelling.

FIGURE 23-15   Laceration to the neck.

Cervical Spine Trauma

Severe blunt trauma and, in some cases, gunshot wounds to the neck may cause vertebral fracture and cervical spine instability. The wounds may cause pressure on the spinal cord, cord contusion, or severing of the cord. Such injuries will likely cause bilateral paresthesia, anaesthesia, weakness (paresis), or paralysis, generally at and below the dermatome controlled by the peripheral nerve branch leaving the vertebral column at the level of the injury. Neurogenic shock from these injuries may cause hypotension from vasodilation. (This is discussed in Chapter 24, "Spinal Trauma.") Blunt trauma may disrupt and injure the muscles and connective tissues of the region and result in serious pain and limited motion.

Other Neck Trauma

The neck may also demonstrate subcutaneous emphysema due to tension pneumothorax (air pushed into the skin from intrathoracic pressure that migrates to the neck) or from tracheal injury in the neck. Penetrating trauma may involve the esophagus, perforating it and permitting gastric contents or undigested material to enter the fascia. Since the fascia communicates with the mediastinum, this foreign material can physically harm mediastinal structures or provide the medium for infection, which may have devastating results. Deep penetrating trauma may disrupt the vagus nerve, causing tachycardia and gastrointestinal disturbances. More anterior and superficial injuries may damage the thyroid and parathyroid glands.

ASSESSMENT OF HEAD, FACIAL, AND NECK INJURIES

As with all trauma patients, assessment of head, facial, and neck injury patients follows the standard format, including the scene size-up, initial assessment, rapid trauma assessment/focused exam and history, and the detailed assessment as appropriate. Perform ongoing assessments frequently on these patients. With head, facial, and neck injuries, pay special attention to assuring airway patency and monitoring breathing, level of consciousness and orientation, pupillary signs, and blood pressure. With these patients, be sure to consider the need for rapid transport to a trauma center specializing in neurological care.

SCENE SIZE-UP

Analysis of the mechanism of injury is a key part of the assessment of the patient with a possible head, face, or neck injury. During the scene size-up, consider the circumstances of injury and identify the nature and extent of forces that caused the injury. In a vehicle crash, for example, look for evidence of head impact such as the characteristic spider-web windshield. Look also for deformity of the upper steering wheel, which suggests head or neck trauma or the use of the shoulder belt without the lap belt. Identify the direction of the forces causing injury and anticipate what body structures the forces may have damaged. In motorcycle impacts, remember that helmet use reduces head injury by about 50 percent but does not spare the neck from cervical spine injury. In shootings, try to determine the caliber and type of weapon, the distance from the gun to the patient, and the approximate angle of the bullet's entry into the patient's body.

With other types of impacts, try to determine what forces were involved and how they were directed to the head, face, and neck. Use this information to anticipate injuries to the brain, airway, and sense organs. Remember that many signs of head injury may be masked by the patient's use of alcohol or other drugs, by the nature of the injury, and/or by the slow development of the wound process. Consequently, a good analysis of the MOI and the resulting indexes of suspicion are very important. Your thorough analysis must enable you to describe both the incident scene and the mechanism of injury to the attending physician at the emergency department. Remember that the mechanism of injury can often give a better indication of the seriousness of the injury than the patient's signs and symptoms.

Rule out scene hazards, and request any additional resources needed at the scene as soon as you can. Use of gloves is the minimum level of BSI protection when approaching the potential head, face, and neck injury patient. Serious head injuries pose real risks of exposure to blood or other fluids propelled by air movement or by arterial or heavy venous bleeding. Anticipate such exposures, and don splash and eye protection when contacting any patient with significant trauma to the head, face, or neck.

INITIAL ASSESSMENT

As you approach, form an initial impression of the patient's condition. Is the patient alert? Does the patient show any signs of anxiety? If there is any reason to suspect that the head or neck sustained serious impact, provide immediate manual immobilization of the head and cervical spine (Figure 23-16). Quickly determine the patient's level of consciousness and then orientation to time, place, and persons early in the initial assessment. While determining the patient's level of orientation may add a few seconds to the initial assessment, assessing trends in orientation can be critical to rapid identification of a brain injury patient. Be alert to the patient's facial skin color, respiratory effort, and to pupil luster and level of responsiveness throughout the initial assessment as these factors can help you recognize internal head injury. As you gather information about the patient, continue to build and modify your general patient impression and your index of suspicion for head injury.

Apply a cervical collar at the end of the initial assessment and maintain manual head immobilization until the patient is fully immobilized to a short spine board, KED, or long spine board with a cervical immobilization device. If there are any significant injuries to the neck, do not apply the collar until you complete the assessment and provide needed care. While the cervical collar provides some neck stabilization, it does not completely immobilize the region, and its placement may be delayed so long as manual immobilization is continued.

While determining the patient's level of orientation may add a few seconds to the initial assessment, assessing trends in orientation can be critical to rapid identification of a brain injury patient.

FIGURE 23-16   If spinal injury is suspected, immediately immobilize the head and neck manually.

If the patient is wearing a helmet, consider whether or not to remove it as described in Chapter 24, "Spinal Trauma." A patient's use of a helmet reduces the likelihood of soft tissue injury and skull and facial fracture. Helmet use can also significantly reduce the incidence of brain injury, but do not be lulled into a false sense of security by the absence of outward signs of trauma. Be watchful for the early signs of internal brain injury, and be sure to inform the emergency department staff that the patient was wearing a helmet. Also alert them to any signs of impact or helmet damage suggestive of the forces of trauma that the patient experienced.

Airway

Then move quickly to evaluate the airway. Examine the face and neck for any deformity, swelling, hemorrhage, foreign bodies, or other signs of injury that may threaten the airway. Suction and insert an oral or nasal airway as necessary. Listen for unusual or changing voice patterns as they may be indicative of airway injury and developing edema. Swelling can quickly occlude the airway, and any hemorrhage can complicate airway maintenance as the patient loses consciousness and the gag reflex. Anticipate vomiting, possibly without warning. Assure that the airway is structurally sound and that the mandible supports the tongue well enough to keep it out of the airway. Have a large-bore suction catheter and strong suction ready to remove any fluids, and consider positioning the patient to enhance airway drainage (left lateral recumbent position) if doing so is not contraindicated by injuries. If the patient does not display a gag reflex or has an altered level of consciousness, consider early insertion of an endotracheal tube.

If there is a serious neck injury, check the structural integrity of the trachea. If the trachea is open to the environment, keep the wound clear of blood to prevent aspiration, and seal the wound unless the patient's upper airway is blocked. If an impaled object obstructs the airway, remove it, anticipating that heavy bleeding may then threaten the airway. Blunt wounds may crush the cartilage of the trachea, permitting it to close with the reduced pressure during inspiration. This type of crushing injury may require surgical opening of the trachea by needle or surgical cricothyrotomy to assure air exchange.

Breathing

Closely monitor breathing to assure that the patient is moving an adequate volume of air. Determine the rate of respirations and their rhythm. Estimate the amount of air moved with each breath, and from those numbers determine the minute volume:

$$\text{Minute volume} = \text{Tidal volume} \times \text{Respiratory rate}$$

If the patient is breathing less than 12 times per minute, moving less than 500 mL of air with each breath, or has a minute volume of less than 6 liters, consider overdrive ventilation. Remember that head injury is likely to produce erratic breathing patterns and that hypoxia and carbon dioxide retention both contribute to morbidity and mortality with brain injury. Ventilate at 12 to 20 full breaths per minute with a volume of between 800 and 1000 mL. Do not hyperventilate the patient if you suspect brain injury. Hyperventilation will blow off carbon dioxide and cause vasoconstriction, further decreasing cerebral perfusion.

Apply oxygen via nonrebreather mask with a flow of 12 to 15 liters per minute, to assure inspiration of high concentrations. It is advisable to apply pulse oximetry to monitor oxygenation. Attempt to keep oxygen saturation above 95 percent.

Circulation

A slow and strong (bounding) pulse may be an early sign of building intracranial pressure.

Begin to monitor the patient's pulse rate and its rhythm early in your care and continue to do so frequently thereafter. A slow and strong (bounding) pulse may be an early sign of building intracranial pressure. Apply an ECG monitor and watch for rhythm disturbances. Quickly look for any hemorrhage from the head, face, and neck and control any moderate to severe bleeding with direct pressure and bandaging. Be cautious of open neck wounds because they may present a risk for air embolism. Cover any such wounds quickly with occlusive dressings and secure them in place.

At the end of the initial assessment, you must determine whether to perform a rapid trauma assessment followed by gathering of vital signs and the patient history or to perform a focused history and physical exam followed by gathering of vital signs. With most head, face, and neck injury patients, you will perform a rapid trauma assessment because of the high likelihood of airway, vascular, special sense organ, or central nervous system injuries in these regions. If there is no significant mechanism of injury and injuries appear minor and superficial, perform an exam focused on the specific area(s) of injury.

RAPID TRAUMA ASSESSMENT

The rapid trauma assessment calls for performance of a quick and directed head-to-toe examination of a patient with a significant mechanism of injury. When head, facial, or neck injury is suggested in such a patient, pay particular attention to the procedures described below as you carry out the assessment. Manage any life-threatening injuries and conditions as you find them during the rapid trauma assessment. If the patient shows any signs of pathology within the cranium, consider rapid transport. Brain injury patients can deteriorate quickly, but rapid neurosurgical intervention can frequently alleviate life-threatening problems.

Head

Look at, then sweep, each region of the skull, feeling for deformity and bleeding with the more sensitive tips of your fingers. Interlock your fingers to sweep the posterior head, and look at your gloves to check for any blood that indicates hemorrhage there. If you find any moderate or serious hemorrhage, apply direct pressure unless you suspect skull fracture. Control the hemorrhage with gentle pressure around the wound and place a loose dressing over it. Palpate gently for any deformities, being careful, however, not to palpate the interior of open wounds (Figure 23-17).

Shine a penlight into the external auditory canal and look for signs of escaping cerebrospinal fluid. This fluid loss may be difficult to notice early during assessment, so observe carefully. If blood or fluid drains from the auditory canal, cover the ear with a gauze dressing to permit fluid to move outward while providing a barrier to keep contaminants from entering. If the fluid drains on a gauze dressing or other fabric, look for the halo sign. However, you should presume (regardless of the presence or absence of halo sign) that any fluid draining from the ear contains cerebrospinal fluid. Examine the pinnae for injury and, after you complete the rapid trauma assessment, bandage and dress as needed.

If you observe a skull deformity, palpate such a closed wound very gently. Try to determine the probability of skull fracture before swelling makes this determination more difficult. Cover any open wounds with dressings to restrict blood flow and prevent further contamination. The signs of basilar skull fracture—bilateral periorbital ecchymosis and retroauricular ecchymosis (raccoon eyes and

Bilateral periorbital ecchymosis and retroauricular ecchymosis are very late signs of basilar skull fracture and are not likely to be recognizable during field assessment and care.

FIGURE 23-17 Carefully inspect and palpate the head for bleeding and other signs of injury.

Battle's sign)—are very late indications of this injury and are not likely to be recognizable during field assessment and care.

Head injury may cause patient seizures. Seizures are serious complications because they may compromise the airway and respirations, increase the intracranial pressure, and exacerbate any existing brain injury. If you observe a seizure or the patient or bystanders describe one as you gather the history, find out as much about the episode as you can and be prepared to describe the seizure in detail, including its origin and progression, to the attending physician. Protect the seizing patient from further injury and be especially watchful of the airway. Consider the administration of diazepam, which reduces electrical impulse transmission across the cerebrum and may limit seizure activity.

Face

Study the patient's facial features carefully, looking for asymmetry, swelling, discoloration, or deformity. Palpate the facial region including the brow ridge, nasal region, cheek, maxilla, and mandible searching for any deformity, instability, or crepitus that suggest fracture and for any signs of soft tissue swelling (Figure 23-18). Palpate the maxilla and attempt, gently, to move it from left to right. It should be firmly attached to the facial bones and should display no crepitus. Do likewise with the mandible. It should be solid yet very mobile from left to right and up and down. Note and investigate any patient report of pain during your palpation and movement. Open the mouth and examine for any signs of trauma, excessive secretions and bleeding, or swelling. All teeth should be firmly in place (loose teeth may suggest mandibular fracture). Find any displaced teeth and prepare them for transport with the patient or suspect that missing teeth may have been aspirated. Assure that the mandible is intact and supports the airway.

Carefully examine the eyes. In general, eye reactivity and luster reflect the oxygenation status of the brain. Watch for bright and sparkling eyes and briskly reactive pupils. Shine a bright light into the eyes—or in bright sunlight, shade them—and watch for sluggishness, non-reactivity, and constriction (or dilation). Assure that reactivity is bilateral. Note that both eyes should respond to changes in light intensity affecting only one eye (**consensual reactivity**). Both eyes should gaze together and, at rest, directly forward. Watch for a down and out gaze. Usually, an affected pupil is on the same side (ipsilateral) as a head

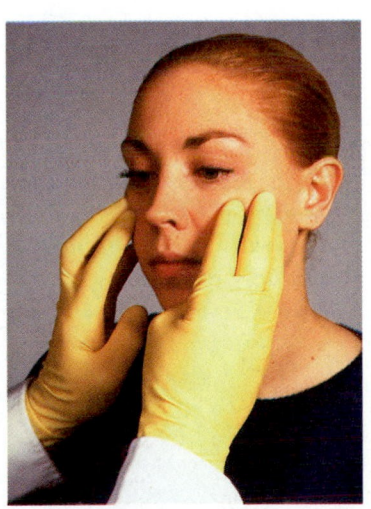

FIGURE 23-18 Carefully palpate the facial bones.

Restricted eye movement suggests eye muscle entrapment or nerve compression or injury and paralysis.

injury. If the patient is conscious and alert, have him follow your finger up and down, left and right, with each eye. Watch for and note any limited eye movement. Restricted eye movement suggests eye muscle entrapment and nerve compression or injury and paralysis.

Carefully examine the pupil, iris, and conjunctiva. The pupil and iris should be round, the anterior chamber clear, and the sclera free of accumulating blood. Check for contact lenses, especially in the unconscious patient. If they are noted, remove them carefully.

Neck

Any penetration of the lateral neck muscles should heighten your index of suspicion for a serious neck injury.

Examine the anterior, lateral, and posterior neck for signs of injury including swelling, discoloration, wounds, blood loss, or frothy blood. Frothy blood is likely caused by bleeding in association with a tracheal injury and suggests serious airway compromise. Palpate the region, feeling for any changes in skin tension, deformities, or unusual masses underneath. Crepitus beneath the skin may be associated with subcutaneous emphysema from a tracheal or chest injury or a tracheal or laryngeal fracture. Identify the thyroid cartilage, beneath and posterior to the mandible. Palpate it, the cricoid cartilage, then the trachea. Assure they are not deformed by trauma and remain midline in the neck. Visually examine the depth of neck wounds to anticipate those that may involve jugular or carotid blood vessels, and cover any open wounds with occlusive dressings.

While carrying out the rapid trauma assessment, question the responsive patient about headaches and increased light sensitivity (photophobia), which are common symptoms of head injury. Also question the patient about his or her memory of the events preceding and following the injury to identify retrograde and anterograde amnesia. Note any repetitive questioning by the patient (inability to establish short-term memory) and any unusual behavior or confusion. Ask if the patient has any unusual fullness in the throat and any difficulty swallowing. Ask about any visual disturbances such as double vision (diplopia) and blurred vision that may indicate eye muscle entrapment. Inquire about visual acuity (the ability to distinguish objects) both near and far, and note reports of any restriction to vision, which the patient might describe as a curtain drawn across the field of view. Patient complaints of eye pain are also important and may suggest conjunctival or corneal injury. You may also note patient complaints about focal deficits. Examine any area of paresthesia, anesthesia, weakness, or paralysis, noting the borders of the area and whether it is unilateral or bilateral. Question the patient frequently to identify any increase or decrease in awareness and any changes in injury symptoms.

Question the head, face, or neck injury patient frequently to identify any increase or decrease in awareness and any changes in injury symptoms.

Complete the rapid trauma assessment by examining the rest of the body, paying particular attention to any region where the mechanism of injury suggests serious injury and in which the patient complains of serious symptoms. While examining the extremities, look for any signs of decreased muscle tone, flaccid muscles, diminished sensation or muscle strength, and determine if any unusual findings are bilateral or unilateral and where the deficit begins. Then gather the balance of the patient history, determine the patient's Glasgow Coma Scale score, and take a set of the patient's vital signs.

Glasgow Coma Scale Score

Determine the patient's best eye opening, motor, and verbal responses using the Glasgow Coma Scale (GCS). The Glasgow Coma Scale awards the patient points for different responses, with a total score that will range between 3 and 15 points (see Table 23-1). The scale is a moderately good predictor of head injury severity. A patient with a score of between 13 and 15 is considered to have a mild head in-

Table 23-1 GLASGOW COMA SCALE

Eye Opening

Spontaneous	4
To verbal command	3
To pain	2
No response	1

Verbal Response

Oriented and converses	5
Disoriented and converses	4
Inappropriate words	3
Incomprehensible sounds	2
No response	1

Motor Response

Obeys verbal commands	6
Localizes pain	5
Withdraws from pain (flexion)	4
Abnormal flexion in response to pain (decorticate rigidity)	3
Extension in response to pain (decerebrate rigidity)	2
No response	1

jury. A score between 9 and 12 indicates moderate injury, while a score of 8 or less represents severe head injury. Most patients with GCS of 8 or less are in a coma.

When assessing eye-opening response, award 1 point for no response, 2 for eye opening in response to pain, 3 for response to verbal command, and 4 for spontaneous eye opening. With verbal response, award 1 point for no sound or response, 2 points for incomprehensible, garbled sounds, 3 points for inappropriate words and speech that makes no sense, 4 points for confused or disoriented speech, and 5 for clear and oriented speech. With motor response, award 1 point for no movement or response, 2 points for decerebrate posturing, 3 points for decorticate posturing, 4 points for purposeful motion (withdrawal of a body part from pain), 5 points for purposeful movement (of the hand) to localize pain, and 6 for following simple verbal commands. The lowest GCS value is 3, which represents a completely unresponsive patient. The maximum GCS value is 15, which represents the fully conscious and alert patient.

Record the best response for each of the GCS criteria (for example, as E_3, V_4, M_5) and note any differences, either from side-to-side or in the upper versus lower extremities. Also note the eye signs along with the Glasgow Coma Scale score results because they help identify the existence and nature of the patient's brain injury.

Patients with a Glasgow Coma Scale score of 8 or less should be immediately intubated.

Vital Signs

Carefully monitor the vital signs for evidence of increasing intracranial pressure. Identify and record the pulse rate and strength. Note the blood pressure and especially the pulse pressure. Lastly, note the respiratory pattern. The vital signs change with increasing ICP or injury to the brainstem. Be watchful for a slowing pulse rate, increasing systolic blood pressure, and the development of erratic respirations (Cheyne-Stokes, central neurologic hyperventilation, or ataxic respirations), which together are known as Cushing's reflex.

At the conclusion of the rapid trauma assessment, determine the need for rapid transport.

At the conclusion of the rapid trauma assessment, determine the need for rapid transport. A history of head trauma coupled with any history of unconsciousness, a degradation in the level of orientation or consciousness, or any vital sign suggestive of brain injury requires rapid transport to the closest appropriate facility. If such signs and symptoms of brain injury exist, begin rapid transport and contact medical direction for approval to transport to the nearest neurocenter. Significant airway threats and uncontrolled hemorrhage are also indicators for rapid transport. Carefully monitor other head, face, and neck injury patients during further assessment and care for any signs of increasing intracranial pressure or expanding lesions. Identify the wounds and other injuries you have found or suspect and prioritize them for care.

FOCUSED HISTORY AND PHYSICAL EXAM

If your head, face, or neck injury patient has no significant mechanism of injury and no other indications of serious injury, perform a focused history and physical exam, concentrating on the area of injury. During your assessment, however, carefully observe for any signs of a diminished level of consciousness or orientation or any evidence of previous unconsciousness or airway or vascular restriction or compromise. If you discover any of these things, complete a rapid trauma assessment and consider the patient for rapid transport to the appropriate facility. Remember, the signs of significant brain injury may not develop for some time or may be masked by drug or alcohol use or by the patient's anxiety. It is always better to err on the side of more intensive patient care.

Direct the focused history and physical exam to the areas of specific patient complaint and to areas where the mechanism of injury suggests injury. Use the assessment techniques—inspection, palpation, etc.—suggested for the rapid trauma assessment.

When you have completed the focused assessment, obtain a set of baseline vital signs and gather a patient history. Then provide emergency care for the injuries you have found and prepare the patient for transport.

With superficial wounds to the head, face and neck, apply dressings and bandages as for minor soft tissue injuries but be alert for hemorrhage into the airway and vomiting that may follow it and for any signs of progressive swelling that may restrict the airway. Watch also for open neck wounds that may permit air to enter the jugular vein. Cover such wounds with occlusive dressings held firmly in place.

Inspect any soft tissue head, facial, or neck injury very carefully before bandaging it and be prepared to describe the injury to the attending emergency department physician or nurse so they do not have to remove and replace dressings and bandages unnecessarily.

DETAILED ASSESSMENT

You will normally perform a detailed assessment for the head, face, and neck injury patient during transport and only if and when you have cared for all other serious injuries. The detailed assessment is an in-depth, head-to-toe assessment searching for any other signs or symptoms suggestive of injury. Use your skills of questioning, inspection, palpation, and—as appropriate—auscultation, to search out these additional injuries. Look for signs of neurologic deficit in the extremities, including flaccidity, paresthesia, anesthesia, weakness, and paralysis. Remember that early in the course of trauma, serious injuries may be masked by other more painful ones, by patient anxiety, and by drug and alcohol use. Careful evaluation is required to identify injuries at this stage of patient care.

ONGOING ASSESSMENT

Perform ongoing assessments every 5 minutes for patients with potentially serious injuries. Be especially alert for slowing of the pulse, increasing systolic blood pressure (an increasing pulse pressure), and development of deeper, more rapid, or erratic respirations. Carefully observe the patient for changes in the level of consciousness and orientation as well. Finally, watch the eyes for signs of cerebral hypoxia—they become dull and lackluster—or of increasing intracranial pressure—one pupil becomes sluggish, non-reactive, then dilated. Note any changes in any element of patient presentation, and track any trends to identify whether the patient's condition is deteriorating, improving or remaining the same.

Watch pulse oximetry and blood pressure readings to assure that the patient becomes neither hypoxic nor hypovolemic. Both of these conditions are associated with increased mortality and morbidity when associated with brain injury. If you notice any sign of deterioration, provide rapid transport.

A slowing pulse rate, increasing systolic blood pressure, and the development of erratic respirations are signs of increasing intracranial pressure.

If the patient's eyes become dull and lackluster, it is a sign of cerebral hypoxia; if one pupil becomes sluggish, non-reactive, then dilated, that indicates intracranial injury.

HEAD, FACIAL, AND NECK INJURY MANAGEMENT

The management priorities for the patient sustaining head, face, or neck trauma include care directed at maintaining the patient's airway and breathing, assuring circulation through hemorrhage control, addressing or taking steps to avoid hypoxia and/or hypovolemia, and providing appropriate medications. Once these priorities have been attended to, you may dress and care for minor head, facial, and neck wounds.

AIRWAY

The airway is one of the most important care priorities with head, face, and neck injury patients. Head, face, and neck injury can leave patients unable to control the airway due either to an altered mental status or to damaged airway structures. In addition, soft tissue trauma to the airway may cause edema that can quickly progress from restriction of the airway to its complete obstruction. Vigilant attention to the airway and aggressive airway care are the only means of assuring that the airway of these patients remains protected and patent. Airway management techniques appropriate for such patients include suctioning, patient positioning, oral and nasal airway insertion, endotracheal intubation, and cricothyrotomy. (You can review these techniques in Chapter 8, "Airway Management and Ventilation.")

Vigilant attention to the airway and aggressive airway care are vital with head, facial, and neck injury patients.

Suctioning

Airway tissues are extremely vascular, bleed profusely, and swell quickly. Soft tissue injury may cause significant hemorrhage that can compromise the airway in two ways. First, the sheer volume of blood may block the airway. Note that aspiration of blood is more often responsible for hypoxia than physical obstruction of the airway, so be certain to suction as necessary in order to remove blood from the airway.

Secondly, blood is a gastric irritant that frequently induces emesis. If a large volume of blood is swallowed, the patient may vomit, thus endangering the airway. In addition, vomiting is common with head injury patients because emesis is a frequent result of brain injury or increasing intracranial pressure. Vomiting often occurs without warning (without nausea) and can be projectile in nature.

Vomiting is especially dangerous with head injury patients because they commonly have a depressed or absent gag reflex. Gastric contents are very acidic and will quickly damage the tissues of the lower airway if aspirated. Aspiration of gastric contents is associated with a high patient mortality. Be ready to suction aggressively as needed in any patients with nasal, oral, or head trauma. Use a large-bore catheter or a suction hose without a tip to clear the airway of any blood or emesis.

Patient Positioning

Consider placing the patient in a position that protects the airway early in your care (during the initial assessment). The best position for the patient with suspected head injury is on the left side with the head turned slightly and facing downward, the left lateral recumbent position. Remember, of course, that head injury patients require spinal precautions. Maintain manual immobilization until the patient is secured to a long spine board, and then be prepared to turn patient and board as a unit to facilitate airway drainage.

It is unlikely that suction alone will evacuate all emesis from the oral cavity before the unconscious or semiconscious patient attempts an inspiration. If the patient experiencing serious oral, nasal (epistaxis), or facial bleeding is conscious and alert and no serious spinal injury is suspected, have the patient sit leaning forward to promote drainage and keep fluids from flowing into the posterior airway. If the patient has sustained an open neck injury with the danger of air embolism, place the patient on a spine board in the Trendelenburg position, with the lower part of the patient's body elevated about 12 inches. Otherwise, position the patient with potential brain injury by elevating the head of the spine board to about 30 degrees to reduce both external hemorrhage and intracranial pressure.

Oropharyngeal and Nasopharyngeal Airways

Oro- and nasopharyngeal airways each have advantages and disadvantages when used with head, face, and neck injury patients. The nasal airway does not trigger the gag reflex as easily as the oral airway and is better tolerated by the semiconscious patient. Because there is less stimulation of the gag reflex, there is also a reduction in transient increases in intracranial pressure and in the chances of increasing the severity of head injury. One hazard of nasal airway use is the possible insertion of the tube directly into the cranium through a fracture of the posterior nasal border. Always insert the nasal airway straight back, through the largest of the nares (nostrils), and use only gentle force in its introduction. If you suspect basilar skull fracture, use an oral airway or endotracheal intubation to establish and maintain the airway.

While the oral and nasal airways help to keep the respective pharynxes open, they can represent threats to the airway. The ends of the tubes sit just superior to the opening of the larynx. If a patient vomits, which frequently happens with brain injury, the vomitus is blocked from exiting the patient's mouth through the airway and remains just at the laryngeal opening. With the next breath, the patient can aspirate the gastric contents, which may have serious consequences. Whenever an oral or nasal airway is in place, monitor the patient's airway carefully and be prepared to remove the airway and evacuate any emesis.

Intubate early in the care of the unresponsive patient, and consider intubation for any patient with a reduced level of consciousness.

Endotracheal Intubation

Endotracheal intubation is the most definitive method of assuring a clear and patent airway in the head injury patient. Intubate early in the care of the unresponsive patient, and consider intubation for any patient with a reduced level of consciousness. Techniques useful in caring for head injury patients include orotracheal, digital, nasotracheal, retrograde, directed, and rapid sequence intubation.

Orotracheal Intubation Orotracheal, or oral, intubation is the most common and usually the most successful technique for placing an endotracheal tube (Figure 23-19). It does, however, pose some hazards for head, face, and neck injury patients. All patients who sustain serious injuries in these regions require spinal immobilization. Immobilization, however, limits the movement of the patient's head during intubation attempts, restricting you from manually bringing the oral opening, pharynx, and trachea in line. The result is often an inability to visualize the vocal folds and watch the endotracheal tube pass into the trachea, seriously reducing the chances of a successful oral intubation.

To improve visualization during oral intubation with spinal immobilization, employ a technique called Sellick's maneuver. Apply pressure directed posteriorly to the cricoid ring with the thumb and index finger, moving it downward toward the vertebral column. This brings the trachea more in line with the oral cavity and pharynx and compresses the esophagus, thus reducing the likelihood of vomitus entering the upper airway during intubation. Exercise caution to prevent the pressure from flexing the cervical spine. Be aware that Sellick's maneuver may not align the airway enough to permit visualized oral intubation.

Attempts at endotracheal intubation can increase the parasympathetic (vagal) tone. This, in turn, may increase intracranial pressure and lower the heart rate or increase the severity of other cardiac dysrhythmias already induced by the brain injury. Therefore, carry out the intubation rapidly. If possible, have the most experienced care provider attempt the procedure to reduce both intubation time and vagal stimulation. Also consider use of a pharmacologic agent, such as a topical anesthetic spray, to reduce both vagal stimulation and the retching associated with stimulation of the gag reflex.

Digital Intubation Another technique that may be effective when intubating a patient undergoing spinal precautions is digital intubation. In this procedure, the endotracheal tube is positioned without visualization; instead, the tube is directed into the trachea from the base of the tongue by the intubator's fingers. This is a procedure best attempted by a paramedic with long thin fingers.

A slightly smaller than usual endotracheal tube is shaped by a stylet into a "J" configuration. The patient's mouth is held open with a bite block while the you insert the first two fingers of one hand and "walk" them back along the tongue to its base. Use these fingers to locate and lift the epiglottis. Advance the tube with your other hand along the back of the tongue and direct it with your fingers past the epiglottis and toward the tracheal opening. Continue to advance the endotracheal tube with slight anterior pressure along the posterior surface of the epiglottis for about 1 1/2 to 2 1/2 inches. Remove the stylet and carefully confirm tube placement in the trachea, not the esophagus.

Nasotracheal Intubation A third procedure for intubation of the patient with possible spinal injury is nasotracheal, or nasal, intubation. Insert the endotracheal tube into the largest of the nares. Then direct it posteriorly, curving it toward the floor of the nasal cavity. Advance the tube the length of an oral airway (the distance between the earlobe and the corner of the mouth). At this point, slowly continue insertion while you, with your ear at the endotracheal tube opening, listen for the sounds of respirations. Gently manipulate the tube until the respiratory sounds are loudest and then advance it during inspiration. The tube should pass directly into the trachea. The technique can be made somewhat easier using an endotracheal tube with a directable tip (such as an Endotrol). With this device, a small cord connected to the tube's end permits the user to increase or decrease the tube's curve.

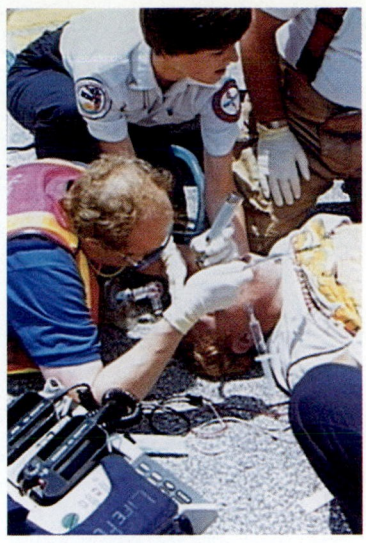

FIGURE 23-19 Oral intubation is difficult in the patient with facial trauma because landmarks may be distorted, blood may flow into the airway, and the head must remain in the neutral position.

If possible, have the most experienced care provider attempt intubation to reduce both the length of the procedure and vagal stimulation.

The disadvantages to nasal intubation include the necessity of having a breathing patient and a quiet environment, and the danger of inserting the tube through a fractured cribiform plate and into the skull. The procedure has a lower rate of success than either oral or digital intubation. Nasal intubation also tends to raise intracranial pressure more than oral intubation because it generally takes longer and more aggressively stimulates the posterior nasal and oral pharynxes.

Retrograde Intubation Retrograde intubation is a process in which a wire is introduced through the cricothyroid membrane into the larynx, then the pharynx, and then out through the mouth. The process begins with the placement of a catheter through the cricothyroid membrane, directed superiorly. A flexible wire is advanced through the catheter toward the oral opening. A laryngoscope may be inserted to visualize the oral cavity and identify the advancing wire. When you see the wire, use the McGill forceps to retrieve it. Then advance an endotracheal tube over the wire down to the thyroid cartilage. When the tube reaches the larynx, withdraw the wire and advance the tube into the trachea.

Directed Intubation In some cases of serious facial or upper neck trauma, as in a shotgun blast, the landmarks of the upper airway are disrupted or destroyed. In such cases, obtaining and maintaining an airway may be extremely difficult. Use strong suction over the area, and use the laryngoscope to attempt to visualize the elements of the oro- and laryngopharynx. If you cannot see airway landmarks themselves, look for bubbling air escaping from the trachea with expirations. If you believe you are close to the tracheal opening and can visualize the area, have an assistant compress the chest to induce bubbling. Attempt to pass the endotracheal tube along the route of bubbles and into the trachea. With this technique, it is critically important to confirm proper placement of the endotracheal tube.

Rapid Sequence Intubation Occasionally, a patient who is responsive or whose teeth are clenched (trismus) needs intubation. Such cases might involve brain injury patients or patients with serious oral trauma with the risk of swelling and progressive airway obstruction. Rapid sequence intubation is a medication-facilitated procedure that paralyzes the conscious or semiconscious patient to permit intubation. A sedative/amnestic is administered to sedate the patient and reduce anxiety. Then a quick-acting paralytic agent is given to induce muscle relaxation, including the muscles of the oral and pharyngeal cavities. The patient must then be intubated and positive pressure ventilations provided quickly because the paralytic agent paralyzes all skeletal muscles, including those associated with breathing. The paralytic also eliminates the gag reflex and the patient's ability to maintain the airway.

The drugs most commonly used for this procedure are the paralytics succinylcholine, pancuronium, and vecuronium and the sedatives diazepam, midazolam, and morphine. Sedative antagonists are frequently used to reverse the effects of these drugs when given and include flumazenil (for diazepam or midazolam) and naloxone (for morphine). (See Chapter 8, "Airway Management and Ventilation.")

The process for rapid sequence intubation begins with reconfirmation of the indications: a patient experiencing muscle spasm (trismus) or who has an intact gag reflex (semiconscious or conscious patient) and who needs a protected airway. Apply Sellick's maneuver and ventilate or be ready to ventilate the patient as needed. Premedicate the patient with the sedative and then administer the paralytic quickly. When the muscles relax and/or the gag reflex ceases, have the most experienced care provider attempt oral or digital intubation.

Confirmation of Tube Placement Once the endotracheal tube is inserted using one of the techniques described above, confirm its proper placement in the trachea. This is especially important when the tube has been placed blindly. Auscul-

Confirmation of tube placement is especially important when the tube has been placed blindly.

tate, at a minimum, the axillae and the over the epigastrium. (Good breath sounds at the axillae reflect good ventilation to the distal alveoli.) Watch carefully for good, symmetrical chest wall excursion with each ventilation. If you hear good breath sounds bilaterally, detect no epigastric sounds, and see the chest wall move equally with each breath, the tube is most likely in the trachea. Inflate the cuff of the tube and hyperventilate the patient for a short period of time. Use an end-tidal CO_2 monitor, pulse oximetry, and observation of the patient's skin color to help confirm and monitor proper and continuing endotracheal tube placement. Remember that the endotracheal tube may dislodge from the trachea during any movement of the patient, as from the ground to the stretcher or as the stretcher is loaded into the ambulance. Reconfirm proper tube placement frequently.

Cricothyrotomy

In some cases of face and neck trauma, the region may be so distorted or blocked that oral and nasal intubation are impossible. Here the only potential for providing a life-saving airway may be opening a surgical pathway for the air. There are two forms of this procedure: the needle cricothyrostomy and the surgical cricothyrotomy. Consult your protocols and medical direction to identify whether these advanced airway procedures or the other procedures already described may be used in your system.

With needle cricothyrostomy, one or more large-bore catheters are inserted into the cricothyroid membrane to provide a temporary airway. This technique permits only limited air exchange and does not sustain the patient. Inspirations can be enhanced by oxygen-powered ventilation (termed transtracheal jet insufflation); however, exhalations are not adequate and the patient cannot be sustained by the technique for more than several minutes.

With surgical cricothyrotomy, an incision and opening is made in the cricothyroid membrane to provide an emergency airway. The soft tissue covering the membrane that separates the thyroid and cricoid cartilages is then held open by a small oral airway or a shortened #6 endotracheal tube. The chief dangers associated with surgical cricothyrotomy are serious bleeding from the soft tissue surrounding the site (and that bleeding's threat to the airway) and damage to the thyroid and parathyroid glands just below the incision site.

To begin either the needle or surgical cricothyrotomy, don gloves, goggles, and gown. Then briskly cleanse the upper anterior neck with an alcohol swab in concentric circles outward from the base of the thyroid cartilage. Set out the needed equipment including a large-bore (14-gauge or larger) over-the-needle catheter and a syringe for the needle procedure or a sharp scalpel and a small oral airway or shortened endotracheal tube for the surgical cricothyrotomy. Palpate upward along the trachea, reaching the cricoid cartilage, then the thyroid cartilage, and the membrane in between them, the cricothyroid membrane. The first solid structure you feel as you palpate up the trachea is the cricoid ring. Just above it and before the next hard ring is the cricothyroid membrane (Figure 23-20).

For the needle cricothyrostomy, attach the catheter to the syringe and perforate the cricothyroid membrane by inserting the needle into the skin and membrane until you feel a "pop." Advance the catheter a few centimeters over the needle and then withdraw the needle. When using a single large-bore catheter, remove the tube from a 6.0 pediatric endotracheal tube and connect it to the catheter hub. Attach the bag and valve and ventilate or use a high-flow transtracheal jet insufflation device. Use of a demand valve is not acceptable since the pressure of its oxygen flow is insufficient to adequately ventilate the patient through the needle. Give the patient a very long time to exhale as the airway is now extremely restricted. Normally, expiration through the catheter takes about four times longer than inspiration. Watch carefully for chest rise and good breath sounds.

If you hear good breath sounds bilaterally, detect no epigastric sounds, and see the chest wall move equally with each breath, the tube is most likely in the trachea.

Endotracheal intubation should be confirmed by the three different methods described in Chapter 8.

Give the patient who has received a needle crichothyrostomy a very long time to exhale because the airway is now extremely restricted.

Placing a second needle adjacent to the first needle will help facilitate exhalation.

Hyoid bone —

Thyroid cartilage —

Cricoid cartilage —

— Epiglottis

— Thyroid gland

— Cricothyroid membrane

— Trachea

For the surgical cricothyrotomy, insert the blade of a sterile scalpel into the skin and the cricothyroid membrane until you feel a "pop." Enlarge the opening, as needed, to accept the shortened endotracheal tube. Introduce an endotracheal tube, cut to about 4 inches in length and bent to a sharp curve, through the surgical opening. Ventilate the patient with a bag-valve-mask device using a child-sized mask or connect the bag and valve to the endotracheal tube and seal the area with sterile dressings. You may have to close the patient's mouth and nose or otherwise seal the upper airway opening to assure that the air reaches the lungs. If the airway obstruction is partial, open the mouth and nose during expiration to enhance the flow of air outward, especially when using needle cricothyrotomy.

BREATHING

Assurance of breathing is an important priority with any patient, but it becomes extremely critical with the head-injured patient. Not only is reduced air exchange a problem, but excessive air exchange and the excessive depletion of carbon dioxide can also endanger the patient. Providing supplemental oxygenation and appropriate ventilation are essential with such patients.

Oxygen

Any patient who has sustained a significant head injury or who displays any indication of lowered level of consciousness, orientation, or arousal is a candidate for high flow, high concentration oxygen.

Any patient who has sustained a significant head injury or who displays any indication of lowered level of consciousness, orientation, or arousal is a candidate for high flow, high concentration oxygen. Administer oxygen at a rate of 12 to 15 liters per minute via a nonrebreather mask with a patient who is moving an adequate respiratory volume. If the patient is not breathing adequately, supplement any positive pressure ventilations with oxygen via reservoir, again flowing at 12 to 15 liters per minute.

Ventilations

Provision of a good supply of oxygen is critical to the head injury patient, but so too is the removal of carbon dioxide. Assess the patient's respiratory status and, if the patient is not moving a normal volume of air, employ overdrive respiration.

Ventilate 12 to 20 times per minute with full breaths (about 800 to 1000 mL). Be careful not to hyperventilate the patient because doing so reduces carbon dioxide levels in the blood and significantly reduces the cerebral blood flow. Endotracheal intubation makes ventilations easier and more efficient. Be careful not to accidentally hyperventilate the head injury patient once the tube is in place. Monitor the oxygen saturation with pulse oximetry to maintain a level of 95 percent or greater.

CIRCULATION

Your care of the patient with head, facial, and neck injury includes both control of any serious hemorrhage and support of the body's attempts to maintain blood pressure and cerebral circulation.

Hemorrhage Control

Head and facial hemorrhage is usually easy to control because most of these injuries are to the tissues that lie over facial and cranial bones. Direct pressure is commonly an effective means of controlling such bleeding, though you should take care not to put pressure directly on suspected skull or facial fractures. Wrap bandaging circumferentially, but be careful to keep the airway clear and give the patient the freedom to rid himself of vomitus should emesis occur. Watch the airway and be prepared to suction aggressively to limit danger from aspiration. Suctioning can also assure that the patient does not swallow large volumes of blood, stimulating emesis. Permit the conscious and alert patient with no suspected spinal injury who is suffering epistaxis to sit leaning forward, allowing the blood to drain. This positioning keeps blood from flowing down the pharynx and entering the esophagus.

An open neck injury carries the risk of air entering the external jugular during strong inspiration, leading to cerebral embolism with stroke-like symptoms. Seal any open neck wound with an occlusive dressing held firmly in place by bandaging and tilt the patient's body head down on a backboard or stretcher, if possible. Carefully evaluate any other open wounds for frothy blood suggestive of tracheal involvement, seal those wounds with occlusive dressings, and monitor respirations.

Blunt trauma to the neck may produce the equivalent of compartment syndrome. Fasciae in the region compartmentalize muscle and anatomic structures and permit pressures to rise with rapid edema or blood accumulation. Any sign of neck edema or hematoma is an indication for rapid transport. Monitor the patient's skin tension and level of consciousness while en route to the hospital.

Severe hemorrhage associated with open neck wounds can lead quickly to hypovolemia and shock. Control the blood loss by using a dressing and gloved fingers to apply direct pressure to the source of bleeding. You may have to maintain digital pressure throughout prehospital care because application of circumferential bandaging may restrict the airway and circulation.

Blood Pressure Maintenance

Another component of circulation care for the head, face, and neck injury patient is guarding against hypotension. The brain is very dependent upon receiving a continuous supply of oxygenated circulation. Any interruption of the supply, such as might be caused by hypotension in response to increasing intracranial pressure, will rapidly prove fatal. Care for the patient in whom you suspect increased intracranial pressure with aggressive fluid resuscitation, even though the patient's other injuries might not suggest that step. For example, the patient with penetrating chest trauma might not receive aggressive fluid resuscitation until the systolic blood pressure drops to below 60 mmHg. If that patient also has a head injury with increasing intracranial pressure, waiting for the blood pressure to drop to that level would be life threatening. Hence, provide rapid fluid (electrolyte) administration, application of a PASG, and other shock care measures well before the blood pressure reaches 60 mmHg.

HYPOXIA

It is very important to monitor the patient with a head injury at all times in order to quickly identify and correct any hypoventilation. Hypoxia can further damage central nervous system tissue already affected by direct injury. If someone else is delivering ventilations, frequently monitor both that person's performance as well as the patient's oxygen saturation levels. Care providers often find it difficult to determine accurate ventilation rates while bag-valve-masking during the emergency. Assure that the patient is well oxygenated before any intubation attempt and hyperventilated for a short time after intubation. Also be watchful for interruptions in ventilations that might occur during patient movement or when changing ventilation providers.

HYPOVOLEMIA

Like hypoxia, hypovolemia and the associated hypotension reduce oxygen transport to the brain. This condition also reduces both circulation through the brain and the blood's ability to remove the products of metabolism. Since brain tissue is especially sensitive to oxygen deprivation, with head injury patients who have already suffered some damage to brain tissue, any further circulatory loss might prove devastating. The problems of hypovolemia and hypotension are compounded if there is any increase in intracranial pressure. Such an increase further restricts cerebral blood flow, and the body's autoregulatory mechanisms cannot compensate in a pre-existing state of hypotension.

Provide aggressive fluid resuscitation for any patient with significant head injury in whom you suspect brain injury and who shows signs of shock compensation.

Provide aggressive fluid resuscitation for any patient with significant head injury in whom you suspect brain injury and who shows signs of shock compensation—rapid, thready pulse, slowed capillary refill, lowered level of consciousness, anxiety, or restlessness. Insert two large-bore catheters and administer lactated Ringer's solution or normal saline at a wide-open rate through non-restrictive trauma IV tubing. Administer 1,000 mL of an isotonic solution, followed by additional boluses as needed to maintain a blood pressure between 90 and 100 mmHg. Consider application of a PASG and carefully monitor the vital signs to assure the blood pressure remains above 90 mmHg.

MEDICATIONS

Several medications may be useful in the care of the head injury patient. These medications include oxygen, diuretics (mannitol, furosemide), paralytics (succinylcholine, pancuronium, vecuronium) sedatives (diazepam, midazolam, morphine), dextrose, thiamine, and topical anesthetic sprays.

Oxygen is the primary first-line drug used in the care of the patient with suspected head injury.

Oxygen

Oxygen is the primary first-line drug used in the care of the patient with suspected head injury. Administration of high flow oxygen provides a high inspired oxygen level and facilitates both diffusion through the alveolar and capillary walls and the highest oxygen uptake by the hemoglobin of the red blood cells. Oxygen saturation is important for the head injury patient because the brain is acutely dependent upon a good supply of oxygen. There are no contraindications nor side effects of concern for use of oxygen during prehospital emergency care. (Note, however, that hyperventilation is contraindicated in head injury patients because it reduces circulating CO_2 levels.)

Administer oxygen via a nonrebreather mask at a flow rate of between 12 and 15 liters per minute for the patient who is breathing adequately. If the patient is receiving positive pressure ventilations, supplement the ventilations with 12 to 15 liters per minute of oxygen flowing into the reservoir. Monitor oxygen administration using the pulse oximeter, and keep the saturation level above 95 percent. Also monitor skin color, respiratory excursion, orientation, and anxiety to assure the patient is well oxygenated.

Diuretics

Mannitol Mannitol is a large glucose molecule that does not leave the bloodstream because of its size. It is an osmolar diuretic that draws water from body tissue into the bloodstream. Mannitol then is eliminated by the kidneys and, as it leaves the kidneys, takes both water and sodium with it, reducing the body's fluid load. Mannitol is especially effective in drawing fluid from the brain, thereby reducing cerebral edema and intracranial pressure. Although very effective in reducing cerebral edema, mannitol may reduce the intracranial pressure associated with intracranial hemorrhage. This may result in increased hemorrhage and, ultimately, more serious brain damage. Mannitol is contraindicated in patients with hypovolemia or hypotension because of its diuretic properties and in patients with a recent history of congestive heart failure because it transiently raises the cardiovascular fluid volume. Mannitol may be most useful in the patient who develops a dilated pupil during care or one who has pupillary dilation and a normal or elevated blood pressure.

Mannitol should only be used in the prehospital setting based upon a consensus agreement with local neurosurgeons and the EMS system medical director.

Mannitol is usually supplied in a single-use vial with a concentration of 20 percent. It is given as a single slow bolus (over 5 minutes) of 1 gm/kg of the patient's weight. It is very hypertonic and forms crystals at low temperatures (below 45°F). It can be reconstituted with rewarming and gentle agitation, although it should always be administered through an in-line filter to assure no particulate matter enters the bloodstream. Flush the IV line before and after the administration of mannitol to reduce the risk of precipitation.

Furosemide Furosemide (Lasix®) is a loop diuretic that inhibits the reabsorption of sodium in the kidneys. It results in the increased secretion of water and electrolytes, including sodium, chloride, magnesium, and calcium. Furosemide also causes venous dilation and a reduced cardiac preload. It is often given in combination with mannitol to increase the rate of diuresis. While it does not remove fluid from cerebral edema as well as mannitol, it does cause a more rapid fluid elimination by the kidneys. Furosemide is generally contraindicated in pregnant patients because it may cause fetal abnormalities. Since, like mannitol, furosemide causes diuresis, use with caution, if at all, in patients with hypotension secondary to hypovolemia.

Furosemide often comes in a pre-loaded syringe or a single-use vial and is given as a slow IV bolus or IM injection. It is administered at a dose of about 0.5 to 1.0 mg/kg, frequently in doses of either 40 or 80 mg. Administer the medication very slowly, over 1 to 2 minutes.

Paralytics

Paralytics are drugs that paralyze the skeletal muscles, permitting intubation in patients with whom the procedure would otherwise be impossible. Administration is a part of the rapid sequence intubation procedure, in which you must quickly sedate, paralyze, then intubate the patient while assuring the patient is well oxygenated and the airway remains clear. Rapid sequence intubation uses diazepam, midazolam, or morphine sulfate to sedate the patient; in some cases, atropine sulfate to limit muscle fasciculations; and succinylcholine chloride, pancuronium bromide, or vercuronium to paralyze the patient.

Succinylcholine   Succinylcholine (Anectine®) is an ultra-short-acting depolarizing skeletal muscle relaxant. It acts upon cholinergic receptors to cause the muscles to contract (depolarize). This action produces **fasciculations,** individual muscle contractions seen beneath the skin. Succinylcholine induces complete paralysis in 30 to 60 seconds and persists for about 2 to 3 minutes with IV administration. Onset of paralysis occurs in 75 seconds to 3 minutes with IM administration. Succinylcholine is frequently administered to achieve temporary paralysis for the intubation of patients with muscle tone, spasms, or seizures that may otherwise prevent the procedure. Succinylcholine paralyzes the muscles of respiration, so care providers must be immediately ready to intubate and ventilate the patient when the drug takes effect. Succinylcholine does not affect the patient's level of consciousness, cerebration, anxiety, or pain perception, so its use should follow the administration of a sedative/amnestic agent. Succinylcholine increases ICP, may induce vomiting, and should be used with caution, if at all, in cases of head injury. Because it slightly increases intraoccular pressure, it is contraindicated for patients with penetrating eye injuries and should be used with caution in patients who are taking digitalis.

Succinylcholine is administered rapidly in a dosage of 1 to 1.5 mg/kg IV. It may be given IM if necessary. In that case, it is usually supplied in a single-use vial with 10 mL of a 20 mg/mL solution. Storage of succinylcholine requires refrigeration. If the patient is conscious, succinlycholine is given after a sedative/amnestic to sedate the patient during the procedure. Frequently 0.5 mg of atropine is administered prior to succinylcholine to halt the fasciculations.

Pancuronium and Vecuronium   Pancuronium (Pavulon®) and vecuronium (Norcuron®) are nondepolarizing skeletal muscle relaxants. They induce paralysis without causing muscle contractions and fasciculations. Pancuronium is a longer acting agent, taking from 3 to 5 minutes to become effective with effects lasting for from 30 to 60 minutes. It is not used frequently in prehospital care and must be refrigerated for maximum shelf life. Vecuronium is a more effective agent with a more rapid onset (less than 1 minute) and shorter duration (25 to 40 minutes). It also has fewer cardiovascular side effects than either succinylcholine or pancuronium. Like succinylcholine, pancuronium and vecuronium are used to paralyze patients with muscle tone, spasms, or seizures in order to permit endotracheal intubation. They also do not have any effect on the level of consciousness, cerebration, anxiety, or pain perception, so their use should follow administration of a sedative/amnestic agent.

Pancuronium comes in single-use vials or pre-loaded syringes containing 1 mg/mL. It is administered by rapid IV bolus of 0.04 to 0.1 mg/kg. Vecuronium is administered rapidly in a dose of 0.08 to 0.1 mg/kg IV. Vecuronium comes as 10 mg vials of powder that must be reconstituted with saline (either 5 or 10 mL) prior to administration.

---

* **fasciculations** involuntary contractions or twitchings of muscle fibers.

It is important to remember that neuromuscular blockers do not affect the patient's level of consciousness. All conscious patients should be sedated before administration of one of these agents.

Sedatives

Diazepam Diazepam (Valium®) is a benzodiazepine with both anti-anxiety and muscle relaxant qualities. In prehospital care, it is often used to premedicate patients to facilitate intubation. Diazepam is also a potent anti-convulsant. It is administered in a slow IV bolus of 5 to 10 mg, not to exceed 5 mg/minute, into a large vein. Diazepam is rather fast acting, with IV effects occurring almost immediately and reaching peak effectiveness in 15 minutes. Its duration is from 15 to 60 minutes. Do not mix diazepam with any other drugs, and flush the IV line before and after administration. Administer it as close to the IV catheter as possible. Do not inject it into a plastic IV bag because diazepam is readily absorbed by plastic, which quickly reduces its concentration.

Diazepam is usually supplied in single-use vials or preloaded syringes containing 2 mL of a 5 mg/mL solution (10 mg). Administer 5 to 10 mg IV every 10 to 15 minutes to a maximum of 30 mg. When an IV line is not immediately available, diazepam may be administered rectally for seizures with effects occurring as quickly as by IV.

The effects of diazepam (and midazolam) may be reversed by the administration of flumazenil. Usually, 2 mL of a 0.1 mg/mL solution is given IV (over 30 seconds) with a second dose repeated at 60 seconds. Be careful in its administration as flumazenil may precipitate seizures in the head injury patient.

Midazolam Midazolam (Versed®) is a benzodiazepine similar to diazepam though it is three to four times more potent. Onset of its effects occurs within 3 to 5 minutes. Administration of midazolam may cause cardiorespiratory arrest, and the drug does not protect against increasing intracranial pressure that follows succinylcholine and pancuronium administration. Midazolam is frequently paired with vecuronium to achieve rapid sedated paralysis. It may cause vomiting and nausea and many of the signs and symptoms of head injury.

Administer midazolam very slowly in small increments (at no more than 1 mg/min) titrated to the desired effect or the maximum administration of 2.5 mg. Midazolam is supplied in 2, 5, and 10 mL vials of a 1 mg/mL concentration and may be mixed in the same syringe with morphine, meperidine, or atropine or diluted with normal saline.

Morphine Morphine (Duramorph®, Astramorph PF®) is an opium alkaloid used to relieve pain (narcotic analgesic), to sedate, and to reduce anxiety. It may mask the signs and symptoms of head injury and mildly increase intracranial pressure. It also reduces vascular volume and cardiac preload by increasing venous capacitance and thus may decrease blood pressure in the hypovolemic patient. Its major side effects are respiratory depression and possible nausea and vomiting.

Morphine is available in 10 mL single-use vials or Tubex® units of a 1 mg/mL solution or as 1mL of a 10 mg/mL solution vial for dilution with 9 mL normal saline. Administer a 5 to 10 mg bolus, slowly IV, and repeat as necessary every few minutes until effective.

Naloxone (Narcan®) is a narcotic antagonist that can quickly reverse the effects of narcotics and should be available anytime you use morphine sulfate. Naloxone is administered IV bolus of 0.4 to 2 mg, repeated every 2 to 3 minutes until effective (up to 10 mg). Naloxone is a shorter acting drug than morphine, so repeat doses may be necessary.

Atropine

Atropine is an anticholinergic (parasympatholytic) agent sometimes administered as part of a rapid sequence intubation routine. It has the ability to reduce parasympathetic (vagal) stimulation associated with intubation attempts and the resultant decrease in heart rate. Atropine may reduce oral and airway secretions and limit the fasciculations associated with administration of succinylcholine. Atropine may cause pupillary dilation and other CNS signs frequently associated with head injury—headache, nausea, vomiting, and blurred vision.

Atropine is available in many concentrations from 0.05 and 0.1 mg/mL preloaded syringes to 10 mL vials of 1 mg/ml solution. For emergency administration, its usual form is 10 mL preloaded syringes of 0.1 mg/mL concentration. Atropine is usually administered as a 0.5 mg bolus for rapid sequence intubation.

Dextrose

The empiric use of dextrose in the head-injured patient is contraindicated.

In general, both hypoglycemia and hyperglycemia are detrimental to the patient with head injury. In the past, dextrose was given routinely to patients who were unresponsive with an undetermined cause. However, current practice calls for identifying the blood glucose level on all unresponsive patients, especially those with a possible history of chronic alcoholism or diabetes. If significant hypoglycemia is found, administer 25 mg of glucose and 100 mg of thiamine.

Dextrose is supplied in preloaded syringes containing 50 mL of a 0.5 mg/mL (50 percent) solution (D50W). It is to be administered slowly through a large vein because it is a very hypertonic solution. In severe cases of hypoglycemia, a second dose may be administered.

Thiamine

Thiamine, more commonly known as vitamin B_1, is a substance obtained from diet and needed for body metabolism. Thiamine is essential for the processing of glucose through Kreb's cycle, from which the body gains its life-sustaining energy. In malnourished patients (like the chronic alcoholic), thiamine is depleted and the body tissue cannot obtain energy from glucose. The brain is especially affected since it does not store energy sources.

Thiamine is supplied in 1 mL single-use ampules, vials, and preloaded syringes containing a 100 mg/mL solution. It is administered IV bolus or IM. It should be administered before or with glucose.

Topical Anesthetic Spray

Topical sprays use an anesthetic agent, such as xylocaine or benzocaine, to anesthetize the oral and pharyngeal mucosa. This reduces the gag reflex, making endotracheal intubation easier and reducing the impact retching has on intracranial pressure. The agent is sprayed into the oral pharynx where it is rapidly absorbed by mucosal tissue. It inhibits nerve sensation, thereby reducing the gag reflex. The effects of the agent are immediate (within 15 seconds), remain local, and last for about 15 minutes. These agents are usually supplied in 2-ounce aerosol spray cannisters with long, hollow extension tubes to direct the spray down the throat. The agent is applied by directing a spray of the material into the posterior oral cavity and pharynx. While topical anesthetic sprays permit easier intubation and reduce the associated vagal effects, they also reduce the patient's ability to remove fluids from the airway and increase the danger of aspiration.

TRANSPORT CONSIDERATIONS

There are special considerations to observe when transporting the patient with serious head injury to the hospital. Limit any external stimulation such as the use of red lights and sirens and try to achieve a smooth ride. Stimulation may further agitate the patient, increase intracranial pressure, and induce seizures.

Be cautious in considering the head injury patient as a candidate for air medical service transport. While the time saved by helicopter transport may be very important, the head injury patient is prone to seizures, especially with the physical stimulation (noise and vibration) associated with this mode of transport. Seizures aboard any type of aircraft are very dangerous. If you elect to transport by air, assure that the patient is firmly secured to a long spine board (including feet and hands) and that his airway is protected by endotracheal intubation.

When transporting head injury patients, limit external stimulation, such as the use of red lights and sirens, and try to provide a smooth ride.

EMOTIONAL SUPPORT

Identify someone to remain with the patient with the specific role of calming and reassuring him during care and transport. Have that person continuously reorient the patient to his environment. Remember, head injury patients may have trouble remembering events preceding and immediately following the incident as well as have difficulty laying down short-term memory. The person assigned the role should describe what happened to the patient and help the patient remain oriented to the current location and what is happening. This simple step aids greatly in reducing the patient's anxiety and in helping a return to a normal level of orientation.

Head injury patients may be very confused, distressed, abusive, or even combative. Do not take their behavior personally. Maintain a professional demeanor and provide emotional support during assessment, care, and transport.

SPECIAL INJURY CARE

There are certain types of head, face, and neck trauma that deserve special care. They include scalp avulsion, injury to the pinna of the ear, eye injury, dislodged teeth, and impaled objects.

Scalp Avulsion

Avulsion occurs when a glancing blow tears the scalp's border and releases a flap of scalp. The flap may remain in anatomic position, fold back exposing the cranium, or may be torn completely free. If the avulsion uncovers the cranium, cover both the open wound and the undersurface of the exposed scalp flap with a large bulky dressing. Also place padding under the fold of the scalp to prevent a sharp kinking along its border. If the region is seriously contaminated, remove gross contamination and rinse the area with normal saline before applying the dressings. Scalp avulsions tend to heal very well unless grossly contaminated or the circulation to the flap is severely disrupted.

Pinna Injury

Serious injury to the pinna, or exposed portion of the ear, often results from glancing blows and trauma, like a tearing or avulsion injury, that disrupts its structure. Such an injury is best treated by placing the pinna in as close to its anatomic position as possible. Then place a dressing between the head and medial surface of the injured ear and cover the exposed ear with a sterile dressing. Finally, bandage the dressed injury firmly to the head.

Eye Injury

Care for eye injuries involves careful assessment and protective care. Most eye wounds or injuries are best cared for by applying soft dressings to cover the closed, injured eye. The other eye, even if uninjured, is also dressed and the dressings on both eyes are held in place with gentle bandaging. This technique prevents sympathetic motion (one eye moving with the other) which may cause additional damage to the injured eye. If the eye injury is an open wound or torn eyelid, consider using a sterile dressing soaked in normal saline to reduce the pain and discomfort and prevent evaporative loss of lacrimal fluid. Place the patient in the supine position if other injuries do not prevent it.

If the patient complains of eye pain without apparent injury, suspect corneal abrasion or laceration, possibly caused by an object embedded in the conjunctiva or sclera. Gently invert the eyelid and examine for any small embedded object (Figure 23-21a and b). If you observe one, you may attempt to remove it with a saline-moistened cotton swab. Even if you successfully remove the object, the patient is likely to continue reporting pain and the sensation of the impaled object. As with apparent wounds, cover both eyes with soft dressings and loose bandaging.

If the eye is avulsed or has an impaled object in it, cover the eye and the object with a cup or other protective material and again dress and bandage both eyes. If the patient is combative or has a significantly reduced level of consciousness, secure his hands together and then to his waist or belt. This prevents accidental dislodging of the protective dressing and possible aggravation of the eye injury.

(a)

(b)

FIGURE 23-21 To remove particles from the white of the eye, (a) pull down the lower lid while the patient looks up or (b) pull up the upper lid while the patient looks down. (c) You can use a moistened suction cup to remove hard lenses.

(c)

Eye injuries and the loss of eyesight in one or both eyes can create anxiety in most patients. Be sure to calm and reassure the patient and explain in advance your actions as you move the patient from the scene to the ambulance and to the hospital.

If, during the assessment, you observe that the patient is wearing contact lenses and there is any risk that he may become unresponsive, have the patient remove the lenses. If the patient is already unresponsive, try removing the lenses yourself with a contact removal suction cup (Figure 23-21c). This miniature suction cup seals against the contact lens and allows easy removal. Alternatively, lift the eyelid, which may cause the lens to dislodge, or, with the eye closed, gently push the lens into the corner of the eye. Keep the lens you remove in a contact lens case where it should be soaked in a contact lens or sterile saline solution.

Dislodged Teeth

Locate any teeth that may have been dislodged by trauma and transport them to the hospital with the patient. Rinse the teeth in normal saline and wrap them in saline-soaked gauze for transport to the emergency department. If a tooth is largely intact, it may be successfully reimplanted.

Impaled Objects

Any object impaled in the head, face, or neck should be left in place and dressed and bandaged to assure that it does not move about during care and transport. Use bulky dressings to stabilize the object. Secure the patient's hands if there is a danger that he may dislodge the object. Only if the object obstructs or seriously threatens the airway should you consider its removal. In such cases, removal will likely increase the associated hemorrhage and possibly damage adjoining structures, but the patency of the airway is essential.

Removal of objects that pass through the patient's cheek pose the least danger for removal. With such a wound, you have ready access to both of its sides, and the wound involves no critical structures or organs. Nevertheless, expect increased hemorrhage from the wound, have dressings ready, and be prepared to apply direct pressure as soon as the object is removed.

ʃUMMARY

The head, face, and neck contain very special and important structures—key elements of the central nervous system, the airway, the alimentary canal, and major organs of sensation. Serious trauma to the region endangers these structures and demands special assessment and care. During the scene size-up, identify possible mechanisms of injury and the injuries they suggest. Confirm the injuries during the initial and rapid trauma assessments. Identify your patient's level of consciousness and orientation early, and watch the eyes carefully for signs of cerebral hypoxia and increasing intracranial pressure. Assure that the spine is immobilized and the airway is clear and protected from aspiration and physical obstruction. Administer high concentration oxygen and ventilate, as necessary, being careful not to under- or overventilate the patient. Secure rapid transport for the patient with possible intracranial hemorrhage or serious lesion. Once the central nervous system, the airway, and breathing are protected, address skeletal structure fractures, minor bleeding, and open wounds. During all your care for the patient with injury to the head, face, or neck, provide emotional support.

CHAPTER 24

Spinal Trauma

Objectives

After reading this chapter, you should be able to:

1. Describe the incidence, morbidity, and mortality of spinal injuries in the trauma patient. (pp. 1069–1070)

2. Describe the anatomy and physiology of spinal structures and structures related to the spine, including the cervical spine, thoracic spine, lumbar spine, sacrum, coccyx, spinal cord, nerve tracts, and dermatomes. (see Chapter 3)

3. Predict spinal injuries based on mechanism of injury. (pp. 1070–1073)

4. Describe the pathophysiology of spinal injuries. (pp. 1073–1076)

5. Identify the need for rapid intervention and transport of the patient with spinal injuries. (pp. 1077–1082)

6. Describe the pathophysiology of traumatic spinal injury related to:
   - Spinal shock (p. 1075)
   - Neurogenic shock (pp. 1075–1076)
   - Quadriplegia/paraplegia (pp. 1074–1075)
   - Incomplete and complete cord injury (pp. 1074–1075)
   - Cord syndromes:
     – Central cord syndrome (p. 1075)

Continued

INTRODUCTION TO SPINAL INJURIES

A spinal cord injury can both threaten life and induce serious, lifelong disability. Each year more than 15,000 permanent spinal cord injuries occur, most commonly in men aged from 16 to 30. Auto and other vehicle crashes account for almost half these spinal cord injuries (48 percent) with falls (21 percent), penetrating injuries (15 percent), and sports-related injuries (14 percent) also contributing significantly to the total. Further, of all patients who suffer neurologic deficit from trauma, some 40 percent have experienced cord injury. The remaining patients with neurologic deficits have suffered injuries that disrupt the spinal or peripheral nerve roots along their course.

Spinal cord injury is an especially devastating type of trauma. The spinal cord consists of highly specialized central nervous system tissue and does not repair itself when seriously injured. Permanent injury to it affects the body's major communications pathways and control over the lower extremities (paraplegia) or both upper and lower extremities (quadriplegia). Spinal cord injuries also affect the body's control over internal organs and the body's internal environment (homeostasis). A patient with a serious spinal injury is left less able to care for himself, will have a significantly altered lifestyle, and will face increased expenses associated with care and support. In fact, lifelong care costs for the victim of a permanent spinal cord injury may well exceed $1 million dollars. This figure does not include the patient's lost earning power due to the disability.

Of all patients who suffer neurologic deficit from trauma, some 40 percent have experienced spinal cord injury.

As with most trauma, the best form of care is prevention. Recent advances in motor vehicle and highway design have helped reduce the incidence of spine injury in its most common category, motor vehicle trauma. Proper use of lap and shoulder belts further reduces the incidence of spinal cord injury, as do programs to reduce drinking and driving. Education programs aimed at teaching safe practices also reduce the potential for spinal cord injury. These programs can foster such behaviors as not diving into unknown waters, developing good physical conditioning, and wearing protective equipment in sports. Following good safety practices in the workplace and in the home can also reduce both temporary and permanent spinal column and cord injury.

PATHOPHYSIOLOGY OF SPINAL INJURY

If you understand how the events of trauma impact the spinal cord and body systems, you will be better prepared to anticipate and recognize spinal column and cord injuries. Traumatic events may cause immediate and devastating injury to the cord with no chance for the patient's recovery. Such events may also cause damage to bones or ligaments, resulting in spinal column instability and providing the potential for cord injury during patient care and transport. By understanding the mechanism of injury and the spinal problems it may produce (the pathophysiology), you can more quickly recognize and better protect the patient with spinal cord trauma.

MECHANISMS OF SPINAL INJURY

The mechanisms of injury that affect the spinal column and cord include extremes of normal motion such as flexion, extension, rotation, and lateral bending (Figure 24-1). Damaging mechanisms also include stresses along the axis of the spine: axial loading and distraction. Finally, spinal injury may occur as a direct result of either blunt or penetrating trauma or as an indirect effect of trauma, when an expanding mass (edema or hematoma) compresses the cord or when a disruption in the blood supply damages it.

Extremes of Motion

Hyperextension or hyperflexion bend the spine forcibly, most commonly in the cervical or lumbar regions. A classic example of an extension injury mechanism is a rear-impact auto crash. The patient's head remains stationary while the upper torso moves rapidly and abruptly forward with the auto. The heavy head moves backwards and hyperextends the neck. The hyperextension places compressing forces on the posterior vertebral structures (the spinous processes, laminae, and pedicles) and stretching forces on the anterior vertebral ligaments. Extremes of extension may cause disk disruption, compression of the interspinous ligaments, and fracture of the posterior vertebral elements. If the forces are great enough, ligaments may tear or the vertebra may fracture, resulting in instability and bone displacement.

In frontal impact crashes, the shoulder strap may restrain the body while the head continues its forward travel. The attachment of the neck restrains the head and flexes the spine with the movement. The process is frequently forceful enough to cause a patient to literally "kiss the chest" (sometimes demonstrated by the patient's lipstick print on the shirt front). Extreme flexion may lead to wedge fractures of the anterior vertebral bodies, stretching or rupture of the posterior longitudinal and interspinous ligaments, compression injury to the cord, fracture of the pedicle(s), and disruption of the intervertebral disks with dislocation of the vertebrae.

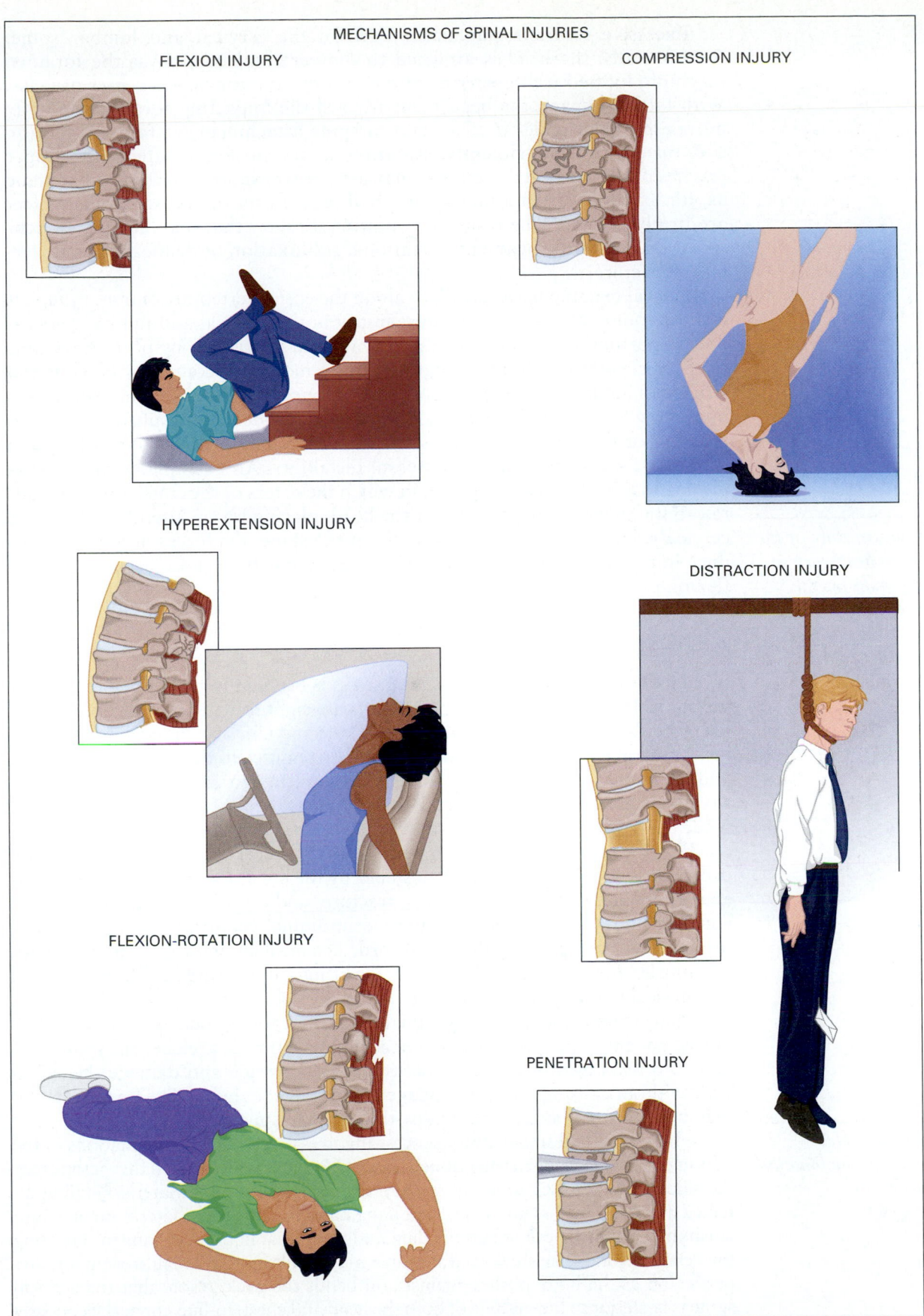

FIGURE 24-1 Mechanisms causing spinal injury.

Excessive rotation may occur both in the cervical and lumbar spine. Anatomically, the head is attached to the vertebral column at the foramen magnum, located well posterior of the midline and the head's center of mass. With lateral impact, the head turns toward the impacting force as the body moves out from under it. The cervical spine attachment restrains its motion and turns the head violently. Rotation injury normally affects the upper reaches of the cervical region, but may also be transmitted to the lumbar spine as, for example, when a tackled football player's thorax twists while his feet are firmly planted. The result is a rotational injury that may include stretching or tearing of the ligaments, rotational subluxation or dislocation, and vertebral fracture.

Lateral bending may take place along the entire vertebral column, though it is most common and likely to cause injury in the cervical and lumbar regions. As one portion of the body moves sideways and the remaining portion remains fixed, the spine absorbs the energy. The movement may compress the vertebral structures inducing compression fracture on one side of the column (toward the impact) while it tears ligaments on the opposite side. The result may be compression of the vertebral pedicles with bone fragments driven into the spinal foramen, torn ligaments, and vertebral instability. An example of this mechanism is a lateral-impact auto crash in which the forces of the crash move the thorax to the side and out from under the head, placing severe lateral stress on the cervical spine. Because of the structure of the spine, the forces necessary to induce injury from lateral bending are generally less than those needed to cause flexion/extension injury.

Axial Stress

Axial loading occurs as compressional stress is brought to bear along the axis of the spine. It may occur when a person lifts a weight too great for the strength of his or her lumbar spine or when a person falls and lands on his or her heels. The resulting force is transmitted up the lower extremities to the pelvis, the sacrum, and the lumbar spine. Another frequent mechanism of axial loading injury is the shallow water dive. In this case, the diver impacts the pool bottom with the head while the weight of the lower portion of the body drives the thorax into the head, crushing the cervical spine. This mechanism also occurs in auto crashes, when an occupant is propelled into the windshield by the crash forces. With these mechanisms, impact is likely to compress, fracture, and crush the vertebrae and herniate (rupture) disks, releasing their semi-liquid centers into the vertebral foramina and compressing the spinal cord. The most common sites of axial loading injuries are between T-12 and L-2 (for lifting injuries and heel-first falls) and the cervical region (for head impacts).

Distraction is the opposite of axial loading. A force, such as gravity applied during hanging or at the end of a bungee jumper's travel, stretches the spinal column and tears ligaments. The process may also stretch and damage the spinal cord without causing physical damage to the spinal column. The upper cervical region is most commonly affected by this mechanism of injury.

Often the actual spinal injury process involves complicated combinations of the various injury mechanisms mentioned above. Hanging may suspend the victim from the side of the head, causing injury from distraction and severe lateral bending directed at the C-1/C-2 region (causing a hangman's fracture). The lateral-impact auto crash may produce both lateral bending and rotational injury mechanisms affecting the cervical spine. The shallow water dive may result in both axial loading and hyperflexion as the body pushes against and bends the neck. (Note that the cervical spine is posterior to the midline of both the head and chest. In-line impacts frequently cause the head and neck to flex as the body pushes forward.)

Be aware of the distinctions among connective tissue, skeletal, and spinal cord injuries. Connective tissue and skeletal injuries do not necessarily result in spinal cord injuries. They do, however, represent potential instability of the spinal column and the danger that any subsequent motion, even normal motion, may result in spinal cord injury. Spinal cord injury can also occur without noticeable injury to the ligaments, disks, and vertebra of the spinal column. This is why, whenever a patient shows any sign of spine injury or has experienced a mechanism that suggests the possibility of spine injury, you must provide immediate manual immobilization and full mechanical immobilization as soon as possible. Maintain immobilization during all of your assessment, care, and transport.

Connective tissue and skeletal injuries represent potential instability of the spinal column and the danger that any subsequent motion may result in spinal cord injury

Other Mechanisms of Injury

Other mechanisms of spine injury can involve both direct blunt and penetrating trauma. Kinetic forces may be directed at the spine when objects strike the spine posteriorly (or laterally in the neck) or when a person falls on or is thrown against an object (as in a blast). Penetrating injuries caused by objects like knives and ice-picks or by missiles like blast fragments and bullets may also apply the forces of trauma directly to the spinal column. The penetrating object may harm vertebral ligaments, fracture vertebral structures, drive bone fragments directly into the spinal cord, or directly damage the cord itself. However, unlike blunt trauma, penetrating injury rarely results in ligamentous instability of the vertebral column.

As a result of trauma, tissues adjacent to the spinal cord may swell or otherwise encroach upon the vertebral foramen. With the close tolerance between the interior surfaces of the vertebral foramen and the cord, this swelling may place pressure on the cord, producing direct compression injury and halting blood flow through the compressed tissues. Such injury may also involve the spinal nerve roots that exit the vertebral column close to the injury.

Electrocution, on rare occasions, can cause spinal injury. The extreme and uncontrolled muscular contractions associated with it can tear tendons and ligaments and fracture vertebrae, resulting in column instability and possible spinal cord injury.

A direct injury to the spinal or vertebral blood vessels or any soft tissue or skeletal injury and the swelling associated with them may decrease the circulation to portions of the cord. This will likely result in tissue ischemia and compromise of cord function.

The coccygeal region of the spinal column can also be injured. Although it contains neither the spinal cord nor many peripheral nerve roots, injury to the region can be painful. Such injuries are usually related to direct blunt trauma, for example, "falling on one's tailbone."

RESULTS OF TRAUMA TO THE SPINAL COLUMN

Spinal injuries may damage the musculoskeletal components of the spinal column, injure the spinal cord, or both. Spinal column injury alone may damage the ligaments and skeletal elements of the column, damaging its integrity and endangering the spinal cord. Injury to the cord may endanger or destroy the ability of the central nervous system to communicate with the body distal to the injury.

Column Injury

The spine is subject to numerous types of injury. The forces of trauma or the stresses of heavy lifting may tear tendons, muscles, and ligaments, resulting in pain and a reduction in the stability of the vertebral column. Those forces may cause movement of the vertebrae from their normal position, a subluxation (partial or incomplete dislocation), or dislocation. The injury process may fracture the spinous or transverse processes, the pedicles, the laminae, or the vertebral bodies. Trauma, especially axial loading, may damage the intervertebral disks. These injuries are to the connective or skeletal tissues of the vertebral column. They may or may not be associated with injury to the spinal cord itself.

Several sites along the spinal column are especially subject to injury. The cervical region accounts for over half of all spinal injuries, with the atlas/axis (C-1/C-2) joint being most frequently involved. This is due to the very delicate nature of the two vertebrae, the mobility of the joint, and the great weight of the head it supports. C-7 is also injured frequently because it is located at the transition between the flexible cervical spine and the more rigid thoracic spine.

Similar injuries occur at the transition point between the thoracic and lumbar vertebrae (T-12/L-1), again due to the differences between the rigid thoracic spine and the flexible lumbar spine. The lumbosacral area (L-5/S-1) likewise is injured because the pelvis immobilizes the sacral spine. Spinal injuries not associated with the cervical spine are about equally divided between the thoracolumbar and lumbosacral regions.

Remember that the spinal cord ends at the L-1/L-2 region. Below this point, the spinal nerve roots extend until they exit the spinal column. These spinal nerve roots are more mobile than the cord and less likely to be injured within the spinal foramen during spinal column injury.

Cord Injury

The spinal cord can be injured through the mechanisms discussed earlier. Those injuries can be further described as either primary or secondary. A primary injury is one directly associated with the insult and its effects occur immediately. For example, a primary injury may be caused by cord compression, stretching, or a direct injury. A secondary injury results, as the initial injury causes swelling or ischemia, further injuring the cord tissue. It may also occur as an unstable spinal column is moved about and causes physical injury to the spinal cord. Primary and secondary injuries to the spinal cord can include concussion, contusion, compression, laceration, hemorrhage, and transection.

Concussion Concussion of the cord, like a cerebral concussion (see Chapter 23, "Head, Facial, and Neck Trauma"), causes a temporary and transient disruption of cord function. Without associated injuries, cord concussion generally does not produce any residual deficit.

Contusion Spinal cord contusion is simply a bruising of the cord. It is associated with some tissue damage, vascular leakage, and swelling. If blood crosses the blood-brain barrier, more significant edema may occur. But, in general, this injury is likely to repair itself with limited residual effects or none at all. The resolution of a cord contusion and its associated signs and symptoms is likely to take longer than is the case with a concussion.

Compression Spinal cord compression may occur secondary to the displacement of a vertebra, through herniation of an intervetebral disk, from displacement of a vertebral bone fragment, or from swelling of adjacent tissue. The pressure caused by these mechanisms results in restricted circulation, ischemic damage, and possibly physical damage to the cord.

Laceration Cord laceration can occur as bony fragments are driven into the vertebral foramen or the cord is stretched to the point of tearing. Laceration is likely to result in hemorrhage into the cord tissue, swelling due to the injury, and disruption of some portions of the cord and their associated communication pathways. In very minor lacerations, some recovery may be expected. Severe lacerations usually result in permanent neurologic deficit.

Hemorrhage Spinal cord hemorrhage, often associated with a contusion, laceration, or stretching injury, produces injury by disruption of the blood flow, application of pressure from accumulating blood, and irritation by blood passing across the blood-brain barrier. Some of the arteries supplying the cord may affect circulation distant from the injury and result in ischemic injury above the level of physical injury.

Transection A cord **transection** is an injury that partially or completely severs the spinal cord. In a complete transection, the cord is totally cut and the potential to send and receive nerve impulses below the site of injury is lost. With transection injuries below the beginning of the thoracic spine, the results include incontinence and paraplegia, while injuries to the cervical spine cause quadriplegia, incontinence, and partial or complete respiratory paralysis.

Incomplete cord transection involves only a portion of the cord, and some spinal tracts remain intact. There is potential for some recovery of function. There are three particular types of incomplete spinal cord transection: anterior cord syndrome, central cord syndrome, and Brown-Séquard's syndrome.

Anterior cord syndrome is caused by bony fragments or pressure compressing the arteries that perfuse the anterior cord. The cord is damaged by vascular disruption and its potential for recovery is poor. The injury generally involves loss of motor function and of sensation to pain, light touch, and temperature below the injury site. The patient is likely to retain motion, positional, and vibration sensation.

Central cord syndrome is usually related to hyperextension of the cervical spine, as might occur with a forward fall and facial impact. It is often associated with a pre-existing degenerative disease, such as arthritis, that has narrowed the vertebral canal. This syndrome results in motor weakness, more likely affecting the upper rather than the lower extremities, and possible bladder dysfunction. Of the three syndromes, central cord syndrome has the best prognosis for recovery.

Brown-Séquard's syndrome is usually caused by a penetrating injury that affects one side of the cord (hemitransection). The damage to one side results in sensory and motor loss to that side (ipsilateral) of the body. Pain and temperature perception are lost on the opposite (contralateral) side of the body because of the switching of the associated nerves that occurs as they enter the spinal cord. This injury is rare and is usually associated with some recovery, except in cases of direct penetrating trauma.

Spinal Shock

Spinal shock is a temporary insult to the cord that affects the body below the level of injury. The affected area becomes flaccid and without feeling, and the patient is unable to move the extremities or other musculature (flaccid paralysis). There is frequently a loss of bowel and bladder control and, in the male, priapism (a prolonged, non-sexual penile erection). Body temperature control is affected, and hypotension is often present due to vasodilatation. Spinal shock is often a transient problem if the cord is not seriously damaged.

Neurogenic Shock

Neurogenic (or spinal-vascular) shock results when injury to the spinal cord disrupts the brain's ability to exercise control over the body. The interruption of signals limits vasoconstriction, most noticeably in the skin below the level of injury. Lack of sympathetic tone permits the arteries and veins to dilate, expanding the vascular space, resulting in a relative hypovolemia. With the reduced cardiac preload, the atria

* **transection** a cutting across a long axis; a cross-sectional cut.

* **anterior cord syndrome** condition that is caused by bony fragments or pressure compressing the arteries of the anterior spinal cord and resulting in loss of motor function and sensation to pain, light touch, and temperature below the injury site.

* **central cord syndrome** condition usually related to hyperflexion of the cervical spine that results in motor weakness, usually in the upper extremities and possible bladder dysfunction.

* **Brown-Séquard's syndrome** condition caused by partial cutting of one side of the spinal cord resulting in sensory and motor loss to that side of the body.

Spinal shock is a temporary form of neurogenic shock that presents with hypotension, bradycardia, and the signs and symptoms of cord injury.

fail to fill adequately, and their contraction does not stretch the walls of the ventricles. This reduces the strength of contraction (Frank-Starling reflex) and cardiac output. The problem is further compounded as the autonomic nervous system loses its sympathetic control over the adrenal medulla. It can then no longer control the release of epinephrine and norepinephrine. These hormones are responsible for increasing the heart rate against direct parasympathetic stimulation. Their absence restricts the increase in heart rate that normally follows reduced cardiac preload and falling blood pressure. The result of all these factors is a patient in relative hypovolemia. In addition, it is difficult for the patient to maintain blood pressure with a reduced cardiac output when the body is unable to increase peripheral vascular resistance through vasoconstriction. The patient in neurogenic shock is thus likely to present with a slow heart rate, low blood pressure, and shock-like symptoms (cool, moist, and pale skin) above the cord injury, and warm, dry, and flushed skin below the injury, as well as with priapism in the male.

Autonomic Hyperreflexia Syndrome

Autonomic hyperreflexia syndrome is associated with the body's resolution of the effects of neurogenic shock. It occurs in patients well after the initial spinal injury as the body begins to adapt to the problems associated with loss of neurologic control below the injury. After a time, the vascular system adjusts to the lack of sympathetic stimulation and the blood pressure moves toward normal. However, the body now does not respond to increases in blood pressure with vasodilation below the cord injury so only bradycardia results. Autonomic hyperreflexia syndrome is most commonly associated with injuries at or above T-6. The syndrome presents with sudden hypertension, as high as 300 mmHg, bradycardia, pounding headache, blurred vision, and sweating and flushing of the skin above the point of injury. Nasal congestion, nausea, and bladder and rectum distention are also frequently present in autonomic hyperreflexia syndrome.

Other Causes of Neurologic Dysfunction

Not all injuries that result in neurologic dysfunction affecting a dermatome or myotome are related to spinal cord injuries. An injury may occur anywhere along a nerve impulse's path of travel. For example, the C-7 nerve root travels from just below the seventh cervical vertebra through the shoulder, arm, and forearm before innervating the little finger. It may be injured by a vertebral fracture, soft tissue injury and swelling, a shoulder, arm, or forearm fracture, penetrating trauma, or compartment syndrome.

Any of the injuries described above will interrupt sensory impulses to the brain from the little finger region and motor signals to the region from the brain (to initiate movement and maintain muscle tone). The most obvious difference between nerve root injury and spinal cord injury is the size of the region affected. Remember, however, that an injury that is currently affecting only a single dermatome may have created a vertebral column instability that threatens the entire cord.

There are also several non-traumatic processes that affect the spinal cord. Refer to Chapter 29 for further information on them.

The obvious difference between nerve root and spinal cord injury is that in the former a single dermatome is affected while in the latter multiple dermatomes are affected.

ASSESSMENT OF THE SPINAL INJURY PATIENT

Put special emphasis on your analysis of the mechanism of injury with a potential spinal injury patient.

Assessment and care for the patient with a potential spinal injury begins with special emphasis on the analysis of the mechanism of injury. During this analysis, consciously try to identify or rule out the likelihood of spinal injury.

This is important because the patient who has suffered serious trauma may have other injuries that are much more painful and more obvious and that may distract you from the less obvious signs of spinal injury. Also, a seriously injured trauma patient may have a reduced level of consciousness due to intoxication or to other processes such as shock or head injury and thus be an unreliable reporter of the symptoms of spinal injury. For these reasons, you should consider the mechanism of injury to be the most critical indicator of spinal injury.

Scene Size-up

Analyze the mechanism of injury very carefully to identify what forces were transmitted to the patient and from which direction they came (Figure 24-2). Identify the likely movements of the spine during the crash or impact and determine if severe flexion, extension, lateral bending, rotation, axial loading, or distraction was likely. Also, assure that direct forces of blunt or penetrating trauma did not involve the spine. Be especially concerned about high-speed motor vehicle crashes, falls from greater than three times the patient's height, any serious blunt injuries above the shoulders, and any penetrating wounds close to or directed toward the spine. Also maintain a high level of suspicion regarding athletic injuries, in which blunt and twisting forces are often transmitted to the spine. If there is any reason to suspect spinal injury, be prepared to employ immediate cervical immobilization as you begin the initial assessment.

FIGURE 24-2   Often the mechanism of injury will suggest the potential for spinal column injury.

Examine the scene to determine whether the patient used a helmet or other protective gear. Remember that helmets reduce the likelihood of head injury but neither increase nor decrease the likelihood of neck injury. Whenever a patient wearing a helmet sustains moderate or severe head impact, suspect spine injury and employ spinal precautions. Also, bring the helmet to the emergency department with the patient or relate the damages it displayed to the emergency department physician.

Even if the incident does not appear to involve a significant mechanism of injury or forces directed at the spine, look for and assure that there are no signs or symptoms of spinal injury during your early assessment. If you are unclear about the mechanism of injury or the potential for spinal involvement, always err on the side of protecting the patient. Full spinal precautions cause some patient discomfort and extend your time at the scene, but failure to provide needed immobilization may result in an unnecessary, devastating, and lifelong patient disability or even in death. Generally, a patient sustaining any serious injury receives immediate manual spinal immobilization, thereafter maintained by mechanical immobilization from your first moments at his side until arrival at the emergency department.

INITIAL ASSESSMENT

As you approach the patient, begin to develop a general impression, determine the patient's mental status, rule out the likelihood of spinal injury or apply cervical spine precautions, and begin assessment of the ABCs. The general impression and mental status determination identify the patient's general condition and level of consciousness. Suspect and treat any trauma or possible trauma patient who is not conscious and alert and fully oriented to time, place, person and his own person as though that patient has a spinal injury. Consider employing spinal precautions for any intoxicated or head-injured patients, any with significant injuries above the shoulders, any with painful injuries, or any one subject to the "fight-or-flight" response. Be aware that these circumstances can distract from or mask the symptoms of spine injury.

Firmly apply manual immobilization to hold the patient's head in the neutral, in-line position before proceeding with the remaining assessment and care. (Many sources in prehospital emergency care refer to the process of manually holding the head in the in-line and neutral position as "manual stabilization," while others refer to it as "manual immobilization." While both terms accurately describe the action, this volume will refer to the procedure as "manual immobilization.") Manual immobilization should continue from the moment you arrive at the patient's side and suspect spinal injury until the patient receives full mechanical immobilization to a long spine board with a cervical immobilization device (or vest-type immobilization device). It is best if the care giver responsible for the overall assessment and care of the patient does not hold the manual immobilization. A well-trained EMT-Basic or First Responder may best provide this immobilization.

Neutral, in-line positioning is very important in the care of a spinal injury patient as it maintains the best orientation of the spinal column and the greatest clearance between the cord and the interior of the spinal foramen. This positioning permits the best circulation and thus lessens the impact of local injury and edema. As your assessment progresses, gently and smoothly move any body segment that is out of alignment toward alignment as you examine it. If the patient feels any increase in pain or if you feel resistance to movement, immobilize the head and neck or other portion of the body in the position achieved. Do not continue movement as doing so may compromise the spinal cord. Maintain the patient's head and body using manual immobilization until you can secure the position with full mechanical immobilization using the spine board, firm padding, and a cervical immobilization device.

If you are unclear about the mechanism of injury or the potential for spinal involvement, always err on the side of overprotecting the patient.

Provide any patient sustaining a serious injury with immediate manual spinal immobilization, followed by full mechanical immobilization from your first moments at his side until arrival at the emergency department.

Once you assess the neck, consider applying a cervical collar. While the collar does not prevent flexion/extension, rotation, or lateral bending, it does limit cervical motion. However, manual immobilization of the head and neck is adequate until time and patient priorities permit you to apply the collar. Manual immobilization must continue even after a cervical collar has been applied until full mechanical immobilization is achieved.

As you move on to assess the airway, be sure that the patient's head remains in the neutral, in-line position. The airway is more difficult to control when you are required to observe spinal precautions. Be ready to carefully log roll the patient if he vomits or, if necessary, to drain the upper airway of fluids. Have adequate suction ready and anticipate the possible need to clear the airway during transport should vomiting occur. To prepare for this, secure the patient firmly to a spine board and immobilize him well enough to permit 90-degree rotation of the board.

If advanced airway procedures are indicated, consider orotracheal intubation with spinal precautions or digital intubation. Have the patient's head held firmly in the neutral, in-line position as you attempt to identify airway features and insert the endotracheal tube. Anticipate that landmarks will be hard to visualize because the head cannot be brought into the sniffing position and the upper airway aligned. During the procedure, be careful not to displace the jaw anteriorly beyond the point at which it begins to lift the neck (extension) or to permit any rotation of the head. Digital intubation has the benefit of not requiring any displacement of the head and neck, although it takes a provider skilled in the procedure who has long fingers to direct the tube properly.

After using any modified or blind intubation technique like those just described, be very careful to assure proper tube placement by assessing for the presence of good chest excursion and bilaterally equal breath sounds and the absence of epigastric sounds with ventilation. Check the depth of tube placement by noting the number on the side of the tube and secure the tube firmly. Monitor both the tube's depth and the breath sounds frequently during your care and transport. Using the pulse oximeter or capnometer can help assure that your patient remains effectively oxygenated.

Quickly evaluate your patient's respiratory effort. In the potential spinal injury patient, watch the motion of the chest and abdomen carefully. They should rise and fall together. Exaggerated movement of the abdomen and limited chest excursion with motion opposite to that of the abdomen suggest diaphragmatic breathing. For such a patient, provide positive pressure ventilation coordinated with the patient's respiratory effort (overdrive ventilation) and employ spinal precautions immediately. Your assistance will make breathing more effective and less energy consuming. Use pulse oximetry to continuously evaluate the effectiveness of respirations.

During your check of the patient's circulation status, monitor the pulse carefully. Be very watchful of patients with bradycardia, especially when it is likely that they may be experiencing hypovolemia and shock. This bradycardia may be relative—for example, if a patient has a normal heart rate in the presence of low blood pressure and hypovolemia when a tachycardia might be expected. As you scan the body for other signs of vascular injury or shock, watch for warm and dry skin in the lower extremities while the upper portions of the body show the cool, clammy skin associated with hypovolemic compensation. This is an indication of neurogenic injury and possible shock secondary to spinal cord damage. Spinal cord injury may also induce paralysis and anesthesia below the lesion, reducing the pain or other symptoms of blood loss into an abdominal or extremity injury.

RAPID TRAUMA ASSESSMENT

Once the initial assessment is complete, determine the need for the rapid trauma assessment or the focused physical exam and history. In patients with suspected or likely spinal column or cord injury, move directly to the rapid trauma assessment

Manual immobilization must continue even after a cervical collar has been applied and until it is maintained with mechanical immobilization.

Be very watchful for patients with bradycardia, especially when it is likely that they may be experiencing hypovolemia and shock.

• PAIN   Unprovoked pain in area of injury, along spine, in lower legs.

• TENDERNESS   Gentle touch of area may increase pain.

• DEFORMITY (rare)   There may be abnormal bend or bony prominence.

• SOFT TISSUE INJURY   Injury to the head, neck, or face may indicate
cervical spine injury. Injury to shoulders, back,
and abdomen may indicate thoracic or lumbar
spine injury. Injury to extremities may indicate
lumbar or sacral spine injury.

• PARALYSIS   Inability to move or inability to feel sensation in some part of
body may indicate spinal fracture with cord injury.

• PAINFUL MOVEMENT   Movement may cause or increase pain. Never try
to move the injured area.

• ALSO: Loss of bowel or bladder control, priapism,
impaired breathing.

FIGURE 24-3   Provide immediate and continuing manual immobilization of the
patient with possible spine injury while assessing for additional signs and symptoms.

(Figure 24-3). Even if such patients are otherwise stable, consider rapid trauma assessment, expeditious employment of spinal precautions, and immediate transport to the trauma center. These patients are likely to deteriorate and to need neurological intervention.

During the rapid trauma assessment, palpate the entire posterior spine. Feel for any deformity, pain, crepitus, unusual warmth, or tenderness from C-1 through L-5. It may be beneficial to repeat palpation of the spine from L-5 to C-1 as pain or tenderness may be difficult to identify in the presence of other painful injuries when minor tenderness may be the only symptom of significant vertebral column instability.

Continue your exam, inspecting each distal extremity and evaluating both motor and sensory function. If there is any limb injury, perform what spinal assessment you can while working around the injuries and assuring that you do not cause further harm to the limb.

For each upper extremity, test finger abduction/adduction (T-1) by having the patient spread the fingers of the hand while you squeeze the second, third, and fourth fingers together. You should meet with bilaterally equal and moderate resistance to your effort. Test finger or hand extension (C-7) by having the patient hold the fingers and/or wrists fully extended. Place pressure against the back of the fingers while you hold the forearm immobile. Again, you should meet bilaterally equal and moderate resistance. Finally, have the patient squeeze your first two fingers in his hand and assure that the grip is firm and bilaterally equal (Figure 24-4).

To assess for limb sensation, first ask about any abnormal feelings in the limb—inability to move (paralysis), weakness, numbness (anesthesia), tingling (paresthesia), or pain. Have the patient close both eyes and check the ability to distinguish between sensations of pain and light touch. To check pain reception (the spinothalamic tract), use the retracted tip of a ballpoint pen or another pointed object not likely to cause injury to induce slight point pain. To check for light touch (involving several tracts), use a cotton swab or a gentle touch with the pad of a finger. Responses to both pain and touch stimulation should be bilateral and equal.

Also test motor and sensory function for the lower extremities (Figure 24-5). Place your hand against the ball of the patient's foot and have him push firmly against it (plantar flexion, S-1 and S-2). Then place your hand on top of the toes and have the patient pull the toes and foot upwards (dorsiflexion, L-5). To evaluate pain sensation, use the same techniques you used in testing the upper extremities. Lower limb strength and sensations should be present and bilaterally equal.

During the full body exam, look for any line of demarcation between normal sensation and paresthesia or anesthesia and any differences in muscle tone. Begin the exam with the feet, and work up the body toward the head. Try not to alarm the patient because if he recognizes that your touch is not felt, his anxiety may increase. Use a sharp object not likely to cause injury, like a ballpoint pen with tip retracted, and move upward. Note the level at which the patient first identifies sensation or pain and relate it to the dermatomes. You might mark the level at which sensation is first noticed on the patient with a pen so that you can compare the results of later tests with your initial results.

Also evaluate the myotomes to determine the level of muscular control. Suspect muscle flaccidity if a body area has muscle masses with a more relaxed tone than the rest of the body. These neurologic signs give you a good indication of the level of spinal cord disruption. Examine both sides of the body as there may be differences from side to side both in sensation and in levels of voluntary and involuntary (muscle tone) motor activity.

You may also perform a test for Babinski's sign (Figure 24-6). Stroke the lateral aspect of the bottom of the foot and watch for the movement of the toes and great toe. Fanning of the toes and dorsiflexion (lifting) of the great toe is a positive sign and suggests injury along the pyramidal (descending spinal) tracts.

If discrete areas of nervous deficit exist, relate them to an injury along the nerve pathway or suspect injury to the spinal nerve root as it emerges from the

FIGURE 24-4 Compare grip strength bilaterally.

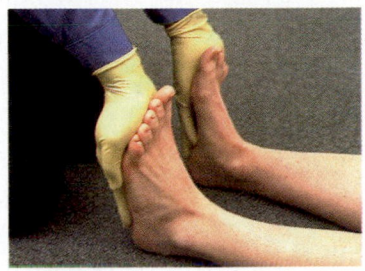

FIGURE 24-5 Compare lower limb strength bilaterally.

FIGURE 24-6 Test for Babinski's sign.

spinal column. A nerve root injury suggests the possibility of a vertebral column injury and the need for spinal immobilization. Also consider that the source of a deficit may be peripheral nerve damage related to soft tissue or skeletal damage along its pathway to the affected area. Again, try to identify the associated dermatome and myotome and, thus, the likely location of the lesion along the spinal column, spinal root, or peripheral nerve.

Another sign of spinal injury is priapism. This prolonged, possibly painful erection of the male genitalia is due to unopposed parasympathetic stimulation. Disruption of the sympathetic (thoracolumbar) pathways during a cervical spinal injury can produce this sign. In many cases, the pain sensation is lost due to disruption of the sensory pathways to the brain.

Occasionally, the patient with mid-cervical spine injury presents with the "hold-up" position. Left on their own, the patient's arms rise to a position above the shoulders and head. This occurs because the injury paralyzes the adductor and extensor muscles while the patient maintains control over the abductors and flexors. Without the opposition of the adductors and extensors, normal muscle tone impulses or any attempt by the patient to move the limb cause it to move toward the flexed position. With such cases, simply tie the patient's wrists to his belt to hold the limbs down for transport.

If the patient does not show any signs or symptoms of spinal injury and the mechanism of injury does not suggest spinal injury, ask the patient to gently move his neck. If the patient experiences any pain or discomfort or shows any neurological deficit, employ spinal precautions and consider transport to a neurocenter for further evaluation. Also examine the extremities for signs of neurologic impairment. If any are found, immediately employ spinal precautions.

Vital Signs

Any signs of abnormally low blood pressure, slow heart rate, or absent, diaphragmatic, or shallow respirations suggest possible spinal cord injury.

Evaluate the vital signs carefully in the patient with suspected spinal injury. Any signs of abnormally low blood pressure, slow heart rate, or absent, diaphragmatic, or shallow respirations indicate possible spinal cord injury.

Body temperature is an important consideration when evaluating the potential spinal injury patient. Spine injury patients are subject to fluctuations in body temperature related to ambient temperature changes. This is because those patients lose the ability to control the skin's heat conservation/dissipation function below the lesion. While this does not result in an obvious sign in the patient, that patient is highly susceptible to body temperature fluctuations. Cover the patient with blankets in all but the warmest environments and monitor the patient's temperature carefully.

At the conclusion of the rapid trauma assessment, consider the patient with any sign, symptom, or mechanism of injury suggestive of vertebral column or spinal cord injury for rapid transport to a nearby neurocenter or trauma center. Employ full spinal precautions, monitor for neurogenic shock, and perform frequent ongoing patient assessments.

ONGOING ASSESSMENT

For the ongoing assessment, repeat the elements of the initial assessment, take vital signs, and re-evaluate any signs or symptoms of spinal cord injury every 5 minutes (Figure 24-7). Monitor carefully for any changes in neurologic signs, including the levels of orientation, responsiveness, sensation, and motor function. Observe also for any changes in the dermatomes and myotomes affected by the injury. Look for any improvement or deterioration. Watch for a slowing pulse rate or a constant pulse rate in the presence of falling blood pressure. Watch for a dropping blood pressure without signs of shock compensation. Remember that

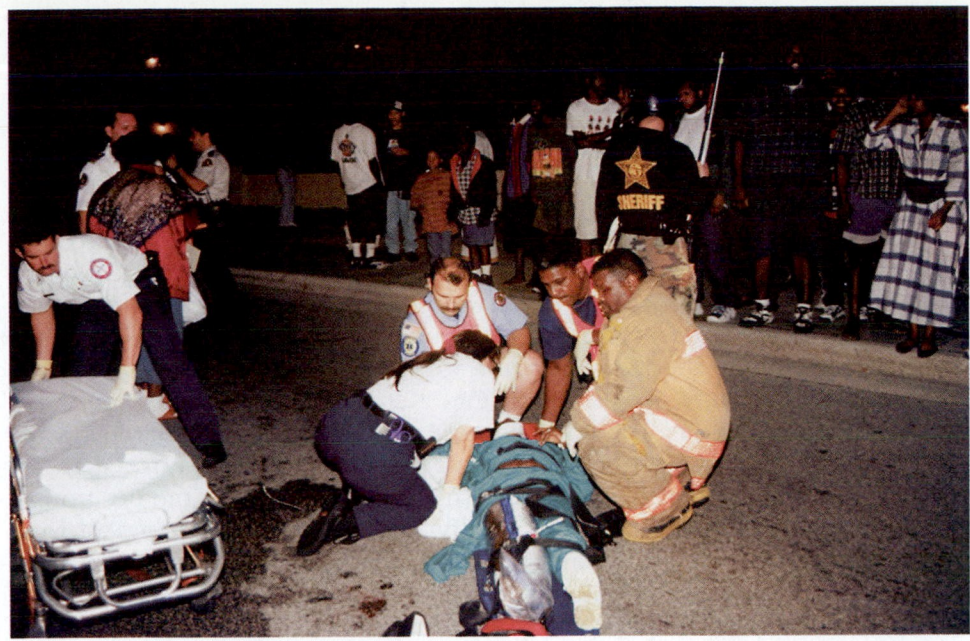

FIGURE 24-7 Repeat the ongoing assessment every 5 minutes with seriously injured patients.

spinal column injury may not produce any overt associated neurologic signs or symptoms yet may still threaten the spinal cord if the patient is moved without proper precautions.

MANAGEMENT OF THE SPINAL INJURY PATIENT

Spinal injury care steps (spinal precautions) performed during the initial assessment include moving the patient to the neutral, in-line position, maintaining that position with manual immobilization until the patient is fully immobilized by mechanical means, and applying the cervical collar once the neck assessment is complete. The remaining steps in management of the spinal injury patient are related to maintaining the neutral, in-line position while moving the patient to the long spine board and then firmly securing him to the board for transport to the hospital.

These skills have but one major objective: maintaining the neutral, in-line position. Although this might seem a simple objective, it is not. Remember that the spine is a chain of 33 small, rather delicate bones, which is attached to other skeletal members only at the head, thorax, and pelvis. These skeletal attachments may transmit forces that attempt to flex, extend, rotate, compress, distract, and laterally bend the spine during any patient movement. The procedures and devices discussed below are intended to assure that the patient remains in the neutral, in-line position throughout care, movement, and transport.

Constantly calm and reassure the patient with suspected spinal injury. Spinal injury can produce extreme anxiety in patients because of the severity of its effects and their potentially lifelong implications. The application of spinal precautions can compound this anxiety. The patient must endure complete immobilization on a rigid and relatively uncomfortable device, the long spine board. He will be unable to move and protect himself during the processes of immobilization, assessment,

Spinal precautions have one major objective: maintaining the patient in a neutral, in-line position.

care, and transport to the hospital. To alleviate some of the anxiety, be sure to communicate frequently with the patient. Tell the patient why you are employing spinal precautions and explain, in advance, what you will be doing in each step of the process. Do what you can to make the patient comfortable and to provide assurance that you and your team are caring for his needs.

SPINAL ALIGNMENT

The first step of the spinal precautions process is to bring the patient from the position in which he is found into a neutral, in-line position adequate for assessment, airway maintenance, and spinal immobilization. This process involves moving the patient to the supine position with the head facing directly forward and elevated 1 to 2 inches above the ground. Remember that the spine curves in an "S" shape through its length. This leaves the head displaced forward when the posterior thorax and buttocks (supporting the pelvis) rest on a firm, flat surface. Also remember that the neutral position (also known as the position of function) is generally with the joints halfway between the extremes of their motion. In spinal positioning, this means the hips and knees should be somewhat flexed for maximum comfort and minimum stress on the muscles, joints, and spine. For complete spinal immobilization, consider placement of a rolled blanket under the knees.

It is also important to assure there are no distracting or compressing forces on the spine. If the patient is seated or standing, support the head to leave only a portion of the head's weight on the spine. Be careful not to lift the entire head as this places a distracting force on the spine. Lastly, bring the spine into line by aligning the nose, navel, and toes to assure that there is no rotation along the spine's length. The head must face directly forward and the shoulders and pelvis must be in a single plane with the body. This neutral, in-line positioning allows for the greatest spacing between the cord and inner lumen of the spinal foramen. Neutral, in-line positioning both reduces pressure on the cord and increases circulation to and through it, an especially important consideration in the presence of injury. There are many techniques for moving and immobilizing the potential spine injury patient; whichever you employ, always focus on obtaining and then maintaining neutral, in-line positioning. Doing this assures you the best opportunity to protect the vertebral column and the spinal cord of the patient during your time at his side.

The only contraindications to moving the potential spine injury patient from the position in which he is found to the neutral, in-line position are as follows: when movement causes a noticeable increase in pain; when you meet with noticeable resistance during the procedure; when you identify an increase in neurologic signs as you move the head; or when the patient's spine is grossly deformed. Pain and resistance both suggest that the alignment process may be moving the injury site and thus may be causing further injury. When you meet with resistance or increased pain during any positioning of the head or spine, immobilize the patient as he lies. The same rule applies when you note an increase in the signs of neurologic injury in the patient with movement of the spine. Finally, in cases of severe deformity of the spine, do not move the patient because any movement will further compromise the column and cord. Use whatever padding and immobilization devices are necessary to accommodate the patient's positioning and assure that no further movement occurs.

Assure that any movement of the patient during assessment or care is toward alignment. If, for example, the patient is lying twisted on the ground when you find him, assess the exposed areas, then move the patient toward alignment. If the patient is found prone, assess the patient's posterior surfaces

Move any body segment that is out of alignment toward alignment as you examine it, but if the patient feels any increase in pain or if you feel resistance to movement, immobilize the head and neck or other portion of the body in the position achieved.

before you log roll him (to a long spine board) for further assessment and care. Never move a patient twice before you complete your mechanical immobilization, if possible.

MANUAL CERVICAL IMMOBILIZATION

The typical trauma patient is found either seated (as in an auto) or lying on the ground. For the seated patient, initially approach from the front and carefully direct the patient not to move or turn his head. It is an almost reflexive act to turn to listen when we hear someone speak to us from behind. Such movement is dangerous in the potential spine injury patient. Ask your patient to keep his head immobile and explain to the patient that a care giver is going to position him- or herself behind the patient to immobilize the spine.

Then the assigned care giver should move behind the patient and bring his or her hands up along the patient's ears, using the little fingers to catch the mandible and the medial aspect of the heels of the hand to engage the mastoid region of the skull (Figure 24-8). Gentle pressure inward engages the head and prevents it from moving. A gentle lifting force of a few pounds helps takes some of the weight of the head off the cervical spine, but care should be taken not to lift the head or apply any traction to this critical region. The patient's head should then be moved slowly and easily to a position in which the eyes face directly forward and along a line central to and perpendicular to the shoulder plane.

If there is no access to the seated patient from behind, employ the same techniques of movement and immobilization from in front with the little fingers engaging the mastoid region while the heels of the hand support the mandible. When approaching from the patient's side, place one hand under the mandible while using the other to support the occiput (Figure 24-9).

If the patient is supine, support the head by placing your hands along the lateral and inferior surfaces of the head. Position the little fingers and heels of the hands just lateral to the occipital region of the skull to support the head. With gentle inward pressure, hold the patient's head immobile and prevent flexion/extension, rotation, and lateral bending motion. Lift the head gently off the ground to approximate the neutral position, usually 1 to 2 inches for the adult. (If the surface on which the patient is found is not flat, adjust the height accordingly.) Position a small adult's or a large child's head at about ground level. Elevate the shoulders of infants or very small children because of their proportionally larger heads. Apply no axial pressure by either pushing or pulling the head toward or away from the body.

FIGURE 24-8 Bring the head to the neutral in-line position and maintain manual immobilization until the head, neck, and spine are mechanically immobilized.

FIGURE 24-9 When you cannot access the patient from behind to apply manual immobilization, use alternative hand placement.

If a patient is found prone or on the side, position your hands according to the patient's position. If it will be some time until the patient can be moved to the supine position, place your hands so that they are comfortable during cervical immobilization. You should then reposition your hands just before the patient is moved to the final position. If the time until moving the patient to the supine position is expected to be short, place your hands so they will be properly positioned at the conclusion of the move. This may involve initially twisting your hands into a relatively uncomfortable position.

Assessment, care, and patient movement may require the care giver holding immobilization to reposition his or her hands. To accomplish this, another care giver supports and immobilizes the patient's head and neck by bringing his or her hands in from an alternate position. This care giver places one hand under the patient's occiput while the other hand holds the jaw. Once the head is stable, have the original care giver reposition his or her hands, reassume immobilization, and then have the second care giver remove his or her hands.

CERVICAL COLLAR APPLICATION

A cervical collar by itself does not immobilize the cervical spine.

Always assure that the cervical collar is correctly sized for the patient or choose another one.

After a potential spinal injury patient has been manually immobilized, consider the application of the cervical collar. Apply the collar as soon as the neck is fully assessed, generally during the rapid trauma assessment. The cervical collar is only an adjunct to full cervical immobilization and should never be considered to provide immobilization by itself. The collar does limit cervical spine motion and reduce the forces of compression (axial loading), but it does not completely prevent flexion/extension, rotation, or lateral bending.

To apply the cervical collar, size it to the patient according to the manufacturer's recommendations. Position the device under the chin and against the chest. Contour it over the shoulders and secure it firmly behind the neck. Be sure the Velcro® closures remain clear of sand, dirt, fabric, or the patient's hair and make a secure seal behind the neck (Figure 24-10). The collar should fit snugly around the neck but not place pressure against its anterior surface (carotid and jugular blood vessels and trachea). The collar should direct a limiting force against the jaw and occiput to restrict any flexion/extension of the head and neck. Assure that the collar does not seriously limit the movement of the jaw, as this could prevent the patient from ridding himself of vomitus. Once the cervical collar is in place, do not release or relax manual cervical immobilization until the patient is fully immobilized either with a vest-type immobilization device or to a long spine board with a cervical immobilization device.

FIGURE 24-10 Properly place and secure the cervical collar on suspected spinal injury patients.

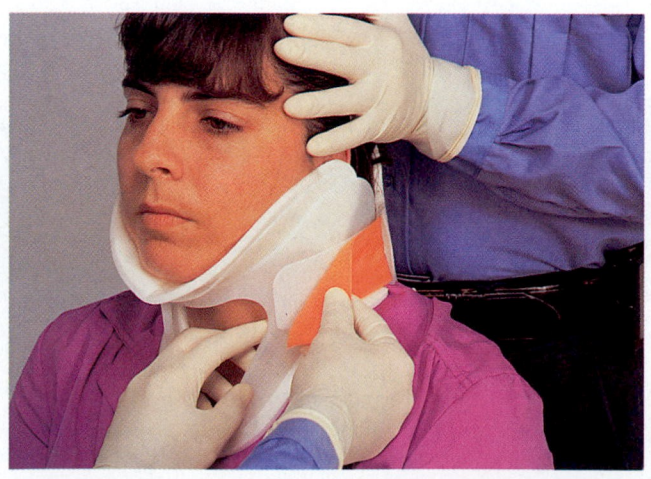

STANDING TAKEDOWN

Often at vehicle crash sites, you will find patients walking around when the mechanisms of injury suggest the potential for spinal injuries. These patients must receive spinal precautions, even though they are found standing. Your objective in such cases is to bring the patient to a fully supine position for further assessment, care, immobilization, and transport.

To accomplish this, employ a standing takedown procedure that maintains the spine in axial alignment. Have the patient remain immobile while a care giver approaches from the rear and assumes manual cervical immobilization. Quickly assess any areas that will be covered by the cervical collar or long spine board. Apply a cervical collar and place a long spine board behind and against the patient, with the care giver holding immobilization spreading his or her arms to accommodate the board. Position two other care givers, one on each side of the spine board, and have each place a hand under the patient's axilla and with it grasp the closest (preferably next higher) handhold on the board. The team should then move the patient and spine board backward, tilting the patient on his heels until the patient and board are supine (Figure 24-11).

During the move, the hands in the handholds support the thorax while the care giver holding cervical immobilization rotates his or her hands against the patient's head without either flexing or extending the head and neck as the patient moves from standing to supine. During this maneuver, the hands holding the patient's head must move from grasping the mastoid and mandible (standing) to grasping the lateral occiput (supine). This is not easy, as the head must rotate while the care giver's hands remain in the same relative position. As with all movement procedures, the care giver at the patient's head should be in control and direct the process.

Once the patient and board are on the ground, continue to maintain manual immobilization while assessing and caring for the patient. Then provide mechanical immobilization to the long spine board before moving the patient to the ambulance.

FIGURE 24-11   The standing takedown.

HELMET REMOVAL

Helmet removal may be a tricky endeavor. You should familiarize yourself with the types of helmets used by sporting teams in your area (e.g. high-school football).

Helmet use in contact sports, bicycling, skateboarding, in-line skating, and motorcycling has increased over the past decade. While these devices offer significant protection for the head during impact, they have not proven to reduce spine injuries. Their use also complicates spinal injury care for prehospital care providers. Many helmets are of the partial variety (such as those worn while bicycling and skateboarding) and are easy to remove at the trauma scene. Some motorcycle and sports helmets, however, fully enclose the head and are very difficult to remove in the field. These helmets are also very difficult to secure to the spine board because of their spherical shapes. Further, most full helmets do not hold the head firmly within, so even fixing the helmet securely to the spine board does not result in effective cervical immobilization. Some newer contact sport helmets contain air bladders that expand and firmly hold the head in position within the helmet. These helmets immobilize the head well, but they are still difficult to firmly secure to a spine board. Consequently, most full-enclosure helmets must be removed to assure adequate spinal immobilization.

The helmet must be removed if you find any of the following conditions:

- The helmet does not immobilize the patient's head within.
- You cannot securely immobilize the helmet to the long spine board.
- The helmet prevents airway care.
- The helmet prevents assessment of anticipated injuries.
- There are, or you anticipate, airway or breathing problems.
- Helmet removal will not cause further injury.

During helmet removal, have a care giver initially stabilize the cervical spine by manually stabilizing the helmet. Remove the face mask, if present, either by unscrewing it or by cutting it off, if possible. Remove or retract any eye protection or visor and unfasten or cut away any chin strap as well. Be careful not to manipulate the helmet or otherwise transmit movement to the patient through the helmet. Then have another care giver immobilize the head by sliding his or her hands under the helmet and placing them along the sides of the head, supporting the occiput, or by placing one hand on the jaw and the other on the occiput. This care giver should choose the hand placement that works best for him or her and can be accommodated by the helmet. The care giver holding the helmet should then grasp the helmet and spread it slightly to clear the ears by pulling laterally just below and anterior to the ear enclosure. That care giver then rotates the helmet to clear the chin, counter-rotates it to clear the occiput, and then rotates it to clear the nose and brow ridge (Figure 24-12). The clearance is usually very tight with a well-fitted helmet.

Execute the procedure above slowly and carefully to prevent head and neck motion and to minimize patient discomfort. For helmets with air bladders, use the same procedure, but empty the bladder after someone stabilizes the head and before you begin the removal. Helmet removal is a complicated skill that you must practice frequently before you can employ it successfully in the field.

MOVEMENT OF THE SPINAL INJURY PATIENT

Once you assess and provide the essential care for a patient with a potential spinal injury, plan the movement to the long spine board carefully. If any step of assessment or patient care requires patient movement, consider moving the patient onto the long spine board. Movement techniques suitable for moving the spinal injury patient to the long spine board include the log roll, straddle slide,

FIGURE 24-12 Helmet removal.

rope-sling slide, orthopedic stretcher lift, application of a vest-type device (or short spine board), and rapid extrication. Choose a technique that affords the least spinal movement for the conditions and equipment at hand. Also select your movement technique and adjust its steps to accommodate the patient's particular injuries.

A key factor in all movement techniques for the patient with potential spinal injury is the coordination of the move. It is essential that you move the patient as a unit with his head facing forward and in a plane with the shoulders and hips. This can best be accomplished if the care giver at the head controls and directs the move. He or she is able to see the other rescuers and has a focused and limited function (holding the head), which permits that person to evaluate what the other care givers are doing. The care giver at the head directs the move by counting a cadence such as, "Move on four—one, two, three, four." A four count is preferable as it gives the other care givers a good opportunity to anticipate the actual start of movement. All moves must be slowly executed and well coordinated among care givers.

Consider what the final positioning of the patient will be when you choose a spinal movement technique. Most spinal injury patients are best served with supine positioning on a long spine board. However, a patient with a thoracic spine injury is frequently placed in a prone position on a soft stretcher. With this patient, other positioning, such as supine on a firm spine board, puts pressure on the injury site from the body's weight and any movement is more likely to cause motion of the injury site and compound any damage.

Choose a spinal movement technique that affords the least spinal movement.

The care giver at the head directs and controls the movement of the patient with a suspected spinal injury.

A four-count is a preferable cadence as it gives a good opportunity to anticipate the start of the move.

Log Roll

The log roll can be used to rotate the patient 90 degrees, insert the long spine board, and then roll the patient back. It can also be used to roll the patient 180 degrees from prone to supine or vice versa.

As you begin the 90-degree roll, assure manual spinal immobilization and apply a cervical collar. Notice that anatomically the shoulders are wider than the hips and legs. To provide a uniform roll, extend the patient's arm above his or her head. Then place a bulky blanket between the legs (with its bulkiest portion between the feet) and tie the legs together. This reduces pelvic movement and lateral bending of the lumbar spine.

It takes four care givers to perform the log roll for a spinal injury patient (Figure 24-13). One care giver holds the head, while one kneels at the patient's shoulder with the knees tight against the patient's chest. The third care giver kneels at the patient's hip with the knees tight against the patient's hip. The

FIGURE 24-13 The 4-person log roll.

last care giver kneels at the patient's knees with the knees tight against the patient's knees.

The care givers reach across the patient and around the opposite shoulder, hip, and knee, respectively, and grasp the patient firmly. On a count initiated by the care giver at the head, the team, in unison, rolls the patient against their knees and up to a 90-degree angle. With a free hand, the care giver at the knees (or an additional care-giver) slides a long spine board under the patient from the patient's side or the foot end. The board should be positioned tightly against the patient so that the head, torso, and pelvis will eventually rest solidly on the board. Then, at the count of the care giver at the head, the team rolls the patient back 90 degrees onto the board.

The 180-degree log roll begins with placement of the long spine board between the care givers and the patient, with the board resting at an angle on the care givers' thighs. The care givers reach across the board and grasp the patient as for the 90-degree log roll. The care giver at the head must be careful to anticipate the turning motion and position his or her hands so they will be comfortably positioned at the end of the roll. On the count of the care giver at the head, the team rolls the patient past 90 degrees until he is positioned against the tilted long spine board. Then they reposition their hands against the other (lower) side of the patient and slowly back their thighs out from under the patient until the board rests on the ground.

Straddle Slide

Another technique effective for moving the patient with potential spinal injury is the straddle slide. In this procedure, three care givers are positioned at the patient's head, shoulders, and pelvis, while a fourth prepares to insert the long spine board from either the patient's head or feet. The care giver at the head holds cervical immobilization and guides the lift with a cadence. The second care giver straddles the patient (facing the patient's head) and grasps the shoulders. The third care giver straddles the patient (facing the head) and grasps the pelvis. All the care givers keep their feet planted widely enough apart to permit the insertion of the long spine board. At the direction of the care giver at the head, the three care givers lift the patient just enough to permit the fourth care giver to negotiate the long spine board underneath the patient. (Note: If the board is to be inserted from the patient's feet, the care giver inserting the board lifts the patient's feet with one hand and slides the board into place with the other.) On a signal from the care giver at the head, the team gently lowers the patient to the long spine board.

Rope-Sling Slide

A continuous ring or length of thick rope or other material can be used to help slide a supine patient, using axial traction, onto a long spine board. One care giver holds cervical immobilization, while another places the rope across the patient's chest and under his arms. The rope is tied together (with a cravat) behind the patient's neck and brought out between the legs of the first care giver. A long spine board is placed between the legs of the care giver holding cervical stabilization. The second care giver positions him- or herself at the head end of the spine board with the board resting on his thighs (this provides a small angle to more easily drag the patient onto the board). The second caregiver then pulls on the two strands of rope, guiding the patient onto the spine board as directed by the care giver at the head. The care giver holding cervical immobilization moves backwards as the patient is moved onto the spine board. (The care giver at the head may crouch or kneel to the patient's side to hold immobilization.) The care giver at the head must be careful to move smoothly with the care giver pulling axial traction. That person must assure that the head moves with the body and does not pull against it.

Orthopedic Stretcher

The orthopedic stretcher, also known as the scoop stretcher, is a valuable device for positioning the patient on the spine board or helping to secure the patient to the long spine board. To apply the device, lengthen it to accommodate the patient's height and then separate it into its two halves. Maintain cervical immobilization while you gently negotiate each half of the stretcher under the patient from the sides and connect them at the top, then bottom. Be careful not to entrap the patient's skin or body parts while positioning the stretcher, especially on uneven ground. Once the device is connected, you may use the stretcher to lift the patient to the waiting spine board. Orthopedic stretchers are usually not rigid enough to use by themselves as transport devices for spinal injury patients. Rather, they are most effective in moving patients to the long spine board, where they may remain as an adjunct to full immobilization, or you may disconnect the halves, remove them, and immobilize the patient to the long spine board in the normal way.

Vest-Type Immobilization Device (and Short Spine Board)

A specialized piece of EMS equipment that may be used with some spinal injury patients is the vest-type immobilization device (Figure 24-14). This device immobilizes the patient's head, shoulders, and pelvis to a rigid board so that you can move the patient from a seated position, as in an automobile, to a fully supine position. The vest-type device comes as a commercially made device that usually has the needed strapping already attached. The device is usually constructed of thin, rigid wood or plastic strips embedded in a vinyl or fabric vest. It is then wrapped and secured around the patient to provide immobilization. An alternative to the vest-type device is the short spine board, a cut-out piece of rigid plywood to which you attach strapping and padding. The basic principles of application are the same with both short-board and vest-type devices.

To apply the vest-type device, manually immobilize the patient's cervical spine and apply a cervical collar while the device is being readied for application. If the patient is positioned against a soft seat (as in an automobile),

FIGURE 24-14 A vest-type immobilization device.

gently move the patient's shoulders and head a few inches forward to permit insertion of the vest. The care giver holding cervical immobilization directs and coordinates the move, while a second care giver guides and controls shoulder motion. Negotiate the device behind the patient by either inserting the head portion under and through the arms of the care giver providing cervical immobilization, or angling it, base first, then moving it behind the patient's back. Position the device vertically so the chest appendages fit just under the arms. This positioning permits you to fasten the straps and secure the shoulders without any upward or downward movement of the device. First, secure the device to the chest and pelvis with strapping and assure that the vest is immobile. Tighten the straps firmly, but be sure that they do not inhibit respiration. Secure the thigh straps as they hold the hips and thighs in the flexed position, limiting lumbar motion. Then fill the space between the occiput and the device with non-compressible padding to assure neutral positioning. Secure both the brow ridge and chin to the device with straps, but be very careful to allow for vomiting by the patient and subsequent clearing of the airway or be prepared to cut the chin strap immediately if vomiting occurs. Tie the patient's wrists together.

The vest-type immobilization device is not meant to lift the patient but rather to facilitate rotating him on the buttocks and then to tilt the patient to the supine position for further spinal immobilization (Figure 24-15). Once the patient is positioned on the long spine board, gently and carefully release the thigh straps and slowly and gently extend the hips and knees. If after transfer to the spine board the patient's head remains firmly affixed to the vest-type device, leave the vest on the patient and secure the vest to the long spine board since doing this effectively secures both head and torso. If the head becomes loose during the transfer, reapply manual cervical immobilization, secure the torso with strapping, and secure the head with a cervical immobilization device.

Rapid Extrication

Applying a vest-type immobilization device is a time-consuming process. Often the circumstances of the emergency, either issues of scene safety or the need for rapid transport to the trauma center, preclude spending the time required for standard spinal immobilization. In such cases, use a rapid extrication procedure.

The vest-type device is not meant to lift the patient but rather to facilitate rotating and tilting the patient to the supine position.

FIGURE 24-15 The vest-type immobilization device is not intended for lifting the patient, but for pivoting him or her.

With whatever personnel are available, stabilize the patient's spine, shoulders, pelvis, and legs with the patient's nose, navel, and toes kept in line. Assure that care givers are coordinated and understand what movement is to take place. One care giver, usually at the patient's head, should direct the move, counting a cadence to permit the crew to work together (Figure 24-16). Assure that personnel involved in the extrication move the patient maintaining the alignment of the patient's nose, naval, and toes. Then, on the leader's count, they should move the patient from a seated or other position to a waiting spine board.

Remember the objectives of spinal movement and stabilization: keep the spine in the neutral, in-line position by keeping the patient's eyes facing directly forward and keeping the shoulders and pelvis in a plane perpendicular to that of the gaze. Be sure to prevent any flexion/extension, rotation, or lateral bending.

While the technique of rapid extrication does not provide maximum protection for the spine, it does permit rapid movement of the patient with a spinal injury when other considerations demand it. Use the procedure only when your patient cannot afford the time it would take for normal spinal movement techniques. Rapid extrication from the confined space of a wrecked automobile is difficult at best. Plan your move carefully and execute the rapid extrication by carefully explaining the process and individual responsibilities to your team members.

During all movement of a spinal injury patient, keep the spine in the neutral, in-line position by keeping the patient's eyes facing directly forward, and the shoulders, pelvis, and toes in the same plane.

FIGURE 24-16 Rapid extrication of a patient with a spinal injury.

Management of the Spinal Injury Patient **1093**

FIGURE 24-17 Immobiliza-
tion of a spinal injury patient
to a long spine board with a
cervical immobilization device
in place.

Final Patient Positioning

Centering the patient on the board is essential to assuring that the patient's spine remains in-line and he is effectively immobilized. Accomplish this by placing team members at the patient's head, shoulders, pelvis, and feet. The care givers then place one hand on each side of the patient and prepare to move the patient toward the center of the board. On a cadence signaled by the care giver at the head, they slide the portion of the patient that is out of alignment to an in-line position, centered on the long spine board.

Long Spine Board

The long spine board is simply a reinforced flat, firm surface designed to facilitate immobilization of a patient in a supine or prone position (Figure 24-17). While the board may immobilize patients with multi-system trauma, pelvic and lower limb fractures, and many other types of trauma, it is primarily designed for patients with spine injuries. The board has several hand and strap holes along its lateral borders. Using nylon web strapping, you can immobilize a patient with almost any combination of injuries to the board firmly enough to permit rotating the patient and board 90 degrees to clear the airway in case of vomiting.

Secure the patient to the board with the strapping, immobilizing and holding the shoulders and pelvis firmly to the board. Such strapping may cross the body and capture the shoulder and pelvic girdles. Assure that you firmly immobilize the patient to prevent lateral motion as well as cephalad (head-ward) and caudad (tail-ward) motion. Be sure that the pressure created by strapping does not come to bear on the central abdomen. That would cause forced extension of the lumbar spine. Immobilize the lower legs and feet with strapping or cravats. Tie the legs together, and place a rolled blanket under the patient's knees to immobilize them in a slightly flexed position.

Long spine board immobilization is made more effective by use of the cervical immobilization device (CID). This device is made up of two soft, padded lateral pieces that bracket the patient's head, maintaining its position, and a base plate that permits you to easily secure the device to the board. The base plate is affixed to the long spine board before the patient is moved to it. Once you position the patient on the board, fill the void between the occiput and the CID base plate with firm, non-compressible padding. Use no padding for the small adult or older child, and pad the shoulders in the young child or infant to assure proper spinal positioning. While a care giver maintains manual immobilization of the head, bring the lateral components of the CID against the sides of the patient's head. Use medial pressure to hold them against the head and the head in position. Then affix the lateral CID components to the Velcro® of the CID base plate. Secure the head in position and to the long spine board using forehead and chin straps or tape. Make sure the strapping catches the brow ridge and the mandible or the upper portion of the collar. The properly secured CID must hold the patient's head in the neutral position without movement while not placing undue pressure on the neck or restricting jaw movement (in case of vomiting). Be careful that the straps do not flex, extend, or rotate the head. Bulky blanket rolls, placed on each side of the head and secured both to the head and the board will also effectively immobilize the head to the long spine board.

The long spine board does have drawbacks. Its firm surface places extreme pressure on the skin and tissues covering the ischial tuberosities and the shoulder blades. If a patient remains immobilized to the board for more than a couple of hours, ulceration injuries are likely to result.

The board also tends to encourage care givers to immobilize the patient directly to it in a non-neutral position. In a proper neutral position, the head should be elevated about 1 to 2 inches above the board's surface and the knees should be bent at 15 to 30 degrees. This positioning relieves pressure on the cervical spine, lumbar spine, hips, and knees and increases patient comfort. You can obtain proper knee positioning by placing folded blankets under the patient's knees. Also pad under the curves of the back. Do not over-pad; just fill the voids at the small of the back and neck with bulky soft dressing material.

A device that is now showing merit for spinal immobilization is the full-body vacuum splint. Like the vacuum splints for the limbs discussed in Chapter 22, "Musculoskeletal Trauma," the full-body splint uses small plastic beads that maintain their position in the reduced pressure after air is evacuated from the splint. To apply the vacuum splint, place the patient on the flattened device and shape it around him. Evacuating the air causes the device to form to the contours of the patient's body and maintain immobilization.

Immobilize the adult patient to the long spine board with the head elevated 1–2 inches, the knees slightly flexed, and with limited padding at the small of the back and the space behind the neck.

Diving Injury Immobilization

Patients injured in shallow water dives are often paralyzed with the impact. They must rely on others to protect their airways and remove them from the water. When carried out by untrained bystanders, however, these activities may compound any spinal injury. If you are present when such an incident occurs, be sure to carefully control any patient motion while he is still in the water. If necessary, turn him to a supine position, assuring that the nose, navel, and toes remain in a single plane and that the eyes face directly forward. You may accomplish this by sandwiching the patient's chest between your forearms while your arms and shoulders cradle the head. Once the patient is in the supine position, water provides an almost neutral buoyancy and, if the water is calm, helps to immobilize the patient. Move the patient by pulling on the shoulders while you cradle the head, in the neutral position, with the forearms. Float a long spine board under the patient to lift and carry him from the water.

MEDICATIONS

There are several conditions in which you may use medications to treat spinal injury patients, if permitted by your system's protocols. These conditions include spinal cord injury, neurogenic shock, and the combative patient.

Medications and Spinal Cord Injury

The initial physical injury to the spinal column or cord can be further compounded by the processes of inflammation and swelling. Certain naturally occurring drugs, called steroids, reduce the body's response to injury and thereby reduce the associated swelling and the resulting pressure on the cord. Methylprednisolone (Solu-Medrol®) and dexamethasone (Decadron®, Hexadrol®) are the most commonly used steroids in the prehospital setting for spinal injury patients.

Due to the high doses of steroids used in spinal injury therapy, many services prepare and carry "ready kits" containing multiple vials and all other materials needed for steroid administration.

Both methylprednisolone and dexamethasone are synthetic glucocorticoids with the potent anti-inflammatory properties of the naturally occurring adrenal cortical steroids. They reduce both capillary dilation and permeability. They do not, however, have the salt-retaining characteristic of other glucocorticoids. Dexamethasone is about 5 times more potent than and has a half-life (3 to 4.5 hours) about that of methylprednisolone. These medications are administered within the first 8 hours after an injury (possibly in the field).

Very high dose methylprednisolone (Solu-Medrol) therapy has been found to be effective in decreasing the severity of spinal cord injury. Improvement in motor, pin, and touch sensation has been reported when the drug is started within 8 hours of injury. Methylprednisolone is first administered as a 30 mg/kg loading dose given over 15 minutes as soon as possible after the injury. This should be followed by a 5.4 mg/kg/hour drip administered over the next 23 hours. The total amount of methylprednisolone required to achieve this protocol is significant. Because of this, many EMS services and emergency departments prepare a spinal injury "ready kit" that contains all of the required drug and administration supplies. Methylprednisolone must be reconstituted prior to use. Once reconstituted, it must be used within 48 hours or discarded. Some neurosurgeons will request the administration of dexamethasone (Decadron). It is usually administered at a dose of 4–24 milligrams with doses as high as 100 milligrams occasionally ordered.

Medications and Neurogenic Shock

The loss of sympathetic control leads to both a relaxation of the blood vessels (vasodilation) below the level of the lesion and the inability of the body to increase the heart rate. This expanded vascular system leads to a relative hypovolemia and lower blood pressure. The problem is further compounded as the heart, without sympathetic stimulation and in the presence of this relative hypovolemia, displays a normal or bradycardic heart rate. Frequently, the hypovolemia is treated with a fluid challenge, followed by careful use of a vasopressor such as dopamine. The slow heart rate is treated with atropine to reduce any parasympathetic stimulation.

The use of the PASG to combat the relative hypovolemia of neurogenic shock is somewhat controversial. The compression of the lower extremities and abdomen may counteract the vasodilation associated with the shock state, but research has not yet proven the garment's use contributes to a better outcome. Follow local protocols and consult with medical direction before using the device.

The initial treatment for hypovolemia from suspected neurogenic shock is by fluid challenge. Establish an IV with a 1,000 mL bag of lactated Ringer's solution or normal saline, a non-restrictive administration set, and a large-bore IV catheter. Administer 250 mL of solution quickly, monitor the blood pressure and heart rate, and auscultate the lungs for signs of developing pulmonary edema (crackles). If the patient responds with an increasing blood pressure, a slowing heart rate, and signs of improved perfusion, consider a second bolus, or monitor the patient and administer a second bolus if the patient's signs and symptoms begin to deteriorate. If the patient does not improve with the fluid challenge, consider vasopressor therapy, as allowed by your protocols.

Dopamine (Intropin®) is a naturally occurring catecholamine that, in addition to its own actions, causes the release of norepinephrine. Dopamine increases cardiac contractility and hence cardiac output and, at higher doses, increases peripheral vascular resistance, venous constriction, cardiac preload, and blood pressure. While there are no contraindications for dopamine use in the emergency setting, its common side effects include tachydysrhythmias, hypertension, headache, nausea, and vomiting.

Dopamine is frequently packaged as either a premixed solution containing 800 or 1600 mcg/mL or as a 5 mL vial containing 200 or 400 mg of drug. Vial contents are added to 250 mL of D5W to yield a concentration of either 800 or 1600 mcg/mL. Dopamine is very light sensitive and once mixed should be discarded after 24 hours. If the solution is either pink or brown, discard it. Dopamine's onset of action is about 5 minutes and its half life is around 2 minutes; hence, it is administered via a continuous infusion. It should be run piggyback through an already well-established IV line as infiltration can cause tissue necrosis. It is administered initially at 2.5 mcg/kg/min., then titrated to an increase in blood pressure or a maximum of 120 mcg/kg/min. (Vasoconstriction usually begins at doses above 10 mcg/kg/min.)

Interruption of the sympathetic pathways by spinal cord injury causes unopposed parasympathetic stimulation and bradycardia (or at least prevents the compensatory tachycardia that occurs with decreased cardiac preload). The net result is a decrease in cardiac output. Atropine is administered to block the parasympathetic impulse that might contribute to slow the heart rate.

Atropine is an anticholinergic agent most frequently used for symptomatic bradycardia and heart blocks in the myocardial infarction patient. It is sometimes helpful in increasing the heart rate of patients with upper spinal cord injury due to unopposed vagal stimulation. It acts by inhibiting the actions of acetylcholine, the major parasympathetic neurotransmitter. Atropine has a quick onset of action and a half life of just over 2 hours. It is available for emergency use in 5 and 10 mL preloaded syringes containing a concentration of 0.5 mg/mL. Atropine is administered rapidly in 0.5 mg (1 mL) intravenous doses every 3 to 5 minutes, up to a maximum of 2 mg. The only expected side effects in the emergency setting are dry mouth, blurred vision, and, possibly, tachycardia.

Medications and the Combative Patient

Frequently the patient who has sustained potentially serious spine injury has also sustained head injury, is intoxicated, or is otherwise very uncooperative or combative. In some of these cases, sedatives may be indicated to reduce anxiety and because the patient actively resists spinal precautions. Consider using meperidine (Demerol®) or diazepam (Valium®) to calm the patient. In extreme circumstances, consider use of the paralytics mentioned in Chapter 23, "Head, Facial, and Neck Trauma" in the discussion of facilitated intubation to paralyze the patient. Whenever you use these agents, you must carefully monitor the patient's level of consciousness and respirations. With use of paralytics, you must provide continuing ventilation for the patient during the action of the drug. Sedatives and paralytics should only be administered as permitted by your system's protocols and under the close and direct supervision of an on-line medical direction physician.

When giving a neuromuscular blocker to a conscious patient with spinal injury, always use a sedative/hypnotic first.

SUMMARY

Spinal injury is a frequent consequence of serious trauma and likely to induce serious disability or death. Injury to the spinal column may occur with only minimal signs and patient symptoms. So prehospital care for any patient with a significant mechanism of injury or any trauma patient with a reduced level of consciousness must include spinal precautions. Throughout patient assessment, immobilization, and movement, provide emotional support and calming reassurance to lower patient anxiety, and carefully monitor level of consciousness.

CHAPTER 25

Thoracic Trauma

Objectives

After reading this chapter, you should be able to:

1. Describe the incidence, morbidity, and mortality of thoracic injuries in the trauma patient. (p. 1100)
2. Discuss the anatomy and physiology of the thoracic organs and structures. (see Chapter 3)
3. Predict thoracic injuries based on mechanism of injury. (pp. 1101–1103)
4. Discuss the pathophysiology of, assessment findings with, and the management and need for rapid intervention and transport of the patient with chest wall injuries, including:
   a. Rib fracture (pp. 1104–1105, 1127)
   b. Flail segment (pp. 1106–1107, 1127)
   c. Sternal fracture (p. 1106)

5. Discuss the pathophysiology of, assessment findings with, and management and need for rapid intervention and transport of the patient with injury to the lung, including:
   a. Simple pneumothorax (pp. 1108–1109)
   b. Open pneumothorax (pp. 1109–1110, 1127–1128)
   c. Tension pneumothorax (pp. 1110–1111, 1128–1130)
   d. Hemothorax (pp. 1111–1112, 1130)
   e. Hemopneumothorax (p. 1112)
   f. Pulmonary contusion (pp. 1112–1113)

Continued

6. Discuss the pathophysiology of, findings of assessment with, and management and need for rapid intervention and transport of the patient with myocardial injuries, including:
   a. Myocardial contusion (pp. 1114–1115, 1130)
   b. Pericardial tamponade (pp. 1115–1116, 1130)
   c. Myocardial rupture (p. 1116)
7. Discuss the pathophysiology of, findings of assessment with, and management and need for rapid intervention and transport of the patient with vascular injuries, including injuries to:
   a. Aorta (pp. 1117, 1130)
   b. Vena cava (pp. 1117–1118)
   c. Pulmonary arteries/ veins (pp. 1117–1118)
8. Discuss the pathophysiology of, findings of assessment with, and management and need for rapid intervention and transport of patients with diaphragmatic, esophageal, and tracheobronchial injuries. (pp. 1118–1119, 1131)
9. Discuss the pathophysiology of, findings of assessment with, and management and need for rapid intervention and transport of the patient with traumatic asphyxia. (pp. 1119, 1131)
10. Differentiate between thoracic injuries based on the assessment and history. (pp. 1119–1125)
11. Given several preprogrammed and moulaged thoracic trauma patients, provide the appropriate scene size-up, initial assessment, rapid trauma or focused physical exam and history, detailed exam, and ongoing assessment and provide appropriate patient care and transportation. (pp. 1119–1131)

INTRODUCTION TO THORACIC INJURY

The thoracic cavity contains many vital structures including the heart, great vessels, esophagus, **tracheobronchial tree**, and lungs. Trauma to any one of these structures could lead to a life-threatening event. Twenty-five percent of all motor vehicle deaths are due to thoracic trauma (about 12,000 per year in the U.S.). The majority of these deaths are secondary to injury to the heart and great vessels. In addition, abdominal injuries are also common in patients with traumatic chest injury and can cause significant **co-morbidity.**

The incidence of blunt thoracic trauma has increased with the development of the modern automobile (Figure 25-1). Together with the development of a national highway system, more people are traveling greater distances, at greater speeds, and roadways are becoming more congested. This allows for an increased incidence of motor vehicle collisions (MVCs) and thus an increase in the incidence of thoracic injuries and subsequent deaths, as most blunt thoracic trauma deaths are MVC related. An increase in penetrating trauma has also been observed in urban areas associated with violent crime. The weapons used in violent crime in years past were likely to be of the "Saturday night special" variety, cheap small-caliber revolvers often producing just single wounds. The weapons of choice now are more likely to be large-caliber semi-automatic or automatic weapons that increase the likelihood of multiple missile injuries. With multiple wounds, there is a higher likelihood of injury to vital structures and therefore a higher mortality. Many advances in the treatment of penetrating thoracoabdominal trauma have been made in recent wars, and the incidence of mortality from these wounds has decreased from 8 to 40 percent in World War II to 3 to18 percent today.

Prevention efforts include gun control legislation, firearm safety courses, seatbelt laws, and better design of automobiles including passive restraint systems such as airbags. Statistics indicate that these efforts have already decreased the incidence of these injuries and the related morbidity and mortality.

In this chapter, we will discuss thoracic trauma in relation to penetrating and blunt injury. These mechanisms have more clinical significance than simple injury categories. Certain injuries are almost exclusively associated with one type of chest trauma but unlikely with the other. For example, pericardial tamponade is almost exclusively associated with penetrating thoracic trauma while cardiac rupture is almost exclusively caused by blunt thoracic trauma. By considering the mechanism of injury, understanding the pathology of the various injuries, and by being aware of the patient's physical signs of injury and symptoms, you will be better able to predict, identify and treat potential life threats.

FIGURE 25-1 An example of blunt trauma to the chest. *(Courtesy of Edward T. Dickinson, MD)*

PATHOPHYSIOLOGY OF THORACIC TRAUMA

Thoracic trauma is classified into two major categories by mechanism; blunt and penetrating. It is important to examine these injury mechanisms and their effects on the organs of the thorax.

BLUNT TRAUMA

Blunt thoracic trauma is injury resulting from kinetic energy forces transmitted through the tissues. These injuries may be further subdivided by mechanism into blast, crush (compression), and deceleration injuries.

Blast injuries result from an explosive chemical reaction that creates a pressure wave travelling outward from the epicenter. This pressure wave causes tissue disruption by dramatic compression and then decompression as the wave passes. In the thorax, this action may tear blood vessels and disrupt the alveolar tissue. These injuries may lead to hemorrhage, pneumothoraces, and air embolism (air entering the disrupted pulmonary vasculature and subsequently returning to the central circulation). Other injuries associated with a blast mechanism can include disruption of the tracheobronchial tree and traumatic rupture of the diaphragm. When the blast occurs in a confined space, the pressure wave may be contained and accentuated. The result is an increase in the incidence and severity of the associated injuries.

Crush injuries occur when the body is compressed between an object and a hard surface. This leads to direct injury or disruption of the chest wall, diaphragm, heart, or tracheobronchial tree. If the victim remains pinned between two objects, significant restriction in ventilation and venous return may occur, also known as traumatic asphyxia.

Deceleration injuries occur when the body is in motion and impacts a fixed object as, for example, the chest against the steering column in a front-end collision (Figure 25-2). This impact causes a direct blunt injury to the chest wall while the internal organs of the thoracic cavity continue in motion. The organs and structures then impact with the internal surface of the thoracic cavity and may be compressed as more posterior structures collide with them. If the organ or structure has points of fixation, as with the aorta at the ligamentum arteriosum, the force of the organ moving against this point of fixation (shear force) can lead to a traumatic disruption. These sudden deceleration and shear forces can cause

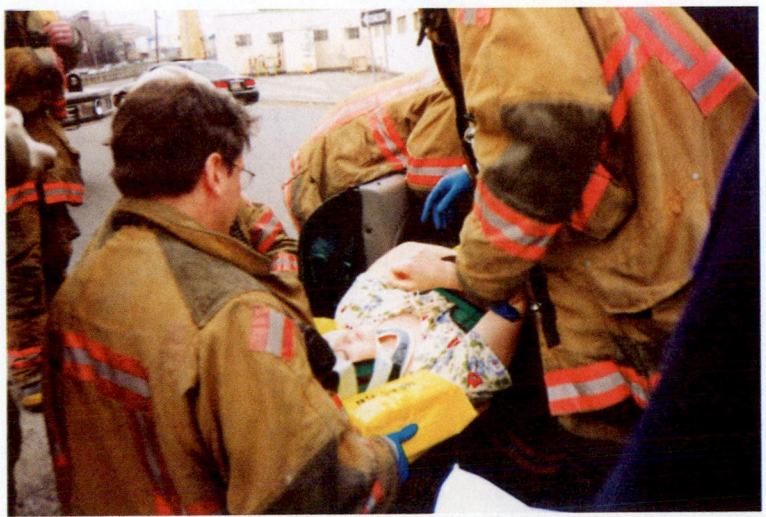

FIGURE 25-2 Frontal impact auto crashes frequently result in chest trauma.

disruption of the myocardium, great vessel, lung, trachea, and bronchi. The rapid compression of the chest, especially against a closed glottis, may also cause alveolar and tracheobronchial rupture and pneumothorax.

The age of the blunt trauma victim may affect the trauma received and its seriousness. The cartilaginous nature of the pediatric thorax spares the infant or child from rib fractures but more easily transmits the energy of trauma to the vital organs below. The result is more minor signs of injury, few rib fractures, and a greater incidence of serious internal injury. The geriatric patient responds very differently to blunt chest trauma. That patient will suffer more frequent rib fracture than the younger adult due to calcification of the skeletal system. Though the greater incidence of rib fracture may somewhat protect the underlying organs, pre-existing disease and the progressive reduction of respiratory and cardiac reserves result in a greater morbidity and mortality from serious chest trauma.

PENETRATING TRAUMA

Penetrating thoracic trauma induces injury as an object enters the chest and causes either direct trauma or secondary injury from transmitted kinetic energy forces related to the cavitational wave of high velocity projectiles. Penetrating chest trauma can be subdivided into three categories: low energy, high energy, and shotgun wounds.

Low energy wounds are those caused by arrows, knives, handguns, and other relatively slow moving objects (Figure 25-3). They cause injury by direct contact or very limited creation of temporary cavities. The injury that occurs from this type of wound is related to the direct path that the missile or object takes.

The age of the blunt trauma victim may affect the seriousness of the trauma received.

FIGURE 25-3 Penetrating (stab) wound to the chest.

High energy wounds are caused by military and hunting rifles (and some high-powered handguns at close range) that fire missiles at very high velocity. Their velocity gives the projectile very high kinetic energy. As the projectile passes through tissue, it creates a shock wave, tissue movement (including compression and stretching), and a large temporary cavity. These wounds cause extensive tissue damage perpendicular to the track of the projectile.

Shotgun wounds are classified according to the distance between the victim and the shotgun. A smaller gauge (a larger caliber) of shotgun and a larger size of shot also increase the effective range and penetrating power of the weapon and its potential to cause tissue damage. Type I injuries are those where the target is greater than 7 meters from the gun barrel at discharge. The pellets usually penetrate the skin and subcutaneous tissue but rarely penetrate the deep fascia to cause body cavity penetration. Type II injuries occur at a distance of 3 to 7 meters and often permit the pellets to penetrate the deep fascia with internal organ injury possible. Type III injuries occur at a distance of less than 3 meters and usually involve massive tissue destruction and life-threatening injury.

Penetrating thoracic trauma is often related to the structures involved. Lung tissue is very resilient when impacted by high energy projectiles. The "spongy" nature of the air-filled alveoli absorbs the energy of cavitation and reduces the size of the temporary cavity and injury associated with the compression and stretching. The great vessels and heart (if it is distended with blood) respond much differently. The fluid transmits the kinetic energy very well and may result in cardiac or vessel rupture. With slower moving projectiles or the heart in diastole the result may be a simple penetration. While a projectile tends to move in a straight line, it is easily deflected by contact with a rib, clavicle, scapula, or the spinal column. Contact with skeletal structures may also fragment the projectile, increasing the rate of energy exchange and the seriousness of injury. Penetrating trauma frequently leads to pneumothorax, which may be bilateral, depending on the track of the missile or knife. Table 25-1 lists common injuries associated with penetrating thoracic trauma.

Shotgun wounds within 3 meters of the discharging barrel cause serious tissue destruction and are frequently life threatening.

Table 25-1	INJURIES ASSOCIATED WITH PENETRATING THORACIC TRAUMA

Closed pneumothorax

Open pneumothorax (including sucking chest wound)

Tension pneumothorax

Pneumomediastinum

Hemothorax

Hemopneumothorax

Laceration of vascular structures, including the great vessels

Tracheobronchial tree lacerations

Esophageal lacerations

Penetrating cardiac injuries

Pericardial tamponade

Spinal cord injuries

Diaphragmatic penetration/laceration/rupture

Intra-abdominal penetration with associated organ injury

CHEST WALL INJURIES

Chest wall injuries are by far the most common injuries encountered in blunt chest trauma.

Chest wall injuries are by far the most common injuries encountered in blunt chest trauma. As previously discussed, an intact and moving chest wall is necessary to develop the pressures essential for air movement into and out of the lungs (the bellows effect). Chest wall injury may disrupt this motion and result in respiratory insufficiency. Closed injuries of the chest wall include contusions, rib fractures, sternal fractures/dislocations, and flail chest. Open injuries to the chest wall are almost entirely due to penetrating trauma and are often associated with deep structure injury in addition to disruption of the changing intrathoracic pressure necessary for respiration.

Chest Wall Contusion

Chest wall contusion is the most common result of blunt injury to the thorax.

Chest wall contusion is the most common result of blunt injury to the thorax. The injury damages the soft tissue covering the thoracic cage and causes pain with respiratory effort. Like contusions elsewhere, contusion of the chest wall may present with erythema initially, then ecchymosis. The discoloration may outline the object that caused the trauma, may outline the ribs as the soft tissue is trapped between the ribs and the offending agent, or may outline a combination of both. The most noticeable symptom of chest wall contusion is pain, made worse with deep breathing and possibly resulting in reduced chest expansion. The area will be tender at the contusion site, and you may observe decreased chest wall movement due to pain. You may auscultate limited breath sounds because of decreased air movement due to limited chest expansion.

The pain of chest wall contusion and associated limiting of deep inspiration may lead to hypoventilation. Hypoventilation may not be apparent in a young, otherwise healthy, individual and may not pose a significant life threat due to the individual's significant pulmonary reserves. The aged patient, however, often has pre-existing medical problems, little pulmonary reserve, and does not tolerate this injury as well. Such a patient quickly becomes hypoxemic (low oxygen levels in the blood) without proper respiratory support. In a pediatric patient, the ribs are very flexible, resist fracture, and easily transmit the forces of trauma. The result may be chest wall contusion and internal injury without rib fracture.

Content Review

SIGNS AND SYMPTOMS OF CHEST WALL INJURIES

Blunt or penetrating trauma to chest
Erythema
Ecchymosis
Dyspnea
Pain on breathing
Limited breath sounds
Hypoventilation
Crepitus
Paradoxical motion of chest wall

Rib Fracture

Rib fractures are found in more than 50 percent of cases of significant chest trauma from blunt mechanisms.

Rib fractures are found in more than 50 percent of cases of significant chest trauma from blunt mechanisms. Rib fractures are likely to occur at the point of impact or along the border of the object that impacts the chest (Figure 25-4). Fractures may also occur at a location remote from the injury site. The thoracic cage is a hollow cylinder that has some flex to it. As the compressional force of blunt trauma deforms the thorax, the ribs flex and may fracture at their weakest point, the posterior angle (along the posterior axillary line).

Ribs 4 through 8 are the most commonly fractured.

Ribs 4 through 8 are the most commonly fractured as they are least protected by other structures and are firmly fixed at both ends (to the spine and sternum). It takes great force to fracture the first three ribs because the shoulder, scapula, and the heavy musculature of the upper chest protect them. Their fracture is frequently associated with severe intrathoracic injuries (tracheobronchial tree injury, aortic rupture, and other vascular injuries), especially if multiple ribs are involved. Fracture of these ribs results in a mortality of up to 30 percent due to the associated injuries. Ribs 9 through 12 are less firmly attached to the sternum, are relatively mobile, and are thus less likely to fracture. However, they better transmit the energy of trauma to internal organs and may

FIGURE 25-4   Rib fractures.

Ribs 1–3 are well protected by shoulder bones and muscles.

Great force is required for sternal fractures.

Ribs 4–8 are most frequently fractured.

Ribs 9–12 are relatively mobile and fracture less frequently.

permit intra-abdominal injury without fracture. Fractures of ribs 9 through 12 are frequently associated with serious trauma and splenic or hepatic injury.

The incidence and significance of rib fracture varies with age. The pediatric patient has very cartilaginous ribs that bend easily. The ribs resist fracture and transmit kinetic forces to the thoracic and abdominal structures underneath. The pediatric patient hence has a decreased incidence of rib fracture and an increase in the incidence of underlying injury. The geriatric patient, on the other hand, has ribs that are calcified, less flexible, and more easily fractured. The geriatric patient is also more likely to have co-morbidity like COPD, which reduces respiratory reserves and compounds the effects of rib injury. If multiple rib fractures are noted in a young adult, they are probably associated with severe trauma and may lead to significant pain, splinting, hypoventilation, and inadequate cough. They also are likely to be associated with significant internal injuries. The mortality associated with rib fractures increases with the number of fractures, extremes of age (the very young or very old), and associated chronic respiratory or cardiac problems, especially in the elderly trauma victim.

The rib fracture is likely to be associated with an overlying chest wall contusion and presents with those signs and symptoms. The fracture site may also demonstrate a grating sensation (crepitus) as the bone ends move against each other, either during chest wall movement or during direct palpation. The pain associated with rib fracture is greater than that with chest wall contusion and will more greatly limit respiratory excursion. This reduced chest wall excursion frequently leads to hypoxia, hypoventilation, and muscle spasms at the fracture site. Hypoventilation can result in a progressive collapse of alveoli called atelectasis. This collapse reduces the lung surface available for gas exchange and contributes to hypoxia. These atelectatic segments also may become filled with blood or tissue fluid due to the injury and set the stage for secondary infection such as pneumonia. While pneumonia does not develop in the emergency setting, it is the cause of a significant mortality in blunt chest injury patients. Serious internal injuries may also result as the jagged rib ends move about and lacerate structures beneath them. Laceration of the intercostal arteries may result in hemothorax, while damage to the intercostal nerves may result in a neurologic deficit. Fracture and displacement of the lower ribs may injure the liver (right) or spleen (left).

In pediatric patients, more flexible ribs permit more serious internal injury before they fracture.

Rib fracture mortality increases with the number of fractures, extremes of age, and associated disease.

Sternal Fracture and Dislocation

Sternal fractures and dislocations are usually associated with blunt anterior chest trauma. Sternal fracture results only from severe impact, as this region of the chest is well supported by the ribs and clavicles. The most likely mechanism is a direct blow, a fall against a fixed object, or the blunt force of the sternum against the steering wheel or dashboard in a motor vehicle crash. The overall incidence of sternal fracture in thoracic trauma patients is between 5 and 8 percent. However, the mortality associated with it is between 25 and 45 percent due to underlying myocardial contusion, cardiac rupture, pericardial tamponade, and pulmonary contusion. If the surrounding ribs or costochondral joints are disrupted, the injury may result in a flail chest. The injury results in a noticeable deformity and possible crepitus with chest wall movement or palpation.

Dislocation at the sternoclavicular joint is uncommon and also requires significant force. It too may occur with blunt trauma to the anterior chest or with a lateral compression mechanism, as in side impact collisions or falls with the patient landing on the shoulder. The clavicle may dislocate from the sternum in one of two ways, anteriorly or posteriorly. The anterior dislocation creates a noticeable deformity anterior to the manubrium. The posterior dislocation displaces the head of the clavicle behind the sternum where it may compress or lacerate underlying great vessels or compress or injure the trachea and esophagus. Tracheal compression may result in stridor and voice change, though any deformity is more difficult to identify except that the shoulder may noticeably displace anteriorly and medially.

Flail Chest

Flail chest is a segment of the chest that becomes free to move with the pressure changes of respiration. The condition occurs when three or more adjacent ribs fracture in two or more places (Figure 25-5). It is one of the most serious chest wall injuries as it is often associated with severe underlying pulmonary injury (contusion) and it reduces the volume of respiration and increases the

FIGURE 25-5 Flail chest occurs when three or more adjacent ribs fracture in two or more places.

effort associated with it. This underlying injury adds to mortality in serious thoracic trauma (between 20 and 40 percent), as does age, head injury, shock, and other associated injuries. The most common mechanisms of injury causing flail chest are blunt traumas from falls, motor vehicle crashes, industrial accidents, and assaults.

The flail segment created by this injury is no longer a controlled component of the chest wall and bellows system. Increasing intrathoracic pressure associated with expiration moves the flail segment outward while the rest of the chest moves inward, pushing air under the moving segment that would normally be exhaled. This reduces the change in chest volume caused by the breathing effort as well as the volume of air expired and draws the mediastinum toward the injury. During inspiration, the intrathoracic pressure falls as the respiratory muscles move the chest wall outward and the diaphragm drops caudally (tail-ward). The reduced pressure draws the flail segment inward. The lung beneath it moves away from the inward-moving segment, reducing the volume of air moving into the thorax and displacing the mediastinum away from the injury. In summary, the injury produces a segment of the chest wall that moves in opposition of the chest's normal respiratory effort (paradoxical movement), it reduces the volume of air moved with each breath, and it displaces the mediastinum toward and then away from the injury site with each breath (Figure 25-6). In flail chest, the patient takes more energy to move less air and the respiratory volume is further reduced as the rib fracture pain produces a natural splinting of the chest.

It takes tremendous energy to create these six fracture sites (three or more ribs fractured in two or more places) and, accordingly, flail chest is often associated with serious internal injury. In addition, the movement of the flail segment, which is opposite to the rest of the chest wall is damaging to surrounding tissue. With each breath, the bone fracture sites move against one another causing further muscle damage, soft tissue damage, and pain. Small flail segments may go undetected as the associated intercostal muscle spasm naturally splints the segment. With time however, these muscles suffer further injury and fatigue and the flail segment's paradoxical movement may become more and more apparent.

Positive pressure ventilation of the patient with flail chest reverses the mechanism that causes the paradoxical chest wall movement, restores the tidal volume, and reduces the pain of chest wall movement. It accomplishes this by pushing the chest wall and the flail segment outward with positive pressure. Passive expiration then may cause both the flail segment and the rest of the chest to move inward, again, together.

Over time, the muscles splinting the flail segment will fatigue, and paradoxical respiration will become more evident.

Inspiration   Expiration

FIGURE 25-6 Paradoxical movement of the chest wall seen in flail chest.

PULMONARY INJURIES

Pulmonary injuries are injuries to lung tissue or injuries that damage the system that holds the lung to the interior of the thoracic cavity. They include the simple pneumothorax, open pneumothorax, tension pneumothorax, hemothorax, and pulmonary contusion.

Simple Pneumothorax

Simple **pneumothorax** (also known as closed pneumothorax) occurs when lung tissue is disrupted and air leaks into the pleural space (Figure 25-7). While there may be an external, and possibly penetrating, wound, there is no communication between the pleural space and the atmosphere. The pressure within the thorax does not exceed normal expiratory pressures and there is no associated mediastinal shift. As more and more air accumulates in the pleural space, the lung collapses. With lung collapse, the alveoli collapse (atelectisis) and blood flowing past the collapsed alveoli does not exchange oxygen and carbon dioxide. As more and more of the alveoli collapse, this condition, called ventilation/perfusion mismatch becomes more pronounced and begins to lower the blood oxygen level (hypoxemia). This soon becomes life endangering, especially if there are other associated injuries or shock.

Simple pneumothorax can occur with penetrating and blunt mechanisms. Blunt trauma may cause a pneumothorax when a rib fracture directly punctures the lung. Another mechanism may cause alveolar rupture from a sudden increase in intrathoracic pressure as the chest impacts the steering column with fully expanded lungs and a closed glottis (much like a paper bag filled with air and compressed suddenly between two hands). The incidence of pneumothorax in serious thoracic trauma is between 10 and 30 percent and its morbidity is related to the amount of atelectisis and the degree of perfusion mismatch. Penetrating trauma to the chest is frequently associated with simple pneumothorax, or with an injury that allows air to enter the pleural space through an external wound (open pneumothorax).

> **Content Review**
>
> **SIGNS AND SYMPTOMS OF PNEUMOTHORAX**
> Trauma to chest
> Chest pain on inspiration
> Hyperinflation of chest
> Diminished breath sounds on affected side

FIGURE 25-7 Simple (closed) pneumothorax.

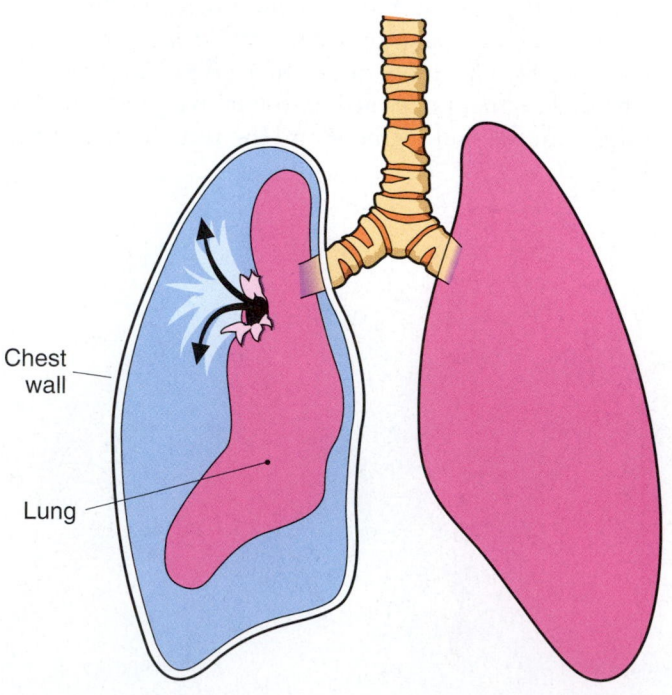

Chest wall

Lung

A simple pneumothorax reduces the efficiency of respiration and quickly leads to hypoxia. The hypoxia and increase in blood levels of CO_2 cause the medulla to increase the respiratory rate (tachypnea) and volume. If only a very small portion of the lung is involved, there may be no apparent signs or symptoms. A larger pneumothorax may cause mild dyspnea, or complete lung collapse may result in severe dyspnea and hypoxia. The signs, symptoms, and significance of simple pneumothorax increase with pre-existing disease. Pneumothorax may produce local chest pain with respiration as the pleurae become irritated (pleuritic pain). The pathology may cause the chest to hyperinflate and breath sounds to diminish on the affected side (usually in the extremes of the upper and lower lung first). A small pneumothorax involving collapse of less than 15 percent of the affected lung may be difficult to detect clinically and requires only supportive measures. Often the small pneumothorax will seal itself and the air in the pleural cavity will be absorbed. A larger pneumothorax is often clinically apparent and requires more aggressive therapy such as high flow oxygen and chest tube placement (in the emergency department).

Open Pneumothorax

Open pneumothorax is most commonly noted in military conflicts when a high-velocity bullet creates a significant wound in the chest wall (usually the exit wound). Recently use of high-velocity assault weapons has become more common in civilian settings and thus the frequency of these injuries is on the increase. Another cause of open pneumothorax is a shotgun blast at close range with an associated large wound to the chest wall. This chest wall disruption leads to the free passage of air between the atmosphere and the pleural space (Figure 25-8). Air is drawn into the wound as the chest moves outward and the diaphragm moves downward during inspiration. The internal thoracic pressure drops and air rushes through the wound and into the chest cavity. This air replaces the lung tissue and permits its collapse and results in a large functional dead space. The inspiratory effort of the intact side of the chest draws the mediastinum toward it and away from

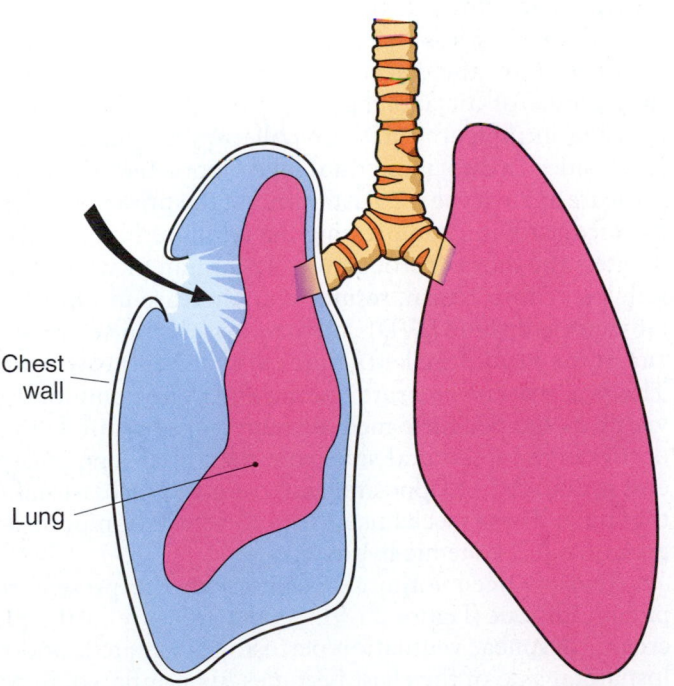

FIGURE 25-8 Open pneumothorax (sucking chest wound).

Chest wall

Lung

the injury. This prevents the uninjured lung from fully inflating. On exhalation, the contracting chest wall and rising diaphragm increase the internal pressure and force air outward through the wound. This movement of air into and out of the chest through the wound is the cause of the "sucking" sound that leads to the wound's common name, "sucking chest wound."

For air movement to occur through the opening in the chest wall, the opening must be at least 2/3 the diameter of the trachea. Remember, the size of the trachea is about the size of the patient's little finger. This must be the size of the opening into the chest, not the size of the wound. The thickness and resiliency of the chest wall often closes the wound to air movement unless it is quite large. Then the remaining defect may permit the free movement of air and create an open pneumothorax.

The open pneumothorax can be recognized by the large open wound to the thorax and the characteristic air movement (or sound) it produces. Air passage through the wound and the wound's associated hemorrhage may produce frothy blood around the opening, another characteristic of the open pneumothorax. The patient is likely to experience severe dyspnea, and possibly hypovolemia from associated injury and hemorrhage. The patient's condition is further compromised because the reduced intrathoracic pressures developed during inspiration do not complement venous return to the heart as they do with the intact thorax and respiratory effort.

Tension Pneumothorax

Tension pneumothorax is an open or simple pneumothorax that generates and maintains a pressure greater than atmospheric pressure within the thorax. It may be caused by a traumatic mechanism and injury or possibly by positive pressure ventilation of a patient with chest trauma or congenital defect affecting the respiratory tree. Tension pneumothorax may also occur as an open pneumothorax is sealed and an internal injury or defect permits the build-up of pressure.

Tension pneumothorax occurs because the mechanism of injury (either the external wound, or the internal injury) forms a one-way valve. Air flows into the pleural space through the defect during inspiration as the pressure within the pleural space is less than atmospheric. With expiration, the increasing pleural pressure closes the defect and does not permit air to escape. With each breath, the volume of air and the pressure within the pleural space increase. The increasing intrapleural pressure collapses the lung on the ipsilateral (same or injury) side, causes intercostal and suprasternal bulging, and begins to exert pressure against the mediastinum. As the pressure continues to build, it displaces the mediastinum, compressing the uninjured lung and crimping the vena cava as it enters the thorax through the diaphragm or where it attaches to the heart. This reduces venous return, results in an increase in venous pressure, causes the jugular veins to distend (JVD), and narrows the pulse pressure. Tracheal shift may occur as the mediastinal structures are pushed away from the increasing pressure. This is a very late and rare finding and more commonly seen in the young trauma victim as the pediatric mediastinum is more mobile than the adult's. Atelectasis occurs in the ipsilateral side from the initial lung collapse and on the contralateral (uninjured or opposite) side from the mediastinal shift and compression of that lung. These mechanisms lead to ventilation/perfusion mismatch, further hypoxemia and systemic hypoxia.

Tension pneumothorax begins with the presentation of a simple or open pneumothorax (Figure 25-9). As the pressure in the pleural space begins to increase, dyspnea, ventilation/perfusion mismatch, and hypoxemia develop. The ipsilateral side of the chest becomes hyperinflated, hyperresonant to percussion,

---

For air movement to occur through the opening in the chest wall, the opening must be at least 2/3 the diameter of the trachea.

＊ **tension pneumothorax** buildup of air under pressure within the thorax. The resulting compression of the lung severely reduces the effectiveness of respirations.

Tension pneumothorax is a serious and immediate life threat.

Apprehension,
agitation

Increasing cyanosis,
air hunger
(ventilation severely
impaired)

Possible
subcutaneous
emphysema

Shock; skin
cold, clammy

Distended neck veins

Trachael displacement
toward uninjured side

Hyperresonant
percussion note;
breath sounds ↓
or absent

FIGURE 25-9 Physical
findings of tension
pneumothorax.

and respiratory sounds become very faint, then absent. The pressure may cause the intracostal tissues to bulge. The opposite or contralateral side of the chest becomes somewhat dull to percussion, with progressively fainter respiratory sounds as the tension pneumothorax becomes worse. Severe hypoxia results in cyanosis, diaphoresis, and an altered mental status while the increased intrathoracic pressure reduces venous return and may cause JVD and hypotension. If the condition is not quickly recognized and promptly treated, it may lead to death.

Tension pneumothorax is a serious and immediate life threat. It is corrected by relieving the intrapleural pressure by inserting a needle through the chest wall to convert the tension pneumothorax to an open pneumothorax. If a valve is added to the decompression needle, it may permit only the escape of air during respiration. If there is no continuing internal defect, this may progressively re-expand the collapsed lung and return effective respiration.

Hemothorax

Hemothorax is simply the accumulation of blood in the pleural space due to internal hemorrhage. It can be very minor and not detectable in the field or, when associated with serious or great vessel injury, may result in rapid patient deterioration. Serious hemorrhage may displace a complete lung, accumulate over 1,500 mL of blood quickly and produce a mortality rate of 75 percent, with most (2/3) of those dying at the scene. Hemothorax is primarily a blood loss problem as each side of the thorax may hold up to 3,000 mL of blood (or half the total blood volume). However, the blood lost into the thorax reduces the tidal volume and efficiency of respiration in a patient who has already suffered trauma and is likely to move quickly into shock.

Tension pneumothorax is a serious and immediate life threat.

* **hemothorax** blood within the pleural space.

Pathophysiology of Thoracic Trauma **1111**

FIGURE 25-10 Physical findings of massive hemothorax.

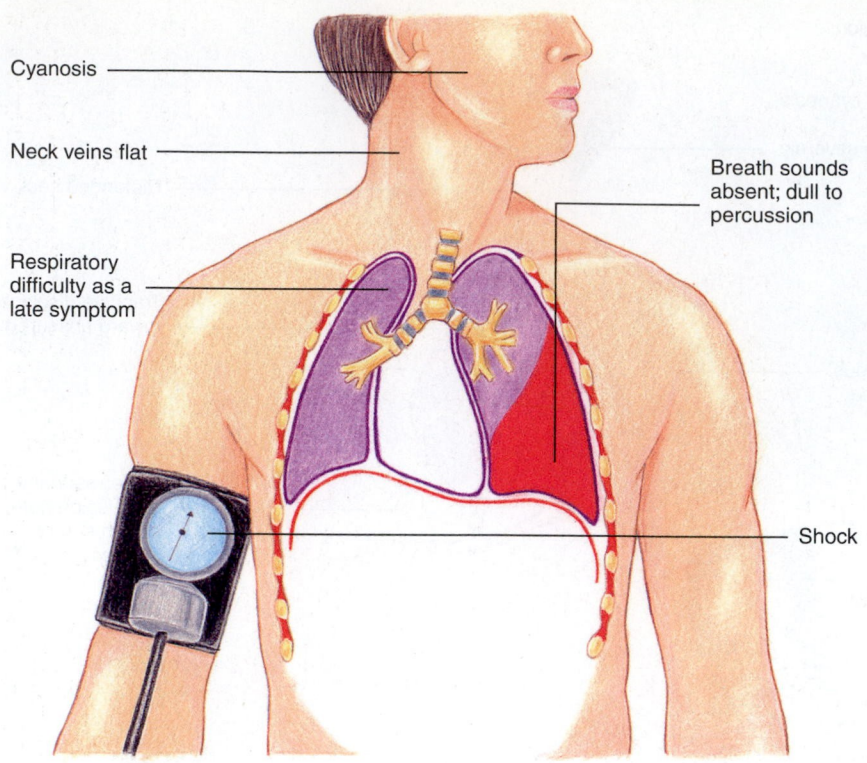

Cyanosis

Neck veins flat

Respiratory difficulty as a late symptom

Breath sounds absent; dull to percussion

Shock

---

* hemopneumothorax condition where air and blood are in the pleural space.

SIGNS AND SYMPTOMS OF HEMOTHORAX

Blunt or penetrating chest trauma
Signs and symptoms of shock
Dyspnea
Dull percussive sounds over site of injury

Hemothorax is frequently associated with rib fractures and can be associated with either blunt or penetrating mechanisms. It often accompanies pneumothorax (a **hemopneumothorax**) and occurs 25 percent of the time with penetrating trauma. Hemorrhage into the pleural space may occur from a lung laceration (most common) or laceration of the intercostal arteries, pulmonary arteries, great vessels, or internal mammary arteries. The intercostal arteries can bleed at a rate of 50 mL/min. The bleeding into the chest is more rapid than would occur elsewhere because the pressure within the chest is often less than atmospheric pressure (Laplace's law). The blood lost into the hemothorax contributes to hypovolemia and displaces lung tissue. If the accumulation is significant, it may cause significant hypovolemia and shock, hypoxemia, respiratory distress, and respiratory failure.

The patient with hemothorax will have either a blunt or penetrating injury like those associated with open or simple pneumothorax. The patient may also display the signs and symptoms of shock and some respiratory distress (Figure 25-10). The blood pools in the lower chest in the seated patient or posterior chest in the supine patient. The lungs present with normal percussion and breath sounds except directly over the accumulating fluid. There the lung percussion is very dull and breath sounds are very distant, if they can be heard at all.

Pulmonary Contusion

Pulmonary contusions are simply soft tissue contusions affecting the lung. They are present in 30 to 75 percent of patients with significant blunt chest trauma and are frequently associated with rib fracture. Pulmonary contusions range in severity from very limited, minor, and unrecognizable injuries, to those that are extensive and quickly life threatening. They result in a mortality rate of between 14 and 20 percent of serious chest trauma patients.

There are two specific mechanisms of injury that allow the transfer of energy to the pulmonary tissue and result in pulmonary contusions. They are deceleration and the pressure wave associated with either passage of a high velocity bullet or explosion. Deceleration injury occurs as the moving body strikes a fixed object. A common example of this mechanism is chest impact with the steering wheel during an auto crash. As the chest wall contacts the wheel and stops, the lungs continue forward, compressing and stretching the alveolar tissue or shearing it from the relatively fixed tracheobronchial tree. This causes disruption at the alveolar/capillary membrane leading to microscopic hemorrhage and edema. The second mechanism, the pressure wave of an explosion or bullet's passage, dramatically compresses and stretches the lung tissue. Due to the nature of the lung tissue (air-filled sacs surrounded by delicate and vascular membranes), the passage of this pressure is partially reflected at the gas/fluid (alveolar/capillary) interface. This leaves small, flame-shaped areas of disruption throughout the membrane leading to microhemorrhage and edema (called the Spalding effect). Pulmonary contusion is not generally associated with low speed penetration of the chest and laceration of the lung tissues and structures.

The overall magnitude of pulmonary injury depends on the degree of deformity or stretch, and the velocity at which it occurs. Similar pulmonary contusions may result from different mechanisms. For example, an AK-47 round fired at 2,300 ft/sec striking body armor and deforming the chest wall instantaneously by 1–2 cm (high velocity) may cause pulmonary contusions similar to chest impact during an MVA where the chest is deformed 50 percent as it strikes the steering wheel at 50 ft/sec (low velocity).

Microhemorrhage into the alveolar tissue associated with pulmonary contusion may be extensive and result in up to 1,000 to 1,500 mL of blood loss. This hemorrhage into the tissue of the alveoli also causes irritation, initiates the inflammation process, and causes fluid to migrate into the region. The accumulation of fluid in the alveolar/capillary membrane (pulmonary edema) progressively increases its dimension and decreases the rate at which gases, and especially oxygen, can diffuse across it. The fluid accumulation also stiffens the membrane, makes the lung less compliant, and increases the work necessary to move air in and out of the affected tissue.

The thickening wall reduces the efficiency of respiration and results in hypoxemia, while the stiffening makes respiration more energy consuming. The development of edema also increases the pressure necessary to move blood through the capillary beds. This increases the pressure within the pulmonary vascular system (pulmonary hypertension) and the workload of the right heart. In combination, these effects lead to atelectasis, hypovolemia, ventilation/perfusion mismatch, hypoxemia, hypotension and, possibly, respiratory failure and shock. Although isolated pulmonary contusions can occur, they are frequently associated with chest wall injury and injuries elsewhere (87 percent of the time).

The patient with pulmonary contusion presents with a mechanism of injury and evidence of blunt or penetrating chest impact. While the associated injuries may display immediate signs and symptoms (as in the pain of a rib fracture), the signs and symptoms of the pulmonary contusion take time to develop. The patient will likely complain of increasing dyspnea, demonstrate increasing respiratory effort, and show the signs of hypoxia. Oxygen saturation may gradually fall as the pathology develops. Careful auscultation of the chest may reveal increasing crackles and fainter breath sounds. Serious pulmonary contusion may cause **hemoptysis** (coughing up blood) and the signs and symptoms of shock.

Cardiovascular Injuries

Cardiovascular injuries are the subset of thoracic trauma that leads to the most fatalities. They include myocardial contusion, pericardial tamponade, myocardial aneurysm or rupture, aortic aneurysm or rupture, and other vascular injuries.

* **hemoptysis** coughing of blood that has origin in the respiratory tract.

Cardiovascular injuries are the subset of thoracic trauma that leads to the most fatalities.

FIGURE 25-11 Myocardial contusion most frequently affects the right atrium and ventricle as they collide with the sternum.

Myocardial Contusion

Myocardial contusion is a frequent result of trauma and may occur in 76 percent of all serious chest trauma. It carries a high mortality rate and occurs most commonly with severe blunt anterior chest trauma. Here, the chest is struck by or strikes an object. The heart, which is relatively mobile within the chest, impacts the inside of the anterior chest wall and then may be compressed between the sternum and the thoracic spine as the thorax flexes with impact. The resulting contusion will most likely affect the right atrium and right ventricle (Figure 25-11). This is related to the heart's position in the chest, rotated somewhat counterclockwise and presenting the right atrium and ventricle surfaces toward the sternum.

The cardiac contusion is similar to a contusion in any other muscle tissue. The injury disrupts the muscle cells and microcirculation, resulting in muscle fiber tearing and damage, hemorrhage, and edema. The injury may reduce the strength of cardiac contraction and reduce cardiac output. Because of the automaticity and conductivity of the cardiac muscle, contusion may also disturb the cardiac electrical system. If the injury is serious, it may lead to hematoma, hemoperitoneum (blood in the peritoneal sac), and necrosis and may result in cardiac irritability, ectopic (irregularly occurring) beats, and conduction system defects such as bundle branch blocks and dysrrhythmias. If the injury is very extensive, it may lead to tissue necrosis (death), decreased ventricular compliance, congestive heart failure, cardiogenic shock, myocardial aneurysm, and acute or delayed myocardial rupture. In contrast to a myocardial infarction from coronary artery disease, the cellular damage from myocardial contusions heals with less scarring and there is no progression of the injury in the absence of associated coronary artery disease.

The patient experiencing myocardial contusion will have a history of significant blunt chest trauma, most likely affecting the anterior chest. The patient will likely complain of chest or retrosternal pain, very much like that of myocardial infarction and may have associated chest injuries such as anterior rib or sternal fractures. Cardiac monitoring most frequently reveals sinus tachycardia (though

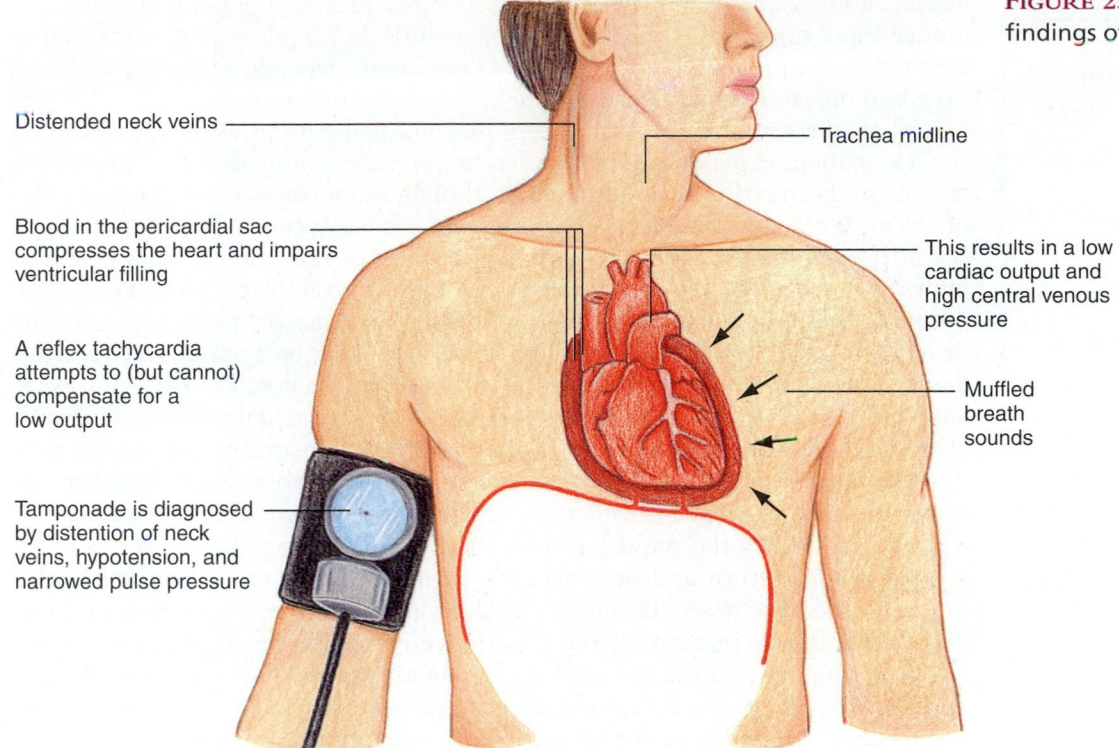

FIGURE 25-12   Physical findings of cardiac tamponade.

Distended neck veins

Trachea midline

Blood in the pericardial sac compresses the heart and impairs ventricular filling

This results in a low cardiac output and high central venous pressure

A reflex tachycardia attempts to (but cannot) compensate for a low output

Muffled breath sounds

Tamponade is diagnosed by distention of neck veins, hypotension, and narrowed pulse pressure

it may be caused by pain, hypovolemia, or hypoxia from associated chest injury). Other dysrhythmias associated with myocardial contusions are atrial flutter or fibrillation, premature atrial or ventricular contractions, tachydysrhythmias, bradydysrhythmias, bundle branch patterns, T wave inversions, and ST segment elevations. A pericardial friction rub and murmur may be auscultated over the **precordium** but is more likely to occur weeks after the injury and is associated with the development of an inflammatory pericardial effusion.

 precordium area of the chest wall overlying the heart.

Pericardial Tamponade

Pericardial tamponade is a restriction to cardiac filling caused by blood (or other fluid) within the pericardial sac. It occurs in less than 2 percent of all serious chest trauma patients and is almost always related to penetrating injury. Gunshot wounds are the most frequent mechanism and carry a high overall mortality, though they often result in rapid hemorrhage through the myocardial wall and then out the defect in the pericardium. The frequency of gunshot wound mortality is probably related to the depth of injury, the degree of cardiac tissue damage caused by the cavitational wave, and a more rapid progression of the pathology.

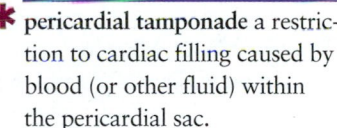 **pericardial tamponade** a restriction to cardiac filling caused by blood (or other fluid) within the pericardial sac.

The pathology of pericardial tamponade begins with a tear in a superficial coronary artery or penetration of the myocardium. Blood seeps into the pericardial space and accumulates (Figure 25-12). The fibrous pericardium does not stretch and the accumulating blood exerts pressure on the heart. The pressure limits cardiac filling, first affecting the right ventricle where the pressure of filling is the lowest. This restricts venous return to the heart, increases venous pressure, and causes jugular vein distention. The reduced right ventricular output limits outflow to the pulmonary arteries and then venous return to the left heart. The result is a decreasing cardiac output and systemic hypotension. The pressure exerted by the blood in the pericardium also restricts the flow of blood through the coronary arteries and to the myocardium. This may result in myocardial ischemia and

Content Review

SIGNS AND SYMPTOMS OF
PERICARDIAL TAMPONADE

Dyspnea and possible
 cyanosis
Jugular venous distention
Weak, thready, pulse
Decreasing blood pressure
Shock
Narrowing pulse pressure

infarct. It takes about 200 to 300 mL of blood to exert the pressure necessary to induce frank tamponade, while removing as little as 20 mL may provide significant relief. The progression of pericardial tamponade depends on the rate of blood flow into the pericardium. It may occur very rapidly and result in death before the arrival of emergency medical services or may gradually progress over hours.

The patient experiencing pericardial tamponade will likely have penetrating trauma to the anterior or posterior chest, though blunt trauma can also cause this problem. While the trajectories of missiles and knife blades are difficult to predict, consider pericardial tamponade with any thoracic or upper abdominal penetrating wound, especially if it is over the precordium (central lower chest). Pericardial tamponade will diminish the strength of pulses, decrease the pulse pressure, and distend the jugular veins (JVD). The patient will likely be agitated, tachycardic, diaphoretic, and ashen in appearance. Cyanosis may be noted in the head, neck, and upper extremities. Heart tones may be muffled or distant sounding. Beck's triad (JVD, distant heart tones, and hypotension) is indicative of pericardial tamponade but may not be recognized early in the injury's progression. Another sign of pericardial tamponade is Kussmaul's sign, the decrease or absence of JVD during inspiration. As the patient inspires, the reduced intrathoracic pressure increases venous return and decreases the pressure the accumulating pericardial fluid exerts on the heart. This then translates to a better venous return and cardiac output during inspiration and the effect then seen in the jugular veins.

Other findings during pericardial tamponade may include pulsus paradoxus and electrical alternans. **Pulsus paradoxus** is a drop in systolic blood pressure of greater than 10 mmHg as the patient inspires during the normal respiratory cycle. (Normally the systolic blood pressure drops just slightly with each inspiration.) Pulsus paradoxus results because cardiac output increases with the minimal relief of the tamponade associated with the reduced intrathoracic pressure of inspiration. **Electrical alternans,** which is only rarely seen in acute pericardial tamponade, is noted on the cardiac rhythm strip as the P, QRS, and T amplitude decreasing with every other cardiac cycle. In profound pericardial tamponade, the heart displays a rhythm without producing a pulse (PEA).

Myocardial Aneurysm or Rupture

Myocardial **aneurysm** or rupture occurs almost exclusively in extreme blunt thoracic trauma as in automobile collisions. It also has been reported in cases where the blunt forces are not extreme, such as a result of CPR. The condition can affect any of the heart's chambers, the interatrial septum, the interventricular septum, or involve the valves and their supporting structures. Multiple heart chambers or structures are involved 30 percent of the time. Aneurysm and delayed myocardial rupture also occur secondary to necrosis from a myocardial infarction, repaired penetrating injury, or myocardial contusion. Necrosis usually develops around two weeks after the injury as inflammatory cells degrade the injured cells, weakening the tissue, and leading to aneurysm of the ventricular wall and/or subsequent rupture. Rupture can also occur with high velocity projectile injury as the bullet impacts the distended heart chamber.

The patient who experiences myocardial rupture will likely have suffered serious blunt or penetrating trauma to the chest and may have severe rib or sternal fracture. Specific symptoms may depend upon the actual pathology. The victim may have the signs and symptoms of peircardial tamponade if the rupture is contained within the pericardial sac. If the pathology only affects the valves, the patient may present with the signs and symptoms of right or left heart failure. If there is myocardial aneurysm, rupture may be delayed. When it happens, the patient will suddenly present with the absence of vital signs or the signs and symptoms of pericardial tamponade.

* **pulsus paradoxus** drop of greater than 10 mmHg in the systolic blood pressure during the inspiratory phase of respiration that occurs in patients with pericardial tamponade.

* **electrical alternans** alternating amplitude of the P, QRS and T waves on the ECG rhythm strip as the heart swings in a pendulum-like fashion within the pericardial sac during tamponade.

* **aneurysm** a weakening or ballooning in the wall of a blood vessel.

Traumatic Aneurysm or Rupture of the Aorta

Aortic aneurysm and rupture are extremely life-threatening injuries resulting from either blunt or penetrating trauma. The aorta is most commonly injured by blunt trauma, carries an overall mortality of 85 to 95 percent, and is responsible for 15 percent of all thoracic trauma deaths. Aneurysm and rupture are usually associated with high-speed automobile crashes (most commonly lateral impact) and in some cases with high falls. Unlike myocardial rupture, a significant number, possibly as high as 20 percent, of these victims will survive the initial insult and aneurysm. Some 30 percent of these initial survivors will die in 6 hours if not treated, increasing to about 50 percent at 24 hours, and just under 70 percent by the end of the first week. It is this subset of patients that survive the initial impact and are alive at the scene that you can benefit the most by recognizing the potential injury and then by rapidly extricating, packaging, and transporting the patients to the trauma center.

Traumatic rupture of the thoracic aorta is almost always fatal.

The aorta is a large high-pressure vessel that provides outflow from the left ventricle for distribution to the body. It is relatively fixed at three points as it passes through the thoracic cavity and, because of this, experiences shear forces secondary to severe deceleration of the chest. The areas of fixation are the aortic annulus where the aorta joins the heart, the aortic isthmus where it is joined by the ligamentum arteriosum, and the diaphragm where it exits the chest (see Table 25-2). Traumatic dissecting aneurysm occurs infrequently to the ascending aorta and, most commonly, to the descending aorta. With severe deceleration, shear forces separate the layers of the artery, specifically the interior surface (the tunica intima) from the muscle layer (the tunica media). This allows blood to enter and, because it is under great pressure, it begins to dissect the aortic lining like a bulging inner tube. It is likely to rupture if it is not surgically repaired.

Serious lateral chest impact carries a high incidence of dissecting aortic aneurysm.

The patient with aortic rupture will be severely hypotensive, quickly lose all vital signs, and die unless moved into surgery immediately. Dissecting aortic aneurysm progresses more slowly, though the aneurysm may rupture at any moment. The patient will probably have a history of a high fall or severe auto impact and deceleration. Lateral impact is an especially high risk factor for aortic aneurysm. The patient may complain of severe tearing chest pain that may radiate to the back. The patient may have a pulse deficit between the left and right upper extremities and/or reduced pulse strength in the lower extremities. Blood pressure may be high (hypertension) due to stretching of sympathetic nerve fibers present in the aorta near the ligamentum arteriosum, or the pressure may be low due to leakage and hypovolemia. Auscultation may reveal a harsh systolic murmur due to turbulence as the blood exits the heart and passes the disrupted blood vessel wall.

OTHER VASCULAR INJURIES

The pulmonary arteries and vena cava are other thoracic vascular structures that can sustain injury during chest trauma. Their injury, and the resulting hemorrhage, may cause significant hemothorax, possibly leading to hypotension and respiratory insufficiency. The blood may also flow into the mediastinum and

Table 25-2	INCIDENCE AND ANATOMIC LOCATION OF TRAUMATIC AORTIC RUPTURE	
Aortic annulus		9%
Aortic isthmus		85%
Diaphragm		3%
Other		3%

compress the great vessels, esophagus, and heart. Penetrating trauma is the primary cause of injury to the pulmonary arteries and vena cava.

The patient with pulmonary artery or vena cava injuries will likely have a penetrating wound to the central chest or elsewhere with a likelihood of central chest involvement. These injuries present with the signs and symptoms of hypovolemia and shock and result in hemothorax or hemomediastinum and then the signs and symptoms associated with those pathologies.

OTHER THORACIC INJURIES

Traumatic Rupture or Perforation of the Diaphragm

Traumatic rupture or perforation of the diaphragm can occur in both high-pressure blunt thoracoabdominal trauma as well as in penetrating trauma. Incidence is estimated from 1 to 6 percent of all patients with multiple trauma. It is more common in patients sustaining penetrating trauma to the lower chest, which has as much as a 30 to 40 percent incidence of abdominal organ and tissue involvement. Remember that during expiration the diaphragm may move superiorly to the level of the 4th intercostal space (nipple level) anteriorly and the 6th intercostal space posteriorly. Any penetrating injuries at these levels or below may penetrate the diaphragm. Diaphragmatic perforation and herniation occur most frequently on the left side because assailants are most frequently right handed and the size and solid nature of the liver protect the diaphragm on the right. The liver is also unlikely to herniate through the torn diaphragm unless the injury is sizeable.

If traumatic diaphragmatic rupture occurs, the abdominal organs may herniate through the defect into the thoracic cavity causing strangulation or necrosis of the bowel, restriction of the ipsilateral lung, and displacement of the mediastinum. Mediastinal displacement occurs when the displaced abdominal contents place pressure on the lung and mediastinal structures, moving them toward the contralateral side through much the same mechanism as is seen in tension pneumothorax.

Diaphragmatic rupture presents with signs and symptoms similar to tension pneumothorax, including, dyspnea, hypoxia, hypotension, and JVD. The patient will have a history of blunt abdominal trauma or penetrating trauma to the lower thorax. The abdomen may appear hollow, and bowel sounds may be noted in one side of the thorax (most commonly the left). The patient may be hypotensive and hypoxic if the herniation is extensive. The patient may complain of upper abdominal pain, though this symptom is often overshadowed by other injuries. Diaphragmatic rupture may be recognized at the time of injury or may be missed if not extensive and present with delayed herniation months to years later.

Suspect diaphragmatic perforation with any penetrating injury to the lower thorax.

Traumatic Esophageal Rupture

Traumatic esophageal rupture is a rare complication of blunt thoracic trauma. The incidence of it related to penetrating trauma of the thorax is somewhat higher but still only about 0.4 percent. Since the esophagus is rather centrally located within the chest, its injury usually coincides with other mediastinal injuries. (Esophageal rupture may also be the result of medical problems such as violent emesis, carcinoma, anatomic distortion, or gastric reflux.) Esophageal rupture carries a 30 percent mortality, even if quickly recognized, and mortality is much greater if this injury is not diagnosed promptly. The life threat from esophageal rupture is related to material entering the mediastinum as it passes down the esophagus or as emesis comes up. This results in serious infection or chemical irritation and serious damage to the mediastinal structures. Air may also enter the mediastinum through an esophageal rupture, especially during positive pressure ventilations.

The patient with espophageal rupture will probably have deep penetrating trauma to the central chest and may complain of difficult or painful swallowing, pleuritic chest pain, and pain radiating to the mid back. The patient may also display subcutaneous emphysema around the lower neck.

Tracheobronchial Injury (Disruption)

Tracheobronchial injury is a relatively rare finding in thoracic trauma with an incidence of less than 3 percent in patients with significant chest trauma. It may occur from either a blunt or a penetrating injury mechanism and carries a relatively high mortality similar to esophageal rupture of 30 percent. In contrast to patients with esophageal rupture who usually die days after injury, 50 percent of patients with tracheobronchial injury die within 1 hour of injury. Disruption can occur anywhere in the tracheobronchial tree but is most likely to occur within 2.5 cm of the carina.

The patient with disruption of the trachea or mainstem bronchi is generally in respiratory distress with cyanosis, hemoptysis, and, in some cases, massive subcutaneous emphysema. The patient may also experience pneumothorax and possibly, tension pneumothorax. Intermittent positive pressure ventilation drives air into the pleura or mediastinum and makes the condition worse.

Traumatic Asphyxia

Traumatic asphyxia occurs when severe compressive force is applied to the thorax and leads to backwards flow of blood from the right heart into the superior vena cava and into the venous vessels of the upper extremities. (Traumatic asphyxia is not as much a respiratory problem as it is a vascular problem.) Traumatic asphyxia engorges the veins and capillaries of the head and neck with desaturated venous blood, turning the skin in this region a deep red, purple, or blue. The back flow of blood damages the microcirculation in the head and neck, producing petechiae (small hemorrhages under the skin) and stagnating blood above the point of compression. The back flow may damage cerebral circulation, resulting in numerous small strokes in the older patient whose venous vessels are not very elastic. If flow restriction continues, toxins and acids accumulate in the blood and may have a devastating effect when they return to the central circulation with the release of pressure. If the thoracic compression continues, it restricts venous return and may prevent the victim from ventilating. This results in hypotension, hypoxemia, and shock. Death may follow rapidly. Extrication of the patient may result in rapid hemorrhage from the injury site with release of the pressure. Release of the compression may likewise result in rapid patient deterioration and death.

The traumatic asphyxia patient will have suffered a severe compression force to the chest that is likely to continue until extrication. The result of the compression, the back flow of blood and restricted blood flow, will be dramatic and cause the classical discoloration of the head and neck regions. The face appears swollen, the eyes bulge, and there are numerous conjunctival hemorrhages. The patient may have severe dyspnea related to the compression and injuries associated with severe chest impact. Once the pressure is released, the patient may show the signs of hypovolemia, hypotension, and shock as well as signs related to any co-existing respiratory problems.

You must be ready to immediately handle the complications of traumatic asphyxia as soon as the patient is released from entrapment.

ASSESSMENT OF THE THORACIC TRAUMA PATIENT

The proper assessment of the patient with a severe chest injury mechanism is critical to anticipating injury and providing the correct interventions. While the approach to this patient follows the standard format for assessment, special considerations regarding chest trauma occur during the scene size-up, initial assessment, and especially during the rapid trauma assessment. The ongoing assessment is also critical for monitoring the thoracic trauma patient for the progression of injuries sustained during serious chest trauma.

SCENE SIZE-UP

Chest injury care, like that for any other serious trauma, requires body substance isolation procedures with gloves as a minimum. Consider a face shield if you will be attending to the airway and a gown for splash protection with serious penetrating thoracic trauma. Assure the scene is safe, including protection from the assailant, if penetrating trauma is suspected.

Examine the mechanism of injury carefully and try to determine if the central chest (heart, great vessels, trachea, and esophagus) might be in the pathway of penetrating trauma. In gunshot injuries, determine the type of weapon, caliber, distance between the gun barrel and the victim, and the probable pathway of the projectile. Determine the direction of blunt trauma impact as it may also have a bearing on which organs sustain injury. Anterior impact may rupture lung tissue and contuse the lung and heart. Lateral impact may tear the aorta as the heart displaces laterally and stresses the aorta's ligamentous attachments.

INITIAL ASSESSMENT

During the initial assessment, determine the patient's mental status and the status of the airway, breathing, and circulation. Intervene as necessary to correct life threatening conditions. It is during the initial assessment that you will first identify the signs and symptoms of serious chest trauma. Be especially watchful for any dyspnea, asymmetrical, paradoxical, or limited chest movement, hyperinflation of the chest, or an abdomen that appears hollow. Notice any general patient color reflective of hypoxia such as cyanosis or an ashen discoloration. Look for distended jugular veins, costal or suprasternal retractions, and the use of accessory muscles of respiration.

<table>
<tr><td>

Administer ventilations with care in the patient with chest trauma.

</td></tr>
</table>

Assure that ventilation is adequate and administer high flow oxygen by nonrebreather mask. Administer any positive pressure ventilations with care as thoracic injury may weaken the lung tissue and make the patient prone to pneumothorax or tension pneumothorax. Aggressive (or even cautious) ventilations may induce these problems. Be suspicious of internal hemorrhage and initiate at least one large-bore intravenous catheter and line in anticipation of hypovolemia, hypotension, and shock. With anterior blunt or penetrating trauma that may involve the heart, attach the ECG electrodes and monitor for dysrrhythmias. Attach a pulse oximeter and monitor oxygen saturation to evaluate the effectiveness of respiration. If there is any mechanism suggesting serious trauma to the chest or any physical signs of either hypoventilation or hypovolemia compensation, perform the rapid trauma assessment with a special focus on the chest and prepare for rapid patient transport to the trauma center.

RAPID TRAUMA ASSESSMENT

During the rapid trauma assessment you will examine the patient's chest in detail, carefully observing, questioning about, palpating, and auscultating the region.

Observe

Observe the chest for evidence of impact. Look for the erythema that develops early in the contusion process, especially as it outlines the ribs or forms a pattern reflecting the contours of the object the chest hit. Look carefully for penetrating trauma and try to determine the angle of entry and depth of penetration. Also look for exit wounds. Lateral chest injury is likely to involve the lungs, while a pathway of energy through the central chest is likely to involve the heart, great vessels, trachea, or esophagus. Injury to the mediastinal structures is also likely to result in serious hemorrhage, hypovolemia, and shock. Look for intercostal and suprasternal retractions as well as external jugular vein distention. Remember, JVD is present in supine normotensive patients and may be exaggerated in them or may continue when the patient is moved to the seated position if venous pressure is elevated.

Watch chest movement carefully during respiration. The chest should rise and the abdomen should fall smoothly with inspiration and return to position during expiration. Any limited motion, either bilaterally or unilaterally, suggests a problem. Watch for the paradoxical motion of flail chest. That movement will be limited due to muscle spasm during early care, but continued motion will further damage the surrounding soft tissue and the intracostal muscles will fatigue. This will lead to a more obvious paradoxical motion and greater respiratory embarrassment with time. Look, too, for any hyperinflation of one side of the chest and any deformity that may exist from rib fracture, sternal fracture or dislocation, or subcutaneous emphysema. Assess the volume of air effectively moved with each breath and assure that the minute volume is greater than 6 liters. If not, consider overdrive ventilation with the bag-valve mask. Examine any open wound for air movement in or out, which is indicative of an open pneumothorax. Observe the patient's general color. If a patient's skin is dusky, ashen, or cyanotic, suspect respiratory compromise. If the head and neck are red, dark red, or blue, suspect traumatic asphyxia.

Question

Question the patient about any pain, pain on motion, pain with breathing effort (pleuritic pain), or dyspnea. Note if the pain is crushing, tearing, or is described otherwise by the patient. Have the patient describe the exact location of the pain, its severity, and any radiation of the pain. Question about other sensations and carefully monitor the patient's level of consciousness and orientation.

Palpate

Palpate the thorax carefully, feeling for any signs of injury (Figure 25-13). Feel for any swelling, deformity, crepitus, or the crackling of subcutaneous emphysema. Compress the thorax between your hands with pressure directed inward.

You may have to rely on your palpation skills to assess chest injuries when scene noise is excessive.

FIGURE 25-13 Carefully palpate the thorax of a patient with a suspected injury to the region.

FIGURE 25-14   Place your hands on the lower thorax and let them rise and fall with respiration.

Then apply downward pressure on the mid-sternum. Such pressure will flex the ribs and should elicit pain from any fracture site along the thorax. (Apply pressure only if you are unsure of chest injury. If you suspect rib or sternal fracture, provide appropriate care but do not aggravate the injury.) Rest your hands on the lower thorax and let the chest lift your hands with inspiration and let them fall with expiration (Figure 25-14). The motion should be smooth and equal. If not, determine the nature of any asymmetry.

Auscultate

Auscultate all lung lobes, both anteriorly and posteriorly (Figure 25-15). Listen for both inspiratory and expiratory air movement and note any crackles, indicating edema from contusion or congestive heart failure, or any diminished breath sounds, suggesting hypoventilation. Compare one side to the other and one lobe to another. Be sensitive for distant or muffled respiratory or heart sounds.

FIGURE 25-15   Auscultate all lung lobes, both anteriorly and posteriorly.

FIGURE 25-16   Percuss all lung lobes, listening for a dull response or hyperresonance.

Percuss

Percuss the chest and note the responses (Figure 25-16). Determine if the area percussed is normal, hyperresonant, or dull. A dull response suggests collecting blood or other fluid, while hyperresonance suggests air or air under pressure as in a pneumothorax or tension pneumothorax.

Your findings from the rapid trauma assessment may suggest an injury or multiple injuries. Identify the likely cause of the signs and symptoms you find and suspect and anticipate the worst. You are likely to note clear evidence of chest wall injury and some signs of internal injuries if they exist. As mentioned earlier, blunt and penetrating trauma present with different typical injuries.

Blunt Trauma Assessment

In blunt trauma, you commonly find slight discoloration of the surface of the chest reflective of contusions. The contusions also cause the patient pain, generally in an area or region, and somewhat limit respiration. As the impact energy increases, it may cause fractures of ribs 4 through 9 and a greater possibility of underlying injury. If the upper ribs or ribs 10 through 12 fracture, suspect serious underlying injury. Sternal fracture takes great energy and is also associated with a higher incidence of internal injury. Rib fractures generate a point-specific pain (at the fracture site) and crepitus upon deep breathing or your flexing of the patient's chest during the rapid trauma assessment. That pain may further limit chest excursion during respiration. As the energy of trauma and the seriousness of chest trauma increase, more ribs may fracture, causing a flail chest. Remember that a flail chest's paradoxical motion is initially limited by muscular splinting and grows more noticeable and causes more respiratory distress as time since the collision increases.

In blunt injury to the chest, you must anticipate and assess for additional signs suggesting internal injury. Signs specific for lung injury include increasing dyspnea, signs of hypoxemia, accessory muscle use, and intracostal and suprasternal retractions. Auscultation will help you differentiate between pulmonary contusion and pneumothorax. Contusions demonstrate progressively increasing crackles, while pneumothorax presents with diminished breath sounds on the ipsilateral side. Further, with pneumothorax the affected side may be hyperinflated and resonant to percussion. If the pneumothorax progresses to tension pneumothorax, you will likely note progressing dyspnea and hypoxia, use of accessory muscles, distended jugular veins, tracheal shift toward the contralateral side (a late finding), and hyperresonance of the ipsilateral chest on percussion. Subcutaneous emphysema may develop, especially if the lung defect was caused by or is associated with a rib fracture that disturbs the integrity of the parietal pleura. Hemothorax is noticeable due to the vascular loss, more so than for the respiratory component of the pathology. Suspect it if you find the signs of hypovolemia associated with blunt chest trauma. Hemothorax, when sizeable, may cause dyspnea and a lung field that is dull to percussion.

Blunt mediastinal injury will probably affect the heart, great vessels, and trachea. Heart injury may present with chest pain similar to that of the myocardial infarction and, if serious enough, with the signs of heart failure or cardiogenic shock. The ECG may reveal tachycardia, bradycardia, cardiac irritability, and, in cases of severe cardiac contusion, may demonstrate ST elevation. Cardiac rupture presents with the signs of sudden death, while pericardial tamponade is unlikely in blunt chest trauma. Injury to the great vessels (aneurysm) is most frequently associated with lateral impacts or feet-first high falls and may produce a tearing chest pain and pulse deficits in the extremities. If the aneurysm ruptures, rapidly progressing hypovolemia, hypotension, shock, and death ensue. Tracheobronchial injury results in rapidly developing pneumomediastinum or pneumothorax and possible subcutaneous emphysema, hemoptysis, dyspnea, and hypoxia. Positive pressure ventilations may increase the development and severity of signs. Traumatic asphyxia presents with jugular vein distention, discoloration of the head and neck, severe dyspnea, and possibly the signs of hypovolemia and shock.

Penetrating Trauma Assessment

Remember, the severity of internal injury associated with penetrating trauma may be great despite seemingly minor entrance and/or exit wounds.

Penetrating injury displays a different set of signs associated with different injuries. Inspect a chest wound for frothy blood or sounds of air exchange with respirations (open pneumothorax). Remember that a wound needs to be rather large (high-velocity bullet exit wound or close-range shotgun blast) for these signs to occur. A penetrating wound, however, commonly induces a simple pneumothorax with its associated signs and symptoms. A hyperinflated chest, distended jugular veins, tracheal shift away from the injury, distant or absent breath sounds, hyperresonance to percussion, and severe dyspnea and hypotension suggest tension pneumothorax. The pressure of tension pneumothorax may push air outward through a penetrating wound or cause subcutaneous emphysema around the wound. Some degree of hemothorax is likely to be associated with penetrating chest trauma and, if extensive, may reveal diminished or absent breath sounds and a chest region that is dull to percussion. Hemothorax also causes or significantly contributes to hypovolemia and shock.

Penetrating trauma to the heart is likely to cause pericardial tamponade and present with jugular vein distention, distant heart sounds, and hypotension (Beck's triad). Pulsus paradoxus may be present and jugular filling may occur with inspiration (Kussmaul's sign), and both are indicative of pericardial tamponade. Heart sounds are distant, pulses are weak, and the patient experiences increasing hypotension and shock (Figure 25-17). Penetrating trauma to the heart may also cause myocardial rupture and associated pericardial tamponade or immediate death (Figure 25-18). The patient demonstrates vital signs that fall precipitously as the vascular volume is pumped into the mediastinum.

ONGOING ASSESSMENT

Continuous reassessment of the patient with chest injury is essential as deterioration may occur within a matter of seconds.

While the ongoing assessment simply repeats elements of the initial assessment, the taking of vital signs, and examination of any injury signs discovered during earlier assessment, it takes on great importance for the patient with chest trauma. With any serious chest impact or any penetrating injury to the chest, observe the respiratory depth, rate, and symmetry of effort. Auscultate the lung fields for equality and

FIGURE 25-17 Penetrating stab wound to the chest involving the heart.

FIGURE 25-18 Stab wound that penetrated the pericardium.

crackles and monitor the distal pulses, oxygen saturation, skin color, and blood pressure for signs of progressing hypovolemia (Figure 25-19). If any signs change between assessments, search out the cause and rule out progressing chest injury. Be especially suspicious of developing tension pnuemothorax, pericardial tamponade, extensive and evolving pulmonary contusion, and hypovolemia associated with hemothorax. If any of these is found, institute the appropriate management steps.

MANAGEMENT OF THE CHEST INJURY PATIENT

The general management of the patient with significant chest injury focuses on assuring good oxygenation and adequate respiratory volume and rate. Administer high flow oxygen using the nonrebreather mask. Assure the airway is patent and consider endotracheal intubation if there is any significant loss in the level of consciousness or orientation. Consider intubation early in your care, as patients with thoracic trauma are likely to get worse with time. Rapid sequence intubation may be needed for the combative patient. Endotracheal intubation also makes ventilation of the flail chest or pulmonary contusion patient easier.

General management of the patient with serious chest trauma requires assurance of good oxygenation and adequate respiratory volume and rate.

Management of the Chest Injury Patient **1125**

Carefully evaluate the minute volume of the patient (breaths per minute times volume) and if it is less than 6,000 mL consider overdrive ventilation. Bag-valve mask the conscious patient with severe dyspnea at a rate of 12 to 16 full breaths per minute, trying to match the patient's respiratory rate. Closely monitor pulse oximetry, level of consciousness, and skin color. Bag-valve masking may also be beneficial for the patient with serious rib fractures and flail chest. The positive pressure displaces the chest outward, reducing the movement of the fracture site and moving the flail segment with the chest. It may also be beneficial to the patient who is exhausted from the increased breathing effort associated with pulmonary contusion. In this case, the ventilations help push any fluids back into the vascular system to relieve edema. Remember, however, that positive pressure ventilations change the dynamics of respiration from a less than atmospheric to a greater than atmospheric process and may exacerbate respiratory problems like tracheobronchial injury, pneumothorax, and tension pneumothorax.

Anticipate heart and great vessel compromise with thoracic injury and be ready to stabilize the patient's cardiovascular system. Initiate at least one large-bore IV site if the patient has a serious mechanism of chest trauma and place two lines if there are any signs of hypovolemia or compensation. Be prepared to administer fluids quickly if the patient's blood pressure begins to fall. Use of the PASG is contraindicated for penetrating chest trauma as it may increase the rate and volume of blood loss and disrupt the clotting process. The PASG should be used only in blunt chest trauma and then only when the blood pressure drops below 60 mmHg or the pulses disappear.

IV fluid infusion for the patient with chest trauma should be conservative. Rapid fluid administration may increase the rate of hemorrhage and dilute the clotting factors, further adding to the problem. Additional fluid also increases the edema associated with pulmonary contusion, increasing the rate and extent of its development. Anytime you administer fluids to the chest trauma patient, auscultate all lung fields carefully and reduce the fluid resuscitation rate whenever you hear respiratory crackles or the patient's dyspnea increases.

Care is specific for thoracic injuries including rib fractures, sternoclavicular dislocation, flail chest, open pneumothorax, tension pneumothorax, hemothorax, cardiac contusion, pericardial tamponade, aortic aneurysm, tracheobronchial injury, and traumatic asphyxia.

Remember, aggressive fluid resuscitation in the patient with chest trauma can result in hemodilution and loss of clotting factors.

RIB FRACTURES

Rib fractures, either isolated or associated with other respiratory injuries, may produce pain that significantly limits respiratory effort and leads to hypoventilation. In these patients you may consider administering analgesics to grant greater patient comfort and improve chest excursion. Assure that the patient is hemodynamically stable, that there is no associated abdominal or head injury, and that the patient is fully conscious and oriented. Consider administration of diazepam, morphine sulfate, meperidine, or nalbuphine as described in Chapter 22, "Musculoskeletal Trauma." Note that use of nitrous oxide is contraindicated in chest trauma as the nitrogen may migrate into a pneumothorax or tension pneumothorax.

STERNOCLAVICULAR DISLOCATION

Supportive therapy with oxygen is usually all that is required for an isolated sternoclavicular dislocation. However, hemodynamic instability indicates associated injuries requiring rapid transport to the trauma center with aggressive resuscitation measures instituted en route. If you suspect posterior sternoclavicular dislocation and note the patient to be in significant respiratory distress that is not effectively treated with initial airway maneuvers and high flow oxygen, then consider dislocation reduction. Place the patient in the supine position with a sandbag between the shoulder blades. The sandbag helps to pull the shoulders backward and moves the head of the clavicle laterally and away from the trachea. Do not perform this procedure for the multiple-trauma patient due to the probability of spine injury. An alternative reduction method is to place the patient supine and grasp the clavicle near the sternum. Pull it upward and laterally, directly perpendicular to the sternum. This distracts the clavicle forward, alleviating its impingement of the airway.

FLAIL CHEST

Place the patient on the side of injury if spinal immobilization is not required, or secure a large and bulky dressing with bandaging against the flail segment to stabilize it (Figure 25-20). Employ high flow oxygen therapy, monitor oxygen saturation with pulse oximetry, and monitor cardiac activity with the ECG. If there is significant dyspnea, evidence of underlying pulmonary injury, or signs of respiratory compromise, these measures will not suffice. Then consider endotracheal intubation, positive pressure ventilations, and high flow oxygen. Positive pressure ventilations internally splint the flail segment, expand atelectatic areas of the lung, and also treat underlying pulmonary contusion. Use of sandbags to support the flail segment is not indicated because it may diminish chest movement, adding to hypoventilation, atelectasis, and subsequent hypoxemia. Rapid transport to the trauma center is indicated as this injury, its complications, and associated injuries are life threatening.

Consider early intubation of the patient with flail chest, especially when oxygenation remains impaired despite the provision of high flow oxygen.

OPEN PNEUMOTHORAX

Support the patient with open pneumothorax by administering high flow oxygen and monitoring oxygen saturation and respiratory effort. If you find a penetrating

FIGURE 25-20 Flail chest should be treated with administration of oxygen and gentle splinting of the flail segment with a pillow or pad.

injury, cover it with a sterile occlusive dressing (sterile plastic wrap) taped on three sides (Figure 25-21). This process converts the open pneumothorax into a closed pneumothorax, prevents further aspiration of air, and relieves any building pressure (tension pneumothorax) through the valve-like dressing. If the dyspnea diminishes somewhat but still continues, provide positive pressure ventilations and intubate as indicated. Carefully monitor the patient when you employ intermittent positive pressure ventilation because its use may lead to a tension pneumothorax. If after the dressing has been applied, the patient has progressive breathing difficulty, appears to be hypoventilating and hypoxemic, has decreasing breath sounds on the injured side and increasing jugular distention, remove the occlusive dressing. If you hear air rush out and the patient's respirations improve, reseal the wound, monitor respiration carefully, and again remove the dressing if any respiratory signs or symptoms redevelop. If removing the dressing does not relieve the increasing signs and symptoms, suspect and treat for tension pneumothorax.

TENSION PNEUMOTHORAX

Confirm possible tension pneumothorax by auscultating the lung fields for diminished breath sounds, percussing for hyperresonnace, and observing for severe dyspnea, hyperinflation of the chest, and jugular vein distention. Successful treatment depends on rapid recognition of this condition and then pleural decompression. As you prepare to decompress the affected (ipsilateral) side, apply high flow oxygen if the airway is intact and the patient is able to demonstrate adequate ventilatory effort.

FIGURE 25-21 By taping the occlusive dressing on three sides, you create a flutter valve that helps to prevent tension pneumothorax.

On inspiration, dressing seals wound, preventing air entry

Collapsed lung

Expiration allows trapped air to escape through untaped section of dressing

Provide ventilations with the bag-valve mask and supplemental oxygen and intubate if the patient is unable to maintain an airway or continues to show signs/symptoms of hypoxemia on high flow oxygen. Perform needle thoracentesis by inserting a 14-gauge intravascular catheter into the 2nd intercostal space, midclavicular line on the side of the thorax with decreased breath sounds and hyperinflation (Figure 25-22). Attach a syringe filled with sterile water or saline to the needle hub of the catheter. Then advance the catheter through the chest wall while maintaining gentle traction on the syringe plunger. Assure you enter the thoracic cavity by passing the needle just over the rib. The intercostal artery, vein, and nerve pass just under each rib and may be injured if the needle's track is too high. As you enter the pleural space, you will feel a pop and note bubbling air through the fluid in the syringe. Advance the catheter into the chest and then withdraw the needle and syringe.

If the patient remains symptomatic, place a second or third catheter to more rapidly facilitate decompression. Secure the catheter in place with tape, being careful not to block the port or kink the catheter. Leaving the catheter open to air converts the tension pneumothorax into a simple pneumothorax and stabilizes the patient. You may create a flutter valve by cutting the finger off a latex glove, making a small perforation in its tip, and securing it to the catheter hub. Monitor the patient's respirations and breath sounds for a recurring tension pneumothorax. If signs and symptoms again appear, decompress the chest again. Frequently, the initial catheter will clog or kink and necessitate replacement by another.

Tension pneumothorax is an occasional complication of multiple trauma. Always assess for it and decompress the chest when indicated.

2nd rib

The intercostal vessels and nerves are located at the inferior borders of the ribs.

To avoid damaging the intercostal neurovascular bundle with needle or catheter, follow the upper border of the 3rd rib in entering the pleural space.

3rd rib

Lung   Parietal pleura

Midclavicular line

Sternum

Angle of Louis

Lung

Heart

Ribs

Diaphragm

Pleural space

FIGURE 25-22   Needle decompression of a tension pneumothorax.

Management of the Chest Injury Patient   **1129**

Rapidly transport the patient to the trauma center for definitive treatment (usually with a chest tube). Be cautious in using IV crystalloid infusion if the patient is hemodynamically stable. An underlying pulmonary contusion may lead to edema, which is made worse with overaggressive fluid therapy. If your patient remains hypotensive after chest decompression and respirations do not become adequate, consider the possibility of internal hemorrhage and the need for (conservative) fluid resuscitation. If respirations do not dramatically improve, assess for a contralateral tension pneumothorax or pericardial tamponade as the cause.

HEMOTHORAX

Treat the patient with suspected hemothorax with oxygen administration and respiratory support, as needed. Initiate two large-bore intravenous catheters, readied to infuse large volumes of fluid. Be conservative in fluid administration. Maintain blood pressure (between 90–100 mmHg) but do not attempt to return it to pre-injury levels. Carefully listen to breath sounds during any infusion because the increasing vascular volume may increase the edema and congestion of pulmonary contusion. It may also increase the pressure, rate, and volume of internal hemorrhage. If the pulmonary contusion is extensive and the patient cannot be adequately oxygenated by high flow oxygen, positive pressure ventilations are indicated and may limit further edema that contributes to the injury

MYOCARDIAL CONTUSION

In serious frontal impact collisions, suspect myocardial contusion and administer high flow oxygen. Monitor cardiac electrical activity and watch for tachycardias, bradycardias, ectopic beats, and conduction defects. Establish an IV line in the event that antidysrhythmics (such as lidocaine) are needed, and monitor the patient for great vessel injury. Employ the pharmacological care measures recommended for advanced cardiac life support (Chapter 28, "Cardiology"). Rapidly transport the patient to the trauma center for further evaluation and continued monitoring.

PERICARDIAL TAMPONADE

If pericardial tamponade is suspected, consider diverting to the closest hospital with a physician-staffed emergency department where emergency pericardiocentesis can be performed.

Maintain a high index of suspicion for pericardial tamponade in the patient with central thoracic penetrating trauma. While there is little prehospital care other than the administration of oxygen and some IV fluids to maximize venous return, definitive care is to remove some of the fluid accumulating in the pericardial sac. This action is rarely permitted in the field; hence the patient needs to be transported as rapidly as possible to the emergency department. Note that a relatively simple procedure can relieve this problem and can be adequately administered by an emergency physician. If a physician-staffed emergency department is closer to you than the trauma center, it may be the best choice for the patient with pericardial tamponade. After the pericardiocentesis is performed, the patient may then be directed to the closest trauma center.

AORTIC ANEURYSM

Care for the patient with dissecting aortic aneurysm is gentle but rapid transport to the trauma center. Any jarring during extrication, assessment, care, packaging, or transport increases the risk of rupture and rapidly fatal exsanguination. Initiate IV therapy en route, but be very conservative in fluid administration. Mild hypotension may be protective of the injury site. If the aneurysm ruptures, as indicated by an immediate deterioration in vital signs, provide rapid administration of fluids. Anxiety and its effect on cardiac output and blood pressure may increase the likelihood of aneurysm rupture. Place a special emphasis on calming and reassuring the patient during very gentle care and transport.

TRACHEOBRONCHIAL INJURY

Support the tracheobronchial injury patient with oxygen and clear the airway of blood and secretions. If you are unable to maintain a patent airway or adequately oxygenate the patient, then intubate the trachea and provide positive pressure ventilations. Observe the patient carefully for the development of a tension pneumothorax, which may result as a complication of positive pressure ventilations, and treat as previously prescribed. Provide rapid transport as soon as the patient can be extricated and stabilized. This is important because these patients can rapidly destabilize and then require emergency surgical intervention.

TRAUMATIC ASPHYXIA

Administer oxygen and support the airway and respiration of the traumatic asphyxia patient. This may require using positive pressure ventilations with the bag-valve mask to assure adequate ventilation during the entrapment and possibly thereafter. Establish two large-bore IV lines for rapid infusion of crystalloid in anticipation of rapidly developing hypovolemia with chest decompression. Once the compressing force is removed, the direct effects of traumatic asphyxia spontaneously resolve; however, serious internal hemorrhage may begin. Prepare to transport immediately after release from entrapment because the patient will likely have severe coexisting injuries.

If the patient remains entrapped for a prolonged time, consider the administration of sodium bicarbonate. Prolonged stagnant blood flow and a hypoxic cellular environment may cause accumulation of metabolic acids. As the compression is released, this blood returns to the central circulation, much as it does with entrapped limbs during crush injury. Consider the administration of 1 mEq/kg of sodium bicarbonate just before or during decompression of the chest if entrapment has lasted more than 20 minutes. Employ this therapy as discussed in Chapter 20, "Soft-Tissue Trauma."

SUMMARY

Thoracic trauma by either blunt or penetrating mechanisms has a great potential for posing a threat to a patient's life. In fact, 25 percent of all traumatic deaths are secondary to injuries in this region. In assessing these patients, the mechanism of injury, when considered along with the clinical findings, may help in differentiating among the many possible injuries. The assessment, in turn, helps guide your interventions and determines the need for rapid extrication and transport. Aggressive airway management, oxygenation, ventilation, and fluid resuscitation, when indicated, can make the difference between the patient's survival or death. Specific interventions, such as pleural decompression or stabilization of a flail segment, can also affect mortality and morbidity from chest trauma. Understanding the pathologic processes affecting the chest during trauma and employing proper assessment and care measures will assure the best possible outcome for your patients.

CHAPTER 26

Abdominal Trauma

Objectives

After reading this chapter, you should be able to:

1. Describe the epidemiology, including morbidity/mortality, for patients with abdominal trauma as well as prevention strategies to avoid the injuries. (p. 1134)

2. Apply the epidemiologic principles to develop prevention strategies for abdominal injuries. (p. 1134)

3. Describe the anatomy and physiology of the abdominal organs and structures. (see Chapter 3)

4. Predict abdominal injuries based on blunt and penetrating mechanisms of injury. (pp. 1135–1143)

5. Describe open and closed abdominal injuries. (pp. 1135–1138)

6. Identify the need for rapid intervention and transport of the patient with abdominal injuries based on assessment findings. (pp. 1143–1149)

7. Explain the pathophysiology of solid and hollow organ injuries, abdominal vascular injuries, pelvic fractures, and other abdominal injuries. (pp. 1138–1143)

8. Describe the assessment findings associated with and the management of solid and hollow organ injuries,

Continued

Objectives Continued

abdominal vascular injuries, pelvic fractures, and other abdominal injuries. (pp. 1143–1151)

9. Differentiate between abdominal injuries based on the assessment and history. (pp. 1143–1149)

10. Given several pre-programmed and moulaged abdominal trauma patients, provide the appropriate scene size-up, initial assessment, rapid trauma or focused physical exam and history, detailed exam, and ongoing assessment and provide appropriate patient care and transportation. (pp. 1143–1151)

INTRODUCTION TO ABDOMINAL TRAUMA

The abdominal cavity is one of the body's largest cavities and contains many vital organs essential to life. Serious direct or secondary injury may damage these vital organs. In addition, large volumes of blood can be lost in the cavity before the loss becomes evident. In the abdomen, however, injury does not always present as dramatically as it does elsewhere in the body. Injury often occurs without overt signs because few skeletal structures protect the abdomen. The signs of transmitted injury—deformity, swelling, and the discoloration of contusions—take time to develop and are not often seen in the prehospital setting. These considerations make the anticipation of possible abdominal injuries and careful abdominal assessment critical for the patient with trauma to this region.

Over the past decade, the relative mortality and morbidity for the various abdominal injuries has declined due to improved surgical and critical care techniques. Reduced injury-to-surgery times have also contributed to this decline as EMS systems have recognized the necessity of rapid surgical intervention. The severity of injuries and the number of deaths associated with blunt trauma have also decreased thanks to improvements in highway design and vehicle structure and to a greater use of seat belts and other safety practices. However, the overall mortality and morbidity from penetrating trauma is on the rise due to the increasing violence in our society, most specifically, in the growing use and power of handguns. Penetrating trauma is approaching trauma associated with auto accidents as the number-one trauma killer. Nowhere is this more apparent than with injuries to the abdomen.

Prevention of abdominal injuries, as with most other types of trauma, is the best way to reduce mortality and morbidity. As noted, highway and vehicle design improvements and the following of safety practices at home and in the workplace play important roles in reducing both the incidence and seriousness of abdominal injury.

There remains room for further improvements in safety practices, however. For example, many people still do not use seat belts. Failure to use the seat belt increases the incidence of abdominal injury secondary to impact with the steering wheel, dash, or other parts of the auto's interior and of impact after ejection. (Side impact air bags have the potential to reduce the incidence of pelvic fracture and internal abdominal injuries frequently associated with this mechanism of injury.)

One area of special concern is the proper application of the auto lap belt. If the belt rides too high on the abdomen, with deceleration the belt directs forces both to the contents of the abdominal cavity and to the lumbar spine. Severe compression may result in serious associated abdominal injury. Proper placement, in which the belt rests on the iliac crests, transmits the forces of severe deceleration to the pelvis and the body's skeletal structure, thus sparing the abdominal contents and the spine from injury. Proper positioning of seat belts is especially important with children.

Mortality and morbidity associated with penetrating trauma can also be reduced by reducing violence in the society and by reducing the availability of hand guns.

PATHOPHYSIOLOGY OF ABDOMINAL INJURY

MECHANISM OF INJURY

Unlike the other major body containers (skull, spine, and thorax), the abdomen is bound by muscles rather than skeletal structures. This results in a freer transmission of the energy of trauma to the internal organs and structures. Concurrently, the overt physical signs of this energy transmission are limited.

Penetrating trauma imparts its energy directly to the tissues touched by the offending object (Figure 26-1) or, as with high-velocity projectiles (from handguns, shotguns, and rifles), transmits energy and injury some distance from the projectile pathway. The bullet injury process causes damage as the projectile contacts tissue, sets that tissue and surrounding tissue in motion, then compresses and stretches surrounding tissue. The projectile adds to the damage as it draws debris and contaminants into the wound, causing wound infection and poor healing. The disruption of tissue from penetrating trauma may permit uncontrolled hemorrhage, organ damage, the spillage of hollow organ contents, and, eventually, irritation of the abdominal lining, the peritoneum. Gunshot wounds to the abdomen, especially those from rifles, high-powered handguns, and shotguns at close range impart tremendous energy to the tissue and organs of the region and tend to cause a mortality and morbidity about ten times greater than that associated with the lower velocity stab wounds. When penetrating trauma induces injury, it affects the liver 40 percent of the time, the small bowel about 25 percent of the time, and the large bowel about 10 percent of the time. Injuries to the spleen, kidneys, and pancreas follow in decreasing order of incidence.

Because the abdomen is bound by muscles rather than skeletal structures, there is a freer transmission of the energy of trauma to the internal organs and structures.

Penetrating trauma most frequently involves the liver and small bowel.

FIGURE 26-1   Stab wound to the right upper quadrant.

FIGURE 26-2   Blunt trauma to the left lower quadrant.

A special type of penetrating trauma is induced by a blast from a shotgun. The shotgun delivers numerous round pellets (called shot) through the hollow gun barrel. The aerodynamics of the shot and the rapid expansion of their distribution (the pattern) cause the energy of impact to decrease rapidly the farther the projectiles move from the barrel. Generally, shotgun blasts at short range (under 3 yards) are extremely lethal. Between 3 and 7 yards, the penetration of the projectiles is great but often survivable. At distances greater than 7 yards, the depth of penetration and subsequent injury fall off quickly. These parameters change somewhat with the decreasing gauge size (gun barrel diameter) and the size of the projectiles. (See Chapter 18, "Penetrating Trauma.")

Blunt trauma to the abdomen produces the least visible signs of injury and causes trauma through three mechanisms: deceleration, compression, and shear (Figure 26-2). As the exterior of the abdomen decelerates (or accelerates) during impact, its contents slam into one another in a chain reaction. They are first injured by the force changing their velocity, then by the forces of compression, as they are trapped between the impacting energy and the more posterior organs. The entire contents of the cavity may be compressed between the force impacting the anterior abdominal cavity and the spinal column. Shear forces induce damage when one part of an organ is free to move while another part is restricted by the forces of trauma or by ligamentous or vascular attachments. Blunt trauma is responsible for about 40 percent of the incidences of splenic injury and a little more than 20 percent of hepatic (liver) injury. The bowel and kidneys are the next most frequently injured abdominal structures in blunt trauma.

Blast injuries to the abdomen involve both blunt and penetrating mechanisms. Shrapnel and debris propelled by the blast act as projectiles and create penetrating trauma. However, because of the irregular shapes of the objects and their poor aerodynamic properties, they tend to produce serious injury only in

Blunt trauma most frequently involves the spleen and liver.

close proximity to the blast's center. The pressure wave generated by the explosion causes blunt trauma as it dramatically compresses and relaxes air-filled organs and is likely to contuse organs or rupture them. Since the stomach and bowel are only occasionally distended with air, they are neither as frequently nor as seriously injured as the lungs by the blast pressure wave. Abdominal injury is a secondary concern with blast injury patients.

Careful evaluation of the mechanism of injury, including identification of the force and direction of impact as it relates to the abdomen, is important to anticipating injuries within the region. Pay special attention to the potential for seat belt injury or direct injury as the abdomen impacts the steering wheel in a vehicle crash, impacts with objects or the ground during a fall, or is struck during an assault. Remember that the early presentation of a contusion will likely be a simple reddening (erythema) of the affected area. Hence it is critically important to carefully analyze the mechanism of injury, identify a high index of suspicion for intra-abdominal injury, and investigate the abdomen for signs and symptoms of injury. The abdominal wall, hollow organs, solid organs, vascular structures, mesentery, and peritoneum all respond differently to trauma.

INJURY TO THE ABDOMINAL WALL

Any injury to the contents of the abdomen must disrupt or be transmitted through the abdominal wall. Since the skin and muscular lining of the abdomen are more resistant to injury than many of the internal organs, they are likely to be uninjured or minimally injured by blunt trauma forces that cause serious injury within. Even when injured, the skin and underlying muscle may only show erythema during the first hour or so. The more visible discoloration of ecchymosis and noticeable swelling require several hours to develop. Penetrating wounds may also be difficult to assess properly because the musculature and skin tension close the wound opening. Bullet and knife wounds look especially small and may appear much less lethal than they are.

Penetrating abdominal injury may permit abdominal contents to protrude through the opening. This type of injury, called an **evisceration,** occurs most frequently through the anterior abdominal wall and is usually associated with a large and deep laceration. The omentum and/or small bowel are most likely to protrude. The evisceration endangers the protruding bowel because of compromised circulation and the drying of this delicate intra-abdominal tissue. However, replacing the protrusion risks introducing bacteria into the peritoneal space. If the bowel is torn, there is the additional danger of its contents leaking into the peritoneal space if it is replaced.

Penetrating trauma to the thorax, buttocks, flanks, and back may also enter the abdomen and injure its contents. The abdominal organs extend well into the thorax and move up to the nipple line, anteriorly, and to the tips of the scapulae, posteriorly, during deep expiration. Injury to the lower portion of the chest may lacerate the diaphragm and injure the stomach, liver, spleen, or gallbladder. The flank, back, and buttock muscles are thick and resist penetrating trauma very well. However, deep wounds in these locations can penetrate into the abdominal cavity and cause injury to adjacent organs. High-powered projectiles, especially those from hunting or military rifles, may have enough energy to deflect when striking bone and enter the abdomen from as far away as a proximal extremity wound.

Tears in the diaphragm may also disrupt the abdominal container. These tears may occur when the patient holds his or her breath just before an impact or with penetrating injury to the lower thorax or upper abdomen. Not only may such an injury compromise the important role of the diaphragm in respiration, but it may also permit or force abdominal contents (like those of the stomach, liver, or a portion of the small bowel) to enter the thoracic cavity. This reduces

With trauma to the abdomen, the discoloration of ecchymosis and noticeable swelling require several hours to develop.

* **evisceration** a protrusion of organs from a wound.

the volume of the thoracic cage available during respiration and compromises the blood supply to the herniated organs. Diaphragmatic injury occurs from stab injuries most frequently on the left side because this is where right-handed assailants strike. Gunshot wounds affect both sides equally. Small tears are unlikely to permit abdominal contents to enter the thorax nor are they likely to greatly effect respiration. Large tears are more likely to do both.

INJURY TO THE HOLLOW ORGANS

Hollow organs like the stomach, small bowel, large bowel, rectum, urinary bladder, gallbladder, and pregnant uterus may rupture with compression from blunt forces, especially if the organ is full and distended. They may also tear as penetrating objects disrupt their structure. (The small bowel is the most frequently injured hollow abdominal organ during penetrating trauma because it rests anteriorly and just beneath the thin anterior abdominal muscles and omentum.) Damage to the hollow organs results in hemorrhage and in the spillage of their contents into the retroperitoneal, peritoneal, or pelvic spaces. The jejunum, ileum, colon, and rectum contain progressively higher bacterial concentrations, and their rupture and the subsequent leakage of material into the abdomen will likely induce severe but delayed infection (called sepsis). The other hollow organs are more likely to release contents that cause a chemical irritation of the abdominal lining. The urinary bladder will release urine, the gallbladder, bile, and the stomach and duodenum, chyme, which is acidic and rich in digestive enzymes. Injury to the hollow organs may result in frank blood in the stool (**hematochezia**), blood in emesis (**hematemesis**), and blood in the urine (**hematuria**).

INJURY TO THE SOLID ORGANS

Solid organs such as the spleen, liver, pancreas, and kidneys are also subject to blunt and penetrating trauma. These organs are especially dense and are not held together as strongly as the more muscular hollow organs of the body. They are prone to contuse, resulting in organ damage and minimal bleeding, or to rupture (also referred to as "fracture"). If the organ's capsule remains intact, it will limit the hemorrhage. However, if the capsule is disrupted by penetrating trauma or torn by the mechanism of blunt trauma, unrestricted hemorrhage may result.

The spleen is especially well protected by the lower ribs, the back and flank muscles, and the spinal column. It is not, however, protected by a strong peritoneal capsule and is very fragile in nature. It may be injured with severe abdominal compression, blunt left flank trauma, or penetrating injury to the region (Figure 26-3). The spleen then bleeds profusely, frequently resulting in shock and a life threat to the patient. The blood loss may accumulate against the diaphragm (especially in the supine patient) and result in referred pain to the left shoulder region.

The pancreas is central to the upper abdomen, somewhat less delicate than the spleen, and well protected from blunt trauma by its location deep in the central abdominal cavity. Penetrating trauma may lacerate its structure and permit blood and digestive enzymes to flow into the abdominal cavity. These digestive juices may actually begin to digest pancreatic and surrounding tissues, leading to severe internal injury. Pancreatic injury does sometimes result from severe blunt trauma to the upper abdomen that compresses the spleen between the trauma force and the vertebral column. This may occur when a patient impacts a steering wheel or the handlebars of a motorcycle during a crash. Such a patient frequently complains of upper abdominal pain that may radiate to the back.

The kidneys are equally well protected by their location deep in the abdominal cavity. They are somewhat more resistant to injury than the pancreas, have a more substantial serous capsule, and are attached by large renal arteries to the

* **hematochezia** blood in the stool.

* **hematemesis** the vomiting of blood.

* **hematuria** blood in the urine.

FIGURE 26-3   Penetrating trauma to the spleen.

FIGURE 26-4 Rupture of the liver.

aorta. They are most frequently injured with trauma to the flanks. Renal injury may result in regional (back or flank) pain as well as hematuria.

The liver is the largest single organ within the abdomen. Being a peritoneal organ, it is surrounded by the strong visceral peritoneum, which resists injury and will hold the organ together if injured. The liver is firmer than both the spleen and pancreas and is somewhat protected by the inferior border of the thorax. When the forces of trauma are directed to this region, however, they are likely to damage the liver, especially if they induce lower rib fracture on the right side (Figure 26-4). The liver is restrained from forward motion by the ligamentum teres. During severe deceleration, the weight of the liver forces it into the ligament, causing shear forces, laceration, and hemorrhage. Liver injury often presents with tenderness along the right lower border of the thoracic cage and, as blood accumulates against the diaphragm, pain in the upper right shoulder.

INJURY TO THE VASCULAR STRUCTURES

Arteries and veins within the abdomen are prone to injury with serious consequences. The abdominal aorta and its major tributaries can be injured by direct blunt or penetrating trauma or may be injured as abdominal organs decelerate and pull on their vascular attachments during an auto crash or similar impact. Penetrating trauma does not frequently involve the very large vessels of the abdomen, but when the aorta or other major artery is damaged, internal hemorrhage can be severe. The vena cava and its tributaries can likewise be injured. Most vascular injuries (97 percent) are associated with penetrating trauma. As blood accumulates in the abdomen of a supine patient, it will come to rest against the diaphragm. There it irritates the muscular structure and produces a referred pain in the shoulder region. However, other signs of significant hemorrhage may be limited.

Vascular injury in the peritoneal, retroperitoneal, and pelvic spaces can be serious for several reasons. These spaces are easily expandable, and hemorrhage may continue without the increase in pressure exerted by surrounding tissue that would occur if the vascular injury were within a mass of muscle elsewhere in the body. Without this pressure, both the rate and volume of blood loss do not diminish. These spaces also contain organs that require significant circulation supplied by rather large arterial and venous vessels. The dynamic nature of the abdomen and its anatomic size mean that a greater volume of blood can be accommodated there before its presence becomes noticeable. Further, due to vagal stimulation caused by the presence of blood in the perotineal cavity, an increasing heart rate may not be present.

Most vascular trauma is associated with penetrating injury.

INJURY TO THE MESENTERY AND BOWEL

The mesentery provides the bowel with circulation, innervation, and attachment. Blunt injury occurs as the mesentery stretches during impact. This type of injury occurs most frequently at points of relative immobility as at the duodenal/jejunal juncture (where the small bowel is affixed by the ligament of Trietz) or where the small bowel joins the large bowel at the ileocecal junction. Injury involving the mesentery may disrupt blood vessels supplying the bowel and eventually cause ischemia, necrosis, and possible rupture. Mesenteric injuries do not usually bleed profusely because the peritoneal layers contain the hemorrhage. Deceleration or compression may tear or rupture the full bowel. With penetrating trauma, the omentum is frequently disrupted and the bowel may be torn anywhere along its length, though tears to the small bowel (jejunum and ileum) are the most likely because of its central and anterior location. Expect a tear to release bowel contents into the peritoneal space, but remember that signs and symptoms of such release are delayed. The duodenum is less frequently injured because of its location deep within the abdomen. Penetrating trauma to the lateral abdomen is likely to injure the large bowel (ascending colon on the right and descending colon on the left).

INJURY TO THE PERITONEUM

* peritonitis inflammation of the peritoneum caused by chemical or bacterial irritation.

* rebound tenderness pain on release of the examiner's hands, allowing the patient's abdominal wall to return to its normal position; associated with peritoneal irritation.

* guarding protective tensing of the abdominal muscles by a patient suffering abdominal pain; may be a voluntary or involuntary response.

The peritoneum is the very delicate and sensitive lining of the anterior abdominal cavity. Its inflammation, called **peritonitis,** can be caused by two major mechanisms, bacterial and chemical irritation. Bacterial peritonitis is an irritation due to infection, which is often released into the space by a torn bowel or open wound. It takes the bacteria between 12 and 24 hours to grow in sufficient numbers to produce the inflammation and hence the condition is usually not apparent during prehospital care. Chemical peritonitis occurs more rapidly than bacterial peritonitis because the caustic nature of digestive enzymes and acids (from the stomach or duodenum), and, to a lesser degree, urine, quickly irritate the peritoneum and induce the inflammatory response. Blood does not induce peritoneal inflammation, and hence serious hemorrhage into the peritoneal cavity will not, by itself, cause this condition.

Peritonitis is a progressive process that presents with characteristic signs and symptoms. It usually begins with a slight tenderness at the location of injury. Over time, the area of inflammation expands, as does the area of tenderness. Any jarring of the abdomen, as occurs with percussion or when you quickly release the pressure of deep palpation, causes a twinge of pain (**rebound tenderness**). In response to pain induced by any movement of the irritated abdominal tissue, the anterior abdominal muscles contract, even in the unconscious patient. This is called **guarding.** If the pain becomes severe, the abdominal muscles assume an extreme contraction and leave the abdominal wall with a rigid, board-like feel. When assessing the abdomen, be aware that local muscle injury caused by trauma may result in local or regional abdominal muscle tenderness and spasm that mimics peritonitis. Tenderness or frank pain from the physical injury may co-exist with the signs of peritonitis.

INJURY TO THE PELVIS

A pelvic fracture represents a serious skeletal injury, serious and often life threatening hemorrhage, and potential injury to the organs within the pelvic space. These organs—the ureters, bladder, urethra, female genitalia, prostate, rectum, and anus—can all be injured by the severe kinetic forces, the crushing nature of the injury, or by displaced bone fragments. Pelvic fracture can also cause serious injury to the pregnant uterus. Pelvic hemorrhage and fracture have been discussed in Chapter 22, "Musculoskeletal Injuries."

Sexual assault may also injure the reproductive structures located internally in the female and externally in the male. Direct trauma to the external female genitalia or injury caused by objects inserted into the vagina may tear the soft tissues of this region. Since these tissues are both very sensitive and vascular, the injury may bleed heavily and be very painful. The same is true for the male genitalia, though they are more prone to accidental injury because of their more external location.

INJURY DURING PREGNANCY

Trauma is the number one killer of pregnant females. Penetrating abdominal trauma alone accounts for as much as 36 percent of overall maternal mortality. Gunshot wounds to the abdomen of the pregnant female also account for fetal mortality rates of between 40 and 70 percent. In blunt trauma, auto collisions are the leading cause of maternal and fetal mortality and morbidity. Proper seat belt placement can significantly reduce injury to the pregnant mother and fetus, while improper placement increases the incidence of both uterine rupture and separation of the placenta from the wall of the uterus. Unrestrained mothers in serious auto collisions are four times more likely to suffer fetal mortality.

The physiologic changes associated with pregnancy protect both the mother and her abdominal organs. With the increasing size of the uterus, most of the abdominal organs are displaced higher in the abdomen (Figure 26-5). This generally protects them, unless blunt or penetrating trauma impacts the upper abdomen. If that happens, then the injury may involve numerous organs with increased morbidity and mortality. Direct penetrating injury to the central and lower abdomen of the late pregnancy mother often spares her from serious injury; the resulting injury, however, often damages the uterus and endangers the fetus.

Trauma is the number one killer of pregnant females and penetrating abdominal trauma alone accounts for as much as 36 percent of overall maternal mortality.

FIGURE 26-5   Changing dimensions of the pregnant uterus. Numbers represent weeks of gestation.

The late term female is at additional risk of vomiting and possible aspiration. Increasing uterine size increases intra-abdominal pressure, while the hormones of pregnancy relax the cardiac sphincter (the valve that prevents reflux of the stomach contents). The bladder is displaced superiorly early in pregnancy and then becomes more prone to injury and, when injured, bleeds more heavily.

The increasing size and weight of the uterus and its contents have several effects on the mother, especially when trauma strikes. The uterus of a supine patient in late pregnancy may compress the inferior vena cava and reduce the venous return to the heart. This may induce hypotension in the uninjured patient and have severe consequences in the hemorrhaging trauma patient. The increased intra-abdominal pressure along with the compression of the inferior vena cava by the uterus raise venous pressure in the pelvic region and lower extremities. This pressure engorges the vessels and increases the rate of venous hemorrhage from pelvic fracture or lower extremity wounds.

The increased maternal vascular volume (up by 45 percent) helps protect the mother from hypovolemia. However, this protection does not extend to the fetus because fetal blood flow is affected well before there are changes in the maternal blood pressure or pulse rate. In fact, it may take a maternal blood loss of between 30 and 35 percent before changes in maternal blood pressure or heart rate are evident. Therefore, it becomes very important to assure early and aggressive resuscitation of the potentially hypotensive pregnant mother.

In the pregnant female, the thick and muscular uterus contains both the developing fetus and amniotic fluid. This container is strong, distributing the forces of trauma uniformly to the fetus and thereby reducing chances for injury. Significant blunt trauma may cause the uterus to rupture or penetrating trauma may perforate or tear it. The dangers of severe maternal hemorrhage and disruption of the blood supply to the fetus present life threats to both. The potential release of amniotic fluid into the abdomen is also of great concern. The risk of uterine and fetal injury increases with the length of gestation and is greatest during the third trimester of pregnancy.

If an open wound to the uterus does occur, there may be added risk to the mother (in addition to hemorrhage) if she is Rh negative and the fetus is Rh positive. Penetrating or severe blunt trauma may permit some fetal/maternal blood mixing and lead to compatibility problems. Frank uterine rupture is a rare complication of trauma, but it does occur with severe blunt impact, pelvic fracture, and—very infrequently—with stab or shotgun wounds.

Blunt trauma to the uterus may cause the placenta to detach from the uterine wall because the placenta is rather inelastic while the uterus is very flexible. This condition, called **abruptio placentae**, presents a life-threatening risk to both mother and fetus because the separation permits both maternal and fetal hemorrhage (Figure 26-6). More frequently than not, this hemorrhage is contained within the uterus and does not extend to the vaginal outlet. Blunt trauma may also cause the premature rupture of the amniotic sac (breaking of the "membranes" or "bag of waters") and may induce an early labor.

INJURY TO PEDIATRIC PATIENTS

Another special patient with regard to abdominal injuries is the child. Children have poorly developed abdominal musculature and a reduced anterior/posterior diameter. The rib cage is more cartilaginous and flexible and more likely to transmit injury to the organs beneath. These factors increase the incidence of pediatric abdominal injury, especially to the liver, spleen, and kidney. Children also compensate very well for blood loss and may not show any signs or symptoms until

While a pregnant mother is somewhat protected from hypovolemia, the fetus is not so protected.

* **abruptio placentae** a condition in which the placenta separates from the uterine wall.

ABRUPTIO PLACENTA

Trapped blood

Placenta

Bleeding may be minimal

FIGURE 26-6 Abruptio placenta.

they have lost over half of their blood volume. This is especially important with abdominal injuries, because a great volume of blood may be lost into the abdomen with little pain or noticeable distention.

ASSESSMENT OF THE ABDOMINAL INJURY PATIENT

Assessment of the patient who has sustained abdominal trauma is somewhat abbreviated because definitive care for such injury is often surgical intervention. Hence, it is imperative that you quickly assess the patient and, if indications of serious abdominal injury exist, that you package and transport him or her expeditiously. Assessment of the abdominal injury patient is like that for any trauma patient, with pertinent and significant information gained during the scene size-up, initial assessment, rapid trauma assessment (or focused exam and history), and serial ongoing assessments.

SCENE SIZE-UP

Assure that the scene is safe for you, fellow rescuers, bystanders, and the patient. Be ready to use appropriate body substance isolation procedures before moving to the patient's side. Also determine the number of expected patients and need for additional EMS, police, fire, and other service personnel.

For the patient who has sustained abdominal injury, the analysis of the mechanism of injury is the most important element of the scene size-up and possibly of the entire assessment. However, forming an index of suspicion for individual abdominal injuries is very difficult because the signs and symptoms are, for the most part, limited and non-specific. In fact, more than 30 percent of patients with serious abdominal injury may present with no specific signs or symptoms of abdominal injury whatsoever. Additionally, other less life-threatening but more painful injuries may overshadow signs and symptoms of the patient's abdominal injury. Also, those signs and symptoms that are present may become less specific in nature with time and the progressive nature of peritonitis. Lastly, the patient's reporting of his or her condition may be unreliable due to the effects of alcohol or drug ingestion, head injury, or shock.

If the patient has suffered blunt trauma, identify the strength and direction of the forces and where on the body they were delivered. Focus your observation and palpation on that site during the initial and rapid trauma assessments and place your highest suspicion of injury there. Begin to develop a list of possible organs injured (the index of suspicion) and the immediate and delayed effects they will have on the patient's condition. In serious blunt trauma or deep penetrating trauma, expect internal and uncontrolled hemorrhage.

If the patient was involved in an auto crash, identify if seat belts were used and if they were used properly (Figure 26-7). Remember that improper placement (above the iliac crests) may increase the likelihood of abdominal compression (and lumbar spine) injury. Lack of seat belt use increases the incidence and severity of all types of injuries, including abdominal injury. Examine the vehicle interior for signs of impact like the deformity of a bent steering wheel, a deflated airbag, or a structural intrusion into the passenger compartment. Frontal impact is most likely to compress the abdomen, injuring the liver and spleen and possibly rupturing distended hollow organs like the stomach and bladder. Right side impact frequently induces liver, ascending colon, and pelvic injury, while left side impact induces splenic,

For the patient who has sustained abdominal injury, the analysis of the mechanism of injury is the most important element of the scene size-up and possibly of the entire assessment.

FIGURE 26-7 Use the mechanism of injury to identify where signs of injury might be found—for example, contusions resulting from compression by a seat belt.

descending colon, and pelvic injuries. Pedestrians, and especially children, are likely to sustain lower abdominal injury, especially if the vehicle impacts the patient's midsection. It is important to determine the velocity of impact and the distance the patient was thrown. Motorcyclists and, to a lesser degree, bicyclists are likely to sustain abdominal injury as they are propelled forward while the handlebars restrain the pelvis and lower abdomen. In assaults and other isolated impacts, be observant for left flank impact and splenic or renal damage and right-side impact causing renal or hepatic (liver) injury. If the impact involves the superior abdomen, suspect liver, stomach, spleen, and pancreatic injury, while impact to the middle or lower abdomen will likely damage the small bowel, kidneys, and bladder.

With a patient who has experienced penetrating trauma, determine the nature of the offending agent. If it is a knife, arrow, or impaled object, determine the probable angle and depth of insertion (Figure 26-8). Do not move or remove the impaled object.

FIGURE 26-8 Analyze the mechanism of a penetrating trauma in an attempt to determine the probable angle and depth of the wound.

With gunshot wounds, determine whether the weapon was a handgun, shotgun, or rifle, the distance from the gun to the victim, and the gun's caliber. Also determine the number of shots fired, if possible, and the angle from which the gun was fired. Be prepared to examine the flanks, the buttocks, and the back for any sign of additional or exit wounds. Attempt to estimate the amount of blood lost at the scene and communicate this, with the other information listed above, to the emergency department physician.

Gunshot wounds provide a challenge to assessment. The damage done does not correlate well to the appearance of the entrance or exit wound. It is more related to the bullet's kinetic energy (velocity and mass) as it enters the body and to its energy exchange characteristics as it travels into and through tissue. Low-velocity bullets cause little damage beyond the bullet's actual path. However, these projectiles are easily deflected from their paths by contact with clothing, bone, or, in some cases, soft tissue. They also carry pieces of clothing and other debris into the body and do not tend to pass through the body.

High-velocity weapons and the wounds they cause were once seen only in the military setting, but now more powerful handguns are causing similar wounds and internal injuries in the civilian life. Their projectiles cause injury well beyond the bullet's path and injure tissue as the projectile creates a cavity and compresses and stretches neighboring tissue (cavitation). The wounding process also draws debris into the wound, where the damaged and devitalized (without circulation) tissue forms a good medium for bacterial growth. The wounding process may create secondary projectiles as the bullet hits bone, breaks it apart, and then drives the fragments into adjacent tissue. The high-velocity bullet may also fragment and transmit its injuring potential to several pathways.

With either significant blunt or any penetrating trauma to the abdomen, suspect serious and continuing internal hemorrhage. Be especially watchful of the patient during your assessment and initiate shock care at the first signs and symptoms of hypoperfusion. These signs and symptoms include diminishing level of consciousness or orientation, increasing anxiety or restlessness, thirst, increasing pulse rate, decreasing pulse pressure, and increasing capillary refill time.

Information you gather at the scene is invaluable to the attending emergency department physician. That information, however, will be unavailable unless you document it carefully and report it upon your arrival at the hospital. Doing this is essential to assuring that the patient receives the best care in both the prehospital and in-hospital settings.

The internal damage done by a bullet does not correlate well to the appearance of the entrance or exit wound.

With significant blunt or penetrating trauma, suspect serious and continuing internal hemorrhage.

INITIAL ASSESSMENT

As you begin the initial assessment, carefully note your patient's level of consciousness and orientation as well as any indication that he or she may be affected by alcohol, drugs, head injury, or shock. These agents and conditions reduce the reliability of your patient's reporting of the signs and symptoms of abdominal injury. Any decrease in the level of orientation or consciousness should alert you to the need to maintain a higher index of suspicion for abdominal injury and to perform more careful initial and rapid trauma assessments. The patient may also complain of dizziness or lightheadedness when moving from a supine to a seated or standing position. (Do not ask the patient to move: however, he may have moved on his own before your arrival.) Any of these signs and symptoms should lead you to suspect hypovolemia, possibly from an abdominal injury. Use your initial evaluation as a baseline against which to trend any changes in the patient's level of consciousness or orientation.

As you evaluate airway, breathing, and circulation, be observant for any associated signs and symptoms of hypovolemia, especially if they occur early in your care or are out of proportion with the obvious or expected injuries. Note any rapid shallow respirations, diminished pulse pressure, rapid pulse rate, slow capillary refill time, or thirst. Limited chest movement may be due to the pain of peritonitis or blood irritating the diaphragm. Shallow respirations may be due to abdominal contents in the thorax from a ruptured diaphragm. Be prepared to protect the airway because abdominal trauma patients are likely to vomit.

RAPID TRAUMA ASSESSMENT

Perform the usual full rapid trauma assessment, but if you have developed a high index of suspicion for abdominal injury, pay particular attention to that region. Carefully examine the abdomen for evidence of injury as suggested by the mechanism of injury or by signs or symptoms observed during the initial assessment. When you suspect that the patient has received blunt trauma, look carefully over the entire abdominal surface for the slight reddening of erythema or minor abrasions associated with superficial soft tissue injury. Remember that any trauma must pass through the exterior of the abdomen before it can do damage within.

Quickly examine the anterior surface of the abdomen and then flanks, then carefully and gently log roll the patient to examine the back, looking for any signs of injury, erythema, ecchymosis, contusions, or open wounds, including eviscerations and impaled objects (Figure 26-9). Also look at the abdomen's general shape and any signs of distention. Visualize the inguinal area for signs of injury or hemorrhage. Jeans may contain hemorrhage without any indication of the accumulation so should be cut away or removed to assess this region when injury is suspected. Remember that the abdominal cavity can contain a very large volume of blood (on the order of 1.5 liters) before it becomes noticeably distended. In obese patients the volume of blood loss may be even greater before distention is visible. Also be aware that the signs and symptoms of hemoperitoneum or retroperitoneal hemorrhage are minimal.

Visualize and palpate the pelvis for signs of injury or instability. Apply gentle pressure directed posteriorly, then medially, on the iliac crests, then place pressure downward on the symphysis pubis. If you note any crepitus or instability, suspect pelvic fracture and both injury to the organs of the lower abdomen and

The abdomen may contain up to 1.5 liters of blood before distention becomes noticeable.

FIGURE 26-9 Examine the abdomen for signs of injury.

severe internal hemorrhage. If you already suspect pelvic injury, do not test or apply any pressure and be very careful during movement to the ambulance and transport to the hospital. Any manipulation of the fracture site may restart or increase hemorrhage.

Question the patient about pain or discomfort in each quadrant, then palpate the quadrants individually, leaving any quadrant with anticipated injury or patient complaint of pain to last. If you palpate an injured quadrant first, the pain may lead the patient to guard during any remaining palpation. Feel for any spasm or guarding as you palpate, then note any patient report of pain when you quickly release the pressure of your palpation (rebound tenderness). If you palpate an abdomen that is board hard, expect injury to the pancreas, duodenum, or stomach, especially if the time since the injury has been short.

Also note any unusual pulsations in the abdomen. You may visualize some pulsing in the thin, young, healthy, athletic patient, but most patients will not have any visible or palpable pulses in the abdomen. Abnormal pulsation suggests arterial injury. Injuries to the thorax or pelvis also suggest abdominal injury, especially if there are lower rib fractures or the pelvic ring is unstable. Auscultation is not recommended during assessment of the abdominal trauma patient. It takes a great deal of time to adequately listen for bowel sounds, and their presence or absence neither confirm nor rule out possible injury.

Abnormal pulsations in the abdomen suggest arterial injury.

When evaluating the patient with penetrating trauma to the abdomen, look carefully at the entrance wound, and note its appearance, size, and depth. Point-blank discharge of a gun against tissue will introduce the barrel exhaust into the wound created by the bullet. You may notice powder debris and the crackling of subcutaneous emphysema. Look for contamination and any signs of serious blood loss. Then examine the patient for an exit wound. Exit wounds may look more "blown out" in nature and are generally larger and more serious in appearance than entrance wounds. Count the number of entry and exit wounds and note whether they are paired or if an inequality suggests that some projectiles did not exit. The wounds from a projectile may be very small and difficult to see, while still carrying the potential to cause lethal injury. Anticipate the injuries that occurred as the object or bullet sped into and through the body, but remember that it is not uncommon for a bullet to alter its path. Be suspicious of any projectile wound in the proximal extremities because the projectile may travel along the limb and into the body's interior. Also keep in mind that a bullet wound to the thorax may then deflect and penetrate the abdomen, or vice versa.

Auscultation is not recommended during assessment of the abdominal trauma patient.

While performing the rapid trauma assessment, carefully question the patient about the characteristics of any pain he feels and ask specifically about any abdominal sensations or other symptoms. Serious injury may result while the patient feels limited pain or injury sensation, especially when other more painful injuries elsewhere might be distracting them. The evaluation of abdominal pain from the patient's complaint may, however, be subjective as patients often vary in their response to pain. In the male, retroperitoneal pain may be referred to the testicular region. Thirst may be one of the few symptoms of abdominal injury as significant hemorrhage draws down the body's blood volume. Be sure to record any symptoms in the patient's own words and assure these comments and your findings are documented on the prehospital care report and reported to the attending physician.

When investigating the rest of the patient history, give special consideration to the last oral intake. The bladder, bowel, and stomach are much more likely to rupture if full and distended. Ask about when the patient last ate or drank and how much he consumed. Relate the intake to the type of impact received, especially blunt trauma to the trunk.

Any patient with a history of significant blunt or any penetrating trauma to the torso is a candidate for rapid transport to the trauma center.

Conclude the rapid trauma assessment by gathering a set of baseline vital signs.

At the end of the rapid trauma assessment, re-evaluate the patient's priority for transport. The potential for an abdominal injury must factor into this determination. Remember that serious internal hemorrhage from blunt or penetrating trauma frequently occurs with few overt signs and symptoms. Any patient with a history of significant blunt or any penetrating trauma to the torso is a candidate for rapid transport to the trauma center. Always err on the side of providing more patient care and early transport rather than underestimating the seriousness of trauma to the abdomen.

Special Assessment Considerations with Pregnant Patients

If the patient you are treating is pregnant, pay special attention to the abdomen and the possibility of injury. Remember that the maternal blood volume is increased by up to 45 percent in the third trimester and blood loss can exceed 30 percent before the normal signs and symptoms of hypovolemia reveal themselves. Watch for the earliest signs of shock. Assure that the uterus does not compress the vena cava by placing the noticeably pregnant mother in the left lateral recumbent position. If spinal injury is also suspected, immobilize her firmly to the spine board and, when placed on the stretcher, rotate her onto her left side. Carefully evaluate the maternal vital signs and remember that the fetus is likely to experience distress before the mother shows any signs of hypotension or hypoperfusion.

Place the late pregnancy patient on her left side to prevent compression of the inferior vena cava.

Trauma to the abdomen in late pregnancy may cause several specific uterine injuries and requires careful assessment. The normal uterus will be firm and round to palpation. It will be palpable above the iliac crests after the first 12 weeks of pregnancy and progress upward in the abdominal cavity until it reaches the costal border at about 32 weeks. Your palpation may result in tenderness and muscular contractions of the uterus, which are normal secondary to uterine contusions. These contractions will often be self-limiting; however, any tenderness, pain, or contractions should raise your suspicions of abruptio placentae. The mother may complain of cramping, generally related to palpable uterine contractions and, in some cases, experience vaginal hemorrhage. Abruptio placentae represents a serious risk to the fetus and mother and is a true emergency requiring rapid transport.

Palpation of the uterus that reveals an asymmetrical uterus or permits you to recognize the irregular features of the fetus suggests uterine rupture. This condition may also present with uterine contractions, but the fundus of the uterus is not palpable and the mass does not harden with the contractions.

If uterine rupture or abruptio placentae are suspected or if you suspect any serious injury to the abdomen of the pregnant patient, determine the mother's Rh status and report it to the emergency department. Alert the emergency department well before your arrival if you are transporting a pregnant mother who was injured by trauma. This allows department personnel to prepare for the special monitoring necessary for both the mother and fetus.

ONGOING ASSESSMENT

The ongoing assessment is an essential part of the continuing care process for the patient with possible abdominal injury. During it, you will look for the signs of progressing abdominal injury or continuing hemorrhage. Perform it every 5 minutes in patients with any significant suggestion of abdominal injury. Often the progressive nature of peritonitis leads to greater and greater patient complaints or may make abdominal signs and symptoms more evident as you care for and reduce the pain of other injuries. The signs of ongoing hemorrhage are equally progressive and may not clearly present until well into your patient care.

Pay close attention to the signs of hidden hemorrhage during ongoing assessments of the patient with potential abdominal injury. Watch the blood pressure, pulse rate, capillary refill time, and the patient's appearance and level of consciousness and orientation. A decrease in the difference between the systolic and diastolic blood pressures (the pulse pressure) suggests the body is compensating for shock. An increasing pulse rate (especially if the strength of the pulse is diminishing), and an increasing capillary refill time both suggest hypovolemic compensation. Also observe for the skin becoming cool, clammy, cyanotic, or ashen, and watch for pulse oximetry readings that become more erratic. A change in either the level of consciousness, or more subtly, a lowering of the patient's orientation suggests the brain is being hypoperfused. These findings all indicate the body is employing increasing levels of shock compensation. If you cannot account for a continuing blood loss elsewhere, suspect internal and continuing abdominal hemorrhage. Subtle changes may be the only apparent signs of gradually worsening shock.

Another sign of continuing blood loss from an abdominal hemorrhage is aggressive fluid resuscitation that appears ineffective. Note your patient's response to fluid resuscitation. If his or her vital signs do not improve and all external hemorrhage is controlled, suspect continuing internal hemorrhage.

Another sign of continuing blood loss from an abdominal hemorrhage is aggressive fluid resuscitation that appears ineffective.

MANAGEMENT OF THE ABDOMINAL INJURY PATIENT

Management of the patient with abdominal injuries is supportive, with the major emphasis on bringing the patient to surgery as quickly as possible. Prehospital care centers on rapid packaging and transport and aggressive fluid resuscitation, as needed. Specific care steps for the abdominal injury patient include proper positioning, general shock care, fluid resuscitation, PASG application, and care for specific injuries (open wounds and eviscerations).

The patient with minor or severe abdominal pain should be positioned for comfort (unless the positioning is contraindicated by suspicion of spinal injury). Flex the patient's knees to relax the abdominal muscles, and if the injuries permit, place the patient in the left lateral recumbent position to maintain knee flexure and the relaxed state of the abdominal muscles, and facilitate the clearing of emesis from the airway.

Assure good ventilation and consider early administration of high flow oxygen for the abdominal injury patient. The pain associated with peritonitis or diaphragmatic irritation may reduce respiratory excursion, adding to the potential for early shock development in these patients.

Control any moderate or serious external hemorrhage with direct pressure and bandaging. Minor bleeding may be controlled during transport if at all.

When a serious mechanism of injury is found and the patient does not present with the signs and symptoms of shock, act in anticipation of it. Start a large-bore IV line with trauma tubing and 1,000 mL of lactated Ringer's solution or normal saline. Be prepared to run it wide open to deliver a bolus of 250 mL of fluid if any signs of shock develop. Monitor the pulse rate and blood pressure. If the pulse does not slow and the pulse pressure does not rise, consider a second bolus. Institute a second line with a non-flow-restrictive saline lock using a large-bore catheter. Use this access if the patient's blood pressure begins to drop. Do not delay transport to initiate any IV access. Start the IV access en route to the hospital if necessary. Prehospital infusion is usually limited

Content Review

MANAGEMENT OF THE ABDOMINAL INJURY PATIENT

Position the patient properly.
Assure oxygenation and ventilation.
Control external bleeding.
Be prepared for aggressive fluid resuscitation.
Apply PASG if not contraindicated.

When a serious mechanism of injury is found and the patient does not present with the signs and symptoms of shock, act in anticipation of it.

to 3,000 mL of fluid. Titrate your administration rate to maintain a systolic blood pressure of 90 mmHg and assure that you do not run out of fluid during field care and transport.

As you should with all serious trauma patients, communicate frequently with the abdominal injury patient to reduce anxiety and provide emotional support. Also watch for any changes in the patient's description of the pain or injury's character or intensity. Be wary of patient hypothermia, especially when providing aggressive fluid resuscitation. Provide ample blankets, keep the patient compartment of the vehicle warm, take patient complaints of being cold seriously, and warm infusion fluids when possible. Hypothermia is a special consideration with pediatric patients because they have a disproportionately large body surface area to body volume and will rapidly loose heat to the environment.

Cover any exposed abdominal organs with a dressing moistened with sterile saline. Be careful to keep the region clean and do not replace any exposed organs. Cover the wet dressing with a sterile occlusive dressing like clear plastic wrap to keep the site as clean as possible and yet retain the moisture. If the transport is lengthy, check the dressing from time to time and remoisten as necessary.

Stabilize impaled objects to prevent further injury and reduce associated hemorrhage.

Another wound that deserves special attention is the impaled object. Do all that you can to keep the object from moving and do not remove it from the victim. Any motion causes further injury, disrupts the clotting mechanisms, and continues the hemorrhage. Removal may withdraw the object from a blood vessel, thereby permitting increased internal and uncontrollable hemorrhage. Pad around the object with bulky trauma dressings and wrap around the trunk with soft, self-adherent roller bandaging to secure it firmly. Apply direct pressure around the object if hemorrhage is anything but minor. If the object is too long to accommodate during transport or it is affixed to an immovable object, attempt to cut it. Use a saw, cutter, or torch, but be very careful to assure that vibration, jarring, and heat are not transmitted to the patient.

Carefully observe and care for penetrating wounds that may traverse both the abdominal and thoracic cavities. If the wound is large and may have penetrated the diaphragm or otherwise entered the thoracic cavity, seal the wound with an occlusive dressing taped on three sides to permit the release of the build-up of air pressure that occurs in a tension pneumothorax. Be especially watchful of respiratory excursion and effort.

The PASG is indicated for the patient with abdominal injury and the early signs of shock. However, it should not be used if there is concurrent penetrating trauma to the chest. The PASG applies circumferential pressure to the abdominal cavity, thereby raising intra-abdominal pressure and reducing the rate of intra-abdominal hemorrhage. Its use is generally contraindicated (inflate the leg sections only) in females in late pregnancy, abdominal evisceration patients, or patients with impaled objects. If the patient with an evisceration experiences a blood pressure below 60 mmHg, consider inflating the abdominal section of the garment as the risks associated with injury to the exposed bowel are less than those of profound hypotension. Incrementally inflate the PASG to maintain blood pressure and pulse rate, not to return them to pre-injury levels.

Inflate the PASG in increments to maintain blood pressure and pulse, not to return them to pre-injury levels.

MANAGEMENT OF THE PREGNANT PATIENT

Special care is offered to the pregnant patient because of the anatomic and physiologic changes induced by pregnancy. Place the late-term mother, when possible, in the left lateral recumbent position. This assures that the weight of the uterus does not compress the vena cava, reduce blood return to the heart, and cause hypotension. It also facilitates airway care. Administer high flow oxygen early in your care because the mother's respiratory reserve volume is diminished, because the work necessary for her to move air is greater because of the increased intra-abdominal pressure, and because the fetus is especially susceptible to hypoxia. If necessary, employ intermittent positive pressure ventilation early in your care. Also consider aggressive airway care. The pregnant mother is prone to vomiting and aspiration. If she has a significantly reduced level of consciousness, consider rapid sequence intubation.

Maintain a high index of suspicion for internal hemorrhage since the increased blood volume of the third-term mother may permit an increased blood loss before the signs and symptoms of hypovolemia become evident. The fetus may be at risk early in the blood loss, well before the mother displays any signs. Initiate IV therapy early, but remember that pregnancy induces a relative anemia and that aggressive fluid resuscitation may further dilute the erythrocyte concentrations and lead to ineffective circulation. Consider using the PASG, inflating the leg sections first. Use of the PASG may be beneficial for the patient in early pregnancy (first-term) as the pressure of the trouser is well distributed within the uterus by the amniotic fluid. However, for the late-term pregnant patient, use of the PASG's abdominal segment is contraindicated because the pressure of the garment may push the uterus more firmly against the inferior vena cava, reducing venous return to the heart, and increasing the effects of hypovolemia.

Use of the PASG's abdominal compartment is contraindicated for late-term pregnant patients.

Summary

Blunt or penetrating abdominal trauma can result in serious organ damage and life-threatening hemorrhage. Concurrently, the signs of injury are limited, nonspecific, and do not reflect the seriousness of abdominal pathology. It is thus very important that your assessment carefully determine the mechanism of injury and the region of the abdomen it affects. This information must be communicated to the emergency department to assure its personnel acknowledge the significance of your first-hand knowledge of the mechanism of injury.

Care for significant abdominal injury is rapid transport to the trauma center. Most significant abdominal injury results in serious internal bleeding or organ injury that can neither be cared for nor stabilized in the prehospital setting. Further, the definitive care for the patient with serious abdominal injury is provided via surgery. The patient must be transported to a facility capable of providing immediate surgical intervention when needed. This is a trauma center. Prehospital care is supportive of the airway and breathing, and preventive for shock.

The pregnant patient with abdominal injury deserves special attention because her vascular volume is increased and she will likely not show the signs of shock until the fetus is at risk. Careful observation while preparation for rapid transport to the trauma center is in order. If any of the slightest signs of hypoperfusion is noted, initiate aggressive fluid resuscitation.

DIVISION 4

MEDICAL EMERGENCIES

CHAPTER 27

Pulmonology

Objectives

After reading this chapter, you should be able to:

1. Discuss the epidemiology of pulmonary diseases and pulmonary conditions. (p. 1155)
2. Identify and describe the function of the structures located in the upper and lower airway. (see Chapter 3)
3. Discuss the physiology of ventilation and respiration. (see Chapter 3)
4. Identify common pathological events that affect the pulmonary system. (pp. 1158–1161)

5. Compare various airway and ventilation techniques used in the management of pulmonary diseases. (pp. 1173–1195)
6. Review the use of equipment utilized during the physical examination of patients with complaints associated with respiratory diseases and conditions. (pp. 1167–1168, 1170–1172)
7. Identify the epidemiology, anatomy, physiology, pathophysiology, assess-

Continued

INTRODUCTION

According to one U.S. study, respiratory complaints accounted for over 28 percent of all EMS calls. Over 200,000 people die each year as a result of respiratory emergencies. Several factors increase the risk of developing respiratory disease. Intrinsic risk factors are those within or influenced by the patient. The most important of these is genetic predisposition. For example, bronchial asthma, **chronic obstructive pulmonary disease (COPD)**, and lung cancer are more common in those who have family members with these diseases.

Certain respiratory conditions are increased in patients with underlying cardiac or circulatory problems. Cardiac conditions that result in ineffective pumping of blood tend to cause pulmonary edema. Cardiac and circulatory diseases may allow blood to pool in the large veins of the pelvis and lower extremities, causing pulmonary emboli. Stress may increase the severity of any respiratory complaint and can precipitate acute episodes of asthma or COPD.

Extrinsic risk factors are those that are external to the patient. The most important of these is cigarette smoking. There is a strong link between cigarette smoking and the development of pulmonary diseases such as lung carcinoma and COPD. Also, diseases such as pneumonia and pulmonary emboli are more likely in patients who smoke. Finally, cigarette smoking has been implicated as a risk factor in the development of cardiac disease. In any case, underlying lung damage caused by cigarette smoking worsens virtually all lung disorders.

Another key extrinsic risk factor is environmental pollutants. The prevalence of COPD is markedly increased in areas with high environmental pollutants, as are the number and severity of acute attacks of asthma and COPD.

This chapter explores the pathophysiology of respiratory disease and how to integrate this knowledge with your assessment findings to develop a field impression and manage the patient with respiratory problems.

The most important intrinsic factor in the development of respiratory disorders is genetic predisposition. The most important extrinsic factor is smoking.

* chronic obstructive pulmonary disease (COPD) a disease characterized by a decreased ability of the lungs to perform the function of ventilation.

PHYSIOLOGICAL PROCESSES

The major function of the respiratory system is to exchange gases with the environment. Oxygen is taken in while carbon dioxide is eliminated, a process known as gas exchange.

Oxygen is vital to our bodies, allowing us to generate the energy that drives our many body functions. Oxygen from the atmosphere diffuses into the bloodstream through the lungs. Oxygen is then available for use in cellular metabolism by the body's 100 trillion cells. Waste products, including carbon dioxide, produced by cellular metabolism, must be eliminated from the body. In the lungs, carbon dioxide is exchanged for oxygen and the carbon dioxide is excreted from the lungs.

Three important processes allow gas exchange to occur:

- Ventilation
- Diffusion
- Perfusion

Ventilation

Ventilation is the mechanical process of moving air in and out of the lungs. In order for ventilation to occur, several body structures must be intact, including the chest wall, the nerve pathways, the diaphragm, the pleural cavity, and the brainstem.

Ventilation is divided into two phases: inspiration and expiration. During inspiration, air is drawn into the lungs. During expiration, air leaves the lungs. These phases of ventilation depend on changes in the volume of the thoracic cavity, as discussed in Chapter 3.

Diffusion

Diffusion is the process by which gases move between the alveoli and the pulmonary capillaries. Remember that gases tend to flow from areas in which there is a high concentration of gas into an area of low concentration. The normal concentration of oxygen in the alveoli is 104 mmHg as opposed to a concentration of 40 mmHg in the pulmonary arterial circulation. Therefore, oxygen will move from the oxygen-rich alveoli into the oxygen-poor capillaries in response to the gradient that exists in the concentration of gases. As the red blood cells move through the pulmonary capillaries, they become enriched with oxygen. Less oxygen will pass into the bloodstream as the gradient between alveolar and capillary oxygen concentration decreases.

Similarly, carbon dioxide passes out of the blood in response to a gradient that exists between the concentration of carbon dioxide in the blood in the pulmonary capillaries (45 mmHg) and in the alveoli (40 mmHg). By the time blood leaves the pulmonary capillaries, it has a dissolved concentration of oxygen of 104 mmHg and a carbon dioxide concentration of 40 mmHg.

The respiratory membrane, which normally measures 0.5 to 1.0 micrometer in thickness, must remain intact for gas exchange to occur. Any disorder that damages the alveoli or allows them to collapse will impede oxygen from entering the body and will reduce carbon dioxide elimination. Changes in the respiratory membrane or any increase in the interstitial space will also impede the process of diffusion. For example, fluid accumulation in the interstitial space as the result of pulmonary edema or pneumonia will prevent proper diffusion of gases. Finally the endothelial lining of the capillaries must be intact for exchange of oxygen and carbon dioxide to occur. Diseases that produce thickening of the endothelial lining will also interfere with the process of diffusion.

Content Review

PROCESSES OF GAS EXCHANGE

Ventilation
Diffusion
Perfusion

---

* **ventilation** the mechanical process of moving air in and out of the lungs.

* **diffusion** the movement of molecules through a membrane from an area of greater concentration to an area of lesser concentration.

There are certain measures that you can take to address problems with lung diffusion. Providing the patient with high concentrations of oxygen is one simple step that can be utilized. Remember that the concentration gradient provides the driving force in moving oxygen into the capillaries. Therefore, the larger the difference between the concentration of oxygen in the alveoli and the capillaries, the greater the diffusion of oxygen into the bloodstream. Similarly, when fluid accumulation or inflammation is the underlying cause of the thickening of the interstitial space within the alveoli, medications such as diuretic agents or anti-inflammatory drugs (corticosteroids, antibiotics) are given to reduce fluid and inflammation.

Provide oxygen to a patient with a lung diffusion problem to increase the concentration gradient that drives oxygen into the capillaries. When fluid accumulation or inflammation is present, consider administering diuretics or antiinflammatory drugs.

Perfusion

One additional process that occurs in the lungs is **perfusion.** Lung perfusion is the circulation of blood through the lungs or, more specifically, the pulmonary capillaries. Lung perfusion is dependent on three conditions:

* Adequate blood volume
* Intact pulmonary capillaries
* Efficient pumping of blood by the heart

For perfusion to proceed effectively, there must be an adequate volume of blood in the bloodstream. Equally important is the concentration of **hemoglobin,** which is the transport protein that carries oxygen in the blood. Remember that oxygen is transported in the bloodstream in one of two ways: bound to hemoglobin or dissolved in the plasma. Under normal conditions, less than 2 percent of all oxygen is transported dissolved in plasma (this is what is measured by the PO_2), whereas more than 98 percent is carried by hemoglobin.

Hemoglobin has some unique properties. It is made up four iron-containing heme molecules and a protein-containing globin portion. Oxygen molecules bind to the heme portion of the hemoglobin molecule. As oxygen binds to hemoglobin, its structure changes so that it more readily binds additional oxygen molecules. Similarly, as fully oxygen-bound hemoglobin begins to release oxygen, it more readily sheds additional oxygen. The relationship is described by the *oxygen dissociation curve* (Figure 27-1). You can see that with between 10 and 50 mmHg, there is a marked increase in the saturation of hemoglobin. However, as the PO_2 increases above 70 mmHg, there is only a small change in the saturation of hemoglobin which is already near 100 percent.

* perfusion the circulation of blood through the capillaries.

* hemoglobin the transport protein that carries oxygen in the blood.

FIGURE 27-1 Oxygen dissociation curve.

Changes in the body temperature, the blood pH, and the PCO_2 can all alter the oxygen dissociation curve. Within the tissues, as hemoglobin becomes bound with carbon dioxide, it loses its affinity for oxygen. As a result, more oxygen is released and is thus available to cells for metabolism (called the Bohr effect).

Carbon dioxide is transported from the cells to the lungs in one of three ways:

- As bicarbonate ion
- Bound to the globin portion of the hemoglobin molecule
- Dissolved in plasma (measured as PCO_2)

The greatest portion of CO_2 produced during metabolism in cells is converted into bicarbonate ion. As the CO_2 is released into the capillaries, it enters the red blood cell where an enzyme (carbonic anhydrase) combines carbon dioxide with water to form two ions, hydrogen (H^+) and bicarbonate (HCO_3^-). Bicarbonate is then released from the red blood cell and transported in plasma. In the lungs, the reverse process takes place, producing water and carbon dioxide. The carbon dioxide then diffuses into the alveoli where it is eliminated during exhalation.

The carbon dioxide that is bound to hemoglobin is released in the lung because of the lower concentration of this gas in the alveoli. Additionally, as the heme portion of the hemoglobin molecule becomes saturated with oxygen, more carbon dioxide is released (called the Haldane effect). Finally, the approximately 10 percent of carbon dioxide that is dissolved in the plasma flows into the alveoli due to the gradient that exists between the concentration of gases (PCO_2 of 45 mmHg in pulmonary artery versus 40 mmHg in the alveoli).

For perfusion to take place, in addition to having adequate blood volume, the pulmonary capillaries must be able to transport blood through all portions of the lung tissue. These vessels must be open and not occluded, or blocked. For example, a pulmonary embolism will occlude the pulmonary artery in which it lodges, making that artery unavailable for perfusion of the portion of the lung it usually supplies with blood. Finally, the heart must pump efficiently in order to push blood effectively through the pulmonary capillaries to perfuse the lung tissues.

In order to maintain perfusion, you must ensure that the patient has an adequate circulating blood volume. In addition, take all the necessary steps to improve the pumping action of the heart. For example, in patients with acute pulmonary edema the use of diuretic agents reduces the blood return (preload) to an ineffectively pumping heart and improves cardiac efficiency.

The entire system we have just discussed provides for **respiration,** which is the exchange of gases between a living organism and its environment. Pulmonary respiration occurs in the lungs when the respiratory gases are exchanged between the alveoli and the red blood cells in the pulmonary capillaries through the respiratory membranes. Cellular respiration, on the other hand, occurs in the peripheral capillaries. It involves the exchange of the respiratory gases between the red blood cells and the various tissues. Many of the principles of gas exchange that occur in the lungs are reversed in the tissues, with oxygen being released to the cells and carbon dioxide accumulating in the plasma and red blood cells.

PATHOPHYSIOLOGY

Remember that many disease states affect the pulmonary system and interfere with its ability to acquire the oxygen required for normal cellular metabolism. Additionally, respiratory diseases limit the body's ability to get rid of waste

In order to maintain perfusion, ensure that the patient has an adequate circulating blood volume. Also, take all necessary steps to improve the pumping action of the heart.

* respiration the exchange of gases between a living organism and its environment.

products such as carbon dioxide. Your understanding of normal anatomy and physiology—ventilation, diffusion, and perfusion—will aid in understanding the mechanism of each disease process and will direct you toward the appropriate corrective actions. Ultimately, any disease process that impairs the pulmonary system will result in a derangement in ventilation, diffusion, perfusion, or a combination of these processes.

DISRUPTION IN VENTILATION

Diseases that affect ventilation will result in obstruction of the normal conducting pathways of the upper or lower respiratory tract, impairment of the normal function of the chest wall, or abnormalities involving the nervous system's control of ventilation.

Upper and Lower Respiratory Tracts

Disease states that affect the upper respiratory tract will result in obstruction of air flow to the lower structures. Upper airway trauma, for example, produces both significant hemorrhage and swelling. Infections of the upper airway structures, including epiglottitis, soft tissue infections of the neck, tonsillitis, and abscess formation within the pharynx (peritonsillar abscess and retropharyngeal abscess), can all obstruct air flow. Similarly, lower airway obstruction may be produced by trauma, foreign body aspiration, mucus accumulation (as in asthmatics), smooth muscle constriction (in asthma and COPD), and airway edema produced by infection or burns.

Chest Wall and Diaphragm

As you read earlier, the chest wall and diaphragm are mechanical components that are essential for normal ventilation. Traumatic injuries to these areas will disrupt the normal mechanics causing loss of negative pressure within the pleural space. This occurs in patients with **pneumothorax,** including open pneumothorax, tension pneumothorax, or **hemothorax.** Infectious processes such as empyema (pus accumulation in the pleural space) or inflammatory conditions produce similar effects. Chest wall injuries including rib fractures or **flail chest** and diaphragmatic rupture limit the patient's ability to expand the thoracic cavity. Certain neuromuscular diseases, such as muscular dystrophy, multiple sclerosis, or amyotrophic lateral sclerosis (ALS or Lou Gehrig's Disease), impair muscular function so as to limit the ability to generate a negative pressure within the chest cavity.

Nervous System

Finally, any disease process that impairs the nervous system's regulation of breathing may also alter ventilation. Central nervous system depressants such as alcohol, benzodiazepines, or barbiturates, alone or in combination, can alter the brain's response to important signals such as rising PCO_2. Similarly, stroke, diseases, or injuries that involve the respiratory centers within the central nervous system can change the normal ventilatory pattern. In fact, certain abnormal respiratory patterns are produced by specific brain injury (Figure 27-2).

- *Cheyne-Stokes respirations* describes a ventilatory pattern with progressively increasing tidal volume, followed by a declining volume,

* **pneumothorax** a collection of air in the pleural space, causing a loss of the negative pressure that binds the lung to the chest wall. In an *open pneumothorax,* air enters the pleural space through an injury to the chest wall. In a *closed pneumothorax,* air enters the pleural space through an opening in the pleura that covers the lung. A *tension pneumothorax* develops when air in the pleural space cannot escape, causing a build-up of pressure and collapse of the lung.

* **hemothorax** a collection of blood in the pleural space.

* **flail chest** one or more ribs fractured in two or more places, creating an unattached rib segment.

FIGURE 27-2 Abnormal respiratory patterns.

Normal

Cheyne-Stokes breathing

Kussmaul's

Central neurogenic hyperventilation

Ataxic (Biot's) pattern

Apneustic pattern

---

* **apnea** absence of breathing.

separated by periods of **apnea** at the end of expiration. This pattern is typically seen in older patients with terminal illness or brain injury.

- *Kussmaul's respirations* are deep, rapid breaths that result as a corrective measure against conditions such as diabetic ketoacidosis that produce metabolic acidosis.

- *Central neurogenic hyperventilation* also produces deep, rapid respirations that are caused by strokes or injury to the brainstem. In this case, there is loss of normal regulation of ventilatory controls and respiratory alkalosis is often seen.

- *Ataxic (Biot's) respirations* are characterized by repeated episodes of gasping ventilations separated by periods of apnea. This pattern is seen in patients with increased intracranial pressure.

- *Apneustic respiration* is characterized by long, deep breaths that are stopped during the inspiratory phase and separated by periods of apnea. This pattern is a result of stroke or severe central nervous system disease.

Also remember that damage to the major peripheral nerves that supply the diaphragm and intercostal muscles, the phrenic nerve, and intercostal nerves will also affect normal ventilatory mechanics. Traumatic disruption of the phrenic nerve during chest surgery, with penetrating trauma, or by neoplastic (cancerous, tumorous) invasion of the nerve can paralyze the diaphragm on the side of involvement.

DISRUPTION IN DIFFUSION

Other disease states can disrupt the diffusion of gases. Any change in the concentration of oxygen in the alveoli, such as occurs when a person ascends to high altitudes, can limit the diffusion of oxygen and produce **hypoxia.** Similarly, any disease that alters the structure or patency of the alveoli will limit diffusion. Destruction of alveoli by certain environmental pathogens such as asbestos or coal (black lung disease), in patients with COPD, or with inhalation injury reduces the capacity of the lungs to diffuse gases.

> **✱ hypoxia** state in which insufficient oxygen is available to meet the oxygen requirements of the cells.

Finally, disease states that alter the thickness of the respiratory membrane will limit the diffusion of gases. The most common cause of this alteration is accumulation of fluid and inflammatory cells in the interstitial space. Fluid can accumulate in the interstitial space if high pressure within the pulmonary capillaries forces fluid out of the circulatory system. This is seen in patients with left-sided heart failure (cardiogenic causes) and is due to increased venous pressure as a result of poor functioning of the left ventricle. Patients with pulmonary hypertension have high resting pressures in the pulmonary circulation which ultimately leads to fluid accumulation in the interstitial space, causing right heart failure.

Similar effects can be produced by changes in the permeability (or leakiness) of the pulmonary capillaries (non-cardiogenic causes). Permeability can be affected by adult respiratory distress syndrome, asbestosis and other environmental pathogens, near-drowning, prolonged hypoxia, and inhalation injury. Also remember that disease states that alter the pulmonary capillary endothelial lining, such as advanced atherosclerosis or vascular inflammatory states, can affect diffusion.

DISRUPTION IN PERFUSION

As detailed earlier, any alteration in appropriate blood flow through the pulmonary capillaries will limit normal gas exchange in the lungs. Any disease state that reduces the normal circulating blood volume, such as trauma, hemorrhage, dehydration, shock or other causes of hypovolemia, will limit normal perfusion of the lungs. Remember that hemoglobin is the major transport protein for oxygen and plays a significant role in the elimination of carbon dioxide. Therefore, any reduction in the normal circulating hemoglobin will also affect perfusion. All causes of anemia, a condition in which the number of red blood cells or amount of hemoglobin in them is below normal, must be considered. Such causes include acute blood loss, iron or vitamin deficiency, malnutrition, and anemia from chronic disease states.

Remember that blood must be available to all of the lung segments for maximum gas exchange to occur. When an area of lung tissue is appropriately ventilated but no capillary perfusion occurs, available oxygen is not moved into the circulatory system. This is referred to as a *pulmonary shunting.* In patients with pulmonary embolism, a blockage of a division of the pulmonary artery by a clot prevents perfusion of the lung segments supplied by that branch of the artery. As a result, there may be significant shunt with return of unoxygenated blood to the pulmonary venous circulation.

ASSESSMENT OF THE RESPIRATORY SYSTEM

Assessment of the respiratory system is a vital aspect of prehospital care. You must quickly assess the airway and ventilation status during the initial assessment. If the patient's complaints suggest that the respiratory system is involved in the patient's problem, the focused history and physical examination should be directed to this aspect of the assessment.

If the patient's complaints suggest respiratory system involvement, direct the focused history and physical examination to this aspect.

SCENE SIZE-UP

When you approach the scene, you should consider two major questions: (1) Is the scene safe to approach the patient? and (2) Are there visual clues that might provide information regarding the patient's medical complaint?

When you approach the scene, consider: (1) Is the scene safe? and (2) Are there visual cues to the patient's medical complaint?

Remember that there are several hazards that may result in respiratory complaints by the patient that are also potentially dangerous for emergency care providers. Certain gases and toxic products that are causing respiratory complaints from your patient may also present a significant risk to you. Carbon monoxide, for example, is a colorless and odorless gas that may be present in quantities enough to overcome unsuspecting emergency care personnel. Other toxins from incomplete combustion produced in fires or industrial processes pose a similar risk. Recent incidents involving chemical agents such as saran gas or biologic agents like anthrax highlight the need for emergency care providers to be aware of hazards to themselves as well as to their patient.

You should also be aware that there are certain rescue environments in which the concentration of available oxygen is significantly reduced. This would include areas such as grain silos, enclosed storage containers, or any enclosed space in which there is an active fire. You must take the appropriate precautions before entering such environments, including the use of your own supplemental oxygen supply.

In any situation where you believe there is a hazard to you as a care provider, make sure that the scene is appropriately secured before you enter. If specific protective items such as hazardous materials suits, self-contained breathing apparatus, or supplemental oxygen are needed, make sure they are available before you attempt to care for your patient. Similarly, if other personnel such as fire suppression units or hazmat teams are required, contact dispatch and have them available on scene before putting yourself at risk.

Once it is safe to enter the scene, look for clues that will provide information regarding the patient's complaints. Do you see evidence of cigarette packs or ashtrays to suggest that the patient or family members are smokers? Look for any home nebulizer machines or supplemental oxygen tanks that may suggest a patient with underlying COPD or asthma. If the patient is a small child, look for small items lying around the house that could suggest potential ingested foreign bodies. Using your eyes, ears, and nose can lead you to several important clues that are useful as you begin your assessment of the patient.

INITIAL ASSESSMENT

General Impression

Take the following considerations and steps to help form your initial impression of the patient's respiratory status:

Content Review

GENERAL IMPRESSION OF RESPIRATORY STATUS
Position
Color
Mental status
Ability to speak
Respiratory effort

- *Position.* Consider the patient's position. Patients with respiratory diseases tend to tolerate an upright posture better than lying flat. In-

FIGURE 27-3   Tripod position.

dications of severe respiratory distress include a patient who is sitting upright with feet dangling over the side of the bed. In the most severe cases, the patient will assume the "tripod" position in which the patient leans forward and supports his weight with the arms extended (Figure 27-3).

- *Color.* Patients with severe respiratory distress display **pallor** and **diaphoresis. Cyanosis** is a late finding and may be absent even with significant hypoxia. Peripheral cyanosis (bluish discoloration involving only the distal extremities) is not a specific finding and is also found in patients with poor circulation. Peripheral cyanosis reflects the slowing of blood flow and increased extraction of oxygen from red blood cells. Central cyanosis (involving the lips, tongue, and truncal skin) is a more ominous finding seen in hypoxia.

- *Mental Status.* Briefly assess the patient's mental status. The hypoxic patient will become restless and agitated. Confusion is seen with both hypoxia (deficiency of oxygen) and hypercarbia (excess of carbon dioxide). When respiratory failure is imminent, the patient will appear severely lethargic and somnolent. The eyelids will begin to droop and the head will bob with each respiratory effort.

- *Ability to Speak.* Assess the patient's ability to speak in full, coherent sentences. Determine the ease with which the patient can discuss symptoms. Patients with respiratory distress will be able to speak only 1 to 2 words before they need to pause to catch their breath. Rambling, incoherent speech indicates fear, anxiety, or hypoxia.

- *Respiratory Effort.* As we have already described, normal ventilation is an active process. However, the use of accessory muscles in the neck (scalenes and sternocleidomastoids) and visible contractions of the intercostal muscles indicate significant breathing effort.

✱ **pallor** paleness.

✱ **diaphoresis** sweatiness.

✱ **cyanosis** bluish discoloration of the skin due to an increase in reduced hemoglobin in the blood. The condition is directly related to poor ventilation.

Assessment of the Respiratory System   **1163**

As you form your general impression, also make specific note of any of the following signs of respiratory distress

nasal flaring excessive widening of the nares with respiration.

- **Nasal flaring**
- Intercostal muscle retraction
- Use of the accessory respiratory muscles
- Cyanosis
- Pursed lips
- **Tracheal tugging**

tracheal tugging retraction of the tissues of the neck due to airway obstruction or dyspnea.

Your initial assessment of the patient is directed at identification of any life-threatening conditions resulting from compromise of airway, breathing, or circulation (the ABCs). Because this chapter concerns the respiratory system, we will focus here on assessment of airway and breathing.

Airway

Any significant abnormality in the respiratory tract must be viewed as potentially life threatening.

Remember that oxygen is one of the most basic necessities for life, and the respiratory system is responsible for supplying it to the body tissues. As a result, any significant abnormality in the respiratory tract must be viewed as potentially life threatening.

After quickly forming your general impression, immediately focus on the patient's airway. When assessing the airway, keep these principles in mind:

- Noisy breathing nearly always means partial airway obstruction.
- Obstructed breathing is not always noisy.
- The brain can survive only a few minutes in **asphyxia.**
- Artificial respiration is useless if the airway is blocked.
- A patent airway is useless if the patient is apneic.
- If you note airway obstruction, do not waste time looking for help or equipment. Act immediately.

asphyxia a decrease in the amount of oxygen and an increase in the amount of carbon dioxide as a result of some interference with respiration.

If the airway is compromised, quickly institute basic airway management techniques. Once you have secured a patent airway, ensure that the patient has adequate ventilation.

If the airway is compromised, quickly institute basic airway management techniques. Once you have secured a patent airway, ensure that the patient has adequate ventilation. Your initial assessment of the respiratory system should be brief and directed. A more detailed examination should be conducted once you have been able to establish that an immediate threat to life does not exist.

Breathing

The following signs should suggest a possible life-threatening respiratory problem in adults. They are listed in order from most ominous to least severe.

dyspnea difficult or labored breathing; a sensation of "shortness of breath."

- Alterations in mental status
- Severe central cyanosis
- Absent breath sounds
- Audible stridor
- 1-to-2-word **dyspnea** (need to breathe between every word or two)
- **Tachycardia** $\geq$ 130 beats per minute
- Pallor and diaphoresis

tachycardia rapid heart rate.

- The presence of intercostal and sternocleidomastoid retractions
- Use of accessory muscles

If any of these signs are present, you should direct your efforts toward immediate resuscitation and transport of the patient to a medical facility.

FOCUSED HISTORY AND PHYSICAL EXAMINATION

History

The history and physical exam should be directed at problem areas as determined by the patient's chief complaint or primary problem. Patients with respiratory diseases will often present with a complaint of "shortness of breath" (dyspnea). Obtain a SAMPLE history. If the chief complaint suggests respiratory disease, ask the OPQRST questions including the following questions about the current symptoms. The answers to these or similar questions will provide you with a pertinent patient history.

If a patient complains of dyspnea, obtain a SAMPLE history. If the chief complaint suggests respiratory disease, ask the OPQRST questions about current symptoms.

How long has the dyspnea been present?

Was the onset gradual or abrupt?

Is the dyspnea better or worse by position? Is there associated orthopnea or paroxysmal nocturnal dyspnea?

Has the patient been coughing?

   If so, is the cough productive?

   What is the character and color of the sputum?

   Is there any hemoptysis (coughing up of blood)?

Is there any chest pain associated with the dyspnea?

   If so, what is the location of the pain?

   Was the onset of pain sudden or slow?

   What was the duration of the pain?

   Does the pain radiate to any area?

   Does the pain increase with respiration?

Are there associated symptoms of fever or chills?

What is the patient's past medical history?

Has the patient experienced wheezing?

Is the patient or close family member a smoker?

✱ **orthopnea** dyspnea while lying supine.

✱ **paroxysmal nocturnal dyspnea** short attacks of dyspnea that occur at night and interrupt sleep.

✱ **hemoptysis** expectoration of blood from the respiratory tree.

It is also important to ask the patient if he has ever experienced similar symptoms in the past. Patients with chronic medical conditions such as COPD or asthma can usually relate the severity of their current presenting complaints to other episodes that they have experienced. Question the patient or family about prior hospitalizations for respiratory disease. In particular, you should try to determine whether the patient required care in the intensive care unit (ICU) for breathing problems. Ask if the patient has ever required endotracheal intubation and ventilatory support. Consider patients who have been previously intubated to be potentially seriously ill and approach them with great caution.

Similarly, it is important to ask the patient if he already has a known respiratory disease. The most common reason for a call to emergency care personnel is a worsening of an already present respiratory disease. This is very typical for patients with COPD, asthma, or lung cancer. If you are not familiar with the patient's diagnosis (for example, alpha-2 anti-trypsin deficiency), try to determine if the disease is affecting the process of ventilation, diffusion, or perfusion.

Continue history taking by determining:

What current medications is the patient taking? (Pay particular attention to oxygen therapy, oral bronchodilators, corticosteroids, and antibiotics.)

Does the patient have any allergies?

A good history of medication use is essential and may provide useful clues to the diagnosis. If time permits, gather the patient's current medications and transport them with the patient. This is a great benefit to the Emergency Department personnel who will be evaluating the patient. Pay particular attention to any medications that suggest pulmonary disease. These would include inhaled or oral sympathomimetics such as albuterol and related agents that are used to treat diseases such as COPD or asthma. Also ask about steroid preparations, which are also used in these conditions. Other common medications used by patients with COPD or asthma include cromolyn sodium, methylxanthines like theophylline, and antibiotic agents.

Also ask about drugs used for cardiac conditions, since cardiac patients often present with dyspnea. Nitrates, calcium channel blockers, diuretic agents, digoxin, and anti-dysrhythmic agents are all commonly used by patients with cardiac disease.

Finally, inquire about medication allergies. This is important information, since it helps to avoid administering agents to which the patient is allergic. Also, it's possible that a specific medication may be the cause of an allergic reaction that has resulted in upper airway edema and respiratory complaints.

Physical Examination

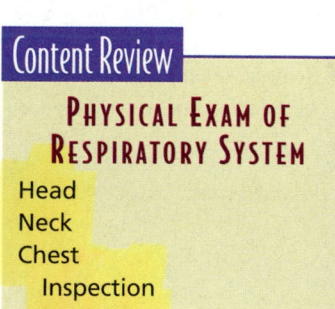

Content Review

PHYSICAL EXAM OF RESPIRATORY SYSTEM

Head
Neck
Chest
   Inspection
   Palpation
   Percussion
   Auscultation
Extremities

First address the patient's head and neck. Look at the lips. Pursed lips indicate significant respiratory distress. This is the patient's way of maintaining positive pressure during expiration and preventing alveolar collapse. Also examine the nose, mouth, and throat for any signs of swelling or infection that might be causing upper airway obstruction.

Occasionally, the patient may also produce sputum, which can suggest an underlying cause of the patient's complaints. An increase in the amount of sputum produced suggests infection of the lungs or bronchial passages (bronchitis). Thick, green or brown sputum is characteristic of these infections. On the other hand, thin, yellow or pale-gray sputum is more typical of inflammation or an allergic cause. Pink, frothy sputum is a sign of severe pulmonary edema. Truly bloody sputum (hemoptysis) may be seen with cancer, tuberculosis, and bronchial infection.

Assess the neck for signs of swelling or infection. Remember to look at the jugular veins for evidence of distention (Figure 27-4). This occurs when the right side of the heart is not pumping blood effectively, causing a "back-up" in the venous circulation. Such findings are often accompanied by left-sided heart failure and pulmonary edema.

Physical examination of the respiratory system should follow the standard steps of patient assessment: *inspection, palpation, percussion,* and *auscultation.*

- *Inspection.* Inspection should include an examination of the anterior-posterior dimensions and general shape of the chest. An

FIGURE 27-4   Jugular vein distention.

increased anterior-posterior diameter is suggestive of chronic obstructive pulmonary disease (COPD). Inspect the chest for symmetrical movement. Any asymmetry may be suggestive of trauma. A paradoxical movement (moving in a fashion opposite to that expected) is suggestive of flail chest. Note any chest scars, lesions, wounds, or deformities.

- *Palpation.* Palpate the chest, both front and back, for any abnormalities. Note any tenderness, crepitus, or subcutaneous emphysema. Palpate the anterior chest first, then the posterior. Inspect your gloved hands for blood each time they are removed from behind the patient's chest. In some instances, it may be appropriate to evaluate tactile fremitus, the vibration felt in the chest during speaking. When evaluating tactile fremitus, compare one side of the chest with the other. Simultaneously, palpate the trachea for tracheal deviation, which is suggestive of a tension pneumothorax.

- *Percussion.* If indicated, quickly percuss the chest. Limit percussion to suspected cases of pneumothorax and pulmonary edema. A hollow sound on percussion is often indicative of pneumothorax or emphysema. In contrast, a dull sound is indicative of pulmonary edema, hemothorax, or pneumonia. Remember, however, that percussion may be of little value in the noisy environment typical of most emergency scenes.

- *Auscultation.* Auscultate the chest. Begin by listening to the patient without a stethoscope and from a distance. Note any loud stridor, wheezing, or cough. If possible, the patient should be in the sitting position and the chest auscultated in a symmetrical pattern. When the patient cannot sit up, auscultate the anterior and lateral parts of the chest. Each area should be auscultated for one respiratory cycle.

✱ **crepitus** crackling sounds.

✱ **subcutaneous emphysema** presence of air in the subcutaneous tissue.

✱ **tactile fremitus** vibratory tremors felt through the chest by palpation.

✱ **tracheal deviation** any position of the trachea other than midline.

Assessment of the Respiratory System   **1167**

Normal breath sounds heard during auscultation can be characterized according to the following descriptions.

Normal Breath Sounds

- Bronchial (or tubular)
  - Loud, high-pitched breath sounds heard over the trachea
  - Expiratory phase lasts longer than inspiratory phase
- Bronchovesicular
  - Softer, medium-pitched breath sounds heard over the mainstem bronchi (below clavicles or between scapulae)
  - Expiratory phase and inspiratory phase equal
- Vesicular
  - Soft, low-pitched breath sounds heard in the lung periphery

While the patient breathes in and out deeply with the mouth open, note any abnormal breath sounds and their location. Many terms are used to describe abnormal breath sounds. The following list includes some of the more common terms.

Abnormal Breath Sounds

- *Snoring.* Occurs when the upper airway is partially obstructed, usually by the tongue.
- *Stridor.* Harsh, high-pitched sound heard on inspiration and characteristic of an upper airway obstruction such as croup.
- *Wheezing.* Whistling sound due to narrowing of the airways by edema, bronchoconstriction, or foreign materials.
- *Rhonchi.* Rattling sounds in the larger airways associated with excessive mucus or other material.
- *Crackles* (also called *rales*). Fine, moist crackling sounds associated with fluid in the smaller airways.
- *Pleural Friction Rub.* Sounds like dried pieces of leather rubbing together; occurs when the pleura become inflamed, as in pleurisy.

Also examine the extremities. Look for peripheral cyanosis, which may indicate hypoxia. Examine the extremities for swelling, redness, and a hard, firm cord indicating a venous clot. This may suggest a possible cause for pulmonary embolism. Look for clubbing of the fingers (Figures 27-5a and b), suggesting long-standing hypoxemia. This is typical of patients with COPD or cyanotic heart disease. Finally, the patient may demonstrate *carpopedal spasm* in which the fingers and toes are contracted in flexion. This is found in patients with hyperventilation and is caused by transient shifts in the blood calcium concentration caused by changes in the serum CO_2 and pH levels.

Vital Signs

The patient's vital signs may also provide information regarding the severity of the respiratory complaints. In general, tachycardia (rapid heart rate) is a very non-specific finding, seen with fear, anxiety, and fever. In patients with respiratory complaints, however, tachycardia may also indicate hypoxia. Remember that the patient may have recently used sympathomimetic drugs such as albuterol, which will accelerate the patient's heart rate. These same drugs will ele-

FIGURE 27-5 (a) Inspect for finger clubbing. Any clubbing may indicate chronic respiratory or cardiac disease. (b) Characteristics of finger clubbing include large fingertips and a loss of the normal angle at the nail bed.

(a)

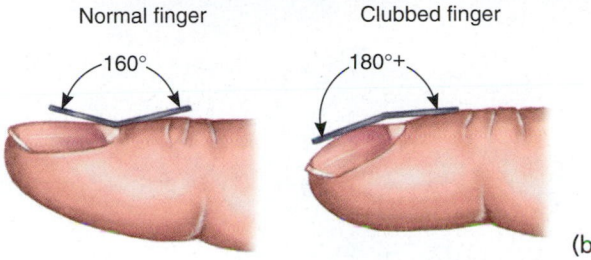

Normal finger   Clubbed finger

160°   180°+

(b)

vate the patient's blood pressure as well. During your assessment of the blood pressure, a patient will occasionally exhibit *pulsus paradoxus,* a drop in the systolic blood pressure of 10 mmHg or more with each respiratory cycle. Pulsus paradoxus is associated with chronic obstructive pulmonary disease (COPD) and cardiac tamponade. As a rule, however, you should not take the time to look for pulsus paradoxus.

A change in a patient's respiratory rate may be one of the earliest indicators of respiratory disease. The patient's respiratory rate can be influenced by several factors, including respiratory difficulty, fear, anxiety, fever, and underlying metabolic disease. Assume that an elevated respiratory rate in a patient with dyspnea is caused by hypoxia. Although fluctuations in the respiratory rate are common, a persistently *slow* rate indicates impending respiratory arrest.

Continually reassess the patient's respiratory rate during the time that you are caring for the patient. Trends in the respiratory rate (for example, an increasing rate) can give you an overall assessment of the effectiveness of any intervention

Assume that an elevated respiratory rate in a patient with dyspnea is caused by hypoxia. A persistently slow rate indicates impending respiratory arrest.

Constantly reassess the patient's respiratory rate and pattern.

you have made. Also assess the patient's respiratory pattern. The normal respiratory pattern (eupnea) is steady, even breaths occurring 12 to 20 times per minute with an expiratory phase that lasts between 3 to 4 times the inspiratory phase. **Tachypnea** describes a respiratory pattern with a rate that exceeds 20 breaths per minute. **Bradypnea** describes a respiratory pattern with a rate slower than 12 breaths per minute. Also, look for any abnormal respiratory patterns (e.g., Cheyne-Stokes, Kussmaul, or other) that were discussed earlier in the chapter.

* tachypnea rapid respiration.

* bradypnea slow respiration.

Diagnostic Testing

Three diagnostic measurements are of value in assessing the patient's respiratory status: *pulse oximetry, peak flow,* and *capnometry.*

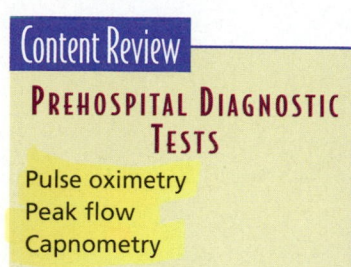

Content Review

PREHOSPITAL DIAGNOSTIC TESTS

Pulse oximetry
Peak flow
Capnometry

- *Pulse Oximetry.* Pulse oximetry offers a rapid and accurate means for assessing oxygen saturation. The pulse oximeter can be quickly applied to a finger or earlobe. The pulse rate and oxygen saturation can be continuously recorded. Use of the pulse oximeter, if available, is encouraged for any patient complaining of dyspnea or respiratory problems (Figure 27-6). Remember that the pulse oximetry reading may

FIGURE 27-6 Sensing unit for pulse oximetry. This device transmits light through a vascular bed, such as in the finger, and can determine the oxygen saturation of red blood cells. To use the pulse oximeter, it is only necessary to turn the device on and attach the sensor to a finger. The desired graphic mode on the oximeter should be selected. The oxygen saturation and pulse rate can be continuously monitored.

FIGURE 27-7 Wright Spirometer for determining Peak Expiratory Flow Rate (PEFR).

be difficult to obtain in a patient with peripheral vasoconstriction (as in sepsis or hypothermia). It may also be inaccurate under conditions in which an abnormal substance like carbon monoxide binds to hemoglobin, since the instrument measures the saturation of hemoglobin without indicating what substance has saturated it.

The oxygen saturation measurement obtained through pulse oximetry is abbreviated as SaO_2 (oxygen saturation). When pulse oximetry first came into use, some authors abbreviated the oxygen saturation measurement as SpO_2. However, this was sometimes confused with the PaO_2 obtained during blood gas measurement. Because of this, SaO_2 has become the preferred abbreviation.

- *Peak Flow.* Small portable hand-held devices are available for use in determining the patient's peak expiratory flow rate (PEFR). The normal expected peak flow rate is based on the patient's sex, age, and height. Remember that the measurement of the peak expiratory flow rate is somewhat effort dependent; you must have a cooperative patient who understands the use of the device in order to get an accurate reading.

The PEFR is obtained using a Wright Spirometer (Figure 27-7), which is inexpensive and easy to use. Place the disposable mouth piece into the meter. First have the patient take in the deepest possible inspiration. Then encourage the patient to seal his lips around the device and forcibly exhale. The peak rate of exhaled gas is recorded in liters per minute. This should be repeated twice, with the highest reading recorded as the patient's PEFR (Table 27-1).

- *Capnometry.* Devices are now available that detect carbon dioxide at the end of the expiratory phase. If gases are sampled at the end of an endotracheal tube, the level of measured carbon dioxide is

Table 27-1	SPIROMETRY AND PEAK FLOW VALUES FOR ADULTS		
FEV$_1$ Severity	FEV$_1$ (Liters)	FVC (%)	Peak Flow (Liters/Min)
Normal	4.0–6.0 L	80–90%	550–650 (Male)
			400–500 (Female)
Mild	3.0 L	70%	300–400
Moderate	1.6 L	50%	200–300
Severe	0.6 L	40%	100

FIGURE 27-8 End-tidal CO$_2$ devices: (a) electronic (b) colormetric.

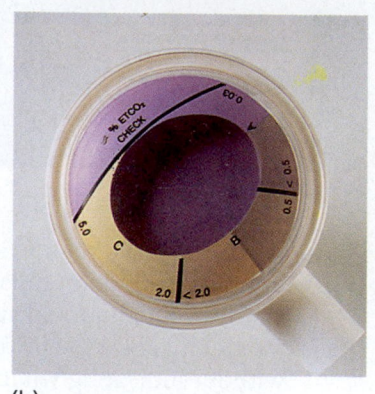

(a)

(b)

highest at the end of expiration. This is referred to as end-tidal CO$_2$ measurement. The fact that carbon dioxide is detected assumes that the metabolic processes of the body are active in producing CO$_2$ and that this gas is adequately exchanged in the lungs. Remember that almost no carbon dioxide is present in the esophagus and stomach. As a result, none would be detected by capnometry if the endotracheal tube is improperly placed into the esophagus. However, even a properly placed capnometry device will not detect CO$_2$ if the patient is in cardiac arrest.

Although several devices are available that measure the level of carbon dioxide during the entire ventilatory cycle (as a continuous waveform called *capnography*), most devices are used primarily in the out-of-hospital setting to assure the proper position of the endotracheal tube in the trachea. These devices, called end-tidal CO$_2$ detectors, focus only on the presence or absence of carbon dioxide in the sampled gas (*capnometry*). If the endotracheal tube becomes dislodged from its proper position, there is an almost immediate change in the readings from the end-tidal CO$_2$ device. This is in contrast to measurement of pulse oximetry which may take several minutes to reflect the hypoxia produced by tube dislodgement.

Two types of devices are commonly used for capnometry. The first device gives a numerical read-out of the level of carbon dioxide detected by the device (Figure 27-8a). The other device relies upon a color change produced by carbon dioxide to demonstrate the presence of the gas during exhalation (Figure 27-8b).

MANAGEMENT OF RESPIRATORY DISORDERS

The following sections will address the pathophysiology, assessment, and management of the more common respiratory disorders encountered in prehospital care. The discussion begins with a look at some general principles that can and should be applied to ALL respiratory emergencies.

MANAGEMENT PRINCIPLES

In cases of acute respiratory insufficiency, several principles should guide your actions in the prehospital setting. These include:

Principles of management for respiratory disorders include (1) Give first priority to the airway, and (2) Always provide oxygen to patients with respiratory distress or the possibility of hypoxia, including patients with COPD.

- The airway always has first priority. In trauma victims who may have associated cervical spine injuries, protect and maintain the airway without extending the neck.
- Any patient with respiratory distress should receive oxygen.
- Any patient whose illness or injury suggests the possibility of hypoxia should receive oxygen.
- If there is a question whether oxygen should be given, as in chronic obstructive pulmonary disease (COPD), administer it. *Oxygen should never be withheld from a patient suspected of suffering hypoxia.*

Keep these precautions in mind as you read through the descriptions of pathophysiology, assessment, and management of respiratory disorders frequently encountered in the field

SPECIFIC RESPIRATORY DISEASES

UPPER-AIRWAY OBSTRUCTION

The most common cause of upper-airway obstruction is the relaxed tongue. In an unconscious patient in the supine position, the tongue can fall into the back of the throat and obstruct the upper airway. Additionally, the upper airway can become obstructed by such common materials as food, dentures, or other foreign bodies. A typical example of upper-airway obstruction is the "cafe coronary," which tends to occur in middle-aged or elderly patients who wear dentures. These people often are unable to sense how well they have chewed their food. Thus, they accidentally inhale a large piece of food (often meat) that obstructs their airway. Concurrent alcohol consumption is often implicated in the "cafe coronary." Also, obstruction of the upper airway can be the result of facial or neck trauma, upper-airway burns, and allergic reactions. In addition, the upper airway can become blocked by an infection that causes swelling of the epiglottis (epiglottitis) or subglottic area (croup).

Content Review

COMMON CAUSES OF AIRWAY OBSTRUCTION
Tongue
Foreign matter
Trauma
Burns
Allergic reaction
Infection

Assessment

Assessment of the patient with an upper-airway obstruction varies, depending upon the cause of the obstruction and the history of the event. The unresponsive patient should be evaluated for snoring respirations, possibly indicating tongue or denture obstruction. If confronted by a patient suffering a "cafe coronary," determine whether the victim can speak. Speech indicates that, at present, the obstruction is incomplete. If the victim is unresponsive and has been eating, strongly suspect a food bolus lodged in the trachea. If a burn is present or suspected, assume laryngeal edema until proven otherwise.

Patients who may be having an allergic reaction to food or medications will often report an itching sensation in the palate followed by a "lump" in the throat. The situation may progress to hoarseness, inspiratory stridor, and complete obstruction. Pay particular attention to the presence of urticaria (hives). Intercostal muscle retraction and use of the strap muscles of the neck for breathing suggest attempts to ventilate against a partially closed airway.

Management

Management of the obstructed airway is based on the nature of the obstruction. Blockage by the tongue can be corrected by opening the airway, using either the head-tilt, chin-lift, the jaw-thrust, or the modified jaw-thrust maneuver. The airway can be maintained by employing either a nasopharyngeal or oropharyngeal airway. If possible, remove obstructing foreign bodies using the following basic airway maneuvers.

Conscious Adult In an adult patient who is conscious:

1. Determine if there is a complete obstruction or poor air exchange. Ask the patient: "Are you choking?" "Can you speak?" If the patient can speak, he should be asked to produce a forceful cough to expel the foreign body.

2. If the patient has complete obstruction or poor air exchange, provide up to five abdominal thrusts in rapid succession. If the thrusts prove unsuccessful, repeat until the obstruction is relieved or the patient becomes unconscious. In very obese or pregnant patients, use chest thrusts in lieu of abdominal thrusts.

Unconscious Adult If the patient is unconscious or loses consciousness:

1. Use the head-tilt, chin lift, the jaw-thrust, or the modified jaw-thrust maneuver in an attempt to open the airway.

2. Pinch the patient's nostrils and attempt to give two ventilations. If the attempts to ventilate fail, reposition the head and repeat attempt. If this fails . . .

3. Straddle the patient and administer up to five abdominal thrusts in quick succession. If this fails . . .

4. Try the tongue-jaw lift and, if the foreign body is seen, attempt finger sweeps. If successful, resume ventilation. If unsuccessful . . .

5. Continue the abdominal thrusts and finger sweeps, while preparing the laryngoscope and the Magill forceps. Visualize the airway with the laryngoscope. If the foreign body can be seen, grasp it with the Magill forceps and remove. Once removed, begin ventilation and administer supplemental oxygen.

In cases of airway obstruction caused by laryngeal edema (e.g., anaphylactic reactions, angioedema), establish the airway by the head-tilt, chin-lift, the jaw-thrust, or triple-airway maneuver. Then administer supplemental oxygen. Attempt bag-valve-mask ventilation. Often, air can be forced past the obstruction and the patient adequately ventilated using this technique. Next, start an IV with a crystalloid solution and administer subcutaneous epinephrine. Then administer diphenhydramine (Benadryl). Transtracheal ventilation may be required if the patient does not respond to the treatments described. See Chapter 42 for pediatric techniques.

NON-CARDIOGENIC PULMONARY EDEMA/ADULT RESPIRATORY DISTRESS SYNDROME

Adult respiratory distress syndrome (ARDS) is a form of pulmonary edema that is caused by fluid accumulation in the interstitial space within the lungs. Patients with *cardiogenic* pulmonary edema have a poorly functioning left ventricle. This leads to increases in hydrostatic pressure and fluid accumulation in the intersti-

* adult respiratory distress syndrome (ARDS) form of pulmonary edema that is caused by fluid accumulation in the interstitial space within the lungs.

tial space. In patients with ARDS, however, fluid accumulation occurs as the result of increased vascular permeability and decreased fluid removal from the lung tissue. This occurs in response to a wide variety of lung insults including:

- Sepsis, particularly with gram-negative organisms
- Aspiration
- Pneumonia or other respiratory infections
- Pulmonary injury
- Burns
- Inhalation injury
- Oxygen toxicity
- Drugs such as aspirin or opiates
- High altitude
- Hypothermia
- Near-drowning
- Head injury
- Emboli from blood clot, fat, or amniotic fluid
- Tumor destruction
- Pancreatitis
- Procedures such as cardiopulmonary bypass or hemodialysis
- Other insults such as hypoxia, hypotension, or cardiac arrest

The mortality in patients who develop ARDS is quite high, approaching 70 percent. While many patients die as the result of respiratory failure, many succumb to failure of several organ systems, including the liver and kidneys.

Pathophysiology

ARDS is a disorder of lung diffusion that results from increased fluid in the interstitial space. Each of the underlying conditions cited above results in the inability to maintain a proper fluid balance in the interstitial space. Severe hypotension, significant hypoxemia as the result of cardiac arrest, drowning, seizure activity or hypoventilation, high altitude exposure, environmental toxins and endotoxins released in septic shock—all can cause disruption of the alveolar-capillary membrane. Increases in pulmonary capillary permeability, destruction of the capillary lining, and increases in osmotic forces all act to draw fluid into the interstitial space and contribute to interstitial edema. This increases the thickness of the respiratory membrane and limits diffusion of oxygen. In advanced cases, fluid also accumulates in the alveoli, causing loss of surfactant, collapse of the alveolar sacs, and impaired gas exchange. This results in a significant amount of pulmonary shunting with unoxygenated blood returning to the circulation. The result is significant hypoxia.

Assessment

Specific clinical symptoms are related to the underlying cause of ARDS. For example, patients who develop ARDS as the result of sepsis will have symptoms related to their underlying infection. Determine if there is a history of prolonged hypoxia, head or chest trauma, inhalation of gases, or ascent to a high altitude without prior acclimation, all of which can suggest an underlying cause for the respiratory complaints.

With ARDS, symptoms are related to the underlying cause.

Patients with ARDS experience a gradual decline in their respiratory status. In rare cases, a seemingly healthy patient has a sudden onset of respiratory failure and hypoxia. Such a presentation is characteristic of patients with high altitude pulmonary edema (HAPE).

Dyspnea, confusion, and agitation are often found in patients with non-cardiogenic pulmonary edema. Patients may also report fatigue and reduced exercise ability. Symptoms such as orthopnea, paroxysmal nocturnal dyspnea, or sputum production are not commonly reported but may be seen.

The prominent physical findings are generally those associated with the underlying lung insult. Tachypnea and tachycardia are often found in association with ARDS. Crackles (rales) are audible in both lungs. Wheezing may also be heard if there is any element of bronchospasm. Severe tachypnea, central cyanosis, and signs of imminent respiratory failure are seen in severe cases. Pulse oximetry will demonstrate low oxygen saturations in those patients with advanced disease. In those patients requiring ventilatory support, a decreased lung compliance will be noted. (It will require more operator force to deliver an adequate lung volume.)

Management

Management of the patient's underlying medical condition is the hallmark of treatment for ARDS.

Oxygen supplementation is essential for all ARDS patients.

* positive end-expiratory pressure (PEEP) a method of holding the alveoli open by increasing expiratory pressure. Some bag-valve units used in EMS have PEEP attachments. Also EMS personnel sometimes transport patients who are on ventilators with PEEP attachments.

Specific management of the patient's underlying medical condition is the hallmark of treatment for this disorder. Treatment of gram negative sepsis with appropriate antibiotics, removal of the patient from any inciting toxin, or rapid descent to a lower altitude in patients with HAPE are the most important therapies for this condition. The patient will usually tolerate an upright position with the legs dangling off the cart.

Since the hypoxia seen in ARDS is the result of diffusion defects, oxygen supplementation is essential for all patients with this condition. Establish intravenous access, but provide fluids only if hypovolemia exists. Establish cardiac monitoring. Suctioning of lung secretions is often required to maintain airway patency.

Use positive pressure ventilation to support any ARDS patient who demonstrates signs of respiratory failure. Use bag-valve-mask ventilation for initial respiratory support but note that these patients generally require endotracheal intubation and support using a mechanical ventilator for early management. **Positive end expiratory pressure (PEEP)** is often required to maintain patency of the alveoli and adequate oxygenation. Diuretics and nitrates, which are used in patients with cardiogenic pulmonary edema, are usually not helpful in patients with ARDS. Your medical director may occasionally order corticosteroids for patients with ARDS/non-cardiogenic pulmonary edema. Corticosteroids are thought to stabilize the alveolar-capillary membrane, although clinical studies have not demonstrated any benefit to their use.

Maintain cardiac monitoring and pulse oximetry throughout transport of the patient. Transport patients to a facility capable of advanced hemodynamic monitoring (including Swan-Ganz catheter) and mechanical ventilation support.

OBSTRUCTIVE LUNG DISEASE

Obstructive lung disease is widespread in our society. The most common obstructive lung diseases encountered in prehospital care are asthma, emphysema, and chronic bronchitis (the last two are often discussed together as chronic obstructive pulmonary disease, or COPD). Asthma afflicts 4-5 percent of the U.S. population and COPD is found in 25 percent of all adults. Chronic bronchitis alone affects one in five adult males. Patients with COPD have a 50 percent mortality within 10 years of the diagnosis.

Content Review

OBSTRUCTIVE LUNG DISEASES

Emphysema
Chronic bronchitis
Asthma

Although asthma may have a genetic predisposition, COPD is known to be directly caused by cigarette smoking and environmental toxins. Other factors have been shown to precipitate symptoms in patients who already have obstructive airway disease. Intrinsic factors include stress, upper respiratory infections, and exercise. Extrinsic factors include tobacco smoke, drugs, occupational hazards (chemical fumes, dust, etc.), and allergens such as foods, animal danders, dusts, and molds.

Obstructive lung diseases all have abnormal ventilation as a common feature. This abnormal ventilation is a result of obstruction that occurs primarily in the bronchioles. Several changes occur within these air conduits. Bronchospasm (sustained smooth muscle contraction) occurs, which may be reversed by beta adrenergic receptor stimulation. Agents such as terbutaline, albuterol, and epinephrine are used to accomplish this stimulation. Increased mucus production by goblet cells that line the respiratory tree also contribute to obstruction. This effect may be worsened by the fact that in many patients, the cilia are destroyed, resulting in poor clearance of excess mucus. Finally, inflammation of the bronchial passages results in the accumulation of fluid and inflammatory cells. Depending on the underlying cause, some elements of bronchial obstruction are reversible, whereas others are not.

During inspiration, the bronchioles will naturally dilate, allowing air to be drawn into the alveoli. As the patient begins to exhale, the bronchioles constrict. When this natural constriction occurs—in addition to the underlying bronchospasm, increased mucus production, and inflammation that exist in patients with obstructive airway disease—the result is significant air trapping distal to the obstruction. This is one of the hallmarks of obstructive lung disease. This section will discuss each of these disease processes—emphysema, chronic bronchitis, and asthma—detailing the pathophysiology, assessment, and treatment.

EMPHYSEMA

Emphysema results from destruction of the alveolar walls distal to the terminal bronchioles. It is more common in men than in women. The major factor contributing to emphysema in our society is cigarette smoking. Significant exposure to environmental toxins is another contributing factor.

Pathophysiology

Continued exposure to noxious substances, such as cigarette smoke, results in the gradual destruction of the walls of the alveoli. This process decreases the alveolar membrane surface area, thus lessening the area available for gas exchange. The progressive loss of the respiratory membrane results in an increased ratio of air to lung tissue. The result is diffusion defects. Additionally, the number of pulmonary capillaries in the lung is decreased, thus increasing resistance to pulmonary blood flow. This condition ultimately causes pulmonary hypertension, which in turn may lead to right-heart failure, **cor pulmonale,** and death (Figure 27-9).

* **cor pulmonale** hypertrophy of the right ventricle resulting from disorders of the lung.

Emphysema also causes weakening of the walls of the small bronchioles. When the walls of the alveoli and small bronchioles are destroyed, the lungs lose their capacity to recoil and air becomes trapped in the lungs. Thus, residual volume increases while vital capacity remains relatively normal. The destroyed lung tissue (called *blebs*) results in alveolar collapse. To counteract this effect, patients tend to breathe through pursed lips. This creates continued positive pressure similar to PEEP (positive end-expiratory pressure) and prevents alveolar collapse.

As the disease progresses, the PaO_2 further decreases, which may lead to increased red blood cell production and **polycythemia** (an excess of red blood cells

* **polycythemia** an excess of red blood cells.

Increased resistance

Right ventricular hypertrophy

FIGURE 27-9 Chronic obstructive pulmonary disease of long standing can cause pulmonary hypertension, which in turn may lead to cor pulmonale.

resulting in an abnormally high hematocrit). The $PaCO_2$ also increases and becomes chronically elevated, forcing the body to depend upon hypoxic drive to control respirations. Finally, remember that emphysema is characterized by irreversible airway obstruction.

Patients with emphysema are more susceptible to acute respiratory infections, such as pneumonia, and to cardiac dysrhythmias. Chronic emphysema patients ultimately become dependent on bronchodilators, corticosteroids, and, in the final stages, supplemental oxygen.

Assessment

Emphysema is rarely associated with a cough except in the morning.

The patient with emphysema may report a history of recent weight loss, increased dyspnea on exertion, and progressive limitation of physical activity. Unlike chronic bronchitis, discussed in subsequent sections, emphysema is rarely associated with a cough, except in the morning. Question the patient about cigarette and tobacco usage. This is generally reported in pack/years. Ask the number of cigarette packs (20 cigarettes/pack) smoked per day and the number of years the patient has smoked. Multiply the number of packs smoked per day by the number of years. For example, a man who has smoked 2 packs per day for 15 years would have a 30 pack/year smoking history. Medical problems related to smoking, such as emphysema, chronic bronchitis, and lung cancer, usually begin after a patient surpasses a 20 pack/year history, although this can vary significantly.

Emphysema patients usually have a barrel chest, are often thin, and have a pink color ("pink puffers").

Physical exam of the emphysema patient usually reveals a barrel chest evidenced by an increase in the anterior/posterior chest diameter. You may also note decreased chest excursion with a prolonged expiratory phase and a rapid resting respiratory rate. Patients with emphysema are often thin since they must use a significant amount of their caloric intake for respiration. They tend to be pink in color due to polycythemia (excess of red blood cells) and are referred to as "pink puffers." Emphysema patients often have hypertrophy of the accessory respiratory muscles (Figure 27-10).

The patient will often involuntarily purse his lips to create continuous positive airway pressure. Clubbing of the fingers is common. Breath sounds are usually diminished. Wheezes and rhonchi may or may not be present, depending on the amount of obstruction to air flow. The patient may exhibit signs of right-heart failure as evidenced by jugular vein distention, peripheral edema, and hepatic congestion. Signs of severe respiratory impairment in all patients with obstructive lung disease include confusion, agitation, somnolence, 1-to-2-word dyspnea, and use of accessory muscles to assist ventilation.

Management

Although emphysema differs in the disease process from chronic bronchitis, the two respiratory disorders share several of the same symptoms and pathophysiology. As a result, you will treat the two disorders in a similar manner. The discussion of management of emphysema will be taken up with chronic bronchitis. (See next section.)

CHRONIC BRONCHITIS

Chronic bronchitis results from an increase in the number of the goblet (mucus-secreting) cells in the respiratory tree (Figure 27-11). It is characterized by the production of a large quantity of sputum. This often occurs after prolonged exposure to cigarette smoke.

Pathophysiology

Unlike emphysema, in chronic bronchitis the alveoli are not severely affected and diffusion remains normal. Gas exchange is decreased because there is lowered

FIGURE 27-11 Chronic mucus production and plugging of the airways occur in chronic bronchitis.

Mucus production

alveolar ventilation, which ultimately results in hypoxia and hypercarbia. Hypoxia may increase red blood cell production, which in turn leads to polycythemia (as occurs in emphysema). Increased $PaCO_2$ levels may lead to irritability, somnolence, decreased intellectual abilities, headaches, and personality changes. Physiologically, an increased $PaCO_2$ causes pulmonary vasoconstriction, resulting in pulmonary hypertension and, eventually, cor pulmonale. Unlike emphysema, the vital capacity is decreased, while the residual volume is normal or decreased.

Assessment

The patient with chronic bronchitis often will have a history of heavy cigarette smoking, but the disease may also occur in nonsmokers. There may also be a history of frequent respiratory infections. In addition, these patients usually produce considerable quantities of sputum daily. Clinically, the patient is described as having a productive cough for at least three months per year for two or more consecutive years.

Patients with chronic bronchitis tend to be overweight and can be cyanotic. Because of this, they are often referred to as "blue bloaters." This can be contrasted with the "pink puffer" image of emphysema patients described above. Auscultation of the thorax often will reveal rhonchi due to occlusion of the larger airways with mucus plugs. The patient may also exhibit signs and symptoms of right-heart failure such as jugular vein distention, ankle edema, and hepatic congestion.

Management

The primary goals in the emergency management of the patient with either emphysema or chronic bronchitis are to relieve hypoxia and reverse any bronchoconstriction that may be present. However, many of these patients are dependent upon hypoxic respiratory drive. As a result, the supplemental administration of oxygen may decrease respiratory drive and inhibit ventilation. You

Chronic bronchitis is usually associated with a productive cough and copious sputum production.

Chronic bronchitis patients tend to be overweight and are often cyanotic ("blue bloaters").

Content Review

EMPHYSEMA AND CHRONIC BRONCHITIS: MANAGEMENT GOALS
Relieve hypoxia
Reverse bronchoconstriction

must continually monitor the patient and be prepared to assist ventilations if signs of respiratory depression develop.

The first step in treating a patient suffering an exacerbation of emphysema or chronic bronchitis is to establish an airway. Then place the patient in a seated or semi-seated position to assist the accessory respiratory muscles. Apply a pulse oximeter and determine the blood oxygen saturation (SaO_2). Administer supplemental oxygen at a low flow rate while maintaining an oxygen saturation above 90 percent. A nasal cannula can often be used, but you must constantly monitor the respiratory rate and depth as well as oxygen saturation. Alternatively, you may use a Venturi mask at a low concentration (24–35 percent). If hypoxia or respiratory failure is evident, then increase the concentration of delivered oxygen. Be prepared to support the ventilation with bag-valve-mask assistance. Intubation may be required if respiratory failure is imminent.

Establish an intravenous line with lactated Ringer's or normal saline at a "to keep open" rate. More aggressive fluid administration is suggested if there are signs of dehydration present. This may also aid in loosening thick mucus secretions. Then, if ordered by medical direction, administer a bronchodilator medication, such as albuterol, metaproterenol or ipratropium bromide, through a small volume nebulizer or particle inhaler (Rotohaler). Corticosteriods are also commonly used in the early management of patients with COPD.

Administer oxygen to the COPD patient who needs it to relieve hypoxia. Since this may decrease the respiratory drive in the COPD patient, monitor the patient and be prepared to assist ventilations if necessary.

ASTHMA

Asthma is a common respiratory illness that affects many persons. Although deaths from other respiratory diseases are steadily declining, deaths from asthma have significantly increased during the last decade. Most of the increased asthma deaths have occurred in patients who are 45 years of age or older. In addition, the death rate for black asthmatics has been twice as high as for their white counterparts. Approximately 50 percent of patients who die from asthma do so before reaching the hospital. Thus, EMS personnel are frequently called upon to treat patients suffering an asthma attack. Prompt recognition followed by appropriate treatment can significantly improve the patient's condition and enhance his chance of survival.

Pathophysiology

Asthma is a chronic inflammatory disorder of the airways. In susceptible individuals, this inflammation causes symptoms usually associated with widespread but variable air flow obstruction. In addition to air flow obstruction, the airway becomes hyperresponsive. The air flow obstruction and hyperresponsiveness are often reversible with treatment. These conditions may also reverse spontaneously.

Asthma may be induced by one of many different factors. These factors, commonly referred to as "triggers" or "inducers," vary from one individual to the next. In allergic individuals, environmental allergens are a major cause of inflammation. These may occur both indoors and outdoors. In addition to allergens, asthma may be triggered by cold air, exercise, foods, irritants, stress, and certain medications. Often, a specific trigger cannot be identified. Extrinsic triggers tend predominantly to affect children, whereas intrinsic factors trigger asthma in adults.

Within minutes of exposure to the offending trigger, a two-phase reaction occurs. The first phase of the reaction is characterized by the release of chemical mediators such as histamine. These mediators cause contraction of the bronchial smooth muscle and leakage of fluid from peribronchial capillaries. This results in both bronchoconstriction and bronchial edema. These two factors can significantly decrease expiratory air flow causing the typical "asthma attack."

Often, the asthma attack will resolve spontaneously in 1–2 hours or may be aborted by the use of inhaled bronchodilator medications such as albuterol. However, within 6–8 hours after exposure to the trigger, a second reaction occurs. This late phase is characterized by inflammation of the bronchioles as cells of the immune system (eosinophils, neutrophils, and lymphocytes) invade the mucosa of the respiratory tract. This leads to additional edema and swelling of the bronchioles and a further decrease in expiratory air flow.

The second phase reaction will not typically respond to inhaled beta-agonist drugs such as metaproterenol or albuterol. Instead, anti-inflammatory agents such as corticosteroids are often required. It is important to point out that the severe inflammatory changes seen in an acute asthma attack do not develop over a few hours or even a few days. The inflammation will often begin several days or several weeks before the onset of the actual asthma attack.

Assessment

Begin the initial prehospital assessment of the asthmatic by considering immediate threats to the airway, breathing, or circulation. Then turn your attention to the focused history and physical examination.

The most common presenting symptoms of asthma are dyspnea, wheezing, and cough. Wheezing results from turbulent air flow through the inflamed and narrowed bronchioles. Many asthmatics will have a persistent cough. This is primarily due to hyperresponsiveness of the airway. It is important to point out that some asthmatics do not wheeze. Instead, their initial presentation may be a frequent and persistent cough. As asthma severity increases, the patient may exhibit hyperinflation of the chest due to trapping of air in the alveoli. In addition, tachypnea (rapid respiration) will occur. The patient may start to use accessory muscles to aid respiration.

Symptoms of a severe asthma attack include 1-to-2-word dyspnea (the inability to complete a phrase or sentence without having to stop to breathe), pulsus paradoxus (a drop of systolic blood pressure of 10 mmHg or more with inspiration), tachycardia, and decreased oxygen saturation on pulse oximetry. As hypoxia develops the patient may become agitated and anxious.

When conducting the focused history and physical examination, start by obtaining a brief patient history. Most asthmatics will report that they suffer from asthma. In addition, the patient's home medications may help confirm a history of asthma. Common asthma medications include inhaled beta-agonists (albuterol, metaproterenol), inhaled corticosteroids (betamethasone, beclomethasone), inhaled cromolyn sodium, and inhaled anticholinergics (ipratropium bromide). Often the patient will be taking oral bronchodilators such as theophylline or may be taking oral corticosteroids (prednisone).

Determine when symptoms started and what the patient has taken in an attempt to abort the attack. Also, find out whether the patient is allergic to any medications. Question the patient about hospitalizations for asthma. If the patient has been hospitalized, ask whether the patient has ever required intubation and mechanical ventilation. A prior history of intubation and mechanical ventilation should heighten your index of suspicion. Similarly, an asthmatic who is on continuous corticosteroid therapy is also a high-risk patient.

After you obtain the pertinent history, perform a brief physical examination. Place particular emphasis on the chest and neck. Examination of the chest should begin with inspection. Note any increase in the diameter of the chest that may indicate air trapping. Also, note the use of accessory muscles, including retraction of the intercostal muscles or use of the strap muscles of the neck. Following inspection, palpate the chest, noting any deformity, crepitus, or asymmetry. Next, auscultate the posterior chest. Note any abnormal breath sounds such as wheezing or rhonchi. Listen to the symmetry of breath sounds. Unilateral wheezing may indicate an aspirated foreign body or a pneumothorax.

Obtain accurate vital signs. One of the most important vital signs is the respiratory rate. An increase in the respiratory rate is one of the earliest symptoms of a respiratory problem. Many EMS personnel inaccurately measure the respiratory rate. The easiest method is to simply place your fingers on the patient's radial artery as if you were measuring the pulse rate. This will make the patient think you are obtaining the pulse rate, and he will not alter his breathing pattern. Measure the respiratory rate for at least 30 seconds. At the same time, note any alterations in the respiratory pattern. Pulse oximetry is an excellent adjunct to respiratory assessment. It will provide you with data regarding the oxygen saturation status (SaO_2) as well as an audible measure of the pulse rate.

EMS systems should be able to measure the Peak Expiratory Flow Rate (PEFR). (Review Figure 27-9 and Table 27-1.) The PEFR is a reliable indicator of air flow. If possible, measure peak flow rates to determine the severity of an asthma attack and the degree of response to treatment. The more severe the asthma attack, the lower will be the PEFR.

Management

Treatment of asthma is designed to correct hypoxia, reverse any bronchospasm, and treat the inflammatory changes associated with the disease. Administer oxygen at a high concentration (100 percent). Establish intravenous access and place the patient on an ECG monitor. Direct initial treatment at reversing any bronchospasm present. The most commonly used drugs are the inhaled beta-agonist preparations such as albuterol (Ventolin, Proventil) in conjunction with ipratropium bromide (Atrovent). These can be easily administered with a small volume, oxygen-powered nebulizer. Monitor the patient's response to these medications by noting improvement in PEFR and pulse oximetry readings.

Many asthmatic patients will wait before summoning EMS. The longer the time interval from the onset of the asthma attack until treatment, the less likely it will be that bronchodilator medications will work. Often, after a prolonged asthma attack, the patient may become fatigued. A fatigued patient can quickly develop respiratory failure and subsequently require intubation and mechanical ventilation. Always be prepared to provide airway and respiratory support for the asthmatic.

Special Cases

While most cases of asthma conform to the preceding descriptions, you may run into several special cases in the field. Asthma conditions that require special concern include status asthmaticus and asthmatic attacks in children.

Status Asthmaticus *Status asthmaticus* is a severe, prolonged asthma attack that cannot be broken by repeated doses of bronchodilators. It is a serious medical emergency that requires prompt recognition, treatment, and transport. The patient suffering status asthmaticus frequently will have a greatly distended chest from continued air trapping. Breath sounds, and often wheezing, may be absent. The patient is usually exhausted, severely acidotic, and dehydrated. The management of status asthmaticus is basically the same as for asthma. *Recognize that respiratory arrest is imminent and be prepared for endotracheal intubation.* Transport immediately and continue aggressive treatment en route.

Asthma in Children Asthma in children is common. The pathophysiology and treatment are essentially the same as in adults, with altered medication dosages.

Several additional medications are used in the treatment of childhood asthma. (Asthma in children is discussed in greater detail in Chapter 42.)

UPPER RESPIRATORY INFECTION (URI)

Infections involving the upper airway and respiratory tract are among the most common infections for which patients seek medical attention. Although these conditions are rarely life-threatening, upper respiratory infections can make many existing pulmonary diseases worse or lead to direct pulmonary infection. The best defense against the spread of upper respiratory infection is common practices such as good hand washing and covering the mouth during coughing and sneezing. Attention to such details is important when caring for patients with underlying pulmonary disease or those who are immunosuppressed (HIV infection, cancer) because URIs are more severe in these populations. Because of the prevalence of such infections, complete protection is impossible.

Pathophysiology

Remember that the upper airway begins at the nose and mouth, passes through the pharynx and ends at the larynx. Other related structures are the paranasal sinuses and the eustachian tubes that connect the pharynx and the middle ear. In addition, several collections of lymphoid tissue found in the pharynx (palatine, pharyngeal, and lingual tonsils) produce antibodies and provide immune protection.

The vast majority of upper respiratory infections (URIs) are caused by viruses. A variety of bacteria may also produce infection of the upper respiratory tract. The most significant is Group A streptococcus, which is the causative organism in "strep throat" and accounts for up to 30 percent of URIs. This bacteria is also implicated in sinusitis and middle ear infections. Up to 50 percent of patients who have pharyngitis (inflammation of the pharynx) are not found to have a viral or bacterial cause. Fortunately, most URIs are self-limiting illnesses that resolve after several days of symptoms.

Assessment

The major symptoms of URI are dependent upon the portion of the upper respiratory tract that is predominantly affected (Table 27-2). Patients with URIs will often have accompanying symptoms such as fever, chills, myalgias (muscle pains), and fatigue.

Remember that any child with suspected epiglottitis (see Chapter 42) should be supported in a position of comfort. Do not attempt examination of the throat as this may produce severe laryngospasm. Adults do occasionally also develop epiglottitis, but this is generally a more benign condition.

Support the child with suspected epiglottitis in a position of comfort. Do not attempt examination of the throat, which may produce severe laryngospasm.

Management

In most cases, the diagnosis and treatment of upper respiratory conditions is based on the history and physical findings. Patients with pharyngitis are often diagnosed by obtaining a throat culture that confirms the presence of a bacterial cause of symptoms. A rapid test is also available. In patients with sinusitis and otitis media, treatment is based on a presumed bacterial cause.

As with other medical conditions, focus your attention on the patient's airway and ventilation. Generally, no intervention is required except in children with epiglottitis and in some complicated upper respiratory infections where a collection of pus may occlude the airway. Give oxygen supplementation to any patient who has underlying pulmonary disease.

In URI, as with other medical conditions, focus attention on the patient's airway and ventilation. Give supplemental oxygen to any patient with underlying pulmonary disease.

Table 27-2 LOCATIONS AND SIGNS AND SYMPTOMS OF UPPER RESPIRATORY INFECTIONS

Structure	Infection	Symptoms	Signs
Nose	Rhinitis	Runny nose, congestion, sneezing	Rhinorrhea
Pharynx	Pharyngitis	Sore throat, pain on swallowing	Erythematous pharynx, tonsil enlargement, pus on tonsils, cervical lymph node enlargement
Middle Ear	Otitis Media	Ear pain, decreased hearing	Red, bulging eardrum, pus behind ear drum, lymph node enlargement in front of or behind ear
Larynx	Laryngitis	Sore throat, hoarseness, pain on speaking	Red pharynx, hoarse quality to voice, cervical lymph node enlargement
Epiglottis	Epiglottitis	Sore throat, drooling, ill appearing	Upright position, drooling, ill appearing
Sinuses	Sinusitis	Headache, congestion	Tenderness over the sinuses, worsening of pain with leaning forward, yellow nasal discharge

Most upper respiratory infections are treated symptomatically. Acetaminophen or ibuprofen is prescribed for fever, headache, and myalgias. Encourage patients to drink plenty of fluids. Salt water gargles may be used for throat discomfort. Decongestants and antihistamines may be used to reduce mucus secretion. Encourage patients being treated with antibiotics for bacterial causes of URI to continue these agents.

In some patients with asthma or COPD, a URI may produce a worsening of their underlying medical condition. Use inhaled bronchodilators and corticosteroid agents according to local protocols or on advice of medical direction. Transport patients with underlying medical conditions to a health care facility capable of continued evaluation and management of the underlying condition. Continue appropriate monitoring with pulse oximetry and ECG during transport.

PNEUMONIA

Pneumonia is an infection of the lungs and a common medical problem, especially in the aged and those infected with the human immunodeficiency virus (HIV). In fact, pneumonia is one of the leading causes of death in both groups of patients and is the fifth leading overall cause of death in the U.S.

Patients with HIV infection and those on immune suppressive therapy (cancer patients) are at high risk of developing pneumonia. In addition, the very young and very old are at higher risk of acquiring pneumonia because of ineffective protective mechanisms. Other risk factors include a history of alcoholism, cigarette smoking, and exposure to cold temperatures.

Pathophysiology

Pneumonia is a collection of related respiratory diseases caused when a variety of infectious agents invade the lungs. Mucus production and the action of respiratory tract cilia play a role in protecting the body against bacterial invasion. When considering which patients are at risk, the unifying concept is that there is a defect in mucus production, ciliary action, or both.

Bacterial and viral pneumonias are the most frequent, although fungal and other forms of pneumonia do exist. More unusual forms of pneumonia are seen in those patients who are currently or recently have been hospitalized where they are exposed to a more unusual variety of microorganisms. This is referred to as hospital-acquired pneumonia. (Cases that develop in the out-of-hospital setting are described as community-acquired pneumonia.)

The infection begins in one part of the lung and often spreads to nearby alveoli. The infection may ultimately involve the entire lung. As the disease progresses, fluid and inflammatory cells collect in the alveoli, and alveolar collapse may occur. Pneumonia is primarily a ventilation disorder. Occasionally, the infection will extend beyond the lungs into the bloodstream and to more distant sites in the body. This systemic spread may lead to septic shock.

Assessment

A patient with pneumonia will generally appear ill. He may report a recent history of fever and chills. These chills are commonly described as "bed shaking." There is usually a generalized weakness and malaise. The patient will tend to complain of a deep, productive cough and may expel yellow to brown sputum, often streaked with blood. Many cases involve associated **pleuritic** chest pain. Therefore, pneumonia should be considered in any patient who presents complaining of chest pain, especially if accompanied by fever and/or chills. In pneumonia involving the lower lobes of the lungs, a patient may complain of nothing more than upper abdominal pain.

Physical examination will commonly reveal fever, tachypnea, tachycardia, and a cough. Respiratory distress may be present. Auscultation of the chest usually demonstrates crackles (rales) in the involved lung segment, although wheezes or rhonchi may be heard. There usually is decreased air movement in the areas filled with infection. Percussion of the chest may reveal dullness over these areas. *Egophony* (a change in the spoken "E" sound to an "A" sound on auscultation) may also be noted.

In the forms of pneumonia involving viral, fungal, and rare bacterial causes, the typical symptoms described above are not seen. Instead, these patients may report a non-productive cough with less prominent lung findings. Systemic symptoms such as headache, malaise, fatigue, muscle aches, sore throat, and abdominal complaints including nausea, vomiting, and diarrhea are more prominent. Fever and chills are not as impressive as in bacterial pneumonia.

Management

Pneumonia is generally diagnosed on the basis of physical examination, X-ray findings, and laboratory cultures. Therefore, diagnosis in the field is unlikely. The primary treatment is antibiotics to which the causative organism is susceptible. In the field, however, antibiotics are not indicated and treatment is purely supportive.

Place the patient in a comfortable position, and administer high-flow oxygen. Use pulse oximetry to assess the patient's oxygen requirements. In severe cases, ventilatory assistance is needed and endotracheal intubation may be required. Establish intravenous access and base fluid resuscitation on the patient's hydration status. Administering fluids for dehydration is appropriate, but over-hydration can also worsen the respiratory condition. Medical direction may

* **pleuritic** sharp or tearing, as a description of pain.

Consider pneumonia in any patient complaining of chest pain, especially if accompanied by fever and/or chills.

Field management of suspected pneumonia is purely supportive. Place the patient in a position of comfort and administer high-flow oxygen.

sometimes order a breathing treatment with a beta agonist, particularly if wheezing is present. Because patients with pneumonia often have some bronchospasm, these drugs will afford the patient some symptomatic relief. Give antipyretic agents such as acetaminophen or ibuprofen to reduce a high fever. Also, a cool, moistened wash cloth may soothe the patient.

Remember to be extremely careful when caring for the patient over age 65 with suspected pneumonia. These patients have high mortality and complication rates. Transport them to a facility capable of handling the significant complications associated with the disease for this population.

LUNG CANCER

Lung cancer (neoplasm) is the leading cause of cancer-related death in the U.S. in both men and women. Most patients with lung cancer are between the ages of 55 and 65 years. There is a high mortality rate for patients with lung cancer after only one year with the disease.

There are currently four major types of lung cancer based on the predominant cell type. Twenty percent of cases involve only the lung tissue. Another 35 percent involve spread to the lymphatic system, and 45 percent have distant metastases (cancer cells spreading to other tissues). In those cases where there is lung tissue invasion, the primary problem is disruption of diffusion. In some larger cancers, there may also be alterations in ventilation by obstruction of the conducting bronchioles.

Cigarette smoking has long been known to be a risk factor for development of lung cancer. Environmental exposure to asbestos, hydrocarbons, radiation, and fumes from metal production have also been identified as risk factors. Finally, home exposure to radon has been implicated in the development of lung cancer. Preventive strategies include educating teenagers about the dangers of cigarette smoking and encouraging current smokers to quit. Implementing environmental safety standards that reduce the risk of exposure to such substances as asbestos will also reduce the risk of lung cancer. Finally, cancer screening of populations at risk is encouraged.

Pathophysiology

Although cancers that start elsewhere in the body can spread to the lungs, the vast majority of lung cancers are caused by carcinogens (cancer-producing substances) from cigarette smoking. A small portion of lung cancers are caused by inhalation of occupational agents such as asbestos and arsenic. These substances irritate and adversely affect the various tissues of the lung, ultimately leading to the development of abnormal (cancerous) cells.

There are four major types of lung cancers depending upon the type of lung tissue involved. The most common type of lung cancer is referred to as *adenocarcinoma*. This cancer arises from glandular-type (i.e. mucus-producing) cells found in the lungs and bronchioles. The next most frequently encountered type of lung cancer is *small cell carcinoma* (also called "oat cell" carcinoma). Small cell carcinoma arises from bronchial tissues. The third type of lung cancer is referred to as *epidermoid carcinoma*. Finally, *large cell carcinoma* is the fourth major type of lung cancer. Like small cell carcinoma, epidermoid and large cell carcinomas typically arise from the bronchial tissues. Lung cancers generally have a bad prognosis with most patients dying within a year of the diagnosis.

Assessment

As with other respiratory diseases, your first priority is to address signs of severe respiratory distress. Look for altered mental status, 1-to-2-word dyspnea, cyanosis, hemoptysis, and hypoxia as documented by pulse oximeter. Severe uncontrolled hemoptysis can be a particularly life-threatening presentation.

Patients with lung cancer will present with a variety of complaints, depending on whether they are related to direct lung involvement, invasion of local structures, or metastatic spread. Patients with localized disease will present with cough, dyspnea, hoarseness, vague chest pain, and hemoptysis. Fever, chills, and pleuritic chest pain are seen in patients who develop pneumonia. Symptoms related to local invasion include pain on swallowing (dysphagia), weakness or numbness in the arm, and shoulder pain. Metastatic symptoms are related to the area of spread and include headache, seizures, bone pain, abdominal pain, nausea, and malaise.

Physical findings are non-specific. Patients with advanced disease have profound weight loss and cachexia (general physical wasting and malnutrition). Crackles (rales), rhonchi, wheezes, and diminished breath sounds may be heard in the affected lung. Venous distention in the arms and neck may be present if there is occlusion of the superior vena cava (called *superior vena cava syndrome*).

Management

Administer supplemental oxygen as needed based on the clinical status and pulse oximetry measurement. Support the patient's ventilation as needed and intubate as necessary. Be attentive, however, for any Do Not Resuscitate order or other advance directive, such as a living will, and follow your local protocol regarding these legal instruments. Consult medical direction if questions arise.

Initiate an IV of 0.9% normal saline and provide fluids if signs of dehydration are present. Follow your local protocol regarding the access of permanent indwelling catheters that many cancer victims have in place.

Out-of-hospital drug therapy consists of bronchodilator agents and corticosteroids when signs of obstructive lung disease are present. Continue any prescribed antibiotics. Transport the patient and monitor mental status, vital signs, and oxygen status, as appropriate. Be prepared to provide emotional support for both the patient and family during transport.

TOXIC INHALATION

Inhalation of toxic substances into the respiratory tract can cause pain, inflammation, or destruction of pulmonary tissues. Significant inhalations can affect the ability of the alveoli to exchange oxygen, thus resulting in hypoxemia.

Pathophysiology

The possibility of inhalation of products toxic to the respiratory system should be considered in any dyspneic patient. Causes of toxic inhalation include superheated air, toxic products of combustion, chemical irritants, and inhalation of steam. Each of these agents can result in upper airway obstruction due to edema and laryngospasm. In such cases, bronchospasm and lower-airway edema may additionally appear. In severe inhalations, disruption of the alveolar/capillary membranes may result in life-threatening pulmonary edema.

Assessment

When assessing the patient with possible toxic inhalation exposure, determine the nature of the inhalant or the combusted material. Several products can result in the formation of corrosive acids or alkalis that irritate and damage the airway. These include:

When assessing the patient with possible toxic inhalation, determine the nature of the inhalant or combusted material.

- Ammonia (ammonium hydroxide)
- Nitrogen oxide (nitric acid)
- Sulfur dioxide (sulphurous acid)
- Sulfur trioxide (sulfuric acid)
- Chlorine (hydrochloric acid)

It is also crucial to determine the duration of the exposure, whether the patient was in an enclosed area at the time of the exposure, or if he experienced a loss of consciousness. Loss of consciousness may cause the airway to became vulnerable as a result of the loss of airway protective mechanisms.

During physical examination, pay particular attention to the face, mouth, and throat. Note any burns or particulate matter. Next, auscultate the chest for the presence of any wheezes or crackles (rales). Wheezing may indicate bronchospasm, while crackles may suggest pulmonary edema.

Management

After assuring the safety of rescue personnel, remove the patient from the hazardous environment. Next, establish and maintain an open airway. Remember that the airway is often irritable and attempts at endotracheal intubation may result in laryngospasm, completely obstructing the airway. Laryngeal edema, as evidenced by hoarseness, brassy cough, and stridor is ominous and may require prompt endotracheal intubation. Administer humidified oxygen at high concentration. As a precaution, start an IV of a crystalloid solution to provide rapid venous access. Transport promptly.

CARBON MONOXIDE INHALATION

Carbon monoxide is an odorless, tasteless, colorless gas produced from the incomplete burning of fossil fuels and other carbon-containing compounds. Carbon monoxide can be encountered in industrial sites, such as mines and factories. It is present in the environment in various concentrations primarily because of automotive exhaust emissions. Most poisonings occur from automobile emissions and home-heating devices used in poorly ventilated areas. Carbon monoxide is often used in suicide attempts. In addition, it is a particular hazard for fire-fighters and rescue personnel.

Pathophysiology

Carbon monoxide exposure is potentially life-threatening because it easily binds to the hemoglobin molecule. It has an affinity for hemoglobin 200 times that of oxygen. Once bound, receptor sites on the hemoglobin can no longer transport oxygen to the peripheral tissues. The result is hypoxia at the cellular level and, ultimately, metabolic acidosis. Additionally, carbon monoxide binds to iron-containing enzymes within the cells, leading to worsening cellular acidosis.

Content Review

TOXIC INHALATION: MANAGEMENT SEQUENCE

- Assure safety of rescue personnel
- Remove patient from toxic environment
- Maintain an open airway
- Provide humidified, high concentration oxygen.

Assessment

When confronted by a patient suffering possible carbon-monoxide poisoning, determine the source of exposure, its length, and the location. Less time is required to develop a significant exposure in a closed space compared to one in an area that is fairly well ventilated.

Signs and symptoms of carbon-monoxide poisoning include headache, nausea and vomiting, confusion, agitation, loss of coordination, chest pain, loss of consciousness, and even seizures. On physical examination, the skin may be cyanotic or it may be bright cherry red (a very late finding). There may be other signs of hypoxia such as peripheral cyanosis or confusion.

Management

Content Review

CARBON MONOXIDE INHALATION: MANAGEMENT SEQUENCE

Assure safety of rescue personnel
Remove patient from exposure site
Maintain an open airway
Provide high concentration oxygen.

Upon detection of carbon monoxide poisoning, first assure the safety of rescue personnel, then remove the patient from the site of exposure. Assure and maintain the airway. Administer supplemental oxygen at the highest possible concentration. If the patient is breathing spontaneously, apply a *tight-fitting* nonrebreather mask. If respiratory depression is noted, assist respirations. If shock is present, treat. Prompt transport is essential.

Hyperbaric oxygen therapy may be used in the treatment of severe carbon monoxide poisoning. Many EMS systems have protocols established whereby patients suffering carbon monoxide poisoning are transported to hospitals with hyperbaric oxygen therapy facilities. Hyperbaric oxygen increases the PaO_2, thus promoting increased oxygen uptake and displacement of the carbon monoxide from the hemoglobin.

PULMONARY EMBOLISM

A pulmonary embolism is a blood clot (thrombus) or some other particle that lodges in a pulmonary artery, effectively blocking blood flow through that vessel. This condition is potentially life threatening because it can significantly decrease pulmonary blood flow, thus leading to hypoxemia (inadequate levels of oxygen in the blood). Pulmonary thromboembolism accounts for 50,000 deaths annually in the U.S. In fact, one in five cases of sudden death are caused by pulmonary emboli. The great majority of patients with pulmonary emboli survive; only one in ten cases of documented pulmonary emboli result in death.

The incidence of pulmonary emboli is increased in certain populations. Any condition that results in immobility of the extremities can increase the risk of thromboembolism. Such conditions include recent surgery, long-bone fractures (with immobilization in casts or splints), bedridden condition, or prolonged immobilization as with long distance travel. Venous pooling that occurs during pregnancy can also lead to pulmonary emboli. Certain disease states increase the likelihood of blood clot formation. These include cancer, infections, thrombophlebitis, atrial fibrillation, and sickle cell anemia. Also, the incidence of thromboembolic disease is increased in patients taking oral birth control pills, particularly among smokers.

Pathophysiology

Sources of pulmonary emboli include air embolism, such as can occur during the placement of a central line; fat embolism, which can occur following a fracture; amniotic fluid embolism; and blood clots. It is also possible for a foreign body (such as part of a venous catheter) to become dislodged in the venous circulation. The vast majority of cases, however, are caused by blood clots that develop in the deep venous system of the lower extremities.

As a rule, a significant amount of blood passes through the veins of the lower extremity. During normal use of our legs, muscular contractions propel the blood through the venous system with the aid of valves that are present in the lower extremity veins. This action prevents blood from flowing backward through the venous system. When there is infection, venous injury, or any other condition that leads to pooling of blood in the deep veins of the lower extremity, clot formation occurs. If a portion of the clot becomes dislodged, it will pass through the right side of the heart and become lodged in the pulmonary vasculature.

When a pulmonary embolism occurs, the blockage of blood flow through the affected artery causes the right heart to pump against increased resistance. This results in an increase in pulmonary capillary pressure. The area of the lung supplied by the occluded pulmonary vessel can no longer effectively function in gas exchange since it receives no effective blood supply. The major derangement in patients with pulmonary emboli is a perfusion disorder. The involved lung segment is still ventilated, producing a ventilation-perfusion mismatch.

Assessment

Signs and symptoms of a patient suffering a pulmonary embolism will vary, depending upon the size and location of the obstruction. The patient suffering acute pulmonary embolism may report a sudden onset of severe unexplained dyspnea, which may or may not be associated with pleuritic chest pain. The patient may also report a cough which is usually not productive but may occasionally produce blood (hemoptysis). There may be a recent history of immobilization such as hip fracture, surgery, or debilitating illness.

The physical examination may reveal labored breathing, tachypnea, and tachycardia. In massive pulmonary emboli, there may be signs of right-heart failure such as jugular venous distention and, in some cases, falling blood pressure. In many cases, auscultation of the chest may reveal no significant lung findings, although rare crackles (rales) and wheezing may be noted. Occasionally, a pleural friction rub (leathery sound heard with inspiration) may be heard.

Always examine the extremities. In up to 50 percent of cases, findings suggestive of deep venous thrombosis will be evident. These include a warm, swollen extremity with a thick cord palpated along the medial thigh and pain upon palpation or when extending the calf.

In extreme cases, the patient may present with extreme confusion as the result of hypoxia, severe cyanosis, profound hypotension, and even cardiac arrest. Physical examination may reveal petechiae (small hemorrhagic spots) on the arms and chest wall in these cases.

Management

As with all respiratory conditions, your first priorities are the airway, breathing, and circulation. Remember that a large pulmonary embolism may lead to cardiac arrest. Perform CPR if needed.

If you suspect a patient is suffering a pulmonary embolism, establish and maintain an airway. Assist ventilations as required. Administer supplemental oxygen at the highest possible concentration. Endotracheal intubation may be required.

Establish an IV of lactated Ringer's or normal saline at a "to keep open" rate. The diagnosis of pulmonary embolism is often difficult and requires a high index of suspicion. Remember that patients with suspected pulmonary embolism may

The patient with acute pulmonary embolism may have a sudden onset of severe unexplained dyspnea, with or without pleuritic chest pain.

With suspected pulmonary embolism, always examine the extremities. In up to 50 percent of cases, findings suggestive of deep venous thrombosis will be evident.

With pulmonary embolism, as with all respiratory conditions, your first priorities are the airway, breathing, and circulation. Remember that a large pulmonary embolism may lead to cardiac arrest. Be prepared to perform CPR if needed.

require a significant amount of care. This disorder has a high complication rate and a significant mortality. Carefully monitor the patient's vital signs and cardiac rhythm. Quickly transport the patient to a facility with the capabilities to care for the critical needs of the patient. Treatment in the hospital setting may include the use of various medications such as thrombolytic agents and blood thinners like heparin.

SPONTANEOUS PNEUMOTHORAX

A **spontaneous pneumothorax** is defined as a pneumothorax that occurs in the absence of blunt or penetrating trauma. Spontaneous pneumothorax is a common clinical condition, with 18 cases occurring for every 100,000 population. There is also a high recurrence rate. Fifty percent of patients will have a recurrent episode within two years.

There is a 5:1 ratio of male to female patients with spontaneous pneumothorax. Other risk factors include a tall, thin stature and a history of cigarette smoking. This disorder tends to develop in patients between the ages of 20 and 40 years. Patients with COPD have a higher incidence of spontaneous pneumothorax, presumably because of the presence of thinned lung tissue (blebs) that may rupture.

Pathophysiology

The primary derangement is one of ventilation as the negative pressure that normally exists in the pleural space is lost. This prevents proper expansion of the lung in concert with the chest wall. A pneumothorax occupying 15–20 percent of the chest cavity is generally well tolerated by the patient unless there is significant underlying lung disease.

Assessment

The patient with a spontaneous pneumothorax presents with a sudden onset of sharp, pleuritic chest or shoulder pain. Often, the symptoms are precipitated by coughing or lifting. Dyspnea is commonly reported. The degree of symptoms is not strictly related to the size of the pneumothorax.

The physical examination is usually not impressive. Decreased breath sounds on the involved side may be difficult to note. They may be best heard at the lung apex. Even more subtle is hyper-resonance to percussion of the chest. Occasionally, the patient may have subcutaneous emphysema, which may be palpated as a crackling under the skin overlying the chest. Tachypnea, diaphoresis, and pallor are also seen. Cyanosis is rarely found.

Management

Use the patient's symptoms and pulse oximetry readings as guides to therapy. For most cases of spontaneous pneumothorax, supplemental oxygen is all that is required. Ventilatory support and endotracheal intubation are rarely required.

Be very careful when managing patients with a spontaneous pneumothorax who require positive pressure ventilation by mask or endotracheal tube. They are at risk for the development of a *tension pneumothorax*. You may note that the patient will become physically difficult to ventilate. Hypoxia, cyanosis, and hypotension may also develop. In addition to the usual signs of a pneumothorax, the patient will develop jugular vein distention and deviation of the trachea away from the pneumothorax. Needle decompression of a tension pneumothorax may be required.

Other management measures should include placing the patient in a position of comfort. Reserve intravenous access and electrocardiographic monitoring for

Table 27-3	CAUSES OF HYPERVENTILATION SYNDROME
Acidosis	Interstitial pneumonitis, fibrosis, edema
Beta-adrenergic agonists	Metabolic disorders
Bronchial asthma	Methyxanthine derivatives
Cardiovascular disorders	Neurologic disorders
Central nervous system infection or tumors	Pain
Congestive heart failure	Pregnancy
Drugs	Pneumonia
Fever, sepsis	Progesterone
Hepatic failure	Psychogenic or anxiety hypertension
High altitude	Pulmonary disease
Hypotension	Pulmonary emboli, vascular disease
Hypoxia	Salicylate

patients with significant symptoms or severe underlying respiratory disease. Carefully monitor such patients during transport.

HYPERVENTILATION SYNDROME

Hyperventilation syndrome is characterized by rapid breathing, chest pains, numbness, and other symptoms usually associated with anxiety or a situational reaction. However, as shown in Table 27-3, many serious medical problems can cause hyperventilation. To avoid improper treatment, consider hyperventilation to be indicative of a serious medical problem until proven otherwise.

Consider hyperventilation indicative of a serious medical problem until proven otherwise.

Pathophysiology

Hyperventilation syndrome frequently occurs in anxious patients. The patient often senses that he cannot "catch his breath." The patient will then begin to breathe rapidly. Hyperventilation in a purely anxious patient results in the excess elimination of CO_2, causing a respiratory alkalosis. This increases the amount of bound calcium, producing a relative hypocalcemia. This results in cramping of the muscles of the feet and hands, which is called *carpopedal spasm*.

Assessment

With a hyperventilating patient, you may elicit a history of fatigue, nervousness, dizziness, dyspnea, chest pain, and numbness and tingling around the mouth, hands, and feet. The physical examination will reveal an anxious patient with tachypnea and tachycardia. As noted above, spasm of the fingers and feet may also be present. If the patient has a history of seizure disorder, the hyperventilation episode may precipitate a seizure. Other symptoms are related to the underlying cause of the hyperventilation syndrome.

Management

The primary treatment for hyperventilation is reassurance. Instruct the patient to reduce his respiratory rate and depth.

The primary treatment for hyperventilation syndrome is reassurance. Instruct the patient to voluntarily reduce his respiratory rate and depth of breathing. Mechanisms that will assist in increasing the PCO_2, such as breath holding or breathing into a paper bag, are discouraged in prehospital care. Hyperventilating patients require oxygen. Allowing them to rebreathe into a paper bag can be deadly. Many EMS systems permit paramedics to use rebreathing techniques only on physician order. It is important to exclude other medical causes before determining that a patient is hyperventilating. Check the oxygen saturation by applying a pulse oximeter. Do not withhold oxygen.

The hyperventilating patient can often present a dilemma for prehospital personnel. Although anxiety is the most common cause of hyperventilation, other more serious diseases can present in exactly the same manner. For example, pulmonary embolism or acute myocardial infarction can exhibit symptoms similar to hyperventilation syndrome.

CENTRAL NERVOUS SYSTEM DYSFUNCTION

Central nervous system dysfunction, with the exception of drug overdose and massive stroke, is a relatively rare cause of respiratory emergencies. However, always consider the possibility of central nervous system dysfunction in any dyspneic patient.

Pathophysiology

Central nervous system dysfunction can be a causative factor in respiratory depression and arrest. Causes include head trauma, stroke, brain tumors, and various drugs. Several medications, such as narcotics and barbiturates, make the respiratory centers in the brain less responsive to increases in $PaCO_2$. These agents also depress areas of the brain responsible for initiating respirations.

Assessment

The assessment of patients with central nervous system dysfunction should follow the same approach as for any respiratory emergency. However, you should be alert for non-respiratory system problems such as CNS trauma or drug ingestion. Be careful to note any variation in the respiratory pattern, which can be an indication of central nervous system dysfunction.

Management

If central nervous system dysfunction is suspected, establish and maintain an open airway. If respiratory depression is noted or if respirations are absent, initiate mechanical ventilation. Administer supplemental oxygen, and establish an IV of normal saline at a "to keep open" rate. Direct specific therapy at the underlying problem, if it is known.

DYSFUNCTION OF THE SPINAL CORD, NERVES, OR RESPIRATORY MUSCLES

Several disease processes can affect the spinal cord, nerves, and/or respiratory muscles. Dysfunction of these structures can lead to hypoventilation and progressive hypoxemia.

Pathophysiology

Numerous disorders can interfere with respiratory function. These include spinal cord trauma, polio, amyotrophic lateral sclerosis (ALS or Lou Gehrig's Disease), and myasthenia gravis. Viral infections, in certain cases, can cause dysfunction

Except in the case of drug overdose or massive stroke, central nervous system dysfunction is rarely the cause of respiratory emergencies.

With suspected central nervous system dysfunction, establish and maintain an open airway. If respiratory depression is noted or respirations are absent, initiate mechanical ventilation with supplemental oxygen and establish an IV of normal saline at a "to keep open" rate.

Disorders that affect the spinal cord, nerves, or respiratory muscles and can interfere with respiratory function include spinal cord trauma, polio, ALS, myasthenia gravis, and tumors that impinge on the spinal cord.

of the nervous system. An example of this is *Guillian-Barré Syndrome (GBS)*. In GBS, the myelin-covering of the nerve is damaged resulting in relative loss of nerve impulse conduction. This affects virtually every peripheral nerve. Approximately 30% of patients with GBS will require ventilatory assistance, as the nerves that stimulate respiration are impaired.

Certain tumors can impinge on the spinal cord, depressing respiratory function. These disorders result in an inability of the respiratory muscles to contract normally, thus causing hypoventilation. Tidal volume and minute volume are decreased. You should also be aware that patients with these disorders do not have the ability to generate an adequate cough reflex and as a result, are at risk of developing pneumonia.

Assessment

Patients with possible dysfunction of the spinal cord, nerves, or respiratory muscles may have a history of trauma that is not readily apparent. Always question the patient about injuries or falls. If there is any doubt about a possible injury, act accordingly and immobilize the cervical spine. Also, inquire about signs of symptoms that may suggest a problem with the peripheral nerves. These include such findings as numbness, pain, or sensory dysfunction. The assessment of patients with possible dysfunction of the spinal cord, nerves, or respiratory muscles should follow the same approach as for any respiratory emergency. However, be alert for subtle findings that may indicate a problem with the peripheral nervous system. Always be ready to protect the airway and support ventilation if the patient has symptoms of possible airway obstruction or respiratory failure.

Management

Management of spinal cord and respiratory muscle dysfunction is purely supportive. Establish an airway, and provide ventilatory support. If myasthenia gravis is present and if transport time is long, the physician may request the administration of one of several agents effective in treating such patients.

> *Management of spinal cord and respiratory muscle dysfunction is purely supportive.*

SUMMARY

Respiratory emergencies are commonly encountered in prehospital care. It is important to recognize that all respiratory disorders may produce derangements in ventilation, perfusion, or diffusion. Recognition and treatment must be prompt. Understanding the underlying cause of the respiratory disorder can guide therapy. The primary treatment is to correct hypoxia. Necessary steps include establishing and maintaining the airway, assisting ventilations as required, and administering supplemental oxygen. Appropriate pharmacological agents may be subsequently ordered by medical direction.

> *No matter the underlying cause of respiratory dysfunction, the primary treatment is to establish and maintain the airway, administer oxygen, and assist ventilations as required.*

CHAPTER 28

Cardiology

Objectives

After reading Part 1 of this chapter, you should be able to:

1. Describe the incidence, morbidity, and mortality of cardiovascular disease. (p. 1201)
2. Discuss prevention strategies that may reduce the morbidity and mortality of cardiovascular disease. (p. 1201)
3. Identify the risk factors most predisposing to coronary artery disease. (p. 1201)
4. Describe the anatomy of the heart, including the position in the thoracic cavity, layers of the heart, chambers of the heart, and location and function of cardiac valves. (pp. 1202–1203; also see Chapter 3)
5. Identify the major structures of the vascular system, the factors affecting venous return, the components of cardiac output, and the phases of the cardiac cycle. (pp. 1202–1203; also see Chapter 3)
6. Define preload, afterload, and left ventricular end-diastolic pressure and relate each to the pathophysiology of heart failure. (see Chapter 3)

Continued

38. Identify additional hazards that interfere with artificial pacemaker function. (p. 1275)

39. Recognize the complications of artificial pacemakers as evidenced on an ECG. (pp. 1274–1275)

Part 2: Assessment and Management of the Cardiovascular Patient (begins on p. 1280)

After reading Part 2 of this chapter, you should be able to:

40. Identify and describe the components of the focused history as it relates to the patient with cardiovascular compromise. (pp. 1282–1286)

41. Identify and describe the details of inspection, auscultation, and palpation specific to the cardiovascular system. (pp. 1286–1290)

42. Identify and define the heart sounds and relate them to hemodynamic events in the cardiac cycle. (pp. 1288–1289)

43. Describe the differences between normal and abnormal heart sounds. (pp. 1288–1289)

44. Define pulse deficit, pulsus paradoxus, and pulsus alternans. (pp. 1289, 1320)

45. Identify the normal characteristics of the point of maximal impulse (PMI). (p. 1289)

46. Based on field impressions, identify the need for rapid intervention for the patient in cardiovascular compromise. (pp. 1280–1290)

47. Describe the incidence, morbidity, and mortality associated with myocardial conduction defects. (pp. 1302, 1314)

48. Identify the clinical indications, components, and the function of transcutaneous and permanent artificial cardiac pacing. (pp. 1274–1275, 1302, 1304–1305)

49. Explain what each setting and indicator on a transcutaneous pacing system represents and how the settings may be adjusted. (pp. 1304–1305)

50. Describe the techniques of applying a transcutaneous pacing system. (pp. 1304–1305)

51. Describe the characteristics of an implanted pacemaking system. (pp. 1274–1275)

52. Describe the epidemiology, morbidity, mortality, and pathophysiology of angina pectoris. (pp. 1307, 1310)

53. Describe the assessment and management of a patient with angina pectoris. (pp. 1310–1312)

54. Identify what is meant by the OPQRST of chest pain assessment. (pp. 1282–1283)

55. List other clinical conditions that may mimic signs and symptoms of coronary artery disease and angina pectoris. (pp. 1307, 1310)

56. Identify the ECG findings in patients with angina pectoris. (pp. 1310–1311)

57. Based on the pathophysiology and clinical evaluation of the patient with chest pain, list the anticipated clinical problems according to their life-threatening potential. (pp. 1307, 1310)

58. Describe the epidemiology, morbidity, mortality, and pathophysiology of myocardial infarction. (pp. 1312–1313)

59. List the mechanisms by which a myocardial infarction may be produced from traumatic and nontraumatic events. (p. 1312)

60. Identify the primary hemodynamic changes produced in myocardial infarction. (pp. 1312–1313)

61. List and describe the assessment parameters to be evaluated in a patient with a suspected myocardial infarction. (pp. 1312–1313)

62. Identify the anticipated clinical presentation of a patient with a suspected acute myocardial infarction. (pp. 1313–1315)

63. Differentiate the characteristics of the pain/discomfort occurring in angina pectoris and acute myocardial infarction. (pp. 1313–1314)

64. Identify the ECG changes characteristically seen during evolution of an acute myocardial infarction. (p. 1314)

65. Identify the most common complications of an acute myocardial infarction. (pp. 1312–1315)

66. List the characteristics of a patient eligible for thrombolytic therapy. (pp. 1314–1317)

67. Describe the "window of opportunity" as it pertains to reperfusion of a myocardial injury or infarction. (pp. 1314–1315)

68. Based on the pathophysiology and clinical evaluation of the patient with a suspected acute myocardial infarction, list the anticipated clinical problems according to their life-threatening potential. (pp. 1313–1317)

69. Specify the measures that may be taken to prevent or minimize complications in the patient suspected of myocardial infarction. (pp. 1315–1317)

70. Describe the most commonly used cardiac drugs in terms of therapeutic effect and dosages, routes of administration, side effects, and toxic effects. (pp. 1295–1296)

71. Describe the epidemiology, morbidity, mortality, and physiology associated with heart failure. (pp. 1318–1320)

72. Identify the factors that may precipitate or aggravate heart failure. (pp. 1318–1319)

73. Define acute pulmonary edema and describe its relationship to left ventricular failure. (p. 1318)

74. Differentiate between early and late signs and symptoms of left ventricular failure and those of right ventricular failure. (p. 1319)

75. Define and explain the clinical significance of paroxysmal nocturnal dyspnea, pulmonary edema, and dependent edema. (pp. 1319–1320)

76. List the interventions prescribed for the patient in acute congestive heart failure. (pp. 1320–1321)

77. Describe the most commonly used pharmacological agents in the management of congestive heart failure in terms of therapeutic effect, dosages, routes of administration, side effects, and toxic effects. (pp. 1295–1296, 1321)

78. Define and describe the incidence, mortality, morbidity, pathophysiology, assessment, and management of the following cardiac related problems (pp. 1321–1332):
    • Cardiac tamponade
    • Hypertensive emergency
    • Cardiogenic shock
    • Cardiac arrest

79. Identify the limiting factor of pericardial anatomy that determines intrapericardiac pressure. (p. 1321)

80. Describe how to determine if pulsus paradoxus, pulsus alternans, or electrical alternans is present. (pp. 1320–1322)

81. Explain the essential pathophysiological defect of hypertension in terms of Starling's law of the heart. (pp. 1319, 1324–1325)

82. Rank the clinical problems of patients in hypertensive emergencies according to their sense of urgency. (p. 1323)

83. Identify the drugs of choice for hypertensive emergencies, cardiogenic shock, and cardiac arrest, including their indications, contraindications, side effects, route of administration, and dosages. (pp. 1295–1296, 1324, 1327, 1328–1329)

84. Describe the major systemic effects of reduced tissue perfusion caused by cardiogenic shock. (pp. 1324–1325)

85. Explain the primary mechanisms by which the heart may compensate for a diminished cardiac output and describe their efficiency in cardiogenic shock. (pp. 1324–1325)

86. Identify the clinical criteria and progressive stages of cardiogenic shock. (pp. 1324–1325)

87. Describe the dysrhythmias seen in cardiac arrest. (p. 1328)
88. Explain how to confirm asystole using the 3-lead ECG. (p. 1328)
89. Define the terms *defibrillation* and *synchronized cardioversion*. (pp. 1297, 1299)
90. Specify the methods of supporting the patient with a suspected ineffective implanted defibrillation device. (p. 1298)
91. Describe resuscitation and identify circumstances and situations where resuscitation efforts would not be initiated. (pp. 1328–1332)
92. Identify communication and documentation protocols with medical direction and law enforcement used for termination of resuscitation efforts. (pp. 1329–1332)
93. Describe the incidence, morbidity, mortality, pathophysiology, assessment, and management of vascular disorders including occlusive disease, phlebitis, aortic aneurysm, and peripheral artery occlusion. (pp. 1332–1336)
94. Identify the clinical significance of claudication and presence of arterial bruits in a patient with peripheral vascular disorders. (pp. 1332–1336)
95. Describe the clinical significance of unequal arterial blood pressure readings in the arms. (p. 1335)
96. Recognize and describe the signs and symptoms of dissecting thoracic or abdominal aneurysm. (pp. 1333–1335)
97. Differentiate between signs and symptoms of cardiac tamponade, hypertensive emergencies, cardiogenic shock, and cardiac arrest. (pp. 1321–1328)
98. Utilize the results of the patient history, assessment findings, and ECG analysis to differentiate between, and provide treatment for, patients with the following conditions (pp. 1280–1336):
    - cardiovascular disease
    - chest pain
    - in need of a pacemaker
    - angina pectoris
    - a suspected myocardial infarction
    - heart failure
    - cardiac tamponade
    - a hypertensive emergency
    - cardiogenic shock
    - cardiac arrest
99. Based on the pathophysiology and clinical evaluation of the patient with chest pain, characterize the clinical problems according to their life-threatening potential. (pp. 1307, 1310)
100. Given several preprogrammed patients with cardiac complaints, provide the appropriate assessment, treatment, and transport. (pp. 1280–1336)

INTRODUCTION

According to current estimates, more than 60 million Americans have some form of **cardiovascular disease (CVD). Coronary heart disease (CHD)**, a type of CVD, is the single largest killer of Americans. Each year, on average, 466,000 people die of CHD. Approximately 225,000 of them, a little more than half, die before ever reaching the hospital. Another way of looking at the impact of coronary heart disease is this: An American will suffer a nonfatal heart attack every 29 seconds. About once every minute, an American will die from CHD. These deaths are usually sudden and often due to lethal cardiac rhythm disturbances that result in cardiac arrest.

Sudden death from CHD is often preventable. To decrease the chances of sudden death, the patient must recognize the signs and symptoms early and seek health care. Then, the health care system must provide definitive care promptly, usually within the first hour after the onset of symptoms.

Public education about CHD has focused on two strategies. The first is to educate the public about the risk factors for the development of CHD. This program encourages patients to modify their lifestyle to minimize these risk factors. A variety of factors have been *proven* to increase the risk of cardiovascular disease. These include:

- Smoking
- Older age
- Family history of cardiac disease
- Hypertension (high blood pressure)
- Hypercholesterolemia (excessive cholesterol in the blood)
- Carbohydrate intolerance (diabetes mellitus)
- Cocaine use
- Male gender

Factors that are *thought* to increase the risk of coronary heart disease include:

- Diet
- Obesity
- Oral contraceptives (birth control pills)
- Sedentary lifestyle
- Type A personality (competitive, aggressive, hostile)
- Psychosocial tensions (stress)

The second component of public education is to teach recognition of the signs and symptoms of heart attack. Patients can only benefit from medical intervention if they recognize the signs and symptoms and promptly access the health care system. Patients are encouraged to access the EMS system early. As a paramedic, you will treat patients who already have developed the manifestations of cardiac disease. This will be an opportunity for you to further serve your patients by teaching preventive strategies, including early recognition of symptoms, education, and alteration of lifestyle.

This chapter discusses the advanced prehospital care of cardiovascular emergencies. First, we will review the pertinent anatomy and physiology, and then we will use that knowledge to discuss assessing, recognizing, and treating cardiovascular disorders.

More than 60 million Americans have some form of cardiovascular disease.

* **cardiovascular disease (CVD)** disease affecting the heart, peripheral blood vessels, or both.

* **coronary heart disease (CHD)** a type of CVD; the single largest killer of Americans.

Part 1: Cardiovascular Anatomy and Physiology, ECG Monitoring, and Dysrhythmia Analysis

REVIEW OF CARDIOVASCULAR ANATOMY AND PHYSIOLOGY

Cardiac anatomy and physiology were discussed in detail in Chapter 3. The following is a brief review of that information.

CARDIOVASCULAR ANATOMY

The heart is located in the center of the chest in the *mediastinum*. It is a muscular organ, consisting of three tissue layers: *endocardium* (the innermost layer that lines the chambers), *myocardium* (the middle layer with its unique ability to generate and conduct electrical impulses, causing the heart to contract), and *pericardium* (the protective sac surrounding the heart).

The heart (Figure 28-1) contains four chambers – two superior, the *atria*, and two inferior, the *ventricles*. Valves control the flow of blood through the heart:

FIGURE 28-1 Blood flow through the heart.

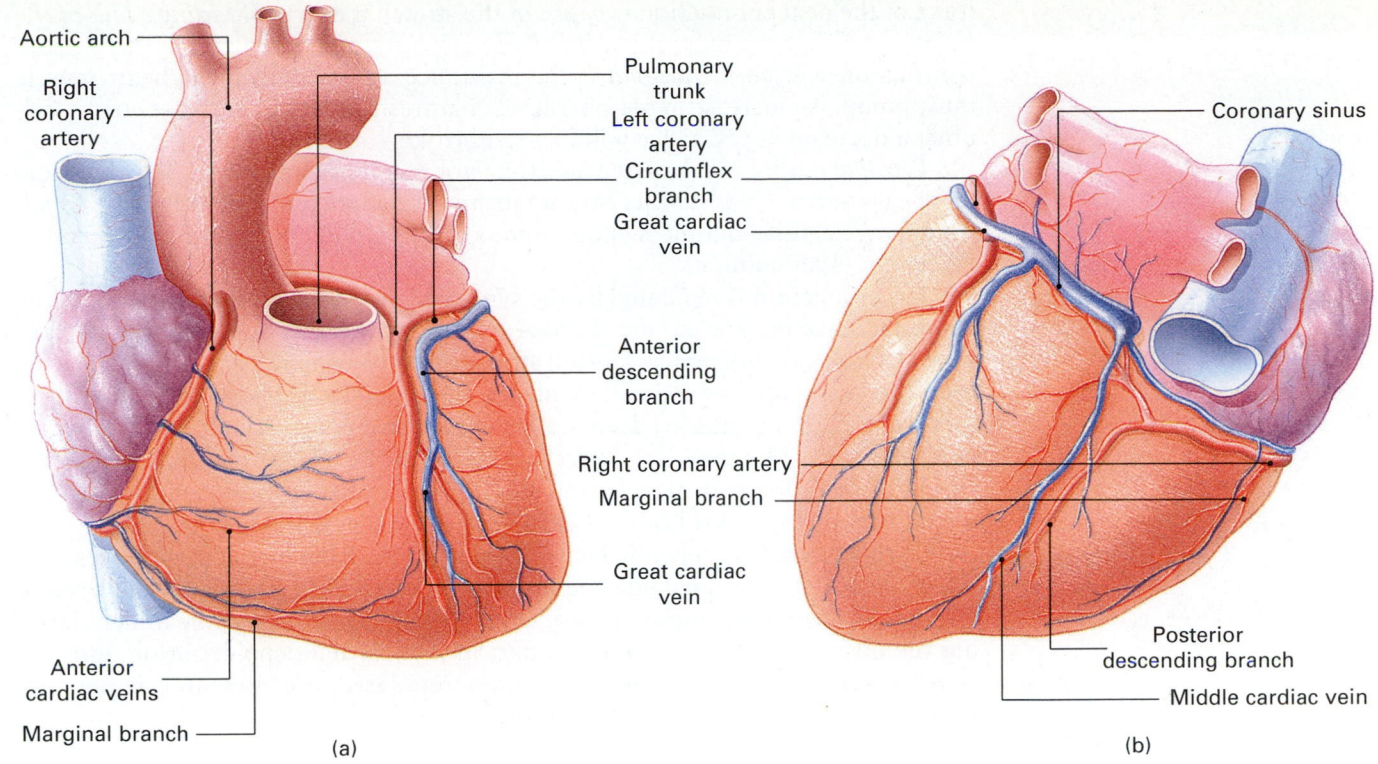

FIGURE 28-2 The coronary circulation: (a) anterior; (b) posterior.

the *mitral valve* between the left atrium and ventricle; the *tricuspid valve* between the right atrium and ventricle; the *aortic valve* between the left ventricle and aorta; the *pulmonary valve* between the right ventricle and pulmonary artery.

The right atrium receives deoxygenated blood from the body via the *superior* and *inferior venae cavae*. The right ventricle sends the deoxygenated blood to the lungs via the *pulmonary artery*. Oxygenated blood is returned from the lungs to the *left atrium* via the *pulmonary veins*. The left ventricle pumps the oxygenated blood to the body via the *aorta*. Oxygenated blood is pumped from the heart to the tissues via the *arteries,* and deoxygenated blood is transported from the tissues back to the heart via the *veins*. The *capillaries* connect arteries and veins. The exchange of oxygen and carbon dioxide with the body tissues takes place through the very thin capillary walls.

The heart receives its nutrients from the *coronary arteries* (Figure 28-2) that originate in the aorta and spread over the heart. The *left coronary artery* supplies the left ventricle, interventricular septum, part of the right ventricle, and the conduction system. Its two main branches are the *anterior descending artery* and *circumflex artery*. The *right coronary artery* supplies a portion of the right atrium and right ventricle and part of the conduction system. Its two major branches are the *posterior descending artery* and *marginal artery*.

CARDIAC PHYSIOLOGY

The *cardiac cycle* consists of *diastole,* the relaxation phase that takes place at the end of a cardiac contraction, and *systole,* the contraction phase. Normally, when the heart contracts each ventricle ejects about two-thirds of the blood it contains (the *ejection fraction*). The amount of blood ejected, known as the *stroke volume,* averages 70 ml. The stroke volume depends on three factors: preload, cardiac contractility, and afterload. *Preload* is the end-diastolic volume and influences the force of the next contraction because of the stretch it exerts. (*Starling's law of the heart* states that the more myocardial muscle is stretched, the greater its force of contraction will be.) *Afterload* is the resistance against which the heart muscle must pump. An increase in peripheral vascular resistance will decrease stroke volume; a decrease in resistance will increase stroke volume.

Cardiac output is calculated as stroke volume times heart rate. Since the normal heart rate is 60–100 beats per minute and the average stroke volume is 70 ml, the average cardiac output is about 5 liters (5000 milliliters) per minute (70 ml $\times$ 70 bpm = 4900 ml/min).

Heart function is regulated by the sympathetic and parasympathetic nervous components of the autonomic nervous system, working in opposition to one another to maintain a balance. During stress, the sympathetic system dominates to raise the heart rate and increase contractile force. During sleep, the parasympathetic system dominates to decrease heart rate and contractile force. The terms *chrontotropy* (referring to heart rate), *inotropy* (referring to contractile strength), and *dromotrpy* (referring to rate of nervous impulse conduction) describe autonomic control of the heart.

Cardiac function depends heavily on electrolyte balances. Electrolytes that affect cardiac function include sodium (Na^+), calcium (Ca^{++}), potassium (K^+), chloride (Cl^-), and magnesium (Mg^{++}). Sodium plays a major role in depolarizing the myocardium. Calcium takes part in myocardial depolarization and myocardial contraction. Potassium influences repolarization. Research is ongoing into the roles of magnesium and chloride.

ELECTROPHYSIOLOGY

Within the cardiac muscle fibers are special structures called *intercalated discs*. These discs connect cardiac muscle fibers and conduct electrical impulses quickly from one muscle fiber to the next. Thus, when one cell becomes excited, the action potential spreads rapidly across the entire group of cells, resulting in a coordinated contraction. This functional unit is a *syncytium*. The heart has two syncytia—the *atrial syncytium* and the *ventricular syncytium*. The atrial syncytium contracts from superior to inferior, so that the atria express blood to the ventricles. The ventricular syncytium contracts from inferior to superior, expelling blood from the ventricles into the aorta and pulmonary arteries. An impulse can be conducted from the atria to the ventricles only through the *atrioventricular (AV) bundle*.

Cardiac muscle functions according to an "all-or-none" principle. That is, if a single muscle fiber becomes *depolarized*, the action potential will spread through the whole syncytium. Stimulating a single atrial fiber will thus completely depolarize the atria, and stimulating a single ventricular fiber will completely depolarize the ventricles.

Cardiac Depolarization

Normally, an ionic difference exists on the two sides of a cell membrane. The cell's sodium-potassium pump expels sodium (Na^+) from the cell, leaving the inside of the cell more negatively charged than the outside. This difference is called the *resting potential*. When the myocardial cell is stimulated, the membrane changes to allow positively charged sodium ions to rush into the cell, giving the inside of the cell a greater positive charge than the outside. This change of membrane polarity is the *action potential*. After the influx of sodium, a slower influx of calcium ions (Ca^{++}) increases the positive charge inside the cell.

This change from the resting potential (when the inside of the cell is more negatively charged) to a relatively more positive charge inside the cell is called *cardiac depolarization*. Once depolarization occurs in a muscle fiber, it is transmitted throughout the entire syncytium, via the intercalated discs, until the entire muscle mass is depolarized. Contraction of the muscle follows depolarization. The cell membrane remains permeable to sodium for only a fraction of a second. Thereafter, sodium influx stops and potassium escapes from inside the cell. This returns the charge inside the cell to normal (negative). In addition, sodium is actively pumped outside the cell, allowing the cell to *repolarize* and return to its normal resting state.

Understanding the process of cardiac depolarization is critical to understanding and interpreting electrocardiograms (ECGs).

The Cardiac Conductive System

The cardiac conductive system stimulates the ventricles to depolarize in the proper direction. It initiates an impulse, spreads it through the atria, transmits it to the apex of the heart, and thence stimulates the ventricles to depolarize from inferior to superior. The conduction system relies on specialized conductive fibers that transmit the depolarization potential through the heart very quickly.

To accomplish their task, the cardiac conductive cells have:

- *Excitability* The cells can respond to an electrical stimulus.
- *Conductivity* The cells can propagate the electrical impulse from cell to cell.
- *Automaticity* Each conductive cell can depolarize without any outside impulse (called self-excitation). Generally, the cell with the fastest rate of discharge, becomes the heart's pacemaker. Usually, this is the sinoatrial (SA) node; however, if one pacemaker cell fails to discharge, then the cell with the next fastest rate becomes the pacemaker.
- *Contractility* The cells have the ability to contract.

Internodal atrial pathways connect the SA node to the AV node (Figure 28-3). These internodal pathways conduct the depolarization impulse to the atrial muscle mass and through the atria to the AV junction. The AV junction (the "gatekeeper") slows the impulse and allows the ventricles time to fill. Then, the impulse passes through the AV junction into the AV node and on to the AV fibers, which conduct the impulse from the atria to the ventricles. In the ventricles the AV fibers form the *bundle of His*.

The bundle of His subsequently divides into the right and left bundle branches. The *right bundle branch* delivers the impulse to the apex of the right ventricle. From there the *Purkinje system* spreads it across the myocardium. The *left bundle branch* divides into *anterior and posterior fascicles* that also ultimately terminate in the Purkinje system. At the same time that the impulse is transmitted to the right ventricle, the Purkinje system spreads it across the mass of the myocardium. Repolarization predominantly occurs in the opposite direction.

Each conductive system component has an intrinsic rate of self-excitation (SA node 60–100 bpm; AV node 40–60 bpm; Purkinje system 15–40 bpm).

SA node

Internodal atrial pathways

AV node

AV junction

Bundle of His

Interventricular septum

Left bundle branch

Right bundle branch

Purkinje fibers

Purkinje system

FIGURE 28-3 The cardiac conductive system.

ELECTROCARDIOGRAPHIC MONITORING

One of your most important skills as a paramedic will be obtaining and interpreting ECG rhythm strips.

* **rhythm strip** electrocardiogram printout.

One of your most important skills as a paramedic will be obtaining and interpreting electrocardiographic (ECG) **rhythm strips.** Your patient's subsequent treatment will be based upon rapid, accurate interpretation of these strips. At first, rhythm strips may seem very difficult to read, for only through classroom instruction and repeated practice can you master their interpretation. Nor will every rhythm strip you encounter be a "textbook" example; you must be comfortable with all possible variants. With practice and a systematic approach, however, you will soon be skilled in their interpretation. This section presents basic information about ECG monitoring, as well as recognizing and interpreting dysrhythmias.

THE ELECTROCARDIOGRAM

* **electrocardiogram (ECG)** the graphic recording of the heart's electrical activity. It may be displayed either on paper or on an oscilloscope.

The **electrocardiogram (ECG)** is a graphic record of the heart's electrical activity. However, it tells you nothing about the heart's pumping ability, which you must evaluate by pulse and blood pressure.

The body acts as a giant conductor of electricity, and the heart is its largest generator of electrical energy. Electrodes on the skin can detect the total electrical activity within the heart at any given time. The electrical impulses on the skin surface have a very low voltage. The ECG machine amplifies these impulses and records them over time on ECG graph paper or a monitor. *Positive impulses* appear as *upward* deflections on the paper, *negative impulses* as *downward* deflections. The absence of any electrical impulse produces an *isoelectric line*, which is flat.

* **artifact** deflection on the ECG produced by factors other than the heart's electrical activity.

Artifacts are deflections on the ECG produced by factors other than the heart's electrical activity. Common causes of artifacts include:

- Muscle tremors
- Shivering
- Patient movement
- Loose electrodes
- 60 hertz interference
- Machine malfunction

It is important for ECGs to be free of artifacts. When an artifact is present, you must first try to eliminate it before recording the ECG. Loose electrodes should be replaced. Occasionally, patients may be quite diaphoretic, thus preventing the electrodes from adhering well to the skin. In these cases, you may need to wipe the skin and apply tincture of Benzoin before applying the electrode.

ECG Leads

You can obtain many views of the heart's electrical activity by monitoring the voltage change through *electrodes* placed at various places on the body surface. Each pair of electrodes is a *lead*. In the hospital, 12 leads are normally used. As a rule, most EMS systems use only 3 leads in the field. In fact, one lead alone is adequate for detecting life-threatening dysrhythmias. With the advent of thrombolytic therapy and computer interpretation, however, 12-lead ECGs are becoming more common in the field, especially in rural EMS systems.

The three types of ECG leads are bipolar, augmented, and precordial. **Bipolar leads,** the kind most frequently used, have one positive electrode and one negative electrode. Any electrical impulse moving toward the positive electrode will cause a positive (upward) deflection on the ECG paper. Any electrical impulse moving toward the negative electrode will cause a negative (downward) deflection. The absence of a positive or negative deflection means either that there is no electrical impulse or that the impulse is moving perpendicular to the lead. Leads I, II, and III, commonly called *limb leads,* are bipolar. They are the most frequently used leads in the field. Table 28-1 lists their placement sites.

These three bipolar leads form **Einthoven's triangle,** named after Dr. Willem Einthoven, who invented the ECG machine (Figure 28-4). The direction from the negative to the positive electrode is the lead's *axis.* Each lead shows a different axis of the heart. Lead I, at the top of Einthoven's triangle, has an axis of 0°. Lead II forms the right side of the triangle and has an axis of 60°. Lead III forms the left side of the triangle and has an axis of 120°.

The bipolar leads provide only three views of the heart. **Augmented,** or **unipolar, leads** provide additional views that are sometimes useful. Although these leads evaluate different axes than the bipolar leads, they utilize the same electrodes. They do this by electronically combining the negative electrodes of two of the bipolar leads to obtain an axis. These augmented leads are designated aVR, aVL, and aVF. The letter *a* indicates that the lead is augmented. The letter *V* identifies it as a unipolar lead. The *R, L,* and *F* identify the extremity on which the lead is placed (R = right arm, L = left arm, and F = left foot).

In addition, six **precordial leads** can be placed across the surface of the chest to measure electrical cardiac activity on a horizontal axis. These leads help in viewing the left ventricle and septum. They are designated V_1 through V_6, with the letter *V* identifying them as unipolar leads.

Content Review

ECG LEADS

- Bipolar (Limb)
- Augmented (Unipolar)
- Precordial

✱ **bipolar limb leads** electrocardiogram leads applied to the arms and legs that contain two electrodes of opposite (positive and negative) polarity; leads I, II, and III.

✱ **Einthoven's triangle** the triangle around the heart formed by the bipolar limb leads.

✱ **augmented limb leads** another term for unipolar limb leads (see definition below), reflecting the fact that the ground lead is disconnected, which increases the amplitude of deflection on the ECG tracing.

✱ **unipolar limb leads** electrocardiogram leads applied to the arms and legs, consisting of one polarized (positive) electrode and a nonpolarized reference point that is created by the ECG machine combining two additional electrodes; also called augmented limb leads; leads aVR, aVL, and aVF.

✱ **precordial (chest) leads** electrocardiogram leads applied to the chest in a pattern that permits a view of the horizontal plane of the heart; leads V1, V2, V3, V4, V5, and V6.

Table 28-1 BIPOLAR LEAD PLACEMENT SITES

Lead	Positive Electrode	Negative Electrode
I	Left arm	Right arm
II	Left leg	Right arm
III	Left leg	Left arm

Figure 28-4 Einthoven's triangle as formed by Leads I, II, and III.

Routine ECG Monitoring

Whether in the ambulance, emergency department, or coronary care unit, routine ECG monitoring generally uses only one lead. The most common monitoring leads are either Lead II or the *modified chest lead 1* (MCL$_1$). Of these, Lead II is used more frequently because most of the heart's electrical current flows toward its positive axis. This gives the best view of the ECG waves and best depicts the conduction system's activity. MCL$_1$ is a special monitoring lead that some systems use selectively to help determine the origin of abnormal complexes such as premature beats. To avoid confusion, we will use Lead II as the monitor lead throughout this text.

Einthoven's triangle offers a basis for placing the leads. Usually you should place the electrodes on the chest wall instead of the extremities. This helps to reduce artifacts from arm movement. (If you use the arms, place the lead as high as possible on the extremity to decrease movement.) Make certain the skin is clean and free of hair before you place the electrodes on the chest wall. For Lead II, the positive electrode is usually placed at the apex of the heart on the chest wall (or on the left leg), the negative electrode below the right clavicle (or on the right arm). The third electrode, the ground, is placed somewhere on the left, upper chest wall (or on the left arm).

> *Lead II gives the best view of the ECG waves and best depicts the conduction system's activity.*

FIGURE 28-5 Recording of the ECG.

A single monitoring lead can provide considerable information, including:

- The rate of the heartbeat
- The regularity of the heartbeat
- The time it takes to conduct the impulse through the various parts of the heart

A single lead cannot provide the following information:

- The presence or location of an infarct
- Axis deviation or chamber enlargement
- Right-to-left differences in conduction or impulse formation
- The quality or presence of pumping action

ECG Graph Paper

ECG graph paper is standardized to allow comparative analysis of ECG patterns. The paper moves across the stylus at a standard speed of 25 mm/sec (Figure 28-5). The *amplitude* of the ECG *deflection* is also standardized. When properly calibrated, the ECG stylus should deflect two large boxes when one millivolt is present. Most machines have calibration buttons, and a calibration curve should be placed at the beginning of the first ECG strip. Many machines do this automatically when they are first turned on.

The ECG graph is divided into a grid of light and heavy lines. The light lines are 1 mm apart, and the heavy lines are 5 mm apart. The heavy lines thus enclose large squares, each containing twenty-five of the smaller squares formed by the lighter lines (Figure 28-6). The following relationships apply to the horizontal axis.

1 small box = 0.04 sec

1 large box = 0.20 sec (0.04 sec × 5 = 0.20 sec)

These increments measure the duration of the ECG complexes and time intervals. The vertical axis reflects the voltage amplitude in millivolts (mV). Two large boxes equal 1.0 mV.

FIGURE 28-6 The ECG paper and markings.

In addition to the grid, ECG paper has time interval markings at the top. These marks are placed at three-second intervals. Each three-second interval contains 15 large boxes (0.2 sec × 15 boxes = 3.0 sec). The time markings measure heart rate.

RELATIONSHIP OF THE ECG TO ELECTRICAL EVENTS IN THE HEART

The ECG tracing's components reflect electrical changes in the heart (Figure 28-7).

- *P wave.* The first component of the ECG, the P wave corresponds to atrial depolarization. On Lead II, it is a positive, rounded wave before the QRS complex (Figures 28-8 to 28-12).
- *QRS complex.* The QRS complex reflects ventricular depolarization. The *Q wave* is the first negative deflection after the P wave; the *R wave* is the first positive deflection after the P wave; and the *S wave* is the first negative deflection after the R wave. Not all three waves are always present, and the shape of the QRS complex can vary from individual to individual (Figure 28-13).

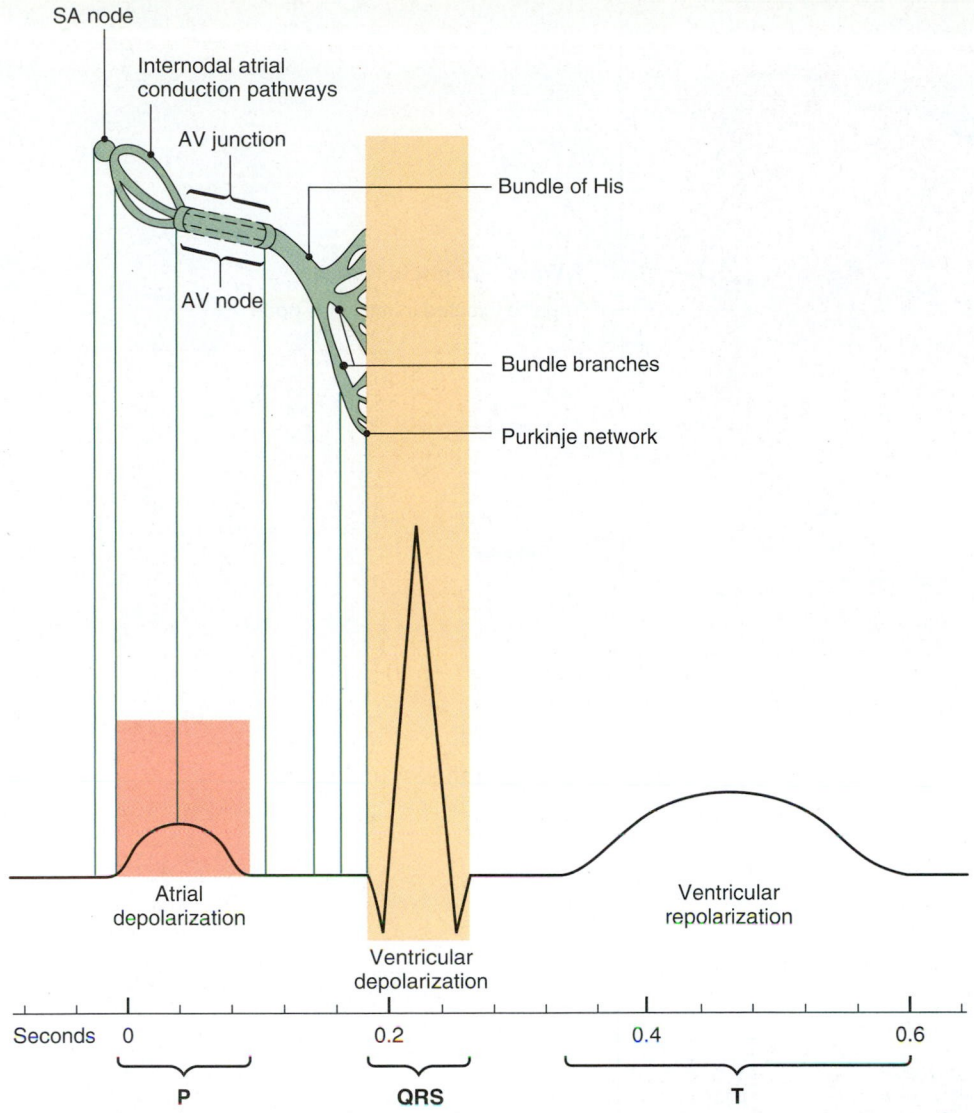

FIGURE 28-7   Relationship of the ECG to electrical activities in the heart.

- *T wave.* The T wave reflects repolarization of the ventricles. Normally positive in Lead II, it is rounded and usually moves in the same direction as the QRS complex (Figure 28-14).
- *U wave.* Occasionally, a U wave appears. U waves follow T waves and are usually positive. U waves may be associated with electrolyte abnormalities, or they may be a normal finding.

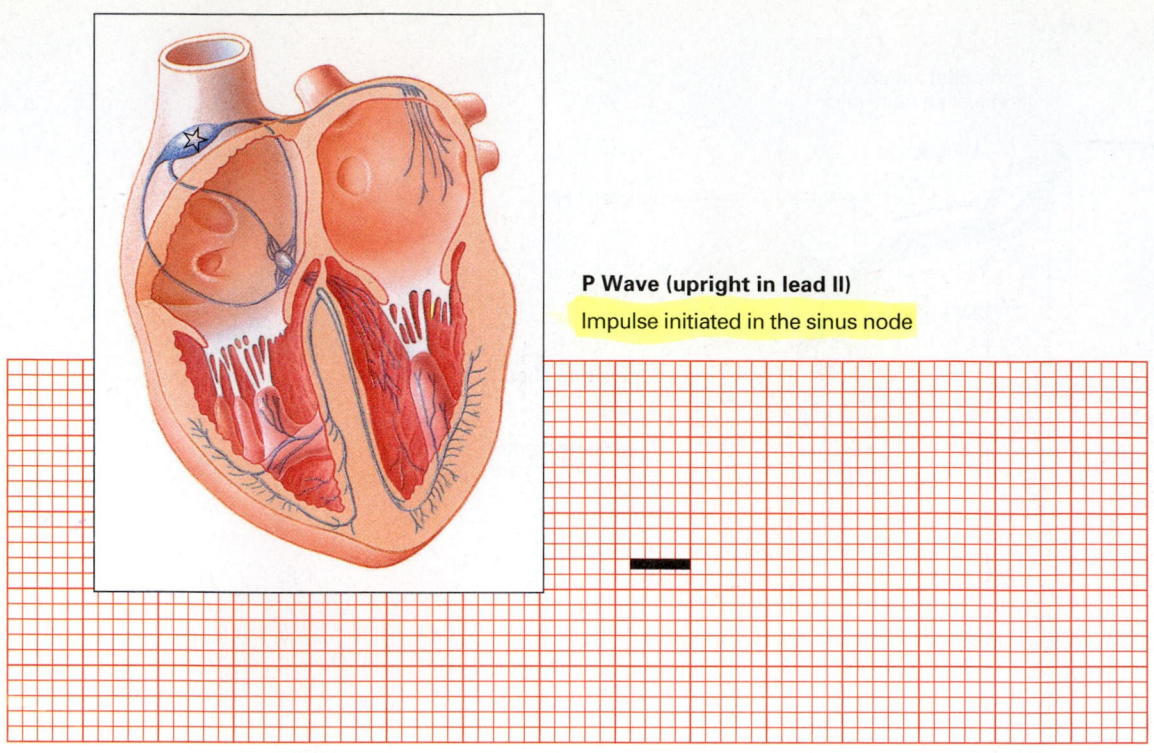

P Wave (upright in lead II)

Impulse initiated in the sinus node

FIGURE 28-8   Impulse initiation in the SA node.

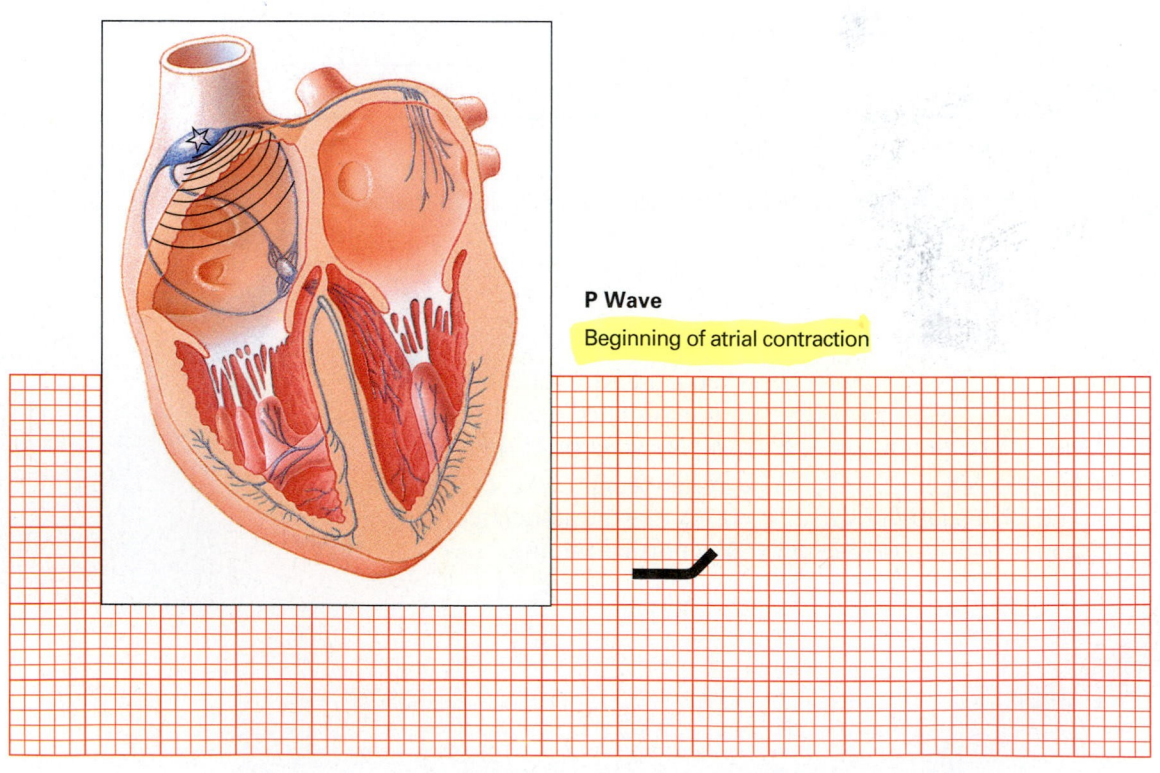

P Wave

Beginning of atrial contraction

FIGURE 28-9   Beginning of atrial contraction.

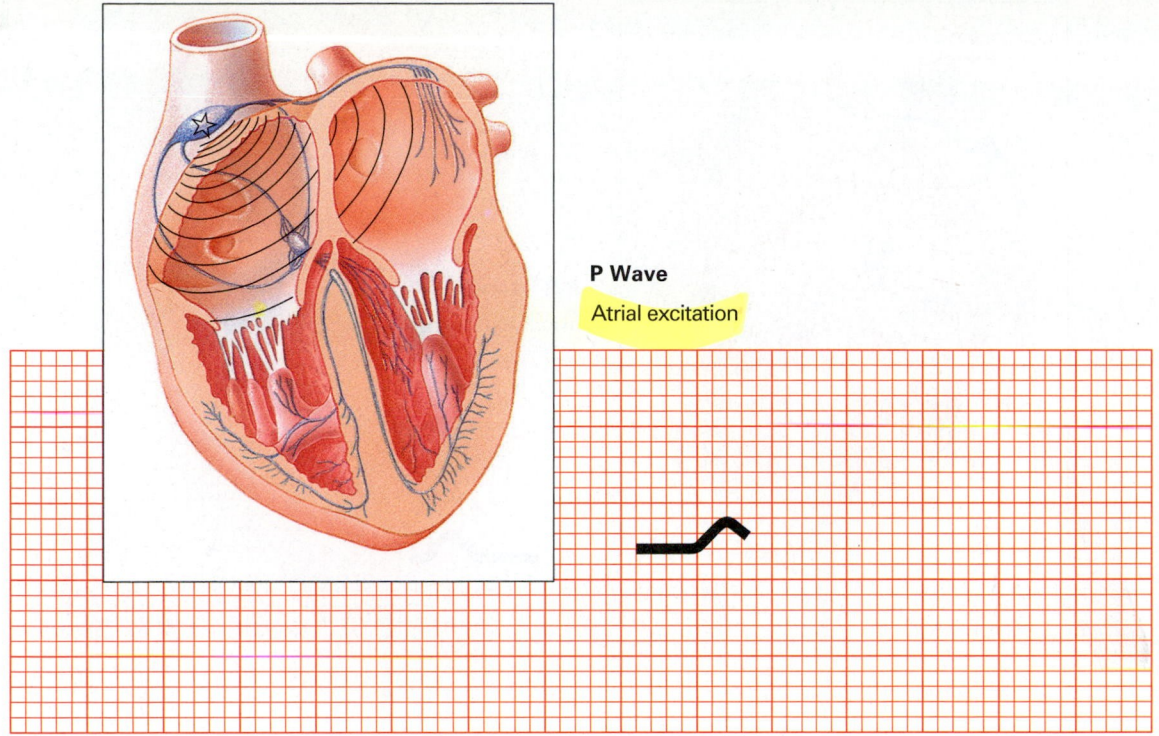

P Wave

Atrial excitation

FIGURE 28-10   Atrial excitation.

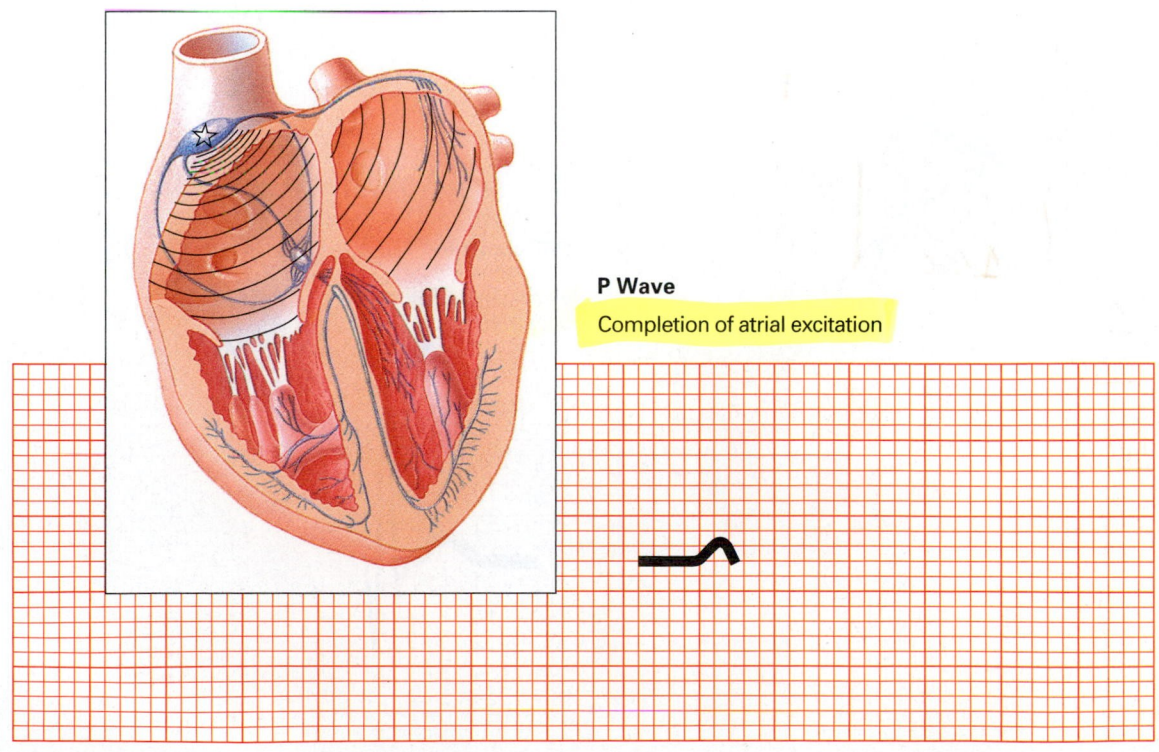

P Wave

Completion of atrial excitation

FIGURE 28-11   Completion of atrial excitation.

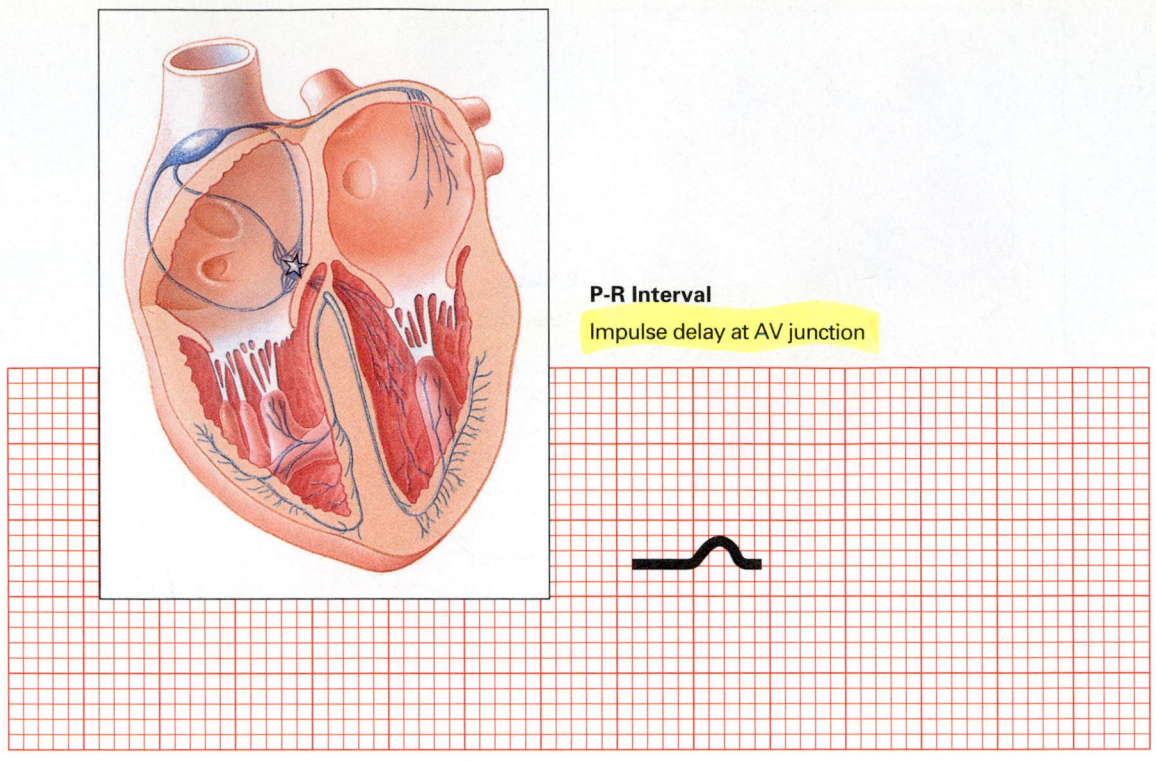

P-R Interval

Impulse delay at AV junction

FIGURE 28–12   Impulse delay at the AV junction.

QRS complex

Electrical excitation
of the ventricles

FIGURE 28–13   Electrical excitation of the ventricles.

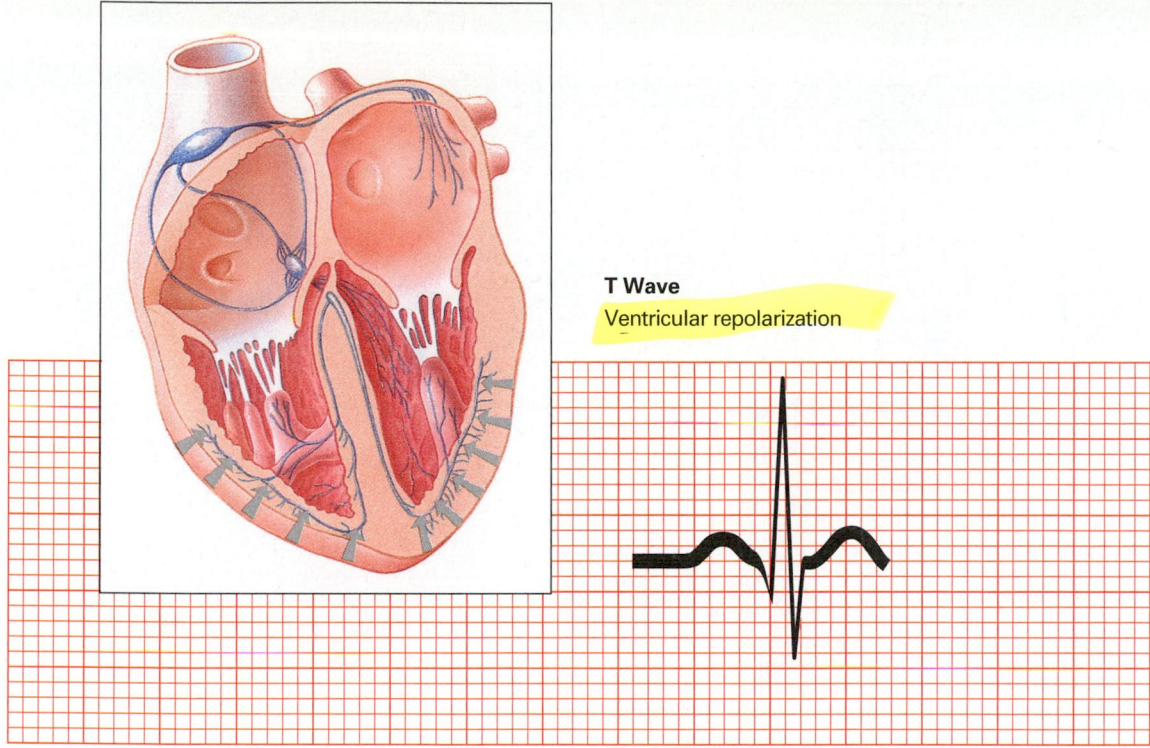

T Wave
Ventricular repolarization

FIGURE 28-14 Ventricular repolarization.

In addition to the wave forms described above, the ECG tracing reflects these important time intervals (Figure 28-15):

- *P-R interval (PRI) or P-Q interval (PQI).* The P-R interval is the distance from the beginning of the P wave to the beginning of the QRS complex. It represents the time the impulse takes to travel from the atria to the ventricles. Occasionally, the R wave is absent, in which case this interval is called the P-Q interval. The terms P-R interval and P-Q interval may be used interchangeably.

- *QRS interval.* The QRS interval is the distance from the first deflection of the QRS complex to the last. It represents the time necessary for ventricular depolarization.

- *S-T segment.* The S-T segment is the distance from the S wave to the beginning of the T wave. Usually it is an isoelectric line; however, it may be elevated or depressed in certain disease states such as ischemia.

A normal P-R interval is 0.12-0.20 second. A short PRI lasts less than 0.12 second; a prolonged PRI lasts longer than 0.20 second. A prolonged PRI indicates a delay in the AV node. A normal QRS complex lasts between 0.08 and 0.12 second. A value of less than 0.12 second means that the ventricles depolarized in a normal length of time.

The **QT interval** represents the total duration of ventricular depolarization. A normal QT interval is 0.33–0.42 second. QT intervals and heart rate have an inverse relationship: increases in heart rate usually decrease the QT interval, while decreases in heart rate usually prolong it. A **prolonged QT interval** is thought to be related to an increased risk of certain ventricular dysrhythmias and sudden death.

Content Review

ECG TIME INTERVALS
- P-R Interval
- QRS Interval
- S-T Segment

Content Review

NORMAL INTERVAL DURATIONS
- PR   0.12–0.20 sec
- QRS 0.08–0.12 sec
- QT   0.33–0.42 sec

✱ **QT interval** period from the beginning of the QRS to the end of the T wave.

✱ **prolonged QT interval** QT interval greater than .44 second.

FIGURE 28-15   The ECG.

The all-or-none nature of myocardial depolarization results in an interval when the heart cannot be restimulated to depolarize. From our earlier discussion you will recall that during this time the myocardial cells have not yet repolarized and cannot be stimulated again (Figure 28-16). This **refractory period** has two parts, an **absolute refractory period** and a **relative refractory period.** During the absolute refractory period stimulation produces no depolarization whatsoever. This usually lasts from the beginning of the QRS complex to the apex of the T wave. During the relative refractory period, a sufficiently strong stimulus may produce depolarization. This usually corresponds to the T wave's down slope.

S-T Segment Changes   The S-T segment is usually an isoelectric line. Myocardial infarctions, which are caused by lack of blood flow to a part of the heart, produce changes in this line. The affected area is then electrically dead and cannot conduct electrical impulses. Myocardial infarctions usually follow this sequence:

1. Ischemia (lack of oxygen)
2. Injury
3. Necrosis (cell death, infarction)

* **refractory period** the period of time when myocardial cells have not yet completely repolarized and cannot be stimulated again.

* **absolute refractory period** the period of the cardiac cycle when stimulation will not produce any depolarization whatever.

* **relative refractory period** the period of the cardiac cycle when a sufficiently strong stimulus may produce depolarization.

FIGURE 28-16   Refractory periods of the cardiac cycle.

Table 28-2	OVERVIEW OF ECG LEAD GROUPINGS
Leads	**Portion of the heart examined**
I and aVL	The left side of the heart in a vertical plane
II, III, and aVF	The inferior (diaphragmatic) side of the heart
aVR	The right side of the heart in a vertical plane
V_1 and V_2	The right ventricle
V_3 and V_4	The intraventricular septum and the anterior wall of the left ventricle
V_5 and V_6	The anterior and lateral walls of the left ventricle

Each of these stages results in distinct S-T segment changes. Ischemia causes S-T segment depression or an inverted T wave. The inversion is usually symmetrical. Injury elevates the S-T segment, most often in the early phases of a myocardial infarction. As the tissue dies, a significant Q wave appears. As we noted earlier, small, insignificant Q waves may show up in normal ECG tracings. A significant Q wave is at least one small square wide, lasting 0.04 second, or is more than one-third the height of the QRS complex. Q waves may also indicate extensive transient ischemia.

Lead Systems and Heart Surfaces Using the various ECG leads is comparable to waiting for a train at a railroad crossing. You will want to know how long you have to wait (in other words, how long is the train), but you can only see the front of the train. If you had cameras at other viewpoints, you could see how long the train actually was. Similarly, by combining the different ECG leads you can view different parts of the heart.

Leads V_1–V_4 view the anterior surface of the heart. Leads I and aVL view the lateral surface of the heart. The inferior surface of the heart can be visualized in leads II, III, and aVF. These leads can show ischemia, injury, and necrotic changes and can provide information about the corresponding heart surface (Table 28-2). For example, significant S-T elevation in V_1–V_4 may indicate anterior involvement, while elevation in II, III, and aVF may indicate inferior involvement.

Medical procedures (angioplasty) and drugs (thrombolytics) can treat acute myocardial infarction. The earlier they are initiated, the better the patient's potential outcome. Earlier identification in the field of patients with AMI will allow for earlier interventions, but the 12-lead ECG's role in out-of-hospital care remains unresolved. Its use may not be appropriate in many EMS settings. Individual EMS medical directors will determine the application and use of the 12-lead ECG in their specific EMS settings.

Earlier identification in the field of patients with AMI will allow for earlier intervention.

INTERPRETATION OF RHYTHM STRIPS

The key to interpreting rhythm strips is to approach each strip logically and systematically. Attempts to nonanalytically "eyeball" the strip often lead to incorrect interpretations. Your approach to rhythm strip interpretation should include the following basic criteria.

The key to interpreting rhythm strips is to approach each strip logically and systematically.

- Always be consistent and analytical.
- Memorize the rules for each dysrhythmia.
- Analyze a given rhythm strip according to a specific format.
- Compare your analysis to the rules for each dysrhythmia.
- Identify the dysrhythmia by its similarity to established rules.

Use ECG calipers to measure ECG tracings to assure accuracy and to avoid misinterpretation.

The health care profession uses several standard formats for ECG analysis. We will use the following five-step procedure:

1. Analyze the rate.
2. Analyze the rhythm.
3. Analyze the P-waves.
4. Analyze the P-R interval.
5. Analyze the QRS complex.

Analyzing Rate The first step in ECG strip interpretation is to analyze the heart rate. Usually this means the ventricular rate; however, if the atrial and ventricular rates differ, you must calculate both. The normal heart rate is 60–100 beats per minute. A heart rate greater than 100 beats per minute is a **tachycardia.** A heart rate less than 60 beats per minute is a **bradycardia.** You can use any of the following methods to calculate the rate.

* *Six-Second Method.* Count the number of complexes in a six-second interval. Mark off a six-second interval by noting two three-second marks at the top of the ECG paper. Then multiply the number of complexes within the six-second strip by ten.
* *Heart Rate Calculator Rulers.* Commercially available heart rate calculator rulers allow you to determine heart rates rapidly. Always use them according to the accompanying directions, since variations occur among different manufacturers. Also learn a manual method so you can still calculate rates if you forget your ruler.
* *R-R Interval.* The R-R interval is related directly to heart rate. The R-R interval method is accurate only if the heart rhythm is regular. You can calculate it in the following ways:
  – Measure the duration between R waves in seconds. Divide this number into 60, giving the heart rate per minute.
    Example: 60 ÷ 0.65 second = 92 (heart rate)
  – Count the number of large squares within an R-R interval, and divide the number of squares into 300.
    Example: 300 ÷ 3.5 large boxes = 86 (heart rate)
  – Count the number of small squares within an R-R interval, and divide the number of squares into 1,500.
    Example: 1,500 ÷ 29 small boxes = 52 (heart rate)
* *Triplicate Method.* Another method, also useful only with regular rhythms, is to locate an R wave that falls on a dark line bordering a large box on the graph paper. Then assign numbers corresponding to the heart rate to the next six dark lines to the right. The order is: 300, 150, 100, 75, 60, and 50. The number corresponding to the dark line closest to the peak of the next R wave is a rough estimate of the heart rate.

Pick one of the above methods and become comfortable with it. Use it to determine the rate on all strips that you look at.

Analyzing Rhythm The next step is to analyze the rhythm. First, measure the R-R interval across the strip. Normally, the R-R rhythm is fairly regular. Some

---

* **tachycardia** a heart rate greater than 100 beats per minute.

* **bradycardia** a heart rate less than 60 beats per minute.

minimal variation, associated with respirations, should be expected. If the rhythm is irregular, note whether it fits one of the following patterns.

- Occasionally irregular (only one or two R-R intervals on the strip are irregular)
- Regularly irregular (patterned irregularity or group beating)
- Irregularly irregular (no relationship among R-R intervals)

Analyzing P Waves The P waves reflect atrial depolarization. Normally, the atria depolarize away from the SA node and toward the ventricles. In Lead II, this appears as a positive, rounded P wave. When analyzing the P waves, ask yourself the following questions:

- Are P waves present?
- Are the P waves regular?
- Is there one P wave for each QRS complex?
- Are the P waves upright or inverted (compared to the QRS complex)?
- Do all the P waves look alike?

Analyzing the P-R Interval The P-R interval represents the time needed for atrial depolarization and conduction of the impulse up to the AV node. Remember, the normal P-R interval is 0.12-0.20 sec (three to five small boxes). Any deviation is an abnormal finding. The P-R interval should be consistent across the strip.

Analyzing the QRS Complex The QRS complex represents ventricular depolarization. When evaluating the QRS complex, ask yourself the following questions:

- Do all of the QRS complexes look alike?
- What is the QRS duration?

Remember, the QRS duration is usually 0.04–0.12 sec. Anything longer than 0.12 sec (three small boxes) is abnormal.

DYSRHYTHMIAS

On a normal ECG, the heart rate is between 60 and 100 beats per minute. The rhythm is regular (both P-P and R-R). The P waves are normal in shape, upright, and appear only before each QRS complex. The P-R interval lasts 0.12-0.20 sec and is constant. The QRS complex has a normal morphology, and its duration is less than 0.12 sec. All of these factors indicate a **normal sinus rhythm** (Figure 28-17a). Any deviation from the heart's normal electrical rhythm is a **dysrhythmia.** The absence of cardiac electrical activity is **arrhythmia.** The causes of dysrhythmias include:

- Myocardial ischemia, necrosis, or infarction
- Autonomic nervous system imbalance
- Distention of the chambers of the heart (especially in the atria, secondary to congestive heart failure)
- Blood gas abnormalities, including hypoxia and abnormal pH
- Electrolyte imbalances (Ca^{++}, K^+, Mg^{++})

Content Review

NORMAL SINUS RHYTHM
- Rate 60–100
- Rhythm: regular
- P waves: normal, upright, only before each QRS complex
- PR interval: 0.12–0.20 sec
- QRS Complex
  —Morphology: normal
  —Duration: <.12 sec

* **normal sinus rhythm** the normal heart rhythm.

* **dysrhythmia** any deviation from the normal electrical rhythm of the heart.

* **arrhythmia** the absence of cardiac electrical activity; often used interchangeably with dysrhythmia.

- Trauma to the myocardium (cardiac contusion)
- Drug effects and drug toxicity
- Electrocution
- Hypothermia
- CNS damage
- Idiopathic events
- Normal occurrences

Dysrhythmias in the healthy heart are of little significance. No matter what the etiology or type of dysrhythmia, treat the patient and his symptoms, not the dysrhythmia. You will hear this repeated over and over: Treat the patient, not the monitor.

MECHANISM OF IMPULSE FORMATION

Several physiologic mechanisms can cause cardiac dysrhythmias. The depolarization impulse is normally transmitted forward (*antegrade*) through the conductive system and the myocardium. In certain dysrhythmias, however, the depolarization impulse is conducted backwards (*retrograde*).

Ectopic Foci One cause of dysrhythmias is *enhanced automaticity*. This condition results when **ectopic foci** (heart cells other than the pacemaker cells) automatically depolarize, producing **ectopic** (abnormal) **beats.** Premature ventricular contractions and premature atrial contractions are examples of ectopic beats. Ectopic beats can be intermittent or sustained.

Reentry *Reentry* may cause isolated premature beats, or *tachydysrhythmias*. It occurs when ischemia or another disease process alters two branches of a conduction pathway, slowing conduction in one branch and causing a unidirectional block in the other. An antegrade depolarization wave travels slowly through the branch with ischemia and is blocked in the branch with a unidirectional block. After the depolarization wave goes through the slowed branch, it enters the branch with the unidirectional block and is conducted retrograde back to the branch's origin. By now the tissue is no longer refractory, and stimulation occurs again. This can result in rapid rhythms such as paroxysmal supraventricular tachycardia or atrial fibrillation.

CLASSIFICATION OF DYSRHYTHMIAS

Dysrhythmias can be classified in any number of ways. Some of the classification methods include:

- Nature of origin (changes in automaticity versus disturbances in conduction)
- Magnitude (major versus minor)
- Severity (life-threatening versus non-life-threatening)
- Site of origin

Classifying dysrhythmias by site of origin is closely related to basic physiology and, thus, is easy to understand. This approach divides dysrhythmias into the following categories:

- Dysrhythmias originating in the SA node
- Dysrhythmias originating in the atria

Treat the patient, not the monitor.

---

* **ectopic focus** nonpacemaker heart cell that automatically depolarizes; *pl.* ectopic foci.

* **ectopic beat** cardiac depolarization resulting from depolarization of ectopic focus.

- Dysrhythmias originating within the AV junction
- Dysrhythmias sustained in or originating in the AV junction
- Dysrhythmias originating in the ventricles
- Dysrhythmias resulting from disorders of conduction

DYSRHYTHMIAS ORIGINATING IN THE SA NODE

Dysrhythmias originating in the SA node most often result from changes in autonomic tone. However, disease can exist in the SA node itself. Dysrhythmias that originate in the SA node include:

- Sinus bradycardia
- Sinus tachycardia
- Sinus dysrhythmia
- Sinus arrest

Sinus Bradycardia

Description: Sinus bradycardia results from slowing of the SA node.

Etiology: Sinus bradycardia may result from any of the following conditions.

- Increased parasympathetic (vagal) tone
- Intrinsic disease of the SA node
- Drug effects (digitalis, propranolol, quinidine)
- Normal finding in healthy, well-conditioned persons

Rules of Interpretation/Lead II Monitoring (Figure 28-17b):

Rate—less than 60
Rhythm—regular
Pacemaker site—SA node
P waves—upright and normal in morphology
P-R interval—normal (0.12–0.20 sec and constant)
QRS complex—normal (0.04–0.12 sec)

Clinical Significance: The decreased heart rate can cause decreased cardiac output, hypotension, angina, or CNS symptoms. This is especially true for rates slower than 50 beats per minute. The slow heart rate may also lead to atrial ectopic or ventricular ectopic rhythms. In a healthy athlete, sinus bradycardia may have no clinical significance.

Treatment: Treatment is generally unnecessary unless hypotension or ventricular irritability is present (Figure 28-18). Remember, treat your patient and not the monitor. If treatment is required, administer a 0.5 mg bolus of atropine sulfate. Repeat every 3–5 minutes until you have obtained a satisfactory rate or have given 0.04 mg/kg of the drug. If atropine fails, consider transcutaneous cardiac pacing (TCP), if available.

FIGURE 28–17A Normal sinus rhythm.

FIGURE 28–17B Sinus bradycardia.

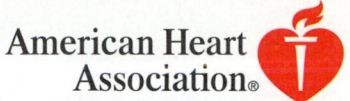

BRADYCARDIA ALGORITHM

Bradycardia
- **Slow** (absolute bradycardia = rate <60 bpm)
  or
- **Relatively slow** (rate less than expected relative to underlying condition or cause)

Primary ABCD Survey
- Assess ABCs
- Secure airway noninvasively
- Ensure monitor/defibrillator is available

Secondary ABCD Survey
- Assess secondary ABCs (invasive airway management needed?)
- Oxygen–IV access–monitor–fluids
- Vital signs, pulse oximeter, monitor BP
- Obtain and review 12-lead ECG
- Obtain and review portable chest x-ray
- Problem-focused history
- Problem-focused physical examination
- Consider causes (differential diagnoses)

Serious signs or symptoms?
Due to the bradycardia?

No

Yes

Type II second-degree AV block
or
Third-degree AV block?

Intervention sequence
- **Atropine** 0.5 to 1.0 mg
- **Transcutaneous pacing** if available
- **Dopamine** 5 to 20 µg/kg per minute
- **Epinephrine** 2 to 10 µg/min
- **Isoproterenol** 2 to 10 µg/min

No

Yes

Observe

- Prepare for transvenous pacer
- If symptoms develop, use transcutaneous pacemaker until transvenous pacer placed

FIGURE 28–18   Management of bradycardia. Reproduced with permission from *Guidelines 2000 for Cardiopulmonary Resuscitation and Emergency Cardiovasular Care,* ©2000, Copyright American Heart Association.

FIGURE 28-19 Sinus tachycardia.

Sinus Tachycardia

Description: Sinus tachycardia results from an increased rate of SA node discharge.

Etiology: Sinus tachycardia may result from any of the following:

- Exercise
- Fever
- Anxiety
- Hypovolemia
- Anemia
- Pump failure
- Increased sympathetic tone
- Hypoxia
- Hyperthyroidism

Rules of Interpretation/Lead II Monitoring (Figure 28-19):

Rate—greater than 100
Rhythm—regular
Pacemaker site—SA node
P waves—upright and normal in morphology
P-R interval—normal
QRS complex—normal

Clinical Significance: Sinus tachycardia is often benign. In some cases, it is a compensatory mechanism for decreased stroke volume. If the rate is greater than 140 beats per minute, cardiac output may fall because ventricular filling time is inadequate. Very rapid heart rates increase myocardial oxygen demand and can precipitate ischemia or infarct in diseased hearts. Prolonged sinus tachycardia accompanying acute myocardial infarction (AMI) is often an ominous finding suggesting cardiogenic shock.

Treatment: Treatment is directed at the underlying cause. Hypovolemia, fever, hypoxia, or other causes should be corrected.

FIGURE 28-20   Sinus dysrhythmia.

Sinus Dysrhythmia

Description: *Sinus dysrhythmia* often results from a variation of the R-R interval.

Etiology: Sinus dysrhythmia is often a normal finding and is sometimes related to the respiratory cycle and changes in intrathoracic pressure. Pathologically, sinus dysrhythmia can be caused by enhanced vagal tone.

Rules of Interpretation/Lead II Monitoring (Figure 28-20):

Rate—60–100 (varies with respirations)
Rhythm—irregular
Pacemaker site—SA node
P waves—upright and normal in morphology
P-R interval—normal
QRS complex—normal

Clinical Significance: Sinus dysrhythmia is a normal variant, particularly in the young and the aged.

Treatment: Typically, none required.

● **Arrest or block**

FIGURE 28-21   Sinus arrest.

Sinus Arrest

Description: *Sinus arrest* occurs when the sinus node fails to discharge, resulting in short periods of cardiac standstill. This standstill can persist until pacemaker cells lower in the conductive system discharge (escape beats) or until the sinus node resumes discharge.

Etiology: Sinus arrest can result from any of the following conditions.

- Ischemia of the SA node
- Digitalis toxicity
- Excessive vagal tone
- Degenerative fibrotic disease

Rules of Interpretation/Lead II Monitoring (Figure 28-21):

Rate—normal to slow, depending on the frequency and duration of the arrest

Rhythm—irregular

Pacemaker site—SA node

P waves—upright and normal in morphology

P-R interval—normal

QRS complex—normal

Clinical Significance: Frequent or prolonged episodes may compromise cardiac output, resulting in syncope (fainting) and other problems. There is always the danger of complete cessation of SA node activity. Usually, an escape rhythm develops; however, cardiac standstill occasionally can result.

Treatment: If the patient is asymptomatic, observation is all that is required. If the patient is extremely bradycardic or symptomatic, administer a 0.5 mg bolus of atropine sulfate. Repeat every 3–5 minutes until you have obtained a satisfactory rate or have administered 0.04 mg/kg of the drug. If atropine fails, consider transcutaneous cardiac pacing (TCP), if available.

FIGURE 28-22   Wandering atrial pacemaker.

Dysrhythmias Originating in the Atria

Dysrhythmias can originate outside the SA node in the atrial tissue or in the internodal pathways. Ischemia, hypoxia, atrial dilation, and other factors can cause atrial dysrhythmias. Dysrhythmias originating in the atria include:

- Wandering atrial pacemaker
- Multifocal atrial tachycardia
- Premature atrial contractions
- Paroxysmal supraventricular tachycardia
- Atrial flutter
- Atrial fibrillation

Wandering Atrial Pacemaker

Description: Wandering atrial pacemaker is the passive transfer of pacemaker sites from the sinus node to other latent pacemaker sites in the atria and AV junction. Often more than one pacemaker site will be present, causing variation in R-R interval and P wave morphology.

Etiology: Wandering atrial pacemaker can result from any of the following conditions:

- A variant of sinus dysrhythmia
- A normal phenomenon in the very young or the aged
- Ischemic heart disease
- Atrial dilation

Rules of Interpretation/Lead II Monitoring (Figure 28-22):

Rate—usually normal

Rhythm—slightly irregular

Pacemaker site—varies among the SA node, atrial tissue, and the AV junction

P waves—morphology changes from beat to beat; P waves may disappear entirely

P-R interval—varies; may be less than 0.12 sec, normal, or greater than 0.20 sec

QRS Complex—normal

Clinical Significance: Wandering atrial pacemaker usually has no detrimental effects. Occasionally, it can be a precursor of other atrial dysrhythmias such as atrial fibrillation. It sometimes indicates digitalis toxicity.

Treatment: If the patient is asymptomatic, observation is all that is required. If the patient is symptomatic, consider adenosine or verapamil.

FIGURE 28–23 Multifocal atrial tachycardia.

Multifocal Atrial Tachycardia

Description: Multifocal atrial tachycardia (MAT) is usually seen in acutely ill patients. Significant pulmonary disease is seen in about 60 percent of these patients. Certain medications used to treat lung disease (such as theophylline) may worsen the dysrhythmia. Three different P waves are noted, indicating various ectopic foci.

Etiology: Multifocal atrial tachycardia can result from any of the following conditions:

- Pulmonary disease
- Metabolic disorders (hypokalemia)
- Ischemic heart disease
- Recent surgery

Rules of Interpretation/Lead II Monitoring (Figure 28-23):

Rate—more than 100

Rhythm—irregular

Pacemaker site—ectopic sites in atria

P waves—organized, discrete nonsinus P waves with at least three different forms

P-R interval—varies

QRS complex—may be less than 0.12 sec, normal, or greater than 0.20 sec, depending on the AV node's refractory status when the impulse reaches it

Clinical Significance: Frequently these patients are acutely ill; this dysrhythmia may indicate a serious underlying medical illness.

Treatment: Treatment of the underlying medical disease usually resolves the dysrhythmia. Specific antidysrhythmic therapy is frequently not needed.

FIGURE 28-24 Premature atrial contractions.

Premature Atrial Contractions

Description: Premature atrial contractions (PACs) result from a single electrical impulse originating in the atria outside the SA node, which in turn causes a premature depolarization of the heart before the next expected sinus beat. Because it depolarizes the atrial syncytium, this impulse also depolarizes the SA node, interrupting the normal cadence. This creates a **noncompensatory pause** in the underlying rhythm.

Etiology: A premature atrial contraction can result from any of the following conditions:

- Use of caffeine, tobacco, or alcohol
- Sympathomimetic drugs
- Ischemic heart disease
- Hypoxia
- Digitalis toxicity
- No apparent cause (idiopathic)

Rules of Interpretation/Lead II Monitoring (Figure 28-24):

Rate—depends on the underlying rhythm

Rhythm—depends on the underlying rhythm; usually regular except for the PAC

Pacemaker site—ectopic focus in the atrium

P waves—the P wave of the PAC differs from the P wave of the underlying rhythm. It occurs earlier than the next expected P wave and may be hidden in the preceding T wave.

P-R interval—usually normal; can vary with the location of the ectopic focus. Ectopic foci near the SA node will have a P-R interval of 0.12 sec or greater, whereas ectopic foci near the AV node will have a P-R interval of 0.12 sec or less.

QRS complex—usually normal; may be greater than 0.12 sec if the PAC is abnormally conducted through partially refractory ventricles. In some cases, the ventricles are refractory and will not depolarize in response to the PAC. In these cases, the QRS complex is absent.

Clinical Significance: Isolated PACs are of minimal significance. Frequent PACs may indicate organic heart disease and may precede other atrial dysrhythmias.

Treatment: If the patient is asymptomatic, observation is all that is required in the field. If the patient is symptomatic, administer oxygen via a nonrebreather mask and start an IV line. Contact medical direction.

* noncompensatory pause pause following an ectopic beat where the SA node is depolarized and the underlying cadence of the heart is interrupted.

FIGURE 28-25   Paroxysmal supraventricular tachycardia.

Paroxysmal Supraventricular Tachycardia

Description: *Paroxysmal supraventricular tachycardia (PSVT)* occurs when rapid atrial depolarization overrides the SA node. It often occurs in paroxysm with sudden onset, may last minutes to hours, and terminates abruptly. It may be caused by increased automaticity of a single atrial focus or by reentry phenomenon at the AV node.

Etiology: Paroxysmal supraventricular tachycardia may occur at any age and often is not associated with underlying heart disease. It may be precipitated by stress, overexertion, smoking, or ingestion of caffeine. It is, however, frequently associated with underlying atherosclerotic cardiovascular disease and rheumatic heart disease. PSVT is rare in patients with myocardial infarction. It can occur with accessory pathway conduction such as Wolff-Parkinson-White syndrome.

Rules of Interpretation/Lead II Monitoring (Figure 28-25):

Rate—150–250 per minute

Rhythm—characteristically regular, except at onset and termination

Pacemaker site—in the atria, outside the SA node

P waves—the atrial P waves differ slightly from sinus P waves. The P wave is often buried in the preceding T wave. The P wave may be impossible to see, especially if the rate is rapid. Turning up the speed of the graph paper or oscilloscope to 50 mm/sec spreads out the complex and can help identify P waves.

P-R interval—usually normal; however, it can vary with the location of the ectopic pacemaker. Ectopic pacemakers near the SA node will have P-R intervals close to 0.12 sec, whereas ectopic pacemakers near the AV node will have P-R intervals of 0.12 sec or less.

QRS complex—normal

Clinical Significance: Young patients with good cardiac reserves may tolerate PSVT well for short periods. Patients often sense PSVT as palpitations. However, rapid rates can cause a marked reduction in cardiac output because of inadequate ventricular filling time. The reduced diastolic phase of the cardiac cycle can also compromise coronary artery perfusion. PSVT can precipitate angina, hypotension, or congestive heart failure.

FIGURE 28-26 Management of tachycardia. Reproduced with permission from *Guidelines 2000 for Cardiopulmonary Resuscitation and Emergency Cardiovascular Care,* ©2000, Copyright American Heart Association.

Treatment: If the patient is not tolerating the rapid heart rate, as evidenced by hemo-dynamic instability, attempt the following techniques in this order (Figure 28-26).

1. Vagal maneuvers. Ask the patient to perform a Valsalva maneuver. This is a forced expiration against a closed glottis, or the act of "bearing down" as if to move the bowels. This results in vagal stimulation, which may slow the heart. If this is unsuccessful, attempt carotid artery massage, if the patient is eligible. Do not attempt carotid artery massage in patients with carotid **bruits** or known cerebrovascular or carotid artery disease.

2. Pharmacological therapy. Adenosine (Adenocard) is very safe and highly effective in terminating PSVT, especially if its etiology is reentry. Administer 6 mg of adenosine by rapid IV bolus over 1–3 sec through the medication port closest to the patient's heart or central circulation. (Adenosine has a very short half-life, and you must immediately follow administration with a bolus of normal saline to allow the medication to reach its site of action while it is still effective.) If the patient does not convert after 1–2 minutes, administer a second bolus of 12 mg over 1–3 sec in the medication port closest to the patient's heart or central circulation. If this fails and the patient has a normal blood pressure, then look again at the width of the cardiac QRS. If it appears to be a narrow complex rhythm with a normal blood pressure, medical direction may request the administration of verapamil 2.5–5.0 mg. This can be repeated once in 15–30 minutes, if needed, at a dose of 5–10 milligrams. Verapamil is contraindicated in patients with a history of bradycardia, hypotension, or congestive heart failure. Do not use it with intravenous beta blockers; use it with caution in patients on chronic beta blocker therapy. Hypotension following verapamil administration can often be reversed with 0.5–1.0 gm of calcium chloride administered intravenously.

3. Electrical therapy. If the ventricular rate is greater than 150 beats per minute, or if the patient is hemodynamically unstable, use synchronized cardioversion (described later in the chapter). If time allows, sedate the patient with 5–10 mg of diazepam or 2-5 mg of midazolam (Versed) IV. Apply synchronized DC countershock of 100 joules. If this is unsuccessful, repeat the countershock at increased energy as ordered by medical direction. DC countershock is contraindicated if you suspect digitalis toxicity as the PSVT's cause.

* **bruit** the sound of turbulent blood flow through a vessel; usually associated with atherosclerotic disease.

FIGURE 28-27 Atrial flutter.

Atrial Flutter

Description: Atrial flutter results from a rapid atrial reentry circuit and an AV node that physiologically cannot conduct all impulses through to the ventricles. The AV junction may allow impulses in a 1:1 (rare), 2:1, 3:1, or 4:1 ratio or greater, resulting in a discrepancy between atrial and ventricular rates. The AV block may be consistent or variable.

Etiology: Atrial flutter may occur in normal hearts, but it is usually associated with organic disease. It rarely occurs as the direct result of an MI. Atrial dilation, which occurs with congestive heart failure, is a cause of atrial flutter.

Rules of Interpretation/Lead II Monitoring (Figure 28-27):

Rate—atrial rate is 250–350 per minute. Ventricular rate varies with the ratio of AV conduction.

Rhythm—atrial rhythm is regular; ventricular rhythm is usually regular, but can be irregular if the block is variable

Pacemaker site—sites in the atria outside the SA node

P waves—flutter (F) waves are present, resembling a sawtooth or picket-fence pattern. This pattern is often difficult to identify in a 2:1 flutter. However, if the ventricular rate is approximately 150, suspect 2:1 flutter.

P-R interval—usually constant but may vary

QRS complex—normal

Clinical Significance: Atrial flutter with normal ventricular rates is generally well tolerated. Rapid ventricular rates may compromise cardiac output and result in symptoms. Atrial flutter often occurs in conjunction with atrial fibrillation and is referred to as "atrial fib-flutter."

Treatment: Treatment is indicated only for rapid ventricular rates with hemodynamic compromise (review Figure 28-26).

1. Electrical therapy. Immediate cardioversion is indicated in unstable patients—those with a heart rate greater than 150 and associated chest pain, dyspnea, a decreased level of consciousness, or hypotension. If time allows, sedate the patient with 5–10 mg of diazepam (Valium) or 2-5 mg of midazolam (Versed) IV. Then apply synchronized DC countershock of 100 joules. If this is unsuccessful, repeat the countershock at increased energy as recommended by AHA guidelines.

2. Pharmacological therapy. Occasionally you may use pharmacological therapy in stable patients with atrial flutter, especially if the rapid heart rate is causing congestive heart failure. Several medications slow the ventricular rate. The most frequently used is diltiazem (Cardizem). In addition, you may use verapamil, digoxin, beta blockers, procainamide, and quinidine. Procainamide and quinidine are often used to convert atrial flutter back to a sinus rhythm. Consult medical direction or refer to local protocols concerning pharmacological therapy for atrial flutter.

FIGURE 28-28   Atrial fibrillation.

Atrial Fibrillation

Description: *Atrial fibrillation* results from multiple areas of reentry within the atria or from multiple ectopic foci bombarding an AV node that physiologically cannot handle all of the incoming impulses. AV conduction is random and highly variable.

Etiology: Atrial fibrillation may be chronic and is often associated with underlying heart disease such as rheumatic heart disease, atherosclerotic heart disease, or congestive heart failure. Atrial dilation occurs with congestive heart failure and often causes atrial fibrillation.

Rules of Interpretation/Lead II Monitoring (Figure 28-28):

Rate—atrial rate is 350–750 per minute (cannot be counted); ventricular rate varies greatly depending on conduction through the AV node.

Rhythm—irregularly irregular

Pacemaker site—numerous ectopic foci in the atria

P waves—none discernible. Fibrillation (f) waves are present, indicating chaotic atrial activity.

P-R interval—none

QRS complex—normal

Clinical Significance: In atrial fibrillation, the atria fail to contract and the so-called atrial kick is lost, thus reducing cardiac output 20–25 percent. There is frequently a *pulse deficit* (a difference between the apical and peripheral pulse rates). If the rate of ventricular response is normal, as often occurs in patients on digitalis, the rhythm is usually well tolerated. If the ventricular rate is less than 60, cardiac output can fall. Suspect digitalis toxicity in patients taking digitalis with atrial fibrillation and a ventricular rate less than 60. If the ventricular response is rapid, coupled with the loss of atrial kick, cardiovascular decompensation may occur, resulting in hypotension, angina, infarct, congestive heart failure, or shock.

Treatment: Treatment is indicated only for rapid ventricular rates with hemodynamic compromise (review Figure 28-26).

1. **Electrical therapy.** Immediate cardioversion is indicated in unstable patients—those with heart rates greater than 150 and associated chest pain, dyspnea, a decreased level of consciousness, or hypotension. If time allows, sedate the patient with 5–10 mg of diazepam (Valium) or 2-5 mg of midazolam (Versed) IV. Then apply synchronized DC countershock of 100 joules. If this is unsuccessful, repeat the countershock at increased energy as ordered by medical direction.

2. **Pharmacological therapy.** Occasionally you will use pharmacological therapy in stable patients with atrial fibrillation, especially if the rapid heart rate is causing congestive heart failure. Several medications slow the ventricular rate. The most frequently used is diltiazem (Cardizem). In addition, verapamil, digoxin, beta blockers, procainamide, and quinidine can be used. Procainamide and quinidine are used to convert atrial fibrillation to a normal sinus rhythm. Atrial fibrillation is a documented risk factor for the development of stroke. As the atria fibrillate, they dilate. This allows for stagnation of blood flow within the atria and subsequent clot development. Because of this, it is sometimes prudent to administer an anticoagulant (heparin or warfarin [Coumadin]) to these patients to prevent stroke. Consult medical direction or refer to local protocols concerning pharmacological therapy of atrial fibrillation.

Patients with accessory pathways, such as in Wolff-Parkinson-White syndrome, who develop atrial flutter or atrial fibrillation, present special concerns. Usually, the electrical impulse reaches the ventricles via the accessory tract, via the AV node (normal conduction pathway), or via both. If the patient's refractory period is short in his accessory tract, more atrial impulses will be conducted down the accessory tract than through the AV node. This will result in a wide QRS complex. Rapid atrial rates occur with atrial fibrillation and flutter and can cause rapid ventricular rates. These rhythms, which have a wide complex, may resemble ventricular tachycardia. Excessive stimulation of the ventricles may actually precipitate ventricular fibrillation.

Verapamil will decrease conduction through the AV node and may shorten the refractory period of the accessory tract. Because of this, however, verapamil may accelerate the ventricular response rate and may precipitate ventricular tachycardia and ventricular fibrillation. Wolff-Parkinson-White, and the other pre-excitation syndromes, are presented in more detail later in this chapter.

DYSRHYTHMIAS ORIGINATING WITHIN THE AV JUNCTION (AV BLOCKS)

Two potential problems in the AV junction (or AV node) may result in dysrhythmias. One is an atrioventricular (AV) block, in which the electrical impulse is slowed or blocked as it passes through the AV node. The other is dysrhythmias due to a malfunction of AV junctional cells themselves.

The AV junction is an important part of the conductive system, serving two important physiological purposes (Figure 28-29). First, it effectively slows the impulse between the atria and the ventricles to allow for atrial emptying and ventricular filling. Second, it serves as a back-up pacemaker if the SA node or cells higher in the conductive system fail to fire. Part of the AV tissues function as a pacemaker node and other parts serve as the junction between the atria and the ventricles.

FIGURE 28-29 Organization of the AV node.

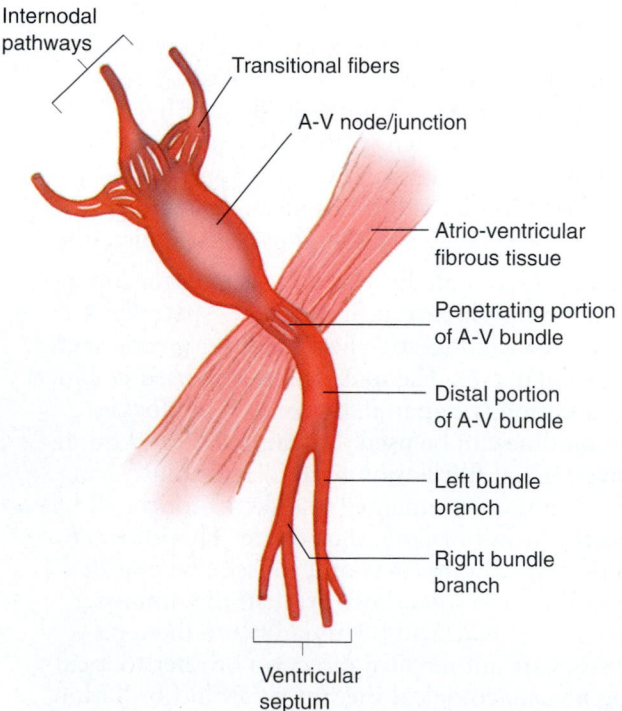

Internodal pathways

Transitional fibers

A-V node/junction

Atrio-ventricular fibrous tissue

Penetrating portion of A-V bundle

Distal portion of A-V bundle

Left bundle branch

Right bundle branch

Ventricular septum

The internodal fibers that blend to form the AV junction are called *transitional fibers*. These small fibers slow the impulse. The transitional fibers then blend into the AV junction. The lower portion of the AV node penetrates the fibrous tissue that separates the atria from the ventricles. This part of the node also slows impulse conduction. After penetrating the fibrous band, the AV node then becomes the AV bundle, which is also called the bundle of His. The bundle of His subsequently divides into the left and right bundle branches.

Atrioventricular Blocks

An *AV block* delays or interrupts impulses between the atria and the ventricles. These dysrhythmias can be caused by pathology of the AV junctional tissue or by a physiological block, such as occurs with atrial fibrillation or flutter. Their causes include AV junctional ischemia, AV junctional necrosis, degenerative disease of the conductive system, and drug toxicity (particularly from digitalis).

AV blocks can be classified according to the site or the degree of the block. Blocks may occur at the following sites:

- At the AV node
- At the bundle of His
- Below the bifurcation of the bundle of His

Our discussion classifies AV blocks by the following degrees (traditional classification):

- First-degree AV block
- Type I second-degree AV block
- Type II second-degree AV block (Mobitz II, or Infranodal)
- Third-degree AV block

Partial block

FIGURE 28–30 First-degree AV block.

First-Degree AV Block

Description: A first-degree AV block is a delay in conduction at the level of the AV node rather than an actual block. First-degree AV block is not a rhythm in itself, but a condition superimposed upon another rhythm. The underlying rhythm must also be identified (for example, sinus bradycardia with first-degree AV block).

Etiology: AV block can occur in the healthy heart. However, ischemia at the AV junction is the most common cause.

Rules of Interpretation/Lead II Monitoring (Figure 28-30):

Rate—depends on underlying rhythm

Rhythm—usually regular; can be slightly irregular

Pacemaker site—SA node or atria

P waves—normal

P-R interval—greater than 0.20 sec (diagnostic)

QRS complex—usually less than 0.12 sec; may be bizarre in shape if conductive system disease exists in the ventricles

Clinical Significance: First-degree block is usually no danger in itself. However, a newly developed first-degree block may precede a more advanced block.

Treatment: Generally, no treatment is required except observation, unless the heart rate drops significantly. If possible, avoid drugs that slow AV conduction, such as lidocaine and procainamide.

Partial block

Complete block

FIGURE 28-31   Type I second-degree AV block.

Type I Second-Degree AV Block

Description: A *type I second-degree AV block* (also called *second-degree, Mobitz I*; or *Wenckebach*), is an intermittent block at the level of the AV node. It produces a characteristic cyclic pattern in which the P-R intervals become progressively longer until an impulse is blocked (not conducted). The cycle is repetitive, and the P-P interval remains constant. The ratio of conduction (P waves to QRS complexes) is commonly 5:4, 4:3, 3:2, or 2:1. The pattern may be constant or variable.

Etiology: Low-grade AV blocks (First-degree and Second-degree Mobitz I) can occur in the healthy heart. However, ischemia at the AV junction is the most common cause. Increased parasympathetic tone and drugs are also common etiologies.

Rules of Interpretation/Lead II Monitoring (Figure 28-31):

Rate—atrial rate is unaffected; the ventricular rate may be normal or slowed

Rhythm—atrial rhythm is typically regular; ventricular rhythm is irregular because of the nonconducted beat

Pacemaker site—SA node or atria

P waves—normal; some P waves are not followed by QRS complexes

P-R interval—becomes progressively longer until the QRS complex is dropped; the cycle then repeats

QRS complex—usually less than 0.12 sec; may be bizarre in shape if conductive system disease exists in the ventricles

Clinical Significance: If beats are frequently dropped, second-degree block can compromise cardiac output by causing problems such as syncope and angina. This block is often a transient phenomenon that occurs immediately after an inferior wall myocardial infarction.

Treatment: Generally, no treatment other than observation is required. If possible, avoid drugs that slow AV conduction, such as lidocaine and procainamide. If the heart rate falls and the patient becomes symptomatic, administer 0.5 mg of atropine IV. Repeat every three to five minutes until you have obtained a satisfactory rate or have given 0.04 mg/kg of the drug. If atropine fails, consider transcutaneous cardiac pacing (TCP), if available.

Partial block

Complete block

FIGURE 28-32   Type II second-degree AV block.

Type II Second-Degree AV Block

Description: A *type II second-degree AV block* (also called *second-degree, Mobitz II;* or *infranodal*) is an intermittent block characterized by P waves that are not conducted to the ventricles, but without associated lengthening of the P-R interval before the dropped beats. The ratio of conduction (P waves to QRS complexes) is commonly 4:1, 3:1, or 2:1. The ratio may be constant or may vary. A 2:1 Mobitz II block is often indistinguishable from a 2:1 Mobitz I block.

Etiology: Second-degree AV block, Mobitz II, is usually associated with acute myocardial infarction and septal necrosis.

Rules of Interpretation/Lead II Monitoring (Figure 28-32):

Rate—atrial rate is unaffected; ventricular rate is usually bradycardic

Rhythm—regular or irregular, depending upon whether the conduction ratio is constant or varied

Pacemaker site—SA node or atria

P waves—normal; some P waves are not followed by QRS complexes

P-R interval—constant for conducted beats; may be greater than 0.21 sec

QRS complex—may be normal; however, it is often greater than 0.12 sec because of abnormal ventricular depolarization sequence

Clinical Significance: A Mobitz II block can compromise cardiac output, causing problems such as syncope and angina if beats are frequently dropped. Since this block is often associated with cell necrosis resulting from myocardial infarction, it is considered much more serious than Mobitz I. Many Mobitz II blocks develop into full AV blocks.

Treatment: Pacemaker insertion is the definitive treatment. In the field, administer medications if stabilization is required. If the heart rate falls and the patient becomes symptomatic, administer 0.5 mg of atropine IV. Repeat every three–five minutes until you have obtained a satisfactory rate or have given 0.04 mg/kg of the drug. Use atropine with caution in patients who have high-grade blocks (second-degree Mobitz II and third-degree). The atropine may accelerate the atrial rate, but it may also worsen the AV nodal block. Consider transcutaneous cardiac pacing (TCP), if available. If the patient remains symptomatic, do not delay application of TCP while waiting for IV access or for atropine to take effect.

Complete block

FIGURE 28-33   Third-degree AV block.

Third-Degree AV Block

Description: A *third-degree AV block*, or *complete block*, is the absence of conduction between the atria and the ventricles resulting from complete electrical block at or below the AV node. The atria and ventricles subsequently pace the heart independently of each other. The sinus node often functions normally, depolarizing the atrial syncytium, while the escape pacemaker, located below the atria, paces the ventricular syncytium.

Etiology: Third-degree AV block can result from acute myocardial infarction, digitalis toxicity, or degeneration of the conductive system, as occurs in the elderly.

Rules of Interpretation/Lead II Monitoring (Figure 28-33):

> Rate—atrial rate is unaffected. Ventricular rate is 40–60 if the escape pacemaker is junctional, less than 40 if the escape pacemaker is lower in the ventricles.
>
> Rhythm—both atrial and ventricular rhythms are usually regular
>
> Pacemaker site—SA node and AV junction or ventricle
>
> P waves—normal. P waves show no relationship to the QRS complex, often falling within the T wave and QRS complex.
>
> P-R interval—no relationship between P waves and R waves
>
> QRS complex—greater than 0.12 sec if pacemaker is ventricular; less than 0.12 second if pacemaker is junctional

Clinical Significance: Third-degree block can severely compromise cardiac output because of decreased heart rate and loss of coordinated atrial kick.

Treatment: Pacemaker insertion is the definitive treatment. In the field, administer medications if stabilization is required. If the heart rate falls and the patient becomes symptomatic, administer 0.5 mg of atropine IV. You can repeat this every 3–5 minutes until you have obtained a satisfactory rate or have given 0.04 mg/kg of the drug. Use atropine with caution in patients with high-grade blocks (second-degree Mobitz II and third-degree). The atropine may accelerate the atrial rate, but it may also worsen the AV nodal block. Consider transcutaneous cardiac pacing (TCP), if available. If the patient remains symptomatic, do not delay application of TCP while waiting for IV access or for atropine to take effect. Never use lidocaine to treat third-degree heart block with ventricular escape beats.

Never use lidocaine to treat third-degree heart block with ventricular escape beats.

FIGURE 28-34   Premature junctional contractions.

DYSRHYTHMIAS SUSTAINED OR ORIGINATING IN THE AV JUNCTION

Dysrhythmias can originate within the AV node. The location of the pacemaker site will dictate the morphology of the P wave. Ischemia, hypoxia, and other factors have been identified as causes. Dysrhythmias originating in the AV junction include:

- Premature junctional contractions
- Junctional escape complexes and rhythm
- Accelerated junctional rhythm
- Paroxysmal junctional tachycardia

All dysrhythmias that originate in the AV junction have in common the following ECG features:

- Inverted P waves in Lead II, resulting from retrograde depolarization of the atria. The P wave's relation to QRS depolarization depends on the relative timing of atrial and ventricular depolarization. The P wave can occur before the QRS complex, if the atria depolarize first; after the QRS, if the ventricles depolarize first; or during the QRS, if the atria and ventricles depolarize simultaneously. Depolarization of the atria during ventricular depolarization masks the P wave. Some atrial complexes that originate near the AV junction can also result in inverted P waves.
- P-R interval of less than 0.12 sec
- Normal QRS complex duration

Premature Junctional Contractions

Description: Premature junctional contractions (PJCs) result from a single electrical impulse originating in the AV node that occurs before the next expected sinus beat. A PJC can result in either a **compensatory pause** or noncompensatory pause, depending on whether the SA node is depolarized. A noncompensatory pause occurs if the premature beat depolarizes the SA node and interrupts the heart's normal cadence. A compensatory pause occurs only if the SA node discharges before the premature impulse reaches it.

Etiology: A premature junctional contraction can result from any of the following conditions:

- Use of caffeine, tobacco, or alcohol
- Sympathomimetic drugs
- Ischemic heart disease
- Hypoxia
- Digitalis toxicity
- No apparent cause (idiopathic)

Rules of Interpretation/Lead II Monitoring (Figure 28-34):

Rate—depends on the underlying rhythm

Rhythm—depends on the underlying rhythm, usually regular except for the PJC

Pacemaker site—ectopic focus in the AV junction

P waves—inverted; may appear before or after the QRS complex. P waves can be masked by the QRS complex or be absent.

P-R interval—if the P wave occurs before the QRS complex, the P-R interval will be less than 0.12 sec; if the P wave occurs after the QRS complex, then technically it is an R-P interval

QRS complex—usually normal; may be greater than 0.12 sec if the PJC is abnormally conducted through partially refractory ventricles

Clinical Significance: Isolated PJCs are of minimal significance. Frequent PJCs indicate organic heart disease and may be precursors to other junctional dysrhythmias.

Treatment: If the patient is asymptomatic, only observation is required in the field.

✳ **compensatory pause** the pause following an ectopic beat where the SA node is unaffected and the cadence of the heart is uninterrupted.

FIGURE 28-35 Junctional escape complex and rhythm.

Junctional Escape Complexes and Rhythms

Description: A *junctional escape beat,* or *junctional escape rhythm,* is a dysrhythmia that results when the rate of the primary pacemaker, usually the SA node, is slower than that of the AV node. The AV node then becomes the pacemaker. The AV node usually discharges at its intrinsic rate of 40–60 beats per minute. This is a safety mechanism that prevents cardiac standstill.

Etiology: Junctional escape rhythm has several etiologies, including increased vagal tone, which can result in SA node slowing; pathological slow SA node discharge; or heart block.

Rules of Interpretation/Lead II Monitoring (Figure 28-35):

Rate—40–60 per minute

Rhythm—irregular in single junctional escape complex; regular in junctional escape rhythm

Pacemaker site—AV junction

P waves—inverted; may appear before or after the QRS complex. The P waves can be masked by the QRS or be absent.

P-R interval—if the P wave occurs before the QRS complex, the P-R interval will be less than 0.12 sec. If the P wave occurs after the QRS complex, technically it is an R-P interval.

QRS complex—usually normal; may be greater than 0.12 sec

Clinical Significance: The slow heart rate can decrease cardiac output, possibly precipitating angina and other problems. If the rate is fairly rapid, the rhythm can be well tolerated.

Treatment: If the patient is asymptomatic, only observation is required in the field. Treatment is unnecessary unless hypotension or ventricular irritability is present. If treatment is required, administer a 0.5 mg bolus of atropine sulfate. Repeat every three–five minutes until you have obtained a satisfactory rate or have given a total of 0.04 mg/kg of the drug. If atropine fails, consider transcutaneous cardiac pacing (TCP), if available.

FIGURE 28-36   Accelerated junctional rhythm.

Accelerated Junctional Rhythm

Description: An *accelerated junctional rhythm* results from increased automaticity in the AV junction, causing the AV junction to discharge faster than its intrinsic rate. If the rate becomes fast enough, the AV node can override the SA node. Technically, the rate associated with an accelerated junctional rhythm is not a tachycardia. However, when compared to the intrinsic rate of the AV junctional tissue (40–60 beats per minute), it is considered accelerated.

Etiology: Accelerated junctional rhythms often result from ischemia of the AV junction.

Rules of Interpretation/Lead II Monitoring (Figure 28-36):

Rate—60–100 per minute

Rhythm—regular

Pacemaker site—AV junction

P waves—inverted; may appear before or after the QRS complex. P waves may be masked by the QRS or be absent.

P-R interval—if the P wave occurs before the QRS complex, the P-R interval will be less than 0.12 sec. If it occurs after the QRS, technically it is an R-P interval.

QRS complex—normal

Clinical Significance: An accelerated junctional rhythm is usually well tolerated. However, since ischemia is often the etiology, the patient should be monitored for other dysrhythmias.

Treatment: Prehospital treatment generally is unnecessary.

Paroxysmal Junctional Tachycardia

Description: *Paroxysmal junctional tachycardia (PJT)* develops when rapid AV junctional depolarization overrides the SA node. It often occurs in *paroxysms* (attacks with sudden onset), may last minutes or hours, and terminates abruptly. It may be caused by increased automaticity of a single AV nodal focus or by a reentry phenomenon at the AV node. Paroxysmal junctional tachycardia is often more appropriately called *paroxysmal supraventricular tachycardia (PSVT),* since the rapid rate may make it indistinguishable from paroxysmal atrial tachycardia.

Etiology: Paroxysmal junctional tachycardia may occur at any age and may not be associated with underlying heart disease. Stress, overexertion, smoking, or ingestion of caffeine may precipitate it. However, it is frequently associated with underlying atherosclerotic heart disease (ASHD) and rheumatic heart disease. PJT rarely occurs with myocardial infarction. It can occur with accessory pathway conduction, as in Wolff-Parkinson-White syndrome.

FIGURE 28-37   Paroxysmal junctional tachycardia.

Rules of Interpretation/Lead II Monitoring (Figure 28-37):

Rate—100–180 per minute

Rhythm—characteristically regular, except at onset and termination of paroxysms

Pacemaker site—AV junction

P waves—if present, P waves are inverted. They can occur before, during, or after the QRS complex. Turning up the speed of the graph paper or oscilloscope to 50 mm/sec spreads out the complex and aids in identifying P waves.

P-R interval—if the P wave occurs before the QRS complex, the P-R interval will be less than 0.12 sec. If it occurs after the QRS complex, technically it is an R-P interval.

QRS complex—normal

Clinical Significance: Young patients with good cardiac reserve may tolerate PJT well for a short time. The patient often will sense PJT as palpitations. However, rapid rates can preclude adequate ventricular filling time and markedly reduce cardiac output. The reduced diastolic phase of the cardiac cycle can also compromise coronary artery perfusion. PJT can precipitate angina, hypotension, or congestive heart failure.

Treatment: If the patient is not tolerating the rapid heart rate, as evidenced by hemodynamic instability, attempt the following techniques in this order:

1. Vagal maneuvers. Ask the patient to perform a Valsalva maneuver. This is a forced expiration against a closed glottis, or "bearing down" as if to move the bowels. This results in vagal stimulation, which may slow the heart. If this is unsuccessful, attempt carotid artery massage if the patient is eligible. (Do not attempt carotid artery massage in patients with carotid bruits or known cerebrovascular or carotid artery disease.)

2. Pharmacological therapy. Adenosine (Adenocard) is relatively safe and highly effective in terminating PJT. This is especially true if its etiology is reentry. Administer 6 mg of adenosine by rapid IV bolus over one to three seconds through the medication port closest to the patient's heart or central circulation. If the patient does not convert after one to two minutes, administer a second bolus of 12 mg over one to three seconds in the medication port closest to the patient's heart or central circulation. If this fails, and the patient has a normal blood pressure, medical direction may request the administration of verapamil. Verapamil is contraindicated in patients with a history of bradycardia, hypotension, or congestive heart failure. Do not use it with intravenous beta blockers; use it with caution in patients on chronic beta blocker therapy. Hypotension that occurs following verapamil administration can often be reversed with 0.5–1.0 gm of calcium chloride administered intravenously.

3. Electrical therapy. If the ventricular rate is greater than 150 beats per minute or the patient is hemodynamically unstable, use synchronized cardioversion. If time allows, sedate the patient with 5–10 mg of diazepam (Valium) or 2–5 milligrams of midazolam (Versed) IV. Apply synchronized DC countershock of 100 joules. If this is unsuccessful, repeat the countershock at increased energy as ordered by medical direction. DC countershock is contraindicated if you suspect digitalis toxicity as the cause of the PJT.

FIGURE 28-38 Ventricular escape complexes and rhythms (idioventricular rhythms).

DYSRHYTHMIAS ORIGINATING IN THE VENTRICLES

Some dysrhythmias originate within the ventricles. The pacemaker site will dictate the morphology of the QRS complex. Many factors, including ischemia, hypoxia, and medications, have been identified as causes. Dysrhythmias originating in the ventricles include:

- Ventricular escape complexes and rhythms
- Accelerated idioventricular rhythm
- Premature ventricular contraction
- Ventricular tachycardia
- Related dysrhythmia
- Ventricular fibrillation
- Asystole
- Artificial pacemaker rhythm

ECG features common to all dysrhythmias that originate in the ventricles include:

- QRS complexes of 0.12 sec or greater
- Absent P waves

Ventricular Escape Complexes and Rhythms

Description: A *ventricular escape beat* (*ventricular escape rhythm* or *idioventricular rhythm*) results either when impulses from higher pacemakers fail to reach the ventricles or when the discharge rate of higher pacemakers becomes less than that of the ventricles (normally 15–40 beats per minute). Ventricular escape rhythms serve as safety mechanisms to prevent cardiac standstill.

Etiology: Ventricular escape complexes and ventricular rhythms have several etiologies, including slowing of supraventricular pacemaker sites or high-degree AV block. They are frequently the first organized rhythms seen following successful defibrillation.

Rules of Interpretation/Lead II Monitoring (Figure 28-38):

Rate—15–40 per minute (occasionally less)

Rhythm—the rhythm is irregular in a single ventricular escape complex. Ventricular escape rhythms are usually regular unless the pacemaker site is low in the ventricular conductive system. Such placement makes regularity unreliable.

Pacemaker site—ventricle

P waves—none

P-R interval—none

QRS complex—greater than 0.12 sec and bizarre in morphology

Clinical Significance: The slow heart rate can significantly decrease cardiac output, possibly to life-threatening levels. The ventricular escape rhythm is a safety mechanism that you should not suppress. Escape rhythms can be perfusing or nonperfusing.

Treatment: Treatment depends on whether the escape rhythm is perfusing or nonperfusing. If it is perfusing, the object of treatment is to increase the heart rate. Administer a 0.5 mg bolus of atropine sulfate. Repeat every 3–5 minutes until you have obtained a satisfactory rate or have given 0.04 mg/kg of the drug. If atropine fails, consider transcutaneous cardiac pacing (TCP), if available. If the rhythm is nonperfusing, follow the pulseless electrical activity (PEA) protocol. This includes airway stabilization and CPR. Place an IV line, and administer 1 mg of epinephrine 1:10,000 IV. Direct treatment at correcting the primary problem (hypovolemia, hypoxia, cardiac tamponade, acidosis, or others). Consider a fluid challenge.

Accelerated Idioventricular Rhythm

Accelerated idioventricular rhythm is an abnormally wide ventricular dysrhythmia that usually occurs during an acute myocardial infarction. It is a sub-type of ventricular escape rhythm. Typically the rate is 60–110 beats per minute. The patient does not require treatment unless he becomes hemodynamically unstable. If this occurs, treat the ventricular focus with atropine or overdrive pacing. The principal action should be aggressive treatment of the underlying myocardial infarction as indicated, including appropriate prehospital care.

FIGURE 28-39 Premature ventricular contractions.

Premature Ventricular Contractions

Description: A *premature ventricular contraction* (PVC, or *ventricular ectopic*) is a single ectopic impulse arising from an irritable focus in either ventricle that occurs earlier than the next expected beat. It may result from increased automaticity in the ectopic cell or a reentry mechanism. The altered sequence of ventricular depolarization results in a wide and bizarre QRS complex and may additionally cause the T wave to occur in the direction opposite the QRS complex.

A PVC does not usually depolarize the SA node and interrupt its rhythm. That is, it does not interrupt the heart's normal cadence. The pause following the PVC is fully *compensatory*. Occasionally, an **interpolated beat** occurs when a PVC falls between two sinus beats without interrupting the rhythm.

If more than one PVC occurs, each can be classified as unifocal or multifocal. Because the PVC's morphology depends on the ectopic pacemaker's location, two PVCs of different morphologies imply two different pacemaker sites (multifocal). PVCs with the same morphology imply one pacemaker site (unifocal). If the **coupling interval** (the distance between the preceding beat and the PVC) is constant, the PVCs are most likely unifocal.

PVCs often occur in patterns of group beating. These include:

- *Bigeminy*—every other beat is a PVC
- *Trigeminy*—every third beat is a PVC
- *Quadrigeminy*—every fourth beat is a PVC

✱ **interpolated beat** a PVC that falls between two sinus beats without effectively interrupting this rhythm.

✱ **coupling interval** distance between the preceding beat and the PVC.

These terms can be applied to PACs and PJCs as well.

Repetitive PVCs are two consecutive PVCs without a normal complex in between. They can occur in groups of two (couplets) or three (triplets). More than three consecutive PVCs are often considered ventricular tachycardia.

PVCs can trigger lethal dysrhythmias such as ventricular fibrillation if they fall within the relative refractory period (the so-called R on T phenomenon). They are often classified by their relationship to the previous normal complex.

Etiologies: Etiologies for PVCs include

- Myocardial ischemia
- Increased sympathetic tone
- Hypoxia
- Idiopathic causes
- Acid-base disturbances
- Electrolyte imbalances
- Normal variant

Rules of Interpretation/Lead II Monitoring (Figure 28-39):

Rate—depends on underlying rhythm and rate of PVCs

Rhythm—interrupts regularity of underlying rhythm; occasionally irregular

Pacemaker site—ventricle

P waves—none; however, a normal sinus P wave (interpolated P wave) sometimes appears before a PVC.

P-R interval—none

QRS complex—greater than 0.12 sec and bizarre in morphology

Clinical Significance: Patients often sense PVCs as "skipped beats." In a patient without heart disease, PVCs may be insignificant. In patients with myocardial ischemia, PVCs may indicate ventricular irritability and may trigger lethal ventricular dysrhythmias. PVCs are often classified as malignant or benign. Malignant PVCs have at least one of the following traits:

- More than 6 PVCs per minute
- R on T phenomenon
- Couplets or runs of ventricular tachycardia
- Multifocal
- Associated chest pain

With most PVCs, the ventricles do not adequately fill. Because of this, you will usually not feel a pulse during the PVCs themselves. Frequent PVCs may reduce cardiac output.

PVCs can be described in terms of the Lown grading system for premature beats. The higher the grade, the more serious the ectopy:

Grade 0 = No premature beats

Grade 1 = Occasional (< 30 per hour) PVCs

Grade 2 = Frequent (> 30 per hour) PVCs

Grade 3 = Multiform (multifocal)

Grade 4 = Repetitive (couplets, salvos of 3 consecutive) PVCs

Grade 5 = R on T phenomenon

FIGURE 28-40 Ventricular tachycardia.

Treatment: If the patient has no history of cardiac disease and no symptoms, and if the PVCs are nonmalignant, no treatment is required. If the patient has a prior history of heart disease or symptoms, or if the PVCs are malignant, administer oxygen and place an IV line. If the patient is symptomatic, administer lidocaine at a dose of 1.0–1.5 mg/kg of body weight. Give an additional lidocaine bolus of 0.5–0.75 mg/kg every 5–10 minutes, if necessary, until you have given a total of 3.0 mg/kg of the drug. If the PVCs are effectively suppressed, start a lidocaine drip beginning at a rate of 2-4 mg/min. Reduce the dose in patients with decreased cardiac output (those with CHF or shock, for instance), in patients who are age 70 or greater, or in patients who have hepatic dysfunction. Give these patients a normal bolus dose first, followed by half the normal infusion. If the patient is allergic to lidocaine, or if you have given a maximum dose of lidocaine (3.0 mg/kg), consider procainamide or bretylium.

Ventricular Tachycardia

Description: Ventricular tachycardia (VT) consists of three or more ventricular complexes in succession at a rate of 100 beats per minute or more. This rhythm overrides the heart's normal pacemaker, and the atria and ventricles are asynchronous. Sinus P waves may occasionally be seen, dissociated from the QRS complexes. In *monomorphic VT* the complexes all appear the same; in *polymorphic VT* they have different sizes and shapes. One example of a polymorphic VT is *torsade de pointes.*

Etiology: As with PVCs, etiologies for ventricular tachycardia include:

- Myocardial ischemia
- Increased sympathetic tone
- Hypoxia
- Idiopathic causes
- Acid-base disturbances
- Electrolyte imbalances

Rules of Interpretation/Lead II Monitoring (Figure 28-40):

Rate—100–250 (approximately)

Rhythm—usually regular; can be slightly irregular

Pacemaker site—ventricle

P waves—if present, not associated with the QRS complexes

P-R interval—none

QRS complex—greater than 0.12 sec and bizarre in morphology

Clinical Significance: Ventricular tachycardia usually results in poor stroke volume, which, coupled with the rapid ventricular rate, may severely compromise cardiac output and coronary artery perfusion. Whether ventricular tachycardia is perfusing or nonperfusing dictates the type of treatment. Ventricular tachycardia may eventually deteriorate into ventricular fibrillation.

Treatment: If the patient is perfusing, as evidenced by the presence of a pulse, administer oxygen and place an IV line. Administer lidocaine at a dose of 1.0–1.5 mg/kg body weight intravenously. Administer additional doses of 0.5–0.75 mg/kg, until you have given a total of 3.0 mg/kg. If this treatment is unsuccessful, attempt to administer procainamide at 20–30 mg/minute to a maximum of 17 mg/kg. If procainamide fails, consider other second-line agents. Amiodarone (Cordarone) is becoming increasingly popular in the treatment of ventricular tachycardia. In the United States, it is primarily a second-line agent to lidocaine. In several of the Commonwealth countries, amiodarone is considered first-line treatment. The dose is 150–300 mg intravenously. Use synchronized cardioversion if the patient becomes unstable, as evidenced by chest pain, dyspnea, or systolic blood pressure of less than 90 mm/kg.

If the patient's condition is unstable, as evidenced by an altered level of consciousness or falling blood pressure, initiate cardioversion immediately after placing an IV line and administering oxygen. If time allows, sedate the patient first. The treatment plan is illustrated in the protocol (review Figure 28-26).

If the patient is nonperfusing, follow the protocol for ventricular fibrillation.

Torsade de Pointes *Torsade de pointes* is a polymorphic ventricular tachycardia that differs in appearance and cause from ventricular tachycardia in general. Torsade is most commonly caused by the use of certain antidysrhythmic drugs, including quinidine (Quinidex), procainamide (Pronestyl), disopyramide (Norpace), flecanide (Tambocor), sotolol (Betapace), and amiodarone (Cordarone). These agents' effects all seem to be exacerbated by the coadministration of certain nonsedating antihistamines, most notably aztemizole (Hismanol) and terfenadine (Seldane) and, in addition, the azole antifungal agents and macrolide antibiotics; erythromycin (PCE), azithromycin, (Zithromax), and clarithramycin (Biaxin). Any of these agents increase the likelihood of the patient's developing *torsade de pointes.*

FIGURE 28-41   Torsade de pointes.

The morphology of the QRS varies from beat to beat (hence the term *torsade de pointes,* which means "twisting on a point"). In addition, the QT interval is markedly increased to 600 milliseconds or more. Torsade will usually occur in bursts that are not sustained. During the "breaks" from these bursts you should examine the rhythm strip for a prolonged Q-T interval. The QRS rate is usually between 166 and 300 beats per minute, and the R-R interval varies in an irregularly irregular pattern. The QRS complexes are wide and change in size over the span of several complexes (Figure 28-41). Attempting treatment of *torsade de pointes* with the antidysrhythmics usually used for the treatment of ventricular tachycardia can have disastrous consequences. Therefore, recognition of *torsade de pointes* as a separate dysrhythmia is essential. Treatment is 1–2 grams of magnesium sulfate placed in 100 ml of D_5W and administered over 1–2 minutes. This can be repeated every 4 hours with close monitoring of the deep tendon reflexes. Amiodarone (Cordarone) has proven effective in the treatment of torsade. Correct any underlying electrolyte problems, especially hyperkalemia.

Figure 28-42 Ventricular fibrillation.

Ventricular Fibrillation

Description: Ventricular fibrillation is a chaotic ventricular rhythm usually resulting from the presence of many reentry circuits within the ventricles. There is no ventricular depolarization or contraction.

Etiology: A wide variety of causes have been associated with ventricular fibrillation. Most cases result from advanced coronary artery disease.

Rules of Interpretation/Lead II Monitoring (Figure 28-42):

Rate—no organized rhythm

Rhythm—no organized rhythm

Pacemaker site—numerous ectopic foci throughout the ventricles

P waves—usually absent

P-R interval—absent

QRS complex—absent

Clinical Significance: Ventricular fibrillation is a lethal dysrhythmia. The absence of cardiac output or an organized electrical pattern results in cardiac arrest.

Treatment: Ventricular fibrillation and nonperfusing ventricular tachycardia are treated identically. Initiate CPR. Follow this with DC countershock at 200 joules. If this is unsuccessful, repeat at 200–300 joules. If still unsuccessful, repeat at 360 joules. Subsequently, control the airway and establish an IV line. Epinephrine 1:10,000 or vasopressin are the drugs of first choice; administer every 3–5 minutes as required. If unsuccessful, consider second-line agents such as lidocaine, amiodarone, procainamide, or possibly magnesium sulfate.

FIGURE 28-43 Asystole.

Asystole

Description: Asystole *(cardiac standstill)* is the absence of all cardiac electrical activity.

Etiology: Asystole may be the primary event in cardiac arrest. It is usually associated with massive myocardial infarction, ischemia, and necrosis. Resulting from heart blocks when no escape pacemaker takes over, asystole is often the final outcome of ventricular fibrillation.

Rules of Interpretation/Lead II Monitoring (Figure 28-43):

> Rate—no electrical activity
>
> Rhythm—no electrical activity
>
> Pacemaker site—no electrical activity
>
> P waves—absent
>
> P-R interval—absent
>
> QRS complex—absent

Clinical Significance: Asystole results in cardiac arrest. The prognosis for resuscitation is very poor.

Treatment: Treat asystole with CPR, airway management, oxygenation, and medications. If you have any doubt about the underlying rhythm, attempt defibrillation. Medications include epinephrine, atropine, and in certain situations, sodium bicarbonate (Figure 28-44).

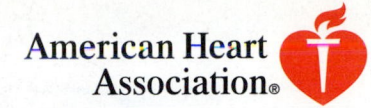

Asystole

↓

Primary ABCD Survey

Focus: *basic CPR and defibrillation*

- **Check** responsiveness
- **Activate** emergency response system
- **Call** for defibrillator

A **Airway:** open the airway
B **Breathing:** provide positive-pressure ventilations
C **Circulation:** give chest compressions
C **Confirm** true asystole
D **Defibrillation:** assess for VF/pulseless VT; shock if indicated

Rapid scene survey: is there any evidence that personnel should ***not*** attempt resuscitation (e.g., DNAR order, signs of death)?

↓

Secondary ABCD Survey

Focus: *more advanced assessments and treatments*

A **Airway:** place airway device as soon as possible
B **Breathing:** confirm airway device placement by exam plus confirmation device
B **Breathing:** secure airway device; purpose-made tube holders preferred
B **Breathing:** confirm effective oxygenation and ventilation
C **Circulation:** confirm true asystole
C **Circulation:** establish IV access
C **Circulation:** identify rhythm → monitor
C **Circulation:** give medications appropriate for rhythm and condition
D **Differential Diagnosis:** search for and treat identified reversible causes

↓

Transcutaneous pacing
If considered, perform immediately

↓

Epinephrine 1 mg IV push,
repeat every 3 to 5 minutes

↓

Atropine 1 mg IV,
repeat every 3 to 5 minutes
up to a total of 0.04 mg/kg

↓

Asystole persists
Withhold or cease resuscitation efforts?
- Consider quality of resuscitation?
- Atypical clinical features present?
- Support for cease-efforts protocols in place?

FIGURE 28-44   Management of asystole. Reproduced with permission from *Guidelines 2000 for Cardiopulmonary Resuscitation and Emergency Cardiovasular Care,* ©2000, Copyright American Heart Association.

Complete block

PACEMAKER

FIGURE 28-45   Artificial pacemaker rhythm.

Artificial Pacemaker Rhythm

Description: An *artificial pacemaker rhythm* results from regular cardiac stimulation by an electrode implanted in the heart and connected to a power source. The pacemaker lead may be implanted in any of several locations in the heart, although it is most often placed in the right ventricle (ventricular pacemaker) or in both the right ventricle and the right atria (dual-chambered pacemaker.)

Fixed-rate pacemakers fire continuously at a preset rate, regardless of the heart's electrical activity. *Demand pacemakers* contain a sensing device and fire only when the natural heart rate drops below a set rate. In these cases, the pacemaker acts as an escape rhythm.

Ventricular pacemakers stimulate only the right ventricle, resulting in a rhythm that resembles an idioventricular rhythm. *Dual-chambered pacemakers,* commonly called *AV sequential pacemakers,* stimulate the atria first and then the ventricles. They are most beneficial for patients with marginal cardiac output who need the extra atrial kick to maintain cardiac output.

Pacemakers are usually inserted into patients who have chronic high-grade heart block or sick sinus syndrome or who have had episodes of severe symptomatic bradycardia.

Rules of Interpretation/Lead II Monitoring (Figure 28-45):

Rate—varies with the preset rate of the pacemaker

Rhythm—regular if pacing constantly; irregular if pacing on demand

Pacemaker site—depends on electrode placement

P waves—none produced by ventricular pacemakers. Sinus P waves may be seen but are unrelated to the paced QRS complexes. Dual-chambered pacemakers produce a P wave behind each atrial spike. A pacemaker spike is an upward or downward deflection from the baseline, which is an artifact created each time the pacemaker fires. The pacemaker spike tells you only that the pacemaker is firing. It reveals nothing about ventricular depolarization.

P-R interval—if present, varies

QRS complex—the QRS complexes associated with pacemaker rhythms are usually longer than 0.12 sec and bizarre in morphology. They often resemble ventricular escape rhythms. A QRS complex should follow each pacemaker spike. If so, the pacemaker is said to be "capturing." With demand pacemakers, some of the patient's own QRS complexes may appear. A pacemaker spike should not be associated with these complexes.

Problems with Pacemakers: Although rare, pacemakers can have problems. One cause is battery failure. Most pacemaker batteries have relatively long lives. The cardiologist can check them and usually replaces them before problems arise. If a battery fails, however, no pacing will occur and the patient's underlying rhythm, which may be bradycardic or asystolic, may return.

Occasionally, a pacemaker can *run away*. This condition, rarely seen with new pacemakers, results in a rapid discharge rate. Runaway pacemaker usually occurs when the battery runs low; newer models compensate for this by gradually increasing rate as their batteries run low.

Demand pacemakers can fail to shut down when the patient's intrinsic heart rate exceeds the rate set for the device. Thus the pacemaker competes with the patient's natural pacemaker. Occasionally, a paced beat can fall in the absolute or relative refractory period, precipitating ventricular fibrillation.

Finally, pacemakers can fail to capture if the leads become displaced or the battery fails. In such cases, pacemaker spikes are usually present without P waves or QRS complexes. Bradycardia often results.

Considerations for Management: Always examine any unconscious patient for a pacemaker. Battery packs are usually palpable under the skin, often in the shoulder or axillary region. Treat bradydysrhythmias, asystole, and ventricular fibrillation from pacemaker failure as in any other patient. You may use lidocaine to treat ventricular irritability without fear of suppressing ventricular response to the pacemaker. Defibrillate patients with pacemakers as usual, but do not discharge the paddles directly over the battery pack. If external cardiac pacing is available, you can use it until definitive care is available. Transport pacemaker failure patients promptly without prolonged field stabilization. Definitive care consists of battery replacement or temporary pacemaker insertion.

Use Of A Magnet: Applying a magnet over the pulse generator inhibits all sensing and sets the pacemaker to a predetermined rate (usually 70). The patient should carry a card with information about his particular pacemaker, since these rates are manufacturer and model dependent. Use the magnet only for short periods to avoid the unlikely development of a serious dysrhythmia (including ventricular fibrillation). The indicator for magnet use is a runaway pacemaker.

Table 28-3	SUGGESTED TREATMENT FOR UNDERLYING CAUSES OF PULSELESS ELECTRICAL ACTIVITY
Condition	**Treatment (if allowed by local protocols)**
Hypovolemia	Fluids
Cardiac tamponade	Pericardiocentesis
Tension pneumothorax	Needle thoracostomy
Hypoxemia	Intubation/Oxygen
Acidosis	Sodium bicarbonate

PULSELESS ELECTRICAL ACTIVITY

Formerly termed electrical mechanical dissociation, *pulseless electrical activity (PEA)* essentially means that electrical complexes are present, but with no accompanying mechanical contractions of the heart. PEA is a perfect example of why you should treat the patient, not the monitor. Your monitor may show a textbook perfect, normal sinus rhythm, but the patient may be pulseless.

Causes of PEA include:

- Hypovolemia
- Cardiac tamponade
- Tension pneumothorax
- Hypoxemia
- Acidosis
- Massive pulmonary embolism
- Ventricular wall rupture

Administer epinephrine 1 mg every three to five minutes and treat the underlying cause(s). Table 28-3 shows suggested treatment for the different underlying causes. Early treatment can potentially reverse some of these conditions; therefore, prompt recognition and initiation of therapy are essential. Treatment for pulseless electrical activity is summarized in Figure 28-46.

DYSRHYTHMIAS RESULTING FROM DISORDERS OF CONDUCTION

Several dysrhythmias result from improper conduction through the heart. The three general categories of conductive disorders include:

- Atrioventricular blocks (discussed earlier in a separate section)
- Disturbances of ventricular conduction
- Pre-excitation syndromes

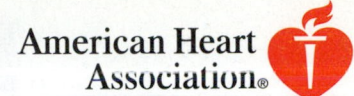

Pulseless Electrical Activity
(**PEA** = rhythm on monitor, without detectable pulse)

Primary ABCD Survey

Focus: *basic CPR and defibrillation*

- **Check** responsiveness
- **Activate** emergency response system
- **Call** for defibrillator
- A **Airway:** open the airway
- B **Breathing:** provide positive-pressure ventilations
- C **Circulation:** give chest compressions
- D **Defibrillation:** assess for and shock VF/pulseless VT

Secondary ABCD Survey

Focus: *more advanced assessments and treatments*

- A **Airway:** place airway device as soon as possible
- B **Breathing:** confirm airway device placement by exam plus confirmation device
- B **Breathing:** secure airway device; purpose-made tube holders preferred
- B **Breathing:** confirm effective oxygenation and ventilation
- C **Circulation:** establish IV access
- C **Circulation:** identify rhythm → monitor
- C **Circulation:** administer drugs appropriate for rhythm and condition
- C **Circulation:** assess for occult blood flow ("pseudo-EMD")
- D **Differential Diagnosis:** search for and treat identified reversible causes

Review for most frequent causes

- **H**ypovolemia
- **H**ypoxia
- **H**ydrogen ion — acidosis
- **H**yper-/hypokalemia
- **H**ypothermia

- "**T**ablets" (drug OD, accidents)
- **T**amponade, cardiac
- **T**ension pneumothorax
- **T**hrombosis, coronary (ACS)
- **T**hrombosis, pulmonary (embolism)

Epinephrine 1 mg IV push,
repeat every 3 to 5 minutes

Atropine 1 mg IV (if PEA rate is ***slow***),
repeat every 3 to 5 minutes as needed, to a total
dose of 0.04 mg/kg

FIGURE 28-46 Management of pulseless electrical activity (PEA). Reproduced with permission from *Guidelines 2000 for Cardiopulmonary Resuscitation and Emergency Cardiovasular Care,* ©2000, Copyright American Heart Association.

Disturbances of Ventricular Conduction

✳ **aberrant conduction** conduction of the electrical impulse through the heart's conductive system in an abnormal fashion.

✳ **bundle branch block** a kind of interventricular heart block in which conduction through either the right of left bundle branches is blocked or delayed.

Disturbances in conduction of the depolarization impulse are not limited to the AV node. Problems can arise within the ventricles as well. **Aberrant conduction** is a single supraventricular beat conducted through the ventricles in a delayed manner. **Bundle branch block** is a disorder in which all supraventricular beats are conducted through the ventricles in a delayed manner. Either the left or right bundle branch can be involved. If both branches are blocked, then a third-degree AV block exists. These complexes originate above the ventricles and should be distinguished from pure ventricular rhythms, which can have a similar QRS morphology. An *incomplete bundle branch block* has a normal QRS complex; a complete block has a wide QRS complex.

One of the two known causes of ventricular conduction disturbances is ischemia or necrosis of either the right or left bundle branch, rendering it incapable of conducting the impulse to the ventricle. The second is either a premature atrial contraction or a premature junctional contraction that reaches the ventricles or one of the bundle branches, usually the right, when it is still refractory. This often happens in atrial fibrillation because of the irregular rhythm's varying speed of repolarization.

The ECG features of ventricular conduction disturbances include a QRS complex longer than 0.12 sec because the blocked side of the heart is depolarized much more slowly than the unaffected side. The impulse passes much more slowly through the myocardium than through the rapid electrical conduction pathway. The QRS morphology is often bizarre. It can be notched or slurred, reflecting rapid depolarization through the normal conductive system and slow depolarization through the myocardium on the blocked side.

Ventricular conduction disturbances sometimes complicate ECG rhythm strip interpretation. In these cases, supraventricular beats can have abnormally wide QRS complexes. If you suspect a conduction system disturbance relating to supraventricular beats, then it is prudent to inspect some of the other leads in order to determine the problems.

Although exceptions do occur, supraventricular tachycardias caused by disturbances in conduction usually differ in several ways from wide complex tachycardias originating in the ventricles:

- A changing bundle branch block suggests supraventricular tachycardia (SVT) with aberrancy.
- A trial of carotid sinus massage may slow conduction through the AV node and may terminate a reentrant SVT or slow conduction with other supraventricular tachydysrhythmias. These maneuvers will have no effect on ventricular tachycardias.
- AV dissociation, also known as AV block, indicates a ventricular origin of the dysrhythmia.
- A full compensatory pause, usually seen after a ventricular beat, indicates ventricular tachycardia.
- Fusion beats suggest ventricular tachycardia.
- A QRS duration of longer than 0.14 sec usually indicates VT.

The patient's history may also help to differentiate the etiologies of wide complex tachycardias. In older patients with a history of myocardial infarction, congestive heart failure, or coronary artery disease, these dysrhythmias most likely have a ventricular origin.

When in doubt, treat the patient as if he has the more lethal dysrhythmia, ventricular tachycardia. In either case, use cardioversion if the patient is unstable; it is effective for both ventricular and supraventricular tachycardias.

Pre-Excitation Syndromes

Pre-excitation syndromes involve premature ventricular excitation by an impulse that bypasses the AV node. The most common of these is *Wolff-Parkinson-White (WPW) syndrome*. WPW occurs in approximately 3 of every 1,000 persons. It is characterized by a short P-R interval, generally less than 0.12 sec, and a long QRS duration, generally more than 0.12 sec. Additionally, the upstroke of the QRS often has a slur, called the *delta wave* (Figure 28-47). In WPW, conduction of the depolarization impulse from the atria to the ventricles is abnormal. The **bundle of Kent,** an extra conduction pathway between the atria and ventricles, effectively bypasses the AV node, shortening the P-R interval and prolonging the QRS complex. Most WPW patients are asymptomatic; however, the disorder is associated with a high incidence of tachydysrhythmias, usually through a reentry mechanism. WPW is also frequently associated with organic heart diseases such as atrial septal defects or mitral valve prolapse. Base treatment on the underlying rhythm.

* bundle of Kent an accessory AV conduction pathway that is thought to be responsible for the ECG findings of pre-excitation syndrome.

ECG CHANGES DUE TO ELECTROLYTE ABNORMALITIES AND HYPOTHERMIA

Electrolyte imbalances can cause dysrhythmias that will appear on ECG rhythm strips. Suspect *hyperkalemia* (excessive potassium in the blood) in patients with a history of renal failure who are on dialysis. On an ECG, tall, peaked T waves in the precordial leads are an early sign of hyperkalemia. As the levels increase further, conduction decreases and the PR and QT intervals increase. At very high potassium levels, an idioventricular rhythm may develop and eventually become a classic sine wave (a wave that rises to a maximum positive level and then drops to a maximal negative level). Prominent U waves appear with *hypokalemia* (deficient potassium levels in the blood). Very low levels can widen the QRS complex.

In *hypothermia*, the Osborn wave, or J wave, is apparent. It is a slow, positive deflection at the end of the QRS complex (Figure 28-48). Other ECG changes may include:

- T wave inversion
- PR, QRS, QT prolongation.
- Sinus bradycardia
- Atrial fibrillation or flutter
- AV block
- PVCs
- Ventricular fibrillation
- Asystole

FIGURE 28-47 The delta wave of Wolf-Parkinson-White syndrome.

FIGURE 28-48 The Osborn ("J") wave.

Part 2: Assessment and Management of the Cardiovascular Patient

Part 2 of this chapter will help you build on the information about cardiovascular anatomy (in Chapter 3) and cardiac physiology, electrographic monitoring, and dysrhythmias (in Part 1 of this chapter) as you develop the skills for assessing and managing a patient suffering a cardiovascular emergency.

Part 2 begins with general principles of assessment and management of cardiovascular emergencies and concludes with discussions of a variety of specific conditions and emergencies including angina pectoris, myocardial infarction, heart failure, cardiac tamponade, hypertensive emergencies, cardiogenic shock, cardiac arrest, and cardiovascular emergencies.

ASSESSMENT OF THE CARDIOVASCULAR PATIENT

Airway, breathing, and circulatory problems and shock are always the most critical issues during the first minute of patient care.

The key to providing your cardiovascular patient with the best possible medical care is to take a systematic, step-by-step approach. When you initially contact your patient, always determine the most important problems first. Airway, breathing, circulatory problems, and shock are always the most critical issues during the first minute of patient care. What may have caused any life-threatening problems does not matter at this point. In some instances such as cardiac arrest, your focus during prehospital care may never go beyond these four concerns.

After you have managed any life-threatening problems, the focused history and physical examination will help you form your field diagnosis. Cardiovascular diseases may affect the myocardium, the electrical conductive system, the pericardium, or the blood vessels. They may also involve a combination of these problems or problems associated with other systems, such as diabetes. Diseases of the myocardium include myocardial infarction, heart failure, or cardiogenic shock. In electrical conductive illnesses, the heart rate is either too fast or too slow. Although pericardial emergencies such as pericarditis or pericardial tamponade are usually diagnosed clinically by the physical examination findings, the focused history (blunt/penetrating trauma or recent infection, for example) may help you to recognize them. Vascular problems may include coronary artery occlusion, peripheral venous or arterial occlusion, or pulmonary embolism.

In the field, therapeutic treatments are generally limited to:

- Administering nitrates, aspirin, and analgesics for symptomatic chest pain
- Treating pulmonary edema
- Giving analgesics in peripheral vascular emergencies

In your on-going assessment, continually reevaluate your initial management. Based on the patient's needs, you will transport him in the appropriate mode to the appropriate facility. As with any patient, your management of the cardiac patient should include patient advocacy as well as communication and emotional support for the patient and his family. You must also effectively communicate the details of your assessment and management to the receiving staff. Additionally, your knowledge of nontransport criteria, education and prevention, proper documentation, and on-going quality assurance will all contribute to providing optimum care.

Your assessment of the patient with a cardiovascular emergency should vary according to the acuity of the situation. Patients with serious illnesses should have a limited, yet focused exam. Patients who are less seriously ill should receive a more comprehensive assessment. It is important to remember that the cardiovascular system affects virtually every other body system. Signs of cardiac disease may initially be evident only in the respiratory system as dyspnea. A comprehensive exam, however, will often reveal subtle findings that point to cardiovascular disease as the cause.

SCENE SIZE-UP AND INITIAL ASSESSMENT

After ascertaining that the scene is safe, begin an initial cardiovascular assessment. This allows you to identify life-threatening problems and set transport priorities. First, determine the patient's level of responsiveness. Is he speaking with you or unresponsive? Then move on to the ABCs. Make sure his airway is patent and free of debris and blood. Suction the airway if appropriate. Next, check the patient's rate and depth of breathing. Listen for the presence or absence of breath sounds. Certain breath sounds such as moist rales should heighten your suspicion of cardiovascular disease. Note the effort or "work" of breathing. If the patient is not breathing, initiate manual ventilation and intubate as soon as possible. Check for the rate and quality of pulses. If no pulse is present, immediately begin cardiopulmonary resuscitation. The skin can indicate the degree of perfusion present. Look for

- Color
- Temperature
- Moisture
- Turgor
- Mobility
- Edema

Finally, check the patient's blood pressure. Is he in shock? Is this a hypertensive emergency? Treat all life-threatening conditions as you find them.

FOCUSED HISTORY

After you have completed your initial cardiovascular assessment and treated life-threatening conditions, proceed with your focused history, using the SAMPLE format (*S*ymptoms, *A*llergies, *M*edications, *P*ast medical history, *L*ast oral intake, and *E*vents preceding the incident).

Common Symptoms

Cardiac disease can manifest itself in several ways. Some common chief complaints and symptoms include:

- Chest pain or discomfort
- Dyspnea
- Cough
- Syncope
- Palpitation

Chest pain is the most common presenting symptom in cases of cardiac disease.

Not all patients who have cardiac disease will have chest pain.

Chest Pain   Chest pain or discomfort that may radiate to the shoulder, neck, jaw, or back is a common symptom of cardiac disease. Always remember, however, that not all patients who have cardiac disease will have chest pain. This is especially true in diabetic patients, who may have a myocardial infarction with no pain at all. Also remember that chest pain can be benign and may have no association with cardiac disease. Differentiating between benign and life-threatening chest pain is extremely difficult; do not attempt it in the field. If a cardiac etiology is even a remote possibility, treat the patient accordingly.

Follow the OPQRST acronym to obtain the patient's description of the pain.

- *Onset.* Ask about the onset of the pain. When did it begin? What was the patient doing when it started? If the patient has had chest pain in the past, ask him to compare it to previous episodes. For instance, if he had a major heart attack in the past and tells you his present pain is the same, then strongly suspect that it is also from his heart.
- *Provocation/Palliation.* What provoked the pain? Is it exertional or nonexertional? The relationship of pain to exertion is very important. During exertion, the heart muscle needs more oxygen. If it does not receive the additional oxygen, the muscle becomes ischemic and the patient has pain (angina). He may tell you that he is now walking shorter distances before the pain begins, indicating

lessening blood flow to the heart. Untreated, this may lead to pain at rest and, eventually, infarction. What alleviates the pain (palliation)? Is the pain related to movement or inspiration?

- *Quality.* Ask the patient to describe the quality of the pain. Ask open-ended questions and allow the patient to characterize this symptom in his own words. Common descriptive words include sharp, tearing, pressure, and heaviness.

- *Region/Radiation.* The patient may complain of pain radiating to other regions of his body, most commonly his arms, neck, jaw, and back.

- *Severity.* Ask the patient to rate the pain on a scale of one to ten, with one being very little and ten being the worst pain he has ever felt. This can also be a useful gauge of your management's effectiveness. Some systems will use a pain scale of one to five. Regardless of the scale, it is important that the scale used is standardized in the system. It can be problematic if a paramedic asks a patient to rate his pain on a scale of one to five, but when the patient gets to the hospital, the nurse or doctor is using a scale of one to ten. Although seemingly trivial, this can significantly affect patient care.

- *Timing.* Check the timing of the pain. How long has the pain lasted? Always determine the time the pain began and record it. The onset and duration of pain directly affect decisions about the use of thrombolytic drugs. Is the pain constant or intermittent? Is it getting worse? better? Does it occur at rest or with activity?

Dyspnea Because of the heart's close relationship with the respiratory system, many cardiac patients have dyspnea (labored breathing). Dyspnea is often associated with myocardial infarction and in some patients may be the only symptom. Also, patients with congestive heart failure will experience increased dyspnea when lying down.

When confronted with a dyspneic patient, ask about the following:

- *Duration.* How long has it lasted? Is it continuous or intermittent?
- *Onset.* Was the onset sudden or rapid?
- *Provocation/palliation.* Does anything aggravate or relieve the dyspnea? Is it exertional or nonexertional?
- *Orthopnea.* Does sitting upright give relief?

Cough Frequently, patients who cough have chest pain. Is the cough dry or productive? Did the patient pull a chest muscle during coughing? Try to determine if the coughing results from congestive heart failure.

Other Related Signs and Symptoms Other related signs and symptoms to look for and ask about include:

- *Level of consciousness.* The level of consciousness indicates brain perfusion. An alteration in the level of consciousness can be due to problems within the cardiovascular system.

- *Diaphoresis (perspiration)* Cardiac problems significantly affect the autonomic nervous system. Stimulation of the sympathetic nervous system can result in marked diaphoresis.

- *Restlessness and anxiety.* Restlessness and anxiety are among the earliest symptoms when a patient is experiencing lowered brain perfusion, whether due to decreased oxygenation, decreased blood supply, or both.

- *Feeling of impending doom.* The significant and massive stimulation of the sympathetic nervous system associated with severe cardiovascular emergencies can cause a feeling of impending doom. This is a part of the "fight or flight" response. A patient with a sensation of impending doom can be experiencing a significant cardiovascular event.

- *Nausea and/or vomiting.* Nausea and vomiting are common during cardiovascular events such as myocardial ischemia. This often results from slowed peristalsis due to sympathetic stimulation.

- *Fatigue.* Fatigue is a generalized finding associated with many diseases. In patients with cardiovascular disease, it can be caused by anemia, poor oxygenation, or poor overall cardiovascular system functioning.

- *Palpitations.* Palpitations are a sensation that the heart is beating fast or skipping beats. This can result from tachycardia or simply from increased awareness of the heart's normal function.

- *Edema.* Edema is the accumulation of fluid in third (interstitial) spaces. It accompanies poor cardiac function and often indicates chronic cardiovascular disease.
  - *Extremities.* Ambulatory patients usually will develop edema in the extremities, due to the effects of gravity.
  - *Sacral.* Sacral, or presacral edema, is seen in bed-bound patients. Fluid collects in the lowest part of the patient's body, usually around the sacrum.

- *Headache.* Headache is a factor in cardiovascular disease for several reasons. First, decreased CNS perfusion can result in headaches. These are often severe. Many patients with established heart disease take nitroglycerin or other nitrate drugs. Excess administration of nitrates can cause a severe headache and may indicate worsening heart disease.

- *Syncope.* Syncope is a brief loss of consciousness due to a transient decrease in cerebral blood flow. It occurs in certain cardiac dysrhythmias and in ischemic lesions where blood flow to the heart may be impaired, reducing cardiac output and interrupting CNS perfusion. Severe pain can also cause syncope as well as other forms of psychic stress.

- *Behavioral change.* A behavioral change may very subtly indicate cardiovascular disease. More common in the elderly, it may point to either an acute or chronic decrease in cerebral blood flow.

- *Anguished facial expression.* The pain that accompanies myocardial ischemia can be quite severe. This, coupled with the effects of sympathetic nervous system stimulation, may cause the patient to exhibit anguished facial expressions.

- *Activity limitations.* Decreased cardiac performance can significantly limit a patient's physical activities. These limitations may develop slowly and be considered chronic or develop quickly and be considered acute.

- *Trauma.* Trauma, especially unexplained trauma, can be due to a temporary decrease in CNS perfusion. Unexplained facial injuries or bruises may indicate a cardiovascular problem.

Many of the signs and symptoms of cardiovascular disease can be subtle. Always assess for them and look for any sign or symptom patterns that point to cardiovascular disease.

Allergies

Ask about the patient's allergies. Is he allergic to any medications? Does he have an allergy to X-ray dye (IVP dye)? Try to differentiate between true medication allergies and undesirable side effects of a particular medication. For instance, the patient who tells you he breaks out in hives and stops breathing if he takes penicillin is having an allergic reaction. The patient who says he gets abdominal upset from aspirin is, most likely, experiencing a side effect. If in doubt, withhold the medication and contact medical direction.

If in doubt about a possible medication allergy, withhold the medication and contact medical direction.

Medications

The patient's current use of prescription medications is important. What medications is he currently taking? Has he recently changed any medications? The following drugs may be especially significant:

- Nitroglycerin (Nitrostat)
- Propranolol (Inderal) and other beta blockers
- Digitalis (Lanoxin)
- Diuretics (Lasix, Maxzide, Dyazide)
- Antihypertensives (Vasotec, Prinivil, Capoten)
- Antidysrhythmics (Mexitil, Quinaglute, Tambocor)
- Lipid lowering agents (Mevacor, Lopid)

Also question the patient in detail about his compliance with his medications. Does he take his medications? Does he take the right amount? Does he take them at the right time? With the high cost of medications and limited coverage by prescription plans, more and more patients are not taking their prescriptions. Some may even borrow a friend's medication, a dangerous practice, since it may be the wrong dosage or even the wrong drug.

The patient's use of nonprescription drugs is also important. Ask if he takes any over-the-counter medications. Numerous drugs interact, and you must be aware of all medications the patient is currently taking, prescription or otherwise. Try to bring all drug containers with you to the hospital if doing so will not adversely prolong transport time. This information is very important for the hospital staff. Recreational drug use is another major problem. For example, cocaine causes vasoconstriction of the blood vessels and can lead to myocardial infarction and severe hypertension, often in the absence of coronary artery disease. These effects can last up to two weeks. Even though this question may make you uncomfortable, you must ask it.

Try to bring all of the patient's prescription and nonprescription drug containers to the hospital with you.

Past Medical History

Avoid spending excessive time obtaining a cardiac patient's past medical history. If the patient's condition permits, however, a past medical history may help you determine if his symptoms are attributable to a cardiac condition.

- Does the patient have a history of coronary artery disease, angina, or a previous myocardial infarction? If so, chances are good that his symptoms are cardiac in origin. Comparing his prior symptoms to his present ones is helpful. If he tells you this pain is just like his previous heart attack, then he likely is experiencing another.

- Has the patient had any prior heart problems? Ask about the following:
  - Valvular disease (rheumatic heart disease)
  - Aneurysm
  - Previous cardiac surgery
  - Congenital cardiac anomalies
  - Pericarditis or other inflammatory cardiac disease
  - Congestive heart failure (CHF)
- What other medical problems does the patient have? Ask about the following:
  - Pulmonary disease/COPD
  - Diabetes mellitus
  - Renal (kidney) disease
  - Hypertension
  - Peripheral vascular disease
- Does anyone in the patient's family have cardiac disease? At what age did it first develop? Cardiac disease before the age of 50 in a close relative should heighten your concern about heart disease. If a family member had a cardiac event at a young age, especially sudden death, your patient is also at risk earlier in life. Has anyone in his family died of heart disease? At what age? Also ask if the family has a history of stroke, diabetes, or hypertension.
- Does the patient smoke? Does he know his cholesterol level? These are other modifiable risk factors for cardiac disease.

Last Oral Intake

When was the patient's last oral intake? If the patient ingested a meal high in saturated fats before the onset of symptoms, then gall bladder disease should be considered as a possible etiology. Also inquire if the patient has had an increase in caffeine intake and ask when he last drank a caffeinated beverage.

Events Preceding the Incident

What was the patient doing before the onset of symptoms? Was there emotional upset? Had he just completed a strenuous task such as mowing the yard? Has he recently started a new exercise program? Did the symptoms begin while the patient was having sex? Does the patient take Viagra? The development of chest pain during sexual intercourse is not uncommon. However, patients often will not volunteer this information. Asking about intimate events such as this may be uncomfortable, but it is necessary for optimal patient care.

PHYSICAL EXAMINATION

After addressing any life-threatening problems you find in the initial assessment, begin the physical exam. Be systematic and thorough, and remember to look (inspect), listen (auscultate), and feel (palpate) while performing your detailed examination.

Inspection

During your inspection, look for:

- *Tracheal Position.* The trachea should be midline. Movement toward a side may indicate a pneumothorax. Inspect the neck veins for evidence of jugular vein distention. The internal jugular veins are major vessels. Thus, jugular vein distention often evidences an increase in central venous pressure (Figure 28-49). Pump failure or cardiac tamponade can cause back pressure in the systemic circulation and jugular vein engorgement. Try to have the patient seated at a 45° angle, not lying flat, for this examination. Remember, however, that jugular vein distention is often difficult to assess in an obese patient.

- *Thorax.* Watch the patient breathe. To do this properly, expose the patient's chest wall, maintaining patient privacy if possible. Evidence of labored breathing includes retractions and accessory muscle use. Retractions are visible depressions in the soft tissues between the ribs that occur with increased respiratory effort. Accessory muscle use involves muscles of the neck, back, and abdomen. Normally these muscles play a small role in breathing, but patients with labored breathing put them to greater use. A patient with chronic obstructive pulmonary disease (COPD) may have an increased anteroposterior (AP) diameter and may appear "barrel-chested." Examination of the thorax can provide a great deal of information about the patient, including chronic problems such as COPD. The presence of a sternotomy scar, especially in an older patient, is a significant indicator of heart disease.

- *Epigastrium.* While the chest wall is exposed, inspect the epigastrium. Look for abdominal distention and visible pulsations. This may mean the patient has an aortic aneurysm with dissection or rupture.

- *Peripheral and Presacral Edema.* Chronic back pressure in the systemic venous circulation causes peripheral and presacral edema. These symptoms are most obvious in dependent parts such as the ankles (Figure 28-50). Often in bedridden patients you must inspect and palpate the sacral region for edema. Edema is generally classified as either mild or pitting. To distinguish between them, press firmly on the edematous part. If the depression remains after you remove pressure, the edema is pitting; otherwise it is mild.

- *Skin.* Several changes in the skin can be associated with cardiovascular disease. Pale and diaphoretic skin indicates peripheral vasoconstriction and sympathetic stimulation. It accompanies heart disease and other problems. A mottled appearance often indicates chronic cardiac failure.

- *Subtle Signs Of Cardiac Disease.* Look for subtle indicators of cardiac disease. Observe for signs that a patient is being treated for cardiac problems. These include midsternal scars from coronary artery bypass surgeries, pacemakers, or nitroglycerin skin patches.

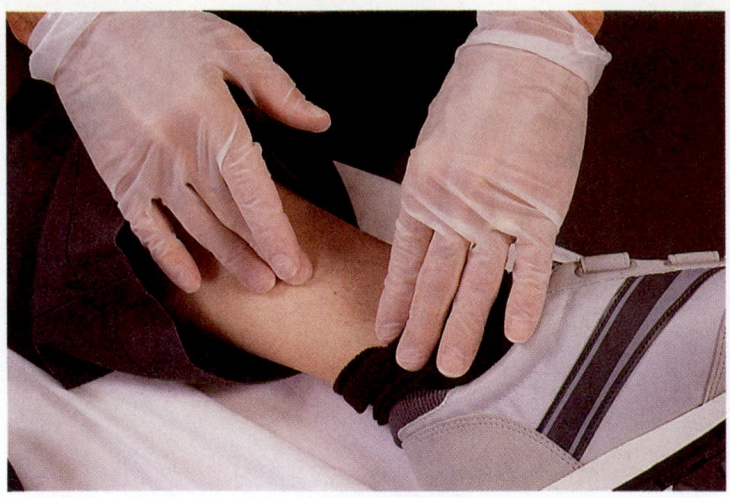

FIGURE 28–50 Check for peripheral edema.

Auscultation

During your inspection listen for:

- *Breath Sounds.* Assessing breath sounds in the cardiac patient is just as important as it is in the respiratory patient. Assess the lung fields for equality. Also listen for *adventitious sounds,* those that arise or occur sporadically or in unusual locations. Such sounds as crackles (rales), wheezes, or rhonchi (whistling or snoring sounds) may indicate pulmonary congestion or edema. Patients with pulmonary edema may also have foamy, blood-tinged sputum from the mouth and nose. In severe cases, this is audible from a distance as an ominous "gurgling" sound.

- *Heart Sounds.* Avoid spending precious time auscultating heart sounds in the field. Background noise from traffic, family members, sirens, and other sources makes it very difficult to hear heart sounds, and the information you obtain generally will not affect patient management. Nonetheless, you should be familiar with normal heart sounds and be able to distinguish abnormal from normal findings (Figure 28-51). The first heart sound (S_1) is produced by closure of the AV valves (tricuspid and mitral)

FIGURE 28–51 Auscultate the chest. Listen for heart sounds.

during ventricular systole. The second heart sound (S_2) is produced by closure of the aortic and pulmonary valves. S_1 and S_2 are normal. Any extra heart sounds are abnormal. The third heart sound (S_3) is associated with congestive heart failure. Occasionally, the skilled listener can hear the fourth heart sound (S_4), which occurs immediately before S_1. It is associated with increased atrial contraction. Ideally, the heart should be examined from the four classic auscultatory sites: aortic, pulmonic, mitral, and tricuspid. The point on the chest wall where the heartbeat can best be heard or felt is known as the point of maximum impulse (PMI). The PMI and examination of the heart are discussed in more detail in Chapter 11, Physical Exam Techniques.

An S_3 heart sound has a cadence like "Kentucky." An S_4 heart sound has a cadence like "Tennessee."

- *Carotid Artery Bruit.* Auscultation of the carotid arteries may reveal bruits (murmurs), which are a sign of turbulent blood flow through a vessel (Figure 28-52). They are audible over all major arteries, including the abdominal aorta. A bruit indicates partial blockage of the vessel, most commonly from atherosclerosis. If you detect a bruit, do not attempt carotid sinus massage. This procedure may dislodge plaque, resulting in stroke or other mishap.

Palpation

During your examination, feel for:

- *Pulse.* Determine the rate and regularity of the pulse (Figure 28-53). Also note the pulse's equality. Any pulse deficit can indicate underlying peripheral vascular disease and should be reported to medical direction.

- *Thorax.* Palpation of the thorax is extremely important as chest wall problems are quite common. These can only be elicited by palpation, which may reveal crepitus. *Crepitus* is a grating sensation that suggests the rubbing of broken bone ends or a "bubble wrap" crackling that suggests subcutaneous emphysema (air in the subcutaneous tissue). Palpapation may also reveal tenderness associated with a chest wall muscle strain, costochondritis (inflammation of the joint where the rib attaches to the sternum), or even rib fractures. It is important to remember that at least

15 percent of patients with acute myocardial infarction will have associated chest wall tenderness.

- *Epigastrium.* Also feel the abdomen for pulsations and distention, which may indicate an abdominal aortic aneurysm.

Physical examination of the chest is an essential aspect of comprehensive prehospital care. Employ the standard techniques of inspection, auscultation, palpation, and occasionally, percussion. Together these skills can provide a great deal of information about chronic problems as well as the ongoing acute episode.

MANAGEMENT OF CARDIOVASCULAR EMERGENCIES

The following section discusses management techniques frequently used in cardiac emergencies. You should also become familiar with your local protocols and procedures, since they vary from system to system.

BASIC LIFE SUPPORT

Basic life support is the primary skill for managing serious cardiovascular problems.

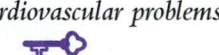

Basic life support is the primary skill for managing serious cardiovascular problems. These include the basic airway maneuvers as well as CPR. Review basic life support techniques frequently to keep your skills at their peak.

ADVANCED LIFE SUPPORT

Most of the procedures that paramedics employ to manage cardiovascular emergencies are considered advanced life support. The number of skills will vary from system to system. Advanced prehospital skills used in managing cardiovascular emergencies include:

- ECG monitoring
- Vagal maneuvers (carotid sinus massage)
- Precordial thump
- Pharmacological management
- Defibrillation

- Synchronized cardioversion
- Transcutaneous cardiac pacing

MONITORING ECG IN THE FIELD

Most systems' primary tool for ECG monitoring in the field is a combination ECG monitor/defibrillator that operates on a direct current (DC) battery source (Procedure 28-1). It has the following parts:

- Paddle electrodes
- Defibrillator controls
- Synchronizer switch
- Oscilloscope
- Paper strip recorder
- Patient cable and lead wires
- Controls for monitoring
- Special features (such as data recorders)

To monitor your patient's ECG, you will place the three limb electrodes on the chest (in left arm, right arm, and left leg positions). Some manufacturers require a fourth lead on the right leg. By placing the three principal electrodes, you can monitor any of the bipolar leads (I, II, or III). On certain machines, you can also monitor the three augmented leads (aVR, aVL, or aVF) through these three electrodes. As a rule, Lead II is usually monitored, as its axis is almost the same as that of the heart. Modified chest lead 1 (MCL_1) is used occasionally and is often better for determining the site of ectopic beats.

You can also monitor your patient through the defibrillator paddles ("quick-look"). The quick-look paddles are more frequently used in cases of cardiac arrest, when there is no time to place chest electrodes. You can also use this system when the patient cable is inoperative. Among the disadvantages of quick-look paddle electrodes are that they tend to pick up more artifacts than chest electrodes and must be held in continuous contact with the chest.

To use quick-look paddles, follow these steps:

1. Turn on oscilloscope power.
2. Apply conducting gel or other medium liberally to the paddle surface.
3. Hold the paddles firmly on the chest wall with the positive electrode on the left lower chest and the negative electrode on the right upper chest. This closely simulates Lead II.
4. Observe the monitor and obtain a tracing if desired.

Chest electrodes vary from manufacturer to manufacturer. Usually to mimic Lead II, you will place the positive electrode on the patient's left lower chest and the negative electrode on his right upper chest. Placement of the ground wire varies. For MCL_1 place the positive electrode on the right lower chest wall and the negative electrode on the left upper chest wall. Again, placement of the ground wire varies. Place the electrodes to avoid large muscle masses, large quantities of chest hair, or anything that keeps the electrodes from resting flat on the skin. Also, avoid placing electrodes where you might have to place defibrillator paddles.

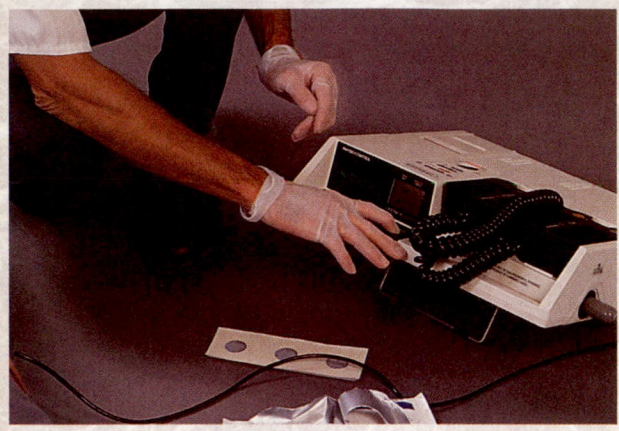

28-1a   Turn on the machine.

28-1b   Prepare the skin.

28-1c   Apply the electrodes.

28-1d   Ask the patient to relax and remain still.

28-1e Check the ECG.

28-1f Obtain a tracing.

28-1g ECG strip.

28-1h Continue ALS care.

To place electrodes follow these steps:

1. Cleanse the skin with alcohol or abrasive pad. This removes dirt and body oil for better skin contact. If chest hair is thick, shave small amounts before placing the electrodes. If the patient is extremely diaphoretic, apply tincture of benzoin.
2. Apply electrodes to the skin surface.
3. Attach wires to the electrodes.
4. Plug the cable into the monitor.
5. Adjust gain or sensitivity to the proper level.
6. Adjust the QRS volume. (The continual beep of the ECG may disturb the patient.)
7. Obtain a baseline tracing.

Poor ECG signals are useless, and you should correct them. Their most common cause is faulty skin contact. Whenever you spot a poor signal, check for the following possible causes:

- Excessive hair
- Loose or dislodged electrode
- Dried conductive gel
- Poor placement
- Diaphoresis

An initially poor tracing may improve as the conductive gel breaks down skin resistance. Other causes of poor tracings include:

- Patient movement or muscle tremor
- Broken patient cable
- Broken lead wire
- Low battery
- Faulty grounding
- Faulty monitor

Obtain a paper printout from each patient you monitor. Be sure to adjust the stylus heat properly. Calibrate each strip when you begin monitoring so that 1 mV deflects the stylus 10 mm (two large boxes).

Again, treat the patient and not the monitor. Always compare the rhythm you see on the monitor with the patient's signs and symptoms. A patient may have a perfect rhythm on the monitor but have no pulse or blood pressure.

VAGAL MANEUVERS

For a stable patient with symptomatic tachycardia, vagal maneuvers sometimes help slow the heart rate. Ask the patient to perform a Valsalva maneuver (bearing down as if attempting to have a bowel movement) or to cough. If these are unsuccessful and the patient is eligible, attempt carotid artery massage. Do not attempt carotid artery massage on patients with carotid bruits or known cerebrovascular or carotid artery disease, as it may precipitate a stroke. Carotid sinus massage is discussed in more detail later in this chapter.

FIGURE 28–54   The precordial thump.

PRECORDIAL THUMP

The precordial thump, a blow to the midsternum with the heel of the fist, can stimulate depolarization within the heart. This is most effective when performed immediately after the onset of ventricular fibrillation or pulseless ventricular tachycardia. On occasion, the precordial thump can cause depolarization of enough ventricular cells to allow resumption of an organized rhythm. Additionally, conversions from ventricular tachycardia, complete AV block, and occasionally, ventricular fibrillation, have been reported. If no defibrillator is immediately available, you may attempt a precordial thump on a pulseless patient who has a witnessed arrest. Since the amount of energy needed to convert ventricular fibrillation increases rapidly with time, a thump is likely to succeed only if delivered early. It is not recommended in pediatric patients.

To deliver a precordial thump strike the midsternum with the heel of your fist from a distance of 10–12 inches (Figure 28-54). To avoid rib fractures and other problems, keep your arm and wrist parallel to the sternum's long axis.

PHARMACOLOGICAL MANAGEMENT

The drugs that you will use to manage cardiovascular emergencies (Table 28-4) generally fall into the categories of antidysrhythmics, sympathomimetics, and drugs used specifically for myocardial ischemia (including thrombolytics), along with other prehospital medications, some of which are used only infrequently. For more detailed information on these types of drugs, see Chapter 6, on pharmacology.

Table 28-4	DRUGS USED TO MANAGE CARDIOVASCULAR EMERGENCIES

Antidysrhythmics

Antidysrhythmic medications control or suppress dysrhythmias.

atropine sulfate	adenosine
lidocaine	amiodarone
procainamide	verapamil
bretylium	

Sympathomimetic Agents

Sympathomimetic agents are similar to the naturally occurring hormones epinephrine and norepinephrine. They duplicate or mimic sympathetic nervous system stimulation.

dopamine	norepinephrine
dobutamine	isoproterenol
epinephrine	

Drugs Used for Myocardial Ischemia

Drugs used to treat myocardial ischemia also act to relieve its pain.

oxygen	morphine sulfate
nitrous oxide	nalbuphine
nitroglycerin	

Thrombolytic Agents

Thrombolytic agents act to break up blood clots blocking a blood vessel

aspirin (not a thrombolytic but inhibits aggregation of platelets)	alteplase (Activase) (tPA)
	reteplase (Retavase)

Other Prehospital Drugs

In some situations, medical direction or local protocol may recommend the following drugs.

furosemide (diuretic)	promethazine (sedative; antihistamine; antiemetic; anticholinergic)
diazepam (sedative-hypnotic; anticonvulsive)	sodium nitroprusside (vasodilator)

Drugs Infrequently Used in the Prehospital Setting

The following are drugs that paramedics who work in the emergency department may encounter and that many patients take on a long-term basis.

digitalis (Digoxin, Lanoxin) (cardiac 1296glycoside: increases cardiac contracile force and cardiac output)

beta blockers (propranolol) (dysrhythmia control)

calcium channel blockers (verapamil, diltiazem, nifedipine) (control supraventricular tachydysrhythmias; help manage hypertension; increase coronary artery perfusion in angina pectoris)

alkalinizing agents (sodium bicarbonate) (occasional use in management of cardiac arrest)

DEFIBRILLATION

Defibrillation is the process of passing a current through a fibrillating heart to depolarize the cells and allow them to repolarize uniformly, thus restoring an organized cardiac rhythm. A critical mass of the myocardium must be depolarized in order to suppress all of the ectopic foci. The critical mass is related to the size of the heart, but it cannot be calculated for a given individual or situation.

The *defibrillator* is an electrical capacitor that stores energy for delivery to the patient at a desired time. It consists of an adjustable high-voltage power supply, energy storage capacitor, and paddles. A current-limiting inductor connects the capacitor to the paddles. Recently, different defibrillation wave forms, most commonly biphasic wave forms, have been utilized to decrease possible tissue damage and to increase battery life. This technology evolved with the development of the compact automated external defibrillators (AEDs).

Most defibrillators use direct current (DC). Alternating current (AC) models should not be used. Direct current is more effective, more portable, and causes less muscle damage. It delivers an electrical charge of several thousand volts over a very short time, generally 4–12 milliseconds. The shock's strength is commonly expressed in energy according to the following formula:

$$\text{energy (joules)} = \text{power (watts)} \times \text{duration (seconds)}$$

The chest wall offers resistance to the electrical charge, which lowers the amount of energy actually delivered to the heart. Therefore, lowering the resistance pathway between the defibrillator paddles and the chest is important. Factors that influence chest wall resistance include:

- Paddle pressure
- Paddle-skin interface
- Paddle surface area
- Number of previous countershocks
- Inspiratory versus expiratory phase at time of countershock

The following factors influence the success of defibrillation.

- *Time until ventricular fibrillation.* In conjunction with effective CPR, defibrillation begun within four minutes after the onset of fibrillation will yield significantly improved resuscitation rates, as compared with defibrillation begun within eight minutes.
- *Condition of the myocardium.* Converting ventricular fibrillation is more difficult in the presence of acidosis, hypoxia, hypothermia, electrolyte imbalance, or drug toxicity. Secondary ventricular fibrillation (ventricular fibrillation that results from another cause) is more difficult to treat than primary ventricular fibrillation.
- *Heart size and body weight.* The effects of heart size and body weight on defibrillation are controversial. Pediatric and adult energy requirements differ, but whether size and energy level settings are related in adults is not clear.
- *Previous countershocks.* Repeated countershocks decrease transthoracic resistance, thereby allowing the defibrillator to deliver more energy to the heart at the same energy level.
- *Paddle size.* Larger defibrillator paddles are thought to be more effective and cause less myocardial damage. The ideal size for adults,

✳ **defibrillation** the process of passing an electrical current through a fibrillating heart to depolarize a critical mass of myocardial cells. This allows them to depolarize uniformly, resulting in an organized rhythm.

however, has not been established. Generally, the paddles should be 10–13 cm in diameter. In infants, 4.5 cm paddles are adequate.

- *Paddle Placement.* For both adults and children in the emergency setting, place the paddles on the chest. Position one paddle to the right of the upper sternum, just below the clavicle. Place the other to the left of the left nipple in an anterior axillary line immediately over the apex of the heart. Do not place paddles over the sternum. Do not place paddles over the generator of an implanted automatic defibrillator or pacemaker, which can damage or disable the device. Place the paddles approximately 5 inches from the generator. The paddles may be marked as apex (positive electrode) and sternum (negative electrode). Although reversing polarity inverts the ECG tracing, it does not affect defibrillation.

- *Paddle-skin interface.* Paddle-skin interface should have as little electrical resistance as possible. Greater resistance decreases energy delivery to the heart and increases heat production on the skin. Many available materials decrease resistance, including gels, creams, pastes, saline-soaked pads, and prepackaged gel pads. Use only creams made specifically for defibrillation, not for ECG monitoring. When using cream, make sure that it does not run and form a bridge between paddles. Never use alcohol-soaked pads; they can ignite.

- *Paddle contact pressure.* The paddle contact pressure is important. Firm, downward pressure decreases transthoracic resistance. Do not lean on the paddles, however; they may slip.

- *Properly functioning defibrillator.* The machine should deliver the amount of energy that it indicates. Therefore, frequent inspection and testing of the machine are necessary. Change and cycle the batteries as the manufacturer directs.

To perform defibrillation, use the following steps (Procedure 28-2):

1. Confirm ventricular fibrillation or pulseless ventricular tachycardia on the cardiac monitor.
2. Place the patient in a safe environment if initially in contact with some electrically conductive material such as metal or water.
3. Apply electrode gel to the paddles, or place commercial defibrillation pads on the patient's exposed thorax.
4. Turn on and charge the defibrillator to 200 joules for the first shock.
5. Ensure that the electrodes are appropriately placed on the patient's thorax with proper pressure.
6. Ensure that no one else is in contact with the patient. Verbally and visually clear everybody, including yourself, before any defibrillation attempt.
7. Deliver a defibrillatory shock by depressing both red buttons simultaneously. (Depressing only one will not deliver a shock.)
8. Reconfirm the rhythm on the monitor screen; if the patient is still in ventricular fibrillation or pulseless ventricular tachycardia, recharge the defibrillator and repeat steps 5–7 at higher energy levels.

Keep in mind the basic energy recommendations for defibrillation. After initially attempting defibrillation at 200 joules in an adult, increase dosage to a maximum of 360 joules in one or two repeat countershocks. The pediatric dosage is generally 2 joules/kg initially, repeated at 4 joules/kg if required.

EMERGENCY SYNCHRONIZED CARDIOVERSION

Synchronized cardioversion is a controlled form of defibrillation for patients who still have organized cardiac activity with a pulse. A synchronizing circuit in the defibrillator interprets the QRS cycle and delivers the electrical discharge during the R wave of the QRS complex. This reduces the likelihood of delivering the cardioversion during the vulnerable period of the QRS cycle, which can precipitate ventricular fibrillation. Synchronizing also permits the use of lower energy levels and reduces the potential for secondary dysrhythmias. Depending on the type of dysrhythmia being treated, as little as 10 joules may be adequate, especially if the origin is atrial.

Indications for emergency synchronized cardioversion in an unstable patient include:

- Perfusing ventricular tachycardia
- Paroxysmal supraventricular tachycardia
- Rapid atrial fibrillation
- 2:1 atrial flutter

The procedure for synchronized cardioversion is the same as for defibrillation. Sedate conscious patients if at all possible. Turn on the synchronizer switch, and verify that the machine is detecting the R waves (Figure 28-55). If not, you may need to reposition the electrodes. Press and hold the discharge buttons until the machine discharges on the next R wave. Some models automatically turn off the synchronizer after a cardioversion and return to defibrillation mode. To give a second synchronized shock, you must depress the synchronizer button again. If ventricular

* **synchronized cardioversion** the passage of an electric current through the heart during a specific part of the cardiac cycle to terminate certain kinds of dysrhythmias.

FIGURE 28-55 Activate the synchronizer.

28-2a   Identify rhythm on the cardiac monitor.

28-2b   Apply electrode gel to the paddles or place commercial defibrillation pads on the patient's exposed thorax.

28-2c   Charge the defibrillation paddles.

28-2d   Reconfirm the rhythm on the cardiac monitor.

28-2e Verbally and visually clear everybody, including yourself, from the cardiac patient.

28-2f Deliver a shock by pressing both buttons simultaneously.

28-2g Reconfirm the rhythm on the cardiac monitor.

fibrillation occurs, you must turn off the synchronizer switch and use the machine in the defibrillation mode, because the heart produces no R wave in ventricular fibrillation and the machine will not discharge. The procedure for synchronized cardioversion is summarized in Figure 28-56.

TRANSCUTANEOUS CARDIAC PACING

Many of the newer cardiac monitor/defibrillators have a built-in cardiac pacing device that enables paramedic units to perform *transcutaneous* (external) cardiac pacing (TCP). Transcutaneous cardiac pacing allows electrical pacing of the heart through the skin via specially designed thoracic electrodes. Before the development of TCP, electrical cardiac pacing required placing an electrode through a major vein or directly into the chest. With TCP, pacing can now be provided in the prehospital setting. This is beneficial in such cases of symptomatic bradycardia as occur with high-degree AV blocks, atrial fibrillation with slow ventricular response, and other significant bradycardias (including asystole). Use transcutaneous pacing if pharmacological intervention has no effect and the patient is hypotensive or hypoperfusing.

To perform external cardiac pacing, follow these steps (Procedure 28-3):

1. Initiate IV, oxygen, and ECG monitoring.
2. Place the patient supine.
3. Confirm symptomatic bradycardia and confirm medical direction order for external cardiac pacing.
4. Apply the pacing electrodes according to the manufacturer's recommendations being sure that they interface well with the skin.
5. Connect the electrodes.
6. Set the desired heart rate on the pacemaker. This will typically range from 60 to 80 beats per minute.
7. Turn the output setting to 0.
8. Turn on the pacer.
9. Slowly increase the output until you note ventricular capture.
10. Check the pulse and blood pressure, and adjust the rate and amperage as medical direction orders.
11. Monitor the patient's response to treatment.

To manage patients in asystole, place the output on its maximum setting. Then decrease the output if capture occurs.

Occasionally, external cardiac pacing may cause patient discomfort. If this occurs, medical direction may request the administration of an analgesic.

Overdrive pacing may deter recurrent tachycardia. This involves increasing the rate above the heart's current rate in order to suppress ventricular ectopy. This is particularly useful in *torsade de pointes*. Failure of transcutaneous pacing is similar to the failure of a permanent pacemaker, as discussed earlier in the section on artificial pacemaker rhythm.

American Heart Association.

Fighting Heart Disease and Stroke

Steps for Synchronized Cardioversion

1. Consider sedation.
2. Turn on defibrillator (monophasic or biphasic).
3. Attach monitor leads to the patient ("white to right, red to ribs, what's left over to the left shoulder") and ensure proper display of the patient's rhythm.
4. Engage the synchronization mode by pressing the "sync" control button.
5. Look for markers on R waves indicating sync mode.
6. If necessary, adjust monitor gain until sync markers occur with each R wave.
7. Select appropriate energy level.
8. Position conductor pads on patient (or apply gel to paddles).
9. Position paddle on patient (sternum-apex).
10. Announce to team members: *"Charging defibrillator—stand clear!"*
11. Press "charge" button on apex paddle (right hand).
12. When the defibrillator is charged, begin the final clearing chant. State firmly in a forceful voice the following chant before each shock:
    - *"I am going to shock on three. One, I'm clear."* (Check to make sure you are clear of contact with the patient, the stretcher, and the equipment.)
    - *"Two, you are clear."* (Make a visual check to ensure that no one continues to touch the patient or stretcher. In particular, do not forget about the person providing ventilations. That person's hands should not be touching the ventilatory adjuncts, including the tracheal tube!)
    - *"Three, everybody's clear."* (Check yourself one more time before pressing the "shock" buttons.)
13. Apply 25 lb pressure on both paddles.
14. Press the "discharge" buttons simultaneously.
15. Check the monitor. If tachycardia persists, increase the joules according to the electrical cardioversion algorithm.
16. **Reset the sync mode after each synchronized cardioversion because most defibrillators default back to unsynchronized mode.** This default allows an immediate shock if the cardioversion produces VF.

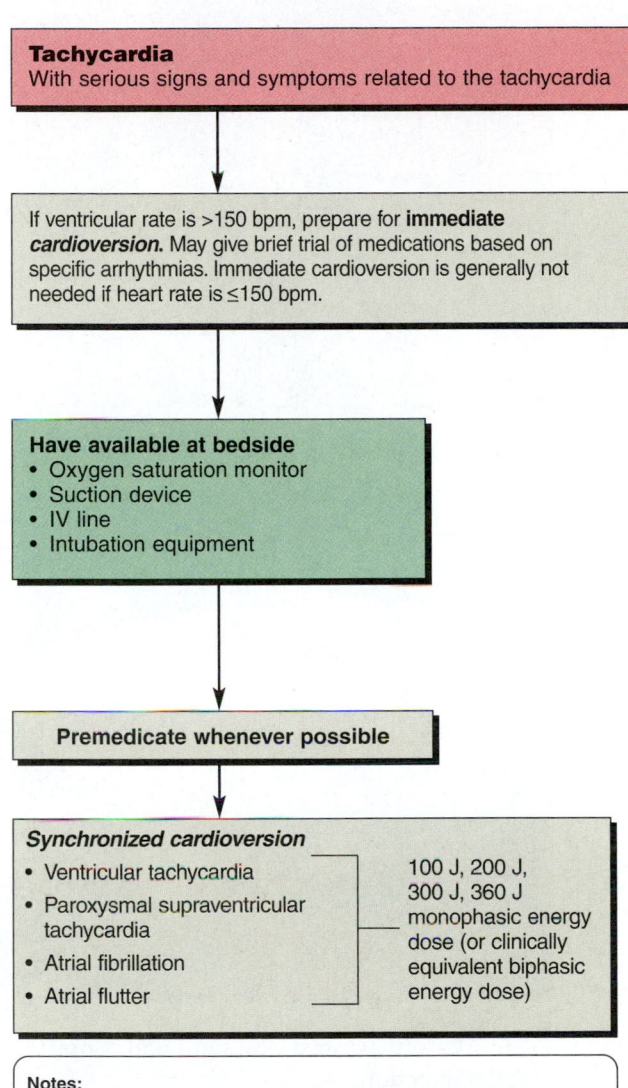

Tachycardia
With serious signs and symptoms related to the tachycardia

↓

If ventricular rate is >150 bpm, prepare for **immediate cardioversion.** May give brief trial of medications based on specific arrhythmias. Immediate cardioversion is generally not needed if heart rate is ≤150 bpm.

↓

Have available at bedside
- Oxygen saturation monitor
- Suction device
- IV line
- Intubation equipment

↓

Premedicate whenever possible

↓

Synchronized cardioversion
- Ventricular tachycardia
- Paroxysmal supraventricular tachycardia
- Atrial fibrillation
- Atrial flutter

100 J, 200 J, 300 J, 360 J monophasic energy dose (or clinically equivalent biphasic energy dose)

Notes:
1. Effective regimens have included a sedative (e.g., **diazepam, midazolam, barbiturates, etomidate, ketamine, methohexital)** with or without an analgesic agent (e.g., **fentanyl, morphine, meperidine).** Many experts recommend anesthesia if service is readily available.
2. Both monophasic and biphasic waveforms are acceptable if documented as clinically equivalent to reports of monophasic shock success.
3. Note possible need to resynchronize after each cardioversion.
4. If delays in synchronization occur and clinical condition is critical, go immediately to unsynchronized shocks.
5. Treat polymorphic ventricular tachycardia (irregular form and rate) like ventricular fibrillation: see ventricular fibrillation/pulseless ventricular tachycardia algorithm.
6. Paroxysmal supraventricular tachycardia and atrial flutter often respond to lower energy levels (start with 50 J).

FIGURE 28–56   Electrical (synchronized) cardioversion algorithm. Reproduced with permission from *Guidelines 2000 for Cardiopulmonary Resuscitation and Emergency Cardiovascular Care,* ©2000, Copyright American Heart Association.

External pacing is of benefit in bradycardias and heart blocks that are symptomatic. The electrodes are placed on the chest as shown. The desired heart rate is selected. The current is then adjusted until "capture" of the heart's conductive system is obtained.

28-3a   Establish an IV line.

28-3b   Place ECG electrodes.

28-3c   Carefully assess vital signs and contact medical direction.

28-3d. If external pacing is ordered, apply the pacing electrodes according to the manufacturer's recommendations.

28-3e Connect the electrodes.

28-3f Select the desired pacing rate and current.

28-3g Monitor the patient's response to treatment.

CAROTID SINUS MASSAGE

Carotid sinus massage can convert paroxysmal supraventricular tachycardia into sinus rhythm by stimulating the baroreceptors in the carotid bodies. This increases vagal tone and decreases heart rate.

To perform carotid sinus massage, have atropine sulfate readily available and use the following technique (Procedure 28-4):

1. Initiate IV, oxygen, and ECG monitoring.
2. Position patient on his back, slightly hyperextending the head.
3. Gently palpate each carotid pulse separately. Auscultate each side for carotid bruits. Do not attempt carotid sinus massage if the pulse is diminished or if carotid bruits are present.
4. Tilt the patient's head to either side. Place your index and middle fingers over one artery, below the angle of the jaw and as high up on the neck as possible.
5. Firmly massage the artery by pressing it against the vertebral body and rubbing.
6. Monitor the ECG and obtain a continuous readout. Terminate massage at the first sign of slowing or heart block.
7. Maintain pressure no longer than 15–20 seconds.
8. If the massage is ineffective, you may repeat it, preferably on the other side of the patient's neck.

Complications of carotid sinus massage include dysrhythmias such as asystole, PVCs, ventricular tachycardia, or fibrillation. In addition, this procedure can interfere with cerebral circulation, causing syncope, seizure, or stroke. Increased parasympathetic tone can cause bradycardias, nausea, or vomiting.

SUPPORT AND COMMUNICATION

As with other emergencies, appropriate support and communication are an integral part of the treatment you provide for your cardiovascular patient. Time permitting, explain your treatment to the patient and his family and offer emotional support as indicated. When rapid transport is necessary, explain why. If the patient refuses transport, you will need to clearly explain the potential consequences, and use every available means to convince him of his need for appropriate treatment. As you transfer care of your patient to the receiving facility staff, you must clearly explain your findings to the receiving nurse or physician in a formal verbal briefing. This briefing should include the patient's vital information, chief complaint and history, physical exam findings, and any treatments rendered. In cardiovascular emergencies, any ECG findings will be especially important to the receiving staff.

MANAGING SPECIFIC CARDIOVASCULAR EMERGENCIES

The following section details the pathophysiology of common cardiovascular emergencies. Each section covers epidemiology, morbidity and mortality, assessment, and management.

ANGINA PECTORIS

Angina pectoris literally means "pain in the chest." This condition, however, is much more complicated than simple pain. Angina occurs when the heart's blood supply is transiently exceeded by myocardial oxygen demands. In other words, during periods of increased oxygen demand, the coronary arteries cannot deliver an adequate amount of blood to the myocardium. This can cause ischemia of the myocardium and chest pain.

As a rule, the reduced blood flow through the coronary arteries results from atherosclerosis. Atherosclerotic plaques can develop throughout the coronary circulation. Some patients may have atherosclerotic lesions that are isolated to one vessel, while others will have diffuse disease involving several vessels. Fixed blockages in the coronary arteries decrease blood flow. Remember that blood flow through a vessel is related to its diameter. Reducing the diameter of a vessel by one-half, as can occur in atherosclerosis, drastically reduces the amount of blood that the vessel can transport.

In addition to atherosclerosis, angina can result from abnormal spasm of the coronary arteries. This disorder, commonly called **Prinzmetal's angina**, *vasospastic angina,* or *atypical angina,* can also lead to inadequate blood flow, causing pain. Approximately two-thirds of the people who have vasospastic angina also have atherosclerotic coronary artery disease. Spasm of the vessel on top of atherosclerotic blockage can cause ischemia. However, one-third of patients with vasospastic angina will have little or no coronary atherosclerosis.

Angina is generally classified as stable or unstable. *Stable angina* occurs during activity, when the heart's oxygen demands are increased. Attacks of stable angina are usually precipitated by physical or emotional stress. They are relatively brief and often respond readily to treatment. *Unstable angina,* on the other hand, occurs at rest and may not respond as readily to treatment. Because unstable angina often indicates severe atherosclerotic disease, it is also called pre-infarction angina. Unstable angina usually indicates that the patient's disease process is worsening.

Angina is not a self-limiting disease. It results from underlying coronary artery disease. If it is untreated and its contributing factors are unchanged, the underlying problem remains even though the pain has resolved. Because of the nature of the episodes, angina is usually progressive (that is, it accelerates in frequency and duration). Myocardial infarction may follow a single episode of angina.

It is important to remember that there are other causes of chest pain. While cardiac ischemia is one of its major causes, chest pain can arise from problems

* **angina pectoris** chest pain that results when blood supply's oxygen demands exceed the heart's.

* **Prinzmetal's angina** variant of angina pectoris caused by vasospasm of the coronary arteries, not blockage per se; also called *vasospastic angina* or *atypical angina.*

28-4a   Assess the patient.

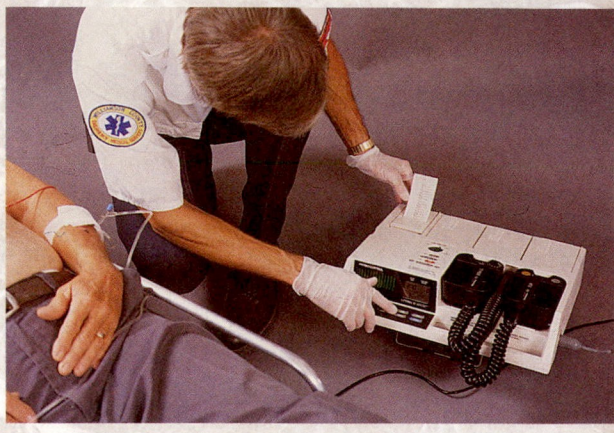

28-4b   Turn on the monitor.

28-4c   Listen to both carotids for the presence of bruits.

28-4d   Start an IV line.

28-4e   Rub either carotid. Wait.

28-4f   Check the rhythm.

28-4g   If unsuccessful, rub the other carotid.

28-4h   Reevalutate the patient.

in the cardiovascular system, the respiratory system, the gastrointestinal system, and the musculoskeletal system. Causes of chest pain include:

- Cardiovascular causes
  - Cardiac ischemia
  - Pericarditis (viral or autoimmune)
  - Thoracic dissection of the aorta
- Respiratory causes
  - Pulmonary embolism
  - Pneumothorax
  - Pneumonia
  - Pleural irritation (Pleurisy)
- Gastrointestinal causes
  - Cholecystitis
  - Pancreatitis
  - Hiatal hernia
  - Esophageal disease
  - Gastroesophageal reflux (GERD)
  - Peptic ulcer disease
  - Dyspepsia
- Musculoskeletal causes
  - Chest wall syndrome
  - Costochondritis
  - Acromioclavicular disease
  - Herpes zoster (shingles)
  - Chest wall trauma
  - Chest wall tumors

Diagnosing the cause of a patient's chest pain can be challenging in the hospital, let alone in the prehospital setting. As frequently occurs in emergency medicine, we look for the worst and hope for the best. Always be prepared to treat patients with chest pain as if they are suffering cardiac ischemia or another major disease process. Once you have excluded these possibilities you can consider less critical causes.

Field Assessment

When you assess an angina patient, remember that weak or absent peripheral pulses indicate potential or pending shock, which you should treat immediately. Changes in skin color such as paleness or cyanosis, or changes in temperature such as cold extremities also suggest shock.

The typical angina patient's chief complaint is a sudden onset of chest discomfort. The pain may radiate, or it may be localized to the chest. Often epigastric pain accompanies the chest pain. The patient with angina, however, often denies having chest pain, largely because he has dealt with this type of chest pain before. Although anginal episodes are common for the patient with a cardiac history, they should be considered significant when EMS is activated.

Angina usually lasts from three to five minutes, sometimes as long as fifteen minutes, and is relieved with rest and/or nitroglycerin. Atypical, or Prinzmetal, angina most often occurs at rest or without a precipitating cause. Prinzmetal angina is often accompanied by S-T segment elevation on the ECG, which can indicate myocardial tissue ischemia.

Labored breathing may or may not be present. After establishing the patency of the patient's airway, auscultate the lungs for congested breath sounds, particularly in the bases. Remember, however, the lungs may be clear. The anginal patient's heart rate and rhythm may be altered. Peripheral pulses should be equal. Typically, the blood pressure will elevate during the episode and normalize afterwards.

The contributing history may indicate that this is the patient's first recognized instance of angina, that it is a recurring event, or that the episodes are increasing in frequency or duration. A recurrence of angina or an increase in its frequency or duration is often the reason an anginal patient calls EMS. Any change in typical anginal pain is significant.

Without prolonging scene time, obtain an ECG tracing. If feasible, a 12-lead ECG is preferred for its additional diagnostic detail. After obtaining and interpreting the tracing, transmit it to the medical facility or medical direction. Typical 12-lead findings in the patient with angina are limited to patterns of ischemia: S-T depression and/or T-wave inversion. After relief of pain, the S-T depression and T-wave inversion generally will return to normal. This can take a few minutes or several hours. Occasionally the patterns may not return to normal.

Many 12-lead monitors have internal computerized pattern identification programs that will identify baseline, certain dysrhythmias, and anomalies that you might otherwise miss. These devices are most often accurate, but they do not always identify everything that may be pertinent. For example, patients experiencing Prinzmetal angina can have S-T segment elevation that dissipates after the pain has been relieved. Never trust the computer interpretation. Always overread the tracing for accuracy or telemeter it to the emergency department. The most common ECG finding in the angina patient is S-T segment depression. S-T segment changes often are not specific, however, and dysrhythmias and ectopy may not be present when the tracing is obtained.

Management

The patient experiencing angina is often apprehensive. Place him at rest in a position of physical and emotional comfort to decrease myocardial oxygen demand. Administer oxygen, generally at a high-flow rate, to increase oxygen delivery to the myocardium. Establish an IV either on scene without delaying transport or en route. If possible, and again without prolonging scene time, obtain and record a 12-lead or 3-lead ECG tracing. This is important because the ECG findings may be normal once the patient is pain free. Measure any S-T segment changes and communicate them to the receiving facility. Because a single anginal episode can be a precursor to a myocardial infarction, anticipate ECG changes such as dysrhythmias and S-T segment elevation.

Administer nitroglycerin sublingually, either as a tablet or a spray. It decreases myocardial work and, to a lesser degree, dilates coronary arteries. If the patient's symptoms persist after one or two doses of nitroglycerin, assume something more serious than angina, such as myocardial infarction. Nifedipine (Procardia), or another calcium channel blocker, is now being used, in addition to nitroglycerin, to manage angina. It is a vasodilator that works through blockade of the slow calcium channels. Consider morphine sulfate for chest pain that does not respond to nitrates or calcium channel blockers.

Patients with first episodes of angina or episodes that medication does not relieve are usually admitted to the hospital for evaluation. There is often a fine line between unstable angina and early myocardial infarction. Immediate transport is indicated if the patient does not feel relief after receiving oxygen and/or nitrates. The absence of relief indicates the patient's underlying disease process may be worsening. If the event is the beginning of a myocardial infarction, *reperfusion* (restoring blood flow to the ischemic tissue) is crucial. Hypotension can occur, especially if the patient has taken nitroglycerin. Its presence indicates transport, because it may lead to hypoperfusion of myocardial tissue. S-T segment changes, especially S-T segment elevation, indicate rapid transport. Transport should be efficient and fast but without lights and sirens unless clinically indicated. The lights and sirens could make the patient apprehensive and increase his pain.

Sometimes, the patient experiencing anginal chest pain will call EMS and then refuse transport after his chest pain is relieved. This may be due to a number of reasons, from denial to the patient's having taken older nitrates, which take longer to work. In any case, strongly encourage immediate evaluation because of the potential serious complications such as MI. Document patient refusal and be sure the patient signs the refusal and understands the potential risks. Encourage the patient to see his cardiologist or private care physician as soon as possible for follow-up.

Explain to the patient and family the reason and necessity for rapid transport, if indicated. Time permitting, also explain your treatment. Upon arrival at the emergency department, inform the physician of your findings—past history, vital signs, labored breathing, relief of pain, no relief of pain, and ECG findings, especially S-T segment findings.

MYOCARDIAL INFARCTION

* **myocardial infarction (MI)** death and subsequent necrosis of the heart muscle caused by inadequate blood supply; also *acute myocardial infarction (AMI)*.

Myocardial infarction (MI) is the death of a portion of the heart muscle from prolonged deprivation of oxygenated arterial blood. MI can also occur when the heart's oxygen demand exceeds its supply over an extended time. Myocardial infarction is most often associated with *atherosclerotic heart disease (ASHD)*. The precipitating event is commonly the formation of a *thrombus*, or blood clot, in a coronary artery already diseased from atherosclerosis. Atherosclerosis places many anginal patients at high risk for a myocardial infarction, especially those suffering from persistent or unstable angina. Myocardial infarction can also result from coronary artery spasm, microemboli (as seen with the recreational use of cocaine), acute volume overload, hypotension (from any cause), or from acute respiratory failure (acute hypoxia). Trauma can also cause myocardial infarction.

The location and size of the infarction depend on the vessel involved and the site of the obstruction (Figure 28-57.) Most infarctions involve the left ventricle. Obstruction of the left coronary artery may result in anterior, lateral, or septal infarcts. Right coronary artery occlusions usually result in infarctions of the inferior wall, posterior wall, or the right ventricle. The actual infarction is often classified as either transmural or subendocardial. In a **transmural infarction**, the entire thickness of the myocardium is destroyed. This lesion is associated with Q-wave changes on the ECG and is occasionally called a pathological Q-wave infarction. **A subendocardial infarction** involves only the subendocardial layer. Because ECG Q-wave changes usually do not accompany this type of infarction, it is often called a *non-Q wave infarction*.

* **transmural infarction** myocardial infarction that affects the full thickness of the myocardium and almost always results in a pathological Q wave in the affected leads.

* **subendocardial infarction** myocardial infarction that affects only the deeper levels of the myocardium; also called non-Q-wave infarction because it typically does not result in a significant Q wave in the affected lead.

Myocardial infarction causes varying degrees of tissue damage. First, following occlusion of the coronary artery, the affected tissue develops ischemia. If the blockage is not relieved and collateral circulation is inadequate, the tissue will infarct and die. In trauma, the usual cause of occlusion is plaque that has broken loose. The infarcted tissue becomes necrotic and eventually forms scar tissue. A ring of ischemic tissue that surrounds the area of infarcted myocardium survives primarily because of collateral circulation. This ischemic area is the site of many dysrhythmias' origins. Cardiogenic shock can develop, typically appearing first as ischemia on the 12-lead ECG (S-T depression or T-wave inversion), followed by injury (S-T elevation), and finally infarction (sometimes a pathological Q wave).

Area of infarct

FIGURE 28-57   Myocardial infarction.

Dysrhythmias are the most common complications of myocardial infarction. They are also the most common direct cause of death resulting from myocardial infarction. Life-threatening dysrhythmias can occur almost immediately and can result in sudden death or death within one hour after the onset of symptoms. Ventricular fibrillation or ventricular tachycardia may present early with myocardial infarction.

In addition to dysrhythmias, the destruction of a portion of the myocardial muscle mass can cause congestive heart failure. Such patients may have right heart failure, left heart failure, or both. *Heart failure* exists if the heart's pumping ability is impaired but the heart can still meet the demands of the body. That is, the heart is inefficient but adequate. If the heart cannot meet the body's oxygen demands, *inadequate tissue perfusion* results in cardiogenic shock. In cardiogenic shock, the heart is both inefficient and inadequate. Another cause of death from MI is *ventricular aneurysm* of the myocardial wall. The damaged portion of the wall weakens and in some cases bursts, resulting in sudden death. *Pump failure* resulting from extensive myocardial damage can also result in death.

The primary strategies in managing a myocardial infarction are pain relief and reperfusion. For reperfusion to be effective, rapid and safe transport is paramount. Maximum efficiency on scene and in transit is the most important care you can provide for the patient suffering an MI.

> *Anticipate life-threatening dysrhythmias while caring for any patient you suspect to be having a myocardial infarction.*
>

Field Assessment

The patient's breathing may or may not be labored. Look for evidence of shock. Check for regularity of the peripheral pulses, which should be equal in the patient experiencing cardiac ischemia. Take the blood pressure; it usually elevates during the episode and normalizes afterwards.

The chief complaint in MI is chest pain. Use the OPQRST mnemonic to determine specifics about the chest pain. Typically, the onset of the chest pain is acute, severe, constant, and unrelenting. Unlike the angina patient, the MI patient's discomfort usually lasts longer than 30 minutes. The pain can radiate to the arms (primarily left), the neck, posterior to the back, or down to the epigastric region of the abdomen. Have the patient rate his pain on a scale of one to ten. Patients with true myocardial ischemia can have severe pain and may rate their chest pain with high numbers such as eight, nine, ten, or above ten. Often they will confirm an acute onset of nausea and vomiting. Neither nitroglycerin nor rest offers much pain relief.

Atypically, a patient may have mild symptoms or minimize his symptoms during your assessment. This is more common in diabetics. The patient can be vague when describing chest pain and may complain of generally not feeling well. You might easily mistake this for angina. This patient generally does not complain of vomiting and may or may not have nausea. He also will rate his pain low on a scale of ten. His vague, general descriptions may arise from many pathological causes. One is that myocardial infarctions generally evolve over 48–72 hours. If the patient is more than 24 hours into the infarction, the pain can be different than it was 12–24 hours after onset.

The patient experiencing chest pains tends to be very frightened, although this is not always the case. "A feeling of impending doom" describes the patient's fright and pain. This pain is so severe and intense that the patient fears death, especially if he is experiencing chest pain for the first time. Ask if this is the patient's first recognized episode of chest pain or a recurring event. A patient who has suffered infarction before or who has chronic angina may be less concerned with his current pain. If it is recurring, are the episodes increasing in frequency or duration? These patients often have angina-like pain with increasing frequency and/or duration. Denial is common among both the patient with a significant cardiac history and the first-time chest-pain sufferer.

After establishing the patient's airway, auscultate lung sounds. They may present clear or with congestion in the bases. The patient suffering a myocardial infarction usually presents with pallor and diaphoresis. Temperature may vary from the norm. Cold skin or extremities indicate shock. Check the heart rate and rhythm, which may be irregular, and check the peripheral pulses for equality, which MI usually does not affect. The patient's blood pressure may be elevated, normal, or lower than normal.

Apply the ECG. First examine the underlying rhythm and potential dysrhythmias. If you are using a 12-lead monitor, examine the S-T segment and Q waves. Check the S-T segment for height, depth, and overall contour. Note changes such as S-T depression, which suggests ischemia or reciprocal changes, or elevation, which suggests injury. A *pathological Q wave*—deeper than 5 mm or wider than 0.04 seconds—can indicate infarcted tissue (necrosis) or extensive transient ischemia.

Cardiac dysrhythmias are the greatest threat to the patient before he arrives at the emergency department. Of the many potential dysrhythmias, the most serious are asystole (confirmed in two leads), pulseless electrical activity (PEA), ventricular fibrillation, and ventricular tachycardia. Other dysrhythmias include narrow or wide-complex tachycardia, heart block, sinus bradycardia, and sinus tachycardia with or without ectopy. Remember, life-threatening dysrhythmias are the leading cause of death among myocardial infarction patients. Anticipate such dysrhythmias while caring for any patient you suspect to be having a myocardial infarction.

After reviewing the patient's ECG tracing, determine if he is a likely candidate for rapid transport and reperfusion. Reperfusion uses thrombolytics such as streptokinase or tPA (Activase) to stop further injury. Used properly, thrombolytics can reperfuse all ischemic tissue and much of the injured myocardial tissue, thus reducing the total damage of a myocardial infarction. They work by destroying blood clots—all clots—which, when lodged in arteries congested with plaque, are the most common cause of acute myocardial infarction. The window of time in which a thrombolytic can be given and be effective is generally considered to be six hours from the onset of symptoms. Occasionally the window will be expanded for a particularly young patient or one who is suffering serious complications. The complications associated with giving thrombolytics include hemorrhage (which can be fatal), allergic reactions, and reperfusion dysrhythmias. Unfortunately, not all myocardial infarctions are caused by blood clots. In addition, many patients have conditions that preclude them from receiving thrombolytics. These include bleeding or clotting disorders, possible blood in the stool, uncontrolled hypertension, recent trauma, recent hemorrhagic stroke, or recent surgery.

Signs of acute injury or pathological Q waves indicate rapid transport for reperfusion, if symptoms began within six hours. Ascertain as near as possible the exact time when the symptoms started, the locations of the ischemia and of the infarction if evidenced on the 12-lead, and any S-T segment changes occurring on the 12-lead. This will help the physician determine quickly if the patient is a candidate for reperfusion. If you are not certain the patient meets local criteria for thrombolytic therapy, assume he does.

After analyzing the patient's rhythm, prepare him for transport. Since reperfusion is the ultimate goal, time is of the utmost importance. Expediently treat any signs of acute ischemia, injury, or infarction. Carefully weigh treating the patient's pain while on scene against rapid transport. Whenever practical treat the patient suffering from a myocardial infarction in transit.

Many EMS systems have a checklist similar to those that emergency departments use to determine if a patient qualifies for thrombolytic therapy. While these checklists vary from area to area, their use has reduced the waiting time for patients who meet the clinical criteria for thrombolytic therapy. Standard information that should be relayed to the emergency department physician or staff includes the time of the pain's onset, S-T segment elevation, and the location of ischemia and infarction on a 12-lead.

If you are not certain the patient meets local criteria for thrombolytic therapy, assume he does.

Whenever practical treat the patient suffering from a myocardial infarction in transit.

Management

Prehospital Management of MI Treatment of the myocardial infarction patient is summarized in Figure 28-58. Keep in mind that the patient experiencing myocardial infarction is often apprehensive. Place him at rest in a position of physical and emotional comfort to decrease myocardial oxygen demand. Administer oxygen, generally at a high-flow rate, to increase oxygen delivery to the myocardium. Establish at least one IV, taking great care not to miss the vein or to have multiple misses, which could jeopardize a patient's chance of receiving thrombolytics.

Administer medications according to written protocols or upon order of medical direction. Remember, always ask the patient if he or she is allergic to any medication before giving any drug. Medications that might be indicated for the patient suspected of myocardial infarction include:

- Aspirin
- Morphine sulfate
- Promethazine (Phenergan)
- Nitroglycerin
- Nitrous oxide (Nitronox)
- Nalbuphine (Nubain)
- Atropine sulfate
- Lidocaine
- Procainamide
- Vasopressin
- Adenosine

ACUTE CORONARY SYNDROME

American Heart Association®
Fighting Heart Disease and Stroke

Assess the initial ECG

The 12-lead ECG is central to triage of ACS in the Emergency Department. Classify patients as being in 1 of 3 syndromes within 10 minutes of arrival.

ST-segment elevation or new LBBB

ST-segment depression/ dynamic T-wave inversion: *strongly suspicious for ischemia*

Nondiagnostic or normal ECG

- ST elevation ≥1 mm in 2 or more contiguous leads
- New or presumably new LBBB (BBB obscuring ST-segment analysis)

- ST depression >1 mm
- Marked symmetrical T-wave inversion in multiple precordial leads
- Dynamic ST-T changes with pain

- ST depression 0.5 to 1.0 mm
- T-wave inversion or flattening in leads with dominant R waves
- Normal ECG

- >90% of patients with ischemic-type chest pain and ST-segment elevation will develop new Q waves or positive serum markers for AMI.
- Patients with hyperacute T waves benefit when AMI diagnosis is certain. Repeat ECG may be helpful.
- Patients with ST depression in early precordial leads who have posterior MI benefit when AMI diagnosis is certain.

High-risk subgroup with increased mortality:
- Persistent symptoms, recurrent ischemia
- Diffuse or widespread ECG abnormalities
- Depressed LV function
- Congestive heart failure
- Serum marker release: positive troponin or CK-MB+

Heterogeneous group: rapid assessment needed by
- Serial ECGs
- ST-segment monitoring
- Serum cardiac markers
Further risk assessment helpful
- Perfusion radionuclide imaging
- Stress echocardiography

- **Reperfusion therapy**
- **Aspirin**
- **Heparin**
  (if using fibrin-specific lytics)
- **β-Blockers**
- **Nitrates** as indicated

- **Antithrombin therapy** with **heparin**
- **Antiplatelet therapy** with **aspirin**
- **Glycoprotein IIb/IIIa inhibitors**
- **β-Blockers**
- **Nitrates**

- **Aspirin**
- Other therapy as appropriate
- Patients with positive serum markers, ECG changes, or functional study: manage as high risk

FIGURE 28–58   Management of acute coronary syndrome. Reproduced with permission from *Guidelines 2000 for Cardiopulmonary Resuscitation and Emergency Cardiovascular Care,* ©2000, Copyright American Heart Association.

Monitor the ECG constantly. Life-threatening dysrhythmias are possible. The patient may need rapid defibrillation or synchronized cardioversion at any moment. Plan to quickly provide defibrillation, cardioconversion, or transcutaneous pacing if needed.

Transport the patient you suspect of a myocardial infarction without delay. Since most myocardial infarction patients are very apprehensive and frightened, you should transport the normotensive patient without lights and sirens. Rapid transport is indicated if the S-T segment has any changes such as depression or elevation or if pathological Q waves present on the 12-lead. If a patient exhibits S-T or Q wave anomalies, has had signs and symptoms less than three hours, or has no relief from medications, consider him a candidate for thrombolytic reperfusion. Hypotension indicates immediate transport, especially if the patient has taken nitroglycerin, because the potential hypoperfusion of myocardial tissue can compound the problem. Other factors that indicate rapid transport are any rhythm abnormalities and the presentation within six hours of the pain's onset.

If the patient is in the early stages of a myocardial infarction, the outcome of refusing transport is likely to be devastating, ranging from extensive, unnecessary myocardial damage to death. Avoid refusal at all cost, using every means at your disposal to convince the patient to be transported. If the patient still refuses, document the fact that the patient was repeatedly warned of the possible outcome and was also aware of the potential for severely decreased lifestyle or death. Have the patient sign to the fact that he understands the implications, and if at all possible, have a witness sign as well.

Explain to the patient and his family the reason and necessity for rapid transport, if indicated, and inform them of your treatment, time permitting. Upon arrival at the emergency department, inform the physician of your findings—past history, vital signs, labored breathing, relief of pain, no relief of pain, and ECG readings, especially S-T segment results.

In-Hospital Management of MI Your understanding of the management of the MI patient after you have delivered him to the emergency department is important. This is especially true if you belong to an EMS system whose paramedics also regularly staff emergency departments.

With the advent of thrombolytic therapy, many hospitals have opened specially designed chest-pain units. These facilities specialize in diagnosing and observing patients with chest pain. In addition to 12-lead ECGs, obtaining cardiac enzyme levels in chest pain patients is routine. Because dead or dying myocardial cells release cardiac enzymes, elevated levels of these enzymes indicate myocardial infarction. The enzyme levels do not increase, however, until the infarction is several hours old, so intervention ideally should occur before the enzymes have a chance to rise. Commonly assayed cardiac enzymes are lactate dehydrogenase (LDH) and creatine phosphokinase (CK). Several newer markers show promise in aiding earlier identification of myocardial injury. These include troponin (I, T, and C), myoglobin, and CK-MB (a type of CK specific for cardiac muscle).

In many chest pain patients, the diagnosis will be readily evident. In many others, however, it will remain unclear. These patients are commonly stratified according to risk. Patients with a low likelihood of cardiac ischemia may be discharged with instructions for follow-up care, which may include diagnostic tools such as stress tests. Patients with a higher likelihood of having myocardial ischemia are usually admitted to the hospital and are typically observed for 24 hours. During the patient's hospitalization, his cardiac enzyme levels are obtained several times, as is his ECG. If the tests all remain negative, the patient will usually see a cardiologist and have a stress test before going home. If the stress test is negative, the cardiologist will work up the problem as an outpatient. If the stress test is positive, additional testing is done prior to discharge. This testing includes nuclear medicine cardiac imaging (Cardiolyte) and, possibly, coronary angiography. Usually, cardiology immediately sees patients who have a high likelihood of cardiac ischemia but nondiagnostic ECGs and enzymes. These patients ordinarily are not observed but are taken directly to the cardiac lab for an angiogram.

Several treatment options are available. Patients with isolated coronary artery lesions may be candidates for percutaneous transluminal coronary angioplasty (PTCA). In these patients, lesions are identified during coronary angiography. A

The trend in emergency cardiac care is rapid cardiac catheterization and therapeutic intervention such as PTCA.

balloon catheter is then inserted into the coronary artery with the lesion. At the level of the lesion, the balloon is inflated, thus increasing the artery's diameter and reducing the relative size of the blockage. Often, the patient will have several lesions. If the arteries do not stay open following angioplasty, another alternative is to place a *stent* in the artery at the site of the lesion. The stent is a hollow tube that keeps the artery open. Patients with severe and diffuse coronary artery disease may not be candidates for angioplasty. The best option for these patients is surgical revascularization of their coronary arteries. The most common operation is the coronary artery bypass graft (CABG), in which grafts are sewn from the aorta to the coronary arteries, thus effectively bypassing the blockage. In younger patients, the surgeon may use the internal mammary artery as the source. Recently, technology has evolved to the point where some bypass grafts can be performed endoscopically. These require only small "keyhole" incisions instead of the classic sternotomy, thus markedly decreasing the pain and the recovery time. Patients whose disease is either too mild or too severe may not be candidates for surgery. These patients are managed with medication alone.

HEART FAILURE

Heart failure is a clinical syndrome in which the heart's mechanical performance is compromised so that cardiac output cannot meet the body's needs. Heart failure is generally divided into left ventricle or right ventricle failure. Its many etiologies include valvular, coronary, or myocardial disease. Dysrhythmias can also cause or aggravate heart failure. Many other factors can contribute to heart failure, such as excess fluid or salt intake, fever (sepsis), hypertension, pulmonary embolism, or excessive alcohol or drug use. It can manifest with exertion in the patient who has an underlying disease or as a progression of the underlying disease.

Left Ventricular Failure Left ventricular failure occurs when the left ventricle fails as an effective forward pump, causing back pressure of blood into the pulmonary circulation, which often results in pulmonary edema. Its causes include various types of heart disease such as MI, valvular disease, chronic hypertension, and dysrhythmias. In left ventricular failure, the left ventricle cannot eject all of the blood that the right heart delivers to it via the lungs. Left atrial pressure rises and is subsequently transmitted to the pulmonary veins and capillaries. When pulmonary capillary pressure becomes too high, it forces the blood plasma into the alveoli, resulting in pulmonary edema. Progressive fluid accumulation in the alveoli decreases the lungs' oxygenation capacity and can cause death from hypoxia. Since MI is a common cause of left ventricular failure, you should consider that all patients with pulmonary edema may have had an MI.

Right Ventricular Failure In right ventricular failure, the right ventricle fails as an effective forward pump, resulting in back pressure of blood into the systemic venous circulation and venous congestion. The most common cause of right ventricular failure is left ventricular failure. This is because myocardial infarction is more common in the left ventricle than in the right and because chronic hypertension affects the left ventricle more adversely than the right. Right ventricular failure's other causes include systemic hypertension, which can affect both sides of the heart and can cause pure right ventricular failure. Pulmonary hypertension and *cor pulmonale* (heart failure due to pulmonary disease) result from the effects of chronic obstructive pulmonary disease (COPD). These problems are related to increased pressure in the pulmonary arteries, which results in right ventricular enlargement, right atrial enlargement, and if untreated, right heart failure.

Pulmonary embolism (PE), a blood clot in one of the pulmonary arteries, also can cause right heart failure. If the clot is large enough to occlude a major vessel, the pressure against which the right ventricle must pump increases. This can

* **heart failure** clinical syndrome in which the heart's mechanical performance is compromised so that cardiac output cannot meet the body's needs.

* **pulmonary embolism (PE)** blood clot in one of the pulmonary arteries.

throw the right ventricle into failure in much the same manner as pulmonary hypertension. In fact, it can be considered an acute form of pulmonary hypertension. Infarct of the right atrium or ventricle, although rare, is another cause of right ventricular failure.

Starling's law of the heart enables heart failure patients to compensate, at least for a time. Starling's law states that the more the myocardial muscle is stretched, the greater will be its force of contraction. Thus, the greater the preload (the volume of blood filling the chamber), the farther the myocardial muscle stretches and the more forceful the cardiac contraction. This has its limits, however. If myocardial muscle is stretched too far, it will not contract properly and the contraction will be weaker. Afterload (the resistance against which the ventricle must contract) also affects stroke volume. An increase in peripheral vascular resistance will decrease stroke volume. The reverse is also true: stroke volume will increase as peripheral vascular resistance decreases.

Congestive Heart Failure In **congestive heart failure (CHF)**, the heart's reduced stroke volume causes an overload of fluid in the body's other tissues. This presents as edema, which can be pulmonary, peripheral, sacral, or ascites (peritoneal edema). Congestive heart failure can manifest in an acute setting as pulmonary edema, pulmonary hypertension, or myocardial infarction. In the chronic setting, it can manifest as cardiomegaly (enlargement of the heart), left ventricular failure, or right ventricular failure. Heart failure can present in a first-time event, as in myocardial infarction, or in multiple events, as in left heart failure. CHF is one of the few diseases still on the rise in America. Approximately 400,000 new cases are diagnosed each year. CHF also is the most common cause of hospitalization in patients over age 65, accounting for approximately 900,000 admissions each year. Mortality is only 5 years in 50 percent of CHF patients. The end stage of this disease involves pulmonary edema and respiratory failure, followed by death. When the CHF patient calls EMS, one thing is clear; Starling's law is no longer allowing the patient to compensate.

Field Assessment

As in all cardiac emergencies, begin your assessment by checking the ABCs and managing any life threats. Often, patients with pulmonary edema will cough up large quantities of clear or pink tinged sputum. Patients with profound pulmonary edema generally have labored breathing, although this may not present until the patient begins to exert himself simply by standing or walking a few steps. Look for any changes or differences in skin color on the patient's arms, face, chest, and back. In profound CHF, mottling is often present.

Focus on the patient's chief complaint. Use the OPQRST mnemonic to elicit the patient's description of symptoms. Patients with pulmonary edema will complain of progressive or acute shortness of breath and will confirm being awakened by shortness of breath (**paroxysmal nocturnal dyspnea, or PND**). If the patient's episodes of PND are becoming more frequent, the disease process usually is worsening.

Often the heart failure patient will confirm progressive accumulation of edema or weight gain over a short time. Because many heart failure patients have an underlying cardiac or prior MI history, they may complain of mild chest pain or generalized weakness. This may be due to a weakened myocardial muscle mass, myocardial ischemia, or current MI.

Determine the patient's current medications. CHF patients are generally prescribed a loop diuretic such as Lasix or Bumex and/or hypertension medication. Many are prescribed digoxin (Lanoxin), which increases the heart's contractile force; many are oxygen dependent and may be on home oxygen. Find out if the patient has been compliant in taking medications; if not, determine how long he has been off medications. Also record and report any over-the-counter medications or herbal medications that the patient is taking, as well as any prescription medications borrowed from someone else.

Unconsciousness or an altered level of consciousness indicates pending respiratory failure. If the patient shows any sign of respiratory failure, immediately assist his breathing with 100 percent oxygen by BVM and prepare to intubate if clinically warranted.

Next assess the patient's breathing. Often, labored breathing, dyspnea, and productive cough appear. Labored breathing is the most common symptom of CHF, and it generally worsens with activity. CHF patients frequently assume the tripod position, sitting upright with both arms supporting the upper body, and confirm PND and pillow orthopnea, the inability to recline in bed without a pillow). Ask the patient how many pillows he sleeps on at night. As a rule, the more pillows, the worse the problem.

Check the skin. CHF patients present with changes in the skin color, such as pallor, diaphoresis, mottling, or signs of cyanosis. Check the peripheral pulses for quality and rhythm. Also check for edema. Edema is usually found in the lower extremities, localized from the ankles to the mid-calf or the knees. Sometimes the edema will be so severe that it obliterates the distal pulses. Check the edematous area for pitting and record its severity on a scale from 0 to 4+. Edema may also be present in the sacral area of the back, especially in the bed-confined, or in the upper quadrants of abdominal cavity. Ascites (abdominal cavity edema or swelling) is very difficult to assess accurately without X-ray or ultrasound. Blood pressure may be elevated in the CHF patient, due to the body's attempt to compensate for decreased cardiac output, but this can change quickly. A decompensating patient can have a normal blood pressure that drops quickly.

The most serious complication of heart failure is pulmonary edema. Untreated pulmonary edema can quickly lead to respiratory failure. This is because the abundant serum fluid in a large portion of the alveoli inhibits oxygen exchange in the lungs and hypoxia ensues. Respiratory failure will quickly lead to death. Patients with severe pulmonary edema present with tachypnea and adventitious lung sounds. Pulmonary edema can present as crackles (rales) at both bases. Rhonchi, which indicates fluid in the larger airways of the lungs, is a sign of severe pulmonary edema. Wheezes in the CHF patient are a sign of the lungs' protective mechanisms, since bronchioles constrict in an attempt to keep additional fluid from entering the lungs. This wheezing in pulmonary edema and congestive heart failure is often called cardiac asthma. This term is confusing, however, and you should avoid using it. Consider wheezes in a geriatric patient to be pulmonary edema until proven otherwise.

Other complications of pulmonary edema are pulsus paradoxus and pulsus alternans. *Pulsus paradoxus* occurs when systolic blood pressure drops more than 10 mmHg with inspiration. This is due to compression of the great vessels or the ventricles. In *pulsus alternans,* the pulse alternates between weak and strong. Pulses may be thready or weak, and jugular vein distention (JVD) might be present. The apical pulse may be abnormal or difficult to auscultate because of abnormalities such as bulges in the heart, a displaced apex, or severe pulmonary edema. The patient may produce frothy sputum with coughing, and cyanosis may present in the late stages of CHF.

Management

In severe CHF with pulmonary edema, obtain pertinent medical history and complete the physical exam while initiating treatment. Reassess all life-threatening conditions and treat them accordingly. Do not have the patient exert himself in any way, including standing up or walking. Do not have the patient lie flat at

Labored breathing is the most common symptom of CHF.

any time. Seat him with his feet dangling. This will promote venous pooling, thus decreasing preload.

Administer high-flow oxygen. If necessary, provide positive-pressure assistance with either a demand valve if the patient can assist or a bag-valve-mask unit if he is unresponsive. When possible, establish an IV at a TKO rate. Consider placing a heparin lock or saline lock. Limiting fluids is imperative; use a minidrip set to avoid accidentally infusing excessive amounts of fluid.

Place ECG electrodes. If the patient is extremely diaphoretic, apply tincture of Benzoin first. Record a baseline ECG and keep the monitor in place throughout care.

Administer medications according to written protocols or on the order of the medical director. Some left ventricular failures result from very rapid dysrhythmias. If you suspect a dysrhythmia as a cause, treat it according to established protocols. Before giving the patient any drug, ask him or his family if he is allergic to any medication. Medications frequently used in left ventricular failure and pulmonary edema include:

- Morphine sulfate
- Nitroglycerin
- Furosemide (Lasix)
- Dopamine (Intropin)
- Dobutamine (Dobutrex)
- Promethazine (Phenergan)
- Nitrous oxide (Nitronox)

Transport the heart-failure patient as a nonemergency unless clinical conditions indicate otherwise. Conditions that indicate emergency transport include hypertension or hypotension, severe respiratory distress or pending respiratory failure, or life-threatening dysrhythmias. Remember that transporting with lights and sirens can increase the conscious patient's anxiety and worsen his condition. If nonemergency transport might compromise the patient's condition, use lights and siren. Place the patient in a position of comfort, but not lying flat.

If the patient refuses transport and is indeed in the early stages of CHF, the outcome is likely to be devastating, leading to worsening signs and symptoms, unnecessary myocardial damage, severe pulmonary edema, and even death. Avoid refusal at all costs, and use every means at your disposal to convince the patient to be transported. If he still refuses, document the fact that you repeatedly warned the patient of the possible outcome.

CARDIAC TAMPONADE

In **cardiac tamponade,** excess fluid accumulates inside the pericardium. (The normal amount of fluid between the visceral pericardium and the parietal pericardium is approximately 25 cc.) This excess fluid causes an increase in intrapericardial pressure that impairs diastolic filling and drastically decreases the amount of blood the ventricles can expel with each contraction. Chest pain or dyspnea is the chief complaint; depending on the underlying cause, the chest pain may be dull or sharp and severe.

Cardiac tamponade's onset may be gradual, as in pericarditis or as in a neoplasm such as benign or malignant cancer. Or it may be acute, as in MI or trauma. All forms of cardiac tamponade involve pericardial effusion of air, pus, serum, blood, or any combination of these four. Gradual onset usually results from an underlying condition, and overlooking or misdiagnosing the tamponade is easy. Renal

✳ cardiac tamponade accumulation of excess fluid inside the pericardium.

disease and hypothyroidism can cause cardiac tamponade, though such instances are rare. Traumatic causes can include CPR and penetrating or nonpenetrating injuries. Whether onset is gradual or acute, cardiac tamponade can lead to death.

Field Assessment

Perform your initial assessment, including the patient's airway, breathing, and circulation. If you suspect cardiac tamponade, limit your history taking to determining the precipitating cause(s). Determine if the cause might be acute trauma such as penetrating or blunt trauma. Has the patient sustained recent trauma, including recent CPR? If you suspect a gradual onset, determine if the patient has recently had an infection or MI. Is he currently having an MI? Does he have a history of renal disease or hypothyroidism? Has he been ill? Use the OPQRST mnemonic to obtain information about the patient's symptoms.

The patient generally will present with dyspnea and orthopnea. Anterior and posterior lung sounds are usually clear. Typically, the pulse is rapid and weak. In the early stages venous pressures are often elevated, as evidenced by jugular vein distention. Blood pressure readings show a decrease in systolic pressure, pulsus paradoxus, and narrowing pulse pressures. Heart sounds are normal early on but then become muffled or faint.

Do not use the ECG, whether monitor quality or 12-lead, to diagnose cardiac tamponade; rather consider it a tool to support your clinical suspicions. The ECG is generally inconclusive, but ectopy is usually a late sign of cardiac tamponade. This is because an effusion easily irritates the heart's epicardial tissue. QRS and T-wave voltages are low, and non-specific T-wave changes occur. S-T segments may elevate. Electrical alternans (weak voltage, then normal) may appear in the P, QRS, T, and S-T segments.

Management

While obtaining any pertinent medical history and completing the physical exam, initiate treatment. Management of cardiac tamponade is primarily supportive, except when you detect shock or low perfusion. Maintain a patent airway and deliver high flow oxygen. If clinically indicated, secure the patient's airway with endotracheal intubation and maintain the patient's circulation with IV support, pharmacological agents, or CPR. Before administering any medication, ask the patient or family if he is allergic to any medications. Medications used in the treatment of cardiac tamponade include:

- Morphine sulfate
- Nitrous oxide (Nitronox)
- Furosemide (Lasix)
- Dopamine (Intropin)
- Dobutamine (Dobutrex)

Rapid transport is indicated for patients with cardiac tamponade. Remember to be supportive of the patient and family throughout your care. Upon arrival at the emergency department, inform the physician of your findings—past history, medications, vital signs, labored breathing, ECG readings, pulsus paradoxus, and shock. The therapy of choice is invasive *pericardiocentesis*, which involves aspirating fluid from the pericardium with a cardiac needle. Unless you have adequate training and local protocol permits you to do so, a physician should perform this procedure.

Always consider the possibility of pericardial tamponade in a patient who received CPR, then later deteriorated.

HYPERTENSIVE EMERGENCIES

A **hypertensive emergency** is a life-threatening elevation of blood pressure. It occurs in one percent or less of patients with hypertension, usually when the hypertension is poorly controlled or untreated. A hypertensive emergency is characterized by a rapid increase in diastolic blood pressure (usually >130 mmHg) accompanied by restlessness, confusion, blurred vision, nausea, and vomiting. It often occurs with **hypertensive encephalopathy,** a condition of acute or subacute consequence of severe hypertension characterized by severe headache, vomiting, visual disturbances (including transient blindness), paralysis, seizures, stupor, and coma. On occasion, this condition may cause left ventricular failure, pulmonary edema, or stroke.

A prior history of hypertension is the precipitating cause of most hypertensive emergencies. In many cases, the patient has not complied with his hypertensive medication or other prescribed drugs. Another cause of hypertensive crisis, toxemia of pregnancy (preeclampsia), can appear at any time between the twentieth week of pregnancy and term delivery. It occurs in five percent of pregnancies and is defined as a blood pressure of at least 140/90 mmHg. Hypertension is a sign of the toxemia, not the cause. Preeclampsia poses a high risk of abruptio placentae and generally progresses to eclampsia (coma and seizures). Left untreated, it progresses to eclampsia and death for the mother and unborn fetus.

Experts estimate that more than 50 million people in the United States are hypertensive patients. Its prevalence increases with age, and it has a higher incidence among blacks, as well as a higher mortality and morbidity. With modern medications, hypertensive encephalopathy has become rare, yet it is still seen in the prehospital setting. Ischemic and hemorrhagic stroke are more common results of severe hypertension. Both hypertensive encephalopathy and stroke (ischemic or hemorrhagic) can have devastating consequences or lead to death if left untreated.

Field Assessment

After making your initial assessment, including airway, breathing, and circulation, conduct your focused history and physical examination. Generally, hypertensive patients have a chief complaint of headache, accompanied by nausea and/or vomiting, blurred vision, shortness of breath, epistaxis (nosebleed), and vertigo (dizziness). However any one of these symptoms might be the patient's only complaint. The patient may be semiconscious or unconscious or seizing. In pregnancy toxemia, the expectant mother usually has edema of the hands or face. Photosensitivity and headache are common complaints.

Determine if the patient has a history of hypertension and if he has been taking medications as prescribed. Often he has been noncompliant, taking medicines only occasionally or not at all. In some situations the patient will borrow someone else's medications or take over-the-counter medications such as herbal medications. He may be on home oxygen.

If left ventricular failure accompanies the hypertension, the lung sounds generally present with pulmonary edema; otherwise they are clear. Often the pulse is strong and at times may be bounding. By definition, hypertension is a systolic pressure greater than 160 mmHg and a diastolic pressure greater than 90 mmHg. Consider signs or symptoms of hypertensive encephalopathy associated with hypertension to be a hypertensive emergency.

The hypertensive patient's level of consciousness may be normal or altered, or he may be unconscious. His skin may be pale, flushed, or normal, cool or warm, moist or dry. Look for edema, either pitting or nonpitting. The patient may confirm PND, orthopnea, vertigo, epistaxis, tinnitus (ringing of the ears), nausea or vomiting, or visual acuities. In addition, he may have seizures or motor/sensory deficits in parts of the body or on one side. ECG findings are generally inconclusive unless the patient has an underlying cardiac condition such as angina or MI.

* **hypertensive emergency** an acute elevation of blood pressure that requires the blood pressure to be lowered within one hour; characterized by end-organ changes such as hypertensive encephalopathy, renal failure, or blindness.

* **hypertensive encephalopathy** a cerebral disorder of hypertension indicated by severe headache, nausea, vomiting, and altered mental status. Neurological symptoms may include blindness, muscle twitches, inability to speak, weakness, and paralysis.

Management

Place the patient in a position of comfort, unless a potential exists for airway compromise, as in stroke. Provide airway and ventilatory support, if clinically indicated. Provide oxygen and base your transport considerations on the patient's clinical presentation. Attempt supportive IV therapy on-scene time or en route. Do not prolong on-scene time to establish an IV. Place pregnant patients on their left side and transport as smoothly and quietly as possible.

In recent years, calcium channel blockers such as nifedipine (Procardia) have been widely used to treat hypertensive emergencies. Now this practice is being questioned because evidence suggests that significantly reducing the patient's blood pressure may actually be harmful. Some systems still use loop diuretics such as Lasix or nitroglycerin to reduce the patient's blood pressure by manipulating preload and afterload. These treatments' effectiveness is also being scrutinized. Follow your local protocols. In severe cases, especially if hypertensive encephalopathy is present, medical direction may order one of the following medications:

* Morphine sulfate
* Furosemide (Lasix)
* Nitroglycerin
* Sodium Nitroprusside (Nipride)
* Labetalol (Trandate, Normodyne)

Explain to the patient and family the reason and necessity for rapid transport, if indicated. Advise the patient who refuses transport of the serious complications that are likely without further medical attention. Stroke, seizures, pulmonary edema, and kidney damage are but a few possible outcomes. Avoid refusal at all costs. As always, use every means at your disposal to convince the patient to be transported. Document refusals as usual.

Upon arrival at the emergency department, inform the physician of your findings—vital signs, history, labored breathing, pulmonary edema, hand or facial edema, and neurological deficits.

CARDIOGENIC SHOCK

Cardiogenic shock, the most severe form of pump failure, is shock that remains after existing dysrhythmias, hypovolemia, or altered vascular tone have been corrected. It occurs when left ventricular function is so compromised that the heart cannot meet the body's metabolic demands and the compensatory mechanisms are exhausted. This usually happens after extensive myocardial infarction, often involving more than 40 percent of the left ventricle, or with diffuse ischemia.

A variety of mechanisms can cause cardiogenic shock, and its onset may be acute or progressive. Among the more common mechanical causes are tension pneumothorax and cardiac tamponade. Both affect ventricular filling, or preload, and tend to manifest acutely. Interference with ventricular emptying, or afterload, as in pulmonary embolism and prosthetic valve malfunction, can also cause cardiogenic shock. Impairments in myocardial contractility, as seen in MI, myocarditis, and recreational drug use, can manifest either progressively or acutely. Trauma, too, can cause cardiogenic shock, secondary to hypovolemia or to significant underlying disease processes such as neurologic, gastroenterologic, renal, or metabolic disorders.

In cardiogenic shock, the body tries to compensate either by increasing the contractile force, by improving preload, by reducing the peripheral resistance, or by all three. In the early stages, a conscious patient presents with obvious signs of shock (cold extremities, weak pulses, and low blood pressure). As Starling's law loses

Elevated blood pressures should only be treated in the prehospital setting if these are associated with end-organ changes.

* **cardiogenic shock** the inability of the heart to meet the metabolic needs of the body, resulting in inadequate tissue perfusion.

Cardiogenic shock is the most severe form of pump failure.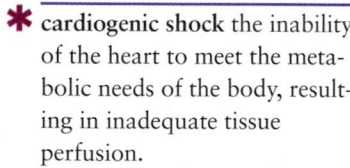

effect, the patient's mental status diminishes and his radial pulses are no longer palpable. Finally, when preload, afterload, and contractility fail to meet vital organ demands, unconsciousness occurs and, if left untreated, the patient will die.

Cardiogenic shock can occur at any age, but it is most often seen as an end-stage event in the geriatric patient, with significant underlying disease(s). Cardiogenic shock's mortality rate is high for geriatric patients following massive MI or septic shock. This is because end-organ damage is so severe or multiple end-organ damage reaches the point that life cannot be sustained.

Cardiogenic shock has a high mortality rate.

Field Assessment

After conducting your initial assessment, including airway, breathing, and circulation, perform your focused history and physical exam. The chief complaint may range from acute onset of chest pain to shortness of breath, altered mental status or unconsciousness, or general weakness; onset may be acute or progressive. Ask about the patient's past medical history and determine if he or she has had any recent trauma. Look for evidence of a hypovolemic cause such as a gastrointestinal bleed, septic shock, and traumatic or nontraumatic internal hemorrhage. Has the patient recently suffered a myocardial infarction? Cardiogenic shock is most often associated with large anterior infarction and/or loss of 40 percent or more of the left ventricle.

The patient's medication history may be important. Large amounts of different cardiac medications may indicate the patient has significant preexisting damage or a compromised but adequate cardiac output. Also, noncompliance with prescribed medications can further insult a preexisting weakened cardiac state, and the use of borrowed or over-the-counter medications can have unpredictable effects.

The altered mental status secondary to decreased cardiac output and unconsciousness common in cardiogenic shock may begin as restlessness and progress to confusion ending in coma. Airway findings include dyspnea, productive cough, or labored breathing. Paroxysmal nocturnal dyspnea, tripoding, adventitious lung sounds, and retractions on inspiration are also common findings. Typical ECG findings include tachycardia and atrial dysrhythmias such as atrial tachycardias. Ectopy is also common.

Myocardial infarction often precedes cardiogenic shock, and symptoms are initially the same as expected with MI; however, as cardiogenic shock develops and compensatory mechanisms fail, hypotension develops. The systolic blood pressure is often less than 80 mmHg. The usual heart rhythm is sinus tachycardia, a reflection of the cardiovascular system's attempts to compensate for the decreased stroke volume. If serious dysrhythmias are present, determining whether they are the cause of the hypotension or the result of the cardiogenic shock may be difficult; therefore, you must correct any major dysrhythmias.

The patient's skin is usually cool and clammy, reflecting peripheral vasoconstriction. Tachypnea is often present, since pulmonary edema is a common complication. Pitting or nonpitting peripheral edema may be present in the lower extremities or in the sacral area and may obliterate peripheral pulses.

Management

To manage the cardiogenic shock patient, place him in a position of comfort if he is hemodynamically stable. If any pulmonary edema is present, the patient may prefer sitting upright, with both legs hanging off the stretcher. Treatment of cardiogenic shock (Figure 28-59) consists mostly of treating the underlying problem (such as MI and CHF) or treating the patient supportively. Remember to

Clinical signs: *Shock, hypoperfusion, congestive heart failure, acute pulmonary edema*
Most likely problem?

Acute pulmonary edema

Volume problem

Pump problem

Rate problem

Bradycardia
See algorithm

Tachycardia
See algorithm

1st — Acute pulmonary edema
• *Furosemide* IV 0.5 to 1.0 mg/kg
• *Morphine* IV 2 to 4 mg
• *Nitroglycerin* SL
• *Oxygen*/intubation as needed

Administer
• *Fluids*
• *Blood transfusions*
• *Cause-specific interventions*
Consider vasopressors

Blood pressure?

Systolic BP
BP defines 2nd line of action
(See below)

Systolic BP
<70 mm Hg
Signs/symptoms
of shock

Systolic BP
70 to 100 mm Hg
Signs/symptoms
of shock

Systolic BP
70 to 100 mm Hg
No signs/symptoms of
shock

Systolic BP
>100 mm Hg

• *Norepinephrine*
0.5 to 30 µg/min IV

• *Dopamine*
5 to 15 µg/kg per
minute IV

• *Dobutamine*
2 to 20 µg/kg per
minute IV

• *Nitroglycerin*
10 to 20 µg/min IV
Consider
• *Nitroprusside* 0.1 to
5.0 µg/kg per minute IV

2nd — Acute pulmonary edema
• **Nitroglycerin/nitroprusside** if BP >100 mm Hg
• **Dopamine** if BP = 70 to 100 mm Hg, signs/symptoms of shock
• **Dobutamine** if BP >100 mm Hg, no signs/symptoms of shock

---

**Further diagnostic/therapeutic
considerations**
• Pulmonary artery catheter
• Intra-aortic balloon pump
• Angiography for AMI/ischemia
• Additional diagnostic studies

FIGURE 28–59   Management of pulmonary edema, hypotension, and shock. Reproduced with permission from *Guidelines 2000 for Cardiopulmonary Resuscitation and Emergency Cardiovascular Care,* ©2000, Copyright American Heart Association.

always treat the rate and rhythm first. Some medications that may be used to treat cardiogenic shock include:

Cardiogenic shock should be aggressively treated, with rapid transport to follow.

- Vasopressors
  - Dopamine (Intropin)
  - Dobutamine (Dobutrex)
  - Norepinephrine (Levophed)

Other useful medications may include:

- Morphine sulfate
- Promethazine (Phenergan)
- Nitroglycerin
- Nitrous oxide (Nitronox)
- Furosemide (Lasix)
- Digitalis, digoxin (Lanoxin)
- Sodium bicarbonate

If the patient refuses transport, follow the general guidelines; however, remember that untreated cardiogenic shock has a grim outcome. No matter how well compensated the patient may appear, true cardiogenic shock will decompensate quickly into irreversible shock. Use every means at your disposal to convince the patient to be transported. If the patient still refuses, document accordingly.

Upon arrival at the emergency department, inform the physician of your findings—vital signs, labored breathing, pulmonary edema, dysrhythmias, or severe shock that remains despite your treatment.

CARDIAC ARREST

Cardiac arrest and sudden death accounts for 60 percent of all deaths from coronary artery disease. **Cardiac arrest** is the absence of ventricular contraction that immediately results in systemic circulatory failure. **Sudden death** is any death that occurs within one hour of the symptoms' onset. At autopsy, actual infarction often is not present. Because severe atherosclerotic disease is common, authorities usually believe that a lethal dysrhythmia is the mechanism of death. The risk factors for sudden death are basically the same as those for atherosclerotic heart disease (ASHD) and coronary artery disease (CAD). In a large number of patients, cardiac arrest is the first manifestation of heart disease. Other causes of sudden death include:

* **cardiac arrest** the absence of ventricular contraction.

* **sudden death** death within one hour after the onset of symptoms.

- Drowning
- Acid-base imbalance
- Electrocution
- Drug intoxication
- Electrolyte imbalance
- Hypoxia
- Hypothermia
- Pulmonary embolism
- Stroke
- Hyperkalemia (high levels of potassium)
- Trauma
- End stage renal disease

Field Assessment

A cardiac arrest patient is unresponsive, apneic, and pulseless. Peripheral pulses are absent. After initiating CPR, place ECG leads. Dysrhythmias found in the cardiac arrest patient include ventricular fibrillation, ventricular tachycardia, asystole, or PEA. If you find asystole, you should confirm it in two or more leads.

Center questions on events prior to the arrest. Did bystanders or EMS personnel witness the arrest? Did bystanders start CPR? How much time passed from the discovery of the arrest until CPR was initiated? From discovery until EMS was activated? These questions all focus on **down time,** the duration from the beginning of the cardiac arrest until effective CPR is established. Often physicians want to know the **total down time,** which is the time from the beginning of the arrest until you deliver the patient to the emergency department. If possible, obtain the patient's past history and medications.

Management

To manage the cardiac arrest patient properly, you must understand the terms *resuscitation, return of spontaneous circulation,* and *survival.*

- **Resuscitation** is the provision of efforts to return a spontaneous pulse and breathing to the patient in cardiac arrest.
- **Return of spontaneous circulation** (ROSC) occurs when resuscitation results in the patient's having a spontaneous pulse. ROSC patients may or may not have a return of breathing, and may or may not survive.
- **Survival** means that the patient is resuscitated and survives to be discharged from the hospital. Many resuscitated patients reach ROSC, but not all resuscitated patients survive.

Begin management of airway, breathing, and circulation simultaneously. When resuscitation is indicated, start CPR immediately. Remember that basic life support is the mainstay of treatment for cardiac arrest. Ventilate the patient with a bag-valve mask and 100 percent oxygen. Intubate or insert an alternative airway as quickly as possible. If changes in the ECG indicate defibrillation or synchronized cardioversion, perform it in conjunction with CPR, stopping CPR only to apply the pads or paddles and to deliver the shock(s). Make sure no one touches the patient when you deliver any shock. If the patient has an internal pacemaker or defibrillator, treat the arrest normally, taking care not to defibrillate over the device.

After establishing CPR and advanced airway management, perform IV access. The site of venipuncture should be as close to the heart as possible—for example, the antecubital area (bend of the forearm and humerus) or the external jugular vein. Follow all intravenous medications with a 30–45 second flush. After each flush, set the IV at a to-keep-open (TKO) drip rate.

Pharmacological agents that might be used in a cardiac arrest setting are:

- Atropine sulfate
- Lidocaine
- Procainamide
- Vasopressin
- Epinephrine
- Norepinephrine
- Isoproterenol

---

* **down time** duration from the beginning of the cardiac arrest until effective CPR is established.

* **total down time** duration from the beginning of the arrest until the patient's delivery to the emergency department.

* **resuscitation** provision of efforts to return a spontaneous pulse and breathing.

* **return of spontaneous circulation** resuscitation results in the patient's having a spontaneous pulse.

* **survival** when a patient is resuscitated and survives to be discharged from the hospital.

Basic life support is the mainstay of prehospital cardiac care.

- Dopamine
- Dobutamine
- Sodium bicarbonate

Management of the successful postcardiac arrest patient generally presents an unusual situation. The patient's blood pressure can return at low, normal, or high readings because of the drugs used in resuscitation. In addition, the pulse can return at bradycardic, normal, or tachycardic rates. Ventricular ectopy is the most serious concern. If the patient presented in ventricular fibrillation or ventricular tachycardia during the arrest, or if ectopy presents in the postarrest, use an antidysrhythmic agent such as lidocaine. The blood pressure may return at low readings. The ideal range of the blood pressure is 80–100 mmHg in the postarrest patient. Do not be concerned if the postarrest patient does not show any signs of response. He has endured a very harsh environment, and recovery, if any, can be slow. The postarrest setting can be unnerving, with the patient's vitals and ECG changing every minute. Approach problems one at a time, and do not be fooled by a return in pulse that fades away while the monitor still has a rhythm (PEA).

Your management of all cardiac arrest patients should follow the American Heart Association guidelines for cardiopulmonary resuscitation and emergency cardiac care. Figure 28-60 summarizes the treatment for ventricular fibrillation or ventricular tachycardia (VF/VT), the cardiac arrest rhythms with the best prognosis for successful resuscitation. Also review the algorithms for asystole (Figure 28-44) and pulseless electrical activity (PEA) (Figure 28-46).

Once you have established advanced life support, move the patient to the MICU as quickly as possible, while taking great care to avoid disrupting IVs, endotracheal intubation, CPR, or pharmacological treatment. Transport the patient to the nearest appropriate facility as safely and as smoothly as possible using lights and siren. Offer emotional support to the patient throughout your care. Upon arrival at the emergency department, inform the physician of your findings, especially down time, total down time, changes in rhythm, or return of pulses.

Postarrest stabilization requires extreme vigilance.

Withholding and Terminating Resuscitation

In some situations, the certainty that the patient will not survive indicates not initiating resuscitation efforts. Rigor mortis, fixed dependent lividity (pooling of the blood), decapitation, decomposition, and incineration are all situations in which you should withhold resuscitation.

In addition, withhold resuscitation efforts if the patient has an out-of-hospital advanced directive. A physician must sign and date the advanced directive, and it must state conditions that apply to the patient at the time of the arrest. For example, the directive may state that resuscitation should be withheld if the patient has an end-stage terminal illness. Each state and many local regions treat advanced directives differently. Review local protocol and medical direction before you might have to decide whether to honor an advanced directive.

In other instances, poor prognosis and survivability of many cardiac arrest patients makes termination of resuscitation a consideration. Some of the *inclusion* criteria for termination of resuscitation are:

- 18 years old or older
- Arrest is presumed cardiac in origin and not associated with a treatable cause such as hypothermia, overdose, or hypovolemia
- Successful and maintained endotracheal intubation
- ACLS standards have been applied throughout the arrest

FIGURE 28–60 Management of ventricular fibrillation and pulseless ventricular tachycardia (VF/VT). Reproduced with permission from *Guidelines 2000 for Cardiopulmonary Resuscitation and Emergency Cardiovascular Care,* ©2000, Copyright American Heart Association.

- On-scene ALS efforts have been sustained for 25 minutes, or the patient remains in asystole through four rounds of ALS drugs
- Patient's rhythm is asystolic or agonal when the decision to terminate is made, and this rhythm persists until the resuscitation efforts are actually terminated
- Victims of blunt trauma who present in asystole or develop asystole on scene

Depending on local protocol, the *exclusion* criteria for termination of resuscitation may include:

- Under 18 years old
- Etiology that could benefit from in-hospital treatment (such as hypothermia)
- Persistent or recurring ventricular tachycardia or fibrillation
- Transient return of a pulse
- Signs of neurological viability
- Arrest witnessed by EMS personnel
- Family or responsible party opposed to termination

Criteria that should not be considered as either inclusionary or exclusionary:

- The patient's age if 18 or over (for example, geriatric)
- Down time before EMS arrival
- Presence of a nonofficial do-not-resuscitate (DNR) order
- Quality-of-life evaluations by EMS

Review local protocol and medical direction before attempting termination of resuscitation. Most systems use documented protocols and direct communication with an on-line medical director or physician to approve or deny termination of resuscitation. The medical director or physician may base his decision on the following information:

Review local protocol and medical direction before attempting termination of resuscitation.

- Medical condition of the patient
- Known etiological factors
- Therapy rendered
- Family's presence and appraisal of the situation
- Communication of any resistance or uncertainty on the part of the family
- Maintain continuous documentation, including the ECG

The family should receive grief support. This requires EMS personnel or a community agency to be in place soon after termination of resuscitation. EMS personnel deal not only with the living or viable but also with the families of lost loved ones, especially when they have witnessed the death. Many systems employ assigned personnel to support the family after termination of resuscitation. In other systems, paramedics on the scene provide support until a predetermined person from another local agency can arrive. Although this supportive role can be uncomfortable, it will be part of your job.

Law enforcement regulations require that all local, state, or federal laws pertaining to a death be followed. These, too, may vary from region to region, but their basic principles are the same. The officer discusses the death certificate with the attending physician. He will determine if the event or patient requires assignment to a medical examiner, if the nature of the death is suspicious in any way, or if the physician is at all hesitant to sign the death certificate. The officer also may be required to assign the patient to a medical examiner if he does not have a physician. Check with local law enforcement agencies to determine their protocol.

PERIPHERAL VASCULAR AND OTHER CARDIOVASCULAR EMERGENCIES

In addition to cardiac arrest, MI, and hypertension emergencies, other common cardiovascular emergencies involve the arterial and venous systems. Such disorders are generally classified as traumatic or nontraumatic. Nontraumatic vascular emergencies typically arise from preexisting conditions or from a disease process.

Atherosclerosis

* **atherosclerosis** a progressive, degenerative disease of the medium-sized and large arteries.

The major underlying factor in many cardiovascular emergencies is **atherosclerosis,** a progressive degenerative disease of the medium-sized and large arteries. Atherosclerosis affects the aorta and its branches, the coronary arteries, and the cerebral arteries, among others. It results from fats (lipids and cholesterol) deposited under the tunica intima (inner lining) of the involved vessels. The fat causes an injury response in the tunica intima, which subsequently damages the tunica media (middle layer) as well. Over time, calcium is deposited, causing plaques, where small hemorrhages can occur. These hemorrhages in turn lead to scarring, fibrosis, larger plaque build-up, and aneurysm. The involved arteries can become completely blocked, either by additional plaque, by a blood clot, or by an aneurysm that results from tearing in the arterial wall.

* **arteriosclerosis** a thickening, loss of elasticity, and hardening of the walls of the arteries from calcium deposits.

The results of atherosclerosis are evident in many disease processes. First, disruption of the vessel's intimal surface destroys the vessel's elasticity. This condition, **arteriosclerosis,** can cause hypertension and other related problems. Second, atherosclerosis can reduce blood flow through the affected vessel; common manifestations include angina pectoris and intermittent **claudication.** Frequently, thrombosis will develop, totally obstructing the vessel or the tissues it supplies. Myocardial infarction is a classic example of this process.

* **claudication** severe pain in the calf muscle due to inadequate blood supply. It typically occurs with exertion and subsides with rest.

Aneurysm

Aneurysm is a nonspecific term meaning dilation of a vessel. The types of aneurysm include:

* **aneurysm** the ballooning of an arterial wall, resulting from a defect or weakness in the wall.

- Atherosclerotic
- Dissecting
- Infectious
- Congenital
- Traumatic

Most aneurysms result from atherosclerosis and involve the aorta, because the blood pressure there is the highest of any vessel in the body. An aneurysm occurs when blood surges into the aortic wall through a tear in the aortic tunica intima. Infectious aneurysms are most commonly associated with syphilis and are rare. Congenital aneurysms can occur with several disease states such as Marfan's syndrome, a hereditary disease that affects the connective tissue. Aortic aneurysm occurs in people with this disease because it involves the connective tissue within the

Right kidney

Aorta

Aneurysm

Inferior
vena cava

FIGURE 28–61 Rupture of an abdominal aortic aneurysm.

vessel wall. Those affected may experience sudden death, usually from spontaneous rupture of the aorta, often at a fairly young age.

Abdominal Aortic Aneurysm Abdominal aortic aneurysm commonly results from atherosclerosis and occurs most frequently in the aorta, below the renal arteries and above the bifurcation of the common iliac arteries (Figure 28-61). It is ten times more common in men than in women and most prevalent between ages 60 and 70.

Signs and symptoms of an abdominal aneurysm include:

- Abdominal pain
- Back and flank pain
- Hypotension
- Urge to defecate, caused by the retroperitoneal leakage of blood

Dissecting Aortic Aneurysm Degenerative changes in the smooth muscle and elastic tissue of the aortic media cause most **dissecting aortic aneurysms.** This can result in hematoma and, subsequently, aneurysm. The original tear often results from **cystic medial necrosis,** a degenerative disease of connective tissue often associated with hypertension and to a certain extent, aging. Predisposing factors include hypertension, which is present in 75–85 percent of cases. It occurs more frequently in patients older than 40–50, although it can occur in younger individuals, especially pregnant women. A tendency for this disease also runs in families.

Of dissecting aortic aneurysms, 67 percent involve the ascending aorta. Once dissection has started, it can extend to all of the abdominal aorta as well as its branches, including the coronary arteries, aortic valve, subclavian arteries, and carotid arteries. The aneurysm can rupture at any time, usually into the pericardial or pleural cavity.

✳ **Dissecting aortic aneurysm** aneurysm caused when blood gets between and separates the layers of the aortic wall.

✳ **cystic medial necrosis** a death or degeneration of a part of the wall of an artery.

Acute Pulmonary Embolism

Acute pulmonary embolism occurs when a blood clot or other particle lodges in a pulmonary artery and blocks blood flow through that vessel. Pulmonary emboli may be composed of air, fat, amniotic fluid, or blood clots. Factors that predispose a patient to blood clots include prolonged immobilization, *thrombophlebitis* (inflammation and clots in a vein), use of certain medications, and atrial fibrillation.

✳ **acute pulmonary embolism** blockage that occurs when a blood clot or other particle lodges in a pulmonary artery.

When a pulmonary embolism blocks the blood flow through a vessel, the right heart must pump against increased resistance, which in turn increases pulmonary capillary pressure. The area of the lung supplied by the occluded vessel then stops functioning, and gas exchange decreases.

The signs and symptoms of pulmonary embolism depend upon the size of the obstruction. The patient suffering acute pulmonary embolism may report a sudden onset of severe and unexplained dyspnea that may or may not be associated with chest pain. He may have a recent history of immobilization from a hip fracture, surgery, or other debilitating illness.

Acute Arterial Occlusion

* **acute arterial occlusion** the sudden occlusion of arterial blood flow.

An **acute arterial occlusion** is the sudden occlusion of arterial blood flow due to trauma, thrombosis, tumor, embolus, or idiopathic means. Emboli are probably the most common cause. They can arise from within the chamber (*mural emboli*), from a thrombus in the left ventricle, from an atrial thrombus secondary to atrial fibrillation, or from a thrombus caused by abdominal aortic atherosclerosis. Arterial occlusions most commonly involve vessels in the abdomen or extremities.

Vasculitis

* **vasculitis** inflammation of blood vessels.

Vasculitis is an inflammation of blood vessels. Most vasculitis stems from a variety of rheumatic diseases and syndromes. The inflammatory process is usually segmental, and inflammation within the media of a muscular artery tends to destroy the internal elastic lamina. Necrosis and hypertrophy (enlarging) of the vessel occur, and the vessel wall has a high likelihood of breaching, leaking fibrin and red blood cells into the surrounding tissue. This potentially can lead to partial or total vascular occlusion and subsequent necrosis.

Noncritical Peripheral Vascular Conditions

Several peripheral vascular conditions are not immediately life threatening but often require prehospital care. They include peripheral arterial atherosclerotic disease, deep venous thrombosis, and varicose veins.

* **peripheral arterial atherosclerotic disease** a progressive degenerative disease of the medium-sized and large arteries.

Peripheral Arterial Atherosclerotic Disease Peripheral arterial atherosclerotic disease is a progressive degenerative disease of the medium-sized and large arteries. It affects the aorta and its branches, the brachial and femoral peripheral arteries, and the cerebral arteries. For reasons unknown it does not affect coronary arteries. It is a gradual, progressive disease, often associated with diabetes mellitus. In extreme cases, significant arterial insufficiency may lead to ulcers and gangrene. Occlusion of the peripheral arteries causes chronic and acute ischemia.

In the chronic setting, intermittent claudication (diminished blood flow in exercising muscle) produces pain with exertion. It occurs most commonly with the calf, but can affect any leg muscle. Rest initially relieves this pain. When the disease progresses, however, the pain presents even at rest. The extremity usually appears normal, but pulses will be reduced or absent. As the ischemia worsens, the extremity becomes painful, cold, and numb, and ulceration, gangrene, and necrosis may be present. There is no edema.

In the acute setting, arterial occlusion from an embolus, aneurysm, or thrombosis occurs. The patient experiences a sudden onset of pain, coldness, numbness, and pallor. Pulses are absent distal to the occlusion. Acute occlusion may cause severe ischemia with motor and sensory deficits. Edema is not present.

* **deep venous thrombosis** a blood clot in a vein.

Deep Venous Thrombosis Deep venous thrombosis is a blood clot in a vein. It most commonly occurs in the larger veins of the thigh and calf. Predisposing factors include a recent history of trauma, inactivity, pregnancy, or varicose veins.

The patient frequently complains of gradually increasing pain and calf tenderness. Often the leg and foot are swollen because of occluded venous drainage. Leg elevation may alleviate the signs and symptoms. In some cases, the patient may be asymptomatic. Gentle palpation of the calf and thigh may reveal tenderness and, on occasion, cord-like clotted veins. Dorsiflexion of the foot may cause Homan's sign, discomfort behind the knee. This is associated with deep venous thrombosis. The skin may be warm and red.

Varicose Veins Varicose veins are dilated superficial veins, usually in the lower extremities. Predisposing factors include pregnancy, obesity, and genetics. Signs and symptoms include the visible distention of the leg veins, lower leg swelling and discomfort (especially at the end of the day), and skin color and texture changes in the legs and ankles. If the condition is chronic, venous stasis ulcers, a noncritical condition, can develop. Venous stasis ulcers can rupture, but direct pressure usually can control the bleeding, which occasionally is significant.

* varicose veins dilated superficial veins, usually in the lower extremity.

General Assessment and Management of Vascular Disorders

Occlusion of any vessel can result in ischemia, injury, and necrosis of the affected tissue. Depending on the tissue or organ involved, untreated occlusion can cause severe disability or death. In pulmonary occlusion, hypotension and cardiac collapse can ensue quickly, and death can occur rapidly. In cerebral occlusion, debilitating seizures, paralysis, or death can occur. Mesenteric occlusion can cause necrosis, giving rise to sepsis. Or it can affect vital organs, causing a slow and agonizing death. Pulmonary embolus, aortic aneurysm, and some acute arterial occlusions can produce a hypoperfusion state, and death can be rapid.

Assessment Begin your assessment by checking airway, breathing, and circulation. Breathing is usually not affected, except in pulmonary embolus and a decompensated state of shock. In decompensated shock resulting from aneurysm, arterial occlusion, or pulmonary embolus, breathing may be labored. Circulation may be compromised or absent distal to the affected area. Check circulation for the Five Ps

- Pallor
- Pain
- Pulselessness
- Paralysis
- Paresthesia

Check the skin for pallor or mottling distal to the affected area. Skin temperature may appear normal systemically but cool or cold at the affected area, or it may be systemically cool and clammy, as occurs in decompensated shock.

Determine the patient's chief complaint. Depending on the type of vascular emergency, the patient may complain of a sudden or gradual onset of discomfort, and the pain may be localized. Use the OPQRST acronym to elicit the patient's description of symptoms and pain. Is the pain in the chest, abdomen, or extremity? Does it radiate or is it localized? Was its onset gradual or sudden? If there is claudication, is it relieved with rest?

Conduct your focused history and physical exam. Determine the contributing history. This may well be the patient's first recognized event, or it may be a recurrence. Patients with a prior vascular emergency are prone to reoccurrences. They may report an increase in the frequency or duration of events. Breath sounds may be clear to auscultation. Alterations in the heart rate and rhythm may occur with pulmonary embolus and aortic aneurysm. Unequal bilateral blood pressures may indicate a high thoracic aneurysm. Peripheral pulses may be diminished or absent in the affected extremity with arterial occlusion or peripheral arterial atherosclerotic

> **Content Review**
>
> **THE FIVE PS OF ACUTE ARTERIAL OCCLUSION**
> Pallor
> Pain
> Pulselessness
> Paralysis
> Paresthesia

disease. Bruits may be audible over the affected carotid artery. The skin may be cool, moist, or dry, reflecting diminished circulation to the affected area or extremity. ECG findings generally do not contribute to vascular emergency treatment. If dysrhythmias or ectopy are present, treat them accordingly.

Management Managing the patient with a vascular emergency is mostly supportive. Place the patient in a position of comfort. Give oxygen by nonrebreather mask if you suspect pulmonary embolus, aortic aneurysm, or arterial occlusion or if any hypotension or a hypoperfusion state presents.

Before administering any drug, ask the patient or his family if he is allergic to any medications. Pharmacological agents that might be used in a vascular emergency include:

- Nitrous oxide (Nitronox)
- Morphine sulfate

Transport the patient as soon as possible. Indications for rapid transport with lights and sirens include any situation in which medications do not relieve the patient's symptoms or in which you suspect pulmonary embolism, aortic aneurysm, or arterial occlusion. Also consider any presentation of hypotension or hypoperfusion to be an emergency and transport the patient rapidly. Report your findings to the emergency department staff.

If the patient refuses transport, advise him that serious complications are likely to occur without further medical attention. Vascular emergencies can reach a point where the patient permanently loses a limb or quickly decompensates into irreversible shock. Some patients will attempt to refuse transport because they have received relief from pain medications. Use every means at your disposal to convince them to be transported. Document refusals according to general guidelines.

PREHOSPITAL ECG MONITORING

Technology has evolved to a point where portable 12-lead ECG monitoring is readily available. Many manufacturers now make 12-lead machines for prehospital care. Most machines have sophisticated electronics, many with ECG diagnostic packages. Some now have a defibrillator/pacer unit. The principles of 12-lead monitoring are similar to those for routine ECG monitoring described earlier in this chapter.

PREHOSPITAL 12-LEAD ECG MONITORING

The following skill sequence details 12-lead prehospital ECG monitoring.

1. Explain what you are going to do to the patient. Reassure him or her that the machine will not shock him.
2. Prepare all of the equipment and assure the cable is in good repair. Check to make sure there are adequate leads and materials for prepping the skin.
3. Prep the skin (Procedure 28-5A). Dirt, oil, sweat, and other materials on the skin can interfere with obtaining a quality tracing. The skin should be cleansed with an appropriate substance. If the patient is diaphoretic, dry the skin with a towel. On very hot days or in situations where the patient is very diaphoretic, tincture of Benzoin can be applied to the skin before attaching the electrode. Occasionally, it may be necessary to

28–5a   Prep the skin.

28–5b   Place the four limb leads according to the manufacturer's recommendations.

Lead V₁ The electrode is at the fourth intercostal space just to the right of the sternum.

Lead V₂ The electrode is at the fourth intercostal space just to the left of the sternum.

Lead V₃ The electrode is at the line midway between leads V₂ and V₄.

Lead V₄ The electrode is at the midclavicular line in the fifth interspace.

Lead V₅ The electrode is at the anterior axillary line at the same level as lead V₄.

Lead V₆ The electrode is at the midaxillary line at the same level as lead V₄.

Angle of Louis

Chest Lead Placement

28–5c   Proper placement of the precordial leads.

28–5d   Place lead V₁.

28–5e   Place lead V₂.

28–5f   Place lead V₄.

28–5g Place lead V₃.

28–5h Place lead V₅.

28–5i Place lead V₆.

28–5j Ensure that all leads are attached.

28–5k Turn on the machine.

28–5l Check the quality of the tracing being received from each channel.

28–5m Record the tracing.

28–5n Examine the tracing.

28–5o Transmit the tracing to the receiving hospital.

slightly abrade the skin to obtain a good interface. Patients with a lot of body hair may need to have the area immediately over the electrode site shaved to assure good skin/electrode interface.

4. Place the four limb leads according to the manufacturer's recommendations (Procedure 28-5B).

5. Following placement of the limb leads, prepare for placement of the precordial leads. Procedure 28-5C illustrates proper placement of the precordial leads.

6. First, place Lead V_1 by attaching the positive electrode to the right of the sternum at the fourth intercostal space (Procedure 28-5D.)

7. Next, place Lead V_2 by attaching the positive electrode to the left of the sternum at the fourth intercostal space (Procedure 28-5E).

8. Next, place Lead V_4 by attaching the positive electrode at the mid-clavicular line at the fifth intercostal space (Procedure 28-5F).

9. Next, place Lead V_3 by attaching the positive electrode in a line midway between Lead V_2 and Lead V_4 (Procedure 28-5G).

10. Next, place Lead V_5 by attaching the positive electrode at the anterior axillary line at the same level as V_4 (Procedure 28-5H).

11. Finally, place V_6 by attaching the positive electrode to the mid-axillary line at the same level as V_4 (Procedure 28-5I).

12. Assure that all leads are attached (Procedure 28-5J).

13. Turn on the machine (Procedure 28-5K).

14. Check to assure all leads are properly attached and a good tracing is being received from each channel (Procedure 28-5L).

15. Record the tracing (Procedure 28-5M).

16. Examine the tracing. Do not completely rely on the machine's interpretation of the tracing. If necessary, confirm with medical direction (Procedure 28-5N).

17. Provide the tracing to the receiving hospital (Procedure 28-5O). If you do not start thrombolytic therapy in the field, you can reduce the door-to-needle time by providing a quality 12-lead tracing to the emergency department staff as soon as the patient arrives.

18. Perform patient pass-off to the hospital personnel.

19. Restock equipment for next call.

20. Compare field interpretation with emergency department and cardiology interpretation.

SUMMARY

Cardiovascular disease is the number one cause of death in the United States and Canada. Many deaths from heart attack occur within the first twenty-four hours—frequently within the first hour. With the advent of thrombolytic therapy, time is of the essence when managing the patient with suspected ischemic heart disease. EMS plays an ever-increasing role in the early recognition of patients suffering coronary ischemia. In certain areas, EMS provides definitive care by initiating thrombolytic therapy in the field. This is especially important in cases where transport times can be long. With cardiovascular disease, EMS can truly mean the difference between life and death.

CHAPTER 29

Neurology

Objectives

After reading this chapter, you should be able to:

1. Describe the incidence, morbidity, and mortality of neurological emergencies. (p. 1341)
2. Identify the risk factors most predisposing to diseases of the nervous system. (pp. 1357, 1361–1362, 1366, 1367, 1375)
3. Discuss the anatomy and physiology of the nervous system. (see Chapter 3)
4. Define and discuss the epidemiology (including the morbidity/mortality and preventative strategies), pathophysiology, assessment findings, and management for the following neurologic problems:

a. Coma and altered mental status (pp. 1354–1356)
b. Seizures (pp. 1361–1366)
c. Syncope (pp. 1366–1367)
d. Headache (pp. 1367–1368)
e. Neoplasms (pp. 1369–1371)
f. Abscess (p. 1371)
g. Stroke (pp. 1356–1361)
h. Intracranial hemorrhage (pp. 1358–1359)
i. Transient ischemic attack (pp. 1359–1361)
j. Degenerative neurological diseases (pp. 1371–1374)

Continued

INTRODUCTION

Nervous system conditions and diseases affect millions of lives in the United States. Strokes attack a half million people every year, of whom 150,000 die. Epilepsy affects 2.5 million people, or approximately one percent of the U.S. population. An additional 50,000 Americans are diagnosed with Parkinson's disease each year. These are only a few examples of the impact of nervous system disorders. Millions of people are also affected by headache, multiple sclerosis, syncope, neoplasm, and other nervous system emergencies, all of which you will learn about in this chapter.

Many conditions, diseases, and injuries can cause nervous system disorders. Such disorders may be caused by internal or external factors. Modern advances and clinical studies continue to yield new medications and treatments for many conditions. Paramedics should maintain a solid knowledge of the nervous system and remain familiar with current trends and advancements in treating the neurological patient.

This chapter provides an overview of the common neurological conditions that may be encountered in the prehospital setting. It discusses the relevant pathophysiology of the nervous system, assessment techniques, and the recommended prehospital management. Figure 29–1 provides an overview of the central and perpheral nervous systems.

FIGURE 29-1   Overview of the nervous system.

PATHOPHYSIOLOGY

A firm grasp of the pathophysiology of nontraumatic neurologic emergencies is essential in order for the paramedic to provide appropriate and timely emergency care.

ALTERATION IN COGNITIVE SYSTEMS

Consciousness is a condition in which an individual is fully responsive to stimuli and demonstrates awareness of the environment. The ability to respond to stimuli is dependent upon an intact reticular activating system (RAS). Cognition and the ability to respond to the environment rely upon an intact cerebral cortex. Therefore, altered forms of consciousness can result from dysfunction or interruption of the central nervous system.

CENTRAL NERVOUS SYSTEM DISORDERS

An alteration in mental status is the hallmark sign of central nervous system (CNS) injury or illness.

✳ **coma** a state of unconsciousness from which the patient cannot be aroused.

An alteration in mental status is the hallmark sign of central nervous system (CNS) injury or illness. Any alteration in mental status is abnormal and warrants further examination. Alterations may vary from minor thought disturbances to unconsciousness. Unconsciousness, also called **coma**, is a state in which the patient cannot be aroused, even by powerful external stimuli. There are generally two mechanisms capable of producing alterations in mental status:

- *Structural lesions.* Structural lesions (e.g., tumors, contusions) depress consciousness by destroying or encroaching upon the substance of the brain. Examples of causes of structural lesions include:
  - Brain tumor (neoplasm)
  - Degenerative disease
  - Intracranial hemorrhage
  - Parasites
  - Trauma

- *Toxic-metabolic states.* Toxic-metabolic states involve either the presence of circulating toxins or metabolites or the lack of metabolic substrates (oxygen, glucose, or thiamine). These states produce diffuse depression of both sides (hemispheres) of the cerebrum, with or without depression within the brainstem. Various causes of toxic-metabolic states include:
  - Anoxia (lack of oxygen)
  - Diabetic ketoacidosis
  - Hepatic failure
  - Hypoglycemia
  - Renal failure
  - Thiamine deficiency
  - Toxic exposure (e.g., cyanide, organophosphates)

Within the two general mechanisms (structural lesions and toxic metabolic states), there are many difficult-to-classify causes of altered mental status. Some of the more common causes are listed in the following four general categories:

- Drugs
  - Depressants (including alcohol)
  - Hallucinogens
  - Narcotics
- Cardiovascular
  - Anaphylaxis
  - Cardiac arrest
  - Stroke
  - Dysrhythmias
  - Hypertensive encephalopathy
  - Shock
- Respiratory
  - COPD
  - Inhalation of toxic gas
  - Hypoxia
- Infectious
  - AIDS
  - Encephalitis
  - Meningitis

CEREBRAL HOMEOSTASIS

The autonomic nervous system (ANS) maintains cerebral homeostasis (internal balance) and regulates and coordinates the body's vital functions, such as blood pressure, temperature regulation, respiration, and metabolism. It can be strongly affected by emotional influences, resulting in blushing, palpitations, clammy hands, and dry mouth.

PERIPHERAL NERVOUS SYSTEM DISORDERS

Peripheral neuropathy is any malfunction or damage of the peripheral nerves. It can affect muscle activity, sensation, reflexes, or internal organ function. The disorder can involve a single nerve, a *mononeuropathy,* or multiple nerves, known as *polyneuropathy.*

Mononeuropathy is usually caused by localized conditions such as trauma, compression, or infections. Fractured bones, for example, may lacerate or compress

✱ **peripheral neuropathy** any malfunction or damage of the peripheral nerves. Results may include muscle weakness, loss of sensation, impaired reflexes, and internal organ malfunctions.

Peripheral neuropathy can affect muscle activity, sensation, reflexes, or internal organ function.

a nerve; excessively tight tourniquets may compress and injure a nerve; and infections such as herpes zoster may affect a single segment of an afferent nerve. Another common example is carpal tunnel syndrome, a compression-type neuropathy. It is caused by compression of the median nerve that travels through the flexor tendon canal of the lower arm. Carpal tunnel syndrome can cause pain or motor dysfunction in the fingers innervated by the median nerve.

Polyneuropathy is characterized by demyelination or degeneration of peripheral nerves. It leads to sensory, motor, or mixed sensorimotor deficits. A number of conditions, such as immune disorders, toxic agents, and metabolic disorders are known causes of polyneuropathy. One example of a polyneuropathy is Guillian-Barré syndrome, which is characterized by rapidly worsening muscle weakness of the limbs that can sometimes lead to paralysis. Diabetes is one of the major causes of peripheral neuropathy. It usually affects the distal nerves of the hands and feet in the classic "stocking and glove" distribution.

Autonomic Nervous System Disorders

Disorders affecting the ANS are frequently a result of another condition. Since the control of the body's internal environment is vested in the ANS, most conditions that affect the integrity of an individual are accompanied by some changes in autonomic nervous system functioning.

GENERAL ASSESSMENT FINDINGS

Assessment of the neurological system is often difficult. Many of the signs and symptoms of nervous system dysfunction are subtle. As you conduct the scene size-up and begin the initial assessment, form a general impression of the patient and evaluate mental status before assessing the ABCs. If your initial assessment causes you to suspect nervous system dysfunction, this will prompt you to place particular emphasis on the neurological examination during the focused history and physical exam.

During the initial assessment, be alert to any signs of nervous system dysfunction. If present, these will prompt you to place particular emphasis on the neurological evaluation during the focused history and physical exam.

SCENE SIZE-UP AND INITIAL ASSESSMENT

A great deal of crucial information can be obtained while approaching the patient. Size up the scene and the surroundings as well as the patient to form a general impression. Is there evidence of toxic exposure or trauma? Look for clues that can indicate a patient's condition, such as:

General Appearance

- Is the patient conscious?
- Alert?
- Confused?
- Sitting upright?

Speech

- Can the patient speak?
- Clear and coherent?
- Full sentences?
- Slurred speech?

Skin

- Color (pink, pale, cyanotic?)
- Temperature (warm, hot, cool?)
- Moisture (diaphoretic, clammy?)

Facial drooping present?

Posture/Gait

- Upright?
- Leaning?
- Staggered?
- Steady gait?

Next, quickly check the patient's mental status through the "AVPU" method.

- **A** = The patient is alert and aware of his surroundings. A patient alert and orientated to time, place, person, and one's own person, is said to be "alert and oriented times four." Remember, no patient is "oriented" unless he has answered the questions that the paramedic has to ask.
- **V** = The patient responds to verbal stimuli. The patient responds when talked to, perhaps in a loud voice. Note if the patient delivers the answers normally or sluggishly. Also observe whether the patient has purposeful or uncoordinated movements.
- **P** = The patient responds to painful stimuli. The patient responds when tactile stimulation is used, such as a sternal rub, a squeeze of the trapezius muscle, or pinching the thenar (thumb) web space.
- **U** = The patient is unresponsive. The patient is not alert and does not respond to verbal or painful stimuli.

Assessment of cerebral functioning also includes assessing the patient's emotional status. If the patient is conscious, you can detect changes in the following:

Mood

- Is the patient's affect natural or is the patient irritable, anxious, or apathetic?
- Does the patient appear depressed? manic? happy? solemn? reserved?

Thought

- What is the patient's thought pattern? Is it logical? appropriate? scattered?

Perception

- How does the patient perceive his surroundings? Are his interactions appropriate?

Judgment

- Is the patient using reasonable and sound judgment? Is he logical?

Memory and Attention

- Is short-term memory present? long-term memory? Question family members or caregivers to obtain this information.
- Does the patient maintain conversation? pay attention? repeatedly ask or answer questions?

Any alteration from the patient's normal mental status or mood should be considered significant and warrants additional assessment.

Once a patient's level of consciousness is determined, place the greatest emphasis on maintenance of the airway. If the patient is unconscious, assume that a cervical spine injury exists and treat it appropriately. Use the modified jaw-thrust maneuver to open the airway. Once opened, insert the appropriate airway adjunct. In unresponsive patients, the tongue may be occluding the airway. In such cases, you may need only to place an oropharyngeal or nasopharyngeal airway to maintain the airway. If the patient tolerates an oropharyngeal airway, consider intubation.

Vigilantly monitor the airway in any patient with central nervous system injury. It is essential to observe for respiratory arrest that can result from increased intracranial pressure. Remain alert for an absent gag reflex and vomiting. In addition, blood from facial injuries and possible aspiration of gastric contents further threaten the patient's airway.

Observe the patient for any signs and symptoms of inadequate or impaired breathing or the presence of any abnormal respiratory patterns. Remember, the body's "breathing center" is located in the brain. Certain neurological conditions can cause these areas to malfunction and limit the patient's ability to breathe.

Complete assessment of the body's circulatory status is also a crucial part of the initial assessment. Evaluation of the heart rate, rhythm, and ECG pattern can shed light on the body's overall state of perfusion. Observe the patient's skin color, temperature, and moisture for abnormal findings such as cyanosis and moisture. A healthy adult's skin is usually warm, dry, and pink.

FOCUSED HISTORY AND PHYSICAL EXAM

Following completion of the initial assessment and correction of any immediate threats to the patient's life, turn your attention to the focused history and physical exam. This assessment should include an accurate history and a physical exam, including vital signs. Remember that any indications of nervous system dysfunction should cause you to place particular emphasis on neurological evaluation. Neurological evaluation will be detailed under "Nervous System Status" later in this chapter.

History

A thorough, accurate history of a patient is crucial in determining the current problem and subsequent treatment of a patient. One of the first steps in obtaining a thorough history involves attempting to determine whether the neurological problem is traumatic or medical. Clarification will help determine the plan for subsequent prehospital treatment. The initial history may not be easy to obtain because of the patient's altered mental status. In these cases, it is critical for you to obtain information from family, friends, or other bystanders, if available.

If the neurological emergency is due to trauma, ask the following questions:

- When did the incident occur?
- How did the incident occur, or what is the mechanism of injury?

- Was there any loss of consciousness?
- Was there evidence of incontinence? (Incontinence suggests loss of consciousness.)
- What is the patient's chief complaint?
- Has there been any change in symptoms?
- Are there any complicating factors?

If there is no evidence of a traumatic cause of the neurological emergency, ask the following questions to determine the nature of illness:

- What is the chief complaint?
- What are the details of the present illness, or the nature of the illness?
- Is there a pertinent underlying medical problem such as:
  – Cardiac disease
  – Chronic seizures
  – Diabetes
  – Hypertension
- Have these symptoms occurred before?
- Are there any environmental clues? These may include:
  – Evidence of current medications
  – Medic-Alert identification
  – Alcohol bottles or drug paraphernalia
  – Chemicals, hazardous materials

Physical Examination

The physical examination of a patient with a neurological emergency should include the standard head-to-toe examination and a more detailed neurological assessment. Pay particular attention to the pupils, respiratory status, and spinal evaluation.

Face A patient's ability to smile, frown, and wrinkle his forehead indicates an intact facial nerve (cranial nerve VII). If the patient is conscious, test these abilities. Note any drooping or facial paralysis.

Eyes The pupils are controlled by the oculomotor nerve (cranial nerve III). This nerve follows a long course through the skull and is easily compressed by brain swelling. While slight pupillary inequality is normal, abnormal pupils can be an early indicator of increasing intracranial pressure. If both pupils are dilated and do not react to light, the patient probably has a brainstem injury or has suffered serious brain anoxia. If the pupils are dilated but still react to light, the injury may be reversible. However, the patient must be transported quickly to an emergency facility capable of treating central nervous system injuries. A unilaterally dilated pupil that remains reactive to light may be the earliest sign of increasing intracranial pressure. The patient with altered mental status who presents with or develops a unilaterally dilated pupil is in the "immediate transport" category. Constricted, or pinpoint, pupils suggest a toxic etiology for the altered mental status.

A common method of assessing extraocular movement is to have the patient follow finger movements. For example, ask the patient to follow your finger to the extreme left, then up, then down. Repeat the same motions to the extreme right. These positions are referred to as the *cardinal positions of gaze*. Because extraocular movements are controlled by cranial nerves III (oculomotor), IV (trochlear), and VI (abducens), inability to look in all directions with both

FIGURE 29-2 Respiratory patterns seen with CNS dysfunction.

eyes can be an early indication of a central nervous system problem. This is particularly important in the indication of facial trauma.

When examining a patient's pupils, it is important to check for contact lenses. Contact lenses, if present, should be removed and placed into their container or a saline solution and transported with the patient.

Nose/Mouth In the presence of facial paralysis, drooping of the patient's mouth may occur. Pay particular attention to any of these changes that may potentially compromise the patient's airway. A common way to assess for mouth droop is to ask the patient to smile. Also, ask the patient to "show your teeth." Both maneuvers will help determine whether there is any degree of facial drooping.

Respiratory Status Respiratory derangement can occur with CNS illness or injury. Any of five abnormal respiratory patterns may commonly be observed (Figure 29-2):

* *Cheyne-Stokes respiration.* A breathing pattern characterized by a period of apnea lasting 10–60 seconds, followed by gradually increasing depth and frequency of respirations.

✱ **Cheyne-Stokes respiration** a breathing pattern characterized by a period of apnea lasting 10-60 seconds, followed by gradually increasing depth and frequency of respirations.

- *Kussmaul's Respiration.* Rapid, deep respirations caused by severe metabolic and CNS problems.
- *Central Neurogenic Hyperventilation.* Hyperventilation caused by a lesion in the central nervous system, often characterized by rapid, deep, noisy respirations.
- *Ataxic Respirations.* Poor respirations due to CNS damage, causing ineffective thoracic muscular coordination.
- *Apneustic Respirations.* Breathing characterized by prolonged inspiration unrelieved by expiration attempts. This is seen in patients with damage to the upper part of the pons.

Several other respiratory patterns are also possible, depending on the injury. A patient's respirations can be affected by so many factors—fear, hysteria, chest injuries, spinal cord injuries, or diabetes—that they are not as useful as other signs in monitoring the course of CNS problems. Just before death, the patient may present with central neurogenic hyperventilation.

It is important to remember that the level of carbon dioxide ($PaCO_2$) in the blood has a critical effect on cerebral vessels. The normal blood $PaCO_2$ is 40 mmHg. Increasing the $PaCO_2$ causes cerebral vasodilatation, while decreasing it results in cerebral vasoconstriction. If the patient is poorly ventilated, the $PaCO_2$ will increase, causing even further vasodilatation with a subsequent increase in intracranial pressure. Hyperventilation can decrease the $PaCO_2$ effectively causing vasoconstriction of the cerebral vessels. This will assist in minimizing brain swelling. Therefore, hyperventilate any patient who is suspected of having increased intracranial pressure at a rate of 20 breaths per minute. It is important to avoid *excessively* hyperventilating a patient so as to prevent decreasing $PaCO_2$ levels to dangerously low levels.

Cardiovascular Status Patients suffering from a neurological event are also likely to suffer changes to the cardiovascular system. Vigilant assessment of a patient's vital signs is necessary to observe these changes. Look for these changes:

- *Heart rate.* A heart rate that is too fast (tachycardia), too slow (bradycardia), or irregular (dysrhythmias).
- *ECG/rhythm.* Development of any changes to the ECG rhythm, including S-T segment changes, the onset of bradycardia, tachycardia, or potentially lethal dysrhythmias, such as ventricular fibrillation or ventricular tachycardia.
- *Bruits.* The sound of turbulent blood flow through the carotid arteries, known as a *bruit,* may be indicative of atherosclerotic disease and decreased blood flow to the brain.
- *Jugular venous distention (JVD).* Increased jugular venous pressure, known as jugular venous distention, may be present, indicating that the heart is not pumping effectively.

Nervous System Status To evaluate nervous system status, take into account sensorimotor status, motor system status, and the status of the cranial nerves.

Sensorimotor Evaluation The purpose of sensorimotor evaluation is to document loss of sensation and/or motor function. To initially assess the patient with a possible spinal injury, perform these steps:

1. If the patient is unconscious, determine the response to voice, gentle tactile stimulation, and then, if necessary, pain.
2. Evaluate the spine for pain and tenderness.

* **Kussmaul's respiration** rapid deep respirations caused by severe metabolic and CNS problems.

* **central neurogenic hyperventilation** hyperventilation caused by a lesion in the central nervous system, often characterized by rapid, deep, noisy respirations.

* **ataxic respiration** poor respirations due to CNS damage, causing ineffective thoracic muscular coordination.

* **apneustic respiration** breathing characterized by a prolonged inspiration unrelieved by expiration attempts, seen in patients with damage to the upper part of the pons.

FIGURE 29-3 Patient with decorticate posturing.

3. Observe for bruises on the spine.
4. Observe for deformity of the spine.
5. Note any incontinence.
6. Check for circulation, motor function, and sensation in each extremity. Does the patient have feeling in his hands and feet? Ask the patient to wiggle his toes and push them against resistance. Compare both sides. Check bilateral grip strength. If the patient is unconscious, pain response should be observed. If the unconscious patient withdraws or localizes to the pinching of fingers and toes, there is intact sensation and motor function. This is a sign of normal or only minimally impaired cortical function.

A patient with a suspected spinal cord injury will require full spinal immobilization on a long spine board. See Chapter 24 for a discussion of traumatic spinal cord injury.

Both **decorticate posturing** (arms flexed, legs extended) and **decerebrate posturing** (arms and legs extended) are ominous signs of deep cerebral or upper brainstem injury (Figures 29-3 and 29-4). Flaccid paralysis usually indicates spinal cord injury.

Motor System Status   A thorough examination of the motor system of the body includes an assessment of muscle tone, strength, flexion, extension, coordination, and balance. Assess the patient for the following:

* *Muscle Tone.* Are the patient's muscles firm? Or, is atrophy present?
* *Strength.* Does the patient have adequate muscle strength? Or is weakness present? Does the patient have strong and equal grip strength?
* *Flexion/Extension.* Can the patient flex, extend, and move extremities adequately?

✱ **decorticate posture** characteristic posture associated with a lesion at or above the upper brainstem. The patient presents with the arms flexed, fists clenched, and legs extended.

✱ **decerebrate posture** sustained contraction of extensor muscles of the extremities resulting from a lesion in the brainstem. The patient presents with stiff and extended extremities and retracted head.

FIGURE 29-4 Patient with decerebrate posturing.

Glasgow Coma Scale

Eye Opening	Spontaneous	4	
	To Voice	3	
	To Pain	2	
	None	1	
Verbal Response	Oriented	5	
	Confused	4	
	Inappropriate Words	3	
	Incomprehensible Words	2	
	None	1	
Motor Response	Obeys Commands	6	
	Locailzes Pain	5	
	Withdraw (Pain)	4	
	Flexion (Pain)	3	
	Extension (Pain)	2	
	None	1	
Glasgow Coma Score Total			

TOTAL GLASGOW COMA SCALE POINTS

13 – 15 = 5

9 – 12 = 4

6 – 8 = 3

4 – 5 = 1

Conversion = Approximately One - Third Total Value

Neurologic Assessment

FIGURE 29-5 Glasgow Coma Scale.

- *Coordination.* Are the patient's gait and movements steady and smooth? Can the patient touch finger to nose?
- *Balance.* Can the patient stand or sit upright without becoming dizzy?

Cranial Nerves Status As you learned earlier, twelve pairs of cranial nerves extend from the lower surface of the brain. Each pair is designated by a Roman numeral from I to XII. Proper and intact functioning of these nerves may be assessed during a complete neurological examination as detailed in, Chapter 11, "Physical Exam Techniques." Review Figure 3-72 in Chapter 3, which outlines the cranial nerves and their functions.

Further Mental Status Assessment For patients with an altered mental status or those who are unresponsive, the **Glasgow Coma Scale (GCS)** is a simple tool that can be used to evaluate and monitor the patient's condition. While it is used most commonly in trauma situations, the scale can also be a valuable tool for monitoring a medical patient's status (Figure 29-5). The scale includes three components:

- Eye opening
- Verbal response
- Motor response

✳ Glasgow Coma Scale (GCS) tool used in evaluating and quantifying the degree of coma by determining the best motor, verbal, and eye-opening response to standardized stimuli.

A number is applied to each of the components based on the patient's condition. The total score can serve as an indicator of survival. The lowest GCS score possible is 3; the highest possible score is 15. The GCS can also be used as a predictor of long-term morbidity and mortality. The following are examples of the predictive value of the GCS system:

A patient with a total score of:	Has an estimated:
8 or better	94% favorable outcome
5, 6, 7	50% favorable (adult), 90% (children)
3.4	10% favorable outcome
5, 6, 7 who drop a grade	0% favorable outcome
5, 6, 7 who improve to more than 7	80% favorable outcome

Vital Signs

Vital signs are crucial in following the course of neurological problems. Such signs can indicate changes in intracranial pressure. Increased intracranial pressure is characterized by the following changes in vital signs, sometimes collectively referred to as **Cushing's reflex:**

* Increased blood pressure
* Decreased pulse
* Decreased respirations
* Increased temperature

A patient in the early stages of increased intracranial pressure usually exhibits a decrease in pulse rate and an increase in blood pressure and temperature. Later, if the intracranial pressure continues to rise without correction, the pulse will increase, the blood pressure will fall, and the body temperature will remain elevated. Dysrhythmias may be seen with increased intracranial pressure. Continuous ECG monitoring and pulse oximetry, if available, should be utilized to spot early signs of CNS lesions. Table 29-1 compares vital signs of a patient in shock with those of a patient with head injury and increased intracranial pressure. Remember, if you suspect that a patient has a CNS injury, take and record vital signs every five minutes.

Additional Assessment Tools

Additional technological tools may be useful in assessing and monitoring the neurological patient. Such tools should be used as adjuncts to a complete patient assessment, and they should not be relied upon as sole indicators of a patient's

* **Cushing's reflex** a collective change in vital signs (increased blood pressure and temperature and decreased pulse and respirations) associated with increasing intracranial pressure.

Table 29-1	COMPARISON OF VITAL SIGNS IN SHOCK AND INCREASED INTRACRANIAL PRESSURE	
Vital Signs	**Shock**	**Increased ICP**
Blood pressure	Decreased	Increased
Pulse	Increased	Decreased
Respirations	Increased	Decreased
Level of Consciousness	Decreased	Decreased

condition. Paramedics should continue to base their clinical decisions on a patient's entire presentation. Use such instruments as the end-tidal CO_2 detector, pulse oximeter, and blood glucometer to gain further insight into a patient's condition.

End-Tidal CO_2 Detector The end-tidal CO_2 detector monitors the amount of carbon dioxide being exhaled by a patient while being ventilated. This device works on the premise that during exhalation CO_2 should be detected. In the apneic patient with a suspected neurological injury, the device can be used to monitor the effectiveness of the assisted ventilations. Monitoring the levels of CO_2 can assure that ventilation rate and quality are appropriate for decreasing the increased intracranial pressure.

Pulse Oximeter The pulse oximeter is an effective tool for monitoring a patient's general state of perfusion. Any patient with a pulse oximetry reading of less than 90 percent is likely to be hypoxic. In a patient who has suffered a stroke, altered mental status, or syncope, the oximeter can be a useful adjunct in monitoring a patient's condition. It can also monitor the effectiveness of airway management techniques.

Blood Glucometer A common cause of an altered mental status or focal neurological deficits is hypoglycemia. Determining the blood glucose level is often a crucial step in caring for the neurological patient. Use the glucometer to obtain an accurate blood glucose level. See Chapter 30 for a discussion of this procedure. Documented hypoglycemia should be treated with a bolus of 50% dextrose.

Geriatric Considerations in Neurological Assessment

The neurological system of the geriatric patient is susceptible to systemic illness and is often affected by other body disorders. In addition, certain neurological changes such as pupil sluggishness, loss of overall body strength, and muscle atrophy occur naturally with the aging process. Slowing of nerve conduction is another characteristic often seen in the geriatric patient. Such slowing may indicate that a little more time is necessary to obtain a complete neurological history.

The level of consciousness and overall mental status of a geriatric patient is evaluated by assessing judgment, memory, affect, mood, orientation, speech, and grooming. Interviewing family members about the patient's normal state may reveal any change in mental status. Common neurological problems of the older patient include headache, low back pain, dizziness, weakness, loss of balance, disorders like Parkinson's disease, and vascular emergencies like stroke.

ONGOING ASSESSMENT

Any patient suffering from a neurological emergency should be reassessed every five minutes during your care and during transportation. Constantly re-evaluate and monitor the patient's airway and neurological system.

MANAGEMENT OF SPECIFIC NERVOUS SYSTEM EMERGENCIES

The primary treatment for nervous system emergencies in the field is supportive. Most conditions will not be "cured" in the prehospital setting but symptoms may

The primary treatment for nervous system emergencies in the field is supportive.

be reduced or controlled. Make a strong effort to make the patient comfortable and to reduce any of the existing symptoms. Follow these steps:

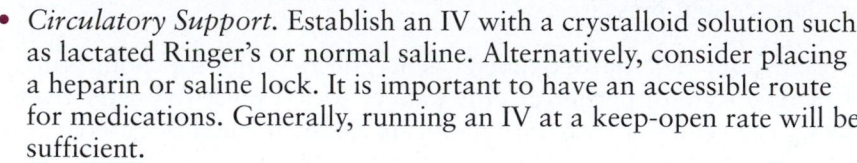

The major concerns in any CNS emergency are always the airway, breathing, circulation, and, if indicated, C-spine control.

- *Airway and Breathing.* Properly position any patient that you suspect has a neurological emergency and protect the airway. If there is known or possible trauma, maintain C-spine immobilization. Administer oxygen via a nonrebreather mask. If the patient is breathing inadequately or is apneic, initiate ventilatory assistance. If an airway problem is detected, first apply basic airway maneuvers such as head positioning or the modified jaw-thrust maneuver. Intubate, if indicated.

- *Circulatory Support.* Establish an IV with a crystalloid solution such as lactated Ringer's or normal saline. Alternatively, consider placing a heparin or saline lock. It is important to have an accessible route for medications. Generally, running an IV at a keep-open rate will be sufficient.

- *Pharmacological Interventions.* Medications are available to alleviate signs and symptoms in patients with neurological emergencies. Medications include dextrose, thiamine, naloxone, and diazepam.

- *Psychological Support.* Patients suffering from a nervous system emergency, acute or chronic, are likely also to suffer anxiety. Neurological deficits of any kind are frightening experiences. Provide the patient with emotional support and explain the treatment regimen. In most cases, it is appropriate to explain to the patient what is occurring and why. Careful explanation and emotional support will help allay anxiety and apprehension.

- *Transport Considerations.* Assess, provide emergency care, and package the patient as quickly and safely as possible. Rapidly transport any patient with a neurological deficit or altered mental status to an appropriate emergency department, equipped with a computerized tomography (CT) or magnetic resonance imaging (MRI) scanner and facilities capable of managing strokes with thrombolytic therapy. Modern medicine has seen the development of new advances in pharmacological and surgical interventions that are only available in the hospital setting.

There are numerous causes of nervous system emergencies. The more common nontraumatic nervous emergencies encountered in the prehospital setting include altered mental status, seizures, stroke, transient ischemic attacks (TIA), and headache. The following discussion details the assessment and management of these frequently encountered nontraumatic nervous system emergencies.

ALTERED MENTAL STATUS

When evaluating a patient, you may find mnemonic devices useful as assessment aids. A mnemonic that may help you remember some of the common causes of altered mental status is "AEIOU-TIPS."

A = Acidosis, alcohol
E = Epilepsy
I = Infection
O = Overdose
U = Uremia (kidney failure)
T = Trauma, tumor, toxin

I = Insulin (hypoglycemia or diabetic ketoacidosis)

P = Psychosis, poison

S = Stroke, seizure

Make an effort through history-taking and patient assessment to determine the underlying cause of the altered level of consciousness. Oftentimes, however, a clear cause will not be evident and cannot be determined in the prehospital setting.

Assessment

Using the AVPU method discussed earlier, determine the patient's level of consciousness. Unresponsive patients require vigilant monitoring and protection of the airway. Use information from family, friends, or other bystanders to try to determine the underlying cause of unconsciousness. Perform a physical exam to uncover any hidden injuries, signs, or symptoms.

Management

Your initial priority is to assure that the patient's airway is open and cervical spine is immobilized (in cases of suspected head/neck injury). Simultaneously secure the patient's airway and administer supplemental oxygen. If the patient is breathing inadequately, support respirations. An unresponsive patient requires an appropriate airway adjunct. Then assess the patient's circulatory status. Evaluate the patient's heart rate, blood pressure, and monitor the cardiac rhythm.

After the above are completed, perform the following steps:

- Establish an IV of normal saline or lactated Ringer's at a keep-open rate or place a heparin or saline lock.
- Determine the blood glucose level using a reagent strip or glucometer. A serum glucose determination will assist in determining if the altered mental status is due to hypoglycemia.
- If the blood glucose level is low, administer 50 percent dextrose. This will mediate hypoglycemia, which may be the cause of the altered mental status. Even if the patient is an uncontrolled diabetic whose body is not producing enough insulin, hyperglycemia produced by administration of glucose will do limited harm in the short time before arrival at the hospital. If, however, the patient is hypoglycemic, for example from too much insulin or missing a meal, the administration of glucose can be life-saving, and the patient may respond immediately. For the alcoholic patient who is hypoglycemic, the glucose may be life-saving as well. For more information or diabetic emergencies, see Chapter 30.
- Administer naloxone if the patient is suspected of having a narcotic overdose. Naloxone, a narcotic antagonist, has proven effective in the management and reversal of overdose caused by narcotics or synthetic narcotic agents. For more information, see Chapter 34.
- If the patient is a suspected alcoholic, consider the administration of 100 mg of thiamine (vitamin B_1). It is required for the conversion of pyruvic acid to acetyl-coenzyme-A (an important step in normal metabolism). Without this conversion, a significant amount of energy available in glucose cannot be obtained. The brain is extremely sensitive to thiamine deficiency. For more information, see Chapter 34.

Chronic Alcoholism Chronic alcoholism interferes with the intake, absorption, and use of thiamine. A significant percentage of alcoholics have thiamine deficiency that can cause Wernicke's syndrome or Korsakoff's psychosis. **Wernicke's syndrome** is an acute but reversible encephalopathy (brain disease) characterized by ataxia, eye muscle weakness, and mental derangement. Of even greater concern is **Korsakoff's psychosis,** characterized by memory disorder. Once established, Korsakoff's psychosis may be irreversible. Paramedics should follow local protocols. If ordered by medical direction, administer 100 mg of thiamine IV or IM.

Increased Intracranial Pressure If an increase in intracranial pressure is likely, as occurs in a closed head injury, hyperventilate the patient at 20 breaths per minute. Decreasing the carbon dioxide level will cause cerebral vasoconstriction and will help minimize brain swelling. Use caution not to over-hyperventilate, which could decrease CO_2 levels to dangerously low levels. Medical direction may order administration of the osmotic diuretic mannitol (Osmotrol). Mannitol causes diuresis, eliminating fluid from the intravascular space through the kidneys. Many authorities feel that its oncotic effect also causes a fluid shift from the substance of the brain to the circulation, thus reducing brain edema. As with all drugs, follow local protocols.

STROKE AND INTRACRANIAL HEMORRHAGE

Stroke, also called a "brain attack," is a general term that describes injury or death of brain tissue usually due to interruption of cerebral blood flow. The term "brain attack" is used because it compares the physiology of a stroke with that of a heart attack. In both cases, oxygen deprivation causes damage to the affected tissue.

The term "brain attack" also reflects recent trends in the treatment of a stroke, which in many cases now parallels the treatment available for heart attack. Prior to 1995, prehospital care of the stroke patient was considered primarily supportive. Since then, modern medicine has discovered new therapies and has realized the importance of early intervention. Now, early recognition and rapid transport to the hospital are identified as crucial to improving the outcome for stroke patients. The National Institute of Neurological Disorders and Stroke (NINDS) suggests transport to an emergency facility with the capability to respond to a stroke patient quickly, such as a facility equipped with computed tomography (CT) and neurological services.

In addition, studies have proven that *tissue plasminogen activator (tPA,)* and other thrombolytic agents used in the treatment of heart attack, are also effective in treating certain occlusive strokes. NINDS stresses that the use of thrombolytic agents in strokes is approved by the Food and Drug Administration and is encouraged in a certain patient population. Stroke patients who may be candidates for the thrombolytic therapy must receive definitive treatment within 3 hours of onset. Because of the possibility of intervention with thrombolytics, it is crucial to determine the exact time of the onset of symptoms as accurately as possible. In addition, it is essential that the public be aware of the signs and symptoms of stroke so that EMS can be notified. Therefore, extensive public education is necessary in achieving early recognition of symptoms and appropriate intervention and treatment. Transportation to an emergency facility is crucial in achieving the best possible outcome for these patients.

Strokes are the third most common cause of death and, in middle-aged and older patients, are a frequent cause of disability. Therefore the public, particularly those with a history of atherosclerosis (hardening of the arteries), heart disease, or hypertension, should be educated on the signs and symptoms of stroke as well as the need to contact EMS at the outset of symptoms. Likewise, paramedics must understand stroke as a serious, potentially life-threatening condition that warrants rapid recognition and prompt transport.

FIGURE 29-6 Etiologies of stroke.

Normal
Artery

Atheromatorus
Artery

Embolus

Hemorrhage

Strokes can be divided into two broad categories: those caused by occlusion (blockage) of an artery and those caused by hemorrhage from a ruptured cerebral artery (Figure 29-6):

- *Occlusive Strokes.* An occlusive stroke occurs when a cerebral artery is blocked by a clot or other foreign matter. This results in *ischemia,* an inadequate blood supply to the brain tissue, and progresses to *infarction,* the death of tissues as a result of cessation of blood supply. In infarction, the tissue that has died will swell, causing further damage to nearby tissues, which only have a marginal blood supply. If swelling is severe, *herniation* (protrusion of brain tissue from the skull through the foramen magnum, the narrow opening at the base of the skull) may result. Occlusive strokes are classified as either embolic or thrombotic, depending on the cause.

  - *Embolic Strokes.* An *embolus* is a solid, liquid, or gaseous mass carried to a blood vessel from a remote site. The most common emboli are clots (thromboemboli) which usually arise from diseased blood vessels in the neck (carotid) or from abnormally contracting chambers in the heart. Atrial fibrillation often results in atrial dilation, a precursor to the formation of clots. Other types of emboli that may cause occlusion in cerebral blood vessels are air, tumor tissue, and fat. Embolic strokes occur suddenly and may be characterized by severe headaches.

  - *Thrombotic Strokes.* A *cerebral thrombus* is a blood clot that gradually develops in and obstructs a cerebral artery. As a person ages, atheromatous plaque deposits can form on the inner walls of arteries. The buildup causes a narrowing of the arteries and reduces the amount of blood that can flow through them. This process is known as atherosclerosis. Once the arteries are narrowed, platelets adhere to the roughened surface and can create a blood clot that blocks the blood flow through the cerebral artery. This ultimately results in brain tissue death. Unlike the embolic stroke, the signs and symptoms of thrombotic stroke develop gradually. This type of stroke often occurs at night and is characterized by a patient awakening with altered mental status and/or loss of speech, sensory, or motor function.

(a)

(b)

FIGURE 29-7   (a) Intracerebral hemorrhage (b) Subarachnoid hemorrhage.

- *Hemorrhagic Strokes.* Hemorrhagic strokes are usually categorized as being within the brain (intracerebral) (Figure 29-7a) or in the space around the outer surface of the brain (subarachnoid) (Figure 29-7b). Onset is often sudden and marked by a severe headache. Most intracranial hemorrhages occur in the hypertensive patient when a small vessel deep within the brain tissue ruptures. Subarachnoid hemorrhages most often result from congenital blood vessel abnormalities or from head trauma. Congenital abnormalities include aneurysms (weakened vessels) and arteriovenous malformations (collections of abnormal blood vessels). Aneurysms tend to be on the surface and may hemorrhage into the brain tissue or the subarachnoid space. Arteriovenous malformations may be within the brain, in the subarachnoid space, or both. Hemorrhage inside the brain often tears and separates normal brain tissue. The release of blood into the cavities within the brain that contain cerebrospinal fluid may paralyze vital centers. If blood in the subarachnoid space impairs drainage of cerebrospinal fluid, it may cause a rise in the intracranial pressure. Herniation of brain tissue may then occur.

Assessment

Signs and symptoms of a stroke will depend upon the type of stroke and the area of the brain damaged. Areas commonly affected are the motor, speech, and sensory centers. The onset of symptoms will be acute, and the patient may experience unconsciousness. There may be stertorous breathing (laborious breathing accompanied by snoring) due to paralysis of a portion of the soft palate. Respiratory expiration may be puffs of air out of the cheeks and mouth. The patient's pupils may be unequal, with the larger pupil on the side of the hemorrhage. Paralysis will usually involve one side of the face, one arm, and one leg. The eyes often will be turned away from the side of the body paralysis. The patient's skin may be cool and clammy. Speech disturbances, or aphasia, may also be noted.

Signs and symptoms of a stroke include:

- Facial drooping
- Headache
- Confusion and agitation
- Dysphasia (difficulty in speaking)
- Aphasia (inability to speak)
- Dysarthria (impairment of the tongue and muscles essential to speech)
- Vision problems such as monocular blindness (blindness in one eye) or double vision
- Hemiparesis (weakness on one side)
- Hemiplegia (paralysis on one side)
- Paresthesia (numbness or tingling)
- Inability to recognize by touch
- Gait disturbances or uncoordinated fine motor movements
- Dizziness
- Incontinence
- Coma

Predisposing factors that may contribute to the stroke include hypertension, diabetes, abnormal blood lipid levels, oral contraceptives, sickle cell disease, and some cardiac dysrhythmias (e.g., atrial fibrillation).

Distinguishing Transient Ischemic Attacks (TIAs) Some patients may have transient stroke-like symptoms known as **TIAs**, or **transient ischemic attacks.** These indicate temporary interference with the blood supply to the brain, producing symptoms of neurological deficit. These symptoms may last for a few minutes or for several hours but usually resolve within 24 hours. After the attack, the patient will show no evidence of residual brain or neurological damage. The patient who experiences a TIA may, however, be a candidate for an eventual stroke. In fact, one third of TIA patients suffer a stroke soon thereafter.

The onset of a transient ischemic attack is usually abrupt. The specific signs and symptoms depend upon the area of the brain affected. Any one or a

✱ transient ischemic attack (TIA) temporary interruption of blood supply to the brain.

combination of stroke symptoms may be present. In fact, it is virtually impossible to determine whether such a neurological event is due to a stroke or to a TIA in the prehospital setting.

The most common cause of a TIA is carotid artery disease. Other causes can be a small embolus, decreased cardiac output, hypotension, overmedication with antihypertensive agents, or cerebrovascular spasm.

While obtaining the history of the patient suspected of sustaining a TIA, you should try to collect information on or take note of the following factors:

- Previous neurological symptoms
- Initial symptoms and their progression
- Changes in mental status
- Precipitating factors
- Dizziness
- Palpitations
- History of hypertension, cardiac disease, sickle cell disease, or previous TIA or stroke

Management

Care for the stroke or TIA patient emphasizes early recognition, supportive measures, rapid transport, and notification of the emergency department (Figure 29-8). Aggressive airway management is a priority in caring for these patients. Field management of the stroke patient generally includes the following procedures:

- Assure scene safety, including body substance isolation.
- Establish and maintain an adequate airway. Have suction equipment readily available. Control of the patient's airway is a priority. Brain damage can affect a patient's ability to swallow and maintain an open airway.
- If patient is apneic or if breathing is inadequate, provide positive pressure ventilations at a rate of 20 per minute. Hyperventilation of the stroke patient will eliminate excessive CO_2 levels. Avoid overzealous hyperventilation that may lower CO_2 levels to detrimentally low levels causing profound cerebral vasoconstriction.
- If breathing is adequate, administer oxygen via a nonrebreather mask at 15 liters per minute.
- Complete a detailed patient history.
- Keep the patient supine or in the recovery position. If the patient has congestive heart failure, he could be maintained in a semi-upright position, if necessary.
- If an altered mental status is present or there is potential for airway compromise, place the patient in the left lateral recumbent, or recovery position.
- Determine the blood glucose level.
- Start an IV of normal saline or lactated Ringer's at a keep-open rate or place a heparin or saline lock. (Avoid dextrose solutions that may increase intracranial pressure due to increased osmotic effects.) If hypoglycemia is present, consider the administration of 50 percent dextrose by intravenous push.
- Monitor the cardiac rhythm.
- Protect the paralyzed extremities.

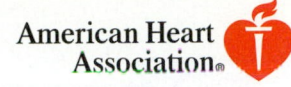

SUSPECTED STROKE ALGORITHM

American Heart Association
Fighting Heart Disease and Stroke

Suspected Stroke

EMS assessments and actions
Immediate assessments performed by EMS personnel include
- *Cincinnati Prehospital Stroke Scale* (includes difficulty speaking, arm weakness, facial droop)
- *Los Angeles Prehospital Stroke Screen*
- Alert hospital to possible stroke patient
- Rapid transport to hospital

✓ Detection
✓ Dispatch
✓ Delivery

✓ Door

Immediate general assessment: <10 minutes from arrival
- Assess ABCs, vital signs
- Provide **oxygen** by nasal cannula
- Obtain IV access; obtain blood samples (CBC, electrolytes, coagulation studies)
- Check blood sugar; treat if indicated
- Obtain 12-lead ECG; check for arrhythmias
- Perform general neurological screening assessment
- Alert Stroke Team: neurologist, radiologist, CT technician

Immediate neurological assessment: <25 minutes from arrival
- Review patient history
- Establish onset (<3 hours required for fibrinolytics)
- Perform physical examination
- Perform neurological examination:
  ✓ Determine level of consciousness *(Glasgow Coma Scale)*
  ✓ Determine level of stroke severity *(NIH Stroke Scale or Hunt and Hess Scale)*
- Order urgent noncontrast CT scan (door-to-CT scan performed: goal <25 minutes from arrival)
- Read CT scan (door-to-CT read: goal <45 minutes from arrival)
- Perform lateral cervical spine x-ray (if patient comatose/history of trauma)

Does CT scan show intracerebral or subarachnoid hemorrhage?

✓ Data   No   Yes

Probable acute ischemic stroke
- Review for CT exclusions: are any observed?
- Repeat neurological exam: are deficits variable or rapidly improving?
- Review fibrinolytic exclusions: are any observed?
- Review patient data: is symptom onset now >3 hours?

Consult neurosurgery

Blood on LP

No to all of above

If high suspicion of subarachnoid hemorrhage remains despite negative findings on CT scan, perform lumbar puncture. Fibrinolytic therapy is contraindicated following a lumbar puncture.

Initiate actions for acute hemorrhage
- Reverse any anticoagulants
- Reverse any bleeding disorder
- Monitor neurological condition
- Treat hypertension in awake patients

✓ Decision

Patient remains candidate for fibrinolytic therapy?   No   No blood on LP

✓ Drug   Yes

- Review risks/benefits with patient and family: If acceptable —
Begin fibrinolytic treatment (door-to-treatment goal <60 minutes):
- Monitor neurological status: emergent CT if deterioration
- Monitor BP; treat as indicated
- Admit to critical care unit
- No anticoagulants or antiplatelet treatment for 24 hours

- Initiate supportive therapy as indicated
- Consider admission
- Consider anticoagulation
- Consider additional conditions needing treatment
- Consider alternative diagnoses

William Hornyak

- Give the patient reassurance—all procedures should be explained. The patient may be unable to speak but still may be able to hear and understand.
- Rapidly transport without excessive movement or noise to an appropriate medical facility.

SEIZURES AND EPILEPSY

A **seizure** is a temporary alteration in behavior due to the massive electrical discharge of one or more groups of neurons in the brain. Seizures in any individual may be caused by stresses to the body, such as hypoxia, or a rapid lowering of

✳ **seizure** a temporary alteration in behavior due to the massive electrical discharge of one or more groups of neurons in the brain. Seizures can be clinically classified as generalized or partial.

blood sugar. Febrile seizures can occur in young children with sudden elevations in body temperature. Structural diseases of the brain such as tumors, head trauma, toxic eclampsia, and vascular disorders also cause seizures. The most common cause is *idiopathic epilepsy*. The term *idiopathic* means "without a known cause." The terms *epilepsy* or *epileptic* indicate nothing more than the potential to develop seizures in circumstances that would not induce them in most individuals. Seizures can provoke a great deal of anxiety in both yourself and bystanders.

To assess seizures quickly under such conditions, you need to be thoroughly familiar with their various forms.

Types of Seizures

Seizures can be clinically classified as generalized or partial. **Generalized seizures** begin as an electrical discharge in a small area of the brain but spread to involve the entire cerebral cortex, causing widespread malfunction. **Partial seizures** may remain confined to a limited portion of the brain, causing localized malfunction, or may spread and become generalized.

Generalized Seizures Generalized seizures include tonic-clonic and absence seizures. Another type, pseudoseizures, may mimic generalized seizures.

- *Tonic-Clonic.* A **tonic-clonic seizure**, also known as a *grand mal seizure*, is a generalized motor seizure, producing a loss of consciousness. It typically includes a **tonic** (increased tone) **phase**, characterized by tensed, contracted muscles, and a **clonic phase**, characterized by rhythmic jerking movements of the extremities. During the seizure episode, a patient's intercostal muscles and diaphragm become temporarily paralyzed, interrupting respirations and producing cyanosis. The patient's neck, head, face, and eye muscles may also jerk. Once respirations resume, there may be copious amounts of oral secretions (frothing) present. Incontinence is also common during a seizure. Agitation or confusion, drowsiness, or coma may also follow the seizure.

  Tonic-clonic seizures have a specific progression of events. It is descriptively convenient to refer to this progression as ranging from warning phase to period of recovery. However, not all seizure patients experience all of these events.
  - *Aura.* An aura is a subjective sensation preceding seizure activity. The aura may precede the attack by several hours or by only a few seconds. An aura may be of a psychic or a sensory nature, with olfactory, visual, auditory, or taste hallucinations. Some common types include hearing noise or music, seeing floating lights, smelling unpleasant odors, feeling an unpleasant sensation in the stomach, or experiencing tingling or twitching in a specific body area. Not all seizures are preceded by an aura.
  - *Loss of Consciousness.* The patient will become unconscious at some point after the aura sensations, if any.
  - *Tonic Phase.* This is a phase of continuous muscle tension, characterized by contraction of the patient's muscles.
  - *Hypertonic Phase.* The patient experiences extreme muscular rigidity, including hyperextension of the back.
  - *Clonic Phase.* The patient experiences muscle spasms marked by rhythmic movements, The patient's jaw usually remains clenched, making airway management difficult.
  - *Post Seizure.* The patient remains in a coma.
  - *Postictal.* The patient may awaken confused and fatigued. He may complain of a headache and may experience some neurological

deficit. In many cases, patients will be in this postictal state upon the arrival of paramedic crews. There may be evidence of incontinence, which supports the likelihood that seizure activity has taken place.

- *Absence.* An **absence seizure,** also called a *petit mal seizure,* is a brief, generalized seizure that usually presents with a 10– to 30–second loss of consciousness or awareness, eye or muscle fluttering, and an occasional loss of muscle tone. Loss of consciousness may be so brief that the patient or observers may be unaware of the episode. Absence seizures are idiopathic disorders of early childhood and rarely occur after age twenty. Children who suffer frequent absence seizures are often accused of day dreaming or inattentiveness. Absence seizures may not respond to normal treatment modalities.

- *Pseudoseizures.* Pseudoseizures, also called "hysterical seizures," stem from psychological disorders. The patient presents with sharp and bizarre movements that can often be interrupted with a terse command, such as "stop it!" The seizure is usually witnessed, and there will not be a postictal period. Very rarely do patients experiencing a pseudoseizure injure themselves.

Partial Seizures Partial Seizures may be either simple or complex.

- *Simple Partial Seizures.* **Simple partial seizures,** also sometimes called focal motor, focal sensory, or Jacksonian seizures, are characterized by chaotic movement or dysfunction of one area of the body. When there is abnormal electrical discharge from a specific portion of the brain, only those functions served by that area will have dysfunction. Simple partial seizures involve no loss of consciousness and begin as localized tonic/clonic movements. They frequently spread and can progress to generalized tonic-clonic seizures. Therefore, it is crucial that you document how such seizures begin and the course that they subsequently take.

- *Complex Partial Seizures.* **Complex partial seizures,** sometimes called temporal lobe or psychomotor seizures, are characterized by distinctive auras. They include unusual smells, tastes, sounds, or the tendency of objects to look either very large and near or small and distant. Sometimes a seizure patient may visualize scenes that look very familiar (*deja vu*) or very strange. A metallic taste in the mouth is a common psychomotor seizure aura. These are focal seizures, lasting approximately 1–2 minutes. The patient experiences a loss of contact with his surroundings. Additionally, the patient may act confused, stagger, perform purposeless movement, or make unintelligible sounds. He may not understand what is said. The patient may even refuse medical aid. Some patients develop automatic behavior or show a sudden change in personality, such as abrupt explosions of rage.

Assessment

Your initial contact with the patient and bystanders will offer a unique opportunity to obtain a history that may influence your plan of management. What an untrained observer calls a seizure may be a simple fainting spell. Therefore, you need to ascertain exactly what the patient may recall or what bystanders witnessed.

Many other problems can mimic or suggest a seizure. These include migraine headaches, cardiac dysrhythmias, hypoglycemia after exercise or drug ingestion, and the tendency to faint when rising from a supine or sitting position (orthostatic hypotension). Hyperventilation, meningitis, intracranial hemorrhage, or certain tranquilizers can cause stiffness of the extremities. Decerebrate movements,

✳ **absence seizure** type of generalized seizure with sudden onset, characterized by a brief loss of awareness and rapid recovery.

✳ **simple partial seizure** type of partial seizure that involves local motor, sensory, or autonomic dysfunction of one area of the body. There is no loss of consciousness.

✳ **complex partial seizure** type of partial seizure usually originating in the temporal lobe characterized by an aura and focal findings such as alterations in mental status or mood.

A good history will be important in distinguishing a seizure from other conditions that may mimic seizure.

Table 29-2	DIFFERENTIATION BETWEEN SYNCOPE AND GENERALIZED TONIC-CLONIC SEIZURE
Syncope	**Seizure**
Usually begins in a standing position	May begin in any position
Patient will usually remember a warning of fainting (feeling of weakness or dizziness)	May begin without warning or may be preceded by an aura
Jerking motions usually not present	Jerking motions present during unconsciousness
Patient regains consciousness almost immediately on becoming supine	Patient remains unconscious during seizure, remains drowsy during postictal period

if present, may be caused by increased intracranial pressure. If you are unsure whether the patient has had a seizure, it may be more harmful than beneficial to administer an anticonvulsant medication.

It is also important to try to distinguish between syncope and true seizure (Table 29-2). Syncope patients sometimes have a short initial period of seizure-like activity (usually less than one minute), but this is not followed by a postictal state. The most common cause of fainting is vasovagal syncope associated with fatigue, emotional stress, or cardiac disease. Syncope will be discussed in greater detail later in this chapter.

When obtaining a history, remember to include the following points:

- History of seizures. This data should include length of any past seizure; whether it was generalized or focal; presence of auras, incontinence, or trauma to the tongue.
- Recent history of head trauma.
- Any alcohol and/or drug abuse.
- Recent history of fever, headache, or stiff neck.
- History of diabetes, heart disease, or stroke.
- Current medications. Most chronic seizure patients take anticonvulsant medication on a regular basis. Common anticonvulsant medications include phenytoin (Dilantin), phenobarbital, carbamazepine (Tegretol), and valproic acid (Depakote).

The physical examination of the seizure patient should include the following steps:

- Note any signs of head trauma or injury to the tongue.
- Note any evidence of alcohol and/or drug abuse.
- Document dysrhythmias.

Management

Remember that seizures tend to provoke anxiety in patients, families, and paramedics. From a medical standpoint, however, most of these situations only require managing the airway and preventing the patient from injuring himself. Because the patient may become hypo- or hyperthermic if exposed, protecting body temperature is also crucial. Field management of the seizure patient generally includes the following procedures:

- Assure scene safety.
- Maintain the airway. Do not force objects between the patient's teeth—this includes padded tongue blades. Pushing objects into the patient's mouth may cause him to vomit or to aspirate. It can also cause laryngospasm.

The prime concerns in seizure management are control of the airway and prevention of injury.

- Administer high-flow oxygen.
- Establish intravenous access. Initiate normal saline or lactated Ringer's solution at a keep-open rate. Do not use dextrose solutions; emergency department personnel may later administer phenytoin (Dilantin), which is incompatible with dextrose solutions.
- Determine the blood glucose level. If hypoglycemic, administer 50 percent dextrose.
- Never attempt to restrain the patient. This may injure him. However, protect the patient from hitting objects in the environment (Figure 29-9). [Note: If there is evidence of head trauma, C-spine immobilization must be considered as in any other head injury.]
- Maintain body temperature.
- Position the patient on his left side after the clonic-tonic phase (Figure 29-10).
- Suction, if required.
- Monitor cardiac rhythm.
- If seizure is prolonged (> 5 minutes), consider an anticonvulsant.
- Provide a quiet, reassuring atmosphere.
- Transport the patient in the supine or lateral recumbent position.

FIGURE 29-9 Protection of a seizing patient.

Status Epilepticus

Status epilepticus is a series of two or more generalized motor seizures without an intervening return of consciousness. The most common cause in adults is failure to take prescribed anticonvulsant medications. Status epilepticus is a major emergency since it involves a prolonged period of apnea, which in turn can cause hypoxia of vital brain tissues. These seizures may result in respiratory arrest, severe metabolic and respiratory acidosis, extreme hypertension, increased intracranial pressure, serious elevations in body temperature, fractures of the long bones and spine, necrosis of the cardiac muscle, and severe dehydration.

The most valuable intervention is to protect the patient from airway obstruction and deliver 100 percent oxygen. Preferably this should be accomplished by bag-valve-mask assistance, since the normal ventilatory mechanisms of the patient are seriously impaired and air exchange is generally ineffective. Once the airway is maintained and ventilations are being assisted, take the following steps:

- Start an IV of normal saline at a keep-open rate.
- Monitor cardiac rhythm.

✳ status epilepticus series of two or more generalized motor seizures without any intervening periods of consciousness.

Status epilepticus—two or more generalized motor seizures with no intervening return of consciousness—is a life-threatening emergency.

FIGURE 29-10 Place a seizing patient with no suspected spine injury on her left side.

- Administer 25 gms of 50 percent dextrose IV push, if hypoglycemia is present.
- Administer 5–10 mg diazepam IV push for an adult. (Diazepam is a sedative and anticonvulsant that depresses the spread of seizure activity across the motor cortex of the brain.)
- Continue to monitor the airway. Some patients may require large doses of diazepam. Always have flumazenil (Romazicon) available in case it is needed to reverse any significant respiratory depression caused by diazepam. Remember, administration of flumazenil may result in the return of seizures. It should only be used when absolutely necessary.

SYNCOPE

* syncope transient loss of consciousness due to inadequate flow of blood to the brain with rapid recovery of consciousness upon becoming supine; fainting.

As discussed earlier, **syncope** (fainting) is a neurological condition characterized by the sudden, temporary loss of consciousness caused by insufficient blood flow to the brain, with recovery of consciousness almost immediately upon becoming supine. Nearly half of all Americans will experience at least one episode of syncope during their lifetime. According to the National Institutes of Health, syncope accounts for three percent of all emergency department visits.

Assessment

Focus on what caused the patient to faint, or lose consciousness. The causes of syncope can be classified into these three general categories:

- *Cardiovascular* conditions, such as dysrhythmias or mechanical problems—A heart rate that is too fast or too slow, or an abnormally functioning heart valve may trigger hypoxia in the brain and subsequent fainting.
- *Non-cardiovascular* disease, such as metabolic, neurological, or psychiatric conditions—Hypoglycemia, a transient ischemic attack, or an anxiety attack can all be causes of syncope.
- *Idiopathic,* or unknown, cause—Oftentimes, the cause of a patient's syncope remains unknown despite careful assessment and diagnostic tests.

Syncope involves rapid recovery of consciousness. If a patient does not regain consciousness within a few moments, it is NOT syncope, but something more serious.

Syncope can occur in all ages from the very young to the very old. Symptoms may include feeling faint, dizziness, lightheadedness, or a loss of consciousness without warning. Keep in mind, however, that the definition of syncope includes rapid recovery of consciousness (usually less than a minute). If a patient does not spontaneously regain consciousness within a few moments, it is NOT syncope—it is something more serious.

Management

When caring for someone who has fainted, it is important to attempt to identify the underlying cause and treat it. If no cause can be identified, anyone who loses consciousness should be transported to an appropriate emergency department and evaluated. Field management of the syncopal patient generally includes the following procedures:

- Assure scene safety.
- Establish and maintain an adequate airway.
- Administer high-flow oxygen and assist ventilations when required.
- Check circulatory status (heart rate, blood pressure, cardiac rhythm).

- Check and continuously monitor mental status.
- Start an IV of normal saline or lactated Ringer's at a keep-open rate.
- Determine the blood glucose level.
- Monitor the cardiac rhythm.
- Reassure the patient.
- Transport the patient to an emergency department.

HEADACHE

Headache can seriously disrupt a person's life. Nearly 45 million Americans suffer from chronic headaches. Of these, approximately 17 million suffer migraine headaches. An estimated 4 billion dollars is spent annually on over-the-counter pain relievers for headache.

Headache pain can be acute (sudden onset) or chronic (constant or recurring), generalized (all over) or localized (in one specific area) and can range from mild to severe. In some cases the cause is known. In others it is not. The most common types of headache can be classified into three categories:

- *Vascular.* Vascular headaches include migraines and cluster headaches. *Migraines* can last from several minutes to several days. They can be characterized by an intense or throbbing pain, photosensitivity (sensitivity to light), nausea, vomiting, and sweats. Migraines are frequently unilateral (on one side of the head) and may be preceded by an aura. *Cluster* headaches usually occur as a series of one-sided headaches that are sudden, intense, and may continue for 15 minutes to 4 hours. Symptoms may include nasal congestion, drooping eyelid, and an irritated or watery eye. Migraines occur more commonly in women, while cluster headaches generally occur in men.
- *Tension.* A significant percentage of headaches are tension headaches. Most personnel in the emergency medical field have, at one time or another, suffered from a tension headache. Sometimes such headaches occur on a daily basis. Sufferers often awake in the morning with a mild headache that gets worse during the course of the day. The tension headache produces a dull, achy pain that feels like a forceful pressure is being applied to the neck and/or head.
- *Organic.* A third, less common category includes organically caused headaches. They occur in individuals suffering from tumors, infection, or other diseases of the brain, eye, or other body system.

A continuous throbbing headache (often predominantly over the occiput) with fever, confusion, and nuchal rigidity (stiffness of the neck) are classic signs and symptoms of *meningitis.* Be alert for these features while assessing patients complaining of headache, particularly those who have also been complaining of nausea, vomiting, or rash. Chapter 11 provides further discussion on meningitis and other infectious diseases.

Assessment

In addition to pain, those suffering from a headache of any type may also complain of nausea, vomiting, blurred vision, dizziness, weakness, or watery eyes. A complete and thorough history of the patient's headache is crucial to its treatment. Determine as much as you can about the pain, including:

- What was the patient doing during the onset of pain?
- Does anything provoke, or worsen, the pain (light, sound, or movement)?

When assessing a patient complaining of headache, ascertain any associated signs and symptoms, such as nausea, vomiting, blurred vision, dizziness, weakness, or watery eyes.

- What is the quality of the pain? (Is it throbbing? crushing? tension?)
- Does the pain radiate to the neck, arm, back, or jaw?
- What is the severity of the pain (On a scale of 1–10, how does the patient rate the pain?)
- How long has the headache been present? (acute vs. chronic?)

Headache of acute onset or of a changing pattern demands immediate attention. A sudden onset of pain, description of the pain as "the worst headache in my life," or changes in the pattern of pain should all be considered characteristics of potential serious conditions, such as intracranial hemorrhage.

Management

Treatment for a victim of headache is supportive. Field management of the headache patient generally includes the following:

- Assure scene safety.
- Establish and maintain an adequate airway.
- Place the patient in a position of comfort. Patients will often place themselves in a position that best alleviates the symptoms, such as lying flat in a dark room.
- Administer high-flow oxygen and assist ventilations when required.
- Start an IV of normal saline or lactated Ringer's at a keep-open rate.
- Determine the blood glucose level.
- Monitor the cardiac rhythm.
- Reassure the patient.
- Consider antiemetics or pain control measures. Migraine headaches typically are accompanied by nausea and vomiting. Antiemetic medications, such as prochlorperazine (Compazine), have proven extremely effective in terminating migraine headaches as well as the accompanying nausea and vomiting. The current pharmacological approach to migraines first includes abortive agents such as sumatriptan (Imitrix) and prochlorperazine (Compazine). If these agents fail, then small doses of analgesics should be considered.
- Ensure a calm, quiet environment. Dimming the interior ambulance lights will help comfort the headache patient with photosensitivity.
- Transport the patient to an emergency department.

"WEAK AND DIZZY"

A frequent problem that paramedics encounter is the patient who is "weak and dizzy" or "weak all over." Generalized weakness and dizziness, although vague, can be symptoms of many diseases. Furthermore, the feeling of being weak or the feeling of being dizzy can be quite disconcerting, especially to the elderly.

Assessment

Obtain a more detailed history of the illness. Has the patient ever had symptoms like this before? Has he had vomiting and/or diarrhea? Has there been a change in his medication regimen recently or has he taken a new medication in the last 72 hours?

Patients with weakness and/or dizziness should receive a focused assessment including a neurological examination. Be alert for the presence of nystagmus (a constant, involuntary, cyclical motion of the eyeball), which can indicate a CNS or inner ear problem. Assess the various muscle groups to try and determine whether the weakness reported by the patient is localized or diffuse. Be alert for potential causes. These can be neurological, respiratory, cardiovascular, endocrine, or infectious. Many viral illnesses will cause a feeling of malaise in the early stages. Inner ear infections (labyrinthitis) often will cause dizziness, especially with sudden movements of the head. Mild volume depletion (dehydration) can cause both weakness and dizziness. Sometimes the dizzy patient will become nauseated or may actually vomit.

Management

While assessing the patient, provide supportive care. This includes:

- Assure scene safety.
- Establish and maintain an adequate airway.
- Place the patient in a position of comfort, generally with head elevated. Avoid sudden or exaggerated movement of the head as it can exacerbate symptoms.
- Administer high-flow oxygen.
- Start an IV of normal saline or lactated Ringer's at a keep-open rate. Consider a fluid bolus if the patient appears dehydrated.
- Check the blood glucose level.
- Monitor the cardiac rhythm.
- Consider the administration of an antiemetic. Often, antiemetics such as dimenhydrinate (Dramamine, Gravol) are helpful in treating dizziness and nausea. If the patient is nauseated or vomiting, consider promethezine (Phenergan) or prochlorperazine (Compazine).
- Ensure a calm, quiet environment.
- Reassure the patient.
- Transport the patient to an emergency department.

NEOPLASMS

Brain and spinal cord tumors are abnormal growths of tissue found inside the skull or the bony spinal column. The term **neoplasm** is used to describe the new growth of a tumor (as contrasted to those present at birth, known as congenital tumors). Neoplasms that affect the central nervous system occur in 40,000 Americans per year.

* neoplasm literally meaning "new form"; a new or abnormal formation; a tumor.

Neurological neoplasms can be divided into two main categories. *Benign* (non-cancerous) *tumors* are those composed of cells that grow similarly to normal cells, grow relatively slowly, and are confined to one location. *Malignant* (cancerous) *tumors* are those with growth very different from that of normal cells. They grow quickly and spread easily to other sites within the body.

Benign neoplasms in most parts of the body are not particularly harmful. Such tumors within the brain or spinal cord, however, pose a greater threat. Because the nervous system is contained within the rigid confines of the skull and spinal column, abnormal growth can place pressure on tissues and impair function. Any tumor located near any of the vital structures of the brain may seriously threaten the ability to breathe, move, or regulate other bodily functions.

Malignant tumors in most parts of the body have a tendency to spread, or *metastasize*. Most brain tumors are metastases from cancer that started somewhere else in the body. For example, breast cancers often metastasize to the brain. These metastases can grow in a single area of the brain or in several areas. However, tumors that originate in the brain or spinal cord rarely spread to other sites in the body. There are numerous types of brain tumors, which must be diagnosed in a medical facility through the use of CT or MRI scan. The cause of most tumors—and most cancers—remains imcompletely known.

Assessment

Central nervous system neoplasms present with many signs and symptoms. The clinical manifestations a patient exhibits will depend on the size, type, and the location of the tumor. As a paramedic, it is not your role to diagnose such new tumors. Instead, you will likely be called to care for someone with a previously diagnosed tumor. Or, perhaps you will be asked to assess a patient with one or more of these common signs and symptoms of a neoplasm:

- Headache (often severe and recurring frequently)
- New seizures in an adult with no history of a seizure disorder
- Nausea
- Vomiting
- Behavioral or cognitive changes
- Weakness or paralysis of one or more limbs or a side of the face
- Change in sensation of one or more limbs or a side of the face
- Lack of coordination
- Difficulty walking or unsteady gait
- Dizziness
- Double vision

Be alert for any of the classic signs and symptoms of a brain or spinal cord tumor. Obtain a thorough medical history. In addition to the SAMPLE questions, ask about the following:

- What is the state of the patient's general health?
- Has the patient had any seizure activity, headache, or nosebleed?

Ask about the type and timing of prior treatment, such as:

- Surgery for removal of a tumor
- Chemotherapy
- Radiation therapy
- Holistic therapy
- Experimental treatments

Management

Treatment of a patient with a neoplasm is primarily supportive.

Treatment of a patient with a neoplasm is primarily supportive. You should attempt to alleviate the patient's anxiety and to reduce his symptoms. Field management of the patient with a neoplasm generally includes the following:

- Assure scene safety.
- Establish and maintain an adequate airway.
- Place the patient in a position of comfort, generally with head elevated.
- Administer high-flow oxygen and assist ventilations when required.
- Start an IV of normal saline or lactated Ringer's at a keep-open rate or a saline or heparin lock.
- Monitor the cardiac rhythm.
- Consider narcotic analgesia if medical direction approves.

- Consider diazepam if seizure activity is present.
- Anti-inflammatories (dexamethasone) and diuretics may be requested by medical direction.
- Ensure a calm, quiet environment.
- Reassure the patient.
- Transport the patient to an emergency department.

BRAIN ABSCESS

A **brain abscess** is a collection of pus localized in an area of the brain. Brain abscesses are uncommon, accounting for two percent of all intracranial masses. Signs and symptoms are similar to those of a neoplasm and include headache, lethargy, hemiparesis, seizures, nuchal rigidity, nausea, and vomiting. Frequently there is also fever. Paramedic management of a patient with an abscess is supportive and similar to that for a neoplasm or meningitis.

* **brain abscess** a collection of pus localized in an area of the brain.

DEGENERATIVE NEUROLOGICAL DISORDERS

A collection of diseases that selectively affect one or more functional systems of the central nervous system are known as **degenerative neurological disorders.** They generally produce symmetrical and progressive involvement of the central nervous system, affect similar areas of the brain, and produce similar clinical signs and symptoms.

* **degenerative neurological disorders** a collection of diseases that selectively affect one or more functional systems of the central nervous system.

Types of Degenerative Neurological Disorders

Alzheimer's Disease   Alzheimer's disease is perhaps the most important of all the degenerative neurological disorders because of its frequent occurrence and devastating nature. It is the most common cause of dementia in the elderly. Alzheimer's disease results from death and disappearance of nerve cells in the cerebral cortex. This causes marked atrophy of the brain. Initially, patients will have problems with short-term memory. This will usually progress to problems with thought and intellect. The patient will develop a shuffling gait and will have stiffness of the body muscles. As the disease progresses, the patient will develop aphasia (inability to speak) and psychiatric disturbances. In the final stages the patient may become nearly decorticate, losing all ability to think, speak, and move.

* **Alzheimer's disease** a degenerative brain disorder; the most common cause of dementia in the elderly.

Muscular Dystrophy   Muscular dystrophy (MD) refers to a group of genetic diseases characterized by progressive muscle weakness and degeneration of the skeletal or voluntary muscle fibers. The heart and other involuntary muscles, are affected in some types of MD. There are several forms of MD, the most common of which is Duchenne. Some forms begin in childhood while others do not appear until middle age. The prognosis of MD varies depending on the type and progression of the disorder.

* **muscular dystrophy** a group of genetic diseases characterized by progressive muscle weakness and degeneration of the skeletal or voluntary muscle fibers.

Multiple Sclerosis   Multiple sclerosis (MS) refers to an unpredictable disease of the central nervous system. MS involves inflammation of certain nerve cells followed by demyelination, or the destruction of the myelin sheath, which is the fatty insulation surrounding nerve fibers of the brain and spinal cord. When the myelin sheath is damaged, the nerves are unable to properly conduct impulses. An estimated 300,000 to 400,000 Americans are presently diagnosed with MS. Most MS sufferers are women and first experience symptoms between the ages of 20 and 40.

The disease is known to involve an autoimmune attack against myelin. Signs and symptoms include weakness of one or more limbs, sensory loss, paresthesias, and changes in vision. Symptoms can wax and wane over years, and range from mild to severe. Severe cases can be debilitating, rendering a patient unable to care for himself.

* **multiple sclerosis** disease that involves inflammation of certain nerve cells followed by demyelination, or the destruction of the myelin sheath, which is the fatty insulation surrounding nerve fibers.

Dystonias The **dystonias** are a group of disorders characterized by muscle contractions that cause twisting and repetitive movements, abnormal postures, or freezing in the middle of an action. Such movements are involuntary and sometimes painful. They may affect a single muscle, a group of muscles, or the entire body.

Early symptoms of dystonia include a deterioration in handwriting, foot cramps, or a tendency of one foot to drag after walking or running. These initial symptoms can be mild and may be noticeable only after prolonged exertion, stress, or fatigue. In many cases, they become more noticeable and widespread over time. In other individuals, there is little or no progression.

Parkinson's Disease **Parkinson's disease** belongs to a group of conditions known as motor system disorders. James Parkinson, a British physician who published a paper on what he called "the shaking palsy," first described the disease in 1817. In his paper, Dr. Parkinson described the major symptoms of the disease that would later bear his name. Since then, scientists have been searching diligently for a cause and subsequent cure.

In the 1960s, researchers identified that a naturally occurring chemical crucial to muscle activity, dopamine, is lower in victims of Parkinson's. This discovery led to the first successful treatment of the disease.

Today, more than a half million Americans are affected with Parkinson's with more than 50,000 new cases being reported every year. It affects men and women in almost equal numbers and it knows no social, economic, or geographic boundaries. The average age of onset is 60 years and it usually does not occur in patients less than 40 years old.

Parkinson's is a chronic and progressive disorder. It has four main characteristics:

- *Tremor.* Sometimes called "pill rolling," the typical tremor is a rhythmic back-and-forth motion of the thumb and forefinger. It usually begins in the hand and may progress to an arm, a foot, or the jaw.
- *Rigidity.* Most Parkinson's patients suffer rigidity, or resistance to movement. All muscles have an opposing muscle. In the healthy adult, one muscle contracts while the opposing muscle relaxes. In Parkinson's, the balance of this opposition is disturbed, leading to rigidity.
- *Bradykinesia.* Normal, spontaneous, and autonomic movement is slowed and sometimes lost. Such loss of movement is unpredictable. While one moment the patient can move easily, the next moment he cannot.
- *Postural Instability.* Impaired balance and coordination cause patients to develop a forward or backward lean, stooped posture, and the tendency to fall easily.

Victims of Parkinson's may also be plagued with depression, a slowing or "shuffling" gait, a stiff or "stone-like" face, and dementia.

Central Pain Syndrome **Central pain syndrome** is a condition that results from damage or injury to the brain, brainstem, or spinal cord. It is characterized by intense, steady pain described as burning, aching, tingling, or a "pins and needles" sensation. The syndrome may develop weeks, months, or years after an injury to the CNS. It occurs in patients who have had strokes, multiple sclerosis, limb amputations, or spinal cord injuries. Pain medications generally provide no relief for victims of central pain syndrome. Patients rely upon sedation and other methods to keep the central nervous system free from stress.

One type of chronic pain is known as trigeminal neuralgia, or *tic douloureux*. It is caused by abnormal electrical conduction along the trigeminal nerve (cranial nerve V). The condition is characterized by episodes of facial pain that are brief, yet intense. The fear of such an episode is often debilitating. Patients are treated with medications such as the anti-convulsant carbamazepine (Tegretol). In select cases, surgical interventions may be used.

Bell's Palsy Bell's palsy is the most common form of facial paralysis. It results from inflammatory reaction of the facial nerve (cranial nerve VII). The condition affects roughly 40,000 Americans every year. It is characterized by one-sided facial paralysis, the inability to close the eye, pain, tearing of the eyes, drooling, hypersensitivity to sound, and impairment of taste.

Although, the specific cause is often unknown, some causes have been identified. They are head trauma, herpes simplex virus, and Lyme disease. Treatment is usually aimed at protecting the eye. Corticosteroids may be prescribed for inflammation when pain is severe. Most patients recover within three months.

Amyotrophic Lateral Sclerosis Amyotrophic lateral sclerosis (ALS), also known as Lou Gehrig's disease, is a progressive degeneration of specific nerve cells that control voluntary movement. Characterized by weakness, loss of motor control, difficulty speaking, and cramping, the disease eventually weakens the diaphragm, which leads to breathing problems. ALS belongs to a class of disorders known as motor neuron diseases. It affects 20,000 Americans with 5,000 new cases being reported each year.

There is currently no cure for ALS. There is also no effective therapy. However, the FDA has approved riluzole, the first drug that has been shown to prolong the lives of ALS patients. The prognosis continues to be poor. Most patients die within three to five years of being diagnosed usually as a result of pulmonary infection.

Myoclonus Myoclonus is a term that refers to the temporary, involuntary twitching or spasm of a muscle or group of muscles. It is generally considered not a diagnosis but a symptom. It is usually one of several symptoms of a variety of nervous system disorders such as multiple sclerosis, Parkinson's, or Alzheimer's. Some simple examples of myoclonus include hiccups or muscle twitching. Pathologic myoclonus can distort normal movement and limit a person's ability to eat, walk, and talk.

Treatment of myoclonus consists of medications to reduce symptoms. Many of these drugs are also used to treat epilepsy, such as barbiturates, clonazepam, phenytoin, and sodium valproate.

Spina Bifida Spina bifida (SB) is a neural defect that results from the failure of one or more of the fetal vertebrae to close properly during pregnancy. This leaves a portion of the spinal cord unprotected. The spinal opening can usually be repaired shortly after birth, but the nerve damage is permanent. Long term effects include physical and mobility impairments, and most individuals also have some form of learning disability. The three most common types of SB are:

- *Myelomeningocele*—the severest form and one in which the spinal cord and the meninges protrude from an opening in the spine.
- *Meningocele*—characterized by the normal development of the spinal cord, but the meninges protrude through a spinal opening.
- *Occulta*—the mildest form and one in which one or more vertebrae are malformed and covered by a layer of skin.

There is presently no cure for spina bifida. Treatment includes surgery, medications, and physiotherapy. With proper care, most children with SB live into adulthood.

Poliomyelitis Poliomyelitis (polio) is an infectious, inflammatory viral disease of the central nervous system that sometimes results in permanent paralysis. It is characterized by fatigue, headache, fever, vomiting, stiffness of the neck, and pain to the hands and feet. New cases in the United States are rare. A vaccine developed in the 1950s caused the number of cases to decline from 50,000 to only a

---

❋ **Bell's palsy** one-sided facial paralysis with an unknown cause characterized by the inability to close the eye, pain, tearing of the eyes, drooling, hypersensitivity to sound, and impairment of taste.

❋ **amyotrophic lateral sclerosis (ALS)** progressive degeneration of specific nerve cells that control voluntary movement characterized by weakness, loss of motor control, difficulty speaking, and cramping. Also called *Lou Gehrig's disease*.

❋ **myoclonus** temporary, involuntary twitching or spasm of a muscle or group of muscles.

❋ **spina bifida (SB)** a neural defect that results from the failure of one or more of the fetal vertebrae to close properly during the first month of pregnancy.

❋ **poliomyelitis (polio)** infectious, inflammatory viral disease of the central nervous system that sometimes results in permanent paralysis.

few per year. Thousands of pre-vaccine survivors of the disease are alive today. Many of these require supportive care.

Assessment of Degenerative Neurological Disorders

When you encounter a patient with a degenerative neurological disorder, use your assessment and history-taking skills to determine the patient's chief complaint. You may be called to treat someone with an exacerbation (flare up) of one of the degenerative diseases or someone with an unrelated complaint. In either case, it is important to conduct an initial assessment, correct any life-threatening problems, and find out exactly what prompted the call to EMS.

Management of Degenerative Neurological Disorders

When caring for a patient with a degenerative neurological disease, make treating the chief complaint a priority. Do not allow the patient's underlying condition to cloud a more serious problem.

When caring for a patient with a degenerative neurological disease, make treating the chief complaint a priority. Do not overlook the patient's underlying condition, but don't allow it to cloud a more serious problem. After performing an initial assessment and managing any life-threatening conditions, manage the chief complaint. While providing care, consider the following about patients who suffer from a degenerative neurological disorder:

- *Mobility.* The ability to walk and move about freely is often taken for granted by many of us. Neurological patients often lack this ability and require assistance.
- *Communication.* Certain neurological disorders will affect a patient's ability to speak clearly and distinctly. Take the necessary time to ensure open communication. Speak with bystanders and family members to assist in gaining a thorough history.
- *Respiratory Compromise.* Exacerbations of ALS and other conditions may affect the ability to breathe. Treat any breathing problem as a priority.
- *Anxiety.* Coping with a debilitating disease is a strenuous and taxing task. Dealing with the ongoing battles with a neurological condition will cause stress—and anxiety. Approach the patient and his family with compassion and care.

The following steps may be appropriate, depending on the patient's chief complaint:

- Determine the blood glucose level. A serum glucose determination will assist in determining if an altered mental status is due to hypoglycemia.
- Establish an IV of normal saline or lactated Ringer's at a keep-open rate.
- Monitor the cardiac rhythm.
- Transport to an emergency department.

BACK PAIN AND NONTRAUMATIC SPINAL DISORDERS

Back pain is one of the most common reasons people seek health care. Millions and millions of health care dollars are spent each year on the treatment of back pain. Back pain can be classified as either traumatic or non-traumatic in origin. Many patients will develop chronic back pain. Chronic back pain is a significant cause of disability and lost time from work. EMS is occasionally called to treat persons with back pain. These calls can be due to a new injury or exacerbation of chronic back pain. In addition, some patients will develop back pain without an identifiable injury.

Low Back Pain

Back pain can be felt anywhere along the spinal column. However, low back pain (LBP) is the most common back-pain complaint. It is a common, yet debilitating condition. Low back pain is defined as back pain felt between the lower rib cage and the gluteal muscles, often radiating to the thighs.

Both chronic and new-onset low back pain are increasingly common. This complaint of low back pain is the cause of great amount of lost work time in the United States. Between 60 and 90 percent of the population experience some form of low back pain at some time in their life. Men and women are equally affected, although women over 60 years of age report low back pain symptoms more often, most likely as a result of post-menopausal osteoporosis. Occupations that involve exposure to vibrations from vehicles or machinery and those that require repetitious lifting are often implicated in low back pain. As a paramedic, you yourself are particularly at risk for back problems.

About one percent of acute low back pain results from sciatica, which causes severe pain along the path of the sciatic nerve, down the back of the thigh and inner leg. This is sometimes accompanied by motor and sensory deficits such as muscle weakness. Sciatica may be caused by compression or trauma to the sciatic nerve or its roots, often resulting from a herniated intervertebral disk or osteoarthrosis of the lumbosacral vertebrae. It may also be caused by inflammation of the sciatic nerve from metabolic, toxic, or infectious causes.

Pain occurring at the level of L-3, L-4, L-5, and S-1 may be due to inflammation of the interspinous bursae. Low back pain may also result from inflammation or sprains or strains of the muscles and ligaments that attach to the spine or from vertebral fractures. Additional causes of back pain include tumors, inflammation of the synovial sacs, rising venous pressure, degenerative joint disease, abnormal bone pressure, problems with spinal mobility, and inflammation caused by infection (osteomyelitis).

In fact, however, most low back pain is idiopathic. That is, the cause may be difficult or impossible to diagnose, even by a physician or in a hospital setting. This makes treatment of many cases of low back pain frustrating and sometimes unsuccessful.

Causes of Nontraumatic Spinal Disorders and Back Pain

Spinal problems may be caused by trauma, but many spinal disorders have nontraumatic causes. Nontraumatic spinal injuries most often result from three causes:

- Degeneration or rupture of the disks that separate the vertebrae
- Degeneration or fracture of the vertebrae
- Cyst or tumor that impinges on the spine

The type and degree of pain that results from these conditions differs from person to person.

Disk Injury The cartilaginous disks that separate the vertebrae may rupture as a result of injury or may rupture or degenerate as part of the process of aging. Degeneration may cause a narrowing of the disk that compromises spinal stability. Degenerative disk disease is more common in patients over 50 years of age.

A herniated disk occurs when the gelatinous center of the disk (the *nucleus pulposa*) extrudes through a tear in the tough outer capsule (the *anulus fibrosa*). The pain that results from these conditions usually results from pressure on the spinal cord or muscle spasm at the site. The intervetebral disks themselves have no innervation. Herniation may be caused by degenerative disk disease, by trauma, or by improper lifting. Improper lifting is the most common cause. Men aged 30 to 50 years are more prone to disk herniation than women. Herniation most commonly affects the disks at L-4, L-5, and S-1 but may also occur in C-5, C-6, and C-7.

Vertebral Injury The vertebrae themselves may break down (vertebral spondylolysis), especially the lamina or vertebral arch between the articulating facets (the areas where adjoining vertebrae contact one another). Heredity is thought to be a significant factor in the development of spondylolysis. Rotational fractures are common at these sites. Spinal fractures are frequently associated with osteoporosis (brittle bones), which tends to develop in many elderly persons.

Cysts and Tumors A cyst or tumor along the spine or intruding into the spinal canal may cause pain by pressing on the spinal cord, by causing degenerative changes in the bone, or by interrupting blood supply. The specific manifestations depend on the location and the type of the cyst or tumor.

Other Medical Causes Back pain can also be caused by medical conditions associated with neither traumatic nor nontraumatic spinal injury. For example, back pain may manifest as referred pain from disorders such as diabetic neuropathy, renal calculus, abdominal aortic aneurysm, and many other conditions such as those discussed in this chapter. It would be a mistake to assume that all back complaints are related to the spinal cord, the vertebrae, the intervetebral disks, or the muscles and ligaments surrounding the vertebrae.

Assessment

Assessment of back pain is based on the patient's chief complaint, the history, and the physical exam. When the complaint is low back pain, a precise diagnosis is likely to be difficult. Preliminary diagnosis may be based on a history of risk factors, such as an occupation requiring repetitive lifting, exposure to vibrations from vehicles or industrial machinery, or a known history of osteoporosis.

The complaint of low back pain often involves radiation of the pain from the gluteus to the thigh, leg, and foot. Usually there is history of slow onset over several weeks to months and the patient has called for your help secondary to an increase in pain and the lack of relief from warm compresses or over-the-counter analgesics. The patient may or may not recall a particular incident that has caused this "low back pain;" direct trauma is very rarely a contributing factor in this type of pain.

Just because low back pain is a common complaint that can be hard to diagnose, do not dismiss this type of complaint as "not real pain." A complete history and physical exam by a physician are necessary to determine the cause of any back pain. Diagnosis will often depend on the results of a CT or MRI scan, electromyelography, or other in-hospital testing.

In the prehospital setting, the important task is to determine if the patient's pain is caused by a life-threatening or a non-life-threatening condition. A good patient history will help in this determination. A history of work or play involving lifting or twisting and a sudden onset of pain, often associated with straining, coughing, or sneezing, may point to a mechanical type of muscle or ligament injury. A gradual onset of pain may point instead to a chronic condition such as degenerative disk disease or tumor development. The presence of associated neurological deficit may also point to a more serious underlying cause. When the complaint is back pain, be sure to inquire about prior back surgery, physical therapy, and time lost from work.

Location of the injury may be revealed by a limited range of motion in the lumbar spine, tenderness on palpation at the location of the injury, alterations in sensation, pain, and temperature at the site, pain or paresthesia below the injury (in the upper extremities with cervical injury, symptoms increasing with neck motion, with possible slight motor weakness in the biceps and triceps; similar symptoms in the lower extremities with injury to the thoracic or lumbar spine).

Keep in mind that you are very unlikely to be able to determine the cause of your patient's back pain in the field. Primarily, you need to gather information from the history and physical exam that you will report to the receiving physician and that will help you determine what degree of immobilization, if any, will be necessary during transport.

Management

Prehospital management of back pain is primarily aimed at decreasing any pain or discomfort caused by moving the patient and keeping a watchful eye for signs and symptoms of any serious underlying disorder.

Should C-spine precautions be taken with the patient complaining of back pain? Should this patient be immobilized to a long back board or a vacuum-type stretcher? These questions are best answered, "It depends." First you must consider trauma as a possible cause of the patient's pain. If there is no recent mechanism of injury, consider whether the patient has a possible history of osteoporosis or another disease that might lead to spinal fracture. In these cases, consider immobilizing the patient.

If trauma and possible fracture are ruled out, you may still undertake C-spine precautions and immobilization, because the less movement a patient is put through the more comfortable he will feel. Long-board or vacuum-stretcher immobilization may be the best mode of transportation. If in doubt, immobilize, remembering the injunction to "do no harm."

Some patients with back pain and back spasms may require parenteral analgesics and parenteral diazepam before they can even lie on the stretcher. Contact medical direction regarding analgesic and muscle relaxant therapy.

Conduct ongoing assessment en route with special attention to the airway, breathing, vital signs, and the possible presence or development of motor and sensory deficits that may indicate a critical condition and that can adversely affect the patient's breathing effort.

Prehospital management of back pain is primarily aimed at decreasing pain and discomfort. Follow local protocols regarding immobilization of a patient with back pain.

Summary

Nervous system emergencies include a complex variety of illnesses and injuries. A thorough patient assessment and medical history will help guide your care and will prove invaluable for subsequent hospital management.

Initial field management is directed at ensuring an adequate airway and ventilation. The brain requires a constant supply of oxygen, glucose, and vitamins. After 10–20 seconds without blood flow, the patient becomes unconscious. Significant loss of oxygen (anoxia) or low blood sugar (hypoglycemia) can cause coma or seizures. Supply high-flow oxygen to patients with neurological disorders. Administer dextrose to any neurological patient with hypoglycemia.

Neurological injuries and illnesses often require treatment as soon as possible to prevent progressive damage. Patients suffering from an altered level of consciousness, stroke (brain attack), transient ischemic attack, seizures, and syncope require early intervention and transportation to the closest appropriate facility.

You will also be called to care for patients suffering from a headache, neoplasm, a degenerative neurological disorder, or a complaint of back pain. These conditions may be relatively minor, or indicative of a much more serious underlying condition. They too require a complete patient assessment, medical history, and supportive care.

Care for the neurological patient may simply be supportive. In other cases, you should provide drug therapy or other interventions to limit or reduce the presenting symptoms. Airway management remains a priority in caring for any patient with an alteration in neurological function.

CHAPTER 30

Endocrinology

Objectives

After reading this chapter, you should be able to:

1. Describe the incidence, morbidity, and mortality of endocrinologic emergencies. (pp. 1380–1381, 1383–1384, 1388–1389)

2. Identify the risk factors that predispose a person to endocrinologic disease. (pp. 1383, 1388–1389, 1392, 1393)

3. Discuss the anatomy and physiology of the endocrine system. (see Chapter 3)

4. Discuss the pathophysiology, assessment findings, need for rapid intervention and transport, and management of endocrinologic emergencies. (pp. 1380–1393)

5. Describe osmotic diuresis and its relationship to diabetes mellitus. (p. 1383)

6. Describe the pathophysiology of adult and juvenile onset diabetes mellitus. (pp. 1383–1384)

7. Differentiate between the pathophysiology of normal glucose metabolism and diabetic glucose metabolism. (pp. 1381–1383)

8. Describe the mechanism of ketone body formation and its relationship to ketoacidosis. (pp. 1382, 1384–1386)

Continued

INTRODUCTION

The *endocrine system* is an important body system that includes eight major glands (Table 30-1). Closely linked to the nervous system, it controls numerous physiological processes. Unlike the nervous system, which exerts its control through nervous impulses, the endocrine system controls the body through specialized chemical messengers called **hormones.** The fundamental structural units of the endocrine system are the **endocrine glands.** Each endocrine gland produces one or more hormones. (An example of an endocrine gland is the pancreas.) The endocrine glands are the chief focus of this chapter.

Endocrine glands differ from other glands in that they are ductless. Instead of releasing hormones through ducts to a local site, they secrete their hormones directly into capillaries to circulate in the blood throughout the body. In contrast, the majority of glands are **exocrine glands,** which release their chemical products through ducts and tend to have a local effect. For example, the salivary glands are a type of exocrine gland. The salivary glands are located near the pharynx and secrete digestive enzymes, such as amylase, into the pharynx.

Keep in mind these important points about endocrine glands:

- In contrast to the exocrine glands, whose effects tend to be localized, endocrine glands tend to have widespread effects.

✱ **hormone** chemical substance released by a gland that controls or affects processes in other glands or body systems.

✱ **endocrine gland** gland that secretes chemical substances directly into the blood; also called a *ductless gland.*

✱ **exocrine gland** gland that secretes chemical substances to nearby tissues through a duct; also called a *ducted gland.*

The effects of exocrine glands tend to be localized, while the effects of endocrine glands tend to be widespread.

Table 30-1	THE MAJOR ENDOCRINE GLANDS	
Hypothalamus	Thymus
Pituitary	Pancreas
Thyroid	Adrenals
Parathyroid	Gonads

- The hormones released by endocrine glands typically act on distant tissues. They exert a very specific effect on their target tissues.
- Some hormones, such as insulin, have many target organs. Other hormones have only a few target organs.
- Through the release of hormones, the endocrine system plays an important role in regulating body function.

As noted above, the principal product of an endocrine gland is a hormone. The term *hormone* comes from the Greek for "to set in motion," and hormones keep in motion, or regulate, numerous vital cell processes. For example, the hormones insulin and glucagon enable the body to maintain a stable blood glucose level, both after and between meals. This is an example of **homeostasis,** the natural tendency of the body to maintain an appropriate internal environment in the face of changing external conditions. Hormones such as growth hormone and thyroid hormone regulate **metabolism.** Metabolism encompasses all the cellular processes that produce the energy and molecules needed for growth or repair. In addition, hormones such as estrogen and testosterone regulate the sexual development of puberty and the subsequent reproductive function of adulthood.

Many people have endocrine disorders involving excessive or deficient hormone function. Some common conditions, such as hypothyroidism, are readily controlled by hormone replacement medication. Other hormonal disorders may have a more difficult course. You will find that the hormonal disorder diabetes mellitus is commonly involved in medical emergencies encountered in the prehospital setting.

ENDOCRINE DISORDERS AND EMERGENCIES

The most common endocrine emergencies you should expect to treat will involve complications of diabetes mellitus. This section explains the pathophysiology of diabetes and its complications, including ketoacidosis and hypoglycemia, as a basis for discussion of field management. In addition, the section covers endocrine emergencies involving disorders of the thyroid and adrenal glands.

DISORDERS OF THE PANCREAS

Diabetes Mellitus

The disease **diabetes mellitus** is marked by inadequate insulin activity in the body. As noted earlier, insulin is critical to maintaining normal blood glucose levels. Glucose is important for all cells, but it is especially important for brain cells. In fact, glucose is the *only* substance that brain cells can readily and efficiently use as an energy source. In addition, insulin enables the body to store energy as glycogen, protein, and fat.

Diabetes mellitus, or sugar diabetes, is not only a serious disease but also a common and ancient one. Over 8 million Americans have been diagnosed with diabetes,

* **homeostasis** the natural tendency of the body to keep the internal environment and metabolism steady and normal.

* **metabolism** the sum of cellular processes that produce the energy and molecules needed for growth and repair.

* **diabetes mellitus** disorder of inadequate insulin activity, due either to inadequate production of insulin or to decreased responsiveness of body cells to insulin.

and U.S. health experts believe nearly the same number of Americans may be living with undiagnosed diabetes. The disease was named in ancient times by Greek physicians who noted that affected persons produced large volumes of urine that attracted bees and other insects, hence diabetes (meaning "to syphon," or "to pass through") for excessive urine production and mellitus (meaning "honey sweet") for the presence of sugar in the urine. If you remember that mellitus means sweet and insipidus means neutral, you will remember the common trait and the major distinctions in the presentations of untreated diabetes insipidus and diabetes mellitus.

Before presenting pathophysiology, we will examine in detail the normal body handling of glucose. The discussion of glucose metabolism will focus on events at the molecular and cellular level, whereas the discussion on regulation of blood glucose will focus on events in the blood and in major target tissues such as liver, fat cells, and kidneys.

Glucose Metabolism You learned in the chapter introduction that metabolism is the sum of the processes that produce the energy and molecules needed for cell growth or repair. The word *metabolism* comes from the Greek for "to change." Two kinds of change take place within a cell. One kind builds complex molecules from simpler ones. The synthesis of glycogen from glucose is an example. The other kind breaks down complex molecules into simpler ones. The breakdown of glucose into carbon dioxide, water, and energy (in the form of adenosine triphosphate, or ATP) is an example.

The building processes within a cell are collectively called **anabolism.** The prefix *ana-* comes from the Greek for "up," and anabolic pathways build molecules of higher complexity. Breakdown processes are collectively called **catabolism.** The prefix *cata-* comes from the Greek for "down," and catabolic pathways produce molecules of lower complexity. Anabolic pathways usually require energy to drive them, and catabolic pathways often release energy as part of the process. In other words, anabolic activity uses energy while catabolic activity produces energy.

Look at the summary of effects of insulin and glucagon in Table 30-2. When materials are abundant after meals and blood glucose is high, insulin enables cells to use glucose directly and to store energy as glycogen, protein, and fat. Insulin stimulates anabolic pathways. In contrast, glucagon is the dominant hormone during periods of low blood glucose. It stimulates catabolic pathways to produce usable energy from the body's stores.

In order for anabolic pathways to proceed, insulin must first exert its stimulatory effects. Insulin acts by binding to receptors in the outer cell membrane. These receptors are proteins whose structure reacts specifically with insulin. When insulin is bound to a receptor, it changes the permeability of the membrane

✱ **anabolism** the constructive or "building up" phase of metabolism.

✱ **catabolism** the destructive or "breaking down" phase of metabolism.

Table 30-2	SUMMARY OF GLUCOSE METABOLISM

Hormonal Effects of Insulin and Glucagon

Insulin	Glucagon
Dominant hormone when blood glucose level is high	Dominant hormone when blood glucose level is low
Major Effects on Target Tissues	*Major Effects on Target Tissues*
all cells: ↑ uptake glucose	
liver: ↑ production of glycogen, protein, fat	liver: ↑ glycogenolysis → glucose
liver, fat: ↑ production of fats	liver: ↑ gluconeogenesis (protein, fat → glucose)

such that glucose enters the cell far more readily. The rate at which glucose can be transported into cells can be increased tenfold or more by the action of insulin. Without insulin activity, the amount of glucose that can enter cells is far too small to meet average body energy demands. Note the two requirements for insulin effectiveness:

1. There must be sufficient insulin circulating in the bloodstream to satisfy cellular needs.
2. Insulin must be able to bind to body cells in such a way that adequate levels of stimulation occur.

The importance of these two requirements will become clear when you learn about the two types of diabetes mellitus.

Sometimes the body cannot use glucose as a primary energy source. In diabetes, this occurs when insufficient insulin activity exists for blood glucose to be taken in and used by cells. Other conditions, such as a high-fat, low-carbohydrate diet or starvation (which can occur in conjunction with some eating disorders) cause depletion of body stores of carbohydrate. Under any of these conditions, the body slowly switches from glucose to fat as the primary energy source. Adipose cells break down fats into their component free fatty acids, and the blood concentration of fatty acids rises considerably.

Most of the fatty acid is used directly by body cells as an energy source. Some is taken in by liver cells. In the liver, catabolism of fatty acids produces acetoacetic acid. When more acetoacetic acid is released from the liver than can be used by body cells, it accumulates in the blood along with two closely related substances, acetone and β-hydroxybutyric acid. These three substances are collectively called **ketone bodies,** and their presence in biologically significant quantity in the blood is called **ketosis.** This catabolic state is significant in the context of the emergency condition called diabetic ketoacidosis, or diabetic coma.

Regulation of Blood Glucose Homeostasis of blood glucose is remarkably effective. If you draw venous blood samples from a group of healthy persons, you'll find that fasting blood glucose (generally done after an overnight fast) is usually between 80 to 90 mg glucose/dL blood. In the first hour or so after a meal, blood glucose may increase to about 120 to 140 mg/dL before falling toward the fasting, or baseline, level. The principal tissues involved in homeostasis are the alpha and beta tissues of the islets of Langerhans (producing glucagon and insulin, respectively) and the liver—as shown in Table 30-2. Liver disease, even in the presence of normal pancreatic function, can cause significant disturbances in glucose homeostasis.

A blood glucose level lower than baseline (often defined as less than 80 mg/dL) reflects **hypoglycemia,** or low blood sugar. Similarly, a blood glucose level higher than that expected shortly after a meal (often defined as greater than 140 mg/dL when drawn in a setting other than directly following a meal) reflects **hyperglycemia,** or high blood sugar. Both terms indicate the blood glucose level only, not the cause of the abnormality.

The last factor to consider in discussing regulation of blood glucose is the role of the kidneys. When blood is filtered through the glomeruli of the kidneys, glucose, along with water and many other small molecules, passes from the blood into the proximal tubule. Water, glucose, and other useful materials are then reabsorbed, while waste products that are not reabsorbed become part of the urine, which will be excreted from the body. The amount of glucose that is reabsorbed depends on the blood level of glucose that already exists. Reabsorption of glucose is essentially complete at blood glucose levels up to about 180 mg/dL. Above that level, glucose begins to be lost in urine.

* **ketone bodies** compounds produced during the catabolism of fatty acids, including acetoacetic acid, β-hydroxybutyric acid, and acetone.

* **ketosis** the presence of significant quantities of ketone bodies in the blood.

* **hypoglycemia** deficiency of blood glucose. Sometimes called *insulin shock*. Hypoglycemia is a medical emergency.

* **hyperglycemia** excessive blood glucose.

Glucose loss in urine can lead to dehydration, which has its physiologic basis in osmosis. Osmosis is the tendency of water molecules to migrate across a semipermeable membrane such that the concentrations of particles approach equivalence on both sides. Our example is the cell membranes that form the boundaries between the tubules of the kidney and the capillaries that surround them.

When glucose spills into urine, the osmotic pressure, or concentration of particulates, rises inside the kidney tubule to a level higher than that of the blood. Water follows glucose into urine to cause a marked water loss termed **osmotic diuresis**, which is the basis of the excessive urination characteristic of untreated diabetes. The term **diuresis** alone refers to increased formation and secretion of urine. The presence of glucose in urine, **glycosuria**, creates the sweet urine that added *mellitus* to *diabetes*.

Last, you should note that whenever the flow rate of fluid inside the kidney tubules rises, as in osmotic diuresis, an increase in excretion of potassium occurs. This leads to the potential for significant hypokalemia and its effects, including cardiac dysrhythmias.

Type I Diabetes Mellitus When we discussed the elements essential to normal insulin activity, the first was the presence of adequate amounts of insulin in the body. *Type I diabetes mellitus* is characterized by very low production of insulin by the pancreas. In many cases, no insulin is produced at all. Type I diabetes is commonly called juvenile-onset diabetes because of the average age at diagnosis. The term *insulin-dependent diabetes mellitus (IDDM)* is also used because patients require regular insulin injections to maintain glucose homeostasis. This type of diabetes is less common than is Type II diabetes, but it is more serious. Diabetes is regularly among the ten leading causes of death in the United States, and Type I diabetes accounts for most diabetes-related deaths.

Heredity is an important factor in determining which persons will be predisposed to development of Type I diabetes. The cause of Type I diabetes is often unclear. However, viral infection, production of autoantibodies directed against beta cells, and genetically determined early deterioration of beta cells are all possible. The immediate cause of the disease is destruction of beta cells.

In untreated Type I diabetes, blood glucose levels rise because, without adequate insulin, cells cannot take up the circulating sugar. Hyperglycemia in the range of 300 to 500 mg/dL is not uncommon. As glucose spills into urine, large amounts of water are lost, too, through osmotic diuresis. Catabolism of fat becomes significant as the body switches to fatty acids as the primary energy source. Overall, this pathophysiology accounts for the constant thirst (polydipsia), excessive urination (polyuria), ravenous appetite (polyphagia), weakness, and weight loss associated with untreated Type I diabetes. Ketosis can occur as the result of fat catabolism, and it may proceed to frank diabetic ketoacidosis, a medical emergency that you will encounter in the field and that will be discussed later in this chapter.

Type II Diabetes Mellitus The second requirement for proper insulin activity is insulin binding such that adequate stimulation of cells occurs. Type II diabetes mellitus is associated with a moderate decline in insulin production accompanied by a markedly deficient response to the insulin that is present in the body. Type II diabetes is also called adult-onset diabetes or *non-insulin-dependent diabetes mellitus (NIDDM)*.

Heredity may play a role in predisposition. In addition, obese persons are more likely to develop Type II diabetes, and obesity probably plays a role in development of the disease. Increased weight (and increased size of fat cells) causes a relative deficiency in the number of insulin receptors per cell, which makes fat cells less responsive to insulin. This type of diabetes is far more common than is

* **osmotic diuresis** greatly increased urination and dehydration that results when high levels of glucose cannot be reabsorbed into the blood from the kidney tubules and the osmotic pressure of the glucose in the tubules also prevents water reabsorption.

* **diuresis** formation and secretion of large amounts of urine.

* **glycosuria** glucose in urine, which occurs when blood glucose levels exceed the kidney's ability to reabsorb glucose.

Content Review

SYMPTOMS OF UNTREATED DIABETES MELLITUS
Polydipsia
Polyuria
Polyphagia
Weakness
Weight loss

Type I diabetes, accounting for about 90 percent of cases of diabetes mellitus. It is also less serious.

Untreated Type II diabetes typically presents with a lower level of hyperglycemia and fewer major signs of metabolic disruption. For instance, glucose use is usually sufficient to keep the body from switching to fats as the primary energy source. Thus, diabetic ketoacidosis is uncommon in these patients. However, a complication called hyperglycemic hyperosmolar nonketotic coma can occur, and you may see it as a medical emergency. It is discussed later in this chapter.

Medical treatment of Type II diabetes is less intensive than that required for Type I diabetes. Initial therapy often consists of dietary change and increased exercise in an attempt to improve body weight. If nonpharmacological therapy is insufficient to bring blood glucose levels down to the normal range, oral hypoglycemic agents may be prescribed. These drugs stimulate insulin secretion by beta cells and promote an increase in the number of insulin receptors per cell. In some cases, however, control may eventually require use of insulin.

* **diabetic ketoacidosis** complication of Type I diabetes due to decreased insulin intake. Marked by high blood glucose, metabolic acidosis, and, in advanced stages, coma. Ketoacidosis is often called diabetic coma.

Diabetic Ketoacidosis (Diabetic Coma)

Diabetic ketoacidosis is a serious, potentially life-threatening complication associated with Type I diabetes. It occurs when there is profound insulin deficiency coupled with increased glucagon activity. It may occur as the initial presentation of severe diabetes, as a result of patient noncompliance with insulin injections, or as the result of physiologic stress such as surgery or serious infection. Some of the major characteristics of diabetic ketoacidosis are listed in Tables 30-3 and 30-4.

Table 30-3 DIABETIC EMERGENCIES

Diabetic Ketoacidosis	Hyperglycemic Hyperosmolar Nonketotic (HHNK) Acidosis	Hypoglycemia
Common Causes	**Common Causes**	**Common Causes**
Cessation of insulin injections	Physiologic stress (such as infection or stroke) producing hyperglycemia and a noncompensated diuresis, modulated by both insulin and glucagon activity	Excessive administration of insulin
Physiologic stress (such as infection or surgery) that causes release of catecholamines, potentiating glucagon effects and blocking insulin effects		Excess insulin for dietary intake
		Overexertion, resulting in lowered blood glucose level
Signs and Symptoms	**Signs and Symptoms**	**Signs and Symptoms**
Polyuria, polydipsia, polyphagia	Polyuria, polydipsia, polyphagia	Weak, rapid pulse
Warm, dry skin and mucous membranes	Warm, dry skin and mucous membranes	Cold, clammy skin
Nausea/vomiting	Orthostatic hypotension	Weakness, uncoordination
Abdominal pain	Tachycardia	Headache
Tachycardia	Decreased mental function or frank coma	Irritable, agitated behavior
Deep, rapid respirations (Kussmaul's respirations)		Decreased mental function or bizarre behavior
Fruity odor on breath		Coma (severe cases)
Fever (if associated with infection)		
Decreased mental function or frank coma		
Management	**Management**	**Management**
Fluids, insulin as directed	Fluids, insulin as directed	Dextrose

Table 30-4 DIAGNOSTIC SIGNS BY SYSTEM FOR DIABETIC EMERGENCIES

System	Diabetic Emergency		
	Diabetic Ketoacidosis	*HHNK Coma*	*Hypoglycemia*
Cardiovascular			
Pulse	Rapid	Rapid	Normal
Blood Pressure	Low	Normal to Low (may be affected by position, or orthostatic)	Normal
Respiratory			
Respiration rate	Exaggerated air hunger	Normal, unlabored	Normal or shallow
Breath odor	Acetone (sweet fruity)	None	None
Nervous			
Headache	Absent	None	Present
Mental state	Restlessness/ unconsciousness	Lethargy/ unconsciousness	Apathy, irritability/ unconsciousness
Tremors	Absent	Absent	Present
Convulsions	None	Possible	In late stages
Gastrointestinal			
Mouth	Dry	Dry	Drooling
Thirst	Intense	Excessive	Absent
Vomiting	Common	Common	Uncommon
Abdominal pain	Frequent	Common	Absent
Ocular			
Vision	Dim	Normal	Double vision (diplopia)

Pathophysiology Reread the discussion of ketosis in the prior section on Glucose Metabolism. Diabetic ketoacidosis reflects amplification of the same physiologic mechanisms as ketosis.

In the initial phase of diabetic ketoacidosis, profound hyperglycemia exists because of lack of insulin. Body cells cannot take in glucose. The compensatory mechanism for low glucose levels within cells, gluconeogenesis, only contributes more blood glucose. The consequent loss of glucose in the urine, accompanied by loss of water through osmotic diuresis, produces significant dehydration.

As the body switches to fat-based metabolism, the blood level of ketones rises. The ketone load accounts for the observed acidosis. By the time the characteristic decrease in pH from about 7.4 to about 6.9 has occurred, the patient is hours from death if left untreated.

Signs and Symptoms The onset of clinically obvious diabetic ketoacidosis is slow, lasting from 12 to 24 hours. In the initial phase, signs of diuresis appear, including increased urine production and dry, warm skin and mucous membranes. The individual often has excessive hunger and thirst, coupled with a progressive sense of general malaise. Volume depletion induces tachycardia and feelings of physical weakness.

As ketoacidosis develops, a major compensatory mechanism for acidosis appears: the rapid, deep breathing pattern termed *Kussmaul's respirations,* which helps expel carbon dioxide, CO_2, from the body (Figure 30-1). The breath itself may have a fruity or acetone-like smell as some blood acetone is expelled through the lungs. The blood profile not only includes hyperglycemia and acidic pH, but also electrolyte abnormalities. Low bicarbonate levels reflect loss of acid-base buffer via Kussmaul's respirations. Low potassium levels may be

The presence of a sweet, fruity odor on the patient's breath is a hallmark of diabetic ketoacidosis.

FIGURE 30–1   Kussmaul's respirations.

Type of respiration	Diagram	Discussion
Normal		16-20/min; regular in rhythm; ratio of respiratory rate to pulse rate is 1:4
Kussmaul's respiration		Increase in both rate and depth. Associated with diabetic ketoacidosis

found secondary to diuresis, with marked hypokalemia increasing the risk for cardiac dysrhythmias or death. Over time, mental function declines and frank coma may occur. A fever is not characteristic of ketoacidosis. If present, it is a signal of infection.

Assessment and Management The approach used with the patient suffering from diabetic ketoacidosis is essentially the same as with any other patient who has mental impairment or is unconscious. First, complete your initial assessment of airway, breathing, and circulation. Then complete a focused history and physical exam. Look for a Medic-Alert bracelet and/or insulin in the refrigerator. Obtain a history from any bystanders. The sweet, fruity odor of ketones occasionally can be detected in the breath. If possible, complete the rapid test for blood glucose level. It is not uncommon for patients with ketoacidosis to have blood glucose levels well in excess of 300 mg/dL.

Focus field management on maintenance of the ABCs and fluid resuscitation to counteract dehydration. In such cases, draw a red top tube (or the tube specified by local protocols) of blood. Following blood sampling, administer one to two liters of normal saline per protocol. If transport time is lengthy, the medical direction physician may request intravenous or subcutaneous administration of regular insulin.

If the blood glucose level cannot be quickly determined, draw a red top tube of blood for analysis and start an IV of normal saline. Following this, administer 50 ml (25 grams) of 50 percent dextrose solution. The additional glucose load will not adversely affect the ketoacidotic patient because it is negligible compared with the quantity present in the body. If the patient were hypoglycemic, however, the additional glucose might be sufficient to protect brain cells from damage. If the patient is a known alcoholic, consider administering 100 mg of thiamine.

Expedite transport to an appropriate facility for definitive therapy.

Hyperglycemic Hyperosmolar Nonketotic (HHNK) Coma

* **hyperglycemic hyperosmolar nonketotic (HHNK) coma** complication of type II diabetes due to inadequate insulin activity. Marked by high blood glucose, marked dehydration, and decreased mental function. Often mistaken for ketoacidosis.

Hyperglycemic hyperosmolar nonketotic (HHNK) coma is a serious complication associated with Type II diabetes. Typically, both insulin and glucagon activity are present. HHNK coma develops when two conditions occur: Sustained hyperglycemia causes osmotic diuresis sufficient to produce marked dehydration, and water intake is inadequate to replace lost fluids. Dialysis, high-osmolarity feeding supplements, infection, and certain drugs can also be associated with development of HHNK coma. Some characteristics of HHNK coma are listed in Tables 30-3 and 30-4.

Pathophysiology As sustained hyperglycemia develops, glucose spills into the urine, causing osmotic diuresis and resultant dehydration. The level of hyperglycemia is often much higher than the levels seen in ketoacidosis (up to 1000 mg/dL). However, insulin activity in patients with HHNK coma prevents significant production of ketone bodies. Inadequate fluid replacement results in characteristic signs and symptoms.

The mortality rate for HHNK coma is higher than that for ketoacidosis, ranging from 40 to 70 percent. The higher mortality rate may be due to the lack of early signs and symptoms that bring patients with ketoacidosis to the attention of family or health care professionals. The mortality rate of HHNK is also high because it primarily affects the elderly.

Signs and Symptoms The onset of HHNK coma is even slower than that of ketoacidosis, with development often occurring over several days. Early signs include increased urination and increased thirst. Subsequent volume depletion can result in orthostatic hypotension when the patient gets out of bed, along with other signs such as dry skin and mucous membranes as well as tachycardia. The patient may become lethargic, confused, or enter frank coma. Kussmaul's respirations are rarely seen because of the lack of acidosis.

Assessment and Management The approach used with the patient suffering from HHNK coma is essentially the same as with any other patient who has mental impairment or is unconscious. It is often difficult in the field to distinguish diabetic ketoacidosis from HHNK coma. Therefore, the prehospital treatment of both emergencies is identical (see earlier discussion of management of ketoacidosis) and transportation should be expedited.

Hypoglycemia (Insulin Shock)

Hypoglycemia, or low blood glucose, is a medical emergency. It can occur when a patient takes too much insulin, eats too little to match an insulin dose, or overexerts and uses almost all available blood glucose. As the period of hypoglycemia lengthens, the risk rises that brain cells will be permanently damaged or killed due to lack of glucose. You have learned that brain cells can adapt to use fats as an energy source. Note, however, that this adaptation requires hours to develop, and the switch to fat-based metabolism cannot correct any damage already incurred. This is why every second counts in treating hypoglycemia.

Pathophysiology Hypoglycemia, or insulin shock, reflects high insulin and low blood glucose. Regardless of the reason for low blood sugar, insulin causes almost all remaining blood glucose to be taken up by cells. Because of the high level of insulin, glucagon may be ineffective in raising blood glucose levels. In prolonged fasts, almost half the glucose normally produced through gluconeogenesis is of renal origin. This activity is stimulated by epinephrine. Diabetic patients with kidney failure may be predisposed to hypoglycemia because of lack of renal gluconeogenesis.

Signs and Symptoms The signs and symptoms of hypoglycemia are many and varied. Altered mental status is the most important. In the earliest stages of hypoglycemia, the patient may appear restless or impatient or complain of hunger. As blood glucose falls lower, he may display inappropriate anger (even rage) or display a bizarre behavior. Sometimes the patient may be placed in police custody for such behavior or be involved in an automobile accident.

＊ **hypoglycemia** deficiency of blood glucose.

Hypoglycemia is a true medical emergency that requires prompt intervention to prevent permanent brain injury.

Hypoglycemia virtually never occurs outside the setting of diabetes mellitus.

hypoglycemic seizure seizure that occurs when brain cells aren't functioning normally due to low blood glucose.

*All ALS vehicles **must** have the capability of rapidly determining a patient's blood glucose level.*

hyperthyroidism excessive secretion of thyroid hormones resulting in an increased metabolic rate.

thyrotoxicosis condition that reflects prolonged exposure to excess thyroid hormones with resultant changes in body structure and function.

hypothyroidism inadequate secretion of thyroid hormones resulting in a decreased metabolic rate.

myxedema condition that reflects long-term exposure to inadequate levels of thyroid hormones with resultant changes in body structure and function.

Graves' disease endocrine disorder characterized by excess thyroid hormones resulting in body changes associated with increased metabolism; primary cause of *thyrotoxicosis.*

Physical signs may include diaphoresis and tachycardia. If blood glucose falls to a critically low level, the patient may have a **hypoglycemic seizure** or become comatose.

In contrast to diabetic ketoacidosis, hypoglycemia can develop quickly. A clear change in mental status can occur without warning. Always consider hypoglycemia when encountering a patient with bizarre behavior. Review Tables 30-3 and 30-4 for additional information.

Assessment and Management In suspected cases of hypoglycemia, perform the initial assessment quickly. Look for a Medic-Alert bracelet. If possible, determine the blood glucose level. Because of the urgency of this emergency, most paramedic units need to have the capability to perform this task or to rush a blood sample along with the patient.

If the blood glucose level is less that 60 mg/dL, draw a red top tube of blood and start an IV of normal saline. Next, administer 50 to 100 milliliters (25 to 50 grams) of 50 percent dextrose intravenously. If the patient is conscious and able to swallow, complete glucose administration with orange juice, sugared sodas, or commercially available glucose pastes.

If blood glucose cannot be obtained and the patient is unconscious, start an IV of normal saline and administer 50 to 100 milliliters (25 to 50 grams) of 50 percent dextrose. Expedite transport to a medical facility. If you suspect alcoholism, also administer 100 mg of thiamine.

When an IV cannot be started, hypoglycemic patients may improve following the administration of glucagon. This is a much slower process and will only work if there are adequate stores of glycogen available. Glucagon must be reconstituted immediately prior to administration. A dose of 0.5 to 1.0 mg intramuscularly is usually adequate.

DISORDERS OF THE THYROID GLAND

You are more likely to see thyroid dysfunction as part of the medical history than as an emergency. However, you may see patients with acute complications of thyroid disorders. The most common of these are:

- **Hyperthyroidism**—the presence of excess thyroid hormones in the blood.
- **Thyrotoxicosis**—a condition that reflects prolonged exposure of body organs to excess thyroid hormones, with resultant changes in structure and function. Thyrotoxicosis is generally caused by *Graves' disease.*
- **Hypothyroidism**—the presence of inadequate thyroid hormones in the blood.
- **Myxedema**—a condition that reflects long-term exposure to inadequate levels of thyroid hormones, with resultant changes in structure and function.

Graves' Disease

Over 95 percent of cases of thyrotoxicosis are due to **Graves' disease.** Roughly 15 percent of Graves' disease patients have a close relative with Graves', which suggests a strong hereditary role in predisposition to the disorder. In addition,

Graves' disease is about six times more common in women than in men, with onset typically in young adulthood (20s and 30s).

Pathophysiology Graves' disease has an autoimmune origin. Autoantibodies are generated that stimulate thyroid tissue to produce excessive amounts of thyroid hormones. The resultant changes in organ function are either responses to excess thyroid hormones or responses to the autoantibodies themselves.

Signs and Symptoms Signs and symptoms of Graves' disease include agitation, emotional changeability, insomnia, poor heat tolerance, weight loss despite increased appetite, weakness, dyspnea, and tachycardia or new-onset atrial fibrillation in the absence of a cardiac history. Nervous system symptoms tend to be more common in younger adults, whereas serious cardiovascular symptoms tend to predominate in older individuals. Prolonged reaction of orbital tissues with the pathological thyroid-stimulating autoantibodies can cause exophthalmos (protrusion of the eyeballs), whereas interaction of autoantibodies with thyroid tissue often produces diffuse goiter (a generally enlarged thyroid gland) (Figure 30-2).

FIGURE 30-2 Generalized enlargement of the thyroid gland (goiter).

Assessment and Management Cardiac dysfunction is probably the most likely context within which an emergency call may arise from thyrotoxicosis (usually caused by Graves' disease, as noted earlier). Use of β-adrenergic blockers such as propranolol may temporarily reduce cardiac stress, but make sure the patient does not have heart failure before considering use. Glucocorticoid therapy (namely, dexamethasone) is sometimes helpful in quickly reducing the level of circulating T_4.

Thyrotoxic Crisis ("Thyroid Storm")

Thyrotoxic crisis, or "thyroid storm," is a life-threatening emergency that can be fatal within as few as 48 hours if untreated. It is usually associated with severe physiologic stress (e.g., trauma, infection), less often with psychological stress. You may also encounter thyroid storm secondary to overdose of thyroid hormone in a hypothyroid individual.

Pathophysiology The mechanisms underlying thyrotoxic crisis are poorly understood. An acute increase in the levels of thyroid hormones does not appear to be the cause. It is more likely that thyroid storm is caused by a shift of thyroid hormone in the blood from the protein-bound (biologically inactive) to the free (biologically active) state.

Signs and Symptoms The signs and symptoms associated with thyrotoxic crisis reflect the patient's extreme hypermetabolic state and increased activity of the sympathetic nervous system. The syndrome is characterized by high fever (106°F/41°C or higher), irritability, delirium or coma, tachycardia, hypotension, vomiting, and diarrhea. A less severe presentation may also occur, with slight fever and marked lethargy.

Assessment and Management In the presence of the above-mentioned signs and symptoms of thyrotoxic crisis, field management is largely focused on supportive care: oxygenation, ventilatory assistance, fluid resuscitation, and cardiac monitoring. Glucocorticoids and β-adrenergic blockers may be helpful. Transport should be expedited for definitive therapy that blocks the high blood levels of thyroid hormones.

Hypothyroidism and Myxedema

Hypothyroidism can be congenital or acquired. Both sexes can be affected. The recent increase in incidence of hypothyroidism in middle-aged women may reflect better diagnostics, a true rise in incidence, or both. Advanced myxedema in middle-aged and elderly individuals is the condition you are most likely to see as part of a medical emergency, so we will focus most attention on myxedema and the uncommon complication of myxedema coma.

Pathophysiology Hypothyroidism creates a low metabolic state, and early signs reflect poor organ function and poor response to challenges such as exercise or infection. Over time, untreated severe hypothyroidism causes the additional sign of myxedema: a thickening of connective tissue in the skin and other tissues, including the heart. Patients with myxedema may progress into a hypothermic, stuporous state called **myxedema coma,** which can be fatal if respiratory depression occurs. Triggers for progression include infection, trauma, a cold environment, or exposure to central nervous system depressants such as alcohol or certain drugs.

✱ **thyrotoxic crisis** toxic condition characterized by hyperthermia, tachycardia, nervous symptoms, and rapid metabolism; also known as *thyroid storm.*

✱ **myxedema coma** life-threatening condition associated with advanced myxedema, with profound hypothermia, bradycardia, and electrolyte imbalance.

FIGURE 30-3 Doughy, edematous skin typical of myxedema.

Signs and Symptoms Early signs of hypothyroidism may be subtle. Symptoms may be as slight as fatigue and slowed mental function attributed falsely to aging. Typically, patients with hypothyroidism or myxedema show lethargy, cold intolerance, constipation, decreased mental function, or decreased appetite with increased weight. In addition, the relaxation stage of deep tendon reflexes (DTRs) is slowed. The classic appearance of myxedema is an unemotional, puffy face, thinned hair, enlarged tongue, and pale, cool skin that looks and feels like dough (Figure 30-3). Myxedema coma may be difficult to identify. Note if the history is consistent with hypothyroidism, and look for the physical appearance of myxedema. Other signs include profound hypothermia (temperatures as low as 75°F/24°C are not uncommon), low amplitude bradycardia, and carbon dioxide retention.

Assessment and Management The presence of the described signs and symptoms may alert you to the possible presence of myxedema. Keep in mind that heart failure due to the combination of age, atherosclerosis, and myxedematous enlargement is not uncommon, so focus on maintenance of ABCs and close monitoring of cardiac and pulmonary status. Most patients with myxedema coma require intubation and ventilatory assistance. Active rewarming is contraindicated due to risk of cardiac dysrhythmias and cardiovascular collapse secondary to vasodilatation. Although IV access is important, limit fluids because fluid and electrolyte imbalance is common. Expedite transport to an appropriate facility for definitive treatment.

While most patients experiencing myxedema coma require intubation and ventilatory assistance, active rewarming is contraindicated due to risk of cardiac dysrhythmias and cardiovascular collapse secondary to vasodilation.

✳ Cushing's syndrome pathological condition resulting from excess adrenocortical hormones. Symptoms may include changed body habitus, hypertension, vulnerability to infection.

✳ Addison's disease endocrine disorder characterized by adrenocortical insufficiency. Symptoms may include weakness, fatigue, weight loss, hyperpigmentation of skin and mucous membranes.

DISORDERS OF THE ADRENAL GLANDS

Two disorders of the adrenal cortex can play a part in medical emergencies or complicate responses to trauma. **Cushing's syndrome** is caused by excessive adrenocortical activity. In contrast, **Addison's disease** is caused by deficient adrenocortical activity. Reread the earlier section where we discussed the anatomy and physiology of the adrenal glands to remind yourself how critical these hormones are to metabolic processes and to salt and water balance.

Hyperadrenalism (Cushing's Syndrome)

Cushing's syndrome is a relatively common disorder of the adrenals. It usually affects middle-aged persons, with women affected more often than men. Excess cortisol can be due to abnormalities in the anterior pituitary or adrenal cortex. It can also be due to treatment with glucocorticoids, such as prednisone. Check the history to note any steroid treatment for nonendocrine conditions such as COPD, asthma, and cancer or rheumatologic disorders.

Pathophysiology Long-term exposure to excess glucocorticoids, primarily cortisol, produces numerous changes. Metabolically, cortisol is an antagonist to insulin. Gluconeogenesis is prominent, with profound protein catabolism. The body's handling of fats is altered: Atherosclerosis and hypercholesterolemia are common. Over time, diabetes mellitus also may develop. Cortisol's mineralo-corticoid activity causes sodium retention and increased blood volume. Increased vascular sensitivity to catecholamines occurs, and this may also be a contributor to hypertension. Potassium loss through the kidneys may cause hypokalemia. Cortisol's anti-inflammatory and immunosuppressive properties predispose to infection.

Signs and Symptoms Regardless of the cause, the presenting signs and symptoms are the same. The earliest sign is weight gain, particularly through the trunk of the body, face, and neck. A "moon-faced" appearance often develops (Figure 30-4). The accumulation of fat on the upper back is occasionally referred to as a "buffalo hump." Skin changes are also very common and may be an early clue to potential problems. These include thinning to an almost transparent appearance, a tendency to bruise easily, delayed healing from even minor wounds, and development of facial hair among women (hirsutism). Mood swings and impaired memory or concentration are also common.

Assessment and Management Although it is unlikely you will see a patient with acute hyperadrenal crisis, you are likely to encounter patients who exhibit signs and symptoms of Cushing's syndrome. Remember that these patients have a higher incidence of cardiovascular disease, including hypertension and stroke. Pay particular attention to skin preparation when starting IV lines because of skin fragility and susceptibility to infection. Observations indicative of Cushing's syndrome should be noted in your report and relayed to hospital staff.

FIGURE 30-4 Facial features of Cushing's syndrome.

Adrenal Insufficiency (Addison's Disease)

Addison's disease is due to cortical destruction. Addison's has become less common as former leading causes of Addison's, such as tuberculosis, have come under control. Currently, over 90 percent of Addison's disease cases are due to autoimmune disease. As with Graves' disease, another autoimmune disorder, heredity plays a prominent role in predisposition. In fact, patients with Addison's are more likely than average to have other autoimmune disorders, including Graves' disease. Persons with Addison's may be tipped into metabolic failure called **Addisonian crisis** by acute stresses such as infection or trauma.

Pathophysiology Destruction of the adrenal cortex results in minimal production of all three classes of hormones: glucocorticoids, mineralocorticoids, and androgens. Low mineralocorticoid activity is key to the changes of Addison's: It causes major disturbances in water and electrolyte balance. Increased sodium excretion in urine causes low blood volume, and potassium retention can cause hyperkalemia and ECG changes. Many cases of adrenal insufficiency are due to therapy with steroids such as prednisone. Such therapy can completely suppress normal adrenal function. Sudden cessation of the drug may trigger symptoms of Addison's disease or even an Addisonian crisis, with cardiovascular collapse.

Signs and Symptoms Addison's disease is characterized by changes related to low corticosteroid activity: progressive weakness, fatigue, decreased appetite, and weight loss. Hyperpigmentation of the skin and mucous membranes, particularly in sun-exposed areas, is also characteristic. Include Addisonian crisis in your list of possible causes of unexplained cardiovascular collapse, particularly if the history suggests primary Addison's or Addison's secondary to drug therapy. Many patients will have gastrointestinal problems such as vomiting or diarrhea, which will exacerbate electrolyte imbalances, low blood volume, and hypotension and increase the potential for cardiac dysrhythmias.

Assessment and Management The patient may reveal the presence of Addison's disease during the history, or the signs and symptoms just discussed may lead you to suspect the presence of Addison's. Focus emergency management on maintenance of the ABCs and close monitoring of cardiac and oxygenation status as well as blood glucose level. Hypoglycemia poses its own threat. Assess blood glucose levels and administer 25–50 grams of 50% dextrose to patients with blood glucose levels less than 50 mg/dL or those with altered mental status. Obtain a baseline 12-lead ECG to check for dysrhythmias related to electrolyte imbalance. Be aggressive in fluid resuscitation. Follow your local protocol or contact medical direction for specific orders based on your patient's presentation. Expedite transport to an appropriate facility.

 Addisonian crisis form of shock associated with adrenocortical insufficiency and characterized by profound hypotension and electrolyte imbalances.

$\int$UMMARY

In conjunction with the nervous system, the endocrine system regulates body functions. The vast majority of endocrine emergencies involve complications of diabetes mellitus such as hypoglycemia or ketoacidosis. Other endocrine emergencies tend to be rare and will more likely be part of the history rather than the emergency. In the field, you should always suspect diabetes when patients present with unexplained changes in mental status. Hypoglycemia, the most urgent diabetic emergency, must be quickly treated to prevent serious nervous system damage. When the exact type of diabetic emergency is undetermined, treat for hypoglycemia. Treatment of diabetic ketoacidosis is primarily a hospital procedure.

CHAPTER 31

Allergies and Anaphylaxis

Objectives

After reading this chapter, you should be able to:

1. Describe the incidence, morbidity and mortality of anaphylaxis. (p. 1305)
2. Identify the risk factors most predisposing to anaphylaxis. (p. 1305)
3. Discuss the anatomy and physiology of the organs and structures related to anaphylaxis. (pp. 1396–1398)
4. Discuss the pathophysiology of allergy and anaphylaxis. (pp. 1396–1399)
5. Describe the common routes of substance entry into the body. (pp. 1398–1399)
6. Define allergic reaction, anaphylaxis, antigen, antibody and natural and acquired immunity. (pp. 1396–1399)
7. List common antigens most frequently associated with anaphylaxis. (pp. 1396–1397)
8. Discuss human antibody formation. (pp. 1396–1398)
9. Describe the physical manifestations of anaphylaxis. (pp. 1399–1401, 1403–1404)

Continued

Objectives Continued

10. Identify and differentiate between the signs and symptoms of an allergic reaction and anaphylaxis. (pp. 1403–1404)
11. Explain the various treatment and pharmacological interventions used in the management of allergic reactions and anaphylaxis. (pp. 1401–1404)
12. Correlate abnormal findings in assessment with the clinical significance in the patient with an allergic reaction or anaphylaxis. (pp. 1399–1401, 1403–1404)
13. Given several pre-programmed and moulaged patients, provide the appropriate assessment, care and transport for the allergic reaction and anaphylaxis patient. (pp. 1395–1404)

INTRODUCTION

An **allergic reaction** is an exaggerated response by the immune system to a foreign substance. Allergic reactions can range from mild skin rashes to severe, life-threatening reactions that involve virtually every body system. The most severe type of allergic reaction is called **anaphylaxis**. Anaphylaxis is a life-threatening emergency that requires prompt recognition and specific treatment by paramedics. The emergency treatment of anaphylaxis is one area of prehospital care where advanced life support measures often mean the difference between life and death. Anaphylaxis can develop within seconds and cause death just minutes after exposure to the offending agent. Fortunately, there are several emergency medications available that can reverse the adverse effects of anaphylaxis.

The first complete description of anaphylaxis was reported in 1902 by Portier and Richet. Portier and Richet were French immunologists who were attempting to immunize dogs against the toxin of the deadly sea anemone (sea flower). They were injecting small, non-lethal quantities of the toxin into the animals in hopes of stimulating immunity to the toxin. However, when the animals received secondary injections of sub-lethal quantities of the toxin, at a time when it might be expected that they would be immune, the dogs developed shock and died. Richet called this dramatic and unexpected phenomenon *anaphylaxis*, which means the opposite of "phylaxis" or protection.

Anaphylaxis results from exposure to a particular substance that sets off a biochemical chain of events that can ultimately lead to shock and death. The exact incidence of anaphylaxis is unknown. However, an estimated 400–800 deaths annually in the United States are attributed to anaphylaxis. Injected penicillin and bee and wasp *(Hymenoptera)* stings are the two most common causes of fatal anaphylaxis. Approximately 100–500 deaths per year are attributed to the parenteral administration of penicillin. Approximately 25–40 persons die each year from *hymenoptera* stings. Fortunately, the incidence of anaphylaxis appears to be declining. This is presumably due to better recognition and treatment, as well as the availability of numerous potent antihistamines.

---

* **allergic reaction** an exaggerated response by the immune system to a foreign substance.

* **anaphylaxis** an unusual or exaggerated allergic reaction to a foreign protein or other substance. Anaphylaxis means the opposite of "phylaxis" or protection.

Anaphylaxis is the most severe form of allergic reaction and is often life threatening.

---

* *Hymenoptera* any of an order of highly specialized insects such as bees and wasps.

PATHOPHYSIOLOGY

* **immune system** the body system responsible for combating infection.

* **immune response** complex of events within the body that works toward the destruction or inactivation of pathogens, abnormal cells, or foreign molecules.

* **pathogen** a disease-producing agent or invading substance.

* **toxin** any poisonous chemical secreted by bacteria or released following destruction of the bacteria.

* **cellular immunity** immunity resulting from a direct attack of a foreign substance by specialized cells of the immune system.

* **humoral immunity** immunity resulting from attack of an invading substance by antibodies.

* **antibody** principal agent of a chemical attack of an invading substance.

* **immunoglobulin** alternative term for antibody.

* **antigen** any substance that is capable, under appropriate conditions, of inducing a specific immune response.

* **primary response** initial, generalized response to an antigen.

The immune system is the principal body system involved in allergic reactions. However, other body systems are also affected by an allergic reaction. These include *the cardiovascular system, the respiratory system, the nervous system,* and *the gastrointestinal system,* among others. To fully appreciate the complexity of allergic and anaphylactic reactions, it is first necessary to review the anatomy and physiology of the immune system as it relates to the immune response.

THE IMMUNE SYSTEM

The **immune system** is a complicated body system responsible for combating infection. Components of the immune system can be found in the blood, the bone marrow, and the lymphatic system.

The **immune response** is a complex cascade of events that occurs following activation by an invading substance, or **pathogen.** The goal of the immune response is the destruction or inactivation of pathogens, abnormal cells, or foreign molecules such as **toxins.** The body can accomplish this through two mechanisms, cellular immunity and humoral immunity. **Cellular immunity** involves a direct attack of the foreign substance by specialized cells of the immune system. These cells physically engulf and deactivate or destroy the offending agent. **Humoral immunity,** on the other hand, is much more complicated. Humoral immunity is basically a chemical attack of the invading substance. The principal chemical agents of this attack are **antibodies,** also called **immunoglobulins (Igs).** Antibodies are a unique class of chemicals that are manufactured by specialized cells of the immune system called *B cells.* There are five different classes of antibodies: IgA, IgD, IgE, IgG, and IgM.

The humoral immune response begins with exposure of the body to an antigen. An **antigen** is defined as any substance capable of inducing an immune response (Table 31-1). Most antigens are proteins. Following exposure to an antigen, antibodies are released from cells of the immune system. These antibodies attach themselves to the invading substance to facilitate removal of that substance from the body by other cells of the immune system.

If the body has never been exposed to a particular antigen, the response of the immune system is different than if it has been previously exposed to the particular antigen. The initial response to an antigen is called the **primary response.**

Table 31-1   AGENTS THAT MAY CAUSE ANAPHYLAXIS

Antibiotics and other drugs

Foreign proteins (e.g., horse serum. Streptokinase)

Foods (nuts, eggs, shrimp)

Allergen extracts (allergy shots)

Hymenoptera stings (bees, wasps)

Hormones (Insulin)

Blood Products

Aspirin

Non-steroidal anti-inflammatory drugs (NSAIDs)

Preservatives (sulfiting agents)

X-ray contrast media

Dextran

Following exposure to a new antigen, several days are required before both the cellular and humoral components of the immune system respond. Generalized antibodies (IgG and IgM) are first released to help fight the antigen.

At the same time, other components of the immune system begin to develop antibodies specific for the antigen. These cells also develop a *memory* of the particular antigen. If the body is exposed to the same antigen again, the immune system responds much faster. This is called the **secondary response**. As a part of the secondary response, antibodies specific for the offending antigen are released. Antigen-specific antibodies are much more effective in facilitating removal of the offending antigen than the generalized antibodies released during the primary response.

Immunity may be either *natural* or *acquired*. **Natural immunity,** also called *innate immunity,* is genetically predetermined. It is present at birth and has no relation to previous exposure to a particular antigen. All humans are born with some innate immunity.

Acquired immunity develops over time and results from exposure to an antigen. Following exposure to a particular antigen, the immune system will produce antibodies specific for the antigen. This protects the organism as subsequent exposure to the same antigen will result in a vigorous immune response. **Naturally acquired immunity** normally begins to develop after birth and is continually enhanced by exposure to new pathogens and antigens throughout life. For example, a child contracts chicken pox (varicella) at age 18 months. Following the infection, the child's immune system creates antibodies specific for the varicella virus. Repeated exposure to the varicella virus usually will not result in another infection. In fact, it is not unusual for a patient exposed to varicella to develop lifelong immunity to the infection.

Induced active immunity, also called *artificially acquired immunity,* is designed to provide protection from exposure to an antigen at some time in the future. This is achieved through vaccination and provides relative protection against serious infectious agents. In vaccination, an antigen is injected into the body so as to generate an immune response. This results in the development of antibodies specific for the antigen and provides protection against future infection. Most vaccines contain antigenic proteins from a particular virus or bacterium. Later, when the individual is actually exposed to the pathogen, the immune response will be vigorous and will often be enough to prevent the infection from developing.

An example of a vaccine commonly used is the DPT (diphtheria/pertussis/tetanus) vaccine. This vaccine contains antigenic proteins from the bacteria that cause diphtheria, whooping cough, and tetanus. The vaccine is administered at several intervals during the first five years of life. It provides protection against infection from these bacteria. Some vaccinations will impart lifelong immunity while others must be periodically followed with a "booster dose" to assure continued protection.

Acquired immunity can be either *active* or *passive*. **Active immunity** occurs following exposure to an antigen and results in the production of antibodies specific for the antigen. Most vaccinations result in the development of active immunity. However, it takes some time for a patient to develop specific antibodies. In certain cases, it is necessary to administer antibodies to provide protection until the active immunity can kick in. The administration of antibodies is referred to as **passive immunity.** There are two types of passive immunity. *Natural passive immunity* occurs when antibodies cross the placental barrier from the mother to the infant so as to provide protection against embryonic or fetal infections. *Induced passive immunity* is the administration of antibodies to an individual to help fight infection or prevent diseases. An example of the clinical use of both active and passive immunity is the regimen used for the prevention of tetanus.

* **secondary response** response by the immune system that takes place if the body is exposed to the same antigen again; in secondary response, antibodies specific for the offending antigen are released.

* **natural immunity** genetically predetermined immunity that is present at birth; also called *innate immunity.*

* **acquired immunity** immunity that develops over time and results from exposure to an antigen.

* **naturally acquired immunity** immunity that begins to develop after birth and is continually enhanced by exposure to new pathogens and antigens throughout life.

* **induced active immunity** immunity achieved through vaccination given to generate an immune response that results in the development of antibodies specific for the injected antigen; also called *artificially acquired immunity.*

* **active immunity** acquired immunity that occurs following exposure to an antigen and results in the production of antibodies specific for the antigen.

* **passive immunity** acquired immunity that results from administration of antibodies either from mother to the infant across the placental barrier (natural passive immunity) or through vaccination (induced passive immunity).

Most persons who are from developed countries have typically received some form of tetanus vaccination during their life. These persons typically have some antibodies to tetanus and often need nothing more than a tetanus booster. However, some persons have never received any sort of tetanus vaccination. When these persons seek treatment for a tetanus-prone wound, they must receive prophylaxis for tetanus in addition to care for their wound. This is best achieved by the provision of both passive and active immunity. To provide immediate protection, the patient is administered antibodies specific for tetanus (tetanus immune globulin (TIG) Hypertet®). Then, they are administered a tetanus vaccination (Td or Dt). The tetanus immune globulin (TIG) provides passive immunity until such time as the body's immune system can respond to the tetanus vaccination with the development of antibodies specific for tetanus. This should be followed by periodic tetanus boosters until such time as the patient's immunization program is complete.

ALLERGIES

The initial exposure of an individual to an antigen is referred to as **sensitization.** Sensitization results in an immune response. Subsequent exposure induces a much stronger secondary response. Some individuals can become hypersensitive (overly sensitive) to a particular antigen. **Hypersensitivity** is an unexpected and exaggerated reaction to a particular antigen. In many instances, hypersensitivity is used synonymously with the term **allergy.** There are two types of hypersensitivity reactions, delayed and immediate.

Delayed and Immediate Hypersensitivity

Delayed hypersensitivity is a result of *cellular immunity* and therefore does not involve antibodies. Delayed hypersensitivity usually occurs in the hours and days following exposure and is the sort of allergy that occurs in normal people. Delayed hypersensitivity most commonly results in a skin rash and is often due to exposure to certain drugs and chemicals. The rash associated with poison ivy is an example of delayed hypersensitivity.

When people use the term "allergy" they are usually referring to **immediate hypersensitivity** reactions. Examples of immediate hypersensitivity reactions include hay fever, drug allergies, food allergies, eczema, and asthma. Some persons have an allergic tendency. This allergic tendency is usually genetic, meaning it is passed from parent to child and is characterized by the presence of large quantities of IgE antibodies. An antigen that causes release of the IgE antibodies is referred to as an **allergen.** Common allergens include:

- Drugs
- Foods and food additives
- Animals
- Insects (*Hymenoptera* stings) and insect parts
- Fungi and molds
- Radiology contrast materials

Allergens can enter the body through various routes. These include oral ingestion, inhalation, topically, and through injection or envenomation. The vast majority of anaphylactic reactions result from injection or envenomation.

Parenteral penicillin injections are the most common cause of fatal anaphylactic reactions. Insect stings are the second most frequent cause of fatal

* **sensitization** initial exposure of a person to an antigen that results in an immune response.

* **hypersensitivity** an unexpected and exaggerated reaction to a particular antigen. It is used synonymously with the term *allergy.*

* **allergy** a hypersensitive state acquired through exposure to a particular allergen.

* **delayed hypersensitivity reaction** a hypersensitivity reaction that takes place after the elapse of some time following reexposure to an antigen. Delayed hypersensitivity reactions are usually less severe than immediate reactions.

* **immediate hypersensitivity reaction** a hypersensitivity reaction that occurs swiftly following reexposure to an antigen. Immediate hypersensitivity reactions are usually more severe than delayed reactions. The swiftest and most severe of such reactions is anaphylaxis.

* **allergen** a substance capable of inducing allergy of specific hypersensitivity. Allergens may be protein or non-protein, although most are proteins.

anaphylactic reactions. Insects in the order *Hymenoptera* are the most frequent offending insects. There are three families in this order: fire ants *(Formicoidea)*; wasps, yellow jackets, and hornets *(Vespidae)*; and the honey bees *(Apoidea)*. All produce a unique venom, although there are similar components in each. Honey bees often will leave their stinger embedded in the victim following a sting.

Following exposure to a particular allergen, large quantities of IgE antibodies are released. These antibodies attach to the membranes of **basophils** and **mast cells**—specialized cells of the immune system which contain chemicals that assist in the immune response. When the allergen binds to IgE attached to the basophils and mast cells, these cells release histamine, heparin, and other substances into the surrounding tissues. Histamine and other substances are stored in *granules* found within the basophils and mast cells. In fact, because of this feature, basophils and mast cells are often called *granulocytes*. The process of releasing these substances from the cells is called *degranulation*. This release results in what people call an *allergic reaction* which can be very mild or very severe.

The principal chemical mediator of an allergic reaction is histamine. **Histamine** is a potent substance that causes bronchoconstriction, increased intestinal motility, vasodilation, and increased vascular permeability. Increased vascular permeability causes the leakage of fluid from the circulatory system into the surrounding tissues. A common manifestation of severe allergic reactions and anaphylaxis is angioneurotic edema. **Angioneurotic edema**, also called *angioedema,* is marked edema of the skin and usually involves the head, neck, face, and upper airway. Histamine acts by activating specialized histamine receptors present throughout the body.

There are two classes of histamine receptors. H_1 receptors, when stimulated, cause bronchoconstriction and contraction of the intestines. H_2 receptors cause peripheral vasodilation and secretion of gastric acids. The goal of histamine release is to minimize the body's exposure to the antigen. Bronchoconstriction decreases the possibility of the antigen entering through the respiratory tract. Increased gastric acid production helps destroy an ingested antigen. Increased intestinal motility serves to move the antigen quickly though the gastrointestinal system with minimal absorption of the antigen into the body. Vasodilation and capillary permeability help remove the allergen from the circulation where it has the potential to do the most harm.

ANAPHYLAXIS

Anaphylaxis usually occurs when a specific allergen is injected directly into the circulation. This is the reason anaphylaxis is more common following injections of drugs and diagnostic agents and following bee stings. When the allergen enters the circulation, it is distributed widely throughout the body. The allergen interacts with both basophils and mast cells, resulting in the massive dumping of histamine and other substances associated with anaphylaxis. The principal body systems affected by anaphylaxis are the cardiovascular system, the respiratory system, the gastrointestinal system, and the skin. Histamine causes widespread peripheral vasodilation as well as increased permeability of the capillaries. Increased capillary permeability results in marked loss of plasma from the circulation. People sustaining anaphylaxis can actually die from circulatory shock.

Also released from the basophils and mast cells is a substance called **slow-reacting substance of anaphylaxis (SRS-A)**. This causes spasm of the bronchial smooth muscle, resulting in an asthma-like attack and occasionally asphyxia. SRS-A potentiates the effects of histamine, especially on the respiratory system.

* **basophil** type of white blood cell that participates in allergic responses.

* **mast cell** specialized cell of the immune system which contains chemicals that assist in the immune response.

* **histamine** a product of mast cells and basophils that causes vasodilation, capillary permeability, bronchoconstriction, and contraction of the gut.

* **angioneurotic edema** marked edema of the skin that usually involves the head, neck, face, and upper airway; a common manifestation of severe allergic reactions and anaphylaxis.

* **slow-reacting substance of anaphylaxis (SRS-A)** substance released from basophils and mast cells that causes spasm of the bronchiole smooth muscle, resulting in an asthma-like attack and occasionally asphyxia.

ASSESSMENT FINDINGS IN ANAPHYLAXIS

The signs and symptoms of anaphylaxis begin within 30–60 seconds following exposure to the offending allergen. In a small percentage of patients the onset of signs and symptoms may be delayed over an hour. The signs and symptoms of anaphylaxis can vary significantly. The severity of the reaction is often related to the speed of onset. Reactions that develop very quickly tend to be much more severe.

A rapid and focused assessment is crucial to the early detection and treatment of anaphylaxis. Patients suffering an anaphylactic reaction often have a sense of impending doom. This sense of impending doom is often followed by development of additional signs and symptoms.

If the patient's condition permits, a brief history should be gathered, including previous allergen exposures and reactions. If possible, try to determine how quickly symptoms started and how severe they were.

Next, quickly evaluate the patient's level of consciousness. Upper airway problems, including laryngeal edema, may result in the patient being unable to speak. As the emergency progresses, the patient will become restless. As cardiovascular collapse continues, the patient will exhibit a decreased level of consciousness. If untreated, this may continue to unresponsiveness.

As noted earlier, a common manifestation of anaphylaxis is angioneurotic edema, involving the face and neck. Laryngeal edema is also a frequent complication and can threaten the airway. Initially, laryngeal edema will cause a hoarse voice. As the edema worsens, the patient may develop stridor. Finally, this all may lead to complete airway obstruction from either massive laryngeal edema, laryngospasm, or pharyngeal edema, or a combination of any of these.

The respiratory system is significantly involved in an anaphylactic reaction. Initially, the patient will become tachypneic. Later, as lower airway edema and bronchospasm develop, respirations will become labored as evidenced by retractions, accessory muscle usage, and prolonged expirations. Wheezing, resulting from bronchospasm and edema of the smaller airways, is a common manifestation and may be so pronounced that it can be heard without the aid of a stethoscope. Ultimately, anaphylaxis can result in markedly diminished lung sounds, which reflect decreased air movement and hypoventilation.

The skin is typically involved early in severe allergic reactions and anaphylaxis. Generally, a fine red rash will appear diffusely on the body. As histamine is released, fluid will diffuse from leaky capillaries, resulting in urticaria. **Urticaria**, also called "hives," is a wheal and flare reaction characterized by red, raised bumps which may appear and disappear across the body (Figure 31-1). As cardiovascular collapse and dyspnea progresses, the patient will become diaphoretic. This may, if untreated, progress to cyanosis and pallor.

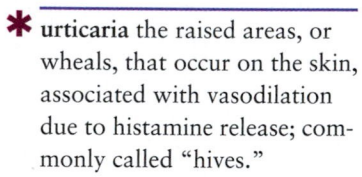

* urticaria the raised areas, or wheals, that occur on the skin, associated with vasodilation due to histamine release; commonly called "hives."

FIGURE 31-1   Hives are red, itchy blotches, sometimes raised, that often accompany an allergic reaction.

The effect of histamine on the gastrointestinal system is pronounced. Initially, the patient may note a rumbling sensation in the abdomen as gastrointestinal motility increases. On physical examination, this may be evident as hyperactive bowel sounds. Later, nausea, vomiting, and diarrhea develop as the body tries to rid itself of the offending allergen.

The vital signs will vary depending on the severity and stage of the severe allergic or anaphylactic reaction. Initially there will be an increase in both the heart and respiratory rate. As airway edema and dyspnea occurs, the respiratory rate can fall—an ominous finding. The blood pressure will fall when significant capillary leakage and peripheral vasodilation occurs. This will often result in a reflex tachycardia as the body attempts to compensate for the fall in blood pressure. Very late in anaphylaxis the heart rate will fall. This too should be considered a very ominous sign.

State of the art advanced prehospital care of anaphylaxis includes use of all available monitoring devices. These include the cardiac monitor, the pulse oximeter, and, if the patient is intubated, an end-tidal carbon dioxide detector. As anaphylaxis progresses, the end-tidal carbon dioxide level may climb due to the development of both respiratory and metabolic acidosis, which results in increased carbon dioxide elimination.

MANAGEMENT OF ANAPHYLAXIS

When responding to a patient with an anaphylactic reaction, first assure that the scene is safe to approach. The presence of chemicals or patrolling bees can pose a risk to EMS personnel as well as to the patient and bystanders. If the patient is still in contact with the agent causing the reaction, he should be moved a safe distance away. Honey bees often leave their stinger behind during a sting. If present, the stinger should be removed by scraping the skin with a fingernail or scalpel blade.

Always consider the possibility of trauma in anaphylaxis. If there is any suspicion of coincidental trauma, stabilize the cervical spine. It is not uncommon for people to fall or otherwise injure themselves as they try to escape from wasps and bees. Signs and symptoms of trauma may be masked by those of anaphylaxis.

PROTECT THE AIRWAY

Position the patient and protect the airway. Administer oxygen via a nonrebreather mask. If the patient is hypoventilating or apneic, initiate ventilatory assistance. If an airway problem is detected, first apply basic airway maneuvers such as head positioning or the modified jaw-thrust maneuver. Use oropharyngeal and nasopharyngeal airways with caution as they can cause laryngospasm. If the patient is having severe airway problems, consider early endotracheal intubation to prevent complete occlusion of the airway. It is important to remember that the glottic opening may be smaller than expected due to laryngeal edema. Also, the larynx will be very irritable, and any manipulation of the airway may lead to laryngospasm. Ideally, the most experienced member of the crew should perform endotracheal intubation, as only one attempt may be possible. Have available equipment for placement of a surgical airway, such as a needle cricothryotomy, in case it is needed.

Establish an IV as soon as possible with a crystalloid solution such as lactated Ringer's or normal saline. Remember that patients suffering anaphylaxis are volume depleted due to histamine-mediated third spacing of fluid. If the patient is hypotensive, administer fluids wide open. If time allows, place a second IV line.

ADMINISTER MEDICATIONS

The primary treatment for anaphylaxis is pharmacological. If the necessary drugs cannot be administered in the field, then the patient should be transported to the emergency department immediately. Emergency medications used in the treatment of anaphylaxis include oxygen, epinephrine, antihistamines, corticosteroids, and vasopressors. Occasionally, inhaled beta agonists, such as albuterol, may be required.

Oxygen Oxygen is always the first drug to administer to a patient with an anaphylactic reaction. Administer high-concentration oxygen with a nonrebreather mask or similar device. If mechanical ventilation is required, attach supplemental oxygen to assure as high an oxygen delivery as possible.

Epinephrine is the primary drug for management of anaphylaxis.

Epinephrine The primary drug for use in treatment of severe allergic reactions and anaphylaxis is epinephrine. Epinephrine is a sympathetic agonist. It causes an increase in heart rate, an increase in the strength of the cardiac contractile force, and peripheral vasoconstriction. It can also reverse some of the bronchospasm associated with anaphylaxis. Epinephrine also reverses much of the capillary permeability caused by histamine. It acts within minutes of administration. In severe anaphylaxis, characterized by hypotension and/or severe airway obstruction, administer epinephrine 1:10,000 intravenously. Epinephrine 1:10,000 contains 1 milligram of epinephrine in 10 milliliters of solvent. The standard adult dose is 0.3–0.5 mg; child dose is 0.01 mg/kg. The effects of intravenous epinephrine wear off in 3–5 minutes, so repeat boluses may be required. In severe cases of sustained anaphylaxis, medical direction may order the preparation and administration of an epinephrine drip.

Antihistamines Antihistamines are second-line agents in the treatment of anaphylaxis. They should only be given following the administration of epinephrine. Antihistamines block the effects of histamine by blocking histamine receptors. They do not displace histamine from the receptors. They only block additional histamine from binding. They also help reduce histamine release from mast cells and basophils. Most antihistamines are non-selective and block both H_1 and H_2 receptors. Others are more selective for either H_1 or H_2 receptors.

Diphenhydramine (Benadryl) is probably the most frequently used antihistamine in the treatment of allergic reactions and anaphylaxis. It is non-selective and acts on both H_1 and H_2 receptors. The standard dose of diphenhydramine is 25–50 milligrams intravenously or intramuscularly. It should be administered slowly when given intravenously. The pediatric dose of diphenhydramine is 1–2 milligrams per kilogram of body weight. Other non-selective antihistamines frequently used are hydroxyzine (Atarax, Vistaril) and promethazine (Phenergan). Hydroxyzine is a potent antihistamine, but it can only be administered intramuscularly. Promethazine can be administered intravenously or intramuscularly, but does not appear to be as potent as diphenhydramine.

Selective histamine blockers are primarily H_2 blockers used to treat ulcer disease. Blockage of the H_2 receptors decreases gastric acid secretion. However, H_2 receptors are also present in the peripheral blood vessels. Administration of H_2 blockers conceivably will reverse some of the vasodilation associated with anaphylaxis. The two most frequently used H_2 blockers are cimetidine (Tagamet) and ranitidine (Zantac). Typically, 300 milligrams of cimetidine or 50 milligrams of ranitidine are administered by slow IV push (over 3–5 minutes). Some recent studies have questioned the effectiveness of H_2 blockers in the treatment of allergic reactions. Also, these agents are more expensive than the non-selective antihistamines.

Corticosteroids Corticosteroids are important in the treatment and prevention of anaphylaxis. Although they are of little benefit in the initial stages of treatment they help suppress the inflammatory response associated with these emergencies. Commonly used corticosteroids include methylprednisolone (Solu-Medrol), hydrocortisone (Solu-Cortef), and dexamethasone (Decadron).

Vasopressors Severe and prolonged anaphylactic reactions may require the use of potent vasopressors to support blood pressure. Use these medications in conjunction with first line therapy and adequate fluid resuscitation. Commonly used agents include dopamine, norepinephrine, and epinephrine. These medications are prepared as infusions and are continuously administered to support blood pressure and cardiac output.

Beta Agonists Many patients with severe allergic reactions and anaphylaxis will develop bronchospasm, laryngeal edema, or both. In these cases, an inhaled beta agonist can be useful. The most frequently used beta agonist in prehospital care is albuterol (Ventolin, Proventil). Although usually used in the treatment of asthma, these agents will help reverse some of the bronchospasm and laryngeal edema associated with anaphylaxis. Give the adult patient 0.5 milliliters of albuterol in 3 milliliters of normal saline via a hand-held nebulizer. Children should receive 0.2–0.5 milliliters of albuterol based on their weight. Other beta agonists, such as metaproterenol (Alupent) and isoetharine (Bronkosol) may be used instead of albuterol.

Other Agents Other drugs occasionally used in the treatment of anaphylaxis include aminophylline and cromolyn sodium. Aminophylline is a bronchodilator unrelated to the beta agonists. It can be administered by slow intravenous infusion to treat the bronchospasm associated with anaphylaxis. Although cromolyn sodium (Intal) is not used in the treatment of allergic reactions and anaphylaxis, it is used in their prevention. Cromolyn sodium helps to stabilize the membranes of the mast cells, thus reducing the amount of histamine and other mediators released when these cells are stimulated.

OFFER PSYCHOLOGICAL SUPPORT

A severe allergic or anaphylactic reaction is a harrowing experience for the patient. Although it is essential to work fast, prehospital crews should provide the patient emotional support and explain the treatment regimen. Caution patients about the potential side effects of administered medications. For example, epinephrine will often cause a rapid heart rate, anxiety, and tremulousness. Likewise, the antihistamines may cause a dry mouth, thirst, and sedation. Careful explanation and emotional support will help allay patient anxiety and apprehension.

ASSESSMENT FINDINGS IN ALLERGIC REACTION

Many patients you will be called to treat will be suffering from forms of allergic reaction less severe than anaphylaxis. An allergic reaction, as contrasted with an anaphylactic reaction, will have a more gradual onset with milder signs and symptoms and the patient will have a normal mental status (Table 31-2).

MANAGEMENT OF ALLERGIC REACTIONS

Common manifestations of mild (non-anaphylactic) allergic reactions include itching, rash, and urticaria. Patients with simple itching and non-urticarial rashes may be treated with antihistamines alone. In addition to antihistamines, epinephrine is often necessary for the treatment of urticaria.

Any patient suffering an allergic reaction who exhibits dyspnea or wheezing should receive supplemental oxygen. This should be followed by subcutaneous epinephrine 1:1,000. Lesser allergic reactions that are not accompanied by hypotension or airway problems can be adequately treated with epinephrine 1:1,000 administered subcutaneously (Figure 31-2). Epinephrine 1:1,000 contains 1 milligram of

Table 31-2	SIGNS AND SYMPTOMS OF ALLERGIC AND ANAPHYLACTIC REACTIONS
Mild Allergic Reaction	**Severe Allergic Reaction or Anaphylaxis**
Onset: Gradual	*Onset:* Sudden (30-60 seconds but can be more than an hour after exposure)
Skin/Vascular system: Mild flushing, rash, or hives	*Skin/vascular system:* Severe flushing, rash, or hives; angioneurotic edema to the face and neck
Respiration: Mild bronchoconstriction	*Respiration:* Severe bronchoconstriction (wheezing), laryngospasm (stridor), breathing difficulty
GI system: Mild cramps, diarrhea	*GI system:* Severe cramps, abdominal rumbling, diarrhea, vomiting
Vital signs: Normal to slightly abnormal	*Vital signs:* Increased pulse early, may fall in late/severe case; increased respiratory rate early, falling respiratory rate late; falling blood pressure late
Mental status: Normal	*Mental status:* Anxiety, sense of impending doom, may decrease to confusion and to unconsciousness
	Other Clues: Symptoms occur shortly after exposure to parenteral penicillin, *Hymenoptera* sting (fire ant, wasp, yellow-jacket, hornet, bee), or ingestion of foods to which patient is allergic such as nuts or shellfish
	Ominous signs: Respiratory distress, signs of shock, falling respiratory rate, falling pulse rate, falling blood pressure

Note: Not all signs and symptoms will be present in every case.

epinephrine in 1 milliliter of solvent. When administered into the subcutaneous tissue, the drug is absorbed more slowly and the effect prolonged. The subcutaneous dose is the same as the intravenous dose (0.3–0.5 milligram). The subcutaneous route should not be used in severe anaphylaxis. Many physicians prefer to give epinephrine 1:1,000 intramuscularly, because this has a faster rate of onset although a shorter duration of action.

FIGURE 31-2 Epinephrine being administered to a pediatric patient.

SUMMARY

Fortunately, severe allergies and anaphylaxis are uncommon. However, when they do occur, they can progress quickly and result in death in minutes. The central physiological action in anaphylaxis is the massive release of histamine and other mediators. Histamine causes bronchospasm, airway edema, peripheral vasodilation, and increased capillary permeability. The prehospital treatment of anaphylaxis is intended to reverse the effects of these agents.

The primary, and most important, drug used in the treatment of anaphylaxis is epinephrine. Epinephrine helps reverse the effects of histamine. It also supports the blood pressure and reverses detrimental capillary leakage. Following the administration of epinephrine, potent antihistamines should be used to block the adverse effects of the massive histamine release. Inhaled beta agonists are useful in cases of severe bronchospasm and airway involvement. Intravenous fluid replacement is crucial in preventing hypovolemia and hypotension.

The key to successful prehospital management of anaphylaxis is prompt recognition and treatment.

CHAPTER 32

Gastroenterology

Objectives

After reading this chapter, you should be able to:

1. Describe the incidence, morbidity and mortality of gastrointestinal emergencies. (p. 1407)

2. Identify the risk factors most predisposing to gastrointestinal emergencies. (pp. 1407–1408)

3. Discuss the anatomy and physiology of the gastrointestinal system. (see Chapter 3)

4. Discuss the pathophysiology of abdominal inflammation and its relationship to acute pain. (pp. 1408–1409)

5. Define somatic, visceral, and referred pain as they relate to gastroenterology. (pp. 1408–1409)

6. Differentiate between hemorrhagic and nonhemorrhagic abdominal pain. (pp. 1409, 1411)

7. Discuss the signs and symptoms and differentiate between local, general, and peritoneal inflammation relative to acute abdominal pain. (pp. 1408–1409)

8. Describe the questioning technique and specific questions when gathering a focused history in a patient with abdominal pain. (pp. 1409–1410)

9. Describe the technique for performing a comprehensive physical

Continued

INTRODUCTION

Gastrointestinal emergencies account for over 500,000 emergency visits and hospitalizations every year, approximately 5 percent of all visits to the emergency department. Of that number, more than 300,000 are due to gastrointestinal bleeding. These figures will probably increase as more and more people treat themselves with over-the-counter medications and delay seeing a physician until their symptoms become severe. Perhaps more important, the numbers will rise as the general population ages. In the last few years the number of patients over 60 years of age included in these statistics has risen from approximately three percent to more than 45 percent.

GENERAL PATHOPHYSIOLOGY, ASSESSMENT, AND TREATMENT

Gastrointestinal (GI) emergencies usually result from an underlying pathologic process that can be predicted by evaluating numerous risk factors. These risk factors are commonly known to physicians; most are self-induced by patients. They

Content Review

GASTROINTESTINAL DISEASE RISK FACTORS

- Excessive alcohol consumption
- Excessive smoking
- Increased stress
- Ingestion of caustic substances
- Poor bowel habits

✱ **visceral pain** dull, poorly localized pain that originates in the walls of hollow organs.

✱ **peritonitis** inflammation of the peritoneum, which lines the abdominal cavity.

✱ **somatic pain** sharp, localized pain that originates in walls of the body such as skeletal muscles.

✱ **referred pain** pain that originates in a region other than where it is felt.

include excessive alcohol consumption, excessive smoking, increased stress, ingestion of caustic substances, and poor bowel habits. The wide variety of risk factors and potential causes requires the emergency care provider to complete a thorough focused history and physical examination before making a field diagnosis, along with assessing the seriousness of the emergency and the need for any prevention strategy to minimize organ damage.

GENERAL PATHOPHYSIOLOGY

Pain is the hallmark of the acute abdominal emergency. The three main classifications of abdominal pain are visceral, somatic, and referred. **Visceral pain** originates in the walls of hollow organs such as the gallbladder or appendix, in the capsules of solid organs such as the kidney or liver, or in the visceral peritoneum. Three separate mechanisms can produce this pain—inflammation, distention (being stretched out or inflated), and ischemia (inadequate blood flow). Because these processes progress at varying rates, they likewise can cause varying intensities, characteristics, and locations of pain.

Inflammation, distention, and ischemia all transmit a pain signal from visceral afferent neural fibers back to the spinal column. Because the nerves enter the spinal column at various levels, visceral pain usually is not localized to any one specific area. Instead, it is often described as very vague or poorly localized, dull, or crampy. The body most often responds to this vague pain with sympathetic stimulation that causes nausea and vomiting, diaphoresis, and tachycardia.

Organs that consist of hollow viscera can frequently cause visceral pain, e.g., the gallbladder (cholecystitis) and the small and large intestines. Many hollow organs first cause visceral pain when they become distended and then cause a different, more specific type of pain (somatic pain, described below) when they rupture or tear. For example, appendicitis initially presents with vague periumbilical abdominal pain that is classified as visceral. If the appendix ruptures it can spill its contents into the peritoneal cavity, causing bacterial **peritonitis** and generating somatic pain. Various microbes associated with pelvic inflammatory diseases can also cause bacterial peritonitis.

Somatic pain, as contrasted to visceral pain, is a sharp type of pain that travels along definite neural routes (determined by the dermatomes, or tissue blocks, present during embryonic development) to the spinal column. Because these routes are clearly defined, the pain can be localized to a particular region or area. As previously noted, bacterial and chemical irritations of the abdomen commonly cause somatic pain. Bacterial irritation can originate from a perforated or ruptured appendix or gallbladder. Chemical irritation of the abdomen can result from leakage of acidic juices from a perforated ulcer or from an inflamed pancreas. Whether the cause is bacterial or chemical, the resulting peritonitis can lead to sepsis and even death. The degree of pain is initially proportional to the spread of the irritant through the abdominal cavity. Somatic pain allows the examiner to locate the specific area of irritation, providing valuable information.

The third type of pain, referred pain, is not a true pain-producing mechanism. As its name implies, **referred pain** originates in a region other than where it is felt. Many neural pathways from various organs pass through or over regions where the organ was formed during embryonic development. For example, the afferent neural pathways that originate in the diaphragm enter the spinal column at the cervical enlargement at the fourth cervical vertebra. Therefore, patients who have an inflammation or injury of the diaphragm often feel pain in their necks or shoulders. One of the most significant hemorrhagic emergencies, the dissecting abdominal aortic artery, produces referred pain felt between the shoulder blades. Some common nonhemorrhagic emergencies are associated with referred-pain patterns, too. Appendicitis often presents with periumbilical pain, whereas pneumonia can cause pain below the lower margin of the rib cage.

GENERAL ASSESSMENT

Your assessment of a patient who complains of abdominal discomfort or whom you suspect of having an abdominal pathology is similar to a trauma assessment with an expanded history. Do not approach the patient until you and your partner have determined the scene to be free and clear of any apparent dangers. Always take appropriate body substance isolation measures, including gloves, eyewear, mask, and disposable body gown to prevent contamination. As you approach the patient, survey the scene for potential evidence of your patient's problem. Medication bottles, alcohol containers, ashtrays, and buckets with emesis or sputum, for instance, can provide valuable information.

Scene Size-up and Initial Assessment

As you approach, look for mechanisms of injury to help determine whether the call is medical or trauma. If you suspect trauma, always immobilize the cervical spine as you assess the adequacy of the patient's airway and his level of responsiveness. In the vast majority of medical patients you can check responsiveness and airway patency by asking the patient his name and chief complaint (why he called the ambulance today) and noting the answers. You can further evaluate the rate, depth, and quality of the patient's respirations fairly rapidly and without great difficulty. As you evaluate the respiratory functions, quickly palpate a pulse and check skin color, temperature, and circulation, including signs of bleeding and capillary refill. If you discover a life-threatening condition during the initial assessment, treat it and then rapidly continue the assessment to identify any other life threats.

History and Physical Exam

Once you have completed the initial assessment and dealt with any life threats, conduct the focused history and physical examination. Your ability to obtain a history from the patient will depend on his level of responsiveness. In some cases, you may detect deterioration of the patient's mental status over time as you take the history.

History An accurate and thorough history can provide invaluable information. After you conduct the SAMPLE history (*s*ymptoms, *a*llergies, *m*edications, *p*ast medical history, *l*ast oral intake, and *e*vents), you can take a more thorough, focused history, exploring the chief complaint, the history of the present illness, the past medical history, and the current health status. The history of the present illness and the past medical history will be especially helpful in sorting the multitude of signs and symptoms and piecing together a clear picture of the underlying pathophysiology.

The history of the present illness and the past medical history will be especially helpful in piecing together a clear picture of the underlying gastrointestinal pathophysiology.

History of the present illness Your OPQRST-ASPN history for gastrointestinal patients should address the following specific concerns:

- *Onset.* When did the pain first start? Was the onset very sudden or gradual? Sudden onsets of abdominal pain are generally caused by perforations of abdominal organs or capsules. Gradual onset of pain usually is associated with the blockage of hollow organs.

- *Provocation/Palliation.* What makes the pain worse? What makes the pain better? If the pain lessens when the patient draws his legs up to his chest or lies on his side, it usually indicates peritoneal inflammation, which is often of GI origin. If walking relieves the pain, the cause may be in the GI or urinary systems—perhaps an obstruction of the gallbladder or a stone caught in the renal pelvis or ureter.

- *Quality.* How would you describe the pain: dull, sharp, constant, intermittent? Localized, tearing pain is usually associated with the rupture of an organ. Dull, steadily increasing pain may indicate a bowel obstruction. Sharp pain, particularly in the flank, may indicate a kidney stone.

- *Region/radiation.* Does the pain travel to any other part of your body? Radiated pain, or pain that seems to change location, is common because it involves the same neural routes as referred pain. Pain referred to the shoulder or neck is usually associated with an irritation of the diaphragm, such as happens with cholecystitis.

- *Severity.* On a scale of 1 to 10, with 10 representing the worst pain possible, how would you rate the pain you are feeling now? The severity of pain usually worsens as the pathology (ischemia, inflammation, or stretching) of the organ advances.

- *Time.* When did the pain first start? Estimation of the pain's time of onset is important to determine its possible causes. Any abdominal pain lasting over six hours is considered a surgical emergency and needs to be evaluated in the emergency department.

- *Associated Symptoms.* Have you experienced any associated nausea and or vomiting with the discomfort? If yes, try to determine the content, color, and smell of the vomitus. Ask if the vomitus contained any bright red blood, "coffee grounds," or clots. Determining if your patient has an active gastrointestinal bleed is imperative.

    Have you experienced any changes in bowel habits—constipation or diarrhea—associated with this discomfort/pain? Question the patient further to determine if there have been any changes in feces such as a tarry, foul-smelling stool. Changes in bowel morphology, color, or smell can be the only indication of such conditions as a lower GI hemorrhage, gastritis, or bleeding diverticula.

    Have you had an associated loss of appetite or weight loss? Patients who have an acute abdomen usually have an associated loss of appetite.

- *Pertinent Negatives.* The absence of symptoms associated with GI function or the presence of symptoms related to urinary function may mean the problem originates in the urinary system. Pain in the lowest part of the abdomen, the pelvis, can be due to problems in the reproductive system. Last, remember that an inferior myocardial infarction (MI) can irritate the diaphragm and generate its referred-pain pattern. Be sure to check for cardiovascular history when this pain pattern (pain in shoulder and/or neck area) is present.

Keep in mind the information that your SAMPLE history gave you about your patient's last oral intake. It can help you to differentiate the possible causes of your patient's pain if the problem is in the GI system.

Not all abdominal emergencies result in abdominal pain. Some may cause chest pain. This, typically, is referred pain. Common gastrointestinal emergencies that can cause chest pain include: gastroesophageal reflux, gastric ulcers, duodenal ulcers, and, in some cases, gall bladder disease. When confronted by a patient with chest pain, always consider the gastrointestinal system as a possible cause.

Past medical history   Have you ever experienced this same type of pain or discomfort before? If the patient answers yes, then investigate whether he saw a physician for the problem and how it was diagnosed. Commonly, patients have been treated for the complaint in the past and the pain is a flare-up of an old problem.

Physical Examination While you are conducting the history you can also begin the physical examination. Your patient's general appearance and posture strongly suggest his apparent state of health and the severity of his complaint. Usually patients with severe abdominal pathology lie as still as possible, often in the fetal position. They do not writhe around on the floor or cry out, because doing so increases the pain. You also should continually monitor the patient's level of consciousness for any subtle changes that indicate early signs of shock.

Take a complete set of vital signs to establish a baseline for further evaluation and treatment. These include pulse, respiratory rate, blood pressure, and pulse oximetry. You can also ascertain additional important information such as body temperature.

Visually inspect the abdomen before palpating it, auscultating it, or moving the patient. Remove the patient's clothing as necessary to freely visualize the entire abdomen. Distention of the abdomen may be an ominous sign. It can be caused by a build-up of free air due to an obstruction of the bowel. If the distention is caused by hemorrhage, the patient has lost a large amount of his circulating volume, for the abdomen can hold from four to six liters of fluid before any noticeable change in abdominal girth occurs. Other signs of fluid loss include periumbilical ecchymosis (**Cullen's sign**) and ecchymosis in the flank (**Grey-Turner's sign**).

Auscultating the abdomen usually provides little helpful information because bowel sounds are heard throughout this area. If you auscultate the abdomen, you must do so before palpating it. Listen for at least two minutes in each quadrant, beginning with the quadrant farthest from the affected area and auscultating the affected area last. Like auscultation, percussion requires a quiet environment and an experienced clinician. It too provides little or no useful information and, therefore, is not routinely performed in the field.

Palpating the abdomen, on the other hand, can give you a plethora of information. It can define the area of pain and identify the associated organs. Before palpating, ask the patient to point to where he is experiencing the most discomfort. Then work in reverse order, palpating that area last. Palpate the abdomen with a gentle pressure, feeling for muscle tension or its absence, as well as for masses, pulsations, and tenderness beneath the muscle. If you identify a pulsating mass, stop palpating at once; the increase in pressure may cause the affected blood vessel or organ to rupture.

GENERAL TREATMENT

Once you have completed the initial assessment and the focused history and physical examination, you can address treatment and transport. Your highest priority when treating a patient with abdominal pain is to secure and maintain his airway, breathing, and circulation. Be prepared to suction the airway of vomitus and blood. High-flow oxygenation and aggressive airway management may be indicated, depending on your patient's status. Monitor circulation by placing the patient on a cardiac monitor and frequently assessing his blood pressure. Measurement of the hematocrit will give an indirect measure of blood loss.

Establish a large-bore IV line in patients who complain of abdominal discomfort for use if emergency blood transfusion becomes necessary. You can use the IV for pharmacological intervention or to replace volume lost to hemorrhage or dehydration. In general, the need to avoid masking any abdominal pain for further evaluation will limit your pharmacological interventions to palliative agents such as antiemetics. Place the patient in a comfortable position and provide emotional reassurance based on your field assessment, any conversation with hospital staff or

Usually patients with severe abdominal pathology lie as still as possible, often in the fetal position.

Distention of the abdomen may be an ominous sign.

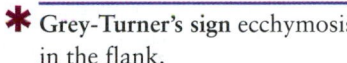

* **Cullen's sign** ecchymosis in the periumbilical area.

* **Grey-Turner's sign** ecchymosis in the flank.

If you auscultate the abdomen, you must do so before palpating it.

Palpating the abdomen can give you a plethora of information.

Your highest priority when treating a patient with abdominal pain is to secure and maintain his airway, breathing, and circulation.

* **upper gastrointestinal bleeding** bleeding within the gastrointestinal tract proximal to the ligament of Treitz.

* **ligament of Treitz** ligament that supports the duodenojejunal junction.

* **Mallory-Weiss tear** esophageal laceration, usually secondary to vomiting.

family, and knowledge of estimated transport time. Keep your voice and actions quiet and collected. Calm, as well as anxiety, are transmitted easily to patients and family. How you transport the patient will depend on his physiological status. Normally, gentle but rapid transport is sufficient. Remember that persistent abdominal pain lasting longer than six hours is classified as a surgical emergency and always requires transport. In all cases, be sure to maintain monitoring of mental status and vital signs and to give nothing by mouth. Bring vomitus to the emergency department for evaluation.

SPECIFIC ILLNESSES

The gastrointestinal (GI) tract is essentially one long tube divided structurally and functionally into different parts. Three other organs, the liver, gallbladder, and pancreas, are intimately associated with it, as is the small structure called the vermiform appendix, which protrudes from the first portion of the large intestine. Collectively, these organs are called the GI, or digestive, system. The GI system converts food into nutrient molecules that individual cells can use, and it excretes solid wastes from the body.

UPPER GASTROINTESTINAL DISEASES

For convenience, clinicians often divide the GI tract broadly into the upper and lower GI tracts. The upper GI tract consists of the mouth, esophagus, stomach, and duodenum, the latter being the first part of the small intestine. Physical digestion of food and some chemical digestion take place here. As food passes through the lower GI tract, consisting of the remainder of the small intestine and the large intestine, nutrients are absorbed into the blood and solid wastes are formed and excreted.

Upper Gastrointestinal Bleeding

Upper gastrointestinal bleeding can be defined as bleeding within the gastrointestinal tract proximal to the **ligament of Treitz,** which supports the duodenojejunal junction, the point where the first two sections of the small intestine (the duodenum and the jejunum) meet.

Upper gastrointestinal bleeds account for over 300,000 hospitalizations per year. The mortality rate has remained fairly steady at approximately 10 percent over the past years. Many factors contribute to this high mortality. First, the number of patients who treat their symptoms with home remedies and over-the-counter medications is increasing rapidly. Many of these patients come under medical care only when their disease has caused significant damage, such as large-scale hemorrhage from an ulcerated lesion. Second, the overall age of the population is increasing. The infirmities of age and its greater likelihood of coexisting illnesses, such as hypertension, atherosclerosis, diabetes, and substance abuse (including abuse of medications), make this older population more vulnerable to the effects of upper gastrointestinal bleeds. The mortality rate is highest in those over 60 years of age. One prevention strategy for the field is to check for such coexisting problems, especially in elderly patients, and to treat accordingly. In particular, look at the history and physical for evidence of tobacco or alcohol use, or both.

The six major identifiable causes of upper GI hemorrhage, in descending order of frequency, are peptic ulcer disease, gastritis, variceal rupture, **Mallory-Weiss syndrome** (esophageal laceration, usually secondary to vomiting), esophagitis, and duodenitis. Peptic ulcer disease accounts for approximately 50 percent of upper GI bleeds, with gastritis accounting for an additional 25 percent. Overall, irritation or erosion of the gastric lining of the stomach causes more than 75 percent of upper

GI bleeds. Most cases of upper GI bleeding are chronic irritations or inflammations that cause minimal discomfort and minor hemorrhage. Physicians can manage these conditions on an outpatient basis; however, if a peptic ulcer erodes through the gastric mucosa, if the esophagus is lacerated in Mallory-Weiss syndrome, or if varices (often secondary to alcoholic liver damage) rupture, an acute-onset, life-threatening, and difficult-to-control hemorrhage can result.

Upper GI bleeds may be obvious, or they may present quite subtly. Most often patients will complain of some type of abdominal discomfort ranging from a vague burning sensation to an upset stomach, gas pain, or tearing pain in the upper quadrants. Because blood severely irritates the GI system, most cases present with nausea and vomiting. If the bleeding is in the upper GI tract, the patient may experience **hematemesis** (bloody vomitus) or, if it passes through the lower GI tract, **melena.** The partially digested blood will turn the stool black and tarry. For melena to be recognizable, approximately 150 cc of blood must drain into the GI tract and remain there for from five to eight hours. Blood in emesis may be bright red (new, fresh blood) or look like coffee grounds (old, partially digested blood).

Upper GI bleeding may be light or it may be brisk and life threatening. Patients who suffer a rupture of an esophageal varix or a tear or disruption in the esophageal or gastric lining may vomit copious amounts of blood. These hemorrhages can cause the classic signs and symptoms of shock, including alteration in mental status, tachycardia, peripheral vasoconstriction, diaphoresis (sweating producing pale, cool, clammy skin), and hemodynamic instability. Besides shock, the vomitus itself can compromise the airway, resulting in impaired respirations, aspiration, and ultimately, respiratory arrest.

A frequently employed clinical indicator is the tilt test, which indicates if the patient has orthostatic hypotension (a 10-mmHg change in blood pressure or a 20-bpm change in heart rate when the patient rises from supine to standing). Hypotension suggests a decreased circulating volume. The human body can compensate for a circulating volume deficit of approximately 15 percent before clinical indicators such as the tilt test show positive results. Thus, those patients whose systolic blood pressure drops 10 mmHg or whose heart rate increases 20 bpm or more need aggressive fluid resuscitation.

When evaluating the patient and his laboratory values, remember that the hematocrit might be within normal ranges when the patient is in the early phase of an acute hemorrhage. The key prevention strategy is to identify subtle indicators and treat the condition before it worsens. More general complaints include malaise, weakness, syncopal (fainting) and near-syncopal (lightheaded) spells, tachycardia, and indigestion.

Your patient's general appearance may be the best indicator of his condition's severity. Because the hemorrhage is internal and histories are often misleading, you must perform a thorough physical examination. The patient may present doubled over in pain or lying very still. The latter is usually an ominous sign that any movement causes extreme pain. If you place the patient supine, be alert to the possibility of vomitus compromising the airway. Patients with a history of GI problems may have scars from past surgeries.

Examination in cases of suspected hemorrhage may be very helpful. Abdominal inspection may show symmetric distention or bulging in one region of the abdomen. Ecchymosis may be present if much blood has been lost into the abdominal cavity. If auscultation is subsequently performed, bowel sounds may be absent if the bleeding is severe or they may be hyperactive if the bleeding is minimal.

Prehospital treatment of an upper gastrointestinal bleed centers on maintaining a patent airway, oxygenation, and circulatory status. Place the patient in the left lateral recumbent or high semi-Fowler's position to prevent aspiration. To maximize the remaining hemoglobin molecules' carrying capability, administer

If an ulcer erodes through the gastric mucosa, if the esophagus tears, or if varices rupture, an acute, life-threatening, and difficult-to-control hemorrhage can result.

* **hematemesis** bloody vomitus.

* **melena** dark, tarry, foul smelling stool indicating the presence of partially digested blood.

The key to managing an acute hemorrhage is to recognize its subtle indicators early and treat the condition before it worsens.

Content Review

UPPER GI DISEASES
Esophageal varices
Acute gastroenteritis
Chronic gastroenteritis
Peptic ulcers

✱ **Sengstaken-Blakemore tube**
three-lumen tube used in
treating esophageal bleeding.

✱ **esophageal varix** swollen vein
of the esophagus.

> *When varices rupture and
> hemorrhage, the mortality rate
> is over 35 percent.*

✱ **portal** pertaining to the flow
of blood into the liver.

✱ **cirrhosis** degenerative disease
of the liver.

high-flow oxygenation via a nonrebreather mask to all patients with a suspected gastrointestinal bleed.

Establish two large-bore (14–16 gauge) IVs in any patient whom you suspect of having a gastrointestinal bleed. Start one with blood tubing for possible transfusion and one with volume-replacement 0.9% NaCl. Base fluid resuscitation on the patient's condition and response to the treatment. In general you can administer a 20 cc/kg fluid bolus to begin treating hemorrhagic hypovolemia.

Once the patient reaches the emergency department, treatment may include gastric decompression and lavage with a nasogastric tube, further fluid/blood resuscitation, endoscopy, **Sengstaken-Blakemore tube** placement, antacid and histamine antagonist administration, or immediate surgery.

Esophageal Varices

An **esophageal varix** is a swollen vein of the esophagus. Often these varices rupture and hemorrhage. When they do, the mortality rate is over 35 percent.

The cause of esophageal varices usually is an increase in **portal** pressure (portal hypertension). The blood flows from the abdominal organs, through the portal vein, and into the liver, where nutrients are absorbed into liver tissue and numerous compounds are detoxified and returned to the blood. From the liver, blood courses directly into the inferior vena cava through the hepatic veins. Blood flow through the liver ordinarily encounters little, if any, resistance. Damage to that organ, however, can impede circulation, causing blood to back up into the left gastric vein and, from there, into the esophageal veins. The dramatically higher pressure in these normally low-pressure pathways causes the esophageal veins to dilate and emerge from their sheaths (to evaginate, or "outpocket"). These small evaginations are called esophageal varices (Figure 32-1). As they become engorged, the varices continue to dilate outward under extreme pressure until they rupture, causing massive hemorrhage. They may also erode through the submucosal layer and directly into the esophagus.

The primary causes of esophageal varices are the consumption of alcohol and the ingestion of caustic substances. Alcoholic liver cirrhosis accounts for two-thirds of cases of esophageal varices. Over time, alcohol consumption can cause a degenerative process known as **cirrhosis** of the liver. Cirrhosis results in fatty deposits and fibrosis in the liver parenchymal tissue, thus obstructing portal

FIGURE 32-1. Esophageal varices occur when the esophageal veins dilate and emerge from their sheaths.

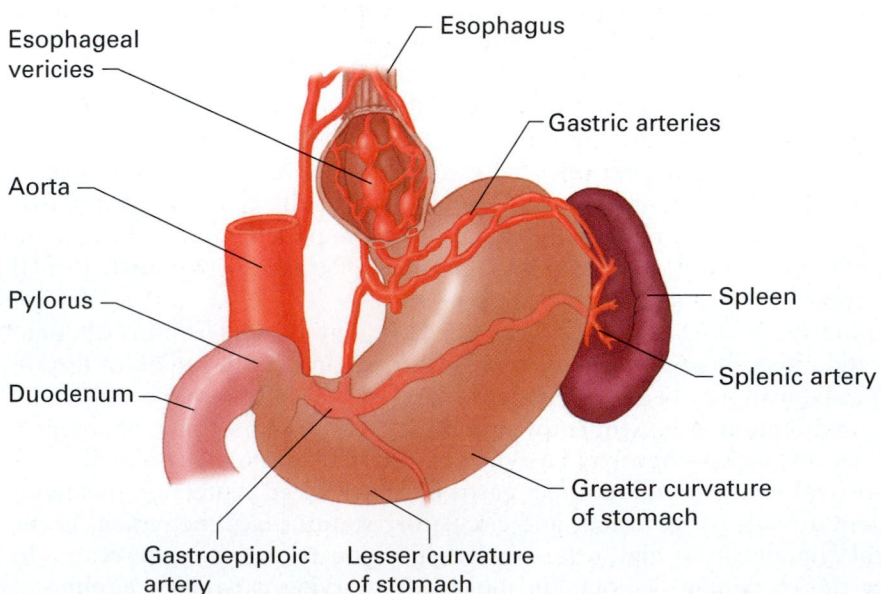

blood flow. Consequently, esophageal varices are common in the United States and the Western Hemisphere in general, where the alcohol consumption rate is high. In fact, cirrhosis is one of the leading causes of death in the Western Hemisphere. Caustic substances such as battery acid or drain cleaners can erode the esophagus from the inside out, causing hemorrhage of a vessel. Caustic ingestion, along with variceal formation due to viral hepatitis and erosive esophagitis accounts for the remaining one-third of cases of esophageal varices.

Patients suffering from leaking or ruptured esophageal varices often present initially with painless bleeding and signs of hemodynamic instability. They may complain of hematemesis with bright red blood, dysphagia (difficulty swallowing), and a burning or tearing sensation as the varices continue to bleed, irritating the lining of the esophagus. The hematemesis can be very forceful and copious if the hemorrhage is large. Clotting time increases because the high portal pressure backs up blood into the spleen, destroying platelets. The patient may exhibit the classic signs of shock, including an increased pulse, increased respirations, and cool, clammy, diaphoretic skin, possibly associated with an altered level of consciousness and hypotension.

Because paramedics cannot tamponade the bleeding in the prehospital setting, your care should focus on aggressive airway management, intravenous fluid resuscitation, and rapid transport to the emergency department. Airway management is a top priority. You may need to suction emesis frequently and diligently from the airway. Orotracheal intubation also may be needed to maintain airway patency. To maximize oxygenation, administer high-flow oxygen via a nonrebreather mask. If the patient shows signs and symptoms of shock, place him in the shock position and begin fluid resuscitation. If the patient continues to hemorrhage, management in the emergency department might include the use of a Sengstaken-Blakemore tube to tamponade the bleeding, endoscopic cauterization, or sclerotherapy (injection of a thrombus-forming drug into the vein itself).

Prehospital placement of nasogastric tubes should be avoided in cases of suspected esophageal varices.

Acute Gastroenteritis

Acute gastroenteritis is defined as inflammation of the stomach and intestines with associated sudden onset of vomiting and/or diarrhea. It affects from three to five million people yearly worldwide and affects approximately 20 percent of all hospitalized patients. The pathologic inflammation causes hemorrhage and erosion of the mucosal and submucosal layers of the gastrointestinal tract. This inflammation and erosion can in turn damage the villi inside the intestine, which absorb water and nutrients. The water that healthy villi normally would absorb now moves through the bowel at an increased rate. Dehydration secondary to diarrhea is a common cause of death in developing nations but is seen far less frequently in the United States. Adequate volume replacement is your major prehospital prevention strategy to minimize the likelihood of hypovolemia, or even possible hypovolemic shock.

Individuals who abuse alcohol and tobacco are at high risk for gastritis (inflammation of the stomach) and gastroenteritis (inflammation of the stomach and intestines). A wide variety of chemical agents and incidents can lead to acute gastritis. One of the most common is the use of nonsteroidal anti-inflammatory drugs such as aspirin, which break down the mucosal surfaces of the stomach and GI tract. Other causes include excessive alcohol intake and tobacco use; alcohol and nicotine have the same irritating effect on the mucosa as nonsterodial anti-inflammatory drugs. Stress, chemotherapeutic agents, and the ingestion of acidic or alkalotic agents can also cause acute gastroenteritis. Both systemic infection (salmonellosis) and infection from ingested pathogens (staphylococcus) can cause infectious acute gastroenteritis.

* **acute gastroenteritis** sudden onset of inflammation of the stomach and intestines.

As the name implies, the onset of acute gastroenteritis is rapid and usually severe. The swift movement of fluid through the gastrointestinal tract causes multiple problems. First, and most obvious, diarrhea is almost always associated with this condition. Approximately 7–9 liters of fluid (secretions and ingested fluids) normally move through the GI tract every 24 hours. Of that, less then 2 percent, or approximately 100 ml, is lost in the stool. With acute gastroenteritis, the GI tract expels the fluid that normally would be absorbed. This fluid loss leads to dehydration, which can cause severe hypovolemia in pediatric, geriatric, and previously compromised patients. Besides appearing watery, the stool might show either melena or **hematochezia**, the latter bright red blood from erosion of the lining of the lower GI tract. Along with the changes in stool, patients may have bouts of hematemesis, fever, nausea and vomiting, and general malaise. Due to dehydration and hemorrhage, the patient can be hemodynamically unstable; the exam may show hypotension, tachycardia, and pale, cool, and clammy skin. The patient may appear restless or show decreased mental status. If dehydration is severe, he can develop chest pain and cardiac dysrhythmias from electrolyte disturbances. The patient may complain of widespread and diffuse abdominal pain that is not specific to any one region. Visible distention is relatively unlikely unless significant gas has built up within the intestines; palpation will probably reveal tenderness throughout the abdomen.

Treatment for acute gastroenteritis is mainly supportive and palliative. Keep the patient positioned with head forward or face to the side to minimize the likelihood of aspiration should vomiting occur. Be prepared to clear the airway of vomit or secretions. Maintaining adequate oxygenation is also a high priority. When there is no significant blood loss, the circulatory system's oxygen-carrying capabilities remain intact. You can establish adequate supplemental oxygenation with a nasal cannula at 2–4 lpm. Rehydration is the next step in treating your patient. If he is conscious and alert, oral fluid rehydration may be appropriate. The easiest and quickest route, however, is IV fluid administration. In the prehospital setting, the fluid of choice is either 0.9% NaCl or lactated Ringer's solution to replace the patient's circulating volume. In-hospital treatment will switch the fluid to D_5/LR or D_5/NS to replace electrolytes. Pharmacological treatment can involve antiemetics such as prochlorperazine (Compazine) or promethazine (Phenergan). Additional replacement of electrolytes such as potassium may be needed. Offer emotional support during transport. Exercise extreme caution and use BSI throughout patient contact to prevent any spread of infectious disease.

Chronic Gastroenteritis

Chronic gastroenteritis is inflammation of gastrointestinal mucosa marked by long-term mucosal changes or permanent mucosal damage. Unlike acute gastroenteritis, chronic gastroenteritis is due primarily to microbial infection. The most prevalent pathogen in the United States is the *Helicobacter pylori* bacillus. Other bacteria that can cause chronic gastroenteritis include *Escherichia coli*, *Klebsiella pneumoniae*, *Enterobacter*, *Campylobacter jejuni*, *Vibrio cholerae*, *Shigella*, and *Salmonella*. Many of these bacteria can be found as part of normal enteric flora, and effective vaccination against pathogenic strains has not been possible. *Shigella* and *Salmonella* are not part of the normal spectrum of intestinal flora. Viral pathogens include the Norwalk virus and rotavirus. Among the parasitic causes are the protozoa *Giardia lamblia*, *Cryptosporidium parvum*, and *Cyclosporidium cayetenis*.

All of these microbes and their associated gastric disorders are far more common in underdeveloped countries. They are transmitted via the fecal-oral route or through infected food or water. Fecal-oral transmission can occur whenever people practice poor personal hygiene or food handling techniques. Local water supplies can become contaminated during natural disasters that disrupt normal water distribution and sewage treatment practices. In such instances, people from outside the endemic area may be more vulnerable to infection than is the local population. *Cyclosporidium* infection reportedly can be contracted by swimming in contaminated water.

Gastroenteritis patients commonly present with nausea and vomiting, fever, diarrhea, abdominal pain, cramping, anorexia (loss of appetite), lethargy, and in severe cases, shock. Usually the intensity of signs and symptoms reflects the degree of microbial contamination. On the other hand, infection with *H. pylori*, the most common infectious gastroenteritis in the United States, often presents with common signs such as heartburn, abdominal pain, and on endoscopic examination, gastric ulcers.

When in contaminated conditions, be sure to decontaminate the drinking water or use a different water source; when in doubt about the reliability of the water, drink only beverages that have been brisk boiled or disinfected. Make sure proper sanitation and preparation of foods is maintained. Handwashing and BSI will protect most EMS providers and prevent transmitting the organism further. To avoid transmitting the disease to patients, health care providers should not work when they are ill.

Prehospital treatment involves protecting yourself and the patient from further contamination, monitoring the ABCs, and transport. Medical treatment of infectious gastroenteritis will require identification of the offending organism. Some of the causative microorganisms are sensitive to antibiotics, but for most the patient will be supported while the disease takes its natural path.

Peptic Ulcers

Peptic ulcers are erosions caused by gastric acid (Figure 32-2). They can occur anywhere in the gastrointestinal tract; terminology is based on the portion of the GI tract affected. Duodenal ulcers most frequently occur in the proximal portion of the duodenum; gastric ulcers occur exclusively in the stomach. Overall, peptic ulcers occur in males four times more frequently than in females, and duodenal ulcers occur from two to three times more frequently than do gastric ulcers. Current statistics place the number of peptic ulcers at 4–5 million, with approximately 500,000 new cases diagnosed yearly. Those patients who are more likely to have gastric ulcers are over 50 years old and work in jobs requiring physical activity. Their pain usually increases after eating or with a full stomach and they usually have no pain at night. Duodenal ulcers are more common in patients from 25 to 50 years old who are executives or leaders under high stress. There is also some familial tendency toward duodenal ulcer, suggesting genetic predisposition. Patients with duodenal ulcers commonly have pain at night or whenever their stomach is empty. Thus, it is important in taking the focused history to get family history and a reliable estimate of the patient's last oral intake. Measurement of hematocrit may substantiate any suspicions of chronic or acute hemorrhage.

Nonsteroidal anti-inflammatory medications (aspirin, Motrin, Advil, Naprosyn), acid-stimulating products (alcohol, nicotine), or *Helicobacter pylori* bacteria are the most common causes of peptic ulcers. To help break down food boluses, the stomach secretes hydrochloric acid. One of the enzymes that control this secretion is pepsinogen. The hydrochloric acid helps to convert pepsinogen into its active form, pepsin. Between them, the pepsin and the hydrochloric acid can make the digestive enzymes very irritating to the GI tract's mucosal lining. Ordinarily, mucous gland secretions protect the stomach's mucosal barrier from these irritants. But when nonsteroidal anti-inflammatory medications, acid stimulators, or *H. pylori* damage the barrier, the mucosa is exposed to the highly acidic fluid, and peptic ulcers result. Prostaglandin, an important locally acting hormone, decreases the stimulation for blood flow through the gastric mucosa, thus allowing its further destruction. Treatment strategies in the prehospital setting focus on antacid treatment and support of any complications such as hemorrhage.

Helicobacter pylori is associated with gastric and duodenal ulcers.

* **peptic ulcer** erosion caused by gastric acid.

Esophagus · Lower esophageal sphincter · Gastric antrum

Pylorus

Duodenal ulcer

Gastric ulcer

Duodenal ulcer

Duodenum

FIGURE 32-2. Peptic ulcer.

The recent discovery that *Helicobacter pylori* bacteria appear in over 80 percent of gastric and duodenal ulcers has enabled physicians to treat the disease by eliminating its cause with antacids and antibiotics, rather than merely treating its symptoms. Definitive treatment includes tamponade of any bleed, possibly by surgical resection, and antibiotic therapy along with histamine blockers and antacids. If medical therapy fails and the problem persists, it may require surgical resection of the vagus nerve (vagotomy) to reduce the stimulation for acid secretion.

A blocked pancreatic duct can also contribute to duodenal ulcers. As chyme passes through the pyloric sphincter from the stomach into the duodenum, the pancreas secretes an alkalotic solution laden with bicarbonate ions that neutralize the acidic hydrogen ions in the chyme. If the pancreatic duct is blocked, however, the acidic chyme can cause ulcerations throughout the intestine. One other cause of duodenal ulcers is **Zollinger-Ellison syndrome**, in which an acid-secreting tumor provokes the ulcerations.

Findings on clinical examination of a patient with peptic ulcer can vary. Chronic ulcers can cause a slow bleed with resulting anemia. Visual inspection of the abdomen is usually helpful only if significant hemorrhage has occurred, in which case the same signs of ecchymosis and distention are found as in other causes of upper GI bleeding. On palpation, pain may be localized or diffuse. These patients often have relief of pain after eating or coating their GI tract with a liquid such as milk.

Acute, severe pain is probably due to a rupture of the ulcer into the peritoneal cavity causing hemorrhage. Depending on the ulcer's location, the patient may

✱ **Zollinger-Ellison syndrome** condition that causes the stomach to secrete excessive amounts of hydrochloric acid and pepsin.

have hematemesis or may have melena-colored stool. Bouts of nausea and vomiting due to the irritation of the mucosa are common. If the ulcer has eroded through a highly vascular area, massive hemorrhage can occur. Along with the signs of hemorrhage on visual inspection, these patients will appear very ill and have signs of hemodynamic instability such as pale, cool, and clammy skin, tachycardia, decreased blood pressure, and possibly, altered mental status. Most patients will lie still to decrease the pain. They may have surgical scars from previous ulcer repair. Bowel sounds will usually be absent.

Treatment for peptic ulcers depends on the severity of the patient's pain. Those who have abdominal pain or hemodynamic instability may require comfortable positioning and psychological support, high-flow oxygen, IV access for fluid resuscitation and pharmacological administration, and rapid transport. Common medications to reduce the mucosal irritation include histamine blockers such as Zantac and Pepcid and antacids such as Carafate.

LOWER GASTROINTESTINAL DISEASES

The lower GI tract consists of the jejunum and ileum of the small intestine and the entire large intestine, the rectum, and the anus. As digestive fluid moves through the small intestine (approximately 6 meters long), nutrients are absorbed into the blood. Water is absorbed and solid wastes formed in the large intestine, also called the large bowel or colon, which is roughly 1.5 meters long.

Lower GI Bleeding

Lower gastrointestinal bleeding is defined as bleeding in the GI tract distal to the ligament of Treitz. Lower GI hemorrhages most frequently occur in conjunction with chronic disorders and anatomic changes associated with advanced age. The most common cause is diverticulosis, which is most prevalent in elderly people. Other causes are colon lesions (cancer or benign polyps), rectal lesions (hemorrhoids, anal fissures, anal fistulas), and inflammatory bowel disorders such as ulcerative colitis and Crohn's disease. These chronic disorders and diverticulosis rarely result in a massive hemorrhage such as that which can occur in the esophagus or stomach.

Your assessment of patients with suspected lower GI bleeds will be identical to your assessment of those with suspected upper GI bleeds. After you complete your initial assessment and treat all life-threatening conditions, you can conduct your focused history and physical examination. First, ask the patient whether this is a new complaint or a chronic problem. If a chronic problem, check the abdomen visually for scars from previous surgery. Frequent complaints with lower GI bleeding include cramping pain that may be described as like a muscle cramp or like gas pain, nausea and vomiting, and changes in stool. Melenic stool usually indicates a slow GI bleed. If the stool contains bright red blood, the hemorrhage either is very large (thus passing through the intestines before melenic change can occur) or has occurred in the distal colon. In the latter case, hemorrhoids or rectal fissures are possible causes. The abdominal exam will show findings similar to those for a bleeding peptic ulcer. If the abdomen has the distention or ecchymosis characteristic of significant hemorrhage, check for signs of early shock such as pale, cool, and clammy skin, tachycardia, decreased blood pressure, and possibly, altered mental status. Because most patients with lower GI bleeds have not lost significant amounts of blood, they will present with hemodynamic stability, including warm dry skin, on physical exam.

How you manage the patient with a lower GI bleed will depend on his physiological status. Watch his airway and oxygenation status closely. If hypoventilation or inadequate respirations develop, administer high-flow oxygenation via a nonrebreather mask or positive pressure ventilation. Establish IV access and fluid resuscitation based on your patient's hemodynamic status. If you find a

Content Review

LOWER GI TRACT

Jejunum

Ileum

Large intestine

Rectum

Anus

✱ **lower gastrointestinal bleeding**
bleeding in the gastrointestinal tract distal to the ligament of Treitz.

Content Review

MAJOR CAUSES OF LOWER GI HEMORRHAGE

• Diverticulosis
• Colon lesions
• Rectal lesions
• Inflammatory bowel disorder

Lower gastrointestinal bleeding is usually chronic and rarely results in exsanguinating hemorrhage.

drop in hematocrit along with other signs of significant blood loss be especially sure that one IV line is of sufficiently large bore for emergency transfusion. Place him in a comfortable position, offer psychological support, and transport him for further examination. If hemodynamic instability develops during transport, consider use of the pneumatic anti-shock garment (PASG) if directed in local protocols.

Ulcerative Colitis

Ulcerative colitis is classified as an idiopathic inflammatory bowel disorder (IBD), that is, one of unknown origin. The inflammatory (ulcerative) process creates a continuous length of chronic ulcers in the mucosal layer of the colon; extension of the ulcers into the submucosal layer is uncommon. As ulcers heal, granular tissue replaces the ulcerations, thickening the mucosa. Approximately 75 percent of all ulcerative colitis involves the rectum or rectosigmoid portion of the large intestine. The inflammatory process usually starts in the rectum and then extends proximally into the colon, sometimes affecting the entire large intestine. If it spreads throughout the entire colon it is called **pancolitis;** if limited to the rectum, it is called **proctitis.**

Though ulcerative colitis is relatively unusual in Africa or Asia, its occurrence in the Western Hemisphere is increasing rapidly. In the United States, more than ten thousand new cases are diagnosed each year. It most frequently strikes people between the ages of 20 and 40 years. While researchers have not found a specific pathogen or cause of ulcerative colitis, they have determined many different contributing factors—psychological, allergic and other immunological, toxic, environmental, immunological, and infectious. Current research has found that the release of cytokines can cause an overwhelming inflammatory response in the submucosa much like the release of histamines during anaphylaxis.

Acute ulcerative colitis is difficult to differentiate from other causes of lower gastrointestinal bleeding. Because of its insidious presentation, diagnosing, tracking, and treating ulcerative colitis may require hematocrit and hemoglobin results, guaiac analyses of the stool, and endoscopic examinations. The severity of ulcerative colitis's signs and symptoms is usually related directly to the extent and severity of current inflammation in the colon. In patients with mild signs and symptoms, the disease often is isolated in one distal segment of the GI tract. Severe presentations, on the other hand, normally involve the entire colon.

Typically, ulcerative colitis presents as a recurrent disorder with occasional bloody diarrhea or stool containing mucus. Accompanying the stool abnormalities are **colicky** abdominal pain (cramping), nausea and vomiting, and occasionally, fever (suggesting infection) or weight loss (suggesting severe or longer-term colonic dysfunction). The cramping is usually limited to the lower quadrants, depending on the extent of colonic involvement, and it occurs when hypertrophic muscles lying beneath the submucosa prevent the colon from stretching in response to pressure from its contents. These patients will typically appear restless due to abdominal discomfort but will not show signs of hemodynamic instability (that is, skin will be warm and dry rather than cool and clammy).

More severe cases may present with bloody diarrhea and intense colicky abdominal pain, electrolyte derangements due to fluid loss through the colon, ischemic damage to the colon itself, or, eventually, perforation of the bowel. Often these patients present with signs and symptoms of hypovolemic shock such as pale, cool, clammy skin, hypotension, and tachycardia. Such patients with advanced disease and ongoing hemorrhage may have distention or ecchymosis on the skin and may show guarding of the lower quadrants during the physical examination. Significant hemorrhage is common in patients with ulcerative colitis.

Your management of the patient with ulcerative colitis will depend on his physiological status. If he presents with signs and symptoms of hypovolemic

pancolitis ulcerative colitis spread throughout the entire colon.

proctitis ulcerative colitis limited to the rectum.

colic acute pain associated with cramping or spasms in the abdominal organs.

Patients with ulcerative colitis are at increased risk of developing colon cancer.

shock, administer high-flow oxygen and circulatory support including intravenous access and fluid resuscitation. If your patient has bouts of nausea and vomiting, you must diligently manage his airway to prevent aspiration of vomitus. Additional management may include antiemetics and antispasmodic medications. Transport any patient who presents with lower GI bleeding or colicky pain to the emergency department for diagnostic evaluation.

Transport any patient who presents with lower GI bleeding or colicky pain to the emergency department for diagnostic evaluation.

Crohn's Disease

Crohn's disease, along with ulcerative colitis, is the other idiopathic inflammatory bowel disorder in humans. It is more common in the Western Hemisphere, with from 20,000 to 30,000 new cases reported annually in the United States. This disease, which strongly tends to run in families, is most prevalent among white females, those under frequent stress, and in the Jewish population.

Unlike ulcerative colitis, which affects the large intestine, Crohn's disease can occur anywhere from the mouth to the rectum. Between 35 and 45 percent of less severe cases involve the small intestine only; approximately 40 percent involve the colon itself. Severe cases of Crohn's disease may involve any portion of the GI tract, causing a variety of problems ranging from diarrhea to intestinal and perianal abscesses and fistulas (the latter, abnormal passages connecting two internal organs or different lengths of intestine). Complete intestinal obstruction, a surgical emergency, can also occur. Significant lower GI bleeding, on the other hand, is rare with Crohn's disease.

As the pathologic inflammation begins, it damages the innermost layer of tissue, the mucosa. Granulomas then form and further break down the mucosal and submucosal layers. The affected section of intestinal wall eventually becomes rubbery and nondistendable due to hypertrophy and fibrosis of the muscles underlying the submucosa. The patchwork-quilt formation of granulomas, fibrosis, and hypertrophy also decreases the intestine's internal diameter, resulting in fissures (incomplete tears) in the mucosa and possibly deeper into the submucosa as food boluses pass through. If a tear extends into the blood vessels in the submucosal layer, small bleeds result. The same pathologic pattern of ulceration and scarring can lead to creation of fistulas, most commonly between lengths of small intestine, or to obstruction of the small bowel. Increased suppressor T-lymphocyte activity suggests an immune-mediated role in the inflammatory process.

Crohn's patients' clinical presentations can vary drastically as the disease progresses, and prehospital diagnosis is difficult or next to impossible. Common signs and symptoms include GI bleeding, recent weight loss, intermittent abdominal cramping/pain, nausea and vomiting, diarrhea, and fever. Onset of a flareup in disease activity is usually rapid, often requiring a visit to the emergency department or physician's office. Abdominal pain cannot be localized to any specific quadrant since the disease can affect any portion of the small intestine and often affects more than one. The physical exam is also nonspecific and nonlocalized, with diffuse tenderness the most commonly found sign. Absence of bowel sounds in a patient with Crohn's disease strongly suggests intestinal obstruction, a surgical emergency.

Because the vast majority of patients with Crohn's disease are hemodynamically stable, prehospital treatment is largely palliative. Your management depends on the patient's physiological status. If he has bouts of nausea and vomiting you must diligently manage the airway to prevent aspiration of vomitus. Additional management may include antiemetics and antispasmodic medications. Particularly if he presents with signs and symptoms of obstruction or significant hemorrhage, administer high-flow oxygenation and circulatory support including intravenous access and fluid resuscitation. As always, calmly and quietly inform the patient of all measures taken and offer psychological support en route to the emergency facility.

* **Crohn's disease** idiopathic inflammatory bowel disorder associated with the small intestine.

Prehospital diagnosis of Crohn's disease is next to impossible because the patient's clinical presentations can vary drastically as the disease progresses.

Diverticulitis

Diverticulitis is a relatively common complication of diverticulosis. **Diverticulosis** a condition characterized by the presence in the intestine of **diverticula,** small outpouchings of mucosal and submucosal tissue that push through the outermost layer of the intestine, the muscle. Colonic diverticula are far more common in developed countries such as the United States and increase markedly in prevalence with increased age. They are present in more than half of patients over 60 years of age. Diverticulitis is an inflammation of diverticula secondary to infection. Unlike diverticulosis, it is symptomatic; patients will complain of lower left-sided pain (because most diverticula are in the sigmoid colon); exam and testing will show fever and an increased white blood cell count.

The pathogenesis of an acquired diverticulum is twofold. First, stool passes sluggishly through the colon, a condition associated with the relatively low fiber diets common in developed countries. The colon responds with muscle spasms that increase bulk movement by raising the pressure on the contents inside the colon and pushing the fecal material forward. Second, the outermost layer of colon tissue is made up of fibrous bands of muscle wrapped around one another. Among them are muscles called the teniae coli. Nerves and blood vessels enter the colon through small openings within the teniae coli. These openings become weakened with age, and the increased pressure of muscle spasms can cause the inner layers of tissue, the mucosa and submucosa, to herniate through the openings, forming diverticula.

These diverticula commonly trap small amounts of fecal material, including sunflower seeds, popcorn fragments, okra seeds, sesame seeds, and others. The entrapped feces may allow bacteria other then the normal flora to grow and cause an infection. The problem is compounded when the diverticula become inflamed, causing diverticulitis. Complications secondary to diverticulitis include possible hemorrhage or larger perforations of the colon wall through which the infected fecal contents can spill into the peritoneal cavity and cause peritonitis.

The most common presentation of diverticulitis is colicky pain associated with a low-grade fever, nausea and vomiting, and tenderness upon palpation. The pain is usually localized to the lower left side because the sigmoid colon is involved in 95 percent of reported cases. Thus diverticulitis is often called left-sided appendicitis. If the diverticula begin to bleed significantly, the usual signs and symptoms associated with severe lower GI bleeding may be present: cool, clammy skin, tachycardia, and diaphoresis. Bleeding diverticula can also result in bright red and bloody feces (hematochezia) because of their close proximity to the rectum. Patients may additionally complain of the perception that they cannot empty their rectums, even after defecation.

The most common presentation of diverticulitis is colicky pain—usually on the lower left side—associated with a low-grade fever, nausea and vomiting, and tenderness upon palpation.

The presence of diverticuli in the colon is common in the elderly. Some patients with diverticuli will develop bleeding, while others will develop an infection (diverticulitis).

Prehospital treatment for diverticulitis is mainly supportive. Measures to counter hypovolemic shock will only be needed when significant hemorrhage has occurred. Monitor the patient's airway and oxygenation and provide supplemental oxygen if needed. Establish intravenous access and begin fluid resuscitation if the patient is hemodynamically unstable. Antiemetics (Phenergan or Vistaril) may comfort the patient. Treatment in the hospital includes antibiotic therapy, endoscopy, and radiological tests to locate the diverticula. Long-term treatment includes implementing a high fiber diet to stimulate daily bowel movements.

Hemorrhoids

Hemorrhoids are small masses of swollen veins that occur in the anus (external) or rectum (internal). They frequently develop during the fourth decade of life. Most hemmorhoids are idiopathic (of unknown cause), although they can result from pregnancy or protal hypertension. External hemorrhoids often result from lifting a heavy object. Other causes of hemorrhoids include straining at defecation and a diet low in fiber. Overall, hemorrhoids are very common, particularly in persons over the age of 50 years. Their morbidity is low in most cases; one marked exception is in alcoholic patients with cirrhosis of the liver.

Internal hemorrhoids most often involve the inferior hemorrhoidal plexus and vasculature. They commonly bleed during the process of defecation due to straining and then thrombose into closed state again. External hemorrhoids result from thrombosis of a vein, often following lifting or straining, causing bright red bleeding with a bowel movement. The increased venous pressure sometimes causes the vessels to erode and bleed spontaneously, which increases the risk of infection. Rarely do hemorrhoids cause a significant hemorrhage.

Patients with hemorrhoids commonly call for emergency care because of bright red bleeding and pain on defecation. Physical assessment usually reveals a hemodynamically stable patient with relatively normal appearance (warm, dry skin, perhaps with slight tachycardia consistent with anxiety) who bleed with defecation. Visual examination of the stool may reveal gross bleeding. Treatment for hemorrhoids depends on the patient's condition. Most frequently, emotional reassurance and transport are all that is needed; however, you should remain alert to the possibility that the bleeding could be from a lower GI bleed, potentially resulting in uncontrolled hemorrhage. Either significant hemorrhage or bleeding hemorrhoids in an alcoholic patient warrant closer monitoring and transport for immediate follow-up.

Bowel Obstruction

Bowel obstructions are blockages of the hollow space, or lumen, within the small and large intestines. Obstructions can be either partial or complete. An obstructed bowel segment can be catastrophic if not rapidly diagnosed and treated. Of this malady's many different causes, **hernias, intussusception, adhesions,** and **volvulus** are the four most frequent, accounting for over 70 percent of all reported cases (Figure 32-3). Other common causes are foreign bodies, gallstones, tumors, adhesions from previous abdominal surgery, and bowel **infarction.** The most common location for obstructions is the small intestine, due to its smaller diameter and its greater length, flexibility, and mobility.

The obstruction may be chronic, as with tumor growth or adhesion progression, or its onset may be sudden and acute, as with obstruction by a foreign body. Chronic obstruction usually results in a decreased appetite, fever, malaise, nausea and vomiting, weight loss, or if rupture occurs, peritonitis. Acute-onset pain may follow ingestion of a foreign body. Pain might also be due to a strangulated hernia, one that has rotated through the muscle wall of the abdomen such that blood flow is suddenly cut off (the herniated tissue has been "strangulated") and ischemia, or even infarction, of tissue occurs. Patients with bowel obstruction will frequently vomit, with the vomitus often containing a significant amount of bile. Severe bowel obstructions may result in the patient's vomiting material that looks and smells like feces. All of these findings suggest a bowel obstruction.

These patients present with diffuse visceral pain, usually poorly localized to any one specific location. They may be hemodynamically unstable due to necrosis within an organ, and you may see signs and symptoms of shock (pale, cool, clammy skin, tachycardia, alterations in level of consciousness, and hypotension). Visual inspection may reveal distention, peritonitis, or free air within

Rarely do hemorrhoids cause a massive hemorrhage.

* **bowel obstruction** blockage of the hollow space within the intestines.

An obstructed bowel segment can be catastrophic if not rapidly diagnosed and treated.

* **hernia** protrusion of an organ through its protective sheath.

* **intussusception** condition that occurs when part of an intestine slips into the part just distal to itself.

* **adhesion** union of normally separate tissue surfaces by a fibrous band of new tissue.

* **volvulus** twisting of the intestine on itself.

* **infarction** area of dead tissue caused by lack of blood.

FIGURE 32-3. The most common causes of bowel obstruction: (a) hernia (b) intussusception (c) adhesion (d) volvulus.

the abdomen secondary to rupture of a strangulated segment of intestine. Look for scars left from previous surgery, as well as for the ecchymosis indicating that significant hemorrhage has occurred into the abdominal cavity. In the earliest phase of acute obstruction, bowel sounds may be present as a high-pitched obstruction sound. In most cases, however, bowel sounds will be greatly reduced or absent. Palpation will reveal tenderness. Be careful to palpate very lightly if you suspect obstruction, as additional pressure may bring about rupture of the obstructed segment.

The treatment for a patient with an obstructed bowel is based on physiological and psychological support during expedited transport to an appropriate facility. Measures include airway management, oxygenation via a nonrebreather mask at 15 lpm, position of comfort or shock position, and fluid resuscitation to prevent shock.

ACCESSORY ORGAN DISEASES

As you learned earlier in this chapter, the GI tract has three closely associated organs, the liver, gallbladder, and pancreas, as well as the small structure called the vermiform appendix. Accessory organ emergencies can arise in all four locations.

Appendicitis

Appendicitis is an inflammation of the vermiform appendix, located at the junction of the large and small intestines (the ileocecal junction). Appendicitis occurs in approximately 10 to 20 percent of the population in the United States, and it is most common in young adults. Acute appendicitis is the most common surgical emergency you will encounter in the field, mostly in older children and young adults. There are no particular risk factors.

The appendix has no known anatomic or physiologic function; most of its tissue is lymphoid in type. It lies just inferior to the ileocecal valve and the first section of the ascending colon. Depending on the individual patient, it may be in the retroperitoneal, pelvic, or abdominal cavity. The appendix can become inflamed, and if left untreated it can rupture, spilling its contents into the peritoneal cavity and setting up peritonitis.

The pathogenesis of appendicitis is most often due to obstruction of the appendiceal lumen by fecal material. The shape and location of the appendix make it particularly vulnerable to obstruction by feces or other material such as food particles or tumor. This inflames the lymphoid tissue and often leads to bacterial or viral infection that ulcerates the mucosa. The inflammation also causes the appendix's internal diameter to expand, which can block the appendicular artery and cause thrombosis. With its blood supply cut off, the appendix becomes ischemic, and infarction and necrosis of tissue follows. At this point the vessel walls often weaken to the point of rupture, spilling the appendiceal contents into the peritoneal cavity.

Appendicitis is frequently misdiagnosed due to the wide variety of signs and symptoms that can accompany it. Mild or early appendicitis causes diffuse, colicky pain often associated with nausea and vomiting and sometimes a low-grade fever. Often the pain is initially located in the periumbilical region. Due to appendiceal blockage, the patient usually loses his appetite. As the appendix continues to dilate the pain will localize in the right lower quadrant. A common site of pain is **McBurney's point,** 1½ to 2 inches above the anterior iliac crest along a direct line from the anterior crest to the umbilicus (Figure 32-4). Once the appendix ruptures the pain becomes diffuse due to development of peritonitis.

❋ **appendicitis** inflammation of the vermiform appendix at the juncture of the large and small intestines.

Appendicitis is evaluated in the emergency department and eventually treated in the operating room more frequently than any other abdominal emergency.

❋ **McBurney's point** common site of pain from appendicitis, one to two inches above the anterior iliac crest in a direct line with the umbilicus.

Physical assessment will find a patient who appears to be in discomfort. The abdominal exam will reveal tenderness or guarding around the umbilicus or right lower quadrant. Do not repeatedly palpate for rebound tenderness. The pressure that this procedure exerts can cause an inflamed appendix to rupture.

Prehospital care for appendicitis includes placing the patient in a position of comfort, giving psychological support, diligently managing his airway to prevent aspiration, establishing intravenous access, and transporting him. In most cases the appendix will not have ruptured, and the patient will remain hemodynamically stable. Monitor as you would for bowel obstruction, and treat any complications such as tachycardia or other signs of shock as they arise.

Cholecystitis

Cholecystitis is an inflammation of the gallbladder. Cholelithiasis (the formation of gallstones), which causes 90 percent of cholecystitis cases, occurs in approximately 15 percent of the adult population in the United States, with over one million new cases diagnosed annually. There are two types of gallstones, cholesterol-based and bilirubin-based. Cholesterol-based stones are far more common and are associated with a specific risk profile: obese, middle-aged women with more than one biological child.

Definitive treatment of acute cholecystitis includes antibiotic therapy, laparoscopic surgery, lithotripsy (ultrasound treatment to break up the stones), and surgery if the other, less invasive, therapies fail. With the advent of laparoscopic surgery, mortality has fallen to less then 1 percent, with an overall morbidity of approximately 6 percent.

Cholecystitis caused by gallstones can be chronic or acute. The liver produces bile, the primary vehicle for removing cholesterol from the body. The bile travels down the common bile duct to empty into the small intestine at the sphincter of Oddi. The sphincter of Oddi opens when chyme exits the stomach through the cardiac sphincter. When the sphincter of Oddi closes, the flow of bile backs up into the gallbladder via the cystic duct. The bile remains in the gallbladder until the sphincter of Oddi opens again.

The bile can become supersaturated and calculi—stone-like masses based on bilirubin, cholesterol, or both—form. These calculi travel down the cystic duct, frequently lodging in the common bile duct. When they obstruct the flow of bile, gallbladder inflammation and irritation result. The bile salts subsequently attack the mucosal membrane lining the gallbladder, leaving the underlying epithelial tissue without protection. Prostaglandins are also released, further irritating the epithelial wall. As irritation continues, the inflammation grows, increasing intraluminal pressure and ultimately reducing blood flow to the epithelium.

Other causes of cholecystitis include acalculus cholecystitis (cholecystitis without associated stones) and chronic inflammation caused by bacterial infection. Acalculus cholecystitis usually results from burns, sepsis, diabetes, and multiple organ failure. Chronic cholecystitis resulting from a bacterial infection (*Escherichia coli* and enterococci) presents with an inflammatory process similar to cholelithiasis.

An inflamed gallbladder usually causes an acute attack of upper right quadrant abdominal pain. The inflammation can cause an irritation of the diaphragm with referred pain in the right shoulder. If the gallstones are lodged in the cystic duct, the pain may be colicky, due to expansion and contraction of the duct. Often the pain occurs after a meal that is high in fat content because of the secondary release of bile from the gallbladder. The right subcostal region may be tender because of abdominal muscle spasms. Patients may experience extreme pain as the epithelium in the gallbladder erodes away. Sympathetic stimulation because of the pain may cause pale, cool, clammy skin. If peritonitis occurs, the skin may be warm due to increased blood flow to the inflamed peritoneum. Nausea and vomiting are common, due to cystic duct spasm.

Visual inspection may reveal scars from previous gallstone surgeries, but distention and ecchymosis are rarely seen. Palpation may reveal either diffuse right-sided tenderness or point tenderness under the right costal margin, a positive **Murphy's sign**.

Prehospital treatment of the patient with acute cholecystitis is mainly palliative. Place the patient in the position of comfort, maintain his ABCs, ensuring adequate oxygenation, and finally establish intravenous access. Pain medications commonly used include meperidine (Demerol) and butorphanol (Stadol). Morphine is contraindicated because it is believed to cause spasms of the cystic duct.

Pancreatitis

Pancreatitis is an inflammation of the pancreas. Its four main categories, based on cause, are metabolic, mechanical, vascular, and infectious. Metabolic causes, specifically alcoholism, account for approximately 80 percent of all cases; consequently, pancreatitis is widespread in the United States, due to the high incidence of alcoholism. Mechanical obstructions caused by gallstones or elevated serum lipids account for another 9 percent. Vascular injuries caused by thromboembolisms or shock, along with infectious diseases, account for the remaining 11 percent. Overall mortality in acute pancreatitis is relatively high, approximately 30–40 percent, mainly due to accompanying sepsis and shock, which lead to multisystem organ failure. In acute pancreatitis, the rate of serious morbidity and mortality has been found to be 14 percent in patients with fewer than three positive findings. The mortality rate exceeded 95 percent when there were three or more positive findings.

The vast bulk of the pancreas's tissue is arranged in glandular structures called *acini* (singular, *acinus*). These cells produce digestive enzymes that empty into the duodenum at the ampulla of Vater, near the junction with the stomach. The other function of the pancreas is endocrine: A small amount of tissue located in isolated islets of tissue secretes the hormones insulin and glucagon. Frequently, gallstones leaving the common bile duct become lodged at the ampulla of Vater and obstruct the pancreatic duct. These obstructions back up pancreatic digestive enzymes into the pancreatic duct and the pancreas itself. The digestive enzymes inflame the pancreas and cause edema, which reduces blood flow, as in the pathogenesis of acute appendicitis. In turn, the decreased blood

Gallbladder pain is located in the right upper quadrant or epigastrium and is collicky in nature. The problem tends to recur unless surgery is performed.

* **Murphy's sign** pain caused when an inflamed gallbladder is palpated by pressing under the right costal margin.

Acute pancreatitis is most often due to alcohol abuse or gallstones.

Content Review

CAUSES OF ACUTE PANCREATITIS

Alcohol abuse
Gallstones
Elevated serum lipids (cholesterol and triglycerides)
Drug-induced

flow causes ischemia and, finally, acinar destruction. This is often called acute pancreatitis based on rapidity of onset.

Acinar tissue destruction causes a second form of pancreatitis, chronic pancreatitis. Acinar tissue destruction commonly occurs due to chronic alcohol intake, drug toxicity, ischemia, or infectious diseases. Alcohol ingestion results in the deposit of platelet plugs in the acinar tissue. The plugs disrupt the enzymes' flow from the pancreas. When digestive juices back up into the pancreas from the ampulla of Vater, the digestive enzymes can become activated and begin to digest the pancreas itself. Morphologically this autodigestion appears as lesions and fatty tissue changes on the pancreas.

As tissue digestion continues, the lesion can erode and begin to hemorrhage. This acute exacerbation of pancreatitis causes intense abdominal pain. Its intensity reflects the number of lesions affected or the degree of acinar tissue death. The pain can be localized to the left upper quadrant or may radiate to the back or the epigastric region. Most patients experience nausea followed by uncontrolled vomiting and retching that can further aggravate the hemorrhage. Visual inspection may reveal previous surgical scars for lesion removal; ecchymosis and swelling of the left upper quadrant may also be present due to hemorrhage or significant organ edema. The patient will appear acutely ill with diaphoresis, tachycardia, and possible hypotension if massive hemorrhaging is involved.

Prehospital treatment is supportive and aimed at maintaining the ABCs by providing high flow oxygenation and establishing intravenous access. Fluid resuscitation with crystalloid may be warranted if the patient appears hemodynamically unstable. Definitive treatment involves gastric intubation and suctioning for emesis control, diagnostic peritoneal lavage, antibiotic therapy, fluid resuscitation, and surgery to remove the blockage.

Hepatitis

Hepatitis involves any injury to hepatocytes (liver cells) associated with an inflammation or infection. Due to its wide range of potential causes, hepatitis has a high mortality rate. Five viruses—hepatitis types A, B, C, D, and E—are the disease's most common causes, resulting in five different kinds of hepatitis that together account for 60–70 percent of all cases. Alcoholic hepatitis, which arises from alcoholic cirrhosis, rather than an infectious agent, is responsible for another 20–30 percent. Trauma and other diseases account for the remaining 10 percent. Factors that increase the risk of contracting hepatitis include, to name a few, crowded, unsanitary living conditions, poor personal hygiene that invites oral-fecal transmission, exposure to blood borne pathogens, and chronic alcohol intake. (Specific risk factors are associated with the different types of hepatitis—A, B, C, D, and E.)

The liver is in the upper right abdominal quadrant. A very vascular organ, it filters and detoxifies blood returning from the abdomen and certain abdominal organs. Its other important functions include synthesizing fatty acids, converting glucose to glycogen, and helping to remove toxic products such as ammonia from the body. Any of the viral pathogens, alcoholic exposure, or trauma can injure the hepatocytes, causing inflammation and, possibly, chronic liver disease. Whatever its cause the results are usually similar. The changes in the liver include enlargement and hypertrophy, fatty changes, loss of architecture, and appearance of lesions and spontaneous hemorrhages. The symptoms' severity can range from mild to complete liver failure and death.

Of the five types of viral hepatitis, hepatitis A (HAV) is probably the best known. Commonly referred to as infectious hepatitis, (HAV) spreads by the oral-fecal route. The disease is self-limiting, usually lasting between two and eight weeks. It rarely causes severe hepatic injury and, thus, has a very low mortality rate. Hepatitis B (HBV), known as "serum hepatitis," is transmitted as a blood borne pathogen that can stay active in bodily fluids outside the body for days. With well over 310 million carriers worldwide, HBV is an epidemic. Its effects may be only minimal, but they can also range to severe liver ischemia and necrosis. Hepatitis C (HCV) is caused by the pathogen most commonly responsible for spreading hepatitis through blood transfusions. Hepatitis C is marked by chronic and often debilitating damage to the liver. Hepatitis D (HDV) is a less common disorder because its pathogen is dormant until activated by HBV. Hepatitis E (HEV) is a waterborne infection that has caused epidemics in Africa, Mexico, and other third-world nations. Its mortality rate for pregnant women is high.

Patients with hepatitis commonly present with symptoms relative to the severity of their disease. Usually they complain of upper right quadrant abdominal tenderness, not relieved by antacids, food, or positioning. They may lose their appetite and become anorexic, usually losing weight. The decrease in bile production changes their stool to a clay color, and increased bilirubin retention causes jaundice, a yellow coloring of the skin, and scleral icterus, a yellowing of the white of the eyes. Other symptoms include severe nausea and vomiting, general malaise, photophobia, pharyngitis, and coughing.

Physical examination will reveal a sick patient, possibly with a jaundiced appearance. Depending on the patient's severity, his positioning can range from standing up and walking around to lying in a fetal position with his knees drawn to his chest. Pain may present in the right upper quadrant or the right shoulder (referred from diaphragmatic irritation). Fever may be secondary to infection or to tissue necrosis. Inspection may yield nonspecific findings. Palpation may reveal an enlarged liver. Skin color and temperature can range from warm and dry (due to the infection) to cool, clammy, and diaphoretic if a hepatic lesion has ruptured and begun to bleed.

Prehospital treatment is mainly palliative. Secure the ABCs and establish intravenous access for fluid resuscitation or antiemetic administration. You must carefully consider any pharmacological administration because the liver breaks down many active drug metabolites. Definitive treatment involves antiviral and anti-inflammatory medications and symptomatic treatment.

Several large fire departments on the Eastern Seaboard of the United States have experienced increased rates of hepatitis C in their personnel. So always take precautions and work closely with your department infection control officer.

> *With well over 310 million carriers worldwide, HBV is an epidemic.*

> *Be wary of HIV, but fear hepatitis B and C. Do not forget to use personal protective equipment (PPE) and body substance isolation (BSI) precautions.*

> *If you suspect hepatitis, you must consider carefully any pharmacological administration because the liver breaks down many active drug metabolites.*

Summary

Abdominal pain can originate from a wide variety of causes, either from the abdominal organs or from areas outside of the abdominal cavity. The prehospital management priorities for the abdominal patient are to establish and maintain his airway, breathing, and circulation. The differential diagnosis can include a multitude of causes that usually cannot be identified without laboratory and radiographic analysis. Airway management is of paramount importance, since patients frequently suffer from severe bouts of nausea and vomiting. Be prepared to turn the patient onto his side if necessary to clear large amounts of vomitus from the airway. Oxygenation usually can be adequately stabilized by placing the patient on high flow oxygen via a nonrebreather mask. Fluid loss, hemorrhage, or sepsis may compromise the circulatory status. You should initiate fluid resuscitation for the hemodynamically unstable patient in the field, but never delay transport. Patients who have abdominal pain lasting over six hours should always be evaluated by a physician.

> *The key to successful treatment of gastrointestinal ailments is prompt recognition, treatment, and rapid transport to the hospital.*

CHAPTER 33

Urology and Nephrology

Objectives

After reading this chapter, you should be able to:

1. Describe the incidence, morbidity, mortality, and risk factors predisposing to urologic and nephrologic emergencies. (pp. 1432–1433, 1439, 1443, 1449, 1451)

2. Discuss the anatomy and physiology of the organs and structures related to the urinary system. (see Chapter 3)

3. Define referred pain and visceral pain as they relate to urology. (p. 1434)

4. Describe the questioning technique and specific questions the paramedic should use when gathering a focused history in a patient with abdominal pain. (pp. 1434–1436)

5. Describe the technique for performing a comprehensive physical examination of a patient complaining of abdominal pain. (pp. 1436–1438)

6. Define acute renal failure. (p. 1439)

7. Discuss the pathophysiology of acute renal failure. (pp. 1439–1441)

8. Recognize the signs and symptoms related to acute renal failure. (pp. 1441–1442)

9. Describe the management of acute renal failure. (pp. 1442–1443)

10. Integrate pathophysiological principles and assessment findings to

Continued

Objectives Continued

formulate a field impression and implement a treatment plan for the patient with acute renal failure. (pp. 1439–1443)

11. Define chronic renal failure. (p. 1443)

12. Discuss the pathophysiology of chronic renal failure. (pp. 1443–1444)

13. Recognize the signs and symptoms related to chronic renal failure. (pp. 1444–1446)

14. Describe the management of chronic renal failure. (pp. 1446–1449)

15. Integrate pathophysiological principles and assessment findings to formulate a field impression and implement a treatment plan for the patient with chronic renal failure. (pp. 1443–1449)

16. Define renal dialysis. (pp. 1446–1449)

17. Discuss the common complications of renal dialysis. (pp. 1447–1448)

18. Define renal calculi. (p. 1449)

19. Discuss the pathophysiology of renal calculi. (p. 1450)

20. Recognize the signs and symptoms related to renal calculi. (p. 1450)

21. Describe the management of renal calculi. (p. 1451)

22. Integrate pathophysiological principles and assessment findings to formulate a field impression and implement a treatment plan for the patient with renal calculi. (pp. 1449–1451)

23. Define urinary tract infection. (p. 1451)

24. Discuss the pathophysiology of urinary tract infection. (pp. 1451–1452)

25. Recognize the signs and symptoms related to urinary tract infection. (pp. 1452–1453)

26. Describe the management of a urinary tract infection. (p. 1453)

27. Integrate pathophysiological principles and assessment findings to formulate a field impression and implement a treatment plan for the patient with a urinary tract infection. (pp. 1451–1453)

28. Apply epidemiology to develop prevention strategies for urologic and nephrologic emergencies. (pp. 1433, 1443)

29. Integrate pathophysiological principles to the assessment of a patient with abdominal pain. (pp. 1433–1438)

30. Synthesize assessment findings and patient history information to accurately differentiate between pain of a urologic or nephrologic emergency and that of another origin. (pp. 1433–1438)

31. Develop, execute, and evaluate a treatment plan based on the field impression made in the assessment. (pp. 1432–1453)

INTRODUCTION

urinary system the group of organs that produces urine, maintaining fluid and electrolyte balance for the body.

urine the fluid made by the kidney and eliminated from the body.

urea waste derived from ammonia produced through protein metabolism.

genitourinary system the male organ system that includes reproductive and urinary structures.

nephrology the medical specialty dealing with the kidneys.

urology the surgical specialty dealing with the urinary/genitourinary system.

renal pertaining to the kidneys.

end-stage renal failure an extreme failure of kidney function due to nephron loss.

dialysis a procedure that replaces some lost kidney functions.

kidney transplantation implantation of a kidney into a person without functioning kidneys.

renal calculi kidney stones.

The **urinary system** performs a number of vital functions. It maintains blood volume and the proper balance of water, electrolytes, and pH (acid-base balance). It ensures that key substances such as glucose remain in the bloodstream, yet it also removes a variety of toxic wastes from the blood. It plays a major role in arterial blood-pressure regulation. In addition, the urinary system controls development of red blood cells, or erythrocytes.

The body eliminates water and other substances removed from blood in the form of the fluid **urine.** The kidneys' regulation of water and other important substances in blood is an example of homeostasis, the body's ability to maintain an appropriate internal environment despite changing conditions. Metabolism, the intracellular processes that generate the energy and materials necessary for cell growth and repair, also creates many waste products. For example, significant amounts of ammonia form in the liver when amino acids are broken down in gluconeogenesis, a process that produces glucose between meals. Ammonia is highly toxic to body cells, particularly brain cells. Liver cells convert the ammonia into **urea,** a less toxic compound. The kidneys remove urea efficiently from the blood and pass it into the urine. Moreover, the urinary system eliminates many foreign chemicals such as drug metabolites.

The urinary system in women is physically distinct from the reproductive system: they share no structures. (Chapters 39 and 40 discuss medical emergencies related to the female reproductive system.) In contrast, the urinary system in men does share some structures with the reproductive system. For instance, both urine and the male reproductive fluid are eliminated from the body through the opening at the tip of the penis. Consequently, the term **genitourinary system** is often used with men. The urinary and reproductive systems' proximity in women and their shared structures in men are due to the common embryonic origin of their tissues.

The most significant medical disorders involving the urinary system affect the kidneys and kidney function. **Nephrology** (from the Greek *nephros,* kidney) is the medical specialty devoted to kidney disorders. **Urology** is the surgical specialty devoted to care of the entire urinary system in women and the genitourinary system in men. We will use nephrology and nephrologic (or the preferred adjective, **renal,** from the Latin *renes,* kidneys) to refer to conditions primarily affecting the kidneys. We will use urology and urologic to refer to conditions that significantly affect other parts of the urinary or genitourinary systems.

Renal and urologic disorders are common, affecting about 20 million Americans. Many disorders are very serious. More than 50,000 Americans die annually from kidney disease. More than 250,000 Americans suffer from the most severe form of long-term kidney failure, **end-stage renal failure.** They require either **dialysis,** a process that artificially performs the most important kidney functions, or **kidney transplantation,** implantation of a kidney from another person, to survive. The leading causes of end-stage renal failure are poorly controlled diabetes mellitus (both type I and type II) and uncontrolled or inadequately controlled hypertension.

Among acute, or sudden-onset, disorders, **renal calculi,** or kidney stones, are very common. More than 500,000 Americans are treated for kidney stones each year. Infections are also common, and they may have different causes in women and men. A woman complaining of burning pain on urination probably has an infection in the urinary system. Men with the same chief complaint may have an infection that arose in the urinary system or as a sexually transmitted disease. Noncancerous enlargement of the prostate gland, or **benign prostatic hypertrophy,** affects about 60 percent of men by age 50 and about 80 percent by age 80. If prostatic hypertrophy obstructs urine flow, a medical emergency involving sharp pain and inability to urinate results.

All of these conditions, as well as others described later, are sufficiently common that you will see them in the field. In any case where existing kidney function may be jeopardized, prehospital care includes **preventive strategies,** or steps to minimize the likelihood of any further loss of function. Our discussion of assessment and management will cover these procedures.

GENERAL MECHANISMS OF NONTRAUMATIC TISSUE PROBLEMS

Both traumatic and nontraumatic problems can affect the urinary system, particularly the kidneys. The kidneys' retroperitoneal location protects them relatively well against injury. Nontraumatic renal and urologic disorders result from four general mechanisms: inflammatory or immune-mediated disease, infectious disease, physical obstruction, or hemorrhage. Traumatic renal and urologic disorders are discussed in Chapter 26. We will discuss nontraumatic disorders later in this chapter.

> **Content Review**
>
> ### MECHANISMS OF NONTRAUMATIC UROLOGIC DISORDERS
>
> - Inflammatory or immune-mediated disease
> - Infectious disease
> - Physical obstruction
> - Hemorrhage

GENERAL PATHOPHYSIOLOGY, ASSESSMENT, AND MANAGEMENT

As you learned in Chapter 32, abdominal emergencies are common. Because of many gastrointestinal (GI) and urologic emergencies' similar presentation, you may have difficulty determining the source of an abdominal problem when pain is the sole complaint. You can often find clues to the eventual diagnosis when you take a focused history and perform the focused physical exam. Before reading further, you may want to review the discussion of GI pathophysiology, assessment, and management in Chapter 32.

Because of many gastrointestinal and urologic emergencies' similar presentation, you may have difficulty determining the source of an abdominal problem when pain is the sole complaint.

PATHOPHYSIOLOGIC BASIS OF PAIN

The nerve fibers that carry pain messages to the brain are triggered by different stimuli. Some are triggered when damage to the epithelial lining of an organ exposes the underlying tissue layer, where the nerve endings are located. Others respond to stretching forces generated when an organ is inflamed or enlarged by internal hemorrhage or obstruction.

Causes of Pain

Bacterial infection damages the epithelial tissue that lines structures such as the urethra and urinary bladder. This damage causes pain that often worsens when urine flows over the affected tissue during urination. Bacteria normally found on the skin can cause infections in women. In men, the same symptom, pain on voiding, is often due to a sexually transmitted disease such as gonorrhea. Distention of a ureter by a renal calculus (kidney stone) causes a sharp pain that may ease or worsen when the stone shifts position inside the ureter.

Types of Pain

The most common types of pain in urologic emergencies are visceral and referred. **Visceral pain** usually arises in hollow structures such as the ureters, urinary bladder, and urethra, or the vas deferens or epididymis in males. Its chief characteristic, an aching or crampy pain felt deep within the body and poorly localized, is due to the relatively low number of nerve fibers in the involved structures. Visceral pain can also be the initial presentation of urinary tract infection or of renal calculi. **Referred pain** is felt in a location other than its site of origin. This occurs when afferent nerve fibers carrying the pain message merge with other pain-carrying fibers at the junction with the spinal cord. If that junction has far more nerve fibers from one or more other locations than from the site of origin, the brain may perceive the pain as coming from those locations rather than the affected one. Pyelonephritis, inflammation associated with kidney infection, is not only associated with pain in the flank, the skin surface closest to the kidney, but sometimes with pain in the neck or shoulder. The referred pain originates in diaphragmatic irritation due to kidney inflammation, but the brain perceives the pain as coming from the area of the neck or shoulder.

ASSESSMENT AND MANAGEMENT

The assessment steps are the same for all abdominal emergencies. Do not try to pinpoint the cause of abdominal pain in the field; diagnosis is often difficult even in the hospital setting. However, you do need to do an assessment to detect and manage life-threatening conditions such as shock and to provide historical and physical information that will be helpful in the hospital.

Scene Size-Up

During scene size-up, look for evidence of a traumatic versus medical cause and for signs of a life-threatening situation, perhaps an observer performing CPR or the presence of blood. Remember to employ personal protective equipment and proper handling.

Initial Assessment

Initial assessment of the patient concentrates on the ABCs of airway, breathing, and circulation, as well as on patient disability (for example, signs of agitation and confused mental state). If the patient is conscious and responsive, ask for the chief complaint.

Focused History

Information about Pain. When the chief complaint is pain or involves pain, initial questions should elicit information about the timing, character, and as-

---

* visceral pain pain arising in hollow organs such as the ureter and bladder.

* referred pain pain felt in a location other than that of its origin.

Do not try to pinpoint the cause of abdominal pain in the field.

Blood always calls for personal protective equipment and proper sample handling on your part.

sociated symptoms of the pain. The OPQRST template is useful for beginning your questions.

- *Onset* When did the pain start, and what were you doing at the time? Visceral pain often arises gradually, with the patient first aware of vague discomfort and only later aware of pain.

- *Provocation/Palliation* What makes the pain worse or better? Increased pain on urination, particularly in light of a fever or history of fever, suggests urinary/genitourinary tract infection. Pain associated with the inability to urinate, particularly in elderly men, points toward urethral obstruction due to prostatic enlargement. Improvement with knees drawn up to the chest points toward peritonitis, whereas improvement with walking may indicate a kidney stone that moved into a less painful position.

- *Quality* What is the pain like? Visceral pain is frequently described as dull or crampy; because many urinary-system structures are hollow, visceral pain is common in these emergencies. Vague discomfort followed by a change to sharp pain localized in the flank, for instance, may indicate ureteral obstruction due to a kidney stone that has moved.

- *Region/Radiation* Where is the pain located, or do you feel pain in several places? Does the pain seem to move from one part of your body to another? Listen for patterns of referred pain such as pain in the lower back and the neck or shoulder, as well as changes in perception of pain on movement of a limb or whole body. In postpubertal women, be sure to ask for menstrual history, particularly if menstrual-like cramps are described or blood is present in the perineal area. (For more on gynecologic and obstetrical emergencies, see Chapters 39 and 40.)

- *Severity* Where is the pain on a scale of 1 to 10? Has the intensity changed over time, and if so, how? Sudden changes to sharp pain, particularly when associated with decreased responsiveness and early signs of shock, may indicate rupture of an internal organ such as the appendix in appendicitis or the fallopian tube in an ectopic pregnancy. Most urologic problems will not show this pattern of abrupt and significant shift in severity and type of pain.

- *Time* How long ago did the pain start? Is it constant or does it come and go? Remember that any case of abdominal pain lasting about 6 hours or longer is considered a surgical emergency until proven otherwise, and the patient should be transported to an appropriate facility. Pelvic visceral pain of long duration and unchanging intensity, particularly if associated with signs suggesting urinary-tract origin such as fever and increased pain on urination, suggests a medical case rather than a surgical one, but you still may need to transport the patient to the hospital. When confronted with an acute abdomen (sudden onset of severe abdominal pain), always err on the side of considering it a potential surgical emergency.

- *Previous history of similar event* Some urologic emergencies such as renal calculus and infection may recur. This makes it especially important to elicit any history of a similar event, the diagnosis at the time, and the treatment given. Because increased risk for renal calculi is genetic in some cases, listen for a history of family members similarly affected.

- *Nausea/Vomiting* As you learned in Chapter 32, severe pain is often associated with autonomic nervous system discharge producing the signs of nausea, possibly with vomiting, along with profuse sweating, clammy skin, and rapid heart rate. Remember that such a presentation does not necessarily indicate that the problem is in the GI system. For instance, the severe pain of a kidney stone can cause this presentation.

- *Changes in bowel habits and stool* Frequent stools, especially if they are diarrheal or contain signs of blood (either melena or hematochezia), suggest a problem in the GI system. Recent constipation may not be relevant except in the context of physical findings.

- *Weight loss* Significant weight loss over a very short period (hours or days) almost always reflects water loss, and signs of dehydration will be evident. Longer-term weight loss may suggest chronic illness or GI dysfunction. Be sure to ask about conditions including diabetes, cardiovascular disease, and cancer, as well as medications and medication changes.

- *Last oral intake* The timing and content of the last meal may indicate an acute, progressive problem (a normal appetite, normal meal) or exacerbation of a long-standing one (poor appetite, small meal). Ask explicitly about fluid intake, because patients may not consider beverages to be food. The timing of the last oral intake is also important if the patient will be undergoing general anesthesia for a surgical procedure.

- *Chest pain* Chest pain, particularly left-sided, does not necessarily indicate a myocardial infarction (MI). Assess whether the pain pattern suggests angina (for example, chest pain associated with radiation to jaw and left arm). Also remember that patients with long-standing or severe diabetes may not show the typical pain pattern of an MI due to diabetic neuropathy (nerve damage), but signs of ischemia may appear on an ECG.

Focused Physical Examination

The focused examination includes forming an overall impression as well as examining the abdomen. Remember that you will not be able to diagnose most cases of abdominal pain in the field. Your job is to gather the historical and physical evidence that can be used in the hospital and to make sure the patient is supported before and during transport.

Appearance In general, any person with significant pain, particularly pain of some duration, will appear uncomfortable. A patient may show discomfort by rigidly maintaining the position of least pain or by constantly pacing if walking helps ease the pain.

Posture Lying with knees drawn to chest suggests peritonitis, which is often of GI origin. Relief with walking suggests visceral pain; kidney stones may shift position during walking, easing the sharp pain. Check visually if the patient who is walking is upright or favoring one side. Someone who looks feverish and walks hunched up, leaning to one side, and complaining of back pain may have a pyelonephritis (kidney infection).

During the focused history and physical exam, your job is to gather the historical and physical evidence that can be used in the hospital and to make sure the patient is supported before and during transport.

Level of Consciousness In the absence of fever, acute-onset decreases in responsiveness often suggest hemorrhage and evolution of hypovolemic shock. Hemorrhage is far more often tied to GI or reproductive (namely, obstetric) emergencies than to urinary system problems. You may see a decreased level of consciousness in sick patients who are undergoing dialysis, the artificial technique that replaces some vital kidney functions, including maintenance of electrolyte balance and removal of wastes. Try to determine if the change in responsiveness is acute or chronic, which may suggest a new problem or an aggravation of preexistent problems.

Apparent State of Health Patients with chronic illness, whether or not it originates in the urinary system, often look ill even without an acute problem. Extreme thinness, pale skin or mucous membranes, or the presence of home health equipment such as a bedside toilet, dialysis machine, or an oxygen tank all suggest chronic problems. In significant emergency states, the patient will usually not be tidy and neatly dressed. If he is, this may suggest that the emergency occurred suddenly, as with a hemorrhage or painful passage of a stone.

Skin Color Pale, dry, cool skin and mucous membranes may suggest chronic anemia such as that found in persons with chronic renal failure. Pale clammy skin suggests severe pain or shock, whereas flushed, dry skin may accompany fever.

Examination of the Abdomen The four components of the abdominal exam are inspection, auscultation, percussion, and palpation.

Always inspect the abdomen first. Note any ecchymotic discoloration or distention, as well as any surgical or traumatic scars. Most nephrologic and urologic emergencies will not show acute abnormalities on exam, whereas a number of GI emergencies will. Auscultation rarely produces a positive finding because bowel sounds are almost always present. Absence of bowel sounds, however, is important and suggests a GI emergency such as bowel obstruction.

Percussion and palpation may be more useful in the field. Percussion of the abdomen or other involved areas may produce clues to the origin of a urologic problem. Pain induced by percussion of the flanks, especially when accompanied by fever, strongly suggests pyelonephritis, or kidney infection. Pain on percussion just above the pelvic rim of the abdomen, especially when accompanied by fever and an increased urge to void, suggests cystitis, bladder infection. Constant, sharp pain increased by percussion of the affected flank may indicate where a kidney stone has lodged in a ureter.

In postpubescent girls and women, abdominal palpation may reveal pregnancy if you feel the firm, muscular mass of the gravid uterus above the pelvic rim. A ruptured ectopic pregnancy is possible when palpation increases pain in the lower quadrant, particularly when accompanied by evidence of hemorrhage or early shock. A vaginal exam is rarely indicated in the field; however, you should check for blood or other discharge at the urethral or vaginal openings. In all cases, ask the patient for the date of her last menstrual period.

Palpation of the lower abdomen may help diagnose acute urinary obstruction in older men due to prostatic enlargement. If enough urine has been retained, you will feel a large (up to roughly the size of a two-liter bottle), painful, fluctuant mass above the pelvic rim of the abdomen. This represents the distended bladder. The male abdominal exam should also include inspection of the penis and scrotum. Purulent discharge from the penis may indicate a sexually transmitted disease (STD). Palpation of the scrotum may detect a testicular mass (remember that testicular cancer is far more common in younger men—the opposite of the age risk for prostatic cancer). Palpable nontesticular masses may be painful (infectious epididymitis) or nonpainful (varicocele, a noninfectious swelling of the epididymis). Ask relevant questions, such as whether

Pain on percussion of the costovertebral angle (CVA—where the last rib meets the lumbar vertebrae) is known as Lloyd's sign and is indicative of pyelonephritis (infection of the kidney and renal pelvis).

swelling has been present for some time (as occurs with a varicocele) or is of recent onset (epididymitis).

Assessment Tools A hematocrit may detect significant or chronic bleeding. If blood is present in underwear or on the perineum itself, consider obtaining a small amount of material from the rectum or penile opening or opening of the vagina to be checked for visible blood or occult bleeding. The latter may help to localize the affected system.

Vital Signs Temperature is important because fever suggests an infectious process. If you found high blood pressure, increased heart rate, or both during the ABC assessment, put those findings into context with other impressions from the exam. For instance, both heart rate and blood pressure commonly increase in someone with severe pain. On the other hand, it is also important to find out the patient's usual readings, if either he or a bystander can tell you. Uncontrolled chronic hypertension is one of the two most common causes of nephron damage and chronic renal failure (with the other cause being diabetes mellitus).

Management and Treatment Plans

Management of the patient with abdominal pain includes general and case-specific elements.

Airway, Breathing, Circulation Field management always starts with the ABCs—airway, breathing, and circulation. Be sure to maintain an open airway and use high-flow oxygen by mask. Be prepared for vomiting in any patient with severe pain, whether or not it is likely of genitourinary origin. Circulatory support is also vital, especially when there is any indication of hemorrhage, dehydration, or shock or the patient appears to have any compromise of renal function. Monitor blood pressure closely, and monitor cardiac status with ECG per local protocol or discussion with medical direction.

In cases of abdominal pain, use analgesics as sparingly as possible.

Pharmacological Interventions Consider placing a large bore IV line for volume replacement or drug administration. Where possible, use a needle of sufficiently large bore for any emergency blood transfusion. In almost all cases involving abdominal pain, the question of **analgesics**, pain-relieving medications, will arise. The positive aspects of analgesic use are that the patient is more comfortable during transport and that pain- or stress-induced tachycardia, hypertension, or both may be abated. On the other hand, analgesics may mask the problem's signs and symptoms, making it very difficult to accurately gauge progression of the pathologic process. Use analgesics as sparingly as possible; local protocol or discussion with medical direction may be advisable.

Nonpharmacological Interventions Remember that patients with an acute abdominal problem are possible surgical cases. Thus, nothing should be given by mouth. Administer fluid or medication only by IV or IM routes. Monitor vital signs closely and look for any change in level of consciousness. Be sure the patient is in a position of relative comfort, but also ensure that the position minimizes risk of aspiration if vomiting occurs.

Transport Considerations Each patient with abdominal pain of greater than 6 hours is considered a surgical emergency until hospital evaluation proves otherwise. Rapidly yet gently transport all such patients. During transportation, talk quietly to the patient, both to calm him and to keep him informed of time until arrival or other pertinent matters. All of your actions, both with the patient and any family or friends in the ambulance, should reflect caring and competence.

RENAL AND UROLOGIC EMERGENCIES

You must know how to respond properly and quickly to each major type of urinary or genitourinary emergency. Prevention strategies, procedures that minimize further loss of any existing kidney function, are vital. Most of this discussion focuses on renal emergencies, those affecting the kidneys. The leading causes of kidney failure are diabetes mellitus (both types) and uncontrolled or inadequately controlled hypertension. Add to that profile the fact that nephron number decreases with age, and you have the general profiles of patients most at risk for significant problems affecting kidney function: older patients, those with diabetes or chronic hypertension, or those with more than one risk factor.

We will discuss three renal emergencies—acute renal failure, chronic renal failure, and renal calculi (kidney stones). We will also discuss one urologic disorder, urinary tract infection, which can affect any or all parts of the urinary/genitourinary system.

ACUTE RENAL FAILURE

Acute renal failure (ARF) is a sudden (often over a period of days) drop in urine output to less than 400–500 ml per day, a condition called **oliguria.** Output may literally fall to zero, a condition called **anuria.** ARF is not uncommon among severely ill, hospitalized patients. It is less common in the field. Noting ARF in the prehospital setting is vital because the condition may be reversible, dependent upon the cause and extent of damage associated with the disorder. Overall mortality is roughly 50 percent, in part because the condition usually appears in significantly injured or ill persons.

Pathophysiology

The three types of ARF are prerenal, renal, and postrenal. The distinct initial pathophysiology of each type determines both the severity of ARF and the likelihood for reversal and preserving renal function. The three types' common point is their clinical presentation: sudden-onset oliguria or anuria. You may wish to reread the summary of kidney physiology before reading about the pathophysiology for each type of ARF.

Prerenal ARF Prerenal ARF begins with dysfunction before the level of the kidney; that is, with insufficient blood supply to the kidneys, or hypoperfusion. Prerenal ARF not only accounts for the highest proportion of ARF cases—40 to 80 percent—but is also often reversible through restoration of proper perfusion. These factors make it extremely important to know conditions associated with increased risk of renal hypoperfusion and to treat the patient quickly and properly. Problems that can trigger prerenal ARF include some common field conditions: hemorrhage, heart failure (MI or CHF), sepsis, and shock (Table 33-1). These triggers decrease renal blood supply through a drop in blood volume, blood pressure, or both. In addition, any anomaly directly affecting blood flow into the kidneys (such as thrombosis of a renal artery or vein) can trigger prerenal ARF through an increase in renal vascular resistance. When renal vascular resistance becomes higher in the renal vessels than in systemic vessels, blood is effectively shunted away from the kidneys.

Normally, the kidneys receive about 20 to 25 percent of cardiac output. This high level of perfusion is essential to sustaining a GFR sufficient to maintain blood volume and composition and to clear wastes such as urea and creatinine from the bloodstream. As GFR drops, less urine forms, and the bloodstream retains water, electrolytes, and wastes such as urea and creatinine. Because the retained electrolytes include H^+ and K^+, metabolic acidosis and hyperkalemia may appear.

* **acute renal failure (ARF)** the sudden-onset of severely decreased urine production.

* **oliguria** decreased urine elimination to 400-500 ml or less per day.

* **anuria** no elimination of urine.

* **prerenal acute renal failure** ARF due to decreased blood perfusion of kidneys.

Prerenal ARF	Renal ARF	Postrenal ARF
Hypovolemia (hemorrhage, dehydration, burns)	Small vessel/glomerular damage (vasculitis—often immune-mediated, acute glomerulonephritis, malignant hypertension)	Abrupt obstruction of both ureters (secondary to large stones, blood clots, tumor)
Cardiac failure (myocardial infarction, congestive heart failure, valvular disease)	Tubular cell damage (acute tubular necrosis—either ischemic or secondary to toxins)	Abrupt obstruction of the bladder neck (secondary to benign prostatic hypertrophy, stones, tumor, clots)
Cardiovascular collapse (shock, sepsis)	Interstitial damage (acute pyelonephritis, acute allergic interstitial reactions)	Abrupt obstruction of the urethra (secondary to inflammation, infection, stones, foreign body)
Renal vascular anomalies (renal artery stenosis, or thrombosis, embolism of renal vein)		

Note: ARF secondary to transplant rejection is considered an immune-mediated form of renal ARF.

If hypoperfusion is prolonged or worsens in degree, two things happen. First, GFR decreases still further, and less filtrate means still less urine formation. Second, the nephron tubular cells become ischemic and active reabsorption and secretion decrease or cease. All of these metabolic effects of decreased nephron function further stress the body, particularly the cardiovascular system, and increase the likelihood that tubular ischemia will advance toward tubular cell death. At this point, the process is renal ARF, not prerenal.

Renal ARF In **renal ARF,** the pathologic process is within the kidney tissue, or renal parenchyma, itself. Three different processes cause renal ARF. The first is injury to small blood vessels (or **microangiopathy**) or glomerular capillaries; the second is injury to tubular cells; the third is inflammation or infection in the interstitial tissue surrounding nephrons (Table 33-1).

Microangiopathy and glomerular injury both result in obstruction of these minute vessels that are a vital part of the blood vessel-tubule structure of the nephron; consequently, nephron function is lost. Microangiopathy and glomerular injury are often immune-mediated and may be associated with systemic immune-mediated diseases such as diabetes mellitus type I and systemic lupus erythematosus. In these cases, ARF involves both preexistent and ongoing (that is, chronic and acute) nephron destruction.

Tubular cell death, or **acute tubular necrosis,** can follow prerenal ARF or can develop directly due to toxin deposition. Along with heavy metals and miscellaneous inorganic and organic compounds, a number of medications (including some antibiotics and cisplatin, an anticancer agent) can cause acute tubular necrosis.

Interstitial nephritis, a chronic inflammatory process also commonly due to toxic compounds including drugs (antibiotics, nonsteroidal anti-inflammatory drugs, diuretics), can also result in renal ARF.

Postrenal ARF The third form of ARF, **postrenal ARF,** originates in a structure distal to the kidney—the ureters, bladder, or urethra. In its earliest phase (before urine has backed up into the kidneys, shutting down further urine formation), postrenal ARF is reversible simply by removing the obstruction that is preventing elimination of urine. Urinary-tract obstruction causes fewer than 5 percent of ARF cases, but like prerenal ARF, it is important to identify be-

✳ renal ARF (renal acute renal failure) ARF due to pathology within the kidney tissue itself.

✳ microangiopathy a disease affecting the smallest blood vessels.

✳ acute tubular necrosis a particular syndrome characterized by the sudden death of tubular cells.

✳ interstitial nephritis an inflammation within the tissue surrounding the nephrons.

✳ postrenal acute renal failure ARF due to obstruction distal to the kidney.

cause the odds of reversal are good. If obstruction is not cleared, renal ARF may develop secondary to nephron and interstitial injury caused by renovascular obstruction.

Because both ureters must be blocked simultaneously for postrenal ARF to develop (assuming two kidneys are present), it is probably the least likely cause of the cases you will see. Far more common will be obstruction of the bladder neck or of the urethra.

Regardless of probable cause, treat ARF aggressively in the field so the patient will have the best chance for recovery.

Assessment

The focused history will often provide clues to the severity and duration of ARF. For instance, if the patient complains of inability to void for a number of hours associated with a feeling of painful bladder fullness, the cause may simply be acute obstruction at the bladder neck or urethra. In contrast, a patient with poor mentation may be unable to give a coherent history, and a family member will tell you that the patient has felt increasingly ill for several days and has not urinated at all within the past twelve hours or so. Questions likely to provide useful information include the following:

- *When was the decrease or absence of urine first noticed, and has there been any observed change in output since the problem was first noted? What was the patient's previous output?* The last question may be useful because patients with chronic renal failure due to inadequate renal function can develop ARF as a complication.

- *Has the patient noted development of edema (swelling) in the face, hands, feet, or torso? How about feelings of heart palpitations or irregular rhythm? Has a family member or friend noticed decreased mental function, lethargy, or overt coma?* If the patient continued to consume fluids after ARF developed, retention of water and Na^+ can lead to visible edema in a relatively short time. Retention of K^+ can lead to hyperkalemia, a condition that can be lethal, especially in a person with previously compromised heart function. Increasingly poor mentation can be a sign of metabolic acidosis.

The focused physical examination may be helpful in assessing the degree of ARF present, the antecedent condition, and any immediate threats to life. Impaired mentation or clear decreases in consciousness in a person with previously good mental function suggest severe ARF and a potential threat to life. In a patient without evidence of shock, cardiovascular findings may include hypertension due to fluid retention, tachycardia, and ECG evidence of hyperkalemia (Figure 33-1). If shock triggered the ARF or has developed more recently, profound hypotension may be present, accompanied by tachycardia and hyperkalemia.

General visual inspection will usually show pale, cool, moist skin; if shock is not present, these findings may still represent homeostatic shunting of blood to the internal organs, including the kidneys. Look for edema in face, hands, and feet (Figure 33-2). Examination of the abdomen will reveal very different findings dependent on the cause of ARF. As with any abdominal complaint, look for scars, ecchymosis, and distention. If the abdomen is distended, note whether the swelling is symmetric. Palpate for pulsing masses, which may indicate an abdominal aortic aneurysm. Auscultation is rarely helpful in renal and urological emergencies, and bowel sounds may be muffled if ascites (fluid

Impaired mentation or clear decreases in consciousness in a person with previously good mental function suggest severe ARF and a potential threat to life.

LOC 55510-3000

25 mm/sec 10.0 mm/mV | F – W 0.50-40

FIGURE 33-1. ECG with signs of hyperkalemia.

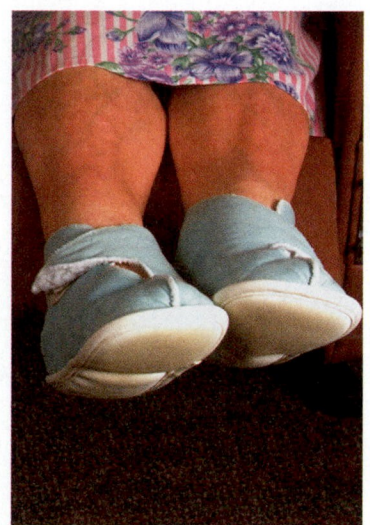

FIGURE 33-2. Edema of the feet consistent with fluid retention in acute renal failure.

Because ARF can lead to life-threatening metabolic derangements, monitoring and supporting the ABCs is vital.

---

within the abdomen) is present. Percussion and palpation findings will depend on the trigger condition.

A hematocrit may be useful if either acute hemorrhage or chronic anemia is suspected (the latter common in patients with cancer or chronic renal failure). Urinalysis can offer useful information very quickly. Proteinuria and glycosuria (urinary protein and glucose, respectively) suggest renal dysfunction. In some infections, notably pyelonephritis, the urine may contain so many white blood cells that they form a visible sediment in the specimen.

Renal function is clinically evaluated by laboratory analysis of the blood. Two frequently used indicators of renal function are the blood urea nitrogen (BUN) level and the serum creatinine. An elevation in either of these two values points toward renal insufficiency or failure. Usually, the ratio of BUN to creatinine (BUN/creatinine ratio) should be less than 20. A BUN/creatinine ratio greater than 20 indicates prerenal or postrenal problems, while a BUN/creatinine ratio of 20 or less indicates a renal problem.

Management

Because ARF can lead to life-threatening metabolic derangements, monitoring and supporting the ABCs is vital. Use high-flow oxygen to maximize breathing efficiency; couple this with circulatory supports such as positioning with head down and legs up to assist blood flow to the brain and internal organs and IV fluid resuscitation (bolus followed by drip) if hypovolemia is present. Patients who undergo peritoneal dialysis may benefit from fluid lavage of the abdomen; consult with medical direction to see if this is an option. Monitor ECG readings closely and adjust supports per local protocol or discussion with medical direction.

The chief prevention strategies are protecting fluid volume and cardiovascular function, as indicated by some of the steps previously noted, and eliminating or reducing exposure to any nephrotoxic agents or medications. If you are unsure whether an antibiotic, analgesic, or other drug is nephrotoxic and you are not in a position to check, discontinue the medication until the patient is at the appropriate care facility.

During transportation, be sure to talk quietly to the patient, both to calm him and to keep him informed of time until arrival or other pertinent matters. As

Table 33-2	CAUSES OF CHRONIC RENAL FAILURE
Type of Tissue Injury	**Examples**
Microangiopathy, glomerular injury	Systemic hypertension, diabetes mellitus, atherosclerosis, glomerulonephritis, systemic lupus erythematosus
Tubular cell injury	Nephrotoxins including analgesics and heavy metals, stones, obstruction at bladder neck or urethra
Interstitial injury	Infections including pyelonephritis, tuberculosis

Note: Congenital disorders resulting in CRF include polycystic disease and renal hypoplasia.

always, your actions should reflect caring competence. Even if the patient is confused or comatose, you should still address him respectfully as you perform procedures and avoid saying anything you do not want him to hear.

CHRONIC RENAL FAILURE

Chronic renal failure (CRF) is inadequate kidney function due to permanent loss of nephrons. Usually, at least 70 percent of the nephrons (healthy norm, 1 million per kidney) must be lost before significant clinical problems develop and the diagnosis is made. Metabolic instability does not occur until about 80 percent or more of nephrons are destroyed. When this point of dysfunction is reached, an individual is said to have developed **end-stage renal failure,** and must have either dialysis or a kidney transplant to survive. Anuria is not necessarily present in either CRF or end-stage renal failure.

> * **chronic renal failure** permanently inadequate renal function due to nephron loss.

Together, diabetes mellitus and hypertension cause more than half of all cases of end-stage renal failure. The death toll from CRF is high: More than 250,000 Americans have end-stage renal failure, and more than 50,000 die yearly from kidney disease. Roughly 30,000 new cases of CRF are diagnosed each year. The number of donor kidneys available in recent years has been sufficient for only about one-third of the persons on the waiting list to receive a kidney.

Pathophysiology

The three pathologic processes that initiate the nephron damage of CRF are the same as those underlying renal ARF: microangiopathy or glomerular capillary injury, tubular cell injury, and inflammation or infection in interstitial tissue (Table 33-2). Although the cause of initial nephron destruction is different for each of the three pathological processes, the same cycle of ongoing nephron damage becomes established: Functional nephrons adapt by increasing glomerular filtration primarily (through decreased vascular resistance in glomerular vessels and hypertrophy of capillary vessels) and by increasing tubular reabsorption and secretion secondarily (through cellular hypertrophy and functional adaptation of tubular cells). After a time, the compensatory changes damage these nephrons, leading to their destruction and initiating adaptive changes in additional, functional nephrons. Most of the damage seems to affect the glomeruli. Under the microscope, surviving nephrons often show dilated, abnormal glomeruli, and nonfunctional nephrons have heavily scarred glomeruli or no visible glomeruli, only sclerotic tissue.

*reduced nephron mass the decrease in number of functional nephrons that causes chronic renal failure.

*reduced renal mass the decrease in kidney size associated with chronic renal failure.

*isosthenuria the inability to concentrate or dilute urine relative to the osmolarity of blood.

*glucose intolerance the body cells' inability to take up glucose from the bloodstream.

*uremia the syndrome of signs and symptoms associated with chronic renal failure.

This characteristic loss of nephrons, or **reduced nephron mass,** is also visible at the level of gross anatomy as shrunken, scarred kidneys, or **reduced renal mass.** Physiologically, each of the kidney's four major functions is highly disturbed or absent, depending upon the degree of renal failure:

- *Maintenance of blood volume with proper balance of water, electrolytes, and pH.* In CRF, active transport in the tubules decreases significantly or ceases. Filtrate simply passes through the tubules, leading to characteristic **isosthenuria,** the inability to concentrate or dilute urine. As overall GFR falls over time, retention of Na^+ and water increases, causing a high-volume stress on the cardiovascular system. Retention of K^+ can lead to dangerous hyperkalemia, and retention of H^+ can lead to equally dangerous metabolic acidosis. Hypocalcemia is also common. It results from several causes, including renal retention of phosphate ions (with higher levels of serum phosphate facilitating Ca^{++} absorption into bone) and lack of renal production of Vitamin D.

- *Retention of key compounds such as glucose with excretion of wastes such as urea.* Glucose and other substances that normally are actively reabsorbed are also lost in urine as filtrate flows passively through the nephron. Any hypoglycemic effect is overshadowed, however, by the significant hyperglycemic effect (**glucose intolerance**) in most patients due to cellular resistance to insulin. The wastes urea and creatinine accumulate in blood almost in direct proportion to the number of nephrons lost. In fact, the general syndrome of signs and symptoms caused by severe CRF is termed **uremia,** for this characteristic buildup of blood urea.

- *Control of arterial blood pressure.* The renin-angiotensin loop is disrupted; even small amounts of renin can lead to severe hypertension. Hypertension may also develop due to retention of Na^+ and water. Cardiac decompensation, with hypotension and tachycardia, can develop suddenly, especially if cardiac function has been independently impaired.

- *Regulation of erythrocyte development.* Because erythropoietin is no longer produced in normal quantities (or at all, in some end-stage patients), chronic anemia develops. Anemia is another cardiac stressor, and it can contribute to cardiac failure.

Assessment

During the focused history and physical exam, you will probably find many characteristics of uremia in patients with CRF and end-stage disease. Table 33-3 lists some of these signs and symptoms, which affect nearly every organ system. Many of the listed problems can precipitate shock or other major physiologic instability; this is one reason you must always be alert when dealing with patients with CRF or end-stage disease, even when they initially appear stable. In addition, this list is by no means exhaustive. Kidney failure affects almost every organ and major function in the body.

The focused history will typically show GI symptoms such as anorexia and nausea, sometimes with vomiting. The patient's mentation as he speaks is an important clue to CNS impairment. Signs may be as subtle as anxiety or mood swings or as immediately serious as seizures or coma.

Always be alert for shock or other major physiologic instability when dealing with CRF or end-stage disease, even when the patient initially appears stable.

Table 33-3 COMMON ELEMENTS OF UREMIC SYNDROME

System	Pathophysiology	Clinical Sign/Symptom
Fluid/Electrolyte	Water/Na^+ retention	Edema, arterial hypertension[1]
	K^+ retention	Hyperkalemia[1]
	H^+ retention	Metabolic acidosis
	PaO_2 retention	Hyperphosphatemia/hypocalcemia[1]
Cardiovascular/Pulmonary	Fluid volume overload	Ascites, pulmonary edema
	Arterial hypertension	Congestive heart failure, accelerated atherosclerosis
	Dysfunctional fat metabolism; retention urea, other wastes	Pericarditis
Neuromuscular		
Central Nervous System	Retention urea, other wastes	Headache, sleep disorders, impaired mentation, lethargy, coma, seizures
Skeletal Muscle	Retention urea, other wastes; hypocalcemia	Muscular irritability and cramps, muscle twitching
Gastrointestinal (GI)	Retention urea, other wastes	Anorexia, nausea, vomiting
	Impaired hemostasis	Peptic ulcer, GI bleeding
Endocrine-Metabolic	Low vitamin D, other factors	Osteodystrophy
	Cellular resistance to insulin	Glucose intolerance
	Mechanisms unclear	Poor growth and development, delayed sexual maturation[2]
Dermatologic	Chronic anemia	Pallor skin, mucous membranes
	Retention urea, pigments	Jaundice, uremic frost
	Clotting disorders	Ecchymoses, easy bleeding
	Secondary hyperparathyroidism	Pruritus, scratches
Hematologic	Lack of renal erythropoeitin	Chronic anemia
	Impaired platelet function and prothrombin consumption	Impaired hemostasis, with easy bleeding, bruising; splenomegaly
Immunologic	Lymphopenia, general leukopenia	Vulnerability to infection

[1]Although relatively uncommon, fluctuations to the other extreme (example, hypokalemia) may occur if oral intake is poor over prolonged period or during or after dialysis treatment.

[2]Primarily seen in children, adolescents, young adults.

Your general impression before the focused physical exam is likely to note marked abnormalities. Skin will typically be pale, moist, and cool. Scratches and ecchymoses are common skin changes associated with CRF. Mucous membranes may also be very pale, dependent on the degree of anemia. Jaundice may be present, dependent on the degree of retention of urea and other pigmented metabolic wastes. A skin condition called uremic frost appears when excessive amounts of urea are eliminated through sweat. As the sweat dries, a white 'frosty' dust of urea may appear on the skin.

The major organ systems often show significant abnormalities on direct examination (Table 33-3). Because of the failure of vital urinary system functions, cardiovascular stress can be enormous. Either hypertension or hypotension may occur, dependent on the degree of fluid retention (retention detectable as peripheral edema or pulmonary edema) and the level of cardiac function; tachycardia is common with both presentations. ECG findings may include a dysrhythmia secondary to hyperkalemia. Metabolic acidosis, when present, compounds the effects of hyperkalemia. Pericarditis is also common, and a rub may be heard on chest auscultation. Neuromuscular abnormalities, in addition to impaired mentation, include muscle cramps and "restless legs syndrome," as well as muscle twitching or tonic-clonic or other forms of seizure.

Your abdominal exam will reveal many abnormalities. The challenge is to begin separating (by exam and history) chronic findings from those of recent onset or aggravated by the emergency that led to your call. For instance, you know that ecchymoses on the abdomen or flank may suggest acute hemorrhage. You may find a patient with ecchymoses scattered over the body surface. Look for evidence of new abdominal ecchymoses versus older bruises or a clear history of recent onset as signs of a current problem. Be sure to note abdominal contour, including the presence of symmetric distention or localized bulges, scars, and ecchymoses before the exam and to clearly document the pre-exam appearance. Findings on auscultation, percussion, and palpation will depend on the presenting problem.

The hematocrit and urinalysis generally have less value in CRF than in ARF. A hematocrit is useful only if you know the patient's baseline value, and recent changes in the amount of urinary output may be more significant than the content. The exceptions are blood (red blood cells) in urine, which is always a significant finding on dipstick analysis, and visible amounts of white blood cells, which suggest significant infection.

In CRF emergencies, the challenge is to separate chronic findings from those of recent onset or aggravated by the emergency that led to your call.

Management

Immediate Management As with ARF, CRF can lead to life-threatening complications, so monitoring and supporting the ABCs is vital. Use high-flow oxygen to maximize breathing efficiency. Couple this with circulatory supports such as positioning with the head down and the legs up to support blood flow to the brain and internal organs. Consider a small IV bolus for fluid resuscitation if hypovolemia is evident. Indications for fluid lavage (in peritoneal dialysis patients) are the same as those for patients with ARF. Monitor the ECG readings closely and adjust supports according to your local protocol or discussion with medical direction.

The chief prevention strategies are regulation of fluid volume and cardiovascular function and major electrolyte disturbances (for example, use of a vasopressor in hypotension and administration of bicarbonate for partial correction of acidosis, respectively) and elimination or reduction of exposure to any nephrotoxic agents or medications. Although uncommon, severe swings in electrolyte levels may occur during and after dialysis, so be cautious about replacement measures in the field in these patients. Err on the side of conservative treatment except for clearly life-threatening complications. If you are unsure whether a drug is nephrotoxic and you are not in a position to check, discontinue it until the patient is at the emergency department.

In CRF, err on the side of conservative treatment except for clearly life-threatening complications.

Expedite transportation to an appropriate facility in the same manner appropriate for patients with ARF. Be sure to talk quietly to the patient, both to calm him and to keep him informed of the time until arrival or other pertinent matters. If the patient is confused, ask short orientation questions periodically to assess lucidity and level of consciousness.

Long-term Management Renal dialysis, the artificial replacement of some of the kidney's most critical functions, is a fact of life for most patients with CRF and end-stage disease. Although dialysis is necessary for survival, it is not without risk.

 renal dialysis artificial replacement of some critical kidney functions.

One risk that you have already learned about is the possibility of physiologically destabilizing shifts in blood volume and composition and arterial blood pressure.

Dialysis was first developed about 30 years ago. Since then, two different technologies, hemodialysis and peritoneal dialysis, have been refined. Both rely on the same physiologic principles: osmosis and equalization of osmolarity across a semipermeable membrane such as that of the renal nephron. (You may wish to reread the explanation of osmosis in this chapter's physiology section before reading further.) In dialysis, the patient's blood flows past a semipermeable membrane that has a special cleansing fluid on the other side that is hypo-osmolar to blood for a number of impurities (such as urea, creatinine) and critical substances (such as Na^+, K^+, H^+). As the blood flows over the membrane, these substances in blood move into the hypo-osmolar solution, called the **dialysate,** and their concentrations in blood are thus reduced. The effect of dialysis is to temporarily lessen or eliminate volume overload and toxically high blood concentrations of electrolytes, urea, and other substances.

In **hemodialysis** (*hemo*=blood, *dia*=across, *lysis*=separation), the patient's blood is passed through a machine that contains an artificial membrane and the dialysate solution. Vascular access is required in order to achieve the necessary blood flow of 300 to 400 ml/minute. Often, a superficial, internal fistula is created surgically by anastamosing an artery and vein in the lower forearm. If the required healthy artery and vein are not available, surgeons can insert a special vascular graft made of artificial material between an artery and vein (Figure 33-3). If creating such a fistula is not possible, an indwelling catheter may need to be placed in the internal jugular vein. Because hemodialysis can be performed in settings including outpatient clinics and at home, you may see patients both between and during hemodialysis sessions. The three most common complications relate to vascular access. Two of the three complications are bleeding from the needle puncture site and local

✱ **dialysate** the solution used in dialysis that is hypo-osmolar to many of the wastes and key electrolytes in blood.

✱ **hemodialysis** a dialysis procedure relying on vascular access to the blood and on an artificial membrane.

FIGURE 33-3.   Vascular access for hemodialysis. (a) arteriovenous fistula; (b) artificial graft between artery and vein.

FIGURE 33-4. Peritoneal dialysis.

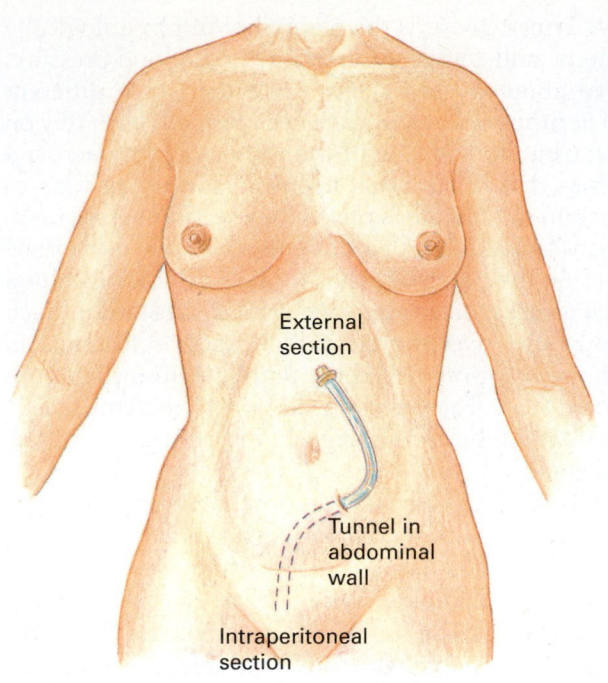

External section

Tunnel in abdominal wall

Intraperitoneal section

* **peritoneal dialysis** a dialysis procedure relying on the peritoneal membrane as the semipermeable membrane.

infection. The third is the narrowing or closing of the internal fistula. Under normal flow conditions, the internal fistula will have a palpable thrill (vibration), or bruit, due to the relatively high-volume turbulent flow from artery into vein. If the fistula narrows significantly or closes, however, this vibration is lost. The leading complications that require hospitalization are thrombosis, infection, and aneurysm development. They are particularly common in patients with grafts of artificial material.

Peritoneal dialysis uses the peritoneal membrane within the patient's abdomen as the semipermeable dialysis membrane, and dialysate solution is introduced and removed from the abdominal cavity via an indwelling catheter (Figure 33-4). This simpler technique, which used to be significantly less effective than hemodialysis, has been improved greatly in recent years. Currently, many patients practice either chronic peritoneal lavage (intermittent cycles in which dialysate is introduced, allowed to remain for an extended period, and then removed) or continuous peritoneal lavage (in which dialysate is introduced via a closed system that allows the patient to remain ambulatory during dialysis). Peritoneal dialysis avoids some of the risk of fluid and electrolyte shifts seen during hemodialysis, but its success requires additional physical characteristics (such as healthy vasculature around the peritoneum). The most common complication is infection in the catheter, the abdominal tunnel containing the catheter, or the peritoneum itself. The incidence of peritonitis is about one episode per year, so you may find its signs in these patients.

Both forms of dialysis have complications not related to vascular access in common. They include hypotension, shortness of breath, chest pain, and neurologic abnormalities ranging from headache to seizure or coma. If the patient is hypotensive, check for dehydration, hemorrhage, or infection. Shortness of breath and chest pain may reflect cardiac dysrhythmias (often secondary to hyperkalemia) or may be without identifiable cause. Be aware that these patients, many of whom have cardiac compromise, are at higher risk for ischemia or MI

FIGURE 33-5. Sectioned kidney with kidney stones.

during these periods. Neurologic abnormalities may occur before, during, or after treatment. In most cases they represent neurotoxicity of accumulated blood urea; in some cases rapid removal of urea from blood causes an osmotic diuresis from brain tissue with a resulting increase in intracranial pressure. Benzodiazepines may be useful in patients who develop seizures.

RENAL CALCULI

Kidney stones, or *renal calculi* (singular, *calculus*), represent crystal aggregation in the kidney's collecting system (Figure 33-5). This condition is also called nephrolithiasis (from Greek *lithos,* stone). Kidney stones affect about 500,000 persons each year. Brief hospitalization is common due to the severity of pain as a stone travels from the renal pelvis, through the ureter, to the bladder, and is eliminated in urine. If necessary, additional inpatient treatment may include shock-wave lithotripsy, a procedure that uses sound waves to break large stones into smaller ones. Overall morbidity and mortality are low, however, unless a complication such as hemorrhage or urinary-tract obstruction results. Stones form more commonly in men than women, although the ratio varies for types of stones with different compositions. Certain stones also occur in familial patterns, suggesting hereditary factors. Another risk factor for calculus formation is immobilization due to surgery or injury, with the latter including immobilization secondary to paraplegia or other paralysis syndromes that involve the absence of motor impulses, sensation, or both. Last, the use of certain medications, including anesthetics, opiates, and psychotropic drugs, increases the risk for stones.

Kidney stones occur more frequently in summer and fall.

Pathophysiology

Stones may form in metabolic disorders such as gout or primary hyperparathyroidism, which produce excessive amounts of uric acid and calcium, respectively. More often, they occur when the general balance between water conservation and dissolution of relatively insoluble substances such as mineral ions and uric acid is lost and excessive amounts of the insolubles aggregate into stones. The problem boils down to "too much insoluble stuff" and urine "too concentrated," a situation that may more likely arise with change in diet, climate, or physical activity.

Stones consisting of calcium salts (namely, calcium oxalate and calcium phosphate) are by far the most common. These compounds are found in from 75 to 85 percent of all stones. Calcium stones are from two to three times more common in men than in women, and the average age at onset is between 20 and 30 years. Their formation frequently runs in families, and anyone who has had a calcium stone is at fairly high risk to form another within two to three years.

Struvite stones (chemically denoted $MgNH_4PO_4$) are also common, representing about 10 to 15 percent of all stones. The pathophysiology of struvite stones differs from that of calcium stones. Their formation is associated with chronic urinary tract infection (UTI) or frequent bladder catheterization. The association with bacterial UTI makes struvite stones much more common in women than in men. These stones can grow to fill the renal pelvis, producing a characteristic "staghorn" appearance on X-rays.

Far less common are stones made of uric acid or cystine. Uric acid stones form more often in men than in women and tend to occur in families; about half of all patients with uric acid stones have gout. Cystine stones are the least common. They are associated with excess levels of cystine in filtrate and are probably due at least in part to hereditary factors, as they often run in families.

Assessment

The focused history almost always centers on pain. (Kidney stones are generally conceded to be among the most painful of human medical conditions.) Typically, the patient first notes discomfort as a vague, visceral pain in one flank. Within 30 to 60 minutes it progresses to an extremely sharp pain that may remain in the flank or migrate downward and anteriorly toward the groin. Migrating pain indicates that the stone has passed into the lowest third of the ureter. Stones that lodge in the lowest part of the ureter, within the bladder wall, often cause characteristic bladder symptoms such as frequency during the day or during the night (nocturia), urgency, and painful urination. Because these latter three symptoms far more frequently suggest bladder infection, making the probable diagnosis may be difficult, particularly in women. Visible hematuria is not uncommon in urine specimens taken during passage of a stone. Fever, however, is not typical unless infection is present. Whenever kidney stones are suspected, be sure to get the patient's personal medical history and family history, because both will often provide useful information.

The physical exam will almost always reveal someone who is very uncomfortable. The patient may be agitated or physically restless; walking sometimes reduces the pain. Vital signs will vary with level of discomfort, with highest blood pressure and heart rate associated with greatest pain. Skin will typically be pale, cool, and clammy. Abdominal examination may be difficult, depending on the patient's ability to remain still. First inspect the abdomen for contour and symmetry. Auscultation and percussion are generally useful only in ruling out GI conditions. Palpation results will vary and may depend, in part, on whether pain is so great that muscle guarding is present, making palpation of underlying structures impossible.

Whenever kidney stones are suspected, be sure to get the patient's personal medical history and family history.

Many male patients with kidney stones present with testicular pain on the affected side.

Management

As always, management begins with the ABCs. Positioning should center on comfort, but be prepared for vomiting due to the severe pain, especially if the patient's last meal was within several hours. Consider analgesia en route to the hospital, according to your local protocol and your perception of the patient's condition. Use narcotics cautiously if a GI condition is at all possible or if mentation is impaired. If the pain is in the initial, intermittent, colicky phase, consider coaching pain management through breathing techniques similar to those used for women in labor. An IV line is useful for volume replacement or drug administration. The usual prevention strategy, if kidney function is adequate, is IV fluid to promote urine formation and movement through the system. Transport is the same as that for other abdominal conditions, i.e., position of comfort and supportive care.

Parenteral narcotic analgesics or ketorolac (Toradol) should be considered for the patient with renal colic.

URINARY TRACT INFECTION

Urinary tract infection, or UTI, affects the urethra, bladder, or kidney, as well as the prostate gland in men. UTIs are extremely common, accounting for over 6 million office visits yearly. Almost all UTIs start with pathogenic colonization of the bladder by bacteria that enter through the urethra. Thus, females in general are at higher risk because of their relatively short urethra. Other groups at risk for UTI are paraplegic patients or patients with nerve disruption to the bladder, including some diabetic persons. Any condition that promotes **urinary stasis** (incomplete urination with urine remaining in the bladder that may serve as nutrition for pathogens) places a person at higher risk. Pregnant women often have urinary stasis due to pressure from the gravid uterus. People with neurological impairment (some patients with spina bifida or with diabetic neuropathy, for example) also tend to have urinary stasis, which predisposes them to infection. The use of instrumentation in patients who require bladder catheterization places them at even higher risk of UTIs.

Morbidities such as scarring, abscesses, or eventual development of CRF are most likely in persons with anatomic abnormalities of the urinary system or chronic calculi (the latter acting as a focus for continuing infection and inflammation), those who are immunocompromised, or those who have renal disease due to diabetes mellitus or another condition.

✱ **urinary tract infection (UTI)** an infection, usually bacterial, at any site in the urinary tract.

✱ **urinary stasis** a condition in which the bladder empties incompletely during urination.

Pathophysiology

UTIs are generally divided into those of the lower urinary tract, namely, urethritis (urethra), cystitis (bladder), and prostatitis (prostate gland), and those of the upper urinary tract, pyelonephritis (kidney).

Lower UTIs are far more common than upper UTIs, for two reasons. First, seeding of infection via the bloodstream is rare. Second, asymptomatic bacterial colonization of the urethra, especially in females, is very common, and can predispose a person to infection by other, pathogenic bacteria.

In females, infection may begin when Gram-negative bacteria normally found in the bowel (that is, the enteric flora) colonize the urethra and bladder. Symptomatic **urethritis,** inflammation secondary to urethral infection, is very uncommon. More often you will see joint symptomatic infection of the urethra and bladder (urethritis and **cystitis,** respectively). Sexually active females are at higher risk, which may be attributed to use of contraceptive devices or agents, to the introduction of enteric flora during intercourse, or both. Recently, homosexually active men who engage in anal sex have also been found to be at higher risk for bacterial cystitis, possibly due to introduction of enteric bacterial flora during

✱ **urethritis** an infection and inflammation of the urethra.

✱ **cystitis** an infection and inflammation of the urinary bladder.

intercourse. In any case, sexually active persons who suffer from urinary stasis are at even higher risk for infection. Persons who urinate after intercourse might lower their risk because voiding eliminates some bacteria. The pathophysiology for persons using bladder catheterization probably differs only in that pathogenic bacteria are introduced directly into the bladder via the catheter. In general, the likelihood that active cystitis will develop, that antibiotic treatment will clear such infections, and that reinfection will occur are all determined by the interplay of the pathogen's virulence, the size of its colony, its sensitivity to antibiotic treatment, and the strength of the host's local and systemic immune functions.

Prostatitis, inflammation of the prostate gland, in our context, denotes inflammation secondary to bacterial infection, as well as any general inflammatory condition. Men with acute bacterial prostatitis, the closest parallel to acute cystitis in women, also tend to show evidence of joint urethritis, and the same bowel flora tend to be involved. The major difference between acute bacterial prostatitis and acute cystitis is the much lower incidence of prostatitis among men who do not require bladder catheterization.

Upper UTIs usually evolve from infection that spreads upward into the kidney. **Pyelonephritis** is an infectious inflammation of the renal parenchyma: nephrons, interstitial tissue, or both. Acute pyelonephritis is ten times more common in women than in men. Its incidence is highest in pregnancy and during periods of sexual activity, reflecting the epidemiology of lower UTIs. If the infection of pyelonephritis persists, intrarenal or perinephric abscesses may occur, but these complications are uncommon. **Intrarenal abscesses** form within the renal parenchyma. If they rupture and spill their contents into the adjacent fatty tissue, **perinephric abscesses** may result. From 20 to 60 percent of patients who develop perinephric abscesses have a clear predisposing factor such as renal calculi, anatomic abnormalities of the kidney, history of urologic surgery or injury, or diabetic renal disease.

Urinary tract infections may be community-acquired or nosocomial. Among **community-acquired infections,** Gram-negative enteric bacteria predominate. In fact, *E. coli* accounts for roughly 80 percent of infections in persons without the complicating factors of bladder catheterization, renal calculi, or anatomic abnormalities. In **nosocomial infections,** cases acquired in an inpatient setting or related to catheterization, *Proteus, Klebsiella,* and *Pseudomonas* are commonly identified. Less common, but still important, are sexually transmitted pathogens (among women and men) such as *Chlamydia* and *N. gonorrhoeae.* Fungi such as *Candida* are rarely seen except in catheterized or immunocompromised patients or patients with diabetes mellitus.

Assessment

The focused history of lower UTI typically centers on three symptoms: painful urination, frequent urge to urinate, and difficulty in beginning and continuing to void. Pain often begins as visceral discomfort that progresses to severe, burning pain, particularly during and just after urination. The evolution of pain corresponds roughly to the degree of epithelial damage caused by the pathogen. In both men and women, pain is often localized to the pelvis and perceived as in the bladder (in women) or bladder and prostate (in men). The patient may complain of a strong or foul odor in the urine. Many women will give a history of similar episodes, which may or may not have been diagnosed or treated. Patients with pyelonephritis are more likely to feel generally ill or feverish. They typically complain of constant, moderately severe or severe pain in a flank or lower back (just under the rib cage). Pain may be referred to the shoulder or neck. The triad of urgency, pain, and difficulty may or may not be present or included in the past history.

*✱ **prostatitis** infection and inflammation of the prostate gland.*

*✱ **pyelonephritis** an infection and inflammation of the kidney.*

*✱ **intrarenal abscess** a pocket of infection within kidney tissue.*

*✱ **perinephric abscess** a pocket of infection in the layer of fat surrounding the kidney.*

*✱ **community-acquired infection** an infection occurring in a non-hospitalized patient who is not undergoing regular medical procedures, including the use of instruments such as catheters.*

*✱ **nosocomial infection** an infection acquired in a medical setting.*

On physical exam, patients with UTI appear restless and uncomfortable. Typically, patients with pyelonephritis appear more ill and are far more likely to have a fever. Skin will often be pale, cool, and moist (in lower UTI) or warm and dry (in febrile upper UTI). Vital signs will vary with the degree of illness and pain, but in an otherwise healthy individual they should not be far from the norms. Inspect and auscultate the abdomen to document findings, but neither procedure is likely to be very useful, as visible appearance and bowel sounds are usually within normal limits. Percussion and palpation will probably reveal painful tenderness over the pubis in lower UTI and at the flank in upper UTI. Lloyd's sign, tenderness to percussion of the lower back at the costovertebral angle (CVA), indicates pyelonephritis.

Management

UTI management should center on the ABCs and circulatory support. If pain is severe, help the patient to a comfortable position, but consider the risk of aspiration during vomiting. Analgesics should be considered as with renal calculi; they will probably be needed only for severely painful cases of pyelonephritis. Consider nonpharmacological pain management with breathing and relaxation techniques. The best prevention technique is hydration to increase blood flow through the kidneys and to produce a more dilute urine. In many cases, this is better accomplished by IV administration, which eliminates the risk of vomiting and satisfies the guidelines for possible surgical cases. Expedite transport to an appropriate facility.

The patient with acute pyelonephritis will usually appear quite ill. The patient with cystitis, on the other hand, will be uncomfortable but will not appear toxic.

Summary

The urinary system (1) maintains blood volume and the proper balance of water, electrolytes, and pH; (2) enables the blood to retain key substances such as glucose and removes a variety of toxic wastes from the blood; (3) plays a major role in regulation of arterial blood pressure; and (4) controls maturation of red blood cells. Kidney nephrons produce urine. Homeostasis through urine production is responsible for the first two functions and assists in the third, regulating blood pressure, by producing renin, the enzyme through which blood pressure is controlled. Other kidney cells produce erythropoietin, the hormone that stimulates red blood cell maturation.

Renal and urologic emergencies typically present as an acute abdomen. The most common are acute renal failure (ARF), chronic renal failure (CRF, with the subset of end-stage renal disease), and renal calculi. Both ARF and CRF may present with life-threatening complications and impaired function of other systems. Be prepared for apparently stable patients to acutely develop destabilizing complications (often, cardiovascular). Urinary tract infections, or UTIs, are divided into those of the lower urinary tract (urethra, bladder, and prostate in men) and those of the upper urinary tract (kidney). Both types of infection can present with considerable pain, but pyelonephritis is the more serious, with fever likely and complications including abscesses possible.

Because renal function is often lowered in the elderly and in persons with hypertension or diabetes, consider it potentially impaired in all of these patients. The best prevention strategies are to minimize the likelihood of prerenal failure by protecting blood volume and blood pressure and to investigate possible postrenal urinary tract obstruction.

CHAPTER 34

Toxicology and Substance Abuse

Objectives

After reading this chapter, you should be able to:

1. Describe the incidence, morbidity, and mortality of toxic and drug abuse emergencies. (p. 1456)
2. Identify the risk factors most predisposing to toxic emergencies. (p. 1456)
3. Discuss the anatomy and physiology of the organs and structures related to toxic emergencies. (pp. 1457–1458)
4. Describe the routes of entry of toxic substances into the body. (pp. 1457–1458)
5. Discuss the role of Poison Control Centers in the United States. (pp. 1456–1457)
6. Discuss the pathophysiology, assessment findings, need for rapid intervention and transport, and management of toxic emergencies. (pp. 1456–1495)
7. List the most common poisonings, pathophysiology, assessment findings, and management of poisoning by ingestion, inhalation, absorption, injection, and overdose. (pp. 1457–1495)
8. Define the following terms:
   a. Substance or drug abuse (p. 1488)
   b. Substance or drug dependence (p. 1488)
   c. Tolerance (p. 1488)
   d. Withdrawal (p. 1489)
   e. Addiction (p. 1488)
9. List the most commonly abused drugs (both by chemical name and by street names). (pp. 1490–1491)
10. Describe the pathophysiology, assessment findings, and management of commonly used drugs. (pp. 1488–1495)
11. List the clinical uses, street names, pharmacology, assessment findings, and

Continued

management for patients who have taken the following drugs or been exposed to the following substances:

a. Cocaine (pp. 1465, 1468, 1489–1490)
b. Marijuana and cannabis compounds (p. 1491)
c. Amphetamines and amphetamine-like drugs (pp. 1490, 1491)
d. Barbiturates (pp. 1490, 1491)
e. Sedative-hypnotics (p. 1491)
f. Cyanide (p. 1491)
g. Narcotics/opiates (p. 1490)
h. Cardiac medications (pp. 1469–1470)
i. Caustics (p. 1470)
j. Common household substances (pp. 1470–1471)
k. Drugs abused for sexual purposes/sexual gratification (p. 1492)
l. Carbon monoxide (pp. 1468–1469)
m. Alcohols (p. 1490)
n. Hydrocarbons (pp. 1471–1472)
o. Psychiatric medications (pp. 1472–1475)
p. Newer anti-depressants and serotonin syndromes (p. 1474)
q. Lithium (pp. 1474–1475)
r. MAO inhibitors (p. 1473)
s. Non-prescription pain medications (1) Nonsteroidal antiinflammatory agents (2) Salicylates (3) Acetaminophen (pp. 1475–1477)
t. Theophylline (p. 1477)
u. Metals (pp. 1477–1478)
v. Plants and mushrooms (pp. 1479–1480)

12. Discuss common causative agents or offending organisms, pharmacology, assessment findings, and management for a patient with food poisoning, a bite, or a sting. (pp. 1478–1488)

13. Given several scenarios of poisoning or overdose, provide the appropriate assessment, treatment, and transport. (pp. 1455–1495)

INTRODUCTION

Toxicology is the study of **toxins** (drugs and poisons) and antidotes and their effects on living organisms. Toxicological emergencies result from the ingestion, inhalation, surface absorption, or injection of toxic substances that then exert their adverse effects on the body's tissues and metabolic mechanisms. Theoretically all toxicological emergencies can be classified as poisoning. However, in this discussion, the term *poisoning* will be used to describe exposure to non-pharmacological substances. The term *overdose* will be used to describe exposure to pharmacological substances, whether the overdose is accidental or intentional. Substance abuse, although technically a form of poisoning, will be addressed separately.

In this chapter we will discuss various aspects of toxicological emergencies as they apply to prehospital care. We will establish general treatment guidelines for each type of toxic exposure, then address the specific issues surrounding some of the more common substances involved. Because the field of toxicology is rapidly changing, it is virtually impossible for a paramedic to remain up to date on treatment guidelines for each type of toxic exposure. Specific treatment should be supervised by medical direction in association with a Poison Control Center. This plan ensures that the patient receives the most current level of care available.

* **toxicology** study of the detection, chemistry, pharmacological actions, and antidotes of toxic substances.

* **toxin** any chemical (drug, poison, or other) that causes adverse effects on an organism that is exposed to it.

EPIDEMIOLOGY

Over the years, the occurrence of toxicological emergencies has continued to increase in number and severity. The following figures reveal the high potential for toxic substance involvement on an EMS call.

- The American Association of Poison Control Centers estimates over 4 million poisonings occur annually.
- Ten percent of all emergency department visits and EMS responses involve toxic exposures.
- Seventy percent of accidental poisonings occur in children under the age of 6 years.
- A child who has experienced an accidental ingestion has a 25 percent chance of another, similar ingestion within one year.
- Eighty percent of all attempted suicides involve a drug overdose.

Although over half of all poisonings occur in children aged 1–5, they are generally accidental and relatively mild, accounting for only ten percent of hospital admissions for poisoning and only five percent of the fatalities. EMS personnel must be aware that more serious poisonings, especially in children older than 5, may represent intentional poisoning by parents or caretakers. Unfortunately, poisoning due to drug experimentation and suicide attempts are also becoming a common consideration in older children.

Adult poisonings and overdoses, although less frequent, account for 90 percent of hospital admissions for toxic substance exposure. They also account for 95 percent of the fatalities in this category. Most adult poisonings and overdoses are intentional. Intentional poisonings and overdoses can be due to illicit drug use, alcohol abuse, attempted suicide, and "suicidal gesturing" in which the patient is making a cry for help but may miscalculate and take a type or amount of toxin that does actually cause injury. More rarely, intentional poisoning can result from attempted homicide or chemical warfare. Accidental poisonings are increasingly caused by exposure to chemicals and toxins on the farm or in the industrial workplace. More often they are the result of idiosyncratic (individual hypersensitivity) reactions or dosage errors when taking prescribed medications, but these usually do not require medical attention.

POISON CONTROL CENTERS

Poison Control Centers have been set up across the United States and Canada to assist in the treatment of poison victims and to provide information on new products and new treatment recommendations. They are usually based in major medical centers and teaching hospitals and serve a large population. Almost all Poison Control Centers now have computer systems to rapidly access information.

Poison Control Centers are usually staffed by physicians, toxicologists, pharmacists, nurses, or paramedics with special training in toxicology. These experts provide information to callers 24 hours a day, seven days a week. They update information regularly and offer the most current treatment guidelines.

Memorize the number of the nearest Poison Control Center and access it routinely. There are several advantages to this. First, the Poison Control Center can help you immediately determine potential toxicity based on the type of agent, amount and time of exposure, and physical condition of the patient. Second, the

Memorize the number of the nearest Poison Control Center and access it routinely for information regarding a poisoning or overdose.

most current, definitive treatment can sometimes be started in the field. Finally, the Poison Control Center can notify the receiving hospital of current treatment and recommendations even before arrival of the patient.

ROUTES OF TOXIC EXPOSURE

In order to have a destructive effect, poisons must gain entrance into the body. The four portals of entry are *ingestion, inhalation, surface absorption,* and *injection*. It is important to note that, regardless of the portal of entry, toxic substances have both immediate and delayed effects.

INGESTION

Ingestion is the most common route of entry for toxic exposure. Frequently ingested poisons include:

- Household products
- Petroleum-based agents (gasoline, paint)
- Cleaning agents (alkalis and soaps)
- Cosmetics
- Drugs (prescription, non-prescription, illicit)
- Plants
- Foods

Immediate toxic effects of ingestion of corrosive substances, such as strong acids or alkalis, can involve burns to the lips, tongue, throat, and esophagus. Delayed effects result from absorption of the poison from the gastrointestinal tract. Most absorption occurs in the small intestine, with only a small amount being absorbed from the stomach. Some poisons may remain in the stomach for up to several hours, because the intake of a large bolus of poison can retard absorption. Aspirin ingestion is a classic example of this. When a patient ingests a large number of aspirin tablets, the tablets can bind together to form a large bolus that is difficult to remove or break down.

INHALATION

Inhalation of a poison results in rapid absorption of the toxic agent through the alveolar-capillary membrane in the lungs. Inhaled toxins can irritate pulmonary passages, causing extensive edema and destroying tissue. When these toxins are absorbed, wider systemic effects can occur. Causative agents can appear as gases, vapors, fumes, or aerosols. Common inhaled poisons include:

- Toxic gases
- Carbon monoxide
- Ammonia
- Chlorine
- Freon
- Toxic vapors, fumes, or aerosols
- Carbon tetrachloride
- Methyl chloride
- Tear gas

Content Review

ROUTES OF TOXIC EXPOSURE
- Ingestion
- Inhalation
- Surface absorption
- Injection

It is important to remember that toxic substances have both immediate and delayed effects.

✱ ingestion entry of a substance into the body through the gastrointestinal tract.

✱ inhalation entry of a substance into the body through the respiratory tract.

- Mustard gas
- Nitrous oxide

SURFACE ABSORPTION

Surface absorption is the entry of a toxic substance through the skin or mucous membranes. This most frequently occurs from contact with poisonous plants such as poison ivy, poison sumac, and poison oak. Many toxic chemicals may also be absorbed through the skin. **Organophosphates,** often used as pesticides, are easily absorbed through dermal contact.

INJECTION

Injection of a toxic agent under the skin, into muscle, or into a blood vessel results in both immediate and delayed effects. The immediate reaction is usually localized to the site of the injection and appears as red, irritated, edematous skin. An allergic or anaphylactic reaction can also appear (see Chapter 31). Later, as the toxin is distributed throughout the body by the circulatory system, delayed systemic reactions can occur.

Other than intentional injection of illicit drugs, most poisonings by injection result from the bites and stings of insects and animals. Most insects that can sting and bite belong to the class *Hymenoptera,* which includes honey bees, hornets, yellow jackets, wasps, and fire ants. Only the females in this group can sting. In addition, spiders, ticks, and other arachnids, such as scorpions, are notorious for causing poisonings by injection. Higher animals that bite and sting include snakes and certain marine animals. Marine animals with venomous stings include jellyfish (especially the Portuguese man-of-war), stingrays, anemones, coral, hydras, and certain spiny fish.

GENERAL PRINCIPLES OF TOXICOLOGIC ASSESSMENT AND MANAGEMENT

Although specific protocols for managing toxicological emergencies may vary, certain basic principles apply to most situations. Keep in mind the importance of recognizing the poisoning promptly. Have a high index of suspicion if circumstances suggest involvement of a toxin in the emergency.

SCENE SIZE-UP

Always begin assessment with a thorough evaluation of the scene. Take note of where you are and who is around you. Be alert for any potential danger to you, the rescuer. Remember, despite your natural urge to immediately assess and treat the patient, if you are incapacitated you will not be able to help anyone and you will become a patient yourself. In toxicological emergencies there are specific hazards to keep in mind.

- Patients who are suicidal may have the potential for violence. They are often intoxicated, may act irrationally, and will not always be cooperative or happy to see you. Therefore, look for signs of overdose such as empty pill bottles and used needles or other drug paraphernalia. Never put your hand blindly into a patient's pocket as it may contain used needles.

- Chemical spills and hazardous material emergencies can quickly incapacitate any individuals who are nearby. Make sure you have the proper clothing and equipment needed for the particular emergency. Distribute this gear to rescuers who have been trained in their use.

Rescuer safety takes particular priority during scene size-up for a toxicological emergency.

INITIAL ASSESSMENT

After the scene size-up, perform the standard initial assessment. Form a general impression and quickly assess mental status. Assessment of the ABCs is critical in toxicological emergencies because airway and respiratory compromise are common complications. This can be due to direct airway injury, pulmonary injury, profuse secretions, or decreased respiratory effort secondary to altered mental status. After assessing the ABCs, set a transport priority for the patient.

HISTORY, PHYSICAL EXAM, AND ONGOING ASSESSMENT

For responsive patients, start by obtaining a history. It is important to find out not only what toxin the patient was exposed to but when the exposure took place, since toxic effects develop over time. Then proceed to a focused physical exam with full vital signs. With unresponsive patients, start with a rapid head-to-toe exam. Be alert for signs of trauma inconsistent with the suspected intoxication. Then proceed to obtain a history from relatives or other bystanders. Relay this information to the local Poison Control Center. They will advise you on the most current protocol for treatment. Be aware of your local policy, which will outline whether you can initiate this protocol or whether you must first contact on-line medical direction. Never delay supportive measures or immediate transport to the hospital based on a delay in contacting or obtaining information from the Poison Control Center.

It is important to find out not only what toxin the patient was exposed to but when the exposure took place, since toxic effects develop over time.

A detailed physical exam can be performed en route if time and the patient's condition permit. Ongoing assessment is essential for these patients. Poisoned patients can deteriorate suddenly and quickly. Repeat the initial assessment and vitals and re-evaluate every five minutes for critical/unstable patients and every fifteen minutes for stable patients.

Never delay supportive measures or immediate transport based on a delay in contacting the Poison Control Center.

TREATMENT

Decontamination

Once you have initiated supportive treatment (airway control, breathing assistance, and IV fluids), proceed to a mode of treatment that is specific to toxicological emergencies: decontamination. **Decontamination** is the process of minimizing toxicity by reducing the amount of toxin absorbed into the body. There are three steps to decontamination.

* decontamination the process of minimizing toxicity by reducing the amount of toxin absorbed into the body.

1. *Reduce intake of toxin.* This means that you must remove a person from an environment where they are inhaling toxic fumes, or you must properly remove a stinger and sac from someone stung by a bee. A classic example involves a person who has had organophosphates spilled on him. The patient's clothes must be removed and the skin cleaned with soap and water to reduce absorption of the toxins.

2. *Reduce absorption of toxin once in the body.* This usually applies to ingested toxins, which wait in the stomach and intestines while the body absorbs them into the blood stream.

> **Content Review**
>
> **PRINCIPLES OF DECONTAMINATION**
> - Reduce intake
> - Reduce absorption
> - Enhance elimination

In the past, syrup of ipecac was used to induce vomiting in order to empty the stomach. **Use of syrup of ipecac is no longer acceptable.** Studies consistently show that the use of syrup of ipecac to induce emesis reduces absorption by only 30 percent. This still leaves 70 percent of the toxin to be absorbed and cause injury. Vomiting also limits the use of other oral agents that are more effective for decontamination (e.g., activated charcoal) or oral antidotes (e.g., N-Acetylcysteine). There is also an increased risk of aspiration with vomiting, which makes induction of vomiting a procedure with minimal usefulness and high risk. Although ipecac may have some minor role in home management of some pediatric poisonings, it has generally become an obsolete treatment.

Gastric lavage ("pumping the stomach") has also been found to be of limited use. This process involves passing a tube into the stomach and repeatedly filling and emptying the stomach with water or saline in hopes of removing the ingested poison. Most studies have shown that gastric lavage removes almost no poisons from the stomach unless it is initiated within one hour of the ingestion. Possible complications, such as aspiration or perforation, make this procedure a risk without much benefit. Except in limited situations with ingestions of highly toxic substances that do not bind to charcoal and for which there is no antidote, gastric lavage has become an uncommon decontamination procedure.

The most effective and widely used method of reducing absorption of toxins is **activated charcoal.** Because of its extremely large surface area, it can adsorb, or bind, molecules from the offending toxin and prevent their absorption into the bloodstream.

3. *Enhance elimination of toxin.* Cathartics, such as sorbitol (often mixed with activated charcoal), increase gastric motility, thereby shortening the amount of time toxins stay in the gastrointestinal tract to be absorbed. Cathartics must be used cautiously, since there is controversy regarding their effectiveness. Cathartics should not be used in pediatric patients because of the potential to cause severe electrolyte derangements.

Whole bowel irrigation is another method of enhancing elimination. Using a gastric tube, polyethylene glycol electrolyte solution is administered continuously at 1–2 L/hr until the rectal effluent is clear or objects recovered. This technique seems effective with few complications and is therefore gaining popularity. Its availability, however, is limited to a few centers.

Antidotes

Finally, if indicated, the appropriate antidote should be administered. An **antidote** is a substance that will neutralize a specific toxin or counteract its effect on the body. There are not many antidotes (Table 34-1), and they will rarely be 100 percent effective. Most poisonings will not require the administration of an antidote.

The specific actions you take when dealing with toxicological emergencies will be dictated by consultation with medical direction, by protocols obtained from the Poison Control Center, and by your local policy and procedures on initiating these protocols.

* **gastric lavage** removing an ingested poison by repeatedly filling and emptying the stomach with water or saline via a gastric tube; also known as "pumping the stomach."

* **activated charcoal** a powder, usually pre-mixed with water, that will adsorb (bind) some poisons and help prevent them from being absorbed by the body.

* **whole bowel irrigation** administration of polyethylene glycol continuously at 1–2 L/hr through a nasogastric tube until the effluent is clear or objects are recovered.

* **antidote** a substance that will neutralize a specific toxin or counteract its effect on the body.

Specific actions in a toxicological emergency will be dictated by consultation with medical direction, protocols from the Poison Control Center, and local policy on initiating these protocols.

Table 34-1 | ANTIDOTES FOR TOXICOLOGICAL EMERGENCIES

Toxin	Antidote	Adult Dosage (Pediatric Dosage)
Acetaminophen	N-Acetylcysteine	Initial: 140 mg/kg
Arsenic	*see* Mercury, Arsenic, Gold	
Atropine	Physostigmine	Initial: 0.5–2 mg IV
Benzodiazepines	Flumazenil	Initial: 0.2 mg q 1 min to total of 1–3 mg
Carbon Monoxide	Oxygen	
Cyanide	Amyl nitrite	Inhale crushed pearl for 30 seconds, then oxygen for 30 seconds
	then sodium nitrite	10 mL of 3% sol'n over 3 min IV (Pediatric: 0.33 mL/kg)
	then sodium thiosulfate	50 mL of 25% sol'n over 10 min IV (Pediatric: 1.65 mL/kg)
Ethylene glycol	Fomepizole (or as methyl alcohol)	Initial: 15 mg/kg IV
Gold	*see* Mercury, Arsenic, Gold	
Iron	Defroxamine	Initial: 10–15 mg/kg/hr IV
Lead	Edetate calcium disodium	1 amp/250 mL D5W over 1 hr
	or Dimercaptosuccinic acid (DMSA)	250 mg PO
Mercury, Arsenic, Gold	BAL (British anti-Lewisite)	5 mg/kg IM
	DMSA	250 mg PO
Methyl alcohol	Ethyl alcohol +/− dialysis	1 mL/kg of 100% ethanol IV
Nitrates	Methylene blue	0.2 mL/kg of 1% sol'n IV over 5 min
Opiates	Naloxone	0.4–2.0 mg IV
Organophosphates	Atropine	Initial: 2–5 mg IV
	Pralidoxime (Protopam)	Initial: 1 g IV

SUICIDAL PATIENTS AND PROTECTIVE CUSTODY

Before leaving a suicidal patient who claims to have been "just kidding," consider the legal ramifications. You may be charged later with patient abandonment. At the same time, be aware of protective custody laws in your state. Always involve law enforcement personnel in these cases and involve them early. Only law enforcement personnel can place a patient in protective custody and ultimately consent to treatment.

Involve law enforcement early in any possible suicide case.

INGESTED TOXINS

Poisoning by ingestion is the most common route of poisoning you will encounter in prehospital care. It is essential to initiate the following principles of assessment and treatment promptly.

Assessment

It takes time for an ingested toxin to make its way from the gastrointestinal system into the circulatory system. Therefore, you need to find out not only what was ingested but when it was ingested. Following are some general guidelines for managing patients who have ingested toxins as well as information about specific substances.

History Begin your history by trying to find out the type of toxin ingested, the quantity of the toxin, the time elapsed since ingestion, and whether the patient took any alcohol or other potentiating substance. Also ask the patient about drug habituation or abuse and underlying medical illnesses and allergies. Remember that in cases of poisoning, inaccuracies creep into nearly half the histories because of drug-induced confusion, patient misinformation, or deliberate patient attempts at deception.

The following questions will help you to develop a relevant history.

- What did you ingest? (Obtain pill containers and any remaining contents, samples of the ingested substance, or samples of vomitus. Bring them with the patient to the emergency department.)
- When did you ingest the substance? (Time is critical for decisions regarding lab tests and the use of gastric lavage and/or antidotes.)
- How much did you ingest?
- Did you drink any alcohol?
- Have you attempted to treat yourself (including inducing vomiting)?
- Have you been under psychiatric care? If so, why? (Answers may indicate a potential for suicide.)
- What is your weight?

Physical Examination Because the history can be unreliable, the physical examination is extremely important. It has two purposes: (1) to provide physical evidence of intoxication and (2) to find any underlying illnesses that may account for the patient's symptoms or that may affect the outcome of the poisoning. As you complete the initial assessment and rapid physical exam, pay attention to the following patient features:

- *Skin.* Is there evidence of cyanosis, pallor, wasting, or needle marks? Flushing of the skin may indicate poisoning with an anticholinergic substance. Staining of the skin may occur from chronic exposure to mercuric chloride, bromine, or similar chemicals.
- *Eyes.* Constriction or dilation of the pupils can occur with various types of poisons (e.g., marijuana, methamphetamines, narcotics). Ask about impaired vision, blurring of vision, or coloration of vision.
- *Mouth.* Look for signs of caustic ingestion, presence of the gag reflex, the amount of salivation, any breath odor, or the presence of vomitus.
- *Chest.* Breath sounds may reveal evidence of aspiration, atelectasis, or excessive pulmonary secretions.
- *Circulation.* Cardiac examination may give clues as to the type of toxin ingested. For example, the presence of tachydysrhythmias (e.g., from methamphetamine) or bradydysrhythmias (e.g., from organophosphates) may suggest specific toxins.
- *Abdomen.* Abdominal pain may result from poisoning by salicylates, methyl alcohol, caustics, or botulism toxin.

You can frequently expect to encounter patients who have ingested more than one toxin. This may be the result of a suicide attempt or of experimentation with illicit drugs. Such multiple ingestions present a diagnostic and therapeutic dilemma. Signs and symptoms may be inconsistent with a single diagnosis, and

In cases of poisoning, histories are often unreliable because of drug-induced confusion, patient misinformation, or deliberate deception.

attempted treatment may produce unexpected results. A common example of this is the "speedball" (heroin mixed with cocaine). If the narcotic overdose is treated, the rescuer is often presented with a patient who is now in a cocaine-induced catecholamine crisis (tachycardia, hypertension, seizures). In such cases, or if you cannot identify what the patient has ingested, consult medical direction and/or the Poison Control Center according to your local protocols.

Management

Prevent Aspiration As previously discussed, initiation of supportive measures (maintaining airway, breathing, and circulation) is top priority in the treatment of the poisoned patient. Aspiration is a frequent complication of poisoning, resulting from an altered level of consciousness and a decreased gag reflex. Preventing aspiration must be one of your major objectives. If insertion of an endotracheal tube is necessary, nasotracheal intubation is preferred in patients who have a gag reflex.

Poisoning is a situation where rapid sequence intubation (RSI) may be required (see Chapter 8). It is not uncommon to encounter a patient with altered mental status who is vomiting. The prevention of aspiration is a primary concern, but attempts at endotracheal intubation fail because the patient will "clamp down" his teeth. In these situations, it is often prudent to use RSI to quickly control and maintain the airway. This is far superior to waiting for the patient to deteriorate to the point where an endotracheal tube can be placed without the aid of neuromuscular blockers. Remember, most poisoning patients will have compromised respiration or circulation, so routinely give high-flow oxygen.

Administer Fluids and Drugs Once you have assured the ABCs, establish intravenous access. An IV of lactated Ringer's or normal saline at a to-keep-open rate is recommended for all potentially dangerous ingestions. In addition to volume replacement with a crystalloid solution, conduct cardiac monitoring and repeat assessments, including frequent monitoring of vital signs.

Many EMS systems still utilize an empiric therapeutic regimen for comatose patients consisting of $D_{50}W$, naloxone (Narcan), and thiamine (Vitamin B_1). This so-called "coma cocktail" should not be used. Instead, treatment should be guided by objective patient information obtained on scene. If immediate determination of blood glucose levels is available (glucometer and chemstrips), withhold the administration of $D_{50}W$ until determination of hypoglycemia is made. If indicated, use 25–50 g of $D_{50}W$ IV push. If narcotic intoxication is suspected (respiratory depression or pinpoint pupils), give 1–2 mg of naloxone IV push. Naloxone reverses the effects of narcotic intoxication. If chronic alcoholism is suspected, consider administration of 100 mg of thiamine IV to address possible encephalopathy. Do not give these medications empirically!

Follow these supportive measures with the decontamination procedures outlined earlier. Often, decontamination is performed in the emergency department rather than on scene or during transport. This also applies to the use of most antidotes. There are exceptions, of course, and each case needs to be treated individually. Consult the Poison Control Center and medical direction according to your local protocols.

Do Not Induce Vomiting As mentioned earlier, induction of vomiting is no longer an accepted routine intervention for patients who have ingested toxins. It is still important to contact the Poison Control Center about this, since, in rare cases of pediatric ingestion, induction of vomiting may play some role. However, for the overwhelming majority of cases, inducement of vomiting is not required and may even be contraindicated.

Maintaining airway, breathing, and circulation is top priority in treating a poisoned patient. Preventing aspiration must be one of your major objectives.

INHALED TOXINS

Toxic inhalations can be self-induced or the result of accidental exposure from such sources as house fires or industrial accidents. Commonly abused inhaled toxins include: paint (and other hydrocarbons), Freon, propellants, glue, amyl nitrite, butyl nitrite, and nitrous oxide. The general guidelines for assessment and management of toxicological emergencies apply to inhaled toxins, but the following provides some specifics.

Assessment

Inhaled toxic substances produce signs and symptoms primarily in the respiratory system. These symptoms are particularly severe in patients who have inhaled chemicals and propellants concentrated in paper or plastic bags. Patients who inhale paint or propellants are often referred to as "huffers." Look for the presence of paint on the upper or lower lip. "Huffers," who report it to be more potent, often prefer gold paint. The presence of paint on the upper or lower lips should alert you to the possibility of inhalant abuse. The sniffing of paint, propellants, or hydrocarbons has become an epidemic problem in many developing countries. This is particularly true in the lower socioeconomic groups, most notably the legions of street children in Latin and South America. "Huffing" can lead to serious, irreversible brain damage. As the toxins are inhaled, oxygen is gradually displaced from the respiratory system, producing a relative hypoxia. Signs and symptoms of aerosol inhalation include:

- *Central nervous system:* dizziness, headache, confusion, seizures, hallucinations, coma
- *Respiratory:* tachypnea, cough, hoarseness, stridor, dyspnea, retractions, wheezing, chest pain or tightness, rales or rhonchi
- *Cardiac:* dysrhythmias

Management

Your first priority in any inhalation emergency is personal safety, then removal of the patient from the toxic environment.

Your first priority in the case of toxin inhalation is to remove the patient from the source as soon as it is safe to do so. Then follow these guidelines:

- Safely remove the patient from the poisonous environment. In doing so, take the following essential precautions:
  - Wear protective clothing.
  - Use appropriate respiratory protection.
  - Remove the patient's contaminated clothing.
- Perform the initial assessment, history, and physical exam.
- Initiate supportive measures.
- Contact the Poison Control Center and medical direction according to your local protocols.

SURFACE-ABSORBED TOXINS

Many poisons, including organophosphates, cyanide, and other toxins, can be absorbed through the skin and mucous membranes.

Assessment and Management

Signs and symptoms of absorbed poisons can vary depending on the toxin involved. See the discussion of specific toxins in the sections that follow. Whenever you suspect absorption of a toxin (especially cyanide or organophosphates), take the following steps:

- Safely remove the patient from the poisonous environment. It is essential that you follow these guidelines:
  - Wear protective clothing.
  - Use appropriate respiratory protection.
  - Remove the patient's contaminated clothing.
  - Perform the initial assessment, history, and physical exam.
  - Initiate supportive measures.
  - Contact the Poison Control Center and medical direction according to your local protocols.

Your first priority in any surface-absorbed poisoning emergency is personal safety, then removal of the patient from the toxic environment.

SPECIFIC TOXINS

To recognize and implement the proper procedure in a given poisoning, you must be familiar with the signs and symptoms that a particular toxin will trigger. Often, you may not be able to identify the exact toxin a patient has been exposed to, but usually a group of toxins will have very similar manifestations and effects and will require similar interventions. Similar toxins with similar signs and symptoms are organized into **toxidromes** (toxic syndromes), which make remembering the details of their effects much simpler. Study the toxidromes listed in Table 34-2.

The following sections address specific toxins commonly encountered. While the standard toxicological emergency procedures, discussed earlier, apply to all of these toxins, pay close attention to variations in treatment. Variations include specific procedures you must perform in a particular case or a poisoning in which an antidote is available or immediately necessary. Management of injected toxins, drug overdose, and substance abuse will be covered later in the chapter.

✱ **toxidrome** a toxic syndrome; a group of typical signs and symptoms consistently associated with exposure to a particular type of toxin.

CYANIDE

Cyanide can enter the body by a variety of routes. It is present in many commercial and household items that can be either ingested or absorbed—rodenticides, silver polish, and fruit pits and seeds (apricots, cherries, pears, and so on). It also can be inhaled, especially in fires that release cyanide from products containing nitrogen. A roomful of burning plastics, silks, or synthetic carpeting can also be a roomful of cyanide-filled smoke. Cyanide also forms in patients on long-term sodium nitroprusside therapy. Suicidal patients have been known to take cyanide salt. Regardless of the entry route, cyanide is an extremely fast-acting toxin. Once cyanide enters the body, it acts as a *cellular asphyxiant*. It inflicts its damage by inhibiting an enzyme vital to cellular use of oxygen.

Signs and Symptoms

Signs and symptoms of cyanide poisoning include:

- A burning sensation in the mouth and throat
- Headache, confusion, combative behavior
- Hypertension and tachycardia followed by hypotension and further dysrhythmias
- Seizures and coma
- Pulmonary edema

| Table 34-2 | TOXIC SYNDROMES |

Toxidromes	Toxin			Signs and Symptoms

Anticholinergic	Belladonna alkaloids
	  Atropine (hyoscyamine)
	  Belladonna alkaloid mixtures: belladonna
	    leaf, fluid extract, tincture
	  Homatropine
	  Methscopolamine
	  Methylatropine nitrate
	  Plants: *Atropa belladonna, Datura stramonium,*
	    Hyoscyamus niger, Amanita muscaria
	    or *pantherina*
	  Scopolamine (I-hyoscine)
				Dry skin and mucous
				  membranes
				Thirst
				Dysphagia
				Vision blurred for near objects
				Fixed dilated pupils
				Tachycardia
				Sometimes hypertension
				Rash, like scarlet fever
				Hyperthermia, flushing
				Urinary urgency and retention

	Synthetic anticholinergics			Lethargy
	Adiphenine	Isopropamide	Pipenzolate	Confusion to restlessness, excitement
	Anisotropine	Mepenzolate	Piperiodolate	Delirium, hallucinations
	Cyclopentolate	Methantheline	Poldine	Ataxia
	Dicyclomine	Methixene	Propantheline	Seizures
	Diphemanil	Oxyphenonium	Thiphenamil	Respiratory failure
	Eucatropine	Oxyphencyclimine	Tridihexethyl	Cardiovascular collapse
	Glycopyrrolate	Pentapiperide	Tropicamide	
	Hexocyclium			
	Incidental anticholinergics			
	Antihistamines	Benactyzine	Phenothiazines	
	Tricyclic antidepressants			

Acetylcholinesterase inhibition	Organophosphates
	  TEPP
	  OMPA
	  Dipterex
	  Chlorthion
	  Di-Syston
	  Co-ral
	  Phosdrin
	  Parathion
	  Methylparathion
	  Malathion
	  Systox
	  EPN
	  Diazinon
	  Guthion
	  Trithion
				Sweating, constricted pupils,
				  lacrimation, excessive
				  salivation, wheezing, cramps,
				  vomiting, diarrhea, tenesmus,
				  bradycardia *or* tachycardia,
				  hypotension *or* hypertension,
				  blurred vision, urinary
				  incontinence
				
				Striated muscle: cramps,
				  weakness, twitching, paralysis,
				  respiratory failure, cyanosis,
				  arrest
				
				Sympathetic ganglia:
				  tachycardia, elevated blood
				  pressure
				
				CNS effects: anxiety, restlessness
				  ataxia, seizures, insomnia,
				  coma, absent reflexes,
				  Cheyne-Stokes respirations,
				  respiratory and circulation
				  depression

Cholinergic	Acetylcholine
	Area catechu
	Carbachol
	Clitocybe dealbata
		Betel nut
		Bethanechol
		Pilocarpine
		Pilocarpus species
			Methacholine
			Muscarine
				Sweating, constricted pupils,
				  lacrimation, excessive
				  salivation, wheezing, cramps,
				  vomiting, diarrhea, tenesmus,
				  bradycardia *or* tachycardia,
				  hypotension *or* hypertension,
				  blurred vision, urinary
				  incontinence

Continued

Table 34-2   TOXIC SYNDROMES (CONTINUED)

Toxidromes	Toxin			Signs and Symptoms
Extrapyramidal	Acetophenazine Butaperazine Carphenazine Chlorpromazine Haloperidol	Mesoridazine Perphenazine Piperacetaxine Promazine	Thioridazine Thiothixene Trifluoperazine Triflupromazine	Parkinsonian Dysphagia, eye muscle spasm, rigidity, tremor, neck spasm, shrieking, jaw spasm, laryngospasm
Hemoglobinopathies	Carbon monoxide Methemoglobin			Headache, nausea, vomiting, dizziness, dyspnea, seizures, coma, death Cutaneous blisters, gastroenteritis Epidemic occurrence with carbon monoxide Cyanosis, chocolate blood with non-functional hemoglobin
Metal fume fever	Fumes of oxides of: Brass Cadmium Copper Zinc	Iron Magnesium Mercury	Nickel Titanium Tungsten	Chills, fever, nausea, vomiting, muscular pain, throat dryness, headache, fatigue, weakness, leukocytosis, respiratory disease
Narcotic	Alphaprodine Anileridine Codeine Cyclazocine Dextromethorphan Dextromoramide Diacetylmorphine Dihydrocodeine Dihydrocodeinone Dipipanone Diphenoxylate (Lomotil)	Ethylmorphine Ethoheptazine (meperidene metabolite) Fentanyl Heroin Hydromorphone Levorphanol Meperidine Methadone Metopon Morphine	Normeperidene Opium Oxycodone Oxymorphone Pentazocine Phenazocine Piminodine Propoxyphene Racemorphan	CNS depression Pinpoint pupils Slowed respirations Hypotension Response to naloxone Pupils may be dilated and excitement may predominate Normeperidine: tremor, CNS excitation, seizures
Sympathomimetic	Aminophylline Amphetamines Caffeine *Catha edulus* (Khat) Cocaehylene Cocaine Dopamine	Ephedrine Epinephrine Fenfluramine Levarterenol Metaraminol Methamphetamine Methcathinone	Methylphenidate (Ritalin) Pemoline Phencyclidine Phenmetrazine Phentermine	CNS excitation Seizures Hypertension Hypotension with caffeine Tachycardia
Withdrawal	Alcohol Barbiturates Benzodiazepines Chloral hydrate	Cocaine Ethchlorvynol Glutethimide Meprobamate	Methaqualone Methyprylon Opiods Paraldehyde	Diarrhea, large pupils, piloerection, hypertension, tachycardia, insomnia, lacrimation, muscle cramps, restlessness, yawning, hallucinations Depression with cocaine

Adapted from Done AK. *Poisoning—A Systematic Approach for the Emergency Department Physician.* Presented Aug. 6–9, 1979, at Snowmass Village, CO, Symposium sponsored by Rocky Mountain Poison Center. Used by Permission.

FIGURE 34-1 Cyanide antidote kit.

Management

First safely remove the patient from the source of exposure. To prevent inhalation, always wear breathing equipment when entering the scene of a fire. Initiate supportive measures immediately. Follow this with the cyanide antidote kit (Figure 34-1). This kit contains amyl nitrite ampules, a sodium nitrite, and a sodium thiosulfate solution. Adding nitrites to blood converts some hemoglobin to *methemoglobin*, which allows cyanide to bind to it. Thiosulfate then binds with the cyanide to form thiocyanate, a nontoxic substance readily excreted renally. Because cyanide is rapidly toxic, you must administer the cyanide antidote kit without delay. If your unit carries this kit, familiarize yourself with its contents and use.

CARBON MONOXIDE

Carbon monoxide (CO) is an odorless, tasteless gas that is often the byproduct of incomplete combustion. Because of its chemical structure, it has more than 200 times the affinity of oxygen to bind with the red blood cell's hemoglobin (producing carboxyhemoglobin). Once this molecule has bound with hemoglobin, it is very resistant to removal and causes an effective hypoxia. Because of the variability of the signs and symptoms, people usually ignore CO poisoning until very toxic levels occur. Common circumstances for CO poisoning include improperly vented heating systems or the use of a small barbecue to heat a house or camper. Symptoms of early poisoning are very similar to those of the flu. Be alert for CO poisoning in multiple patients living together in a poorly heated and vented space, having "flulike" symptoms.

Signs and Symptoms

Signs and symptoms of CO poisoning include:

- Headache
- Nausea, vomiting
- Confusion or other altered mental status
- Tachypnea

FIGURE 34-2 Hyperbaric chamber.

Management

Because of the difficulty in removing CO from hemoglobin, definitive treatment is often performed in a hyperbaric chamber (Figure 34-2). In this specially designed environment, oxygen under several atmospheres of pressure surrounds the body. This increases oxygenation of available hemoglobin. In field settings, take the following supportive steps:

- Ensure safety of rescue personnel.
- Remove the patient from the contaminated area.
- Begin immediate ventilation of the area.
- Initiate supportive measures. High-flow oxygen by nonrebreather is critical in this setting.

CARDIAC MEDICATIONS

The list of cardiac medications grows almost daily. Many classes of these drugs exist, including antidysrythmics, beta blockers, calcium channel blockers, glycosides, ACE inhibitors, and so on. Generally these medications regulate heart function by decreasing heart rate, suppressing automaticity, and/or reducing vascular tone. Overdoses of these drugs can be intentional but are more often due to errors in dosage.

Signs and Symptoms

In overdose quantities, signs and symptoms of cardiac medication poisoning include:

- Nausea and vomiting
- Headache, dizziness, confusion
- Profound hypotension
- Cardiac dysrhythmias (usually bradycardia)
- Heart conduction blocks
- Bronchospasm and pulmonary edema (especially beta blockers)

Management

Initiate standard toxicological emergency assessment and treatment immediately. Be aware that severe bradycardia may not respond well to atropine; therefore, you may need to use an external pacing device. Some cardiac medications do have antidotes that may help with severe adverse effects. These include calcium for calcium channel blockers, glucagon for beta blockers, and Digoxin-specific Fab (Digibind) for digoxin. Contact medical direction before giving these antidotes.

CAUSTIC SUBSTANCES

Caustic substances are either **acids** or **alkalis** (bases) that are found in both the home and the industrial workplace. Approximately 12,000 exposures occur annually with 150 major complications or deaths. Strong caustics can produce severe burns at the site of contact and, if ingested, cause tissue destruction at the lips, mouth, esophagus, and other areas of the gastrointestinal tract.

Strong *acids* have a pH less than 2. They are found in plumbing liquids such as drain openers and bathroom cleaners. Contact with strong acids usually produces immediate and severe pain. This is a result of tissue coagulation and necrosis. Often this type of contact injury will produce *eschar* at the burn site, which will act like a shield and prevent further penetration or damage to deeper tissues. If ingested, acids will cause local burns to the mouth and throat. Because of the rapid transit through the esophagus, the esophagus is not usually damaged. More likely, the stomach lining will be injured. Immediate or delayed hemorrhage can occur and may be associated with perforation. Pain is severe and usually due to direct injury and spasm from irritation. Absorption of acids into the vascular system will occur quite readily, causing a significant acidemia, which will need to be managed along with the direct local effects.

Strong *alkaline* agents typically have a pH greater than 12.5. They can be in solid or liquid form (such as in Drano or Liquid Plumber) and are routinely found around the house. These agents cause injury by inducing liquefaction necrosis. Pain is often delayed, which allows for longer tissue contact and deeper tissue injury before the exposure is even recognized. Solid alkaline agents can stick to the oropharynx or esophagus. This can cause perforation, bleeding, and inflammation of central chest structures. Liquid alkalis are more likely to injure the stomach because they pass quickly through the esophagus. Within 2–3 days of exposure, complete loss of the protective mucosal tissue can occur, followed by either gradual healing and recovery or further bleeding, necrosis, and stricture formation.

Signs and Symptoms

Signs and symptoms of caustic injury include:

- Facial burns
- Pain in the lips, tongue, throat, or gums
- Drooling, trouble swallowing
- Hoarseness, stridor, or shortness of breath
- Shock from bleeding, vomiting

Management

Assessment and intervention must be aggressive and rapid to minimize morbidity and mortality. Take precautions to prevent injury to rescuers. Initiate standard toxicological emergency assessment and treatment, but pay particular attention to establishing an airway. Injury to the oropharynx and larynx may make airway

*acid a substance that liberates hydrogen ions (H^+) when in solution.

*alkali a substance that liberates hydroxyl ions (OH^-) when in solution; a strong base.

control and ventilation very difficult and may even require cricothyrotomy. Since caustics will not adsorb to activated charcoal, there is no indication to administer it. In the past, rescuers often gave water or milk to dilute any ingested caustics but there is controversy as to whether this is beneficial. Rapid transport to the emergency department is essential.

HYDROFLUORIC ACID

Hydrofluoric (HF) acid deserves special attention because it is extremely toxic and can be lethal despite the appearance of only moderate burns on skin contact. HF acid penetrates deeply into tissues and is inactivated only when it comes in contact with *cations* such as calcium. Calcium fluoride is formed by this inactivation and settles in the tissue as a salt. The removal of calcium from cells causes a total disruption of cell functioning and can even cause bone destruction as calcium is leeched out of the bones. Death has been reported from exposure of < 2.5% body surface area to a highly concentrated solution.

Hydrofluoric acid is used to clean glass in lab settings and for etching glass in art.

Signs and Symptoms

Signs and symptoms of HF acid exposure include:

- Burning at site of contact
- Trouble breathing
- Confusion
- Palpitations
- Muscle cramps

Management

Management includes:

- Ensure the safety of rescue personnel.
- Initiate supportive measures.
- Remove exposed clothing.
- Irrigate the affected area with water thoroughly.
- Immerse the affected limb in iced water with magnesium sulfate, calcium salts, or benzethonium chloride.
- Transport immediately for definitive care.

ALCOHOL

See the section on Alcohol Abuse later in this chapter.

HYDROCARBONS

Hydrocarbons are organic compounds composed of mostly carbon and hydrogen. They include such common recognizable names as kerosene, naphtha, turpentine, mineral oil, chloroform, toluene, and benzene. These chemicals are found in common household products such as lighter fluid, paint, glue, lubricants, solvents, and aerosol propellants. Toxicity from hydrocarbons can occur through any route, including ingestion, inhalation, or surface absorption.

Signs and Symptoms

Signs and symptoms of hydrocarbon poisoning will vary with the type and route of exposure but may include:

- Burns due to local contact
- Wheezing, dyspnea, hypoxia, and pneumonitis from aspiration/inhalation
- Headache, dizziness, slurred speech, ataxia (irregular and difficult-to-control movements), and obtundation (dulled reflexes)
- Foot and wrist drop with numbness and tingling
- Cardiac dysrhythmias

Management

Recent studies have shown that very few poisonings with hydrocarbons are serious, and less than one percent require physician intervention. If you know the exact chemical that the patient has been exposed to and the patient is asymptomatic, medical direction may suggest that the patient can be left at home. On the other hand, a few hydrocarbon poisonings can be very serious. Any patient who is symptomatic, does not know what he has taken, or who has taken a hydrocarbon that requires gastrointestinal decontamination (halogenated or aromatic hydrocarbons) must be treated using standard toxicological emergency procedures. Since charcoal will not bind hydrocarbons, this may be one of the few cases in which gastric lavage can be useful.

TRICYCLIC ANTIDEPRESSANTS

* **therapeutic index** the maximum tolerated dose divided by the minimum curative dose of a drug; the range between curative and toxic dosages; also called *therapeutic window*.

Tricyclic antidepressants were once commonly used to treat depression. Close monitoring was required because these medications have a narrow **therapeutic index,** meaning that a relatively small increase in dose can quickly lead to toxic effects. The very nature of their use, treating depression, presents a dilemma because the patients most seriously in need of treatment may also be the most likely to attempt to take an overdose. Deaths due to antidepressant overdose have dropped significantly in recent years since the development and rapid acceptance of safer agents unrelated to tricyclics. However, tricyclic antidepressants are still used for various clinical problems such as chronic pain or migraine prophylaxis and may still be responsible for more deaths due to intentional overdose than any other medication. Common agents include amitriptyline (Elavil), amoxapine, clomipramine, doxepin, imipramine, nortriptyline.

Signs and Symptoms

Signs and symptoms of tricyclic antidepressant toxicity include:

- Dry mouth
- Blurred vision
- Urinary retention
- Constipation

Late into an overdose, more severe toxicity may produce:

- Confusion, hallucinations
- Hyperthermia

- Respiratory depression
- Seizures
- Tachycardia and hypotension
- Cardiac dysrhythmias (heart block, wide QRS, *Torsades de pointes*)

Management

Toxicity from tricyclic antidepressants requires immediate initiation of standard toxicological emergency procedures. Cardiac monitoring is critical since dysrhythmias are the most common cause of death. If you suspect a mixed overdose with benzodiazepines, do *not* use Flumazenil, since it may precipitate seizures. If significant cardiac toxicity occurs, sodium bicarbonate can be used as an additional therapy. Contact medical direction as necessary.

If you suspect a mixed overdose with benzodiazepines, do not *use Flumazenil, since it may precipitate seizures.*

MAO INHIBITORS

Monoamine oxidase inhibitors (MAOIs) have been used, although rarely, to treat depression. Recently they have been used, on a limited basis, to treat obsessive-compulsive disorders. They are relatively unpopular because of a narrow therapeutic index, multiple-drug interactions, serious interactions with foods containing *tyramine* (for example, red wine and cheese), and high morbidity and mortality when taken in overdose. These drugs inhibit the breakdown of neurotransmitters such as norepinephrine and dopamine while increasing the availability of the components needed to make even more neurotransmitters. When taken in overdose, MAOIs can be extremely dangerous, although symptoms may not appear for up to 6 hours.

Signs and Symptoms

Signs and symptoms of MAOI overdose include:

- Headache, agitation, restlessness, tremor
- Nausea
- Palpitations
- Tachycardia
- Severe hypertension
- Hyperthermia
- Eventually bradycardia, hypotension, coma, and death occur

New MAOIs have recently entered the marketplace. These next-generation drugs are reversible, less toxic, and do not have the same reactions with food as the older MAOIs. Data is not yet available on the outcome of patients overdosing with these newer agents.

Management

No antidote exists for MAOI overdose because the inhibition is not reversible except with newer drugs. Therefore, institute standard toxicological emergency procedures as soon as possible. If necessary, give symptomatic support for seizures and hyperthermia using benzodiazepines. If vasopressors are needed, use norepinephrine.

NEWER ANTIDEPRESSANTS

In recent years, several new agents have been developed to treat depression. Because of their high safety profile in therapeutic and overdose amounts, these drugs have been widely accepted and have virtually replaced tricyclic antidepressants.

Recently introduced drugs include trazodone (Desyrel), bupropion (Wellbutrin), and the large group of very popular *selective serotonin re-uptake inhibitors,* or SSRIs, (Prozac, Luvox, Paxil, Zoloft). SSRIs prevent the re-uptake of serotonin in the brain, theoretically making it more available for brain functions. The true mechanism by which these drugs treat depression is unclear.

Signs and Symptoms

When these drugs are taken in overdose, usually the signs and symptoms are mild. Occasionally trazodone and buproprion will cause CNS depression and seizures, but deaths are very rare and have only been reported in mixed overdoses with multiple ingestions. More commonly, signs and symptoms of overdose with the newer antidepressant agents include:

- Drowsiness
- Tremor
- Nausea and vomiting
- Sinus tachycardia

SSRIs are now also associated with *serotonin syndrome.* This syndrome is caused by increased serotonin levels and is often triggered by increasing the dose of SSRI or adding a second drug such as Demerol, codeine, dextromethorphan (cough syrup), or other antidepressants. Signs and symptoms of serotonin syndrome include:

- Agitation, anxiety, confusion, insomnia
- Headache, drowsiness, coma
- Nausea, salivation, diarrhea, abdominal cramps
- Cutaneous piloerection, flushed skin
- Hyperthermia, tachycardia
- Rigidity, shivering, incoordination, myoclonic jerks

Management

Overdose with these new antidepressants is not as life threatening as with previous agents unless other drugs or alcohol are taken simultaneously. Consequently, treat overdoses with the standard toxicological emergency procedures. Also have the patient discontinue all serotonergic drugs and implement supportive measures. Benzodiazepines or beta blockers occasionally are used to improve patient comfort, but these are rarely given in the field.

LITHIUM

In the treatment of bipolar (manic-depressive) disorder, no other drug has been proven to be more effective than lithium. It is unclear how lithium exerts its therapeutic effect. However, like tricyclic antidepressants, lithium has a narrow therapeutic index which results in toxicity during normal use and in overdose situations.

Signs and Symptoms

Signs and symptoms of lithium toxicity include:

- Thirst, dry mouth
- Tremor, muscle twitching, increased reflexes
- Confusion, stupor, seizures, coma
- Nausea, vomiting, diarrhea
- Bradycardia, dysrhythmias

Management

Treat lithium overdose with mostly supportive measures. Use the standard toxicological emergency procedures, but remember that activated charcoal will not bind lithium and need not be given. Alkalinizing the urine with sodium bicarbonate and osmotic diuresis using mannitol may increase elimination of lithium, but severe toxic cases require hemodialysis.

SALICYLATES

Salicylates are some of the more common drugs taken in overdose, largely due to the fact that they are readily available over the counter. The most recognizable forms are aspirin, oil of wintergreen, and some prescription combination medications.

Aspirin in large doses can cause serious consequences. About 300 mg/kg is required to cause toxicity. In such amounts, salicylates inhibit normal energy production and acid buffering in the body. This results in a metabolic acidosis, which further injures other organ systems.

Signs and Symptoms

Signs and symptoms of salicylate overdose include:

- Rapid respirations
- Hyperthermia
- Confusion, lethargy, coma
- Cardiac failure, dysrhythmias
- Abdominal pain, vomiting
- Pulmonary edema, ARDS (adult respiratory distress syndrome)

Chronic overdose symptoms are somewhat less severe and do not tend to include abdominal complaints. It is difficult to distinguish chronic overdose from very early acute overdose or early overdose that has progressed past the abdominal irritation stage.

Management

In all cases, salicylate poisoning should be treated using standard toxicological emergency procedures. Activated charcoal definitely reduces drug absorption and should be used. If possible, find out the time of ingestion, since blood levels measured at the right time can indicate the expected degree of injury. Most symptomatic patients will require generous IV fluids and may need urine alkalinization with sodium bicarbonate. Severe cases may require dialysis.

ACETAMINOPHEN

Due to its few side effects in normal dosages, acetaminophen (e.g., paracetamol, Tylenol) is one of the most common drugs in use today. It is used to treat fever and/or pain and is a common ingredient in hundreds of over-the-counter preparations. It can be also obtained by prescription in combination with various other drugs.

In large doses, however, acetaminophen can be a very dangerous pharmaceutical. A dose of 150 mg/kg is considered toxic and may result in death due to injury to the liver. A highly reactive byproduct of acetaminophen metabolism is responsible for most adverse effects, but this is usually avoided by the body's detoxification system. When large amounts of acetaminophen enter the system, the detoxification system is overwhelmed and gradually depleted, leaving the toxic metabolite in the circulation to cause hepatic necrosis.

Signs and Symptoms

Signs and symptoms of acetaminophen toxicity appear in four stages.

Stage 1	½ hour to 24 hours	Nausea, vomiting, weakness, fatigue
Stage 2	24–48 hours	Abdominal pain, decreased urine, elevated liver enzymes
Stage 3	72–96 hours	Liver function disruption
Stage 4	4–14 days	Gradual recovery or progressive liver failure

Management

Treat acetaminophen overdose with standard toxicological emergency procedures. Find out the time of ingestion since blood levels taken at the right time can predict the potential for injury. An antidote called N-acetylcysteine (NAC, Mucomyst) is available and highly effective. However, NAC is usually administered based on clinical and laboratory studies and is rarely given in the prehospital setting.

OTHER NON-PRESCRIPTION PAIN MEDICATIONS

Non-steroidal anti-inflammatory drugs (NSAIDs) are another group of medications that are readily available and are often overdosed. Common examples include naproxen sodium, indomethacin, ibuprofen, and ketorolac (Toradol).

Signs and Symptoms

The presentation of toxicity caused by NSAIDs varies greatly but can include:

- Headache
- Ringing in the ears (tinnitus)
- Nausea, vomiting, abdominal pain
- Swelling of the extremities
- Mild drowsiness
- Dyspnea, wheezing, pulmonary edema
- Rash, itching

Management

There is no specific antidote for NSAID toxicity. Use general overdose procedures, including supportive care as soon as possible and transport to the emergency department for observation and any necessary symptomatic treatment.

THEOPHYLLINE

Theophylline belongs to a group of medications called xanthines. It is usually used for patients with asthma or COPD because of its moderate bronchodilation and mild anti-inflammatory effects. Like other drugs with a narrow therapeutic index and high toxicity, theophylline has become less popular recently and therefore is not implicated in as many overdose injuries as in the past.

Signs and Symptoms

Symptoms of theophylline toxicity include:

- Agitation
- Tremors
- Seizures
- Cardiac dysrhythmias
- Nausea and vomiting

Management

Theophylline can cause significant morbidity and mortality. In overdose situations, it is essential that you institute toxicological emergency procedures immediately. In fact, theophylline is on the small list of drugs that have significant *entero-hepatic circulation*. This means that multiple doses of activated charcoal over time will continuously remove more and more of the drug from the body. Treat any dysrhythmias according to ACLS procedures.

METALS

With the exception of iron, overdose of heavy metals is a rare occurrence. Other possible involved metals include lead, arsenic, and mercury. All metals affect numerous enzyme systems within the body and therefore present with a variety of symptoms. Some also have direct local effects when ingested and when accumulated in various organs.

Iron

The body only requires small amounts of iron on a daily basis to maintain a sufficient store for enzyme and hemoglobin production. Excess amounts are easily obtained from nonprescription supplements and multi-vitamins. Children have a tendency to accidentally overdose on iron by taking too many candy-flavored chewable vitamins containing iron. To determine the amount of iron ingested, you must calculate the amount of elemental iron present in the type of pill ingested. Symptoms occur when more than 20 mg/kg of elemental iron are ingested.

Signs and Symptoms Excess iron will cause gastrointestinal injury and possible shock from hemorrhage, especially if it forms *concretions* (lumps of iron formed when tablets fuse together after being swallowed). Patients with significant iron ingestions will often have visible tablets or concretions in the stomach or small intestine when x-rayed. Other signs and symptoms of iron ingestion include:

- Vomiting (often hematemesis), diarrhea
- Abdominal pain, shock
- Liver failure
- Metabolic acidosis with tachypnea
- Eventual bowel scarring and possible obstruction

Management It is essential to initiate standard toxicological emergency procedures immediately. Since iron tends to inhibit gastrointestinal motility, pills sit longer in the stomach and may possibly be easier to remove through gastric lavage. Because activated charcoal will not bind iron (or any metals), it should not be used. Deferoxamine, a chelating agent, may be used in iron overdose as an antidote since it binds to iron so that less is moved into cells and tissues to cause damage.

Lead and Mercury

Both lead and mercury are heavy metals found in varying amounts in the environment. Lead was often used in glazes and paints before the toxic potential of such exposure became apparent. Mercury is a contaminant from industrial processing but is also found in thermometers and temperature-control switches in most homes. Chronic and acute exposures are possible with both metals.

Signs and Symptoms Signs and symptoms of heavy metal toxicity include:

- Headache, irritability, confusion, coma
- Memory disturbance
- Tremor, weakness, agitation
- Abdominal pain

Management Chronic poisoning can cause permanent neurological injury, which makes it imperative that the proper agencies monitor heavy metal levels in the environment of a patient who has presented with toxicity. Learn to recognize the signs of heavy metal toxicity and institute standard toxicology emergency procedures as needed. Activated charcoal will not bind heavy metals but various chelating agents (DMSA, BAL, CDE) are available and may be used in definitive management in the hospital.

CONTAMINATED FOOD

Food poisoning is caused by a spectrum of different factors. For example, bacteria, viruses, and toxic chemicals notoriously produce varying levels of gastrointestinal distress. The patient may present with nausea, vomiting, diarrhea, and diffuse abdominal pain.

Bacterial food poisonings range in severity. Bacterial **exotoxins** (secreted by bacteria) or **enterotoxins** (exotoxins associated with gastrointestinal diseases, including food poisoning) cause the adverse GI complaints noted previously. Food contaminated with other bacteria such as *Shigella, Salmonella,* or *E. coli* can produce even more severe gastrointestinal reactions, often leading to electrolyte imbalance and hypovolemia. *Clostridium botulinum,* the world's most toxic poison, presents as severe respiratory distress or arrest. The incubation of this toxin can range from 4 hours to 8 days. Fortunately, botulism rarely occurs, except in cases of improper food storage methods such as canning.

* **exotoxin** a soluble poisonous substance secreted during growth of a bacterium.

* **enterotoxin** an exotoxin that produces gastrointestinal symptoms and diseases such as food poisoning.

A variety of seafood poisonings are a result of specific toxins found in dinoflagellate contaminated shellfish such as clams, mussels, oysters, and scallops and can produce a syndrome referred to as *paralytic shellfish poisoning*. This condition can lead to respiratory arrest in addition to standard gastrointestinal symptoms.

Increased fish consumption by North Americans has also increased the number of cases of poisonings from toxins found in many commonly eaten fish. *Ciguatera (bony fish) poisoning* most frequently turns up in fish caught in the Pacific Ocean or along the tropical reefs of Florida and the West Indies. Ciguatera normally takes 2–6 hours to incubate and may produce myalgia and paresthesia. *Scombroid (histamine) poisoning* results from bacterial contamination of mackerel, tuna, bonitos, and albacore. Both types of poisoning cause the common gastrointestinal symptoms. Scombroid poisoning will present with an immediate facial flushing as histamines cause vasodilation.

Signs and Symptoms

As mentioned above, signs and symptoms of food poisoning may include:

- Nausea, vomiting, diarrhea, abdominal pain
- Facial flushing, respiratory distress (with some seafood poisonings)

Management

Except for botulism, food poisoning is rarely life threatening. Treatment, therefore, is largely supportive. In suspected cases of food poisoning, contact poison control and medical direction, and take the following steps.

- Perform the necessary assessment.
- Collect samples of the suspected contaminated food source.
- Perform the following management actions:
  - Establish and maintain the airway.
  - Administer high-flow oxygen.
  - Intubate and assist ventilations, if appropriate.
  - Establish venous access.
- Consider the administration of antihistamines (especially in seafood poisonings) and antiemetics.

POISONOUS PLANTS AND MUSHROOMS

Plants, trees, and mushrooms contribute heavily to the number of accidental toxic ingestions. While the vast majority of plants are nontoxic, many of the popular decorative houseplants can present a danger to children, who frequently ingest non-food items. Most Poison Control Centers distribute pamphlets that identify toxic household plants. (These pamphlets will help "poison proof" the home.)

It is impossible to cover all the toxic plants and mushrooms. Few rescuers are trained as botanists, and they find it difficult to identify the offending material. Mushrooms are particularly difficult to identify from small pieces. Additionally, most people recognize mushrooms and other plants by common names rather than by the nomenclature of scientific species. A general approach is to obtain a sample of the plant, if possible. Try to find a full leaf, stem, and any flowers.

Since many ornamental plants contain irritating chemicals or crystals, examine the patient's mouth and throat for redness, blistering, or edema. Identify other abnormal signs during the focused physical exam.

Mushroom poisonings generally fall into two categories: people seeking edible mushrooms and accidental ingestions by children. Fortunately, few of the

FIGURE 34-3 Poisonous mushrooms from *Amanita* and *Galerina* class.

many mushroom species possess extremely dangerous toxins. Toxic mushrooms fall into seven classes. *Amanita* and *Galerina* belong to the deadly *cyclopeptide* group (Figure 34-3). (*Amanita* accounts for over 90 percent of all deaths.) These mushrooms produce a poison that is extremely toxic to the liver, with a mortality rate of about 50 percent.

Signs and Symptoms

Signs and symptoms of poisonous plant ingestion include:

- Excessive salivation, lacrimation (secretion of tears), diaphoresis
- Abdominal cramps, nausea, vomiting, diarrhea
- Decreasing levels of consciousness, eventually progressing to coma

Management

For guidance on the treatment of plant poisonings, call the Poison Control Center. If contact cannot be made, use the procedures outlined under treatment of food poisoning earlier.

INJECTED TOXINS

Although we generally think of intentional or accidental drug overdoses as sources of injected poisons, the most common source for these poisonings is the animal kingdom. Bites and stings from a variety of insects, reptiles, and animals are among the most common injuries sustained by humans. Further injury can result from bacterial contamination or from a reaction produced by an injected substance.

GENERAL PRINCIPLES OF MANAGEMENT

The general principles of field management for bites and stings include:

- Protect rescue personnel—the offending organism may still be around.
- Remove the patient from danger of repeated injection, especially in the case of yellow jackets, wasps, or hornets.

In the case of a bite or sting, remember to protect rescue personnel. The offending organism may still be around.

- If possible, identify the insect, reptile, or animal that caused the injury and bring it to the emergency department along with the patient (if it can be done safely).
- Perform an initial assessment and rapid physical exam.
- Prevent or delay further absorption of the poison.
- Initiate supportive measures as indicated.
- Watch for anaphylactic reaction (see Chapter 5).
- Transport the patient as rapidly as possible.
- Contact the Poison Control Center and medical direction according to your local protocols.

INSECT BITES AND STINGS

Insect Stings

Many people die from allergic reactions to the stings from an order of insects known as *Hymenoptera*. As mentioned earlier, *Hymenoptera* includes wasps, bees, hornets, and ants. Only the common honeybee leaves a stinger. Wasps, yellow jackets, hornets, and fire ants sting repeatedly until removal from contact.

In most cases of insect bite, local treatment is all that is necessary. Unless an allergic reaction occurs, most patients will tolerate the isolated *Hymenoptera* sting.

Signs and Symptoms Signs and symptoms include:

- Localized pain
- Redness
- Swelling
- Skin wheal

Idiosyncratic reactions to the toxin may occur, resulting in a progressing localized swelling and edema. This is not an allergic reaction, however, if it responds well to an antihistamine such as diphenhydramine hydrochloride. The major problem resulting from a *Hymenoptera* sting is an allergic reaction or anaphylaxis. Signs and symptoms of allergic reaction include the following:

- Localized pain, redness, swelling, and a skin wheal
- Itching or flushing of the skin, rash
- Tachycardia, hypotension, bronchospasm, or laryngeal edema
- Facial edema, uvular swelling

Management For *Hymenoptera* stings, take the following supportive measures:

- Wash the area.
- Gently remove the stinger, if present, by scraping without squeezing the venom sac.
- Apply cool compresses to the injection site.
- Observe for and treat allergic reactions and/or anaphylaxis. (See Chapter 31.)

Brown Recluse Spider Bite

The brown recluse spider lives in the southern and midwestern states. It is found in large numbers in Tennessee, Arkansas, Oklahoma, and Texas. It has also been reported in Hawaii and California.

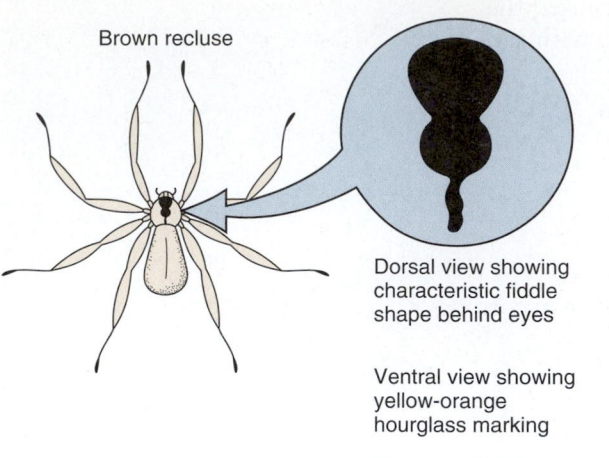

Brown recluse

Dorsal view showing characteristic fiddle shape behind eyes

Ventral view showing yellow-orange hourglass marking

FIGURE 34-4 Brown recluse spider.

The brown recluse is about 15 mm in length. It generally lives in dark, dry locations and can often be found in and around the house. There is a characteristic violin-shaped marking on the back, giving the spider its nickname, "fiddleback spider" (Figure 34-4). Another identifying feature is the presence of six eyes (three pairs in a semicircle), instead of the eight eyes common to most spiders.

Signs and Symptoms Brown recluse spider bites are usually painless. Not uncommonly, bites occur at night while the patient sleeps. Most victims are unaware they have been bitten until the local reaction starts. Initially a small erythematous macule surrounded by a white ring forms at the site (Figure 34-5). This usually appears within a few minutes of the bite. Over the next eight hours localized pain, redness, and swelling develop. Tissue necrosis at the site occurs over days to weeks (Figure 34-6). Other symptoms include chills, fever, nausea and vomiting, joint pain and in severe situations, bleeding disorders (disseminated intravascular coagulation).

Management Treatment is mostly supportive. Since there is no antivenin, the emergency department treatment consists of antihistamines to reduce systemic reactions and possible surgical excision of necrotic tissue.

FIGURE 34-5 Brown recluse spider bite 24 hours after bite. Note the bleb and surrounding white halo. (Courtesy of Scott and White Hospital and Clinic.)

FIGURE 34-6 Brown recluse spider bite 4 days after the bite. Note the spread of erythema and early necrosis. (Courtesy of Scott and White Hospital and Clinic.)

Black Widow Spider Bites

Black widow spiders live in all parts of the continental United States. They are usually found in woodpiles or brush. The female spider is responsible for bites and can be easily identified by the characteristic orange hourglass marking on her black abdomen (Figure 34-7). The venom of the legendary black widow is very potent, causing excessive neurotransmitter release at the synaptic junctions.

Signs and Symptoms Signs and symptoms of black widow spider bites start as immediate localized pain, redness, and swelling. Progressive muscle spasms of all large muscle groups can occur and are usually associated with severe pain. Other systemic symptoms include nausea, vomiting, sweating, seizures, paralysis, and decreased level of consciousness.

Black Widow dorsal view

FIGURE 34-7 Black widow spider.

Management Prehospital treatment is mostly supportive. It is important to reassure the patient. IV muscle relaxants may be necessary for severe spasms. With physician order you may use diazepam (2.5–10 mg IV) or calcium gluconate (0.1–0.2/kg of 10 percent solution IV). Note that calcium chloride is not effective and should not be used. Since hypertensive crisis is possible, monitor blood pressure carefully. Antivenin is available, so transfer the patient to the emergency department as soon as possible.

Scorpion Stings

There are many species of scorpion in the United States (Figure 34-8). All can sting, causing localized pain, but only one, the bark scorpion, has caused fatalities. These arthropods live mostly in Arizona and adjacent areas of California, Nevada, New Mexico, and Texas. There have been no deaths in Arizona from scorpion stings since 1970.

Scorpions move mostly at night, hiding in the day under debris and buildings. The venom they inject is stored in a bulb at the end of the tail. If provoked the scorpion will sting with its tail, injecting only a small amount of poison.

Signs and Symptoms The bark scorpion's venom acts on the nervous system, producing a burning and tingling effect without much evidence of injury initially. Gradually this progresses to numbness. Systemic effects are more pronounced with slurred speech, restlessness (hyperactivity in 80 percent of children), muscle twitching, salivation, abdominal cramping, nausea and vomiting, and seizures.

Management Begin treatment by reassuring the patient. Apply a constricting band above the wound site no tighter than a watchband to occlude lymphatic flow only. Avoid the use of analgesics, which may increase toxicity and potentiate the venom's effect on airway control. Transport the patient to the emergency department if systemic symptoms develop. Antivenin is available but is an unlicensed goat-serum-derived product found in Arizona only. It can produce allergic or anaphylactic reactions and should be used only in severe cases.

SNAKEBITES

There are several thousand snakebites each year in the United States. Fortunately, these bites result in very few deaths. The signs and symptoms of snakebite depend upon the snake, the location of the bite, and the type and amount of venom injected.

FIGURE 34-8 Scorpion.

FIGURE 34-9   Venomous snakes in the United States.

There are two families of poisonous snakes native to the United States (Figure 34-9). One family (*Crotalidae*) includes the pit vipers. Common pit vipers are cottonmouths (water moccasins), rattlesnakes, and copperheads. Pit vipers are so named because of the distinctive pit between the eye and the nostril on each side of the head. These snakes have elliptical pupils, two well-developed fangs, and a triangular-shaped head. Only the rattlesnake, the most common pit viper, has rattles on the end of its tail.

The second family of poisonous snakes is the *Elapidae*, or coral snake, which is a distant relative of the cobra. Several varieties of coral snakes are found in the United States, primarily in the southwest. Because it is a small snake and has small fangs, the coral snake cannot readily attach itself to a large surface, such as an arm or leg. The coral snake has round eyes, a narrow head, and no pit. It has characteristic yellow-banded red and black rings around its body. Several nonpoisonous snakes, such as the King Snake, mimic this coloration pattern. Keep in mind a helpful mnemonic: "red touch yellow, kill a fellow; red touch black, venom lack." This rhyme indicates the distinctive pattern of the coral snake—a pattern that signals danger.

Pit Viper Bites

Pit viper venom contains hydrolytic enzymes that are capable of destroying proteins and most other tissue components. These enzymes may produce destruction of red blood cells and other tissue components and may affect the body's blood clotting system within the blood vessels. This will produce infarction and tissue necrosis, especially at the site of the bite.

A severe pit-viper bite can result in death from shock within 30 minutes. However, most deaths from pit-viper bites occur from 6 to 30 hours after the bite, with 90% occurring within the first 48 hours.

Signs and Symptoms   Signs and symptoms of pit viper bite include:

- Fang marks (often little more than a scratch mark or abrasion)
- Swelling and pain at the wound site
- Continued oozing at the wound site
- Weakness, dizziness, or faintness
- Sweating and/or chills
- Thirst
- Nausea and vomiting
- Diarrhea
- Tachycardia and hypotension

- Bloody urine and gastrointestinal hemorrhage (late)
- Ecchymosis
- Necrosis
- Shallow respirations progressing to respiratory failure
- Numbness and tingling around face and head (classic)

Management In treating a person who has been bitten by a pit viper, the primary goal is to slow absorption of the venom. Remember, about 25% of all rattlesnake bites are "dry" and no venom is injected. The amount of venom a pit viper injects varies significantly. It is helpful to try to classify the degree of envenomation:

Degree of Envenomation	Signs and Symptoms
None	None (either local or systemic)
Minimal	Swelling
	Pain
	No systemic symptoms
Moderate	Progressive swelling
	Mild systemic symptoms
	– paresthesias
	– nausea and vomiting
	– unusual tastes
	– mild hypotension
	– mild tachycardia
	– tachypnea
Severe	Swelling (spreading rapidly)
	Severe pain
	Systemic symptoms
	– altered mental status
	– nausea and vomiting
	– hypotension (systolic <80)
	– severe tachycardia
	– severe respiratory distress
	Blood oozes freely from puncture wounds

Antivenin is available for the various common pit vipers found in the United States. However, antivenin should only be considered for severe cases where there is marked envenomation as evidenced by severe systemic symptoms. In some cases, people become more ill from the antivenin than they do from the snakebite itself. Routine emergency treatment of pit viper bites includes the following steps:

- Keep the patient supine.
- Immobilize the limb with a splint.
- Maintain the extremity in a neutral position. Do not apply constricting bands.

Initiate supportive care using the following guidelines:

- Apply high-flow oxygen.
- Start IV with crystalloid fluid.
- Transport the patient to the emergency department for management, which may include the administration of antivenin.
- DO NOT apply ice, cold pack, or freon spray to the wound.
- DO NOT apply an arterial tourniquet.
- DO NOT apply electrical stimulation from any device in an attempt to retard or reverse venom spread.

Coral Snake Bites

The venom of the coral snake contains some of the enzymes found in pit viper venom. However, because of the presence of neurotoxin, coral snake venom primarily affects nervous tissue. The classic, severe coral snake bite will result in respiratory and skeletal muscle paralysis.

Signs and Symptoms After the bite of a coral snake, there may be no local manifestations or even any systemic effects for as long as 12–24 hours. Signs and symptoms of a coral snake bite include:

- Localized numbness, weakness, and drowsiness
- Ataxia
- Slurred speech and excessive salivation
- Paralysis of the tongue and larynx (produces difficulty breathing and swallowing)
- Drooping of eyelids, double vision, dilated pupils
- Abdominal pain
- Nausea and vomiting
- Loss of consciousness
- Seizures
- Respiratory failure
- Hypotension

Management Treatment in cases of suspected coral snake bites includes the following steps:

- Wash the wound with copious amounts of water.
- Apply a compression bandage and keep the extremity at the level of the heart.
- Immobilize the limb with a splint.
- Start an IV using crystalloid fluid.
- Transport the patient to the emergency department for administration of antivenin.
- DO NOT apply ice, cold pack, or freon sprays to the wound.
- DO NOT incise the wound.
- DO NOT apply electrical stimulation from any device in an attempt to retard or reverse venom spread.

FIGURE 34-10   Stingray.

MARINE ANIMAL INJECTION

Although most dangerous marine life prefer warm, tropical waters, some can be found in more northern waters. With the large number of people who flock to beaches and coastal recreation areas every year, the number of injuries from marine life has increased moderately. The most common encounters occur while the person is walking on the beach but can also happen while wading in shallow waters or scuba diving in deeper waters. Injection of toxins from marine life can result from stings of jellyfish and corals or from punctures by the bony spines of animals such as sea urchins and stingrays (Figure 34-10). All venoms of marine animals contain substances that produce pain out of proportion to the size of the injury. These poisonous toxins are unstable and heat sensitive. Heat will relieve pain and inactivate the venom.

Both fresh water and salt water contain considerable bacterial and viral pollution. Therefore, secondary infection is always a possibility in injuries from marine animals. Particularly severe and life-threatening infections can be inflicted by a number of organisms. In all cases of marine-acquired infections, *Vibrio* species must be considered.

Signs and Symptoms Signs and symptoms of marine animal injection include:

- Intense local pain and swelling
- Weakness
- Nausea and vomiting
- Dyspnea
- Tachycardia
- Hypotension or shock (severe cases)

Management In suspected cases or marine animal injection, take the following steps:

- Establish and maintain the airway.
- Apply a constricting band between the wound and the heart no tighter than a watchband to occlude lymphatic flow only.
- Apply heat or hot water (110°–113°F).
- Inactivate or remove any stingers.

✱ **substance abuse** use of a pharmacological substance for purposes other than medically defined reasons.

✱ **addiction** compulsive and overwhelming dependence on a drug; an addiction may be physiological dependence, a psychological dependence, or both.

✱ **tolerance** the need to progressively increase the dose of a drug to reproduce the effect originally achieved by smaller doses.

SUBSTANCE ABUSE AND OVERDOSE

Substance abuse, the use of a pharmacological substance for purposes other than medically defined reasons, is a very serious problem in our nation. Drugs are abused because they stimulate a feeling of euphoria in the abuser. Eventually, abusers begin to crave the feeling the drug gives them and therefore develop a *dependence* on the drug, also called **addiction.** An addiction exists when a person repeatedly uses and feels an overwhelming need to obtain and continue using a particular drug. Becoming accustomed to the use of the drug is called *habituation.* *Physiological dependence* is the resulting condition if removal of the drug causes adverse physical reactions. There can also be *psychological dependence,* in which use of the drug is required to prevent or relieve tension or emotional stress. With continued use, **tolerance** develops, which means that the abuser must use increasingly larger doses to get the same effect.

Attempts to stop the drug can trigger a psychological or physical reaction known as **withdrawal.** Withdrawal reactions can be quite unpleasant and severe. In some cases (especially with alcohol), withdrawal can be severe enough to cause death. These reactions further strengthen the victim's dependence on the drug. At this point the abuser may begin to withdraw from regular activities. He may have conflicts with family, friends, and coworkers as his personality and priorities change. Often the abuser will be involved in criminal activities to support the habit. The abuser has formed an addiction at the point when the substance abuse begins to affect some part of his life. This includes affecting the abuser's health, work, or relationships. Also, the abuser begins to act in a manner so as to seek out the drug he abuses.

The National Institute on Drug Abuse performed a survey to estimate national use and exposure to illicit drugs. The results were astounding.

* 28 million Americans used illicit drugs at least once.
* 14.5 million use illicit drugs regularly.
* 20 million Americans have tried cocaine.
* 860,000 people use cocaine weekly.
* 11.6 million use marijuana regularly.
* 770,000 use hallucinogens such as PCP or LSD regularly.
* 2.5 million have used heroin.

The use of illicit drugs has fluctuated in recent years. Most recently, heroin has regained popularity, especially among middle to upper class teenagers and young adults. Beyond hurting themselves, substance abusers are 18 times more likely to be involved in criminal activities. These include violent crimes as well as theft to support drug habits. (The Secretary of Health and Human Services has estimated that cocaine is a $65 billion per year industry.)

In general terms, **drug overdose** refers to poisoning from a pharmacological substance, either legal or illegal. This can occur by accident, miscalculation, changes in the strength of a drug, suicide, polydrug use, or recreational drug usage. Many overdose emergencies seen in the field occur in the habitual drug abuser. It is most difficult to obtain a good history in these cases. However, if the paramedic is familiar with street-drug slang, a more accurate history may be obtained. It is imperative that the paramedic maintain a nonjudgmental attitude in these cases, even though this may be difficult.

The presentation of the drug overdose will vary based on the substance used. Management should be the same as for any ingested, inhaled, or injected poison. Poison control should be contacted for additional direction.

DRUGS OF ABUSE

Drugs Commonly Abused

Drugs of abuse are both common and dangerous. These drugs all have various signs and symptoms and require supportive treatment and general toxicological emergency management. Refer to Table 34-3 for further details on what you may find on assessment and the interventions required.

Remember these specific guidelines for patients who have taken the following drugs:

* *Alcohol*—May require thiamine and $D_{50}W$ for hypoglycemia.
* *Cocaine*—Benzodiazepines (diazepam) may be needed for sedation and to treat seizures. Beta blockers are absolutely contraindicated

* **withdrawal** referring to alcohol or drug withdrawal in which the patient's body reacts severely when deprived of the abused substance.

* **drug overdose** poisoning from a pharmacological substance in excess of that usually prescribed or that the body can tolerate.

Table 34-3 COMMON DRUGS OF ABUSE

Drug	Signs and Symptoms	Routes	Prehospital Management
Alcohol beer whiskey gin vodka wine tequila	CNS depression Slurred speech Disordered thought Impaired judgment Diuresis Stumbling gait Stupor Coma	Oral	ABCs Respiratory support Oxygenate Establish IV access Administer 100 mg thiamine IV ECG monitor Check glucose level Administer $D_{50}W$, if hypoglycemic
Barbiturates thiopental phenobarbital primidone	Lethargy Emotional lability Incoordination Slurred speech Nystagmus Coma Hypotension Respiratory depression	Oral IV	ABCs Respiratory support Oxygenate Establish IV access ECG monitor Contact Poison Control—may order bicarbonate
Cocaine crack rock	Euphoria Hyperactivity Dilated pupils Psychosis Twitching Anxiety Hypertension Tachycardia Dysrhythmias Seizures Chest pain	Snorting Injection Smoking (freebasing)	ABCs Respiratory support Oxygenate ECG monitor Establish IV access Treat life-threatening dysrhythmias Seizure precautions: diazepam 5–10 mg
Narcotics heroin codeine meperidine morphine hydromorphone pentazocine Darvon Darvocet methadone	CNS depression Constricted pupils Respiratory depression Hypotension Bradycardia Pulmonary edema Coma Death	Oral Injection	ABCs Respiratory support Oxygenate Establish IV access *Administer 1–2 mg naloxone IV or endotracheally as ordered by medical direction until respirations improve. Larger than average doses (2–5 mg) have been used in the management of Darvon overdose and alcoholic coma ECG monitor

*With the advent of the opiate antagonist naloxone, narcotic overdosage became easier to manage. It is possible to titrate this effective medication to increase respirations to normal levels without fully awakening the patient. In the case of narcotics addicts, this prevents hostile and confrontational episodes.

Continued

because unopposed alpha receptor stimulation can cause cardiac ischemia, hypertension, and hyperthermia.

- *Narcotics/Opiates*—Naloxone is effective in reversing respiratory depression and sedation, but be careful, since it may trigger a withdrawal reaction in chronic opiate abusers.
- *Amphetamines*—Use benzodiazepines (diazepam) for seizures and in combination with haloperidol for hyperactivity.

Table 34-3 COMMON DRUGS OF ABUSE (CONTINUED)

Drug	Signs and Symptoms	Routes	Prehospital Management
Marijuana grass weed hashish	Euphoria Dry mouth Dilated pupils Altered sensation	Smoked Oral	ABCs Reassure the patient Speak in a quiet voice ECG monitor if indicated
Amphetamines Benzedrine Dexedrine Ritalin "speed"	Exhilaration Hyperactivity Dilated pupils Hypertension Psychosis Tremors Seizures	Oral Injection	ABCs Oxygenate ECG monitor Establish IV access Treat life-threatening dysrhythmias Seizure precautions: diazepam 5–10 mg
Hallucinogens LSD STP mescaline psilocybin PCP**	Psychosis Nausea Dilated pupils Rambling speech Headache Dizziness Suggestibility Distortion of sensory perceptions Hallucinations	Oral Smoked	ABCs Reassure the patient "Talk down" the "high" patient Protect the patient from injury Provide a dark, quiet environment Speak in a soft, quiet voice Seizure precautions: diazepam 5–10 mg

**While PCP was originally an animal tranquilizer, it manifests hallucinogenic properties when used by humans. In addition to bizarre delusions, it can cause violent and dangerous outbursts of aggressive behavior. The rescuer is advised to remain safe when attempting to treat this type of overdose. PCP patients have been known to have almost superhuman strength and high pain tolerance.

Drug	Signs and Symptoms	Routes	Prehospital Management
Sedatives Seconal Valium Librium Xanax Halcion Restoril Dalmane Phenobarbital	Altered mental status Hypotension Slurred speech Respiratory depression Shock Bradycardia Seizures	Oral	ABCs Respiratory support Oxygenate Establish IV access ECG monitor Medical direction may order naloxone
Benzodiazepines* Valium Librium Xanax Halcion Restoril Dalmane Centrax Ativan Serax	Altered mental status Slurred speech Dysrhythmias Coma	Oral	ABCs Respiratory support Oxygenate Activated charcoal as ordered by medical Direction Establish IV access ECG monitor Contact poison control

***Deaths due to pure benzodiazepine are rare. Minor toxicity ranges are 500–1,500 mg. A benzodiazepine antagonist (Romazicon) is available (IV dosage 1–10 mg or infusion 0.5 mg/hr). It may cause seizures in a benzodiazepine dependent patient.

- *Hallucinogens*—Use benzodiazepines for seizures and in combination with haloperidol for hyperactivity.
- *Benzodiazepines*—Use flumazenil to counteract adverse effects. Be careful not to trigger a withdrawal syndrome with seizures.
- *Barbiturates*—Forced diuresis and alkalinization of the urine improve elimination of barbiturates from the body.

Drugs Used for Sexual Purposes

There are a number of drugs that deserve mention as a separate category. These drugs are used to stimulate and enhance the sexual experience, but without medically approved indications for such use. *Ecstasy,* also called *MDMA,* is one such drug. Ecstasy is a modified form of methamphetamines and has similar, although milder effects. It is very popular in today's university and nightclub environments.

Use of Ecstasy initially causes anxiety, nausea, tachycardia, and elevated blood pressure, followed by relaxation, euphoria, and feelings of enhanced emotional insight. No definitive data exists as to whether the experience of sexual intercourse is improved. Studies show that prolonged use may cause brain damage. Some deaths from MDMA ingestion have been reported. These cases present with confusion, agitation, tremor, high temperature, and diarrhea. No specific treatment exists. Standard supportive measures should be initiated.

Rohypnol (flunitrazepam) is another drug abused for sexual purposes. Illegal in the United States, it is commonly called the "date rape drug," since it can be secretly slipped into a woman's drink. This drug is a strong benzodiazepine like diazepam, lorazepan, and midazolam. The resulting sedation and amnesia allows the perpetrator to rape the victim. Treatment is the same as for any benzodiazepine, but consequences of the sexual assault require attention as well.

ALCOHOL ABUSE

Alcohol is the most common substance of abuse in the United States and most of the world. Almost 75 percent of Americans have at least one drink per year. The average American consumes 2.5 gallons of pure ethanol every year. Alcohol has been linked to 5 percent of deaths in the United States. Alcoholism costs over $100 billion per year due to lost work time and medical costs to treat complications and injuries. Alcoholism progresses in much the same way as drug dependence, discussed earlier.

PHYSIOLOGICAL EFFECTS

Alcohol (ethyl alcohol, or ethanol) depresses the central nervous system, potentially to the point of stupor, coma, and death. In patients with severe liver disease, metabolism of alcohol may become impaired, which increases the course and severity of intoxication. At low doses, alcohol has excitatory and stimulating effects, thus depressing inhibitions. At higher doses alcohol's depressive effect is more obvious. Alcohol abuse and dependence is called *alcoholism.* It is a major problem, contributing to highway traffic fatalities, drownings, burns, trauma, and drug overdoses.

Alcohol is completely absorbed from the stomach and intestinal tract in approximately 30 to 120 minutes after ingestion. Once absorbed, alcohol is distributed to all body tissues and fluids, with concentrations of alcohol in the brain rapidly approaching the alcohol level in the blood.

Some alcoholics will drink methanol (wood alcohol) or ethylene glycol (a component of antifreeze) if ethanol is unavailable. Ingestion of these chemicals can cause blindness or death.

In addition, alcohol causes a peripheral vasodilator effect on the cardiovascular system, resulting in flushing and a feeling of warmth. In cold conditions, alcohol's dilation of the blood vessels results in an increased loss of body heat. The diuretic effect seen when large amounts of alcohol are ingested is due to the inhibition of *vasopressin,* which is the hormone responsible for the conservation of body fluids. Without vasopressin, an increase in urine flow occurs. The "dry mouth syndrome" experienced after alcohol consumption may be the result of alcohol-induced cellular dehydration.

In addition, methanol will also cause visual disturbances, abdominal pain, and nausea and vomiting even at low doses. In fact, death has been reported after ingestion of only 15 mL of a 40 percent solution. Occasionally patients will complain of headache or dizziness and may even present with seizures and obtundation. Ethylene glycol ingestion has similar symptoms, but the CNS effects such as hallucinations, coma, and seizures are more pronounced in the early stages.

GENERAL ALCOHOLIC PROFILE

The classic alcoholic portrayed in movies is an unkempt, continually intoxicated street person who is completely non-functional. Although alcoholics of this type exist, it would be a grave error to consider this the typical picture of someone dependent on alcohol. More commonly, alcoholism is characterized by impaired control over drinking, preoccupation with the drug ethanol, use of ethanol despite adverse consequences, and distortions in thinking, such as denial. This is the definition used by the National Council on Alcoholism and Drug Dependence. Obviously, this definition applies to many people, including many functional people at all levels of society who have masked their addiction well. Take note of these warning signs, which may indicate alcohol abuse:

Most alcoholics are not unkempt street people but are functional people at all levels of society who are able to mask their addiction.

- Drinks early in the day
- Prone to drink alone and secretly
- Periodic binges (may last for several days)
- Partial or total loss of memory ("blackouts") during period of drinking
- Unexplained history of gastrointestinal problems (especially bleeding)
- "Green tongue syndrome" (using chlorophyll-containing substances to disguise the odor of alcohol on the breath)
- Cigarette burns on clothing
- Chronically flushed face and palms
- Tremulousness
- Odor of alcohol on breath under inappropriate conditions

CONSEQUENCES OF CHRONIC ALCOHOL INGESTION

Alcohol has many deleterious effects on the body. Chronic abuse can be devastating, effecting every organ system as shown in Figure 34-11. Some of the more common effects include:

- Poor nutrition
- Alcohol hepatitis
- Liver cirrhosis with subsequent esophageal varices
- Loss of sensation in hands and feet
- Loss of cerebellar function (balance and coordination)
- Pancreatitis
- Upper gastrointestinal hemorrhage (often fatal)
- Hypoglycemia
- Subdural hematoma (due to falls)
- Rib and extremity fractures (due to falls)

FIGURE 34-11 The chronic alcoholic.

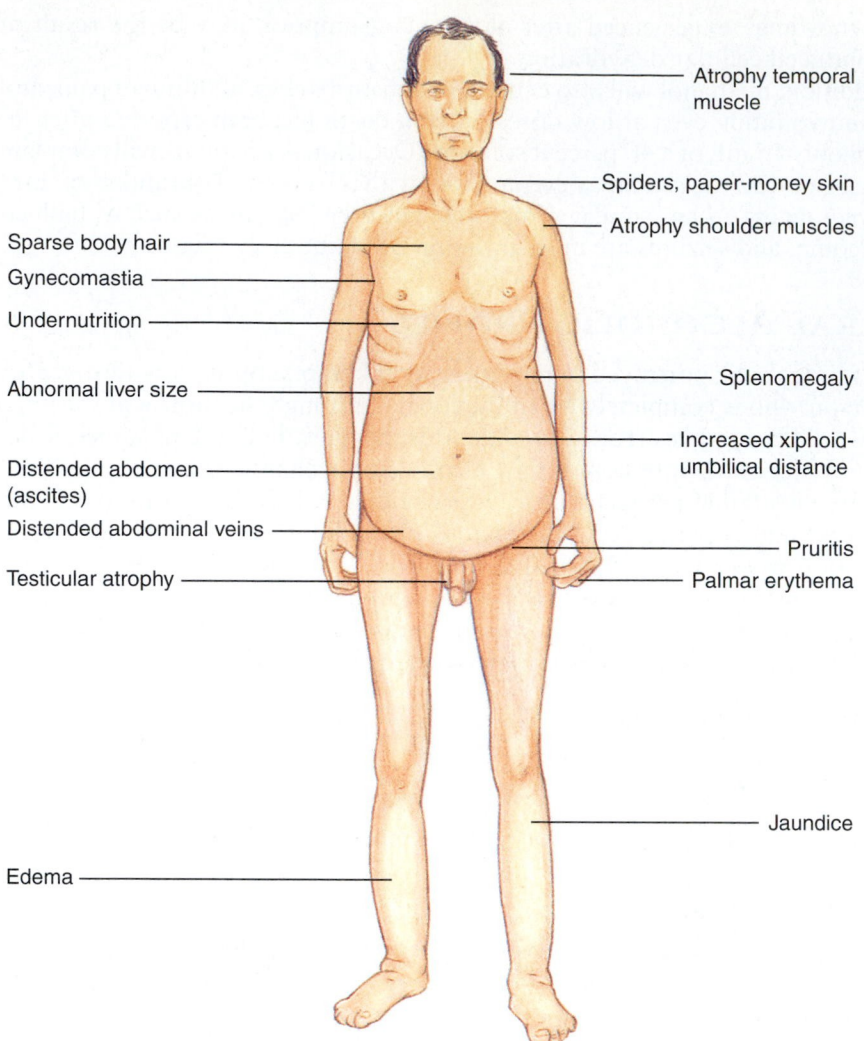

Atrophy temporal muscle

Spiders, paper-money skin

Atrophy shoulder muscles

Sparse body hair

Gynecomastia

Undernutrition

Abnormal liver size

Splenomegaly

Increased xiphoid-umbilical distance

Distended abdomen (ascites)

Distended abdominal veins

Pruritis

Testicular atrophy

Palmar erythema

Jaundice

Edema

Conditions such as subdural hematomas, sepsis, and other diseases may mimic signs and symptoms of alcohol intoxication. For example, ketoacidosis produces an odor similar to alcohol on the breath.

❋ delirium tremens (DTs) disorder found in habitual and excessive users of alcoholic beverages after cessation of drinking for 48–72 hours. Patients experience visual, tactile, and auditory disturbances. Death may result in severe cases.

Keep in mind that conditions such as subdural hematomas, sepsis, and other life-threatening disease processes may mimic the signs and symptoms of alcohol intoxication. For example, diabetic ketoacidosis produces a breath odor that can easily be confused with the odor of alcohol.

Withdrawal Syndrome

The alcoholic may suffer a withdrawal reaction from either abrupt discontinuation of ingestion after prolonged use or from a rapid fall in blood-alcohol level after acute intoxication. Alcohol withdrawal can be potentially fatal. Withdrawal symptoms can occur several hours after sudden abstinence and can last up to 5 to 7 days. Seizures (sometimes called "rum fits") may occur within the first 24–36 hours of abstinence. **Delirium tremens (DTs)** usually develops on the second or third day of the withdrawal. Delirium tremens is characterized by a decreased level of consciousness during which the patient hallucinates and misinterprets nearby events. Seizures and delirium tremens are ominous signs. There is a significant mortality from delirium tremens. Medical direction may order diazepam in severe cases.

Signs and Symptoms Signs and symptoms of withdrawal syndrome include:

- Coarse tremor of hands, tongue, and eyelids
- Nausea and vomiting

- General weakness
- Increased sympathetic tone
- Tachycardia
- Sweating
- Hypertension
- Orthostatic hypotension
- Anxiety
- Irritability or a depressed mood
- Hallucinations
- Poor sleep

Management Alcohol intoxication, whether acute or chronic, should not be underestimated as a toxic emergency problem. In cases of suspected alcohol abuse, take the following steps.

- Establish and maintain the airway.
- Determine if other drugs are involved.
- Start an IV using lactated Ringer's or normal saline.
- Chemstrip and administer 25 g of $D_{50}W$ if hypoglycemic.
- Administer 100 mg of thiamine intravenously or intramuscularly.
- Maintain a sympathetic attitude and reassure the patient of help.
- Transport to the emergency department for further care.

Do not underestimate alcohol intoxication as a toxic emergency.

SUMMARY

Clearly, there is much to remember when dealing with toxicological emergencies. To effectively manage these situations you must focus on three things.

- *Recognize the poisoning promptly.* In other words, you must have a high index of suspicion when circumstances suggest a toxin may be involved.
- *Be thorough in your initial assessment and evaluation of the patient.* This will facilitate your efforts to identify the toxin and the measures needed to control the situation.
- *Initiate the standard treatment procedures required for all toxicological emergencies.* Beyond the usual concern for rescuer safety and rapid implementation of ABCs and supportive measures, consider the methods needed to minimize any further exposure to the toxin, decontaminate the patient from the toxins already involved, and finally administer any useful antidote if one exists for the particular toxin.

If you remember these three steps, you will be equipped to handle most toxicological emergencies promptly and efficiently.

CHAPTER 35

Hematology

Objectives

After reading this chapter, you should be able to:

1. Identify the anatomy and physiology of the hematopoietic system. (see Chapter 3)
2. Discuss the following: (see Chapter 3)
   - plasma
   - red blood cells (erythrocytes)
   - hemoglobin
   - hematocrit
   - white blood cells (leukocytes)
   - platelets, clotting, and fibrinolysis
   - hemostasis
3. Identify the following: (see Chapter 4)
   - inflammatory process
   - cellular and humoral immunity
   - alterations in immunological response
4. Identify blood groups. (pp. 1498–1499)
5. List erythrocyte disorders. (pp. 1506–1508)
6. List leukocyte disorders. (pp. 1509–1510)
7. List platelet and clotting disorders. (pp. 1511–1512)

Continued

INTRODUCTION

Hematology is the study of the blood and the blood-forming organs. It exemplifies the way that multiple organ systems interact to maintain homeostasis, the normal balance of body functions. Hematological disorders are common and include red blood cell disorders, white blood cell disorders, platelet disorders, and coagulation problems. Although these disorders are common, they rarely are the primary cause of a medical emergency. They usually accompany other ongoing disease processes. Some hematological diseases are genetic in origin. Hemophilia A is a classic example. It is a sex-linked disease that causes abnormally low levels of an essential blood clotting protein (Factor VIII). It affects approximately 1–2 persons per 10,000 in the United States. Some hematological diseases are more common in certain ethnic groups. For example, among the population as a whole, sickle cell anemia is relatively uncommon. However, among African-Americans specifically, 8 percent of the population has sickle cell trait. In addition to their primary effects, hematological disorders may predispose patients to infection and intolerance to exercise, hypoxia, acidosis, and blood loss.

Patients with hematological problems often complain of signs and symptoms that do not point directly to a specific disease process. Careful examination and history taking may be necessary to further clarify the diagnosis. Often, however, laboratory findings will be needed to confirm the diagnosis. Thus, the final diagnosis of patients for whom you provide prehospital care is often not immediately apparent. You must use your assessment skills to recognize and treat injuries, pain, and instabilities, while formulating a field impression that enables you to anticipate further complications and thus enhance patient outcome and survivability. Because of this, it is essential that you have a good understanding of the basic pathophysiological processes of your patients' disease, including hematological disorders.

* **hematology** the study of blood and the blood-forming organs.

FIGURE 35-1   Blood transfusion.

BLOOD PRODUCTS AND BLOOD TYPING

A blood transfusion is the transplantation of blood or a component of blood from one person to another. It is accomplished by IV infusion (Figure 35-1). Various types of transfusions are given for various purposes (Table 35-1).

In the 1800s when patients received blood from others, some had a reaction that led to multiple organ failure and death. Karl Landsteiner discovered the reason for this was reaction **antigens,** proteins on the surface of the donor's red blood cells that the patient's body recognized as "not self." Following transfusion, antibodies in the patient's own blood attacked the foreign antigens present in the transfused blood. Landsteiner named the antigens A and B and the opposing antibodies anti-A and anti-B. Someone with A antigen on his red blood cells would have anti-B antibodies. His blood type would be A. Someone with B antigens on the red blood cell surface would have anti-A antibodies; his type would be B. Some people's red blood cells have both antigens on their surface but neither antibody. Their blood type is AB. Others have neither antigen but both antibodies; their blood type is O (for zero antigens, but pronounced "Oh"). Blood type is an inherited trait. Approximately 45 percent of the United States population has type O, 39 percent type A, 11 percent type B, and 5 percent type AB.

Since only the antibodies recognize and attack foreign tissue, a person with no antibodies (type AB) can receive any blood type in an emergency, and the body will not attack the cells. So a person with type AB blood is called a *universal recipient.* Conversely, blood with no antigens to any other blood group type (type O) would not trigger a reaction, as the recipient's blood recognizes nothing "foreign." So people with type O blood are called *universal donors.*

Crossmatching blood involves checking samples from both donor and recipient to ensure the greatest compatibility. If a donor's blood does not clump together, or agglutinate, when mixed with the recipient's blood, they are compatible. Reliance on the universal donor and recipient concept is useful only in an emergency, when there is no time to check samples.

✳ **antigen** protein on the surface of a donor's red blood cells that the patient's body recognizes as "not self."

Content Review

BLOOD TYPES

- A
- B
- AB
- O

Table 35-1 TYPES OF TRANSFUSIONS

Type of Transfusion	Contents	Use
Whole blood	All cells, platelets, clotting factors, and plasma	Replace blood loss from hemorrhage
Packed red blood cells (PRBCs)	Red blood cells and some plasma	Replace red blood cells in anemic patients
Platelets	Thrombocytes and some plasma	Replace platelets in a patient with thrombocytopenia
Fresh frozen plasma (FFP)	Plasma, a combination of fluids, clotting factors, and proteins	Replace volume in a burn patient or in hypovolemia secondary to low oncotic pressure
Clotting factors	Specific clotting factors needed for coagulation	Replace factors missing due to inadequate production as in hemophilia

Blood transfusion is not as simple as that, however. Approximately 40 years after the discovery of A and B antigens, Landsteiner and A.S. Weiner observed another antigen present on red blood cells. Research leading to this antigen's discovery used rhesus monkey blood, so the antigen was called the Rh factor. If a person has the Rh factor, he is Rh positive; if not, he is Rh negative. As many as 500 other lesser antigens have since been identified but they usually do not cause the severe hemolytic reaction seen in the patients sensitized to the Rh factor. *Erythroblastosis fetalis*, more commonly called hemolytic disease of the newborn, can lead to a fatal hemolytic reaction in neonates. In this disease, the mother who is Rh⁻ is sensitized by previous exposure to the Rh antigen during a previous pregnancy with an Rh⁺ child or from a previous blood transfusion. Therefore, if she subsequently becomes pregnant with an Rh⁺ child, the mother produces antibodies that attack the fetus's red blood cells, leading to a severe and often fatal hemolytic reaction. Fortunately, the incidence of hemolytic disease of newborns has been declining due to the administration of Rh immune globulin (RhoGAM) to mothers. This inhibits formation of anti-Rh antibodies. Additionally, transfusions in *utero* or fetal exchange transfusions immediately after birth can diminish or eliminate the likelihood of infant death.

TRANSFUSION REACTIONS

There are many types of transfusion reactions. One, hemolytic transfusion reaction, occurs when a donor's and recipient's blood are not compatible. Antigens on the donor's red blood cells trigger a response from the antibodies in the recipient's blood. The antibodies attach to the red blood cells, which are then *hemolyzed*, or taken up by the fixed macrophages of the spleen's reticuloendothelial system.

Signs and symptoms of a hemolytic transfusion reaction may include facial flushing, hyperventilation, tachycardia, and a sense of dread. Hives may appear on the skin, and the patient may develop chest pain, wheezing, fever, chills, and cyanosis. Flank pain may occur as small clots begin to clog the microvasculature of the kidneys, which can lead to kidney failure requiring dialysis. The damage can be permanent.

If you are caring for a patient receiving a blood transfusion and he develops what you believe to be a hemolytic reaction, stop the transfusion immediately.

If a patient receiving a blood transfusion develops what you believe to be a hemolytic reaction, stop the transfusion immediately.

Change all associated IV tubing and initiate IV therapy with normal saline or lactated Ringer's solution. Administer a bolus as necessary to maintain good perfusion and blood pressure. Furosemide (Lasix) is often administered to promote diuresis. Low dose dopamine (2–5 mcg/kg/minute) should be considered along with the IV fluid to help maintain adequate renal perfusion. If you observe evidence of an allergic reaction, you can give diphenhydramine (Benadryl) 25–50 mg IV to help with some of the histamine-mediated effects such as itching or hives. In extreme cases of anaphylactic reaction, you may need to administer IV epinephrine if the patient is hypotensive or demonstrates severe bronchospasm.

The most common transfusion reaction is the febrile nonhemolytic reaction. It is caused by sensitization to antigens on the white blood cells, platelets, or plasma proteins. Signs and symptoms include headache, fever, and chills. As with any other transfusion reaction, always stop the transfusion before attempting to treat it. After stopping the blood product, change all tubing, and initiate normal saline IV. Patients are often given diphenhydramine (Benadryl) and an antipyretic (ibuprofen, acetaminophen) for the fever. No further treatment may be necessary, as this reaction rarely progresses to more serious complications. However, close observation is required to exclude development of a hemolytic reaction. In the event of any transfusion reaction, return all blood bags, tubing, and filters to the blood bank for analysis. Medical direction may order you to take blood and urine samples.

Because blood transfusion adds fluid to the system, a patient may experience signs and symptoms of circulatory overload. In fact, signs and symptoms are the same as those for left ventricular failure and may include pulmonary edema, dyspnea, and chest pain. Hypotension is not usually a problem, and you may treat the patient successfully by slowing the heart rate and administering diuretics.

GENERAL ASSESSMENT AND MANAGEMENT

In general, patients with disorders of the hematopoietic system may present with a variety of complaints and physical findings. Patients with infection, white blood cell abnormalities (immunocompromised and prone to infection), or transfusion reactions may present with febrile symptoms. Subsequently, these patients may develop hemodynamic instability as infection progresses to sepsis or as the transfusion reaction leads to a hemolytic reaction, renal failure, and disseminated intravascular coagulation (DIC). Acute hemodynamic compromise can also be found in patients with anemia secondary to acute blood loss, coagulation defects, or autoimmune disease. These disease processes may not be easily differentiated in the field and often require significant laboratory testing to confirm the diagnosis. In most cases, however, if you obtain a careful history, you will have a good working diagnosis.

Most hematopoietic disorders are chronic conditions that present with acute exacerbation when the patient is exposed to an additional stress such as infection or trauma. Treatment of patients with disorders of the hematopoietic system, in most cases, is supportive. Some patients may have hemodynamic instability from blood or fluid loss. These patients may require intravenous fluids to support end-organ perfusion and prevent shock. In addition, they should receive oxygen therapy to prevent hypoxia from poor perfusion and diminished oxygen carrying capacity of the blood. It is important to recognize the need for rapid transport in patients with hemodynamic instability who may require transfusion or other definitive care measures. Always contact medical direction for questions or problems.

SCENE SIZE-UP

Assessment of the patient with a possible hematopoietic abnormality begins the same as for any other patient. Perform a scene size-up and take BSI precautions. During your approach, form a general impression of the patient. Is the patient a trauma or medical patient? In how much distress is the patient?

INITIAL ASSESSMENT

Complete an initial assessment for life threats. Determine responsiveness and assess the airway, breathing, and circulation. Alterations in the hematopoietic system may present as life-threatening bleeds or overwhelming infections with septic shock. Do not spend time obtaining a complete set of vital signs during the initial assessment. Check the ABCs and quickly determine your priority for transport. Critical or unstable patients should be considered candidates for expeditious transport.

FOCUSED HISTORY AND PHYSICAL EXAM

Next, complete a focused history and physical exam. Use your general impression to choose a format for a responsive or unresponsive medical patient or trauma patient with significant or nonsignificant mechanism of injury. Each format follows a sequence of history gathering and examination designed to meet the needs of that particular patient. Trauma patients and unresponsive medical patients often present life-threatening problems that are noted in your initial assessment.

SAMPLE History

For a responsive medical patient, obtain a SAMPLE history and perform a physical exam. Obtain a set of vital signs and place the pulse oximeter. Keep in mind that an anemic patient will have increased heart and respiratory rates as his body attempts to compensate for less oxygen reaching the tissues. Ask for the chief complaint—why did the patient call for assistance? What signs or symptoms (SAMPLE) accompanied or preceded the complaint? Pay attention to generalized complaints such as fatigue, lethargy, malaise, apprehension, or confusion. These may indicate inadequate oxygen delivery to the tissues. Have there been any unusual skin changes such as coloring or bruising? Does the patient complain of itching? Inquire about lymph node enlargement (swollen glands), sore throat, or pain upon swallowing. These may indicate infection.

Any change in the blood's ability to deliver oxygen to the body will appear in the cardiovascular and respiratory systems. Note dyspnea, palpitations, and dizziness with changes in the patient's position. Patients with hematological problems may suffer syncope. Did the patient have a syncopal episode or is he just weak? Syncope can be due to several factors but is often related to a sudden change in position in a patient who has a marked anemia. Bleeding abnormalities may be disguised as gastrointestinal upset. Ask about overt bleeding with vomiting or diarrhea, but do not overlook complaints of nausea or anorexia, vomiting of "coffee ground" material, or having black tarry or cranberry, sticky, odoriferous stools. Many patients will notice bleeding of the gums when they brush their teeth. This can, on occasion, be hard to control. Atraumatic bleeding of the gums almost always points to an underlying hematologic abnormality. Ask about changes in urination, hematuria (blood in the urine), and alterations in the usual menstrual pattern in females. Keep in mind that hematological disorders are often diagnosed when the patient seeks assistance for another medical condition.

> *Keep in mind that hematological disorders are often diagnosed when the patient seeks assistance for another medical condition.*
>
>

Determine any allergies (SAMPLE). Be sure to ask about use of prescription or over-the-counter medications (SAMPLE). Make note of the patient's medication, dose, and the condition for which he takes the medication. Also, if time allows, note the dosing schedule of the medications. Ask about compliance. Does the patient take medication as prescribed? When was the last dose taken? Medications that may indicate an alteration in the hematologic system, or that might make the patient more susceptible to an alteration in the system, include pain relievers, antibiotics, anticoagulants, hormones, and medications for heart disease, arthritis, and seizures.

When asking about past medical history (SAMPLE), make note of surgeries such as a splenectomy, heart-valve replacement, or placement of long-term venous-access devices. Ask about bloodborne infections such as HIV or hepatitis B or C. Make note of liver or bone marrow disease or cancers. Include questions about family history such as hemophilia, sickle cell disease, cancer, or death at an early age that was not trauma related. Inquire also about social habits such as smoking, alcohol consumption, IV drug use, or long-term exposure to chemicals or radiation.

If you find a significant history, ask about the last episode of an incident or last use of a medication. Remember to include the usual questions about last oral intake (SAMPLE). Also, inquire about any unusual events (SAMPLE) that preceded the onset of the complaint such, as the start of a new medication, recent transfusion, fall, or injury.

Physical Exam

When performing the physical exam, evaluate each system methodically as you would in any other patient. If the history suggests a hematopoietic problem, look for potential pathology during the physical exam that may confirm your working diagnosis and be a clue to developing complications.

- *Nervous system* Always evaluate the nervous system in any patient with a suspected hematological problem. First, note the patient's level of consciousness using the AVPU system. Be alert for other nervous system disorders. Many patients with hematological problems will complain of being "weak and dizzy." Try to clarify this further. Is the patient fatigued, weak all over, or does he have focal weakness? Is he dizzy or is he suffering true vertigo? Both can be associated with hematological problems such as anemia. Ask if the patient has any numbness or motor deficits. Pernicious anemia can cause sensory deficits that are often unilateral. Try to determine whether the patient had a syncopal episode. What were the patient's condition and position immediately prior to the syncopal episode? Many of the hematological diseases, especially the autoimmune diseases, will affect the eye. Always examine the eyes for abnormalities. Question the patient about any visual disturbances or visual loss. In addition to the autoimmune diseases, sickle cell anemia is notorious for causing eye problems.

- *Skin* Note the patient's skin color (Figure 35-2). Jaundice (yellow skin) may indicate liver disease or hemolysis of red blood cells, while a florid (reddish) appearance is often associated with polycythemia. Patients with anemia typically exhibit pallor. Observe for petechiae (tiny red dots in the skin), purpura (large purplish blotches related to multiple hemorrhages into the skin), and bruising. Inquire about pruritus (itching). Patients with hematological disorders often develop pruritus. Some hematological problems, such as sickle cell

A

Petechiae – Reddish-purple spots, diameter less than 0.5 cm

B

Purpura – Reddish-purple blotches, diameter more than 0.5 cm

C

FIGURE 35-2   Abnormal skin colors: A) jaundice, B) petechiae, C) purpura.

anemia, cause the destruction of red blood cells. This results in hemoglobin's spilling into the circulatory system. Macrophages then break down the hemoglobin. The iron is removed and transported to the bones or liver. The porphyrin portion of the hemoglobin is subsequently converted into bilirubin, which is taken up by the liver. An excess of bilirubin, either from liver disease or from the breakdown of hemoglobin associated with the hemolytic anemias, can cause pruritis. Often, patients will develop itching over a bruise. As the hemoglobin breaks down within the bruise, the localized accumulation of bilirubin causes the itching. This is most common 1–2 weeks after the bruise occurs. When examining the skin, be alert for any evidence of prolonged bleeding. The patient may have several bandages over relatively minor wounds where he could not stop the bleeding.

- *Lymphatic* The lymphatic system is affected early in hematopoietic diseases, especially those of the immune system. During your physical exam, pay particular attention to the lymph nodes. Palpate the lymph nodes of the neck, clavicle, axilla, and groin. Note any enlargement. Compare sides. Splenomegaly (an enlarged spleen) is also often present, but this can be hard to examine in the field.

- *Gastrointestinal* The gastrointestinal effects of hematological problems can be quite varied. Epistaxis (nosebleed) is common. The nasal mucosa is quite vascular as it warms and humidifies the inhaled air. A slight crack in the nasal mucosa can result in brisk bleeding. This is a particular problem in people with blood clotting abnormalities, as stopping the bleeding is very difficult for them. These patients may swallow a great deal of blood and may become nauseated. Also, blood acts as a cathartic (laxative). Patients who swallow even moderate amounts of blood will often report loose bowel movements. These are often dark (melena). Blood present in emesis may be bright red or appear like coffee grounds.

Bleeding gums are often associated with a decreased platelet count.

Bleeding of the gums is one of the earliest findings of hematological problems. Patients with blood clotting abnormalities and low platelet levels will often develop atraumatic bleeding of the gums. Any patient with bleeding gums requires a detailed investigation for a possible hematological disorder. Gingivitis (infection of the gums) can be due to poor hygiene, disease, or both. However, chronic gingivitis should cause increased suspicion of a hematological disorder, especially involving the immune system. Also, gingivitis increases a patient's risk of developing sepsis. Slight trauma, such as brushing the teeth, can cause the bacteria to enter the circulatory system, resulting in generalized sepsis. Always note the presence of gingivitis when examining for bleeding gums. Ulcerations of the gums and oral mucosa are typically due to viral diseases. These infections are more common in immunosuppressed patients. Thrush (yeast infection in the mouth) in adults is almost always associated with AIDS. (Thrush in children is common and not a reason for concern.)

An oral yeast infection in an adult is commonly associated with AIDS.

The liver plays a major role in manufacturing many of the substances required for blood clotting. Liver disease can slow blood clotting. This is most evident in a prolonged prothrombin (PT) time. Also, as the liver fails, the bilirubin level will increase, resulting in jaundice. Thus, any patient with jaundice should be evaluated for liver disease.

Abdominal pain is not uncommon in persons with hematological disease. Two of the major organs associated with the hematopoeitic system, the liver and spleen, are in the abdomen. Problems with the spleen, liver, or both can lead to abdominal pain. Splenomagaly is common in hematological problems, as the spleen is active in the removal of abnormal or aged red cells. In some of the anemias, especially the hemolytic anemias, the spleen can become markedly enlarged. Patients with sickle cell anemia will often develop splenic infarcts as sickled cells accumulate and block blood supply to parts of the spleen. By the time children with sickle cell disease are 5 years of age, they are virtually asplenic (without a spleen), as the disease has completely infarcted their spleen. Because the spleen is not functional, these patients are placed at increased risk of infection, especially by encapsulated bacteria.

- *Musculoskeletal* Many hematopoietic problems are autoimmune in nature. That is, a problem develops in which the immune system has trouble determining which tissues are self and which are nonself. Autoimmune diseases such as rheumatoid arthritis result from the body's immune system attacking various tissues in the joints. This can cause arthralgia (pain and swelling of the joints). Autoimmune diseases tend to affect more than one joint, whereas infectious processes tend to affect only a single joint. Patients with blood clotting disorders such as hemophilia will often develop hemarthrosis (bleeding into a joint) with only minor trauma. This can result in an extremely swollen, discolored, and painful joint. Always inquire about joint pain and examine the major joints in any patient suspected of having hematopoietic disease.

- *Cardiorespiratory* The effects of hematopoietic problems on the cardiorespiratory system are varied. Patients with anemia will often develop dyspnea, tachycardia, and chest pain from the increased cardiac work caused by the anemia. In severe cases, patients can develop high-output heart failure, where the heart works excessively hard to compensate for a profound anemia. If untreated, heart failure and pulmonary edema can result. Patients with bleeding disorders may report expectorating blood with coughing. This can be due to small tears in the respiratory mucosa from the coughing. Normally, these heal quickly. Patients with bleeding disorders, however, will continue to bleed, resulting in potential airway obstruction and, in severe cases, shock. Always auscultate for breath sounds. Note crackles or rhonchi indicative of heart problems or infection.

Be alert for high-output heart failure in patients with severe anemia.

- *Genitourinary* The genitourinary effects of hematopoietic problems are typically due to bleeding disorders or infection. Bleeding disorders can cause hematuria (blood in the urine) and blood in the scrotal sac in males. A woman who still has her uterus may develop menorrhagia (heavy menstrual bleeding) or frank vaginal bleeding (dysfunctional uterine bleeding). Immunocompromised patients are at increased risk for developing genitourinary infections. These can range from recurrent urinary tract infections to severe sexually transmitted diseases. Sickle cell anemia, especially in the later stages, can cause priapism. This is a prolonged, painful erection due to obstruction of the blood vessels that drain the penis and allow for detumescence. Sickle cell disease is the most common cause of priapism in the emergency setting. All of these require additional evaluation in the emergency department. Detailed evaluation of the genitourinary system is not appropriate for field settings.

Sickle cell disease is a common cause of priapism in the emergency setting.

GENERAL MANAGEMENT OF HEMATOPOIETIC EMERGENCIES

Pay close attention to the airway and ventilation status of patients experiencing any alteration in the hematopoietic system. Place the patient on high-concentration supplemental oxygen and monitor breathing for difficulty or fatigue. Be ready to assist ventilations with a bag-valve mask.

Assess the circulatory system. Consider fluid volume replacement, but remember that crystalloid solutions cannot carry oxygen. Too much fluid can "dilute" the blood and reduce its capacity per unit volume to carry oxygen. Be alert for dysrhythmias and treat accordingly. Based on your assessment and evaluation, create the optimum environment for the blood to perform its tasks of oxygen delivery and waste product removal. Creating such an environment may

Pay close attention to the airway and ventilation status of patients experiencing any alteration in the hematopoietic system.

include giving the patient aspirin to inhibit platelet aggregation or ventilating the patient to compensate for acidosis and to allow oxygen to unload from hemoglobin at the tissues.

Transport the patient to the appropriate facility, provide comfort measures including analgesia, and provide psychological support to both the patient and his family.

MANAGING SPECIFIC PATIENT PROBLEMS

Remember that many hematological problems occur in conjunction with other illnesses.

The rest of this chapter will detail the more common hematopoietic diseases that you might encounter in prehospital care. Again, it is important to remember that many hematological problems occur in conjunction with other illnesses. For example, someone with a cancer or significant renal disease quite commonly will have a coexisting anemia. In the following sections we will first examine diseases of the red blood cells. These are the most common hematological problems encountered. Second, we will look at the white blood cell diseases. These include the leukemias, lymphomas, and similar illnesses. Finally, we will present diseases of the platelets and blood coagulation disorders.

DISEASES OF THE RED BLOOD CELLS

Red blood cell diseases result in too many red blood cells, too few red blood cells, or improperly functioning red blood cells. An excess of red blood cells is called **polycythemia**. Although uncommon, several conditions can cause polycythemia. An inadequate number of red blood cells or inadequate hemoglobin within the red blood cells is called **anemia**. Anemia is common, and several types are frequently encountered. Finally, red blood cell function can be impaired. Most commonly, this is due to problems with either hemoglobin structure and function or with the red blood cell membrane. Problems with red blood cell function include the thallasemias and sickle cell anemia.

* **polycythemia** an excess of red blood cells.

* **anemia** an inadequate number of red blood cells or inadequate hemoglobin within the red blood cells.

Content Review

DISEASES OF THE RED BLOOD CELLS
- Anemia
- Sickle cell disease
- Polycythemia

Anemias

The most common diseases of the red blood cells are the anemias. Anemia is typically classified as a hematocrit of less than 37 percent in women or less than 40 percent in men. Most patients with anemia will remain asymptomatic until the hematocrit drops below 30 percent. The decreased hematocrit in anemia is due to a reduction in the number of red blood cells or in the amount or quality of hemoglobin in the red blood cells. Anemia is actually a sign of an underlying disease process that is either destroying red blood cells and hemoglobin or decreasing the production of red blood cells and hemoglobin. Blood loss, either acute or chronic, also can cause anemia. Anemia can be a self-limited disease or it can be a lifelong illness requiring periodic transfusions. Anemias that result from the destruction of red blood cells are called hemolytic anemias. These can be hereditary or acquired. Examples of hereditary hemolytic anemias include sickle cell anemia, thalassemia, and glucose-6-phosphate dehydrogenase deficiency (G6PD). Acquired hemolytic anemias can result from immune system disorders, drug effects, or environmental effects. Anemias caused by inadequate red blood cell production include such problems as iron deficiency anemia, pernicious anemia, and anemia of chronic disease. Table 35-2 shows the numerous types of anemia, all of which must be confirmed by laboratory diagnosis.

Anemia is a sign, not a disease process in itself. Since the red blood cells' primary purpose is to transport oxygen, anemia results in hypoxia. The signs and symptoms of anemia vary, depending upon the rapidity of its onset and

Table 35-2 TYPES OF ANEMIA

Cause	Type	Pathophysiology
Inadequate production of red blood cells	Aplastic	Failure to produce red blood cells
	Iron deficiency	Iron is primary component of hemoglobin
	Pernicious	Vitamin B_{12} is necessary for correct red blood cell division during its development
	Sickle cell	Genetic alteration causes production of a hemoglobin that changes shape of red blood cell to a C, or sickle, in low oxygen states
Increased red blood cell destruction	Hemolytic	Body destroys red blood cells at greater rate than production; red blood cell parts interfere with blood flow
Blood cell loss or dilution	Chronic disease	Hemorrhage leads to cell loss while excessive fluid leads to a dilution of red blood cell concentration

upon the patient's age and underlying general health. A mild anemia may not exhibit signs or symptoms until the body is stressed, as during exercise. Then a mild dyspnea, fatigue, palpitations, and syncope may be present. Chronic anemias may present signs or symptoms of pica (the craving of unusual substances such as clay or ice), headache, dizziness, ringing in the ears, irritability or difficulty concentrating, pallor, and tachycardia. Angina pectoris can be an important indicator.

If anemia develops rapidly, the body does not have time to compensate for the change. Signs and symptoms of shock may be present, including postural hypotension and decreased cardiac output, resulting in a shunting of blood away from the periphery to the heart, lungs, and brain. Compensatory mechanisms can cause diaphoresis, pallor, cool skin, anxiety, thirst, and air hunger. If the anemia's onset is slower, the body can adjust to oxygen's reduced availability with a right shift of the oxyhemoglobin dissociation curve and an increase in plasma volume.

Prehospital treatment of anemia is primarily symptomatic. Direct your attention at maximizing oxygenation, stemming blood loss, and transporting to a medical facility for treatment of the cause. Start volume replacement if there is evidence of dehydration.

Sickle Cell Disease

Sickle cell anemia, often termed "sickle cell disease," is a disorder of red blood cell production. Normal hemoglobin is very flexible, and the red blood cell can pass easily through the tiny capillaries. Sickle hemoglobin has an abnormal chemical sequence that gives red blood cells a C, or sickle, shape when oxygen levels are low (Figure 35-2). Patients with sickle cell disease will have a chronic anemia that results from destruction of abnormal red blood cells (hemolytic anemia). The average

 sickle cell anemia an inherited disorder of red blood cell production, so named because the red blood cells become sickle-shaped when oxygen levels are low.

Normal red blood cell

Sickle cell

FIGURE 35-3   A normal red blood cell contrasted with a sickle cell.

life span of sickled red blood cells is 10–20 days compared to 120 days for normal red blood cells. In addition, sickled red blood cells increase the blood's viscosity, leading to sludging and obstruction of the capillaries and small blood vessels. Blockage of blood flow to various tissues and organs is common and usually occurs following a period of stress. This process, called a vasoocclusive crisis, is characteristic of sickle cell anemia. Because of the vasoocclusive crisis, tissues and organs are eventually damaged. Adult sickle cell patients often have multiple organ problems, including cardiopulmonary disease, renal disease, and neurological disorders.

Sickle cell disease is inherited. It primarily affects African-Americans although other ethnic groups can be affected. These include Puerto Ricans and people of Spanish, French, Italian, Greek, and Turkish heritage. If both parents carry a gene for sickle cell anemia, the chances are one in four that the child will have normal hemoglobin. The chances are two in four that he will have both normal hemoglobin and sickle hemoglobin, which is referred to as *sickle cell trait*. The chances are one in four that he will have only sickle hemoglobin (no normal hemoglobin.) This condition is referred to as *sickle cell disease*.

Patients with sickle cell disease will develop three types of problems. *Vasoocclusive crises* cause musculoskeletal pain, abdominal pain, priapisms, pulmonary problems, renal crises (renal infarctions), and central nervous system crises (cerebral infarctions). In addition, they will develop *hematological crises* that consist of a fall in the hemoglobin level, sequestration of red blood cells in the spleen, and problems with bone marrow function. In severe cases, the bone marrow can shut down, causing an aplastic crisis. These are usually self-limited. Finally, sickle cell patients often develop *infectious crises*. They are functionally immunosuppressed, and the loss of splenic function makes them particularly vulnerable to encapsulated bacteria. Infections become common and are often the cause of death in sickle cell anemia.

Prehospital care for patients in sickle cell crisis is primarily supportive. Begin high-flow oxygen to saturate as much hemoglobin as possible. Initiate IV therapy with an isotonic crystalloid solution. These patients are often dehydrated and hydration will sometimes help with the vasoocclusive process. Venous access is sometimes difficult in older patients with sickle cell disease due to the large number of IV starts they have required in their lifetime. Placing a central line is occasionally necessary. Vasoocclusive crises can be extremely painful. Start analgesic therapy in the field, if possible. Often these patients will require large amounts of narcotics for pain control. Always consult medical direction if there is a question regarding management. Transport is indicated.

Polycythemia

* **polycythemia** an abnormally high hematocrit.

Polycythemia is an abnormally high hematocrit. It is due to excess production of red blood cells. Polycythemia is a relatively rare disorder and typically occurs in patients 50 years of age or older. It can occur secondarily to dehydration. The increased red blood cell load increases the patient's risk of thrombosis. Most deaths from polycythemia are due to thrombosis.

Polycythemia's signs and symptoms vary. The principal finding is a hematocrit of 50 percent or greater. The patient will usually have an increased number of white blood cells and platelets. However, the large number of red blood cells may cause a platelet dysfunction. This can result in bleeding abnormalities such as epistaxis, spontaneous bruising, and gastrointestinal bleeding. Patients with polycythemia may complain of headache, dizziness, blurred vision, itching, and gastrointestinal disease. Severe cases can result in congestive heart failure.

The prehospital treatment of polycythemia is supportive. Assure that the airway and breathing are adequate. Administer supplemental oxygen as required. Initiate an IV with an isotonic crystalloid solution. The principal treatment is phlebotomy, which removes excess red blood cells.

Content Review

SICKLE CELL CRISES
• Vasoocclusive
• Hematological
• Infectious

DISEASES OF THE WHITE BLOOD CELLS

The white blood cells are the body's principal defense system. Problems with white blood cells typically result from too few white blood cells (**leukopenia**), too many white blood cells (**leukocytosis**), or improper white blood cell function. The neutrophil is the main blood component protecting against a bacterial or fungal reaction. A reduction in the number of neutrophils (**neutropenia**) predisposes the patient to bacterial and fungal infections.

Leukopenia/Neutropenia

The status of the white blood cells is easily determined by obtaining a complete blood count. A normal white blood cell count ranges from 5,000 to 9,000 per cubic millimeter of blood. A decrease in the number of white blood cells indicates a problem with white-blood-cell production in the marrow or destruction of white blood cells. Because bacterial infections pose a major risk to humans, an absolute neutrophil count is a better indicator of the immune system's status. The prehospital treatment of leukopenia/neutropenia is supportive. Pay special attention to preventing infection in the patient, as his immune system is overstressed or may be functioning inadequately.

Leukocytosis

Leukocytosis is an increase in the number of circulating white blood cells. This occurs when the body is exposed to an infectious agent or is particularly stressed. Following exposure, the immune system is stimulated and the marrow and spleen start releasing white blood cells to help the body fight infection. A white blood cell count between 10,800 and 23,000 per cubic millimeter of blood is characteristic of a bacterial infection. During periods of stress, immature neutrophils may be released into the circulation. These differ from mature neutrophils in that they have a segmented nucleus. These cells are referred to as "bands" or "segs." An increase in the number of bands is indicative of a significant bacterial infection. Causes of leukocytosis include bacterial infection, rheumatoid arthritis, DKA, leukemia, pain, and exercise. Viral infections tend to have little effect on the white blood cell count or, in some cases, actually cause a decrease in the white blood cell count. A white blood cell count greater than 30,000 per cubic millimeter is called a *leukemoid reaction*. A white blood cell count this high indicates a problem with excess white blood cell production. Any patient with a significantly elevated white blood cell count should be evaluated for possible leukemia.

Leukemia

Leukemias are cancers of hematopoietic cells. Precursors of white blood cells in the bone marrow begin to replicate abnormally. The cells proliferate initially in the bone marrow and then spread to the peripheral blood. Leukemias affect approximately 13 in 100,000 persons. They are classified by the type of cell or cells involved. The most common types of leukemia are:

- Acute lymphocytic leukemia (ALL)
- Acute myeologenous leukemia (AML)
- Chronic lymphocytic leukemia (CLL)
- Chronic myelogenous leukemia (CML)
- Hairy cell leukemia

---

* **leukopenia** too few white blood cells.

* **leukocytosis** too many white blood cells.

> **Content Review**
>
> **DISEASES OF THE WHITE BLOOD CELLS**
> - Leukopenia/Neutropenia
> - Leukocytosis
> - Leukemia
> - Lymphoma

* **neutropenia** a reduction in the number of neutrophils.

* **leukemia** a cancer of the hematopoietic cells.

Discussion of the pathology of the various leukemias is not within the scope of this text. ALL is primarily a disease of children and young adults. CML occurs in both children and adults. AML, CLL, and hairy cell leukemia tend to occur in the sixth and seventh decades of life. Medicine has made significant advances in the treatment of leukemia. Treatments such as chemotherapy, radiation therapy, and bone marrow transplantation have resulted in cures of certain types of leukemias. The treatment of pediatric leukemia is one of the great successes of modern medicine. More than 50 percent of pediatric patients with ALL live a normal life with the disease in remission or cured. Infections are a common complication of leukemia, primarily due to the low number of circulating neutrophils. Deaths from leukemias are typically secondary to infection or bleeding.

The signs and symptoms of leukemia vary. Most patients will have a moderate to severe anemia as the cancerous cell production overwhelms the bone marrow. Thrombocytopenia (an abnormal decrease in platelets) is common for the same reason. Many leukemia patients will present with bleeding, usually due to the thrombocytopenia. With the initial presentation, leukemia patients will appear acutely ill. They will be febrile and weak, usually due to a secondary infection. Various lymph nodes may be enlarged. Patients often have a history of weight loss and anorexia. In addition, liver and spleen enlargement are typical, resulting in a sensation of abdominal fullness or abdominal pain. The sternum may be tender, secondary to the increased bone marrow activity. Fatigue is a common complaint.

The prehospital treatment of the patient with leukemia is primarily supportive. Place the patient in a position of comfort. Administer supplemental oxygen via a nonrebreather mask. Initiate an IV with an isotonic crystalloid solution such as lactated Ringer's or normal saline. Consider a fluid bolus if the patient is dehydrated. If the patient is having pain secondary to the leukemia, consider administration of an analgesic. Remember, leukemia patients are at increased risk of developing infection. Employ proper isolation techniques.

Employ proper isolation techniques for leukemia patients, who are at increased risk of developing infection.

Lymphomas

Lymphomas are cancers of the lymphatic system. Malignant lymphoma is typically classified as follows:

* Hodgkin's lymphoma
* Non-Hodgkin's lymphoma

✱ **lymphoma** a cancer of the lymphatic system.

Malignant lymphoma is classified by the cell type involved, which indicates the stem cell from which the malignancy arises. In the United States, each year approximately 40,000 persons are diagnosed with non-Hodgkin's lymphoma, and 7,500 are diagnosed with Hodgkin's lymphoma. The long-term survival rate is much better with Hodgkin's lymphoma. In fact, many patients with Hodgkin's lymphoma who have been treated with radiation, chemotherapy, or both are considered cured.

The most common presenting sign of non-Hodgkin's lymphoma is painless swelling of the lymph nodes. The majority of patients with Hodgkin's lymphoma typically have no related symptoms. Patients with lymphoma may report fever, night sweats, anorexia, weight loss, fatigue, and pruritis. Treat patients with lymphomas symptomatically. Place the patient in a position of comfort. Administer supplemental oxygen via a nonrebreather mask. Initiate an IV with an isotonic crystalloid solution such as lactated Ringer's or normal saline. Consider a fluid bolus if the patient is dehydrated. If the patient is having pain secondary to the lymphoma, consider administration of an analgesic. As with leukemia patients, lymphoma patients are at increased risk of developing infection. Employ proper isolation techniques.

Lymphoma patients are at increased risk of developing infection. Use proper isolation techniques.

DISEASES OF THE PLATELETS/ BLOOD CLOTTING ABNORMALITIES

Various disorders can affect the platelets or the body's blood clotting system. Some of these are hereditary, while others may be acquired. Examples of platelet abnormalities include thrombocytosis (increased platelets) and thrombocytopenia (reduced platelets). Various disorders can affect the coagulation system. These include hemophilia A, hemophilia B (Christmas disease), and others.

Thrombocytosis

Thrombocytosis is an increase in the number of platelets, usually due to increased platelet production (essential thrombocytosis). It is also seen in polycythemia vera where both red blood cells and platelets are increased. Thrombocytosis often complicates chronic myelogenous leukemia. Thrombcytosis can be secondary to other disorders such as malignant diseases, hemolytic anemias, acute hemorrhage, and autoinflammatory diseases. Most patients with thrombocytosis are asymptomatic. Prehospital treatment is supportive.

✳ **thrombocytosis** an abnormal increase in the number of platelets.

Thrombocytopenia

Thrombocytopenia is an abnormal decrease in the number of platelets. It is due to decreased platelet production, sequestration of platelets in the spleen, destruction of platelets, or any combination of the three. Many drugs can induce thrombocytopenia. *Acute idiopathic thrombocytopenia purpura (ITP)* results from destruction of platelets by the immune system. It is most commonly seen in children following a viral infection. ITP is characterized by easy bruising, bleeding, and a falling platelet count. Chronic ITP usually occurs in adult women and is often associated with autoimmune disease. Prehospital treatment is supportive.

✳ **thrombocytopenia** an abnormal decrease in the number of platelets.

Hemophilia

Hemophilia is a blood disorder in which one of the proteins necessary for blood clotting is missing or defective. A deficiency of factor VIII is called hemophilia A. A deficiency of factor IX is known as hemophilia B (Christmas disease). Hemophilia A is the most common inherited disorder of hemostasis. The severity of the disease is directly related to the amount of circulating factor VIII available. Patients are classified as mild, moderate, or severe, based upon the amount of circulating factor VIII. Hemophilia B is more rare, but also more severe, than hemophilia A.

When a person with hemophilia is injured, the bleeding will take longer to stop because the body cannot form stable fibrin clots. Simple trauma such as nosebleeds or tooth extractions can lead to prolonged, occasionally life-threatening bleeds. In extensive trauma such as pelvic fractures blood loss can be overwhelming. A common problem with hemophilia is hemarthrosis (bleeding into the joint space). This can result from even the most minor trauma. Eventually, repeated bleeding episodes will lead to permanent joint damage.

Hemophilia is a sex-linked, inherited bleeding disorder. The gene with the defective information is carried on the X chromosome. Females have two X chromosomes, one from their mother and one from their father. If one chromosome has the defective gene and the other does not, the disease is not expressed. Females who have one X chromosome containing the defective gene are referred to as carriers. Males, however, have an X chromosome from their mother and a Y chromosome from their father. If that X chromosome carries

✳ **hemophilia** a blood disorder in which one of the proteins necessary for blood clotting is missing or defective.

the defective gene, males will express the disease. Hemophilia A affects approximately 1 in 10,000 males. A female, on the other hand, can inherit hemophilia only if she receives two X chromosomes that express the disease. That is, she must be the offspring of a carrier mother and a father with hemophilia.

The signs and symptoms of hemophilia include numerous bruises, deep muscle bleeding characterized as pain or a "pulled muscle," and the joint bleeding called hemarthrosis. Most patients will be aware of their diagnosis and will tell you. Some may wear Medic-Alert bracelets or similar devices.

Hemophiliacs can be treated in the hospital with infusions of factor VIII. In addition to factor VIII, some hemophiliacs will require blood transfusions due to bleeding from trauma. Unfortunately, before blood and blood products were routinely tested, transfusions infected many hemophiliacs with the human immunodeficiency virus, hepatitis B, and/or hepatitis C.

Prehospital treatment of the patient with hemophilia should be comprehensive. The normal hemostatic mechanisms of vasoconstriction and platelet aggregation will still occur, but the platelet plug will not be stable, due to the deficiency of factor VIII. Thus, you should be attentive to prolonged bleeding or possible rebleeds. The hemophiliac is at risk of both. Administer supplemental oxygen via a nonrebreather mask and initiate IV therapy with an isotonic crystalloid such as normal saline. Be careful to help prevent additional trauma, which can result in further hemorrhage. If the patient sustained a joint injury with resultant hemarthrosis, splinting the extremity will sometimes help control pain. Occasionally, analgesics will be required.

If your patient has hemophilia, be especially careful to help prevent additional trauma, which can result in further hemorrhage.

Von Willebrand's Disease

* **von Willebrand's disease** condition in which the vWF component of factor VIII is deficient.

Factor VIII actually consists of several components. One of these components is factor VIII:vWF, also called von Willebrand's factor. In **von Willebrand's disease,** this component of factor VIII is deficient. It is produced by the endothelial cells and is necessary for normal platelet adhesion. Thus, in addition to the clotting problem, platelet function is abnormal in patients with von Willebrand's disease. While the disease is inherited, it is not sex linked, equally affecting both females and males. A sign of this disease is excessive bleeding, primarily after surgery or injury. It is not associated with the deep muscle or joint bleeding of hemophilia, nor is it usually as serious, although nosebleeds, excessive menstruation, and gastrointestinal bleeds can occur. Prehospital treatment is supportive. Aspirin is generally contraindicated as it further inhibits platelet aggregation, thus exacerbating the disease. Definitive treatment is the administration of von Willebrand factor.

OTHER HEMATOPOIETIC DISORDERS
Disseminated Intravascular Coagulation

* **disseminated intravascular coagulation (DIC)** a disorder of coagulation caused by systemic activation of the coagulation cascade.

Disseminated intravascular coagulation (DIC), also called consumption coagulopathy, is a disorder of coagulation caused by systemic activation of the coagulation cascade. Normally, inhibitory mechanisms localize coagulation to the affected area. A combination of protein inhibitors, rapid blood flow, and absorption of the fibrin clot restricts circulating free thrombin to the site of coagulation. In DIC, circulating thrombin cleaves fibrinogen to form fibrin clots throughout the circulation. This can cause widespread thrombosis and, occasionally, end-organ ischemia. Bleeding is the most frequent sign of DIC and is due to the reduced fibrinogen level, consumption of coagulation factors, and thrombocytopenia. DIC most commonly results from sepsis, hypotension, obstetric complications, severe tissue injury, brain injury, cancer, and major hemolytic transfusion reactions. The disease is quite grave. Its signs include oozing blood at venipuncture and wound sites. The patient may exhibit a purpuric rash, often over the chest and abdomen. Minute hemorrhages may be noted just under the skin. Prehospital care is symptomatic. The DIC patient may be hemodynamically unstable and may require IV fluids. Definitive treatment includes the administration of fresh frozen plasma and platelets.

Multiple Myeloma

Multiple myeloma is a cancerous disorder of plasma cells. Plasma cells are a type of B cell responsible for producing immunoglobulins (antibodies). The disease is rarely found in persons under the age of 40. Approximately 14,000 new cases are diagnosed each year. Usually, multiple myeloma begins with a change or mutation in a plasma cell in the bone marrow. These cancerous plasma cells crowd out healthy cells and lead to a reduction in blood cell production. The patient then becomes anemic and prone to infection.

The first sign of multiple myeloma often is pain in the back or ribs. The diseased marrow weakens the bones and *pathological fractures* (those occurring with minimal or no trauma) may occur. The resulting anemia leads to fatigue, and reduced platelet production places the patient at risk for bleeding. Laboratory evaluation will reveal an elevation in the level of a circulating antibody or part of an antibody (light chain). This is due to the proliferation of plasma cells. Despite this, the patient is at increased risk of infection, as the plasma cells do not secrete specific antibodies in response to infection. In addition, the calcium level is often elevated due to bone destruction. This can lead to renal failure.

Treatment of multiple myeloma includes chemotherapy, radiation, and bone marrow transplants. Prehospital care is supportive. Establish an IV of isotonic crystalloid solution. Consider a fluid bolus if there are symptoms of dehydration. Multiple myeloma can be very painful due to the proliferation of the plasma cells and destruction of the marrow. Consider analgesics if pain is severe. A pathological fracture in a patient with multiple myeloma is very painful, and you should start analgesic therapy if so indicated.

* **multiple myeloma** a cancerous disorder of plasma cells.

SUMMARY

Hematology is the study of the blood and blood-forming organs. Hematological disorders include red blood cell disorders, white blood cell disorders, platelet disorders, and coagulation problems. Problems can also be caused when the body has an immunological response to antigens present on red blood cells from a foreign donor. Although hematological disorders are common, they are seldom the primary reason for an emergency call. Rather, they are likely to accompany another ongoing disease process.

The signs and symptoms that accompany hematological problems seldom point directly to the underlying disease. Generally, lab findings are necessary to clarify the diagnosis. However, an understanding of hematological pathophysiology is important to understanding the disease process your patient may be undergoing and to helping you to form a field impression and make appropriate decisions about emergency care.

CHAPTER 36

Environmental Emergencies

Objectives

After reading this chapter, you should be able to:

1. Define "environmental emergency." (p. 1516)
2. Describe the incidence, morbidity, and mortality associated with environmental emergencies. (p. 1535)
3. Identify risk factors most predisposing to environmental emergencies. (p. 1516)
4. Identify environmental factors that may cause illness or exacerbate a preexisting illness or complicate treatment or transport decisions. (p. 1516)
5. Define "homeostasis" and relate the concept to environmental influences. (pp. 1516–1517)
6. Identify normal, critically high, and critically low body temperatures. (pp. 1518–1519, 1520)
7. Describe several methods of temperature monitoring. (p. 1519)
8. Describe human thermal regulation, including system components, substances used, and wastes generated. (pp. 1517–1520, 1527)
9. List the common forms of heat and cold disorders. (pp. 1521–1534)

Continued

INTRODUCTION

The *environment* can be defined as all of the surrounding external factors that affect the development and functioning of a living organism. Human beings obviously depend on the environment for life. But they also must be protected from its extremes. When factors such as temperature, weather, terrain, and atmospheric pressure act on the body, they can create stresses that the body is unable to compensate for. A medical condition caused or exacerbated by such environmental factors is known as an **environmental emergency.**

Environmental emergencies include a variety of conditions such as heatstroke, hypothermia, drowning or near-drowning, altitude sickness, nuclear radiation, and diving accidents or barotraumas, among others. Such emergencies often call for special rescue resources.

Although environmental emergencies can affect anyone, several risk factors predispose certain individuals to developing environmental illnesses. These factors include:

* Age—Very young children and older adults do not tolerate environmental extremes very well.
* Poor general health
* Fatigue
* Predisposing medical conditions
* Certain medications—either prescription or over-the-counter

Environmental factors must also be considered when determining the risk for environmental emergencies. For example, climate in a particular place may vary greatly from moment to moment. Areas where change in temperature can be drastic over the course of the day may catch unwary individuals off guard. For example, desert areas can have temperatures of 105° F during the day but drop below freezing at night, placing unprepared travelers in a difficult situation. Temperatures in parts of southern Alberta can change drastically when the Chinook winds kick up. Other considerations include the current season, local weather patterns, atmospheric pressures (high altitude or underwater), and the type of terrain, which can cause injury or hinder rescue efforts.

As a paramedic, you will frequently be called upon to treat medical emergencies related to environmental conditions. It is critical that you understand the particular conditions that prevail in your region. If you live in a mountain area, near large caves, in an area with swift moving water, or in a resort area where diving is prominent, you need to be familiar with the specialized rescue resources these situations may require and the particular environmental emergencies they may cause. Understanding their causes and underlying pathophysiologies can help you recognize these emergencies promptly and manage them effectively.

Although many environmental factors can result in medical emergencies, this chapter will focus primarily on problems related to temperature extremes, drowning or near-drowning, diving emergencies, high altitude illness, and nuclear radiation.

HOMEOSTASIS

In order for the human body to function properly, it must interact with the environment to obtain oxygen, nutrients, and other necessities, but it must also avoid being damaged by extreme external environmental conditions. The process of maintaining constant suitable conditions within the body is called **homeostasis.** Various body systems respond in an effort to maintain the correct core and peripheral temperature, oxygen level, and energy supply to maintain life.

* environmental emergency a medical condition caused or exacerbated by the weather, terrain, atmospheric pressure, or other local factors.

* homeostasis the natural tendency of the body to maintain a steady and normal internal environment.

The following sections address how the body attempts to maintain these normal settings and what happens when certain environmental conditions exceed the ability of the body to compensate.

PATHOPHYSIOLOGY OF HEAT AND COLD DISORDERS

MECHANISMS OF HEAT GAIN AND LOSS

The body gains and loses heat in two ways, from within the body itself and by contact with the external environment.

The body receives heat from or loses it to the environment via the thermal gradient. The **thermal gradient** is the difference in temperature between the environment (the ambient temperature) and the body. The ambient temperature is usually different from body temperature. If the environment is warmer than the body, heat flows from the environment to the body. If the body is warmer than the environment, heat flows from the body to the environment. Other environmental factors, including wind and relative humidity (the percentage of water vapor in the air), also affect heat gain and loss.

The mechanisms by which heat is generated within the body and by which heat is gained or lost to the environment are discussed in more detail in the following sections.

✳ **thermal gradient** the difference in temperature between the environment and the body.

THERMOGENESIS (HEAT GENERATION)

The amount of heat in the body continually fluctuates as a result of the heat generated or gained and the heat lost. The body gains heat from both external and internal sources. In addition to the heat the body absorbs from the environment, the body also generates heat through energy-producing chemical reactions (metabolism).

The creation of heat is called **thermogenesis.** There are several types of thermogenesis. One is *work-induced thermogenesis* that results from exercise. Our muscles need to create heat because warm muscles work more effectively than cold ones. One way muscles can produce heat is by shivering. Another type, *thermoregulatory thermogenesis,* is controlled by the endocrine system. The hormones norepinephrine and epinephrine can cause an immediate increase in the rate of cellular metabolism, which in turn increases heat production. The last type, metabolic thermogenesis, or *diet-induced thermogenesis,* is caused by the processing of food and nutrients. When a meal is eaten, digested, absorbed, and metabolized, heat is produced as a by-product of these activities.

✳ **thermogenesis** the production of heat, especially within the body.

THERMOLYSIS (HEAT LOSS)

The heat generated by the body is constantly lost to the environment. This occurs because the body is usually warmer than the surrounding environment. The transfer of heat into the environment occurs through the following mechanisms (Figure 36-1):

- **Conduction.** Direct contact of the body's surface to another, cooler object causes the body to lose heat by conduction. Heat flows from higher temperature matter to lower temperature matter.
- **Convection.** Heat loss to air currents passing over the body is called convection. Heat, however, must first be conducted to the air before being carried away by convection currents.
- **Radiation.** An unclothed person will lose approximately 60 percent of total body heat by radiation at normal room temperature. This

✳ **conduction** moving electrons, ions, heat, or sound waves through a conductor or conducting medium.

✳ **convection** transfer of heat via currents in liquids or gases.

✳ **radiation** transfer of energy through space or matter.

Respiration

Evaporation
Body heat
lost by
evaporation
of perspiration

Convection
Body heat
lost to
air

Radiation
Body heat
lost to
nearby
objects
without
touching
them

Conduction
Body heat
lost to
nearby
objects
through
touch

FIGURE 36-1   Heat loss by the body.

✱ **evaporation** change from liquid to a gaseous state.

✱ **respiration** the exchange of gases between a living organism and its environment.

✱ **thermoregulation** the maintenance or regulation of a particular temperature of the body.

✱ **core temperature** the body temperature of the deep tissues, which usually does not vary more than a degree or so from its normal 37° C (98.6° F).

heat loss is in the form of infrared rays. All objects not at absolute zero temperature will radiate heat into the atmosphere.

- **Evaporation.** Evaporation is the change of a liquid to vapor. Evaporative heat loss occurs as water evaporates from the skin. Additionally, a great deal of heat loss occurs through evaporation of fluids in the lungs. Water evaporates from the skin and lungs at approximately 600 mL/day.

- **Respiration.** Respiration combines the mechanisms of convection, radiation, and evaporation. It accounts for a large proportion of the body's heat loss. Heat is transferred from the lungs to inspired air by convection and radiation. Evaporation in the lungs humidifies the inspired air (adds water vapor to it). During expiration this warm, humidified air is released into the environment, creating heat loss.

THERMOREGULATION

Thermoregulation is the maintenance or regulation of temperature. The body temperature of the deep tissues, commonly called the **core temperature**, usually does not vary more than a degree or so from its normal 98.6° (37° C). A naked person can be exposed to an external environment ranging anywhere from 55° F to 144° F and still maintain a fairly constant internal body temperature. This characteristic of warm-blooded animals is called *steady-state metabolism.* The various biochemical reactions occurring within the cell are most efficient when the body temperature is within this narrow temperature range.

Evaluation of peripheral body temperature can be measured by touch or by taking the temperature by oral or axillary means. Core body temperatures can be measured using tympanic or rectal thermometers.

The body maintains a balance between the production and loss of heat almost entirely through the nervous system and negative feedback mechanisms. The **hypothalamus,** located at the base of the brain, is responsible for temperature regulation. It functions as a thermostat, controlling temperature through the release of neurosecretions (secretions produced by nerve cells). When the hypothalamus senses an increased body temperature, it shuts off the mechanisms designed to create heat, for example, shivering. When it senses a decrease in body temperature, the hypothalamus shuts off mechanisms designed to cool the body, for example, sweating. Because the action involved requires stopping, or negating, a process, it is called a **negative feedback** system.

When the heat regulating function of the hypothalamus is disrupted, the result can be an abnormally high or low body temperature. At the extremes, such abnormal temperatures can result in death (Figure 36-2).

Thermoreceptors

Although the hypothalamus plays a key role in body temperature regulation, temperature receptors in other parts of the body also help to moderate temperatures. There are thermoreceptors in the skin and certain mucous membranes (peripheral thermoreceptors) as well as in certain deep tissues of the body (central thermoreceptors). The skin has both cold and warm receptors. Because cold receptors outnumber warm receptors, peripheral detection of temperature consists mainly of detecting cold rather than warmth. Deep body temperature receptors lie mostly in the spinal cord, abdominal viscera, and in or around the great veins. These receptors are exposed to the body's core temperature rather than the peripheral temperature. They also respond mainly to cold rather than warmth. Both peripheral and central thermoreceptors act to prevent lowering of the body temperature.

Metabolic Rate

The **basal metabolic rate (BMR)** is the metabolism that occurs when the body is completely at rest. It is the rate at which the body consumes energy just to maintain itself—the rate of metabolism that maintains brain function, circulation, and cell stability. Any additional activity that the body performs demands energy consumption beyond that supported by the basal rate, metabolizing more nutrients and releasing more calories (units of heat). The rate of metabolism that supports this additional activity is called an **exertional metabolic rate.**

The body continually adjusts the metabolic rate in order to maintain the temperature of the core (where the crucial structures like the heart and brain are located). The body also achieves temperature maintenance by dilating some blood vessels and constricting others so that the blood carries the excess heat from the core to the periphery where it is close to the skin. This allows heat to dissipate through the skin into the environment.

Content Review

MECHANISMS OF HEAT DISSIPATION

Sweating
Vasodilation

MECHANISMS OF HEAT CONSERVATION

Shivering
Vasoconstriction

✱ **hypothalamus** portion of the diencephalon producing neurosecretions important in the control of certain metabolic activities, including body temperature regulation.

✱ **negative feedback** homeostatic mechanism in which a change in a variable (here, core temperature) ultimately inhibits the process that led to the shift.

✱ **basal metabolic rate (BMR)** rate at which the body consumes energy just to maintain stability; the basic metabolic rate (measured by the rate of oxygen consumption) of an awake, relaxed person 12 to 14 hours after eating and at a comfortable temperature.

✱ **exertional metabolic rate** rate at which the body consumes energy during activity. It is faster than the basic metabolic rate.

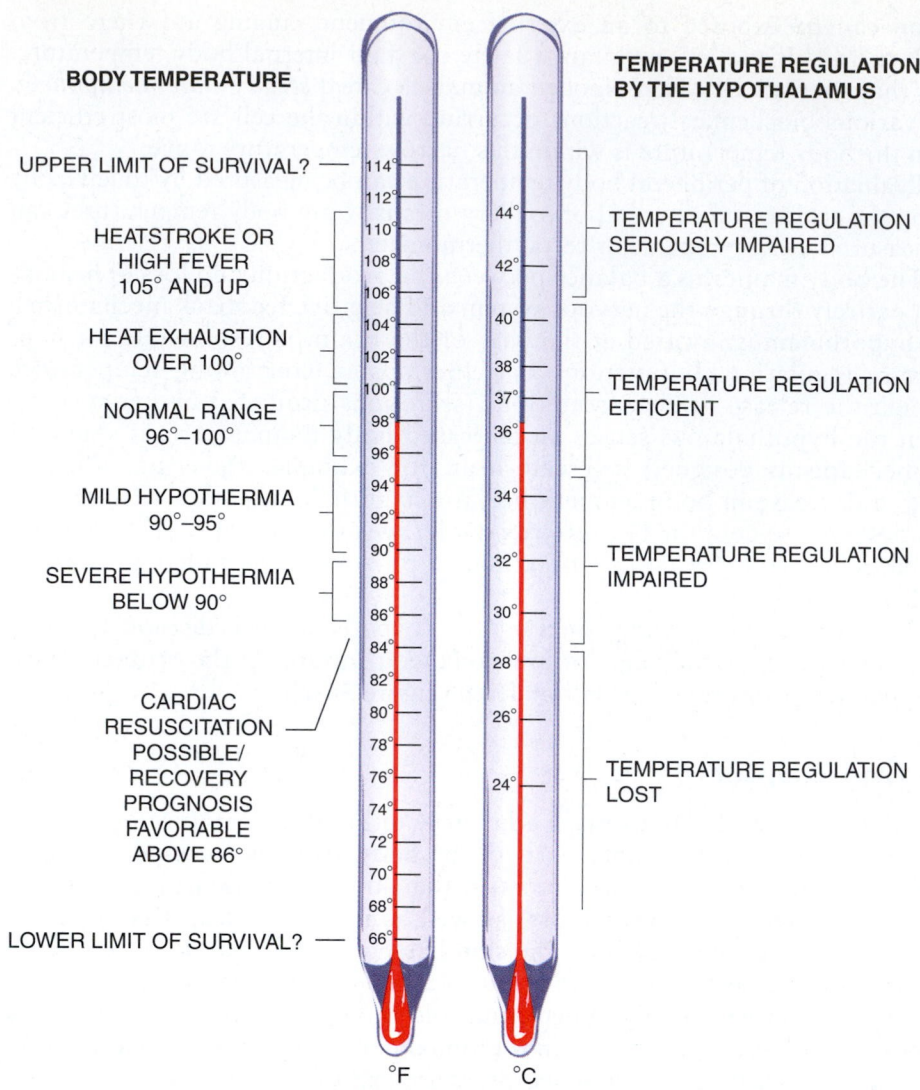

BODY TEMPERATURE

TEMPERATURE REGULATION
BY THE HYPOTHALAMUS

UPPER LIMIT OF SURVIVAL? — 114°

112°

HEATSTROKE OR
HIGH FEVER
105° AND UP
110°
108°
106°

44°

42°

TEMPERATURE REGULATION
SERIOUSLY IMPAIRED

HEAT EXHAUSTION
OVER 100°
104°
102°
100°

40°

38°
37°

TEMPERATURE REGULATION
EFFICIENT

NORMAL RANGE
96°–100°
98°
96°

36°

MILD HYPOTHERMIA
90°–95°
94°
92°
90°

34°

32°

TEMPERATURE REGULATION
IMPAIRED

SEVERE HYPOTHERMIA
BELOW 90°
88°
86°

30°

84°
82°

28°

CARDIAC
RESUSCITATION
POSSIBLE/
RECOVERY
PROGNOSIS
FAVORABLE
ABOVE 86°
80°
78°
76°
74°

26°

24°

TEMPERATURE REGULATION
LOST

72°
70°
68°

LOWER LIMIT OF SURVIVAL? — 66°

°F   °C

FIGURE 36-2   Temperature regulation by the hypothalamus.

Conversely, when the environment is too cold, *counter-current heat exchange* is used to shunt warm blood away from the superficial veins near the skin and back into the deep veins near the core to keep vital structures warm. Another body response that counters a cold environment is shivering, a physical activity that increases metabolism and generates heat.

It is important to note that these various mechanisms can create a difference between the core body temperature and the peripheral body temperature. Core temperature is the crucial measurement since, as noted, the core is where the major organs are located. Therefore, it is important in any heat-related or cold-related emergency to obtain a core temperature reading such as from the rectum. Oral and axillary temperatures may provide convenient approximations in some situations but may lead to incorrect interventions if relied upon for treatment of the patient with an environmental illness.

HEAT DISORDERS

Disruption of the body's normal thermoregulatory mechanisms can produce a number of heat illnesses, such as hyperthermia and fever. **Heat illness** is increased *core body temperature (CBT)* due to inadequate thermolysis.

HYPERTHERMIA

Hyperthermia is a state of unusually high body temperature, specifically the core body temperature. Hyperthermia is usually caused by heat transfer from the external environment that the body cannot compensate for. Occasionally it is caused by excessive generation of heat within the body.

As the body attempts to eliminate this excessive heat, you will see the general signs of thermolysis (heat loss). These signs are caused by the body's two chief methods of heat dissipation, sweating (which leads to evaporative heat loss) and vasodilation (which allows the blood to carry heat to the periphery for dissipation through the skin). These include:

- Diaphoresis (sweating)
- Increased skin temperature
- Flushing

As heat illness progresses, you will also note signs of thermolytic inadequacy (the failure of the body's thermoregulatory mechanisms to compensate adequately):

- Altered mentation
- Altered level of consciousness

Hyperthermia can manifest as heat cramps, heat exhaustion, or heatstroke, which will be discussed in following sections.

PREDISPOSING FACTORS

Age, general health, and medications are predisposing factors in hyperthermia. Factors that may contribute to a susceptibility to hyperthermia include:

- *Age of the patient*—Pediatric and geriatric populations can tolerate less variation in temperature and their heat regulating mechanisms are not as responsive as those of young adult and adult populations.
- *Health of the patient*—Diabetics can become hyperthermic more easily because they develop **autonomic neuropathy.** This condition damages the autonomic nervous system, which may interfere with thermoregulatory input and with vasodilation and perspiration, which normally dissipate heat.
- *Medications*—Various medications can affect body temperature in the following ways:
  – *Diuretics* predispose to dehydration, which worsens hyperthermia.
  – *Beta blockers* interfere with vasodilation and reduce the capacity to increase heart rate in response to volume loss and may also interfere with thermoregulatory input.
  – *Psychotropics and antihistamines,* such as antipsychotics and phenothiazines, interfere with central thermoregulation.

* **heat illness** increased core body temperature due to inadequate thermolysis.

* **hyperthermia** unusually high core body temperature.

Content Review

HEAT DISORDERS
Hyperthermia
Heat cramps
Heat exhaustion
Heatstroke

* **autonomic neuropathy** condition that damages the autonomic nervous system, which usually senses changes in core temperature and controls vasodilation and perspiration to dissipate heat.

* acclimatization the reversible changes in body structure and function by which the body becomes adjusted to a change in environment.

- *Level of acclimatization*—**Acclimatization** is the process of becoming adjusted to a change in environment. In response to an environmental change, reversible changes in body structure and function take place that help to maintain homeostasis.
- *Length of exposure*
- *Intensity of exposure*
- *Environmental factors* such as humidity and wind

PREVENTIVE MEASURES

Ideally, prevention of heat disorders is preferable to treating an illness already in progress. Measures to prevent hyperthermia include the following:

- Maintain adequate fluid intake, remembering that thirst is an inadequate indicator of dehydration.
- Allow time for gradual acclimatization to being out in the heat. Acclimatization results in more perspiration with lower salt concentration and increases body-fluid volume.
- Limit exposure to hot environments.

SPECIFIC HEAT DISORDERS

Inevitably, you will be required to respond to heat-related emergencies: heat cramps, heat exhaustion, or heatstroke. Heat cramps and heat exhaustion result from dehydration and depletion of sodium and other electrolytes. Heatstroke, a far more serious and potentially life-threatening condition, results from the failure of the body's thermoregulatory mechanisms.

Signs and symptoms and emergency care procedures for heat cramps, heat exhaustion, and heatstroke are discussed in the following sections.

Heat (Muscle) Cramps

* heat cramps acute painful spasms of the voluntary muscles following strenuous activity in a hot environment without adequate fluid or salt intake.

Heat cramps are muscle cramps caused by overexertion and dehydration in the presence of high atmospheric temperatures. Sweating occurs as sodium (salt) is transported to the skin. Because "water follows sodium," water is deposited on the skin surface where evaporation occurs, aiding in the cooling process. Since sweating involves not only the loss of water but also the loss of electrolytes (such as sodium), intermittent cramping of skeletal muscles may occur. Heat cramps are painful but are not considered to be an actual heat illness.

Signs and Symptoms The patient with heat cramps will present with cramps in the fingers, arms, legs, or abdominal muscles. He will generally be mentally alert with a feeling of weakness. He may feel dizzy or faint. Vital signs will be stable. Body temperature may be normal or slightly elevated. The skin is likely to be moist and warm.

Treatment Treatment of the patient with heat cramps is usually easily accomplished:

1. *Remove the patient from the environment.* Place the patient in a cool environment such as a shaded area or the air conditioned back of the ambulance.

In the case of severe cramps:

2. *Administer an oral saline solution* (approximately 4 teaspoons of salt to a gallon of water) or a sports drink. Do NOT administer salt tablets, which are not absorbed as readily and may cause stomach irritation and ulceration or hypernatremia. *If the patient is unable to take fluids orally, an IV of normal saline may be needed.*

Some EMS systems recommend massaging the painful muscles. Application of moist towels to the patient's forehead and over the cramped muscles may also be helpful.

Heat Exhaustion

Heat exhaustion, which is considered to be a mild heat illness, is an acute reaction to heat exposure. It is the most common heat-related illness seen by prehospital personnel. An individual performing work in a hot environment will lose 1 to 2 liters of water an hour. Each liter lost contains 20 to 50 milliequivalents of sodium. The resulting loss of water and sodium, combined with general vasodilation, leads to a decreased circulating blood volume, venous pooling, and reduced cardiac output.

Dehydration and sodium loss due to sweating account for the presenting symptoms. However, these signs and symptoms are not exclusive to heat exhaustion. Instead, they mimic those of an individual suffering from fluid and sodium loss from any of a number of other causes. A history of exposure to high environmental temperatures is needed to obtain an accurate assessment.

If not treated, heat exhaustion may progress to heatstroke.

Signs and Symptoms Signs and symptoms that you may encounter include increased body temperature (over 100° F or 37.8° C), skin that is cool and clammy with heavy perspiration, breathing that is rapid and shallow, and a weak pulse. There may be signs of active thermolysis such as diarrhea and muscle cramps. The patient will feel weak and, in some cases, may lose consciousness. There may be central nervous system (CNS) symptoms such as headache, anxiety, paresthesia, and impaired judgment or even psychosis.

Treatment Prehospital management of the patient with heat exhaustion is aimed at immediate cooling and fluid replacement. Steps include:

1. *Remove the patient from the environment.* Place the patient in a cool environment such as a shaded area or the air-conditioned ambulance.

2. *Place the patient in a supine position.*

3. *Administer an oral saline solution* (approximately 4 teaspoons of salt to a gallon of water) or a sports drink. Do NOT administer salt tablets, which are not absorbed as readily and may cause stomach irritation and ulceration or hypernatremia. *If the patient is unable to take fluids orally, an IV of normal saline may be needed.*

4. *Remove some clothing and fan the patient.* Remove enough clothing to cool the patient without chilling him. Fanning increases evaporation and cooling. Again, be careful not to cool the patient to the point of chilling. If the patient begins to shiver, stop fanning and perhaps cover the patient lightly.

5. *Treat for shock, if shock is suspected.* However, be careful not to cover the patient to the point of overheating him.

* **heat exhaustion** a mild heat illness; an acute reaction to heat exposure.

Symptoms should resolve with fluids, rest, and supine posturing with knees elevated. If they do not, consider that the symptoms may be due to an increased core body temperature, which is predictive of impending heatstroke and should be treated aggressively, as outlined in the following section.

Heatstroke

Heatstroke is a true environmental emergency that occurs when the body's hypothalamic temperature regulation is lost, causing uncompensated hyperthermia. This in turn causes cell death and damage to the brain, liver, and kidneys. There is no arbitrary core temperature at which heatstroke begins. However, heatstroke is generally characterized by a body temperature of at least 105° F (40.6° C), central nervous system disturbances, and usually the cessation of sweating.

Signs and Symptoms Sweating is thought to stop due to destruction of the sweat glands or when sensory overload causes them to temporarily dysfunction. However, the patient's skin may be either dry or covered with sweat that is still present on the skin from earlier exertion. In either case, the skin will be hot.

The patient may present with the following signs and symptoms:

- Cessation of sweating
- Hot skin that is dry or moist
- Very high core temperature
- Deep respirations that become shallow, rapid at first but may later slow
- Rapid, full pulse, may slow later
- Hypotension with low or absent diastolic reading
- Confusion or disorientation or unconsciousness
- Possible seizures

Classic heatstroke commonly presents in those with chronic illnesses, with the increased core body temperature due to deficient thermoregulatory function. Predisposing conditions include age, diabetes, and other medical conditions. In this type of heatstroke hot, red, dry skin is common.

Exertional heatstroke commonly presents in those who are in good general health, with the increased core body temperature due to overwhelming heat stress. There is excessive ambient temperature as well as excessive exertion with prolonged exposure and poor acclimatization. In this type of heatstroke you will find that, although sweating has ceased and the skin is hot, moisture from prior sweating may still be present.

If the patient develops heatstroke due to exertion, he may go into severe metabolic acidosis caused by lactic acid accumulation. Hyperkalemia (excessive potassium in blood) may also develop because of the release of potassium from injured muscle cells, renal failure, or metabolic acidosis.

Treatment Prehospital management of the heatstroke patient is aimed at immediate cooling and replacement of fluids. Steps include:

1. *Remove the patient from the environment.* This first step is essential. If you do not remove the patient from the hot environment, any other measures will be only minimally useful. Move the patient to a cool environment, such as the air-conditioned ambulance.

2. *Initiate rapid active cooling.* Body temperature must be lowered to 102° F (39° C). A target of 102° F (39° C) is used to avoid an overshoot. This can be accomplished en route to the hospital.

Remove the patient's clothing and cover the patient with sheets soaked in tepid water. Fanning and misting may also be used if necessary. Refrain from over-cooling, as this may cause reflex hypothermia (low body temperature). This results in shivering, which can raise the core temperature again. Tepid water is used because ice packs and cold-water immersion may affect peripheral thermoreceptors, producing reflex vasoconstriction and shivering.

3. *Administer oxygen.* Administer high-flow oxygen by nonrebreather mask. If respirations are shallow, assist with a bag-valve-mask unit supplied with 100 percent oxygen. Utilize pulse oximetry, if available.

4. *Administer fluid therapy if the patient is alert and able to swallow.*
   - *Oral fluids.* In many cases oral fluid therapy will be all that is needed. Some salt additive is beneficial, but salt tablets should be avoided as they may cause gastrointestinal irritation and ulceration or hypernatremia. There is a very limited need for other electrolytes in oral rehydration.
   - *Intravenous fluids.* Begin 1 to 2 IVs, using normal saline. Initially infuse them wide open.

5. *Monitor the ECG.* Cardiac dysrhythmias may occur at any time. S-T segment depression, non-specific T-wave changes with occasional PVCs, and supraventricular tachycardias are common.

6. *Avoid vasopressors and anticholinergic drugs.* These agents may potentiate heatstroke by inhibiting sweating. They can also produce a hypermetabolic state in the presence of high environmental temperatures and relatively high humidity.

7. *Monitor body temperature.* EMS systems operating in extremely warm climates should carry some device to record the body temperature, whether a simple rectal thermometer or a sophisticated electronic device. Simple glass thermometers generally do not measure above 106° F (41° C) or below 95° F (35° C). This may become significant during long transport when it is essential to detect changes in the patient's condition.

ROLE OF DEHYDRATION IN HEAT DISORDERS

Dehydration often goes hand in hand with heat disorders because it inhibits vasodilation and therefore thermolysis. Dehydration leads to orthostatic hypotension (increased pulse and decreased blood pressure on rising from a supine position) and the following symptoms which may occur along with the signs and symptoms of heatstroke:

- Nausea, vomiting, and abdominal distress
- Vision disturbances
- Decreased urine output
- Poor skin turgor
- Signs of hypovolemic shock

When these signs and symptoms are present, rehydration of the patient is critical. Oral fluids may be administered if the patient is alert and not nauseated. Administration of IV fluids may be necessary, especially if the patient has an altered mental status or is nauseated. It is not uncommon for the adult patient with moderate to severe dehydration to require 2–3 liters of IV fluids (occasionally more!).

Dehydration often goes hand in hand with heat disorders.

Thirst is a poor indication of the degree of dehydration present.

FEVER (PYREXIA)

 pyrexia fever, or above-normal body temperature.

 pyrogen any substance causing a fever, such as viruses and bacteria or substances produced within the body in response to infection or inflammation.

A fever (**pyrexia**) is the elevation of the body temperature above the normal temperature for that person. (An individual person's normal temperature may be one or two degrees above or below 98.6° F or 37° C.) The body develops a fever when pathogens enter and cause infection, which in turn stimulates the production of pyrogens.

Pyrogens are any substances that cause fever, such as viruses and bacteria or substances produced within the body in response to infection or inflammation. They reset the hypothalamic thermostat to a higher level. Metabolism is increased, which produces the elevation of temperature. The increased body temperature fights infection by making the body a less hospitable environment for the invading organism. The hypothalamic thermostat will reset to normal when pyrogen production stops or when pathogens end their attack on the body.

Fever is sometimes difficult to differentiate from heatstroke, and neurological symptoms may present with either, but there is usually a history of infection or illness with a fever. While the heatstroke patient usually has a history of exertion and exposure to high ambient temperatures, this is not always the case. In some cases, heatstroke can be caused by impaired functioning of the hypothalamus without exertion or exposure to ambient heat. Treat for heatstroke if you are unsure which it is.

Although fever may be beneficial, it can be disconcerting to the parents of children with fever. In addition, fever can be uncomfortable for the patient. If the patient is uncomfortable, measures should be taken to treat the fever. Also, if a child has a history of febrile seizures, the fever should be treated. Parents will often have their febrile children wrapped in several layers of clothing or blankets because the child is "cold." These should be removed, leaving only the diaper or underclothes, exposing the child to the ambient air. This will allow a controlled cooling.

Sponge baths and cool-water immersion should not be used. These cause a rapid drop in the body core temperature and result in shivering. This again elevates the core temperature, which complicates the process. Several medications are good antipyretics (that is, they lower body temperature in fever). These include acetaminophen (Tylenol) and ibuprofen (Motrin). Many EMS systems will utilize an antipyretic in the treatment of fever, particularly in pediatric patients. Liquid acetaminophen and ibuprofen are easy to administer and effective. Acetaminophen is also available in a suppository form for patients with active vomiting. These antipyretics are typically dosed based on the patient's weight:

When unsure if the problem is heatstroke or fever, treat for heatstroke.

Do not use sponge baths to cool febrile children.

Consider administering an antipyretic, primarily for patient comfort. This is especially important in services with long tranportation times.

- *Acetaminophen*—15 mg/kg for pediatric patients; adult dose is typically 650 mg
- *Ibuprofen*—10 mg/kg for pediatric patients; adult dose is typically 600–800 mg

These liquid medications should be dosed with syringes as teaspoons are inaccurate measuring devices. EMS services with prolonged transport times should consider the use of antipyretics for patient comfort as well as for the prevention of febrile seizures.

Content Review

COLD DISORDERS
Hypothermia
Frostbite
Trench foot

COLD DISORDERS

Disruption of the body's normal thermoregulation may produce cold-related disorders such as hypothermia, frostbite, and trench foot.

HYPOTHERMIA

Hypothermia is a state of low body temperature, specifically low core temperature. When the core temperature of the body drops below 95° F (35° C), an individual is considered to be hypothermic. Hypothermia can be attributed to inadequate thermogenesis, excessive cold stress, or a combination of both.

MECHANISMS OF HEAT CONSERVATION AND LOSS

Exposure to cold normally triggers compensatory mechanisms designed to conserve and generate heat in order to maintain a normal body temperature. One such mechanism is piloerection (hair standing on end, "goose bumps") to impede air flow across the skin. Shivering and increased muscle tone occur, resulting in increased metabolism. There is peripheral vasoconstriction with an increase in cardiac output and respiratory rate. When these mechanisms can no longer adequately compensate for heat lost from the body surface, the body temperature falls. As the body temperature falls, so do the metabolic rate and cardiac output.

As discussed, major mechanisms of body heat loss are conduction, convection, radiation, evaporation, and respiration. Heat loss can be increased by the removal of clothing (decreased insulation, increased radiation), the wetting of clothing by rain or snow (increased conduction and evaporation), air movement around the body (increased convection), or contact with a cold surface or cold-water immersion (increased conduction).

PREDISPOSING FACTORS

Several factors can contribute to the risk of developing hypothermia. They also contribute to the severity of damage if cold injury occurs. Risk factors that increase the danger of developing hypothermia include:

- *Age of the patient*—Pediatric or geriatric patients cannot tolerate cold environments and have less responsive heat generating mechanisms to combat cold exposure. Elderly persons often become hypothermic in environments that seem only mildly cool to others.

- *Health of the patient*—Hypothyroidism suppresses metabolism, preventing patients from responding appropriately to cold stress. Malnutrition, hypoglycemia, Parkinson's disease, fatigue, and other medical conditions can interfere with the body's ability to combat cold exposure.

- *Medications*—Some drugs interfere with proper heat generating mechanisms. These include narcotics, alcohol, phenothiazines, barbiturates, antiseizure medications, antihistamines and other allergy medications, antipsychotics, sedatives, antidepressants, and various pain medications such as aspirin, acetaminophen, and NSAIDs.

- *Prolonged or intense exposure*—The length and severity of cold exposure have a direct effect on morbidity and mortality.

- *Coexisting weather conditions*—High humidity, brisk winds, or accompanying rain can all magnify the effect of cold exposure on the human body by accelerating the loss of heat from skin surfaces.

PREVENTIVE MEASURES

Certain precautions can decrease the risk of morbidity related to cold injury.

- Dress warmly.
- Get plenty of rest to maximize the ability of heat generating mechanisms to replenish energy supplies.
- Eat appropriately and at regular intervals to support metabolism.
- Limit exposure to cold environments.

DEGREES OF HYPOTHERMIA

Hypothermia can be classified as mild or severe, as follows:

- *Mild*—a core temperature greater than 90° F (32° C) with signs and symptoms of hypothermia
- *Severe*—a core temperature less than 90° F (32° C) with signs and symptoms of hypothermia

Initially some patients may exhibit *compensated* hypothermia. In this case signs and symptoms of hypothermia will be present but with a normal core body temperature, temporarily maintained by thermogenesis. As energy stores from the liver and muscle glycogen are exhausted, the core body temperature will drop.

The onset of symptoms may be *acute,* as occurs when a person suddenly falls through ice into a frigid lake. *Subacute* exposure can occur in situations such as when mountain climbers are trapped in a snowy, cold environment. Finally, *chronic* exposure to cold is a growing problem in our inner cities where homeless people endure frequent and prolonged cold stress without shelter.

In some cases cold exposure is the primary cause of hypothermia, but in others, hypothermia may develop secondary to other problems, such as medical problems. For example, hypothyroidism depresses the body's heat-producing mechanisms. Brain tumors or head trauma can depress the hypothalamic temperature control center, causing hypothermia. Other conditions such as myocardial infarction, diabetes, hypoglycemia, drugs, poor nutrition, sepsis, or old age can also contribute to metabolic and circulatory disorders that predispose to hypothermia. Any patient thought to have hypothermia, but with no history of exposure to a cold environment, should be assessed for any predisposing factors. Evaluate the patient for level of consciousness, cool skin, and shivering. Also, evaluate the rectal temperature. A rectal temperature of less than 95° F (35° C) indicates hypothermia. Key findings at different degrees of hypothermia are summarized in Table 36-1.

Patients who experience body temperatures above 86° F (30° C) will usually have a favorable prognosis. Those with temperatures below 86° F (30° C) show a significant increase in mortality rate. Remember that most thermometers used in medicine do not register below 95° F (35° C). EMS systems in colder areas should carry special thermometers for recording subnormal temperature readings as there is no reliable correlation between signs and symptoms and actual core body temperature.

Services operating in colder environments should carry specialized hypothermia thermometers for cold exposure victims.

Signs and Symptoms

Signs and symptoms of hypothermia are summarized in Table 36-2. Patients experiencing mild hypothermia (core temperature >90° F or 32° C) will generally exhibit shivering. The patient may be lethargic and somewhat dulled

Table 36-1 KEY FINDINGS AT DIFFERENT DEGREES OF HYPOTHERMIA

C°	F°	Clinical Findings
37.6	99.6	Normal rectal temperature
37	98.6	Normal oral temperature
36	96.8	Metabolic rate increased
35	95	Maximum shivering seen
		Impaired judgment
34	93.2	Amnesia
		Slurred speech
33	91.4	Severe clouding of consciousness/apathy
		Uncoordinated movement
32	89.6	Most shivering ceases
		Pupils dilate
31	87.8	Blood pressure may no longer be obtainable
30	86	Atrial fibrillation/other dysrhythmias develop
		Pulse and cardiac output decreased by 33%
29	84.2	Progressive decrease in pulse and breathing
		Progressive decrease in level of consciousness
28	82.4	Pulse and oxygen consumption decreased by 50%
		Severe slowing of respiration
		Increased muscle rigidity
		Loss of consciousness
		High risk of ventricular fibrillation
27	80.6	Loss of reflexes and voluntary movement
		Patients appear clinically dead
26	78.8	No reflexes or response to painful stimuli
25	77	Cerebral blood flow decreased by 66%
24	75.2	Marked hypotension
22	71.6	Maximum risk for ventricular fibrillation
19	66.2	Flat electroencephalogram (EEG)
18	64.4	Asystole
16	60.8	Lowest reported adult survival from accidental exposure
15.2	59.2	Lowest reported infant survival from accidental exposure
10	50	Oxygen consumption 8% of normal
9	48.2	Lowest reported survivor from therapeutic exposure

mentally. (In some cases, however, they may be fully oriented.) Muscles may be stiff and uncoordinated, causing the patient to walk with a stumbling, staggering gait.

Patients experiencing severe hypothermia (core temperature <90° F or 32° C) may be disoriented and confused. As their temperatures continue to fall, they will proceed into stupor and complete coma. Shivering will usually stop, and physical activity will become uncoordinated. Muscles may be stiff and rigid. Continuous cardiac monitoring is indicated for anyone experiencing hypothermia. The ECG

Table 36-2	HYPOTHERMIA: SIGNS AND SYMPTOMS	
Mild		**Severe**
Lethargy		No shivering
Shivering		Dysrhythmias, asystole
Lack of coordination		Loss of voluntary muscle control
Pale, cold, dry skin		Hypotension
Early rise in blood pressure, heart, and respiratory rates		Undetectable pulse and respirations

 J wave ECG deflection found at the junction of the QRS complex and the ST segment. It is associated with hypothermia and seen at core temperatures below 32° C, most commonly in leads II and V$_6$; also called an *Osborn wave*.

will frequently show pathognomonic (indicative of a disease) **J waves,** also called Osborn waves, associated with the QRS complexes (Figure 36-3), but these are not useful diagnostically. Atrial fibrillation is the most common presenting dysrhythmia seen in hypothermia. As the body cools, however, the myocardium becomes progressively more irritable and may develop a variety of dysrhythmias. In severe hypothermia, bradycardia is inevitable.

Ventricular fibrillation becomes more probable as the body's core temperature falls below 86° F (30° C). The severely hypothermic patient requires assessment of pulse and respirations for at least 30 seconds every 1 to 2 minutes.

Treatment for Hypothermia

All victims of hypothermia should have the following care (see also Figure 36-4):

1. *Remove wet garments.*
2. *Protect against further heat loss and wind chill.* Use *passive external warming* methods such as application of blankets, insulating materials, and moisture barriers.
3. *Maintain the patient in a horizontal position.*
4. *Avoid rough handling,* which can trigger dysrhythmias.
5. *Monitor the core temperature.*
6. *Monitor the cardiac rhythm.*

Rewarming is not the mirror image of the cooling process.

Active Rewarming Victims of mild hypothermia may also be rewarmed, using *active external methods.* This includes the use of warmed blankets and/or heat packs placed over areas of high heat transfer with the core: the base of the neck, the axilla,

FIGURE 36-3   ECG tracing showing J wave following the QRS complex as seen in hypothermia.

American Heart Association®

Fighting Heart Disease and Stroke

Initial therapy for all patients
- Remove wet garments
- Protect against heat loss and wind chill (use blankets and insulating equipment)
- Maintain horizontal position
- Avoid rough movement and excess activity
- Monitor core temperature
- Monitor cardiac rhythm

Assess responsiveness, breathing, and pulse

Pulse and breathing present

What is core temperature?

34°C to 36°C (mild hypothermia)
- Passive rewarming
- Active external rewarming

30°C to 34°C (moderate hypothermia)
- Passive rewarming
- Active external rewarming of truncal areas only

<30°C (severe hypothermia)
- Active internal rewarming sequence (see below)

Active internal rewarming
- Warm IV fluids (43°C)
- Warm, humid *oxygen* (42°C to 46°C)
- Peritoneal lavage (KCl-free fluid)
- Extracorporeal rewarming
- Esophageal rewarming tubes

Continue internal rewarming until
- Core temperature >35°C or
- Return of spontaneous circulation or
- Resuscitative efforts cease

Pulse or breathing absent

- Start CPR
- *Defibrillate* VF/pulseless VT up to a **maximum** of 3 shocks (200 J, 200 to 300 J, 360 J or per AED; see VF/VT algorithm and AED algorithm)
- Attempt, confirm, secure airway
- Ventilate with warm, humid *oxygen* (42°C to 46°C)
- Establish IV access
- Infuse warm normal saline (43°C)

What is core temperature?

<30°C   **>30°C**

- Continue CPR
- Withhold IV medications
- Limit shocks for VF/VT to maximum of 3
- Transport to hospital

- Continue CPR
- Give IV medications as indicated (but space at longer than standard intervals)
- Repeat defibrillation for VF/VT as core temperature rises

Notes:
1. This may require needle electrodes through the skin.
2. Many experts think these interventions should be done only in-hospital, though practice varies.
3. Methods include electric or charcoal warming devices, hot water bottles, heating pads, radiant heat sources, and warming beds.
4. Esophageal rewarming tubes are widely used internationally and are expected to become available in the United States.

FIGURE 36-4   Management of hypothermia. Reproduced with permission from *Guidelines 2000 for Cardiopulmonary Resuscitation and Emergency Cardiovascular Care*, ©2000, Copyright American Heart Association.

and the groin. Be sure to insulate between the heat packs and the skin to prevent burning. Intravenous fluid heaters (i.e. Hot I.V.) can be used to warm the IV fluid to 95° to 100° F/ 35° to 38° C. Warmed IV fluids are helpful in treating mild to moderate hypothermia. Heat guns and lights may also be used, but this will most likely take place in the emergency department. Warm water immersion in water between 102° and 104° F (39° to 40° C) may be used but can induce rewarming shock (see below), so this method also has little application in an out-of-hospital setting.

Active rewarming of the severely hypothermic patient is best carried out in the hospital using a prearranged protocol. Most patients who die during rewarming die from ventricular fibrillation, the risk of which is related to both the depth and the duration of hypothermia. Rough handling of the hypothermic patient may also induce ventricular fibrillation. Active rewarming should not be attempted in the field unless travel to the emergency department will take more than 15 minutes.

If such is the case, active internal means may also be used, including the use of warmed (102° to 104° F/38° to 40° C) humidified oxygen, and administration of warmed IV fluids (also warmed to 102° to 104° F/38° to 40° C). This is crucial to prevent further heat loss, but actual heat transferred is minimal, so there is limited contribution to the rewarming effort.

Rewarming Shock While application of warmed blankets is a safe and effective means of rewarming the hypothermic patient, application of external heat, as with heat packs, is usually not recommended in the prehospital setting. For effective rewarming, more heat transference is generally required than is possible with out-of-hospital methods. Additionally, application of external heat may result in *rewarming shock* by causing reflex peripheral vasodilatation. This reflex vasodilation causes the return of cool blood and acids from the extremities to the core. This may cause a paradoxical "afterdrop" core temperature decrease and further worsen core hypothermia. This, in turn, may cause the blood pressure to fall, especially when there is also volume depletion.

If active rewarming is necessary in the prehospital setting, for example when transport is delayed, administration of warmed IV fluids during rewarming can prevent the onset of rewarming shock.

Cold Diuresis Volume depletion can occur as a result of *cold diuresis*. Core vasoconstriction causes increased blood volume and blood pressure, so the kidneys remove excess fluid to reduce the pressure, thus causing diuresis. A warmed IV volume expander (e.g., normal saline) should be used both to prevent rewarming shock and to replace fluid lost from cold diuresis.

The conscious patient who is able to manage his airway may be given warmed, sweetened fluids. Alcohol and caffeine should be avoided.

Resuscitation

There are certain resuscitation considerations when handling cardiac arrest victims with core temperatures below 86° F (30° C).

Basic Cardiac Life Support BLS providers should start cardiopulmonary resuscitation (CPR) immediately, although pulse and respirations may need to be checked for longer periods to detect minimal cardiopulmonary efforts. Use normal chest compression and ventilation rates and ventilate with warmed, humidified oxygen. If an AED is available and ventricular fibrillation is detected, three shocks may be given. Further shocks should be avoided until after rewarming to above 86° F. CPR, rewarming, and rapid transport should immediately follow the three defibrillation attempts.

Advanced Cardiac Life Support Since there is no increased risk of inducing ventricular fibrillation from orotracheal or nasotracheal intubation, ALS

Active rewarming of the severely hypothermic patient should be deferred until the patient is at the hospital unless transport time is long and rewarming is ordered by medical direction.

providers may intubate the patient and ventilate with warmed, humidified oxygen. Drug metabolism is reduced however, so administered medications, such as epinephrine, lidocaine and procainamide may accumulate to toxic levels if used repeatedly in the severely hypothermic victim. In addition, administered drugs may remain in the peripheral circulation. When the patient is rewarmed and perfusion resumes, large, toxic boluses of these medications may be delivered to the central circulation and target tissues. Lidocaine and procainamide may also paradoxically lower the fibrillatory threshold in a hypothermic heart and increase resistance to defibrillation. Bretylium and magnesium sulfate however, may be effective even in hypothermic hearts.

The American Heart Association recommends that, if the patient fails to respond to initial defibrillation attempts or initial drug therapy, subsequent defibrillations or boluses of medication should be avoided until the core temperature is about 86° F (30° C). This is because it is generally impossible to electrically defibrillate a heart that is colder than 86° F. Active core rewarming techniques are the primary modality in hypothermia victims who are either in cardiac arrest or unconscious with a slow heart rate.

Techniques that may be used include the administration of heated, humidified oxygen and warmed intravenous fluids, preferably normal saline, infused centrally at rates of 150 to 200 mL an hour to avoid overhydration. Peritoneal lavage with warmed potassium-free fluid administered 2 L at a time may be used, as may extracorporeal blood warming with partial cardiac bypass. Obviously some of these techniques may only be carried out in a hospital setting.

If the hypothermic cardiac arrest patient fails to respond to initial defibrillation attempts or drug therapy, avoid subsequent defibrillations or medication until the core temperature is about 86° F (30° C). It is generally impossible to defibrillate a heart that is colder than 86° F.

Transportation

When transporting a hypothermic patient, remember that gentle transportation is necessary due to myocardial irritability and that the patient should be kept level or slightly inclined with head down. Contact the receiving hospital for general rewarming options. When determining your destination, consider the availability of cardiac bypass rewarming.

FROSTBITE

Frostbite is environmentally induced freezing of body tissues (Figure 36-5). As the tissues freeze, ice crystals form within and water is drawn out of the cells into the extracellular space. These ice crystals expand, causing the destruction of cells.

✱ **frostbite** environmentally induced freezing of body tissues causing destruction of cells.

FIGURE 36-5 Frostbite.

During this process, intracellular electrolyte concentrations increase, further destroying cells. Damage to blood vessels from ice crystal formation causes loss of vascular integrity, resulting in tissue swelling and loss of distal nutritional flow.

Superficial and Deep Frostbite

Generally, there are two types of frostbite: superficial and deep. **Superficial frostbite** (frostnip) exhibits some freezing of epidermal tissue, resulting in initial redness, followed by blanching. There will also be diminished sensation. **Deep frostbite** affects the epidermal and subcutaneous layers. There is a white appearance and the area feels hard (frozen) to palpation. There is also loss of sensation in deep frostbite.

Frostbite mainly occurs in the extremities and in areas of the head and face exposed to the environment. Subfreezing temperatures are required for frostbite to occur, although they are not necessary to produce hypothermia. Many patients who have frostbite will also have hypothermia.

There can be tremendous variation in how an individual can present with frostbite. For example, some patients feel little pain at onset. Others will report severe pain. A certain degree of compliance may be felt beneath the frozen layer in superficial frostbite, but in deep frostbite, the frozen part will be hard and noncompliant.

Treatment for Frostbite

In treating frostbite, take the following recommended steps:

- Do not thaw the affected area if there is any possibility of refreezing.
- Do not massage the frozen area or rub with snow. Rubbing the affected area may cause ice crystals within the tissues to damage the already injured tissues more seriously.
- Administer analgesia prior to thawing.
- Transport to the hospital for rewarming by immersion. If transport will be delayed, thaw the frozen part by immersion in a 102–104° F (39°–40° C) water bath. Water temperature will fall rapidly, requiring additions of warm water throughout the process.
- Cover the thawed part with loosely applied dry, sterile dressings.
- Elevate and immobilize the thawed part.
- Do not puncture or drain blisters.
- Do not rewarm frozen feet if they are required for walking out of a hazardous situation.

TRENCH FOOT

Trench foot (immersion foot) is similar to frostbite, but it occurs at temperatures above freezing. It is rarely seen in the civilian population. It received its name in World War I, when troops confined to trenches with standing cold water developed progressive symptoms over days. Symptoms are similar to frostbite, but there may be pain. Blisters may form upon spontaneous rewarming.

Treatment of Trench Foot

Treatment of trench foot requires early recognition of developing symptoms and immediate steps to warm, dry, aerate, and elevate the feet. Measures to prevent trench foot are most effective, such as avoiding prolonged exposure to standing water, changing wet socks frequently, and never sleeping in wet boots or socks.

---

* **superficial frostbite** freezing involving only epidermal tissues resulting in redness followed by blanching and diminished sensation; also called *frostnip*.

* **deep frostbite** freezing involving epidermal and subcutaneous tissues resulting in a white appearance, hard (frozen) feeling on palpation, and loss of sensation.

Do not thaw frozen flesh if there is any possibility of refreezing. Do not massage the frozen area or rub it with snow.

* **trench foot** a painful foot disorder resembling frostbite and resulting from exposure to cold and wet, which can eventually result in tissue sloughing or gangrene; also called *immersion foot*.

NEAR-DROWNING AND DROWNING

Drowning is asphyxiation resulting from submersion in liquid. There has been an attempt made to differentiate between the terms drowning and near-drowning. The term *drowning* means that death occurred within 24 hours of submersion, while the term **near-drowning** indicates that death either did not occur or occurred more than 24 hours after submersion.

It is estimated that in the United States, approximately 4,500 persons die annually due to drowning. Many more sustain serious injury due to near-drowning. This makes drowning the third most common cause of accidental death in the United States. Approximately 40 percent of these deaths are in children under 5 years of age. There is a second peak incidence in teenagers and a final third peak in the elderly as a result of accidental bathtub drownings. Approximately 85 percent of near-drowning victims are male, and two-thirds of these do not know how to swim. Most commonly, these situations are due to fresh-water submersion, especially in swimming pools. Unfortunately, alcohol use by the victim or the supervising adult is frequently associated with this type of accident.

It is important to note that other emergency conditions are often associated with near-drowning. If the cause of the submersion is unknown, you must consider the possibility of trauma and treat the patient accordingly.

Frequently the submersion occurs in cold water, causing hypothermia. Hypothermia slows the body's metabolic processes thereby decreasing the need for oxygen. This can have a protective effect on organs and tissues which become hypoxic (low in oxygen) in submersion situations. However, it is important to treat the hypoxia first, once you have initiated rescue.

PATHOPHYSIOLOGY OF DROWNING AND NEAR-DROWNING

As a paramedic, you need to understand the sequence of events in drowning or near-drowning. Following submersion, if the victim is conscious, he will undergo a period of complete apnea for up to three minutes. This apnea is an involuntary reflex as the victim strives to keep his head above water. During this time, blood is shunted to the heart and brain because of the mammalian diving reflex, which is described later in this chapter.

When the victim is apneic, the $PaCO_2$ in the blood rises to greater than 50 mmHg. Meanwhile, the PaO_2 of the blood falls below 50 mmHg. The stimulus from the hypoxia ultimately overrides the sedative effects of the hypercarbia, resulting in central nervous system stimulation.

Dry Versus Wet Drowning

Until unconscious, the victim experiences a great deal of panic. During this stage the victim makes violent inspiratory and swallowing efforts. At this point, copious amounts of water enter the mouth, posterior oropharynx, and stomach, stimulating severe laryngospasm (airway obstruction due to aspirated water) and bronchospasm. In approximately 10 percent of drowning victims, and in a much greater percentage of near-drowning victims, this laryngospasm prevents the influx of water into the lungs. If a significant amount of water does not enter the lungs, it is referred to as a *dry drowning*. Conversely, if a laryngospasm does not occur, and a significant quantity of water does enter the lungs, it is referred to as a *wet drowning*.

The laryngospasm further aggravates the hypoxia, with coma ultimately ensuing. Persistent anoxia (absence of oxygen) results in a deeper coma. Following

* **drowning** asphyxiation resulting from submersion in liquid with death occurring within 24 hours of submersion.

* **near-drowning** an incident of potentially fatal submersion in liquid which did not result in death or in which death occurred more than 24 hours after submersion.

unconsciousness, reflex swallowing continues, resulting in gastric distention and increased risk of vomiting and aspiration. If untreated, hypotension, bradycardia, and death result in a short period.

Drowning and near-drowning are primarily due to asphyxia from airway obstruction in the lung secondary to the aspirated water or the laryngospasm. If, in a near-drowning episode, this process does not end in death, any fluid that has entered the lungs may cause lower-airway disease.

Fresh-Water Versus Saltwater Drowning

You should expect different physiological reactions in cases of fresh-water and saltwater drownings or near-drownings. However, these mechanistic differences do not make any difference in the end metabolic result or in the prehospital management.

Fresh-Water Drowning In fresh-water drowning or near-drowning, the large surface area of the alveoli and small airways allow a massive amount of hypotonic water to diffuse across the alveolar/capillary membrane and into the vascular space. This results in hemodilution, an expansion in blood plasma volume and relative reduction in red blood cell concentration. *Hemodilution* produces a thickening of the alveolar walls with inflammatory cells, hemorrhagic pneumonitis (bleeding lung inflammation), and destruction of surfactant.

Surfactant is a substance in the alveoli responsible for keeping the alveoli open. In drowning, some surfactant is lost when the capillaries of the alveoli are damaged. Plasma proteins then leak back into the alveoli, resulting in the accumulation of fluid in the small airways. This in turn leads to multiple areas of atelectasis—areas of alveolar collapse. Atelectasis causes shunting, which is the return of unoxygenated blood from the damaged alveoli to the bloodstream. In other words, blood is traveling through the lungs without being oxygenated. The result is hypoxemia (inadequate oxygenation of the blood) (Figure 36-6).

Saltwater Drowning In saltwater drowning or near-drowning, the hypertonic nature of sea water, which is 3 to 4 times more hypertonic than plasma, draws water from the bloodstream into the alveoli (Figure 36-6). This produces pul-

> *Although the physiology of fresh-water and saltwater drownings differ, there is no difference in the end result or in prehospital management.*

* **surfactant** a compound secreted by cells in the lungs that regulates the surface tension of the fluid that lines the alveoli, important in keeping the alveoli open for gas exchange.

Alveoli

Fresh water washes away surfactant— alveoli collapse

...ventricular fibrillation usually occurs

Salt water draws fluids from bloodstream

...and pulmonary edema occurs

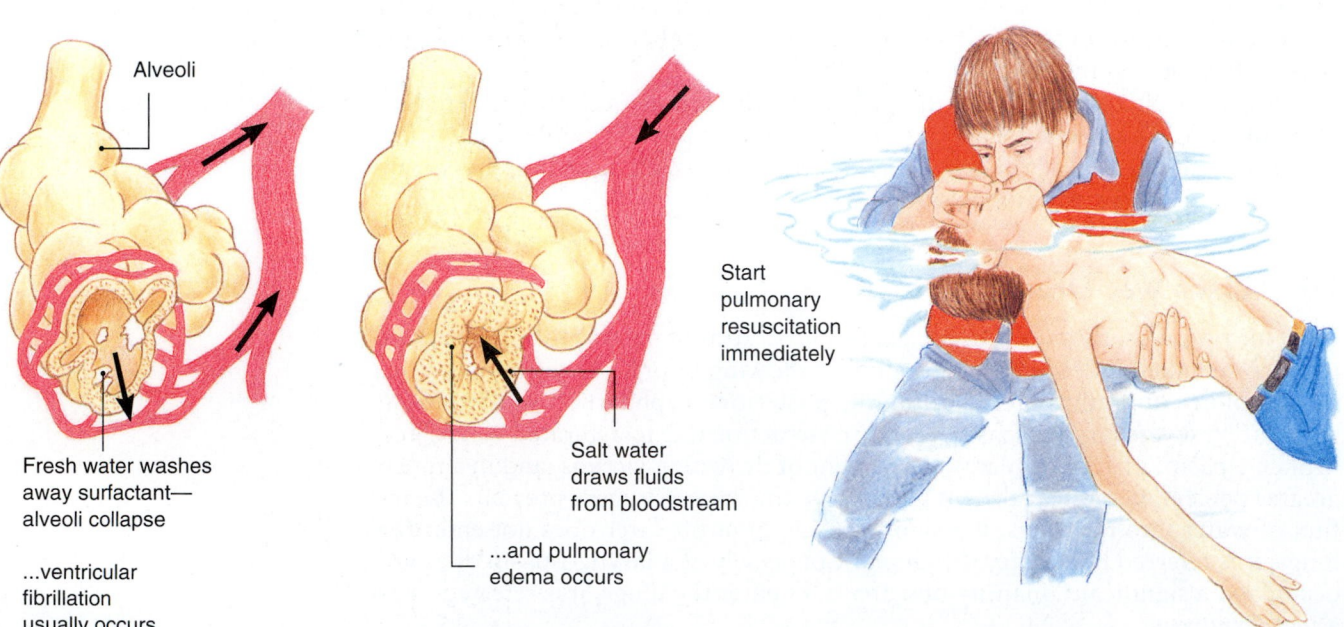

Start pulmonary resuscitation immediately

FIGURE 36-6 Pathophysiological effects of drowning.

monary edema, leading to profound shunting. The result is failure of oxygenation, producing hypoxemia. Additionally, respiratory and metabolic acidosis develop due to the retention of CO_2 and developing anaerobic (without-oxygen) metabolism.

Factors Affecting Survival

A number of factors have an impact on drowning and near-drowning survival rates. These include the cleanliness of the water, the length of time submerged, and the age and general health of the victim. Children have a longer survival time and a greater probability of a successful resuscitation. Even more significant is the water temperature. The concept of developing brain death after four to six minutes without oxygen is not applicable in cases of near-drowning in cold water. Some patients in cold water (below 68° F) can be resuscitated after 30 minutes or more in cardiac arrest. However, persons under water 60 minutes or longer usually cannot be resuscitated.

A possible contribution to survival may be the **mammalian diving reflex.** When a person dives into cold water, he reacts to the submersion of the face. Breathing is inhibited, the heart rate becomes bradycardic, and vasoconstriction develops in tissues relatively resistant to asphyxia. Meanwhile cerebral and cardiac blood flow is maintained. In this way, oxygen is sent and used only where it is immediately needed to sustain life. The colder the water, the more oxygen is diverted to the heart and brain. A common saying in emergency medicine states: "The cold-water drowning victim is not dead until he is warm and dead." In other words, a person who has been submerged in cold water may only seem to be dead, but due to the continued supply of oxygen to the heart and brain may indeed still be alive.

TREATMENT FOR NEAR-DROWNING

Since fresh-water and saltwater near-drownings both involve factors that disrupt normal pulmonary function, initial field treatment must be directed toward correcting the profound hypoxia. Take the following steps:

- Remove the patient from the water as soon as possible. This should be done by a trained rescue swimmer.

- Initiate ventilation while the patient is still in the water. Rescue personnel should wear protective clothing if water temperature is less than 70° F. In addition, attach a safety line to the rescue swimmer. In fast water, it is essential to use personnel specifically trained for this type of rescue.

- Suspect head and neck injury if the patient experienced a fall or was diving. Rapidly place the victim on a long backboard and remove him from the water. Use C-spine precautions throughout care.

- Protect the patient from heat loss. Avoid laying the patient on a cold surface. Remove wet clothing and cover the body to the extent possible.

- Examine the patient for airway patency, breathing, and pulse. If indicated, begin CPR and defibrillation.

- Manage the airway using proper suctioning and airway adjuncts.

- Administer oxygen at a 100 percent concentration.

- Use respiratory rewarming, if available, and if transport time is longer than 15 minutes. (In the past, prophylactic abdominal thrusts

> ✳ **mammalian diving reflex** a complex cardiovascular reflex, resulting from submersion of the face and nose in water, that constricts blood flow everywhere except to the brain.

> *The cold-water drowning victim is not dead until he is warm and dead.*
>

> *Never attempt to rescue a drowning victim unless you have been trained and have the necessary safety equipment.*
>

were used to clear the airway, but there are conflicting recommendations regarding the practice as there is no definitive scientific data to support this maneuver.)

- Establish an IV of lactated Ringer's or normal saline for venous access and run at 75 mL/hr. If indicated, carry out defibrillation.
- Follow ACLS protocols if the patient is normothermic. If the patient is hypothermic, treat him according to the hypothermia protocol presented earlier in the chapter.

Resuscitation is not indicated if immersion has been extremely prolonged (unless hypothermia is present) or if there is evidence of putrefaction (decomposition).

Adult Respiratory Distress Syndrome

All near-drowning patients should be admitted to the hospital for observation since complications may not appear for 24 hours.

More than 90 percent of near-drowning patients survive without *sequelae* (after effects). However, all near-drowning patients should be admitted to the hospital for observation since complications may not appear for 24 hours.

Adult respiratory distress syndrome (ARDS) is one of the more severe post-resuscitation complications, with a high rate of mortality. The physiologic stress of near-drowning causes the lungs to leak fluid into the alveoli. This fluid is loaded with various chemical factors that cause severe inflammation of the tissues and failure of the respiratory system. In addition, some of these patients have problems with pulmonary parenchymal injury, destruction of surfactant, aspiration pneumonitis, or pneumothorax. A number require an extended hospital stay due to renal failure, hypoxia, hypercarbia, and mixed metabolic and respiratory acidosis. The effects of cerebral hypoxia occasionally require treatment throughout hospitalization and beyond.

DIVING EMERGENCIES

* **scuba** abbreviation for *self-contained underwater breathing apparatus*. Portable apparatus that contains compressed air which allows the diver to breathe underwater.

Scuba diving has become an extremely popular recreational sport. Divers wear portable equipment containing compressed air, which allows the diver to breathe underwater. Although scuba diving accidents are fairly uncommon, inexperienced divers have a higher rate of injury. Scuba diving emergencies can occur on the surface, in three feet of water, or at any depth. The more serious emergencies usually occur following a dive. To better assess and care for diving injuries, you need to understand a few principles of pressure.

THE EFFECTS OF AIR PRESSURE ON GASES

Water is an incompressible liquid. Fresh water has a density, or weight per unit of volume, of 62.4 pounds per cubic foot. Saltwater has a density of 64.0 pounds per cubic foot. This density can be equated to pressure, which is defined as the weight or force acting upon a unit area. Thus, a cubic foot of fresh water exerts a pressure ("weight") of 62.4 pounds over an area of one square foot. This measurement is typically stated in pounds per square inch (psi).

Humans at sea level live in an atmosphere of air, which is a mixture of gases. These gases weigh and exert a pressure of 14.7 pounds per square inch (760 mmHg). This pressure, however, may vary within the environment. For example, ascending to an altitude of one mile will decrease the atmospheric pressure by 17 percent to approximately 12.2 pounds.

To understand how air pressure affects diving accidents, you need to look at three physical laws: Boyle's Law, Dalton's Law, and Henry's Law.

Boyle's Law

Boyle's Law states that the volume of a gas is inversely proportional to its pressure if the temperature is kept constant. As you increase pressure, the gas is compressed into a smaller space. For example, doubling the pressure of a gas mixture will decrease its volume by one-half. The pressure of air at sea level is 14.7 lb./sq.in. or 760 mmHg. This pressure is called one "atmosphere absolute" or one "ata." Two ata occur at a depth of 33 feet of water, three ata occur at a depth of 66 feet of water, and so on. Therefore, one liter of air at the surface is compressed to 500 mL at 33 feet. At 66 feet, one liter of air would be compressed to 250 mL.

Dalton's Law

Dalton's Law states that the total pressure of a mixture of gases is equal to the sum of the partial pressures of the individual gases. The air we breathe is a mixture of nitrogen (about 78%), oxygen (about 21%), and carbon dioxide plus traces of argon, helium, and other rare gases (about 1%). Since the pressure of air at sea level is 760 mmHg, the pressure of nitrogen is about 593 mmHg, the pressure of oxygen is about 160 mmHg, and the pressure of carbon dioxide is somewhat less than 4 mmHg—each gas exerting its proportion of the total pressure of the mixture.

At different altitudes above sea level or depths below sea level, the pressure of air will change (less at higher altitudes, more at greater depths), but the component gases will still account for the same proportion of whatever the total pressure is at that level: nitrogen 78%, oxygen 21%, and carbon dioxide less than 1%.

Henry's Law

Henry's Law states that the amount of gas dissolved in a given volume of fluid is proportional to the pressure of the gas above it. When we descend below sea level, and the pressure bearing down on us increases, the gases that make up the air we breathe tend to dissolve in the liquids (mainly blood plasma) and tissues of the body.

Let us compare what happens to the two chief components of the air we breathe—oxygen and nitrogen—when a person descends to greater and greater depths below sea level. Much of the oxygen is used up in the normal metabolism of the cells, leaving only a small amount to be dissolved in the blood and tissues. Nitrogen, however, is an inert gas and, as such, is not used by the body. Therefore, a far greater quantity of nitrogen is available to dissolve in the blood and tissues as a person descends below sea level. In brief, at depths below sea level, oxygen metabolizes but nitrogen dissolves.

When the person ascends toward sea level again, the gases that are dissolved in the blood and tissues, being under less and less pressure, come out of the blood and tissues and, if the ascent is too rapid, form bubbles. To understand this phenomenon, compare the human body to a bottled carbonated soft drink—that is, a liquid in which carbon dioxide gas is dissolved. The gas is kept dissolved in the liquid by the cap on the bottle and a high-pressure gas under the cap, on top of the liquid. When the cap is removed and the pressure is released, the gas bubbles out of the liquid, causing a fizz that will sometimes rise completely out of the bottle.

In the following sections, we will discuss how the phenomena of gases and pressure can cause serious problems for divers.

PATHOPHYSIOLOGY OF DIVING EMERGENCIES

As noted above, gases are dissolved in the diver's blood and tissues under pressure. As the diver goes deeper into the water, pressure increases, causing more gas to dissolve in the blood (Henry's Law). According to Boyle's Law, these gases will have a smaller volume due to the increased ambient pressure. During *controlled* ascent, with decreasing pressure, dissolved gases come out of the blood and tissues slowly, escaping gradually through respiration.

If ascent is *too rapid*, however, the dissolved gases, mostly nitrogen, come out of solution and expand quickly, forming bubbles in the blood, brain, spinal cord, skin, inner ear, muscles, and joints. Once bubbles of nitrogen have formed in various tissues, it is difficult for the body to remove them. The ascending diver who comes to the surface too rapidly, not adhering to safety measures, is at risk of becoming a veritable living bottle of soda.

CLASSIFICATION OF DIVING INJURIES

Scuba diving injuries are due to barotrauma, pulmonary over-pressure, arterial gas embolism, decompression illness, cold, panic, or a combination of these. Accidents generally occur at one of the following four stages of a dive:

- On the surface
- During descent
- On the bottom
- During ascent

Injuries on the Surface

Surface injuries can involve any of several factors. One such factor can be entanglement of lines or entanglement in kelp fields while swimming to the area of the dive. Divers in these situations may panic, become fatigued, even drown. Another factor may be cold water that produces shivering and blackout. Boats in the area are another potential source of injury to the diver. To prevent such accidents, divers will usually mark the area of their dive with a flag. Maritime rules require boat operators to stay clear of a flagged area.

Injuries during Descent

* **barotrauma** injuries caused by changes in pressure. Barotrauma that occurs from increasing pressure during a diving descent is commonly called "the squeeze."

Barotrauma means injuries caused by changes in pressure. Barotrauma during descent is commonly called "the squeeze." It can occur if the diver cannot equilibrate the pressure between the nasopharynx and the middle ear through the eustachian tube. The diver can experience middle ear pain, ringing in the ears, dizziness, and hearing loss. In severe cases, rupture of the eardrum can occur. A diver who has an upper respiratory infection, and who therefore cannot clear the middle ear through the eustachian tube, should not dive. A similar lack of equilibration can occur in the sinuses, producing severe frontal headaches or pain beneath the eye in the maxillary sinuses.

Injuries on the Bottom

* **nitrogen narcosis** a state of stupor that develops during deep dives due to nitrogen's effect on cerebral function; also called "raptures of the deep."

Major diving emergencies while at the bottom of the dive often involve **nitrogen narcosis** (a state of stupor), commonly called "raptures of the deep." This is due to nitrogen's effect on cerebral function. The diver may appear to be intoxicated and may take unnecessary risks. Other emergencies occur when a diver runs low on or out of air. The diver who panics will exacerbate this situation by consuming even more oxygen and producing even more carbon dioxide.

Injuries during Ascent

Serious and life-threatening emergencies, many involving barotrauma, can occur during the ascent. For example, as during descent, an ascending diver may be unable to equilibrate inner ear and nasopharyngeal pressure.

Dives below 40 feet require staged ascent to prevent **decompression illness,** also called "the bends." This condition develops in divers subjected to rapid reduction of air pressure while ascending to the surface following exposure to compressed air, with formation of nitrogen bubbles causing severe pain, especially in the abdomen and the joints.

The most serious barotrauma that occurs during ascent is injury to the lung from **pulmonary over-pressure.** This can occur with a deep dive, or it can occur with a dive of as little as three feet below the surface. The injury results from the diver holding his breath during the ascent. As the diver ascends, the air in the lung, which has been compressed, expands. If it is not exhaled, the alveoli may rupture. If this occurs, the result will be structural damage to the lung and, possibly, **arterial gas embolism (AGE),** an air bubble, or air embolism, that enters the circulatory system from the damaged lung. Another result may be **pneumomediastinum,** the release of gas (air) through the visceral pleura into the mediastinum and pericardial sac around the heart as well as into the tissues of the neck. **Pneumothorax** is possible if the alveoli rupture into the pleural cavity. Air embolism can occur if the air ruptures into the pulmonary veins or arteries and returns to the left atrium and finally into the left ventricle and out into the systemic circulation.

GENERAL ASSESSMENT OF DIVING EMERGENCIES

In the early assessment of diving accidents, all symptoms of air embolism and decompression illness are considered together. Early assessment and treatment of a diving injury is of more importance than trying to distinguish the exact problem. One of your most important tasks in a diving-related injury is elicitation of a diving history or profile. There are several essential factors to consider. These include:

- Time at which the signs and symptoms occurred
- Type of breathing apparatus utilized
- Type of hypothermia protective garment worn
- Parameters of the dive:
    - Depth of dive(s)
    - Number of dives(s)
    - Duration of dive(s)
- Aircraft travel following a dive (in a pressurized cabin?)
- Rate of ascent
- Associated panic forcing rapid ascent
- Experience of the diver, for example, student, inexperienced, or "pro"
- Properly functioning depth gauge
- Previous medical diseases
- Old injuries
- Previous episodes of decompression illness
- Use of medications
- Use of alcohol

✱ **decompression illness** development of nitrogen bubbles within the tissues due to a rapid reduction of air pressure when a diver returns to the surface; also called "the bends."

✱ **pulmonary over-pressure** expansion of air held in the lungs during ascent. If not exhaled, the expanded air may cause injury to the lungs and surrounding structures.

✱ **arterial gas embolism (AGE)** an air bubble, or air embolism, that enters the circulatory system from a damaged lung.

✱ **pneumomediastinum** the presence of air in the mediastinum.

✱ **pneumothorax** a collection of air in the pleural space. Air may enter the pleural space from through an injury to the chest wall or through an injury to the lungs. In a *tension pneumothorax,* pressure builds because there is no way for the air to escape, causing lung collapse.

In a diving emergency, consider all symptoms of air embolism and decompression illness together. Early assessment and treatment are more important than identifying the exact problem.

Table 36-3	FACTORS RELATED TO THE DEVELOPMENT OF DECOMPRESSION ILLNESS

General Factors	Individual Factors
Cold water dives	Age—older individuals
Diving in rough water	Obesity
Strenuous diving conditions	Fatigue—lack of sleep prior to dive
History of previous decompression dive incident	Alcohol—consumption before or after dive
Overstaying time at given dive depth	History of medical problems
Dive at 80 feet or greater	
Rapid ascent—panic, inexperience, unfamiliarity with equipment	
Heavy exercise before or after dive to the point of muscle soreness	
Flying after diving (24 hour wait is recommended)	
Driving to high altitude after dive	

From a quick assessment of the patient's diving profile, you can rapidly determine if the diver is a likely candidate for a pressure disorder.

PRESSURE DISORDERS

Injuries caused by pressure, as noted earlier, are known as *barotrauma*. In the case of diving accidents, most barotrauma results from a pressure imbalance between the external environment and gases within the body. The following sections describe some of the most common forms of barotrauma involved in diving accidents.

Decompression Illness

Decompression illness develops in divers subjected to rapid reduction of air pressure after ascending to the surface following exposure to compressed air. A number of general and individual factors can contribute to the development of decompression illness, or the bends (Table 36-3). Decompression illness results as nitrogen bubbles come out of solution in the blood and tissues, causing increased pressure in various body structures and occluding circulation in the small blood vessels. This occurs in joints, tendons, the spinal cord, skin, brain, and inner ear. Symptoms develop when a diver rapidly ascends after being exposed to a depth of 33 feet or more for a time sufficient to allow the body's tissues to be saturated with nitrogen.

Signs and Symptoms The principal signs and symptoms of decompression illnesses are joint and abdominal pain, fatigue, paresthesias, and CNS disturbances. The nitrogen bubbles produced by rapid decompression are thought to produce obstruction of blood flow and lead to local ischemia, subjecting tissues to anoxic stress. In some cases, this stress may lead to tissue damage.

Treatment Patients with decompression illness usually seek medical treatment within 12 hours of ascent from a dive. Some patients may not seek treatment for as long as 24 hours after the last dive. It is generally safe to assume that signs or symptoms developing more than 36 hours after a dive cannot reasonably be attributed to decompression illness.

FIGURE 36-7 Hyperbaric oxygen chamber used in the treatment of decompression illness.

Decompression illness may require urgent definitive care through **recompression.** This can be accomplished by placing the patient in a **hyperbaric oxygen chamber** (Figure 36-7). There the patient is subjected to oxygen under greater-than-atmospheric pressure to force the nitrogen in the body to re-dissolve, then gradually decompressed to allow the nitrogen to escape without forming bubbles. However, prompt stabilization at the nearest emergency department should be accomplished before transportation to a recompression chamber.

Early oxygen therapy may reduce symptoms of decompression illness substantially. Divers who are administered high concentrations of oxygen have a considerably better treatment outcome. The following list outlines some of the steps in the prehospital management of decompression illnesses.

* Assess the ABCs.
* Administer CPR, if required.
* Administer oxygen at 100 percent concentration with a nonrebreather mask. An unconscious diver should be intubated.
* Keep the patient in the supine position.
* Protect the patient from excessive heat, cold, wetness, or noxious fumes.
* Give the conscious, alert patient nonalcoholic liquids such as fruit juices or oral balanced salt solutions.
* Evaluate and stabilize the patient at the nearest emergency department prior to transport to a recompression chamber. Begin IV fluid replacement with electrolyte solutions for unconscious or seriously injured patients. You may use lactated Ringer's or normal saline. Do not use 5 percent dextrose in water.
* If there is evidence of CNS involvement, administer dexamethasone, heparin, or Valium as ordered by medical direction.

* **recompression** resubmission of a person to a greater pressure so that gradual decompression can be achieved; often used in the treatment of diving emergencies.

* **hyperbaric oxygen chamber** recompression chamber used to treat patients suffering from barotrauma.

Recompression in a hyperbaric oxygen chamber may be required for the patient suspected of suffering decompression illness or an air embolism.

- If air evacuation is used, do not expose the patient to decreased barometric pressure. Cabin pressure must be maintained at sea level, or fly at the lowest possible safe altitude.
- Send the patient's diving equipment with the patient for examination. If that is impossible, arrange for local examination and gas analysis.

Pulmonary Over-Pressure Accidents

Lung overinflation due to rapid ascent is the common cause of a number of emergencies, particularly at shallow depths of less than 6 feet. Air can become trapped in the lungs by mucous plugs, bronchospasm, or simple breath holding. With rapid ascent, ambient pressure drops quickly, causing the trapped air to expand. Air expansion can rupture the alveolar membranes. This can result in hemorrhage, reduced oxygen and carbon dioxide transport, and capillary and alveolar inflammation. Air can also escape from the lung into other nearby tissues and cause pneumothorax and tension pneumothorax, subcutaneous emphysema, or pneumomediastinum.

Signs and Symptoms Divers with this type of condition will complain of substernal chest pain. Respiratory distress and diminished breath sounds are common findings on examination.

Treatment Treatment for this condition is the same as for pneumothorax caused by any other mechanism (see Chapter 27). Rest and supplemental oxygen are important but hyperbaric oxygen is not usually necessary.

Arterial Gas Embolism (AGE)

As described above, a pressure buildup in the lung can damage and rupture alveoli. This can allow air in the form of a large bubble to escape into the circulation. This air embolism, or arterial gas embolism, can travel to the left atrium and ventricle of the heart and out into various parts of the body where it may lodge and obstruct blood flow, causing ischemia and possibly infarct. Such obstruction of blood flow can have devastating effects triggered by cardiac, pulmonary, and cerebral compromise.

Signs and Symptoms Signs and symptoms of air embolism include onset within 2 to 10 minutes of ascent, a rapid and dramatic onset of sharp, tearing pain, and other symptoms related to the organ system affected by blocked blood flow. The most common presentation mimics a stroke with confusion, vertigo, visual disturbances, and loss of consciousness. Although rare, you may also encounter paralysis on one side of the body (hemiplegia), as well as cardiac and pulmonary collapse. If any person using SCUBA equipment presents with neurologic deficits during or immediately after ascent, an air embolism should be suspected. As death or serious disability can result, prompt medical treatment is crucial.

Treatment Management of air embolism includes the following steps:

- Assess ABCs.
- Administer oxygen by nonrebreather mask at 100 percent.
- Place the patient in a supine position.
- Monitor vital signs frequently.
- Administer IV fluids at a TKO rate.
- Administer a corticosteroid agent, if ordered by medical direction.
- Transport to a recompression chamber as rapidly as possible. If air transport is utilized, it is very important to use a pressurized aircraft or to fly at a low altitude.

Pneumomediastinum

As noted earlier, a pneumomediastinum is the release of gas (air) through the visceral pleura into the mediastinum and pericardial sac around the heart. It can result from a pulmonary over-pressure accident during rapid ascent from a dive.

Signs and Symptoms Signs and symptoms of a pneumomediastinum include substernal chest pain, irregular pulse, abnormal heart sounds, reduced blood pressure and narrow pulse pressure, and a change in voice. There may or may not be evidence of cyanosis.

Treatment The field management of pneumomediastinum includes:

- Administer high-concentration oxygen via nonrebreather mask.
- Start an IV lactated Ringer's or normal saline per medical direction.
- Transport to the emergency department.

Treatment generally ranges from observation to recompression for relief of acute symptoms. The patient should be observed for 24 hours for any other signs of lung overpressure. He should not be recompressed unless air embolism or decompression illness is also present.

Nitrogen Narcosis

Nitrogen narcosis develops during deep dives and contributes to major diving emergencies while the diver is at the bottom. With an elevated partial pressure, more nitrogen dissolves in the bloodstream. With higher concentrations of nitrogen in the body, including the brain, the result is intoxication and altered levels of consciousness very similar to the effects of alcohol or narcotic use. Between 70 and 100 feet these effects become apparent in most divers, but at 200 feet most divers become so impaired that they cannot do any useful work. At 300 to 350 feet unconsciousness occurs. The main concern with nitrogen narcosis is the same as with any person who is intoxicated while in a situation requiring alertness and common sense. Impaired judgment during a deep dive can cause accidents and unnecessary risk taking.

Signs and Symptoms Altered levels of consciousness and impaired judgment.

Treatment Treatment simply requires return to a shallow depth since this condition is self resolving on ascent. To avoid this problem altogether in deep dives, oxygen mixed with helium is used, since helium does not have the anesthetic effect of nitrogen.

OTHER DIVING-RELATED ILLNESSES

There are less frequent problems that can occur as a result of SCUBA diving. For example, oxygen toxicity caused by prolonged exposure to high partial pressures of oxygen can cause lung damage or even convulsions. Hyperventilation due to excitement or panic may lead to a decreased level of consciousness or muscle cramps and spasm. This will impair the diver's ability to function properly, possibly leading to injury. Inadequate breathing or faulty equipment may lead to increased CO_2 levels, or *hypercapnia*. This also may cause unconsciousness. Finally, poorly prepared air tanks may be contaminated with other gases, which can increase the risk of hypoxia, narcosis, and accidental injury.

DIVERS ALERT NETWORK (DAN)

Clearly, SCUBA diving has a unique set of potential problems. With the popularity of this activity rising so dramatically, it is important for EMS personnel in popular diving areas to become familiar with recognition and treatment of these problems. If assistance is needed, the Divers Alert Network (DAN) operates a non-profit consultation and referral service in affiliation with Duke University Medical Center. In an emergency, contact (919) 684-8111. For non-emergency situations call (919) 684-2948.

HIGH ALTITUDE ILLNESS

In contrast to illnesses related to diving and high atmospheric pressure, high altitude illnesses are caused by a decrease in ambient pressure. Essentially, high altitude is a low-oxygen environment. As noted in the discussion of Dalton's law, earlier, oxygen concentration in the atmosphere remains constant at 21 percent. Therefore, as you go higher and barometric pressure decreases, the partial pressure of oxygen also decreases (is 21 percent of a lower total pressure). Oxygen becomes less available, triggering a number of related illnesses as well as aggravating pre-existing conditions such as angina, congestive heart failure, chronic obstructive pulmonary disease, and hypertension.

Even in healthy individuals, ascent to high altitude, especially if it is very rapid, can cause illness. It is difficult to predict who will be affected and to what degree. The only predictor is the hypoxic ventilatory response.

Every year millions of visitors to mountains expose themselves to altitudes greater than 2,400 m (8,000 ft.) the altitude at which high altitude illnesses start to become manifest. For reference purposes, Denver, Colorado, is at 1,610 m where there is 17 percent less oxygen than at sea level. Aspen at 2,438 m has 26 percent less oxygen, and at the top of Mount Everest (8,848 m or 29,028 ft.) there is 66 percent less oxygen than at sea level. At *high altitude* (4,900 to 11,500 ft.) the hypoxic environment causes decreased exercise performance, although without major disruption of normal oxygen transport in the body. However, if ascent is very rapid, altitude illness will commonly occur at 8,000 feet and beyond. *Very high altitude* (11,500 to 18,000 ft.) will result in extreme hypoxia during exercise or sleep. It is important to ascend to these altitudes slowly allowing for acclimatization to the environment. *Extreme altitude* beyond 18,000 feet will cause severe illness in almost everyone.

Some of the signs and symptoms of altitude illness are malaise, anorexia, headache, sleep disturbances and respiratory distress that increases with exertion.

PREVENTION

Acclimatization, exertion, sleep, diet, and medication are key considerations in preventing or limiting high altitude medical emergencies. A description of each follows.

Gradual Ascent

To avoid developing high altitude medical problems, it is important to allow a period of acclimatization. Slow, gradual ascent over days to weeks gives the body a chance to adjust to the hypoxic state caused by high altitudes. A person who would normally become short of breath, dizzy, and confused by a rapid drop in oxygen can function quite well if the oxygen level is decreased to the same level gradually over a long period of time. Acclimatization occurs through several mechanisms. They are:

- *Ventilatory Changes.* The *hypoxic ventilatory response (HVR)* is triggered by decreased oxygen. When oxygen is decreased, ventilation increases. This hyperventilation causes a decrease in CO_2, but

High altitude illnesses start to become manifest at altitudes greater than 8,000 ft.

the kidneys compensate by eliminating more bicarbonate from the body. In essence, the body resets its normal ventilation and operating level of CO_2. The process takes 4 to 7 days at a given altitude.

- *Cardiovascular Changes.* The heart rate increases at high altitude, allowing more oxygen to be delivered to the tissues. In addition, peripheral veins constrict, increasing the central blood volume. In response, the central receptors, which sense blood volume, induce a diuresis, which causes concentration of the blood. Unfortunately, pulmonary circulation also constricts in a hypoxic environment. This causes or exacerbates pre-existing hypertension and predisposes to developing high altitude pulmonary edema.

- *Blood Changes.* Within two hours of ascent to high altitude the body begins making more red blood cells to carry oxygen. Over time, this mechanism will significantly compensate for the hypoxic environment. It is this mechanism that fostered the idea of "blood-doping" during athletic competition, especially at high altitudes. Athletes donate their own blood long in advance of a competition at high altitude. This allows them time to rebuild their red blood cells. Just before the competition they receive a transfusion of their own blood to increase their oxygen carrying capacity. This practice is frowned upon by most athletic governing bodies.

Limited Exertion

Clearly, one of the easiest ways to avoid some effects of high altitude is to limit the amount of exertion. By limiting the body's need for oxygen, the effect of oxygen deprivation will be minimized.

Sleeping Altitude

Sleep is often disrupted by high altitude. Hypoxia causes abnormal breathing patterns and frequent awakenings in the middle of the night. Descending to a lower altitude for sleep improves rest and allows the body to recover from hypoxia. This practice will, however, interfere with the process of acclimatization.

High Carbohydrate Diet

Carbohydrates are converted by the body into glucose and rapidly released into the blood stream, providing quick energy. The theory that this is helpful in acclimatizing to high altitude is controversial.

Medications

Two medications will limit or prevent the development of medical conditions related to high altitude. They are:

- *Acetazolamide.* Acetazolamide (Diamox) acts as a diuretic. It forces bicarbonate out of the body, which greatly enhances the process of acclimatization as discussed above. The hypoxic ventilatory response reaches a new set point more quickly. This improves ventilation and oxygen transport with less alkalosis. In addition, the periodic breathing that occurs at high altitude is resolved, thereby preventing sudden drops in oxygen.

- *Nifedipine.* Nifedipine (Procardia, Adalat) is a medication usually used to treat high blood pressure. It causes blood vessels to dilate, preventing the increase in pulmonary pressure that often causes pulmonary edema.

Other treatments are currently under evaluation. Phenytoin (Dilantin), for example, is being studied because of its membrane stabilization effects. Steroids are commonly used but their efficacy is still controversial.

TYPES OF HIGH ALTITUDE ILLNESS

A variety of symptoms occur when the average person ascends rapidly to high altitude. These may range from fatigue and decreased exercise tolerance to headache, sleep disturbance, and respiratory distress. The following section will deal with some of the specific syndromes that will occur.

Acute Mountain Sickness (AMS)

Acute mountain sickness usually manifests in an unacclimatized person who ascends rapidly to an altitude of 2,000 m (6,600 ft.) or greater.

Signs and Symptoms The mild form of acute mountain sickness presents with the following symptoms:

- Lightheadedness
- Breathlessness
- Weakness
- Headache
- Nausea and vomiting

These symptoms can develop from 6 to 24 hours after ascent. More severe cases can develop especially if the person continues to ascend to higher altitudes. These symptoms include:

- Weakness (requiring assistance to eat and dress)
- Severe vomiting
- Decreased urine output
- Shortness of breath
- Altered level of consciousness

Mild AMS is self-limiting and will often improve within 1 to 2 days if no further ascent occurs.

Treatment Treatment of AMS consists of halting ascent, possibly lowering altitude, using acetazolamide (Diamox), and anti-nauseants such as prochlorperazine (Compazine) as necessary. It is not usually necessary to descend to sea level. Supplemental oxygen will relieve symptoms but is usually used only in severe cases. In severe cases oxygen, if available, will help. In addition, immediate descent is the definitive treatment. For very severe cases, hyperbaric oxygen may be necessary.

Definitive treatment of all high altitude illnesses is descent to a lower altitude. Administration of supplemental oxygen is also important.

High Altitude Pulmonary Edema (HAPE)

HAPE develops as a result of increased pulmonary pressure and hypertension caused by changes in blood flow at high altitude. Children are most susceptible, and men are more susceptible than women.

Signs and Symptoms Initially symptoms include dry cough, mild shortness of breath on exertion, and slight crackles in the lungs. As the condition progresses, so will the symptoms. Dyspnea can become quite severe and cause cyanosis. Coughing may be productive of frothy sputum, and weakness may progress to coma and death.

Treatment In the early stages, HAPE is completely and easily reversible with descent and the administration of oxygen. It is therefore critical to recognize the illness early and initiate appropriate treatment. If immediate descent is not possible, supplemental oxygen can completely reverse HAPE but requires 36 to 72 hours. Such a supply of oxygen is rarely available to mountain climbers. In this situation the portable hyperbaric bag can be very useful. This is a sealed bag that can be inflated to 2 psi, which simulates a descent of approximately 5,000 feet. Acetazolamide can be used to decrease symptoms. Medications such as morphine, nifedipine (Procardia), and furosemide (Lasix) have been used with some success, but they carry complications such as hypotension and dehydration and should be used with caution.

High Altitude Cerebral Edema (HACE)

The exact cause of high altitude cerebral edema is not known. It usually manifests as progressive neurological deterioration in a patient with AMS or HAPE. The increased fluid in the brain tissue causes a rise in intracranial pressure.

Signs and Symptoms The symptoms of high altitude cerebral edema include:

- Altered mental status
- Ataxia (poor coordination)
- Decreased level of consciousness
- Coma

Headache, nausea, and vomiting are less common. Occasionally actual focal neurological changes may occur.

Treatment As in all altitude illnesses, definitive treatment is descent to lower altitude. Oxygen and steroids may also help to improve recovery. If descent is not possible, the use of oxygen with steroids and a hyperbaric bag may be sufficient, although often unavailable. If coma develops, it may persist for days after descent to sea level but usually resolves, although sometimes leaving residual disability.

NUCLEAR RADIATION

Injury due to exposure to ionizing radiation occurs infrequently. However, the incidence of radiation emergencies has increased in recent years due to the expansion of nuclear medicine procedures and commercial nuclear facilities.

Keep in mind that radiation emergencies should be handled only by those with proper protective equipment and adequate training.

Radiation emergencies should be handled only by those with proper protective equipment and adequate training.

BASIC NUCLEAR PHYSICS

Radiation is a general term applied to the transmission of electromagnetic or particle energy. This energy can include nuclear energy, ultraviolet light, visible light, infrared, and x-ray. A radioactive substance emits ionizing radiation. Such a substance is referred to as a *radionuclide* or *radioisotope*.

To understand nuclear radiation, you might begin by taking a look at the structure of an atom and by becoming familiar with some of the basic terms associated with nuclear physics. The atom consists of various subatomic particles. These include:

- *Protons.* Positively charged particles that form the nucleus of hydrogen and that are present in the nuclei of all elements. The atomic number of the element indicates the number of protons present.
- *Neutrons.* Subatomic particles that are approximately equal in mass to a proton, but lack an electrical charge. As a free particle, a neutron has an average life of less than 17 minutes.
- *Electrons.* Minute particles with negative electrical charges that revolve around the nucleus of an atom. When emitted from radioactive substances, electrons are called beta particles.

You should also be familiar with the following two basic terms associated with nuclear medicine:

- *Isotopes (radioisotope).* Atoms in which the nuclear composition is unstable. That is, they give off **ionizing radiation.**
- *Half-life.* **Half-life** is the time required for half the nuclei of a radioactive substance to lose its activity due to radioactive decay.

A radioactive substance is one that emits ionizing radiation. There are four types of ionizing radiation. These include:

- *Alpha Particles.* Alpha particles are slow-moving, low-energy particles that usually can be stopped by such things as clothing and paper. When they contact the skin, they only penetrate a few cells deep. Because they can be absorbed (stopped) by a layer of clothing, a few inches of air, or the outer layer of skin, alpha particles usually constitute a minor hazard. However, they can produce serious effects if taken internally by ingestion or inhalation.
- *Beta Particles.* Smaller than alpha particles, beta particles are higher in energy. Although beta particles can penetrate air, they can be stopped by aluminum and similar materials. Beta particles generally cause less local damage than alpha particles, but they can be harmful if inhaled or ingested.
- *Gamma Rays.* Gamma rays are more highly energized and penetrating than alpha and beta particles. The origin of gamma rays is related to that of x-rays. Gamma radiation is extremely dangerous, carrying high levels of energy capable of penetrating thick shielding. Gamma rays easily pass through clothing and the entire body, inflicting extensive cell damage. They also create indirect damage by causing internal tissue to emit alpha and beta particles. Protection from gamma radiation can be provided by lead shielding.
- *Neutrons.* Neutrons are more penetrating than the other types of radiation. The penetrating power of neutrons is estimated to be 3 to 10 times greater than gamma rays, but less than the internal hazard associated with ingestion of alpha and beta particles. Exposure to neutrons causes direct tissue damage. However, in nuclear accidents, neutron exposure is not normally a problem for paramedics because neutrons tend to be present only near a reactor core.

✳ **ionizing radiation** electromagnetic radiation (e.g., x-ray) or particulate radiation (e.g., alpha particles, beta particles, and neutrons) that, by direct or secondary processes, ionizes materials that absorb the radiation. Ionizing radiation can penetrate the cells of living organisms, depositing an electrical charge within them. When sufficiently intense, this form of energy kills cells.

✳ **half-life** time required for half of the nuclei of a radioactive substance to lose activity by undergoing radioactive decay. In biology and pharmacology, the time required by the body to metabolize and inactivate half the amount of a substance taken in.

Table 36-4 DOSE-EFFECT RELATIONSHIPS TO IONIZING RADIATION

Whole Body Exposure

Dose (RAD)	Effect
5–25	Asymptomatic. Blood studies are normal.
50–75	Asymptomatic. Minor depressions of white blood cells and platelets in a few patients.
75–125	May produce anorexia, nausea, and vomiting, and fatigue in approximately 10–20% of patients within two days.
125–200	Possible nausea and vomiting. Diarrhea, anxiety, tachycardia. Fatal to less than 5% of patients.
200–600	Nausea and vomiting, diarrhea in the first several hours, weakness, fatigue. Fatal to approximately 50% of patients within six weeks without prompt medical attention.
600–1,000	Severe nausea and vomiting, diarrhea in the first several hours. Fatal to 100% of patients within two weeks without prompt medical attention.
1,000 or more	"Burning sensation" within minutes, nausea and vomiting within 10 minutes, confusion ataxia, and prostration within one hour, watery diarrhea within 1–2 hrs. Fatal to 100% within short time without prompt medical attention.

Localized Exposure

Dose (RAD)	Effect
50	Asymptomatic.
500	Asymptomatic (usually). May have risk of altered function of exposed area.
2,500	Atrophy, vascular lesion, and altered pigmentation.
5,000	Chronic ulcer, risk of carcinogenesis.
50,000	Permanent destruction of exposed tissue.

EFFECTS OF RADIATION ON THE BODY

Ionizing radiation cannot be seen, felt, or heard. Therefore, a detection instrument is required to measure the radiation given off by the radiation source. The most commonly used device is the *Geiger counter*. The rate of radiation is measured in roentgens per hour (R/hr) or milliroentgens per hour (mR/hr) (1,000 mR = 1R).

The unit of local tissue energy deposition is called *radiation absorbed dose (RAD)*. *Roentgen equivalent in man (REM)* provides a gauge of the likely injury to the irradiated part of an organism. For all practical purposes, RAD and REM are equal in clinical value. When neutrons or other high-energy radiation sources are used, a *quality factor (QF)* is applied to determine the equivalent dose.

Simply stated, ionizing radiation causes alterations in the body's cell, primarily the genetic material (DNA). Depending upon the dosage received, the changes can be in cell division, cell structure, and cellular biochemical activities. Cell damage due to ionizing radiation is cumulative over a lifetime. If a person is exposed to ionizing radiation long enough, there will be a decreased number of white blood cells. Additionally, there may be defects in offspring, an increased incidence of cancer, and various degrees of bone marrow damage.

Detection of the first biological effects of exposure to ionizing radiation occurs at varying times (Table 36-4). Biological effects include:

- *Acute.* Effects appearing in a matter of minutes or weeks.
- *Long-term.* Effects appearing years or decades later.

PRINCIPLES OF SAFETY

Limiting radiation exposure is based on three principles: time, distance, and shielding.

There are three basic principles that allow rescue personnel and patients to limit exposure to ionizing radiation. These are *time*, *distance*, and *shielding*. Determining exposure, absorption, and damage done by radiation requires specialized training. The amount of radiation received by a person depends upon the source of radiation, the length of time exposed, the distance from the source, and the shielding between the exposed person and the source. For example, the amount of radiation at the patient's initial location may be 300 R/hr. If exposure is for 20 minutes, this is the same radiation equivalent as working for one hour at a 100 R/hr scene.

The amount of radiation may drop off rapidly as the patient is decontaminated and moved away from the exposure. The distance from an ionizing radiation source is crucial since exposure is determined by the inverse square relationship. Doubling the distance away from a radiation source reduces the exposure by a factor of four. Conversely, halving the distance to a radiation source increases exposure by a factor of four.

There are basically two types of ionizing radiation accidents—clean and dirty. In a *clean accident,* the patient is exposed to radiation but is not contaminated by the radioactive substance, particles of radioactive dust, or radioactive liquids, gases, or smoke. If he is properly decontaminated before arrival of rescue personnel, there will be little danger, provided the source of the radiation is no longer exposed at the scene. After exposure to ionizing radiation, the patient is not radioactive. Therefore, he poses no hazard to rescue personnel.

In contrast, the *dirty* accident, often associated with fire at the scene of a radiation accident, exposes the patient to radiation and contaminates him with radioactive particles or liquids. The scene may be highly contaminated, although the primary source of radiation is shielded when rescue personnel arrive. Unless you are properly trained in dealing with this type of emergency, you may have to delay rescue procedures until properly trained technical assistance arrives.

Content Review

"CLEAN" RADIATION ACCIDENTS

Patient is exposed to radiation but not contaminated by radioactive particles, liquids, gases, or smoke.

"DIRTY" RADIATION ACCIDENTS

Patient is contaminated by radioactive particles, liquids, gases, or smoke.

MANAGEMENT

In a radiation accident, externally radiated *and* internally contaminated *patients pose little danger to rescue personnel. Provide normal emergency care.* Externally contaminated *patients must be decontaminated before normal emergency care is initiated. Paramedic personnel and equipment must be decontaminated after the call.*

If you find yourself involved in a radioactive emergency, take the following precautionary steps:

- Park the rescue vehicle upwind to minimize contamination.
- Look for signs of radiation exposure. Radioactive packages are marked by clearly identifiable color-coded labels (Figure 36-8).
- Use portable instruments to measure the level of radioactivity. If dose estimates are significant, rotate rescue personnel.
- Normal principles of emergency care should be applied, for example, ABCs, shock management, and trauma care.
- Externally radiated patients pose little danger to rescue personnel. Initiate normal care procedures for injuries other than radiation.
- Internally contaminated patients (who have ingested or inhaled radioactive particles) pose little danger to rescue personnel. Normal care procedures should be undertaken. Collect body wastes. If assisted ventilation is required, use a bag-valve-mask unit or demand valve. If radioactive particles are inhaled, swab the nasal passages and save the swabs.

FIGURE 36-8 Radioactive warning labels.

- Externally contaminated patients (liquids, dirt, smoke) require decontamination. Following decontamination, initiate normal emergency care procedures. Decontamination of paramedic personnel and equipment is required after the call is completed.
- Patients with open, contaminated wounds require normal emergency care procedures. Avoid cross-contamination of wounds.

SUMMARY

Our environment provides us with all that we need to survive and prosper. The extremes of our environment, however, can have significant impact on human metabolism. Our bodies will, of course, compensate for these extremes, but sometimes it is not enough. Sometimes the heat gain or loss is too much. Sometimes the pressure change is too much. As a result, medical illnesses and emergencies arise. These can range from abnormal core body temperatures to decompensation, shock, and even death.

Basic knowledge of common environmental, recreational, and exposure emergencies is necessary in order for you to administer prompt and proper treatment in the prehospital setting. It is not easy to remember this type of information since these problems are not usually encountered on a daily basis. Remember the general principles involved. Remove the environmental influence causing the problem. Support the patient's own attempt to compensate. Finally, select a definitive care location and transport the patient as rapidly as possible.

In every case, remember that you must maintain your own safety. There are too many cases in which paramedics have lost their lives as a result of attempting a rescue for which they were not properly trained. Rapid action is always necessary when performing an environmental rescue. However, common sense must prevail.

CHAPTER 37

Infectious Disease

Objectives

After reading this chapter, you should be able to:

1. Describe the specific anatomy and physiology pertinent to infectious and communicable diseases. (pp. 1557–1561; also see Chapter 4)
2. Define specific terminology identified with infectious/communicable diseases. (pp. 1556–1603)
3. Discuss public health principles relevant to infectious/communicable diseases. (pp. 1556–1557)
4. Identify public health agencies involved in the prevention and management of disease outbreaks. (p. 1557)
5. List and describe the steps of an infectious process. (pp. 1562–1564)
6. Discuss the risks associated with infection. (pp. 1556, 1562–1564)
7. List and describe the stages of infectious diseases. (pp. 1562–1564)
8. List and describe infectious agents, including bacteria, viruses, fungi, protozoans, and helminths (worms). (pp. 1557–1561)

Continued

INTRODUCTION

infectious disease illness caused by infestation of the body by biological organisms.

Infectious diseases are illnesses caused by infestation of the body by biological organisms such as bacteria, viruses, fungi, protozoans, and helminths (worms). Most infectious disease states are not life-threatening and the patient recovers completely. Some types of infection, however, such as human immunodeficiency virus (HIV), hepatitis B virus (HBV), and acute bacterial meningitis, are particularly dangerous and may result in death or permanent disability.

All health care professionals must maintain a strong working knowledge of public health principles and infectious diseases. This is especially true for paramedics, who are often the first to encounter patients with communicable diseases. Early recognition and management of these patients may make a difference in how the patient is treated and may also ensure that care providers take necessary precautions to prevent the spread of the disease to others.

This chapter discusses infectious diseases, including the types of disease-causing organisms, functions of the immune system, and general pathophysiology of infectious diseases. It emphasizes the specific diseases, discussing those that you may encounter during interhospital transports or out-of-hospital care, especially those that you are most likely to encounter in the field.

PUBLIC HEALTH PRINCIPLES

When dealing with infectious diseases, you must consider the impact of the disease process on the community as well as on the infected patient. An infectious agent is a "hazardous material" that can affect large numbers of people.

Epidemiologists, health professionals who study how infectious diseases affect populations, attempt to describe and predict how diseases move from individuals to populations. Through various clinically based studies and statistical techniques, they try to determine how effectively an infectious agent can travel through a population. Using the population of infected individuals as a standard, they attempt to predict those individuals in the larger population who may be most at risk for contracting the infectious agent. Recognizing that risk may be predictable, and not just random, is important. The characteristics of the host, the infectious agent, and the environment may yield clues as to how the infectious agent is transmitted and reveal individuals or populations susceptible to infection.

How a population is identified is important. It may be defined by such parameters as geographic boundary, workplace, school, correctional institution, age group, income level, or ethnic group. All of the characteristics of a certain population are known as its demographics. The population's tendency to expand, decline, or move is important as well. Besides stimulating social and economic progress, the movement of people and animals within and among other societies also provides a vehicle for infectious agents.

index case the individual who first introduced an infectious agent to a population.

To track the progress of infection within a population, epidemiologists work backward through the chain of infection to determine the **index case,** that individual who first introduced the infectious agent to the population. From the index case, they then retrace the chain forward to verify their reconstruction of the infection's pattern.

To gauge a disease's potential impact on the community, paramedics must evaluate the host (patient), what they believe to be the infectious agent, and the environment. Based on that assessment, they may use more aggressive personal protective equipment. They must also consider the patient, those in the patient's immediate environment, and those in the environment where the patient is being transported all to be at risk for infection. On a more personal level, paramedics must appreciate that they and their families could also be at risk.

PUBLIC HEALTH AGENCIES

Local agencies are the first line of defense in disease surveillance and outbreak. Municipal, city, and county agencies, including fire departments, ambulance services, and health departments, must cooperate to monitor and report the incidence and prevalence of disease.

At the state level, a designated agency (health department or board of health, for instance) generally monitors infectious diseases. These agencies may set policies requiring vaccinations and regulate or implement control programs in vector and animal control, food preparation, water, sewer, and other sanitation control programs. State and local laws sometimes require these agencies to meet or exceed federal guidelines and recommendations.

A number of federal agencies are involved in tracking the morbidity and mortality of infectious diseases. The U.S. Department of Health and Human Services (DHHS) Centers for Disease Control and Prevention (CDC) in Atlanta, Georgia, is the most visible federal agency. The CDC monitors national disease data and freely disseminates this information to all health care providers. It sends personnel nationally and internationally to assist with studying, characterizing, and managing serious disease outbreaks. The CDC is also involved in researching infectious diseases. The National Institute for Occupational Safety and Health (NIOSH), also under the aegis of DHHS, works with the U.S. Department of Labor's Occupational Safety and Health Administration (OSHA), in setting standards and guidelines for workplace and worker controls to prevent infectious diseases in the workplace. This level of federal government involvement would not be possible without the leadership of the U.S. Congress in establishing national health policies and in drafting the federal budget.

Other organizations and governmental agencies that might serve as resources to your organization include the Federal Emergency Management Agency (FEMA), the National Fire Protection Association (NFPA), the United States Fire Protection Administration (USFPA), and the International Association of Firefighters (IAFF). These groups develop helpful blueprints for incorporating OSHA, NIOSH, and other standards and guidelines into daily operations.

Local agencies are the first line of defense in disease surveillance and outbreak.

MICROORGANISMS

The vast majority of disease-causing organisms are microscopic (visible only under a microscope). These microorganisms surround us. They are on our skin and in the air we breathe, and they colonize virtually every orifice of our bodies. Some can even live in the highly acidic environment of our stomachs, which destroys other disease-producing microorganisms or deactivates their toxic products. Microorganisms that reside in our bodies without ordinarily causing disease are part of the *host defenses* known as **normal flora**. Normal flora help keep us disease-free by creating environmental conditions that are not conducive to disease-producing microorganisms, or **pathogens.** Competition between colonies of normal flora and pathogens also discourages the survival of pathogens. Common bacterial pathogens include *Staphylococci, Streptococci,* and *Enterobacteriaceae.* Certain viruses, rickettsiae, fungi, and protozoans are also pathogenic.

* **normal flora** organisms that live inside our bodies without ordinarily causing disease.

* **pathogen** organism capable of causing disease.

FIGURE 37-1 Bacteria are single-celled organisms that range in length from one to twenty micrometers.

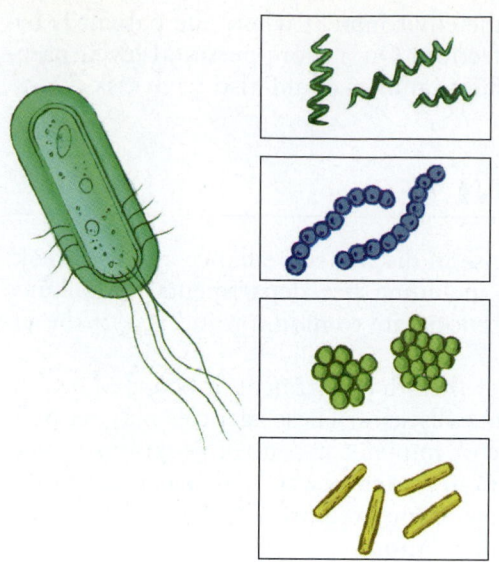

Opportunistic pathogens are ordinarily nonharmful bacteria that cause disease only under unusual circumstances. Most opportunistic pathogens are normal flora. Patients who have a weakened immune system or who are under unusual stress become susceptible to diseases caused by opportunistic organisms. For example, the fungus *Pneumocystis carinii* is usually harmless but can cause a deadly form of pneumonia in patients with HIV. The fungus overwhelms the weakened immune system and begins to reproduce rapidly in the lungs. Left untreated, *Pneumocystis carinii* pneumonia may be fatal. Organ transplant recipients are also at increased risk for infectious diseases because they must take immunosuppressant medications to prevent organ rejection. A more common (and less harmful) opportunistic infection is thrush (oral candidiasis), often seen in patients who take broad spectrum antibiotics. As the antibiotic kills normal bacterial flora in the mouth, the fungus *Candida albicans* grows almost uninhibited on the tongue and in the pharynx, producing a white coating on the mucosa.

BACTERIA

Bacteria are microscopic single-celled organisms that range in length from one to twenty micrometers (Figure 37-1). They are living cells that are classified as *prokaryotes* because they do not have a distinct nuclear membrane and possess only one chromosome in the cytoplasm. Bacteria reproduce independently, but they require a host to supply food and a supportive environment. Some common diseases caused by pathogenic bacteria include sinusitis, otitis media, bacterial pneumonia, pharyngitis (strep throat), tuberculosis, and most urinary tract infections.

Most bacteria are easily identifiable with stains or by their appearance under a microscope. Similar colorfastness indicates similarities in cell wall structure and other anatomic features. The **Gram stain** is the most common method of differentiating bacteria. Bacteria this process turns purple are known as gram-positive bacteria; those it turns red are gram-negative. Because of the similarities in their cell walls, bacteria that stain alike may respond to similar treatments.

* **opportunistic pathogen** ordinarily nonharmful bacterium that causes disease only under unusual circumstances.

* **bacteria** microscopic single-celled organisms that range in length from one to twenty micrometers.

* **Gram stain** method of differentiating types of bacteria according to their reaction to a chemical stain process.

Bacteria are further categorized into groups based on their general appearance: cocci, or spheres, (staphylococcus, streptococcus) are round; rods (*Enterobacter* sp., *E. coli*) are elongated; and spirals (spirochetes, vibrio) are coiled. *Enterobacter* sp. and *E. coli* are gram-negative rods. *Staphylococci* and *streptococci* are gram-positive cocci. Regardless of how bacteria stain or appear under a microscope, it is the specific tissues and organs which are infected that chiefly determine the patient's signs and symptoms.

Pathogenic bacteria may harm their human hosts in a number of ways. Heavy colonization may result in direct damage to tissues as the bacteria feed. Bacteria may also cause indirect damage by releasing toxic chemicals that can have localized or systemic effects. The two general categories of toxins are exotoxins and endotoxins. This classification is no longer based primarily on where they originate, as their names imply, but by their chemical structures. **Exotoxins** are poisonous proteins shed by bacteria during bacterial growth. They stimulate the immune system to form antibodies to these proteins, and they may also be deactivated by chemicals, light, or heat. Exotoxins are more toxic than endotoxins. The infectious agent of toxic shock syndrome, *S. aureus,* releases an exotoxin, as does anthrax, which can be delivered as a biological weapon of mass destruction.

Endotoxins are composed of proteins, polysaccharides (large sugar molecules), and lipids. The immune system cannot form antibodies specific to a particular endotoxin unless both the protein and polysaccharide portions are present. Endotoxins come from the bacterial cell wall and are released when the bacterial cell is destroyed. They are more stable in heat than exotoxins. Only gram-negative bacteria make endotoxins. The skin lesions of meningococcemia and the signs of shock that sometimes accompany it are due to large amounts of endotoxin released by the infectious agent, *N. menningitidis.*

Most bacterial infections respond to treatment with antibiotics that are either **bactericidal** (kill bacteria) or **bacteriostatic** (inhibit bacterial growth or reproduction). Antibiotics are prescribed based on bacterial sensitivity; different antibiotics are required to treat different bacteria. Their administration usually decreases bacterial presence and reduces symptoms. Some types of bacterial infections respond quickly to antibiotics; others take longer. In recent years, a number of bacterial strains have developed resistance to antibiotic therapy, making treatment more difficult. The more a type of bacterium is exposed to an antibiotic, the greater the likelihood of its developing resistance. The overuse of antibiotics in both medical and veterinary settings has contributed to this serious problem. Resistant forms of tuberculosis (mycobacterium) are of particular concern. Antibiotics may now be ineffective against this disease, and its mortality rate is high. The willingness of some physicians to prescribe the newest antibiotics for relatively minor infections and the widespread addition of antibiotics to animal feed have only added to the problem.

Antimicrobial treatment alters the normal flora of the skin, mouth, mucosa, and gastrointestinal tract and often results in colonization of those areas by new microorganisms that resist antibiotics. In some cases, an antibiotic may kill normal flora and allow more virulent and dangerous opportunistic pathogens to multiply freely. This can lead to a secondary infection that is more severe than the original infection being treated. For all of these reasons, antibiotics should be prescribed cautiously.

VIRUSES

Viruses are much smaller than bacteria and can be seen only with an electron microscope (Figure 37-2). Viruses cannot reproduce and carry on metabolism by themselves. Therefore, they are considered to be neither prokaryotes nor eukaryotes.

Content Review

TYPES OF BACTERIA
- Spheres (cocci)
- Rods
- Spirals

✱ **exotoxin** toxic waste products released by living bacteria.

✱ **endotoxin** toxic products released when bacteria die and decompose.

✱ **bactericidal** capable of killing bacteria.

✱ **bacteriostatic** capable of inhibiting bacterial growth or reproduction.

✱ **virus** disease-causing organism that can be seen only with an electron microscope.

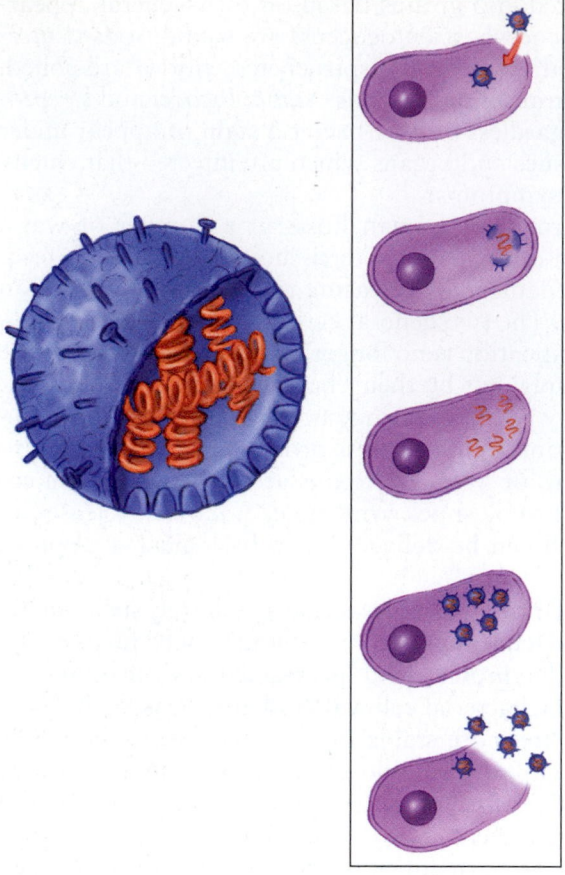

✱ **obligate intracellular parasite** organism that can grow and reproduce only within a host cell.

Instead, viruses are **obligate intracellular parasites;** that is, they can grow and reproduce only within a host cell. Once inside, the virus takes control of the host cell's protein synthesis mechanism and directs it to begin reproducing the virus. The cell then releases new virus particles, which infect nearby cells.

Since viruses "hide" inside the host's cells, they resist antibiotic treatment. Once a virus enters a host cell, it becomes part of that host cell, making selective eradication of the virus virtually impossible, as any treatment capable of killing the virus will generally kill the host cell as well. This is the major obstacle facing researchers as they work to find cures for HIV and other viruses.

Approximately 400 types of viruses have been identified. One frequently encountered viral disorder, the common cold, is caused by a number of different viruses (nearly 200) that all produce similar symptoms. Fortunately, most viral diseases are mild and self-limiting. They run their course until the patient's immune system eventually fights them off. A host is generally susceptible to any particular virus only once. Once a person's immune system develops active immunity against a particular type of virus, it becomes attuned to similar attacking viruses and will destroy them.

OTHER MICROORGANISMS

✱ **prions** particles of protein, folded in such a way that protease enzymes cannot act upon them.

Prions are a new classification of disease-producing agents that microbiologists used to refer to as "slow viruses." They are neither prokaryotes nor eukaryotes but particles of protein, folded in such a way that proteases (enzymes that break down proteins) cannot act upon them. These protein particles accumulate in nervous system and brain tissue, destroying them and giving them a spongy appearance on gross examination. Prions are known to cause progressive, untreatable dementia in Kuru, Creutzfeldt-Jakob disease, mad cow disease, and fatal familial insomnia. Although EMS providers will rarely respond to patients with diseases caused by prions, a general discussion of infectious agents must acknowledge their existence.

Fungi are plant-like microorganisms, most of which are not pathogenic. Yeasts, molds, and mushrooms are types of fungi. Some fungi have a capsule around the cell wall that provides additional protection against phagocytes. While fungi compose a large part of the body's normal flora, they may become pathogenic in patients with compromised immune function, such as those with HIV. Fungi may also lead to disease states in patients taking broad-spectrum antibiotics. As the antibiotics kill off bacteria, the fungi are able to grow uninhibited. Fungi are a common cause of vaginal infections and often cause pneumonia in patients with weakened immune systems.

* **fungus** plant-like microorganism.

Protozoa are single-celled parasitic organisms with flexible membranes and the ability to move. Most protozoa live in the soil and ingest decaying organic matter. Although rarely a cause of disease in humans, they are considered opportunistic pathogens in patients with compromised immune function. These organisms may enter the body by the fecal-oral route or through a mosquito bite. Common diseases caused by protozoa include malaria and forms of gastroenteritis. Protozoa also cause vaginal infections (trichomoniasis) in women with normal immune function.

* **protozoan** single-celled parasitic organism with flexible membranes and the ability to move.

Parasites are common causes of disease where sanitation is poor (generally in developing countries). Occasional cases are seen in this country. Roundworms (ascarides) live in the intestinal mucosa and may reach 30–50 cm in length. Symptoms include abdominal cramping, fever, and cough. Diagnosis usually depends on finding eggs in the patient's stool.

* **parasite** organism that lives in or on another organism.

Pinworms (*Enterobius vermicularis*) are common in the United States and in other civilized countries. It is estimated that 20 percent of children living in temperate climates harbor this disease. These tiny worms (3–10 mm long) live in the distal colon and crawl onto the anal mucosa to lay their eggs, usually when the host is asleep. Although the disease may remain asymptomatic, it is a common cause of anal pruritus (itching) and infection and is easily spread among children, especially in day-care centers. Children may carry the disease home and infect their entire family. This disease is often endemic among institutionalized children. Treatment involves a single dose of an antibiotic (mebendazole); all family members must be treated simultaneously to avoid reinfection.

* **pinworm** parasite that is 3–10 mm long and lives in the distal colon.

Hookworms (*Ancylostoma duodenale, Necator americanus*) are found in warm, moist climates. This parasite infects an estimated 25 percent of the world's population, although it is relatively rare in the United States. The larvae are passed in the stool of infected animals. The disease is most commonly contracted when a barefoot child walks in a contaminated area. The larvae enter through the skin and migrate to the intestines, where they grip and irritate the intestinal wall and feed on blood. Epigastric pain and anemia are possible. Prevention involves wearing shoes; treatment is similar to that for pinworms.

* **hookworm** parasite that attaches to the host's intestinal lining.

Trichinosis (*Trichinella spiralis*) may be contracted by eating raw or inadequately cooked pork products, most commonly sausage. Females burrow into the intestinal wall and produce thousands of living larvae that migrate to skeletal muscle, where each forms a cyst and remains. Symptoms include gastrointestinal disturbances, edema (especially of the eyelids), fever, and a variety of other diffuse and secondary symptoms. If the worms invade the heart, lungs, or brain in large numbers, death may result. Diagnosis is made by finding encysted worms during examination of muscle biopsy. Mebendazole is the antibiotic of choice.

* **trichinosis** disease resulting from an infestation of *Trichinella spriralis*.

Other types of worms such as tapeworms and flukes are rarely encountered in the United States.

CONTRACTION, TRANSMISSION, AND STAGES OF DISEASE

As a paramedic you must understand the relationship between the pathophysiology and the assessment and management of patients with infections or diseases resulting from infections. This knowledge will prepare you for leadership in recognizing infectious diseases and curbing their transmission.

The interactions of host, infectious agent, and environment are the elements of disease transmission. Studying each of these factors individually and then looking for relationships among them often reveals how an infectious agent has been effectively transmitted. Infectious agents exist in all types of **reservoirs**— animals, humans, insects, and the environment. While inhabiting animal or insect reservoirs, they do not cause disease. Their presence at any time in a given environment is affected by their life cycle, by the presence of stressors that may force them outside of their normal reservoirs, and by the climate. The initiation of therapy can sometimes disrupt the life cycle of the infectious agent and may eradicate the infection. When a host and infectious agent come together at the right time and under the right conditions, disease transmission takes place.

Infectious agents may invade hosts through one of two basic mechanisms. The more common is direct transmission from person to person through a cough, sneeze, kiss, or sexual contact. The other mechanism, indirect transmission, can spread organisms in a number of ways. Infected persons often shed organisms into the environment. These organisms come to rest on doorknobs, handrails, computer keyboards, and so on. Other people who contact those surfaces are at risk for contracting the disease. Similarly, microorganisms may be transmitted via food products, water, or even through the soil.

Bloodborne diseases are transmitted by contact with the blood or body fluids of an infected person. They include AIDS, hepatitis B, hepatitis C, hepatitis D, and syphilis. The risk of transmission of bloodborne diseases increases if a patient has open wounds, active bleeding, or increased secretions. Assume that every patient has an infectious bloodborne disease and take precautions to avoid contact with blood and other body fluids.

Some infectious diseases may be transmitted through the air on droplets expelled during a productive cough or sneeze. They include tuberculosis, meningitis, mumps, measles, rubella, and chicken pox (varicella). Other, more common diseases such as the common cold, influenza, and respiratory syncytial virus (RSV) may also be transmitted by the **airborne** route.

Some infectious diseases are transmitted orally (primarily by eating) or by the **fecal-oral route,** in which enteric microorganisms (normally found in the GI system and the feces) are transmitted between potential hosts, as in shaking hands or other social customs, and then having the recipient somehow introduce the infectious agent into his mouth by scratching or eating with his hands. Fecal-oral diseases are prevalent in third world countries or in areas with unsanitary conditions. Hepatitis A, hepatitis E, and other viruses can be transmitted by this route. Foodborne illnesses include food poisoning, certain parasitic infections, and trichinosis.

The risk of infection is considered *theoretical* if transmission is acknowledged to be possible but has not actually been reported. It is considered *measurable* if factors in the infectious agent's transmission and their associated risks have been identified or deduced from reported data. Generally, the risk of disease transmission rises if a patient has open wounds, increased secretions, active coughing, or any ongoing invasive treatment where exposure to an infectious body fluid is likely (Table 37-1). In the prehospital setting, the unpredictable environment and behavior of patients increase the risk of exposure. For example, a patient with a

---

* **reservoir** any living creature or environment (water, soil, etc.) that can harbor an infectious agent.

* **bloodborne** transmitted by contact with blood or body fluids.

* **airborne** transmitted through the air by droplets or particles.

* **fecal-oral route** transmission of organisms picked up from the gastrointestinal tract (e.g., feces) into the mouth.

Generally, the risk of disease transmission rises if a patient has open wounds, increased secretions, active coughing, or any ongoing invasive treatment where exposure to an infectious body fluid is likely.

Table 37-1 MODES OF TRANSMISSION OF INFECTIOUS DISEASES

Disease	Blood-borne	Airborne	Sexual	Indirect	Opportunist	Oral-Fecal
Hepatitis A						✔
Hepatitis B	✔					
Hepatitis C						
HIV	✔		✔			
Influenza		✔	✔	✔		
Syphilis			✔			
Gonorrhea			✔			
Measles		✔				
Mumps		✔				
Strep throat		✔			✔	
Herpes virus	✔		✔	✔		
Food poisoning		✔		✔		✔
Lyme disease	✔					
Pneumonia		✔			✔	

closed head injury and multiple lacerations may be combative, thereby contaminating EMS personnel with blood or other body fluids. Broken windshield glass contaminated with blood may easily penetrate examination gloves and skin. Patients who are violent and aggressive may deliberately bite, scratch, or spit at rescuers. Many EMS patient care activities occur in a closed, poorly ventilated environment such as the back of an ambulance. Thus, you must have available, and routinely use, protective clothing and other barrier devices, as indicated.

Not all exposures to microorganisms from body fluids or infected patients will result in transmission of those agents. Nor are all infectious agents and diseases **communicable** (capable of being transmitted to another host). Communicability depends on several factors. Exposure to an infectious agent may just result in **contamination**, in which the agent exists only on the surface of the host without penetrating it. Penetration of the host implies that **infection** has occurred, but infection should never be equated with disease. Factors that affect the likelihood that an exposed individual will become infected and then actually develop disease include:

- *Correct mode of entry* Certain external barriers in hosts, particularly the skin, make it impossible for infectious agents to establish themselves. Mucous membranes, however, often present an effective point of entry.
- *Virulence* **Virulence** is an organism's strength or ability to infect or overcome the body's defenses. Some organisms, such as the hepatitis B virus (HBV), are very virulent and can remain infectious on a surface for weeks. Others, such as HIV and syphilis, die when exposed to air and light. Some bacteria (Clostridium) may remain dormant in the soil for months and be capable of causing disease if contracted. Infection generally occurs either when a highly virulent microorganism interacts with a normal, intact host or when a less virulent microorganism enters a host with impaired defenses (immunosuppression).

✱ **communicable** capable of being transmitted to another host.

✱ **contamination** presence of an agent only on the surface of the host without penetrating it.

✱ **infection** presence of an agent within the host, without necessarily causing disease.

Content Review

FACTORS AFFECTING DISEASE TRANSMISSION
- Mode of entry
- Virulence
- Number of organisms transmitted
- Host resistance

✱ **virulence** an organism's strength or ability to infect or overcome the body's defenses.

- *Number of Organisms Transmitted (Dose)* For most diseases, a minimum number of organisms must enter the host to cause infection. As a rule, the higher the number, the greater the likelihood of contracting the disease.

- *Host Resistance* **Resistance** is the host's the ability to fight off infection. Several factors affect the host's resistance. They include general health and fitness, genetic predisposition or resistance to infection, nutrition status, recent exposure to stressors, hygiene, and the presence of underlying disease processes. Persons with decreased immune function are at significantly increased risk for contracting infectious diseases. Cigarette smokers and those regularly exposed to secondhand cigarette smoke are also at increased risk.

- *Other Host Factors* The tendency of the host to travel or be in contact with other potential hosts, the age and socioeconomic status of the host, the characteristics of other hosts within the population of which the infected host is a member all effect the likelihood of contracting disease.

PHASES OF THE INFECTIOUS PROCESS

Disease progression varies greatly, depending on the infectious agent and the host. Conditions can manifest themselves in various ways. Once infected with an infectious agent, the host goes through a **latent period** when he cannot transmit the agent to someone else. Following the latent period is a **communicable period** when the host may exhibit signs of clinical disease and can transmit the infectious agent to another host.

The appearance of symptoms often lags after exposure to an infectious disease. The time between exposure and presentation, known as the **incubation period,** may range from a few days, as in the common cold, to months or years, as in HIV/AIDS or hepatitis. Thus, prehospital personnel must be notified if any patient for whom they provide care subsequently develops a life-threatening infectious disease.

Most viruses and bacteria have surface proteins, or **antigens,** that stimulate the body to produce **antibodies.** These antibodies react to or unite with the antigens. The antibodies' presence in the blood indicates exposure to the particular disease that they fight. Although testing for the presence of a specific disease antigen is difficult, laboratory tests can often spot antibodies that are specific for the disease or antigen. For example, they detect the human immunodeficiency virus (HIV) through the presence of antibodies specific to HIV. When a person develops antibodies after exposure to a disease, his previously negative test will be positive and **seroconversion** has occurred. The time between exposure to disease and seroconversion is referred to as the **window phase.** A person in the window phase may test negative even though he is infected. From the standpoint of the immune system response, the window phase is the period when antigen is present but antibody production has not reached detectable levels. The **disease period** is the duration from the onset of signs and symptoms of disease until the resolution of symptoms or death. Keep in mind that the resolution of symptoms does not necessarily imply that the infectious agent has been eradicated.

INFECTION CONTROL

The body protects itself from disease in many ways. At the basic level, skin defends against invading pathogens. Turbulent airflow through the airway and nasal hair assist in capturing foreign bodies. Mucus can trap and kill foreign materials. Coughing and sneezing expel foreign materials. Further, as you learned in Chapter 4 on pathophysiology, the body has a very sophisiticated immune system. The complement and lymphatic systems also assist in fighting infection through inflammatory responses and filtering of body fluids.

To supplement the body's natural defenses against disease, EMS providers must protect themselves from infectious exposures (Figure 37-3). The four phases of infection control in prehospital care include preparation for response, response, patient contact, and recovery.

PREPARATION FOR RESPONSE

Infection control begins long before an emergency call. To ensure proper protection, the EMS agency should implement the following procedures:

- Establish and maintain written standard operating procedures (SOPs) for infection control, and monitor employee compliance.
- Prepare an infection control plan that includes a schedule of when and how to implement OSHA, NIOSH, and CDC pathogen standards and guidelines.
- Provide adequate original and ongoing infection control training to all personnel, including engineering and work practice controls.

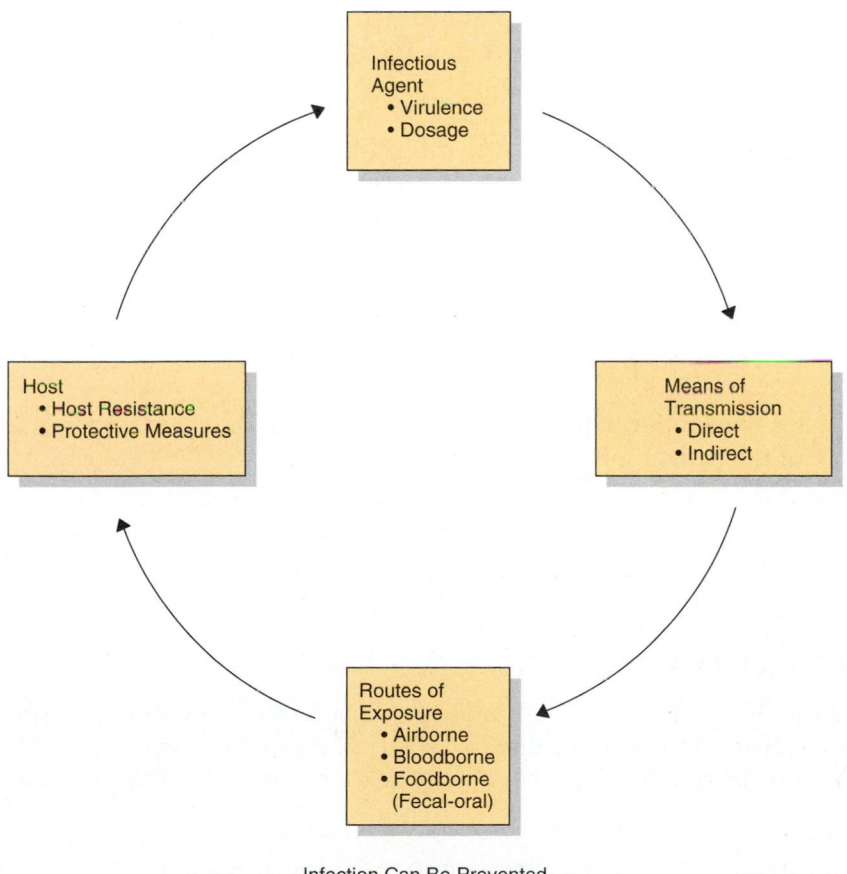

Infection Can Be Prevented by Interrupting the Disease Process

FIGURE 37-3 Interruption of infectious disease transmission is a role of prehospital personnel.

- Ensure that all employees are provided with personal protective equipment (PPE) and that it is fitted appropriately, checked regularly, maintained properly, and can be located easily.
- Ensure that all EMS personnel treat and bandage all personal wounds (e.g., open sores, cuts, or skin breaks) before any emergency response.
- Use disposable supplies and equipment whenever possible. The risk of transmitting disease is generally much lower than when reusing items, even though they have been cleaned or disinfected.
- Assure that all EMS personnel have access to the facilities and supplies needed to maintain a high level of personal hygiene.
- Do not allow EMS personnel to deliver patient care if they exhibit signs or symptoms of an infectious disease.
- Monitor all EMS personnel for compliance with vaccinations and appropriate diagnostic tests (e.g., **PPD**, antibody titers).
- Appoint a designated infectious disease control officer (IDCO) to serve as a contact person for personnel exposed to an infectious disease and monitor the infection control program.
- Identify specific job classifications and work processes in which the possibility of exposure exists.
- Provide haz-mat (hazardous materials) education for employees, including how to locate and interpret material safety data sheets (MSDS) regarding chemicals or chemical mixtures with information on the associated health hazards.

Do not assume that your EMS agency can protect you from exposure to all infectious agents. Your attitude toward protecting yourself against infectious agents is one measure of your professionalism.

✳ PPD purified protein derivative, the substance used in a test for tuberculosis.

RESPONSE

When responding to an EMS call, take the following infection control measures:

- Obtain as much information as possible from dispatch regarding the nature of the patient's illness or injury.
- Prepare for patient contact. Put on gloves and don eye and face protection before patient contact whenever practical.
- Prepare mentally for the call. Think *infection control!*

PATIENT CONTACT

Your contact with a patient, especially at an emergency scene, poses your highest risk for acquiring an infectious disease.

Your contact with a patient, especially at an emergency scene, poses your highest risk for acquiring an infectious disease. Have all personal protective equipment with you before leaving the emergency vehicle, and follow these guidelines:

- Isolate all body substances and avoid any contact with them.
- Wear appropriate personal protective equipment such as gowns, gloves, face shields, masks, protective eyewear, aprons, and similar items.

Table 37-2	GUIDELINES FOR PREVENTION OF TRANSMISSION OF HIV AND HBV TO PREHOSPITAL PERSONNEL			
Task or Activity	**Disposable Gloves**	**Gown**	**Mask**	**Protective Eyewear**
Bleeding control with active bleeding	Yes	Yes	Yes	Yes
Bleeding control with minimal bleeding	Yes	No	No	No
Emergency childbirth	Yes	Yes	Yes	Yes
Blood drawing	Yes	No	No	No
IV insertion	Yes	No	No	No
Endotracheal intubation	Yes	No	Yes	Yes
EOA insertion	Yes	No	Yes	Yes
Oral/nasal suctioning; manually clearing airway	Yes	Yes	Yes	Yes
Handling/cleaning instruments with possible contamination	Yes	Yes	Yes	Yes
Measuring blood pressure	Yes	No	No	No
Giving an injection	Yes	No	No	No
Measuring temperature	Yes	No	No	No
Rescuing from a building fire	Yes	No	No	No
Cleaning back of ambulance after a medical call	Yes	No	No	No

- Allow only necessary personnel to make patient contact. Limit the risk to as few people as possible, thus minimizing exposure.
- Use airway adjuncts such as a pocket mask or bag-valve-mask unit to minimize exposure. Disposable items are preferable.
- Properly dispose of biohazardous waste.
- Use extreme caution with sharp instruments. Utilize retractable IV needles and needleless injection systems when possible. Never bend, recap, or remove contaminated needles. Dispose of all contaminated sharps in properly labeled puncture-resistant containers.
- Never smoke, eat, or drink in the patient compartment of the ambulance. Each service should have strict guidelines regarding the presence of food and drink in the driver compartment during down times. Strictly adhere to OSHA guidelines.
- Do not apply cosmetics, lip balm, or handle contact lenses when a likelihood of exposure exists.

Table 37-2 details specific measures for protection against HIV (human immunodeficiency virus) and HBV (hepatitis B virus) infections.

RECOVERY

Infection control does not end when you deliver the patient to the emergency department. Decontaminating the ambulance and equipment is essential. Take the following steps at the completion of each response:

Infection control does not end when you deliver the patient to the emergency department.

- Wash hands immediately after patient contact. Ample data substantiate that *effective, vigorous* hand washing is superior to some disinfectants. On-scene, you can wipe your hands with a waterless hand-cleansing solution. However, this provides for only partial cleansing because it cannot grossly remove the particles to which microorganisms adhere. Only soap and water can do that. Upon returning to quarters, or at the earliest opportunity, thoroughly wash your hands with soap and warm water, paying attention to the webs between fingers. Overlooking this important habit may result in the inadvertent contamination of personal clothing or anything else that you contact. Such oversight can result in transmitting the disease to family and friends.

- If you sustain a wound and are exposed to the body fluids of others, vigorously wash the wound with soap and warm water immediately, *before* contacting your employer or IDCO.

- Dispose of all biohazardous wastes in accordance with local laws and regulations.

- Place potentially infectious wastes in leak-proof biohazard bags. Bag any soiled linen and label for laundry personnel (Figure 37-4).

- Decontaminate all contaminated clothing and reusable equipment.

- Handle uniforms in accordance with the agency's standard procedures for personal protective equipment.

FIGURE 37-4 Bag all linen and label it infectious.

Decontamination Methods and Procedures

Decontaminate infected equipment according to local protocol and SOPs established by the EMS agency. Perform decontamination in a designated area that is properly marked and secured. The room should have a suitable ventilation system and adequate drainage. Be sure to wear gloves, gowns, boots, protective eyewear, and a face mask. To begin decontamination, remove surface dirt and debris with soap and water. Then disinfect and, if required, sterilize all items. The four levels of decontamination are low-level disinfection, intermediate-level disinfection, high-level disinfection, and sterilization.

Low-Level Disinfection Low-level **disinfection** destroys most bacteria and some viruses and fungi. It does not destroy *Mycobacterium tuberculosis* or bacterial spores. Use low-level disinfection for routine housekeeping and cleaning, as well as for removing visible body fluids. All EPA-registered disinfectants are suitable for low-level disinfection.

Intermediate-Level Disinfection Intermediate-level disinfection destroys *Mycobacterium tuberculosis* and most viruses and fungi. It does not, however, destroy bacterial spores. Use it for all equipment that has come into contact with intact skin such as stethoscopes, splints, and blood pressure cuffs. A 1:10 to 1:100 dilution of water and chlorine bleach is acceptable for intermediate-level disinfection. Hard-surface germicides and EPA-registered disinfectants/chemical germicides are also effective.

High-Level Disinfection High-level disinfection destroys all forms of microorganisms except certain bacterial spores. High-level disinfection is required for all reusable devices that have come into contact with mucous membranes, including laryngoscopes, Magill forceps, and airway adjuncts. For high-level disinfection, immerse objects in an EPA-approved chemical-sterilizing agent for 10 to 45 seconds (depending upon the manufacturer's instructions). Alternatively, immerse the device in hot water (176°–212°F) for 30 minutes.

Sterilization Sterilization destroys all microorganisms and is required for all contaminated invasive instruments. An autoclave that uses pressurized steam or ethylene-oxide gas effectively sterilizes equipment. These methods, however, are rarely available outside of a hospital setting. Alternatively, prolonged immersion (6–10 hours, depending on the manufacturer's instructions) in an EPA-approved chemical-sterilizing agent is usually adequate. Whenever possible, use disposable instruments for invasive procedures.

INFECTIOUS DISEASE EXPOSURES

Infectious disease exposures occur during all hours of a work shift. Since you may not always be able to contact an agency administrator, you need a working knowledge of your agency's standard operating procedures, as well as of the laws and regulations applicable to exposures. The following recommendations will help to ensure that exposure management will protect you, other emergency responders and health care professionals, the agency, and the confidentiality of the patient's information.

Reporting an Infectious Disease Exposure Immediately report exposures of EMS personnel to the designated IDCO, according to local protocol. Report all exposures to blood, blood products, or any potentially infectious material, regardless of their perceived severity. This will permit immediate medical follow-up,

---

❋ decontaminate to destroy or remove pathogens.

Content Review

DECONTAMINATION LEVELS
- Low-level disinfection
- Intermediate-level disinfection
- High-level disinfection
- Sterilization

❋ disinfect to destroy certain forms of microorganisms, but not all.

❋ sterilize to destroy all microorganisms.

Report all exposures to blood, blood products, or any potentially infectious material, regardless of their perceived severity.

including counseling for the EMS provider and identification of the infectious agent. It also enables the IDCO to evaluate the circumstances of the exposure and implement changes to prevent future exposures, if needed. Finally, it facilitates follow-up testing if the source individual consents.

The Ryan White Act The **Ryan White Act** is a federal law that outlines the rights and responsibilities of agencies and health care workers when an infectious disease exposure occurs. Under its provisions, the exposed employee has the right to ask the source patient's infection status, but neither the agency nor the employee can force the source individual to be tested. Employers must also tell their employees what to do if an exposure occurs.

Federal law further mandates that each agency designate an IDCO to whom exposures are reported. This officer coordinates implementation of the exposure control plan and follows local reporting requirements.

Postexposure Employers are required to provide a medical evaluation and treatment for any paramedic or other EMS provider exposed to an infectious disease. The nature of the exposure is assessed based on the route, dose, and nature of the infectious agent. As part of the medical evaluation, employees are entitled to receive counseling about alternatives for treatment, the risks of treatment, signs, symptoms, the possibility of developing disease, and preventing further spread of the potential infection. This includes the available medications, their potential side effects, and their contraindications. Treatment must be in line with current United States Public Health Service recommendations.

After a paramedic is exposed to an infectious disease, he has the option to submit a blood sample for baseline testing. If the employee does not consent to having his blood screened for specific diseases, the blood samples are normally maintained for 90 days in the event that he changes his mind.

The IDCO or other health care professional who specializes in occupational infectious diseases should counsel the exposed employee and obtain informed consent for post-exposure prophylaxis (PEP) based on CDC guidelines. All records related to employee counseling and PEP are forwarded to the IDCO. Vaccines may be made available to the employee if deemed appropriate by an occupational medicine physician.

Confidentiality The IDCO will maintain records of all exposures as required by law. All of these exposure records (like any medical records) are confidential. They must not be released to anyone without express written permission from the employee.

ASSESSMENT OF THE PATIENT WITH INFECTIOUS DISEASE

When assessing a patient, always maintain a high index of suspicion that an infectious agent may be involved. Consider the dispatch information, evaluate the environment for its suitability for transmitting infectious agents, and maintain appropriate BSI. Gloves are the mandatory minimum level of personal protective equipment (PPE) required on every patient contact.

When approaching a patient with a possible infectious disease, look for general indicators of infection such as unusual skin signs, fever, weakness, profuse sweating, malaise, anorexia, and unexplained worsening of existing disease states. If an infection is localized, signs of inflammation may include redness, swelling, tenderness to palpation, capillary streaking, and warmth in the affected area. A rash or other diagnostic skin signs may make identifying an infectious disease much easier.

✳ **Ryan White Act** federal law that outlines the rights and responsibilities of agencies and health care workers when an infectious disease exposure occurs.

Approach every scene with a high index of suspicion that a patient may have an infectious disease.

PAST MEDICAL HISTORY

The patient's past medical history (PMH) may provide valuable clues to his illness. Patients who have AIDS or are taking immunosuppressant medications such as steroids are particularly susceptible to infection. COPD patients, patients with autoimmune diseases, and transplant recipients frequently take steroids and immunosuppressants. Persons with diabetes and other endocrine disorders are also more likely to get infections due to additional stressors on their immune systems. Other conditions that increase the risk for developing infectious diseases include alcoholism, malnutrition, IV drug abuse, malignancy (cancer), and splenectomy (removal of the spleen), as well as artificial heart valves (aortic or mitral) or joints (hip or knee). Any significant increase in emotional stress may also increase a person's risk of significant illness, including infectious diseases.

A patient with a PMH of numerous untreated throat infections who suddenly develops a heart murmur, fever, and malaise may have rheumatic fever, a streptococcal infection that can affect the heart. Such patients are often found in medically underserved areas where access to primary care is difficult or nonexistent. Patients with cancer are at increased risk for acquiring numerous opportunistic infectious diseases. A recently transmitted sexual disease may precede systemic infection. Recent unfinished antibiotic treatment may lead to the proliferation of drug-resistant infectious agents, causing recurrent, persistent bacterial infections or development of other opportunistic infections.

In addition to determining past or current illnesses or diseases, thoroughly investigate the patient's chief complaint and any history of the present illness including:

- When did signs and symptoms begin?
- Is fever present? How has the temperature changed over time?
- Has the patient taken any aspirin, acetaminophen, or other medications?
- Does the patient have any neck pain or stiffness when his head is moved, especially during flexion?
- Has the patient had any difficulty swallowing?
- Has the patient had any previous symptoms or illnesses similar to this one?

THE PHYSICAL EXAMINATION

Physical examination of the patient whom you suspect of having an infectious disease follows the standard format for assessing a medical patient. Determine the patient's level of consciousness and vital signs early on. Increased temperature commonly indicates infection. Significant increases in pulse may occur due to the infection and as a result of elevated body temperature. As a consequence, metabolic needs will increase. The patient will require more oxygen and more nutrients to maintain normal physiologic function. This may be a serious problem for elderly, very young, or debilitated patients with concurrent illnesses that limit their cardiovascular and respiratory reserve.

Hypotension in the patient with an infectious disease may result from dehydration, vasodilation, or both, as in septic shock. In rare cases, infections of the heart muscle (endocarditis) may result in decreased cardiac output (cardiogenic shock). In any case, assess the cause of hypotension and treat it promptly. If the lungs are clear, the judicious use of fluids may be beneficial; if fluid status is not a problem, vasopressors such as dopamine may be necessary.

Dehydration is a common consequence of infectious diseases. Increased body temperature is often accompanied by increased respiratory rate and concomitant

Every EMS unit should have the capability of measuring and monitoring body temperature (e.g., a tympanic thermometer).

fluid loss, of which the patient is often unaware (insensible fluid loss). Vomiting or diarrhea can quickly cause life-threatening dehydration, especially in pediatric patients who have large body surface areas relative to their volume. Electrolyte imbalances often occur with fluid loss. Advances in technology that may soon make the prehospital evaluation of electrolytes cost-effective may be indicated in the setting of significant dehydration. Clinically significant dehydration will usually cause tachycardia and hypotension, but you should be vigilant for more subtle signs that include thirst, poor skin turgor, and a shrunken and furrowed tongue. A history of decreased fluid intake, fever, vomiting, and/or diarrhea should trigger a thorough assessment of fluid status. While performing a physical exam similar to that for any patient with a medical emergency, assess the following:

- Skin for temperature, hydration, color, or rash
- Sclera for icterus
- Reaction to neck flexion (Is nuchal rigidity [neck stiffness] present?)
- Lymph nodes for swelling or tenderness (lymphadenopathy)
- Breath sounds (for adventitious sounds and evidence of consolidation)
- Hepatomegaly (enlargement of the liver)
- Purulent (pus-filled) lesions

SELECTED INFECTIOUS DISEASES

The following section profiles infectious diseases that either may be encountered in the prehospital setting or are commonly known by emergency health care practitioners. The first major category includes diseases of immediate concern to EMS. General profiles of other diseases follow. You should be familiar with the terminology of these profiles, realize which diseases you will more commonly encounter in patients, and know which BSI precautions to employ.

DISEASES OF IMMEDIATE CONCERN TO EMS PROVIDERS

The diseases of immediate concern to EMS providers include HIV, hepatitis, tuberculosis, pneumonia, chickenpox, and bacterial meningitis. They are infectious diseases that have gained notoriety, pose a high risk for communicability and debilitating disease, or are relevant to direct patient care. While most attention focuses on reducing transmission from patient to health care worker, the profiles also consider reverse transmission, because responsible health care workers protect both themselves and their patients. The inclusion of chickenpox may surprise some EMS personnel, but the disease is highly communicable and poses a serious occupational risk for unvaccinated or previously unexposed health care workers.

Human Immunodeficiency Virus

The **human immunodeficiency virus (HIV)** is the most discussed and feared infectious agent of the modern era, especially of the last two decades. The clinical condition that it causes, acquired immune deficiency syndrome (AIDS), is not a disease *per se,* but a collection of signs and symptoms that share common anatomical, physiological, and biochemical derangements in the immune system. Like other viruses, HIV utilizes the host cell's reproductive apparatus to copy it-

Content Review

DISEASES OF IMMEDIATE CONCERN TO EMS PROVIDERS

- HIV
- Hepatitis
- Tuberculosis
- Pneumonia
- Chickenpox
- Meningitis

* **human immunodeficiency virus (HIV)** organism responsible for acquired immune deficiency syndrome (AIDS).

self. HIV is a retrovirus, that is, it normally carries its genetic material in RNA (instead of DNA) and utilizes an enzyme called *reverse transcriptase* (hence the designation "*retro*virus") to use RNA to synthesize DNA. This is the reverse of the usual process of transcription of DNA into RNA. The action of reverse transcriptase enables genetic material from a retrovirus to become permanently incorporated into the DNA of an infected cell. Two types of HIV have been identified, HIV-1 and HIV-2. Most research targets the HIV-1 variant, which has proven much more pathogenic than HIV-2.

The emergence of HIV and AIDS, more than any other infectious process, has increased emergency and health care workers' awareness of the dangers of infectious disease. The worldwide research and educational activities resulting from concern about HIV and AIDS are effective models for teaching health care workers and lay persons about how other infectious diseases are transmitted and for providing personal and community action plans to prevent the spread of infectious agents. Although it is a worldwide epidemic, with an especially high mortality rate in sub-Saharan Africa, AIDS poses a significantly lower *occupational* risk to health care workers in developed countries than other infectious agents.

Pathogenesis In the past five years, we have learned about the dynamics of HIV infection and the development of AIDS. It was first assumed that the virus caused a cellular immune system response and then remained in a dormant phase. The humoral response was known to produce antibodies within one to three months after infection, with clinical disease developing in from one to ten years. For unexplained reasons, the virus would become active, and the worsening clinical signs were attributed to an increasing viral population. The extent of immune cell activity during the incubation phase, reported to be from months to ten years, was not immediately understood.

Research in the mid 1980s and early 1990s determined that HIV specifically targets T-lymphocytes with the CD4 marker, a surface molecule that attaches the virus to the cell, and a better understanding of the cellular immune response and CD4 markers emerged. A reasonably reliable correlation between disease progression and the decrease in CD4 T-lymphocyte count was developed. Physicians could predict the development of specific clinical events as the CD4 count decreased. For example, *Pneumocystis carinii* pneumonia (PCP), an opportunistic AIDS infection, frequently develops when CD4 counts drop to a certain level. The CD4 count thus became a guide to treatment. Its usefulness, however, was limited because it only reflected the immune system's destruction.

Recent advances in molecular biology and more reliable and cost-effective assays of proteins and other biochemical molecules have revealed a tremendous increase in virus production immediately after infection and have shown that the immune system increases its activity to counter it. Eventually the number of immune system cells (T-lymphocytes) offsets the viral load, reflected by the HIV RNA. This equilibrium, or "set point," may take years to establish. Even during the dynamic phase when the equilibrium has not yet been set, measurement of viral load is still the best available indicator of response to therapy and long-term clinical outcome.

Risk to the General Public HIV is transmitted through contact with blood, blood products, and body fluids. The virus has been noted in blood, semen, vaginal secretions, and breast milk. Although not yet reported, tears, amniotic fluid, urine, saliva, and bronchial secretions may theoretically transmit the disease.

The virus can enter the body through breaks in the skin, mucous membranes, the eyes, or by placental transmission. Reports of the transmission rate from mother to infant range from 13 to 30 percent. The virus is most commonly contracted through sexual contact or sharing contaminated needles. Before the initiation of stringent controls in screening donor blood and blood products, hemophiliacs and individuals needing frequent blood transfusions were at increased risk. Other groups initially identified at high risk included IV drug abusers and homosexual or bisexual males. The morbidity of heterosexual transmission of HIV has been steadily increasing, with vaginal and anal sex the primary concerns. The risk of oral sex has not been quantified but is believed to be low. Vector transmission by mosquitoes has been postulated but not yet reported. Coexisting sexually transmitted disease, especially with ulceration, appears to increase the risk of infection in sexual transmission. Ethnicity and gender are not established risk factors, and the period of maximum infectiousness cannot be effectively determined. No recovery from AIDS has ever been reported, although post-exposure prophylaxis has been demonstrated to decrease the severity of disease and delay mortality.

Risk to Health Care Workers Although contact with contaminated blood or body secretions potentially places health care workers at risk, infection from HIV-positive patients has been exceedingly rare, with an estimated probability of from 0.2 to 0.44 percent after exposure to virus-containing blood. Accidental needle-stick injuries are the most frequent source of infection in health care workers.

The risk for effective transmission of HIV to health care workers initially depends on whether the exposure to HIV was percutaneous, mucosal, or cutaneous (to intact skin). Within each of those categories, the risk depends on fluid type. Blood is the most dangerous, followed by fluids that may or may not contain blood: semen, vaginal secretions, and cerebrospinal, synovial, pleural, peritoneal, pericardial, and amniotic fluid. Urine and saliva, unlikely to contain blood, pose a very low risk. Source patients (those possibly infecting health care workers) who are HIV-positive or die within two months after the health care worker's exposure, are considered to increase the risk. The highest risk exposure involves a large volume of blood, high antibody titer against a retrovirus in the source patient, deep percutaneous injury, or actual intramuscular injection.

Clinical Presentation The Centers for Disease Control first established the case definition of what constituted AIDS in 1982. Since then, it has expanded the definition of the syndrome to include other diseases such as extrapulmonary and pulmonary tuberculosis, recurrent pneumonia, wasting syndrome, HIV dementia, and sensory neuropathy. The AIDS patient may first develop a mononucleosis-like syndrome with non-specific signs and symptoms such as fatigue, fever, sore throat, lymphadenopathy (lymph node disease), splenomegaly (enlarged spleen), rash, and diarrhea. Since not all of those signs are present, the situation may seem so trivial that the patient does not seek health care. Many patients develop purplish skin lesions known as Kaposi's sarcoma. Kaposi's sarcoma is a cancerous lesion that was quite rare until the HIV virus appeared. As the disease progresses, many patients develop life-threatening opportunistic infections such as *Pneumocystis carinii* pneumonia. Secondary infections caused by *Mycobacterium tuberculosis* may also be present. As AIDS progresses, it involves the central nervous system; dementia, psychosis, encephalopathy, and peripheral neurological disorders may develop.

Postexposure Prophylaxis There is no cure or vaccine for AIDS. After an exposure to a confirmed HIV-positive source patient, the health care worker should immediately seek evaluation and possible initiation of treatment by an occupational medicine or infectious disease physician. Current CDC recommendations establish two hours as the optimum time within which to start postexposure prophylaxis with triple therapy (two reverse transcriptase inhibitors [AZT and 3TC] and one protease inhibitor [IDV]) as the current standard for comparison. This is because early, aggressive treatment may decrease the viral load and alter the set point. Counseling by the ICDO or a trained occupational infectious disease specialist must supplement the postexposure evaluation as part of the agency's exposure control plan. EMS personnel should not attempt to determine their own risk and need for postexposure prophylaxis. Health care workers have significantly underestimated their own risk and need for medical intervention regarding other infections, and the element of denial in HIV increases that tendency.

Summary of HIV HIV-positive patients generally do not present in life-threatening situations to EMS; however, they pose substantial psychosocial challenges. Despite changes in societal attitudes and increased tolerance of differences, HIV-positive individuals are often marginalized and shunned. Their subsequent feeling of social isolation is often worsened by depression. In spite of this, these patients are usually forthcoming about their infection status when dealing with health care workers. Although a paramedic generally has little to offer in terms of treatment, it is vitally important that care be compassionate, understanding, and nonjudgmental. Take appropriate precautions to prevent disease transmission, but if you truly understand the risk as it applies to you as a health care worker, it should be no barrier to your providing professional and emotionally supportive care, including a caring touch. In the EMS environment, physical isolation of the HIV-positive patient is unjustified.

Universal (Standard) Precautions The CDC, OSHA, and NIOSH recommend universal (standard) precautions for health care workers at increased risk for exposure to HIV and other bloodborne pathogens. Since reliably determining which patients have blood-borne infections is impossible, the following precautions are recommended for all patients.

- All health care workers should routinely use appropriate barrier precautions to prevent exposure of the skin and mucous membranes to any contact with blood, or other body fluids, from any patient. Wear disposable gloves whenever touching blood and body fluids, mucous membranes, or broken skin, handling items or surfaces soiled with blood or body fluids, and performing venipuncture or other vascular access procedures. Change and discard gloves after contact with each patient. To prevent exposure of the mucous membranes of the mouth, nose, and eyes, wear masks and protective eyewear or protective face shields during procedures likely to aerosolize blood or other body fluids. If a glove is torn or a needle-stick occurs, remove the glove and replace it as soon as possible. Discard the needle or instrument and obtain another. Wear gowns or aprons during any procedure likely to generate splashes of bloods or other body fluids.

- Wash your hands (including the webs between your fingers) and other skin surfaces thoroughly with soap and warm water after removal of gloves and especially after contamination with blood or other body fluids.

- Take precautions to prevent injuries caused by needles, scalpels, or other sharp instruments or devices whenever performing procedures, cleaning instruments, or disposing of instruments. To prevent needle-stick injuries, needles should not be recapped, purposely bent, broken by hand, removed from disposable syringes, or otherwise manipulated by hand. Position puncture-resistant containers as close as possible to work areas and place disposable syringes and needles, scalpel blades, and other sharp items in them for disposal.

- Although saliva has not been directly implicated in HIV transmission, use mouthpieces with one way valves or filters, bag-valve-mask devices, and other ventilation devices to avoid mouth-to-mouth contact. Place these resuscitation items where the need for resuscitation is predictable.

- Do not put gloved hands close to your mouth, and avoid wiping your face with your forearms or the backs of your gloved hands. Use clean towels to deal with perspiration.
- If you have exudative or weeping skin lesions, refrain from direct patient care and from handling patient care equipment until the condition resolves.
- Pregnant health care workers are not believed to be at greater risk of HIV infection than health care workers who are not pregnant. If a health care worker develops HIV infection during pregnancy, however, the infant is at risk for transplacental transmission. Therefore, pregnant health care workers should be especially familiar with, and strictly adhere to, precautions to minimize the risk of HIV transmission.
- Disinfection of diagnostic or therapeutic equipment and supplies is mandatory.

Hepatitis

hepatitis inflammation of the liver characterized by diffuse or patchy tissue necrosis.

Hepatitis is an inflammation of the liver caused by viruses, bacteria, fungi, parasites, excessive alcohol consumption, or medications. Viruses are by far the most common cause of hepatitis. The clinical signs and symptoms of hepatitis secondary to viral infection are the same regardless of the type of virus. Initially they include headache, fever, weakness, joint pain, anorexia, nausea and vomiting, and in some cases, right upper quadrant abdominal pain. As disease progresses, the patient may become jaundiced, with fever often resolving at the onset of jaundice. This stage is sometimes marked by a darkened urine and the development of clay-colored stools. The various types of hepatitis are transmitted in specific ways. Hepatitis A, B, C, D, and E represent the greatest potential for communicable disease. Paramedics who practice universal precautions against blood-borne and fecal-oral transmission will drastically reduce their risk of contracting hepatitis through occupational exposure.

Hepatitis A Hepatitis A (infectious or viral hepatitis) is transmitted by the fecal-oral route. The causative agent, hepatitis A virus, is usually found in the stool of infected persons, who may not exercise suitable personal hygiene. After these individuals handle food or contact another individual even as casually as shaking hands, the virus can then be transmitted via contaminated hands, food, water, ice, and eating utensils. Furthermore, the virus can exist on unwashed hands for as long as four hours. Many hepatitis A infections are asymptomatic. They do not present with obvious signs like jaundice and are recognizable only by liver function studies. This is especially true of children, who represent most cases of infection and often transmit the virus to others by close social contact. Sexual contact can also spread the virus. Transmission by needle-stick injury is unlikely and has not been reported.

Diaper changing, especially in day care centers with an infected child, is known to increase risk. Travelers to areas with poor sanitary conditions are also at risk. Two inactivated hepatitis A vaccines (Havrix and Vaqta) provide effective active immunization. Health care workers serving on disaster medical teams to Africa, the Middle East, Central and South America, and Asia should be immunized. Immunization is not generally recommended for health care workers in the United States but may be advised in some areas where hepatitis A prevalence is unusually high. Passive preexposure immunization with immune globulin (gamma globulin) is therefore falling out of favor, but immunization may be used after exposure in selected incidents.

The hepatitis A virus's incubation period averages from three to five weeks, with the greatest probability of transmission in the latter half of that period. Afflicted individuals are most infectious during the first week of symptoms. The disease follows a mild course, is rarely serious, and lasts from two to six weeks.

Hepatitis B The hepatitis B (serum hepatitis) virus is transmitted through direct contact with contaminated body fluids (blood, semen, vaginal fluids, and saliva) and therefore represents a substantial risk to EMS providers. Hepatitis B is much more contagious than HIV. The potential for transmitting hepatitis B following exposure to infected blood ranges from 1.9 to 40.0 percent and by needle stick from 5.0 to 35.0 percent. The incidence of antibodies in hepatitis B in health care workers has been reported to be two to four times greater than in the community at large. Health care workers infected by hepatitis B can develop acute hepatitis, cirrhosis, and liver cancer. From 5.0 to 10.0 percent of infected health care workers may become asymptomatic chronic carriers and pose an infection risk to family and other intimate contacts. The effectiveness of the three series of immunizations has been reported to be close to 90.0 percent in adults and higher in children, but low rates of health care worker compliance with immunization are distressingly common. No clearly identifiable populations are at risk except for those individuals who are exposed to high-risk body fluids in the course of their employment.

In the general populace, sexual transmission of hepatitis B is common. Transmission has also been known to occur with transfusion, dialysis, needle and syringe sharing in IV drug use, tattooing, acupuncture, and communally used razors and toothbrushes. The virus is stable on surfaces with dried, visible blood for more than seven days. Infection of toddlers from household contacts with family member carriers has been reported. Transmission by insect vectors or the fecal-oral route has not been reported.

Serum markers that reflect amounts of antigen or antibody from surface or core molecules of the virus reliably reflect active infection, communicability, the window phase of infection, and peak virus replication levels. A detailed discussion of the clinical significance of these markers and how they guide therapy is beyond the scope of this text.

With as much as is known about hepatitis B's disease process and its consequences, combined with the fact that effective vaccines exist, the number of health care workers who have not been immunized or are unaware of their immune status is alarming. Two vaccines, Recombivax HB and Engerix B, both products of genetic recombinant technology, are available. They are reported to be as effective as the previously available Heptavax, derived from blood plasma, without the risk of HIV transmission or other viral infection. The immunization regimen is a series of three intramuscular injections. Following the initial dose, booster doses are administered at one and six months. After the immunization regimen, antibody assays are obtained to confirm active immunity.

The target antibody titer is 10 milli-international units per ml (10 mIU/ml), with a recommendation to draw for antibody titer from 4 to 6 weeks after the series is completed. An additional booster may be necessary if the individual does not develop adequate antibody levels. The duration of protection is thought to be five years, perhaps longer. The vaccine is safe in pregnancy. Its side effects include local redness, occasional low grade fever, rash, nausea, joint pain, or mild fatigue.

Hepatitis B's incubation period lasts from eight to twenty-four weeks. Joint pain and rash are more common with hepatitis B infection than with other types of hepatitis, but 60 to 80 percent of hepatitis B infections are asymptomatic.

Hepatitis C The prevalence of hepatitis C (HCV) in the United States is believed to be 1.8 percent in the adult population and from 2.7 to 10.0 percent in health care workers. The virus is transmitted primarily by IV drug abuse and sexual contact. Sexual contact, however, does not appear to transmit hepatitis C as effectively as it does hepatitis B. After 1989, effective blood donor screening for hepatitis C practically eliminated the risk of transfusion-associated infection.

All EMS workers should receive the hepatitis B vaccination series.

Fecal-oral transmission and household contact have not been reported as factors in transmission, and no specific groups have been identified to be at greater risk for hepatitis C infection.

Hepatitis C is a chronic condition in about 85 percent of infected people. Because of its chronic nature and its ability to cause active disease years later, it poses a great international public health problem. Antibodies can be produced against hepatitis C and provide the laboratory method for determining infection. However, the antibodies are not effective in eliminating the virus, and their presence does not indicate immunity. The ineffectiveness of antibodies is attributed to the virus's high mutation rate. Consequently, the cellular immune response, which results in the immune system's killing infected cells, is very aggressive and is believed, ironically, to cause most of the associated liver injury.

Hepatitis C infection, formerly called non-A, non-B hepatitis, often causes liver fibrosis, which progresses over decades to cirrhosis and is estimated to develop in about 20 percent of infected individuals. This progression is known to be accelerated in persons older than 50 at the time of initial infection, in those consuming more than 50 grams of alcohol per day, and in men. Cirrhosis has also been known to occur in those who have not consumed alcohol and can worsen to end-stage liver disease with jaundice, ascites, and esophageal varices.

No effective vaccination for hepatitis C exists. Treatment with alpha interferon has had limited success, with about 15–20 percent of patients responding positively, as defined by the liver enzymes' return to normal levels. Another drug, ribavirin (an antiviral), administered orally, is known to potentiate interferon's immune system effects, and researchers are now focusing their efforts on improving the results of combination therapy with ribavirin and alpha interferon.

Hepatitis D seems only to coexist with hepatitis B infection.

Hepatitis D The hepatitis D virus (HDV), formerly called delta hepatitis, depends on a surface antigen of the hepatitis B virus (HBV) to produce its structural protein shell. Thus, HDV infection seems to exist only with a coexisting HBV infection. Immunization against HBV therefore confers immunity to HDV. When a patient who has HBV infection with liver disease develops an overlying HDV infection, mortality rates are very high.

Parenteral HDV transmission occurs similarly to HBV in western Europe and North America. Fortunately, cases in health care workers are extremely rare. Frequent epidemics of nonparenteral transmission occur in central Africa, the Middle East, and the Mediterranean countries. HDV's incubation period has not been determined.

Hepatitis E Hepatitis E (HEV) is transmitted like hepatitis A virus (HAV), through the fecal-oral route, and seems to be associated with contaminated drinking water more commonly than HAV. It occurs primarily in young adults, with highest rates in pregnant women. First described in India, outbreaks have occurred in Russia, Nepal, Southeast Asia, the Middle East, Pakistan, and China. Only six cases were reported in the United States from 1989 to 1992, most likely because of more sanitary sources of drinking water.

Tuberculosis

* tuberculosis (TB) disease caused by a bacterium known as *Mycobacterium tuberculosis* that primarily affects the respiratory system.

Tuberculosis (TB) is the most common preventable adult infectious disease in the world. TB is caused by bacteria known collectively as the *Mycobacterium tuberculosis* complex, which includes *M. tuberculosis, M. bovis,* and *M. africanum.* Other bacteria in the *Mycobacterium* family can cause tuberculosis, particularly in immunocompromised patients. These other types of *Mycobacterium* are referred to as atypicals. It primarily affects the respiratory system, including a highly contagious form in the larynx. Untreated or undertreated, it may spread to other organ systems, causing extrapulmonary TB and other complications.

The disease appeared about 7,000 years ago and peaked in the eighteenth century. The number of new cases in the United States has increased steadily since 1985, in large part because of TB in AIDS patients and in recently arrived immigrants from countries where the disease is prevalent.

The development of multiple drug resistant tuberculosis (MDR-TB) has been known since the late 1940s. Drug resistance occurs when drug-resistant bacteria outgrow drug-susceptible bacteria. These bacteria acquire resistance either because of patient noncompliance with therapy or inadequate treatment regimens. Drug resistance occurs early in therapy, especially when only one drug is used. For this reason, most current CDC recommendations for the initiation of therapy in the United States involve several options for treatment, each calling for multiple medications, including isoniazid (INH), rifampin, pyrazinamide, ethambutol, and streptomycin, among others.

M. tuberculosis is most commonly transmitted through airborne respiratory droplets but may also be contracted by direct inoculation through mucous membranes and broken skin or by drinking contaminated milk. Animal reservoirs for the bacteria include cattle, swine, badgers, and primates. Coughing and other expiratory actions (sneezing, speaking, singing) create bacteria-containing droplets from 5 to 10 microns in size, which susceptible individuals inhale into the alveoli.

The risk of transmitting tuberculosis is not as high as measles. Although the average case infects only about a third of his close contacts, prolonged exposure to a person with active TB is always listed as a risk factor. Communicability varies from case to case. Although a single occupational exposure to a patient with active TB is highly unlikely to transmit the disease to a paramedic, universal precautions against TB should still be employed.

Skin Testing The commonly used purified protein derivative (PPD) skin test effectively identifies candidates for prophylactic drug therapy (to prevent active TB) in large groups of health care workers. It has limited value in guiding individual therapy in those with active TB because a positive PPD indicates previous infection but does not distinguish active from dormant disease. Another health care worker experienced in interpreting the results should read the skin test, rather than the worker tested, because health care workers are known to under-interpret positive results. In addition, the skin test must be interpreted on the basis of the disease's prevalence in the community. A negative test does not rule out active disease, particularly in immunosuppressed individuals or in those who were infected so recently that their immune systems have not yet had time to mount the cellular mediated response that causes a positive PPD.

Most EMS agencies require skin testing at least annually. This may be sufficient, but again, decisions about the frequency of testing should be based on the disease's prevalence in the community. For individuals who have not been previously skin tested or who have no documentation of a negative PPD in the last 12 months, two-step testing may be reasonable. In these individuals, an initial negative test may be due to weak reactivity to the PPD. A second skin test is administered from one to three weeks later. A positive reaction to the second test probably represents a boosted reaction, which means that the individual has been previously infected, and should be evaluated for possible prophylaxis. If the second test is negative, that individual is classified as uninfected. A positive reaction to any subsequent test would represent a new infection by *M. tuberculosis*.

Pathogenesis TB's incubation period is 4–12 weeks. In most people with subclinical infections, immediate disease (primary TB) does not develop because of a cell-mediated immune response. Development of disease normally occurs 6–12 months after infection. Susceptibility to primary infection is increased in persons who are malnourished and those persons whose immune systems are suppressed, such as the elderly, HIV patients, and people taking immunosuppressant drugs. Children less

TB is the most common preventable adult infectious disease in the world. Its incidence in the United States has been rising since 1985.

EMS workers should receive TB screening on an annual basis.

than three years old are at risk because of underdeveloped immune systems, with older children identified at lowest risk. As expected, the aged are at high risk, and the reactivation of latent infections in this age group implies that the immune system has difficulty dealing with the complex nature of the *M. tuberculosis* infection. Once the bacteria enter the lungs, alveolar macrophages attack them and attempt to "wall them off" (forming granulomas) in a localized immune response. For this reason most TB infections do not produce disease. Healed sites leave lesions of calcified areas known as Ghon foci. When Ghon foci combine with lymph nodes, they form a Ghon complex, which creates small, sharply defined shadows on a chest X-ray.

If the macrophages cannot destroy them, the bacteria lie dormant within the macrophages and are then distributed to other sites within the body. They remain dormant until some event, usually a depression of the immune system, triggers their reactivation into secondary TB. The sites of reactivation are greatest in areas of the lung with the highest oxygen tension, the apices or upper lobes. Reactivation in extrapulmonary sites such as lymph nodes, pleura, and pericardium are much more common in HIV-infected persons. In AIDS patients, the disease may spread to the thoracic and lumbar spine, destroying intervertebral disks and adjacent vertebral bodies. TB is also known to lead to subacute meningitis and granulomas in the brain.

Clinical Presentation The signs and symptoms of active TB can be very non-specific and can be manifestations of other clinical conditions. However, a typical list would include chills, fever, fatigue, productive or nonproductive chronic cough, and weight loss. Many patients report night sweats, leaving their bed linens drenched with perspiration. Hemoptysis (expectorating blood) is very suggestive of active TB. Reactivation of dormant TB manifests as signs and symptoms specific to the organ systems involved.

EMS Response Your acceptance of responsibility for protecting yourself from *M. tuberculosis* is the most important step in preventing disease transmission. A proactive, high-index-of-suspicion-driven response is essential. The factors that increase a paramedic's risk of transmission are close and sometimes prolonged contact with the patient. Care and transport are provided in a very small, often ineffectively ventilated, space, and the patient may affect various expiratory actions while in contact with EMS personnel. Placing a mask over the patient, when it does not create undue anxiety or dyspnea, effectively decreases the number of expectorated droplet nuclei. Also, nebulized medications may be administered more safely with a nebulization mask. Use appropriate respiratory precautions while performing CPR and intubation.

You should don a protective respirator upon contact with a patient you suspect may have TB. Your knowledge of the prevalence of TB and the most susceptible populations in your jurisdiction should reinforce your index of suspicion. The most current NIOSH/OSHA standards for protecting health care workers from TB call for N95 **respirators,** which are designed to prevent contaminated air from reaching the health care workers wearing them (Figure 37-5a). High efficiency particulate aspirator (HEPA) respirators (Figure 37-5b) are no longer required in TB, but EMS agencies may opt to continue their use. They are more expensive, bulky, and sometimes difficult to breathe through.

Masks, as opposed to respirators, work primarily as barriers against larger particles and are not certified to prevent contaminated air from reaching the paramedic. However, they effectively prevent the transmission of many airborne pathogens, especially when both provider and patient wear them. They also provide a more comfortable and cost-effective alternative to the routine use of respirators. The extensive terminology and guidelines relative to the design, construction, and classification of various respirators is beyond the scope of this text. EMS agencies and their ICDOs are responsible for educating their

* **respirator** an apparatus worn that cleanses or qualifies the air.

* **mask** a device for protecting the face.

FIGURE 37-5A NIOSH/OSHA standards call for N95 respirators when caring for patients with tuberculosis.

FIGURE 37-5B EMS agencies may opt to use high efficiency particulate aspirator (HEPA) respirators in TB.

personnel in the proper use and application of respirators and for ensuring proper fit and easy access. According to the NIOSH classification, N series respirators provide protection against non-oil-based aerosols, including the droplet nuclei from TB patients. These N type respirators must filter 95 percent of particles that are no larger than 0.3 microns in diameter, hence the designation N 95. This is a very safe standard since the diameter of TB aerosol droplets ranges from 5 to 10 microns. Health care workers' noncompliance causes most respirator failures.

Ventilation systems currently being marketed in selected ambulances claim to effectively recycle and filter enough air to ensure the expulsion of infected droplet nuclei. Such ventilation systems should include HEPA filtration in addition to recycling the patient compartment air volume according to OSHA standards. Do not open patient compartment windows to increase ventilation and dilute the concentration of droplet nuclei. The moving ambulance may create a Bernoulli effect that draws engine exhaust, including carbon monoxide, into the patient compartment.

Postexposure Identification and Management Early identification of exposure and drug prophylaxis, if deemed necessary, are the keys to effectively preventing active TB in health care workers. An occupational medicine physician should assess TB skin test results and determine the appropriateness of chest X-rays, sputum cultures, and a myriad of other diagnostic procedures to confirm infection or the presence of frank disease. The polymerase chain reaction (PCR) test, which eliminates the need to wait for cultures and provides a diagnosis in six hours, may soon become the gold standard for identifying the presence of *M. tuberculosis*.

Pneumonia

Patients with difficulty breathing often confront paramedics with the enigma of differentiating pneumonia from mild exacerbations of congestive heart failure and its more severe form, acute pulmonary edema. The mistaken assumption that a patient has CHF may lead to aggressive treatment that reduces the patient's respiratory drive, dries protective mucous secretions, and contributes to hypotension.

Pneumonia, an acute lung inflammation, is not a single disease but a family of diseases that result from respiratory infection by viruses, bacteria, or fungi. The infectious agent most often associated with pneumonia, and against which the

✱ **pneumonia** acute infection of the lung, including alveolar spaces and interstitial tissue.

pneumococcal vaccine is targeted, is *Streptococcus pneumoniae*, gram-positive spheres found in pairs or chains. Other microorganisms known to cause pneumonia are *Mycoplasma pneumoniae* (primary atypical pneumonia), *H. influenzae*, *Klebsiella pneumoniae*, *M. catarrhalis*, *Legionella*, *S. aureus* in nosocomial infections, and *P. carinii*. These agents are also known to cause meningitis, ear infections, and pharyngitis. In addition to droplet nuclei, the infectious agents are also spread by direct contact and through linens soiled with respiratory secretions.

Those at highest risk for pneumonia are the immunocompromised, patients with sickle cell disease, transplanted organs, cardiovascular disease, diabetes mellitus, kidney disease, multiple myeloma, lymphoma, Hodgkin's disease, those without functioning spleens, and the elderly, particularly those in common residential situations. Low-birth-weight neonates and malnourished infants are very susceptible. In otherwise healthy individuals, susceptibility is increased by a previous respiratory infection like influenza, exposure to inhaled toxins, chronic lung disease, and aspiration (post-alcohol ingestion, near drowning, ingested toxins, or gastric distention from BVM ventilation). When patients contract infectious agents of pneumonia outside of a hospital or other health care institution, they are referred to as cases of community-acquired pneumonia.

History and Assessment Always consider the possibility of community-acquired pneumonia. In geriatric communities where residents live in their own home but may share common social facilities, ask if neighbors recently have been diagnosed with pneumonia or other respiratory infections. Signs and symptoms in previously healthy individuals include an acute onset of chills, high-grade fever, dyspnea, pleuritic chest pain worsened by deep inspiration, and cough, which may be productive with phlegm of various colors. The absence of fever does not rule out pneumonia. Breath sounds may include adventitious lung sounds (crackles, wheezes) and signs of consolidation. When purulent fluids accumulate in many lobes of the lung because of inflammation, alveoli collapse and their acoustic properties change to those of solid tissue, hence the name *consolidation*. Consolidation causes the expiratory sounds in the peripheral lung fields to develop the same duration as inspiration and to be just as loud. Assessment with pulse oximetry may be useful. In geriatric patients, the only presenting sign may be an altered mental status; fever is often absent, and headache, aches and pain, nausea, diarrhea, and nonproductive cough, if present, do not allow you to rule out pneumonia. In children, fever, tachypnea, and retractions are ominous signs but are not specific to pneumonia; this triad of signs, however, reliably indicates respiratory distress secondary to an infectious process in pediatric patients.

Patient Management and PPE Management of the pneumonia patient aims at supporting adequate ventilation and oxygenation, with supplemental oxygen often providing relief. Always consider TB a possibility in any patient with pneumonia and place a mask either on yourself or on your patient.

Immunization and Postexposure Management An effective vaccination exists against most serotypes of *S. pneumoniae* known to cause disease. It is highly recommended for children two years old or younger, for adults over sixty-five years old, and for those without spleens. Routine vaccination of EMS workers is not necessary. In health care settings, health care workers who routinely treat elderly, immunocompromised, or other at-risk patients may be required to be immunized because they pose the risk of patient transmission. Because EMS workers are predominantly healthy, exposure to a single patient with pneumonia generally will not result in infection or disease. A number of antimicrobial agents are effective against the infectious agents known to cause pneumonia. However, multidrug resistant strains have been reported.

Chickenpox

Chickenpox is caused by the varicella zoster virus (VZV). The varicella zoster virus is in the herpesvirus family. Although chickenpox (**varicella**) in pediatrics is considered a self-limited disease that rarely causes severe complications, it is much more lethal in adults. It results in fewer than 100 deaths per year in the United States, but while adults represent only 2 percent of the morbidity, they account for 50 percent of the mortality. Thus, health care workers who have not been immunized against VZV or been exposed to it as children must increase their awareness of this infection and its consequences. It is estimated that 10 percent of adults have not contracted VZV during childhood. VZV is also the infectious agent of shingles (herpes zoster), a painful condition that causes skin lesions along the course of peripheral nerves and dermatome bands. Approximately 15 percent of patients with chickenpox will eventually develop shingles.

Clinical Presentation Chickenpox usually occurs in clusters during winter and spring and presents with respiratory symptoms, malaise, and low-grade fever, followed by a rash that starts on the face and trunk and progresses to the rest of the body, including mucous membranes. The rash may be the first sign of illness, and infected persons may have anywhere from a few to 500 lesions. It is more profuse on the trunk, with less distribution to the extremities and scalp. The fluid-filled vesicles that form the rash soon rupture, forming small ulcers that eventually scab over within one week, at which point the patient is no longer contagious. Transmission occurs through inhalation of airborne droplets and direct contact with weeping lesions and tainted linen. The incubation period is from ten to twenty-one days.

In adults, varicella's most common complication is a VZV pneumonia. A large percentage of adult deaths from VZV occur in immunocompromised patients. The most alarming aspect of adult epidemiology, however, is a significant death rate in previously healthy patients. Therefore, it is important for unexposed or unvaccinated paramedics to be immunized.

Assessing Immunity Most people develop immunity for life after recovery from childhood chickenpox infections. Thus, a history of chickenpox is considered adequate evidence of immunity. An available blood test can determine immunity in those who are unsure about their history or who have not had chickenpox.

Immunization A chickenpox vaccine, Varivax, has been licensed in the United States since 1995, and the Advisory Committee on Immunization Practices (ACIP) of CDC now recommends that all states require children entering day care facilities and elementary school to be vaccinated or have some other evidence of immunity. Such evidence would include a primary care provider's diagnosis of chickenpox, a reliable history of the disease, or blood test confirming immunity. Vaccination is also routinely recommended for all susceptible health care workers. ACIP has also strengthened its recommendations for all other susceptible persons 13 years old or younger to include any adolescents living in the same household with younger children.

The vaccine is administered as one subcutaneous dose in children under age 12 and as two doses in susceptible adolescents and adults. Among vaccinated people 13 years old or older, 78 percent developed protective antibodies, with 99 percent seroconverting after the second dose. Health care workers who receive the vaccination should have their antibody level checked six weeks after the second vaccination.

Patients with active TB, malignant conditions, or those being treated with immunosuppressants should not receive varicella vaccine. Its use in those taking steroids depends on a variety of factors beyond the scope of this discussion. Few

✱ **varicella** viral disease characterized by a rash of fluid-filled vesicles that rupture, forming small ulcers that eventually scab; commonly called *chickenpox*.

adverse effects have been reported through CDC's Vaccine Adverse Events Reporting System (VAERS). The most frequent was rash, with some cases of herpes zoster. No incidents of chickenpox have been reported. Although a few serious adverse effects were reported, no cause and effect relationship was clearly established with the vaccination. The vaccine manufacturer discourages taking aspirin within six weeks after receiving the vaccination.

EMS Response and Postexposure Observe universal precautions and place masks on patients. If a patient only has chickenpox, he should remain at home until the lesions are crusted and dry. If a susceptible paramedic is exposed to chickenpox, postexposure vaccination may be warranted. Recent data indicate that if used within three days, and possibly up to five days, Varivax may be effective in preventing chickenpox or lessening its severity. Varicella–zoster immune globulin (VZIG) is an alternative postexposure prophylaxis. Unlike Varivax, it provides passive immunity, and the most current recommendation for its use is in immunocompromised patients. The use of Acyclovir, which inhibits replication of the virus, within 24 hours of the onset of rash may decrease the disease's severity in adults and adolescents.

Meningitis

Meningitis is an inflammation of the meninges (the membranes protecting the brain and spinal cord) and cerebrospinal fluid, caused by bacterial and viral infections. Meningococcal meningitis (spinal meningitis), caused by *Neisseria meningitidis,* is the disease variant of greatest concern to EMS responders.

Other agents are, or have been, known to cause meningitis. *Streptococcus pneumoniae,* the primary infectious agent of concern in pneumonia, is the second most common cause of pneumonia in adults and the most common cause of otitis media in children. Vaccines have proven very effective, especially in children. *Haemophilus influenzae* type B, a gram-negative rod, was once the leading cause of meningitis in children aged six months to three years. However, with the implementation of effective childhood vaccination against *H. influenzae* since 1981, *N. meningitidis* has become the bacterium most commonly implicated in serious meningitis cases. Viruses and other microorganisms are known to cause meningitis, with similar disease profiles. Enteroviruses are implicated in 90 percent of patients with viral (aseptic) meningitis. In healthy individuals, viral meningitis is a self-limited disease that lasts about seven to ten days.

Transmission Factors *N. meningitidis* asymptomatically colonizes the upper respiratory tract of healthy individuals and is then transmitted by respiratory droplets. Up to 35 percent of the general population may be infected with the bacterium, which is prevented from gaining access to the CSF by the epithelial lining of the pharynx. Almost every human has probably been a carrier at some point in his life. Conversion from carrier to clinical disease is rare in developed countries and occurs in clusters in developing nations. The disease appears to peak in midwinter months with low temperature and humidity. This has been validated by observations of epidemic seasonal variations in the "meningitis belt" of sub-Saharan Africa. Epidemiologists have hypothesized that this pattern may represent a herd immunity, in which host resistance factors may be more a function of the population's general immunity than of the immunity of individuals within that population. One theory that could explain the phenomenon of herd immunity holds that another species within the genus *Neisseria* may be "mistaken" for *N. meningitidis* (a cross reaction), resulting in effective antibody production against the pathogen. Meningococcal meningitis occurs more commonly in some areas of the United States, and the world, for reasons not yet un-

EMS transport of a patient with chickenpox should be followed by extensive decontamination of the ambulance and any equipment used.

meningitis inflammation of the meninges, usually caused by an infection.

derstood. Other factors that have been implicated in transmission of *N. meningitidis* include contacting oral secretions of the index case (kissing, sharing food or drink), crowding, close contact, smoking, and lower socioeconomic status. For the EMS responder, contact with secretions during mouth-to-mask ventilation, intubation, or suctioning would increase the probability of transmission.

Clinical Presentation The incubation period most commonly ranges from two to four days but may last as long as ten days. As with most bacterial infections, signs and symptoms develop rapidly within a few hours or one to two days of exposure and include fever, chills, headache, nuchal rigidity with flexion, arthralgia, lethargy, malaise, altered mental status, vomiting, and seizures. An upper respiratory or ear infection may precede the disease. A characteristic rash may appear and develop into hemorrhagic spots, or petechiae. Roughly 10 percent of patients may develop septic shock. Acute adrenal insufficiency, disseminated intravascular coagulation (DIC), and coma are other consequences. Death can ensue in six to eight hours.

Newborns and infants may seem slow or inactive, vomit, appear irritable, or feed poorly. Fever in newborns should be evaluated with a high index of suspicion for meningococcemia. Rarely, bulging of an open anterior fontanel is seen. In older children, assessment techniques that stretch the inflamed meninges and cause pain may reveal positive Brudzinski's and Kernig's signs. **Brudzinski's sign** is a physical exam finding suggestive of meningitis. Due to irritation of the meninges, flexion of the neck causes flexion of the hips and knees. To test for Brudzinski's sign, have the patient lie supine without a pillow. Flex the neck while observing the hips and knees. Flexion of the hips or knees when the neck is flexed is considered a positive Brudzinski's sign. **Kernig's sign** is likewise suggestive of meningitis. To elicit Kernig's sign, have the patient sit or lie and flex the hips. With the hips flexed, attempt to extend (straighten) the knee. Inability to fully extend the knee is due to meningeal irritation and is considered a positive Kernig's sign. Maternal antibodies protect newborns from meningitis and other infections until up to six months of age (slightly longer in breast fed children). Infants from six months to two years are especially susceptible to meningitis because they no longer have circulating maternal antibodies and their immune systems are immature and incompetent.

Immunization *N. meningitidis* has several serotypes (A, B, C, X, Y, Z, 29-E, W-135), with B and C causing most disease outbreaks in the United States. The A serotype is the most common cause of epidemics in Africa and Asia. An effective vaccine has been developed against the A, C, Y, and W-135 serotypes. Attempts to develop one against the B serotype have so far resulted in weak immune responses. The meningococcal vaccine is not presently recommended for routine immunization of health care workers. Travelers to endemic areas and children younger than two years who are asplenic (without a spleen) or have a certain deficiency in their complement system are candidates for vaccination.

EMS Response and Postexposure Observing universal precautions and using masks on yourself and/or your patients with suspected meningococcal meningitis will adequately protect you against all the infectious agents of meningitis. Postexposure prophylaxis with rifampin, ciprofloxacin (Cipro), or ceftriaxone (Rocephin) is the primary means of preventing meningococcal disease. Prophylaxis should be started within 24 hours after exposure because the rate of effective transmission in close contacts (EMS responders) with the index-case patient has been estimated to be 500–800 times that of the general population. Initiation of chemoprophylaxis 14 days or more after the onset of illness in the index case is of limited or no value. All postexposure medications are easily complied with and have few side effects.

✱ **Brudzinki's sign** physical exam finding in which flexion of the neck causes flexion of the hips and knees.

✱ **Kernig's sign** inability to fully extend the knees with hips flexed.

Effective, vigorous hand washing with soap and warm water after patient contact is the most important personal precaution against disease transmission.

*influenza disease caused by a group of viruses.

Other Job-Related Airborne Diseases

Influenza and colds, rubella, measles, mumps, and respiratory syncytial virus (RSV) are viral infections that may be contracted in the EMS environment. Pertussis, a highly contagious bacterial disease, also poses a risk. These diseases are transmitted by direct inhalation of infected droplets or through exposed mucosal surfaces. Handling contaminated surfaces or objects and subsequently introducing the virus by scratching, wiping, or other activities with unwashed hands (autoinoculation) is another route of transmission. Masks and ventilation are recommended for measles. Precautions against autoinoculation with RSV infections, influenza, and colds include masks, more practically placed on patients, and possibly gloves, gowns, and goggles. Avoid touching your face and areas of broken skin while in contact with the patient. Effective, vigorous hand washing with soap and warm water after patient contact is the most important personal precaution against disease transmission.

Influenza and the Common Cold Influenza is caused by viruses designated types A, B, and C. Within these types are various subtypes that mutate so often that they are identified on the basis of where they were isolated, the culture number, and year of isolation—for instance, A/Japan/305/57. Two glycoproteins, hemagglutinin and neuraminidase, on the outer membrane of an influenza virus determine its virulence. The letters H and N, which denote these two glycoproteins, are often seen in parentheses along with a number, as in A (H1N1). This method of classification helps epidemiologists to more specifically identify a flu virus, since it is based on the immune responses to hemagglutinin and neuraminidase.

Influenza is a leading cause of respiratory disease worldwide, and various strains cause epidemics, mainly during the winter months. It is easily transmittable in crowded spaces such as public transportation vehicles, and can be spread by direct contact. The virus can persist on environmental surfaces for hours, especially in low humidity and cold temperatures. Thus, it has a high potential for transmission by autoinoculation. It is much more serious than the common cold and has caused worldwide epidemics with high mortality rates. The last great epidemic was in 1918, and CDC and the World Health Organization (WHO) closely monitor worldwide disease outbreaks.

Influenza is characterized by the sudden onset of fever, chills, malaise, muscle aches, nasal discharge, and cough. The disease is more serious in the very young, the very old, and those with underlying disease. Its incubation period is from one to three days. Fever generally lasts three to five days. Signs include mild sore throat, nonproductive cough, and nasal discharge. The cough may be severe and of long duration. Secondary infections may occur as the virus damages respiratory epithelial cells, thereby decreasing resistance to other, primarily bacterial, disorders. Severe cases may result in pneumonia, hemorrhagic bronchitis, and death. The uncomplicated disease usually lasts two to seven days and full recovery is the norm.

Management is primarily supportive. Fever may increase body temperature to as high as 105°F. Begin cooling measures for patients with temperatures of 104°F or greater. Increased body temperature may lead to significant insensible fluid loss and dehydration. Determine hydration status early and begin fluid replacement if indicated.

Everyone is susceptible to influenza. Although infection confers resistance after recovery, the influenza viruses mutate so rapidly that protection is effective only against the particular strain or variant from which the person has just recovered. An immunization is available and is recommended for the elderly, those who live or work in correctional institutions, and military recruits. Patients should be immunized between early September and mid-November for maximum effectiveness. The CDC recommends vaccination for EMS personnel to reduce transmission of influenza to patients and to decrease worker absenteeism. EMS responders who are diabetics, especially those requiring frequent medical follow up, are strongly urged to be immunized. Three antiviral drugs, amantadine (Symmetrel), oseltamivir (Tambiflu), and rimantadine (Flumadine), are available for the prevention and treatment of influenza; however, they only work against the type A influenza virus. They are as effective as vaccines when used preventively, and they shorten the illness's duration when used as a treatment. A new agent, zanamavir (Relenza), which is effective against type B, was recently released. However, its use is limited because only 35 percent of influenza cases are type B and because it must be delivered by aerosol nebulizer.

The common cold, or viral rhinitis, is caused by the rhinoviruses, of which there are more than 100 serotypes. Its incidence in the United States rises in fall, winter, and spring, is highest in children younger than five years, and declines in older adults, displaced by more serious diseases. Transmission is by direct contact, airborne droplets, or more importantly, by hands and linen soiled with discharges from infected individuals. The incubation period ranges from 12 hours to 5 days and averages 48 hours. The disease's course is mild, often without fever and generally without muscle aching. Aside from severity, it is often difficult to differentiate from influenza. Mortality has not been reported, but a cold may lead to more serious complications such as otitis media and sinusitis.

Measles Measles (rubeola, hard measles), a systemic disease caused by the measles virus of the genus *Morbilli,* is highly communicable. It is most common in children but may affect older persons who have not had it. Immunity following disease is usually lifelong. Maternal antibodies protect neonates for about four to five months after birth.

Measles is transmitted by inhalation of infective droplets and direct contact. The incubation period ranges from seven to fourteen days, averaging ten. The infected person presents prodromally like a severe cold, with fever, conjunctivitis, swelling of the eyelids, photophobia, malaise, cough, and nasopharyngeal congestion. The fever increases, rising to as high as 104°–106°F, when the rash reaches its maximum. A day or two before the rash develops, Koplik's spots (bluish-white specks with a red halo approximately 1 mm in diameter) appear on the oral mucosa. The red, bumpy (maculopapular) rash normally lasts about six days and spreads from head to feet by the third day. At that point, it appears to thicken on the head and shoulders and then disappear in the same direction as its progression.

Measles is so highly communicable that the slightest contact with an active case may infect a susceptible person. Infectivity is greatest before the prodrome and subsides about four days after the rash appears or as it fades. Everyone should be immunized. Immunization is 99 percent effective in children, for whom vaccination is mandatory since there is no specific treatment. Unimmunized or previously unexposed paramedics should mask their measles patients and be vigilant about handling linens and touching their face during and after the call. Postexposure hand washing is critical.

In otherwise healthy children or adults, uncomplicated measles has a low mortality rate. Potential complications include bacterial pneumonia, eye damage, and myocarditis. The most life-threatening sequela is encephalitis in children and adolescents that causes gradual decreases in mental capacity and muscle coordination.

Mumps The **mumps** virus, a member of the genus *Paramyxovirus,* is transmitted through respiratory droplets and direct contact with the saliva of infected patients. It is characterized by painful enlargement of the salivary glands. Most cases occur in the five- to fifteen-year age group. After a 12–25 day incubation period, mumps presents as a feverish cold that is soon followed by swelling and stiffening of the parotid salivary gland in front of the ear. The condition is often

* measles highly contagious, acute viral disease characterized by a reddish rash that appears on the fourth or fifth day of illness.

* mumps acute viral disease characterized by painful enlargement of the salivary glands.

found bilaterally. The patient may also experience earache and difficulty chewing and swallowing. In most cases, the submaxillary and sublingual glands are very tender to palpation. Most cases resolve spontaneously within one week without intervention.

Mumps occurs in epidemics, with danger of transmission beginning one week before the infected person feels sick and lasting about two weeks. Lifelong immunity is generally conferred after infection, even in the absence of disease (subclinical infection).

Mumps is generally benign and self-limiting; however, complications may occur. In postpubescent patients, inflammation of the testicles (orchitis), breasts (mastitis), or ovaries (oophoritis) may occur, but is of short duration and of no serious consequence. Meningoencephalitis is fairly common but resolves without residual neurological sequelae.

A mumps live-virus vaccine is available and should be administered with measles and rubella vaccines to all children over one year old. Mumps is not easily transmitted, and with standard BSI precautions the risk of contracting the disease is minimal. For the benefit of their patients, EMS workers should not work without an established mumps/measles/rubella (MMR) immunity.

Rubella Rubella (**German measles**) is a systemic viral disease caused by the rubella virus, of the genus *Rubivirus,* transmitted by inhalation of infective droplets. Generally milder than measles, it is characterized by sore throat and low-grade fever, accompanied by a fine pink rash on the face, trunk, and extremities that lasts about 3 days. The incubation period is 12–19 days, with natural infection conferring lifelong immunity, as does immunization. Transfer of maternal antibodies does not confer lifelong immunity but does protect the neonate. There is no specific treatment for rubella. More serious complications that occur in measles do not occur in rubella, but young females sometimes develop a short course of arthritis.

Rubella is devastating to a developing fetus. Mothers infected during the first trimester are at risk for abnormal fetal development, with offspring often developing congenital rubella syndrome and shedding large quantities of virus in their secretions. An infant acquiring this infection *in utero* (in the uterus) is likely to be retarded and suffer eye inflammation, deafness, and congenital heart defects. All females, therefore, should be immunized against rubella before becoming pregnant.

Vaccines for measles, mumps, and rubella are commonly combined in an MMR vaccination, which can be given safely with the varicella vaccine. Immunization is 98–99 percent effective but is not recommended for pregnant women because of a theoretical possibility of birth defects. Health care workers have been identified as the source in numerous outbreaks. For this reason, and for their own protection, all EMS providers should be required to receive the MMR vaccination before they are allowed to work. Immunizations, along with placing a mask on the patient, are an effective method of preventing these diseases.

Respiratory Syncytial Virus Respiratory syncytial virus (RSV) is one of the most common causes of pneumonia and bronchiolitis in infants and young children. In this age group, RSV may be fatal. In older children and adults RSV is less common, and its symptoms are generally milder. RSV is often associated with outbreaks of lower respiratory infections from November to April. If a patient with pneumonia or bronchitis simultaneously contracts this virus, the disease becomes more severe. RSV commonly begins as an upper respiratory infection, and is often misdiagnosed as a simple cold. Children with RSV infection will initially develop a runny nose and nasal congestion. Later, this will spread to lower airway involvement evidenced by wheezing, tachypnea, and signs of respiratory distress. It is a common infection that can be diagnosed by a rapid assay using nasal washings. In winter months, wheezing in children under a year of age should be

* rubella (German measles) systemic viral disease characterized by a fine pink rash that appears on the face, trunk, and extremities and fades quickly.

Paramedics should not be allowed to work until they have received the MMR vaccination.

* respiratory syncytial virus (RSV) common cause of pneumonia and bronchiolitis in children.

presumed to be due to RSV until proven otherwise. High-risk children (those with congenital heart conditions, prematurity, or cancers, for instance) can be treated with the antiviral agent ribavirin (Virazole). However, this treatment is quite expensive and poses a significant risk to unborn babies of pregnant health care workers. Postexposure prophylaxis with Respi-Gam (RSV immune globulin) is also an option.

Pertussis The word *pertussis* means "violent cough." **Pertussis** (whooping cough) is caused by the bacterium *Bordetella pertussis,* affecting the oropharynx in three clinical phases after an incubation period of from six to twenty days. The *catarrhal phase,* characterized by symptoms similar to those of the common cold, lasts from one to two weeks. The *paroxysmal phase,* during which the fever subsides, can last a month or longer. The patient develops a mild cough that quickly becomes severe and violent. Rapid consecutive coughs are followed by a deep, high-pitched inspiration. (This characteristic "whoop" often is not present in infants and adults.) The cough often produces large amounts of thick mucus, and vomiting may also occur. Sustained coughing may lead to increased intracranial pressure and intracerebral hemorrhage. Continually high intrapulmonary pressure and vigorous chest movement may cause pneumothorax. During the *convalescent phase* the frequency and severity of coughing attacks decrease, and the patient is not contagious.

The widespread vaccination of children in a combination diphtheria-pertussis-tetanus vaccine (DTP) caused a dramatic decrease in the incidence of pertussis until the early 1980s. Over the past 20 years, however, its incidence has steadily grown, with the greatest increase in persons aged 5 years or older. This has occurred in spite of unprecedented pertussis vaccination coverage. One factor in the increase may be a waning effectiveness of the vaccine among adolescents and adults vaccinated during childhood. Although disease is likely to confer immunity against pertussis, the duration of that immunity is unknown. Previously immunized and exposed adolescents and adults therefore may be at risk of infection. Thus, booster doses are recommended.

For patients with pertussis, EMS is most likely to be requested during the paroxysmal phase, when the primary treatment will be calming and oxygenating the patient. Anticipate the needs to intubate patients with respiratory failure and to perform chest decompression for those whose coughing paroxysms might have caused a pneumothorax. During the response, remember that pertussis is highly contagious. Fortunately, the communicable period is thought to be greatest before the paroxysmal phase. Transmission occurs via respiratory secretions or in an aerosolized form. Mask the patient and observe standard BSI precautions, including postexposure hand washing.

Everyone is susceptible to *B. pertussis* infection. Routine immunization of EMS workers against pertussis is not yet recommended. Evaluation of pertussis vaccination is ongoing, however, and considering the unknown duration of immunity with past immunization or exposure, adolescent and adult immunization may be recommended in the future. Erythromycin is known to decrease the period of communicability, but can reduce symptoms only if administered before the onset of violent coughing.

Viral Diseases Transmitted by Contact

Mononucleosis and herpex simplex type 1 infections pose little risk to EMS providers who observe BSI precautions and wash their hands after patient contact. Since these diseases cause relatively minor symptoms, patients may not even be aware of their infection status. The public is highly aware of these two diseases, however, so as health care providers, paramedics should be familiar with them.

* **pertussis** disease characterized by severe, violent coughing.

Content Review

PHASES OF PERTUSSIS
- Catarrhal
- Paroxysmal
- Convalescent

Content Review

VIRAL DISEASES TRANSMITTED BY CONTACT
- Mononucleosis
- Herpes Simplex Virus Type 1

Mononucleosis Mononucleosis is caused by the Epstein-Barr virus (EBV). It affects the oropharynx, tonsils, and the reticuloendothelial system (the phagocytes). A four- to six-week incubation period precedes the development of symptoms, which characteristically begin with fatigue. Fever, severe sore throat, oral discharges, and enlarged, tender lymph nodes generally follow several days to weeks later. Splenomegaly (enlargement of the spleen) is present in approximately one-half of patients. The disease is common; over 95 percent of the general population has antibodies to the virus. One half of all children will have contracted it before the age of five years. Infection by EBV generally confers immunity for life.

Mononucleosis is most commonly transmitted through oropharyngeal contact involving the exchange of saliva between an uninfected person and one who has the disease but who is asymptomatic. Kissing is implicated in adolescents and adults, and transmission from care givers to young children is common. Blood transfusions can be a mode of transmission, but with few cases of disease attributed to it. Active disease is most common in those between 15 and 25 years of age. The risk of contracting the disease without close facial contact is minimal. Symptoms generally dissipate within a few weeks, but full recuperation may take several months. There is no specific treatment for mononucleosis, and immunization is unavailable. Corticosteroids are occasionally administered to help minimize tonsillar swelling. Nonsteroidal antiinflammatory drugs (NSAIDs) may provide symptomatic relief.

Herpes Simplex Virus Type 1 There are two types of **herpes simplex virus,** herpes simplex virus type 1 (HSV-1) and herpes simplex virus type 2 (HSV-2). HSV-2 will be discussed in the section on sexually transmitted diseases. HSV-1 is transmitted in the saliva of carriers and commonly infects the oropharynx, face, lips, skin, fingers, and toes. Everyone is susceptible. Infections of health care workers' hands and fingers can result in herpetic whitlow, weeping inflammations at the distal fingers and toes. The incubation period following exposure ranges from two to twelve days. In the oral cavity, fluid-filled vesicles develop into cold sores or fever blisters that soon deteriorate into small ulcers. Fever, malaise, and dehydration may accompany these primary lesions. The lesions usually disappear in two to three weeks. They may recur spontaneously, especially following periods of stress or other illness. Recurrent HSV labialis (lip lesions) may cause problems for many years in some adults.

Although primarily recognized for causing skin and mucous membrane disorders, HSV-1 can cause meningoencephalitis in newborns and aseptic meningitis in adults. A high index of suspicion for HSV-1 in these situations may result in timely treatment with antiviral agents like acyclovir, which is somewhat effective against HSV-1.

Universal precautions, primarily gloves, are absolutely essential, especially if an intimate contact or family member of the EMS worker is afflicted. Breaks in the skin place everyone at greater risk, and may not be visible to the naked eye. Treatment with acylovir (Zovirax) provides relief when used topically or orally. Immunization is not available.

OTHER INFECTIOUS CONDITIONS OF THE RESPIRATORY SYSTEM

The majority of profiles in this section discuss pathological conditions of the airway caused by a variety of infectious agents. They are not diseases, per se. Chapter 42 on pediatrics discusses croup and epiglottitis in greater detail. Hantavirus is included here, although its sites of pathology extend beyond the airways.

Content Review

OTHER INFECTIOUS RESPIRATORY CONDITIONS
- Epiglottitis
- Croup
- Pharyngitis
- Sinusitis
- Hantavirus

Epiglottitis Epiglottitis is an inflammation of the epiglottis and may also involve the areas just above and below it. In children it is a true emergency, usually caused by *H. influenzae,* with an abrupt onset over several hours and without any immediate history of upper respiratory disease. Patients present with one or more of the "four Ds:" dysphonia, drooling, dysphagia, or distress. Epiglottitis can also occur in teenagers and adults. In the older age groups, stridor, sore throat, fever, and drooling usually develop over days, not hours. Due to natural immunity from initial infection, epiglottitis is not known to reoccur in any age group. Increased immunization against *H. influenzae* has reduced the incidence of epiglottitis caused by this bacterium. However, *S. pneumoniae* and *S. aureus* have been implicated as causative agents of epiglottitis.

Croup Croup (laryngotracheobronchitis) is a common cause of acute upper airway obstruction in children. A viral illness characterized by inspiratory and expiratory stridor and a seal-bark-like cough, it is most common in children under the age of three. Although generally not life threatening, croup may create panic in parents and children alike. Viruses implicated in croup include the parainfluenza viruses, rhinoviruses, and RSV. Croup is often preceded by an upper respiratory infection. The child commonly awakens during the night with acute respiratory distress, tachypnea, and retractions. Seasonal outbreaks of this disease are common. Total airway obstruction is rare.

Pharyngitis Pharyngitis is a common infection of the pharynx and tonsils. It may be caused by a virus or bacteria and is characterized by a sudden onset of sore throat and fever. The tonsils and palate become red and swollen, and the cervical lymph nodes enlarge. Headache, neck pain, nausea, and vomiting may also be present. Most cases occur in late winter and early spring. Although this disease may occur in any age group, most cases are seen in five- to eleven-year-olds.

Group A streptococcus (strep throat) causes a particularly serious pharyngitis that, if left untreated, in certain cases, can progress to rheumatic fever. There are several sub-types of Group A streptococcus. One strain causes rheumatic fever. Another strain is responsible for scarlet fever (scarletina). Patients infected with this bacterium may present with a scarlet-colored rash. Because strep throat is very contagious, you should wear a mask when assessing and managing these patients. Although laboratory tests can easily determine which cases of pharyngitis are caused by strep, it is virtually impossible to tell clinically. Assume that all cases of pharyngitis are serious and contagious until proven otherwise. Antibiotics (penicillin, amoxicillin, erythromycin, azithromycin) effectively treat strep throat.

Sinusitis Sinusitis is an inflammation of the paranasal (ethmoid, frontal, maxillary, or sphenoid) sinuses. It occurs when mucus and pus cannot drain and become trapped in the sinus. Sinusitis is usually preceded by a viral upper respiratory infection or exposure to allergens, either of which may cause nasal congestion and blocked sinus passages. Postnasal drip may develop and nasal drainage may be blood-tinged and purulent. As fluids collect in the sinus, a sensation of pressure or fullness generally develops. If left untreated, the condition may become painful, and the infection can cause an abscess or spread into the cranium and attack the brain. Discomfort often worsens when the patient bends forward or when pressure is applied over the affected sinus. Sinusitis is occasionally a causative factor of meningitis. Management includes antibiotics, decongestants, and supportive care. Apply a heat pack directly over the affected sinus to help relieve pain and facilitate drainage.

Hantavirus Hantavirus is a family of viruses carried by rodents such as the deer mouse. Other known carriers are the rice and cotton rats in the southeastern United States and the white-footed mouse of the northeastern states. The common house mouse is not known to carry the virus. Most cases of hantavirus infection have occurred in the southwestern United States, particularly the Four Corners region. Transmission is primarily by inhalation of aerosols created by

Croup is a viral infection that affects the tissues below the glottis, while epiglottitis is a bacterial infection that affects the glottis and the tissue above the glottis.

* **croup** viral illness characterized by inspiratory and expiratory stridor and a seal-bark-like cough.

* **pharyngitis** infection of the pharynx and tonsils.

* **sinusitis** inflammation of the paranasal sinuses.

* **hantavirus** family of viruses that are carried by the deer mouse and transmitted by ticks and other arthropods.

stirring up the dried urine, saliva, and fecal droppings of these rodents. Contamination of food and autoinoculation after handling objects tainted by rodent droppings may also cause transmission. Direct bites are possible routes, but are thought to be rare. Person-to-person transmission is not possible.

The virus causes hantavirus pulmonary syndrome (HPS), to which anyone is susceptible. The initial symptoms are fatigue, fever, and muscle aches, especially of large muscle groups. Headaches, nausea, vomiting, diarrhea, and abdominal pain are also common. Earache, sore throat, and rash are uncommon. Approximately four to ten days later, symptoms of pulmonary edema occur. Patients with fatal infections appear to have severe myocardial depression, which can progress to sinus bradycardia and subsequent electromechanical dissociation, ventricular tachycardia, or fibrillation. Hemodynamic compromise occurs a median of five days after symptoms' onset—usually dramatically within the first day of hospitalization. The only specific treatment is intensive supportive care, and no immunization is available.

EMS responders who find themselves in dusty, unoccupied buildings for extended times should wear face masks to prevent inhaling aerosolized rodent droppings.

GI SYSTEM INFECTIONS

You may on occasion respond to scenes with single or multiple cases of foodborne illness. Although you cannot determine the causative agent outside of the hospital, you must have a basic knowledge of the infectious process and guidelines for assessment, management, and safe handling of these patients. Many EMS personnel are being recruited and volunteering for domestic and international disaster medical teams. In these situations, when the sanitation infrastructure (water treatment and distribution, sewer, animal control, and so forth) are disrupted, GI system infections increase significantly.

Gastroenteritis

✱ gastroenteritis generalized disorder involving nausea, vomiting, gastrointestinal cramping or discomfort, and diarrhea.

Gastroenteritis is a gastrointestinal disorder manifested by nausea, vomiting, gastrointestinal cramping or discomfort, anorexia, and diarrhea. In more advanced cases, which are rare, it can cause lassitude and shock. It is a common disease that many of us in developed countries have experienced. The reference to "stomach flu" in these situations is incorrect, since an influenza of the GI system has not yet been identified. What this distressing and uncomfortable condition usually represents, at least in developed countries, is a viral gastroenteritis. The causative agents may be viruses (Norwalk virus, Rotavirus, and others), bacteria (*E. coli, K. pneumoniae, C. jejuni, E. aerogenes, V. cholerae, Shigella,* and *Salmonella*), and parasites (*G. lamblia, C. parvum, C. cayetensis*). Gastroenteritis is highly contagious via the fecal-oral route, including the ingestion of contaminated food and water. It is especially contagious during natural disasters in epidemic proportions. International travelers into endemic areas are very susceptible, while native populations are generally resistant.

In otherwise healthy persons, gastroenteritis is generally self-limiting and benign; however, in the very young, the very old, or those with preexisting disease, it can be serious and often fatal. Prolonged vomiting and/or diarrhea may result in dehydration and electrolyte disturbances. Patients generally experience painful and severe abdominal cramping, and some develop hypovolemic shock. Always consider dehydration in any patient who presents with signs of gastroenteritis. If a patient has vomited many times or is actively vomiting, has multiple medical problems, is debilitated, or at risk by virtue of age and general health, start an IV with isotonic saline. Pay careful attention to hydration status. If the patient is in shock, the management objectives are no different than for hemorrhagic shock. If the patient is not in shock, the judicious use of fluids is warranted. A good rule of thumb is to replace fluids at approximately the rate they are lost. The World Health Organization and other international disaster response agencies have found oral rehydration very effective in treating fluid loss, even with cholera. Do not feel compelled to pour in IV fluids. If prolonged vomiting or retching is present, administer an antiemetic such as droperidol (Inapsine), prochlorperazine (Compazine), or promethazine (Phenergan). Remember that vehicle movements often aggravate symptoms and increase the probability of vomiting.

With isolated cases of gastroenteritis, compliance with universal precautions and postexposure hand washing are critical to avoiding infection. In times of disaster, EMS responders must be more focused on environmental health and sanitation issues: preparing food, identifying clean sources of water, using mosquito netting while sleeping, and general sanitation. Eat hot foods only and drink hot beverages that have been brisk boiled. Be careful to avoid personal habits that facilitate fecal-oral transmission. Prevention is important because even though antimicrobials may be available to treat isolated cases, resources for treating gastroenteritis during disasters or in developing countries may be limited. In those situations, many people receive symptomatic treatment.

Food Poisoning

Food poisoning is a nonspecific term often applied to gastroenteritis. Food poisoning occurs suddenly and is caused by eating. Diarrhea, vomiting, and gastrointestinal discomfort characterize its more benign presentation. Most cases are caused by bacteria and their toxic products. In the majority of cases, only the GI system is affected, but other systems may be affected in some cases, as with botulism or *Escherichia coli* O157:H7, causing debilitating illness or death. *Clostridium botulinum* produces a very potent neurotoxin that causes flaccid paralysis by blocking the release of acetylcholine at motor end plates and preganglionic autonomic synapses.

E. coli O157:H7, transmitted by the ingestion of uncooked or undercooked ground beef, often causes severe bloody diarrhea and abdominal cramps; sometimes the infection causes nonbloody diarrhea or no symptoms. Drinking unpasteurized milk and swimming in or drinking sewage-contaminated water can also cause infection. Little or no fever is usually present, and the illness resolves in five to ten days. In some persons, particularly children under five years of age and the elderly, the infection can cause a complication called hemolytic uremic syndrome, in which the red blood cells are destroyed and the kidneys fail. About 2–7 percent of infections lead to this complication. In the United States, hemolytic uremic syndrome is the principal cause of acute kidney failure in children, and *E. coli* O157:H7 causes most cases of hemolytic uremic syndrome.

Other bacteria implicated in food poisoning include *Campylobacter, Salmonella, Shigella,* and *Vibrio cholerae.* Microorganisms may be transmitted in other meats that are insufficiently cooked. *Salmonella* is commonly transmitted through incompletely cooked poultry. It may also be spread through contaminated cookware and utensils used in preparation of poultry. Hepatitis A and Norwalk virus are known to have been ingested in undercooked seafood. Bacterial gastrointestinal infections tend to be much more severe than viral gastrointestinal infections. With bacterial infections, the patient will appear more toxic. There is often a history of bloody, foul-smelling diarrhea (especially with shigellosis). The presence of leukocytes in a fecal smear is suggestive of bacterial disease. Ultimately, stool cultures are required to confirm a bacterial cause of gastroenteritis.

Initiate standard advanced life support (ALS) protocols, including assessment of airway and ventilatory status, oxygenation, initiation of an IV, and cardiac

* **food poisoning** nonspecific term often applied to gastroenteritis that occurs suddenly and that is caused by the ingestion of food containing preformed toxins.

monitoring. Fluid resuscitation with isotonic crystalloids is often required. It is not uncommon for an adult with severe gastroenteritis to require 2–3 liters of fluid. In patients with significant vomiting or diarrhea, also consider antiemetics. Constant reassessment of ventilatory status is essential since the neurotoxin in *C. botulinum* ingestion may cause respiratory arrest. Observing universal precautions should protect against foodborne transmission of infectious agents. No immunization against these agents or their toxins exists.

Prevention efforts are the primary means of reducing foodborne illness. Advances in technology may provide better alternatives for food supply surveillance, an aspect of foodborne disease prevention that could be improved. Lawrence Berkeley National Laboratory has developed plastic strips that turn from blue to red in the presence of toxic strains of *E. coli*. This technology's basis could become a prototype for other simple reagent strips that can detect foodborne pathogens.

NERVOUS SYSTEM INFECTIONS

Encephalitis, rabies, tetanus, and Lyme disease all have significant effects on the nervous system. These infectious conditions or diseases do not necessarily pose occupational risks to EMS providers. They are well known to the general public, however, and are very much associated with recreational activities in which EMS responders participate.

Encephalitis

* **encephalitis** acute infection of the brain, usually caused by a virus.

Encephalitis is an inflammation caused by infection of the brain and its structures, usually by viruses such as equine viruses, arboviruses, the rubella virus, or the mumps virus. These viral infections usually result in one of the following:

1. They cause no pathology until they are transported to cerebral neurons, which they invade, and then replicate (the rabies and arthropod-borne viruses, for instance).
2. They first injure nonnervous tissues and then, rarely, invade the cerebral neurons (for example, herpes simplex 1 and varicella-zoster virus).

Bacteria, fungi, or parasites may also cause encephalitis, but the viruses are the predominant infectious agents.

The clinical presentation of encephalitis is similar to that of meningitis since they often coexist. Signs and symptoms include decreased level of consciousness, fever, headache, drowsiness, coma, tremors, and a stiff neck and back. Seizures may occur in patients of any age but are most common in infants. Characteristic neurological signs include uncoordinated and involuntary movements, weakness of the arms, legs, or other portions of the body, or unusual sensitivity of the skin to various types of stimuli.

Treatment is difficult, even when the virus is known. Despite the severity of illness, many patients suffer no long-term neurological deficits; however, as many as 50 percent of children younger than one year may suffer irreversible brain damage after contracting eastern or western equine encephalitis, diseases of horses and mules transmitted to humans by mosquitoes.

Rabies

* **rabies** viral disorder that affects the nervous system.

Rabies is transmitted by the rabies virus, a member of the Rhabdovirus family and *Lyssavirus* genus, which affects the nervous system. It exists in two epidemiological forms: *urban*, propagated chiefly through unimmunized domestic dogs and cats, and *sylvatic,* propagated by skunks, foxes, raccoons, mongooses, coyotes, wolves, and bats. Humans are especially susceptible when bitten by infected animals. The virus is transmitted in the saliva of infected mammals by bites, an opening in the skin, or direct contact with a mucous membrane. It passes along motor and sensory fibers to the spinal ganglia corresponding to the site of invasion, and then to the brain, creating an *encephalomyelitis* that is almost always fatal. Although rare, transmission is also known to occur by inhalation of aerosolized virus, through nasal nerve fibers and mucosa, along the olfactory nerve, and then to the brain. Mammals are highly susceptible to infection. Transmission is known to be affected by the severity of the wound, abundance of the nerve supply close to the wound, the distance to the CNS, the amount and strain of virus, protective clothing, and other undetermined factors. The highly variable incubation period is usually from three to eight weeks but can be as short as nine days (rare) or as long as ten years. It is believed to be dependent on the bite site, with bites to the head and neck generally followed by shorter incubation periods.

Rabies is characterized by a non-specific *prodrome* (symptoms that precede the appearance of a disease) of malaise, headache, fever, chills, sore throat, myalgias, anorexia, nausea, vomiting, and diarrhea. The prodrome typically lasts from one to four days. The next phase, the *encephalitic phase,* begins with periods of excessive motor activity, excitation, and agitation. This is soon followed by confusion, hallucinations, combativeness, bizarre aberrations of thought, muscle twitches and tetany, and seizures. Soon, focal paralysis appears. When left untreated, it can cause death within two to six days. Attempts to drink water may produce laryngospasm, causing the characteristic profuse drooling commonly known as hydrophobia (fear of water).

Rabies in the United States has become more prevalent in the wild. From 1980 to 1999, 58 of the rabies cases diagnosed in the United States have been attributed to bat variants. It is not surprising then, that the CDC has identified wildlife as the most important potential source of infection for humans and domestic animals in this country. In Africa, Asia, and Latin America, dogs remain the major source. Human rabies is rare in the United States, but each year 16,000–39,000 people receive postexposure prophylaxis. This is not a matter of paranoia. The CDC estimates that up to one-third of persons who have contracted rabies cannot accurately relate a history of having been bitten by an animal. Thus, epidemiologists now believe that the inhalation route, once thought to be theoretical, may be more common than previously believed. Human-to-human transmission of rabies is not known to occur; however, paramedics should take BSI precautions to protect themselves from contact with infectious saliva. The use of masks in environments where a patient has been exposed may be prudent, judging from the recent epidemiological evidence in the United States with bats.

When caring for a bite patient, first inspect the site of the wound for bite pattern and the presence of saliva. Then rinse the wound with copious amounts of normal saline to remove saliva and blood. Do not bandage or dress the wound, but allow it to drain freely during transport. Irrigation en route from a 10- or 15-drop/ml IV administration set may be beneficial. If the patient refuses transport to the emergency department, you must inform him of the consequences of the bite and the importance of medical follow up. If time and circumstances permit, ensure that the suspect animal has been secured and contained for transport to the hospital or animal control shelter for subsequent postmortem examination of cerebral tissue.

If you are bitten or exposed to an animal you believe is rabid, take the following measures:

1. Vigorously wash the wound with soap and warm water.
2. Debride and irrigate the wound, and allow it to drain freely on the way to the emergency department.

3. Discuss postexposure prophylaxis with the physician. Consultation with public health officials may be necessary. Unless you have an actual bite from an animal whose behavior is consistent with rabies infection, exposure is a medical urgency, not emergency.

4. Consider the need for tetanus and other antibiotic therapy as the attending physician deems appropriate.

Several alternatives now exist for rabies immunization. Individuals who should be immunized include animal care workers and shelter personnel, those who work outdoors and have frequent contact with wild animals known to transmit rabies.

Tetanus

* **tetanus** acute bacterial infection of the central nervous system.

Tetanus is an acute bacterial infection of the central nervous system. It presents with musculoskeletal signs and symptoms caused by tetanospasmin, an exotoxin of the *Clostridium tetani* bacillus. *C. tetani* is present as extremely durable spores in the soil, street dust, and feces and is in the same genus as *C. perfringens,* the causative organism of gas gangrene. Since *Clostridium* species favor an anaerobic environment, the bacteria are particularly suited to colonizing dead or necrotic tissue. Infection has been contracted through wounds considered too minor to warrant medical attention and through burns. Although puncture wounds are classically associated with *C. tetani* infection, deep lacerations can also be suitable environments. Transmission can even occur by injection of contaminated drugs and surgical procedures, leading to the conclusion that *C. tetani* spores are found everywhere. The incubation period is variable (usually from three to twenty-one days, sometimes from one day to several months) and depends on the wound's severity and location. Generally, a shorter incubation period leads to a more severe illness. The mortality rate increases in direct proportion to age. The general population is susceptible, but incidence is highest in agricultural areas where unimmunized people are in frequent contact with animal feces. The disease is rare in the United States, with fewer than 100 cases reported each year.

Localized tetanus symptoms include rigidity of muscles in close proximity to the injury site. Subsequent generalized symptoms may include pain and stiffness in the jaw muscles and may progress to cause muscle spasm and rigidity of the entire body. Respiratory arrest may result. In children, abdominal rigidity may be the first sign. Rigidity occurs after the toxin is taken up at the myoneural junction and transported to the CNS. The toxin then acts upon inhibitory neurons, which normally suppress unnecessary efferent impulses and muscle movements. The reduction in inhibitory action results in the muscles' receiving more nervous impulses and tetany. Sometimes a sardonic grin, *risus sardonicus,* accompanies the lock jaw and conjures memories of the Cheshire Cat in *Alice in Wonderland.*

EMS responders will rarely encounter this disease, much less recognize its signs and symptoms until they are advanced to the point of tetany. A possible EMS scenario would be the transfer of a patient from a rural community hospital to an urban medical center for intensive care. Universal precautions should provide adequate protection. Masks probably are not necessary unless the infectious agent is unknown. Respiratory arrest is a possibility, so you should consider wearing masks while performing endotracheal intubation. If you incur a wound in the course of treating a patient, wash the wound thoroughly or, if warranted, have it inspected and debrided in the emergency department. Wounds that are cared for within six hours pose a lower risk for growth of anaerobic micro-organisms. Consideration should be given to post exposure prophylaxis with tetanus immune globulin (TIG), diphtheria-tetanus toxoid (Td), or diphtheria-tetanus toxoid, pertussis (DTP).

Immunizations, which generally begin in childhood as DTP vaccinations, include boosters before entering elementary school and every ten years thereafter. A booster administered every ten years is believed to confer effective active immunity. Previous documented infection is not known to confer lifelong immunity.

Lyme Disease

Lyme disease is a recurrent inflammatory disorder accompanied by skin lesions, polyarthritis, and involvement of the heart and nervous system. Caused by the tick-borne spirochete *Borrelia burgdorferi,* similar in shape to the causative organism of syphilis, it is the most commonly reported vector-borne disease in the United States. The tick that carries Lyme disease is very common in the Northeast, the Upper Midwest, and along the Pacific Coast. Deer and mice are both reservoirs of the tick, and the disease is common in people living and recreating near wooded areas with high deer populations. Most infections occur in spring and summer, when tick exposure is most likely. Everyone is susceptible, and natural infection does not appear to confer immunity. The incubation period ranges from three to thirty-two days.

Lyme disease progresses in three stages:

- *Early Localized Stage* A painless, flat, red lesion appears at the bite site. In some patients, a ring-like rash, *erythema migrans (EM),* develops and spreads outward. The outer border remains bright red, with the center becoming clear, blue, or even necrotic. The rash—often called a "bull's eye" rash—usually disappears in time, whether treated or not. At this stage, patients also may complain of headache, malaise, and muscle aches. Although uncommon, the patient's neck may be stiff.

- *Early Disseminated Stage* The spirochete spreads to the skin, nervous system, heart, and joints. More EM lesions develop. CNS sequelae include meningitis, seventh-cranial-nerve Bell's palsy, and peripheral neuropathy. Cardiac abnormalities include conduction defects and myopathy. Arthritis and myalgia are common months after infection. Approximately 8 percent of patients will have some cardiac involvement. The most common manifestations are varying degrees of atrioventricular block (first degree, Wenckebach, and complete heart block). Less commonly, myocarditis and left ventricular dysfunction are seen. Cardiac involvement typically lasts only a few weeks, but can recur.

- *Late Stage (persistent infection)* The late stage can occur months or years after the initial exposure. Although the incidence of cardiac problems is lower, it involves the same neurological complications as second stage, plus encephalopathy with cognitive deficits, depression, and sleep disorders. Monoarthritis of large joints and more than one joint concurrently (polyarthritis) is common.

Development of erythema migrans, the bull's eye rash, usually 3 to 30 days after tick exposure, is presumptive for the diagnosis.

The EMS response to Lyme disease will probably be to treat its clinical consequences, especially those of the disseminated and late stages. ALS treatment is directed toward those consequences, not the infection. Adhere to universal precautions. After responding to calls in heavily wooded areas infested by ticks, always check both your and the patient's clothing, shoes, socks, and body for ticks. Spray the ambulance compartment with an insecticide effective against arthropods. Available antibiotic therapies are effective for the stages of the disease progression.

* **Lyme disease** recurrent inflammatory disorder caused by a tick-borne spirochete.

Content Review

STAGES OF LYME DISEASE
- Early localized
- Early disseminated
- Late

* **sexually transmitted disease (STD)** illness most commonly transmitted through sexual contact.

* **gonorrhea** sexually transmitted disease caused by a gram-negative bacterium.

* **syphilis** bloodborne sexually transmitted disease caused by the spirochete *Treponema pallidum*.

Protection against Lyme disease (LYMErix) is now available as a series of three vaccinations, with the second dose given at one month and the third at twelve. It is recommended for persons aged 15–70 years whose activities result in frequent exposure to tick habitats, and for selected travelers to endemic areas where exposure to tick habitats is anticipated.

SEXUALLY TRANSMITTED DISEASES

Infectious diseases transmitted through sexual contact are known as **sexually transmitted diseases,** or **STDs.** They represent some of the most prevalent communicable diseases. A variety of bacterial (gonorrhea, syphilis, chancroid, chlamydia), viral (HIV, herpes), and parasitic (*Pediculosis, Trichomonas*) infections are spread by this route. Other illnesses that are generally not considered STDs, including hepatitis A, B, C, D, salmonella, and shigella, may also be transmitted through sexual contact. STDs affect the genital organs, often resulting in pathology to reproductive structures. Although EMS responders do not treat these diseases, other emergency health care personnel commonly know the information in the following profiles. Your knowledge of these diseases will put you on a "level playing field" with those other health care workers and bolster your credibility. When you treat or transport patients with STDs, observe universal precautions, avoid contact with lesions and exudates, and wash your hands vigorously after exposure.

Gonorrhea

Gonorrhea, caused by *Neisseria gonorrhoeae,* a gram-negative bacterium, is one of the most commonly diagnosed communicable diseases in the United States. Over one million cases are treated annually. Everyone is susceptible to infection, and although antibodies develop after exposure and confer immunity, they do so only for the specific serotype that caused the infection. Thus, persons contracting gonorrhea would not be immune to penicillinase-producing *N. gonorrhoeae* (PPNG), a strain of *N. gonorrhoeae* known by military personnel during the Vietnam War as black clap. Most commonly seen in males in their early twenties, gonorrhea is transmitted by direct contact with exudates of mucous membranes, primarily from direct sexual contact. In men, the disease presents as painful urination and a purulent urethral discharge. Untreated, it can lead to epididymitis, prostatitis, and urethral strictures. The majority of women contracting the disease have no pain and minimal discharge. In some cases, symptoms include urinary frequency, vaginal discharge, fever, and abdominal pain. Pelvic inflammatory disease (PID) often results after menstruation when bacteria spread from the cervix to the upper genital tract. Affected females are at increased risk for sterility, ectopic pregnancy, abscesses within reproductive structures, and peritonitis.

Gonorrhea may occasionally become systemic, causing sepsis or meningitis. Septic arthritis may result, presenting with fever, pain, swelling, and limited range of motion in one or two joints, sometimes leading to progressive deterioration. In the United States, single dosing is often effective in treating localized gonorrhea (genitourinary only). Treating systemic gonorrhea often involves additional chemotherapy. When gonorrhea infection coexists with chlamydial infections (as is estimated to occur in about 50 percent of gonorrhea patients), two-drug therapy is routinely advised. No immunization is available.

Syphilis

Syphilis is a disease caused by the spirochete *Treponema pallidum*. It is transmitted by direct contact with exudates from other syphilitic lesions of skin and mucous membranes, semen, blood, saliva, and vaginal discharges. It is therefore most commonly contracted through sexual intercourse but also may be transmitted by kissing or close contact with an open lesion. An estimated 30 percent of exposures result in infection. In congenital syphilis, infants contract the disease before birth from an infected mother. Everyone is susceptible to infection. Although the risk of transmission by blood transfusion or needle-stick injury is low, health care workers have been infected after physical examination involving manual contact with a lesion. A gradual immunity does develop after infection, but aggressive antimicrobial therapy may interfere with this natural antibody formation, especially during the primary and secondary stages.

Syphilis is characterized by lesions that may involve virtually any organ or tissue. It usually has cutaneous manifestations with frequent relapses, and it may remain latent for years. The incubation period is three weeks. Syphilis may occur in four stages, depending on how early and aggressively treatment is initiated:

Content Review

STAGES OF SYPHILIS
- Primary
- Secondary
- Latent
- Tertiary

- *Primary syphilis (first stage)* presents as a painless lesion, or chancre. In heterosexual men, the chancre is usually on the penis. In homosexual men, the chancre is often found on the anal canal, rectum, tongue, lips, or other point of entry. The chancre typically occurs three to six weeks after exposure. Nontender enlargement of regional lymph nodes may also occur.

- *Secondary syphilis (second stage),* or the bacteremic stage, begins five to six weeks after the chancre has healed. It is characterized by a maculopapular skin rash (small, red, flat lesions) on the palms and soles, condyloma latum (painless, wart-like lesions on warm, moist skin areas that are very infectious), and cutaneous infection in areas of hair growth causing loss of hair and/or eyebrows. These skin signs last for about six weeks. CNS disease (syphilitic meningitis) and arthritis may occur, as can infections of the eyes and kidneys.

- *Latent syphilis (third stage),* a period when symptoms improve or disappear completely, may last from months to many years. Twenty-five percent of cases may relapse with secondary stage symptoms; however, relapses usually do not occur after four years. Thirty-three percent of cases will progress to tertiary syphilis, and the rest will remain asymptomatic

- *Tertiary syphilis (fourth stage)* is the stage of syphilis that justifies its reputation as a "great imitator." Lesions with sharp borders, called gummas, may appear on skin and bones, causing a deep, gnawing pain. Cardiovascular syphilis may appear, usually ten years after the primary infection, resulting in aortic aneurysms that antibiotic therapy does not reverse. Neurosyphilis is diagnosed when there are neurological signs in seropositive patients. Meningitis may result, with possible spinal cord disease causing loss of reflexes, and reduced sensation of pain and temperature. The spirochetes can also invade the cerebral vessels, causing a stroke. A progressive dementia can also occur during this stage.

EMS responders may treat a variety of clinical complications of syphilis, often without being aware of infection as the primary etiology. ALS is directed toward treating the clinical presentation, which may include seizures, an acute onset of dementia, signs of a stroke, aortic aneurysm, or acute myocardial infarction. Avoid frequent contact with lesions on any part of the patient's body, and pay attention to handwashing technique after patient contact since *T. pallidum* is easily killed by heat, soap, and water.

For presumptive screening after exposure, rapid plasmin reagin (RPR) and venereal disease research labs (VDRL) tests are available. Because RPR or VDRL have fairly high rates of false-positive reactions, more specific tests should always follow. Treatment of primary syphilis is benzathine penicillin, with erythromycin and doxycycline (Vibramycin) as alternatives for patients allergic to penicillin. No immunization is available.

Genital Warts

Genital warts (condyloma acuminatum) are caused by the human papillomavirus (HPV), a DNA virus. To date, research has identified 70 HPV types, with most known to cause specific clinical manifestations. Some of the types known to cause genital warts are associated with cervical cancer. Genital warts are contagious and easily spread. In males, they generally appear as cauliflower-like, fleshy growths on the penis, anus, and mucosa of the anal canal. In females, they usually appear on the labial surfaces. Genital warts are sometimes difficult to distinguish from the condyloma latum seen in the secondary stage of syphilis. HPV has been implicated as a causative factor of cervical cancer in females.

Herpes Simplex Type 2

HSV-2 causes 70–90 percent of all genital herpes cases. Transmission is usually by sexual contact. Everyone is susceptible, but adolescents and young adults are most commonly afflicted. Neonates are often infected during passage down the birth canal. The prevalence of HSV-2 antibody, which does not confer immunity, is greater in lower socioeconomic groups and persons with multiple sex partners. The disease presents as vesicular lesions on the penis, anus, rectum, and mouth of the male depending on sexual activity. Females are sometimes asymptomatic, but can display lesions of the vagina, vulva, perineum, rectum, mouth, and cervix. Recurrent infections in females are often found on the vulva, buttocks, legs, and the perineum. Patients may present with fever and enlarged lymph nodes during the initial infection. Lesions may last up to several weeks before eventually crusting over and healing. The most serious consequence of HSV-2 infection is that painful lesions may recur periodically during the patient's lifetime, significantly diminishing quality of life. Recent evidence suggests that symptomatic treatment with the antiviral agent acyclovir orally, intravenously, or topically, may decrease the incidence of recurrences and lessen the severity of their symptoms. Other treatment alternatives include CO_2 laser removal, cryotherapy (freezing and removal) with liquid nitrogen, electrical cauterization, and interferon. Immunization is not currently available.

Chlamydia

* chlamydia group of intracellular parasites that cause sexually transmitted diseases.

Chlamydia is a genus of intracellular parasites most like gram-negative bacteria. Once thought to be viruses, the chlamydiae are now known to have an inner and outer membrane, to contain both DNA and RNA, and to be susceptible to numerous antibiotics. However, they lack peptidoglycan, a net of polysaccharides found in all true bacterial walls.

From the standpoint of STDs, *Chlamydia trachomatis* is the most clinically significant species, affecting the genital area, eyes, and respiratory system. Everyone is susceptible, and up to 25 percent of men may be carriers. *C. trachomatis* is responsible for roughly 50 percent of all cases of nongonococcal urethritis (NGU) in men, with dysuria and penile discharge common. It is transmitted by sexual activity and by hand-to-hand transfer of eye secretions, causing conjunctivitis. Internationally, this is the leading cause of preventable blindness. Because children are the major reservoir and the common use of infected linen can transmit chlamydia, child care center and school workers should exercise caution in handling blankets, sheets, and towels.

The symptoms are similar to gonorrhea's but less severe, often making the clinical differentiation difficult. In addition, the progression of disease in women is identical, with both causing a mucopurulent discharge that often accompanies cervicitis. Some women may have retrograde infections of the reproductive tract, causing pelvic inflammatory disease. Sterility may result. Newborns may be infected during passage through an infected birth canal, resulting in infant pneumonia or blindness.

No immunization is available, but *C. trachomatis* infection responds to a variety of antimicrobial agents such as tetracycline, doxycycline (Vibramycin), erythromycin (PCE), and orally administered azithromycin (Zithromax). Natural infection is not known to confer immunity.

Another species of Chlamydia, *C. pneumoniae,* has been found in atherosclerotic lesions of patients who have died of myocardial infarction. This has led to speculation about the relationship between *C. pneumoniae* infection and atherosclerosis as an inflammatory process.

Trichomoniasis

Trichomonas vaginalis, a protozoan parasite, is a common cause of vaginitis. In women, the symptoms of **trichomoniasis** include a greenish-yellow vaginal discharge, irritation of the perineum and thighs, and dysuria. This disease is frequently present with gonorrhea. Men are generally asymptomatic carriers of the disease. When present, symptoms include dysuria, urethral discharge, and discomfort in the perineum. The infection is currently treated with metronidazole (Flagyl).

✳ **trichomoniasis** sexually transmitted disease caused by the protozoan *Trichomonas vaginalis.*

Chancroid

Chancroid is a highly contagious ulcer caused by *Haemophilus ducreyi,* a gram-negative bacterium. It is more frequently diagnosed in men, particularly those who have sex with prostitutes. Uncircumcised men are at higher risk. It is spread by direct contact, mostly sexual, with open lesions and pus. Autoinoculation has occurred in infected persons. Its incubation period is typically 3–5 days but may be as long as 14 days.

The disease begins with a painful, inflamed pustule or ulcer that may appear on the penis, anus, urethra, or vulva. It spreads easily to other sites such as breasts, fingers, and thighs. Lymph nodes may become swollen and tender, and fever may be present. Chancroid ulcer is linked with increased risk of HIV infection. Chancroid lesions in children beyond the neonatal period should alert EMS responders to the possibility of reportable child sexual abuse.

Health care workers have contracted the disease by contacting patients' ulcers. Immunization is not available, and infection does not appear to confer immunity. Several effective antimicrobials (for example, erythromycin) are available.

✳ **chancroid** highly contagious sexually transmitted ulcer.

DISEASES OF THE SKIN

EMS responders' interactions with patients or the general public may expose them to contagious skin infections such as impetigo or the ectoparasites lice and scabies. Because the public frequently attempts to consult paramedics about general topics in personal and community health, your knowledge of ectoparasites may enable you to provide education and customer service. As always, use universal precautions and effective postexposure hand washing.

> **Content Review**
>
> **DISEASES OF THE SKIN**
> - Impetigo
> - Lice
> - Scabies

Impetigo

impetigo infection of the skin caused by staphylococci or streptococci.

Impetigo is a very contagious infection of the skin caused by staphylococci or streptococci. The disease begins as a single vesicle that ruptures and forms a thick, honey-colored crust with a yellowish-red center. Lesions most commonly occur on the extremities and joints. Although few patients call an ambulance for this condition, it often appears on patients who seek EMS for other reasons. EMS responders who develop impetigo should not report for work until cleared by their physician. It is easily transmitted by direct skin-to-skin contact, so universal precautions should provide ample protection.

Lice

lice parasitic infestation of the skin of the scalp, trunk, or pubic area.

infestation presence of parasites that do not break the host's skin.

Lice (pediculosis) is a parasitic **infestation** of the skin of the scalp, trunk, or pubic area. Lice infest hosts rather than infect them because they do not break the skin. The three different varieties of infestations are *Pediculus humanus var. capitis* (head lice), *Pediculus humanus var. corporis* (body lice), and *Pthirus pubis* (pubic lice, or crabs). Historically, head lice have been involved in outbreaks of typhus, trench fever in World War I, and relapsing fever. Head and body lice appear similar, both being 3–4 mm long. Head lice are transmitted by sharing of combs or hats and are fairly common among young school-aged children regardless of socioeconomic status. Outbreaks in day care centers and schools are common. Head lice are easily diagnosed by the presence of small, white, oval-shaped eggs (nits) attached to the hair shafts. Nits can be seen with the naked eye but are more easily found with a magnifying glass. Lice themselves are rarely seen. They tend to leave febrile hosts, so high environmental temperatures and crowding favor transmission. Lice have a three-stage life cycle of eggs, nymphs, and adults. Eggs hatch in 7–10 days but cannot hatch below 72°F. The nymph stage lasts about 7–13 days, again depending on temperature, with a total egg to egg cycle of 3 weeks.

Anyone can be infested, and repeated infestations may cause an allergic response. Infestation often occurs on eyebrows and eyelashes, hair, mustaches, and beards. Symptoms are generally limited to severe itching. Body lice often infest clothing along seams close to skin surfaces and attach to the skin only to feed. They can be vectors of bacteria. Red macules, papules, and urticaria commonly appear on the shoulders, buttocks, and abdomen. Pubic lice infest through sexual contact by attaching to hair in the genital and anal regions but can also infest facial hair.

Any EMS responder exposed to a patient with lice may be treated with one of several nonprescription agents. Pyrethrin preparations such as RID are commonly used, but require two applications one week apart because they do not kill eggs. Permethrin agents such as Nix or Elimite theoretically require only a single application because they kill adults and eggs. Lindane 1% shampoo (Kwell) may be used, but it is available only by prescription and is more toxic than the other treatments. Eliminating the eggs by combing the hair is essential. Nits are more easily removed (nit picking) after soaking combs in a white vinegar solution or using a commercial preparation such as the Step 2 Nit Removal System. Separately bagging linen in an occupational setting is unnecessary. At home, however, isolating infested linen and clothing is advisable to avoid exposing uninfested laundry for extended periods. Lice are not known to jump great distances like fleas, so spraying the ambulance's interior close to the cot and the area by the patient's head with an insecticide, preferably one containing premethrin, should be sufficient after a call. Clean and wipe all sprayed areas to remove insecticide residues.

Scabies

Scabies is caused by infestation of a mite (*Sarcoptes scabiei*) that is barely visible without magnification. Exposure to the mite is through close personal contact, from hand holding to sexual relations. The mite can remain viable on clothing or in bedding for up to 48 hours.

Upon attaching to a new host, the female tunnels into the skin within 2.5 minutes and lays up to three eggs a day along the "burrow" in the epidermis. The larvae hatch shortly thereafter, leading to a full grown adult 10 to 20 days later. The adults remain near hair follicles and forage for nourishment with their jaws and the claws of their forelegs.

The primary symptom is intense itching (hence the name "seven-year itch"), usually at night. It generally occurs from two to six weeks after infestation. The irritation results from sensitization to the mite and its droppings. Inflammatory lesions appear as fine, wavy, dark lines, usually not more than one centimeter long. In males they most commonly occur on the webs of the fingers, wrists, elbows, armpits, belt line, thighs, and external genitalia. In females, they most often involve the areolae and nipples, abdomen, and lower portions of the buttocks. In infants, the head, neck, palms, and soles are frequently involved. Older children exhibit patterns similar to adults. Complications are generally due to infections of lesions that are broken by scratching.

Although everyone is susceptible to infection, immunocompromised patients sometimes develop Norwegian scabies, a more severe form of scabies. Persons with previous exposure appear to have fewer mites on subsequent exposures and develop symptoms much sooner (in from one to four days), suggesting an amnestic (remembered) immune system response. Outbreaks of scabies resistant to lindane (Kwell) have been reported in several nursing homes across the country.

Scabies remains communicable until all mites and eggs are destroyed. Because of the long incubation period, all household members and/or close contacts of infested EMS responders should be treated simultaneously. Although some experts recommend that clothing and uniforms worn within two days of treatment, along with towels and bed linen, should be washed in hot water or dry cleaned, this necessity is questionable for most infestations. It is essential, however, for articles contacting patients with Norwegian scabies. Bag and remove all linens from the ambulance immediately after you deliver the patient. To prevent spread of the mite, clean the stretcher and patient compartment as recommended for lice. Remove and decontaminate any clothing that may have contacted the patient.

The scabicides of choice are premethrin cream (Elimite) or lindane (Kwell), which is applied to the skin from the neck down, left on for 8 to 14 hours, and then washed off. This should be repeated within one week. If premethrin is ineffective, 10% crotamiton (Eurax) and ivermectin (Stromectol) are also available.

> ✳ **scabies** skin disease caused by mite infestation and characterized by intense itching.

NOSOCOMIAL INFECTIONS

Hospitalized patients, especially those with compromised immune function, often acquire new infectious diseases. Especially virulent strains of microorganisms may cause these **nosocomial** (hospital acquired) diseases. Bacteria that resist antibiotics are of particular concern. Recently, vancomycin-resistant enterococcus (VRE) and methicillin-resistant *Staphylococcus aureus* (MRSA) have become especially alarming. Both of these organisms can cause severe host damage, and both are difficult to treat. They rapidly colonize patients in whom broad-spectrum antibiotics have eliminated normal flora. Hospitalized patients may also contract resistant strains of tuberculosis that spread easily from patient to patient if protective clothing and hand-washing precautions are not strictly observed.

> ✳ **nosocomial** acquired while in the hospital.

PREVENTING DISEASE TRANSMISSION

Preventing or limiting exposure to infectious or communicable diseases cannot be overemphasized. While some infectious diseases are relatively minor with no long-term effects, others can be very serious and even life threatening. As a paramedic, you must be extremely vigilant during patient contact and take every step possible to ensure your health and safety. Personal accountability is important. Do not go to work if you:

- Have diarrhea
- Have a draining wound or any type of wet lesions. Allow them to dry and crust over before returning to work.
- Are jaundiced
- Have mononucleosis
- Have been exposed to lice or scabies and have not yet been treated
- Have strep throat and have not been taking antibiotics for at least 24 hours
- Have a cold

Keep the following immunizations current: MMR, hepatitis A (if deemed appropriate in your jurisdiction), hepatitis B, DPT, polio, chickenpox, influenza (seasonal), and rabies (if appropriate).

Always approach the scene cautiously with a high index of suspicion. Upon arrival, control the scene to decrease the likelihood of body fluid exposure for everyone present. Observe BSI. Always wear gloves. If there is the remotest possibility of splashing or aerosolization of body fluids, wear protective eyewear or a mask with face shield. If large volumes of blood or other fluids may result from the response, don a gown. When contacting a patient who has or may have active TB, wear the appropriate N95 respirator.

Patients who have coughs, fever, headache, general weakness, recent weight loss, or nuchal rigidity or are taking certain medications may raise your awareness of the potential for contracting an infectious agent. With experience, you will develop your intuition and associate certain symptoms with infectious patients you have treated. Bolster your experience by increasing your knowledge, particularly your clinical acumen in recognizing the immunocompromised patient.

After a call, wash your hands first. Decontaminate and disinfect your equipment and the interior of the ambulance. Using commercially available disinfectants that certify bactericidal activity against *M. tuberculosis* should provide ample disinfection of those infectious agents that pose your greatest occupational risk. Remember that HIV is a fragile virus that any vigorous application of soap and water will kill. Utilize high-level disinfection on airway equipment. If the patient or the situation surrounding the response presents the possibility of lice, scabies, or ticks, spray the gurney and interior of the ambulance with the appropriate insecticide and wipe or mop up any residue. Ensure that linen will not be taken home. If practical, do not wear uniforms home. To discourage that practice, some EMS agencies consider uniforms as PPE. Report any infectious exposure to the IDCO, human resources director, or appropriate designated official.

The topics mandated by OSHA/NIOSH for compliance with published standards and guidelines (that is, bloodborne pathogens and TB) reflect the paramedic's minimum needed knowledge of infectious diseases. Proactive EMS agencies offer their personnel continuing education in infectious diseases that have high incidence or prevalence in the communities they serve. Continuing education sessions should include identification of causative agents, modes of transmission, epidemiological patterns within the community, signs and symptoms, methods to avoid infection, and special postexposure considerations, including postexposure prophylaxis, if appropriate.

To maintain a perspective on personal risk, always consider the interaction of three major factors: infectious agent, host, and environment. Are you aware of the infectious agent's virulence? Do you have some idea of the dose of the organism involved? For example, was a large volume of body fluid involved? How healthy are you? Do you have any chronic medical conditions or take any medications that would classify you as immunocompromised? What was the nature of the exposure? Is it significantly high? The probability of risk is sometimes just a measure of exposure. Not all infectious diseases are communicable. If they are communicable, they may not necessarily pose a high probability of developing disease. The risk and potential for HIV transmission to health care workers may be high, but the probability of transmission, which averages approximately 0.3 percent, is very low.

As you are promoted within your organization, your first additional responsibility may be as a preceptor for a new paramedic or student. You therefore assume responsibility for his well being. Are you familiar with your local protocols and procedures for reporting and recording an exposure? Can you adequately document the circumstances surrounding the exposure to facilitate review by the IDCO, physician, or agency administrator? If you cannot, what kind of a role model are you for that new employee or student?

Paramedics cannot allow their personal prejudices to interfere with providing optimum care for their patients. Patients should not be treated differently because they have an infectious disease that might reflect on their ethnicity, culture, sexual preference, or social status. You should not avoid certain procedures because you find a disease process or its consequences personally repulsive. It is sometimes helpful to think about doing things *for* patients, as opposed to doing things *to* them.

SUMMARY

Over the past thirty years, medical science has made tremendous progress in diagnosing and treating infectious diseases. New vaccines and antibiotics are continually being developed. Advances in laboratory technology, notably the polymerase chain reaction (PCR), have made the presence and identification of microorganisms easier, quicker, and more accurate. Despite these tremendous advances, many infectious diseases cannot be effectively treated. Specific treatments for most viral diseases remain elusive, and each year countless people die from AIDS, hepatitis, pneumonia, sexually transmitted diseases, and other infectious diseases.

EMS can have a significant impact upon the incidence of infectious disease if providers remain knowledgeable, are leaders in public education, and are consistently alert in protecting themselves and their patients. The title of the International Association of Fire Fighters (IAFF) hepatitis B curriculum, *The Silent War,* provides a metaphor for the dilemma of infectious diseases in EMS: EMS personnel deal with few infectious disease emergencies; however, when we do respond to such emergencies, we often are unaware of the disease's presence until after the call. Standard (universal) precautions, often written for clinical and research facilities with more predictable hazards and risks, are increased to body substance isolation (BSI) for emergency health care providers because of the uncertainties of our profession. Constant vigilance and personal accountability are the keys to reducing those risks.

All body fluids are possibly infectious. Universal precautions should be followed at all times.

CHAPTER 38

Psychiatric and Behavioral Disorders

Objectives

After reading this chapter, you should be able to:

1. Define behavior and distinguish among normal behavior, abnormal behavior, and the behavioral emergency. (pp. 1607–1608)
2. Discuss the prevalence of behavioral and psychiatric disorders. (p. 1608)
3. Discuss the pathophysiology of behavioral and psychiatric disorders. (pp. 1608–1609)
4. Discuss the factors that may alter the behavioral or emotional status of an ill or injured individual. (pp. 1608–1609)
5. Describe the medical legal considerations for management of emotionally disturbed patients. (pp. 1626–1627)

6. Describe the overt behaviors associated with behavioral and psychiatric disorders. (pp. 1613–1624)
7. Define the following terms:
   - Affect (p. 1610)
   - Anger (p. 1616)
   - Anxiety (pp. 1615–1616)
   - Confusion (p. 1610)
   - Depression (pp. 1617–1618)
   - Fear (p. 1610)
   - Mental status (p. 1610)
   - Open-ended question (p. 1611)
   - Posture (p. 1610)
8. Describe verbal techniques useful in managing the emotionally disturbed patient. (pp. 1611–1612)

Continued

Objectives Continued

9. List the appropriate measures to ensure the safety of the paramedic, the patient, and others. (pp. 1609–1611, 1626–1627)
10. Describe the circumstances when relatives, bystanders, and others should be removed from the scene. (p. 1610)
11. Describe techniques to systematically gather information from the disturbed patient. (pp. 1612, 1626)
12. Identify techniques for physical assessment in a patient with behavioral problems. (pp. 1612, 1626–1627)
13. List situations in which you are expected to transport a patient forcibly and against his will. (pp. 1626–1627)
14. Describe restraint methods necessary in managing the emotionally disturbed patient. (pp. 1627–1629)
15. List the risk factors and behaviors that indicate a patient is at risk for suicide. (p. 1623)
16. Use the assessment and patient history to differentiate between the various behavioral and psychiatric disorders. (pp. 1609–1624)
17. Given several preprogrammed behavioral emergency patients, provide the appropriate scene size-up, initial assessment, focused assessment, and detailed assessment, then provide the appropriate care and patient transport. (pp. 1607–1629)

INTRODUCTION

A significant difference between behavioral and psychiatric conditions and other types of medical emergencies is that most of your assessment and care will depend on your people skills. You can evaluate a bradycardia with a cardiac monitor and treat it with atropine or a pacing unit. You evaluate the psychiatric patient, on the other hand, by observing his behavior, by gathering information from his family and bystanders, and by interviewing him. Your care, which includes support, calming reassurance, and occasionally restraint, requires interpersonal skills more than diagnostic equipment.

BEHAVIORAL EMERGENCIES

Behavior is a person's observable conduct and activity. A **behavioral emergency** is a situation in which a patient's behavior becomes so unusual, bizarre, threatening, or dangerous that it alarms the patient or another person such as a family member or bystander and requires the intervention of emergency service and/or mental health personnel.

Notice that the definition of behavioral emergency does not use the word *abnormal*. The differentiation between normal and abnormal is largely subjective. What is normal varies based on culture, ethnic group, socioeconomic class, and personal interpretation and opinion. What one person considers normal, another might consider highly abnormal. Generally, however, normal behavior can be defined as behavior that is readily acceptable in a society.

Indications of a behavioral or psychological condition include actions that:

* **behavior** a person's observable conduct and activity.

* **behavioral emergency** situation in which a patient's behavior becomes so unusual that it alarms the patient or another person and requires intervention.

- Interfere with core life functions (eating, sleeping, ability to maintain housing, interpersonal or sexual relations)
- Pose a threat to the life or well-being of the patient or others
- Significantly deviate from society's expectations or norms

PATHOPHYSIOLOGY OF PSYCHIATRIC DISORDERS

Experts estimate that up to 20 percent of the population has some type of mental health problem and that as many as one person in seven will actually require treatment for an emotional disturbance. These problems may be severely disabling and require inpatient care, or the patient may quietly tolerate them with no outward symptoms. That all people with psychiatric conditions exhibit bizarre or unusual behavior is a misconception. The small percentage of patients with psychiatric disorders who publicly exhibit bizarre behavior tends to create this misconception among lay people. In reality, most patients who suffer from disorders such as anxiety, depression, eating disorders, or mild personality disorders function normally on a daily basis, going unnoticed in society. Nonetheless, behavioral and psychiatric disorders incapacitate more people than all other health problems combined. Most patients with mental illness are cared for in outpatient settings such as public mental health centers. Only those with severe psychiatric illnesses remain institutionalized. Because of this, EMS providers are increasingly being called to care for patients with behavioral complaints. A common reason for EMS intervention in psychiatric illness is patients' failure to take their psychiatric medications. When mental health patients such as schizophrenics begin to deteriorate and develop bizarre behavior, more often than not they have not been adhering to their psychiatric medication regimen.

Another common misconception is that all mental patients are unstable and dangerous and that their conditions are incurable. This is simply not true. Research in psychiatry, like other areas in medicine, has made great strides in determining causes and treatments for many psychiatric conditions. Suffering from a mental disorder is not reason for embarrassment or shame, although society often stigmatizes these patients unfairly. The general causes of behavioral emergencies are biological (or organic), psychosocial, and sociocultural. Each of these three possible causes should guide your questioning during the patient interview. Keep in mind, however, that a patient's condition may result from more than one pathological process.

BIOLOGICAL

For many years, medical practitioners have used the terms *biological* and *organic* interchangeably when discussing certain types of psychiatric disorders whose causes are physical rather than purely psychological. They result from disease processes such as infections and tumors or from structural changes in the brain such as those brought on by the abuse of alcohol or drugs (including over-the-counter and prescription medications). It could be argued, however, that even purely psychological conditions originate in the brain and for that very reason are organic. Indeed, many psychiatric conditions do originate from alterations in brain chemistry.

Behavioral emergencies frequently involve biological conditions. Never assume a patient with an altered mental status or unusual behavior is suffering

---

Most patients who suffer from disorders such as anxiety, depression, eating disorders, or mild personality disorders function normally on a daily basis, going unnoticed in society.

✳ **biological/organic** related to disease processes or structural changes.

Never assume a patient with an altered mental status or unusual behavioral is suffering from a purely psychological condition or disease until you have completely ruled out medical conditions and substance abuse.

---

from a purely psychological condition or disease until you have completely ruled out medical conditions and substance abuse.

PSYCHOSOCIAL

Psychosocial (personal) conditions are related to a patient's personality style, dynamics of unresolved conflict, or crisis management methods. These disorders are not attributable to substance abuse or medical conditions.

Environment plays a large part in psychosocial development. Traumatic childhood incidents may affect a person throughout life. Parents or other persons in positions of authority can have a tremendous impact on a child's development. Dysfunctional families, abusive parents, alcohol or drug abuse by parents, or neglect can cause behavioral problems from childhood through adulthood. Such conditions, in addition to—or in combination with genetic predisposition and brain chemistry—form the basis for psychosocial conditions.

* **psychosocial** related to a patient's personality style, dynamics of unresolved conflict, or crisis management methods.

SOCIOCULTURAL

Sociocultural (situational) causes of behavioral disorders are related to the patient's actions and interactions within society and to factors such as socioeconomic status, social habits, social skills, and values. These problems are usually attributable to events that change the patient's social space (relationships, support systems), social isolation, or otherwise have an impact on socialization.

Some events in the lives of children and adults that may cause a profound psychological change are rape, assault, witnessing the victimization of another, death of a loved one, and acts of violence such as war or riots. Events that occur over time may also have an impact on the individual. These include the loss of a job, economic problems such as poverty, and ongoing prejudice or discrimination. Sometimes simply doing anything outside the norms of society can lead to stress and psychological changes.

* **sociocultural** related to the patient's actions and interactions within society.

ASSESSMENT OF BEHAVIORAL EMERGENCY PATIENTS

The assessment and care of behavioral emergency patients is similar to that for other medical conditions. The order of assessment (scene size-up, initial assessment, focused history and physical examination) remains unchanged. Potential medical conditions that mimic behavioral emergencies require you to perform a thorough medical assessment.

Among the differences between your assessment and care of a patient with a medical condition and one with a behavioral emergency is that, as already noted, you actually begin your care at the same time you begin your assessment by developing a rapport with the patient. Interpersonal skills are important for all patients, but perhaps never more than for one who is experiencing a behavioral emergency. Additionally, the focused history and physical exam for a behavioral emergency includes a mental status examination.

SCENE SIZE-UP

As with any call, determining scene safety is of the utmost importance. Approach the scene carefully. If a patient is experiencing a behavioral emergency that is significant enough to warrant EMS, it is most likely significant enough to have law enforcement authorities respond. Most patients experiencing behavioral emergencies

FIGURE 38-1 Approach every patient cautiously. If you determine a potential for violence, request police assistance.

or crises will not attack you; however, those who are behaving unusually, experiencing hallucinations or delusions, or are under the effect of a substance may become violent. Approach every patient cautiously to protect yourself and your crew from injury (Figure 38-1).

Approach every patient cautiously to protect yourself and your crew from injury.

The scene size-up also includes making observations that relate to patient care. Look for evidence of substance use or abuse, for therapeutic medications that may indicate an underlying medical condition (or abuse of that medication), and for signs of violence or destruction of property. Examine the general environmental condition and, when possible, observe the patient from a distance to note any visible behavior patterns or violent behavior.

INITIAL ASSESSMENT

Because many behavioral emergencies are caused by or concurrent with medical conditions, you should be acutely suspicious of life-threatening emergencies. As with any other injury or condition, assess the ABCs and intervene when necessary. Continue to observe the patient for any clues to his underlying condition. Be cautious of any overt behavior such as **posture** or hand gestures. Note any emotional response such as rage, **fear,** anxiety, **confusion,** or anger. Early in the evaluation try to determine the patient's **mental status,** the state of his cerebral functioning. Continue assessing mental status throughout the patient encounter by evaluating his awareness, orientation, cognitive abilities, and **affect** (visible indicators of mood).

* **posture** position, attitude, or bearing of the body.

* **fear** feeling of alarm and discontentment in the expectation of danger.

* **confusion** state of being unclear or unable to make a decision easily.

* **mental status** the state of the patient's cerebral functioning.

* **affect** visible indicators of mood.

Control the scene as soon as possible. Remove anyone who agitates the patient or adds confusion to the scene. Generally, a limited number of people around the patient is best. At times, performing an effective assessment and care may necessitate totally clearing a room or moving the patient to a quiet area. Finally, observe the patient's affect in greater detail. To avoid being grabbed or struck by the patient, stay alert for signs of aggression.

Stay alert for signs of aggression.

FOCUSED HISTORY AND PHYSICAL EXAMINATION

Your examination of a patient experiencing a behavioral emergency is largely conversational. This makes your interpersonal technique very important. Just as starting an IV with poor technique most likely will not establish a patent IV line, interviewing with poor interpersonal skills most likely will not obtain significant information. Remove the patient from the crisis area and limit interruptions. Focus your questioning and assessment on the immediate problem and follow these guidelines:

- *Listen.* Ask open-ended questions (those that require more than a yes or no response). These will encourage your patient to respond in detail and share important information. Listen to the answer. Pay attention. No one likes being ignored. When you need information from a patient, listen.

- *Spend time.* Rushing the patient's answers, cutting him off, or appearing hurried will cause him to "shut down" and stop answering questions.

- *Be assured.* Communicate self-confidence, honesty, and professionalism.

- *Do not threaten.* Avoid rapid or sudden movements or questions that the patient might interpret as threats. Approach him slowly and confidently.

- *Do not fear silence.* Silence can be appropriate. Encourage the patient to tell his or her story, but do not be forceful or antagonizing.

- *Place yourself at the patient's level.* Standing over the patient may be intimidating. Unless you are intentionally attempting to gain a position of authority, crouch, kneel, or sit near the patient. Do not position yourself where you cannot respond appropriately to danger or attack.

- *Keep a safe and proper distance.* The surest way to make a behavioral emergency patient violent is to invade his "personal space" (Figure 38-2). This is an area within an approximately three-foot radius around every person; encroaching upon it causes anxiety. If appropriate, however, you may touch the patient's shoulder or use another consoling touch when he allows.

- *Appear comfortable.* Do not appear uncomfortable—even if you are. Talking to patients about suicide, self-mutilation, or other psychological conditions is difficult. If the patient sees that you are uncomfortable, however, he is unlikely to open up to you. Would you expect a patient to tell you his reasons for attempting suicide when you appear uncomfortable even saying the word? To help, use terms the patient has used. If he says he wanted to "end it all," begin with that. Caregivers

FIGURE 38-2   Avoid invading the patient's personal space, the area within about three feet of the patient.

sometimes hesitate to use the word *suicide* because it might give the patient ideas of suicide. If you are there to care for a suicidal or potentially suicidal patient, however, he has already had those thoughts.

- *Avoid appearing judgmental.* Patients who are experiencing behavioral emergencies may feel strong emotions toward their caregivers. The patient should believe that you are interested in his condition and welfare. Be supportive and empathetic, and avoid judgments, pity, anger, or any other emotions that may damage your relationship with the patient.

- *Never lie to the patient.* Honesty is the best policy. Do not reinforce false beliefs or hallucinations or mislead the patient in any way.

MENTAL STATUS EXAMINATION

As part of the focused history and physical examination for behavioral emergencies, do not overlook any physical or medical complaint. In addition to the medical evaluation, which is covered in depth throughout this and the other volumes of this program, your examination of the patient with psychiatric or behavioral disorders should include a psychological evaluation, also known as a **mental status examination (MSE)**. The components of the MSE include:

✱ mental status examination (MSE), a structured exam designed to quickly evaluate a patient's level of mental functioning.

- *General Appearance.* The patient's appearance can provide important information when looking at his "big picture." Observe hygiene, clothing, and overall appearance.

- *Behavioral Observations.* Observe verbal or nonverbal behavior, strange or threatening appearance, or facial expressions. Note tone of voice, rate, volume, and quality.

- *Orientation.* Does the patient know who he is and who others are? Is he oriented to current events? Can he concentrate on simple questions and answer them?

- *Memory.* Is the patient's memory intact for recent and long-term events?

- *Sensorium.* Is the patient focused? Paying attention? What is his level of awareness?

- *Perceptual Processes.* Are the patient's thought patterns ordered? Does he appear to have any hallucinations, delusions, or phobias?

- *Mood and Affect.* Observe for indicators of the patient's mood. Is it appropriate? What is his prevailing emotion? Depression, elation, anxiety, or agitation? Other?

- *Intelligence.* Evaluate the patient's speech. What is his level of vocabulary? His ability to formulate an idea?

- *Thought Processes.* What is the patient's apparent form of thought? Are his thoughts logical and coherent?

- *Insight.* Does the patient have insight into his own problem? Does he recognize that a problem exists? Does he deny or blame others for his problem?

- *Judgment.* Does the patient base his life decisions on sound, reasonable judgments? Does he approach problems thoughtfully, carefully, and rationally?

- *Psychomotor.* Does the patient exhibit an unusual posture or is he making unusual movements? Patients with hallucinations may react to them. For example, a patient who believes he is covered with insects may be picking at his skin to remove the "bugs."

PSYCHIATRIC MEDICATIONS

Many patients who suffer from psychiatric or behavioral disorders are under the care of a mental health professional and may be taking prescription medications. During the interview and history-taking process, determine whether the patient is taking medications and, if so, what type. The patient's use of such medications can provide clues to his underlying condition. Additionally, if a patient is not taking a medication as directed, his condition may deteriorate. Some schizophrenic patients may receive periodic injections of extremely long-acting antipsychotics (for example, haloperidol deconoate) because of poor compliance. They will often carry an identification card or may report that they "go to the clinic every three weeks for a shot." Types of psychiatric medications are discussed in the pharmacology chapter, Chapter 6.

SPECIFIC PSYCHIATRIC DISORDERS

Almost all psychiatric disorders have two diagnostic elements: symptoms of the disease or disorder and indications that the disease or disorder has impaired major life functions resulting in loss of relationships, a job, or housing or in another significant social problem. To define specific conditions, mental health professionals use the *Diagnostic and Statistical Manual of Mental Disorders,* Fourth Edition (DSM-IV). Published by the American Psychiatric Association (APA), the DSM-IV details diagnostic criteria for all currently defined psychiatric disorders, which are grouped according to the patient's signs and symptoms. The recognized types of behavioral and psychiatric disorders include:

- Cognitive disorders
- Schizophrenia
- Anxiety disorders
- Mood disorders
- Substance-related disorders
- Somatoform disorders
- Factitious disorders
- Dissociative disorders
- Eating disorders
- Personality disorders
- Impulse control disorders

The following summaries of these illnesses' major criteria do not imply that you should diagnose behavioral disorders. Even for skilled psychologists and psychiatrists, diagnosis is complicated by the considerable overlap in symptoms from one disease to another. A patient may actually fit into several categories. You should use the information here only as a guide to better understanding the science of psychiatry and the criteria applied to patients with behavioral emergencies. Knowledge of these terms and conditions will also allow you to communicate better with psychiatric care providers.

COGNITIVE DISORDERS

Psychiatric disorders with organic causes such as brain injury or disease are known as cognitive disorders. This family of disorders includes conditions caused by metabolic disease, infections, neoplasm, endocrine disease, degenerative neurological disease, and cardiovascular disease. They might also be caused by physical or chemical injuries due to trauma, drug abuse, or reactions to prescribed drugs. The specific brain pathology will differ based on the type of disease. Two types of cognitive disorders are delirium and dementia.

Delirium **Delirium** is characterized by a relatively rapid onset of widespread disorganized thought. These patients suffer from inattention, memory impairment, disorientation, and a general clouding of consciousness. In some cases, individuals may experience vivid visual hallucinations. Delirium is characterized by a fairly acute onset (hours or days) and may be reversible. Delirium may be due to a medical condition, substance intoxication, substance withdrawal, or multiple etiologies. Confusion is a hallmark of delirium.

Dementia **Dementia** may be due to several medical problems. Included among the more common causes of dementia are Alzheimer's disease (both early and late onset), vascular problems, AIDS, head trauma, Parkinson's disease, substance abuse, and other chronic problems. Regardless of its cause, dementia involves memory impairment, cognitive disturbance, and pervasive impairment of abstract thinking and judgment. Unlike delirium, dementia usually develops over months and, in many cases, is irreversible.

Dementia involves cognitive deficits manifested by both memory impairment (diminished ability to learn new information or to recall previously learned information) and one or more of the following cognitive disturbances:

* *Aphasia.* Impaired ability to communicate.
* *Apraxia.* Impaired ability to carry out motor activities despite intact sensory function.
* *Agnosia.* Failure to recognize objects or stimuli despite intact sensory function.
* *Disturbance in executive functioning.* Impaired ability to plan, organize, or sequence.

These conditions must significantly impair social or occupational functioning and represent a significant decline from a previous level of functioning. Your approach to patients with either of these conditions should be supportive. Assess and manage any medical complaints or conditions and transport to an appropriate medical facility.

SCHIZOPHRENIA

Schizophrenia is a common mental health problem, affecting an estimated one percent of the United States population. Its hallmark is a significant change in behavior and a loss of contact with reality. Signs and symptoms often include hallucinations, delusions, and depression. The schizophrenic patient may live in his "own world" and be preoccupied with inner fantasies. Although several biological and psychosocial theories attempt to explain the condition and its manifestations, its definitive cause is unknown.

The symptoms of schizophrenia include:

* *Delusions.* Fixed, false beliefs that are not widely held within the context of the individual's cultural or religious group.
* *Hallucinations.* Sensory perceptions with no basis in reality. These are often auditory ("hearing voices").
* *Disorganized speech.* Frequent derailment or incoherence.
* *Grossly disorganized* or **catatonic** *behavior.*
* *Negative symptoms* (**flat affect**).

* **delirium** condition characterized by relatively rapid onset of widespread disorganized thought.

* **dementia** condition involving gradual development of memory impairment and cognitive disturbance.

* **schizophrenia** common disorder involving significant change in behavior often including hallucinations, delusions, and depression.

* **delusions** fixed, false beliefs not widely held within the individual's cultural or religious group.

* **hallucinations** sensory perceptions with no basis in reality.

* **catatonia** condition characterized by immobility and stupor, often a sign of schizophrenia.

* **flat affect** appearance of being disinterested, often lacking facial expression.

A diagnosis of schizophrenia requires that two or more symptoms must each be present for a significant portion of each month over the course of six months. The symptoms must cause a social or occupational dysfunction (decline in social relations or work from the predisease state). Most schizophrenics are diagnosed in early adulthood.

The DSM-IV defines several major types of schizophrenia:

- *Paranoid*. The patient is preoccupied with a feeling of persecution and may suffer delusions or auditory hallucinations.
- *Disorganized*. The patient often displays disorganized behavior, dress, or speech.
- *Catatonic*. The patient exhibits catatonic rigidity, immobility, stupor, or peculiar voluntary movements. Catatonic schizophrenia is exceedingly rare.
- *Undifferentiated*. The patient does not readily fit into one of the categories above.

Your approach to the schizophrenic patient should be supportive and nonjudgmental. Do not reinforce the patient's hallucinations, but understand that he considers them real. Speak openly and honestly with him. Be encouraging yet realistic. Remain alert for aggressive behavior, and restrain the patient if he becomes violent or presents a danger to you, to himself, or to others.

ANXIETY AND RELATED DISORDERS

The group of illnesses known as **anxiety disorders** is characterized by dominating apprehension and fear. These disorders affect approximately two to four percent of the population. Broadly defined, **anxiety** is a state of uneasiness, discomfort, apprehension, and restlessness. More specifically, anxiety disorders fall into three categories: panic disorder, phobia, and posttraumatic stress syndrome.

Panic Attack The DSM-IV does not list **panic attacks** in themselves as a disease. Characterized by recurrent, extreme periods of anxiety resulting in great emotional distress, they are symptoms of disease and are included among the criteria for other disorders (panic disorder, agoraphobia). Panic attacks differ from generalized feelings of anxiety in their acute nature. They are usually unprovoked, peaking within 10 minutes of their onset and dissipating in less than one hour.

The presentation of panic and anxiety may resemble a cardiac or respiratory condition. This presents a dilemma for EMS personnel. Ruling out those conditions is difficult in the prehospital setting; psychiatrists usually diagnose anxiety or panic disorders by excluding known medical conditions. Keys to identifying panic or anxiety in the field are the patient's having a history of the condition and being outside the expected age range for certain cardiac or respiratory illnesses. This, of course, is not to say that young people cannot have myocardial infarction. Many symptoms of panic resemble those of hyperventilation, and some do appear to be correlated, such as the paresthesia from panic being due largely to hyperventilation.

The diagnostic criteria for a panic attack require a discrete period of intense fear or discomfort, during which four or more of the following symptoms develop abruptly and reach a peak within ten minutes:

- Palpitations, pounding heart, or accelerated heart rate
- Sweating
- Trembling or shaking

Content Review

MAJOR TYPES OF SCHIZOPHRENIA
Paranoid
Disorganized
Catatonic
Undifferentiated

* **anxiety disorder** condition characterized by dominating apprehension and fear.

* **anxiety** state of uneasiness, discomfort, apprehension, and restlessness.

* **panic attack** extreme period of anxiety resulting in great emotional distress.

Content Review

ANXIETY RELATED DISORDERS
Panic attack
Phobia
Posttraumatic stress syndrome

- Sensations of shortness of breath or smothering
- Feeling of choking
- Chest pain or discomfort
- Nausea or abdominal distress
- Feeling dizzy, unsteady, lightheaded, or faint
- Derealization (feelings of unreality) or depersonalization (being detached from oneself)
- Fear of losing control or going crazy
- Fear of dying
- Paresthesia (numbness or tingling sensations)
- Chills or hot flashes

Management for anxiety disorders is generally simple and supportive. Show empathy. Assess any medical complaints and manage them appropriately. If the patient experiences hyperventilation, calm and reassure him in order to decrease his respiratory rate to normal. Patients with severe or incapacitating symptoms may benefit from the administration of a sedative. Benzodiazepines, such as diazepam (Valium) and lorazepam (Ativan) can be administered in the prehospital setting. In addition, antihistamines, such as hydroxyzine (Vistaril) and diphenhydramine (Benadryl), have sedative effects and are useful in treating patients with significant anxiety. Consult medical direction in accordance with local protocol and transport to an appropriate medical facility.

Phobias Everyone has some source of fear or anxiety that they consciously avoid. When this fear becomes excessive and interferes with functioning, it is a **phobia**. A phobia, generally considered an intense, irrational fear, may be due to animals, the sight of blood (or injection or injury), situational factors (elevators, enclosed spaces), or environmental conditions (heights or water). Exposure to the situation or item will induce anxiety or a panic attack. Some patients experience extreme phobias that prevent or limit their normal daily activities. For example, a patient suffering from agoraphobia (fear of crowds) may confine himself to his home and avoid ever venturing outdoors. In most patients, however, the phobia is less severe; the patient realizes that his fear is unreasonable, and the anxiety dissipates.

Management for a patient with a phobia is supportive. Understand that the patient's fear is very real. Do not force him to do anything that he opposes. Manage any underlying problems and transport for evaluation.

Posttraumatic Stress Syndrome EMS providers often are particularly interested in **posttraumatic stress syndrome** because their responsibilities may make them susceptible to it. Originally recognized on the battlefields of war, posttraumatic stress syndrome is a reaction to an extreme, usually life-threatening, stressor such as a natural disaster, victimization (rape, for instance), or other emotionally taxing situation. It is characterized by a desire to avoid similar situations, recurrent intrusive thoughts, depression, sleep disturbances, nightmares, and persistent symptoms of increased arousal. The patient may feel guilty for having survived the incident, and substance abuse may frequently complicate his condition.

Treat any posttraumatic stress syndrome patient with respect, empathy, and support, and transport him to an appropriate facility for evaluation.

MOOD DISORDERS

The DSM-IV defines mood as "a pervasive and sustained emotion that colors a person's perception of the world." Common examples of mood alterations include depression, elation, **anger**, and anxiety. The main **mood disorders** are depression and bipolar disorder.

✻ phobia excessive fear that interferes with functioning.

✻ posttraumatic stress syndrome reaction to an extreme stressor.

✻ anger hostility or rage to compensate for an underlying feeling of anxiety.

✻ mood disorder pervasive and sustained emotion that colors a person's perception of the world.

Depression Depression is characterized by a profound sadness or feeling of melancholy. It is common in everyday life and is to be expected following the break-up of a relationship or the loss of a loved one. Most of us have experienced some sort of depression, at least in its mildest form. It is one of the most prevalent psychiatric conditions, affecting from 10 to 15 percent of the population. When depression becomes prolonged or severe, however, it is diagnosed as a *major depressive episode*.

✳ **depression** profound sadness or feeling of melancholy.

Content Review

MOOD DISORDERS

Depression
Bipolar disorder

The symptoms of major depressive disorder include:

- Depressed mood most of the day, nearly every day, as indicated by subjective report or observation by others.
- Markedly diminished interest in pleasure in all, or almost all, activities most of the day nearly every day.
- Significant weight loss (without dieting) or weight gain. A five-percent change in body weight is considered significant.
- Insomnia or hypersomnia nearly every day.
- Psychomotor agitation or retardation every day (observable by others, not just the subjective feeling of the patient).
- Feelings of worthlessness or excessive inappropriate guilt (may be delusional) nearly every day.
- Diminished ability to think or concentrate, or indecisiveness nearly every day.
- Recurrent thoughts of death (not just fear of dying), recurrent suicidal ideation without a specific plan, or a suicide attempt or a specific plan for committing suicide. (Depression greatly increases the risk of suicide.)

The diagnostic criteria for major depressive disorder require that five or more of the symptoms have been present during the same two-week period and represent a change from previous functioning; at least one of the symptoms must be either a depressed mood or loss of interest in pleasure. The condition must cause clinically significant distress or impairment in social, occupational, or other important functions. Further, it must not meet the criteria for a mixed episode (mixtures of mania and depression); it must not be due to the direct physiological effects of a substance such as drug abuse or a medication, or to a general medical condition such as hypothyroidism; finally, it must not be better accounted for by **bereavement**. The acronym *In SAD CAGES* provides a screening mnemonic for major depression.

✳ **bereavement** death of a loved one.

- *In*terest
- *S*leep
- *A*ppetite
- *D*epressed mood
- *C*oncentration
- *A*ctivity
- *G*uilt
- *E*nergy
- *S*uicide

Depression may occur as an isolated condition, but it is often accompanied by other disorders such as substance abuse, anxiety disorders, and schizophrenia.

Depression can also affect a patient without meeting all of the identified clinical criteria. It can affect different people in different ways and is often atypical. Bereavement is one of the situations in which depression is expected. If the depression lasts longer than two months or is accompanied by suicidal ideation or marked functional impairment, it could be classified as a major depressive episode. Depression is more prevalent in females and is spread evenly throughout the life span.

Bipolar Disorder Bipolar disorder is characterized by one or more **manic** episodes (periods of elation), with or without subsequent or alternating periods of depression. In the past, the term *manic-depressive* was used to describe this condition. Bipolar disorder is not particularly common, affecting approximately less than one percent of the population.

Manic-depressive episodes are not the "Jeckyl and Hyde" transformations that television and the movies often portray. However, they often begin suddenly and escalate rapidly over a few days. In contrast to major depressive disorders, bipolar disorders usually develop in adolescence or early adulthood and occur as often in males as in females. Some patients with major depressive episodes will eventually develop a bipolar disorder and experience manic episodes. Commonly patients have several depressive episodes before having a manic episode.

The diagnostic criteria for a manic episode require a distinct period of abnormally and persistently elevated, expansive, or irritable mood lasting for at least one week (or for any duration when hospitalization is necessary). Three or more (four or more if the mood is only irritable) of the following symptoms must have been present to a certain degree and must have persisted during that time:

- Inflated self-esteem or grandiosity
- Decreased need for sleep
- More talkative than usual or pressure to keep talking
- Flight of ideas or subjective experience that thoughts are racing
- Distractibility
- Increase in goal directed activity (socially, at work or school, or sexually) or psychomotor agitation
- Excessive involvement in pleasurable activities that have a high potential for painful consequences (buying sprees, sexual indiscretions, foolish business investments)
- Delusional thoughts (grandiose ideas or unrealistic plans)

The symptoms must not meet the criteria for a mixed episode. The mood disturbance must be severe enough to markedly impair occupational or social functioning, to require hospitalizing the patient to prevent harm to himself or others, or present with psychotic features. As with depression, the symptoms must not be due to the direct physiological effects of a substance or a general medical condition. Patients with bipolar illness are often prescribed lithium (Lithobid, Eskalith) for treatment.

Management of these patients includes maintaining a calm, protective environment. Avoid confronting the manic patient. Never leave a depressed or suicidal patient alone. Assess and manage any other coexisting medical problems, and transport to an appropriate medical facility. Bipolar patients in an extreme manic phase may be overtly psychotic. In these cases, medication with an antipsychotic medication such as haloperidol may be indicated. Always contact medical direction for treatment options.

* **bipolar disorder** condition characterized by one or more manic episodes, with or without periods of depression.

* **manic** characterized by excessive excitement or activity (mania).

Many patients with bipolar disorder are treated with lithium. Lithium has a very narrow therapeutic index, making lithium toxicity a significant complicating factor.

SUBSTANCE RELATED DISORDERS

Substance abuse is a common disorder. Any patient exhibiting symptoms of a psychiatric or behavioral disorder should be screened for substance use and/or abuse. Substance abuse patients may present as being depressed, psychotic, or delirious, and their signs and symptoms may mimic those of many behavioral disorders. The DSM-IV lists substance abuse as a psychiatric disorder; you should consider it a serious condition. Any mood-altering chemical has the potential for abuse. Alcohol is a common part of our culture, but can be abused. The user of a substance may be intoxicated from the effects of the chemical or may be ill from addiction or withdrawal of the chemical. Intoxication, in and of itself, may cause behavioral problems.

Repetitive use of a mood-altering chemical may lead to dependence or addiction. Dependence on a substance is characterized by repeated use of the substance. Dependence may be either psychological, physical, or both. Psychological dependence is a compelling desire to use the substance, inability to reduce or stop use, and repeated efforts to quit. Physical dependence is characterized by the need for increased amounts of the chemical to obtain the desired effect. Also, the presence of withdrawal symptoms when the substance is reduced or stopped is characteristic of physical dependence. All drugs have the potential to cause psychological dependence; many have the potential to cause physical dependence as well.

SOMATOFORM DISORDERS

Somatoform disorders are characterized by physical symptoms that have no apparent physiological cause. They are believed to be attributable to psychological factors. People who suffer from somatoform disorders believe their symptoms are serious and real. The major types of somatoform disorder are:

* *Somatization disorder.* The patient is preoccupied with physical symptoms.
* *Conversion disorder.* The patient sustains a loss of function, usually involving the nervous system (for instance, blindness or paralysis), unexplained by any medical illness.
* *Hypochondriasis.* Exaggerated interpretation of physical symptoms as a serious illness.
* *Body dysmorphic disorder.* A person believes he or she has a defect in physical appearance.
* *Pain disorder.* The patient suffers from pain, usually severe, that is unexplained by a physical ailment.

Somatoform disorders are often difficult to identify and diagnose. They can mimic and be confused with various bona fide physical conditions. Never attribute physical symptoms to a behavioral disorder until medical conditions have been ruled out.

* **somatoform disorder** condition characterized by physical symptoms that have no apparent physiological cause and are attributable to psychological factors.

> ### Content Review
>
> #### SOMATOFORM DISORDERS
> Somatization disorder
> Conversion disorder
> Hypochondriasis
> Body dysmorphic disorder
> Pain disorder

FACTITIOUS DISORDERS

Factitious disorders are sometimes confused with somatoform disorders. They are characterized by the following three criteria:

* An intentional production of physical or psychological signs or symptoms.

* **factitious disorder** condition in which the patient feigns illness in order to assume the sick role.

- Motivation for the behavior is to assume the "sick role."
- External incentives for the behavior (e.g., economic gain, avoiding work, avoiding police) are absent.

While patients suffering from factitious disorders essentially feign their illnesses, that does not preclude the possibility of true physical or psychological symptoms. The disorder is apparently more common in males than in females. In severe cases, patients will go to great length to obtain medical or psychological treatment. Patients with factitious disorders often will voluntarily produce symptoms and will present with a very plausible history. They often have an extensive knowledge of medical terminology and can be very demanding and disruptive. In severe cases (Munchausen syndrome), patients will undergo multiple surgical operations and other painful procedures.

DISSOCIATIVE DISORDERS

Like somatoform disorders, **dissociative disorders** are attempts to avoid stressful situations while still gratifying needs. In a manner, they permit the person to deny personal responsibility for unacceptable behavior. The individual avoids stress by *dissociating* from his core personality. These behavior patterns can be complex but are quite rare. The disorders include:

Psychogenic Amnesia While amnesia is a partial or total *inability* to recall or identify past events, **psychogenic amnesia** is a *failure* to recall. The "forgotten" material is present but "hidden" beneath the level of consciousness.

Fugue State An amnesic individual may withdraw even further by retreating in what is known as a **fugue state.** A patient in a fugue state actually flees as a defense mechanism and may travel hundreds of miles from home.

Multiple Personality Disorder In **multiple personality disorder** the patient reacts to an identifiable stress by manifesting two or more complete systems of personality. While such disorders have received a great deal of attention in television, film, and novels, they are actually quite rare.

Depersonalization Depersonalization is a relatively more frequent dissociative disorder that occurs predominantly in young adults. Patients experience a loss of the sense of one's self. Such individuals suddenly feel "different"—that they are someone else or that their body has taken on a different form. The disorder is often precipitated by acute stress.

EATING DISORDERS

The two classifications of eating disorders are anorexia nervosa and bulimia nervosa. Both generally occur between adolescence and the age of 25. The condition afflicts women more than men at a rate of 20:1.

Anorexia Nervosa Anorexia is the loss of appetite. **Anorexia nervosa** is a disorder marked by excessive fasting. Individuals with this disorder have an intense fear of obesity and often complain of being fat even though their body weight is low. They suffer from weight loss (25 percent of body weight or more), refusal to maintain body weight, and often a cessation of menstruation from severe malnutrition.

Bulimia Nervosa Recurrent episodes of seemingly uncontrollable binge eating with compensatory self-induced vomiting or diarrhea, excessive exercise, or dieting and with a full awareness of the behavior's abnormality characterize **bulimia nervosa.** Individuals often display personality traits of perfectionism, low self-esteem, and social withdrawal.

---

* dissociative disorder condition in which the individual avoids stress by separating from his core personality.

Content Review

DISSOCIATIVE DISORDERS
Psychogenic amnesia
Fugue state
Multiple personality disorder
Depersonalization

* psychogenic amnesia failure to recall, as opposed to inability to recall.

* fugue state condition in which an amnesiac patient physically flees.

* multiple personality disorder manifestation of two or more complete systems of personality.

* depersonalization feeling detached from oneself.

Content Review

EATING DISORDERS
Anorexia nervosa
Bulimia nervosa

* anorexia nervosa psychological disorder characterized by voluntary refusal to eat.

* bulimia nervosa recurrent episodes of binge eating.

The weight loss and body changes experienced by anorexic and bulimic patients can lead to serious physical problems. Starvation and attempts to purge can have drastic consequences such as anemia, dehydration, vitamin deficiencies, hypoglycemia, and cardiovascular problems. In addition to psychological support, prehospital care is likely to include treatment for dehydration and physical problems. Both disorders have a high potential morbidity and mortality.

PERSONALITY DISORDERS

Most adults' personalities are attuned to social demands. Some individuals, however, often seem ill-equipped to function adequately in society. These people might be suffering from a **personality disorder.** Stemming largely from immature and distorted personality development, these personality, or character, disorders result in persistently maladaptive ways of perceiving, thinking, and relating to the world.

The broad category of personality disorder includes problems that vary greatly in form and severity. Although others might describe them as "eccentric" or "troublesome," some patients with personality disorders function adequately. In extreme cases, patients act out against or attempt to manipulate society.

* **personality disorder** condition that results in persistently maladaptive behavior.

Personality Disorder Clusters

The DSM-IV groups similar personality disorders into three broad types, Cluster A, Cluster B, and Cluster C.

Cluster A These individuals often act odd or eccentric. Their unusual behavior can take drastically different forms. This cluster includes the following:

- *Paranoid personality disorder.* Pattern of distrust and suspiciousness.
- *Schizoid personality disorder.* Pattern of detachment from social relationships.
- *Schizotypal personality disorder.* Pattern of acute discomfort in close relationships, cognitive distortions, and eccentric behavior.

Cluster B Individuals often appear dramatic, emotional, or fearful. This cluster includes the following:

- *Antisocial personality disorder.* Pattern of disregard for the rights of others.
- *Borderline personality disorder.* Pattern of instability in interpersonal relationships, self-image, and impulsivity.
- *Histrionic personality disorder.* Pattern of excessive emotions and attention seeking.
- *Narcissistic personality disorder.* Pattern of grandiosity, need for admiration, and lack of empathy.

Cluster C Individuals often appear anxious or fearful. This cluster includes the following:

- *Avoidant personality disorder.* Pattern of social inhibition, feelings of inadequacy, and hypersensitivity to criticism.
- *Dependent personality disorder.* Pattern of submissive and clinging behavior related to an excessive need to be cared for.
- *Obsessive-compulsive disorder.* Pattern of preoccupation with orderliness, perfectionism, and control.

Content Review

PERSONALITY DISORDER CLUSTERS

- Cluster A personality disorders
  —Paranoid
  —Schizoid
  —Schizotypal
- Cluster B personality disorders
  —Antisocial
  —Borderline
  —Histrionic
  —Narcissistic
- Cluster C personality disorders
  —Avoidant
  —Dependent
  —Obsessive-compulsive

Diagnosing a personality disorder requires evaluating the individual's long-term functioning and behavior. In many cases, the individual suffers from multiple disorders. A complete interview, history, and assessment will assist you in determining your approach. Your prehospital care will vary based on the patient's chief complaint and overall presentation.

IMPULSE CONTROL DISORDERS

Related to the personality disorders are the **impulse control disorders.** Recurrent impulses and the patient's failure to control them characterize these disorders. Examples of impulse control disorders include:

- *Kleptomania.* A recurrent failure to resist impulses to steal objects not for immediate use or for their monetary value
- *Pyromania.* A recurrent failure to resist impulses to set fires
- *Pathological gambling.* A chronic and progressive preoccupation with gambling and the urge to gamble
- *Trichotillomania.* A recurrent impulse to pull out one's own hair
- *Intermittent explosive disorder.* Recurrent and paroxysmal episodes of significant loss of control of aggressive responses

Disorders of impulse control may be harmful to the patient and others. Prior to committing the act the patient will have an increasing sense of tension. After the act, he will either have pleasure gratification or release.

SUICIDE

Suicide, simply stated, is when a person intentionally takes his or her own life. Suicide is alarmingly common. It is the ninth leading cause of death overall, and it is the third leading cause in the 15–24-year age group. Suicide rates have risen dramatically in the younger age groups and have also increased significantly in the elderly population. Women attempt suicide more than men, but men—especially those over 55 years of age—are more likely to succeed. Statistically, suicide successes and methods vary widely by race, sex, and culture. The most common methods of suicide (1992) are:

1. Bullet wound (60 percent)
2. Poisoning (18 percent)
3. Strangulation (15 percent)
4. Cutting (1 percent)
5. Other, or unspecified (6 percent)

Assessing Potentially Suicidal Patients

In cases of attempted suicide, many focus on whether the patient really wanted to kill himself. Indeed this question will be at the heart of the patient's future psychiatric care, and information from the paramedic will be crucial to making that determination. But never lose sight of patient care while probing the psychological nature of attempted suicide.

Document observations at the scene of an attempted suicide, especially any detailed suicide plans, suicide notes, and statements by the patient and bystanders.

Perform an appropriate focused history and physical exam concurrently with providing sound psychological care. Mental health professionals are rarely on the scene. It is up to you to document observations at the scene, especially any detailed suicide plans, any suicide notes, and any statements of the patient and bystanders. This information may not be available after the event when the patient receives psychiatric screening at the hospital. Such care and observations at the scene, combined with detailed documentation, are critical to the patient's long-term psychological care.

Risk Factors for Suicide

The risk factors for suicide are numerous. When assessing a patient who has indicated suicidal intentions, screen for any of these risk factors:

- Previous attempts (Eighty percent of persons who successfully commit suicide have made a previous attempt.)
- Depression (Suicide is 500 times more common among patients who are severely depressed than those who are not.)
- Age (Incidence is high between the ages of 15 and 24 years and over the age of 40.)
- Alcohol or drug abuse
- Divorced or widowed (The rate is five times higher than among other groups.)
- Giving away personal belongings, especially cherished possessions
- Living alone or in increased isolation
- The presence of **psychosis** with depression (for example, suicidal or destructive thoughts or hallucinations about killing or death)
- Homosexuality (especially homosexuals who are depressed, aging, alcoholic, or HIV-infected)
- Major separation trauma (mate, loved one, job, money)
- Major physical stresses (surgery, childbirth, sleep deprivation)
- Loss of independence (disabling illness)
- Lack of goals and plans for the future
- Suicide of same-sexed parent
- Expression of a plan for committing suicide
- Possession of the mechanism for suicide (gun, pills, rope)

* **psychosis** extreme response to stress characterized by impaired ability to deal with reality.

Patients who have attempted suicide must be evaluated in a hospital or psychiatric facility. Many people assume that "they were just looking for attention." Applied to the wrong patient, that conjecture may contribute to his death.

AGE-RELATED CONDITIONS

Some behavioral disorders are particularly common among patients at the ends of the age spectrum—the young and the elderly. Your awareness of age-related conditions will help you to assess and interact with these patients.

Crisis in the Geriatric Patient

Common physical problems among the elderly include dementia, chronic illness, and diminished eyesight and hearing. The elderly also experience depression that is often mistaken for dementia. When confronted with an elderly person in a crisis, take the following steps:

- Assess the patient's ability to communicate.
- Provide continual reassurance.
- Compensate for the patient's loss of sight and hearing with reassuring physical contact.

- Treat the patient with respect. Call the patient by name and title, such as "Mrs. Jones." Avoid such terms as "dear," "honey," and "babe."
- Avoid administering medication.
- Describe what you are going to do before you do it.
- Take your time. Do not convey the impression that you are in a hurry.
- Allow family members and friends to remain with the patient if possible.

Crisis in the Pediatric Patient

Behavioral emergencies are not limited to adults. Children also have behavioral crises. While the child's developmental stage will affect his or her behavior, these general guidelines will assist you when confronting an emotionally distraught or disruptive child.

- Avoid separating a young child from his parent.
- Attempt to prevent the child from seeing things that will increase his distress.
- Make all explanations brief and simple, and repeat them often.
- Be calm and speak slowly.
- Identify yourself by giving both your name and your function.
- Be truthful with the child. Telling the truth will develop trust.
- Encourage the child to help with his care.
- Reassure the child by carrying out all interventions gently.
- Do not discourage the child from crying or showing emotion.
- If you must be separated from the child, introduce the person who will assume responsibility for his care.
- Allow the child to keep a favorite blanket or toy.
- Do not leave the child alone, even for a short period.

Always be mindful of every young or elderly patient's uniqueness. Treat him equally and fairly, as you would any other patient.

MANAGEMENT OF BEHAVIORAL EMERGENCIES

Patients who are experiencing behavioral emergencies require both medical and psychological care. In general, take the following measures when you treat a patient who is experiencing a behavioral emergency:

1. Assure scene safety and BSI precautions.
2. Provide a supportive and calm environment.
3. Treat any existing medical conditions.
4. Do not allow the suicidal patient to be alone.
5. Do not confront or argue with the patient.
6. Provide realistic reassurance.
7. Respond to the patient in a direct, simple manner.
8. Transport to an appropriate receiving facility.

Remember to treat the whole patient. Never overlook any serious, or potentially serious, medical complaints while focusing on the psychiatric assessment.

MEDICAL

Patients who are experiencing apparent behavioral emergencies often have concurrent medical conditions—some of which may be responsible for the behavioral problem. Current literature indicates that medical conditions and/or substance abuse cause a much higher proportion of behavioral emergencies than previously believed. Medical care may include treatment for overdose, lacerations, toxic inhalation, hypoxia, or metabolic conditions. Many patients with chronic psychiatric conditions take medications for their illnesses; when abused, those medications have extremely toxic side effects. (See the pharmacology chapter, Chapter 6.) Additionally these patients often live in conditions ranging from substandard housing to the street. This existence may predispose them to other medical problems such as exposure, infections, and untreated illnesses.

PSYCHOLOGICAL

Patients who present with an apparent behavioral emergency also require psychological care. The time you spend developing a rapport with the patient—before, during, and after assessment—is actually a part of the care you provide. In effect, when you begin an assessment you are also beginning your care, and you will continue to perform psychological assessment and care concurrently with medical assessment and care. Be calm and reassuring while you interview your patient.

Since much of your care will be aimed at the psychological problem, you should steer your conversation and actions in that direction. Visualize your patients on a continuum ranging from agitated and out-of-control to introverted and depressed (Figure 38-3). As a paramedic, you will need to defuse the agitated patient and

Never overlook any serious, or potentially serious, medical complaints while focusing on the psychiatric assessment.

The time you spend developing a rapport with the behavioral emergency patient—before, during, and after assessment—is actually a part of the care you provide.

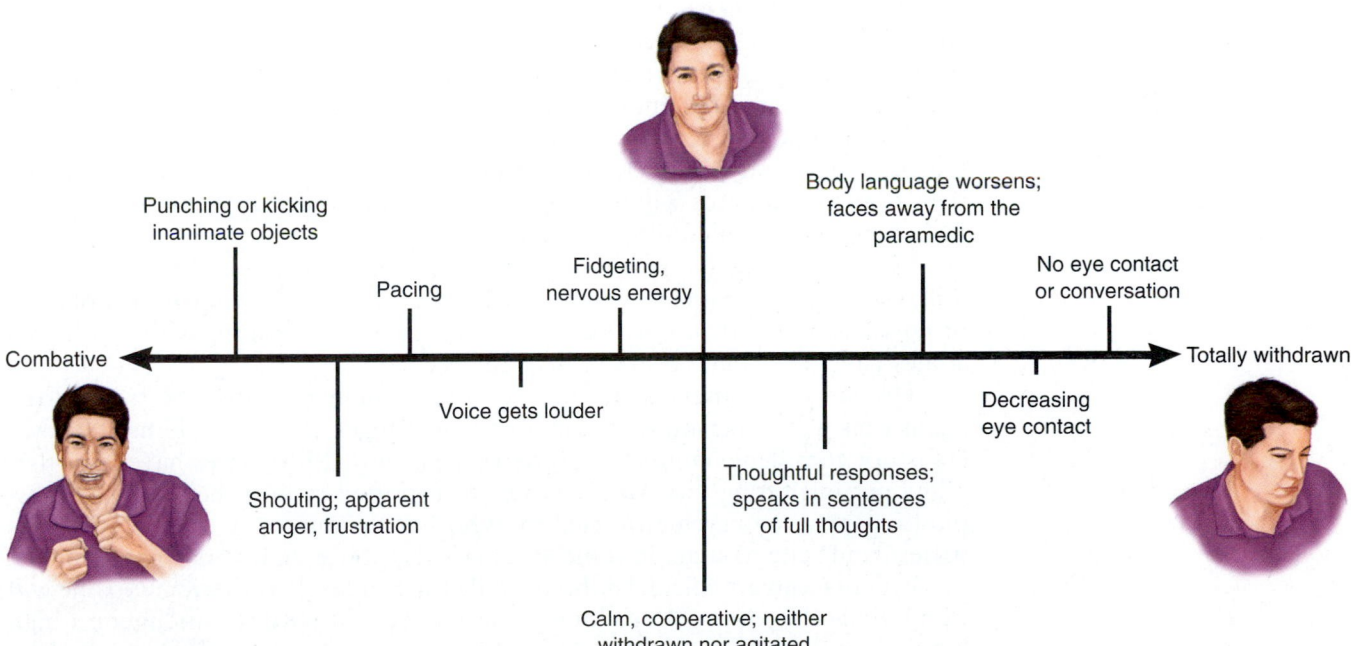

FIGURE 38-3 Continuum of patient responses during behavioral emergency. Whether dealing with an agitated or withdrawn patient, you will use your interpersonal skills to bring him to the calm, cooperative state in the middle of the continuum.

attempt to communicate with the withdrawn patient. These situations especially will require the interviewing skills you learned earlier in this chapter.

As you approach the patient, introduce yourself and state that you want to help, since this might not be intuitively clear to a person with distorted perceptions. As you begin to converse, note how the patient reacts to you. Generally, if he responds appropriately to your actions, you should continue what you are doing. If the patient becomes more agitated or further withdrawn, rethink. Perhaps you are getting too close, talking too fast, or addressing difficult topics too early. Be sure your exit path is not blocked.

Your approach to these patients requires excellent people skills—especially listening and observing. If you do not use these skills, or if you rush or seem disinterested, your care will likely fail. Therapeutic communication, as this interaction has been called, is an art. "Talking down" the behavioral emergency patient requires effort and skill. Some patients, however, will not react favorably even to the best people skills. Extremely withdrawn patients or those with severe psychotic symptoms may never fully respond during the time you spend with them out of the hospital. These patients still deserve quality care and compassion, even when they are uncommunicative or restrained.

Just as we must observe the patient, the patient observes us. Patients may actually be able to "read" us as accurately (or more accurately) than we read them. Perform your assessment and care confidently and competently. If patients sense uneasiness or indecision, they are more likely to act out. Never play along with a patient's hallucinations or delusions. It may seem to be the easiest route, but ultimately it may be harmful. Often the patient will recognize that you are patronizing him. Or the patient may talk of hallucinations or appear delusional, but not fully believe what he says. If you play along, you will lose credibility.

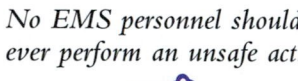

VIOLENT PATIENTS AND RESTRAINT

Who should be responsible for restraining a patient at an emergency scene is sometimes controversial. Many argue that physical restraint is clearly a police responsibility and EMS should not be involved. Others point out the gray areas, such as when the police are 30 minutes away, when only one officer is available, or when a patient is in imminent danger and paramedics must choose to act. One thing is certain: you should know how to control violent situations and restrain patients safely and effectively. Your agency's policies, your safety, and your patient's safety and needs will dictate how you handle individual emergencies. No EMS personnel should ever perform an unsafe act.

Most patients will respond to your care and therefore consent to treatment. Still, you will have patients whom the best interpersonal techniques cannot calm or reassure. If a patient must be legally transported against his will or if he becomes violent en route, restraint may be necessary.

The laws of consent state that no competent person may be transported against his will. A person who is in imminent danger of harming himself or others is not considered competent to refuse transport. Most states have laws that allow persons fitting this criterion to be transported against their will to a hospital or approved psychiatric facility. Who has the authority to determine this varies from state to state. In some areas it is the police, in others a physician.

Patients who are suicidal or homicidal clearly meet this criterion. No one will dispute that the patient with a knife to his wrist or the patient standing on a high ledge about to jump are both potential dangers to themselves. The many others who are on the border require careful evaluation. The patient who stripped off all his clothes in sub-zero weather or the patient who is not oriented enough to stay on the sidewalk and wanders into traffic may also meet the criterion.

Follow medical direction or local protocol when determining who can order a patient transported against his will. Protocols or agency rules may also state whether you should be involved in restraining violent patients. Finally, scene size-up may uncover dangers that you will decide to leave for the police to defuse before providing care. In general, be guided by what is best for the patient.

Paramedics must be intimately familiar with local laws and protocols that apply to patient restraint.

METHODS OF RESTRAINT

The main objective in restraint is to prevent the patient from harming himself or others while simultaneously allowing care providers unimpeded access to perform thorough initial and ongoing assessments, and to provide complete medical treatment. Consider the following general guidelines during restraint:

The main objective in restraint is to restrict the patient's movement in order to stop dangerous behaviors and prevent him from harming himself.

- Use the minimum force needed to restrain the patient. When verbal techniques will work, physical restraint may not be necessary.

- Use appropriate devices to perform restraint. Metal handcuffs may cause injury and should not be used. Thick roller bandages (Kling™, Kerlex™) are considered safer.

- Restraint is not punitive. Patients who are agitated frequently insult you, your partner, even your mother. This is not personal. The patient would make the same comments to anyone else in your position. Remain calm.

- Patients who have been restrained require careful monitoring. Assessment and care are not over when the patient is restrained; they are just beginning.

There are many techniques and devices for restraining the violent patient. Before restraining a person, consider the normal range of motion for the major joints. The arms cannot flail backwards, the legs cannot kick backwards, and the spinal column cannot double over backwards. Also consider the power of each major muscle group. For example, the flexor muscles of the arm are much stronger than the extensor muscles. Whenever possible, position the patient to limit his or her strength and range of motion.

Become familiar with the restraint devices your service employs and periodically refresh your training in their application. Whether using gauze bandages or some form of commercial restraint, you must maintain proficiency in using restraint devices in an effective and safe manner. Many devices must be appropriately decontaminated after each use. Some devices, such as leather restraints, require monthly maintenance to ensure their continued effectiveness. Restraints can also be improvised from common materials as noted below:

- Duct tape may be used as a restraint. Be sure to encircle the wrist or ankle at least twice, and then encircle the anchor area of the stretcher AND the limb at least twice.

- Cravats or triangular bandages are also effective. Tie one cravat around the wrist or ankle and securely knot it into a "bracelet" that will not slip off the limb. Use another cravat to anchor the bracelet to the cot.

- Roller bandages (Kling™, Kerlex™) are safe and effective. Assure that you use thick (6 ply), wide, non-stretch gauze bandages.

When you must restrain a patient, do not attempt to hold him for a long period. This sets up a confrontation and aggravates the situation. It also limits care, because you will be too busy holding the patient to treat him. Continuous restraint also requires more than one paramedic or assistant per patient. Following this sequence of actions will help you to restrain an unarmed patient:

1. Make certain you have adequate assistance; this will reduce the likelihood of injury both to you and to the patient. Prepare your stretcher and restraint equipment in advance. Keep restraints out of the patient's view until you need them.

2. Offer the patient one final opportunity to cooperate.

3. If the patient does not respond to this request, at least two persons, preferably three or four, should move swiftly towards him. He cannot simultaneously focus on multiple paramedics. When four rescuers are present, one person can control each extremity. This prevents the patient from striking and kicking. Keep away from the patient's mouth to avoid being bitten. Your swiftness will minimize the accuracy of a patient's kick or blow. Attempting to restrain a patient with too many rescuers can be confusing and inefficient. Someone should continue talking with the patient throughout the restraining process.

4. When the patient's extremities are physically restrained, move him to a laterally recumbent position on the stretcher, where he can be secured. This prevents him from using his strong abdominal and leg muscles to break free from restraint. If your agency uses the Reeves stretcher to secure patients, be sure that the circumferential wrapping does not restrict the patient's respiratory efforts.

5. Generally once a patient is restrained, keeping him restrained is best. The thought of regaining control of a patient in a moving ambulance by yourself is not pleasant. If the patient calms down, you may try to reduce the discomforts caused by the restraints, but you must keep adequate restraints in place.

6. Monitor the patient carefully during transport.

POSITIONING AND RESTRAINING PATIENTS FOR TRANSPORT

Once the patient is successfully restrained, position him on his side. This dramatically reduces resistance and allows continued airway assessment and maintenance. Adjust the cot to its lowest position to improve stability, avoid lifting, and shorten the distance to the ground in case the patient falls. Do not allow the patient's large muscle groups to work together. For example, restrain one arm at the patient's side and the other above his head. Place a webbed strap across the patient's lumbar region, but do not cinch it too tightly. After applying restraints to the ankles and securing the cot, tie the ankle restraints to one another. Do not remove the restraints until enough personnel are present to control the patient. Always check the distal pulses after placing restraints.

Restraint is not without risk either to the paramedic or to the patient. Improper restraint threatens injury to everyone involved. Occasionally a restrained patient dies. The term for this phenomenon is **restraint asphyxia.** The most common scenario in these cases involves a patient who has struggled violently, either during the restraint process or during a foot pursuit or struggle with police. The patient is eventually captured, restrained, and placed in a hog-tie or hobble restraint. He struggles for a time, then becomes quiet. While police and EMS crews think he is calming down, he is actually in cardiac arrest. Resuscitation attempts are usually unsuccessful. Some experts believe the restraint itself

Patients who are physically restrained must receive frequent and close monitoring. Ideally this should include continuous ECG monitoring and pulse oximetry. Vital signs should be taken at least every 15 minutes, or every 5 minutes if the patient's condition is critical.

✳ restaint asphyxia death from positioning that prevents sufficient intake of oxygen.

Never use hog-tie or hobble restraints.

causes the patient's death. Others believe the combination of restraint, exertion, hyperthermia, and drug or alcohol abuse causes it. To prevent these deaths (and the liability they will bring), never use hog-tie or hobble restraints. Monitor all restrained patients carefully, as noted earlier. Be alert for mental status changes from agitated to calm or sleepy—they may mean hypoxia. Monitor respiratory rate and depth frequently.

CHEMICAL RESTRAINT

Some EMS systems allow the use of antipsychotic medications for controlling acutely psychotic and combative patients. This is especially important for long transports or for aeromedical operations. The most commonly used antipsychotics include haloperidol (Haldol), chlorpromazine (Thorazine) and others. These medications can be very effective in sedating patients who are agitated or hostile. Remember that medications in this class may cause an extrapyramidal system (EPS) reaction. Be prepared for EPS reactions and, if indicated, administer diphenhydramine (Benadryl) or a similar agent. Always consult and follow local protocol regarding use of antipsychotic agents or chemical restraint.

SUMMARY

Calls involving psychiatric and behavioral emergencies will challenge your skills as a paramedic. Differentiating physiological and psychological conditions will try your diagnostic skills, and developing the interview abilities that form the basis of psychiatric assessment and care will test your people skills. Ultimately, you will be called upon to help patients in a time of great need—the time of crisis. Once you determine that the patient is experiencing a purely behavioral emergency your compassion and communication skills rather than medications and procedures will benefit him most.

Situations involving crisis can drain your emotions. Observing a suicide or attempted suicide or struggling with or restraining a patient can take its toll. Take care of yourself before, during, and after these calls.

CHAPTER 39

Gynecology

Objectives

After reading this chapter, you should be able to:

1. Review the anatomic structures and physiology of the female reproductive system. (see Chapter 3)
2. Identify the normal events of the menstrual cycle. (see Chapter 3)
3. Describe how to assess a patient with a gynecological complaint. (pp. 1631–1633)
4. Explain how to recognize a gynecological emergency. (pp. 1631–1633)
5. Describe the general care for any patient experiencing a gynecological emergency. (pp. 1633–1634, 1636)
6. Describe the pathophysiology, assessment, and management of the following gynecological emergencies.

   a. Pelvic inflammatory disease (pp. 1634–1635)
   b. Ruptured ovarian cyst (p. 1635)
   c. Cystitis (p. 1635)
   d. Mittelschmertz (p. 1635)
   e. Endometritis (p. 1635)
   f. Endometriosis (pp. 1635–1636)
   g. Ectopic pregnancy (p. 1636)
   h. Vaginal hemorrhage (p. 1636)
7. Describe the assessment, care and emotional support of the sexual assault patient. (pp. 1637–1639)
8. Given several preprogrammed gynecological patients, provide the appropriate assessment, management, and transportation. (pp. 1631–1639)

INTRODUCTION

The term **gynecology** is derived from Greek, *gynaik,* meaning "woman." Gynecology is the branch of medicine that deals with the health maintenance and the diseases of women and primarily of their reproductive organs. **Obstetrics** is the branch of medicine that deals with the care of women throughout pregnancy. This chapter focuses on the assessment and care of non-pregnant patients with problems of the reproductive system. The assessment and care of the obstetrical patient is the subject of the next chapter.

* **gynecology** the branch of medicine that deals with the health maintenance and the diseases of women, primarily of the reproductive organs.

* **obstetrics** the branch of medicine that deals with the care of women throughout pregnancy.

ASSESSMENT OF THE GYNECOLOGICAL PATIENT

Beyond labor and delivery, the most common emergency complaints of women in the childbearing years are abdominal pain and vaginal bleeding. Abdominal pain is often due to problems of the reproductive organs. In addition to the usual history and physical assessment activities, you will need to ask specific questions pertinent to reproductive function and dysfunction. However, don't allow yourself to get distracted from getting complete past medical histories including chronic medical problems, medications, and allergies.

You may feel uncomfortable asking a patient about her reproductive history, but remember that you are a health care professional who is trying to obtain pertinent information in order to provide the best possible care for your patient. If you conduct yourself in this manner, it should not be uncomfortable for you or your patient. Assess your patient's emotional state. If she is reluctant to discuss her complaint in detail, respect her wishes and transport her to the emergency department where a more thorough assessment can be done.

> **Content Review**
>
> **MOST COMMON EMERGENCY GYNECOLOGICAL COMPLAINTS**
>
> Abdominal pain
> Vaginal bleeding

HISTORY

Use the SAMPLE approach for obtaining additional information about the history of the present illness. If the chief complaint is pain, then use the mnemonic OPQRST to gather more information. Is the patient's pain abdominal or in the pelvic region? Is it localized in a specific quadrant of the pelvis? Is she having her menstrual period? If so, how does the pain she is having now compare with how she usually feels? Some women have severe discomfort during their menstrual periods. This is called **dysmenorrhea.** Others may experience **dyspareunia,** painful sexual intercourse. Does walking or defecation aggravate her pain? What, if anything, alleviates her pain? Does positioning herself on her back or side with her knees bent relieve her discomfort?

You need to determine if there are any associated signs or symptoms that will be helpful in determining what is wrong with your patient. For instance, does your patient report a fever or chills? Is she reporting signs of gastrointestinal problems, such as nausea, vomiting, diarrhea, or constipation? Or perhaps she's complaining of urinary problems, such as frequency, painful urination, or "colicky" urinary cramping. Does she report a vaginal discharge or bleeding? If so, you should obtain information about the color, amount, frequency, or odors associated with either vaginal bleeding or discharge. If she reports vaginal bleeding, how does the amount compare with the volume of her usual menstrual period? Does she report dizziness with changes in position (orthostatic hypotension), syncope, or diaphoresis?

You will need to obtain specific information about her obstetric history. Has she ever been pregnant? *Gravida (G)* is the term used to describe the number of

* **dysmenorrhea** painful menstruation.

* **dyspareunia** painful sexual intercourse.

times a woman has been pregnant, including this one if she is pregnant. How many of those pregnancies ended in the delivery of a viable infant? *Para* or *parity* (P) refers to the number of deliveries. *Abortion* (Ab) refers to any pregnancy that ends before 20 weeks of gestation, regardless of cause. You may see this information recorded in "shorthand," for example, $G_3 P_2 Ab_1$, or gravida 3, para 2, ab 1. This means that she has been pregnant 3 times and had 2 prior deliveries and 1 pregnancy that ended before 20 weeks gestation. These terms refer to the number of pregnancies and deliveries, not the number of infants delivered, so even twins or triplets counts only as one pregnancy and one delivery.

You will also need to obtain a gynecological history. Question the patient about previous ectopic pregnancies, infections, cesarean sections, pelvic surgeries such as tubal ligation, abortions (either elective or therapeutic), and dilation and curettage (D&C) procedures. Also ask the patient about any prior history of trauma to the reproductive tract. It is often helpful to find out whether the patient, if sexually active, has had pain or bleeding during or after sexual intercourse.

It is important to document the date of the patient's last menstrual period, commonly abbreviated LMP (or LNMP for "last normal menstrual period"). Ask whether the period was of a normal length and whether the flow was heavier or lighter than usual. An easy way for women to estimate menstrual flow is by the number of pads or tampons used. She can easily compare this number to her routine usage. It is also important to inquire how regular the patient's periods tend to be. Ask her what form of birth control, if any, she uses. Also, find out if she uses it regularly. Direct questions such as "Could you be pregnant?" are generally unlikely to get an accurate response. Indirect questioning is often more helpful in determining the likelihood of pregnancy, such as "When did your last menstrual period start?" If you suspect pregnancy, inquire about other signs, including a late or missed period, breast tenderness, bloating, urinary frequency, or nausea and vomiting. Until proven otherwise, you should assume that any missed or late period is due to pregnancy even though your patient may deny it.

Contraception, or the prevention of pregnancy, takes many forms. Remember that many contraceptives are medications, so don't forget to ask about their use. With the exception of oral contraceptives ("the pill") and intrauterine devices (IUDs), side effects caused by contraceptives are relatively rare. Oral contraceptives have been associated with hypertension, rare incidents of stroke and heart attack, and possibly pulmonary embolism. IUDs can cause perforation of the uterus, uterine infection, or irregular uterine bleeding. This is especially true for IUDs that have remained in place longer than the time recommended by the manufacturer, which rarely exceeds 2 years.

PHYSICAL EXAM

Physical examination of the gynecological patient is limited in the field. More than at any other time, the patient's comfort level should guide your actions. Respect your patient's modesty and maintain her privacy. This may mean that you need to exclude parents from the room when assessing adolescent patients or that you need to exclude spouses of married patients. Recognizing that most people are not comfortable discussing matters related to sexuality or reproductive organs, take your cues from the patient. Maintain a professional demeanor. Explain all procedures thoroughly so that your patient can understand them prior to initiating any care. Some women may feel more comfortable if they can be cared for by a female paramedic.

As always, the level of consciousness is the best indicator of your patient's status. Assess your patient's general appearance, paying particular attention to the color of her skin and mucous membranes. Cyanosis and pallor may indicate

In the female patient of childbearing age, always document the LMP.

Any patient of reproductive age who still has her uterus should be considered to be pregnant until proven otherwise.

shock or a gas-exchange problem, while a flushed appearance is more indicative of fever.

Remember that vital signs are useful clues to the nature of your patient's problem. Pain and fever tend to cause an increase in pulse and respiratory rates along with a slight increase in blood pressure. Significant bleeding will cause increased pulse and respiratory rates as well as narrowing pulse pressures (the difference between systolic and diastolic pressures). Perform a tilt test to assess for orthostatic changes in her vital signs (a decrease in blood pressure and an increase in pulse rate when the patient rises from a supine or seated position), which again points to significant blood loss.

Assess your patient for evidence of vaginal bleeding or discharge. If possible estimate blood loss. The use of more than two sanitary pads per hour is considered significant bleeding. If serious bleeding is reported or evident, it may be necessary to inspect the patient's perineum. Document the color and character of the discharge, as well as the amount, and the presence or absence of clots. *Do not perform an internal vaginal exam in the field.*

Do not perform an internal vaginal exam in the field.

Pay particular attention to the abdominal examination. Auscultate the abdomen and note whether bowel sounds are absent or hyperactive. Gently palpate the abdomen. Document and report any masses, distention, guarding, localized tenderness, or rebound tenderness. In thin patients, a palpable mass in the lower abdomen may be an intrauterine pregnancy. At three months, the uterus is barely palpable above the symphysis pubis. At four months, the uterus is palpable midway between the umbilicus and the symphysis pubis. At five months (approximately 20 weeks), the uterus is palpable at the level of the umbilicus.

MANAGEMENT OF GYNECOLOGICAL EMERGENCIES

In general, the management of the patient experiencing a gynecological emergency is focused on supportive care. Rely on your initial assessment to guide your decision-making about the need for oxygen therapy or intravenous access. If your patient's status warrants it, administer oxygen or assist ventilation as necessary. As a rule, intravenous access and fluid replacement is usually not indicated. However, if your patient has excessive bleeding or demonstrates signs of shock, then establish at least one large bore IV and administer normal saline at a rate indicated by the patient's presentation. You may also want to initiate cardiac monitoring if your patient is unstable.

General management of gynecological emergencies is focused on supportive care.

Continue to monitor and evaluate serious bleeding. *Do not pack dressings in the vagina.* Discourage the use of tampons to absorb blood flow. If your patient is bleeding heavily, count and document the number of sanitary pads used. If your patient demonstrates signs of impending shock, you may elect to place her in the Trendelenburg position (head lower than feet). The use of a pneumatic anti-shock garment in this situation should be governed by your local protocol. If shock is not a consideration, then position your patient for comfort in the left lateral recumbent position or supine with her knees bent, as this decreases tension on the peritoneum. Analgesics (pain-control medications) are not usually given in the field for gynecological complaints because these drugs tend to mask signs and symptoms of a deteriorating condition and make assessment and diagnosis difficult.

Do not pack dressings in the vagina.

Since it is not appropriate to perform an internal vaginal exam in the field, most patients with gynecological complaints will be transported to be evaluated by a physician. Some problems may require surgical intervention, so you should consider emergency transport to the appropriate facility based on your local protocols.

Psychological support is particularly important when caring for patients with gynecological complaints. Keep calm. Maintain your patient's modesty and privacy. Remember that this is likely to be a very stressful situation for your patient, and she will appreciate your gentle, considerate care.

SPECIFIC GYNECOLOGICAL EMERGENCIES

Gynecological emergencies can be generally divided into two categories—medical and traumatic.

MEDICAL GYNECOLOGICAL EMERGENCIES

Gynecological emergencies of a medical nature are often hard to diagnose in the field. The most common symptoms of a medical gynecological emergency are abdominal pain and/or vaginal bleeding.

Gynecological Abdominal Pain

Pelvic Inflammatory Disease Probably the most common cause of nontraumatic abdominal pain is **pelvic inflammatory disease** (PID). Pelvic inflammatory disease (PID) is an infection of the female reproductive tract that can be caused by a bacterium, virus, or fungus. The organs most commonly involved are the uterus, fallopian tubes, and ovaries. Occasionally the adjoining structures, such as the peritoneum and intestines, also become involved. PID is the most common cause of abdominal pain in women in the childbearing years, occurring in one percent of that population. The highest rate of infection occurs in sexually active women ages 15 to 24. The most common causes of PID are gonorrhea *(Neisseria gonorrhoeae)* or chlamydia *(Chlamydia trachomatis),* although rarely streptococcus or staphylococcus bacteria may cause it. Commonly, gonorrhea or chlamydia progresses undetected in a female until frank PID develops.

Predisposing factors include multiple sexual partners, prior history of PID, recent gynecological procedure, or an IUD. Post-infection damage to the fallopian tubes is a common cause for infertility. PID may be either acute or chronic. If it is allowed to progress untreated, sepsis may develop. Additionally, PID may cause adhesions, in which the pelvic organs "stick together." Adhesions are a common cause of chronic pelvic pain and increase the frequency of infertility and ectopic pregnancies.

While it is possible for a patient with pelvic inflammatory disease to be asymptomatic, most patients with PID complain of abdominal pain. It is often diffuse and located in the lower abdomen. It may be moderate to severe, which occasionally makes it difficult to distinguish it from appendicitis. Pain may intensify either before or after the menstrual period. It may also worsen during sexual intercourse, as movement of the cervix tends to cause increased discomfort. Patients with PID tend to walk with a shuffling gait, since walking often intensifies their pain. In severe cases, fever, chills, nausea, vomiting, or even sepsis may accompany PID. Occasionally, patients have a foul-smelling vaginal discharge, often yellow in color, as well as irregular menses. It is common also to have mid-cycle bleeding.

Generally, on physical examination, the patient with PID appears acutely ill or toxic. The blood pressure is normal, although the pulse rate may be slightly increased. Fever may or may not be present. Palpation of the lower abdomen generally elicits moderate to severe pain. Occasionally, in severe cases, the abdomen will be tense with obvious rebound tenderness. Such cases may be impossible to distinguish from appendicitis in the prehospital setting.

* **pelvic inflammatory disease (PID)** an acute infection of the reproductive organs that can be caused by a bacteria, virus, or fungus.

PID is a major risk factor for pelvic adhesions.

The primary treatment for PID is antibiotics, often administered intravenously over an extended period. Once the causative organism is determined, the sexual partner may also require treatment. In the field, the primary goal is to make the patient as comfortable as possible. Place the patient on the ambulance stretcher in the position in which she is most comfortable. She may wish to draw her knees up toward her chest, as this decreases tension on the peritoneum. *Do not perform a vaginal examination.* If your patient has signs of sepsis, administer oxygen and establish intravenous access.

Ruptured Ovarian Cyst *Cysts* are fluid-filled pockets. When they develop in the ovary, they can rupture and be a source of abdominal pain. When an egg is released from the ovary, a cyst, known as a corpus luteum cyst, is often left in its place. Occasionally, cysts develop independent of ovulation. When the cysts rupture, a small amount of blood is spilled into the abdomen. Because blood irritates the peritoneum, it can cause abdominal pain and rebound tenderness. Ovarian cysts may be found during a routine pelvic examination. However, in the field setting, your patient is likely to complain of moderate to severe unilateral abdominal pain, which may radiate to her back. She may also report a history of dyspareunia, irregular bleeding, or a delayed menstrual period. It is not uncommon for patients to rupture ovarian cysts during intercourse or physical activity. This often results in immediate, severe abdominal pain causing the patient to immediately stop intercourse or other physical activity. Ruptured ovarian cysts may be associated with vaginal bleeding.

Cystitis Urinary bladder infection, or **cystitis**, is a common cause of abdominal pain. Bacteria usually enter the urinary tract via the urethra, ascending into the bladder and ureters. The bladder lies anterior to the reproductive organs and, when inflamed, causes pain, generally immediately above the symphysis pubis. If untreated, the infection can progress to the kidneys. In addition to abdominal pain, your patient may report urinary frequency, pain or burning with urination (**dysuria**), and a low-grade fever. Occasionally the urine may be blood-tinged.

* **cystitis** infection of the urinary bladder.

* **dysuria** painful urination often associated with cystitis.

Mittelschmerz Occasionally, ovulation is accompanied by mid-cycle abdominal pain known as **mittelschmerz.** It is thought that the pain is related to peritoneal irritation due to follicle rupture or bleeding at the time of ovulation. The unilateral lower quadrant pain is usually self-limited and may be accompanied by mid-cycle spotting. While some women may report a low-grade fever, it should be noted that body temperature normally increases at the time of ovulation and remains elevated until the day prior to the onset of the menstrual period. Treatment is symptomatic.

* **mittelschmerz** abdominal pain associated with ovulation.

Endometritis An infection of the uterine lining called **endometritis** is an occasional complication of **miscarriage,** childbirth, or gynecological procedures such as dilatation and curettage (D & C). Commonly reported signs and symptoms include mild to severe lower abdominal pain, a bloody, foul-smelling discharge, and fever (101° to 104° F). The onset of symptoms is usually 48 to 72 hours after the gynecological procedure or miscarriage. These infections often mimic the presentation of PID and can be quite serious if not quickly treated with the appropriate antibiotics. Complications of endometritis may include sterility, sepsis, or even death.

* **endometritis** infection of the endometrium.

* **miscarriage** commonly used term to describe a pregnancy which ends before 20 weeks gestation; may also be called spontaneous abortion.

Endometriosis Endometriosis is a condition in which endometrial tissue is found outside of the uterus. Most commonly it is found in the abdomen and pelvis, although it has been found virtually everywhere in the body, including the central nervous system and lungs. Regardless of its site, the tissue responds to the hormonal changes associated with the menstrual cycle and thus bleeds in a cyclic manner. This bleeding causes inflammation, scarring of adjacent tissues, and the

* **endometriosis** condition in which endometrial tissue grows outside of the uterus.

subsequent development of adhesions, particularly in the pelvic cavity.

Endometriosis is usually seen in women between the ages of 30 to 40 and is rarely seen in postmenopausal women. The exact cause is unknown. The most common symptom is dull, cramping pelvic pain that is usually related to menstruation. Dyspareunia and abnormal uterine bleeding is also commonly reported. Painful bowel movements have also been reported when the endometrial tissue has invaded the gastrointestinal tract. It is not uncommon for endometriosis to be diagnosed when the patient is being evaluated for infertility. Definitive treatment may include medical management with hormones, analgesics, and anti-inflammatory drugs, and/or surgery to remove the excessive endometrial tissue or adhesions from other organs.

Ectopic Pregnancy An **ectopic pregnancy** is the implantation of a fetus outside of the uterus. The most common site is within the fallopian tubes. This is a surgical emergency, because the tube can rupture, triggering a massive hemorrhage. Patients with ectopic pregnancy often have severe unilateral abdominal pain which may radiate to the shoulder on the affected side, a late or missed menstrual period, and, occasionally, vaginal bleeding. Additional discussion of ectopic pregnancy is presented in the next chapter.

* **ectopic pregnancy** the implantation of a developing fetus outside of the uterus, often in a fallopian tube.

Ectopic pregnancy is a life-threatening condition.

Content Review

TREATMENT FOR ABDOMINAL PAIN

Make the patient comfortable.
Transport.

Management of Gynecological Abdominal Pain

Any woman with significant abdominal pain should be treated and transported to the hospital for evaluation. Administer oxygen and establish intravenous access if indicated. Refer to the earlier section on management of gynecological emergencies for additional information.

Non-Traumatic Vaginal Bleeding

Non-traumatic vaginal bleeding is rarely seen in the field unless it is severe. Refer to the earlier section in this chapter on completing a patient history. You should not presume that vaginal bleeding is due to normal menstruation. Occasionally a woman will experience **menorrhagia,** or excessive menstrual flow, but rarely is it the cause for a 911 call. Hemorrhage, regardless of cause, is always potentially life threatening, so be alert for signs of impending shock.

The most common cause of non-traumatic vaginal bleeding is a spontaneous abortion (miscarriage). If it has been more than 60 days since your patient's LMP, you should assume that this is the cause. Vaginal bleeding due to miscarriage is often associated with cramping abdominal pain and the passage of clots and tissue. The loss of a pregnancy, even at a very early phase, is a significant emotional event for your patient, so your kind and considerate care is important. Spontaneous abortion and other causes of bleeding in the obstetric patient will be discussed further in the next chapter. Other potential causes of vaginal bleeding include cancerous lesions, PID, or the onset of labor.

* **menorrhagia** excessive menstrual flow.

The most common cause of nontraumatic vaginal bleeding is spontaneous abortion (miscarriage).

Content Review

TREATMENT FOR VAGINAL BLEEDING

Absorb blood flow, but do not pack the vagina.
Transport.
Initiate oxygen therapy and IV access based on the patient's condition.

Management of Non-Traumatic Vaginal Bleeding

Your field management of patients suffering non-traumatic vaginal bleeding will depend on the severity of the situation and your assessment of the patient's status. Absorb the blood flow. *Do not pack the vagina.* If your patient is passing clots or tissue, save these for evaluation by a physician. Transport your patient in a position of comfort. The initiation of oxygen therapy and intravenous access should be guided by the patient's condition.

TRAUMATIC GYNECOLOGICAL EMERGENCIES

Most cases of vaginal bleeding result from obstetrical problems or are related to the menstrual period. However, trauma to the vagina and perineum can also cause bleeding and abdominal pain.

Causes of Gynecological Trauma

The incidence of genital trauma is increasing, with vaginal injury occurring far more commonly than male genital injury. Gynecological trauma may occur at any age. Blunt trauma occurs more frequently than penetrating trauma. Straddle injury (such as may occur with riding a bicycle) is the most common form of blunt trauma. Vaginal injuries are most often lacerations due to sexual assault. Other causes of gynecological trauma include blunt force to the lower abdomen due to assault or seat-belt injuries, direct blows to the perineal area, foreign bodies inserted into the vagina, self-attempts at abortion, and lacerations following childbirth.

Management of Gynecological Trauma

Injuries to the external genitalia should be managed by direct pressure over the laceration or a chemical cold pack applied to a hematoma. In most cases of vaginal bleeding, the source is not readily apparent. If bleeding is severe or your patient demonstrates signs of shock, establish IV access to maintain intravascular volume and monitor vital signs closely. Blunt force may cause organ rupture leading to the development of peritonitis or sepsis. *Never* pack the vagina with any material or dressing, regardless of the severity of the bleeding. Expedite transport to the emergency department since surgical intervention is often required.

Sexual Assault

Sexual assault continues to represent the most rapidly growing violent crime in America. Over 700,000 women are sexually assaulted annually. Unfortunately, it is estimated that more than 60 percent of all sexual assaults are never reported to authorities. Male victims represent 5 percent of reported sexual assaults. Sexual abuse of children is reported even less frequently. It is estimated that the incidence of sexual abuse in children ranges from 50,000 to 350,000/year. There is no "typical victim" of sexual assault. Nobody, from small children to aged adults, is immune.

Most victims of sexual assault know their assailants. Friends, acquaintances, intimates, and family members commit the vast majority (80 percent) of sexual assaults against women. Acquaintance rape is particularly common among adolescent victims. Sexual assault is a crime of violence, not passion, that is motivated by aggression and a need to control, humiliate, or inflict pain. There are very few predictors of who is capable of committing sexual assault, as age, economic status, and ethnic origins vary widely. Common behavioral characteristics found among rapists include poor impulse control, the need to achieve sexual satisfaction within the context of violence, and immaturity.

The definition of sexual assault varies from state to state. The common element of any definition is sexual contact without consent. Generally, rape is defined as penetration of the vagina or rectum of an unwilling female or the rectum in an unwilling male. In most states, penetration must occur for an act to be classified as rape. Sexual assault also includes oral-genital sex. Regardless of the legal definition, sexual assault is a crime of violence with serious physical and psychological implications.

FIGURE 39-1 If possible, have a female EMT or paramedic accompany the sexual assault victim to the hospital.

Assessment The victim of sexual assault is a unique patient with unique needs. Your patient needs emergency medical treatment and psychological support. Your patient also needs to have legal evidence gathered. *Your* objectivity is essential, as your attitude may affect long-term psychological recovery. As a rule, victims of sexual abuse *should not* be questioned about the incident in the field. Don't ask questions about specific details of the assault. It is not important, from the standpoint of prehospital care, to determine whether penetration took place. Do not inquire about the patient's sexual practices. Confine your questions to the physical injuries the patient received. Even well-intentioned questions may lead to guilt feelings in the patient. Don't ask questions, such as why did you go with him or get in his car.

The psychological response of sexual assault victims is widely variable. The victim of sexual assault may be withdrawn or hysterical. Some use denial, anger, or fear as defense mechanisms. Approach the patient calmly and professionally. Allay the patient's fear and anxiety. Respond to the patient's feelings but be aware of your own. If the patient is incompletely dressed, a cover should be offered. Respect the patient's modesty. Explain all procedures and obtain the patient's permission before beginning them. Avoid touching the patient other than to take vital signs or examine other physical injuries. *Do not* examine the genitalia unless there is life-threatening hemorrhage.

Management In most situations, psychological and emotional support is the most important help you can offer. Maintain a nonjudgmental attitude and assure the patient of confidentiality. If the patient is female, allow her to be cared for by a female EMT or paramedic (if available). If the patient desires, have a female accompany her to the hospital (Figure 39-1). Provide a safe environment, such as the back of a well-lit ambulance. Respond to the patient's feelings and respect the patient's wishes. Unless your patient is unconscious, do not touch the patient unless given permission. Even when your patient appears to have an altered level of consciousness, explain what's going to be done before initiating any treatment.

Preservation of physical evidence is important. When the patient arrives at the hospital, a physician or sexual assault nurse examiner will complete a sexual assault examination to gather physical evidence. To protect this evidence, it is important that you adhere to the following guidelines:

- Consider the patient a crime scene and protect that scene.
- Handle clothing as little as possible, if at all.

Do not ask about specific details of a sexual assault.

Do not examine the external genitalia of a sexual assault victim unless there is a life-threatening hemorrhage.

Psychological and emotional support are the most important elements of care for the sexual assault victim.

- If you must remove clothing, bag separately each item that must be bagged.
- Do not cut through any tears or holes in the clothing.
- Place bloody articles in brown paper bags.
- Do not examine the perineal area.
- If the assault took place within the hour or the patient is bleeding, put an absorbent underpad (e.g., Chux) under the patient's hips to collect that evidence.
- If you cover the patient with a sheet or blanket, turn that over to the hospital as evidence.
- Do not allow patients to change their clothes, bathe, or douche (if female) before the medical examination.
- Do not allow patients to comb their hair, brush their teeth, or clean their fingernails.
- Do not clean wounds, if at all possible.
- If you must initiate care on scene, avoid disruption of the crime scene.

Documentation When completing your patient care report, keep the following documentation guidelines in mind:

- State patient remarks accurately.
- Objectively state your observations of the patient's physical condition, environment, or torn clothing.
- Document any evidence (e.g., clothing, sheets) turned over to the hospital staff and the name of the individual to whom you gave it.
- Do NOT include your opinions as to whether rape occurred.

SUMMARY

Most gynecological emergency patients have either abdominal pain or vaginal bleeding. The patient with abdominal pain should be made comfortable and transported to the emergency department. The management of vaginal bleeding depends on the severity. Minor bleeding should be simply monitored. Severe bleeding should be treated with IV fluids, if indicated.

In the case of sexual assault, you should first determine if any life-threatening physical injuries exist. Second, respect the patient's wishes and offer emotional support. Third, in treating victims of sexual assault, make every effort to preserve physical evidence. As with any type of emergency care, the primary concern is the patient.

CHAPTER 40

Obstetrics

Objectives

After reading this chapter, you should be able to:

1. Describe the anatomic structures and physiology of the reproductive system during pregnancy. (pp. 1641–1645)
2. Identify the normal events of pregnancy. (pp. 1645–1647)
3. Describe how to assess an obstetrical patient. (pp. 1648–1651)
4. Identify the stages of labor and the paramedic's role in each stage. (pp. 1663–1664)
5. Differentiate between normal and abnormal delivery. (pp. 1670–1675)
6. Identify and describe complications associated with pregnancy and delivery. (pp. 1652–1662, 1670–1677)
7. Identify predelivery emergencies. (pp. 1652–1662)
8. State indications of an imminent delivery. (p. 1664)
9. Identify the contents of an obstetrical kit and explain the use of each item. (pp. 1664–1668)
10. Differentiate the management of a patient with predelivery emergencies from a normal delivery. (pp. 1651–1662)

Continued

INTRODUCTION

Pregnancy, childbirth, and the potential complications of each are the focus of this chapter. Pregnancy is a normal, natural process of life that results from ovulation and fertilization. Complications of pregnancy are uncommon, but when they do occur, you must be prepared to recognize them quickly and manage them. Childbirth occurs daily, usually requiring only the most basic assistance. This chapter will prepare you to assess and care for the female patient throughout her pregnancy and delivery of her child.

THE PRENATAL PERIOD

The *prenatal period* (literally "prebirth period") is the time from conception until delivery of the fetus. During this period, fetal development takes place. In addition, significant physiological changes occur in the mother.

ANATOMY AND PHYSIOLOGY OF THE OBSTETRIC PATIENT

As you learned in the previous chapter, the first two weeks of the menstrual cycle are dominated by the hormone estrogen, which causes the endometrium (the inner lining of the uterus) to thicken and become engorged with blood. In response to a surge of luteinizing hormone (LH) and follicle stimulating hormone (FSH), **ovulation,** or release of an egg (ovum) from the ovary, takes place. The egg travels down the fallopian tube to the uterus. If the egg has been fertilized, it becomes implanted in the uterus and pregnancy begins. If the egg has not been fertilized, menstruation (discharge of blood, mucus, and cellular debris from the endometrium) takes place 14 days after ovulation. (The time from ovulation to menstruation is always exactly 14 days. However, the time from menstruation to

* ovulation the release of an egg from the ovary.

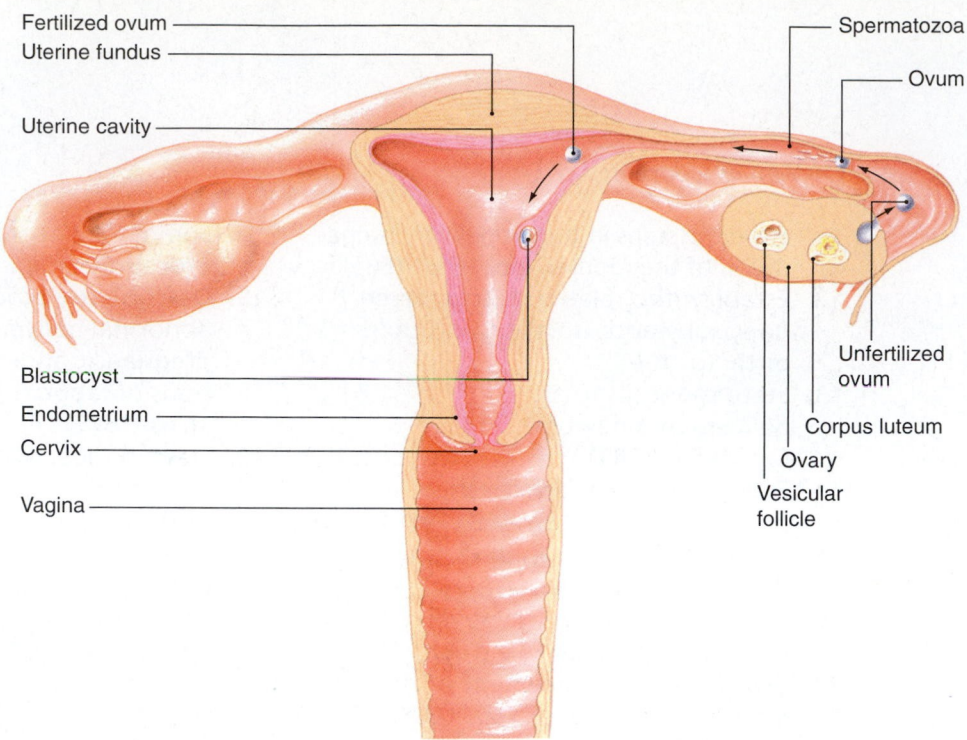

Fertilized ovum
Uterine fundus
Uterine cavity
Blastocyst
Endometrium
Cervix
Vagina
Spermatozoa
Ovum
Unfertilized ovum
Corpus luteum
Ovary
Vesicular follicle

FIGURE 40-1   Fertilization and implantation of the ovum.

the next ovulation may vary by several days from the average of 14 days, which is why it can be difficult for couples to find the optimum time of the month to conceive, or to avoid conceiving, a baby.)

If the woman has had intercourse within 24 to 48 hours before ovulation, fertilization may occur. The male's seminal fluid carrying numerous spermatozoa, or male sex cells, enters the vagina and uterus and travels toward the fallopian tubes. Fertilization, which usually takes place in the distal third of the fallopian tube, occurs when a male spermatozoon fuses with the female ovum (Figure 40-1). After fertilization, the ovum begins cellular division immediately, which continues as it moves through the fallopian tube to the uterus. The ovum then becomes a *blastocyst* (a hollow ball of cells). The blastocyst normally implants in the thickened uterine lining, which has been prepared for implantation by the hormone progesterone, where the fetus and placenta subsequently develop.

Approximately three weeks after fertilization, the placenta develops on the uterine wall at the site where the blastocyst attached (Figure 40-2). The **placenta,** known as the "organ of pregnancy," is a temporary, blood-rich structure that serves as the lifeline for the developing fetus. It transfers heat while exchanging oxygen and carbon dioxide, delivering nutrients such as glucose, potassium, sodium, and chloride, and carrying away wastes such as urea, uric acid, and creatinine. The placenta also serves as an endocrine gland throughout pregnancy, secreting hormones necessary for fetal survival as well as the estrogen and progesterone required to maintain the pregnancy. Additionally, the placenta serves as a protective barrier against harmful substances. (However, some drugs such as narcotics, steroids, and some antibiotics, are able to cross the placental membrane from the mother to the fetus.) When expelled from the uterus following birth of the child, the placenta and accompanying membranes are called the **afterbirth.**

* **placenta** the organ that serves as a lifeline for the developing fetus. The placenta is attached to the wall of the uterus and the umbilical cord.

* **afterbirth** the placenta and accompanying membranes that are expelled from the uterus after the birth of a child.

FIGURE 40-2 Anatomy of the placenta.

The placenta is connected to the fetus by the **umbilical cord,** a flexible, rope-like structure approximately two feet in length and three-quarters of an inch in diameter. Normally, the umbilical cord contains two arteries and one vein. The umbilical vein transports oxygenated blood to the fetus, while the umbilical arteries return relatively deoxygenated blood to the placenta.

The fetus develops within the **amniotic sac,** sometimes called the "bag of waters" (BOW). This thin-walled membranous covering holds the **amniotic fluid** that surrounds and protects the fetus during intrauterine development. The amniotic fluid increases in volume throughout the course of the pregnancy. After the 20th week of gestation, the volume varies from 500 to 1000 cc. The presence of amniotic fluid allows for fetal movement within the uterus and serves to cushion and protect the fetus from trauma. The volume changes constantly as amniotic fluid moves back and forth across the placental membrane. During the latter part of the pregnancy, the fetus contributes to the volume by secretions from the lungs and urination. Although it may rupture earlier, the amniotic sac usually breaks during labor, and the amniotic fluid or "water" flows out of the vagina. This is called *rupture of the membranes (ROM).* It is what has happened when the pregnant woman says, "My water has broken."

Physiologic Changes of Pregnancy

The physiologic changes associated with pregnancy are due to an altered hormonal state, the mechanical effects of the enlarging uterus and its significant vascularity, and the increasing metabolic demands on the maternal system. It is important for you to understand the physiologic changes associated with pregnancy so that you can better assess your pregnant patients.

✳ **umbilical cord** structure containing two arteries and one vein that connects the placenta and the fetus.

✳ **amniotic sac** the membranes that surround and protect the developing fetus throughout the period of intrauterine development.

✳ **amniotic fluid** clear, watery fluid that surrounds and protects the developing fetus.

The Prenatal Period **1643**

FIGURE 40-3 Uterine changes associated with pregnancy.

3 Months

8 Months

Placenta

Cord

Bag of waters

Uterus

Placenta

Cervix

Umbilical cord

Vagina

Pubic bone

Bladder

Cervix

Reproductive System It is understandable that the most significant pregnancy-related changes occur in the uterus. In its non-pregnant state, the uterus is a small pear-shaped organ weighing about 60 g (2 ounces) with a capacity of approximately 10 cc. By the end of pregnancy, its weight has increased to 1000 g (slightly more than 2 pounds) while its capacity is now approximately 5,000 ml (Figure 40-3). Another notable change is that during pregnancy the vascular system of the uterus contains about one-sixth (16 percent) of the mother's total blood volume.

Other changes include the formation of a mucous plug in the cervix that protects the developing fetus and helps to prevent infection. This plug will be expelled when cervical dilatation begins prior to delivery. Estrogen causes the vaginal mucosa to thicken, vaginal secretions to increase, and the connective tissue to loosen to allow for delivery. The breasts enlarge and become more nodular as the mammary glands increase in number and size in preparation for lactation.

Respiratory System As maternal oxygen demands increase, progesterone causes a decrease in airway resistance. This results in a 20 percent increase in oxygen consumption and a 40 percent increase in tidal volume. There is only a slight increase in respiratory rate. The diaphragm is pushed up by the enlarging uterus, resulting in flaring of the rib margins to maintain intrathoracic volume.

Cardiovascular System Various changes take place in the cardiovascular system during pregnancy. Cardiac output increases throughout pregnancy, peaking at 6–7 liters/minute by the time the fetus is fully developed. The maternal blood volume increases by 45 percent and, although both red blood cells and plasma increase, there is slightly more plasma, resulting in a relative anemia. To combat this anemia, pregnant women receive supplemental iron to increase the oxygen-carrying capacity of their red blood cells. Due to the increase in blood volume, the pregnant female may suffer a blood loss of 30–35 percent without a significant change in vital signs. The maternal heart rate increases by 10–15 bpm. Blood pressure decreases slightly during the first two trimesters, then rises to near non-pregnant levels during the third trimester.

Supine hypotensive syndrome occurs when the gravid uterus compresses the inferior vena cava when the mother lies in a supine position, causing decreased venous return to the right atrium, which lowers blood pressure. Current research suggests that the abdominal aorta may also be compressed. The enlarging uterus also may press on the pelvic and femoral vessels, causing impaired venous return from the legs and venous stasis. This may lead to the development of varicose veins, dependent edema, and postural hypotension. Some patients are predisposed to this problem because of an overall decrease in circulating blood volume or because of anemia. Assessment and management of supine hypotensive syndrome will be discussed later in this chapter.

Gastrointestinal System Nausea and vomiting are common in the first trimester as a result of hormone levels and changed carbohydrate needs. Peristalsis is slowed, so delayed gastric emptying is likely and bloating or constipation is common. As the uterus enlarges, abdominal organs are compressed, and the resulting compartmentalization of abdominal organs makes assessment difficult.

Urinary System Renal blood flow increases during pregnancy. The glomerular filtration rate increases by nearly 50 percent in the second trimester and remains elevated throughout the remainder of the pregnancy. As a result, the renal tubular absorption also increases. Occasionally glucosuria (large amounts of sugar in the urine) may result from the kidney's inability to reabsorb all of the glucose being filtered. Glucosuria may be normal or may indicate the development of gestational diabetes. The urinary bladder gets displaced anteriorly and superiorly increasing the potential for rupture. As a result, urinary frequency is common, particularly in the first and third trimesters.

Musculoskeletal System Loosened pelvic joints caused by hormonal influences account for the waddling gait that is often associated with pregnancy. As the uterus enlarges and the mother's center of gravity changes, postural changes take place to compensate for anterior growth, causing low back pain.

FETAL DEVELOPMENT

Fetal development begins immediately after fertilization and is quite complex. The time at which fertilization occurs is called *conception*. Since conception occurs approximately 14 days after the first day of the last menstrual period, it is possible to calculate, with fair accuracy, the approximate date the baby should be born. This estimate is usually made during the mother's first prenatal visit. The normal duration of pregnancy is 40 weeks from the first day of the mother's last menstrual period. This is equal to 280 days, which is 10 lunar months or, roughly, 9 calendar months. This estimated birth date is commonly called the *due date*. Medically, it is known as the **estimated date of confinement (EDC)**. Generally, pregnancy is divided into *trimesters*. Each trimester is approximately 13 weeks, or 3 calendar months, long.

Several different terms are used to describe the stages of development. The *pre-embryonic stage* covers the first 14 days following conception. The *embryonic stage* begins at day 15 and ends at approximately 8 weeks. The period from 8 weeks until delivery is known as the *fetal stage*. As a paramedic you should be familiar with some of the significant developmental milestones that occur during these three periods (Table 40-1). During normal fetal development, the sex of the infant can usually be determined by 16 weeks gestation. By the 20th week, *fetal heart tones (FHTs)* can be detected by stethoscope. The mother also has generally felt fetal movement. By 24 weeks, the baby may be able to survive if born prematurely. Fetuses born after 28 weeks have an excellent chance of survival. By the 38th week the baby is considered *term*, or fully developed.

* **estimated date of confinement (EDC)** the approximate day the infant will be born. This date is usually set at 40 weeks after the date of the mother's last menstrual period (LMP).

Table 40-1	SIGNIFICANT FETAL DEVELOPMENTAL MILESTONES
Pre-embryonic Stage	
2 weeks	Rapid cellular multiplication and differentiation
Embryonic Stage	
4 weeks	Fetal heart begins to beat
8 weeks	All body systems and external structures are formed
	Size: approximately 3 centimeters (1.2 inches)
Fetal Stage	
8–12 weeks	Fetal heart tones audible with Doppler
	Kidneys begin to produce urine
	Size: 8 centimeters (3.2 inches), weight about 1.6 ounces
	Fetus most vulnerable to toxins
16 weeks	Sex can be determined visually
	Swallowing amniotic fluid and producing meconium
	Looks like a baby, although thin
20 weeks	Fetal heart tones audible with stethoscope
	Mother able to feel fetal movement
	Baby develops schedule of sucking, kicking, and sleeping
	Hair, eyebrows, and eyelashes present
	Size: 19 centimeters (8 inches), weight approximately 16 ounces
24 weeks	Increased activity
	Begins respiratory movement
	Size: 28 centimeters (11.2 inches), weight 1 pound 10 ounces.
28 weeks	Surfactant necessary for lung function is formed
	Eyes begin to open and close
	Weighs 2 to 3 pounds
32 weeks	Bones are fully developed but soft and flexible
	Subcutaneous fat being deposited
	Fingernails and toenails present
38–40 weeks	Considered to be full-term
	Baby fills uterine cavity
	Baby receives maternal antibodies

Most of the fetus's organ systems develop during the first trimester. Therefore, this is when the fetus is most vulnerable to the development of birth defects.

FETAL CIRCULATION

The fetus receives its oxygen and nutrients from its mother through the placenta. Thus, while in the uterus, the fetus does not need to use its respiratory system or its gastrointestinal tract. Because of this, the fetal circulation shunts blood around the lungs and gastrointestinal tract.

Inferior vena cava

Liver

Placenta

Umbilical cord

Umbilical vein

Ductus arteriosus

Umbilical artery

Foramen ovale

Left ventricle

Right ventricle

Inferior vena cava

FIGURE 40-4 The maternal-fetal circulation.

The infant receives its blood from the placenta by means of the umbilical vein (Figure 40-4). The umbilical vein connects directly to the inferior vena cava by a specialized structure called the *ductus venosus.* Blood then travels through the inferior vena cava to the heart. The blood enters the right atrium and passes through the tricuspid valve into the right ventricle. It then exits the right ventricle, through the pulmonic valve, into the pulmonary artery. The fetus's heart has a hole between the right and left atria, termed the *foramen ovale,* which allows mixing of the oxygenated blood in the right atrium with that leaving the left ventricle bound for the aorta.

At this time, the blood is still oxygenated. Once in the pulmonary artery, the blood enters the *ductus arteriosus,* which connects the pulmonary artery with the aorta. The ductus arteriosus causes blood to bypass the uninflated lungs. Once in the aorta, blood flow is basically the same as in extrauterine life. Deoxygenated blood containing waste products exits the fetus, after passage through the liver, via the umbilical arteries.

The fetal circulation changes immediately at birth. As soon as the baby takes its first breath, the lungs inflate, greatly decreasing pulmonary vascular resistance to blood flow. Also, the ductus arteriosus closes, diverting blood to the lungs. In addition, the ductus venosus closes, stopping blood flow from the placenta. The foramen ovale also closes as a result of pressure changes in the heart, which stops blood flow from the right to left atrium.

GENERAL ASSESSMENT OF THE OBSTETRIC PATIENT

INITIAL ASSESSMENT

The initial approach to the obstetrical patient should be the same as for the non-obstetrical patient, with special attention paid to the developing fetus. Complete initial assessment quickly. Next, obtain essential obstetric information.

HISTORY

The SAMPLE history will allow you to gain specific information about the mother's situation as well as her pertinent medical history.

General Information

Obtain information about the pregnancy. Ask about gravidity, parity, length of gestation, and EDC. Ask about past gynecological or obstetrical complications and prenatal care. Determine current medications and any drug allergies.

You will want to obtain information about the pregnancy, such as the mother's gravidity and parity, the length of gestation, and the estimated date of confinement (EDC), if known. In addition, you should determine whether the patient has had any cesarean sections or any gynecological or obstetrical complications in the past. It is also important to ascertain whether the patient has had any prenatal care. Determine what type of health care professional (physician or nurse midwife) is providing her care and when she was last evaluated. Ask the patient whether a sonogram examination was done. A sonogram reveals the age of the fetus, the presence of more than one fetus, abnormal presentations, and certain birth defects. A general overview of the patient's current state of health is important. Pay particular attention to current medications and drug and/or medication allergies.

Pre-existing or Aggravated Medical Conditions

Pregnancy aggravates many pre-existing medical conditions and may trigger new ones.

Diabetes Previously diagnosed diabetes can become unstable during pregnancy due to altered insulin requirements. Diabetics are at increased risk of developing preeclampsia and hypertension (discussed later in this chapter). Pregnancy may also accelerate the progression of vascular disease complications of diabetes. It is not uncommon for pregnant diabetics to have problems with fluctuating blood sugar levels, causing hypoglycemic or hyperglycemic episodes. Also, many patients develop diabetes during pregnancy (*gestational diabetes*). Pregnant diabetics cannot be managed with oral hypoglycemic agents because these drugs tend to cross the placenta and affect the fetus. Therefore, all pregnant diabetics are placed on insulin, if their blood sugar levels cannot be controlled by diet alone. It has been shown that maintaining careful control of the mother's blood sugar between 70 and 120 mg/dl reduces risks to mother and fetus.

Diabetes also affects the infant. Infants of diabetic mothers, especially those with poorly controlled blood sugar levels, tend to be large. This complicates delivery. Such infants also may have trouble maintaining body temperature after birth and may be subject to hypoglycemia. Babies born to diabetic mothers are also at increased risk of congenital anomalies (birth defects).

Heart Disease During pregnancy, cardiac output increases up to 30 percent. Patients who have serious pre-existing heart disease may develop congestive heart failure in pregnancy. When confronted by a pregnant patient in obvious or suspected heart failure, inquire about pre-existing heart disease or murmurs. It is important to be aware, however, that most patients develop a quiet systolic flow murmur during pregnancy. This is caused by increased cardiac output and is rarely a source of concern.

Hypertension Hypertension is also aggravated by pregnancy. Generally, blood pressure is lower in pregnancy than in the non-pregnant state. However, women who were borderline hypertensive before becoming pregnant may become dangerously hypertensive when pregnant. Also, many common blood pressure medications cannot be used during pregnancy. In addition, preeclampsia (discussed later in this chapter) may contribute to maternal hypertension. Persistent hypertension may adversely affect the placenta, thus compromising the fetus as well as placing the mother at increased risk for stroke, seizure, or renal failure.

Seizure Disorders Most women with a history of seizure disorders controlled by medication have uneventful pregnancies and deliver healthy babies. However, women who have poorly controlled seizure disorders are likely to have increased seizure activity during pregnancy. Medications to control seizures are commonly administered throughout the pregnancy.

Pregnancy can aggravate pre-existing medical conditions such as diabetes, heart disease, hypertension, seizure disorders, and neuromuscular disorders, and may trigger new ones. (However, a remission of neurological disorder symptoms during pregnancy is not unusual.)

Neuromuscular Disorders Disabilities associated with neuromuscular disorders, such as multiple sclerosis, may be aggravated by pregnancy. However, it is more common that pregnant women enjoy remission of symptoms during pregnancy and a slight increase in relapse rate during the postpartum period. The strength of uterine contractions is not diminished in these patients. Also, their subjective sensation of pain is often less than seen in other patients.

Pain

When the patient complains of pain, determine onset, character, and especially the regularity of occurrence.

If the patient is in pain, try to determine when the pain started and whether its onset was sudden or slow. Also, attempt to define the character of the pain—its duration, location, and radiation, if any. It is especially important to determine whether the pain is occurring on a regular basis.

Vaginal Bleeding

If there is vaginal bleeding, determine events prior to its start. Assess the amount by the number of sanitary pads used and save any clots or passed tissue.

The presence of vaginal bleeding or spotting is a major concern in an obstetrical patient. Ask about events immediately prior to the start of bleeding. You also need to gain information about the color, amount, and duration. To assess the amount of bleeding, count the number of sanitary pads used. If your patient is passing clots or tissue, save this material for evaluation. In addition, question the patient about the presence of other vaginal discharges, as well as the color, amount, and duration.

Active Labor

For a patient in labor, determine if she feels the need to push or move her bowels or if her membranes have ruptured (her "water broke")—all signs of possible imminent delivery.

When confronted with a patient in active labor, assess whether the mother feels the need to push or has the urge to move her bowels. Determine whether the patient thinks her membranes have ruptured. Patients often sense this as a dribbling of water or, in some cases, a true gush of water.

Always protect the patient's modesty.

PHYSICAL EXAMINATION

Physical examination of the obstetric patient is essentially the same as for any emergency patient. However, you should be particularly careful to protect the patient's modesty as well as to maintain her dignity and privacy.

When examining a pregnant patient, first estimate the date of the pregnancy by measuring the *fundal height*. The fundal height is the distance from the symphysis pubis to the top of the uterine fundus. Each centimeter of fundal height roughly corresponds to a week of gestation. For example, a woman with a fundal height of 24 centimeters has a gestational age of approximately 24 weeks. If the fundus is just palpable above the symphysis pubis, the pregnancy is about 12–16 weeks gestation. When the uterine fundus reaches the umbilicus, the pregnancy is about 20 weeks. As pregnancy reaches term, the fundus is palpable near the xiphoid process. If fetal movement is felt when the abdomen is palpated, the pregnancy is at least 20 weeks. Fetal heart tones can be heard by stethoscope at approximately 18–20 weeks. The normal fetal heart rate ranges from 140–160 beats per minute.

Generally, vital signs in the pregnant patient should be taken with the patient lying on her left side. As noted earlier, as pregnancy progresses, the uterus increases in size. Ultimately, when the patient is supine, the weight of the uterus compresses the inferior vena cava, severely compromising venous blood return from the lower extremities. Turning the patient to her left side alleviates this problem. Occasionally, it may be helpful to perform orthostatic vital signs. First, obtain the blood pressure and pulse rate after the patient has rested for five minutes in the left lateral recumbent position. Then repeat the vital signs with the patient sitting up or standing. A drop in the blood pressure level of 15 mmHg or more, or an increase in the pulse rate of 20 beats per minute or more, is considered significant and should be reported and documented. When performing this maneuver, it is always important to be alert for syncope. This procedure should *not* be performed if the patient is in obvious shock.

You may need to examine the genitals to evaluate any vaginal discharge, the progression of labor, or the presence of a *prolapsed cord*, an umbilical cord that comes out of the uterus ahead of the fetus. This can be accomplished simply by looking at the perineum. If, during the physical examination, the patient reports that she feels the need to push, or if she feels as though she must move her bowels, examine her for crowning. **Crowning** is the bulging of the fetal head past the opening of the vagina during a contraction. Crowning is an indication of impending delivery. Examine for crowning only during a contraction. *Do not perform an internal vaginal examination in the field.*

> ✱ **crowning** the bulging of the fetal head past the opening of the vagina during a contraction. Crowning is an indication of impending delivery.

GENERAL MANAGEMENT OF THE OBSTETRIC PATIENT

The first consideration for managing emergencies in obstetric patients is to remember that you are in fact caring for two patients, the mother and the fetus. Fetal well-being is dependent on maternal well-being. Also keep in mind that your calm, professional demeanor and caring attitude will go a long way in reducing the emotional stress during any obstetric emergency. Remember to protect your patient's privacy and maintain her modesty.

The physiologic priorities for obstetric emergencies are identical to those for any other emergency situation. Focus your efforts on maintaining the airway, breathing, and circulation. Administer high-flow, high-concentration oxygen as needed based on the patient's condition. Initiate intravenous access by using a large bore catheter in a large vein and consider fluid resuscitation based on your local protocols. If your patient is bleeding or showing signs of shock, establish two IV lines. Cardiac monitoring is also appropriate. Place your patient in a position of comfort, but remember that left lateral recumbent is preferred after the 24th week.

If pain is the primary complaint, administer analgesics such as morphine. However, analgesics should be used with caution since they can alter your ability to assess a deteriorating condition as well as other changes in patient status and may negatively affect the fetus. Nitrous oxide is the preferred analgesic in pregnancy, but narcotics are acceptable.

When transport is indicated, transport immediately to a hospital that is capable of managing emergency obstetric and neonatal care. Report the situation to the receiving hospital prior to your arrival, as emergency department personnel may want to summon obstetrics department staff to assist with patient care.

> *Do not perform an internal vaginal examination in the field.*
>

> *Always remember that you are caring for two patients, the mother and the fetus.*
>

> *Focus on airway, breathing, and circulation. Monitor for shock. As needed, administer oxygen, initiate IV access, consider fluid resuscitation, and monitor the heart. Place the patient in a position of comfort. The left lateral recumbent position is preferred after the 24th week.*

COMPLICATIONS OF PREGNANCY

Pregnancy is a normal process. However, women who are pregnant are not immune from injury or other health problems. There may also be complications associated with the pregnancy itself.

TRAUMA

Paramedics frequently receive calls to help a pregnant woman who has been in a motor vehicle accident or who has sustained a fall. In pregnancy, syncope occurs frequently. The syncope of pregnancy often results from compression of the inferior vena cava, as described earlier, or from normal changes in the cardiovascular system associated with pregnancy. Also, the weight of the gravid uterus alters the patient's balance, making her more susceptible to falls.

Pregnant victims of major trauma are more susceptible to life-threatening injury than are non-pregnant victims because of the increased vascularity of the gravid uterus. Trauma is the most frequent, non-obstetric cause of death in pregnant women. Some form of trauma, usually a motor vehicle crash or a fall but sometimes physical abuse, occurs in 6–7 percent of all pregnancies. Since the primary cause for fetal mortality is maternal mortality, the pregnant trauma patient presents a unique challenge. The later in the pregnancy, the larger the uterus and the greater the likelihood of injury. All patients at 20 weeks (or more) gestation with a history of direct or indirect injury should be transported for evaluation by a physician.

Transport all trauma patients at 20 weeks or more gestation. Anticipate the development of shock.

Paramedics should *anticipate* the development of shock based on the mechanism of injury rather than waiting for overt signs and symptoms. Due to the cardiovascular changes of pregnancy, overt signs of shock are late and inconsistent. Trauma significant enough to cause maternal shock is associated with a 70–80 percent fetal mortality. In the face of acute blood loss, significant vasoconstriction will occur in response to catecholamine release, resulting in maintenance of a normotensive state for the mother. However, this causes significant uterine hypoperfusion (20–30 percent decrease in cardiac output) and fetal bradycardia.

Generally, the amniotic fluid cushions the fetus from blunt trauma fairly well. However, in direct abdominal trauma, the pregnant patient may suffer premature separation of the placenta from the uterine wall, premature labor, abortion, uterine rupture, and possibly fetal death. The presence of vaginal bleeding or a tender abdomen in a pregnant patient should increase your suspicion of serious injury. Fetal death may result from death of the mother, separation of the placenta from the uterine wall, maternal shock, uterine rupture, or fetal head injury. Any pregnant patient who has suffered trauma should be immediately transported to the emergency department and evaluated by a physician. Trauma management essentials include the following:

- Apply a C-collar to provide cervical stabilization and immobilize on a long backboard.
- Administer high-flow, high-concentration oxygen.
- Initiate two large bore IVs for crystalloid administration per protocol.

- Transport tilted to the left to minimize supine hypotension.
- Reassess frequently.
- Monitor the fetus.

MEDICAL CONDITIONS

The pregnant patient is subject to all of the medical problems that occur in the non-pregnant state. Abdominal pain is a common complaint. It is often caused by the stretching of the ligaments that support the uterus. However, appendicitis and cholecystitis can also occur. Pregnant women are at increased risk of developing gallstones as a result of hormonal influences that delay emptying of the gall bladder. In pregnancy, the abdominal organs are displaced because of the increased mass of the gravid uterus in the abdomen, which makes assessment more difficult. The pregnant patient with appendicitis may complain of right upper quadrant pain or even back pain. The symptoms of acute cholecystitis may also differ from those in non-pregnant patients. Any pregnant patient with abdominal pain should be evaluated by a physician.

> *Any pregnant patient with abdominal pain should be evaluated by a physician.*

BLEEDING IN PREGNANCY

Vaginal bleeding may occur at any time during pregnancy. Bleeding is usually due to abortion, ectopic pregnancy, placenta previa, or abruptio placentae. Generally, the exact etiology of vaginal bleeding during pregnancy cannot be determined in the field. Refer to the earlier discussion in this chapter and your own local protocols for management of obstetric emergencies. Vaginal bleeding is associated with potential fetal loss. Keep in mind that this is a very emotionally stressful situation for your patient, so a professional, caring demeanor is imperative.

Abortion

Abortion, the expulsion of the fetus prior to 20 weeks gestation, is the most common cause of bleeding in the first and second trimesters of pregnancy. The terms "abortion" and "miscarriage" can be used interchangeably. Generally, the lay public think of abortion as termination of pregnancy at maternal request and of miscarriage as an accident of nature. Medically, the term abortion applies to both kinds of fetal loss. Spontaneous abortion, the naturally occurring termination of pregnancy that is often called miscarriage, is most commonly seen between the 12th and 14th weeks of gestation. It is estimated that 10 to 20 percent of all pregnancies end in spontaneous abortion. If the pregnancy has not yet been confirmed, the mother often assumes she is merely having a period with unusually heavy flow.

About half of all abortions are due to fetal chromosomal anomalies. Other causes include maternal reproductive system abnormalities, maternal use of drugs, placental defects, or maternal infections. Although many people believe that trauma and psychological stress can cause abortion, research does not support that belief.

* **abortion** termination of pregnancy before the 20th week of gestation. The term "abortion" refers to both miscarriage and induced abortion. Commonly, "abortion" is used for elective termination of pregnancy and "miscarriage" for the loss of a fetus by natural means. A miscarriage is sometimes called a "spontaneous abortion."

Assessment The patient experiencing an abortion is likely to report cramping abdominal pain and a backache. She is also likely to report vaginal bleeding, which is often accompanied by the passage of clots and tissue. If the abortion was not recent, then frank signs and symptoms of infection may be present. In addition to your routine emergency assessments, assess for orthostatic vital sign changes and ascertain the amount of vaginal bleeding.

Management Place the patient who is experiencing an abortion in a position of comfort. Treat for shock with oxygen therapy and IV access for fluid resuscitation. As mentioned earlier, any tissue or large clots should be retained and given to emergency department personnel. If the abortion occurs during the late first trimester or later, a fetus may be passed. Often, the placenta does not detach, and the fetus is suspended by the umbilical cord. In such a case, place the umbilical clamps from the OB kit on the cord and cut it. Carefully wrap the fetus in linen or other suitable material and transport it to the hospital with the mother.

An abortion is generally a very sad occurrence. Provide emotional support to the parents. This can be a devastating psychological experience for the mother, so avoid saying trite but inaccurate phrases meant to provide comfort. Inappropriate remarks include "You can always get pregnant again" or "This is nature's way of dealing with a defective fetus." Parents who wish to view the fetus should be allowed to do so. Occasionally, Roman Catholic parents may request baptism of the fetus. You can perform this by making the sign of a cross and stating, "I baptize you in the name of the father, the son, and the holy spirit. Amen."

Ectopic Pregnancy

As you learned earlier, the fertilized egg normally is implanted in the endometrial lining of the uterine wall. The term *ectopic pregnancy* refers to the abnormal implantation of the fertilized egg outside of the uterus. Approximately 95 percent are implanted in the fallopian tube. Occasionally (< one percent), the egg is implanted in the abdominal cavity. Current research indicates that the incidence of ectopic pregnancy is one for every 44 live births. Improved diagnostic technology is credited with an increased incidence, as most are detected between the 2nd and 12th week. Ectopic pregnancy accounts for approximately 10 percent of maternal mortality.

Predisposing factors in the development of ectopic pregnancy include scarring of the fallopian tubes due to pelvic inflammatory disease (PID), a previous ectopic pregnancy, or previous pelvic or tubal surgery, such as a tubal ligation. Other factors include endometriosis or use of an intrauterine device (IUD) for birth control.

Assessment Ectopic pregnancy most often presents as abdominal pain, which starts out as diffuse tenderness and then localizes as a sharp pain in the lower abdominal quadrant on the affected side. This pain is due to rupture of the fallopian tube when the fetus outgrows the available space. The woman often reports that she missed a period or that her LMP occurred 4 to 6 weeks ago, but with decreased menstrual flow that was brownish in color and of shorter duration than usual. As the intra-abdominal bleeding continues, the abdomen becomes rigid and the pain intensifies and is often referred to the shoulder on the affected side. The pain is often accompanied by syncope, vaginal bleeding, and shock.

Assume that any female of childbearing age with lower abdominal pain is experiencing an ectopic pregnancy.

Total placenta
previa

Partial placenta
previa

FIGURE 40-5   Placenta previa (abnormal implantation).

Management   Ectopic pregnancy poses a significant life threat to the mother. Transport this patient immediately, since surgery is often required to resolve the situation. Interim care measures should include oxygen therapy and IV access for fluid resuscitation. Trendelenburg position or the use of a pneumatic anti-shock garment may be indicated by your local protocols.

> *Ectopic pregnancy is life-threatening. Transport the patient immediately.*
>

Placenta Previa

Placenta previa occurs as a result of abnormal implantation of the placenta on the lower half of the uterine wall, resulting in partial or complete coverage of the cervical opening (Figure 40-5). Vaginal bleeding, which may initially be intermittent, occurs after the 7th month of the pregnancy as the lower uterus begins to contract and dilate in preparation for the onset of labor. This process pulls the placenta away from the uterine wall, causing bright red vaginal bleeding. Placenta previa occurs in about one of every 250 live births. It is classified as complete, partial, or marginal, depending on whether the placenta covers all or part of the cervical opening or is merely in close proximity to the opening.

Although the exact cause of placenta previa is unknown, certain predisposing factors are commonly seen. These factors include a previous history of placenta previa, multiparity, or increased maternal age. Other factors include the presence of uterine scars from cesarean sections, a large placenta, or defective development of blood vessels in the uterine wall.

Assessment   The patient with placenta previa is usually a multigravida in her third trimester of pregnancy. She may have a history of prior placenta previa or of bleeding early in the current pregnancy. She may report a recent episode of sexual intercourse or vaginal examination just before vaginal bleeding began, or she may not bleed until the onset of labor. The onset of painless bright red vaginal bleeding, which may occur as spotting or recurrent hemorrhage, is the hallmark of placenta previa. In fact, any painless bleeding in pregnancy is considered placenta previa until proven otherwise. The bleeding may or may not be associated with uterine contractions. The uterus is usually soft, and the fetus may be in an unusual presentation. *Vaginal examination should never be attempted, as an examining finger can puncture the placenta, causing fatal hemorrhage.*

The presence of placenta previa may already have been diagnosed with an ultrasound during prenatal care, in which case the mother is anticipating the onset of symptoms. The prognosis for the fetus is dependent on the extent of the previa. Obviously, in profuse hemorrhage the fetus is at risk of severe hypoxia

> *Third-trimester bleeding should be attributed to either placenta previa or abruptio placentae until proven otherwise. Placenta previa usually presents with painless bleeding. Abruptio placentae usually presents with sharp pain, with or without bleeding.*
>

> *Never attempt vaginal examination since an examining finger can puncture the placenta and cause fatal hemorrhage.*
>

| Partial separation (concealed hemorrhage) | Partial separation (apparent hemorrhage) | Complete separation (concealed hemorrhage) |

FIGURE 40-6   Abruptio placentae (premature separation).

and the viability of the placenta is compromised. You should perform your assessment and physical exam as discussed earlier in this chapter.

Management   If the placenta previa was previously diagnosed, your patient may already have been managed by placing her on bed rest. Because of the potential for profuse hemorrhage, you should treat for shock. Administer oxygen and initiate intravenous access. Additionally, continue to monitor the maternal vital signs and FHTs. Since the definitive treatment is delivery of the fetus by cesarean section, it is imperative to transport the patient to a hospital with obstetric surgical capability.

Abruptio Placentae

Abruptio placentae, or the premature separation (abruption) of a normally implanted placenta from the uterine wall, poses a potential life threat for both mother and fetus (Figure 40-6). The incidence of abruptio placentae is one in 120 live births. It is associated with 20 to 30 percent fetal mortality, which rises to 100 percent in cases where the majority of the placenta has separated. Maternal mortality is relatively uncommon, although it rises markedly if shock is inadequately treated. Abruptio placentae is classified as marginal (or partial), central (severe), or complete, as explained below.

Although the cause of abruptio placentae is unknown, predisposing factors include multiparity, maternal hypertension, trauma, cocaine use, increasing maternal age, and history of abruption in previous pregnancy.

Assessment   The presenting signs and symptoms of abruptio placentae vary depending on the extent and character of the abruption. Partial abruptions can be marginal or central. Marginal abruptio is characterized by vaginal bleeding but no increase in pain. In central abruptio, the placenta separates centrally and the bleeding is trapped between the placenta and the uterine wall, or "concealed," so there is no vaginal bleeding. However, there is a sudden sharp, tearing pain and development of a stiff, boardlike abdomen. In complete abruptio placentae there is massive vaginal bleeding and profound maternal hypotension. If the patient is in labor at the time of the abruptio, separation of the placenta from the uterine wall will progress rapidly, with fetal distress versus fetal demise dependent on percentage of separation.

Because of the potential for profuse hemorrhage, always treat the patient with suspected placenta previa for shock. Transport immediately since definitive treatment is delivery by cesarean section.

Signs and symptoms of abruptio placentae vary. With a marginal abruption, there will be bleeding but no pain. With a central abruption, there will be sharp, tearing pain and a stiff, boardlike abdomen. Complete abruption will result in massive hemorrhage.

Management Abruptio placentae is a life-threatening obstetrical emergency. Immediate intervention to maintain maternal oxygenation and perfusion is imperative. Immediately place two large bore intravenous lines and begin fluid resuscitation. Position your patient in the left lateral recumbent position. Transport immediately to a hospital with available surgical obstetric and high-risk neonatal care.

Abruptio placentae is a life-threatening emergency. Treat for shock, including fluid resuscitation, and transport immediately in the left lateral recumbent position.

MEDICAL COMPLICATIONS OF PREGNANCY

As discussed earlier, pregnancy can exacerbate pre-existing medical conditions such as diabetes, heart disease, hypertension, and seizure or neuromuscular disorder.

Hypertensive Disorders

The American College of Obstetricians and Gynecologists has identified four classifications of *hypertensive disorders of pregnancy* (formerly called "toxemia of pregnancy"). They include the following:

- *Preeclampsia and eclampsia*

     Pregnancy-induced hypertension (PIH), which includes preeclampsia and eclampsia, occurs in approximately 5 percent of all pregnancies. Preeclampsia is the most common hypertensive disorder seen in pregnancy. There is a higher incidence among primigravidas, particularly if they are teenagers or over the age of 35. Others at increased risk are diabetics, women with a history of preeclampsia, and those who are carrying multiple fetuses.

     Preeclampsia is a progressive disorder that is usually categorized as mild or severe. Seizures (or coma) develop in its most severe form, known as eclampsia. Preeclampsia is defined as an increase in systolic blood pressure by 30 mmHg and/or a diastolic increase of 15 mmHg over baseline on at least two occasions at least six hours apart. Remember that maternal blood pressure normally drops during pregnancy, so a woman may be hypertensive at 120/80 if her baseline in early pregnancy was 90/66. If there is no baseline blood pressure available then a reading ≥ 140/90 is considered to be hypertensive.

     Preeclampsia is most commonly seen in the last ten weeks of gestation, during labor, or in the first 48 hours postpartum. The exact cause of preeclampsia is unknown. It is thought to be caused by abnormal vasospasm, which results in increased maternal blood pressure and other associated symptoms. Additionally, the vasospasm causes decreased placental perfusion, contributing to fetal growth retardation and chronic fetal hypoxia.

     Mild preeclampsia is characterized by hypertension, edema, and protein in the urine. Severe preeclampsia progresses rapidly with maternal blood pressures reaching 160/110 or higher, while the edema becomes generalized and the amount of protein in the urine increases significantly. Other commonly seen signs and symptoms in the severe state include headache, visual disturbances, hyperactive reflexes, and the development of pulmonary edema, along with a dramatic decrease in urine output.

     Patients who are preeclamptic have intravascular volume depletion, since a great deal of their body fluid is in the third space. Those who develop severe preeclampsia and eclampsia are at increased risk for cerebral hemorrhage, pulmonary embolism, abruptio placentae, disseminated intravascular coagulopathy (DIC), and the development of renal failure.

Content Review

MEDICAL COMPLICATIONS OF PREGNANCY

Hypertensive disorders
Supine hypotensive syndrome
Gestational diabetes

Eclampsia, the most serious manifestation of pregnancy-induced hypertension, is characterized by grand mal (major motor) seizure activity. Eclampsia is often preceded by visual disturbances, such as flashing lights or spots before the eyes. Also, the development of epigastric pain or pain in the right upper abdominal quadrant often indicates impending seizure. Eclampsia can often be distinguished from epilepsy by the history and physical appearance of the patient. Patients who become eclamptic are usually grossly edematous and have markedly elevated blood pressure, while epileptics usually have a prior history of seizures and are usually taking anticonvulsant medications. If eclampsia develops, death of the mother and fetus frequently results. The risk of fetal mortality increases by 10 percent with each maternal seizure.

- *Chronic hypertension*

  Hypertension is considered chronic when the blood pressure is ≥ 140/90 before pregnancy or prior to the 20th week of gestation, or if it persists for more than 42 days postpartum. As a general rule, if the diastolic pressure exceeds 80 mmHg during the second trimester, chronic hypertension is likely. The cause of chronic hypertension is unknown. The goal of management is to prevent the development of preeclampsia.

- *Chronic hypertension superimposed with preeclampsia*

  It is not uncommon for the chronic hypertensive who develops preeclampsia to progress rapidly to eclampsia even prior to the 30th week of gestation. The same diagnostic criteria for preeclampsia are used (systolic blood pressure increases > 30 mmHg over baseline, edema, and protein in the urine).

- *Transient hypertension*

  Transient hypertension is defined as a temporary rise in blood pressure which occurs during labor or early in postpartum and which normalizes within ten days.

Assessment Obtaining an accurate history is extremely important whenever you suspect one of the hypertensive disorders of pregnancy. Question the patient about excessive weight gain, headaches, visual problems, epigastric or right upper quadrant abdominal pain, apprehension, or seizures. On physical exam, patients with PIH or preeclampsia are usually markedly edematous. They are often pale and apprehensive. The reflexes are hyperactive. The blood pressure, which is usually elevated, should be taken after the patient has rested for 5 minutes in the left lateral recumbent position.

Management Definitive treatment of the hypertensive disorders of pregnancy is delivery of the fetus. However, in the field, use the following management tactics to prevent dangerously high blood pressures or seizure activity.

- *Hypertension*

  Closely monitor the patient who is pregnant and has elevated blood pressure without edema or other signs of preeclampsia. Record the fetal heart tones and the mother's blood pressure level.

- *Preeclampsia*

  The patient who is hypertensive and shows other signs and symptoms of preeclampsia, such as edema, headaches, and visual disturbances, should be treated quickly. Keep the patient calm and dim the lights. Place the patient in the left lateral recumbent position and quickly carry out the initial assessment. Begin an IV of normal saline.

With suspected hypertensive disorder, it is critical to obtain an accurate history, including information about weight gain, headaches, visual problems, epigastric or right upper quadrant abdominal pain, apprehension, or seizures.

Preeclampsia and eclampsia are life-threatening. Keep the patient calm. Dim the lights. Place patient in left lateral recumbent position and transport quickly without lights or sirens. Administer magnesium sulfate to control seizures if they occur. Medical direction may request administration of antihypertensive or sedative drugs.

Transport the patient rapidly, without lights or sirens. If the blood pressure is dangerously high (diastolic > 110), medical direction may request the administration of hydralazine (Apresoline) or similar antihypertensives that are safe for use in pregnancy. If the transport time is long, the administration of magnesium sulfate may also be ordered.

- *Eclampsia*

    If the patient has already suffered a seizure or a seizure appears to be imminent, then, in addition to the above measures, administer oxygen and manage the airway appropriately. Administer a bolus dose of magnesium sulfate (2 to 5 g diluted in 50 to 100 mL slow IV push) to control the seizures. If you are unable to control the seizures with magnesium sulfate, you may consider diazepam (Valium) or other sedative. It is important to keep calcium gluconate available for use as an antidote to magnesium sulfate. Also monitor your patient closely for signs (vaginal bleeding or abdominal rigidity) of abruptio placentae or developing pulmonary edema. Transport immediately to a hospital with surgical obstetric and neonatal care availability.

Supine-Hypotensive Syndrome

Supine-hypotensive syndrome usually occurs in the third trimester of pregnancy. Also known as vena caval syndrome, supine hypotensive syndrome occurs when the gravid uterus compresses the inferior vena cava when the mother lies in a supine position (Figure 40-7).

Assessment Supine-hypotensive syndrome usually occurs in a patient late in her pregnancy who has been supine for a period of time. The patient may complain of dizziness, which results from the decrease in venous return to the right atrium and

Vena cava   Sacrum

FIGURE 40-7   The supine-hypotensive syndrome results from compression of the inferior vena cava by the gravid uterus.

consequent lowering of the patient's blood pressure. Question the patient about prior episodes of a similar nature and about any recent hemorrhage or fluid loss. Direct the physical examination at determining whether the patient is volume depleted.

Management If there are no indications of volume depletion, such as decreased skin turgor or thirst, place the patient in the left lateral recumbent position or elevate her right hip. Monitor the fetal heart tones and maternal vital signs frequently. If there is clinical evidence of volume depletion, administer oxygen and start an IV of normal saline. Check for orthostatic changes (a decrease in blood pressure and increase in heart rate when rising from the supine position) and place electrodes for cardiac monitoring. Transport the patient promptly in the left lateral recumbent position

Gestational Diabetes

Diabetes mellitus occurs in approximately 4 percent of all pregnancies. Hormonal influences cause an increase in insulin production as well as an increased tissue response to insulin during the first 20 weeks of gestation. However, during the last 20 weeks placental hormones cause an increased resistance to insulin and a decreased glucose tolerance. This causes catabolism (the "breaking down" phase of metabolism) between meals and during the night. At these times, ketones may be present in the urine because fats are metabolized more rapidly. Further, maternal glucose stores are used up, as they are the sole source of glucose to meet the energy needs of the growing fetus. This is known as the *diabetogenic* (diabetes-causing) *effect of pregnancy*. Gestational diabetes usually subsides after pregnancy.

Routine prenatal care includes screening to detect diabetes throughout the pregnancy. Women who are considered to be at high risk for developing gestational diabetes are given a glucose tolerance test at their first prenatal visit. High risk is associated with maternal age (over 35), obesity, hypertension, family history of diabetes, and history of prior stillbirth.

Management of gestational diabetes requires good prenatal care. The mother will be instructed on diabetic management and the importance of balancing diet and exercise as well as how to monitor her glucose levels and administer insulin. Fetal development will be monitored on an ongoing basis throughout the pregnancy.

Assessment When you encounter a pregnant patient with an altered mental status, consider hypoglycemia as a likely cause. Remember that the clinical signs and symptoms of hypoglycemia are many and varied. An abnormal mental status is the most important. Physical signs may include diaphoresis and tachycardia. If the blood sugar falls to a critically low level, she may sustain a hypoglycemic seizure or become comatose, which poses a potential life threat to the mother and fetus. Obtaining an accurate history of associated signs and symptoms, such as nausea, vomiting, abdominal pain, increased urination, or a recent infection, will allow you to ascertain whether diabetic ketoacidosis might be the cause of your patient's altered mental status. Determine the blood glucose level in addition to obtaining baseline vital signs and FHTs.

Management If the blood glucose level is noted to be less that 60 mg/dl, draw a red-top tube of blood and start an IV of normal saline. Next, administer 50–100 ml (25–50 g) of 50 percent dextrose intravenously. If the patient is conscious and able to swallow, complete glucose administration with orange juice, sugared soft drinks, or commercially available glucose pastes.

If the blood glucose level is in excess of 200 mg/dl, draw a red-top tube (or the tube specified by local protocols) of blood and then establish IV access to administer one to two liters of 0.9 percent sodium chloride per protocol. If transport time is lengthy, medical direction may request intravenous or subcutaneous administration of regular insulin.

Treat supine hypotensive syndrome by placing the patient in the left lateral recumbent position or elevating her right hip. Monitor fetal heart tones and maternal vital signs. If volume depletion is evident, initiate an IV of normal saline.

Consider hypoglycemia when encountering a pregnant patient with altered mental status.

If blood glucose is below 60 mg/dl, draw a red-top tube of blood, start an IV of normal saline, and administer 25 grams of 50 percent dextrose. If blood glucose is above 200 mg/dl, draw a red-top tube of blood and administer 1 to 2 liters of normal saline by IV per protocol.

BRAXTON-HICKS CONTRACTIONS

It is occasionally difficult to determine the onset of labor. As early as the 13th week of gestation, the uterus contracts intermittently, thus conditioning itself for the birth process. It is also believed that these contractions enhance placental circulation. These painless, irregular contractions are known as Braxton-Hicks contractions. As the EDC approaches, these contractions become more frequent. Ultimately, the contractions become stronger and more regular, signaling the onset of labor. Labor consists of uterine contractions that cause the dilation and **effacement** (thinning and shortening) of the cervix. The contractions of labor are firm, fairly regular, and quite painful. Prior to the onset of labor Braxton-Hicks contractions, occasionally called *false labor,* increase in intensity and frequency but do not cause cervical changes.

It is virtually impossible to distinguish false labor from true labor in the field. Distinguishing the two requires repeated vaginal examinations, over time, to determine whether the cervix is effacing and dilating. *Remember: Internal vaginal exams should not be performed in the field.* Therefore, all patients with uterine contractions should be transported to the hospital for additional evaluation.

Braxton-Hicks contractions do not require treatment by the paramedic aside from reassurance of the patient and, if necessary, transport for evaluation by a physician.

* effacement the thinning and shortening of the cervix during labor.

PRETERM LABOR

As you have already learned, normal gestation is 40 weeks and, in terms of fetal development, the fetus is not considered to be full term until the 38th week. True labor that begins before the 38th week of gestation is called *preterm labor* and frequently requires medical intervention. A variety of maternal, fetal, or placental factors may cause this potentially life-threatening situation for the mother and fetus.

- Maternal Factors
  - Cardiovascular disease
  - Renal disease
  - Pregnancy-induced hypertension (PIH)
  - Diabetes
  - Abdominal surgery during gestation
  - Uterine and cervical abnormalities
  - Maternal infection
  - Trauma, particularly blows to the abdomen
  - Contributory factors: history of preterm birth, smoking, and cocaine abuse
- Placental Factors
  - Placenta previa
  - Abruptio placentae
- Fetal Factors
  - Multiple gestation
  - Excessive amniotic fluid
  - Fetal infection

In many cases, physicians attempt to stop preterm labor to give the fetus additional time to develop in the uterus. Prematurity is the primary neonatal health problem in the nation and occurs in 7 to 10 percent of all live births. All of the preterm infant's organ systems are immature to some degree, but lung development is of greatest concern. Although technological advances in the care of preterm infants have improved the prognosis dramatically, the consequences of a preterm birth can last a lifetime.

Assessment When confronted by a patient with uterine contractions, first determine the approximate gestational age of the fetus. If it is less than 38 weeks, then suspect preterm labor. If gestational age is greater than 38 weeks, treat the patient as a term patient, as described later in this chapter.

After determining gestational age, obtain a brief obstetrical history. Then question the mother about the urge to push or the need to move her bowels or urinate. Also ask if her membranes have ruptured. Any sensation of fluid leakage or "gushing" from the vagina should be interpreted as ruptured membranes until proven otherwise. Next, palpate the contractions by placing your hand on the patient's abdomen. Note the intensity and length of the contractions, as well as the interval between contractions.

Commonly reported signs and symptoms of preterm labor include contractions that occur every 10 minutes or less, low abdominal cramping that is similar to menstrual cramps, or a sensation of pelvic pressure. Other complaints such as low backache, changes in vaginal discharge, and abdominal cramping with or without diarrhea may also be reported. Rupture of the membranes is confirmatory for preterm labor.

Management Preterm labor, especially if quite early in the pregnancy, should be stopped if possible. The process of stopping labor, or **tocolysis,** is frequently practiced in obstetrics. However, it is infrequently done in the field.

There are three general approaches to tocolysis. The first is to sedate the patient, often with narcotics or barbiturates, thus allowing her to rest. Often, after a period of rest, the contractions stop on their own. The second approach is to administer a fluid bolus intravenously. The administration of approximately 1 liter of fluid intravenously increases the intravascular fluid volume, thus inhibiting ADH secretion from the posterior pituitary. Since oxytocin and ADH are secreted from the same area of the pituitary gland, the inhibition of ADH secretion also inhibits oxytocin release, often causing cessation of uterine contractions. Ultimately, if the above methods fail, a beta agonist, such as terbutaline or ritodrine, or magnesium sulfate may be administered to stop labor by inhibiting uterine smooth muscle contraction. Current research in tocolysis includes the administration of calcium channel blockers, such as nifedipine, and prostaglandin inhibitors, such as indomethacin. You may also find that a patient with preterm labor has been given corticosteroids to accelerate fetal lung maturity.

As a rule, tocolysis in the field is limited to sedation and hydration, especially if transport time is long. Paramedics may, however, transport a patient from one medical facility to another with beta agonist administration underway. You should therefore be familiar with its use. Commonly associated side effects include being jittery, tachycardia usually described by the patient as palpitations, and occasionally abdominal pain. You will, of course, want to transport your patient to the nearest facility that has neonatal intensive care capabilities. Careful and frequent monitoring of maternal vital signs and FHTs is imperative during tocolysis.

THE PUERPERIUM

The **puerperium** is the time period surrounding birth of the fetus. Childbirth generally occurs in a hospital or similar facility with appropriate equipment. Occasionally, prehospital personnel may be called upon to attend a delivery in the field. Therefore, you should be familiar with the birth process and some of the complications that may be associated with it.

The patient with suspected preterm labor should be transported immediately.

* **tocolysis** the process of stopping labor.

* **puerperium** the time period surrounding the birth of the fetus.

LABOR

Childbirth, or the delivery of the fetus, is the culmination of pregnancy. The process by which delivery occurs is called **labor**, the physiologic and mechanical process in which the baby, placenta, and amniotic sac are expelled through the birth canal. The duration of labor is widely variable.

Prior to the onset of true labor, the head of the fetus descends into the bony pelvis area. The frequency and intensity of the Braxton-Hicks contractions increase in preparation for true labor. Increased vaginal secretions and softening of the cervix occur. Bloody show, pink-tinged secretions, is generally considered a sign of imminent labor as the mucous plug is expelled from the cervix. Labor then usually begins within 24 to 48 hours. Many people also consider the rupture of the membranes as a sign of impending labor. If labor does not begin spontaneously within 12 to 24 hours after rupture, labor will likely require induction because of the risk of infection.

Pressure exerted by the fetus on the cervix causes changes that lead to the subsequent expulsion of the fetus. Muscular uterine contractions increase in frequency, strength, and duration. You can assess the frequency and duration of contractions by placing one hand on the fundus of the uterus. Time contractions from the beginning of one contraction until the beginning of the next. It is important to note whether the uterus relaxes completely between contractions. It is also desirable to monitor fetal heart tones during and between contractions. Occasional fetal bradycardia occurs during contractions, but the heart rate should increase to a normal rate (120–160) after the contraction ends. Failure of the heart rate to return to normal between contractions is a sign of fetal distress.

Labor is generally divided into three stages:

- ***Stage One (Dilatation Stage)***

  The first stage of labor begins with the onset of true labor contractions and ends with the complete dilatation and effacement of the cervix. Early in pregnancy the cervix is quite thick and long, but after complete *effacement* it is short and paper-thin. Effacement usually begins several days before active labor ensues. *Dilatation* is the progressive stretching of the cervical opening. The cervix dilates from its closed position to 10 centimeters, which is considered complete dilation. This stage lasts approximately 8 to 10 hours for the woman in her first labor, the nullipara, and about 5 to 7 hours in the woman who has given birth previously, the multipara. Early in this stage the contractions are usually mild, lasting for 15 to 20 seconds with a frequency of 10 to 20 minutes. As labor progresses, the contractions increase in intensity and occur approximately every 2 to 3 minutes with duration of 60 seconds.

- ***Stage Two (Expulsion Stage)***

  The second stage of labor begins with the complete dilatation of the cervix and ends with the delivery of the fetus. In the nullipara, this stage lasts 50 to 60 minutes, while it takes about half that amount of time for the multipara. The contractions are very strong, occurring every 2 minutes and lasting for 60 to 75 seconds. Often, the patient feels pain in her lower back as the fetus descends into the pelvis. The urge to push or "bear down" usually begins in the second stage. The membranes usually rupture at this time, if they have not ruptured previously. Crowning during contractions is evident as the delivery of the fetus nears. Crowning occurs when the head (or other presenting part of the fetus) is visible at the vaginal opening during a

---

✳ **labor** the time and processes that occur during childbirth; the physiologic and mechanical process in which the baby, placenta, and amniotic sac are expelled through the birth canal.

Content Review

STAGES OF LABOR

Stage one: dilatation
Stage two: expulsion
Stage three: placental

---

contraction and is the definitive sign that birth is imminent. The most common presentation is for the infant to be delivered headfirst, face down (vertex position).

- **Stage Three (Placental Stage)**

    The third and final stage of labor begins immediately after the birth of the infant and ends with the delivery of the placenta. The placenta generally delivers within 5 to 20 minutes. There is no need to delay transport to wait for its delivery. Classic signs of placental separation include a gush of blood from the vagina; a change in size, shape or consistency of the uterus; lengthening of the umbilical cord protruding from the vagina; and the mother's report that she has the urge to push.

MANAGEMENT OF A PATIENT IN LABOR

Probably one of the most important decisions you must make with a patient in labor is whether to attempt to deliver the infant at the scene or to transport the patient to the hospital. It is generally preferable to transport the mother unless delivery is imminent. There are several factors to take into consideration when making this decision. They include the patient's number of previous pregnancies, the length of labor during the previous pregnancies, the frequency of contractions, the maternal urge to push, and the presence of crowning. Some women have rapid labors and may be completely dilated in a short period of time. Also, as mentioned above, multiparas generally have shorter labors than nulliparas. The maternal urge to push or the presence of crowning indicates that delivery is imminent. In such cases, the infant should be delivered at the scene or in the ambulance.

Traditionally, a woman who had previously delivered by a cesarean section was advised to deliver all subsequent infants by cesarean sections. However, current thinking encourages women to attempt vaginal birth after cesarean (VBAC). If your patient has had prenatal care during this pregnancy she has probably already discussed this with her health care provider. The only absolute contraindication for VBAC is a classic vertical uterine incision. However, most cesarean sections done today are done using a low transverse uterine incision. (Note that a horizontal skin incision does not assure that the uterine incision is horizontal.) A labor patient who is opting for VBAC requires no more special care than any other labor patient does.

However, certain factors should prompt immediate transport, despite the threat of delivery. These include prolonged rupture of membranes (> 24 hours), since prolonged time between rupture and delivery often leads to fetal infection; abnormal presentation, such as breech or transverse; prolapsed cord; or fetal distress, as evidenced by fetal bradycardia or meconium staining (the presence of meconium, the first fetal stools, in the amniotic fluid). The presence of multiple fetuses may also contribute to your decision to transport. You will read more about these conditions later in this chapter.

FIELD DELIVERY

If delivery is imminent, you can assist the mother to deliver the baby in the field (Procedure 40-1 and Figures 40-8 through 40-16). Equipment and facilities must be quickly prepared. Set up a delivery area. This should be out of public view, such as in a bedroom or the back of the ambulance. Administer oxygen to the mother via nasal cannula or nonrebreather mask. If time permits, establish intravenous access and administer normal saline at a keep-open rate. Place the patient on her back with knees and hips flexed and buttocks slightly elevated.

Transport the patient in labor unless delivery is imminent. Maternal urge to push or the presence of crowning indicates imminent delivery. Delivery at the scene or in the ambulance will be necessary.

Remember: Childbirth is a normal event. Your primary job will be to assist the mother in the delivery of the child.

FIGURE 40-8 Crowning.

FIGURE 40-9 Delivery of the head.

FIGURE 40-10 External rotation of the head.

FIGURE 40-11 As soon as possible, suction the mouth, then the nose.

FIGURE 40-12 Delivery of the anterior shoulder.

FIGURE 40-13 Complete delivery of the infant.

FIGURE 40-14 Dry the infant.

FIGURE 40-15 Place the infant on the mother's stomach.

FIGURE 40-16 Deliver the placenta and save for transport with the mother and infant.

It should be noted that this position is easier on you than the mother. She may prefer to squat or lie in a semi-Fowler's position with her knees and hips flexed. Either of these positions enables gravity to facilitate the delivery. If time permits, drape the mother with toweling from the OB kit. Place one towel under the buttocks, another below the vaginal opening, and another across the lower abdomen.

Until delivery, the fetal heart rate should be monitored frequently. A drop in the fetal heart rate to less than 90 beats per minute indicates fetal distress and should prompt immediate transport with the mother in the left lateral recumbent position. Coach the mother to breathe deeply between contractions and to push with contractions. If the baby does not deliver after 20 minutes of contractions every 2–3 minutes, *transport immediately.*

Prepare the OB equipment and don sterile gloves, gown, and goggles. If time permits, wash your hands and forearms prior to gloving. As the head crowns, control it with gentle pressure. Providing support to the head and perineum decreases the likelihood of vaginal and perineal tearing and decreases the potential for rapid expulsion of the baby's skull through the birth canal which may cause intracranial injury. Support the head as it emerges from the vagina and begins to turn. If it is still enclosed in the amniotic sac, tear the sac open to permit escape of the amniotic fluid and enable the baby to breathe.

Gently slide your finger along the head and neck to ensure that the umbilical cord is not wrapped around the baby's neck. If it is, try to gently slip it over the shoulder and head. If this cannot be done and it is so wrapped tightly as to inhibit labor, carefully place two umbilical cord clamps approximately 2 inches apart and cut the cord between the clamps. As soon as the infant's head is clear of the vagina, instruct the mother to stop pushing. While supporting the head, suction the baby's mouth, then nose, using a bulb syringe. If meconium-stained fluid is noted, suction the mouth, nares, and pharynx with mechanical suction to prevent aspiration. Then tell the mother to resume pushing, while you support the infant's head as it rotates.

Gently guide the baby's head downward to allow delivery of the upper shoulder. Do not pull! Gently guide the baby's body upward to allow delivery of the lower shoulder. Once the head and shoulders have been delivered, the rest of the body will follow rapidly. Be prepared to support the infant's body as it emerges. Remember to keep the baby at the level of the vagina to prevent over- or undertransfusion of blood from the cord. Never "milk" the cord. Clamp and cut the cord as follows (Figure 40-17). Supporting the baby's body, place the first umbilical clamp approximately 10 centimeters from the baby. Place the second clamp

FIGURE 40-17 Clamp and cut the cord.

approximately 5 centimeters above the first. Then carefully cut the umbilical cord between the clamps. Wipe the baby's face clean of blood and mucus and repeat suctioning of the mouth and nose until the airway is clear. Dry the infant thoroughly and then cover with warm, dry blankets or towels, and position on his side. Record the time of birth.

Usual maternal blood loss with delivery is 1 pint (about 500 cc). Following delivery, if the uterus is contracting normally, the fundus should be at the level of the umbilicus and have the size and consistency of a grapefruit. After birth, the mother's vagina should continue to ooze blood. Do not pull on the umbilical cord. Eventually, the cord will appear to lengthen, which indicates separation of the placenta. The placenta should be delivered and transported with the mother to the hospital. If it does deliver, place it in a plastic biohazard bag and bring it to the hospital for evaluation. Retained placenta may cause maternal hemorrhage or become a source of infection. However, there is no need to delay transport for delivery of the placenta. At this time, massage the uterine fundus by placing one hand immediately above the symphysis pubis and the other on the uterine fundus. Cup the uterus between the two hands and support it. Massage until the uterus assumes a woody hardness. Avoid overmassage. Putting the baby to the mother's breast also stimulates uterine contractions, which will further decrease bleeding.

Following delivery, inspect the mother's perineum for tears. If any tears are present, apply direct pressure. Continuously monitor vital signs. Note the presence of continued hemorrhage and report it to medical direction. In some systems, paramedics may administer oxytocin (Pitocin) to facilitate uterine contraction in the control of postpartum hemorrhage. Oxytocin should only be administered *after* delivery of the placenta has been confirmed. Following stabilization, transport the mother and infant to the hospital.

NEONATAL CARE

✳ **neonate** newborn infant

Care of the **neonate** will be discussed in detail in Chapter 41. Initial care of the neonate has been described in the preceding section. Several additional important considerations regarding routine care of the neonate, APGAR scoring, and neonatal resuscitation are briefly discussed in the following sections.

Routine Care of the Neonate

Support the infant's head and torso, using both hands. Maintain warmth, repeat suctioning of the mouth and nose as needed, and assess using APGAR scoring.

Newborns are slippery and will require both hands to support the head and torso. Position yourself so that you can work close to the surface where you have placed the infant.

Maintain warmth! Cold infants rapidly become distressed infants. Quickly dry the infant with towels, discarding each as it becomes wet. Then cover the infant with a dry receiving blanket or use a commercial warming blanket made of a material such as Thinsulate™.

Repeat suctioning of the mouth and nose as needed until the infant's airway is clear. Generally, suctioning and drying the baby will stimulate respirations, crying, and activity. This should cause the infant to "pink up." (Do not be alarmed if the extremities remain dusky. This is known as *acrocyanosis* and is very common in the first hours of life.) If this is not effective, you may try flicking your finger against the soles of the feet or rubbing gently in a circular motion in the middle of the back (Figure 40-18).

Assess the neonate as soon as possible after birth. The normal neonatal respiratory rate should average 30–60 breaths per minute while the heart rate should be between 100–180 beats per minute. If resuscitation is not indicated, assign APGAR scores. Do not however, delay resuscitative efforts and transport in order to complete APGAR scoring.

FIGURE 40-18 Stimulate the infant as required.

APGAR Scoring

Named for Dr. Virginia Apgar, who developed the assessment tool, the APGAR scoring system is a means of evaluating the status of a newborn's vital functions at 1 minute and 5 minutes after delivery. There are five parameters and each is given a score from a low value of 0 to a normal value of 2. APGAR is an acronym for the names of the five parameters, which are *a*ppearance (skin color), *p*ulse rate, *g*rimace (irritability), *a*ctivity (muscle tone), and *r*espiratory effort (Table 40-2).

The majority of infants are healthy and active and have total scores between 7–10, requiring only routine care. Infants scoring between 4–6 are moderately depressed and require oxygen and stimulation to breathe. Infants scoring 0–3 are severely depressed and require immediate ventilatory and circulatory assistance. By repeating the score at 1 and 5 minutes, it is possible to determine whether intervention has caused a change in infant status.

Neonatal Resuscitation

It is estimated that approximately 6 percent of all neonates born in a hospital require resuscitation. It is likely that this percentage is higher for out-of-hospital deliveries, although the exact numbers are not available. Factors that contribute to the need for resuscitation include prematurity, pregnancy and delivery complications, maternal health problems, or inadequate prenatal care.

If tactile stimulation does not increase the neonate's respiratory rate, immediately assist ventilations using a pediatric bag-valve-mask device attached to high-flow oxygen. Reassess after 15 to 30 seconds. If the respiratory rate is now within normal limits, assess the heart rate. If not, continue ventilations.

If the infant's respirations are below 30 per minute and tactile stimulation does not increase the rate to a normal range, immediately assist ventilations using a pediatric bag-valve-mask with high-flow oxygen. If the heart rate is below 80 and does not respond to ventilations, initiate chest compressions. Transport to a facility with neonatal intensive care capabilities.

Table 40-2	THE APGAR SCORE				
Element	**0**	**1**	**2**	**Score**	
Appearance (skin color)	Body and extremities blue, pale	Body pink, extremities blue	Completely pink		
Pulse rate	Absent	Below 100/min	100/min or above		
Grimace (Irritability)	No response	Grimace	Cough, sneeze, cry		
Activity (Muscle tone)	Limp	Some flexion of extremities	Active motion		
Respiratory effort	Absent	Slow and irregular	Strong cry		
			TOTAL SCORE =		

Assess the heart rate using a stethoscope to auscultate the apical pulse, by feeling the pulse at the base of the umbilical cord, or by palpating the brachial or femoral artery. The heart rate should normally be between 100 and 180 beats per minute with a range of 140 to 160 beats per minute being optimal. If the pulse is 100 or greater with spontaneous respirations, continue assessment. If less than 100, continue positive pressure ventilations. If less than 80 and not responding to ventilations, initiate chest compressions. Continue to reassess respiratory status and heart rate frequently.

Make every effort to expedite transport to a facility capable of providing neonatal intensive care while you continue resuscitative efforts. If you have a long transport time, it may be necessary to initiate vascular access in order to administer medications or fluid resuscitation. The most logical (and easiest) access is the umbilical vein. If this is not feasible, consider peripheral veins or an intraosseous access. While many medications (epinephrine, atropine, lidocaine, and naloxone) can be administered via the endotracheal route, this route is not suitable for fluid resuscitation. During transport, continue to maintain warmth while supporting ventilations, oxygenation, and circulation. Refer to Chapter 41 for more information on neonatal resuscitation.

ABNORMAL DELIVERY SITUATIONS

Breech Presentation

Content Review

ABNORMAL DELIVERIES
Breech presentation
Prolapsed cord
Limb presentation
Occiput posterior

Most infants present head first and face down, which is called the vertex position. Breech presentation is the term used to describe the situation in which either the buttocks or both feet present first. This occurs in approximately 4 percent of all live births. In such presentations, there is an increased risk for delivery trauma to the mother, as well as an increased potential for cord prolapse, cord compression, or anoxic insult for the infant. Although the cause is unknown, breech presentations are most commonly associated with preterm birth, placenta previa, multiple gestation, and uterine and fetal anomalies.

Management Because cesarean section is often required, delivery of the breech presentation is best accomplished at the hospital. However, if field delivery is unavoidable, the following maneuvers are recommended. First, position the mother with her buttocks at the edge of a firm bed. Ask her to hold her legs in a flexed position. She will often require assistance in doing this. As the infant delivers, do not pull on the infant's legs. Simply support them. Allow the entire body to be delivered with contractions while you merely continue to support the infant's body (Figure 40-19).

As the head passes the pubis, apply gentle upward traction until the mouth appears over the perineum. If the head does not deliver, and the baby begins to breathe spontaneously with its face pressed against the vaginal wall, place a gloved hand in the vagina with the palm toward the infant's face. Form a "V" with the index and middle fingers on either side of the infant's nose, and push the vaginal wall away from the infant's face to allow unrestricted respiration (Figure 40-20). If necessary, continue during transport.

Alternatively, you may find that the shoulders, not the head, are the most difficult part to deliver. In that case, allow the body to deliver to the level of the umbilicus. Support the infant's body in your palm while gently extracting approximately 4 to 6 inches of umbilical cord. Be very careful that you do not compress the cord during this extraction. Gently rotate the infant's body so that the shoulders are now in an anterior-posterior position. Apply gentle traction to the body until the axilla become visible. Guide the infant's body upward to deliver the posterior shoulder. Then, guide the neonate downward to facilitate delivery of the anterior shoulder. Now gently ease the head through the birth canal. Continue your care of the mother and infant as you would with a normal delivery.

FIGURE 40-19 Breech delivery.

If the infant starts to breathe with its face pressed against the vaginal wall, form a "V" with the index and middle fingers on either side of the infant's nose and push the vaginal wall away from the infant's face. If necessary, continue during transport.

FIGURE 40-20 Placement of the fingers to maintain the airway in a breech birth.

- Elevate hips, administer oxygen and keep warm
- Keep baby's head away from cord
- Do not attempt to push cord back
- Wrap cord in sterile moist towel
- Transport mother to hospital, continuing pressure on baby's head

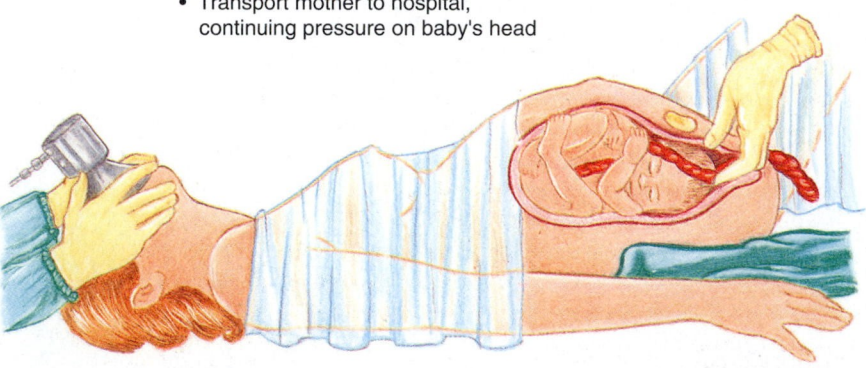

Figure 40-21 Prolapsed cord.

Prolapsed Cord

A *prolapsed cord* occurs when the umbilical cord precedes the fetal presenting part. This causes the cord to be compressed between the fetus and the bony pelvis, shutting off fetal circulation (Figure 40-21). This occurs once in every 250 deliveries. Predisposing factors include prematurity, multiple births, and premature rupture of the membranes before the head is fully engaged. It is a serious emergency, and fetal death will occur quickly without prompt intervention.

Management If the umbilical cord is seen in the vagina, insert two fingers of a gloved hand to raise the presenting part of the fetus off the cord. At the same time, gently check the cord for pulsations, but take great care to insure that you do not compress the cord. Place the mother in a Trendelenburg or knee-chest

If the umbilical cord is seen in the vagina, insert two gloved fingers to raise the fetus off the cord. Place the mother in Trendelenburg or knee-chest position, administer oxygen, and transport immediately. Do not attempt delivery.

FIGURE 40-22 Patient positioning for prolapsed cord.

position (Figure 40-22). Administer high-flow oxygen to the mother and transport her immediately, with the fingers continuing to hold the presenting part off the umbilical cord. If assistance is available, apply a dressing moistened with sterile saline to the exposed cord. *Do not attempt delivery! Do not pull on the cord! Do not attempt to push the cord back into the vagina!*

Limb Presentation

Sometimes, if the baby is in a transverse lie across the uterus, an arm or leg is the presenting part protruding from the vagina. This is seen in less than one percent of births and is more commonly associated with preterm birth and multiple gestation.

Management When examination of the perineum reveals a single arm or leg protruding from the birth canal, a cesarean section is necessary. Under no circumstance should you attempt a field delivery. Do not touch the extremity, as to do so may stimulate the infant to gasp, risking inhalation and aspiration of amniotic fluid. *Do not pull on the extremity or attempt to push it back into vagina!*

Assist the mother into a knee-chest position as is also done when there is a prolapsed cord and administer oxygen via nonrebreather mask. Provide reassurance to the mother. Transport immediately (still in knee-chest position) for emergency cesarean section.

With limb presentation, place the mother in knee-chest position, administer oxygen, and transport immediately. Do not attempt delivery.

Other Abnormal Presentations

Other abnormal presentations can complicate delivery. One of the most common is the *occiput posterior position*. Normally, as the infant descends into the pelvis, its face is turned posteriorly. This is important, as extension of the head assists delivery. However, if the infant descends facing forward, or occiput posterior, its passage through the pelvis is delayed. This presentation occurs most frequently in primigravidas. In multigravidas it usually resolves spontaneously.

The presenting part may also be the face or brow, rather than the crown of the head. Occasionally, during these presentations, the face or brow can be seen high in the pelvis during a contraction. Usually, vaginal delivery is impossible in these cases.

As described earlier for a limb presentation, the fetus can lie transversely in the uterus. In such a case, the fetus cannot enter the pelvis for delivery. If the membranes rupture, the umbilical cord can prolapse, or an arm or leg can enter the vagina. Vaginal delivery is impossible.

Management Early recognition of an abnormal presentation is important. If one is suspected, the mother should be reassured, placed on oxygen, and transported immediately, since forceps or cesarean delivery is often required.

OTHER DELIVERY COMPLICATIONS

Although most deliveries proceed without incident, complications can arise. Therefore, you should be prepared to deal with them.

Multiple Births

Multiple births are fairly rare, with twins occurring approximately once in every 90 deliveries, about 40 percent of those being preterm. Usually, the mother knows or at least suspects the presence of more than one fetus. Multiple births should also be suspected if the mother's abdomen remains large after delivery of one baby and labor continues.

Management Manage this situation with the normal delivery guidelines, recognizing that you will need additional personnel and equipment to manage a multiple birth. In twin births, labor often begins earlier than expected, and the infants are generally smaller than babies born singly. Usually, one twin presents vertex and the other breech. There may be one shared placenta or two placentas. After delivery of the first baby, clamp and cut the cord. Then deliver the second baby. Because prematurity is common in multiple births, low birth weight is common and prevention of hypothermia is even more crucial.

Cephalopelvic Disproportion

Cephalopelvic disproportion occurs when the infant's head is too big to pass through the maternal pelvis easily. This may be caused by an oversized fetus. Large fetuses are associated with diabetes, multiparity, or post-maturity. Fetal abnormalities such as hydrocephalus, conjoined twins, or fetal tumors may make vaginal delivery impossible. Women of short stature or women with contracted pelvises are at increased risk for this problem. If cephalopelvic disproportion is not recognized and managed appropriately, fetal demise or uterine rupture may occur.

Cephalopelvic disproportion tends to develop most frequently in the primigravida. There may be strong contractions for an extended period of time. On physical examination, the fetus may feel large. Also, labor generally does not progress. The fetus may be in distress, as evidenced by fetal bradycardia or meconium staining.

Management The usual management of cephalopelvic disproportion is cesarean section. Administer oxygen to the mother and establish intravenous access. Transport should be immediate and rapid.

Precipitous Delivery

A *precipitous delivery* is a delivery that occurs after less than 3 hours of labor. This type of delivery occurs most frequently in the grand multipara and is associated with a higher-than-normal incidence of fetal trauma, tearing of the umbilical cord, or maternal lacerations.

Management The best way to handle precipitous delivery is to be prepared. Do not turn your attention from the mother. Be ready for a rapid delivery, and attempt to control the infant's head. Once delivered, the baby may have some difficulty with temperature regulation and must be kept warm.

Shoulder Dystocia

A *shoulder dystocia* occurs when the infant's shoulders are larger than its head. This occurs most frequently with diabetic and obese mothers and in post-term pregnancies. In shoulder dystocia, labor progresses normally and the head is delivered routinely. However, immediately after the head is delivered, it retracts back into the perineum because the shoulders are trapped between the symphysis pubis and the sacrum ("turtle sign").

Management If a shoulder dystocia occurs, *do not pull on the infant's head*. Administer oxygen to the mother and have her drop her buttocks off the end of the bed. Then flex her thighs upward to facilitate delivery and apply firm pressure with an open hand immediately above the symphysis pubis. If delivery does not occur, transport the patient immediately.

Meconium Staining

Meconium staining occurs when the fetus passes feces into the amniotic fluid. Between 10 and 30 percent of all deliveries have meconium-stained fluid. It is always indicative of a fetal hypoxic incident. Hypoxia causes an increase in fetal peristalsis along with relaxation of the anal sphincter, causing meconium to pass into the amniotic fluid. In addition to the stress that caused the incident, there is a risk of aspiration of the meconium-stained fluid.

Meconium staining is often associated with prolonged labor but may be seen in term, post-term, and low birth weight infants. The incident may occur a few days prior to delivery or during labor. Some meconium staining is virtually always associated with breech deliveries. This is due to vagal stimulation, which occurs as a result of the pressure of the contracting uterus on the fetus's head.

Evidence of meconium staining is readily observable. Normally the amniotic fluid is clear or possibly light straw-colored. When meconium is present, the color varies from a light yellowish-green to light green or worst case, dark green, which is sometimes described as "pea soup." As a rule, the thicker and darker the color, the higher the risk of fetal morbidity.

Management As noted earlier, once the head of the newborn is out of the birth canal you should suction the mouth and nose on the perineum. If the meconium is thin and light colored no further treatment is required, and you should continue with the delivery and routine care. However, if the meconium is thick, visualize the glottis and suction the hypopharynx and trachea using an endotracheal tube until you have cleared all of the meconium from the newborn's airway. Failure to do so will cause the meconium to be pushed farther into the airway and down into the lungs during the delivery process.

If meconium is thick, visualize the infant's glottis and suction the hypopharynx and trachea using an endotracheal tube until all meconium has been cleared from the airway.

MATERNAL COMPLICATIONS OF LABOR AND DELIVERY

Several maternal problems can arise during and after delivery. These include postpartum hemorrhage, uterine rupture, uterine inversion, and pulmonary embolism.

Postpartum Hemorrhage

Postpartum hemorrhage is the loss of more than 500 cc of blood immediately following delivery. It occurs in approximately 5 percent of deliveries. The most common

---

Content Review

MATERNAL COMPLICATIONS
Postpartum hemorrhage
Uterine rupture
Uterine inversion
Pulmonary embolism

cause of postpartum hemorrhage is *uterine atony,* or lack of uterine muscle tone. This tends to occur most frequently in the multigravida and is most common following multiple births or births of large infants. Uterine atony also occurs after precipitous deliveries and prolonged labors. In addition to uterine atony, postpartum hemorrhage can be caused by placenta previa, abruptio placentae, retained placental parts, clotting disorders in the mother, or vaginal and cervical tears. Occasionally, the uterus fails to return to its normal size during the postpartum period, and postpartum hemorrhage occurs long after the birth, potentially as much as two weeks postpartum.

Assessment of the patient with postpartum hemorrhage should focus on the history and the predisposing factors described above. You must rely heavily on the clinical appearance of the patient and her vital signs. Often, the uterus will feel boggy and soft on physical examination. Vaginal bleeding is usually obvious as a steady, free flow of blood. Counting the number of sanitary pads used is a good way to monitor the bleeding. When postpartum bleeding takes place in the hospital setting the pads are often weighed, since 500 cc of blood weighs approximately one pound. You should also examine the perineum for evidence of traumatic injury, which may be the source of the bleeding.

When there is a loss of more than 500 cc of blood immediately following delivery, administer oxygen and begin fundal massage. Establish two large-bore IVs of normal saline. Treat for shock as necessary. Follow local protocols regarding application of anti-shock trousers.

Management When confronted by a patient with postpartum hemorrhage, complete the initial assessment immediately. Administer oxygen and begin fundal massage. Establish at least one, preferably two, large-bore IVs of normal saline. If shock is evident, apply anti-shock trousers according to your local protocols. Never attempt to force delivery of the placenta or pack the vagina with dressings. In severe cases, medical direction may request the administration of oxytocin (Pitocin). The usual dose is 10 to 20 USP units (20 mg) oxytocin in one liter of normal saline to run at 125 cc/hr titrated to response. If IV access cannot be obtained, an alternative therapy is to administer 10 USP units intramuscularly.

Uterine Rupture

Uterine rupture is the actual tearing, or rupture, of the uterus. It usually occurs with the onset of labor. However, it can also occur before labor as a result of blunt abdominal trauma. During labor, it often results from prolonged uterine contractions or a surgically scarred uterus, such as occurs from previous cesarean sections, especially in those with the classic vertical incision. It can also occur following a prolonged or obstructed labor, as in the case of cephalopelvic disproportion or in conjunction with abnormal presentations. Although it is a rare occurrence, it carries with it an extremely high maternal and fetal mortality rate.

The patient with uterine rupture will complain of excruciating abdominal pain and will often be in shock. Uterine rupture is virtually always associated with the cessation of labor contractions. If the rupture is complete, the pain usually subsides. On physical examination, there is often profound shock without evidence of external hemorrhage, although it is sometimes associated with vaginal bleeding. Fetal heart tones are absent. The abdomen is often tender and rigid and may exhibit rebound tenderness. It is often possible to palpate the uterus as a separate hard mass found next to the fetus.

Management Management is the same as for any patient in shock. Administer oxygen at high concentration. Next, establish two large-bore IVs with normal saline and begin fluid resuscitation. Monitor vital signs and fetal heart tones continuously. Transport the patient rapidly. If the fetus is still viable, the definitive treatment is cesarean section with subsequent repair or removal of the uterus.

Uterine Inversion

Uterine inversion is a rare emergency occurring only once in every 2,500 live births. It occurs when the uterus turns inside out after delivery and extends through the cervix. When uterine inversion occurs, the supporting ligaments and blood vessels supplying blood to the uterus are torn, usually causing profound shock. The average blood loss associated with uterine inversion ranges from 800 to 1,800 cc. Uterine inversion usually results from pulling on the umbilical cord while awaiting delivery of the placenta or from attempts to express the placenta when the uterus is relaxed.

Management If uterine inversion occurs, you must act quickly. First, place the patient in a supine position and begin oxygen administration. *Do not* attempt to detach the placenta or pull on the cord. Initiate two large bore IVs of normal saline and begin fluid resuscitation. Make one attempt to replace the uterus, using the following technique. With the palm of the hand, push the fundus of the inverted uterus toward the vagina. If this single attempt is unsuccessful, cover the uterus with towels moistened with saline and transport the patient immediately.

In the rare occurrence of uterine inversion, begin fluid resuscitation, then make one attempt to replace the uterus. If this fails, cover the uterus with towels moistened with saline and transport immediately.

Pulmonary Embolism

Pulmonary embolism is the presence of a blood clot in the pulmonary vascular system (see Chapter 27). It can occur after pregnancy, usually as a result of venous thromboembolism. It is one of the most common causes of maternal death and appears to occur more frequently following cesarean section than vaginal delivery. Pulmonary embolism may occur at any time during pregnancy. There is usually a sudden onset of severe dyspnea accompanied by sharp chest pain. Some patients also report a sense of impending doom. On physical examination, the patient may show tachycardia, tachypnea, jugular vein distention, and, in severe cases, hypotension.

Management Management of pulmonary embolism consists of administration of high-flow oxygen and ventilatory support as needed. Also establish an IV of normal saline at a keep-open rate. Initiate cardiac monitoring and carefully monitor the patient's vital signs and oxygen saturation while transporting her immediately.

Pulmonary embolism usually presents with sudden severe dyspnea and sharp chest pain. Administer high-flow oxygen and support ventilations as needed. Establish an IV of normal saline. Transport immediately, monitoring the heart, vital signs, and oxygen saturation.

⨍UMMARY

Childbirth is a normal process and obstetrical emergencies are fairly uncommon. However, all pregnant patients are at risk for developing complications, and it is impossible to predict which ones will actually occur. It is therefore important to recognize these complications and act accordingly. Keep in mind that you are caring for two patients, and as long as you remember the priorities of patient care, the situation should go smoothly. Relax and enjoy the opportunity to help bring a new life into the world.

DIVISION 5

SPECIAL CONSIDERATIONS/ OPERATIONS

CHAPTER 41

Neonatology

Objectives

After reading this chapter, you should be able to:

1. Define newborn and neonate. (p. 1681)
2. Identify important antepartum factors that can affect childbirth. (p. 1682)
3. Identify important intrapartum factors that can determine high-risk newborn patients. (p. 1682)
4. Identify the factors that lead to premature birth and low-birth-weight newborns. (pp. 1700, 1704–1705)
5. Distinguish between primary and secondary apnea. (p. 1683)
6. Discuss pulmonary perfusion and asphyxia. (p. 1683)
7. Identify the primary signs utilized for evaluating a newborn during resuscitation. (p. 1685)
8. Identify the appropriate use of the APGAR scale. (pp. 1685–1686)
9. Calculate the APGAR score given various newborn situations. (pp. 7–8; see also Chapter 40)
10. Formulate an appropriate treatment plan for providing initial care to a newborn. (p. 1686)

Continued

INTRODUCTION

Babies pass through stages of physical and emotional development. This chapter concerns itself with babies one month old and under. Babies less than one month old are called **neonates**. Recently born neonates—those in the first few hours of their lives—may also be called **newborns** or *newly born infants* (Figure 41-1).

After an unscheduled delivery in the field, you have two patients to manage—the mother and the baby. You can review information on care of the mother in Chapter 40. The present chapter describes the initial care of newborns, focusing on the special needs of distressed and premature newborns.

＊ **neonate** an infant from the time of birth to one month of age.

＊ **newborn** a baby in the first few hours of its life; also called a *newly born infant.*

After an unscheduled delivery in the field, you have two patients to manage—the mother and the baby.

FIGURE 41-1 Term newborn.

GENERAL PATHOPHYSIOLOGY, ASSESSMENT, AND MANAGEMENT

The care of newborns follows the same priorities as for all patients. You should complete the initial assessment first. Correct any problems detected during the initial assessment before proceeding to the next step. The vast majority of newborns require no resuscitation beyond suctioning the airway, mild stimulation, and maintenance of body temperature. However, for newborns that require additional care, your quick actions can make the difference between life and death.

* **antepartum** before the onset of labor.

* **intrapartum** occurring during childbirth.

EPIDEMIOLOGY

Approximately 6 percent of field deliveries require life support. The incidence of complications increases as the birth weight decreases. About 80 percent of newborns weighing less than 1,500 grams (3 pounds, 5 ounces) at birth require resuscitation. Determine at-risk newborns by considering the **antepartum** and **intrapartum** factors that may indicate complications at the time of delivery (Table 41-1).

Your success in resuscitating these at-risk infants increases with training, ongoing practice, and proper stocking of equipment on board the ambulance. Make sure your ambulance carries a basic OB kit and resuscitation equipment for newborns of various sizes. (See the list under "Resuscitation," later in this chapter.)

Table 41-1	RISK FACTORS INDICATING POSSIBLE COMPLICATIONS IN NEWBORNS	
Antepartum Factors		**Intrapartum Factors**
Multiple gestation		Premature labor
Inadequate prenatal care		Meconium-stained amniotic fluid
Mother's age (<16 or >35)		Rupture of membranes more than 24 hours prior to delivery
History of perinatal morbidity or mortality		Use of narcotics within four hours of delivery
Post-term gestation		Abnormal presentation
Drugs/medications		Prolonged labor or precipitous delivery
Toxemia, hypertension, diabetes		Prolapsed cord or bleeding

Plan transport in advance. Know the type of facilities available in your locality and local protocols governing use of these facilities. A nearby neonatal intensive care unit (NICU) makes the best choice for at-risk newborns. However, if you must transport to a distant NICU, determine whether it might be in the best interests of the infant to transport him or her to the nearest facility for stabilization. Follow local protocols and consult medical direction as needed.

PATHOPHYSIOLOGY

Upon birth, dramatic changes occur within the newborn to prepare it for **extrauterine** life. The respiratory system, which is essentially nonfunctional when the fetus is in the uterus, must suddenly initiate and maintain respirations. While in the uterus, fetal lung fluid fills the fetal lungs. The capillaries and arterioles of the lungs are closed. Most blood pumped by the heart bypasses the nonfunctional respiratory system by flowing through the **ductus arteriosus.**

Approximately one-third of fetal lung fluid is removed through compression of the chest during vaginal delivery. Under normal conditions, the newborn takes its first breath within the first few seconds after delivery. The timing of the first breath is unrelated to the cutting of the umbilical cord. Factors that stimulate the baby's first breath include:

- Mild acidosis
- Initiation of stretch reflexes in the lungs
- Hypoxia
- Hypothermia

With the first breaths, the lungs rapidly fill with air, which displaces the remaining fetal fluid. The pulmonary arterioles and capillaries open, decreasing pulmonary vascular resistance. At this point, the resistance to blood flow in the lungs is now less than the resistance of the ductus arteriosus. Because of this pressure difference, blood flow is diverted from the ductus arteriosus to the lungs, where it picks up oxygen for transport to the peripheral tissues (Figure 41-2).

Soon, there is no need for the ductus arteriosus, and it eventually closes. However, if hypoxia or severe acidosis occurs, the pulmonary vascular bed may constrict again and the ductus may reopen. This will retrigger fetal circulation with its attendant shunting and ongoing hypoxia. (This condition is called **persistent fetal circulation.**) To help the newborn make its transition to extrauterine life, it is very important for the paramedic to facilitate its first few breaths and to prevent ongoing hypoxia and acidosis.

Remain alert at all times to signs of respiratory distress. Infants are susceptible to hypoxemia, which can lead to permanent brain damage. After initial hypoxia, the infant rapidly gasps for breath. If the asphyxia continues, respiratory movements cease altogether, the heart rate begins to fall, and neuromuscular tone gradually diminishes. The infant then enters a period of apnea known as *primary apnea.* In most cases, simple stimulation and exposure to oxygen will reverse bradycardia and assist in the development of pulmonary perfusion.

With ongoing asphyxia, however, the infant will enter a period known as *secondary apnea.* During secondary apnea, the infant takes several last deep gasping respirations. The heart rate, blood pressure, and oxygen saturation in the blood continue to fall. The infant becomes unresponsive to stimulation and will not spontaneously resume respiration on its own. Death will occur unless you promptly initiate resuscitation. For this reason, always assume that apnea in the newborn is secondary apnea and rapidly treat it with ventilatory assistance with oxygen and, when appropriate, chest compressions.

* extrauterine outside the uterus.

Upon birth, dramatic changes take place within the newborn to prepare it for extrauterine life.

* ductus arteriosus channel between the main pulmonary artery and the aorta of the fetus.

The time of a newborn's first breath is unrelated to the cutting of the umbilical cord.

* persistent fetal circulation condition in which blood continues to bypass the fetal respiratory system, resulting in ongoing hypoxia.

Always assume that apnea in the newborn is secondary apnea and rapidly treat it with ventilatory assistance.

FIGURE 41-2 Hemodynamic changes in the newborn at birth.

Air

Fetal lung fluid

Air

1st   2nd   3rd
Breaths

Following birth, the lungs expand as they are filled with air. The fetal lung fluid gradually leaves the alveoli.

Arterioles dilate and blood flow increases

O_2
O_2
O_2 O_2
O_2
Blood

At the same time as the lungs are expanding and the fetal lung fluid is clearing, the arterioles in the lung begin to open, allowing a considerable increase in the amount of blood flowing through the lungs.

Pulmonary blood flow increases

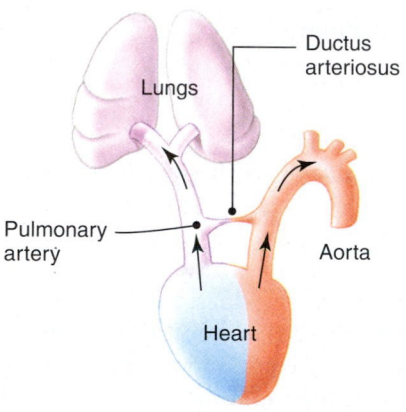

Ductus arteriosus

Lungs

Pulmonary artery

Aorta

Heart

Blood previously diverted through the ductus arteriosus flows through the lungs where it picks up oxygen to transport to tissues throughout the body. Soon there is no need for the ductus and it eventually closes.

Congenital Anomalies

Approximately 2 percent of infants are born with some sort of congenital problem. Congenital problems typically arise from a problem in fetal development. Most fetal development occurs during the first trimester of pregnancy. It is during this time that the developing fetus is most sensitive to environmental factors and substances that can affect normal development.

There are many types of congenital anomalies. These may affect a single organ or structure or may affect many organs or structures. There are several recognized patterns, called *syndromes*, that can occur. It is not within the scope of this text to discuss all the various congenital anomalies. However, there are a few congenital anomalies that can make resuscitation more difficult. For example, some children may be born with a defect in the diaphragm that allows some of the abdominal contents to enter the chest. This abnormality is referred to as a **diaphragmatic hernia.** If you suspect a diaphragmatic hernia, do not treat the infant with bag-valve-mask ventilation. This procedure will distend the stomach, which protrudes into the chest cavity, thus decreasing ventilatory capacity. Instead, immediately intubate the infant. (Diaphragmatic hernia will be discussed in more detail later in this chapter.)

Newborns may have congenital anomalies that make resuscitation more difficult.

✱ **diaphragmatic hernia** protrusion of abdominal contents into the thoracic cavity through an opening in the diaphragm.

Some infants are born with a defect in their spinal cords. In some cases, the spinal cord and associated structures may be exposed. This abnormality is called a **meningomyelocele.** Infants born with a meningomyelocele should not be placed on their backs. Instead, place them on their stomachs or sides and conduct resuscitation in this position, if possible. Cover the spinal defect with sterile gauze pads soaked in warm sterile saline and inserted in a plastic covering.

A newborn may exhibit a defect in the area of the umbilicus. In some cases, the abdominal contents will fill this defect, resulting in an **omphalocele.** If you encounter a newborn with an omphalocele, cover the defect with an occlusive plastic covering to decrease water and heat loss.

Since newborns are obligate nose breathers, **choanal atresia** can cause upper airway obstruction and respiratory distress. Choanal atresia is the most common birth defect involving the nose and is due to the presence of a bony or membranous septum between the nasal cavity and the pharynx. Suspect this condition if you are unable to pass a catheter through either nare into the oropharynx. An oral airway will usually bypass the obstruction.

A fairly common congenital anomaly is cleft lip and cleft palate. During fetal development, the lip and palate come together in the middle forming the oral cavity. Failure of the palate to completely close during fetal development can result in a defect known as **cleft palate.** Cleft palate may also be associated with failure of the upper lip to close. This condition, referred to as **cleft lip,** can make it difficult to obtain an adequate seal for effective mask ventilation. If a child with a cleft lip or cleft palate will require more than brief mechanical ventilation, you should place an endotracheal tube.

Pierre Robin Syndrome is a congenital condition characterized by a small jaw and large tongue in conjunction with a cleft palate. In this condition, the tongue is likely to obstruct the upper airway. A nasal or oral airway usually bypasses the obstruction. If the obstruction cannot be bypassed with a simple airway, then intubation will be necessary, although it can be very difficult to carry out on newborns with this condition.

ASSESSMENT

Assess the newborn immediately after birth. (Ideally, if two paramedics are available, one paramedic attends the mother, while the other attends the newborn.) Make a mental note of the time of birth and then quickly obtain vital signs. Remember that newborns are slippery and will require both hands to support the head and torso. Position yourself so that you can work close to the surface where you have placed the infant.

The newborn's respiratory rate should average 40–60 breaths per minute. If respirations are not adequate or if the newborn is gasping, immediately start positive-pressure ventilation.

Expect a normal heart rate of 150–180 beats per minute at birth, slowing to 130–140 beats per minute thereafter. A pulse rate of less than 100 beats per minute indicates distress and requires emergency intervention.

Evaluate the skin color as well. Some cyanosis of the extremities is common immediately after birth. However, cyanosis of the central part of the body is abnormal, as is persistent peripheral cyanosis. In such cases, administer 100% oxygen until the cause is determined or the condition is corrected.

THE APGAR SCALE

As discussed in Chapter 40, as soon as possible, assign the newborn an **APGAR score** (See Table 40-2 in Chapter 40.) Ideally, try to do this at 1 and 5 minutes after birth. However, if the newborn is not breathing, DO NOT withhold resuscitation in order

* **meningomyelocele** herniation of the spinal cord and membranes through a defect in the spinal column.

* **omphalocele** congenital hernia of the umbilicus.

* **choanal atresia** congenital closure of the passage between the nose and pharynx by a bony or membranous structure.

* **cleft palate** congenital fissure in the roof of the mouth, forming a passageway between oral and nasal cavities.

* **cleft lip** congenital vertical fissure in the upper lip.

* **Pierre Robin Syndrome** unusually small jaw, combined with a cleft palate, downward displacement of the tongue, and an absent gag reflex.

Content Review

APGAR
- Appearance
- Pulse rate
- Grimace
- Activity
- Respiratory effort

* **APGAR scoring** a numerical system of rating the condition of a newborn. It evaluates the newborn's heart rate, respiratory rate, muscle tone, reflex irritability, and color.

If a newborn is not breathing, DO NOT withhold resuscitation until determining the APGAR score.

to determine the APGAR score. The APGAR scoring system helps distinguish between newborns who need only routine care and those who need greater assistance. The system also predicts long-term survival. A score of 0, 1, or 2 is given for each of the above parameters. The minimum total score is 0 and the maximum is 10. A score of 7–10 indicates an active and vigorous newborn that requires only routine care. A score of 4–6 indicates a moderately distressed newborn that requires oxygenation and stimulation. Severely distressed newborns, those with APGAR scores of less than 4, require immediate resuscitation.

TREATMENT

Treatment starts prior to delivery. Begin care by preparing the environment and assembling the equipment needed for delivery and immediate care of the newborn. The initial care of a newborn follows the same priorities as for all patients. Complete the initial assessment first. Correct any problems detected during the initial assessment before proceeding to the next step. The vast majority of term newborns—approximately 80 percent—require no resuscitation beyond suctioning of the airway, mild stimulation, and maintenance of body temperature by drying and warming with blankets.

Establishing the Airway

Airway management is one of the most critical steps in caring for the newborn. During delivery, fluid is forced out of the baby's lungs, into the oropharynx, and out through the nose and mouth. Fluid drainage occurs independently of gravity. As soon as you deliver the newborn's head, suction the mouth and then the nose, using a bulb suction. Always suction the mouth first so that there is nothing for the infant to aspirate if he or she gasps when the nose is suctioned.

Immediately following delivery, maintain the newborn at the same level as the mother's vagina, with the head approximately 15 degrees below the torso. This facilitates the drainage of secretions and helps to prevent aspiration. If there appears to be a large amount of secretions, attach a **DeLee suction trap** to a suction source. As previously explained, suction the mouth first and then the nose (Figure 41-3a). Repeat these steps until the airway is clear. If you detect **meconium,** prepare intubation equipment and a meconium aspirator (Figure 41-3b). (Meconium staining will be discussed in more detail in several later sections of this chapter.)

Drying and suctioning produce enough stimulation to initiate respirations in most newborns. If the newborn does not immediately cry, stimulate it by flicking the soles of its feet or gently rubbing its back (Figure 41-4). DO NOT spank or vigorously rub a newborn baby.

Prevention of Heat Loss

Heat loss can be a life-threatening condition in newborns. Cold infants quickly become distressed infants. Heat loss occurs through evaporation, convection, conduction, and radiation. Most heat loss in newborns results from evaporation. The newborn comes into the world wet, and the amniotic fluid quickly evaporates. Immediately after birth, the newborn's core temperature can drop 1° C (1.8°F) or more from its birth temperature of 38° C (100.4° F).

Loss of heat can also occur through convection, depending upon the temperature of the room and the movement of the air around the newborn. The newborn can lose additional heat through contact with surrounding surfaces (convection) or by radiating heat to colder objects nearby.

FIGURE 41-3a Suctioning of the mouth using flexible suction catheter.

When head is delivered

As soon as the baby's head is delivered (prior to delivery of the shoulders) *the mouth, oropharynx, and hypopharynx should be thoroughly suctioned*, using a 10 Fr. DeLee suction catheter or other flexible suction catheter. Any catheter used should be no smaller than a 10 Fr.

FIGURE 41-3b Intubation for removal of residual meconium.

Following delivery

After delivery of the infant, if a great deal of meconium is present, the trachea should be intubated and any residual meconium removed from the lower airway.

FIGURE 41-4 Stimulate the newborn as required.

FIGURE 41-5 Dry the infant to prevent loss of evaporative heat.

To prevent heat loss, take these steps.

- Dry the newborn immediately to prevent evaporative cooling (Figure 41-5).
- Maintain the ambient temperature—the temperature in the delivery room or ambulance—at a *minimum* of 23–24° C (74–76° F).
- Close all windows and doors.
- Discard the towel used to dry the newborn and swaddle the infant in a warm, dry receiving blanket or other suitable material. Cover the head.
- In colder areas, place well-insulated water bottles or rubber gloves filled with warm water (40°C or 104°F) around the newborn to help maintain a warm body temperature. To avoid burns, do not place these items against the skin. Be sure the newborn is wrapped in a blanket and place the water bottle or rubber glove against the blanket.

Cutting the Umbilical Cord

After you have stabilized the newborn's airway and minimized heat loss, clamp and cut the umbilical cord. You can prevent over- and under-transfusion of blood by maintaining the baby at the same level as the vagina, as previously described. Do not "milk" or strip the umbilical cord, since this increases blood viscosity, or **polycythemia.** Polycythemia can cause cardiopulmonary problems. It can also contribute to excessive red blood cell destruction, which may in turn lead to **hyperbilirubinemia**—an increased level of bilirubin in the blood that causes jaundice.

Apply the umbilical clamps within 30–45 seconds after birth. Place the first clamp approximately 10 cm (4 inches) from the newborn. Place the second clamp about 5 cm (2 inches) farther away than the first. Then cut the cord between the

---

Do not "milk" or strip the umbilical cord.

✳ polycythemia an excess of red blood cells. In a newborn, the condition may reflect hypovolemia or prolonged intrauterine hypoxia.

✳ hyperbilirubinemia an excessive amount of bilirubin—the orange-colored pigment associated with bile—in the blood. In newborns, the condition appears as jaundice. Precipitating factors include maternal Rh or ABO incompatibility, neonatal septis, anoxia, hypoglycemia, and congenital liver or gastrointestinal defects.

two clamps (see Figure 40-17 in Chapter 40). After the cord is cut, inspect it periodically to make sure there is no additional bleeding.

THE DISTRESSED NEWBORN

The distressed newborn can be either full term or premature. (See "Premature Infants" later in this chapter.) The presence of fetal meconium at birth indicates that fetal distress has occurred at some point during pregnancy. If the newborn is simply meconium stained, then distress may have occurred at a remote time. If you see *particulate* meconium, however, distress may have occurred recently and the newborn should be managed accordingly.

Aspiration of meconium can cause significant respiratory problems and should be prevented. Whenever you spot meconium during delivery, do not induce respiratory effort until you have removed the meconium from the trachea by suctioning under direct visualization with the laryngoscope. (There will be more about this topic under "Meconium Stained Amniotic Fluid" later.) Be sure to report the presence of meconium to the medical direction physician.

The most common problems experienced by newborns during the first minutes of life involve the airway. For this reason, resuscitation usually consists of ventilation and oxygenation. Except in special situations, the use of IV fluids, drugs, or cardiac equipment is usually not indicated. (See "Inverted Pyramid for Resuscitation" on the next page.) The most important procedures include suctioning, drying, and stimulating the distressed newborn.

Of the vital signs, fetal heart rate is the most important indicator of neonatal distress. The newborn has a relatively fixed stroke volume. Thus, cardiac output depends more on heart rate. Bradycardia, as caused by hypoxia, results in decreased cardiac output and, ultimately, poor perfusion. A pulse rate of less than 60 beats per minute in a distressed newborn should be treated with chest compressions. In distressed newborns, monitor the heart rate manually. Do not depend on external electronic monitors.

Of the vital signs, fetal heart rate is the most important indicator of neonatal distress.

RESUSCITATION

The vast majority of newborns do not require resuscitation beyond stimulation, maintenance of the airway, and maintenance of body temperature. Unfortunately, it is difficult to predict which newborns ultimately will require resuscitation. Each EMS unit, therefore, should contain a neonatal resuscitation kit with the following items:

- Neonatal bag-valve-mask unit
- Bulb syringe
- DeLee suction trap
- Meconium aspirator
- Laryngoscope with size 0 and 1 blades
- Uncuffed endotracheal tubes (2.5, 3.0, 3.5, 4.0) with appropriate suction catheters
- Endotracheal tube stylet
- Tape or device to secure endotracheal tube
- Umbilical catheter and 10 mL syringe
- Three-way stopcock

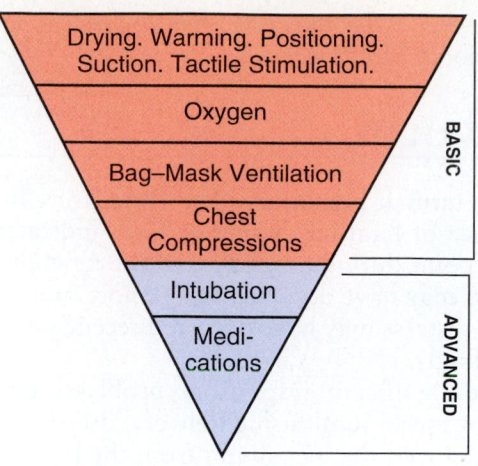

- 20 mL syringe and 8 french feeding tube for gastric suction
- Glucometer
- Assorted syringes and needles
- Towels (sterile)
- Medications:
  - Epinephrine 1:10,000 and 1:1,000
  - Neonatal naloxone (Narcon)
  - Volume expander (lactated Ringer's solution or saline)
  - Sodium bicarbonate (10 mEq in 10 mL)

INVERTED PYRAMID FOR RESUSCITATION

Resuscitation of the newborn follows an inverted pyramid (Figure 41-6). As this pyramid indicates, most distressed newborns respond to relatively simple maneuvers. Few require CPR or advanced life support measures.

The following are steps for the initial care of the newborn. Also see the resuscitation steps illustrated in Procedure 41–1 and Figure 41-7.

Step 1: Drying, Warming, Positioning, Suctioning, and Tactile Stimulation

Resuscitation begins with drying, warming, positioning, suctioning, and stimulating the newborn. Immediately upon delivery, minimize heat loss by drying the newborn. Next, place the newborn in a warm, dry blanket. Make sure the environment is warm and free of drafts.

After you have dried the newborn, place the infant on its back with its head slightly below its body and its neck slightly extended (Figure 41-8). This facilitates drainage of secretions and fluids from the lungs. Place a small blanket, folded to a 2 cm (3/4 inch) thickness, under the newborn's shoulders to help maintain this position.

Next, suction the newborn again, using a bulb syringe or DeLee suction trap. Deep suctioning can cause a **vagal response,** resulting in bradycardia. Because of this, suctioning should last no longer than 10 seconds. If meconium is present, avoid stimulating the infant and visualize the airway with a laryngoscope. Suction the meconium, preferably with a DeLee suction trap. If there is a great deal of meconium,

---

✳ vagal response stimulation of the vagus nerve causing a parasympathetic response.

Suctioning of a newborn should last no longer than 10 seconds.

41-1a Ventilate with 100% oxygen for 15–30 seconds.

41-1b Evaluate heart rate.

41-1c Initiate chest compressions if: HR less than 60, or between 60 and 80 and **not** increasing.

41-1d Evaluate heart rate: Below 80—Continue chest compressions, 80 or above—Discontinue chest compressions.

NORMAL NEWBORN ASSESSMENT AND SUPPORT

Temperature: Dry, warm
Airway: Position, suction
Breathing: Gentle stimulation to cry
Circulation: Pulse rate, color

ASSISTANCE SOME NEWBORNS MAY REQUIRE
(Note: Moving down the list, progressively
fewer patients will require the listed interventions.)

Meconium present and patient has not taken first breath (green/brown staining of birth fluids)	Suction via endotracheal tube while withdrawing and repeat until fluid is clear or patient becomes bradycardic.
Breathing is adequate but central cyanosis persists	Provide 100% oxygen, blow-by method.
Not breathing, or not breathing adequately	Provide stimulation.
Not breathing, or not breathing adequately, after stimulation	Assist ventilations with 100% oxygen *Rate: 40–60/min*
Pulse > 60 bpm but < 100 bpm	Continue assisted ventilations at 40–60/min; perform tracheal intubation.
Pulse < 60 bpm despite assisted ventilations	Continue assisted ventilations, perform endotracheal intubation, and begin chest compressions. *Compression Rate*: 120/min (or 90 compressions + 30 ventilations/min) *Compression/ventilation ratio:* 3:1 (pause for ventilations till intubated)
Pulse remains < 60 bpm with adequate ventilation and chest compressions	Administer epinephrine 0.1 mg/kg first available route (intratracheal, IO, UV, or IV)

FIGURE 41-7 Resuscitation of the newborn. (Adapted from David S. Markenson, *Pediatric Prehospital Care,* Prentice Hall, 2002.)

place an appropriately-sized endotracheal tube (Table 41-2) and suction the meconium directly through the tube. Remove the tube and discard. Do not use the same tube for mechanical ventilation. (See Procedure 41-2.) Following adequate tracheal suctioning, stimulate the newborn by flicking the soles of its feet or rubbing its back.

After carrying out the preceding procedures, assess the newborn as noted below.

Newborn Assessment Parameters

- *Respiratory effort.* The rate and depth of the newborn's breathing should increase immediately with tactile stimulation. If the respiratory response is adequate, evaluate the heart rate next. If the respiratory rate is inadequate, begin positive-pressure ventilation (see Step 3).

Content Review

NEWBORN ASSESSMENT PARAMETERS
- Respiratory effort
- Heart rate
- Color
- APGAR Score

CORRECT

Neck slightly extended

Care should be taken to prevent hyperextension or underextension of the neck since either may decrease air entry.

INCORRECT

Neck hyperextended   Neck underextended

FIGURE 41-8   Positioning the newborn to open the airway.

- *Heart rate.* As noted earlier, heart rate is critical in the newborn. Check the heart rate by listening to the apical area of the heart with a stethoscope, feeling the pulse by lightly grasping the umbilical cord, or feeling either the brachial or femoral pulse. If the heart rate is greater than 100 and spontaneous respirations are present, continue the assessment. If the heart rate is less than 100, immediately begin positive-pressure ventilation (see Step 3).

> **Content Review**
>
> ### NORMAL NEWBORN VITAL SIGNS
> - Respirations 30–60
> - Heart rate 100–180
> - Blood pressure 60–90 systolic
> - Temperature 36.7°–37.8° C (98°–100° F)

Table 41-2	GUIDELINES FOR TRACHEAL TUBE SIZES AND DEPTH OF INSERTION IN THE NEWBORN

Tube Size, mm ID	Depth of Insertion from Upper Lip, cm	Weight, g	Gestation, wk
2.5	6.5–7	<1000	<28
3.0	7–8	1000–2000	28–34
3.5	8–9	2000–3000	34–38
3.5–4.0	> 9	>3000	>38

American Heart Association: *2000 Handbook of Cardiovascular Care for Healthcare Providers*
© 2000, American Heart Association

41-2a   Position the infant.

41-2b   Insert the laryngoscope.

41-2c   Elevate the epiglottis by lifting.

41-2d   Visualize the cords.

41-2e   Suction any meconium present.

41-2f   Insert a fresh tube for ventilation.

41-2g   Remove the laryngoscope.

41-2h   Check proper tube placement.

- *Color.* A newborn may be cyanotic despite a heart rate greater than 100 and spontaneous respirations. If you note central cyanosis, or cyanosis of the chest and abdomen, in a newborn with adequate ventilation and a pulse rate greater than 100, administer supplemental oxygen (see Step 2). Newborns with peripheral cyanosis do not usually need supplemental oxygen UNLESS the cyanosis is prolonged.
- *APGAR score.* Unless resuscitation is required, obtain 1- and 5-minute APGAR scores.

Step 2: Supplemental Oxygen

If central cyanosis is present or the adequacy of ventilation is uncertain, administer supplemental oxygen by blowing oxygen across the newborn's face (Figure 41-9). If possible, the oxygen should be warmed and humidified. Continue oxygen administration until the newborn's color has improved. Although oxygen toxicity is a concern, this condition usually results from prolonged usage over several days. Administration of blow-by oxygen in the prehospital setting will not cause problems. NEVER DEPRIVE A NEWBORN OF OXYGEN IN THE PREHOSPITAL SETTING FOR FEAR OF OXYGEN TOXICITY.

Never deprive a newborn of oxygen in the prehospital setting for fear of oxygen toxicity.

Step 3: Ventilation

Begin positive-pressure ventilation if *any* of the following conditions is present:

- Heart rate less than 100 beats per minute
- Apnea
- Persistence of central cyanosis after administration of supplemental oxygen

FIGURE 41-9 Guidelines for estimating oxygen concentration. Based in oxygen flow rate of 5 liters per minute.

A ventilatory rate of 40–60 breaths per minute is usually adequate. A bag-valve-mask unit is the device of choice. A self-inflating bag of an appropriate size (450 mL is optimal) should be used. Many self-inflating bags have a pressure-limiting pop-off valve that is preset at 30–45 cm H_2O. However, since the initial pressures required to ventilate a newborn may be as high as 60cm/H_2O, you may have to depress the pop-off valve to deactivate it and ensure adequate ventilation. If prolonged ventilation is required, it may be necessary to disable the pop-off valve.

Face masks in various sizes must be available. The most effective ones are designed to fit the contours of the newborn's face and have a low dead space volume (less than 5 mL). When a mask is correctly sized and positioned, it covers the newborn's nose and mouth, but not the eyes.

Endotracheal intubation of a newborn should be carried out in the following situations:

- The bag-valve-mask unit does not work.
- Tracheal suctioning is required (such as in cases of thick meconium).
- Prolonged ventilation will be required.
- A diaphragmatic hernia is suspected.
- Inadequate respiratory effort is found.

Because of the narrowness of the neonatal airway at the level of the cricoid cartilage, always use an *uncuffed* endotracheal tube. (Review Table 41-2.) After inserting it, ensure proper placement by noting symmetrical chest wall motion and equal breath sounds. (Review Procedure 41-2.)

Intubation has several effects in the newborn. First, it bypasses **glottic function.** Second, it eliminates **PEEP**—the physiologic positive end-expiratory pressure created during normal coughing and crying. To maintain adequate functional residual capacity, a PEEP of 2–4 cm/H_2O should be provided when mechanical ventilation is initiated by adding a magnetic-disk PEEP valve to the bag-valve outlet.

Gastric distention, caused by a leak around an uncuffed endotracheal tube, may compromise ventilation of a newborn. This can be minimized by using a properly sized endotracheal tube. If there is significant gastric distension, a **nasogastric tube** or **orogastric tube** should be inserted (through the nose or mouth, then through the esophagus into the stomach) as soon as the airway is controlled. It is recommended that the endotracheal tube be in place before the gastric tube is placed to avoid misplacing the gastric tube into the trachea.

Make sure the newborn is well oxygenated before attempting to insert a gastric tube. To determine the depth of insertion, measure a nasogastric tube from the tip of the nose, around the ear, to below the xiphoid process. Measure an orogastric tube from the lips to below the xiphoid process. Lubricate the end of the tube and pass it gently along the nasal floor or the mouth and into the esophagus. Confirm that the tube is in the stomach by injecting 10 cc of air into the tube and auscultating a bubbling sound, or sound of rushing air, over the epigastrium.

Step 4: Chest Compressions

Initiate chest compressions if *either* of the following conditions exists:

- The heart rate is less than 60 beats per minute.
- The heart rate is between 60 and 80, *but does not increase* with 30 seconds of positive-pressure ventilation and supplemental oxygenation.

✱ glottic function opening and closing of the glottic space.

✱ PEEP positive end-expiratory pressure.

✱ nasogastric tube/orogastric tube a tube that runs through the nose or mouth and esophagus into the stomach, used for administering liquid nutrients or medications or for removing air or liquids from the stomach.

Perform chest compressions by following these steps.

- Encircle the newborn's chest, placing both of your thumbs on the lower one-third of the sternum. If the newborn is very small, you may need to overlap your thumbs. If the newborn is very large, you may need to place the ring and middle fingers of one hand just below the nipple line and perform two-finger compression (Figure 41-10).
- Compress the sternum 1.5–2.0 cm ($\frac{1}{2}$–$\frac{1}{3}$ inch) at a rate of 120 times per minute. Accompany compressions with positive-pressure ventilation. Maintain a ratio of 3 compressions to 1 ventilation.

(A) For a very small newborn, encircle chest with fingers and overlap thumbs on the sternum just below an imaginary line connecting the nipples.

(B) For an average-size newborn, encircle chest with fingers and place thumbs side by side on the sternum just below an imaginary line connecting the nipples.

(C) For an infant that is older or too large to encircle the chest, place middle and ring fingers on sternum one finger-width below imaginary line connecting nipples. Measure distance by first placing, then raising, index finger.

FIGURE 41-10   Position fingers for chest compressions according to the size of the infant.

FIGURE 41-11 The umbilical cord contains two arteries and one vein. The umbilical vein can be accessed for vascular administration of fluids and drugs. The vein is larger than the arteries and has a thinner wall.

- Reassess the newborn after 20 cycles of compressions and ventilations, or at approximately one-minute intervals.
- Discontinue compressions if the spontaneous heart rate exceeds 80.

Step 5: Medications and Fluids

Most cardiopulmonary arrests in newborns result from hypoxia. Because of this, initial therapy consists of ventilation and oxygenation. However, when these measures fail, fluid and medications should be administered. They may also be necessary in cases of persistent bradycardia, hypovolemia, respiratory depression secondary to narcotics, and metabolic acidosis.

Vascular access for the administration of fluids and drugs can most readily be managed by using the umbilical vein. The umbilical cord contains three vessels—two arteries and one vein. The vein is larger than the arteries and has a thinner wall (Figure 41-11). To establish venous access, follow these procedures.

Vascular access for the administration of fluids and drugs can most readily be managed by using the umbilical vein.

- Trim the umbilical cord with a scalpel blade to 1 cm above the abdomen. Be sure to save enough of the umbilical cord stump in case neonatal personnel have to place additional lines.
- Insert a 5 French umbilical catheter into the umbilical vein. Connect the catheter to a three-way stopcock and fill it with saline.
- Insert the catheter until the tip is just below the skin and you note the free flow of blood. (If the catheter is inserted too far, it may become wedged against the liver, and it will not function.)
- After the catheter is in place, secure it with umbilical tape.

If an umbilical vein catheter cannot be placed, some medications can be given via the endotracheal tube. They include atropine, epinephrine, lidocaine, and naloxone. Other options for vascular access are peripheral vein cannulation and intraosseous cannulation. Table 41-3 lists recommended medications and doses for the newborn. Fluid therapy should consist of 10 mL/kg of saline or lactated Ringer's solution given by syringe as a slow IV push.

Table 41-3   NEONATAL RESUSCITATION DRUGS

Medication	Concentration to Administer	Preparation	Dosage/Route*	Total Dose/Infant		Rate/Precautions
Epinephrine	1:10,000	1 mL	0.1–0.3 mL/kg I.V. or I.T.	*weight . . . total mLs* 1 kg 0.1–0.3 mL 2 kg 0.2–0.6 mL 3 kg 0.3–0.9 mL 4 kg 0.4–1.2 mL		Give rapidly.
Volume Expanders	Whole Blood 5% Albumin Normal Saline Lactated Ringer's	40 mL	10 mL/kg I.V.	*weight . . . total mLs* 1 kg 10 mL 2 kg 20 mL 3 kg 30 mL 4 kg 40 mL		Give over 5–10 min.
Sodium Bicarbonate	0.5 mEq/mL	20 mL or two 10-mL prefilled syringes	2 mEq/kg I.V.	*weight . . . total dose . . . mLs* 1 kg 2 mEq 4 mL 2 kg 4 mEq 8 mL 3 kg 6 mEq 12 mL 4 kg 8 mEq 16 mL		Give slowly, over at least 2 min. Give only if infant is being effectively ventilated.
Narcan Neonatal	1.0 mg/mL or 0.4 mg/mL (dilute 1.0 mg in 9mL of Saline)	2 mL	0.1 mg/kg I.V., I.M., S.Q., I.T.	*weight . . . total mLs* (0.1 mg/mL) 1 kg 1.0 mL 2 kg 2.0 mL 3 kg 3.0 mL 4 kg 4.0 mL		Give rapidly.
Dopamine	$6 \times \dfrac{\text{weight (kg)} \times \text{desired dose (mcg/kg/min)}}{\text{desired fluid (mL/hr)}} = $ mg of dopamine per 100 mL of solution		Begin at 5 mcg/kg/min (may increase to 20 mcg/kg/min if necessary) I.V.	*weight . . . total mcg/min* 1 kg 5–20 mcg/min 2 kg 10–40 mcg/min 3 kg 15–60 mcg/min 4 kg 20–80 mcg/min		Give as continuous infusion using an infusion pump. Monitor HR and BP closely. Seek consultation.

From Textbook of Neonatal Resuscitation © 2001, American Heart Association

* I.M. = Intramuscular
  I.T. = Intratracheal
  I.V. = Intravenous
  S.Q. = Subcutaneous

MATERNAL NARCOTIC USE

Maternal abuse of narcotics—either illegal or prescribed—can complicate field deliveries. Maternal narcotic use has been shown to produce low-birth-weight infants. Such infants may demonstrate withdrawal symptoms—tremors, startles, and decreased alertness. They also face a serious risk of respiratory depression at birth.

Naloxone (Narcan), which is extremely safe even at high doses, is the treatment of choice for respiratory depression secondary to maternal narcotic use *within four hours of delivery*. Ventilatory support must be provided prior to administration of naloxone. Because the duration of the narcotics may exceed that of the naloxone, repeat administration as necessary.

Keep in mind, however, that the naloxone may induce a withdrawal reaction in an infant born to *a narcotic-addicted* mother. Medical direction may advise that naloxone NOT be administered if the mother is drug addicted, advising that prolonged ventilatory support be provided instead.

The dosage of naloxone is 0.1 mg/kg. The initial dose may be repeated every 2 to 3 minutes as needed. Naloxone may be given by intravenous, intraosseous, endotracheal, subcutaneous, or intramuscular routes.

As with other newborns, continue all resuscitative measures until the newborn is resuscitated or until the emergency staff assumes care.

Keep in mind that naloxone may induce a withdrawal reaction with an infant born to a narcotic-addicted mother.

NEONATAL TRANSPORT

Healthy newborns should be allowed to begin the bonding process with the mother as soon as possible (Figure 41-12). Distressed newborns, however, must be positioned on their side to prevent aspiration and rapidly transported.

In addition to field deliveries, paramedics are frequently called upon to transport a high-risk newborn from a facility where stabilization has occurred to a neonatal intensive care unit (NICU). The trip may be across the street or across the state. Usually, a pediatric nurse, respiratory therapist, and, often, a physician accompany the newborn. During transport, a paramedic crew will help maintain a newborn's body temperature, control oxygen administration, and maintain ventilatory support. Often, a transport **isolette** with its own heat, light, and oxygen source is available. In such cases, intravenous medications are usually infused through the umbilical vein. The umbilical artery is catheterized as well.

If a self-contained isolette is not available for transport, it is important to keep the ambulance warm. Wrap the newborn in several blankets, keep the infant's head covered, and place hot-water bottles containing water heated to no more than 40° C (104° F) near, but not touching, the newborn. Do not use chemical packs to keep the newborn warm. These can generate excessive heat and may burn the infant.

✳ **isolette** also known as an *incubator*; a clear plastic enclosed bassinet used to keep prematurely born infants warm. The temperature of an isolette can be adjusted regardless of the room temperature. Some isolettes also provide humidity control.

FIGURE 41-12 A healthy newborn can be placed on the mother's abdomen. Write the mother's last name and time of delivery on a tape and place it around the infant's wrist. (Do not allow adhesive to contact the infant's skin.)

SPECIFIC NEONATAL SITUATIONS

Rapid assessment and treatment of a distressed newborn is the key to the infant's survival. The following information will help you to formulate treatment plans for specific emergencies involving newborns. Remember that, unless otherwise directed, it will be necessary to transport these infants to a facility that is able to handle high-risk neonates. A reference card should be available in the ambulance and in the dispatch office that tracks the availability of neonatal unit beds. Whenever possible, keep the parents advised of what is happening and the reason for any treatments being given to the infant. However, do not discuss "chances of survival" with the family or caregivers.

Do not discuss "chances of survival" with a newborn's family or caregivers.

MECONIUM-STAINED AMNIOTIC FLUID

Meconium-stained amniotic fluid occurs in approximately 10–15 percent of deliveries, mostly in post-term or in small-for-gestational-age (SGA) newborns. The mortality rate for meconium-stained infants is considerably higher than the mortality rate for non-stained infants, and meconium aspiration accounts for a significant proportion of neonatal deaths.

Fetal distress and hypoxia can cause the passage of meconium into the amniotic fluid. Meconium is a dark green substance found in the digestive tract of full-term newborns. It arises from secretions of the various digestive glands and amniotic fluid. Either *in utero,* or more often with the first breath, thick meconium is aspirated into the lungs, resulting in small-airway obstruction and aspiration pneumonia. This may produce respiratory distress within the first hours, or even minutes, of life as evidenced by tachypnea, retraction, grunting, and cyanosis in severely affected newborns.

The partial obstruction of some airways may lead to pneumothorax. A pneumothorax may occur in an infant, cause no distress, and require no active treatment. If, however, the infant has significant respiratory distress, then the pneumothorax must be evacuated. If tension pneumothorax has occurred, needle decompression may be required.

An infant born through thin meconium may not require treatment, but depressed infants born through thick, particulate (pea-soup) meconium-stained fluid should be intubated immediately, prior to the first ventilation (Figure 41-13). Aspiration of meconium by a newborn can result in either partial or complete

FIGURE 41-13 Intubate the infant born through particulate, thick meconium immediately—prior to the first ventilation.

airway obstruction. Complete airway obstruction causes atelectasis (collapsed or airless lungs). In addition, some aspects of fetal blood flow resume a right-to-left shunt of blood across the foramen ovale (the opening between the atria of the fetal heart). This results from increased pulmonary pressures. Incomplete obstruction can act as a ball-valve in the smaller airways, thus preventing exhalation. Also, the newborn is at increased risk of developing a pneumothorax.

Before stimulating the infant to breathe, apply suction with a meconium aspirator attached to an endotracheal tube. Connect to suction at 100 cm/H$_2$O or less to remove meconium from the airway. Withdraw the endotracheal tube as suction is applied.

Repeat intubation and suction until the meconium clears, usually not more than two times. Once the airway is clear and the infant is able to breathe on its own, ventilate with 100% oxygen. If the infant is found to be hypotensive, consider a fluid challenge. Remember to warm the infant to prevent hypothermia. The parents will probably question the treatment being performed on the infant. Explain what you are doing and why, without discussing chances of survival. Stress the need for rapid transport to a facility able to handle high-risk infants.

APNEA

Apnea is a common finding in pre-term infants, infants weighing under 1,500 grams (3 pounds, 5 ounces), infants exposed to drugs, or infants born after prolonged or difficult labor and delivery. Typically, the infant fails to breathe spontaneously after stimulation, or the infant experiences respiratory pauses of greater than 20 seconds.

While apnea is usually due to hypoxia or hypothermia, there may be other causative factors. These include:

- Narcotic or central nervous depressants
- Weakness of the respiratory muscles
- Septicemia
- Metabolic disorders
- Central nervous system disorders

Begin management of apnea with tactile stimulation. Flick the soles of the infant's feet or gently rub its back. If necessary, ventilate using a bag-valve mask with the pop-off valve disabled. If the infant still does not breathe on its own, or if it has a heart rate of less than 60 with adequate ventilation and chest compressions, perform tracheal intubation with direct visualization. Gain circulatory access, and monitor the heart rate continuously. If the apnea is due to narcotics administered within the previous four hours, consider naloxone. As noted earlier, however, the use of narcotic antagonists is generally contraindicated if the mother is a drug abuser.

Early and aggressive treatment of apnea usually results in a good outcome. Throughout treatment, keep the infant warm to prevent hypothermia. Also explain procedures to parents and the need for rapid transport.

DIAPHRAGMATIC HERNIA

Diaphragmatic hernias rarely occur. They are seen in approximately 1 out of every 2,200 live births. When they do appear, the **herniation** takes place most often in the posterolateral segments of the diaphragm, and most commonly (90 percent) on the left side. The defect is caused by the failure of the pleurperitoneal canal (foramen of Bochdalek) to close completely. The survival rate for infants

Content Review

CAUSES OF APNEA IN NEWBORNS

- Hypoxia
- Hypothermia
- Narcotics
- Respiratory muscle weakness
- Septicemia
- Metabolic disorder
- Central nervous system disorder

DO NOT utilize narcotic antagonists if the mother is a drug abuser.

* herniation protrusion or projection of an organ or part of an organ through the wall of the cavity that normally contains it.

who require mechanical ventilation in the first 18 to 24 hours is approximately 50 percent. However, if there is no respiratory distress in the first 24 hours of life, the survival rate approaches 100 percent.

Protrusion of abdominal viscera through the hernia into the thoracic cavity occurs in varying degrees. In severe cases, the stomach and a large part of the intestines and the spleen, liver, and kidneys displace the lungs and heart to the opposite side. The lung on the affected side is compressed, causing diminished total lung volume. In at least one-third of patients, pulmonary hypertension is present. With a patent ductus arteriosus, there may be severe right-to-left shunting, further aggravating tissue hypoxia.

Assessment findings may include:

- Little to severe distress present from birth
- Dyspnea and cyanosis unresponsive to ventilations
- Small, flat (scaphoid) abdomen
- Bowel sounds in the chest
- Heart sounds displaced to the right

As soon as you suspect a diaphragmatic hernia, position the infant with its head and thorax higher than the abdomen and feet (Figure 41-14). This will help facilitate the downward displacement of the abdominal organs. Place a nasogastric or orogastric tube and apply low, intermittent suctioning. This will decrease the entrapment of air and fluid within the herniated viscera and will lessen the degree of ventilatory compromise. DO NOT use bag-valve-mask ventilation, which can worsen this condition by causing gastric distention. If necessary, cautiously administer positive-pressure ventilation through an endotracheal tube.

This condition usually requires surgical repair. Explain the possible need for surgery to parents, assuring them that their newborn child will be transported quickly to the facility best able to handle this procedure.

If you suspect a diaphragmatic hernia, DO NOT use bag-valve-mask ventilation, which can worsen the condition by causing gastric distention.

Position of distressed neonate with suspected diaphragmatic hernia.

FIGURE 41-14 If a diaphragmatic hernia is suspected, position the infant with its head and thorax higher than the abdomen and feet to facilitate downward displacement of abdominal organs.

BRADYCARDIA

Bradycardia in the newborn is most commonly caused by hypoxia. However, it may also be due to several other factors, including increased intracranial pressure, hypothyroidism, or acidosis.

In cases of hypoxia, the infant experiences minimal risk if the hypoxia is corrected quickly. In providing treatment, follow the procedures in the inverted pyramid, as discussed earlier. Check for secretions in the airway, check tongue and soft tissue positioning, and check for possible foreign body obstruction. Resist the inclination to treat the bradycardia with pharmacological measures alone. While epinephrine may be necessary, in all likelihood you will be able to correct the problem with suctioning, positioning, administration of oxygen (blow-by or bag-valve mask), or tracheal intubation. Throughout treatment, keep the newborn warm and transport to the nearest facility.

Resist the temptation to treat bradycardia in a newborn with pharmacological measures alone.

PREMATURE INFANTS

A premature newborn is an infant born prior to 37 weeks of gestation or with weight ranging from 0.6 to 2.2 kg (1 pound, 5 ounces to 4 pounds, 13 ounces). Healthy premature infants weighing more than 1,700 grams (3 pounds, 12 ounces) have a survivability and outcome approximately that of full-term infants. The mortality rate decreases weekly as the gestational age surpasses the age of fetal viability. With the technology currently available, fetal viability is considered to be 23–24 weeks of gestation.

Premature newborns are at greater risk of respiratory suppression, head or brain injury caused by hypoxemia, changes in blood pressure, intraventricular hemorrhage, and fluctuations in serum osmolarity. They are also more susceptible to hypothermia than full-term newborns. Reasons premature newborns lose heat more readily include:

- The premature newborn has a relatively large body surface area and comparatively small weight.
- The premature newborn has not sufficiently developed the various control mechanisms needed to regulate body temperature.
- The premature newborn has smaller subcutaneous stores of insulating fat.
- Newborns cannot shiver and must maintain body temperature through other mechanisms.

The degree of immaturity determines the physical characteristics of a premature newborn (Figure 41-15). Premature newborns often appear to have a

FIGURE 41-15 The premature newborn.

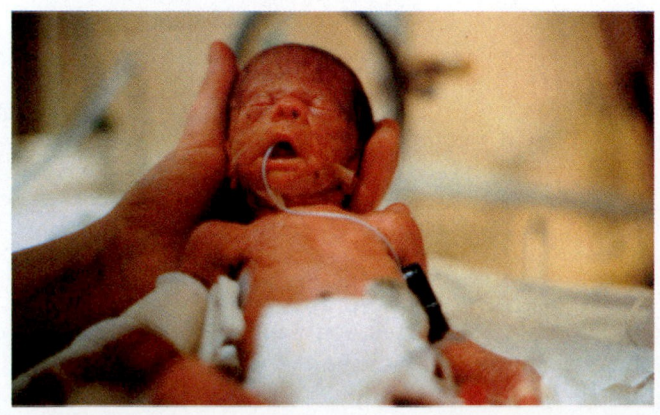

larger head relative to body size. They may have large trunks and short extremities, transparent skin, and few wrinkles.

Prematurity should not be a factor in short-term treatment. Resuscitation should be attempted if there is any sign of life, and the measures of resuscitation should be the same as those for newborns of normal weight and maturity. Maintain a patent airway and avoid potential aspiration of gastric contents. Medical direction may advise administration of epinephrine. Throughout treatment, maintain the newborn's body temperature and transport to a facility with special services for low-birth-weight newborns.

Prematurity should not be a factor in short-term treatment. Resuscitation should be attempted if there is any sign of life.

RESPIRATORY DISTRESS/CYANOSIS

Prematurity is the single most common factor causing respiratory distress and cyanosis in the newborn. The problem occurs most frequently in infants less than 1,200 grams (2 pounds, 10 ounces) and 30 weeks of gestation. Premature infants have an immature central respiratory control center and are easily affected by environmental or metabolic changes. Multiple gestations or prenatal maternal complications may also increase the risk of respiratory distress and cyanosis.

The severely ill newborn with respiratory distress and cyanosis presents a difficult diagnostic challenge. There may be many contributing factors, including lung or heart disease, central nervous system disorders, meconium aspiration, metabolic problems, obstruction of the nasal passages, shock and sepsis, diaphragmatic hernia, and more. Assessment findings include:

- Tachypnea
- Paradoxical breathing
- Intercostal retractions
- Nasal flaring
- Expiratory grunt

Follow the inverted pyramid of treatment, paying particular attention to airway and ventilation. Suction as needed and provide a high concentration of oxygen. Ventilate, as needed, with a BVM. If prolonged ventilation will be required, consider placing an endotracheal tube. Perform chest compressions, if indicated. Sodium bicarbonate may be helpful for prolonged resuscitation. Consider dextrose ($D_{10}W$ or $D_{25}W$) solution if the newborn is hypoglycemic. Maintain body temperature and transport. Be sure to keep the parents informed and provide needed psychological support.

HYPOVOLEMIA

Hypovolemia is the leading cause of shock in newborns. It may result from dehydration, hemorrhage, or third-spacing of fluids. Dehydration is by far the most common cause. Signs of hypovolemia include:

- Pale color
- Cool skin
- Diminished peripheral pulses
- Delayed capillary refill, despite normal ambient temperature
- Mental status changes
- Diminished urination (oliguria)

When you observe these signs, administer a fluid bolus and assess the infant's response. If signs of shock continue, administer a second bolus. Additional boluses should be infused as indicated by repeated assessments. A hypovolemic infant may often need 40 to 60 mL/kg of fluid during the first hour of resuscitation.

Fluid bolus resuscitation consists of 10 mL/kg of an isotonic crystalloid solution, such as Ringer's lactate or normal saline. Administer the bolus over 5 to 10 minutes as soon as intravascular or intraosseous access is obtained. Do not use solutions containing dextrose, as they can produce hypokalemia or worsen ischemic brain injury.

In treating hypovolemia in a newborn, do not use solutions containing dextrose, as they can produce hypokalemia or worsen ischemic brain injury.

SEIZURES

Although seizures occur in a very small percentage of all newborns, they usually indicate a serious underlying abnormality and represent a medical emergency. Prolonged and frequent multiple seizures may result in metabolic changes and cardiopulmonary difficulties.

Neonatal seizures differ from seizures in a child or an adult, because generalized tonic-clonic convulsions normally do not occur during the first month of life. Seizures in neonates include:

- *Subtle seizures.* These seizures consist of chewing motions, excessive salivation, blinking, sucking, swimming movements of the arms, pedaling movements of the legs, apnea, and changes in color.
- *Tonic seizures.* These seizures are characterized by rigid posturing of the extremities and trunk. They are sometimes associated with fixed deviation of the eyes. They occur more commonly in premature infants, especially those with an intraventricular hemorrhage.
- *Focal clonic seizures.* These seizures consist of rhythmic twitching of muscle groups, particularly the extremities and face. They may occur in both full-term and premature infants.
- *Multi focal seizures.* These seizures are similar to focal clonic seizures, except that multiple muscle groups are involved. Clonic activity randomly migrates. These seizures occur primarily in full-term newborns.
- *Myoclonic seizures.* These seizures involve brief focal or generalized jerks of the extremities or parts of the body that tend to involve distal muscle groups. They may occur singly or in a series of repetitive jerks.

Causes of neonatal seizures include sepsis, fever, hypoglycemia, hypoxic-ischemic encephalopathy, metabolic disturbances, meningitis, developmental abnormalities, or drug withdrawal. Assessment findings include a decreased level of consciousness and seizure activities such as those described above. Treatment focuses on airway management and oxygen saturation. With medical direction, consider administration of an anti-convulsant. You might also administer a benzodiazepine (usually lorazepam) for status epilepticus or dextrose ($D_{10}W$ or $D_{25}W$) for hypoglycemia. As with all distressed newborns, maintain body temperature and transport rapidly.

FEVER

Average normal temperature in a newborn is 37.5° C (99.5°F). A rectal temperature of 38.0° C (100.4° F) or higher is considered fever. Neonates do not develop fever as readily as older children. Thus, any fever in a neonate requires extensive evaluation, because it may be caused by life-threatening conditions such as pneumonia, sepsis, or meningitis. Fever may be the only sign of meningitis in a neonate. Because of their immature development, they do not develop the classic symptoms such as a stiff neck. Thus, any neonate with a fever should be considered to have meningitis until proven otherwise.

In assessing a neonate with fever, remember that infants have a limited ability to control their body temperature. As a result, fever can be a serious problem. Assessment findings will probably include the following:

- Mental status changes (irritability/somnolence)
- Decreased feeding
- Skin warm to the touch
- Rashes or *petechia* (small, purplish, hemorrhagic spots on the skin)

Term infants may produce beads of sweat on their brow, but not on the rest of their body. Premature infants will have no visible sweat at all.

Treatment of a neonate with fever will, for the most part, be limited to assuring a patent airway and adequate ventilation. Do not use cold packs, which may drop the temperature too quickly and may also cause seizures. If the newborn becomes bradycardic, provide chest compressions. In the prehospital setting, administration of an antipyretic agent to a neonate is of questionable benefit and should be avoided. Select the appropriate treatment facility, and explain the need for transport to the parents or caregivers.

HYPOTHERMIA

As previously noted, hypothermia presents a common and life-threatening condition for newborns. Adults sometimes fail to realize that a newborn may die because of exposure to temperatures that adults find comfortable. The increased surface-to-volume relationship in newborns makes them extremely sensitive to environmental temperatures, especially right after delivery when they are wet. As a result, it is important to control the four methods of heat loss—evaporation, conduction, convection, and radiation.

In treating hypothermia—a body temperature below 35°C (95° F)—keep in mind that it can also be an indicator of sepsis in the newborn. Regardless of the cause, the increased metabolic demands created by hypothermia can produce a variety of related conditions including metabolic acidosis, pulmonary hypertension, and hypoxemia.

In assessing a hypothermic newborn, remember that they do not shiver. Instead, expect these findings:

- Pale color
- Skin cool to the touch, particularly in the extremities
- **Acrocyanosis**
- Respiratory distress
- Possible apnea
- Bradycardia
- Central cyanosis
- Initial irritability
- Lethargy in later stages

Management focuses on assuring adequate ventilations and oxygenation. Chest compressions may be performed, if necessary. With medical direction, you

Any neonate with a fever should be considered to have meningitis until proven otherwise.

In assessing a neonate with fever, remember that infants have a limited ability to control their body temperature. As a result, fever can be a serious condition.

* acrocyanosis cyanosis of the extremities.

might administer warm fluids through an IV fluid heater. Do not microwave fluids, as there can be a great variation in fluid temperature. Dextrose ($D_{10}W$ or $D_{25}W$) may also be given if the newborn is hypoglycemic. Above all, the newborn must be kept warm. Set the ambulance temperature at 24–26°C (75.2°F–78.8°F). Also remember to warm your hands before touching the newborn. Select the appropriate receiving facility and transport rapidly.

Remember to warm your hands before touching a neonate.

HYPOGLYCEMIA

Newborns are the only age group that can develop severe hypoglycemia and not have diabetes mellitus. Hypoglycemia may be due to inadequate glucose intake or increased glucose utilization. Stress and other factors can also cause the blood sugar to fall, sometimes to a critical level.

Hypoglycemia is more common in premature or small-for-gestational-age (SGA) infants, the smaller twin, and newborns of a diabetic mother, as these infants often have decreased glycogen stores. Hypoglycemia can also develop due to increased glucose utilization. Causes include respiratory illnesses, hypothermia, toxemia, CNS hemorrhage, asphyxia, meningitis, and sepsis. In an older infant, hypoglycemia may be due to an inadequate glucose intake or increased utilization of glucose. Infants receiving glucose infusions can develop hypoglycemia if the infusion is suddenly stopped.

Infants with hypoglycemia may be asymptomatic or they may exhibit symptoms such as apnea, color changes, respiratory distress, lethargy, seizures, acidosis, and poor myocardial contractility.

Persistent hypoglycemia can have catastrophic effects on the brain. The normal newborn's glycogen stores are sufficient to meet glucose requirements for only 8–12 hours. This time frame is diminished in infants with decreased glycogen stores or the presence of other problems where glucose utilization increases. As a result, you should determine the blood glucose on all sick infants. A blood glucose screening test of less than 45 mg/dl indicates hypoglycemia.

Because hypoglycemia can have a catastrophic effect on a neonate's brain, you should determine the blood glucose on all sick infants.

In response to hypoglycemia, the newborn's body will release counter-regulatory hormones such as glucagon, epinephrine, cortisol, and growth hormone. These hormones help raise the blood glucose level by mobilizing glucose stores. In fact, this hormone response may cause transient symptoms of hyperglycemia that may last for several hours. However, when the infant's glucose stores are depleted, the glucose level will again fall.

In assessing hypoglycemic newborns, expect these findings:

- Twitching or seizures
- Limpness
- Lethargy
- Eye-rolling
- High-pitched cry
- Apnea
- Irregular respirations
- Possible cyanosis

Treatment begins with management of the airway and ventilations. Assure adequate oxygenation. Perform chest compressions, if indicated. With medical direction, administer dextrose ($D_{10}W$ or $D_{25}W$). Maintain a normal body temperature in the newborn and transport to the appropriate facility.

VOMITING

Vomiting in a neonate may result from a variety of causes and rarely presents as an isolated symptom. Vomiting (a forceful ejection of stomach contents) is uncommon during the first weeks of life and may be confused with regurgitation (a simple backflow of stomach contents into the mouth, or "spitting up"). Vomiting in the neonate usually occurs because of an anatomic abnormality such as a tracheoesophageal fistula or upper gastrointestinal obstruction. More often, it may be a symptom of some disease such as increased intracranial pressure or an infection. Vomitus containing dark blood often signals a life-threatening illness. Keep in mind, however, that vomiting of mucus—which may occasionally be blood streaked—in the first few hours after birth is not uncommon.

Assessment findings may include a distended stomach, signs of infection, increased ICP, or drug withdrawal. Because vomitus can be aspirated, management considerations focus on assuring a patent airway. If you detect respiratory difficulties or obstruction of the airway, suction or clear vomitus from the airway and assure adequate oxygenation. Fluid administration may be needed to prevent dehydration. Also remember that, as with older patients, vagal stimulation may cause bradycardia in the neonate.

After you have protected the airway, place the infant on its side and transport to an appropriate facility. As with all other situations involving distressed neonates, advise parents or caregivers of steps taken and why.

DIARRHEA

Diarrhea in a neonate can cause severe dehydration and electrolyte imbalances. Although diarrhea may be harder to assess in neonates than in other patients, consider five to six stools per day as normal, especially in breast-fed infants.

Causes of diarrhea in a neonate include:

- Bacterial or viral infection
- Gastroenteritis
- Lactose intolerance
- **Phototherapy**
- **Neonatal abstinence syndrome (NAS)**
- **Thyrotoxicosis**
- Cystic fibrosis

In treating neonates with diarrhea, remember to take appropriate BSI precautions, just as you would do in any situation involving body fluids. Expect to find loose stools, decreased urinary output, and other signs of dehydration such as prolonged capillary refill time, cool extremities, and listlessness or lethargy. It is often difficult for the parents to estimate the number of stools. In such cases, it might be better to inquire about the number of diapers the baby is using.

Management consists of maintenance of airway and ventilations, adequate oxygenation, and chest compressions, if indicated. With medical direction, you might also consider fluid therapy. Explain all treatments to parents or caregivers, and transport the neonate to a facility able to handle high-risk infants.

COMMON BIRTH INJURIES

A **birth injury** occurs in an estimated 2 to 7 of every 1,000 live births in the United States. About 5 to 8 of every 100,000 infants die of birth trauma and 25

---

* photography exposure to sunlight or artificial light for therapeutic purposes. In newborns, light is used to treat hyperbilirubinemia or jaundice.

* neonatal abstinence syndrome (NAS) a generalized disorder presenting a clinical picture of CNS hyperirritability, gastrointestinal dysfunction, respiratory distress, and vague autonomic symptoms. It may be due to intrauterine exposure to heroin, methadone, or other less potent opiates. Non-opiate central nervous system depressants may also cause NAS.

* thyrotoxicosis toxic condition characterized by tachycardia, nervous symptoms, and rapid metabolism due to hyperactivity of the thyroid gland.

In treating a neonate with diarrhea, remember to take appropriate BSI precautions.

* birth injury avoidable and unavoidable mechanical and anoxic trauma incurred by the newborn during labor and delivery.

of every 100,000 die of anoxic injuries. Such injuries account for 2–3 percent of infant deaths. Risk factors for birth injury include:

- Prematurity
- Postmaturity
- Cephalopelvic disproportion
- Prolonged labor
- Breech presentation
- Explosive delivery
- Diabetic mother

Birth injuries take various forms. Cranial injuries may include molding of the head and overriding of the parietal bones, erythema (reddening of the skin), abrasions, ecchymosis (black-and-blue discoloration) and subcutaneous fat necrosis, subconjunctival and retinal hemorrhage, subperiosteal hemorrhage, and fracture of the skull. Intracranial hemorrhage may result from trauma or asphyxia. Often the infant will develop a large scalp hematoma during the birth process. This injury, called *caput succedaneum*, will usually resolve over a week's time. There may be damage to the spine and spinal cord from strong traction exerted when the spine is hyperextended or there is a lateral pull. Other birth injuries include peripheral nerve injury, injury to the liver, rupture of the spleen, adrenal hemorrhage, fractures of the clavicle or extremities, and, of course, hypoxia-ischemia.

Assessment findings may include:

- Diffuse, sometimes ecchymotic, edematous swelling of soft tissues around the scalp
- Paralysis below the level of the spinal cord injury
- Paralysis of the upper arm with or without paralysis of the forearm
- Diaphragmatic paralysis
- Movement on only one side of the face when crying
- Inability to move the arm freely on the side of the fractured clavicle
- Lack of spontaneous movement of the affected extremity
- Hypoxia
- Shock

Management of a newborn or newborn with birth injuries usually centers on protection of the airway, provision of adequate ventilation and oxygen, and, if needed, chest compressions. With medical direction, you may administer medications or take other non-pharmacological steps to support the specific injury. Newborns with birth injuries usually require treatment at specialized facilities. As in the management of other neonatal emergencies, provide professional and compassionate communication to parents or caregivers.

In treating distressed neonates with birth injuries or other critical conditions, provide professional and compassionate communication to the parents or caregivers.

CARDIAC RESUSCITATION, POST RESUSCITATION, AND STABILIZATION

The incidence of neonatal cardiac arrest is related primarily to hypoxia. As previously explained, the outcome will be poor unless you immediately initiate appropriate interventions. As you might expect, cases involving cardiac arrest have an increased chance of brain and organ damage. Risk factors for cardiac arrest in newborns include:

- Bradycardia
- Intrauterine asphyxia
- Prematurity
- Drugs administered to or taken by the mother
- Congenital neuromuscular diseases
- Congenital malformations
- Intrapartum hypoxemia

Cardiac arrest can be caused by primary or secondary apnea, bradycardia, persistent fetal circulation, or pulmonary hypertension. Assessment findings may include peripheral cyanosis, inadequate respiratory effort, and ineffective or absent heart rate.

In managing neonatal cardiac arrest, follow the inverted pyramid for resuscitation. Administer drugs or fluids according to medical direction. Maintain normal body temperature while you transport the distressed newborn to the appropriate facility. This situation will require delicate handling of the parents or caregivers. Explain what is being done for the infant, without entering into the possibilities of survival.

Content Review

CAUSES OF NEONATAL CARDIAC ARREST
- Primary or secondary apnea
- Bradycardia
- Persistent fetal circulation
- Pulmonary hypertension

SUMMARY

After a woman gives birth, you must care for two patients—the mother and her newborn child. The newborn has several special needs, the most important of which are protection of the airway and support of ventilations. The newborn must be kept warm at all times. If assessment reveals a distressed newborn, you should initiate ventilatory support, stimulation, and, if required, CPR. If possible, newborns should be transported to a facility with an NICU. Maintain communications with family members or caregivers, explaining all procedures performed on the newborn.

CHAPTER 42

Pediatrics

Objectives

After reading this chapter, you should be able to:

1. Discuss the paramedic's role in the reduction of infant and childhood morbidity and mortality from acute illness and injury. (pp. 1714–1716)

2. Identify methods/mechanisms that prevent injuries to infants and children. (pp. 1715–1716)

3. Describe Emergency Medical Services for Children (EMSC) and how it can affect patient outcome. (p. 1715)

4. Identify the common family responses to acute illness and injury of an infant or child. (p. 1717)

5. Describe techniques for successful interaction with families of acutely ill or injured infants and children. (p. 1717)

6. Identify key anatomical, physiological, growth, and developmental characteristics of infants and children and their implications. (pp. 1718–1721)

7. Outline differences in adult and childhood anatomy, physiology, and "normal" age-group-related vital signs. (pp. 1721–1725)

8. Describe techniques for successful assessment and treatment of infants and children. (pp. 1726–1736)

9. Discuss the appropriate equipment used to obtain pediatric vital signs. (pp. 1734–1736)

Continued

10. Determine appropriate airway adjuncts, ventilation devices, and endotracheal intubation equipment; their proper use; and complications of use for infants and children. (pp. 1736–1746)
11. List the indications and methods of gastric decompression for infants and children. (pp. 1746–1747, 1748)
12. Define pediatric respiratory distress, failure, and arrest. (pp. 1754–1756)
13. Differentiate between upper airway obstruction and lower airway disease. (pp. 1757–1763)
14. Describe the general approach to the treatment of children with respiratory distress, failure, or arrest from upper airway obstruction or lower airway disease. (pp. 1757–1763)
15. Discuss the common causes and relative severity of hypoperfusion in infants and children. (pp. 1763–1769)
16. Identify the major classifications of pediatric cardiac rhythms. (pp. 1769–1772)
17. Discuss the primary etiologies of cardiopulmonary arrest in infants and children. (pp. 1754–1756, 1763)
18. Discuss age-appropriate sites, equipment, techniques, and complications of vascular access for infants and children. (pp. 1747, 1749–1750)
19. Describe the primary etiologies of altered level of consciousness in infants and children. (pp. 1753–1780, 1785–1786, 1796–1797)
20. Identify common lethal mechanisms of injury in infants and children. (pp. 1780–1783)
21. Discuss anatomical features of children that predispose or protect them from certain injuries. (pp. 1786–1789)
22. Describe aspects of infant and child airway management that are affected by potential cervical spine injury. (pp. 1783, 1785)
23. Identify infant and child trauma patients who require spinal immobilization. (pp. 1752–1753)
24. Discuss fluid management and shock treatment for infant and child trauma patients. (pp. 1764–1768, 1785)

25. Determine when pain management and sedation are appropriate for infants and children. (p. 1785)
26. Define child abuse, child neglect, and sudden infant death syndrome (SIDS). (pp. 1789–1793)
27. Discuss the parent/caregiver responses to the death of an infant or child. (p. 1790)
28. Define children with special health care needs and technology-assisted children. (pp. 1794–1797)
29. Discuss basic cardiac life support (CPR) guidelines for infants and children. (pp. 1736–1741)
30. Integrate advanced life support skills with basic cardiac life support for infants and children. (pp. 1742–1752, 1769–1772)
31. Discuss the indications, dosage, route of administration, and special considerations for medication administration in infants and children. (pp. 1750–1752)
32. Discuss appropriate transport guidelines for low- and high-risk infants and children. (p. 1753)
33. Describe the epidemiology, including the incidence, morbidity/mortality, risk factors, prevention strategies, pathophysiology, assessment, and treatment of infants and children with:
    a. Respiratory distress/failure (pp. 1754–1763)
    b. Hypoperfusion (pp. 1763–1768)
    c. Cardiac dysrhythmias (pp. 1769–1772)
    d. Neurological emergencies (pp. 1771, 1773–1774)
    e. Trauma (pp. 1780–1788)
    f. Abuse and neglect (pp. 1790–1793)
    g. Special health-care needs, including technology-assisted children (pp. 1794–1797)
    h. SIDS (pp. 1789–1790)
34. Given several pre-programmed simulated pediatric patients, provide the appropriate assessment, treatment, and transport. (pp. 1714–1797)

INTRODUCTION

The ill or injured child presents special concerns for prehospital personnel. Current research indicates that more than 20,000 pediatric deaths occur each year in the United States. The leading causes of death are age specific. They include motor vehicle collisions, burns, drownings, suicides, and homicides. These alarming facts become even more troublesome when experts theorize that many of them could have been prevented by early intervention. Tragedies involving children—neonates to adolescents—account for some of the most stressful incidents that you will encounter in EMS practice.

Treatment of pediatric patients presents a number of challenges for the paramedic. Children, especially young ones, often cannot describe what is bothering them or what has happened to them. In addition to the child patient, you must deal with the parents or caregivers. Finally, a child's size often makes routine procedures more difficult. Keep in mind that children are not simply small adults. They have special considerations and needs. This chapter will present the topic of pediatric emergencies as it applies to advanced prehospital care.

Tragedies involving children account for some of the most stressful incidents that you will encounter in EMS practice.

Children are not simply small adults.

ROLE OF PARAMEDICS IN PEDIATRIC CARE

When considering the reduction of pediatric morbidity and mortality, your role as a paramedic centers around two key concepts. First, you must realize that pediatric injuries have become a major health concern. Second, you should remember that children are at a higher risk of injury than adults and that they are more likely to be adversely affected by the injuries that they suffer.

Numerous factors account for the high pediatric injury rates. Some factors, such as geography and weather, cannot be altered. However, other factors, particularly dangers within the home and community, can be eliminated or minimized. As health care professionals, we must all get involved in identifying and implementing methods and mechanisms that prevent injuries to infants and children. Those of us who deliver prehospital care must do more than simply enter the picture after an injury has taken place.

In addition to pediatric injuries, paramedics are often responsible for treating the ill child. There are many aspects of disease and disease processes that are unique to children. It is important that the paramedic be familiar with these, as early intervention is often the key to reduced morbidity and mortality.

CONTINUING EDUCATION AND TRAINING

Your role in improving the health care offered to pediatric patients begins with your own training. Because you will encounter pediatric patients less frequently than adult patients, you have a professional responsibility to maintain and improve upon your pediatric knowledge, particularly your clinical skills. Continuing education programs include:

Because you will encounter pediatric patients less frequently than adult patients, you have a professional responsibility to maintain and improve upon your pediatric knowledge, particularly your clinical skills.

- Pediatric Advanced Life Support (PALS)
- Pediatric Basic Trauma Life Support (PBTLS)
- Advanced Pediatric Life Support (APLS)
- Prehospital Pediatric Care (PPC)

In addition to these programs, you can also attend regional conferences and seminars designed to increase your knowledge of pediatric care. These are often conducted by regional children's hospitals. You can further enhance your clinical skills by spending time in pediatric emergency departments, pediatric hospitals, or pediatric departments in local hospitals. You might also visit the offices of pediatricians or talk with Pediatric Nurse Practitioners—registered nurses who provide primary health care to children.

For self-study, you can choose among many excellent pediatric textbooks currently available or read articles on pediatric care in the various EMS journals. Many good pediatric educational sites are available on the Internet. A particularly useful source of information is the Center for Pediatric Medicine (CPEM), established in 1985 at the New York University Medical Center and Bellevue Hospital. This federally funded center promotes education, research, and development of systems aimed at improving emergency medical services for children in the United States. CPEM has made available the *Teaching Resource for Instructors in Prehospital Pediatrics* (TRIPP), a progressive and comprehensive resource for instructors of prehospital providers. This resource contains a thorough review of prehospital pediatric emergencies.

IMPROVED HEALTH CARE AND INJURY PREVENTION

Funding for CPEM comes largely from a group known as the **Emergency Medical Services for Children (EMSC)**. This federally funded program falls under the management of the Maternal and Child Health Bureau—an agency of the U.S. Department of Health and Human Services. The EMSC was formed for the express purpose of improving the health of pediatric patients who suffer potentially life-threatening illnesses or injuries. This nationally coordinated effort has identified a number of pediatric health care concerns, including:

* Community education
* Data collection
* Quality improvement
* Injury prevention
* Access
* Prehospital care
* Emergency care
* Definitive care
* Finance
* Rehabilitation
* A systems approach to pediatric care
* Ongoing health care from birth to young adulthood

* **Emergency Medical Services for Children (EMSC)** federally funded program aimed at improving the health of pediatric patients who suffer from life-threatening illnesses and injuries.

As a paramedic, you can take part in this national effort by actively participating in programs that promote injury prevention. Let's face it—as prehospital care providers, we see the consequences of pediatric trauma all too often. You can help reduce the rate of injury by taking advantage of opportunities to share "teaching points" in your daily life, both personally and professionally. Take part in, or offer to organize, school or community programs in injury prevention or health care. Engage student interest in the EMS profession by volunteering to speak at "career days," emphasizing those aspects of your job that relate to young people. Use non-urgent ambulance calls as a chance to educate family members or caregivers on the importance of "child-proofing" a home or neighborhood.

Work with appropriate agencies in initiating or conducting safety inspections, block watches, and more.

There has been an increased effort to identify the severity and nature of prehospital pediatric emergencies. Many regions now have both pediatric and trauma registries. These, in addition to standard epidemiological research conducted by local health departments, are dependent on quality prehospital documentation. If your area is participating in a registry program or research study, be sure to obtain and record all required data. Information gained from these registries will help identify the need for more or specialized resources.

GENERAL APPROACH TO PEDIATRIC EMERGENCIES

The approach to the pediatric patient varies with the age of the patient and with the problem being treated. Foremost in approaching any pediatric emergency is consideration of the patient's emotional and physiological development. Care also involves the family members or caregivers responsible for the child. They will demand information, express fears, and, ultimately, give or refuse consent for treatment and/or transport.

COMMUNICATION AND PSYCHOLOGICAL SUPPORT

Treatment of an infant, child, or teenager begins with communication and psychological support.

Treatment of an infant, child, or teenager begins with communication and psychological support. Interaction with pediatric patients and related adults continues throughout assessment and management. When obtaining the medical history of the pediatric patient, you should gather information as quickly and as accurately as possible. The parents and caregivers are often the primary source of information, especially in the case of infants. However, as children become older, they can also be a good source of information. Older children, for example, can often give accurate descriptions of symptoms or other details. Treat pediatric patients with respect, allowing them to express opinions and ask questions. Your listening skills will play an important role in alleviating the fears of child patients. You can even communicate a calm and caring attitude to infants, who respond to touch and voice just like any other human being.

Responding to Patient Needs

As previously mentioned, a child's response to an emergency will vary, depending on the age and emotional maturity of the child. The child's most common response to illness or injury is fear. Common fears of children include:

- Fear of being separated from the parents or caregivers
- Fear of being removed from a family place, such as home, and never returning
- Fear of being hurt
- Fear of being mutilated or disfigured
- Fear of the unknown

These fears may be intensified if the child detects fear or anxiety from the parents or caregivers. The general chaos and panic that often surround pediatric emergency situations may further distress the child.

Remember that children have the right to know what is being done to them. You should be as honest as possible with them. If a procedure such as an IV needle stick will hurt, tell them so. Tell them immediately before performing a procedure. Do not say that a procedure will be painful and then take 5 minutes to prepare the equipment, allowing time for the child's anticipation of pain to build.

Always use language that is appropriate for the age of the child. Medical and anatomical terms that we routinely use may be completely foreign to children. Telling a child that you are going to "apply a cervical collar" means nothing. Instead, tell the child: "I'm going to put this collar around your neck to keep it from moving." "Try to hold your head still." "Tell me if it is too tight." This will involve children in their own care and reduce their feelings of helplessness.

Responding to Parents or Caregivers

As you might expect, the reaction of parents or caregivers to a pediatric emergency will vary. Initial reactions might include shock, grief, denial, anger, guilt, fear, or complete loss of control. Their behavior may change during the course of the emergency. Communication is the key. Preferably only one paramedic will speak with adults at the scene. This will avoid any chance of conflicting information and allow a second paramedic to focus on the child. If parents or caregivers sense your confidence and professionalism, they will regain control and trust your suggestions for care. As with the child, most parents and caregivers feel overwhelmed by fear. They often express their fears in questions such as the following:

"Is my child going to die?"
"Did my child suffer brain damage?"
"Is my child going to be all right?"
"What are you doing to my child?"
"Will my child be able to walk?"

It may be difficult to answer these questions in the prehospital setting. However, the following actions may help allay parents' fears:

- Tell them your name and qualifications.
- Acknowledge their fears and concerns.
- Reassure them that it is all right to feel the way they do.
- Redirect their energies toward helping you care for the child.
- Remain calm and appear in control of the emergency.
- Keep the parents or caregivers informed as to what you are doing.
- Don't "talk down" to them.
- Assure them that everything possible is being done for their child.

If conditions permit, you should allow one of the parents or caregivers to remain with the child at all times. Some family members may be extremely emotional in emergency situations. The child will react more positively to a family member who appears calm and reassuring. If a parent or caregiver is "out of control," have another person take him or her away from the immediate area to settle down. Maintain a reasonable level of suspicion if a child shows a pattern of injuries, some old and some new. In such cases, the parent or caregiver may try to cover up what may be an abusive situation. They may also try to block examination and treatment. (There will be more on potential abuse or neglect later in this chapter.)

GROWTH AND DEVELOPMENT

Children progress through developmental stages on their way to adulthood. You should tailor your approach to the developmental level of your pediatric patient.

Newborns (First Hours after Birth)

Although the terms "newborn" and "neonate" are often used interchangeably, "newborn" refers to a baby in the first hours of extrauterine life. The term "neonate" describes infants from birth to 1 month of age. The method most frequently used to assess newborns is the *APGAR scoring system,* which was described in Chapter 40. Resuscitation of the newborn generally follows the inverted pyramid described in Chapter 41 and the guidelines established in the Neonatal Advanced Life Support (NALS) curriculum.

Neonates (Ages Birth to 1 Month)

The neonate, as noted above (and described in Chapter 41), is an infant up to 1 month of age. This is a major stage of development. Soon after birth, the neonate typically loses up to 10 percent of its birth weight as it adjusts to extrauterine life. This lost weight, however, is ordinarily recovered within 10 days. Gestational age affects early growth. Children born at term (40 weeks) should follow accepted developmental guidelines. Infants born prematurely will not be as developed, either neurologically or physically, as their term counterparts.

The neonatal stage of development centers on reflexes. The neonate's personality also begins to form. The infant is close to the mother and may stare at faces and smile. The mother, and occasionally the father, can comfort and quiet the child. Obviously, the history must be obtained from the parents or caregivers. However, it is also important to observe the child. Common illnesses in this age group include jaundice, vomiting, and respiratory distress. Serious illnesses, such as meningitis, are difficult to distinguish from minor illnesses in neonates. Often, fever is the only sign, although the majority of neonates with fever have minor illnesses (96–97 percent). The few that are seriously ill can be easily missed. For this reason, any fever in a neonate requires extensive evaluation.

The approach to this age group should include several factors. First, the child should always be kept warm. Observe skin color, tone, and respiratory activity. The absence of tears when crying may indicate dehydration. The lungs should be auscultated early during the exam, while the infant is quiet. You might find it helpful to have the child suck on a pacifier during the examination. Allowing the infant to remain in a parent's or caregiver's lap may help keep the child calm.

Infants (Ages 1 to 5 Months)

Infants should have doubled their birth weight by 5 to 6 months of age. They should be able to follow the movements of others with their eyes. Muscle control develops in a cephalo-caudal progression. This means, literally, that development of muscular control begins at the head (cephalo) and moves toward the tail (caudal). Muscular control also spreads from the trunk toward the extremities during this period. The infant's personality at this stage still centers closely on the parents or caregivers. The history must be obtained from these individuals, with close attention to possible illnesses and accidents, including SIDS, vomiting, dehydration, meningitis, child abuse, and household accidents.

Concentrate on keeping these patients warm and comfortable. Allow the infant to remain in the parent's or caregiver's lap. A pacifier or bottle can be used to help keep the baby quiet during the examination.

Infants (Ages 6 to 12 Months)

Infants in this age group may stand or even walk with assistance. They are quite active and enjoy exploring the world with their mouths. In this stage of development, the risk of **foreign body airway obstruction (FBAO)** becomes a serious concern.

Infants 6 months and older have more fully formed personalities and express themselves more readily. They have considerable anxiety toward strangers. They don't like lying on their backs. Children in this age group tend to cling to the mother, though the father "will do" in many cases. Common illnesses and accidents include febrile seizures, vomiting, diarrhea, dehydration, bronchiolitis, car accidents, croup, child abuse, poisonings, falls, airway obstructions, and meningitis.

These children should be examined while sitting in the lap of the parent or caregiver (Figure 42–1). The exam should progress in a toe-to-head order, since starting at the face may upset the child. If time and conditions permit, allow the child to become familiar with you before beginning the examination.

 foreign body airway obstruction (FBAO) blockage or obstruction of the airway by an object that impairs respiration; in the case of pediatric patients, tongues, abundant secretions, and deciduous (baby) teeth are more likely to block airways.

Examine infants and toddlers in a toe-to-head order.

Toddlers (Ages 1 to 3 Years)

Great strides occur in gross motor development during this stage. Children tend to run underneath or stand on almost everything. They seem to always be on the move. As they grow older, toddlers become braver and more curious or stubborn. They begin to stray away from the parents or caregivers more frequently. Yet these remain the only people who can comfort them quickly, and most children will cling to a parent or caregiver if frightened.

At ages 1 to 3 years, language development begins. Often children can understand better than they can speak. Therefore, the majority of the medical history will still come from the parents or caregivers. Remember, however, that you can ask toddlers simple and specific questions.

Accidents of all types are the leading cause of injury deaths in pediatric patients ages 1 to fifteen years. Common accidents in this age group include motor vehicle collisions, homicides, burn injuries, drownings, and pedestrian accidents. Common illnesses and injuries in the toddler age group include vomiting, diarrhea, febrile seizures, poisonings, falls, child abuse, croup, and meningitis. Keep in mind that FBAO is still a high risk for toddlers.

Be cautious when treating toddlers. Approach toddlers slowly and try to gain their confidence. Conduct the exam in a toe-to-head order. The child may be difficult to examine and may resist being touched. Speak quietly and use only simple words. Avoid asking questions that allow the child to say "no." If the situation permits, allow toddlers to hold transitional objects such as a favorite blanket or toy. Be sure to tell the child if something will hurt. If at all possible, avoid procedures on the dominant arm/hand, which the child will try to pull away.

FIGURE 42–1 Infants and young children should be allowed to remain in their mother's arms.

Preschoolers (Ages 3 to 5 Years)

Children in this age group show a tremendous increase in fine and gross motor development. Language skills increase greatly. Children in this age group know how to talk. However, if frightened, they often refuse to speak, especially to strangers. They often have vivid imaginations and may see monsters as part of their world. Preschoolers may have tempers and will express them. During this stage of development, children fear mutilation and may feel threatened by treatment. Avoid frightening or misleading comments.

Preschoolers often run to a particular parent or caregiver, depending upon the occasion. They stick up for the people they love and are openly affectionate. They still seek support and comfort from within the home.

When evaluating children in this age group, question the child first, keeping in mind that imagination may interfere with the facts. The child often has a distorted sense of time, and thus you must rely on the parents or caregivers to fill in the gaps. Common illnesses and accidents in this age group include croup, asthma, poisonings, auto accidents, burns, child abuse, ingestion of foreign bodies, drownings, epiglottitis, febrile seizures, and meningitis.

Treatment of preschoolers requires tact. Avoid baby talk. If time and situation permit, give the child health care choices. Often the use of a doll or stuffed animal will assist in the examination. Allow the child to hold a piece of equipment, such as a stethoscope, and to use it. Let the child sit on your lap. Start the examination with the chest and evaluate the head last. Avoid misleading comments. Do not trick or lie to the child, and always explain what you are going to do.

Do not trick or lie to the child, and always explain what you are going to do.

School-Age Children (Ages 6–12 Years)

Children in this age group are active and carefree. Growth spurts sometimes lead to clumsiness. The personality continues to develop. School-age children are protective and proud of their parents or caregivers and seek their attention. They value peers, but also need home support.

When examining school-age children, give them the responsibility of providing the history. However, remember that children may be reluctant to provide information if they sustained an injury while doing something forbidden. The parents or caregivers can fill in the pertinent details. When assessing children in this age group, it is important to respect their modesty. Be honest and tell the child what is wrong. A small toy may help to calm the child (Figure 42–2). Common illnesses and injuries for this age group include drownings, auto collisions, bicycle accidents, falls, fractures, sports injuries, child abuse, and burns.

Adolescents (Ages 13 to 18)

Adolescence covers the period from the end of childhood to the start of adulthood (age 18). It begins with puberty, roughly age 13 for male children and age 11 for female children. (For this reason, adolescence is often defined as including ages 11 to 18, rather than 13 to 18.) Puberty is highly child specific and can begin at various ages. A female child, for example, may experience her first menstrual period as early as age 7 or 8.

Adolescents vary significantly in their development. Those over age 15 are physically nearer to adults in terms of their vital signs but emotionally may still be children. Regardless of physical maturity, remember that teenagers as a group are "body conscious." They worry about their physical image more than any other pediatric age group. You should tactfully address their stated concerns about body integrity or disfigurement. The slightest possibility of a lasting scar may be a tremendous issue to the adolescent patient.

Although patients in this age are not yet legally adults, most consider themselves to be grown up. They take offense at the use of the word "child." They have a strong desire to be liked by their peers and to be included. Relationships with parents and caregivers may at times be strained as the adolescent demands greater independence. They value the opinions of other adolescents, especially members of the opposite sex. Generally, these patients make good historians. Do not be surprised, however, if their perception of events differs from that of their parents or caregivers.

Common illnesses and injuries in this age group include mononucleosis, asthma, auto collisions, sports injuries, drug and alcohol problems, suicide gestures, sexual abuse. Remember that pregnancy is also possible in female adolescents. When assessing teenagers, remember that vital signs will approach

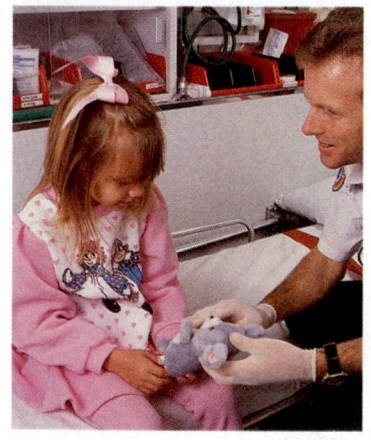

FIGURE 42-2 A small toy may calm a child in the 6–10 year age range.

those of adults. In gathering a history, be factual and address the patient's questions. It may be wise to interview the patient away from the parents or caregivers. Listen to what the teenager is saying, as well as what he or she is *not* saying. If you suspect substance abuse or endangerment of the patient or others, approach the subject with tact and compassion. If you must perform a detailed physical exam, respect the teenager's sense of privacy. If the patient exhibits modesty or bodily shame, have a paramedic of the same sex as the teenager conduct the examination, if possible. Regardless of the situation, provide psychological support and reassurance.

ANATOMY AND PHYSIOLOGY

The differences between the anatomy and physiology of infants and children and that of adults form the basis for the differences in the emergency medical care offered to the two groups (Table 42-1). As previously mentioned, children are not simply small adults. They possess bodies well suited to growth. As a rule, they have healthier organs, a greater ability to compensate for most illnesses, and softer, more flexible tissues. Because you will probably have infrequent contact with pediatric patients, you need to regularly review the physical characteristics that distinguish them from the adult patients that you encounter more often.

Table 42-1 ANATOMICAL AND PHYSIOLOGICAL CHARACTERISTICS OF INFANTS AND CHILDREN

Differences in Infants and Children as Compared to Adults	Potential Effects That May Impact Assessment and Care
Tongue proportionately larger	More likely to block airway
Smaller airway structures	More easily blocked
Abundant secretions	Can block the airway
Deciduous (baby) teeth	Easily dislodged; can block the airway
Flat nose and face	Difficult to obtain good face mask seal
Head heavier relative to body and less-developed neck structures and muscles	Head may be propelled more forcefully than body producing a higher incidence of head injury in trauma
Fontanelle and open sutures (soft spots) palpable on top of young infant's head	Bulging fontanelle can be a sign of increased intracranial pressure (but may be normal if infant is crying); shrunken fontanelle may indicate dehydration
Thinner, softer brain tissue	Susceptible to serious brain injury
Head larger in proportion to body	Tips forward when supine; possible flexion of neck, which makes neutral alignment of airway difficult
Shorter, narrower, more elastic (flexible) trachea	Can close off trachea with hyperextension of neck
Short neck	Difficult to stabilize or immobilize
Abdominal breathers	Difficult to evaluate breathing
Faster respiratory rate	Muscles easily fatigue, causing respiratory distress
Newborns breathe primarily through the nose (obligate nose breathers)	May not automatically open mouth to breathe if nose is blocked; airway more easily blocked
Larger body surface relative to body mass	Prone to hypothermia
Softer bones	More flexible, less easily fractured; traumatic forces may be transmitted to internal organs, causing injuring without fracturing the ribs; lungs easily damaged with trauma
Spleen and liver more exposed	Organ injury likely with significant force to abdomen

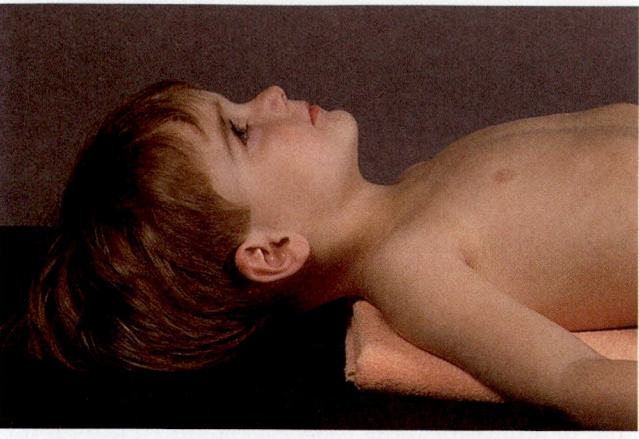

a.

b.

FIGURE 42-3   a. In the supine position, an infant's or child's larger head tips forward, causing airway obstruction. b. Placing padding under the patient's back and shoulders will bring the airway to a neutral or slightly extended position.

Head

The pediatric patient's head is proportionally larger than an adult's and the occipital region is significantly larger. In comparison to their head size, most pediatric patients have small faces and flat noses, which makes it difficult to obtain a good face mask seal.

With infants, pay special attention to the fontanelles—areas of the skull that have not yet fused. The fontanelles allow for compression of the head during childbirth and for rapid growth of the brain during early life. The posterior fontanelle generally closes by 4 months of age. The anterior fontanelle diminishes after 6 months of age and usually closes between 9 and 18 months.

During assessment, always inspect the anterior fontanelle. Normally, it should be level with the surface of the skull or slightly sunken. It also may pulsate. With increased intracranial pressure, as with meningitis or head trauma, the fontanelle may become tight and bulging and pulsations may diminish or disappear. In the presence of dehydration, the anterior fontanelle often falls below the level of the skull and appears sunken.

The heavy head relative to body size places an infant or child at risk of blunt head trauma. In accidents, the head may be propelled more forcefully than the body, resulting in a higher incidence of brain injury. Head size also affects the airway positioning techniques you should use in treating pediatric patients. In general, follow these guidelines:

- In treating seriously injured patients less than 3 years of age, place a thin layer of padding under their back to obtain a neutral position. This will prevent the head from tipping forward when supine, causing flexion of the neck (Figure 42-3).
- In treating medically ill children over 3 years of age, place a folded sheet or towel under the occiput to obtain a sniffing position (neck flexed slightly forward, head extended slightly backward to align pharynx and trachea).

In assessing infants, pay special attention to the fontanelles, especially the anterior fontanelle.

Airway

In managing the airway of an infant or child, keep in mind these anatomical and physiological considerations:

- Pediatric patients have narrower airways at all levels and these are more easily blocked by secretions or obstructions.
- Infants are obligate nose breathers. If their noses are blocked by secretions, for example, they may not automatically "know" to open their mouths to breathe.
- The tongue takes up more space proportionately in a child's mouth and can more easily obstruct breathing in an unconscious patient.
- The trachea is softer and more flexible in a child and can collapse if the neck and head are hyperextended.
- A child's larynx is higher (C-3–C-4) and extends into the pharynx.
- In young children, the cricoid ring is the narrowest part of the airway.
- Infants have an omega-shaped (horseshoe-shaped) epiglottis that extends at a 45-degree angle into the airway. Because epiglottic folds in pediatric patients have softer cartilage than in adults, they can be more floppy, especially in infants.

Take these anatomic and physiological differences into account by following these general procedures: Always keep the nares clear in infants less than 6 months of age. Do not overextend the neck, which may collapse the trachea. Open the airway gently to avoid soft-tissue injury. Because any device placed in the infant's or child's airway further narrows the passage's diameter and may result in localized swelling, consider use of an oral or a nasal airway only after other manual maneuvers have failed to keep the airway open. (There will be more information on pediatric airway management later in this chapter.)

Consider use of an oral or nasal airway in a pediatric patient only after other manual maneuvers have failed to keep the airway open.

Chest and Lungs

In evaluating the chest and lungs of an infant or child, remember that tissues and muscles are more immature than in adults. Chest muscles tire easily, and lung tissues are more fragile. The soft, pliable ribs offer less protection to organs. Expect the ribs to be positioned horizontally and the mediastinum to be more mobile.

Take into account the following anatomical and physiological considerations when assessing the chest and lungs of a pediatric patient:

- Infants and children are diaphragmatic breathers.
- Pediatric patients, especially young infants, are prone to gastric distention.
- Although rib fractures occur less frequently in children, they are not uncommon in cases of child abuse.
- Because of the softness of a child's ribs, greater energy can be transmitted to underlying organs following trauma. As a result, significant internal injury can be present without external signs.
- Pulmonary contusions are more common in pediatric patients who have been subjected to major trauma.
- An infant's or child's lungs are more prone to pneumothorax following barotrauma.

- The mediastinum of a child or infant will shift more with tension pneumothorax than in an adult.
- Thin chest walls in infants and children allow for easily transmitted breath sounds. This may result in perception of breath sounds from elsewhere in the chest, which may cause you to miss a pneumothorax or misplaced intubation.

Abdomen

Note that the liver and spleen, both very vascular organs, are proportionally larger in the pediatric patient than in the adult patient. Abdominal organs lie closer together. Because of the immature abdominal muscles in an infant or child, expect to find more frequent damage to the liver and spleen and more multiple organ injuries than in an adult.

Extremities

Until pediatric patients reach adolescence, they have softer and more porous bones than adults. Therefore, you should treat "sprains" and "strains" as fractures and immobilize them accordingly.

During early stages of development, injuries to the **growth plate** may also disrupt bone growth. Keep this in mind when inserting an intraosseous needle, which could mistakenly pierce the plate. (Intraosseous infusion is discussed later in this chapter.)

* **growth plate** the area just below the head of a long bone in which growth in bone length occurs; the epiphyseal plate.

During the early stages of development, injuries to the growth plate by an intraosseous needle may disrupt bone growth.

Skin and Body Surface Area (BSA)

There are three distinguishing features of the pediatric patient's skin and BSA. First, the skin of an infant or child is thinner than that of an adult. Second, infants and children generally have less subcutaneous fat. Finally, they have a larger body-suface-area-to-weight ratio.

As a result of these features, children risk greater injury from extremes in temperature or thermal exposure. They lose fluids and heat more quickly than adults and have a greater likelihood of dehydration and hypothermia. They also burn more easily and deeply than adults, explaining why burns account for one of the leading causes of death among pediatric trauma patients.

Respiratory System

Although infants and children have a tidal volume proportionately similar to that of adolescents and adults, they require double the metabolic oxygen. They also have proportionately smaller oxygen reserves. The combination of increased oxygen requirements and decreased oxygen reserves makes infants and children especially susceptible to hypoxia.

Cardiovascular System

Infants and children increase their cardiac output by increasing their heart rate. They have a very limited capacity to increase their stroke volume.

Cardiac output is rate dependent in infants and small children. They possess vigorous, but limited, cardiovascular reserves. Although infants and children have a circulating blood volume proportionately larger than adults, their absolute blood volume is smaller. As a result, they can maintain blood pressure longer than an adult but still be at risk of shock (hypoperfusion). In assessing a pediatric patient for shock, keep in mind the following points:

- A smaller absolute volume of fluid/blood loss is needed to cause shock in infants and children.

- A larger proportional volume of fluid/blood loss is needed to cause shock in these same patients.

- As with all categories of patients, hypotension is a late sign of shock. In pediatric patients, it is an ominous sign of imminent cardiopulmonary arrest.

- A child may be in shock despite a normal blood pressure.

- Shock assessment in children and infants is based upon clinical signs of tissue perfusion. (See the later discussion of circulation assessment.)

- Suspect shock if tachycardia is present.

- Monitor the pediatric patient carefully for the development of hypotension.

Once again, remember that children are not small adults. Bleeding that would not be dangerous in an adult may be a serious and life-threatening condition in an infant or child. Shock can develop in the small child who has a laceration to the scalp (with its many blood vessels), or in the 3-year-old who loses as little as a cup of blood. (Management of shock in pediatric patients will be discussed in detail later in the chapter.)

Bleeding that would not be dangerous in an adult may be life-threatening in an infant or child.

Nervous System

The nervous system develops continually throughout childhood. Even so, the neural tissue remains more fragile than in adults. The skull and spinal column, which are softer and more pliable than in adults, offer less protection of the brain and spinal cord. Therefore, greater force can be transmitted to a child's neural tissue with more devastating consequences. These injuries can occur without injury to the skull or to the spinal column. (Treatment of head and neck trauma will be discussed later in the chapter.)

Metabolic Differences

You may have noticed the repeated emphasis on the need to keep neonatal and pediatric patients warm during treatment and transport. The emphasis on warming techniques is based upon the following metabolic considerations:

- Infants and children have a limited store of glycogen and glucose.

- Pediatric patients are prone to hypothermia because of their greater BSA-to-weight ratio.

- Significant volume loss can result from vomiting and diarrhea.

- Newborns and neonates lack the ability to shiver.

To prevent heat loss, always cover the patient's head and maintain adequate temperature controls in the ambulance. Ensure that the ambulance is always stocked with an adequate supply of blankets and, if you live in a cold area, hot water bottles.

GENERAL APPROACH TO PEDIATRIC ASSESSMENT

Priorities in the management of the pediatric patient, as with all patients, are established on a threat-to-life basis. If life-threatening problems are not present, you will complete each of the general steps discussed in the following sections.

BASIC CONSIDERATIONS

Many of the components of the initial patient assessment can be done during a visual examination of the scene. (This is sometimes called the "assessment from the doorway," during which you quickly note signs of an ill child such as lethargy.) Whenever possible, involve the parent or caregiver in efforts to calm or comfort the child. Depending on the situation, you may decide to allow the parent or caregiver to remain with the child during treatment and transport. As previously mentioned, the developmental stage of the patient and the coping skills of the parents or guardians will be key factors in making this decision.

When interacting with parents or other responsible adults, keep in mind the communication techniques suggested earlier. Pay attention to the way in which parents or caregivers interact with the child. Are the interactions appropriate to the emergency? Are family members concerned? Are they angry? Are they overly emotional or entirely indifferent?

From the time of dispatch, you will continually acquire information relative to the patient's condition. As with all patients, personal safety must be your first priority. In treating pediatric patients, follow the same guidelines in approaching the scene as you would with any other patient. Observe for potentially hazardous situations, and make sure you take appropriate BSI precautions. Remember that infants and young children are at especially high risk of an infectious process.

Remember to take appropriate BSI precautions when treating infants and children.

SCENE SIZE-UP

Upon arrival, conduct a quick scene size-up. Dispatch information received en route, as well as your own observations, can provide critical indicators of scene safety. Be aware of the increased anxiety and stress in any situation involving an infant or child. Try to set aside thoughts of your own children and adopt the professional, systematic approach to assessment necessary for scene safety and effective patient management. If you find yourself getting angry or upset, temporarily turn over care to another paramedic until you compose yourself.

As you survey the scene, look for clues to the mechanism of injury (MOI) or the nature of the illness (NOI). These clues will help guide your assessment and determine appropriate interventions. Note the presence of dangerous substances—e.g., medicine bottles, household chemicals, or poisonous plants—that the child may have ingested. Spot environmental hazards such as unprotected stairwells, kerosene heaters, and so on. Identify possible causes of trauma, especially in motor vehicle collisions. Remain alert for evidence of child abuse, particularly in cases in which the injury and history do not coincide. As already mentioned, pay attention to the way parents or caregivers respond to the child and the way the child responds to them.

Keep the child in mind while conducting your scene size-up. Pace your approach to give the child time to adjust to your presence. Speak in a soft voice, using simple words. As soon as you reach the child, position yourself at eye level with the patient and make every effort to win his trust. If the child bonds more readily with one member of the team than another, allow that person to remain with the child and, if possible, to conduct most of the physical exam.

INITIAL ASSESSMENT

The patient's condition determines the course of your initial assessment. An active and alert child will allow for a more comfortable approach, with more time spent on communication with the child and appropriate adults. A critically ill or injured child, however, may require quick intervention and rapid transport. Your choice of action depends upon your general impression of the patient.

General Impression

The major points in forming your general impression are outlined in an assessment tool called the *pediatric assessment triangle*. Many experts recommend this assessment tool as a way of quickly evaluating the level of severity and the need for immediate intervention. It is a rapid "eyes-open, hands-on" approach that allows you to detect a life-threatening situation without the use of a stethoscope, blood pressure cuff, pulse oximeter, or other medical device. The triangle's three components are:

- *Appearance*—focuses on the child's mental status and muscle tone
- *Breathing*—directs attention to respiratory rate and respiratory effort
- *Circulation*—uses skin signs and color as well as capillary refill as indicators of the patient's circulatory status

Vital Functions

After quickly applying the pediatric assessment triangle to form a general impression, you will evaluate vital functions—mental status (level of consciousness) and the ABCs—as they apply to infants and children. Although assessment steps are basically the same as for adults, certain modifications must be made to collect accurate data.

Level of Consciousness Employ the AVPU method (*a*lert, responds to *v*erbal stimuli, responds to *p*ainful stimuli, *u*nresponsive) to evaluate the pediatric patient's level of consciousness. Adjust the techniques for the child's age. With an infant, you may need to shout to elicit a response (perhaps crying) to verbal stimulus. An infant should withdraw from a noxious stimulus. *Never shake an infant or child.*

Airway Assess the airway using the techniques shown in Figures 42-4 to 42-7. If at any point the patient shows little or no movement of air, intervene immediately. Keep this fact in mind: *Airway and respiratory problems are the most common cause of cardiac arrest in infants and young children.*

As you inspect the airway, ask yourself the following questions:

- Is the airway patent?
- Is the airway maintainable with head positioning, suctioning, or airway adjuncts?
- Is the airway *not* maintainable? If so, what action is required? (Airway management techniques are discussed later in this chapter.)

Breathing In assessing the breathing of a pediatric patient, recall the CPR certification courses in which you learned to "Look, Listen, and Feel." *Look* at the patient's chest and abdomen for movement. *Listen* for breath sounds—both normal and abnormal. *Feel* for air movement at the patient's mouth.

Keep in mind that pediatric patients have small chests. For this reason, place the stethoscope near each of the armpits in order to minimize transmitted breath

Never shake an infant or child.

Airway and respiratory problems are the most common cause of cardiac arrest in infants and young children.

FIGURE 42-4 Opening the airway in a child.

Never shake an infant or child.

sounds. When considering the respiratory rate, remember that pain or fear can increase a child's respiratory efforts. Tachypnea, an abnormally rapid rate of breathing, may indicate fear, pain, inadequate oxygenation, or, in the case of neonates, exposure to cold.

If you suspect trauma, check the infant or child for life-threatening chest injuries. Keep in mind that even a minor injury to the chest can interfere with a child's breathing efforts. A chest injury can also interfere with your effort to provide adequate oxygenation or ventilation.

FIGURE 42-5 Head-tilt/chin-lift method.

FIGURE 42-6   Jaw-thrust method.

Your goal is to identify any evidence of compromised breathing. Evaluation of breathing includes assessment of the following conditions:

- *Respiratory Rate.* Tachypnea is often the first manifestation of respiratory distress in infants. Regardless of the cause, an infant breathing at a rapid rate will eventually tire. Keep in mind that a decreasing respiratory rate may be a result of tiring and is not necessarily a sign of improvement. A slow respiratory rate in an acutely ill infant or child is an ominous sign. (Normal respiratory rates are listed in Table 42-2.) In short, be alert for a respiratory rate that is *either* abnormally fast *or* abnormally slow.

- *Respiratory Effort.* The quality of air entry can be assessed by observing for chest rise, breath sounds, stridor, or wheezing. An increased respiratory effort in the infant or child is also evidenced by

FIGURE 42-7   Assessing breathing.

Table 42-2 Normal Vital Signs: Infants and Children*

Normal Pulse Rates (Beats per Minute, at Rest)

Newborn	100 to 180
Infant (0–5 Months)	100 to 160
Infant (6–12 Months)	100 to 160
Toddler (1–3 Years)	80 to 110
Preschooler (3–5 Years)	70 to 110
School Age (6–10 Years)	65 to 110
Early Adolescence (11–14 Years)	60 to 90

Normal Respiration Rates (Breaths per Minute, at Rest)

Newborn	30 to 60
Infant (0–5 Months)	30 to 60
Infant (6–12 Months)	30 to 60
Toddler (1–3 Years)	24 to 40
Preschooler (3–5 years)	22 to 34
School Age (6–10 Years)	18 to 30
Early Adolescence (11–14 Years)	12 to 26

Normal Blood Pressure Ranges (mmHg, at Rest)

	Systolic Approx. 90 plus 2 × age	Diastolic Approx. 2/3 systolic
Preschooler (3–5 Years)	average 98 (78 to 116)	average 65
School age (6–10 Years)	average 105 (80 to 122)	average 69
Early Adolescence (11–14 Years)	average 114 (88 to 140)	average 76

*Adolescents ages 15 to 18 approach the vital signs of adults.

Note: A high pulse in an infant or child is not as great a concern as a low pulse. A low pulse may indicate imminent cardiac arrest. Blood pressure is usually not taken in a child under 3 years of age. In cases of blood loss or shock, a child's blood pressure will remain within normal limits until near the end, then fall swiftly.

nasal flaring and the use of accessory respiratory muscles. (Signs of respiratory effort are listed in Table 42-3.)

- *Color.* Cyanosis is a fairly late sign of respiratory failure and is most frequently seen in the mucous membranes of the mouth and the nail beds. Cyanosis of the extremities alone is more likely due to circulatory failure (shock) than to respiratory failure.

Circulation As mentioned earlier, you should assess a pediatric patient's circulation by first checking the child's color. Keep in mind that the pediatric patient tends to become hypothermic; therefore, you should check the capillary refill time in an area of central circulation, such as the sternum or forehead. (Note that capillary refill time, as discussed later in this chapter, is considered reliable as a sign of perfusion primarily in children less than 6 years of age.) In general, evaluate the following conditions when assessing circulation during the initial assessment:

- *Heart Rate.* As previously mentioned, infants develop sinus tachycardia in response to stress. Thus any tachycardia in an infant or child

Table 42-3	SIGNS OF INCREASED RESPIRATORY EFFORT
Retraction	Visible sinking of the skin and soft tissues of the chest around and below the ribs and above the collarbone
Nasal flaring	Widening of the nostrils; seen primarily on inspiration
Head bobbing	Observed when the head lifts and tilts back as the child inhales and then moves forward as the child exhales
Grunting	Sound heard when an infant attempts to keep the alveoli open by building back pressure during expiration
Wheezing	Passage of air over mucous secretions in bronchi; heard more commonly upon expiration; a low- or high-pitched sound
Gurgling	Coarse, abnormal bubbling sound heard in the airway during inspiration or expiration; may indicate an open chest wound
Stridor	Abnormal, musical, high-pitched sound, more commonly heard on inspiration

requires further evaluation to determine the cause. Bradycardia in a distressed infant or child may indicate hypoxia and is an ominous sign of cardiac arrest. (Normal heart rates are listed in Table 42-2.)

- *Peripheral Circulation.* The presence of peripheral pulses is a good indicator of the adequacy of end-organ perfusion. Loss of central pulses is an ominous sign.

- *End-Organ Perfusion.* End-organ perfusion is most evident in the skin, kidneys, and brain. Decreased perfusion of the skin is an early sign of shock. A capillary refill time of greater than 2 seconds is indicative of low cardiac output. Impairment of brain perfusion is usually evidenced by a change in mental status. The child may become confused or lethargic. Seizures may occur. Failure of the child to recognize the parents' faces is often an ominous sign. Urine output directly relates to kidney perfusion. Normal urine output is 1–2 mL/kg/hr. Urine flow of less than 1 mL/kg/hr is an indicator of poor renal perfusion.

Remember that evaluation of mental status and ABCs during the initial assessment is rapid and not detailed—aimed at discovering and correcting immediate life threats. More thorough measurements will be performed during the focused history and physical exam.

Anticipating Cardiopulmonary Arrest

Your initial assessment—and the repeated assessments that follow—help you to recognize and prevent cardiopulmonary arrest. At each stage of evaluating vital functions, ask yourself this question: *"Does this child have pulmonary or circulatory failure that may lead to cardiopulmonary arrest?"* Early recognition of the physiologically unstable child is one of the main goals of pediatric advanced life support (PALS). Conditions that place a pediatric patient at risk of cardiopulmonary arrest include:

At each stage of evaluating vital functions, ask yourself "Does this child have pulmonary or circulatory failure that may lead to cardiopulmonary arrest?"

- Respiratory rate greater than 60
- Heart rate greater than 180 or less than 80 (under 5 years)
- Heart rate greater than 180 or less than 60 (over 5 years)

- Respiratory distress
- Trauma
- Burns
- Cyanosis
- Altered level of consciousness
- Seizures
- Fever with petechiae (small purple spots resulting from skin hemorrhages)

Evaluate the patient for these conditions throughout assessment and transport. Cardiopulmonary arrest in infants and children is usually not a sudden event. Instead, it is the end result of progressive deterioration in respiratory and cardiac function. Therefore, you need to determine whether the patient's condition is deteriorating or improving. Any decompensation or change in the patient's status will prompt you to perform basic or advanced life support measures, as appropriate.

Transport Priority

Based on your initial assessment, you will assign the patient one of the following transport priorities:

- *Urgent*—Proceed with the rapid trauma assessment, if trauma is suspected, then transport immediately with further assessment and treatment performed en route.
- *Non-urgent*—Complete the focused history and physical exam at the scene, then transport.

Transitional Phase

The way in which the pediatric patient is transferred to EMS care depends entirely on the seriousness of the patient's condition. A transitional phase is intended for the conscious, non-acutely ill child. This phase of assessment allows the infant or child to become familiar with you and the equipment that you will be using. When dealing with the unconscious or acutely ill patient, however, you will skip this phase and proceed directly to the treatment and transport phases of assessment. In essence, you assign the patient an "urgent" status.

FOCUSED HISTORY AND PHYSICAL EXAM

After you have prioritized patient care at the end of the initial assessment, you will obtain a history and perform a physical exam. If the patient has a medical illness, the history will precede the physical exam. If the patient is suffering from trauma, the physical exam will take precedence. If partners are working together, the history and physical exam may be performed simultaneously.

History

Whenever a patient is identified as a priority patient, then the focused history will occur en route to the hospital, after essential treatments or interventions for life-threatening conditions have been performed.

To obtain a history for a pediatric patient, you will probably need to involve a family member or caregiver. Remember, however, that school-age children and adolescents like to take part in their own care. As previously mentioned, you can elicit valuable information from even very young patients. As a general precaution, question older adolescent patients in private, especially about issues such as sexual activity, pregnancy, or illicit drug and alcohol use. If you question adolescents about these subjects in the presence of an adult, they will probably be more reticent for fear of later repercussions.

As with any patient, you will use the history to uncover additional pertinent injuries or medical conditions. The history should center on the chief complaint and past medical history.

To evaluate the nature of the chief complaint, determine each of the following:

- Nature of the illness/injury
- Length of time the patient has been sick/injured
- Presence of fever
- Effects of the illness/injury on patient behavior
- Bowel/urine habits
- Presence of vomiting/diarrhea
- Frequency of urination

The past medical history identifies chronic illnesses, use of medications, and allergies. Be sure to inquire whether the infant or child is currently under a doctor's care. If so, obtain the name of the physician and present it at the receiving hospital. In the case of trauma patients, reconsider the mechanism of injury and the results of your on-scene physical examination (which, as noted earlier, will precede the history in the case of trauma).

Physical Exam

Focused Exam Carry out the physical exam after all life-threatening conditions have been identified and addressed. If there is a significant mechanism of injury or if the patient is unresponsive, perform a complete rapid trauma assessment or rapid medical assessment. Use the toe-to-head approach with the younger child (or begin with the chest and examine the head last) and the head-to-toe approach in the older child. If the injury is minor or if the ill patient is responsive, perform a physical exam that is focused on the affected areas and systems.

Perform the physical exam as described in Volume 2. Depending upon the particular situation, some or all of the following assessment techniques may be appropriate to include in the exam:

- *Pupils.* Inspect the patient's pupils for equality and reaction to light.
- *Capillary Refill.* As noted earlier, this technique is valuable for pediatric patients less than 6 years of age. Blanch the nail bed, base of the thumb, or sole of one of the feet. Remember that normal capillary refill is 2 seconds or less. Recall that this technique is less reliable in cold environments.
- *Hydration.* Note skin turgor, presence of tears and saliva and, with infants, the condition of the fontanelles.
- *Pulse Oximetry.* Use this mechanical device on moderately injured or ill infants and children. Readings will give you immediate information regarding peripheral oxygen saturation and allow you to

Table 42-4	GLASGOW COMA SCALE MODIFICATIONS FOR INFANTS	
Category	**Response**	**Score**
Verbal	Happy, coos, babbles, or cries spontaneously	5
	Irritable crying, but consolable	4
	Cries to pain, weak cry	3
	Moans to pain	2
	None	1
Motor	Spontaneous movement	6
	Withdraws to touch	5
	Withdraws to pain	4
	Abnormal flexion	3
	Abnormal extension	2
	None	1
Eye Opening (same as adult)	Spontaneous	4
	To speech	3
	To pain	2
	None	1

Source: *Adapted from James, H.E., (1986): "Neurological evaluation and support in the child with acute brain insult,"* Pediatric Annals, 15(1): 17.

Content Review

ELEMENTS OF THE GLASGOW COMA SCALE

- Verbal responses
- Motor functions
- Eye movements

In using the Glasgow coma scale with pediatric patients, you will have to make certain modifications. The younger the patient, the more adjustments you will need to make.

Remember that poorly taken vital signs are of less value than no vital signs at all.

follow trends in the patient's pulse rate and oxygenation status. Keep in mind, however, that hypothermia or shock can affect readings.

Glasgow Coma Scale In cases of trauma, you may need to apply the Glasgow coma scale (GCS)—a scoring system for monitoring the neurological status of patients with possible head injuries. The Glasgow coma scale assigns scores based on verbal responses, motor functions, and eye movements.

In using the Glasgow coma scale with pediatric patients, you will have to make certain modifications. The younger the patient, the more adjustments you will need to make. Verbal responses, for example, will not be possible for neonates and infants. However, motor function may be assessed in very young children by observing voluntary movement. Infants under 4 months of age should have a grasp reflex when an object is placed on the palmar surface of their hand. The grasp should be immediate. Children over 3 years of age will follow directions, when encouraged. Sensory function can be observed by the withdrawal reaction from "tickling" the patient. (See Table 42-4 for a modified GCS for infants.)

After you score the GCS for the patient, prioritize the patient according to severity. Guidelines are:

- *Mild*—GCS 13 to 15
- *Moderate*—GCS 9 to 12
- *Severe*—GCS less than or equal to 8

Vital Signs Remember that poorly taken vital signs are of less value than no vital signs at all. The following guidelines will help you obtain accurate pediatric readings. (Review Table 42-2 for normal pediatric vital signs.)

- Take vital signs with the patient in as close to a resting state as possible. If necessary, allow the child to calm down before attempting vital signs. Vital signs in the field should include pulse, respiration, blood pressure, and temperature.

- Obtain blood pressure with an appropriate-sized cuff. The cuff should be two-thirds the width of the upper arm. Note that the pulse pressure (the difference between the systolic and diastolic blood pressure) narrows as shock develops. *Note that hypotension is a late and often sudden sign of cardiovascular decompensation.* Even mild hypotension should be taken seriously and treated quickly and vigorously, since cardiopulmonary arrest is probably imminent.

- Feel for peripheral, brachial, or femoral pulses. There is often a significant variation in pulse rate in children due to varied respirations. Therefore, it is important to monitor the pulse for at least 30 seconds, a full minute if possible.

- It is generally not possible to weigh the child. However, if medications are required, make a good estimate of the child's weight. Often the parents or caregivers can provide a fairly reliable weight from a recent visit to the doctor.

- Observe respiratory rate before beginning the examination. After the examination is started, the child will often begin to cry. It will then be impossible to determine respiratory rate. For an estimate of the upper limit of respiratory rate, subtract the child's age from 40. It is also important to identify respiratory pattern, as well as retractions, nasal flaring, or paradoxical chest movement.

- Measure temperature early in the patient encounter and repeat toward the end. IV fluid and exposure to the environment can cause a drop in core temperature.

- Continue to observe the child for level of consciousness. There may be a wide variety in levels of consciousness and activity during treatment.

Noninvasive Monitoring Modern noninvasive monitoring devices all have their application in pediatric emergency care (Figure 42-8). These may include the pulse oximeter, automated blood pressure devices, self-registering thermometers, and ECGs. To promote the goal of early recognition of cardiopulmonary arrest, every seriously ill or injured child should receive continuous pulse oximetry. This will provide you with essential information regarding the patient's heart rate and peripheral O_2 saturation. It will also help you to monitor the effects of any medications administered. ECG and automated blood pressure/pulse monitor should also be considered. However, these devices may frighten the child. Before applying any monitoring device, explain what you are going to do. Demonstrate the display or

Even mild hypotension should be taken seriously in infants and young children.

Every seriously ill or injured child should receive continuous ECG monitoring.

FIGURE 42-8 If available, noninvasive monitoring, including pulse oximetry and temperature measurement, should be used in prehospital pediatric care.

lights. If the monitoring device makes noise, allow the child to hear the noise before you apply it. Reassure the child that the device will not hurt him.

ONGOING ASSESSMENT

Because a pediatric patient's condition can rapidly change for the better or the worse, it is necessary to repeat relevant portions of the assessment. (For this reason, ongoing assessment is sometimes called "reassessment.") You should continually monitor the patient's respiratory effort, skin color, mental status, temperature, and pulse oximetry. Retake vital signs and compare them with baseline vitals. In general, reassess stable patients every 15 minutes, critical patients every 5 minutes.

GENERAL MANAGEMENT OF PEDIATRIC PATIENTS

The same ABCs that guide the management of adult patients apply to pediatric patients: Your top priorities in treating an infant or child are airway, breathing, and circulation. However, because of the special anatomical and physiological considerations that influence the management of pediatric patients, you need to practice these skills on an ongoing and regular basis.

BASIC AIRWAY MANAGEMENT

In treating the pediatric patient, basic life support (BLS) should be applied according to current standards and protocols. BLS should include maintenance of the airway, artificial ventilation, and if required, chest compressions. (See Table 42-5.) As with all patients, your priority is to assure an open airway. The following modifications of BLS airway skills will ensure that you take into account the clinical implications of the pediatric airway.

Table 42-5	SUMMARY OF BLS MANEUVERS IN INFANTS AND CHILDREN	
Target of Maneuver	**Infant (< 1 year)**	**Child (1 to 8 years)**
Airway		
Open airway	Head tilt/chin lift (unless trauma present)	Head tilt/chin lift (unless trauma present)
	Jaw thrust	Jaw Thrust
Clear foreign body obstruction	Back blows/chest thrusts	Heimlich maneuver
Breathing		
Initial	2 breaths at 1 to 1½ seconds/breath	2 breaths at 1 to 1½ seconds/breath
Subsequent	20 breaths/minute	20 breaths/minute
Circulation		
Pulse check	Brachial/femoral	Carotid
Compression area	Lower third of sternum	Lower third of sternum
Compression width	2 or 3 fingers	Heel of 1 hand
Depth	Approximately ½ to 1 inch (Newborn ½ to ¾ inch)	Approximately 1 to 1½ inches
Rate	At least 100/minute (Newborn 120/minute)	100/minute
Compression-ventilation ratio	5:1 (Newborn 3:1)	5:1

Manual Positioning

Allow the pediatric patient to assume a position of comfort, if possible. When placing the patient in a supine position, avoid hyperextension of the neck. As previously mentioned, infants and small children risk collapsed tracheas from hyperextension of the neck. For trauma patients less than 3 years old, place support under the torso. For supine medical patients 3 years old and older, provide occipital elevation.

Foreign Body Airway Obstruction (FBAO)

Before administering treatment, determine if an airway obstruction is partial or complete. Infants or children with a partial airway obstruction will have a cough, hoarse voice or cry, stridor, or some other evidence that at least some air is passing through the airway. Avoid any maneuvers that will turn a partial obstruction into a complete obstruction. Instead, place the patient in a position of comfort and transport immediately.

In the case of complete airway obstruction, take one of the following age-specific maneuvers:

- *Children.* For children older than 1 year of age, perform a series of abdominal thrusts.
- *Infants.* For infants less than 1 year old, deliver a series of 5 back blows followed by 5 chests thrusts. Inspect the infant's mouth upon completion of each series.

As you recall from the basic CPR courses, never check a pediatric patient's mouth with blind finger sweeps.

Never use blind finger sweeps in a pediatric patient.

Suctioning

Apply suctioning whenever you detect heavy secretions in the nose or mouth of a pediatric patient, especially if the patient has a diminished level of consciousness. You can use a bulb syringe, flexible suction catheter, or rigid-tip suction catheter, depending upon the patient's age or size (Figure 42-9). Make sure that flexible catheters are correctly sized (Table 42-6).

Although pediatric suctioning techniques vary very little from adult suctioning techniques, keep the following modifications in mind:

- Decrease suction pressure to less than 100 mm/Hg in infants.

FIGURE 42-9 Pediatric-size suction catheters. Top: soft suction catheter. Bottom: rigid or hard suction catheter.

Table 42-6	SUCTION CATHETER SIZES FOR INFANTS AND CHILDREN	
Age		**Suction Catheter Size (French)**
Up to 1 Year		8
2 to 6 Years		10
7 to 15 Years		12
16 Years		12 to 14

- Avoid excessive suctioning time (suction less than 10 seconds) in order to decrease the possibility of hypoxia.
- Avoid stimulation of the vagus nerve, which may produce bradycardia. As a general rule, suction no deeper than you can see and for no more than 15 seconds per attempt.
- Frequently check the patient's pulse. If bradycardia occurs, stop suctioning immediately and oxygenate.

Oxygenation

Adequate oxygenation is the hallmark of pediatric patient management.

Adequate oxygenation is the hallmark of pediatric patient management. Methods of oxygen delivery include "blow-by" techniques (especially for neonates) and pediatric-sized nonrebreather masks. Although nonrebreather masks provide the highest concentration of supplemental oxygen, children may resist their use. Try to overcome their fear by demonstrating the use of the mask on yourself (Figure 42-10). Better yet, enlist the support of a parent or caregiver, and ask them to demonstrate the mask. As an alternative, you might place the mask over the face of a stuffed animal.

If the child refuses to accept the nonrebreather mask, resort to high-flow, blow-by oxygen. Some units place oxygen tubing through the bottom of a colorful paper cup and use it to deliver the blow-by supplemental oxygen. Children often find a familiar object less frightening than complicated medical equipment.

FIGURE 42-10   To overcome the child's fear of the nonrebreather mask, try it on yourself or have the parent try it on before attempting to place it on the child.

Airway Adjuncts

As a general rule, use airway adjuncts in pediatric patients only if prolonged artificial ventilations are required. There are two reasons for this. First, infants and children often improve quickly through the administration of 100 percent oxygen. Second, airway adjuncts may create greater complications in children than in adults. Pediatric patients risk soft-tissue damage, vomiting, and stimulation of the vagus nerve.

Use airway adjuncts in pediatric patients only if prolonged artificial ventilations are required.

Oropharyngeal Airways Oropharyngeal airways should be used only in pediatric patients who lack a gag reflex. (Patients with a gag reflex risk vomiting and bradycardia.) Size the airway by measuring from the corner of the mouth to the front of the earlobe. Remember: Oropharyngeal airways that are too small can obstruct breathing; ones that are too large can both block the airway and cause trauma. (For general sizing suggestions, see Table 42-7.)

In placing an oropharyngeal airway, use a tongue blade to depress the tongue and jaw (Figure 42-11). If you detect a gag reflex, continue to maintain an open airway with a manual maneuver (jaw-thrust or head tilt/chin lift) and consider the use of a nasal airway. Remember that with a pediatric patient, the oral airway is inserted with the tip pointing toward the tongue and pharynx.

Table 42-7 EQUIPMENT GUIDELINES ACCORDING TO AGE AND WEIGHT

Equipment	**Age (50th Percentile Weight)**					
	Premie (1–2.5 kg)	**Neonate (2.5–4.0 kg)**	**6 Months (7.0 kg)**	**1–2 Years (10–12 kg)**	**5 Years (16–18 kg)**	**5–10 Years (24–30 kg)**
Airway *Oral*	infant (00)	infant (small) (0)	small (1)	small (2)	medium (3)	medium large (4.5)
Breathing *Self-inflating bag*	infant	infant	child	child	child	child/adult
O₂ ventilation mask	premature	newborn	infant/child	child	child	small adult
Endotracheal tube	2.5–3.0 (uncuffed)	3.0–3.5 (uncuffed)	3.5–4.0 (uncuffed)	4.0–4.5 (uncuffed)	5.0–5.5 (uncuffed)	5.5–6.5 (uncuffed)
Laryngoscope blade	0 (straight)	1 (straight)	1 (straight)	1–2 (straight)	2 (straight or curved)	2–3 (straight or curved)
Suction/stylet (F)	6–8/6	8/6	8–10/6	10/6	14/14	14/14
Circulation *BP cuff*	newborn	newborn	infant	child	child	child/adult
Venous access *Angiocath*	22–24	22–24	22–24	20–22	18–20	16–20
Butterfly needle	25	23–25	23–25	23	20–23	18–21
Intracath	—	—	19	19	16	14
Arm board	6″	6″	6″–8″	8″	8″–15″	15″
Orogastric tube (F)	5	5–8	8	10	10–12	14–18
Chest tube (F)	10–14	12–18	14–20	14–24	20–32	28–38

Reproduced with permission of the American Heart Association.

FIGURE 42-11 Inserting an oropharyngeal airway in a child with the use of a tongue blade.

Nasopharyngeal Airways Use nasopharyngeal airways for those children who possess a gag reflex and who require prolonged artificial ventilations. DO NOT use them on any child with midface or head trauma. You might mistakenly pass the airway through a fracture into the sinuses or the brain.

Size a nasal airway in the same fashion as for adult patients. (Use the outside diameter of the patient's little finger as a measure.) Although nasopharyngeal airways come in a variety of sizes, they are not readily available for infants less than 1 year old. Equipment required for insertion of a nasal airway includes:

- Appropriately sized soft, flexible latex tubing
- Water-based lubricant

When inserting the nasal airway, follow the same basic method as you would in an adult patient. It is important to remember that younger children often have enlarged adenoids (lymphatic tissues in the nasopharynx) which can be easily lacerated when inserting a nasopharyngeal airway. Because of this, always use care when inserting a nasopharyngeal airway in a younger child. If resistance is met, do not force the airway as significant bleeding can result.

Ventilation

Adequate tidal volume and ventilatory rate provide more than just a high oxygen saturation for your patient. Ventilation is a two-way physiological street: Maintenance of appropriate oxygen levels results in appropriate carbon dioxide levels as well. However, you will achieve neither of these clinically important events without tailoring the ventilatory device and technique to your pediatric patient. Important points to remember include the following:

- Avoid excessive bag pressure and volume. Ventilate at an age-appropriate rate, using only enough ventilation to make the chest rise.
- Use a properly sized mask to ensure a good fit. In general, the mask should fit on the bridge of the nose and the cleft of the chin (Figure 42-12).

FIGURE 42-12   In placing a mask on a child, it should fit on the bridge of the nose and the cleft of the chin.

- Obtain a chest rise with each breath.
- Allow adequate time for exhalation.
- Assess BVM ventilation. (Provide 100 percent oxygen by using a reservoir attached to the BVM.)
- Remember that flow-restricted, oxygen-powered ventilation devices are contraindicated in pediatric resuscitation.
- Do not use BVMs with pop-off valves unless they can be readily occluded, if necessary. (Ventilatory pressures required during pediatric CPR may exceed the limit of the pop-off valve.)
- Apply cricoid pressure through application of the Sellick maneuver to minimize gastric inflation and passive regurgitation (Figure 42-13).
- Ensure correct positioning to avoid hyperextension of the neck.

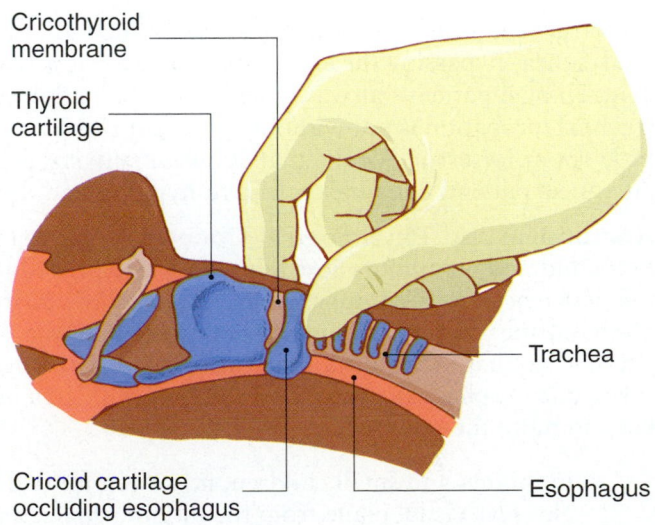

Cricothyroid membrane

Thyroid cartilage

Trachea

Cricoid cartilage occluding esophagus

Esophagus

FIGURE 42-13   In the Sellick maneuver, pressure is placed on the cricoid cartilage, compressing the esophagus. This reduces regurgitation and helps bring the vocal cords into view, which is useful if intubation is to be performed.

ADVANCED AIRWAY AND VENTILATORY MANAGEMENT

As a paramedic, you will be expected to master the advanced life support (ALS) procedures that make you a leader in the EMS system. Your clinical skills will help save the lives of pediatric patients whose respiratory systems have failed so severely that BLS measures are insufficient. When signs of impending cardiopulmonary arrest have been identified (as discussed earlier), you may be called upon to implement the following pediatric advanced life support (PALS) techniques, either in your own unit or in a transfer of care from a BLS unit. The success of these techniques requires knowledge of the procedures that set pediatric skills apart from the advanced life support skills used on adults. (Review the advanced airway skills for adults discussed in Chapter 8.)

Foreign-Body Airway Obstruction

One advantage of being able to perform endotracheal intubation is that it gives you another treatment modality for children with foreign-body airway obstructions. If a child's airway cannot be cleared by basic airway procedures, visualize the airway with the laryngoscope. Often, the obstructing foreign body can be seen. Once visualized, grasp the foreign body with the Magill forceps and remove it. If you cannot remove the foreign body with Magill forceps, try to intubate around the obstruction. This often requires using an endotracheal tube smaller than you would normally choose. However, this will provide an adequate airway until the foreign body can be removed at the hospital. Finally, if the foreign body cannot be removed with Magill forceps, and it is impossible to intubate around it, then you should consider placing a cricothyrotomy needle. This should only be done as a last resort. Be sure to follow local protocols regarding needle cricothyrotomy.

Needle Cricothyrotomy

Needle cricothyrotomy in children is the same as for adult patients (as discussed in Chapter 8). It is important to remember that the anatomical landmarks are smaller and more difficult to identify. For years it was taught that needle cricothyrotomy was contraindicated in children less than one year of age. However, current thinking is that the possible benefit (life) exceeds the risks (bleeding, local tissue damage). Remember, the only indication for cricothyrotomy is failure to obtain an airway by any other method.

Endotracheal Intubation

Endotracheal intubation allows direct visualization of the lower airway through the trachea, bypassing the entire upper airway. It is the most effective method of controlling a patient's airway, whether it be an adult or a child. However, endotracheal intubation is not without complications. It is an invasive technique with little room for error. A tube that is mistakenly sized or misplaced, especially in an apneic patient, can quickly lead to hypoxia and death.

Anatomical and Physiological Concerns Although endotracheal intubation of a child and an adult follow the same basic procedures, the special features of the pediatric airway complicate placement of any orotracheal tube. In fact, variations in the airway size of children discourage the use of certain airways, including esophageal obturator airways (EOA), pharyngeotracheal lumen airways (PtL), and esophageal-tracheal combitubes (ETC). In using an endotracheal tube, keep in mind these points:

- In infants and small children, it is often more difficult to create a single clear visual plane from the mouth, through the pharynx, and

The only indication for cricothyrotomy is failure to obtain an airway by any other method.

Remember: An endotracheal tube that is mistakenly sized or misplaced, especially in the apneic patient, can quickly lead to hypoxia and death.

Alternative airways (EOA, PtL, ETC) cannot be used in children. A properly sized laryngeal mask airway (LMA) can be used in the pediatric patient. However, you should remember that LMAs do not protect the airway from aspiration.

Table 42-8 INFANT/CHILD ENDOTRACHEAL TUBES

Age of Patient	Measurement of the Endotracheal Tube at the Teeth
6 Months to 1 Year	12 cm—teeth to mid-trachea
2 Years	14 cm—teeth to mid-trachea
4 to 6 Years	16 cm—teeth to mid-trachea
6 to 10 Years	18 cm—teeth to mid-trachea
10 to 12 Years	20 cm—teeth to mid-trachea

into the glottis. A straight-blade laryngoscope is preferred, since it provides greater displacement of the tongue and better visualization of the relatively cephalad and anterior glottis. For larger children, a curved blade may sometimes be used. (Review Table 42-7.)

- Variations in the sizes of pediatric airways, coupled with the fact that the narrowest portion of the airway is at the level of the cricoid ring, makes proper sizing of the endotracheal tube crucial. To determine correct size, apply any of the following methods:
  - Use a resuscitation tape, such as the Broselow™ tape, to estimate tube size based on height.
  - Estimate the correct tube size by using the diameter of the patient's little finger or the diameter of the nasal opening.
  - Calculate the correct tube size by using this simple numerical formula:
    (Patient's age in years + 16) ÷ 4 = Tube size

- The depth of insertion can be estimated based on age (Table 42-8). However, the best method of determining depth is direct visualization. Due to the distance between the mouth and the trachea, a stylet is rarely needed to position the tube properly. When a stylet is used, select a malleable yet rigid style.

- Because the pediatric airway narrows at the level of the cricoid cartilage, uncuffed tubes should be used in children younger than 8 years old. The tubes should display a vocal cord marker to ensure correct placement.

- Infants and small children may have greater vagal response than adults. Therefore, laryngoscopy and passage of an endotracheal tube are likely to cause a vagal response, dramatically slowing the child's heart rate and decreasing the cardiac output and blood pressure. As a result, pediatric intubations must be carried out swiftly, accurately, and with continuous monitoring.

Pediatric intubation must be carried out swiftly, accurately, and with continuous monitoring.

Indications The indications for endotracheal intubation in a pediatric patient are the same as those for an adult. They include:

- Need for prolonged artificial ventilations
- Inadequate ventilatory support with a bag-valve mask
- Cardiac or respiratory arrest
- Control of an airway in a patient without a cough or gag reflex
- Necessary for providing a route for drug administration
- Need to gain access to the airway for suctioning

Additionally, if local protocols allow it, endotracheal intubation may be used in a child who is suffering croup or epiglottitis and an increasingly compromised airway.

a.

b.

FIGURE 42-14 Placement of the laryngoscope: a. MacIntosh (curved) blade, b. Miller (straight) blade.

Techniques for Pediatric Intubation To perform endotracheal intubation on a pediatric patient, follow the basic steps in Procedure 42-1. Detailed steps include:

1. While maintaining ventilatory support, hyperventilate the patient with 100 percent oxygen. If time allows, hyperventilate for a full 2 minutes.

2. Assemble and check your equipment. As stated earlier, a straight-blade laryngoscope is preferred. Assorted sizes of endotracheal tubes, both cuffed and uncuffed, should be stocked in the pediatric kit aboard your ambulance.

3. Place the patient's head and neck into an appropriate position. With a pediatric patient, the head should be maintained in a sniffing position.

4. Hold the laryngoscope in your left hand.

5. Insert your laryngoscope blade into the right side of the patient's mouth. With a sweeping action, displace the tongue to the left.

6. Move the blade slightly toward the midline, and then advance it until the distal end is positioned at the base of the tongue (Figure 42-14).

7. Look for the tip of the epiglottis, and place the laryngoscope blade into its proper position. Keep in mind that a child—particularly an infant—has a shorter airway and a higher glottis than an adult. Because of this, you'll see the cords much sooner than you may expect.

8. With your left wrist straight, use your shoulder and arm to lift the mandible and tongue at a 45-degree angle to the floor until the glottis is exposed. Use the little finger of your left hand to apply gentle downward pressure to the cricoid cartilage. This will permit easier visualization of the cords.

42-1a   Hyperventilate the child.

42-1b   Position the head.

42-1c   Insert the laryngoscope and visualize the airway.

42-1d   Insert the tube and ventilate the child.

42-1e   Confirm tube placement.

9. Grasp the endotracheal tube in your right hand. To pass the tube into your patient's mouth, it may be helpful to hold it so that its curve is in a horizontal plane (bevel sideways). Insert the tube through the right corner of the child's mouth.

10. Under direct observation, insert the endotracheal tube into the glottic opening and pass it through until its distal cuff disappears past the vocal cords—approximately 5 to 10 cm. As a tube is advanced, it should be rotated into the proper plane. In some cases, it will be difficult to advance an endotracheal tube at the level of the cricoid. DO NOT force the tube through this region, as it may cause laryngeal edema.

11. Hold the tube in place with your left hand. Attach an infant- or child-size bag-valve device to the 15/22 mm adapter and deliver several breaths.

12. Check for proper tube placement. Watch for chest rise and fall with each ventilation and listen for equal, bilateral breath sounds. There should also be an absence of sounds over the epigastrium with ventilations. Confirm placement with an ETCO$_2$ detector.

13. If the tube has a distal cuff, inflate it with the recommended amount of air.

14. Recheck for proper placement of the tube, and hyperventilate the patient with 100% oxygen.

15. Secure the endotracheal tube with umbilical tape while maintaining ventilatory support.

16. Continue supporting the tube manually while maintaining ventilations. Check periodically to ensure proper tube position. As with adults, allow no more than 30 seconds to pass without ventilating your patient.

> *DO NOT force an endotracheal tube through the cricoid region, as it may cause laryngeal edema.*
>
>

Nasogastric Intubation

If gastric distention is present in a pediatric patient, you may consider placing a nasogastric tube (NG tube). In infants and children, gastric distention may result from overly aggressive artificial ventilations or from air swallowing. Placement of an NG tube will allow you to decompress the stomach and proximal bowel of air. An NG tube can also be used to empty the stomach of blood or other substances. Indications for use of a nasogastric intubation include:

- Inability to achieve adequate tidal volumes during ventilation due to gastric distention
- Presence of gastric distention in an unresponsive patient

As with nasopharyngeal airways, an NG tube is contraindicated in pediatric patients who have sustained head or facial trauma. Because the NG tube might migrate into the cranial sinuses, consider the use of an orogastric tube instead. Other contraindications include possible soft-tissue damage in the nose and inducement of vomiting.

Equipment for placing an NG tube includes:

- Age-appropriate NG tubes
- 20 mL syringe
- Water-soluble lubricant
- Emesis basin
- Tape

- Suctioning equipment
- Stethoscope

In sizing the NG tube, keep in mind the following recommended guidelines:

- Newborn/infant: #8.0 French
- Toddler/preschooler: #10 French
- School-age children: #12 French
- Adolescents: #14-16 French

In determining the correct length, measure the tube from the top of the nose, over the ear, to the tip of the xiphoid process. The steps for inserting the tube can be followed in Procedure 42-2. Keep in mind as you examine these steps that many experts believe that an NG tube should only be inserted when an endotracheal tube is in place. This precaution will prevent misplacement of the tube into the trachea instead of the esophagus. Consult protocols in your area on the use of NG tubes.

NG tube insertion is safest when the airway is protected with an ET tube.

Rapid Sequence Intubation

Advanced airway management may sometimes be indicated in pediatric patients with a significant level of consciousness and the presence of a gag reflex. Examples may include a combative child with head trauma or an adolescent with a drug overdose. In such cases, clenched teeth and resistance may make intubation difficult or impossible. As a result, medical direction may authorize the use of "paralytics" to induce a state of neuromuscular compliance. All skeletal muscles, including the muscles of respiration, respond to these drugs, known as neuromuscular blocking agents. Following their administration, the patient will require mechanical ventilation.

An example of a commonly used neuromuscular blocker is succinylcholine (Anectine). Typically, it is administered at 1–2 mg/kg IV push. It acts in 60–90 seconds and lasts approximately 3–5 minutes. Remember that succinylcholine has no effect on consciousness or pain. Thus, a sedative agent must be used for all children except those who are unconscious. Commonly used drugs include midazolam (Versed), diazepam (Valium), thiopental, and fentanyl. A bite block should be placed to prevent the patient from biting the endotracheal tube. Medical direction may authorize sedation to minimize the emotional trauma to the patient or drugs such as pancuronium or vecuronium if longer paralysis is required.

CIRCULATION

As mentioned earlier, the respiratory and cardiovascular systems are interdependent. In pediatrics, you are encouraged to look at the total child. You should assess the child by assessing the various body systems. For example, instead of simply checking a pulse, you should look for end-organ changes that indicate the effectiveness of respiratory and cardiovascular function. These include such things as mental status, skin color, skin temperature, urine output, and others. There are two problems that lead to cardiopulmonary arrest in children: shock and respiratory failure. Both must be identified and corrected early. The following section will address assessment of the cardiovascular system. Particular emphasis is placed on venous access and fluid resuscitation, as these are essential skills for prehospital ALS personnel who treat pediatric patients.

There are two problems that lead to cardiopulmonary arrest in children: shock and respiratory failure.

Vascular Access

Intravenous techniques for children are basically the same as for adults. (See Chapter 7.) However, additional veins may be accessed in the infant. These include veins of the neck and scalp, as well as of the arms, hands, and feet. The external jugular vein, however, should only be used for life-threatening situations.

In obtaining venous access, the external jugular vein should only be used for life-threatening situations.

42-2a Oxygenate and continue to ventilate, if possible.

42-2b Measure the NG tube from the tip of the nose, over the ear, to the tip of the xiphoid process.

42-2c Lubricate the end of the tube. Then pass it gently downward along the nasal floor to the stomach.

42-2d Ausculate over the epigastrium to confirm correct placement. Listen for bubbling while injecting 10–20 cc of air into the tube.

42-2e Use suction to aspirate stomach contents.

42-2f Secure the tube in place.

a.

b.

FIGURE 42-15 a. Intraosseous administration in the pediatric patient.
b. An intraosseous needle.

Intraosseous Infusion

The use of intraosseous (IO) infusion has become popular in the pediatric patient. (See Figure 42-15a.) This is especially true when large volumes of fluid must be administered, as occurs in hypovolemic shock, and when other means of venous access are unavailable. Certain drugs can be administered intraosseously, including epinephrine, atropine, dopamine, lidocaine, sodium bicarbonate, and dobutamine. Indications for intraosseous infusion include:

- Children less than 6 years old
- Existence of shock or cardiac arrest
- An unresponsive patient
- Unsuccessful attempts at peripheral IV insertion

The primary contraindications for IO infusion include:

- Presence of a fracture in the bone chosen for infusion
- Fracture of the pelvis or extremity fracture in the bone proximal to the chosen site

In performing IO perfusion, you can use a standard 16- or 18-gauge needle (either hypodermic or spinal). However, an intraosseous needle is preferred and significantly better (Figure 42-15b). The anterior surface of the leg below the knee should be prepped with antiseptic solution such as povidone iodine. The needle is then inserted, in a twisting fashion, 1–3 centimeters below the tuberosity. Insertion should be slightly inferior in direction (to avoid the growth plate) and perpendicular to the skin (Figure 42-16). Placement of the needle into the marrow cavity can be determined by noting a lack of resistance as the needle passes through the bony cortex. Other indications include the needle standing upright without support, the ability to aspirate bone marrow into a syringe, or free flow of the infusion without infiltration into the subcutaneous tissues. (See also the discussion of intraosseous infusion in Chapter 7.)

Fluid Therapy

The accurate dosing of fluids in children is crucial. Too much fluid can result in heart failure and pulmonary edema. Too little fluid can be ineffective.

The accurate dosing of fluids in children is crucial. Too much fluid can result in heart failure and pulmonary edema. Too little fluid can be ineffective. The initial dosage of fluid in hypovolemic shock should be 20 mL/kg of an isotonic solution such as lactated Ringer's or normal saline, as soon as IV access is obtained. After the infusion, the child should be reassessed. If perfusion is still diminished, then a second bolus of 20 mL/kg should be administered. A child with hypovolemic shock may require 40–60 mL/kg, while a child with septic shock may require at least 60–80 mL/kg. Fluid therapy should be guided by the child's clinical response.

DO NOT allow a full liter bag of fluid to be directly connected to a small child or infant without having a flow limiter attached.

Intravenous infusions in children should be closely monitored with frequent patient reassessment. Minidrip administration sets, flow limiters, or infusion pumps should be routinely used in pediatric cases.

Medications

Cardiopulmonary arrest in infants and children is almost always due to a primary respiratory problem, such as drowning, choking, or smoke inhalation. The major aim in pediatric resuscitation is airway management and ventilation, as well as replacement of intravascular volume, if indicated. In certain cases, medications may be required. The objectives of medication therapy in pediatric patients include:

- Correction of hypoxemia
- Increased perfusion pressure during chest compressions
- Stimulation of spontaneous or more forceful cardiac contractions
- Acceleration of the heart rate
- Correction of metabolic acidosis

- Suppression of ventricular ectopy
- Maintenance of renal perfusion

The dosages of medications must be modified for the pediatric patient. Tables 42-9 and 42-10 illustrate recommended pediatric drug dosage in advanced cardiac life support.

ELECTRICAL THERAPY

You are less likely to use electrical therapy on pediatric patients than adult patients. This is due to the fact that ventricular fibrillation is much less common

Table 42-9	DRUGS USED IN PEDIATRIC ADVANCED LIFE SUPPORT*	
Drug	**Dose**	**Remarks**
Adenosine	0.1 to 0.2 mg/kg Maximum strength dose 12 mg	Rapid IV bolus
Amiodarone	5 mg/kg IV/IO	Rapid IV bolus
Atropine sulfate	0.02 mg/kg per dose	Minimum dose 0.1 mg Maximum single dose: 0.5 mg in child; 1.0 mg in adolescent
Calcium chloride 10 percent	20 mg/kg per dose	Give slowly
Dopamine hydrochloride	2–10 mcg/kg per minute	Adrenergic action dominates at ≥ 15–20 mcg/kg per minute
Epinephrine *for bradycardia*	IV/IO 0.01 mg/kg (1:10,000) ET: 0.1 mg/kg (1:1,000)	Be aware of effective dose of preservatives administered (if preservatives are present in epinephrine preparation) when high doses are used
for asystolic or pulseless arrest	*First dose:* IV/IO: 0.01 mg/kg (1: 10,000) ET: 0.1 mg/kg (1:1,1000) Doses as high as 0.2 mg/kg may be effective *Subsequent doses:* IV/IO/ET: 0.1 mg/kg (1:1,000) Doses as high as 0.2 mg/kg may be effective	Be aware of effective dose of preservatives administered (if preservatives are present in epinephrine preparation) when high doses are used
Epinephrine infusion	Initial at 0.1 mcg/kg per minute Higher infusion dose used if asystole present	Titrate to desired effect (0.1–1.0 mcg/kg per minute)
Lidocaine	1 mg/kg per dose	Rapid bolus
Lidocaine infusion	20–50 mcg/kg per minute	
Sodium bicarbonate	1 mEq/kg per dose or 0.3 × kg × base deficit	Infuse slowly and only if ventilation is adequate

*IV indicates intravenous route; IO, intraosseous route; ET, endotracheal route.

Table 42-10   PREPARATION OF INFUSIONS

Drug	Preparation*	Dose
Epinephrine	0.6 × body weight (kg) equals milligrams added to diluent† to make 100 mL	Then 1 mL/h delivers 0.1 mcg/kg per minute; titrate to effect
Dopamine/ dobutamine	0.6 × body weight (kg) equals milligrams added to diluent† to make 100 mL	Then 1 mL/h delivers 0.3 mcg/kg per minute; titrate to effect
Lidocaine	120 mg of 40 mg/mL solution added to 97 mL of 5 percent dextrose in water, yielding 1200 mcg/mL solution	Then 1 mL/kg per hour delivers 20 mcg/kg per minute

*Standard concentration may be used to provide more dilute or more concentrated drug solution, but then individual dose must be calculated for each patient and each infusion rate:

$$\text{Infusion Rate (mL/h)} = \frac{\text{Weight (kg)} \times \text{Dose (mcg/kg/min)} \times 60 \text{ min/h}}{\text{Concentration (mcg/mL)}}$$

†Diluent may be 5 percent dextrose in water, 5 percent dextrose in half-normal, normal saline, or Ringer's lactate.

in children than adults. However, you should review and keep the following principles in mind for times when these emergencies arise:

- Administer an initial dosage of 2 joules per kilogram of body weight.
- If this is unsuccessful, increase the dosage to 4 joules per kilogram.
- If this is unsuccessful, focus your attention on correcting hypoxia and acidosis.
- Transport to a pediatric critical care unit, if possible.

C-SPINE IMMOBILIZATION

Any time an infant or child sustains a head injury, assume that a neck injury may also be present.

Spinal injuries in children are not as common as in adults. However, because of a child's disproportionately larger and heavier head, the cervical spine (C-spine) is vulnerable to injury. Any time an infant or child sustains a significant head injury, assume that a neck injury may also be present. Children can suffer a spinal cord injury with no noticeable damage to the vertebral column as seen on cervical spine X-rays. Thus, negative cervical spine X-rays do not necessarily assure that a spinal cord injury does not exist. Because of this, children should remain immobilized until a spinal cord injury has been excluded by hospital personnel. As previously noted, even children secured in a car safety seat can suffer neck injuries if the heads are propelled forward during an accident or sudden stop.

Always make sure that you use the appropriate-sized pediatric immobilization equipment. These supplies may include rigid cervical collars, towel or blanket rolls, foam head blocks, commercial pediatric immobilization devices, vest-type or short wooden backboards, and long boards with the appropriate padding. For pediatric patients found in car seats, you can also use the seat for immobilization. The Kendrick Extrication Device (KED) can be quickly modified to immobilize a pediatric patient. Because of the significant variations in the size of children, you must be creative in devising a plan for pediatric immobilization.

In securing the pediatric patient to the backboard, use appropriate amounts of padding to secure infants, toddlers, and preschoolers in a supine, neutral position. Never use sandbags when immobilizing a pediatric patient's head. If you must tip the board to manage vomiting, the weight of the sand bag may worsen the head injury.

Any time you immobilize a pediatric patient, remember that many children, especially those under age 5, will protest or fight restraint. Try to minimize the emotional stress by having a parent or caretaker stand near or touch the child. Often the child will quit struggling when secured totally in an immobilization device. Ideally, a rescuer or family member should remain with the child at all times to reassure and calm the child, if possible.

TRANSPORT GUIDELINES

In managing a pediatric patient, never delay transport to perform a procedure that can be done en route to the hospital. After deciding upon necessary interventions—first BLS, then ALS—determine the appropriate receiving facility. In reaching your decision, consider three factors:

In managing a pediatric patient, never delay transport to perform a procedure that can be done en route to the hospital.

- Time of transport
- Specialized facilities
- Specialized personnel

If you live in an area with specialized prehospital crews such as Critical Care Crews and Neonatal Nurses, their availability should weigh in your decision as well. Consider whether the patient would benefit by transfer by one of these crews. If so, request support. If not, determine the closest definitive care facility for the infant or child placed in your care. If time allows, continue to reduce the fear involved in transition of care from the family to the hospital. If you have won the trust of the child, and conditions permit, you might allow the patient to sit on your lap en route to the hospital (Figure 42-17). Think of what you would do or say to calm your own child or the child of a close relative or friend.

SPECIFIC MEDICAL EMERGENCIES

As you already realize from your earlier training and experience, a variety of pediatric medical problems can activate the EMS system. Although the majority of childhood medical emergencies involve the respiratory system, other body systems can be involved as well. To help you recognize and treat pediatric medical emergencies, the following sections cover some of the specific conditions you may encounter.

INFECTIONS

Childhood is a time of frequent illnesses because of the relative immaturity of the pediatric immune system. Infectious diseases may be caused by the infection or infestation of the body by an infectious agent such as a virus, bacterium, fungus, or parasite. Most infections are minor and self limiting. There are, however, several infections that can be life-threatening. These include meningitis, pneumonia, and septicemia—a systemic infection (usually bacterial) in the bloodstream.

The impact of an infection upon physiological processes depends upon the type of infectious agent and the extent of the infection. Signs and symptoms also vary, depending upon the type of infection and the time since exposure. Any of the following conditions may indicate the presence of an infection: fever, chills, tachycardia, cough, sore throat, nasal congestion, malaise, tachypnea, cool or clammy skin, petechiae, respiratory distress, poor appetite, vomiting, diarrhea, dehydration, hypoperfusion (especially with septicemia), purpura (purple blotches resulting from hemorrhages into the skin that do not disappear under pressure), seizures, severe headache, irritability, stiff neck, or bulging fontanelle (infants).

The management of infections depends upon the body system or systems affected. Treatment of some of the most common and serious infections will be found in the sections that follow. As a general rule, you should adhere to these guidelines when treating an infectious illness:

- Take all BSI precautions, due to the unknown cause of the infection.
- Become familiar with the common pediatric infections encountered in your area.
- If possible, try to determine which, if any, pediatric infections you have not been exposed to or vaccinated for. For example, if you did not have chicken pox (varicella) or measles (rubeola) as a child, and were not vaccinated for them, then you should consider receiving vaccination for these illnesses. If you encounter a child suspected of having an infectious disease to which you may be susceptible, consider allowing another rescuer to be the primary person to care for the child.

RESPIRATORY EMERGENCIES

Respiratory emergencies constitute the most common reason EMS is summoned to care for a pediatric patient. Respiratory illnesses can cause respiratory compromise due to their affect on the alveolar/capillary interface. Some illnesses are quite minor, causing only mild symptoms, while others can be rapidly fatal. Your approach to the child with a respiratory emergency will depend upon the severity of respiratory compromise. If the child is alert and talking, then you can take a more relaxed approach. However, if the child is ill-appearing and exhibiting marked respiratory difficulty, then you must immediately intervene to prevent respiratory arrest and possible cardiopulmonary arrest.

Severity of Respiratory Compromise

The severity of respiratory compromise can be quickly classified into the following categories:

- Respiratory distress
- Respiratory failure
- Respiratory arrest

Respiratory emergencies in pediatric patients may quickly progress from respiratory distress to respiratory failure to respiratory arrest. You must learn to recognize the phase your patient is in and take the appropriate interventions. Prompt recognition and treatment can literally mean the difference between life and death for an infant or child suffering from respiratory compromise.

Respiratory Distress The mildest form of respiratory impairment is classified as respiratory distress. The most noticeable finding is an increased work of breathing. One of the earliest indicators of respiratory distress is an increase in respiratory rate. Unfortunately, respiratory rate is one of the vital signs that is most often "estimated." As mentioned previously, it is essential to obtain an accurate respiratory rate in children. Ideally, the respiratory rate should be measured for an entire minute. If time does not allow it, or if the child is deteriorating, then the respiratory rate should be measured for at least 30 seconds and multiplied by two to obtain the respiratory rate.

In addition to an increased work of breathing, the child in respiratory distress will initially have a slight decrease in the arterial carbon dioxide tension as the respiratory rate increases. However, as respiratory distress increases, the carbon dioxide tension will gradually increase.

The signs and symptoms of respiratory distress include:

- Normal mental status deteriorating to irritability or anxiety
- Tachypnea
- Retractions
- Nasal flaring (in infants)
- Good muscle tone
- Tachycardia
- Head bobbing
- Grunting
- Cyanosis that improves with supplemental oxygen

If not corrected immediately, respiratory distress will lead to respiratory failure.

Respiratory Failure Respiratory failure occurs when the respiratory system is not able to meet the demands of the body for oxygen intake and for carbon dioxide removal. It is characterized by inadequate ventilation and oxygenation. During respiratory failure, the carbon dioxide level begins to rise as the body is not able to remove carbon dioxide. This ultimately leads to respiratory acidosis.

The signs and symptoms of respiratory failure include:

- Irritability or anxiety deteriorating to lethargy
- Marked tachypnea later deteriorating to bradypnea
- Marked retractions later deteriorating to agonal respirations
- Poor muscle tone
- Marked tachycardia later deteriorating to bradycardia
- Central cyanosis

Respiratory failure is a very ominous sign. If immediate intervention is not provided, the child will deteriorate to full respiratory arrest.

Respiratory Arrest The end result of respiratory impairment, if untreated, is respiratory arrest. The cessation of breathing typically follows a period of bradypnea and agonal respirations.

Prompt recognition of a respiratory emergency in an infant or child can literally mean the difference between life and death.

It is essential that you carefully count the pediatric's respiratory rate for at least 30 seconds, preferably 1 minute.

Signs and symptoms of respiratory arrest include:

- Unresponsivenes deteriorating to coma
- Bradypnea deteriorating to apnea
- Absent chest wall motion
- Bradycardia deteriorating to asystole
- Profound cyanosis

Respiratory arrest will quickly deteriorate to full cardiopulmonary arrest if appropriate interventions are not made. The child's chances of survival markedly decrease when cardiopulmonary arrest occurs.

Management of Respiratory Compromise

The management of respiratory compromise should be based upon the severity of the problem. The goals of management include increasing ventilation and increasing oxygenation. You should try to identify the signs and symptoms of respiratory distress early so that you can intervene before the child deteriorates.

Your initial attention should be directed at the airway. Is it patent? Is it maintainable with simple positioning? Is endotracheal intubation required?

After assessing the airway, assure continued maintenance of the airway by positioning, placement of an airway adjunct (oropharyngeal or nasopharyngeal airway), or endotracheal intubation.

For children in respiratory distress or early respiratory failure, administer oxygen at high flow. Some children will tolerate a nonrebreather mask. Others may not and may require that someone (perhaps a parent) hold blow-by oxygen for them to breathe. If the child fails to improve with supplemental oxygen administration, the patient should be treated more aggressively. Oftentimes it is necessary to separate the parents from the child so that you can provide the necessary care without interruption or distraction.

Pediatric patients with late respiratory failure or respiratory arrest require aggressive treatment. This includes:

- Establishment of an airway
- High-flow supplemental oxygen administration
- Mechanical ventilation with a bag-valve-mask device attached to a reservoir delivering 100% oxygen
- Endotracheal intubation if mechanical ventilation does not rapidly improve the patient's condition
- Consideration of gastric decompression with an orogastric or nasogastric tube if abdominal distension is impeding ventilation
- Consideration of needle decompression of the chest if a tension pneumothorax is thought to be present
- Consideration of cricothyrotomy if complete airway obstruction is present and the airway cannot be obtained by any other method.

In addition to the above, you should obtain venous access. The child should be promptly transported to a facility staffed and equipped to handle critically ill children. While en route, continue to reassess the child. Signs of improvement include an improvement in skin color and temperature. As end-organ perfusion improves, the child will exhibit an increase in pulse rate, an increase in oxygen saturation, and an improvement in mental status. Provide emotional and psychological support to the parents and keep them abreast of the results of your care.

SPECIFIC RESPIRATORY EMERGENCIES

Respiratory problems typically arise from obstruction of a part of the respiratory tract or impairment of the mechanics of respiration. In the following discussion we will present the common pediatric respiratory emergencies based upon the part of the airway they most affect.

Upper Airway Obstruction

Obstruction of the upper airway can be caused by many factors. As previously mentioned, upper airway obstruction may be partial or complete. It can be caused by inflamed or swollen tissues caused by infection or by an aspirated foreign body. Appropriate care depends on prompt and immediate identification of the disorder and its severity. Whenever you find an infant, toddler, or young child in respiratory or cardiac arrest, assume complete upper airway obstruction until proven otherwise.

Croup Croup, medically referred to as *laryngotracheobronchitis*, is a viral infection of the upper airway. It most commonly occurs in children 6 months to 4 years of age and is prevalent in the fall and winter. Croup causes an inflammation of the upper respiratory tract involving the subglottic region. The infection leads to edema beneath the glottis and larynx, thus narrowing the lumen of the airway. Severe cases of croup can lead to complete airway obstruction. Another form of croup called *spasmodic croup* occurs mostly in the middle of the night without any prior upper respiratory infection.

Assessment   The history for croup is fairly classic. Often, the child will have a mild cold or other infection and be doing fairly well until evening. After dark, however, a harsh, barking or brassy cough develops. The attack may subside in a few hours but can persist for several nights.

The physical exam will often reveal inspiratory stridor. There may be associated nasal flaring, tracheal tugging, or retraction. You *should never* examine the oropharynx. Often, in the prehospital setting, it is difficult to distinguish croup from **epiglottitis**. (See Table 42-11 and Figure 42-18.) If epiglottitis is present, examination of the oropharynx may result in laryngospasm and complete airway obstruction. If the attack of croup is severe and progressive, the child may develop restlessness, tachycardia, and cyanosis. Although croup can result in complete airway obstruction and respiratory arrest, this is a rare event.

Management   Management of croup consists of appropriate airway maintenance. Place the child in a position of comfort and administer cool mist oxygen at 4–6 L/minute. Oxygen can be delivered by face mask or blow-by method. If the attack is severe, the medical direction physician may order the administration of racemic epinephrine or albuterol. Some physicians also advocate the use of steroids, because they feel these drugs will shorten the course of the illness.

> *Whenever you find an infant, toddler, or young child in respiratory or cardiac arrest, assume complete upper airway obstruction until proven otherwise.*

* **croup** laryngotracheobronchitis; a common viral infection of young children, resulting in edema of the sub-glottic tissues; characterized by barking cough and inspiratory stridor.

* **epiglottitis** bacterial infection of the epiglottis, usually occurring in children older than age four; a serious medical emergency.

Table 42-11   SYMPTOMS OF CROUP AND EPIGLOTTITIS

Croup	Epiglottitis
Slow onset	Rapid onset
Generally wants to sit up	Prefers to sit up
Barking cough	No barking cough
No drooling	Drooling; painful to swallow
Fever approx. 100–101° F	Fever approx. 102–104° F
	Occasional stridor

a.   b.

FIGURE 42-18   a. Epiglottitis is characterized by inflammation of the epiglottis and supraglottic tissues. b. Croup is characterized by subglottic edema.

In preparing the patient for transport, remember that the journey from the house to the ambulance will often allow the child to breathe cool air. Because cool air causes a decrease in subglottic edema, the child may be clinically improved by the time you reach the ambulance. If appropriate, keep the parent or caregiver with the infant or child. Do not agitate the patient, which could worsen the croup, by administering nonessential measures such as IVs or blood pressure readings.

Epiglottitis   Epiglottitis is an acute infection and inflammation of the epiglottis and is potentially life-threatening. (Recall that the epiglottis is a flap of cartilage that protects the airway during swallowing.) Epiglottitis, unlike croup, is caused by a bacterial infection, usually *Hemophilus influenza* type B. Due to the availability of the *H. flu* vaccination, epiglottitis has become an uncommon occurrence. When it does occur, it tends to strike preschool and school-age children ages 3–7 years.

Assessment   Epiglottitis presents similarly to croup. Often the child will go to bed feeling relatively well, usually with what parents or caregivers consider to be a mild infection of the respiratory tract. Later, the child awakens with a high temperature and a brassy cough. The progression of symptoms can be dramatic. There is often pain upon swallowing, sore throat, high fever, shallow breathing, dyspnea, inspiratory stridor, and drooling (Figure 42-19).

On physical examination, the child will appear acutely ill and agitated. *Never attempt to visualize the airway.* If the child is crying, the tip of the epiglottis can be seen posterior to the base of the tongue. In epiglottitis, the epiglottis is cherry red and swollen. As airway obstruction develops, the child will exhibit retractions, nasal flaring, and pulmonary hyperexpansion. As the epiglottis swells, he may not be able to swallow his saliva and will begin to drool. Often the child will want to remain seated. Patients will often assume the "tripod position" to help maximize their airway. If they lean backward or lie flat, the epiglottis can fall back and completely obstruct the airway.

Management   Management of epiglottitis consists of appropriate airway maintenance and oxygen administration by face mask (Figure 42-20) or the

Never attempt to visualize the airway in patients with epiglottitis.

FIGURE 42-19   Posturing of the child with epiglottitis. Often, there will be excessive drooling.

blow-by technique. Ideally, the oxygen should be humidified to minimize drying of the epiglottis and airway. To reduce the child's anxiety, you might ask the parent or caregiver to administer the oxygen. If the airway becomes obstructed, two-rescuer ventilation with BVM is almost always effective. Make sure that all intubation equipment is available, including an appropriate-sized endotracheal tube. Remember, however, that intubation is contraindicated unless complete obstruction has occurred.

Also, do not intubate in settings with short transport times. If endotracheal intubation is required, it may be necessary to use a smaller endotracheal tube because of narrowing of the glottic opening. If you perform chest compression upon glottic visualization during intubation, a bubble at the tracheal opening may form. This may help to establish upper airway landmarks that are distorted by the disease. As a last resort, consider needle cricothyrotomy per medical direction.

Pediatric patients with epiglottitis require immediate transport. Handle the child gently, since stress could lead to total airway obstruction from spasms of the larynx and swelling tissues. Avoid IV sticks, do not take a blood pressure, and do not attempt to look into the mouth. During transport, allow the child to sit on the lap of the parent or caregiver, if appropriate. Constantly monitor the child, and notify the hospital of any changes in status. Remember, if the patient is maintaining his airway, *do not put anything in the child's mouth*, including a thermometer. At all times, consider epiglottitis a critical condition.

Do not put anything in the mouth of an epiglottitis patient, including a thermometer.

At all times, consider epiglottitis a critical condition.

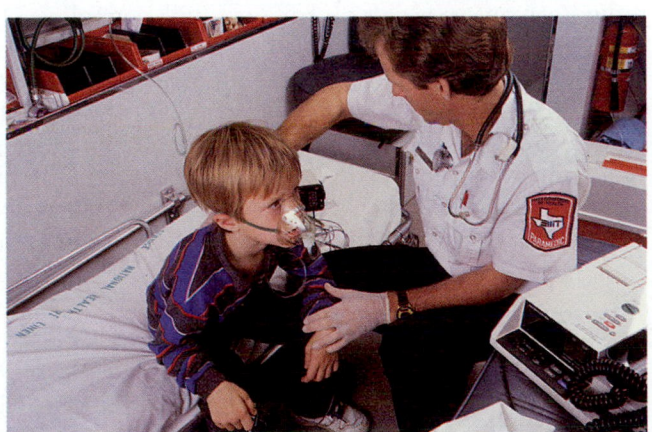

FIGURE 42-20   The child with epiglottitis should be administered humidified oxygen and transported in a comfortable position.

bacterial tracheitis bacterial infection of the airway, subglottic region; in children, most likely to appear after episodes of croup.

Bacterial Tracheitis Bacterial tracheitis is a bacterial infection of the airway, subglottic region. Although the condition is very uncommon, it is most likely to appear following episodes of viral croup. It afflicts mainly infants and toddlers 1–5 years of age.

Assessment In assessing this condition, parents or caregivers will typically report that the child has experienced an episode of croup in the preceding few days. They will also indicate the presence of a high-grade fever accompanied by coughing up of pus and/or mucus. The patient may exhibit a hoarse voice and, if able to talk, the child may complain of a sore throat. A physical examination may reveal inspiratory or expiratory stridor.

Management As with all respiratory emergencies, the child must be carefully monitored since respiratory failure or arrest may be an end result. Carefully manage airway and breathing, providing oxygenation by face mask or blow-by technique. Keep in mind that ventilations may require high pressure in order to adequately ventilate the patient. This may require depressing the pop-off valve of the pediatric bag-valve-mask device, if the valve is present. Consider intubation only in cases of complete airway obstruction. Transport guidelines are similar to those for cases of epiglottitis.

Foreign Body Aspiration Children—especially toddlers and preschoolers ages 1–4—like to put objects into their mouths. As a result, these children are at increased risk of aspirating foreign bodies, especially when they run or fall. In fact, foreign body aspiration is the number one cause of in-home accidental deaths in children under 6 years of age. In addition, many children choke on, or aspirate, food given to them by their parents or other well-meaning adults. Young children have not yet developed coordinated chewing motions in their mouth and pharynx and cannot adequately chew food. Common foods associated with aspiration and airway obstruction in children include hard candy, nuts, seeds, hot dogs, sausages, and grapes. Non-food items include coins, balloons, and other small objects.

Assessment The child with a suspected aspirated foreign body may present in one of two ways. If the obstruction is complete, the child will have minimal or no air movement. If the obstruction is partial, the child may exhibit inspiratory stridor, a muffled or hoarse voice, drooling, pain in the throat, retractions, and cyanosis.

Management Whenever you suspect that a child has aspirated a foreign body, immediately assess the patient's respiratory efforts. If the obstruction is partial, make the child as comfortable as possible and administer humidified oxygen. If old enough, place the child in a sitting position. Do not attempt to look in the mouth. Intubation equipment should be readily available since complete airway obstruction can occur. Transport the child to a hospital, where the foreign body can be removed by hospital personnel in a controlled environment.

If the obstruction is complete, clear the airway with accepted basic life support techniques. Sweep visible obstructions with your gloved finger. Do not perform blind finger sweeps, as this can push a foreign body deeper into the airway. Following BLS foreign body removal procedures, attempt ventilation with a BVM. If unsuccessful, visualize the airway with a laryngoscope. If the foreign body is seen and readily accessible, try to remove it with Magill forceps. Intubate if possible. Continue BLS foreign body removal procedures. If the airway cannot be cleared by routine measures, consider needle cricothyrotomy per medical direction and only as a last resort. Transport following appropriate guidelines, avoiding further agitation of the child.

Content Review

COMMON CAUSES OF UPPER AIRWAY OBSTRUCTIONS
- Croup
- Epiglottitis
- Bacterial tracheitis
- Foreign body aspiration

Lower Airway Distress

As already discussed, suspect lower airway distress when the following conditions exist: an absence of stridor, presence of wheezing during exhalation, and increased work of breathing. Common causes of lower airway distress include respiratory diseases such as asthma, bronchiolitis, and pneumonia. Although infrequent, you may also encounter cases of foreign body lower airway aspiration, especially in toddlers and preschoolers.

Asthma Asthma is a chronic inflammatory disorder of the lower respiratory tract. The disease affects more than 6 million Americans. It occurs before age 10 in approximately 50 percent of the cases, and before age 30 in another 33 percent of cases. The disease tends to run in families. It is also commonly associated with atopic conditions, such as eczema and allergies. Although deaths from other respiratory conditions have been steadily declining, asthmatic deaths have risen significantly in recent decades. Hospitalization of children for treatment of asthma has increased by more than 200 percent over the past 20 years. Because children can readily succumb to asthma, prompt prehospital recognition and treatment are essential.

Pathophysiology Asthma is a chronic inflammatory disorder of the airways, characterized by bronchospasm and excessive mucus production. In susceptible children, this inflammation causes widespread, but variable, airflow obstruction. In addition to airflow obstruction, the airways become hyperresponsive.

Asthma may be induced by one of many different factors, commonly called "triggers." The triggers vary from one child to the next. Common triggers include environmental allergens, cold air, exercise, foods, irritants, emotional stress, and certain medications.

Within minutes of exposure to the trigger, a two-phase reaction occurs. The first phase of the reaction is characterized by the release of chemical mediators such as histamine. These cause bronchoconstriction and bronchial edema that effectively decreases expiratory airflow, causing the classic "asthmatic attack." If treated early, asthma may respond to inhaled bronchodilators. If the attack is not aborted, or does not resolve spontaneously, a second phase may occur. The second phase is characterized by inflammation of the bronchioles as cells of the immune system invade the respiratory tract. This causes additional edema and further decreases expiratory airflow. The second phase is typically unresponsive to inhaled bronchodilators. Instead, antiinflammatory agents, such as corticosteroids, are often required.

As the attack continues, and swelling of the mucous membranes lining the bronchioles worsens, there may be plugging of the bronchi by thick mucus. This further obstructs airflow. As a result, there is an increase in sputum production. In addition, the lungs become progressively hyperinflated, since airflow is more restricted in exhalation. This effectively reduces vital capacity and results in decreased gas exchange by the alveoli, resulting in hypoxemia. If allowed to progress untreated, hypoxemia will worsen, and unconsciousness and death may ensue.

Assessment Asthma can often be differentiated from other pediatric respiratory illnesses by the history. In many cases, there is a prior history of asthma or reactive airway disease. The child's medications may also be an indicator. Children with asthma often have an inhaler or take a theophylline or oral beta agonist preparation.

On physical examination, the child is usually sitting up, leaning forward, and tachypneic. Often, there is an associated unproductive cough. Accessory respiratory muscle usage is usually evident. Wheezing may be heard. However, in a severe attack, the patient may not wheeze at all. This is an ominous finding. Some children will not wheeze, but will cough—often continuously. Generally there is associated tachycardia, and this should be monitored, since virtually all medications used to treat asthma increase the heart rate.

Management The primary therapeutic goals in the asthmatic are to correct hypoxia, reverse bronchospasm, and decrease inflammation. First, it is imperative that you establish an airway. Next, administer supplemental, humidified

* **asthma** a condition marked by recurrent attacks of dyspnea with wheezing due to spasmodic constriction of the bronchi, often as a response to allergens, or by mucous plugs in the arterial walls.

If an asthmatic attack is allowed to progress untreated, hypoxemia will worsen, and unconsciousness and death may result.

In severe asthmatic attacks, the patient may not wheeze at all. This is an ominous finding.

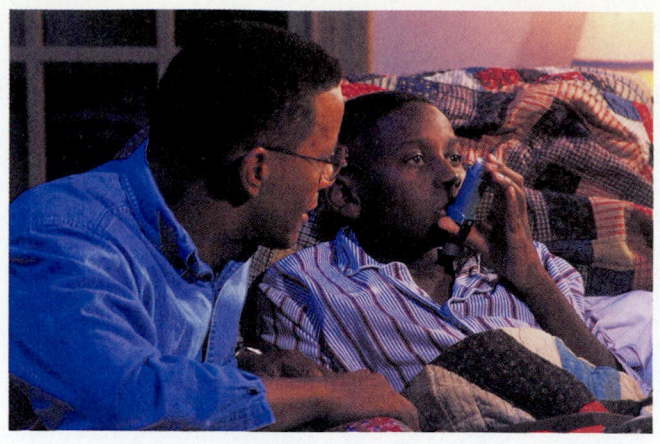

oxygen as necessary. Initial pharmacological therapy is the administration of an inhaled beta agonist (Figure 42-21). All paramedic units should have the capability of administering nebulized bronchodilator medications, such as albuterol, metaproterenol, or isoetharine. Alternatively, a metered-dose inhaler (MDI) may be used. If there is a prolonged transport time, the medical direction physician may also request administration of a steroid preparation.

Status Asthmaticus Status asthmaticus is defined as a severe, prolonged asthma attack that cannot be broken by aggressive pharmacological management. This is a serious medical emergency and prompt recognition, treatment, and transport are required. Often, the child suffering status asthmaticus will have a greatly distended chest from continued air trapping. Breath sounds, and often wheezing, may be absent. The patient is usually exhausted, severely acidotic, and often dehydrated. The management of status asthmaticus is basically the same as for asthma. However, you should recognize that respiratory arrest is imminent and remain prepared for endotracheal intubation. Transport should be immediate, with aggressive treatment continued en route.

Brochiolitis Brochiolitis is a respiratory infection of the medium-sized airways—the bronchioles—that occurs in early childhood. It should not be confused with bronchitis, which is an infection of the larger bronchi. Bronchiolitis is caused by a viral infection, most commonly *respiratory syncytial virus (RSV)*, that affects the lining of the bronchioles.

Bronchiolitis is characterized by prominent expiratory wheezing and clinically resembles asthma. It most commonly occurs in winter in children less than 2 years of age. Bronchiolitis often spreads quickly through day care and preschool facilities. Most children will develop life-long immunity to *RSV* following infection. The exception is the very young infant who has an immature immune system.

Assessment A history is necessary to distinguish bronchiolitis from asthma. Often, with bronchiolitis, there is a family history of asthma or allergies although neither is yet present in the child. In addition, there is often a low-grade fever. A major distinguishing factor is age. Asthma rarely occurs before the age of 1 year, where bronchiolitis is more frequent in this age group.

Your physical examination should be systematic. Pay particular attention to the presence of crackles or wheezes. Also, note any evidence of infection or respiratory distress.

Management Prehospital management of suspected bronchiolitis is much the same as with asthma. Place the child in a semi-sitting position, if old enough, and administer humidified oxygen by mask or blow-by method. Ventilations should be supported as necessary. Equipment for intubation should be readily

Subcutaneous epinephrine or terbutaline may be used when inhaled medications are poorly tolerated or are unavailable.

Status asthmaticus requires immediate transport with aggressive treatment administered en route.

* bronchiolitis viral infection of the medium-sized airways, occurring most frequently during the first year of life.

available. If respiratory distress is present, consider administration of a bronchodilator such as albuterol (Ventolin, Proventil) by small-volume nebulizer. The cardiac rhythm should be constantly monitored. Pulse oximetry, if available, should be used continuously.

Pneumonia Pneumonia is an infection of the lower airway and lungs. It may be caused by either a bacterium or a virus. Pneumonia can occur at any age, but in pediatric patients, it most commonly appears in infants, toddlers, and preschoolers ages 1–5 years. Most cases of pneumonia in children are viral and self-limited. As children get older, they can contract bacterial pneumonias like adults. A pneumonia vaccine is available. However, its use is reserved for patients with an immune system problem or who are asplenic.

Assessment Persons with pneumonia often have a history of a respiratory infection, such as a severe cold or bronchitis. Signs and symptoms include a low-grade fever, decreased breath sounds, crackles, rhonchi, and pain in the chest area. Conduct a systematic assessment of a patient with suspected pneumonia, paying particular attention to evidence of respiratory distress.

Management Prehospital management of pneumonia is supportive. Place the patient in a position of comfort. Assure a patent airway and administer supplemental oxygen via a nonrebreather device. If respiratory failure is present, support ventilations with a bag-valve-mask device. If prolonged ventilation will be required, perform endotracheal intubation. Transport the patient in a position of comfort. Provide emotional and psychological support to the parents.

Foreign Body Lower Airway Obstruction The same pediatric patients that are at risk from upper airway obstruction are at risk for lower airway obstruction. A foreign body can enter the lower airway if it is too small to lodge in the upper airway. The object is often food (nuts, seeds, candy), small toys, or parts of toys. The child will take a deep breath or will fall and accidentally aspirate the foreign body. The foreign body will fall into the lower airway until it reaches the airway that is smaller than the foreign body. Depending upon positioning, the foreign body can act as a one-way valve either trapping air in distal lung tissues or preventing aeration of distal lung tissues, causing a ventilation/perfusion mismatch.

Assessment There will often be a history of the child having a foreign body in the mouth and then it is gone. The parents may be unsure whether the child swallowed it, aspirated it, or simply lost the object. If the object is fairly large and aspirated, then respiratory distress may be present. There is often considerable, often intractable, coughing. The child will be anxious and may have diminished breath sounds in the part of the chest affected by the foreign body. There may be crackles or rhonchi, usually unilateral. In some cases, there may be unilateral wheezing where some air is getting past the object. Unilateral wheezing should be considered to be due to an aspirated foreign body until proven otherwise.

Management The management of an aspirated foreign body is supportive. Place the child in a position of comfort and avoid agitation. Provide supplemental oxygen. Transport the child to a facility that has the capability of performing pediatric fiber-optic bronchoscopy. The bronchoscope can be used to visualize the airway and remove any foreign objects detected.

> **Content Review**
>
> **COMMON CAUSES OF LOWER AIRWAY DISTRESS**
> - Asthma
> - Bronchiolitis
> - Pneumonia
> - Foreign body lower airway obstruction

SHOCK (HYPOPERFUSION)

The second major cause of pediatric cardiopulmonary arrest—after respiratory impairment—is shock. Shock can most simply be defined as inadequate perfusion of the tissues with oxygen and other essential nutrients and inadequate removal of metabolic waste products. This ultimately results in tissue hypoxia and metabolic acidosis. Ultimately, if untreated, cellular death will occur.

PREDISPOSING FACTORS OF PEDIATRIC SHOCK

- Hypothermia
- Dehydration (vomiting, diarrhea)
- Infection
- Trauma
- Blood loss
- Allergic reactions
- Poisoning
- Cardiac events (rare)

When compared with the incidence of shock in adults, shock is an unusual occurrence in children because their blood vessels constrict so efficiently. However, when blood pressure does drop, it drops so far and so fast that the child may quickly develop cardiopulmonary arrest. A number of factors place infants and young children at risk of shock. As mentioned in Chapter 41, newborns and neonates can develop shock as a result of a loss of body heat. Other causes include dehydration (from vomiting and/or diarrhea), infection (particularly septicemia), trauma (especially from abdominal injuries), and blood loss. Less common causes of shock in infants and children include allergic reactions, poisoning, and cardiac events (rare).

The definitive care of shock takes place in the emergency department of a hospital. Because shock is a life-threatening condition in pediatric patients, it is important to recognize early signs and symptoms—or even the possibility of shock in a situation where signs and symptoms have not yet developed. In a situation in which you suspect a possibility of shock, provide oxygen to boost tissue perfusion and transport as quickly as possible. Also, keep the patient in a supine position and take steps to protect the child from hypothermia and agitation that might worsen the condition.

The definitive care of shock takes place in the emergency department of a hospital. However, early detection of shock by EMS personnel makes sure the patient gets to the hospital.

Severity of Shock

Shock is classified by degrees of severity as compensated, decompensated, and irreversible. The child responds to decreased perfusion by increasing heart rate and by increasing peripheral vascular resistance. The child has very little capacity to increase stroke volume. The key to early identification of shock is detecting the subtle signs that result from the body's various compensatory mechanisms.

Compensated Shock Early shock is known as *compensated shock* because the body is able to compensate for decreased tissue perfusion through various physiological mechanisms. In compensated shock, the patient exhibits a normal blood pressure. The signs and symptoms of compensated shock include:

A slight increase in the heart rate is one of the earliest signs of shock.

- Irritability or anxiety
- Tachycardia
- Tachypnea
- Weak peripheral pulses, full central pulses
- Delayed capillary refill (more than 2 seconds in children less than 6 years of age)
- Cool, pale extremities
- Systolic blood pressure within normal limits
- Decreased urinary output

Compensated shock is generally reversible if appropriate treatment measures are instituted. Again, the key to a good outcome is prompt detection of the early signs and symptoms and initiation of therapy based upon this. Management is directed at correcting the underlying problem. High-flow oxygen should be administered and venous access obtained. If the patient is hypovolemic, then fluid replacement should be initiated. If the cause is cardiogenic, then medications should be administered to support cardiac output and increase peripheral vascular resistance. Sometimes definitive care of shock is surgical. However, in these cases, fluid therapy and oxygen administration will help buy time until the patient can be taken to surgery.

Decompensated Shock *Decompensated shock* develops when the body can no longer compensate for decreased tissue perfusion. The hallmark of decompen-

Rapid respiratory rate.

Absence of tears when crying.

Decreased urination.

Delayed capillary refill.

Impaired mental status or unresponsiveness.

Weak or absent peripheral pulse.

Pale, cool, clammy skin.

FIGURE 42-22   Signs and symptoms of shock (hypoperfusion) in a child.

sated shock is a fall in blood pressure (an ominous sign in children). This results in hypoperfusion and inadequate end-organ perfusion. It is important to remember that a child's compensatory mechanisms are quite efficient. Thus, when a child develops decompensated shock, there has been a significant loss of fluid or a significant impairment of cardiac output. The signs and symptoms of decompensated shock (Figure 42-22) include:

- Lethargy or coma
- Marked tachycardia or bradycardia
- Absent peripheral pulses, weak central pulses
- Markedly delayed capillary refill
- Cool, pale, dusky, mottled extremities
- Hypotension
- Markedly decreased urinary output
- Absence of tears

Decompensated shock can become irreversible if aggressive treatment measures are not undertaken. In some cases, it may be irreversible despite the fact that aggressive treatment measures have been provided. Management is directed at treatment of the underlying cause. You should have a low threshold for initiating mechanical ventilation with a bag-valve-mask device and 100% oxygen. Consider intubating the patient if mechanical ventilation will be prolonged.

Irreversible Shock   *Irreversible shock* occurs when treatment measures are inadequate or too late to prevent significant tissue damage and death. Sometimes, blood pressure and pulse can be restored. However, the patient later succumbs due to organ failure. The best treatment for irreversible shock is prevention.

Categories of Shock

There are a number of ways of categorizing shock. Shock can be categorized as *cardiogenic* (caused by impaired pumping power of the heart), *hypovolemic* (caused by decreased blood or water volume), *obstructive* (caused by an obstruction that

The hallmark of decompensated shock is a fall in blood pressure (an ominous sign in children).

The child in decompensated shock is critically ill and will rapidly die without aggressive intervention.

interferes with return of blood to the heart, such as a pulmonary embolism, cardiac tamponade, or tension pneumothorax), and *distributive* (caused by abnormal distribution and return of blood resulting from vasodilation, vasopermeability, or both, as in septic, anaphylactic, or neurogenic shock).

Often, shock is classified into two general categories—cardiogenic and noncardiogenic. As noted above, **cardiogenic shock** results from an inability of the heart to maintain an adequate cardiac output to the circulatory system and tissues. Cardiogenic shock in a pediatric patient is ominous and often fatal. **Noncardiogenic shock** includes types of shock that result from causes other than inadequate cardiac output. Causes may include hemorrhage, abdominal trauma, systemic bacterial infection, spinal cord injury, and others.

Noncardiogenic Shock

Noncardiogenic shock is more frequently encountered in prehospital pediatric care than cardiogenic shock. (Recall that children have a much lower incidence of cardiac problems than adults.) The forms that you will most commonly assess and manage are hypovolemic and distributive shock. (See also the discussion of metabolic problems in children later in the chapter.)

Hypovolemic Shock Hypovolemic shock results from loss of intravascular fluids. In pediatric patients, the most common causes include severe dehydration from vomiting and/or diarrhea and blood loss, usually as a result of trauma. Trauma may include blood loss into a body cavity (particularly the abdomen) or frank external hemorrhage. Children are also at risk of fluid loss as a result of burns, the second leading cause of pediatric deaths in the United States.

Treatment of hypovolemic shock involves administration of supplemental oxygen and establishment of intravenous access. This should be followed by a 20 mL/kg bolus of lactated Ringer's or normal saline. Following the bolus, the child should be reassessed. If signs and symptoms of compensated shock still exist, then administer a second bolus. Some children may require 80–100 mL/kg of fluid, depending upon the volume of fluid lost.

Distributive Shock Distributive shock presents with a marked decrease in peripheral vascular resistance, usually due to a loss of vasomotor tone. In pediatric patients, causes include septicemia from bacterial infection, anaphylactic reaction, and damage to the brain and/or spinal cord. Cardiac output and fluid volume are adequate.

Septic Shock   This condition is caused by sepsis, an infection of the bloodstream by some pathogen, usually bacterial. Sepsis commonly occurs as a complication of an infection at some other site such as pneumonia, an ear infection, or a urinary tract infection. Meningitis is frequently associated with sepsis. The etiology can be varied, as can be the signs and symptoms.

The septic child is critically ill. Septic shock may develop when the pathogen causing the infection releases deadly toxins. These toxins cause peripheral vasodilatation, leading to a drop in blood pressure and decreased tissue perfusion. Sepsis can be rapidly fatal if not promptly identified and treated.

Signs of sepsis include:

- Ill appearance
- Irritability or altered mental status
- Fever
- Vomiting and diarrhea
- Cyanosis, pallor, or mottled skin

* **cardiogenic shock** the inability of the heart to meet the metabolic needs of the body, resulting in inadequate tissue perfusion.

* **noncardiogenic shock** types of shock that result from causes other than inadequate cardiac output.

* **hypovolemic shock** decreased amount of intravascular fluid in the body; often due to trauma that causes blood loss into a body cavity or frank external hemorrhage; in children, can be the result of vomiting and diarrhea.

* **distributive shock** marked decrease in peripheral vascular resistance with resultant hypotension; examples include septic shock, neurogenic shock, and anaphylactic shock.

Sepsis can be rapidly fatal if not promptly identified and treated. Your goal in treating sepsis is to prevent the development of septic shock.

- Nonspecific respiratory distress
- Poor feeding

Signs and symptoms of septic shock include:

- Very ill appearance
- Altered mental status
- Tachycardia
- Capillary refill time greater than 2 seconds
- Hyperventilation, leading to respiratory failure
- Cool and clammy skin
- Inability of child to recognize parents

Your goal in treating sepsis is to prevent the development of septic shock. Supplemental oxygen should be administered and intravenous access obtained. Administer a 20 mL/kg bolus of lactated Ringer's or normal saline. Consider initiating pressor therapy with dopamine. Begin at 2 mcg/kg/minute and gradually increase the dose until the blood pressure improves or there is evidence of improved end-organ perfusion. Definitive treatment includes antibiotics and other therapy. Transport should be rapid with care provided en route.

Anaphylactic Shock Anaphylactic shock results from exposure to an antigen to which the patient has been previously exposed. Milder cases may simply result in an allergic reaction. More severe reactions can impair tissue perfusion. This primarily occurs as a result of the release of histamine and other similar chemicals. Histamine causes peripheral vasodilation and leakage of fluid from the intravascular space into the interstitial space. Anaphylactic shock can be differentiated from a severe allergic reaction by the presence of signs and symptoms of impaired end-organ perfusion. These include:

- Tachycardia
- Tachypnea
- Wheezing
- Urticaria (hives)
- Anxiousness
- Edema
- Hypotension

Treatment of a severe allergic reaction includes administration of subcutaneous epinephrine 1:1,000 and an antihistamine. Treatment of anaphylactic shock includes supplemental oxygen administration and intravenous access. If the patient is exhibiting decompensated shock, administer epinephrine 1:10,000 intravenously and diphenhydramine (Benadryl) intravenously. Patients not exhibiting hypotension may be given an initial dose of epinephrine subcutaneously. If this does not rapidly improve the situation, then an intravenous dose of epinephrine should be considered. Contact medical direction for additional assistance. EMS systems with long transport times may be asked to administer an initial dose of a corticosteroid such as methylprednisolone (Solu-Medrol).

Neurogenic Shock Neurogenic shock is due to sudden peripheral vasodilation resulting from interruption of nervous control of the peripheral vascular system. The most common cause is injury to the spinal cord. Cardiac output and intravascular fluid volume are usually adequate.

Septic shock kills!

The child in septic shock may require pressor therapy (dopamine or epinephrine).

Allergic reactions can usually be managed with subcutaneous epinephrine 1:1,000, while severe allergic reactions require intravenous spinephrine 1:10,000.

Treatment is directed at increasing peripheral vascular resistance. This is primarily through administration of a pressor agent such as dopamine. Care should also include stabilization of the injury and administration of supplemental oxygen.

Cardiogenic Shock

Cardiogenic shock results from inadequate cardiac output. In children, cardiogenic shock usually results from a secondary cause such as near-drowning or a toxic ingestion. Children, unlike adults, rarely have primary cardiac disease. The exceptions are congenital heart disease and cardiomyopathy.

Congenital heart disease is an abnormality or defect in the heart that is present at birth. Many congenital cardiac problems are detected at birth. However, some may not be detected until later in life. Cardiomyopathy causes a decrease in cardiac output due to impairment of cardiac muscle contraction. Dysrhythmias, although rare in children, can cause a decrease in cardiac output. Rapid dysrhythmias may impair ventricular filling and thus cause a decrease in cardiac output. Likewise, slow dysrhythmias may cause decreased cardiac output simply due to their slow rate.

In the following sections we will discuss in more detail congenital heart disease, cardiomyopathy, and dysrhythmias which, as noted, are primary causes of pediatric cardiogenic shock. Remember, however, cardiogenic shock in children most often results from secondary causes.

Congenital Heart Disease

Congenital heart disease is the primary cause of heart disease in children. As noted above, although most congenital heart problems are detected at birth, some problems may not be discovered until later in childhood. A common symptom of congenital heart disease is cyanosis. This occurs when blood going to the lungs for oxygenation mixes with blood bound for other parts of the body. This may result from holes in the internal walls of the heart or from abnormalities of the great vessels.

The child with congenital heart disease may develop respiratory distress, congestive heart failure, or a "cyanotic spell." *Cyanotic spells* occur when oxygen demand exceeds that provided by the blood. They begin as irritability, inconsolable crying, or altered mental status, and progressive cyanosis in conjunction with severe dyspnea. In severe and prolonged cases, seizures, coma, or cardiac arrest may result. Non-cyanotic problems associated with congenital heart disease include respiratory distress, tachycardia, decreased end-organ perfusion, drowsiness, fatigue, and pallor.

Treatment includes the standard primary assessment. Administer oxygen at a high concentration. If necessary, provide ventilatory support. If the patient is having a cyanotic spell, place the child in the knee-chest position facing downward. This will help increase the cardiac return. Apply the ECG monitor, and start an intravenous line at a keep-open rate. Transport immediately.

Cardiomyopathy

Cardiomyopathy is a disease or dysfunction of the cardiac muscle. Although fairly rare, cardiomyopathy can result from congenital heart disease or infection. A frequent cause of infectious cardiomyopathy is Coxsackie virus. Cardiomyopathy causes mechanical pump failure, which is usually biventricular. It often develops slowly and is not detectable until heart failure develops.

The signs and symptoms of cardiomyopathy include early fatigue, crackles, jugular venous distension, engorgement of the liver, and peripheral edema. Later, as the disease progresses, the signs and symptoms of shock can develop.

***

✱ **congenital** present at birth.

Tetralogy of Fallot, a type of congenital heart disease with a right-to-left shunt, is often characterized by cyanotic episodes ("tet" spells) which are relieved by the child squatting.

The prehospital treatment of cardiomyopathy is supportive. Supplemental oxygen should be administered via a nonrebreather mask. Fluids should be restricted. If possible, IV access should be obtained. Severe cases resulting in the development of severe dyspnea should be treated with furosemide and pressor agents (dobutamine, dopamine). The child should be transported to a facility capable of managing critically ill children. Most cases of cardiomyopathy are managed with medication. Definitive care in severe cases may include cardiac transplantation.

Dysrhythmias

Dysrhythmias in children are uncommon. When dysrhythmias occur, bradydysrhythmias are the most common. Supraventricular tachydysrhythmias are uncommon and ventricular tachydysrhythmias are very uncommon. Dysrhythmias can cause pump failure ultimately leading to cardiogenic shock. Children have a very limited capacity to increase stroke volume. The primary mechanism through which they increase cardiac output is through changes in the heart rate. The treatment of dysrhythmias is specific for the dysrhythmia in question.

Tachydysrhythmias Tachydysrhythmias are dysrhythmias in which the rate is greater than the estimated maximum normal heart rate for the child. These can result from primary cardiac disease or from secondary causes. Tachydysrhythmias from any cause are relatively uncommon in children.

Supraventricular Tachycardia True supraventricular tachycardia is a narrow complex tachycardia with a heart rate of 220 per minute or greater. Supraventricular tachycardia is typically due to a problem in the cardiac conductive system. Rarely, it can be due to a secondary cause such as drug ingestion. It is occasionally seen in infants with no prior history. The cause is uncertain but may be due to immaturity of the cardiac conductive system. Rapid heart rates often do not allow time for adequate cardiac filling, eventually causing congestive heart failure and cardiogenic shock.

The signs and symptoms of supraventricular tachycardia include irritability, poor feeding, jugular venous distension, hepatomegaly (enlarged liver), and hypotension. The ECG will show a narrow complex (supraventricular) tachycardia with a rate greater than 220 per minute. Children can often tolerate the rapid rate well.

Prehospital treatment of supraventricular tachycardia depends upon the clinical findings. Children who are tolerating the heart rate (normal blood pressure) and are stable should receive supplemental oxygen and transport. Adenosine should be considered if the child is stable. If the child is exhibiting signs of decompensation (hypotension, mental status change, poor skin color) then synchronized cardioversion should be attempted at initial dose of 0.5 to 1.0 Joules per kilogram of body weight. This can be increased to 2 Joules per kilogram if the initial shock is unsuccessful. The child should be transported to the appropriate facility.

Ventricular Tachycardia with a Pulse Ventricular tachycardia and ventricular fibrillation are exceedingly rare in children. They are occasionally seen following drowning or following a prolonged resuscitation attempt. Unlike adults, where ventricular tachydysrhythmias result from primary heart disease, ventricular tachydysrhythmias in children are almost always due to a secondary cause. The exception is structural, congenital heart disease.

The signs and symptoms of ventricular tachycardia with a pulse include poor feeding, irritability, and a rapid, wide complex tachycardia. Children are unable to tolerate this dysrhythmia very long. They soon develop signs of shock.

The prehospital management of ventricular tachycardia with a pulse include supplemental oxygen and intravenous access. Stable patients who are not hypotensive should be transported. Unstable patients (hypotension) should be aggressively

Wide-complex tachycardia should be treated with amiodarone, procainamide, or lidocaine, if stable. If unstable, go directly to synchronized cardioversion.

treated. Initially, amiodarone, procainamide, or lidocaine should be administered. However, ventricular tachycardia due to structural heart disease often does not respond to antidysrhythmic drugs. If the patient is unstable or deteriorating, administer synchronized cardioversion at 0.5—1.0 Joules/kilogram. This can be increased to 2 Joules/kilograms if needed. Transport emergently and provide care en route.

Bradydysrhythmias Bradydysrhythmias are the most common type of pediatric dysrhythmia. They most frequently result from hypoxia. Although rare, they can also result from vagal stimulation from such causes as marked gastric distension.

The signs and symptoms of bradycardia include a slow, narrow complex rhythm. The child may be lethargic or exhibiting early signs of congestive heart failure.

Stable children with bradydysrhythmias should receive supportive care. Unstable children should be ventilated with a bag-valve-mask unit and 100% oxygen. If the heart rate does not readily increase, consider endotracheal intubation. Perform chest compressions if oxygenation and ventilation do not increase the heart rate. Consider administering epinephrine or atropine down the endotracheal tube until intravenous access can be obtained. Transport emergently with care provided en route. (See the algorithm for treatment of pediatric bradycardia, Figure 42-23.)

Absent Rhythm The absence of a cardiac rhythm is an ominous finding. Most cases are asystole. However, some cases may be a very fine ventricular fibrillation. If necessary, turn up the gain on the ECG to distinguish between the two.

Asystole Asystole is the absence of a rhythm and may be the initial rhythm seen in cardiopulmonary arrest. (Remember, children rarely develop ventricular fibrillation, which is often the precursor to arrest in adults.) Bradycardias can degenerate to asystole if appropriate intervention is not provided. The mortality rate associated with asystole in children is very high.

The child with asystole is pulseless and apneic. The cardiac rhythm is a straight line that should be confirmed in two leads. Treatment is often futile. However, CPR should be initiated. The patient should be intubated and ventilated with 100% oxygen. Chest compressions should be continued. Emergency resuscitative drugs (epinephrine, atropine) should be administered through the endotracheal tube until intravenous access can be obtained. (See the algorithm for pediatric asystole and cardiac arrest, Figure 42-24.)

Ventricular Fibrillation/Pulseless Ventricular Tachycardia Ventricular fibrillation and pulseless ventricular tachycardia are functionally the same rhythm. They are exceedingly rare in children. Causes include electrocution and drug overdoses. The mortality rate is very high.

The child with ventricular fibrillation/pulseless ventricular tachycardia will be pulseless and apneic. The ECG will exhibit a wide complex tachycardia or fibrillation. In unmonitored patients, provide CPR. If the patient was monitored at the time of the arrest, then defibrillate 3 times (2 Joules/kg, then 4 Joules/kg, then repeat at 4 Joules/kg). Ventilate the patient with 100% oxygen and intubate. Continue chest compressions. Resuscitative medications (epinephrine, lidocaine, amiodarone) can be administered down the endotracheal tube until intravenous access can be obtained. Transport as soon as possible.

Pulseless Electrical Activity Pulseless electrical activity (PEA) is the presence of a cardiac rhythm without an associated pulse. This is due to noncardiogenic causes such as hypoxia, pericardial tamponade, tension pneumothorax, trauma, acidosis, hypothermia, hypoglycemia, and others.

The patient with PEA is pulseless and apneic. Resuscitation should be directed toward correcting the underlying cause. The patient should receive CPR, be intubated and ventilated, and given the standard resuscitative medications (epinephrine). Transport should be prompt with care provided en route.

PEDIATRIC BRADYCARDIA ALGORITHM

- BLS Algorithm: Assess and support ABCs as needed
- Provide oxygen
- Attach monitor/defibrillator

Is bradycardia causing severe cardiorespiratory compromise? (poor perfusion, hypertension, respiratory difficulty, altered consciousness)

No

- Observe
- Support ABCs
- Consider transfer or transport to ALS facility

Yes

Perform chest compression
  If despite oxygenation and ventilation:
- Heart rate <60/min in in infant or child *and* poor systemic perfusion

During CPR

Attempt/verify
- Tracheal intubation and vascular access

Check
- Electrode position and contact
- Paddle position and contact
- Pacer position and contact

Give
- Epinephrine every 3 to 5 minutes and consider alternate medications; epinephrine or dopamine infusions

Identify and treat possible causes
- Hypoxemia
- Hypothermia
- Head injury
- Heart block
- Heart transplant (special situation)
- Toxins/poisons/drugs

*Epinephrine**
- IV/IO: 0.01mg/kg (1:10,000; 0.1 mL/kg)
- Tracheal tube: 0.1 mg/kg (1:1000; 0.1 mL/kg)
- May repeat every 3 to 5 minutes at the same dose

*Atropine** 0.02 mg/kg (minimum dose: 0.1 mg)
- May be repeated once

Consider cardiac pacing

If pulseless arrest develops, see Pulseless Arrest Algorithm

*Give atropine first for bradycardia due to suspected increased vagal tone or primary AV block

FIGURE 42-23
Pediatric bradycardia treatment algorithm. Reproduced with permission from *Guidelines 2000 for Cardiopulmonary Resuscitation and Emergency Cardiovasular Care,* ©2000, Copyright American Heart Association.

NEUROLOGICAL EMERGENCIES

Neurological emergencies in childhood are fairly uncommon. However, seizures can and do occur in children. In fact, they are a frequent reason for summoning EMS. In addition to seizures, meningitis tends to show up more often in children than in adults. Although your chances of encountering either of these two conditions are small, both are life threatening and should be promptly identified and treated.

Seizures

Seizures result from an abnormal discharge of neurons in the brain. Many people suffer seizures and it is a common reason why EMS is summoned. People with

FIGURE 42-24 Pediatric asystole treatment algorithm. Reproduced with permission from *Guidelines 2000 for Cardiopulmonary Resuscitation and Emergency Cardiovasular Care,* ©2000, Copyright American Heart Association.

chronic seizure disorders can often control their seizures with medications. A seizure can be an exceptionally scary event for both the parents and the child. This is especially true if the child has never had a seizure before.

Although the etiology for seizures is often unknown, several risk factors have been identified. They include:

- Fever
- Hypoxia
- Infections
- Idiopathic epilepsy (epilepsy of unknown origin)
- Electrolyte disturbances
- Head trauma
- Hypoglycemia
- Toxic ingestions or exposure
- Tumor
- CNS malformations

Seizures in pediatric patients may be either partial or generalized. (Recall that generalized seizures normally do not occur during the first month of life.) Simple partial seizures, sometimes called focal motor seizures, involve sudden jerking of a particular part of the body, such as an arm or a leg. Other characteristics include lip smacking, eye blinking, staring, confusion, and lethargy. There is usually no loss of consciousness. Generalized seizures involve sudden jerking of both sides of the body, followed by tenseness and relaxation of the body. In a generalized seizure, patients typically experience a loss of consciousness.

Keep in mind that children can have **status epilepticus**—a series of one or more generalized seizures without any intervening periods of consciousness. Status epilepticus is a serious medical emergency because it involves a prolonged period of apnea, which in turn can cause hypoxia of vital brain tissues. (For more on seizures and status epilepticus, see Chapter 29.)

Most of the pediatric seizures that you will probably encounter are febrile seizures. **Febrile seizures** are those seizures that occur as a result of a sudden increase in body temperature. They occur most commonly between the ages of 6 months and 6 years. Febrile seizures seem related to the rate at which the body temperature increases, not to the degree of fever. Often, the parents or caregivers will report the recent onset of fever or cold symptoms. The diagnosis of febrile seizure should not be made in the field. All pediatric patients suffering a seizure must be transported to the hospital so that other etiologies can be excluded.

Assessment The history is a major factor in determining seizure type. Febrile seizure should be suspected if the temperature is above 103°F (39.2° C). The history of a previous seizure may suggest idiopathic epilepsy or another CNS problem. However, there is also a tendency for recurrence of febrile seizures in children.

When confronted with a seizing child, determine whether there is a history of seizures or seizures with fever. Has the child had a recent illness? Also, determine how many seizures occurred during the incident. If the child is not seizing upon arrival, elicit a description of the seizure activity. Note the condition and position of the child when found. Question parents, caregivers, or bystanders about the possibility of head injury. A history of irritability or lethargy prior to the seizure may indicate CNS infection. If possible, find out whether the child suffers from diabetes or has recently complained of a headache or a stiff neck. Note any current medications, as well as possible ingestions.

The physical examination should be systematic. Pay particular attention to the adequacy of respirations, the level of consciousness, neurological evaluation,

✳ **status epilepticus** prolonged seizure or multiple seizures with no regaining of consciousness between them.

Status epilepticus is a serious medical emergency because it involves a prolonged period of apnea, which in turn can cause hypoxia of vital brain tissues.

✳ **febrile seizures** seizures that occur as a result of a sudden increase in body temperature; occur most commonly between ages 6 months and 6 years.

The diagnosis of febrile seizure should not be made in the field.

and signs of injury. Also inspect the child for signs of dehydration. Dehydration may be evidenced by the absence of tears or, in an infant, by the presence of a sunken fontanelle.

Management Management of pediatric seizures is essentially the same as for seizing adults. Place patients on the floor or on the bed. Be sure to lay them on their side, away from the furniture. Do not restrain patients, but take steps to protect them from injury. Maintain the airway, but do not force anything, such as a bite stick, between the teeth. Administer supplemental oxygen. Then take and record all vital signs. If the patient is febrile, remove excess layers of clothing, while avoiding extreme cooling. If status epilepticus is present, institute the following steps:

Some medical directors prefer lorazepam (Ativan) as the anticonvulsant of choice for pediatrics.

- Start an IV of normal saline or lactated Ringer's and perform a glucometer evaluation.
- Administer diazepam as follows:
  - *Children 1 month to 5 years:* 0.2–0.5 mg slowly IV push every 2–5 minutes up to a maximum of 2.5 milligrams.
  - *Children 5 years and older:* 1 mg slowly IV push every 2–5 minutes to a maximum of 5 milligrams.
- Contact medical direction for additional dosing. Diazepam can be administered rectally if an IV cannot be established.
- If the seizure appears to be due to fever and a long transport time is anticipated, medical direction may request the administration of acetaminophen to lower the fever. Acetaminophen is supplied as an elixir or as suppositories. The dose should be 15 mg/kg body weight.

As mentioned previously, all pediatric patients should be transported. Reassure and support the parents or caregivers, since this is a very stressful and frightening situation for them.

Meningitis

Meningitis is an infection of the meninges, the lining of the brain and spinal cord. Meningitis can result from both bacteria and viruses. Viral meningitis is frequently called *aseptic meningitis,* since an organism cannot be routinely cultured from CSF fluid. Aseptic meningitis is generally less severe than bacterial meningitis and self-limiting. Bacterial meningitis most commonly results from *Streptococcus pneumoniae, Haemophilus influenza,* and *Neisseria meningitides.* These infections can be rapidly fatal if they are not promptly recognized and treated appropriately.

Assessment Meningitis is more common in children than in adults. Findings in the history that may suggest meningitis include a child who has been ill for one day to several days, recent ear or respiratory tract infection, high fever, lethargy or irritability, a severe headache, or a stiff neck. Infants generally do not develop a stiff neck. They will generally become lethargic and will not feed well. Some babies may simply develop a fever.

On physical examination, the child with meningitis will appear very ill. With an infant, the fontanelle may be bulging or full unless accompanied by dehydration. Extreme discomfort with movement, due to irritability of the meninges, may be present.

Be alert for rapid cardiopulmonary collapse in the child with fulminant meningitis, or severe meningitis with a rapid onset.

Management Prehospital care of the pediatric patient with meningitis is supportive. Rapidly complete the primary assessment and transport the child to the emergency department. If shock is present, treat the child with intravenous fluids (20 mL/kg) and oxygen.

Table 42-12 SIGNS AND SYMPTOMS OF DEHYDRATION

Signs/Symptoms	Mild	Moderate	Severe
Vital Signs			
Pulse	normal	increased	markedly increased
Respirations	normal	increased	tachypneic
Blood pressure	normal	normal	hypotensive
Capillary refill	normal	2–3 seconds	> 2 seconds
Mental Status	alert	irritable	lethargic
Skin	normal	dry and ashen	dry, cool, mottled
Mucous Membranes	dry	very dry	very dry/no tears

GASTROINTESTINAL EMERGENCIES

Childhood gastrointestinal problems almost always present with nausea and vomiting as a chief complaint. As a child gets older, other gastrointestinal system emergencies, such as appendicitis, become more common.

Nausea and Vomiting

Nausea and vomiting are not diseases themselves, but are symptoms of other disease processes. Virtually any medical problem can cause these conditions in an infant or child. The most common causes include fever, ear infections, and respiratory infections. In addition, many viruses and certain bacteria can infect the gastrointestinal system. These infections—collectively known as *gastroenteritis*—readily cause vomiting, diarrhea, or both.

The biggest risks associated with nausea and vomiting in children are dehydration and electrolyte abnormalities. Infants and toddlers can quickly become dehydrated from bouts of vomiting. If diarrhea or fever is also present, fluid loss is further accelerated, worsening the situation. Dehydration in infants and toddlers is more difficult to detect than in older children. (See Table 42-12 for a description of the signs and symptoms of dehydration.)

Treatment of pediatric nausea and vomiting is primarily supportive. If the child is dehydrated and unable to keep oral fluids down, intravenous fluid therapy may be indicated. Severe dehydration, as evidenced by prolonged capillary refill time, should be treated by 20 mL/kg fluid boluses of lactated Ringer's solution or 0.9 percent sodium chloride solution (normal saline).

Diarrhea

Diarrhea is a common occurrence in childhood. Often, what parents call diarrhea is actually loose bowel movements. Generally, 10 or more stools per day is considered diarrhea. As with nausea and vomiting, the main concern associated with diarrhea is dehydration. Most diarrhea is due to viral infections of the gastrointestinal system or secondary to infections elsewhere in the body. However, certain bacterial infections can cause significant, even life-threatening, diarrhea.

Treatment of the child suffering from diarrhea is primarily supportive. If dehydration is evident, administer fluids. Severe dehydration should be treated with 20 mL/kg boluses of intravenous fluids (lactated Ringer's or normal saline).

METABOLIC EMERGENCIES

Metabolic problems are uncommon in children. However, diabetes can occur in very young children. It is rarely diagnosed until the child comes to the hospital in

Vomiting and diarrhea carry the potential for dehydration and electrolyte abnormalities—serious conditions in the pediatric patient.

diabetic ketoacidosis. Diabetic children can have great swings in their blood glucose levels due to diet, growth, and physical activity. Because of this, hypoglycemia and hyperglycemia are possible. It is important to remember that very young children, unlike adults, can develop hypoglycemia without having diabetes. This can occur with severe illnesses such as meningitis and pneumonia. The following section will present the prehospital treatment of pediatric hypoglycemia and hyperglycemia.

Hypoglycemia

Hypoglycemia is an abnormally low concentration of sugar (glucose) in the blood. It is a true medical emergency that must be treated immediately. Without treatment, a low blood sugar may progress to unconsciousness and convulsions.

In the prehospital setting, hypoglycemia in pediatric patients usually occurs in newborn infants and children with Type I diabetes. Diabetic children increase their risk of hypoglycemia through overly strenuous exercise, too much insulin, and dehydration from illness. Non-diabetic children can develop hypoglycemia from physical activity, diet changes, illness, and growth.

In known diabetics or hypoglycemics, preventive steps include:

- Taking extra snacks for extra activity
- Eating immediately after taking insulin if the blood sugar is less than 100 mg/dl
- Eating regular meals
- Regularly monitoring blood sugar
- Eating an extra snack of carbohydrate and protein if the blood sugar is less than 120 mg/dl at bedtime
- Replacing carbohydrates in the meal plan with things like regular soda pop or regular popsicles on days when the child is sick

Assessment Suspect hypoglycemia when the patient exhibits signs and symptoms such as weakness, dizziness, tachypnea, tachycardia, pallor, sweating, tremors, vomiting, or altered mental status. Measure blood glucose with a glucometer, and elicit a history of conditions known to cause hypoglycemia in infants and children. Treatment should be initiated whenever you have a high index of suspicion and/or blood sugar drops below 70 mg/dl.

Management As with all patients, continually monitor the ABCs. Be sure to find out if parents or caregivers have given the patient any glucose tablets, gels, foods (cake icing, honey, maple syrup, sugar, raisins), or drinks (juice, regular soda pop, milk) to correct the situation. If so, find out what was given, how much was given, and when it was given. Take a blood glucose test, if possible.

In the conscious, alert patient, administer oral fluids with sugar or oral glucose. (Amounts are age and/or weight specific, so check with medical direction.) If there is no response, or if the patient exhibits an altered mental status, transport immediately. Consult your medical direction physician on orders for the administration of dextrose or IM glucagon. Twenty-five percent dextrose solution ($D_{25}W$) can be prepared by diluting fifty percent dextrose solution 1:1 with sterile water or saline. It is easier to dose children with this concentration and does not cause as much discomfort as with intravenous administration. Repeat blood glucose tests within 10–15 minutes of infusion or the administration of glucose.

In treating diabetic pediatric patients, remember that most children have been taught about their condition and can participate, in varying degrees, in their care. Most understand how glucometers work, for example, and can hand you a test strip (Figure 42-25). Also, they may be sensitive to their condition. So avoid labeling any tests as "good" or "bad."

FIGURE 42-25 Many diabetic children have home glucometers to test their blood glucose levels. Older children know what the readings mean and will be curious about any glucose testing device that you may use.

Hyperglycemia

Hyperglycemia is an abnormally high concentration of blood sugar. For patients with Type I diabetes, hyperglycemia may lead to dehydration and **diabetic ketoacidosis,** a very serious medical emergency. Left untreated, the condition will deteriorate to coma. Hyperglycemia and diabetic ketoacidosis are the most common findings in new-onset diabetics.

In the prehospital setting, pediatric hyperglycemia is commonly associated with Type I diabetes. Causes include:

- Eating too much food relative to injected insulin
- Missing an insulin injection
- Defective insulin pump, blockage of tubing, or disconnection of insulin pump infusion set
- Illness or stress

Hyperglycemia can occur with other severe illnesses and not necessarily mean that the child is developing diabetes mellitus.

Assessment In cases of hyperglycemia, glucose is spilled into the urine, taking water with it through osmotic diuresis. This can result in a signficant fluid loss with resultant dehydration.

Keep in mind that acidosis results from the accumulation of ketones, a by-product of fat metabolism. A continual increase in the ketones eventually leads to metabolic acidosis, which produces the fruity breath odor commonly associated with hyperglycemia. For other signs and symptoms, see Table 42-13.

As with hypoglycemia, elicit a history to determine causes linked with hyperglycemia. If possible, confirm your suspicions with blood glucose test. A blood sugar reading of greater than 200 mg/dl typically indicates hyperglycemia.

Management Carefully monitor the ABCs and vital signs. If you cannot confirm the presence of hyperglycemia with a blood glucose test, consider administering oral fluids with sugar or oral glucose in case the patient is hypoglycemic. If intravenous access is possible, consider initiating an IV of either normal saline or lactated Ringer's. Administer an IV bolus of 20 mL/kg, and repeat the bolus if the patient's vital signs do not change. Monitor the patient's mental status and be prepared to intubate if the respirations continue to decrease.

Remember this is a potentially life-threatening situation. Consult with medical direction on all actions taken and transport immediately.

✳ **hyperglycemia** abnormally high concentration of glucose in the blood.

✳ **diabetic ketoacidosis** complication of diabetes due to decreased insulin secretion or intake; characterized by high levels of blood glucose, metabolic acidosis, and, in advanced stages, coma; often referred to as diabetic coma.

Diabetic ketoacidosis is a very serious medical emergency, which may quickly deteriorate into coma.

Table 42-13	SIGNS AND SYMPTOMS OF HYPERGLYCEMIA	
Early	**Late**	**Ketoacidosis**
Increased thirst	Weakness	Continued decreased level of consciousness progressing to coma
Increased urination	Abdominal pain	
Weight loss	Generalized aches	Kussmaul respirations (deep and slow)
	Loss of appetite	Signs of dehydration
	Nausea	
	Vomiting	
	Signs of dehydration, except increased urinary output	
	Fruity breath odor	
	Tachypnea	
	Hyperventilation	
	Tachycardia	

POISONING AND TOXIC EXPOSURE

Accidental poisoning or toxic exposure is a common reason for summoning EMS. Pediatric patients account for the majority of poisonings treated by EMS. Most poisonings result from accidental ingestion of a toxic substance, usually by a young child. Toddlers and preschoolers like to taste things, especially colorful objects and substances that look like food or beverages. They also mimic their parents or caregivers, swallowing pills or drinking alcohol "just like Mommy and Daddy." Teenagers on antidepressants are also at risk of misusing or abusing their prescriptions, especially if given a one- or two-month supply of a medication.

Poisonings are the leading cause of preventable death in children under age 5. Because of their immature respiratory and cardiovascular systems, even a single pill can poison or, in some cases, kill a child. Iron-containing supplements are the leading cause of poisonings, especially in toddlers and preschoolers.

The most dangerous rooms in a house in terms of poisons are the kitchen, where household cleaners are stored, and the bathroom, where many people keep their over-the-counter and prescription medications. Garages and utility rooms also contain toxic substances, made more attractive to children when they are poured into everyday containers such as coffee cans, soda bottles, or plastic cups. Living rooms may have poisonous plants and liquor bottles.

The best way to prevent pediatric poisonings is by helping the families in your communities learn how to "poison proof" their homes. You can obtain guidelines from the Food and Drug Administration in Rockville, Maryland. Poisoning prevention should be a major goal of EMS prevention and community education programs.

Assessment Common substances involved in pediatric poisonings include:

- Alcohol, barbiturates, sedatives
- Amphetamines, cocaine, hallucinogens
- Anticholinergic agents (jimson weed, belladonna products)
- Aspirin, acetaminophen
- Lead
- Vitamins and iron-containing supplements
- Corrosives

- Digitalis and beta blockers
- Hydrocarbons
- Narcotics
- Organic solvents (inhaled)
- Organophosphates (insecticides)

Poisoning can cause many different signs and symptoms (Figure 42-26). Narcotics and some of the hydrocarbons can cause respiratory system depression. Digitalis, beta blockers, and many of the antihypertensive agents can cause circulatory depression or collapse. The central nervous system can be impaired by a great many agents, including alcohol, barbiturates, narcotics, cocaine and others. Thought and behavior can be affected by virtually any substance. Common agents include the anticholinergics, alcohol, narcotics, hydrocarbons, and many others.

POSSIBLE INDICATORS OF INGESTED POISONING IN CHILDREN

PAY PARTICULAR ATTENTION TO:

The child who has swallowed a poison before.

The level of responsiveness, including any behavioral changes (clumsiness, drowsiness, coma, convulsions, mental disturbances, confusion)

Skin and mucosa findings (color, temperature of skin, lips, mucous membranes)

Temperature, blood pressure, pulse rate, respiratory alterations

Constriction   Dilation

The size and reaction of pupils (constriction, dilation)

Mouth signs (burns, discoloration, dryness, excessive salivation, stains, characteristic breath odors, pain on swallowing)

Nausea, vomiting (Examine the vomitus. Make note of pill fragments if present.)

Diarrhea (blood present)

FIGURE 42-26   Possible indicators of ingested poisoning in children.

Aspirin, corrosives, and hydrocarbons can irritate or destroy the gastrointestinal system. Acetaminophen can cause liver necrosis and liver failure.

Management Although scenarios vary, take these general steps in managing a pediatric poisoning patient:

Responsive poisoning patient

- Administer oxygen.
- Contact medical direction and/or the poison control center.
- Consider the need for activated charcoal.
- Transport. (Be sure to take all pills, substances, and containers to the hospital.)
- Monitor the patient continuously in case the child suddenly becomes unresponsive.

Unresponsive poisoning patient

- Assure a patent airway. Apply suctioning, if necessary.
- Administer oxygen.
- Be prepared to provide artificial ventilations if respiratory failure or cardiac arrest is present.
- Contact medical direction and/or the poison control center.
- Transport.
- Monitor the patient continuously, and rule out trauma as a cause of altered mental status.

For more on poisonings and toxic exposure, see Chapter 34.

TRAUMA EMERGENCIES

Trauma is the number one cause of death in infants and children. Most pediatric injuries result from blunt trauma. As previously mentioned, children have thinner body walls that allow forces to be more readily transmitted to body contents, increasing the possibility of injury to internal tissues and organs. If you serve in an urban area, you can expect to see a higher incidence of penetrating trauma, mostly intentional and mostly from gunfire or knife wounds. There is also a significant incidence of penetrating trauma outside the cities, mostly unintentional from hunting accidents and agricultural accidents.

MECHANISMS OF INJURY

Children tend to be more susceptible to certain types of injuries than grownups. The following categories describe the most common mechanisms of injury among infants and children.

Falls

Falls are the single most common cause of injury in children (Figure 42-27). Fortunately, serious injury or death from accidental falls is relatively uncommon unless from a significant height. Falls from bicycles account for a significant number of injuries. The incidence of head injuries is declining, primarily because of bicycle safety helmets.

> **Content Review**
>
> **MOST COMMON PEDIATRIC MECHANISMS OF INJURY**
> - Falls
> - Motor vehicle collisions
> - Car vs. pedestrian collisions
> - Drownings and near-drownings
> - Penetrating injuries
> - Burns
> - Physical abuse

Motor Vehicle Collisions

Approximately 25,000 American children die annually from trauma. Approximately one-third of these die from motor vehicle collisions, making motor vehicle collisions the leading cause of traumatic death in children. In addition, motor vehicle collisions are the leading cause of permanent brain injury and the new-onset of epilepsy. Improperly seated children are at increased risk of sustaining injury or death from automobile air bags when they deploy (Figure 42-28). This is an area where EMS prevention strategies can make a difference. Public education

FIGURE 42-28   A deploying airbag can propel a child safety seat back into the vehicle's seat, seriously injuring the child secured in it.

programs on drunk driving, safe driving, air bags, and proper use of children's car seats can be a major focus of EMS personnel. Some states have given paramedics the ability to issue citations for persons who do not correctly buckle their children or place them in child safety seats.

Car vs. Pedestrian Injuries

Car versus child pedestrian injuries are more common in cities where children play close to the street. Car/pedestrian injuries are a particularly lethal form of trauma in children, as their short stature tends to push them down under the car. There are two phases of injury in car versus pedestrian accidents. The first group of injuries occur when the auto contacts the child. Because of the energy present, the child may be propelled away from the car or pushed down underneath the car. It is at this point that the second group of injuries occur as the child contacts the ground or other objects. Head and spinal injuries often occur with the secondary impact. The best treatment for car versus child pedestrian accidents is prevention. This too can be a major area of emphasis for prehospital prevention programs.

Drownings and Near-Drownings

Drowning is the third leading cause of death in children between birth and 4 years of age, with approximately 2,000 deaths occurring in the United States annually. The term *drowning* is used to describe deaths that occur within 24 hours of the accident. *Near-drowning* refers to injuries where the child did not die or where the death occurred more than 24 hours after the injury. Many children who do not die from drowning suffer severe and irreversible brain injuries as a result of anoxia. Approximately 20 to 25 percent of near-drowning survivors exhibit severe neurological deficits. The outcomes are better when the water is cold, as the body's protective mechanisms protect against brain injury.

Again, as with the other injury processes, the best treatment is prevention. EMS systems, in conjunction with local building inspectors, can inspect pools for safety. A pool should be fenced off with a gate that closes automatically. Essential rescue equipment (pole, life saver) should be immediately available and the local emergency number posted. The best time for drowning prevention is late spring and early summer. Encourage parents to enroll their children in water safety classes as soon as possible.

Penetrating Injuries

Until 20 years ago, penetrating injuries in children were fairly uncommon. Since then, an increase in violent crime (although violent crime rates have both risen and fallen within that period) has resulted in an increasing number of children sustaining penetrating trauma. Stab wounds and firearm injuries account for approximately 10–15 percent of all pediatric trauma admissions. The risk of death increases with age. Children are usually innocent victims of crimes perpetrated against adults. However, children are sometimes the intended victims of gunfire and stabbings, as in the shootings that have taken place in schools.

It is important to remember that visual inspection of external injuries does not provide adequate evaluation of internal injuries. This is especially true with high-energy, high-velocity weapons that can cause massive internal injury with only minimal external trauma.

Paramedics can play a major role in preventing pediatric shootings. During public education and community service programs, it is prudent to talk about gun safety, including such measures as using trigger locks or locking weapons in places where children cannot reach them. You might emphasize the fact that children have an uncanny ability to find and gain access to weapons that adults think they have hidden and secured. As with many other pediatric emergencies, the best treatment is prevention.

Burns

Burn injuries are the leading cause of accidental death in the home for children under 14 years of age. Children can sustain both burn injuries and smoke inhalation in house fires. Unsupervised children with matches or cigarette lighters are responsible for many fires that result in pediatric injury.

Fire prevention programs are a major area of emphasis for fire departments. The importance of smoke detectors cannot be overemphasized. Citizens should be encouraged to change the batteries in their smoke detectors when the clock is moved backwards or forwards for daylight savings time. Many fire departments and EMS systems replace smoke detector batteries as a part of their fire prevention program. Part of the fire prevention program should be specifically directed at children. It is especially important to teach children how to exit their house in case fire erupts.

Physical Abuse

Unfortunately, children are at risk for physical abuse by adults and older children. Factors leading to child abuse are known to include social phenomena such as poverty, domestic disturbances, younger-aged parents, substance abuse, and community violence. Paramedics are often the first members of the health care team to come into contact with the abused child. It is very important to not accuse the parents or to confront a suspected abuser. Instead, document all pertinent findings, treatments, and interventions and report these to the proper authorities. (Child abuse is discussed in more detail later in this chapter.)

SPECIAL CONSIDERATIONS

As mentioned previously, children are not small adults. You should keep this in mind and modify treatment accordingly. Specific items to consider include the following:

Airway Control

Special considerations are related to characteristics of the child's airway. These include the following:

- Maintain in-line stabilization in neutral instead of the sniffing position to prevent possible pinching of the trachea (Figure 42-29).
- Administer 100% oxygen to all trauma patients.
- Maintain a patent airway with suctioning and the jaw-thrust maneuver.
- Be prepared to assist ineffective respirations. Remember that airway pressures can be high in children and it may be necessary to depress the pop-off valve to ventilate the child adequately.
- Intubate the child when the airway cannot be maintained, while simultaneously maintaining cervical spine stabilization (Figure 42-30).

FIGURE 42-29 In the pediatric trauma victim, use the combination of jaw-thrust/spine stabilization maneuver to open the airway.

- A gastric tube should be placed following intubation to decompress the stomach.
- Needle cricothyrotomy is rarely indicated for traumatic upper airway obstruction.

Immobilization

Use appropriate-sized pediatric immobilization equipment including:

- Rigid cervical collar
- Towel or blanket roll
- Child safety seat
- Pediatric immobilization device

FIGURE 42-30 Simultaneous cervical spine immobilization and intubation in a pediatric patient.

- Vest-type device (KED)
- Short wooden backboard
- Straps and cravats
- Tape
- Padding

Keep infants, toddlers, and preschoolers supine with the cervical spine in a neutral in-line position by placing padding from the shoulders to the hips. (Review the discussion of pediatric immobilization earlier in this chapter.)

Fluid Management

Management of the airway and breathing takes priority over management of circulation, as circulatory compromise is less common in children than in adults. When obtaining vascular access, remember the following:

- If possible, insert a large-bore intravenous catheter into a peripheral vein.
- Do not delay transport to gain venous access.
- Intraosseous access in children less than 6 years of age is an alternative when a peripheral IV cannot be obtained.
- Administer an initial fluid bolus of 20 mL/kg of lactated Ringer's solution or normal saline.
- Reassess the vital signs and re-bolus with another 20 mL/kg if there is no improvement.
- If improvement does not occur after the second bolus, there is likely to be a significant blood loss that may require surgical intervention. Rapid transport is essential.

Pediatric Analgesia and Sedation

An often overlooked aspect of prehospital pediatric care is pain control. Many pediatric injuries are painful and analgesics are indicated. These include burns, long bone fractures, dislocations, and others. Unless there is a contraindication, pediatric patients should receive analgesics. Commonly used analgesics include meperidene, morphine, and fentanyl. It is best to avoid using the synthetic analgesics (e.g., butorphanol [Stadol], nalbuphine [Nubain]) as their effects on children are unpredictable. Also, certain pediatric emergencies may benefit from sedation. These include such problems as penetrating eye injuries, prolonged rescue from entrapment in machinery, cardioversion, and other painful procedures. Always consult medical direction if you feel pediatric analgesia or sedation may be indicated.

Traumatic Brain Injury

Children, because of the relatively large size of their head and weak neck muscles, are at increased risk for traumatic brain injury. These injuries can be devastating and are often fatal. Early recognition and aggressive management can reduce both morbidity and mortality. Pediatric head injuries can be classified as follows:

- Mild – Glasgow coma score is 13–15
- Moderate – Glasgow coma score is 9–12
- Severe – Glasgow coma score is less than or equal to 8

Traumatic head injuries can cause intracranial bleeding or swelling. This ultimately results in an increase in intracranial pressure. The signs of increased intracranial pressure can be subtle. They include:

- Elevated blood pressure
- Bradycardia
- Rapid, deep respirations progressing to slow, deep respirations
- Bulging fontanelle in infants

Increased intracranial pressure will eventually lead to herniation of a portion of the brain through the foramen magnum. This is an ominous development that is often associated with irreversible injury. Signs and symptoms of herniation include:

- Asymmetrical pupils
- Decorticate posturing
- Decerebrate posturing

Specific management of traumatic head injuries in children is similar to that for adults. As a rule, follow these steps.

- Administer a high concentration of oxygen for mild to moderate head injuries.
- Intubate children with a Glasgow coma score of less than or equal to 8 (severe head injury) and ventilate at a normal rate with 100% oxygen.
- Consider using intravenous or tracheal lidocaine prior to intubation to blunt the rise in intracranial pressure that often occurs in association with this procedure.
- Consider rapid sequence intubation (RSI) for children with a Glasgow coma score of less than or equal to 8 who have too much muscle tone to allow endotracheal intubation.

Consider hyperventilation if there is a deterioration in the child's condition as evidenced by asymmetric pupils, active seizures, or neurological posturing. Children with traumatic head injuries do best at facilities that treat a great number of children and who have pediatric neurosurgeons on staff. Consider diverting to a pediatric trauma facility if a moderate or severe traumatic head injury is present.

SPECIFIC INJURIES

As previously mentioned, more pediatric patients die of trauma than of any other cause. Statistics reveal that nearly 50 percent of these deaths occur within the first hour of injury. The quick arrival of EMS at the scene can literally mean the difference between life and death for a child. Although management of trauma is basically the same for children as adults, anatomical and physiological differences cause pediatric patients to have different patterns of injury.

Head, Face, and Neck

The majority of children who sustain multiple trauma will suffer associated head and/or neck injuries. As previously mentioned, the larger relative mass of the head and lack of neck muscle strength provide for increased momentum in acceleration-deceleration injuries and a greater stress on the cervical spine. The fulcrum of cervical mobility in the younger child is at the C2–C3 level. As a result, nearly 60 to 70 percent of pediatric fractures occur in C1–C2.

Injuries to the head are the most common cause of death in pediatric trauma victims. School-age children tend to sustain head injuries from bicycle accidents, falls from trees, or auto-pedestrian accidents. Older children most commonly suffer head injuries from sporting events. Heads injuries in all age groups may result from abuse.

In treating head injuries, remember that diffuse injuries are common in children, while focal injuries are rare. Because the skull is softer and more compliant in children than in adults, brain injuries occur more readily in infants and young children. Because of open fontanelles and sutures, infants up to an average age of 16 months may be more tolerant to an increase in intracranial pressure and can have delayed signs. (Keep this fact in mind when taking the history of children in the 1-month to 2-year age range.)

Children also frequently injure their faces. The most common facial injuries are lacerations secondary to falls. Young children are very clumsy when they first start walking. A fall onto a sharp object, such as the corner of a coffee table, can result in a laceration. Older children sustain dental injuries in falls from bicycles, skateboard accidents, fights, and sports activities.

Spinal injuries in children are not as common as in adults. However, as noted earlier, a child's proportionally larger and heavier head makes the cervical spine vulnerable to injury. Any time a child sustains a severe head injury, always assume that a neck injury may also be present.

Chest and Abdomen

Most injuries to the chest and abdomen result from blunt trauma. As noted earlier, infants and young children lack the rigid rib cages of adults. Therefore, they suffer fewer rib fractures and more intrathoracic injuries. Likewise, their relatively undeveloped abdominal musculature affords minimal protection to the viscera.

Because of the high mortality associated with blunt trauma, children with significant blunt abdominal or chest trauma should be transported immediately to a pediatric trauma center with appropriate care provided en route.

Injuries to the Chest Chest injuries are the second most common cause of pediatric trauma deaths. Because of the compliance of the chest wall, severe intrathoracic injury can be present without signs of external injury. Pneumothorax and hemothorarax can occur in the pediatric patient, especially if the mechanism of injury was a motor vehicle collision. Tension pneumothorax can also occur in children. The condition is poorly tolerated by pediatric patients and a needle thoracostomy may be lifesaving. Tension pneumothorax presents with the following signs and symptoms:

Children tend to develop pulmonary contusions, sometimes massive, following blunt trauma to the chest.

- Diminished breath sounds over the affected lung
- Shift of the trachea to the opposite side
- A progressive decrease in ventilatory compliance

Keep in mind that children with cardiac tamponade may have no physical signs of tamponade other then hypotension. Also remember that flail chest is an uncommon injury in children. When noted without a significant mechanism of injury, suspect child abuse.

Injuries to the Abdomen Significant blunt trauma to the abdomen can result in injury to the spleen or liver. In fact, the spleen is the most commonly injured organ in children. Signs and symptoms of a splenic injury include tenderness in the left upper quadrant of the abdomen, abrasions on the abdomen, and hematoma of the abdominal wall. Symptoms of liver injury include right upper quadrant abdominal pain and/or right lower chest pain. Both splenic and hepatic injuries can cause life-threatening internal hemorrhage.

In treating blunt abdominal trauma, keep in mind the small size of the pediatric abdomen. Be certain to palpate only one quadrant at a time. In cases of both chest and abdominal trauma, treat for shock with positioning, fluids, and maintenance of body temperature.

Extremities

Extremity injuries in children are typically limited to fractures and lacerations. Children rarely sustain amputations and other serious extremity injuries. An exception includes farm children who are vulnerable to becoming entangled in agricultural equipment.

The most common injuries are fractures, usually resulting from falls. Because children have more flexible bones than adults, they tend to have incomplete fractures such as **bend fractures, buckle fractures,** and **greenstick fractures.** In younger children, the bone growth plates have not yet closed. Some types of growth plate fractures can lead to permanent disability if not managed correctly.

Whenever indicated, perform splinting in order to decrease pain and prevent further injury and/or blood loss. In rare cases, the PSAG may be useful in unstable pelvic fractures with hypotension.

Burns

Burns are the second leading cause of death in children. They are the leading cause of accidental death in the home for children under 14. Burns may be chemical, thermal, or electrical. The most common type of burn injury encountered by EMS personnel is scalding. Children can scald themselves by pulling hot liquids off tables or stoves. In cases of abuse, they can be scalded by immersion in hot water.

Estimation of the burn surface area is slightly different for children than for adults (Figure 42-31). In adults, the "rule of nines" assigns 9 percent of the body surface area (BSA) to each of 11 body regions: the entire head and neck; the anterior chest; the anterior abdomen; the posterior chest; the lower back (posterior abdomen); the anterior surface of each lower extremity; the posterior surface of each lower extremity; and the entirety of each upper extremity. The remaining 1 percent is assigned to the genitalia.

In a child, the head accounts for a larger percentage of BSA while the legs make up a smaller percentage. So for children the rule of nines is modified to take away 8 percent from the lower extremities (2 percent from the front and 2 percent from the back of each leg) plus the 1 percent assigned to the adult genitalia. This 9 percent that is taken from the lower part of the body is reassigned to the head. So whereas the adult's entire head and neck are counted as 9 percent, in the child the anterior head and neck count as 9 percent and the posterior head and neck count as another 9 percent.

You can also use the child's palm as a guide (the "rule of palm"). The palm equals about 1 percent of the body surface area. You can calculate a burn area by estimating how many palm areas it equals. Usually, the rule of nines works best for more extensive burns. The rule of palm works best for less extensive ones.

Management considerations for pediatric burn patients include the following:

- Provide prompt management of the airway, as swelling can develop rapidly.
- If intubation is required, you may need to use an endotracheal tube up to two sizes smaller than normal.
- Thermally burned children are very susceptible to hypothermia. Be sure to maintain body heat.

* **bend fractures** fractures characterized by angulation and deformity in the bone without an obvious break.

* **buckle fractures** fractures characterized by a raised or bulging projection at the fracture site.

* **greenstick fractures** fractures characterized by an incomplete break in the bone.

THE RULE OF NINES

Head and neck 9%

Posterior trunk 18%

Anterior trunk 18%

Each upper extremity 9%

External genitalia 1%

Each lower extremity 18%

9%

14%

18%

14%

18%

9%

Posterior trunk 18%

FIGURE 42-31   The rule of nines helps to estimate the extent of a burn in adults and children. Note the modifications for the child.

- When treating serious electrical burn patients, suspect musculoskeletal injuries and perform spinal immobilization.

SUDDEN INFANT DEATH SYNDROME (SIDS)

Sudden infant death syndrome (SIDS) is defined as the sudden death of an infant during the first year of life from an illness of unknown etiology. The incidence of SIDS in the United States is approximately 2 deaths per 1,000 births. SIDS is the leading cause of death between 2 weeks and 1 year of age. It is responsible for a significant number of deaths between 1 month and 6 months, with peak incidence occurring at 2–4 months.

SIDS occurs most frequently in the fall and winter months. It tends to be more common in males than in females. It is more prevalent in premature and low birthweight infants, in infants of young mothers, and in infants whose mothers did not receive prenatal care. Infants of mothers who used cocaine, methadone, or heroin during pregnancy are at greater risk. Occasionally, a mild upper respiratory infection will be reported prior to the death. SIDS is not caused by external suffocation from blankets or pillows. Neither is it related to allergies to cow's milk or regurgitation and aspiration of stomach contents. It is not thought to be hereditary.

Current theories vary about the etiology of SIDS. Some authorities feel it may result from an immature respiratory center in the brain that leads the child to simply stop breathing. Others think there may be an airway obstruction in the posterior pharynx as a result of pharyngeal relaxation during sleep, a hypermobile mandible, or an enlarged tongue. Studies strongly link SIDS to a prone sleeping position. Soft bedding, waterbed mattresses, smoking in the home, and/or an overheated environment are other potential associations. A small percentage of SIDS may be abuse related.

✱ **sudden infant death syndrome (SIDS)** illness of unknown etiology that occurs during the first year of life, with the peak at ages 2–4 months.

Although research into SIDS continues, the American Academy of Pediatrics suggests that infants be placed supine unless medical conditions prevent this. In addition, the academy urges parents or caregivers to avoid placing infants in overheated environments, overwrapping them with too many clothes or blankets, smoking before and after pregnancy, and filling the crib with soft bedding.

Assessment Infants suffering SIDS have similar physical findings. From an external standpoint, there is a normal state of nutrition and hydration. The skin may be mottled. There are often frothy, occasionally blood-tinged, fluids in and around the mouth and nostrils. Vomitus may be present. Occasionally, the infant may be in an unusual position as a result of muscle spasm or high activity at the time of death. Common findings noted at autopsy include intrathoracic petechiae (small hemorrhages) in 90 percent of cases. There is often associated pulmonary congestion and edema. Sometimes, stomach contents are found in the trachea. Microscopic examination of the trachea often reveals the presence of inflammatory changes.

Management The immediate needs of the family with a SIDS baby are many. Unless the infant is obviously dead, undertake active and aggressive care of the infant to assure the family that everything possible is being done. A first responder or other personnel should be assigned to assist the parents and to explain the procedures. At all points, use the baby's name.

After arrival at the hospital, direct management at the parents or caregivers, since nothing can be done for the child. Allow the family to see the dead child. Expect a normal grief reaction. Initially, there may be shock, disbelief, and denial. Other times, the parents or caregivers may express anger, rage, hostility, blame, or guilt. Often, there is a feeling of inadequacy as well as helplessness, confusion, and fear. The grief process is likely to last for years. SIDS has major long-term effects on family relations. It may also affect you, the on-scene paramedic. If so, do not be reluctant to request a Critical Incident Stress Debriefing.

In SIDS, active and aggressive care of the infant should continue until delivery to the emergency room unless the infant is obviously dead.

At all points in a SIDS case, use the baby's name when speaking with parents or caregivers.

CHILD ABUSE AND NEGLECT

A tragic truth is that some people cause physical and psychological harm to children, either through intentional abuse or through intentional or unintentional neglect. In fact, child abuse is the second leading cause of death in infants less than 6 months of age. An estimated 2,000 to 5,000 children die each year as a result of abuse or neglect.

There are several characteristics common to abused children. Often, the child is seen as "special" and different from others. Premature infants and twins stand a higher risk of abuse than other children. Many abused children are less than 5 years of age. Physically and mentally handicapped children as well as those with other special needs are at greater risk. So are uncommunicative (autistic) children. Boys are more often abused than girls. A child who is not what the parents wanted (e.g., the "wrong" gender) is at increased risk of abuse, too.

PERPETRATORS OF ABUSE OR NEGLECT

Abuse or neglect may be instigated by a parent, a legal guardian, or a foster parent. It can be carried out by a person, an institution, or an agency or program entrusted with custody. Abuse or neglect can also result from the actions of a caretaker, such as a baby-sitter or a "nanny."

The person who abuses or neglects a child can come from any geographic, religious, ethnic, racial, occupational, educational, or socioeconomic background. Despite their diversity, people who abuse children tend to share certain traits. The abuser is usually a parent or a full-time caregiver. When the mother spends the majority of the time with the child, she is the parent most frequently identified as the abuser. Most abusers were abused themselves as children.

Three conditions can alert you to the potential for abuse. They include:

- A parent or adult who seems capable of abuse—especially one who exhibits evasive or hostile behavior
- A child in one of the high-risk categories
- The presence of a crisis, particularly financial stress, marital or relationship stress, or physical illness in a parent or child

TYPES OF ABUSE

Child abuse can take several forms. These forms include:

- Psychological abuse
- Physical abuse
- Sexual abuse
- Neglect (either physical or emotional)

Abused children suffer every imaginable kind of mistreatment. They are battered with fists, belts, broom handles, hair brushes, baseball bats, electric cords, and any other objects that can be used as weapons (Figure 42-32). They are

FIGURE 42-32 An abused child. Note the marks on the legs associated with beatings with an electric wire. The burns on the buttocks are from submersion in hot water. (Courtesy of Scott and White Hospital and Clinic.)

FIGURE 42-33 Burn injury from placing a child's buttocks in hot water as a punishment. (Courtesy of Scott and White Hospital and Clinic.)

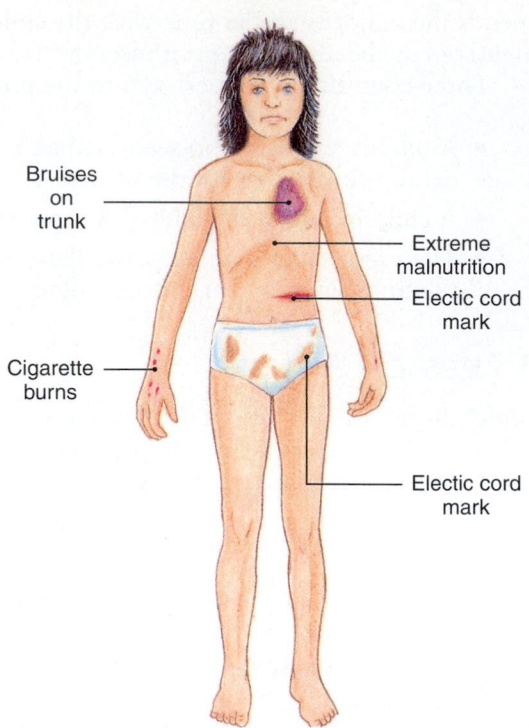

Bruises on trunk

Extreme malnutrition

Electic cord mark

Cigarette burns

Electic cord mark

FIGURE 42-34 The stigmata of child abuse.

FIGURE 42-35 The effects of child abuse, both physical and mental, can last a lifetime. (Courtesy of Scott and White Hospital and Clinic.)

locked in closets, denied food, or deprived of access to a toilet. They are intentionally burned or scalded with anything from hot water to cigarette butts to open flames (Figure 42-33). They are severely shaken, thrown into cribs, pushed down stairs, or shoved into walls. Some are shot, stabbed, or suffocated.

Sexual abuse ranges from adults exposing themselves to children to overt sexual acts to sexual torture. Sexual abuse can occur at any age, and the victims may be either male or female. Generally, the sexual abuser is someone the child knows and, perhaps, trusts. Stepchildren or adopted children face a greater risk for sexual abuse than biological children. Cases in which sexual abuse causes physical harm may get reported. Other cases, especially those with emotional and minor physical injury, may go undetected.

ASSESSMENT OF THE POTENTIALLY ABUSED OR NEGLECTED CHILD

Signs of abuse or neglect can be startling (Figure 42-34). As a guide, the following findings should trigger a high index of suspicion:

- Any obvious or suspected fractures in a child under 2 years of age
- Multiple injuries in various stages of healing, especially burns and bruises (Figure 42-35)
- More injuries than usually seen in children of the same age or size
- Injuries scattered on many areas of the body

- Bruises or burns in patterns that suggest intentional infliction
- Increased intracranial pressure in an infant
- Suspected intra-abdominal trauma in a young child
- Any injury that does not fit with the description of the cause given

Information in the medical history may also raise the index of suspicion. Examples include:

- A history that does not match the nature or severity of the injury
- Vague parental accounts or accounts that change during the interview
- Accusations that the child injured himself intentionally
- Delay in seeking help
- Child dressed inappropriately for the situation
- Revealing comments by bystanders, especially siblings

Suspect child neglect if you spot any of the following conditions:

- Extreme malnutrition
- Multiple insect bites
- Long-standing skin infections
- Extreme lack of cleanliness
- Verbal or social skills far below those you would expect for a child of similar age and background
- Lack of appropriate medical care (Figure 42-36)

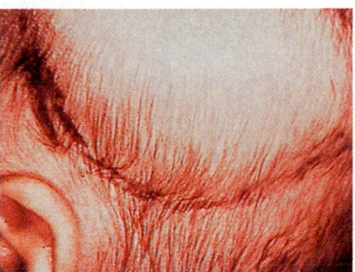

FIGURE 42-36 Child neglect from a lack of appropriate medical care.

MANAGEMENT OF THE POTENTIALLY ABUSED OR NEGLECTED CHILD

In cases of child abuse or neglect, the goals of management include appropriate treatment of injuries, protection of the child from further abuse, and notification of proper authorities. You should obtain as much information as possible, in a nonjudgmental manner. Document all findings or statements in the patient report. Don't "cross-examine" the parents—this job belongs to the police or other authorities. Try to be supportive toward the parents, especially if it helps you to transport the child to the hospital. Remember: Never leave transport to the alleged abuser.

Upon arrival at the emergency department, report your suspicions to the appropriate personnel. Complete the patient report and all available documentation at this time, since delay may inhibit accurate recall of data.

Child abuse and neglect are particularly stressful aspects of emergency medical services. You must recognize and deal with your feelings, perhaps taking them up at a Critical Incident Stress Debriefing.

Never leave transport of an abused child to an alleged abuser.

In many states, prehospital personnel are required by law to report suspected child abuse or neglect to the appropriate authorities.

RESOURCES FOR ABUSE AND NEGLECT

You can contact your local child protection agency for additional information on child abuse. Consider taking a course in the recognition of child abuse and neglect. These are often offered by children's hospitals. The Internet has several sites that provide up-to-date information on child abuse.

INFANTS AND CHILDREN WITH SPECIAL NEEDS

For most of human history, infants and children with devastating congenital conditions or diseases either died or remained confined to a hospital. In recent decades, however, medical technology has lowered infant mortality rates and allowed a greater number of children with special needs to live at home. (See more about home care in Chapter 46.) Some of these infants and children include:

- Premature babies
- Infants and children with lung disease, heart disease, or neurological disorders
- Infants and children with chronic diseases, such as cystic fibrosis, asthma, childhood cancers, cerebral palsy, and others
- Infants and children with altered functions from birth (Examples include cerebral palsy, spina bifida, and other congenital birth defects.)

In caring for these children, family members receive education relative to the special equipment required by the infant or child. Even so, they may feel a great deal of apprehension when care moves from the hospital to the home. As a result, they may summon EMS at the first indication of trouble. This is especially true in the initial weeks following discharge.

COMMON HOME-CARE DEVICES

Devices you might commonly find in the home include tracheostomy tubes, apnea monitors, home artificial ventilators, central intravenous lines, gastric feeding tubes, gastrostomy tubes, and shunts. In treating children with special needs, remember that the parents and caregivers are often very knowledgeable about their children and the devices that sustain their lives. Listen to them. They know their children better than anybody else.

Tracheostomy Tubes

Patients who are on prolonged home ventilators or who have chronic respiratory problems may have surgically placed tubes in the inferior trachea (Figure 42-37). A **tracheostomy** (trach) tube may be utilized as a temporary or a permanent device. Although there are various types of tubes, you might expect some common complications. They include:

* **tracheostomy** a surgical incision in the neck held open by a metal or plastic tube.

- Obstruction, usually by a mucous plug
- Site bleeding, either from the tube or around the tube
- An air leakage
- A dislodged tube
- Infection—a condition that will worsen an already impaired breathing ability

Management steps for a patient with a tracheostomy include:

- Maintaining an open airway
- Suctioning the tube, as needed
- Allowing the patient to remain in a position of comfort, if possible
- Administering oxygen in cases of respiratory distress

FIGURE 42-37 Tracheostomy tubes. Top: plastic tube. Bottom: metal tube with inner cannula.

Inner Cannula

Tracheostomy Tube

Fenestration

- Assisting ventilations in cases of respiratory failure/arrest by:
  - Intubating orally in the absence of an upper airway obstruction
  - Intubating via the **stoma** if there is an upper airway obstruction
- Transporting the patient to the hospital

* **stoma** a permanent surgical opening in the neck through which the patient breathes.

Apnea Monitors

Apnea monitors are used to alert parents or caregivers to the cessation of breathing in an infant, especially a premature infant. Some types of monitors signal changes in heart rate, such as bradycardia or tachycardia. They operate via pads attached to the baby's chest and connected to the monitor by wires. If the device does not detect a breath within a specific time frame or if the infant's heart rate is too slow or too fast, an alarm will sound.

When an apnea monitor is placed in a home, the parents are typically instructed on what to do if the alarm sounds (stimulate the child, provide artificial respirations, and so on). If these fail, EMS may be summoned. Also, nervous parents who have just brought a baby home on an apnea monitor may panic the first couple of times the alarm sounds and call 911. Be patient and kind while instructing them on what to do when the alarm sounds.

Most parents who have infants on apnea monitors have received training in pediatric CPR.

Home Artificial Ventilators

Various configurations exist for home ventilators. Demand ventilators sense rate and quality of a patient's respiration as well as several other parameters, including pulse oximetry. They typically respond to pre-set limits. Other devices provide a constant PEEP (positive end-expiratory pressure) and a set oxygen concentration for the patient.

Two complications commonly result in EMS calls: (1) a device's mechanical failure and (2) shortages of energy during an electrical failure. Treatment typically includes:

- Maintaining an open airway
- Administering artificial ventilations via an appropriately sized BVM with oxygen
- Transporting the patient to a hospital until the home ventilator is working

Central Intravenous Lines

Children who require long-term IV therapy will often have central lines placed into the superior vena cava near the heart. In cases where IV therapy is necessary for only several weeks, PIC (percutaneous intravenous catheter) lines may be placed in the arm and threaded into the superior vena cava. Otherwise the lines are placed through subclavian venipuncture. **Central IV lines** are commonly used to administer intravenous nutrition. antibiotics, or chemotherapy for cancer.

Possible complications for central IV lines include:

* Cracked line
* Infection, either at the site or at more distal aspects of the line
* Loss of patency—e.g., clotting
* Hemorrhage, which can be considerable
* Air embolism

Emergency medical care steps include control of any bleeding through direct pressure. If a large amount of air is in the line, try to withdraw it with a syringe. If this fails, clamp the line and transport. In cases of a cracked line, place a clamp between the crack and the patient. If the patient exhibits an altered mental status following the cracked line, position the child on the left side with head down. Transport the child to the hospital as quickly as possible.

Gastric Feeding Tubes and Gastrostomy Tubes

Children who are not capable of swallowing or eating receive nutrition through either a gastric feeding tube or a gastrostomy tube. (A gastric feeding tube is placed through the nostrils into the stomach. A gastrostomy tube is placed through the abdominal wall directly into the stomach.) These special devices are commonly used in disorders of the digestive system or in situations in which the developmental ability of the patient hinders feeding. Food consists of nutritious liquids.

Possible emergency complications include:

* Bleeding at the site
* Dislodged tube
* Respiratory distress, particularly if a tube feeding backs up into the esophagus and is aspirated into the trachea and lungs
* In the case of diabetics, altered mental status due to missed feedings

Emergency medical care involves supporting the ABCs, including possible suctioning and administration of supplemental oxygen. Patients should be transported to a definitive care facility, either in a sitting position or lying on the right side with the head elevated. The goal is to reduce the risk of aspiration, a serious condition.

Shunts

A **shunt** is a surgical connection that runs from the brain to the abdomen. It removes excess cerebrospinal fluid from the brain through drainage. A subcutaneous reservoir is usually palpable on one side of the patient's head. A pathological rise in intracranial pressure, secondary to a blocked shunt, is a primary complication. Shunt failure may also result when the shunt's connections separate, usually because of a child's growth.

* **central IV line** intravenous line placed into the superior vena cava for the administration of long-term fluid therapy.

* **shunt** surgical connection that runs from the brain to the abdomen for the purpose of draining excess cerebrospinal fluid, thus preventing increased intracranial pressure.

Cases of shunt failure present as altered mental status. The patient may exhibit drowsiness, respiratory distress, or the classic signs of pupil dysfunction or posturing. Be aware that an altered mental status may be caused by infection—a distinction to be made in a hospital setting.

Care steps involve maintenance of an open airway, administration of ventilations as needed, and immediate transport. Shunt failures require correction in the operating room, where the cerebrospinal fluid can be drained or, in rare cases, an infection identified and treated.

GENERAL ASSESSMENT AND MANAGEMENT PRACTICES

Remember that pediatric patients with special needs require the same assessment as other patients. Always evaluate the airway, breathing, and circulation. (Recall that in the initial assessment, "disability" refers to patient's neurological status—not to the child's special need.) If you discover life-threatening conditions in the initial assessment, begin appropriate interventions. Keep in mind that the child's special need is often an ongoing process. In most cases, you should concentrate on the acute problem.

During the assessment, ask pertinent questions of the patient, parent, or caregiver such as: "What unusual situation caused you to call for an ambulance?" As already mentioned, the parent or caregiver is usually very knowledgeable about the patient's condition.

In most cases, the physical examination is essentially the same as with other patients. It is important to explain everything that is being done, even if the patient does not seem to understand. Do not be distracted by the special equipment. Be aware of the help that the patient, parent, or caregiver may be able to provide in handling home-care devices.

In managing patients with special needs, try to keep several thoughts in mind.

- Avoid using the term "disability" (in reference to the child's special need). Instead, think of the patient's many abilities.
- Never assume that the patient cannot understand what you are saying.
- Involve the parents, caregivers, or the patient, if appropriate, in treatment. They manage the illness or congenital condition on a daily basis.
- Treat the patient with a special need with the same respect as any other patient.

Remember that pediatric patients with special needs require the same assessment as other patients.

In most cases, concentrate on the acute problem rather than the ongoing special need.

SUMMARY

Pediatric emergencies can be stressful for both you and the adults responsible for the child's well-being. Most pediatric emergencies result from trauma, respiratory distress, ingestion of poisons, or febrile seizure activity. In addition, you must always be on the lookout for signs and symptoms of child abuse or neglect. The approach and management of pediatric emergencies must be modified for the age and size of the child. Certain skills generally considered routine, such as IV administration, become difficult in the pediatric patient because of size and other factors. It is important to remember that children are not "small adults." They have special considerations—both physical and emotional—that must be managed accordingly.

CHAPTER 43

Geriatric Emergencies

Objectives

After reading this chapter, you should be able to:

1. Discuss the demographics demonstrating the increasing size of the elderly population in the United States. (pp. 1800–1801)
2. Assess the various living environments of elderly patients. (p. 1801)
3. Discuss society's view of aging and the social, financial, and ethical issues facing the elderly. (pp. 1800–1802)
4. Discuss common emotional and psychological reactions to aging, including causes and manifestations. (pp. 1800–1801)
5. Apply the pathophysiology of multi-system failure to the assessment and management of medical conditions in the elderly patient. (p. 1803)
6. Compare the pharmacokinetics of an elderly patient to that of a young patient, including drug distribution, metabolism, and excretion. (pp. 1803–1804)
7. Discuss the impact of polypharmacy, dosing errors, increased drug sensitivity, and medication non-compliance on assessment and management of the elderly patient (pp. 1803–1804)

Continued

8. Discuss the use and effects of commonly prescribed drugs for the elderly patient (pp. 1803–1804, 1840–1841)

9. Discuss the problem of mobility in the elderly, and develop strategies to prevent falls. (pp. 1804–1805)

10. Discuss age-related changes in sensations in the elderly, and describe the implications of these changes for communication and patient assessment. (pp. 1805, 1808–1810)

11. Discuss the problems with continence and elimination in the elderly patient, and develop communication strategies to provide psychological support. (pp. 1805–1806)

12. Discuss factors that may complicate the assessment of the elderly patient. (pp. 1802–1803, 1807–1812)

13. Discuss the principles that should be employed when assessing and communicating with the elderly. (pp. 1805, 1807–1812)

14. Compare the assessment of a young patient with that of an elderly patient. (pp. 1807–1808, 1812–1818)

15. Discuss common complaints of elderly patients. (pp. 1803, 1819–1845)

16. Discuss the normal and abnormal changes of age in relation to the:
    a. Pulmonary system. (pp. 1813–1814)
    b. Cardiovascular system. (pp. 1813, 1814–1815)
    c. Nervous system. (pp. 1815–1816)
    d. Endocrine system. (pp. 1813, 1816)
    e. Gastrointestinal system. (pp. 1813, 1816)
    f. Thermoregulatory system. (pp. 1813, 1817)
    g. Integumentary system. (pp. 1813, 1817)
    h. Musculoskeletal system. (pp. 1813, 1817)

17. Describe the incidence, morbidity/mortality, risk factors, prevention strategies, pathophysiology, assessment, need for intervention and transport, and management for elderly medical patients with:
    a. Pneumonia, chronic obstructive disease, and pulmonary embolism. (pp. 1819–1822)
    b. Myocardial infarction, heart failure, dysrhythmias, aneurysm, and hypertension. (pp. 1822–1827)
    c. Cerebral vascular disease, delirium, dementia, Alzheimer's disease, and Parkinson's disease. (pp. 1827–1831)
    d. Diabetes and thyroid diseases. (pp. 1831–1832)
    e. Gastrointestinal problems, GI hemorrhage, and bowel obstruction. (pp. 1832–1834)
    f. Skin diseases and pressure ulcers. (pp. 1834–1835)
    g. Osteoarthritis and osteoporosis. (pp. 1835–1837)
    h. Hypothermia and hyperthermia. (pp. 1838–1839)
    i. Toxicological problems, including drug toxicity, substance abuse, alcohol abuse, and drug abuse. (pp. 1840–1843)
    j. Psychological disorders, including depression and suicide. (pp. 1843–1845)

18. Describe the incidence, morbidity/mortality, risk factors, prevention strategies, pathophysiology, assessment, need for intervention and transport, and management of the elderly trauma patient with:
    a. Orthopedic injuries. (pp. 1849–1850)
    b. Burns. (pp. 1850–1851)
    c. Head injuries. (p. 1851)

19. Given several pre-programmed simulated geriatric patients with various complaints, provide the appropriate assessment, management, and transport. (pp. 1800–1851)

INTRODUCTION

Aging—the gradual decline of biological functions—varies widely from one individual to another. Most people reach their biological peak in the years before age 30. For practical purposes, however, the aging process does not affect their daily lives until later years. Many of the decrements commonly ascribed to aging are caused by other factors, such as lifestyle, diet, behavior, or environment. The aging process becomes even more complicated if we remember that age-related changes in organ functions also occur at different rates. For example, a person's kidneys may decline rapidly with age, while the heart remains strong or vice versa.

As people age, they actually become less alike, both physiologically and psychologically. Although some functional losses in old age are due to normal age-related changes, many others result from abnormal changes, particularly disease. In assessing and treating older patients, it is important to distinguish, when possible, normal age-related changes from abnormal changes. The purpose of this chapter is to present some of the most common physiological changes associated with aging and the implications of these changes to the quality of EMS care provided to the **elderly**—one of the fastest-growing segments of our population.

Many of the decrements commonly ascribed to aging are caused by other factors, such as lifestyle, diet, behavior, or environment.

* **elderly** a person age 65 or older.

EPIDEMIOLOGY AND DEMOGRAPHICS

The twentieth century—with its tremendous medical and technological advances—witnessed both a reduction in infant mortality rates and an increase in life expectancies. The cumulative effect was a population boom worldwide, with the greatest gains seen among people age 65 or older. During the 1900s, the population of the United States increased threefold, while the number of elderly increased tenfold. The growing number of elderly patients presents a challenge to all health-care services, including EMS, not only in terms of resources, but in the enormous impact that aging has upon our society.

POPULATION CHARACTERISTICS

America is getting older. Between 1960 and 1990, the number of elderly people in the United States nearly doubled. By late 1998, the total reached more than 34 million, with nearly 400,000 people ages 95 and older. As the 2000s opened, demographers talked about the "graying of America," a process in which the number of elderly people is pushing up the average age of the U.S. population as a whole. Reasons for this trend include:

- The mean survival rate of older persons is increasing.
- The birth rate is declining.
- There has been an absence of major wars and other catastrophes.
- Health care and standards of living have improved significantly since World War II.

In 2030, when the post-World War II baby boomers enter their 80s, more than 70 million people will be age 65 or older. By 2040, the elderly will represent roughly 20 percent of the population. In other words, one in five Americans will be age 65 or older.

Not only will the elderly population increase in size, its members will live longer, which in turn will swell the number of the **old-old**. By 2040, the number of people age 85 and over is expected to rise by 17 percent. Whether longer life spans mean longer years of active living or longer years of disease and disability is unknown.

* **old-old** an elderly person age 80 or older.

Gerontology—the study of the effects of aging on humans—is a relatively new science. (The Gerontological Society of America [GSA] was formed in 1945.) Gerontologists still do not fully understand the underlying causes of aging. However, most believe that some form of cellular damage or loss, particularly of nerve cells (neurons), is involved. The result is a general decline in the body's efficiency, such as a reduction in the size and function of most internal organs.

To treat age-related changes, physicians and other health care workers have increasingly specialized in the care of the elderly. This aspect of medicine, known as **geriatrics,** is essential in caring for our aging population.

The demographic changes will also affect your EMS career. Today nearly 36 percent of all EMS calls involve the elderly. The percentage is expected to grow. Therefore, you will need to be familiar with the fundamental principles of geriatrics, especially those related to advanced prehospital care. You will also need to be aware of the social issues that can affect the health and mental well-being of the elderly patients that you will be treating.

SOCIETAL ISSUES

For a typical working person, the post-retirement years can be up to one-third of an average life span. The years include a series of transitions, such as reduced income, relocation, and loss of friends, family members, spouse, or partner.

After years of working and/or raising a family, an elderly person must not only find new roles to fulfill, but in many cases, must overcome the societal label of "old person." A lot of elderly people disprove **ageism**—and all the stereotypes it engenders—by living happy, productive, and active lives (Figure 43-1). Others, however, feel a sense of social isolation or uselessness. Physical and financial difficulties reinforce these feelings and help create an emotional context in which illnesses can occur. Therefore, successful medical treatment of elderly patients involves an understanding of the broader social situation in which they live.

The elderly live in both independent and dependent living environments. Many continue to live alone or with their partner well into their 80s or 90s. The "oldest" old are the most likely to live alone, and, in fact, nearly half of those age 85 and over live by themselves. The great majority of these people—an estimated 78 percent—are women. This is because married men tend to die before their wives, and widowed men tend to remarry more often than widowed women.

* **gerontology** scientific study of the effects of aging and of age-related diseases on humans.

* **geriatrics** the study and treatment of diseases of the aged.

* **ageism** discrimination against aged or elderly people.

Emotional, physical, and/or financial difficulties can help create a context in which illnesses can occur. Successful medical treatment of elderly patients involves an understanding of the broader social context in which they live.

FIGURE 43-1 Many older adults live active lives, participating in sports and exercises popular among people of all ages.
(© The Stock Market Photo Agency.)

Table 43-1   **PREVENTION STRATEGIES FOR THE OLDER PERSON**

Issues	Strategies
Lifestyle	
Exercise:	Weight-bearing and cardiovascular exercise (walking) for 20–30 minutes at least three times a week
Nutrition:	Varies, but generally low fat, adequate fiber (complex carbohydrates), reduced sugar (simple carbohydrates), moderate protein; adequate calcium, especially for women*
Alcohol/tobacco:	Moderate alcohol, if any; abstinence from tobacco
Sleep:	Generally 7–8 hours a night
Accidents	Maintain good physical condition; add safety features to home (handrails, nonskid surfaces, lights, etc.); modify potentially dangerous driving practices (driving at night with impaired night vision, traveling in hazardous weather, etc.)
Medical Health	
Disease/Illness:	Routine screening for hearing, vision, blood pressure, hemoglobin, cholesterol, etc.; regular physical examinations; immunizations (tetanus booster, influenza vaccine, once-in-a-lifetime pneumococcal vaccine)
Pharmacological:	Regular review of prescriptive and over-the-counter medications, focusing on potential interactions and side effects
Dental:	Regular dental checkups and good oral hygiene (important for nutrition and general well-being)
Mental/emotional:	Observe for evidence of depression, disrupted sleep patterns, psychosocial stress; ensure effective support networks and availability of psychotherapy; compliance with prescribed antidepressants

*Vitamin supplements may be required, but should be taken only after other medications are reviewed and in correct dosages. Excessive doses of vitamin A or D, for example, can be toxic.

Prevention and Self-Help

In treating the elderly, remember that the best intervention is prevention.

In treating the elderly, remember that the best intervention is prevention (Table 43-1). The goal of any health-care service, including EMS, should be to help keep people from becoming sick or injured in the first place. As previously mentioned, disease and disability in later life are often linked to unhealthy or unsafe behavior. As a paramedic, you can reduce morbidity among the elderly by taking part in community education programs and by cooperating with agencies or organizations that support the elderly. Some possible resources are described in the following sections.

GENERAL PATHOPHYSIOLOGY, ASSESSMENT, AND MANAGEMENT

* **functional impairment** decreased ability to meet daily needs on an independent basis.

In treating elderly patients, it is important to recall several facts. First, medical disorders in the elderly often present as **functional impairment** and should be treated as an early warning of a possibly undetected medical problem. Second, signs and symptoms do not necessarily point to the underlying cause of the problem or illness. For example, while confusion often indicates a brain disease in younger patients, this may not be the case in an elderly patient. The confused patient may be suffering from a wide range of disorders, including drug toxicity, malnutrition, or accidental hypothermia.

A thorough evaluation must always be done to detect possible causes of an impairment. If identified early, an environmental- or disease-generated impairment can often be reversed. Your success depends upon a knowledge of age-related changes and the implications of these changes for patient assessment and management.

PATHOPHYSIOLOGY OF THE ELDERLY PATIENT

As mentioned, patients become less alike as they enter their elderly years, Even so, certain generalizations can be made about age-related changes and the disease process in the elderly.

Multiple-System Failure

There is no escaping the fact that the body becomes less efficient with age, increasing the likelihood of malfunction. The body is susceptible to all the disorders of young people, but its maintenance, defense, and repair processes are weaker. As a result, the elderly often suffer from more than one illness or disease at a time. On average, six medical disorders may coexist in an elderly person and perhaps even more in the old-old. Neither the patient nor the patient's doctor may be aware of all of these problems. Furthermore, disease in one organ system may result in the deterioration of other systems, compounding existing acute and/or chronic conditions.

Because of concomitant diseases (**comorbidity**) in the elderly, complaints may not be specific to any one disorder. Common complaints of the elderly include: fatigue and weakness, dizziness/vertigo/syncope, falls, headaches, insomnia, **dysphagia,** loss of appetite, inability to void, and/or constipation/diarrhea.

Elderly patients often accept medical problems as a part of aging and fail to monitor changes in their condition. In some cases, such as a silent myocardial infarction, pain may be diminished or absent. In others, an important complaint may seem trivial, such as constipation.

Although many medical problems in the young and middle-aged populations present with a standard set of signs and symptoms, the changes involved in aging lead to different presentations. In pneumonia, for example, the classic symptom of fever is often absent in the elderly. Chest pain and a cough are also less common. Finally, many cases of pneumonia among the elderly are due to aspiration, not infection. The presentation of pneumonia and other diseases commonly found in the elderly will be covered later in the chapter.

Pharmacology in the Elderly

The existence of multiple chronic diseases in the elderly leads to the use of multiple medications. Persons age 65 and older use one-third of all prescriptive drugs in the United States, taking an average of 4.5 medications per day. This does not include over-the-counter medications, vitamin supplements, or herbal remedies.

If medications are not correctly monitored, **polypharmacy** can lead to a number of problems among the elderly. In general, a person's sensitivity to drugs increases with age. When compared to younger patients, the elderly experience more adverse drug reactions, more drug-drug interactions, and more drug-disease interactions. Because of age-related pharmacokinetic changes such as a loss of body fluid and atrophy of organs, drugs concentrate more readily in the plasma and tissues of elderly patients. As a result, drug dosages often must be adjusted to prevent toxicity. (The problem of toxicity will be discussed in more detail later in the chapter.)

In taking a medical history of an elderly patient, remember to ask questions to determine if a patient is taking a prescribed medication as directed. Noncompliance

The elderly often suffer from more than one illness or disease at a time.

* **comorbidity** having more than one disease at a time.

* **dysphagia** inability to swallow or difficulty swallowing.

The existence of multiple chronic disease in the elderly often leads to the use of multiple medications. Keep this in mind throughout the assessment.

* **polypharmacy** multiple drug therapy in which there is a concurrent use of a number of drugs.

In taking a medical history of an elderly patient, remember to ask if the patient is taking a prescribed medication as directed.

with drug therapy, usually underadherence, is common among the elderly. Up to 40 percent do not take medications as prescribed. Factors that can decrease compliance in the elderly include:

- Limited income
- Memory loss due to decreased or diseased neural activity
- Limited mobility
- Sensory impairment (cannot hear/read/understand directions)
- Multiple or complicated drug therapies
- Fear of toxicity
- Child-proof containers (especially with arthritic patients)
- Duration of drug therapy (The longer the therapy, the less likely a patient will stick with it.)

Factors that can increase compliance among the elderly include:

- Good patient-physician communication
- Belief that a disease or illness is serious
- Drug calendars or reminder cards
- Compliance counseling
- Blister-pack packaging or other easy-to-open packaging
- Multi-compartment pill boxes
- Transportation services to pharmacy
- Clear, simple directions written in large type
- Ability to read

Problems with Mobility and Falls

Regular exercise and a good diet are two of the most effective preventive measures for ensuring mobility among the elderly. However, not all elderly take these measures. They may suffer from a severe medical problem, such as crippling arthritis. They may fear for their personal safety, either from accidental injury or intentional injury, such as robbery. Certain medications also may increase their lethargy. Whatever the cause, a lack of mobility can have detrimental physical and emotional effects. Some of these include:

- Poor nutrition
- Difficulty with elimination
- Poor skin integrity
- A greater predisposition for falls
- Loss of independence and/or confidence
- Depression from "feeling old"
- Isolation and lack of a social network

Fall-related injuries represent the leading cause of accidental death among the elderly. Intrinsic factors include a history of repeated falls, dizziness, a sense of weakness, impaired vision, an altered gait, CNS problems, decreased mental status, or use of certain medications. Extrinsic factors include environmental hazards such as slippery floors, a lack of handrails, or loose throw rugs.

In assessing an elderly patient who has fallen, remember that a fall often has multiple causes. An over-medicated patient, for example, trips over a throw rug. A fall may also be a presenting sign of an acute illness, such as a myocardial infarction, or a sign that a chronic illness has worsened. Bear in mind the possibility of physical abuse, especially if the injury does not match the story.

In assessing an elderly patient who has fallen, remember that a fall often has multiple causes.

Communication Difficulties

Most elderly patients suffer from some form of age-related sensory changes. Normal physiological changes may include impaired vision or blindness, impaired or loss of hearing, an altered sense of taste or smell, and/or a lower sensitivity to pain (touch). Any of these conditions can affect your ability to communicate with the patient. For communication strategies, see Table 43-2. (A discussion on the implications of sensory impairment on patient assessment appears later in the chapter.)

Problems with Continence and Elimination

The elderly often find it embarrassing to talk about problems with continence and elimination. They may feel stigmatized, isolated, and/or helpless. When confronted with these problems, DO NOT make a big deal out of them. Respect the patient's dignity, and assure the person that, in many cases, the problem is treatable.

Incontinence The problem of **incontinence** can affect nearly any age group, but is most commonly associated with the elderly. Incontinence may be either urinary or fecal. An estimated 15 percent of the elderly who live at home experience some form of urinary incontinence. Nearly 30 percent of the hospitalized elderly and 50 percent of those living in nursing homes suffer from the same condition. Although fecal, or bowel, incontinence is less common, it seriously impairs activity and may lead to dependent care. Between 16–60 percent of the institutionalized elderly have some kind of fecal incontinence.

* **incontinence** inability to retain urine or feces because of loss of sphincter control or cerebral or spinal lesions.

Incontinence can lead to a variety of conditions such as rashes, skin infections, skin breakdown (ulcers), urinary tract infections, sepsis, and falls or fractures. As mentioned, the condition takes a high emotional toll, on both the patient and the caregiver. Management of incontinence costs billions of dollars each year.

Table 43-2 AGE-RELATED SENSORY CHANGES AND IMPLICATIONS FOR COMMUNICATION

Sensory Change	Result	Communication Strategy
Clouding and thickening of lens in eye	Cataracts; poor vision, especially peripheral vision	Position yourself in front of patient where you can be seen; put hand on arm of blind patient to let patient know where you are; locate a patient's glasses, if necessary.
Shrinkage of structure in ear	Decreased hearing, especially ability to hear high frequency sounds; diminished sense of balance	Speak clearly; check hearing aids as necessary; write notes if necessary; allow the patient to put on the stethoscope, while you speak into it like a microphone.
Deterioration of teeth and gums	Patient needs dentures, but they may inflict pain on sensitive gums, so patient doesn't always wear them	If patient's speech is unintelligible, ask patient to put in dentures, if possible.
Lowered sensitivity to pain and altered sense of taste and smell	Patient underestimates the severity of the problem or is unable to provide a complete pertinent history	Probe for significant symptoms, asking questions aimed at functional impairment.

In general, effective continence requires several physical conditions. These include:

- An anatomically correct GI/GU tract
- Competent sphincter mechanism
- Adequate cognition and mobility

Although incontinence is not necessarily caused by aging, several factors predispose older patients to this condition. As mentioned, the elderly tend to have several medical disorders, each of which may require drug therapy. These disorders and/or the drugs used to treat them may compromise the integrity of either the urinary or bowel tracts. In addition, bladder capacity, urinary flow rate, and the ability to postpone voiding appear to decline with age. Certain diseases, such as diabetes and autonomic neuropathy, may also cause sphincter dysfunction. Diarrhea, or lack of physical sensation, may produce bowel incontinence as well.

Management of incontinence depends upon the cause, which cannot be easily diagnosed in the field. Some cases of incontinence can be managed surgically. In most cases, however, patients use some type of absorptive devices, such as leak-proof underwear or panty liners. Indwelling catheters are less common and may cause infections when used, particularly if not properly managed. Of critical importance is respect for the patient's modesty and dignity.

Elimination Difficulty with elimination can be a sign of a serious underlying condition (Table 43-3). It can also lead to other complications. Straining to eliminate may have serious effects on the cerebral, coronary, and peripheral arterial circulations. In elderly people with cerebrovascular disease or impaired baroreceptor reflexes, efforts to force a bowel movement can lead to a **transient ischemic attack (TIA)** or syncope. In the case of prolonged constipation, the elderly may experience colonic ulceration, intestinal obstruction, and urinary retention.

In assessing a patient with difficulty eliminating, remember to inquire about their medications. Any of the following drugs can cause constipation:

- Opioids
- Anticholinergics (e.g., antidepressants, antihistamines, muscle relaxants, antiparkinsonian drugs)
- Cation-containing agents (e.g., antacids, calcium supplements, iron supplements)
- Neurally active agents (e.g., opiates, anticonvulsants)
- Diuretics

In treating incontinence, remember to respect the patient's modesty and dignity.

Difficulty with elimination can be a sign of a serious underlying condition.

* **transient ischemic attacks (TIA)** reversible interruptions of blood flow to the brain; often seen as a precursor to a stroke.

Table 43-3	POSSIBLE CAUSES OF ELIMINATION PROBLEMS
Difficulty in Urination	**Difficulty with Bowel Movements**
Enlargement of the prostate in men	Diverticular disease
Urinary tract infection	Constipation*
Acute or chronic renal failure	Colorectal cancer

*Constipation may be related to dietary, medical, or surgical conditions. It could also be the result of a malignancy, intestinal obstruction, or hypothyroidism. Treat constipation as a serious medical problem.

ASSESSMENT CONSIDERATIONS

As with all patients, be sure to take appropriate BSI precautions when assessing an elderly patient. Because of the increased risk of tuberculosis in patients who are in nursing homes, consider wearing a HEPA or N-95 respirator. Remain alert to the environment, particularly the temperature of the surroundings and evidence of prescription medications.

In general, assessment of the elderly patient follows the same basic approach used with any patient. However, you need to keep in mind several factors that will improve the quality of your evaluation and make subsequent treatment more successful.

General Health Assessment

As already mentioned, you need to set a context for illness when assessing an elderly patient. When performing a general health assessment, take into account the patient's living situation, level of activity, network of social support, level of independence, medication history (both prescription and non-prescriptive), and sleep patterns.

Pay particularly close attention to the patient's nutrition. Elderly patients often have a decreased sense of smell and taste, which decrease their pleasure in eating. They also may be less aware of internal cues of hunger and thirst. Although caloric requirements generally decrease with age, an elderly patient may still suffer from malnutrition. Conditions that may complicate or discourage eating among the elderly include:

- Breathing or respiratory problems
- Abdominal pain
- Nausea/vomiting, sometimes a drug-induced condition as with antibodies or aspirin
- Poor dental care
- Medical problems, such as hyperthyroidism, hypercalcemia, and chronic infections (e.g., cancer or tuberculosis)
- Medications (e.g., digoxin, vitamin A, fluoxetine)
- Alcohol or drug abuse
- Psychological disorders, including depression and **anorexia nervosa**
- Poverty
- Problems with shopping or cooking

As with any person, nutrition greatly affects a patient's overall health. Because of reasons cited above, patients may suffer from a number of by-products of malnutrition, including vitamin deficiencies, dehydration, and hypoglycemia. Also remember that when a malnourished elderly person is fed, the food may produce yet other side effects, including electrolyte abnormalities, hyperglycemia, aspiration pneumonia, and a significant drop in blood pressure.

Pathophysiology and Assessment

Assessment of the elderly reflects the pathophysiology of this age group. As already mentioned, the chief complaint of the elderly may seem trivial or vague at first. Also, the patient may fail to report important symptoms. Therefore, you should try to distinguish the patient's chief complaint from the patient's primary problem. A patient may report nausea, which is the chief complaint.

> *Because of the increased risk of tuberculosis in the patients who are in nursing homes, consider using a HEPA or N-95 respirator.*
>
>

Content Review

FACTORS IN FORMING A GENERAL ASSESSMENT
- Living situation
- Level of activity
- Network of social support
- Level of independence
- Medication history
- Sleep patterns

✱ anorexia nervosa eating disorder marked by excessive fasting.

Content Review

BY-PRODUCTS OF MALNUTRITION
- Vitamin deficiencies
- Dehydration
- Hypoglycemia

> *Try to distinguish the patient's chief complaint from the primary problems.*
>
>

The primary problem, however, may be the rectal bleeding that the patient neglected to mention.

The presence of multiple diseases also complicates the assessment process. The presence of chronic problems may make it more difficult to assess an acute problem. It is easy to confuse symptoms from a chronic illness with those of an acute condition. When confronted with an elderly patient who has chest pain, for example, it is difficult to determine whether the presence of frequent premature ventricular contractions is acute or chronic. Lacking access to the patient's medical record, you should treat the patient on a "threat-to-life" basis.

Other complications stem from age-related changes in an elderly patient's response to illness and injury. Pain may be diminished, causing both you and the patient to underestimate the severity of the primary problem. In addition, the temperature-regulating mechanism may be altered or depressed. This can result in the absence of fever, or a minimal fever, even in the face of a severe infection. Alterations in the temperature-regulating mechanism, coupled with changes in the sweat glands, also makes the elderly more prone to environmental thermal problems.

Because of the complexity of factors that can affect assessment, you must probe for significant symptoms, and ultimately, the primary problem. Patience, respect, and kindness will elicit the answers needed for a pertinent medical history.

History

You should be prepared to spend more time obtaining histories from elderly patients. You may need to split the interview into sessions. For example, you might need to allow patients time to rest, if they become fatigued during the interview, or you might take a break to talk with caregivers.

When gathering the history, keep in mind the complications that arise from multiple diseases and multiple medications. Medications can be an especially important indicator of the patient's diseases. Therefore, you should find the patient's medications and take them to the hospital with the patient. Try to determine which of the medications, including over-the-counter medications, are currently being taken. In cases of multiple medications, there is an increased incidence of medication errors, drug interactions, and noncompliance.

Communication Challenges As previously mentioned, communications may be more difficult when dealing with the aged. **Cataracts** (Figure 43-2) and **glaucoma** can diminish sight. Blindness, often resulting from diabetes and stroke, is more common in the elderly. The level of anxiety increases when a patient is unable to see his or her surroundings clearly. As a result, you should talk calmly to the visually impaired patient. Yelling does not help. Instead, position yourself so the patient can see or touch you.

Age also affects hearing. Overall hearing decreases and patients may suffer from auditory disorders such as **tinnitus** or **Meniere's disease.** Diminished hearing or deafness can make it virtually impossible to obtain a history. In such cases, try to determine the history from a friend or family member. DO NOT shout at the patient. This will not help if the patient is deaf, and it may distort sounds and make it difficult for the patient who still has some hearing to understand you. Write notes if necessary. If the patient can lip-read, speak slowly and directly toward the patient. Whenever possible, verify the history with a reliable source. Also, because loss of hearing may result from other causes (such as a build up of earwax), confirm whether deafness is a pre-existing condition.

Patients may also have trouble with speech. They find it difficult to retrieve words. They will often speak slowly and exhibit changes in voice quality, which may be a normal age-related change. If a patient has forgotten to put in dentures, politely ask the person to do so.

✱ **cataracts** medical condition in which the lens of the eye loses its clearness.

✱ **glaucoma** medical condition where the pressure within the eye increases.

✱ **tinnitus** subjective ringing or tingling sound in the ear.

✱ **Meniere's disease** a disease of the inner ear characterized by vertigo, nerve deafness, and a roar or buzzing in the ear.

Retina

Choroid

Sclera

Optic nerve

Central artery and vein of retina

Vitreous body Ciliary processes

Tendon of lateral rectus muscle

Conjunctiva

Ciliary body

Iris

Anterior chamber

Cornea

Lens

Cataract

Posterior chamber

Posterior capsule of lens

Tendon of medial rectus muscle

Cataract

CATARACT

FIGURE 43-2 Cataracts, which cloud the lens, can diminish eyesight in the elderly.

To improve your skill at communicating with the elderly, keep these techniques in mind.

- Always introduce yourself.
- Speak slowly, distinctly, and respectfully.
- Speak to the patient first, rather than family members, caregivers, or bystanders.
- Speak face to face, at eye level with eye contact (Figure 43-3).
- Locate the patient's hearing aid or eyeglasses, if needed.
- Allow the patient to put on the stethoscope, while you speak into it like a microphone (Figure 43-4).
- Turn on the room lights.

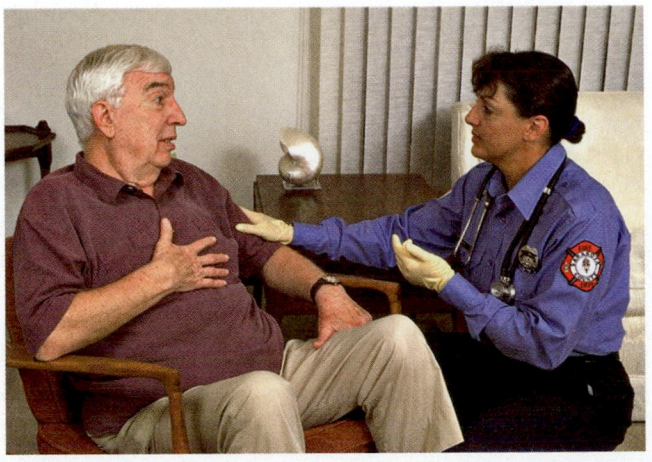

FIGURE 43-3 If possible, talk *to* the elderly patient rather than talking about the patient to others.

FIGURE 43-4 Allow the elderly patient with hearing difficulties to put on the stethoscope while you speak into it like a microphone.

- Display verbal and nonverbal signs of concern and empathy.
- Remain polite at all times.
- Preserve the patient's dignity.
- Always explain what you are doing and why.
- Use your power of observation to recognize anxiety—tempo of speech, eye contact, tone of voice—during the telling of the history.

Altered Mental Status and Confusion Remember that age sometimes diminishes mental status. The patient can be confused and unable to remember details. In addition, the noise of radios, ECG equipment, and strange voices may add to the confusion. Both senility and organic brain syndrome may manifest themselves similarly. Common symptoms include:

- Delirium
- Confusion
- Distractibility
- Restlessness
- Excitability
- Hostility

DO NOT assume that a confused, disoriented patient is "just senile," thus failing to assess for a serious underlying problem.

When confronted with a confused patient, try to determine whether the patient's mental status represents a significant change from normal. DO NOT assume that a confused, disoriented patient is "just senile," thus failing to assess for a serious underlying problem (Figure 43-5). Alcoholism, for example, is more common in the elderly than was once recognized. It can further complicate taking the history.

FIGURE 43-5 DO NOT assume that an altered mental status is a normal age-related change. A number of serious underlying problems may be responsible for changes in consciousness.

Another complication results from depression, which can be mistaken for many other disorders. It can often mimic senility and organic brain syndrome. Depression may also inhibit patient cooperation. The depressed patient may be malnourished, dehydrated, overdosed, contemplating suicide, or simply imagining physical ailments for attention. If you suspect depression, question the patient regarding drug ingestion or suicidal ideation. It is important to remember that suicide is now the fourth-leading cause of death among the elderly in the United States.

Treat depression as a warning sign of substance abuse and/or suicide ideation—both more common among the elderly than previously understood.

Concluding the History After obtaining the history, and if time allows, try to verify the patient's history with a credible source. This will often be less offensive to the patient if done out of his or her presence. While at the scene, it is important to observe the surroundings for indications of the patient's self-sufficiency. Look for evidence of drug or alcohol ingestion or for Medic-Alert or Vial-of-Life items. It is also important to spot signs of abuse or neglect, particularly in dependent living arrangements.

Physical Examination

Certain considerations must be kept in mind when examining the elderly patient. Remember that some patients are often easily fatigued and cannot tolerate a long examination. Also, because of the problems with temperature regulation, the patient may be wearing several layers of clothing, which can make examination difficult. Be sure to explain all actions clearly before initiating the examination, especially to patients with impaired vision. Be aware that the patient may minimize or deny symptoms because of a fear of becoming institutionalized or loss of self-sufficiency.

Try to distinguish signs of chronic disease from an acute problem. Peripheral pulses may be difficult to evaluate, because of peripheral vascular disease and arthritis. The elderly may also have non-pathological crackles (rales) upon lung auscultation. In addition, the elderly often exhibit an increase in mouth breathing and a loss of skin elasticity, which may be easily confused with dehydration. Dependent edema may be caused by inactivity, not congestive heart failure. Only experience and practice will allow you to distinguish acute from chronic physical findings.

Only experience and repeated practice will allow you to distinguish acute from chronic physical findings in the elderly patient.

MANAGEMENT CONSIDERATIONS

As you have read, people become less alike as they age. Therefore, each elderly patient presents a unique challenge in terms of assessment and management. You will need to tailor your management plan to fit a patient's illness, injury, and overall general health. Because of the potential for rapid deterioration among the elderly, you must quickly spot conditions requiring rapid transport. As with any other patient, your first concern is the ABCs. Remain alert at all times for changes in an elderly patient's neurological status, vital signs, and general cardiac status. (Management of specific disorders is covered in other sections of this chapter.)

In general, remember that transport to a hospital is often more stressful to the elderly than to any other age group except for the very young. Avoid lights and sirens in all but the most serious cases, such as when you suspect a pulmonary embolism or bowel infarction. A calm, smooth transport helps to reduce patient anxiety—and the resulting strain on an elderly patient's heart.

Provide emotional support at every phase of the call. Nearly any serious illness or injury in the elderly can provoke a sense of impending doom. Death is a very real possibility to this age group. To help reduce patient fears, keep these guidelines in mind.

- Encourage patients to express their feelings.
- DO NOT trivialize their fears.
- Acknowledge nonverbal messages.
- Avoid questions that are judgmental.
- Confirm what the patient says.
- Recall all you have learned about communicating with the elderly, thus avoiding communication breakdowns.
- Assure patients that you understand that they are adults on an equal footing with their care providers, including you.

SYSTEM PATHOPHYSIOLOGY IN THE ELDERLY

Although aging begins at the cellular level, it eventually affects virtually every system in the body. Age-related changes in the structure and function of organs increase the probability of disease, modify the threshold at which signs and symptoms appear, and affect assessment and treatment of the elderly patient (Table 43-4). You should be familiar with normal systemic changes related to aging so that you can more easily identify the abnormal changes that may point to a serious underlying problem.

Table 43-4 COMMON AGE-RELATED SYSTEMIC CHANGES

Body System	Changes with Age	Clinical Importance
Respiratory	Loss of strength and coordination in respiratory muscles Cough and gag reflex reduced	Increased likelihood of respiratory failure
Cardiovascular	Loss of elasticity and hardening of arteries Changes in heart rate, rhythm, efficiency	Hypertension common Greater likelihood of strokes, heart attacks Great likelihood of bleeding from minor trauma
Neurological	Brain tissue shrinks Loss of memory Clinical depression common Altered mental status common Impaired balance	Delay in appearance of symptoms with head injury Difficulty in patient assessment Increased likelihood of falls
Endocrine	Lowered estrogen production (women) Decline in insulin sensitivity Increase in insulin resistance	Increased likelihood of fractures (bone loss) and heart disease Diabetes mellitus common with greater possibility of hyperglycemia
Gastrointestinal	Diminished digestive functions	Constipation common Greater likelihood of malnutrition
Thermoregulatory	Reduced sweating Decreased shivering	Environmental emergencies more common
Integumentary (Skin)	Thins and becomes more fragile	More subject to tears and sores Bruising more common Heals more slowly
Musculoskeletal	Loss of bone strength (osteoporosis) Loss of joint flexibility and strength (osteoarthritis)	Greater likelihood of fractures Slower healing Increased likelihood of falls
Renal	Loss of kidney size and function	Increased problems with drug toxicity
Genitourinary	Loss of bladder function	Increased urination/incontinence Increased urinary tract infection
Immune	Diminished immune response	More susceptible to infections Impaired immune response to vaccines
Hematological	Decrease in blood volume and/or RBCs	Slower recuperation from illness/injury Greater risk of trauma-related complications

RESPIRATORY SYSTEM

The effects of aging on the respiratory system begin as early as age 30. Age-related changes in the respiratory system include:

- Decreased chest wall compliance
- Loss of lung elasticity
- Increased air trapping due to collapse of the smaller airways
- Reduced strength and endurance of the respiratory muscles

Functionally, by the time we reach age 65, vital capacity may be reduced by as much as 50 percent. In addition, the maximum breathing capacity may decrease by as much as 60 percent, while the maximum oxygen uptake may decrease by as much as 70 percent. These changes ultimately result in decreased ventilation and progressive hypoxemia. Any presence of underlying pulmonary diseases, such as emphysema and chronic bronchitis, further reduces respiratory function.

In addition, there is a decrease in an effective cough reflex and the activity of the cilia—the small hairlike fibers that trap particles and infectious agents. The decline of these two defense mechanisms leave the lungs more susceptible to recurring infection.

Other factors that may affect pulmonary function in the elderly include:

- **Kyphosis**
- Chronic exposure to pollutants
- Long-term cigarette smoking

The management of respiratory distress in elderly patients is essentially the same as for all age groups. Position the patient for adequate breathing, usually upright or sitting. Teach breathing patterns that assist in exhalation, such as "pursed-lip breathing." (Tell patients to pretend they are blowing out a candle with each exhalation.) Use bronchodilators as needed, and provide high concentration supplemental oxygen.

At all points, remain attentive for possible complications, such as **anoxic hypoxemia.** Monitor ventilations closely as an elderly patient can become easily fatigued from any increase in the work of breathing. Remember that many elderly patients with respiratory disease have underlying cardiac disease. With this in mind, drugs such as theophylline and the beta agonists should be used with extreme caution. Monitor cardiovascular status, and administer IV fluids judiciously. DO NOT FLUID OVERLOAD. When infusing fluids, frequently reassess lung sounds to check for the pressure of pulmonary edema.

CARDIOVASCULAR SYSTEM

A number of variables unrelated to aging influence cardiovascular function. They include diet, smoking and alcohol use, education, socioeconomic status, and even personality traits. Of particular importance is the level of physical activity. Even though maximum exercise capacity and maximum oxygen consumption decline with age, a well-trained elderly person can match—or even exceed—the aerobic capacity of an unconditioned younger person.

This said, the cardiovascular system still experiences, in varying degrees, age-related deterioration. The wall of the left ventricle may thicken and enlarge (**hypertrophy**), often by as much as 25 percent. This is even more pronounced if there is associated hypertension. In addition, **fibrosis** develops in the heart and peripheral vascular system, resulting in hypertension, arteriosclerosis, and decreased cardiac function.

The aorta also becomes stiff and lengthens. This results from deposits of calcium and changes in the connective tissue. These changes predispose the aorta to partial tearing, resulting in dissection (thoracic) or aneurysm (abdominal).

As a person ages, the pattern of ventricular filling changes. Less blood enters the left ventricle during early diastole when the mitral valve is open. Therefore, filling and stretch (preload) depend on atrial contraction. Loss of the atrial kick (as will occur with atrial fibrillation) is not well tolerated in the elderly.

Over time, the conductive system of the heart degenerates, often causing dysrhythmias and varying degrees of heart block. Ultimately, the stroke volume declines and the heart rate slows, leading to decreased cardiac output. Because of

---

* kyphosis exaggeration of the normal posterior curvature of the spine.

* anoxic hypoxemia an oxygen deficiency due to disordered pulmonary mechanisms of oxygenation.

In treating respiratory disorders in the elderly patient, DO NOT FLUID OVERLOAD.

* hypertrophy an increase in the size or bulk of an organ.

* fibrosis the formation of fiber-like connective tissue, also called scar tissue in an organ.

this, the heart's ability to respond to stress diminishes. In such situations, expect exercise intolerance—an inability of the heart to meet an exercising muscle's need for oxygen.

To adequately manage complaints related to the cardiovascular system, ask the patient to stop all activity. This reduces the myocardial oxygen demand. DO NOT walk a patient with a cardiovascular complaint to your rig. Take the following basic steps per local protocols.

- Provide high concentration supplemental oxygen.
- Start an IV for medication administration. Medications will vary with the complaint, but may include:
  —Antianginal agents
  —Aspirin
  —Diuretics
  —Antidysrhythmics
- Inquire about age-related dosages.
- Monitor vital signs and rhythm.
- Acquire a 12-lead ECG.
- Remain calm, professional, and empathetic. A heart attack is one of the most fearful situations for the elderly.

DO NOT walk a patient with a cardiovascular disorder to your rig.

NERVOUS SYSTEM

Unlike cells in other organ systems, cells in the central nervous system cannot reproduce. The brain can lose as much as 45 percent of its cells in certain areas of the cortex. Overall, there is an average 10 percent reduction in brain weight from age 20 to age 90. Keep in mind that reductions in brain weight and ventricular size are not well correlated with intelligence, and elderly people may still be capable of highly creative and productive thought. Once again, DO NOT assume that an elderly person possesses less cognitive skill than a younger person. Slight changes that may be expected include:

- Difficulty with recent memory
- Psychomotor slowing
- Forgetfulness
- Decreased reaction times

Although brain size may not have clinical implications in terms in intelligence, it does have implications for trauma. A reduction in brain size leaves room for increased bleeding following a blow to the head, making the elderly more prone to subdural hematomas. In cases of altered mental status, maintain a suspicion of trauma, especially when an accident has been reported.

Whenever you assess an elderly patient for mental status, determine a baseline. Presume your patient to have been mentally sharp unless proven otherwise. (Talk with partners, caregivers, family members, and so on.) Focus on the patient's perceptions, thinking processes, and communication. In questioning an elderly patient, provide an environment with minimal distractions. As already mentioned, ask clear and unhurried questions.

In forming a patient plan, observe for weakness, chronic fatigue, changes in sleep patterns, and syncope or near syncope. If you suspect a stroke, think "brain attack" and assign the patient a priority status. (Additional material on strokes will appear later in the chapter.) Consider blood pressure control per local protocol—but remember that perfusion of the brain tissue depends upon an

In assessing an elderly patient with altered mental status, presume the patient to have been mentally sharp unless proven otherwise.

adequate BP. DO NOT plan to reduce the blood pressure to an average of 120/80 as cerebral blood flow may be diminished. Consider the causes of changes in mental status, keeping in mind the possibility of trauma. Apply oxygen, and monitor ventilations. Depending upon the situation, you may be called on to administer dextrose, thiamine, and naloxone.

ENDOCRINE SYSTEM

Early diagnosis of disorders in the endocrine system offers some of the greatest opportunities to prevent disabilities through appropriate hormonal therapy and/or lifestyle changes. Diabetes mellitus, for example, is extremely common among the elderly. However, normalization of glucose levels—through diet, exercise, and/or drug therapy—can reduce some of the devastating vascular and neurological complications.

In women, menopause—a normal age-related hormonal deficiency—can be similarly treated in a variety of ways, including hormone replacement therapy (HRT). By taking preventive measures, women can reduce and/or delay the incidence of heart disease, bone loss, and possibly Alzheimer's disease.

Thyroid disorders are "clinical masqueraders," especially in the elderly. Common signs and symptoms may be absent or diminished. When signs and symptoms are present, they may be attributed to aging or tied to other diseases, such as cardiovascular, GI, or neuromuscular disorders. However, it has been shown that thyroid disorders, especially hypothyroidism and thyroid nodules, increase with age. (For more on thyroid disorders, see "Metabolic and Endocrine Disorders" later in the chapter.)

With the exception of glucose disorders, most endocrine disorders cannot be easily determined in the field. Many endocrine emergencies will present as altered mental status, especially with insulin-related diseases. Monitor for cardiovascular effects of endocrine changes such as aortic aneurysm in a patient with **Marfan's Syndrome**—a disorder resulting in abnormal growth of distal tissues and a dilatation of the root of the aorta. Also remain alert to blood pressure swings in thyroid disorders such as hyperthyroidism and hypothyroidism.

GASTROINTESTINAL SYSTEM

Age affects the gastrointestinal system in various ways. The volume of saliva may decrease by as much as 33 percent, leading to complaints of dry mouth, nutritional deficiencies, and a predisposition to choking. Gastric secretions may decrease to as little as 20 percent of the quantity present in younger people. Esophageal and intestinal motility also decrease, making swallowing more difficult and delaying digestive processes. The production of hydrochloric acid also declines, further disrupting digestion and, in some adults, contributing to nutritional anemia. Gums atrophy and the number of taste buds decrease, reducing even further the desire to eat.

Other conditions may also develop. **Hiatal hernias** are not age-related per se, but can have serious consequences for the elderly. They may incarcerate, strangulate, or, in the most severe cases, result in massive GI hemorrhage. A diminished liver function, which is associated with aging, can delay or impede detoxification. A common drug toxicity problem for EMS personnel is the use of lidocaine for ventricular arrythmias. (See "Toxicological Emergencies" later in the chapter.) A diminished liver function can also reduce the production of clotting proteins, which in turn leads to bleeding abnormalities.

Complications in the gastrointestinal system can be life-threatening. Use shock protocols as necessary, and remember that not all fluid loss occurs outside the body.

Many endocrine emergencies encountered in the field present as altered mental status, especially with insulin-related disorders.

✳ **Marfan's Syndrome** hereditary condition of connective tissue, bones, muscles, ligaments, and skeletal structures characterized by irregular and unsteady gait, tall lean body type with long extremities, flat feet, stooped shoulders. The aorta is usually dilated and may become weakened enough to allow an aneurysm to develop.

✳ **hiatal hernia** protrusion of the stomach upward into the mediastinal cavity through the esophageal hiatus of the diaphragm.

A diminished liver function, which is associated with aging, can delay or impede detoxification. A common drug toxicity problem for EMS personnel is the use of lidocaine for ventricular arrythmias.

THERMOREGULATORY SYSTEM

The elderly and infants are highly susceptible to variations in environmental temperatures. This occurs in the elderly because of altered or impaired thermoregulatory mechanisms. Aging seems to reduce the effectiveness of sweating in cooling the body. Older persons tend to sweat at higher core temperatures and have less sweat output per gland than younger people. As people age, they also experience deterioration of the autonomic nervous system, including a decrease in shivering and lower resting peripheral blood flow. In addition, the elderly may have a diminished perception of the cold. Drugs and disease can further affect an elderly patient's response to temperature extremes, resulting in hyperthermia or accidental hypothermia.

Environmental emergencies are common causes of EMS calls, especially among the elderly living alone or in poverty. For more on these emergencies, see the discussion of heatstroke, hypothermia, and hyperthermia later in the chapter.

INTEGUMENTARY SYSTEM

As people age, the skin loses collagen, a connective tissue that gives elasticity and support to the skin. Without this support, the skin is subject to a greater number of injuries from bumping or tearing. The lack of support also makes it more difficult to start an IV, as the veins "roll away." Furthermore, the assessment of tenting skin becomes an inaccurate indicator of fluid status in the elderly. Without elasticity, the skin often will remain tented regardless of water balance.

As the skin thins, cells reproduce more slowly. Injury to skin is often more severe than in younger patients and healing time is increased. As a rule, the elderly are at a higher risk of secondary infection, skin tumors, drug-induced eruptions, and fungal or viral infections. Decades of exposure to the sun also makes the elderly vulnerable to melanoma and other sun-related carcinomas (e.g., basal cell carcinoma, squamous cell carcinoma).

MUSCULOSKELETAL SYSTEM

An aging person may lose as much as 2–3 inches of height from narrowing of the intervertebral discs and **osteoporosis.** Osteoporosis is the loss of mineral from the bone, resulting in softening of the bones. This is especially evident in the vertebral bodies, thus causing a change in posture. The posture of the aged individual often reveals an increase in the curvature of the thoracic spine, commonly called kyphosis, and slight flexion of the knee and hip joints. The demineralization of bone makes the patient much more susceptible to hip and other fractures. Some fractures may even occur from simple actions such as sneezing.

> * **osteoporosis** softening of bone tissue due to the loss of essential minerals, principally calcium.

In addition to skeletal changes, a decrease in skeletal muscle weight commonly occurs with age—especially with sedentary individuals. To compensate, elderly women develop a narrow, short gait, while older men develop a wide gait. These changes make the elderly more susceptible to falls and, consequently, a possible loss of independence.

Because of the changes in the musculoskeletal system, simple trauma in the elderly can lead to complex injuries. In treating musculoskeletal disorders, supply supplemental oxygen, initiate an IV line, and consider pain control. Many extremity injuries should be splinted as found because of changes in the bone and joint structure of the elderly. To determine the cause of any injury, be sure to look beyond the obvious. Keep in mind the possibility of underlying medical conditions, drug complications, abuse or neglect, and ingestion of alcohol or drugs.

> *Many extremity injuries should be splinted as found because of changes in the bone and joint structure in the elderly.*
>
>

RENAL SYSTEM

* **nephrons** the functional units of the kidneys.

Aging affects the renal system through a reduction in the number of functioning **nephrons,** which may be decreased by 30–40 percent. Renal blood flow may also be reduced by up to 45 percent, increasing the waste products in the blood and upsetting the fluid and electrolyte balance. Because the kidneys are responsible for the production of erythropoietin (which stimulates the production of red blood cells in the bone marrow) and renin (which stimulates vasoconstriction), a decrease in renal function may result in anemia or hypertension in the older patient.

Prehospital treatment of complaints involving the renal and urinary systems is directed toward adequate oxygenation, fluid status, monitoring output, and pain control. Pay attention to the airway as nausea and vomiting are complications of pain secondary to renal obstruction. Also monitor vital signs to detect changes in blood pressure and pulse.

GENITOURINARY SYSTEM

As people age, they experience a progressive loss of bladder sensation and tone. The bladder does not empty completely and consequently the patient may sense a frequent need to urinate. This urge increases the risk of falls, especially during the middle of the night when lighting is dim or the patient is sleepy. Furthermore, the lack of emptying increases the likelihood of urinary tract infection and perhaps sepsis. In the male, the prostate often becomes enlarged (benign prostatic hypertrophy), causing difficulty in urination or urinary retention. As already mentioned, the elderly also commonly develop, in varying degrees, problems with incontinence.

Treatment for a complaint in the genitourinary system is described in the preceding section on the renal system and in the earlier discussion of incontinence.

IMMUNE SYSTEM

As a person ages, the function of T cells declines, making them less able to notify the immune system of invasion by antigens. A diminished immune response, sometimes called **immune senescence,** increases the susceptibility of the elderly to infections. It also increases the duration and severity of an infection.

* **immune senescence** diminished vigor of the immune response to the challenge and rechallenge by pathogens.

Unless contraindicated, the elderly should receive vaccinations suggested by the Health Department. However, keep in mind that aging impairs the immune response to vaccines. The best prevention is adequate nutrition, infection control measures (e.g., washing hands), and exercise. Recognition and treatment of diseases such as diabetes mellitus, heart failure, thyroid disease, and occult malignancy also reduce the risk and severity of infections. As a paramedic, you should treat alterations in immune status as life threats and seek to prevent exposure of patients to infectious agents. DO NOT transmit an illness—even a mild cold—to an elderly patient.

DO NOT transmit an illness—even a mild cold—to an elderly patient.

HEMATOLOGY SYSTEM

The hematology system is affected by a failure of the renal system to stimulate the production of red blood cells. Nutritional abnormalities may also produce abnormal RBCs. Since there is less body water present in the elderly, blood volume similarly decreases. This makes it difficult for an elderly patient to recuperate from an illness or injury. Intervention must be started early in order to make a lasting difference.

In addition to providing supplemental oxygen, you should prepare for increases in bleeding time. Monitor the elderly patient closely as deterioration is difficult to stop.

COMMON MEDICAL PROBLEMS IN THE ELDERLY

In general, the elderly suffer from the same kinds of medical emergencies as younger patients. However, illnesses may be more severe, complications more likely, and classic signs and symptoms absent or altered. In addition, the elderly are more likely to react adversely to stress and deteriorate much more quickly than young or middle-aged adults. The following are some of the medical disorders that you may encounter.

PULMONARY/RESPIRATORY DISORDERS

Respiratory emergencies are some of the most common reasons elderly persons summon EMS or seek emergency care. Most elderly patients with a respiratory disorder present with a chief complaint of dyspnea. However, coughing, congestion, and wheezing are also common chief complaints.

Many factors can trigger respiratory distress among the elderly (Figure 43-6). Descriptions of the most common ones follow.

Pneumonia

Pneumonia is an infection of the lung. It is usually caused by a bacterium or virus. However, aspiration pneumonia may also develop as a result of difficulty swallowing.

Pneumonia is a serious disease for the elderly. It is the fourth leading cause of death in people age 65 and older. Its incidence increases with age at a rate of 10 percent for each decade beyond age 20. It is found in up to 60 percent of the

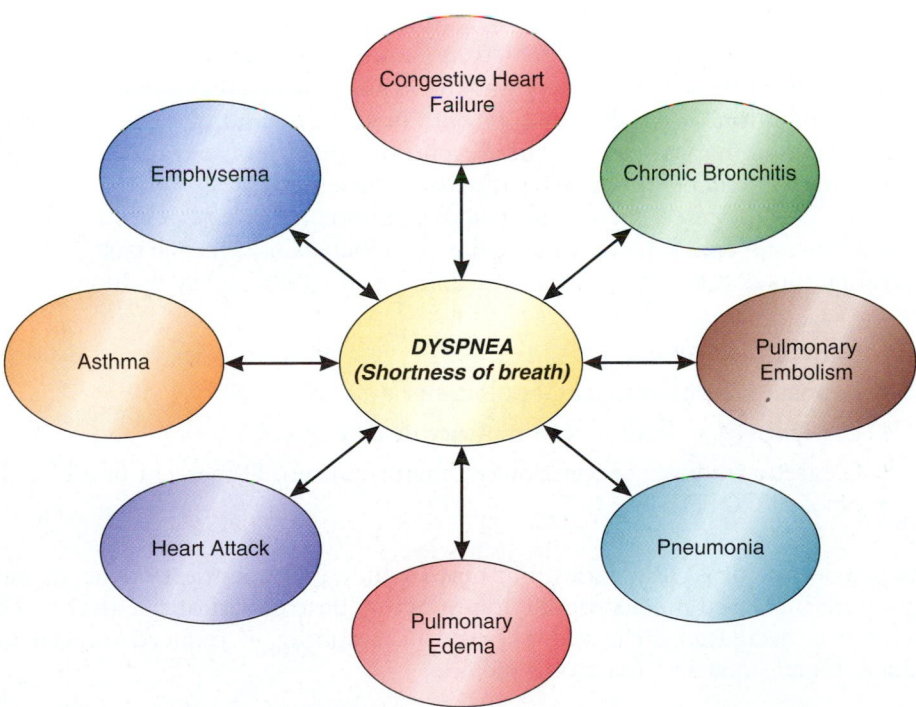

FIGURE 43-6   Dyspnea can be caused by a number of respiratory and cardiac problems in the elderly.

autopsies performed on the elderly. Reasons the elderly develop pneumonia more frequently than younger patients include:

- Decreased immune response
- Reduced pulmonary function
- Increased colonization of the pharynx by gram-negative bacteria
- Abnormal or ineffective cough reflex
- Decreased effectiveness of mucociliary cells of the upper respiratory system

The elderly who are at greatest risk for contracting pneumonia include frail adults and those with chronic, multiple diseases or compromised immunity. Institutionalized patients—either in hospitals or nursing homes—are especially vulnerable because of increased exposure to microorganisms and limited mobility. A patient in an institutional setting is up to 50 times more likely to contract pneumonia than an elderly patient receiving home care.

Common signs and symptoms of pneumonia include increasing dyspnea, congestion, fever, chills, tachypnea, sputum production, and altered mental status. Occasionally, abdominal pain may be the only symptom. Because of thermoregulatory changes, a fever may be absent in an elderly patient.

Prevention strategies include prophylactic treatment with antibiotics. Efforts should also be taken to reduce exposure to infectious patients and to promote patient mobility.

In treating an elderly patient with pneumonia, manage all life threats. Maintain adequate oxygenation. Transport the patient to the hospital for diagnosis, keeping in mind that patients with respiratory disease often have other underlying problems.

Chronic Obstructive Pulmonary Disease

Chronic obstructive pulmonary disease (COPD) is really a collection of diseases, characterized by chronic airflow obstruction with reversible and/or irreversible components. Although each COPD has its own distinct features, elderly patients commonly have two or more types at the same time. COPD usually refers to some combination of emphysema, chronic bronchitis, and, to a lesser degree, asthma. Pneumonia, as well as other respiratory disorders, can further complicate chronic obstructive pulmonary disease in the elderly.

In the United States, chronic obstructive pulmonary disease is among the ten leading causes of death. Its prevalence has been increasing over the past 20 years. Several factors combine to produce the damage of COPD. They include:

- Genetic disposition
- Exposure to environmental pollutants
- Existence of a childhood respiratory disease
- Cigarette smoking, a contributing factor in up to 80 percent of all cases of COPD

The physiology of COPD varies, but may include inflammation of the air passages with increased mucus production or actual destruction of the alveoli. The outcome is decreased airflow in the alveoli, resulting in reduced oxygen exchange. Usual signs and symptoms include:

- Cough
- Increased sputum production

- Dyspnea
- Accessory muscle use
- Pursed-lip breathing
- Tripod positioning
- Exercise intolerance
- Wheezing
- Pleuritic chest pain
- Tachypnea

COPD is progressive and debilitating (Figure 43-7). The patient can often keep the signs and symptoms under control until the body is stressed. When the condition becomes disabling, it is called exacerbation of COPD. This condition can lead rapidly to patient death as hypoxia and hypercapnia alter acid-base balance and deprive the tissues of the oxygen needed for efficient energy production.

The most effective prevention involves elimination of tobacco products and reduced exposure to cigarette smoke (in non-smokers). Recent legislation has sought to keep public places smoke free and to discourage cigarette smoking in the young. Once the disease is present, patients are taught to identify stresses that exacerbate the condition. Appropriate self care includes exercise, avoidance of infections, appropriate use of drugs, and, when necessary, calling EMS.

When confronted with an elderly patient with COPD, treatment is essentially the same as for all age groups. Supply supplemental oxygen and possibly drug therapy, usually for reducing dyspnea.

FIGURE 43-7 The COPD patient may use a nasal cannula with a home oxygen unit.

Pulmonary Embolism

Pulmonary embolism (PE) should always be considered as a possible cause of respiratory distress in the elderly. Although statistics for the elderly are unavailable, approximately 650,000 cases occur annually in the United States alone. Of this number, a pulmonary embolism is the primary cause of death in 100,000 people and a contributing factor in another 100,000 deaths. Nearly 11 percent of PE deaths take place in the first hour and 38 percent in the second hour.

Blood clots are the most frequent cause of pulmonary embolism. However, the condition may also be caused by fat, air, bone marrow, tumor cells, or foreign bodies. Risk factors for developing pulmonary embolism include:

- Deep venous thrombosis
- Prolonged immobility, common among the elderly
- Malignancy (tumors)
- Paralysis
- Fractures of the pelvis, hip, or leg
- Obesity
- Trauma to the leg vessels
- Major surgery
- Presence of a venous catheter
- Use of estrogen (in women)
- Atrial fibrillation

Pulmonary emboli usually originate in the deep veins of the thigh and calf. The condition should be suspected in any patient with the acute onset of dyspnea. Often, it is accompanied by pleuritic chest pain and right heart failure. If the pulmonary embolus is massive, you can expect severe dyspnea, cardiac dysrhythmias, and, ultimately, cardiovascular collapse.

Definitive diagnosis of a pulmonary embolism takes place in a hospital setting. The goals of field treatment are to manage and minimize complications of the condition. General treatment considerations include delivery of high-flow oxygen via mask, maintaining oxygen levels above an SaO_2 of 90 percent. Establishment of an IV for possible administration of medications is appropriate, but vigorous fluid therapy should be avoided, if possible.

Prehospital pharmacological therapy for pulmonary embolism is limited. Upon advice from medical direction, you may administer small doses of morphine sulfate to reduce patient anxiety. After confirming the absence of GI bleeding, medical direction may also prescribe anticoagulants to prevent clot formation and/or to speed clot dissolution. If the administration of a vasopressor is indicated by low blood pressure, then dopamine may be prescribed. In such cases, remember to titrate the dopamine to a desirable blood pressure.

The risk of death from pulmonary embolism is greatest in the first few hours. As a result, rapid transport is essential. Position the patient in an upright position and avoid lifting the patient by the legs or knees, which may dislodge thrombi in the lower extremities. During transport, continue to monitor changes in skin color, pulse oximetry, and changes in breathing rate and rhythm. Your field assessment and interventions can save the patient's life and guide the hospital physician in a direction that will result in an accurate diagnosis and rapid treatment.

The risk of death from pulmonary embolism is greatest in the first few hours. As a result, rapid transport is essential.

Pulmonary Edema

Pulmonary edema is an effusion or escape of serous fluids into the alveoli and interstitial tissues of the lungs. Acute pulmonary edema can develop rapidly in the elderly. Although most commonly associated with acute myocardial infarction, it can also occur due to other factors including pulmonary infections, inhaled toxins, narcotic overdose, pulmonary embolism, and decreased atmospheric pressure.

Pulmonary edema causes severe dyspnea associated with congestion. Other signs and symptoms include rapid labored breathing, cough with blood-stained sputum, cyanosis, and cold extremities. Physical examination usually reveals the presence of moist crackles and accessory muscle use. Severe cases will exhibit rhonchi.

Treatment is directed toward altering the cause of the condition. The existence of pulmonary edema can be life-threatening and is often the symptom of a fatal cardiovascular disease.

The existence of pulmonary edema can be life-threatening and is often the symptom of a fatal cardiovascular disease.

Lung Cancer

North America has the highest incidence of lung cancer in the world. The incidence increases with age, with about 65 percent of all lung cancer deaths occurring among people age 65 and older. The leading cause of lung cancer is cigarette smoking.

Often, progressive dyspnea will be the first presentation of a cancerous lesion. Hemoptysis (bloody sputum), chronic cough, and weight loss are also common symptoms.

Treatment of lung cancer occurs in a hospital setting. However, you may be called to assist in the follow-up home care or, in terminal stages, a hospice. (See Chapter 46 for more information on this subject.)

CARDIOVASCULAR DISORDERS

The leading cause of death in the elderly is cardiovascular disease. Assessment and treatment of cardiovascular disease in the elderly patient is often complicated by non-age-related factors and disease processes in other organ systems. In conducting your history, determine the patient's level of cardiovascular fitness, changes in exercise tolerance, recent diet history, use of medications, and use of cigarettes and/or alcohol. Ask questions about breathing difficulty, especially at night, and evidence of palpitations, flutter, or skipped beats.

In performing the physical exam, look for hypertension and orthostatic hypotension (a decrease in blood pressure and an increase in heart rate when rising from a seated or supine position). Watch for dehydration or dependent edema. When taking an elderly patient's blood pressure, consider checking both arms. Routinely determine pulses in all the extremities. In auscultating the patient, remember that a bruit or noise in the neck, abdomen, or groin indicates a high probability of carotid, aortorenal, or peripheral vascular disease. Keep in mind, too, that heart sounds are generally softer in the elderly, probably because of a thickening of lung tissue between the heart and chest wall.

In evaluating the problem, recall the cardiovascular disorders commonly found in elderly patients. They include angina pectoris, myocardial infarction, heart failure, dysrhythmias, aortic dissection, aneurysm, hypertension, and syncope.

Angina Pectoris

The likelihood of developing angina increases dramatically with age. This is especially true of women, who are estrogen protected until after menopause. Angina is usually triggered by physical activity, especially after a meal, and by exposure to very cold weather. Attacks vary in frequency, from several a day to occasional episodes separated by weeks or months.

Angina pectoris literally means "pain in the chest." However, the pain of angina is actually felt in only about 10–20 percent of elderly patients. The changes in sensory nerves, combined with the myocardial changes of aging, make dyspnea a more likely symptom of angina than pain.

Angina develops when narrowing of coronary vessels due to plaque or vasospasm lead to an inability to meet the oxygen demands of the heart muscle. The heart muscle usually responds by sending out pain signals, which represent a build-up of lactic acid. In an elderly patient, exercise intolerance is a key symptom of angina. In obtaining a history, you should ask the patient about sudden changes in routine. In addition, inquire about any increased stresses on the heart, such as anemia, infection, dysrhythmias, and thyroid changes.

General prevention strategies in the elderly are similar to those in young patients. Blood pressure control, combined with diet, exercise, and smoking modifications reduces the risk in all groups.

Myocardial Infarction

A myocardial infarction (MI) involves actual death of muscle tissue due to a partial or complete occlusion of one or more of the coronary arteries. The greatest number of patients hospitalized for acute myocardial infarction are older than 65. The elderly patient with myocardial infarction is less likely to present with classic symptoms such as chest pain than a younger counterpart. Atypical presentations that may be seen in the elderly include:

- Absence of pain
- Exercise intolerance
- Confusion/dizziness
- Syncope
- Dyspnea—common in patients over age 85
- Neck, dental, and/or epigastric pain
- Fatigue/weakness

In auscultating a patient, remember that a bruit in the neck, abdomen, or groin indicates a high probability of carotid, aortorenal, or peripheral vascular disease.

Keep in mind that heart sounds are generally softer in the elderly, probably because of a thickening of lung tissues between the heart and chest wall.

In an elderly patient, exercise intolerance is a key symptom of angina.

The elderly patient with myocardial infarction is less likely to present with classic symptoms than a younger counterpart.

The mortality rate associated with myocardial infarction and/or resulting complications doubles after age 70. Unlike younger patients, the elderly are more likely to suffer a **silent myocardial infarction.** They also tend to have larger myocardial infarctions. The majority of deaths that occur in the first few hours following a myocardial infarction are due to dysrhythmias.

A myocardial infarction is most commonly triggered by some form of physical exertion or a preexisting heart disease. Because of the high mortality associated with myocardial infarctions in the elderly, early detection and emergency management are critical.

Heart Failure

Heart failure takes place when cardiac output cannot meet the body's metabolic demands. The incidence rises exponentially after age 60. The condition is widespread among the elderly and is the most common diagnosis in hospitalized patients over age 65. The causes of heart failure fall in one of four categories: impairment to flow, inadequate cardiac filling, volume overload, and myocardial failure.

Typical age-related factors, such as prolonged myocardial contractions, make the elderly vulnerable to heart failure. Other factors that place them at risk include:

- Noncompliance with drug therapy
- Anemia
- Ischemia
- Thermoregulatory disorders (hypothermia/hyperthermia)
- Hypoxia
- Infection
- Use of non-steroidal anti-inflammatory drugs

Signs and symptoms of heart failure vary. In most patients, regardless of age, some form of edema exists. However, edema in the elderly can indicate a range of problems, including musculoskeletal injury. Assessment findings specific to the elderly include:

- Fatigue (left failure)
- **Two pillow orthopnea**
- Dyspnea on exertion
- Dry, hacking cough progressing to productive cough
- Dependent edema (right failure)
- **Nocturia**
- Anorexia, **hepatomegaly,** ascites

Nonpharmacologic management of heart failure includes modifications in diet (e.g., less fat and cholesterol), exercise, and reduction in weight, if necessary. Pharmacologic management may include treatment with diuretics, vasodilators, antihypertensive agents, or inotropic agents. Check to see if the patient is already on any of these medications and if the patient is compliant with scheduled doses.

Dysrhythmias

Many cardiac dysrhythmias develop with age. Atrial fibrillation is the most common dysrhythmia encountered.

Dysrhythmias occur primarily as a result of degeneration of the patient's conductive system. Anything that decreases myocardial blood flood can produce a dysrhythmia. They may also be caused by electrolyte abnormalities.

To complicate matters further, the elderly do not tolerate extremes in heart rate as well as a younger person would. For example, a heart rate of 140 in an older patient may cause syncope, while a younger patient can often tolerate a heart rate greater than 180. In addition, dysrhythmias can lead to falls from cerebral hypoperfusion. They can also result in congestive heart failure (CHF) or a transient ischemic attack (TIA).

Treatment considerations depend upon the type of dysrhythmia. Patients may already have a pacemaker in place. In such cases, keep in mind that pacemakers have a low but significant rate of complications such as a failed battery, fibrosis around the catheter site, lead fracture, or electrode dislodgment. In a number of situations, drug therapy may be indicated. Whenever you discover a dysrhythmia, remember that an abnormal or disordered heart rhythm may be the only clinical finding in an elderly patient suffering acute myocardial infarction.

Aortic Dissection/Aneurysms

Aortic dissection is a degeneration of the wall of the aorta, either in the thoracic or abdominal cavity. It can result in an **aneurysm** or in a rupture of the vessel.

Approximately 80 percent of thoracic aneurysms are due to atherosclerosis combined with hypertension. The remaining cases occur secondary to other factors, including Marfan's Syndrome or blunt trauma to the chest. Patients with dissections will often present with tearing chest pain radiating through to the back or, if rupture occurs, cardiac arrest.

The distal portion of the aorta is the most common site for abdominal aneurysms. Approximately 1 in 250 people over age 50 die from a ruptured abdominal aneurysm. The aneurysm may appear as a pulsatile mass in a patient with a normal girth, but lack of an identifiable mass does not eliminate this condition. Patients may present with tearing abdominal pain or unexplained low back pain. Pulses in the legs are diminished or absent and the lower extremities feel cold to the touch. There may be sensory abnormalities such as numbness, tingling, or pain in the legs. The patient may fall when attempting to stand.

Treatment of an aneurysm depends on its size, location, and the severity of the condition. In the case of thoracic aortic dissection, continuous IV infusion and/or administration of drug therapy to lower the arterial pressure and to diminish the velocity of left ventricle contraction may be indicated. Rapid transport is essential, especially for the older patient who most commonly requires care and observation in an intensive care unit.

Hypertension

Hypertension appears to be a product of industrial society. In developed nations, such as the United States, the systolic and diastolic pressures have a tendency to rise until age 60. Systolic pressure may continue to rise after that time, but diastolic pressure stabilizes. Since this rise in blood pressure is not seen in less developed nations, experts believe that hypertension is not a normal age-related change.

Today more than 50 percent of Americans over age 65 have clinically diagnosed hypertension—defined as blood pressure greater than 140/90 mmHg. Prolonged elevated blood pressure will eventually damage the heart, brain, or kidneys. As a result of hypertension, elderly patients are at greater risk for heart failure, stroke, blindness, renal failure, coronary heart disease, and peripheral vascular disease. In men with blood pressure greater than 160/95 mmHg, the risk of mortality nearly doubles.

Content Review

POSSIBLE PACEMAKER COMPLICATIONS

- Failed battery
- Fibrosis around the catheter site
- Lead fracture
- Electrode dislodgment

Remember that an abnormal or disordered heart rhythm may be the only clinical finding in an elderly patient suffering acute myocardial infarction.

* **aortic dissection** a degeneration of the wall of the aorta.

* **aneurysm** abnormal dilation of a blood vessel, usually an artery, due to a congenital defect or a weakness in the wall of the vessel.

Most abdominal aortic aneurysms occur below the renal arteries.

＊ **epistaxis** nosebleed.

＊ **varicosities** an abnormal dilation of a vein or group of veins.

＊ **autonomic dysfunction** an abnormality of the involuntary aspect of the nervous system.

＊ **valsalva maneuver** forced exhalation against a closed glottis, such as with coughing. This maneuver stimulates the parasympathetic nervous system via the vagus nerve, which in turn slows the heart rate.

＊ **Stokes-Adams syndrome** a series of symptoms resulting from heart block, most commonly syncope. The symptoms result from decreased blood flow to the brain caused by the sudden decrease in cardiac output.

＊ **sick sinus syndrome** a group of disorders characterized by dysfunction of the sinoatrial node in the heart.

Hypertension increases with atherosclerosis, which is more common with the elderly than other age groups. Other contributing factors include obesity and diabetes. The condition can be prevented or controlled through diet (sodium reduction), exercise, cessation of smoking, and compliance with medications.

Hypertension is often a silent disease that produces no clinically obvious signs or symptoms. It may be associated with nonspecific complaints such as headache, tinnitus, **epistaxis,** slow tremors, or nausea and vomiting. An acute onset of high blood pressure without any kidney involvement is often a telltale indicator of thyroid disease.

Management of hypertension depends upon its severity and the existence of other conditions. For example, hypertension is often treated with beta-blockers—medications that are contraindicated in patients with chronic obstructive lung disease, asthma, or heart block greater than first degree. Diuretics, another common drug used in treating hypertension, should be prescribed with care for patients on digitalis. Keep in mind that centrally acting agents are more likely to produce negative side effects in the elderly. Unlike younger patients, the elderly may experience depression, forgetfulness, sleep problems, or vivid dreams and/or hallucinations.

Syncope

Syncope is a common presenting complaint among the elderly. The condition results when blood flow to the brain is temporarily interrupted or decreased. It is most often caused by problems with either the nervous system or the cardiovascular system. In general, syncope has a higher incidence of death in elderly patients than in younger individuals. The following are some of the common presentations that you may encounter:

- *Vasodepressor Syncope.* Vasodepressor syncope is the common faint. It may occur following emotional distress, pain, prolonged bed rest, mild blood loss, prolonged standing in warm, crowded rooms, anemia, or fever.

- *Orthostatic Syncope.* Orthostatic syncope occurs when a person rises from a seated or supine position. There are several possible causes. First, there may be a disproportion between blood volume and vascular capacity. That is, there is a pooling of blood in the legs, reducing blood flow to the brain. Causes of this include hypovolemia, venous **varicosities,** prolonged bed rest, and **autonomic dysfunction.** Many drugs, especially blood pressure medicines, can cause drug-induced orthostatic syncope due to the effects of the medications on the capacitance vessels.

- *Vasovagal Syncope.* Vasovagal syncope occurs as a result of a **valsalva maneuver,** which happens during defecation, coughing, or similar maneuvers. This effectively slows the heart rate and cardiac output, thus decreasing blood flow to the brain.

- *Cardiac Syncope.* Cardiac syncope results from transient reduction in cerebral blood flow due to a sudden decrease in cardiac output. It can result from several mechanisms. Syncope can be the primary symptom of silent myocardial infarction. In addition, many dysrhythmias can cause syncope. Dysrhythmias that have been shown to cause syncope include bradycardias, **Stokes-Adams syndrome,** heart block, tachydysrhythmia, and **sick sinus syndrome.**

- *Seizures.* Syncope may result from a seizure disorder or syncope (prolonged) may cause seizure activity. Syncope due to seizures tends to occur without warning. It is associated with muscular jerking or convulsions, incontinence, and tongue-biting. Postictal confusion may follow.

- *Transient Ischemic Attacks.* Transient ischemic attacks occur more frequently in the elderly. They may cause syncope.

NEUROLOGICAL DISORDERS

Elderly patients are at risk for several neurological emergencies. Often, the exact cause is not initially known and may require probing at the hospital.

Many of the neurological disorders that you will encounter in the field will exhibit an alteration in mental status. You may discover a range of underlying causes from stroke to degenerative brain disease. Some of the most common causes of altered mental status include:

- Cerebrovascular disease (stroke or transient ischemic attack)
- Myocardial infarction
- Seizures
- Medication-related problems (drug interactions, drug underdose, and drug overdose)
- Infection
- Fluid and electrolyte abnormalities (dehydration)
- Lack of nutrients (hypoglycemia)
- Temperature changes (hypothermia, hyperthermia)
- Structural changes (dementia, subdural hematoma)

As mentioned, it is often impossible in the field to distinguish the cause of an altered mental status. Even so, you should carry out a thorough assessment. Administer supplemental oxygen. As soon as practical, obtain a blood glucose level to exclude hypoglycemia as a possible cause. Overall, the approach to the elderly patient with altered mental status is the same as with any other patient presenting with similar symptoms.

Cerebrovascular Disease (Stroke/Brain Attack)

Stroke is the third leading cause of death in the United States. Annually, about 500,000 people suffer strokes and about 150,000 die. Incidence of stroke and the likelihood of dying from a stroke increase with age. Occlusive stroke is statistically more common in the elderly and relatively uncommon in younger individuals. Older patients are at higher risk of stroke because of atherosclerosis, hypertension, immobility, limb paralysis, congestive heart failure, and atrial fibrillation. Transient ischemic attacks (TIAs) are also more common in older patients. More than one-third of patients suffering TIAs will develop a major, permanent stroke. As previously mentioned, TIAs are a frequent cause of syncope in the elderly.

Strokes usually fall in one of two major categories. **Brain ischemia**—injury to brain tissue caused by an inadequate supply of oxygen and nutrients—accounts for about 80 percent of all strokes. Brain hemorrhage, the second major category, may be either **subarachnoid hemorrhage** or **intracerebral hemorrhage**. These different patterns of bleeding have different presentations, causes, and treatments. However, together they account for a high percentage of all stroke deaths.

Because of the various kinds of strokes, signs and symptoms can present in many ways—altered mental status, coma, paralysis, slurred speech, a change in

As soon as practical, obtain a blood glucose level to exclude hypoglycemia as a possible cause of altered mental status in an elderly patient.

* **stroke** injury to or death of brain tissue resulting from interruption of cerebral blood flow and oxygenation.

* **brain ischemia** injury to brain tissues caused by an inadequate supply of oxygen and nutrients.

* **subarachnoid hemorrhage** bleeding that occurs between the arachnoid and dura mater of the brain.

* **intracerebral hemorrhage** bleeding directly into the brain.

mood, and seizures. Stroke should be highly suspect in any elderly patient with a sudden change in mental status.

Whenever you suspect a stroke, it is essential that you complete the Glasgow Coma Scale for later comparison in the emergency department. Thrombolytic agents administered to a patient suffering an occlusive (ischemic) stroke can decrease the severity of damage if administered within 3 hours of onset. Rapid transport is essential for avoiding brain damage or limiting its extent. In the case of stroke, "time is brain tissue."

By far the most preferred treatment is prevention of strokes in the first place. Strategies include:

- Control of hypertension
- Treatment of cardiac disorders, including dysrhythmias and coronary artery disease
- Treatment of blood disorders, such as anemia and **polycythemia**
- Cessation of smoking
- Cessation of recreational drugs
- Moderate use of alcohol
- Regular exercise
- Good eating habits

Seizures

Seizures may be easily mistaken for stroke in the elderly. Also, a first-time seizure may occur due to damage from a previous stroke. Not all seizures experienced by the elderly are of the major motor type. Some are more subtle. Many causes of seizure activity in the elderly have been identified. Common causes include:

- Seizure disorder (epilepsy)
- Syncope
- Recent or past head trauma
- Mass lesion (tumor or bleed)
- Alcohol withdrawal
- Hypoglycemia
- Stroke

Often the cause of the seizure cannot be determined in the field. As a result, treat the condition as a life-threatening emergency and transport as quickly as possible to eliminate the possibility of stroke. If the patient has fallen during a seizure, check for evidence of trauma and treat accordingly.

Dizziness/Vertigo

Dizziness is a frightening experience and a frequent complaint of the elderly. The complaint of dizziness may actually mean that the patient has suffered syncope, pre-syncope, light-headedness, or true **vertigo**. Vertigo is a specific sensation of motion perceived by the patient as spinning or whirling. Many patients will report that they feel as though they are spinning. Vertigo is often accompanied with sweating, pallor, nausea, and vomiting. Meniere's disease can cause severe, **intractable** vertigo. It is often, however, associated with a constant "roaring" sound in the ears, as well as ear "pressure."

Whenever you suspect stroke, it is essential that you complete the Glasgow Coma Scale for later comparison in the emergency department.

* **polycythemia** an excess of red blood cells.

Treat seizures in the elderly as a life-threatening condition and transport as quickly as possible to eliminate the possibility of stroke.

* **vertigo** the sensation of faintness or dizziness; may cause a loss of balance.

* **intractable** resistant to cure, relief, or control.

Table 43-5	DISTINGUISHING DEMENTIA AND DELIRIUM*
Dementla	**Delirium**
Chronic, slowly progressive development	Rapid in onset, fluctuating course
Irreversible disorder	May be reversed, especially if treated early
Greatly impairs memory	Greatly impairs attention
Global cognitive deficits	Focal cognitive deficits
Most commonly caused by Alzheimer's disease	Most commonly caused by systemic disease, drug toxicity, or metabolic changes
Does not require immediate treatment	Requires immediate treatment

*These are general characteristics that apply to most, but not all cases. For example, some forms of dementia, such as those caused by hypothyroidism, may be reversed.

Vertigo results from so many factors that it is often hard, even for the physician, to determine the actual cause. Any factor that impairs visual input, inner-ear function, peripheral sensory input, or the central nervous system can cause dizziness. In addition, alcohol and many prescription drugs can cause dizziness. So can hypoglycemia in its early stages. It is virtually impossible to distinguish dizziness, syncope, and pre-syncope in the prehospital setting.

Delirium, Dementia, Alzheimer's Disease

Approximately 15 percent of all Americans over age 65 have some degree of dementia or delirium. **Dementia** is a chronic global cognitive impairment, often progressive or irreversible. The best-known form of dementia is **Alzheimer's disease,** a condition that affects 4 million Americans. **Delirium** is a global mental impairment of sudden onset and self-limited duration. (For differences between dementia and delirium, see Table 43-5.)

Delirium Many conditions can cause delirium. The cause may be either organic brain disease or disorders that occur elsewhere in the body. Delirium in the elderly is a serious condition. According to some estimates, about 18 percent of hospitalized elderly patients with delirium die. Possible etiologies or causes include:

* Subdural hematoma
* Tumors and other mass lesions
* Drug-induced changes or alcohol intoxication
* CNS infections
* Electrolyte abnormalities
* Cardiac failure
* Fever
* Metabolic disorders, including hypoglycemia
* Chronic endocrine abnormalities, including hypothyroidism and hyperthyroidism
* Postconcussion syndrome

The presentation of delirium varies greatly and can change rapidly during assessment. Common signs and symptoms include the acute onset of anxiety, an inability to focus, disordered thinking, irritability, inappropriate behavior, fearfulness, excessive energy, or psychotic behavior such as hallucinations or paranoia. Aphasic

✱ **dementia** a deterioration of mental status that is usually associated with structural neurological disease. It is often progressive and irreversible.

✱ **Alzheimer's disease** a progressive, degenerative disease that attacks the brain and results in impaired memory, thinking, and behavior. It affects 4 million American adults.

✱ **delirium** an acute alteration in mental functioning that is often reversible.

or speaking errors and/or prominent slurring may be present. Normal patterns of eating and sleeping are almost always disrupted.

In distinguishing between delirium and dementia, err on the side of delirium. The condition is often caused by life-threatening, but reversible, conditions. Causes of delirium such as infections, drug toxicity, and electrolyte imbalances generally have a good prognosis if identified quickly and managed promptly.

Dementia Dementia is more prevalent in the elderly than delirium. Over 50 percent of all nursing home patients have some form of dementia. It is usually due to an underlying neurological disease. This mental deterioration is often called "organic brain syndrome," **"senile dementia,"** or "senility." It is important to find out whether an alteration in mental status is acute or chronic. Causes of dementia include:

- Small strokes
- Atherosclerosis
- Age-related neurological changes
- Neurological diseases
- Certain hereditary diseases (e.g., Huntington's disease)
- Alzheimer's disease

Signs and symptoms of dementia include progressive disorientation, shortened attention span, **aphasia** or nonsense talking, and hallucinations. Dementia often hampers treatment through the patient's inability to communicate and exhausts caregivers. In moderate to severe cases, you will need to rely on the caregiver for information. (Remain alert to signs of abuse or neglect, which occurs in a disproportionate number of elderly suffering from dementia.)

Alzheimer's Disease Alzheimer's disease is a particular type of dementia. It is a chronic degenerative disorder that attacks the brain and results in impaired memory, thinking, and behavior. It accounts for more than half of all forms of dementia in the elderly.

Alzheimer's disease generally occurs in stages, each with different signs and symptoms. These stages include:

- *Early Stage.* Characterized by loss of recent memory, inability to learn new material, mood swings, and personality changes. Patients may believe someone is plotting against them when they lose items or forget things. Aggression or hostility is common. Poor judgment is evident.
- *Intermediate Stage.* Characterized by a complete inability to learn new material; wandering, particularly at night; increased falls; loss of ability for self-care, including bathing and use of the toilet.
- *Terminal Stage.* Characterized by an inability to walk and regression to infant stage, including the loss of bowel and bladder function. Eventually the patient loses the ability to eat and swallow.

Families caring for an Alzheimer's patient at home also present signs of stress. Remember to treat both the Alzheimer patient and the family and/or caregivers with respect and compassion. Evaluate the needs of the family and make an appropriate report at your facility. There are support groups available to assist families.

In distinguishing between delirium and dementia, err on the side of delirium. The condition is often caused by life-threatening, but reversible, conditions.

* senile dementia general term used to describe an abnormal decline in mental functioning seen in the elderly; also called "organic brain syndrome" or "multi-infarct dementia."

* aphasia absence or impairment of the ability to communicate through speaking, writing, or signing as a result of brain dysfunction.

Remember to treat both the Alzheimer patient and family and/or caregivers with respect and compassion.

Parkinson's Disease

Parkinson's disease is a degenerative disorder characterized by changes in muscle response, including tremors, loss of facial expression, and gait disturbances. It mainly appears in people over age 50 and peaks at age 70. The disease affects about 1 million Americans, with 50,000 new cases diagnosed each year. It is the fourth most common neurodegenerative disease among the elderly.

The cause of primary Parkinson's disease remains unknown. However, it affects the basal ganglia in the brain, an area that deciphers messages going to muscles. Secondary Parkinson's disease is distinguished from primary Parkinson's disease by having a known cause. Some of the most common causes include:

- Viral encephalitis
- Atherosclerosis of cerebral vessels
- Reaction to certain drugs or toxins, such as antipsychotics or carbon monoxide
- Metabolic disorders, such as anoxia
- Tumors
- Head trauma
- Degenerative disorders, such as **Shy-Drager syndrome**

It is impossible in a field setting to distinguish primary and secondary Parkinson's disease. The most common initial sign of a Parkinson's disorder is a resting tremor combined with a **pill-rolling motion.** As the disease progresses, muscles become more rigid and movements become slower and/or more jerky. In some cases, patients may find their movements halted while carrying out some routine task. Their feet may feel "frozen to the ground." Gaits becomes shuffled with short steps and unexpected bursts of speed, often to avoid falling. Kyphotic deformity is a hallmark of the disease.

Patients with Parkinson's disease commonly develop mask-like faces devoid of all expression. They speak in slow, monotone voices. Difficulties in communication, coupled with a loss of mobility, often lead to anxiety and depression.

There is no known cure for Parkinson's disease, with the exception of drug-induced secondary Parkinson's disorders. Exercise may help maintain physical activity or teach the patient adaptive strategies. In calls involving a Parkinson's patient, observe for conditions that may have involved the EMS system, such as a fall or the inability to move. Manage treatable conditions and transport as needed.

METABOLIC AND ENDOCRINE DISORDERS

As previously mentioned, the endocrine system undergoes a number of age-related changes, which affect hormone levels. The most common endocrine disorders include diabetes mellitus and problems related to the thyroid gland. Of the two, you will more often treat diabetic-related emergencies, particularly hypoglycemia.

Diabetes Mellitus

An estimated 20 percent of older adults have diabetes mellitus, primarily Type II diabetes. Almost 40 percent have some type of glucose intolerance. Reasons that the elderly develop these disorders include:

- Poor diet
- Decreased physical activity
- Loss of lean body mass

---

* **Parkinson's disease** chronic, degenerative nervous disease characterized by tremors, muscular weakness and rigidity, and a loss of postural reflexes.

---

* **Shy-Drager syndrome** chronic orthostatic hypotension caused by a primary autonomic nervous system deficiency.

---

* **pill-rolling motion** an involuntary tremor, usually in one hand or sometimes in both, in which fingers move as if they were rolling a pill back and forth.

- Impaired insulin production
- Resistance by body cells to the actions of insulin

Diagnosis of Type II diabetes usually occurs during routine screening in a physical exam. In some cases, urine tests may register negative because of an increased renal glucose threshold in the elderly. The condition may present, in its early stages, with such vague constitutional symptoms as fatigue or weakness. Allowed to progress, diabetes can result in neuropathy and visual impairment. These manifestations often lead to more aggressive blood testing, which in most cases will reveal elevated glucose levels.

The treatment of diabetes involves diet, exercise, the use of sulfonylurea agents, and/or insulin. Many diabetics use self-monitoring devices to test glucose levels. Unfortunately, the cost of these devices and the accompanying test strips, sometimes discourages the elderly from using them. Elderly patients on insulin also risk hypoglycemia, especially if they accidentally take too much insulin or do not eat enough food following injection. The lack of good nutrition can be particularly troublesome to elderly diabetics. They often find it difficult to prepare meals, fail to enjoy food because of altered taste perceptions, have trouble chewing food, or are unable to purchase adequate and/or the correct food because of limited income.

Management of diabetic and hypoglycemic emergencies for the elderly are generally the same as for any other patient. DO NOT rule out alcohol as a complicating factor, especially in cases of hypoglycemia. In addition, remember that diabetes places the elderly at increased risk of other complications, including atherosclerosis, delayed healing, **retinopathy**, blindness, altered renal function, and severe peripheral vascular disease, leading to foot ulcers and even amputations.

DO NOT rule out alcohol as a complicating factor in cases of hypoglycemia.

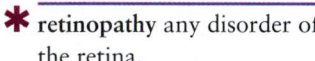

* **retinopathy** any disorder of the retina.

Thyroid Disorders

With normal aging the thyroid gland undergoes moderate atrophy and changes in hormone production. An estimated 2 to 5 percent of people over age 65 experience hypothyroidism, a condition resulting from inadequate levels of thyroid hormones. It affects women in greater numbers than men, and the prevalence rises with age.

Less than 33 percent of the elderly present with typical signs and symptoms of hypothyroidism. When they do, their complaints are often attributed to aging. Common nonspecific complaints in the elderly include mental confusion, anorexia, falls, incontinence, and decreased mobility. Some patients also experience an increase in muscle or joint pain. Treatment involves thyroid hormone replacement.

Hyperthyroidism is less common among the elderly but may result from medication errors such as an overdose of thyroid hormone replacement. The typical symptom of heat intolerance is often present. Otherwise, hyperthyroidism presents atypically in the elderly. Common nonspecific features or complaints include atrial fibrillation, failure to thrive (weight loss and apathy combined), abdominal distress, diarrhea, exhaustion, and depression.

The diagnosis and treatment of thyroid disorders does not take place in the field. Elderly patients with known thyroid problems should be encouraged to go to the hospital for medical evaluation.

GASTROINTESTINAL DISORDERS

Gastrointestinal emergencies are common among the elderly. The most frequent emergency is gastrointestinal bleeding. However, older people will also describe a variety of other gastrointestinal complaints—nausea, poor appetite, diarrhea, and constipation, to name a few. Remember, that like other presenting complaints, these conditions may be symptomatic of more serious diseases. Bowel problems, for example, may point to cancer of the colon or other abdominal organs.

Regardless of the complaint, remember that prompt management of a GI emergency is essential for young and old alike. For the elderly, there is a significant risk of hemorrhage and shock. There is a tendency to take GI patients less seriously than those suffering moderate or severe external hemorrhage. This is a serious mistake. Patients with gastrointestinal complaints should be aggressively managed, especially the elderly. Keep in mind that older patients are far more intolerant of hypotension and anoxia than younger patients. Treatment should include:

- Airway management
- Support of breathing and circulation
- High-flow oxygen therapy
- IV fluid replacement with a crystalloid solution
- PASG placement, if indicated
- Rapid transport

Some of the most critical GI problems that you may encounter in the field will involve internal hemorrhage and bowel obstruction. You may also be called upon to treat **mesenteric infarct**—a serious and life-threatening condition in an elderly patient. The following will help you to recognize each of these gastrointestinal disorders.

GI Hemorrhage

Gastrointestinal bleeding falls into two general categories: upper GI bleed and lower GI bleed.

Upper GI Bleed This form of gastrointestinal bleeding includes:

- *Peptic Ulcer Disease.* Injury to the mucous lining of the upper part of the gastrointestinal tract due to stomach acids, digestive enzymes, and other agents, such as anti-inflammatory drugs.
- *Gastritis.* An inflammation of the lining of the stomach.
- *Esophageal Varices.* An abnormal dilation of veins in the lower esophagus; a common complication of cirrhosis of the liver.
- *Mallory-Weiss Tear.* A tear in the lower esophagus that is often caused by severe and prolonged retching.

Lower GI Bleed Conditions categorized as lower gastrointestinal bleeding include:

- *Diverticulosis.* The presence of small pouches on the colon that tend to develop with age; causes 70 percent of life-threatening lower GI bleeds.
- *Tumors.* Tumors of the colon can cause bleeding when the tumor erodes into blood vessels within the intestine or surrounding organs.
- *Ischemic Colitis.* An inflammation of the colon due to impaired or decreased blood supply.
- *Arterio-Venous Malformations.* An abnormal link between an artery and a vein.

Signs of significant gastrointestinal blood loss include the presence of "coffee ground" emesis; black tar-like stools (**melena**); obvious blood in the emesis or stool; orthostatic hypotension; pulse greater than 100 (unless on beta blockers); and

> *Patients with gastrointestinal complaints should be aggressively managed, especially the elderly.*
>

* **mesenteric infarct** death of tissue in the peritoneal fold (mesentery) that encircles the small intestine; a life-threatening condition.

* **melena** a dark, tarry stool caused by the presence of "digested" free blood.

Bowel Obstruction

Bowel obstruction in the elderly typically involves the small bowel. Causes include tumors, prior abdominal surgery, use of certain medications, and occasionally the presence of vertebral compression fractures. The patient will typically complain of diffuse abdominal pain, bloating, nausea, and vomiting. The abdomen may feel distended when palpated. Bowel sounds may be hypoactive or absent. If the obstruction has been present for a prolonged period of time, the patient may have fever, weakness, shock, and various electrolyte disturbances.

Mesenteric Infarct

Vessels arising from the superior or inferior mesenteric arteries generally serve the bowel. An infarct occurs when a portion of the bowel does not receive enough blood to survive. Certain age-related changes make the elderly more vulnerable to this condition. First, as a person ages, changes in the heart (such as atrial fibrillation) or the vessels (atherosclerosis) predispose the patient to a clot lodging in one of the branches serving the bowel. Second, changes in the bowel itself can promote swelling that effectively cuts off blood flow.

The primary symptom of a bowel infarct is pain out of proportion to the physical exam. Signs include:

- Bloody diarrhea, but usually not a massive hemorrhage
- Some tachycardia, although there may be a vagal effect masking the sign
- Abdominal distention

The patient is at great risk for shock as the dead bowel attracts interstitial and intravascular fluids, thus removing them from use. Necrotic products are released to the peritoneal cavity, leading to a massive infection. The prognosis is poor due, in part, to decreased physiologic reserves on the part of the older patient.

SKIN DISORDERS

Younger and older adults experience common skin disorders at about the same rates. However, age-related changes in the immune system make the elderly more prone to certain chronic skin diseases and infections. They are also more likely to develop **pressure ulcers** (bedsores) than any other age group.

Skin Diseases

Elderly patients commonly complain about **pruritus,** or itching. This condition can be caused by dermatitis (eczema) or environmental conditions, especially during winter (i.e., from hot dry air in the home and cold windy air outside). Keep in mind that generalized itching can also be a sign of systemic diseases, particularly liver and renal disorders. When itching is strong and unrelenting, suspect an underlying disease and encourage the patient to seek medical evaluation.

Slower healing and compromised tissue perfusion in the elderly makes them more susceptible to bacterial infection of wounds, appearing as cellulitis, impetigo, and, in the case of immunocompromised adults, staphylococcal scalded skin. The elderly also experience a higher incidence of fungal infections, partly because of decreases in the cutaneous immunologic response. In addition, they

* **pressure ulcer** ischemic damage and subsequent necrosis affecting the skin, subcutaneous tissue, and often the muscle; result of intense pressure over a short time or low pressure over a long time; also known as pressure sore or bedsore.

* **pruritus** itching; often occurs as a symptom of some systemic change or illness.

Keep in mind that generalized itching can also be a sign of systemic diseases, particularly liver and renal disorders.

suffer higher rates of **herpes zoster** (shingles), which peaks between ages 50 and 70. Although these skin disorders occur in the young, their duration and severity increases markedly with age.

In treating skin disorders, remember that many conditions may be drug-induced. Beta-blockers, for example, can worsen psoriasis, which occurs in about 3 percent of elderly patients. Question patients about their medications, keeping in mind that certain prescription drugs (e.g., penicillins and sulfonamides) and some over-the-counter drugs can cause skin eruptions. Also ask about topical home remedies, such as alcohol or soaps, that may cause or worsen the disorder. Find out if the patient is compliant with prescribed topical treatments. Finally, remember that some drugs and topical medications commonly used to treat skin disorders in the young can worsen or cause other problems for the elderly. Antihistamines and corticosteroids are two to three times more likely to provoke adverse reactions in the elderly than in younger adults.

Pressure Ulcers (Decubitus Ulcers)

Most pressure ulcers occur in people over age 70. As many as 20 percent of patients enter the hospital with a pressure ulcer or develop one while hospitalized. The highest incidence occurs in nursing homes where up to 25 percent of patients may develop this condition.

Pressure ulcers typically develop from the waist down, usually over bony prominences, in bedridden patients. However, they can occur anywhere on the body and with the patient in any position. Pressure ulcers usually result from tissue hypoxia and affect the skin, subcutaneous tissues, and muscle. Factors that can increase the risk of this condition include:

- External compression of tissues (i.e., pressure)
- Altered sensory perception
- **Maceration,** caused by excessive moisture
- Decreased activity
- Decreased mobility
- Poor nutrition
- Friction or shear

To reduce the development of pressures ulcers or to alleviate their condition, you may take these steps.

- Assist the patient in changing position frequently, especially during extended transport, to reduce the length of time pressure is placed on any one point.
- Use a pull sheet to move the patient, reducing the likelihood of friction.
- Reduce the possibility of shearing by padding areas of skin prior to movement.
- Unless a life-treating condition is present, take time to clean and dry areas of excessive moisture, such as urinary or fecal incontinence and excessive perspiration.
- Clean ulcers with normal saline solution and cover with hydrocolloid or hydrogel dressings, if available. With severe ulcers, pack with loosely woven gauze moistened with normal saline.

MUSCULOSKELETAL DISORDERS

The skeleton, as you know, is a metabolically active organ. Its metabolic processes are influenced by a number of factors, including age, diet, exercise, and

✱ herpes zoster an acute eruption caused by a reactivation of latent varicella virus (chicken pox) in the dorsal root ganglia; also known as shingles.

Antihistamines and corticosteroids are two to three times more likely to provoke adverse reactions in the elderly than in younger patients.

✱ maceration process of softening a solid by soaking in a liquid.

Wear and tear is the most common factor leading to osteoarthritis.

hormone levels. The musculoskeletal system is also subject to disease. In fact, musculoskeletal diseases are the leading cause of functional impairment in the elderly. Although usually not fatal, musculoskeletal disorders often produce chronic disability, which in turn creates a context for illness. Two of the most widespread musculoskeletal disorders include **osteoarthritis** and **osteoporosis**.

Osteoarthritis

Osteoarthritis is the leading cause of disability among people age 65 and older. Many experts think the condition may not be one disease but several with similar presentations. While wear and tear as well as age-related changes such as loss of muscle mass predispose the elderly to osteoarthritis, other factors may play a role as well. Presumed contributing causes include:

- Obesity
- Primary disorders of the joint, such as inflammatory arthritis
- Trauma
- Congenital abnormalities, such as hip dysplasia

Osteoarthritis in the elderly presents initially as joint pain, worsened by exercise and improved by rest. As the disease progresses, pain may be accompanied by diminished mobility, joint deformity, and crepitus or grating sensations. Late signs include tenderness upon palpation or during passive motion.

The most effective treatment involves management before the disability develops or worsens. Prevention strategies include stretching exercises and activities that strengthen stress-absorbing ligaments (Figure 43-8). Immobilization, even for short periods, can accelerate the condition. Drug therapy is usually aimed at lessening pain and/or inflammation. Surgery—i.e., total joint replacement—is usually the last resort after more conservative methods have failed.

Osteoporosis

Osteoporosis affects an estimated 20 million Americans and is largely responsible for fractures of the hip, wrist, and vertebral bones following a fall or other injury. Risk factors include:

- *Age.* Peak bone mass for men and women occurs in their third and fourth decades of life and declines at varying rates thereafter. Decreased bone density generally becomes a treatment consideration at about age 50.
- *Gender.* The decline of estrogen production places women at a higher risk of developing osteoporosis than men. Women are more than twice as likely to have brittle bone, especially if they experience early menopause (before age 45) and do not take estrogen replacement therapy.
- *Race.* Whites and Asians are more likely to develop osteoporosis than African Americans and Latinos, who have higher bone mass at skeletal peak.
- *Body Weight.* Thin people, or people with low body weight, are at greater risk of osteoporosis than obese people. Increased skeletal weight is thought to promote bone density. However, weight-bearing exercise can have the same effect.
- *Family History.* Genetic factors—i.e., peak bone mass attainment—and a family history of fractures may predispose a person to osteoporosis.

FIGURE 43-8 Regular stretching and weight-bearing exercises help prevent the development of osteoarthritis. (© The Stock Market Photo Agency.)

- *Miscellaneous.* Late menarche, nulliparity, and use of caffeine, alcohol, and cigarettes are all thought to be important determinants of bone mass.

Unless a bone density test is conducted, persons with osteoporosis are usually asymptotic until a fracture occurs. The precipitating event can be as slight as turning over in bed, carrying a package, or even a forceful sneeze. Management includes prevention of fractures through exercise and drug therapy, such as the administration of calcium, Vitamin D, estrogen, and other medications or minerals. Once the condition occurs, pain management also becomes a consideration.

RENAL DISORDERS

The most common renal diseases in the elderly include renal failure, **glomerulonephritis,** and renal blood clots. These problems may be traced to two age-related factors: (1) loss in kidney size and (2) changes in the walls of the renal arteries and in the arterioles serving the glomeruli. In general, the kidney loses approximately one-third of its weight between the ages of 30 and 80. Most of this loss occurs in the tissues that filter blood. When filtering tissue is gone, blood is shunted from the precapillary side directly to venules on the postcapillary side, thus bypassing any tissue still capable of filtering. The result is a reduction in kidney efficiency. This condition is complicated by changes in renal arteries, which promote the development of renal emboli and thrombi.

With renal changes, elderly patients are more likely to accumulate toxins and medications within the bloodstream. Occasionally, this will be obvious to the patient as he or she experiences a substantial decrease in urine output. More often, however, the elderly are prone to a type of renal failure in which urine output remains normal to high while the kidney remains ineffective in clearing wastes.

Processes that precipitate acute renal failure include hypotension, heart failure, major surgery, sepsis, angiographic procedures (the dye is nephrotoxic), and use of nephrotoxic antibiotics (i.e., gentamycin, tobramycin). Ongoing hypertension also figures in the development of chronic renal failure.

URINARY DISORDERS

Urinary tract infections (UTI) affect as much as 10 percent of the elderly population each year. Younger women generally suffer more UTIs than young men, but in the elderly the distribution is almost even. Most of these infections result from bacteria and easily lead to **urosepsis** due to reduced immune system function among the elderly.

✳ **glomerulonephritis** a form of nephritis, or inflammation of the kidneys; primarily involves the glomeruli, one of the capillary networks that are part of the renal corpuscles in the nephrons.

✳ **urosepsis** septicemia originating from the urinary tract.

A number of factors contribute to the high rate of UTIs among the elderly. They include:

- Bladder outlet obstruction from benign prostatic hyperplasia (in men)
- atrophic vaginitis (in women)
- Stroke
- Immobilization
- Use of indwelling bladder catheters
- Diabetes
- Upper urinary tract stone
- Dementia, with resulting poor hygiene

Signs or symptoms of a UTI range from cloudy, foul smelling urine to the typical complaints of bladder pain and frequent urination. Urosepsis presents as an acute process, including fever, chills, abdominal discomfort, and other signs of septic shock. The septicemia generally begins within 24–72 hours after catheterization or cystoscopy.

Treatment of urosepsis commonly includes placement of a large-bore IV catheter for administration of fluids and parenteral antibiotics. Diagnosis of urosepsis is based on history and other physical findings. Prompt transport is critical. The prognosis for elderly patients with urosepsis is poor, with a mortality rate of approximately 30 percent. Maintenance of fluid balance as well as adequate blood pressure is essential.

Prompt transport is critical for elderly patients with suspected urosepsis, as the condition has a mortality rate of approximately 30 percent.

* **heatstroke** life-threatening condition caused by a disturbance in temperature regulation; in the elderly, characterized by extreme fever and, in extreme cases, delirium or coma.

ENVIRONMENTAL EMERGENCIES

As previously mentioned, environmental extremes represent a great health risk for the elderly. Nearly 50 percent of all **heatstroke** deaths in the United States occur among people over age 50. The elderly are just as susceptible to low temperatures, suffering about 750,000 winter deaths annually, primarily from hypothermia and "winter risks" such as pneumonia and influenza. As you may already know from your EMT experience, thermoregulatory emergencies represent some of the most common EMS calls involving the elderly.

Hypothermia

A number of factors predispose the elderly to hypothermia. These include:

- Accidental exposure to cold
- CNS disorders, including head trauma, stroke, tumors, or subdural hematomas
- Endocrine disorders, including hypoglycemia and diabetes (Patients with diabetes are six times as likely to develop hypothermia as other patients.)
- Drugs that interfere with heat production, including alcohol, antidepressants, and tranquilizers
- Malnutrition or starvation
- Chronic illness
- Forced inactivity as a result of arthritis, dementia, falls, paralysis, or Parkinson's disease
- Low or fixed income, which discourages the use of home heating

- Inflammatory dermatitis
- A-V shunts, which increase heat loss

Signs and symptoms of hypothermia can be slow to develop. Many times, elderly patients with hypothermia lose their sensitivity to cold and fail to complain. As a result, hypothermia may be missed. Nonspecific complaints may suggest a metabolic disorder or stroke. Hypothermic patients may exhibit slow speech, confusion, and sleepiness. In the early stages, patients will exhibit hypertension and an increased heart rate. As hypothermia progresses, however, blood pressure drops and the heart rate slows, sometimes to a barely detectable level.

Remember that the elderly patient with hypothermia often does not shiver. Check the abdomen and back to see if the skin is cool to the touch. Expect subcutaneous tissues to be firm. If your unit has a low-temperature thermometer, check the patient's core temperature. (Regular thermometers often do not "shake down" far enough for an accurate reading.)

As with other medical disorders, prevention is the preferred treatment. However, once elderly patients develop hypothermia, they become progressively impaired. Treat even mild cases of hypothermia, or suspected hypothermia, as a medical emergency. Focus on the rewarming techniques used with other patients and rapid transport. Maintain ongoing assessment to ensure that the hypothermia does not complicate existing medical problems or heretofore untreated disorders. Death most commonly results from cardiac arrest or ventricular fibrillation.

Remember that the elderly hypothermic patient often does not shiver.

Treat even a mild case of hypothermia, or suspected hypothermia, as a medical emergency.

Hyperthermia (Heatstroke)

Age-related changes in sweat glands and increased incidence of heart disease place the elderly at risk of heat stress. They may develop heat cramps, heat exhaustion, or heatstroke. While the first two disorders rarely result in death, heatstroke is a serious medical emergency. Risk factors for severe hyperthermia include:

Heatstroke in the elderly is a serious medical emergency.

- Altered sensory output, which would normally warn a person of overheating
- Inadequate liquid intake
- Decreased functioning of the thermoregulatory center
- Commonly prescribed medications that inhibit sweating such as antihistamines and tricyclic antidepressants
- Low or fixed income, which may result in a lack of air conditioning or adequate ventilation
- Alcoholism
- Concomitant medical disorders
- Use of diuretics, which increase fluid loss

Like hypothermia, early heatstroke may present with nonspecific signs and symptoms, such as nausea, light-headedness, dizziness, or headache. High temperature is the most reliable indicator, but consider even a slight temperature elevation as symptomatic if coupled with an absence of sweating and neurological impairment. Severe hypotension also exists in many critical patients.

Prevention strategies include adequate fluid intake, reduced activity, shelter in an air conditioned environment, and use of light clothing. If hyperthermia develops, however, rapid treatment and transport are necessary.

TOXICOLOGICAL EMERGENCIES

As previously mentioned, aging alters pharmacokinetics and pharmacodynamics in the elderly. Functional changes in the kidneys, liver, and gastrointestinal system slow the absorption and elimination of many medications. In addition, the various compensatory mechanisms that help buffer against medication side effects are less effective in the elderly than these mechanisms are in younger patients.

Approximately 30% of all hospital admissions are related to drug-related illnesses. About 50% of all drug-related deaths occur in people over age 60. Accidental overdoses may occur more frequently in the aged due to confusion, vision impairment, self-selection of medications, forgetfulness, and concurrent drug use. Intentional drug overdose also occurs in attempts at self-destruction. Another complicating factor is the abuse of alcohol among the elderly.

It is essential for the paramedic to be familiar with the range of side effects that can be caused by the polypharmacy (use of multiple medications) of medications taken by geriatric patients. In assessing the geriatric patient, always take these steps:

- Obtain a full list of medications currently taken by the patient, including prescribed medications, over-the-counter medications, and herbal and other dietary supplements.
- Elicit any medications that are newly prescribed. (Some side effects appear within a few days of taking a new medication.)
- Obtain a good past medical history. Find out if your patient has a history of renal or hepatic depression.
- Know your medications, their routes of elimination, and their potential side effects.
- If possible, always take all medications to the hospital along with the patient.

A knowledge of pharmacology is important in all patients. However, it is critical in recognizing potential toxicological emergencies in the geriatric patient. Some of the drugs or substances that have been identified as commonly causing toxicity in the elderly are described in the following sections.

Lidocaine

Lidocaine is used for the treatment of ventricular dysrhythmias. It is also a commonly used local anesthetic. The drug is primarily metabolized by the liver and excreted through the kidneys. In older patients, hepatic impairment can cause elevated lidocaine levels and possible toxicity. It is recommended that the lidocaine dose be reduced by 50 percent in patients greater than 70 years of age.

Beta Blockers

Beta blockers are used as antihypertensives, antidysrhythmics, and for glaucoma. In the elderly, beta blockers can cause depression, lethargy, and orthostatic hypotension. It is important to remember that patients taking beta blockers may not be able to increase their heart rate, which can mask the early findings of shock.

Antihypertensives/Diuretics

Diuretics can cause electrolyte abnormalities. In the elderly, decreased drug clearance can result in hypotension or dehydration. Other types of antihypertensives may affect the elderly differently. Because of this, it is sometimes necessary to reduce the dose or change to a less toxic agent.

Angiotensin-Converting Enzyme (ACE) Inhibitors

ACE inhibitors are popular antihypertensive agents because they have a good safety profile and are well tolerated by most patients. ACE inhibitors are also used to decrease afterload in CHF and pulmonary edema. In the elderly, ACE inhibitors can cause plasma volume reduction and hypotension. Also they have been associated with dizziness, lightheadedness, skin rashes, and cough.

Digitalis (Digoxin, Lanoxin)

Most patients who take digitalis on a regular basis are elderly. The drug is extremely effective at controlling the heart rate in tachydysrhythmias and at increasing cardiac output in CHF. Digitalis toxicity is the most common adverse drug effect that is seen in the elderly. It can cause visual disturbances, nausea, anorexia, abdominal discomfort, headache, and vomiting. Virtually any dysrhythmia can be seen in digitalis toxicity.

Antipsychotics/Antidepressants

Psychoactive medications affect mood, behavior, and other aspects of mental functioning. They are used in the elderly for depression and psychosis. The elderly are more vulnerable to the side effects of these medications and should be closely monitored. Be particularly alert for extrapyramidal system reactions with the antipyschotic medications.

Antiparkinsonion Agents

Drugs used in the treatment of Parkinson's disease can affect other body systems. Common complications include dyskinesia and psychological disturbances (such as hallucinations and nightmares).

Antiseizure Medications

Medications that prevent seizures can cause sedation in the elderly. They can also cause GI distress, headache, lack of coordination, and skin rashes. The doses of these drugs often must be reduced in the elderly.

Analgesics and Anti-Inflammatory Agents

Plain medications, especially the narcotics, can cause sedation, mood changes, nausea, vomiting, and constipation. The anti-inflammatory agents can cause GI distress, including gastritis and peptic ulcers. Elderly patients taking these classes of medications should be closely monitored.

Corticosteroids

Corticosteroids are necessary for the treatment of several diseases seen in the aged, including chronic obstructive pulmonary disease, rheumatoid arthritis, and other inflammatory conditions. These drugs can cause ulcers, hypertension, glaucoma, and increased risk of infection. These side effects are more prevalent in the elderly.

For additional information on pharmacology, pharmacokinetics, and pharmacodynamics, review Chapter 6, Pharmacology. For more information on specific drugs, consult the Brady publication *Drug Guide for Paramedics*.

SUBSTANCE ABUSE

Substance abuse is a widespread problem in the United States. It affects nearly all age groups, including the elderly. Up to 17 percent of Americans over age 60 are addicted to substances. That number is expected to rise as the baby boom generation swells the size of the elderly population.

In general, the factors that contribute to substance abuse among the elderly are different from those of younger people. They include:

- Age-related changes
- Loss of employment
- Loss of spouse or partner
- Multiple prescriptions
- Malnutrition
- Loneliness
- Moving from a long-loved house to an apartment

Like other age groups, the elderly may intentionally abuse substances, to escape pain or life itself. Other times, particularly in the case of prescription drugs, the abuse is accidental. Substance abuse in the elderly may involve drugs, alcohol, or both drugs and alcohol.

Drug Abuse

As previously mentioned, people age 65 and older have more illnesses, consume more drugs, and are more sensitive to adverse drug reactions than younger adults. The sheer number of medications taken by the elderly make them vulnerable to drug abuse. Of the 1.5 billion prescriptions written each year in the United States, more than one-third go to the elderly. People age 65 and older fill an average of 13 prescriptions per year. The elderly also use a disproportionate percentage of over-the-counter drugs.

Polypharmacy, coupled with impaired vision and/or memory, increase the likelihood of complications. The elderly might experience drug-drug interactions, drug-disease interactions, and drug-food interactions.

The elderly who become physically and/or psychological dependent upon drugs (or alcohol) are more likely to hide their dependence and less likely to seek help than other age groups. Common signs and symptoms of drug abuse include:

- Memory changes
- Drowsiness
- Decreased vision/hearing
- Orthostatic hypotension
- Poor dexterity
- Mood changes
- Falling
- Restlessness
- Weight loss

In cases of suspected drug abuse, carefully document your findings. Collect medications for identification at the hospital, where the patient can be evaluated and, if necessary, referred for substance abuse treatment.

Alcohol Abuse

In a national survey, nearly 50 percent of the elderly reported abstinence from alcohol. However, the same survey found that 15 percent of the men and 12 percent of the women interviewed regularly drank in excess of the one-drink-a-day limit suggested by the National Institute on Alcohol Abuse and Alcoholism. Those percentages are expected to rise with the aging of the baby boom generation, which has generally used alcohol more frequently than their predecessors.

The use or abuse of alcohol places the elderly at high risk of toxicity. Physiological changes, such as organ dysfunction, makes older adults more susceptible to the effects of alcohol. Consumption of even moderate amounts of alcohol can interfere with drug therapy, often leading to dangerous consequences. Severe stress and a history of heavy and/or regular drinking predisposes a person to alcohol dependence or abuse in later life.

Unless a patient is openly intoxicated, discovery of alcohol abuse depends on a thorough history. Signs and symptoms of alcohol abuse in the elderly may be very subtle or confused with other conditions. Remember that even small amounts of alcohol can cause intoxication in an older person. If possible, question family, friends, or caregivers about the patient's drinking patterns. Pertinent findings include:

Unless an elderly patient is openly intoxicated, discovery of alcohol abuse often depends upon a thorough history.

- Mood swings, denial, and hostility (especially when questioned about drinking)
- Confusion
- History of falls
- Anorexia
- Insomnia
- Visible anxiety
- Nausea

Treatment follows many of the same steps as for any other patient with a pattern of abusive drinking. DO NOT judge the patient. Evaluate the need for fluid therapy, and keep in mind the possibility of withdrawal. Transport the patient to the hospital for evaluation and referral for treatment. Ideally, these patients will seek support from community organizations such as Alcoholics Anonymous (AA). Many communities have AA groups specifically for senior citizens.

BEHAVIORAL/PSYCHOLOGICAL DISORDERS

When behavioral or psychological problems develop later in life, they are often dismissed as normal age-related changes. This attitude denies an elderly person the opportunity to correct a treatable condition and/or overlooks an underlying physical disorder. Studies have shown that the elderly retain their basic personalities and their adaptive cognitive abilities. In other words, intellectual decline and/or regressive behavior are not normal age-related changes. Unless an organic brain disorder is involved, alterations in behavior should be considered symptomatic of a possible psychological problem.

It is important to keep in mind the emotionally stressful situations facing many elderly people—isolation, loneliness, loss of self-dependence, loss of strength, fear of the future, and more. The elderly also face a higher incidence of secondary depression as a result of neuroleptic medications such as Haldol and Thorazine. Some of the common classifications of psychological disorders related to age include:

- Organic brain syndrome
- Affective disorders (depression)

- Personality disorders (dependent personality)
- Dissociative disorders (paranoid schizophrenia)

As with other people, the emotional well-being of the elderly impacts upon their overall physical health. Therefore, it is important that you note evidence of altered behavior in any elderly patient that you assess and examine. Common signs and symptoms of a psychological disorder include lapses in memory, cognitive difficulty, changes in sleep patterns, fear of death, changes in sexual interest, thoughts of suicide, or withdrawal from society.

In general, management of psychological disorders in the elderly is the same as for other age groups. Two of the most common emotional disturbances that you may encounter in the elderly are depression and suicide.

Depression

Up to 15 percent of the non-institutionalized elderly experience depression. Within institutions, that figure rises to about 30 percent. The incidence of depression among the elderly is expected to rise in the early 2000s as the baby boomers—with their larger numbers and more prevalent depression at an earlier age—enter their 60s.

Some of the general signs and symptoms noted previously may indicate depression. Ask the patient about feelings of sadness or despair. Determine if he or she has suffered episodes of crying. Inquire about past psychological treatment and current stressful events, particularly the death of a loved one. Keep in mind that sensory changes—especially deafness and blindness—may make the patient vulnerable to depression. Serious acute diseases can have the same effect. If the patient recognizes the depression, ask about the duration and any prior bouts. Find out if the patient has been given any medications to treat the depression. If so, check compliance.

Some depressed patients may exhibit **hypochondriasis** (hypochondria). If this condition is a side effect of the depression, the patient will still show some degree of emotional pain and/or **dysphoria.** Although you may not be able to identify hypochondria in the field, remember that the condition is an illness and requires treatment by trained medical personnel.

In general, depressed patients should receive supportive care. Encourage them to talk, delicately raising questions about suicidal thoughts. The seriously depressed patient should be transported to the hospital. Treatment of depression usually entails psychotherapy and/or antidepressants.

Suicide

The highest suicide rates in the United States are among people over age 65, especially men. The elderly account for 20 percent of all suicides, but represent only 12 percent of the total population. Someone over age 65 completes suicide about every 90 minutes. Suicide is the third leading cause of death among the elderly, following falls and car accidents.

Depression is the leading cause for suicide among the elderly. As a group, the elderly are less likely to seek help than the young. They are also less likely to express their anger or sorrow, turning their feelings inward instead. Other stressors that put the elderly at risk of suicide include:

- Chronic illness
- Physical impairment
- Unrelieved pain
- Living in a youth-oriented society

✱ **hypochondriasis** an abnormal concern with one's health, with the false belief of suffering from some disease, despite medical assurances to the contrary; commonly known as hypochondria.

✱ **dysphoria** an exaggerated feeling of depression or unrest, characterized by a mood of general dissatisfaction, restlessness, discomfort, and unhappiness.

Remember that hypochondriasis is an illness, too.

- Family issues
- Financial problems
- Isolation and loneliness
- Substance abuse
- Low serotonin levels (Serotonin declines with age.)
- Bereavement
- Family history of suicide

Suicidal behavior is related to stress. As a paramedic, you should try to evaluate the stress from an elderly patient's point of view, keeping the preceding factors in mind. In cases of a seriously depressed patient, elicit behavior patterns from family, friends, or caregivers. Warning signs may include:

- Loss of interest in activities that were once enjoyable
- Curtailing social interaction, grooming, and self-care
- Breaking from medical or exercise regimens
- Grieving a personal loss ("I don't want to live without him/her.")
- Feeling useless ("Nobody would miss me.")
- Putting affairs in order, giving away things, finalizing a will
- Stock-piling medications or other lethal means of self-destruction, including firearms

Be particularly alert to suicide among the acutely ill. With more patients being returned home to care for themselves, there is a higher incidence of suicide among the terminally ill, especially cancer victims. A lack of post-acute hospital care can be interpreted as a lack of caring in general.

Prevention of suicide among the elderly involves intervention by all levels of society, from family to EMS to hospital workers. It is important to dispel the common myths about aging and age-related diseases. Recognition of warning signs and involvement of appropriate individuals and agencies is critical.

Your first priorities in the management of a suicidal elderly patient are to protect yourself and then to protect the patient from self-harm. To do this, you must gain access to the patient. This may require breaking into a house or room, particularly if the patient is unconscious or can be readily seen. Remember to summon law enforcement personnel as necessary. DO NOT RULE OUT FIREARMS AMONG THE ELDERLY.

If you reach the patient, emergency care has the highest priority secondary to crew safety. Conduct a brief interview with the patient, if possible, to determine the need for further action. DO NOT leave the suicidal patient alone. Administer medications with caution, keeping in mind polypharmacy and drug interactions in the elderly. (Consult with medical direction.) ALL SUICIDAL ELDERLY PATIENTS SHOULD BE TRANSPORTED TO THE HOSPITAL.

DO NOT rule out firearms among the elderly.

All suicidal elderly patients should be transported to the hospital.

TRAUMA IN THE ELDERLY PATIENT

Trauma is the leading cause of death among the elderly. Older patients who sustain moderate to severe injuries are more likely to die than their younger counterparts. Post-injury disability is also more common in the elderly than in the young.

CONTRIBUTING FACTORS

A number of factors contribute to the high incidence and severity of trauma among the elderly. Slower reflexes, arthritis, and diminished eyesight and hearing predispose the elderly to accidents, especially falls. The elderly, because of their physical state and vulnerability, are also at high risk from trauma caused by criminal assault. Purse-snatching, armed robbery, and assault occur all too frequently in the elderly population, especially among those living in urban areas.

Age-related factors that place the elderly at risk of severe injury and complications include:

- Osteoporosis and muscle weakness—increased likelihood of fractures
- Reduced cardiac reserve—decreased ability to compensate for blood loss
- Decreased respiratory function—increased likelihood of **acute respiratory distress syndrome (ARDS)**
- Impaired renal function—decreased ability to adapt to fluid shifts
- Decreased elasticity in the peripheral blood vessels—greater susceptibility to tearing

GENERAL ASSESSMENT

As with any other trauma patient, determine the mechanism of injury. Leading causes of trauma in the elderly include: falls, motor vehicle crashes, burns, assault or abuse, and underlying medical problems such as syncope.

In assessing elderly trauma patients, remember that blood pressure readings may be deceptive. Older patients typically have a higher blood pressure than younger patients. Although a blood pressure of 110/70 may be normal for a 30-year-old, it could represent a low blood pressure, and possibly shock, for an older patient. Elderly trauma patients also may not exhibit an elevated pulse—a common early sign of hypoperfusion. This may be because of a chronic heart disease or the use of medications to treat hypertension or a myocardial infarction. Fractures may also be obscured or concealed because of a diminished sense of pain among the elderly. One of the best indicators of shock in the elderly is an altered mental status or changes in consciousness during assessment. Elderly trauma patients who exhibit confusion or agitation are candidates for rapid transport.

Observing for Abuse/Neglect

Make sure you observe the scene for signs of abuse and neglect. Abuse of the elderly is as big a problem in our society as child abuse and neglect. **Geriatric abuse** is defined as a syndrome in which an elderly person has received serious physical or psychological injury from family members or other caregivers. Abuse of the elderly knows no socioeconomic bounds. It often occurs when an older person is no longer able to be totally independent, and the family has difficulty upholding their commitment to care for the patient. It can also occur in nursing homes and other health care facilities. The profile for the potential geriatric abuser may often show a great deal of life stress. In many cases, there is sleep deprivation, marital discord, financial problems, and work-related problems. As the abuser's life gets in further disarray, and as the patient further deteriorates, abuse may be the outcome.

Signs and symptoms of geriatric abuse and neglect are often obvious (Figure 43-9). Unexplained trauma is usually the primary presentation. The average abused patient is older than 80 and has multiple medical problems, such

---

* acute respiratory distress syndrome (ARDS) respiratory insufficiency marked by progressive hypoxemia, due to severe inflammatory damage.

In assessing elderly trauma patients, remember that blood pressure and pulse readings can be deceptive indicators of hypoperfusion.

* geriatric abuse a syndrome in which an elderly person is physically or psychologically injured by another person.

as cancer, congestive heart failure, heart disease, and incontinence. Senile dementia is often present. In these cases, it can be hard to determine whether the dementia is chronic or acute, especially if there is an increased likelihood of head trauma from abuse.

Whenever you suspect geriatric abuse, obtain a complete patient and family history. Pay particular attention to inconsistencies. *DO NOT confront the family.* Instead, report your suspicions to the emergency department and the appropriate governmental authority. Many states have very strong laws protecting the elderly from abuse or neglect. In fact, many states consider it a criminal offense *not* to report suspected geriatric abuse. These states also offer legal immunity to those who report geriatric abuse, as long as the report is made in good faith.

Many states have laws that require prehospital personnel to report suspected cases of geriatric abuse and/or neglect.

GENERAL MANAGEMENT

The priorities of care for the elderly trauma patient are similar to those for any trauma patient. However, you must keep in mind age-related systemic changes and the presence of chronic diseases. This is especially true of the cardiovascular, respiratory, and renal systems.

Cardiovascular Considerations

Recent or past myocardial infarctions may contribute to the risk of dysrhythmia or congestive heart failure in the trauma patient. In addition, there may be a decreased response of the heart, in adjusting heart rate and stroke volume, to hypovolemia. An elderly trauma patient may require higher than usual arterial pressures for perfusion of vital organs, due to increased peripheral vascular resistance and hypertension. Care must be taken in intravenous fluid administration because of decreased myocardial reserves. Hypotension, hypovolemia, and hypervolemia are poorly tolerated in the elderly patient.

Respiratory Considerations

In managing the airway and ventilation in an elderly trauma patient, you must consider the physical changes that may affect treatment. Check for dentures and determine whether they should be removed. Keep in mind that age-related changes can decrease chest wall movement and vital capacity. Age also reduces the tolerance of all organs for anoxia. Remember, too, that chronic obstructive pulmonary disease is widespread among the elderly.

Make necessary adjustments in treatment to provide adequate oxygenation and appropriate CO_2 removal. It is important to remember that use of 50 percent nitrous oxide (Nitronox) for elderly patients may result in more respiratory depression than would occur in younger patients. Positive pressure ventilation should also be used cautiously. There is an increased danger of resultant alkalosis and rupture of emphysematous bullae, making the elderly more vulnerable to pneumothorax.

Renal Considerations

The decreased ability of the kidneys to maintain normal acid/base balance, and to compensate for fluid changes, can further complicate the management of the elderly trauma patient. Any preexisting renal disease can decrease the kidney's ability to compensate. The decrease in renal function, along with a decreased cardiac reserve, places the elderly injured patient at risk for fluid overload and pulmonary edema. Remember, too, that renal changes allow toxins and medications to accumulate more readily in the elderly.

Transport Considerations

Keep in mind that trauma places an elderly person at increased risk of hypothermia. Ensure that the patient is kept warm at all times.

You may have to modify the positioning, immobilization, and packaging of the elderly trauma patient before transport. Be attentive to physical deformities such as arthritis, spinal abnormalities, or frozen limbs that may cause pain or special care (Figure 43-10a-c). Recall the frailty of an elderly person's skin and avoid creating skin tears or pressure sores. Keep in mind that trauma places an elderly person at increased risk of hypothermia. Ensure that the patient is kept warm at all times.

FIGURE 43-10a   In an elderly patient with curvature of the spine, place padding behind the neck when immobilizing a patient to a long spine board.

FIGURE 43–10b   Additional padding, such as rolled blankets or towels behind the head, may be needed to keep the head in a neutral, in-line position.

FIGURE 43–10c   Secure the patient's head with a head immobilizer device. To prevent spinal damage, maintain manual stabilization until the head is secured.

SPECIFIC INJURIES

The elderly can be subject to a variety of injuries, just like any other age group. The three most common categories of injuries among the elderly include orthopedic injuries, burns, and injuries of the head and spine.

Orthopedic Injuries

As previously mentioned, the elderly suffer the greatest mortality and greatest incidence of disability from falls. Approximately 33 percent of falls in the elderly result in at least one fractured bone. The most common fall-related fracture is a fracture of the hip or pelvis (Figure 43-11). Osteoporosis and general frailty contribute to this. The older patient who has fallen should be assumed to have a hip fracture until proven otherwise. Signs and symptoms of a hip fracture include tenderness over the affected joint and shortening and external rotation of the leg. The patient is unable to bear weight on the affected leg. Those patients who live alone may not be able to get to a phone to summon help. Because of this, they may remain on the floor for a prolonged period of time. This can lead to hypothermia, hyperthermia, and/or dehydration.

> **Content Review**
>
> **COMMON FRACTURES AMONG THE ELDERLY**
> - Hip or pelvis fractures
> - Proximal humerus
> - Distal radius
> - Proximal tibia
> - Thoracic and lumbar bodies

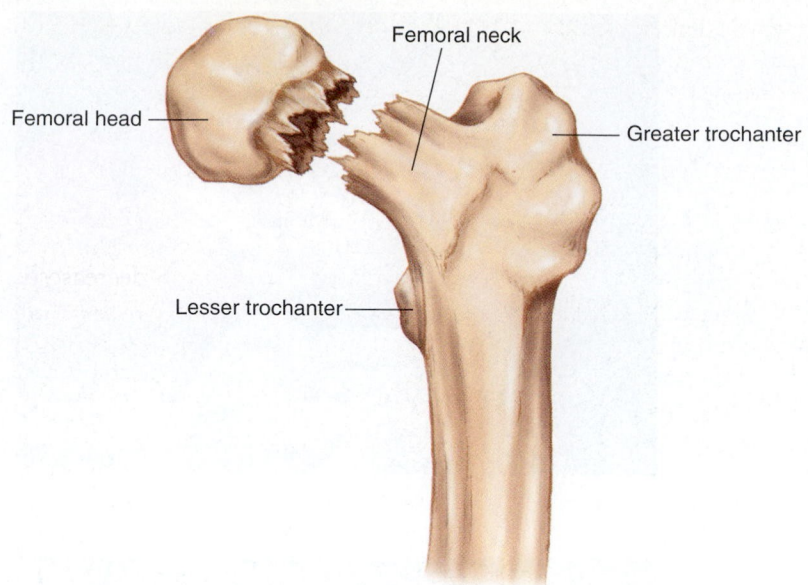

FIGURE 43-11 Subcapital femoral neck fracture. Patients with a displaced femoral neck fracture present with groin pain and a shortened externally rotated leg.

Femoral head

Femoral neck

Greater trochanter

Lesser trochanter

Falls also result in a variety of other stress fractures in the elderly, including fractures of the proximal humerus, distal radius, proximal tibia, and thoracic and lumbar bodies. Falls may also lead to soft-tissue injuries and hot water burns, if the incident occurred in a tub or hot shower.

In treating orthopedic injuries, remember to ask questions aimed at detecting an underlying medical condition. Ask if the patient recalls "blacking out." Remain alert for evidence of potential cardiac emergencies. Package and transport the patient per the general guidelines mentioned earlier.

Burns

People age 60 and older are more likely to suffer death from burns than any other age group except neonates and infants. Several factors help explain the high mortality rate among elderly burn victims. They include:

- Reaction time slows as people age, so the elderly often stay in contact with thermal sources longer than their younger counterparts.
- Pre-existing diseases place the elderly at risk of medical complications, particularly pulmonary and cardiac problems.
- Age-related skin changes (thinning) result in deeper burns and slower healing time.
- Immunological and metabolic changes increase the risk of infection.
- Reductions in physiologic function and the reduced reserve of several organ systems make the elderly more vulnerable to major systemic stress.

Management of elderly burn patients follows the same general procedures as other patients. However, remember that the elderly are at increased risk of shock. Administration of fluids are important to prevent renal tubular damage. Assess hydration in the initial hours after a burn injury by blood pressure, pulse, and urine output (at least 1–2 mL/kg per hour).

In the case of the elderly, complications from a burn may manifest themselves in the days and weeks following the incident. For serious burns to heal, the body may use up to 20,000 calories a day. Elderly patients, with altered metabolisms and complications such as diabetes, may not be able to meet this demand, increasing the chances for infection and systemic failure. Part of your job may be to prepare the family for such a delayed response and to provide necessary psychological support.

Head and Spinal Injuries

As a group, the elderly experience more head injuries, even from relatively minor trauma than their younger counterparts. A major factor is the difference in proportion between the brain and the skull. As mentioned earlier, the brain decreases in size and weight with age. The skull, however, remains constant in size, allowing the brain more room to move, thus increasing the likelihood of brain injury. Because of this, signs of brain injury may develop more slowly in the elderly, sometimes over days and weeks. In fact, the patient may often have forgotten the offending injury.

The cervical spine is also more susceptible to injury due to osteoporosis and spondylosis. **Spondylosis** is a degeneration of the vertebral body. The elderly often have a significant degree of this disease. In addition, arthritic changes can gradually compress the nerve rootlets or spinal cord. Thus, injury to the spine in the elderly makes the patient much more susceptible to spinal cord injury. In fact, sudden neck movement, even without fracture, may cause spinal-cord injury. This can occur with less than normal pain, due to the absence of fracture. Therefore, it is important to provide older patients with suspected spinal injuries, especially those involved in motor vehicle accidents, with immediate manual cervical spinal stabilization at the time of initial assessment.

* spondylosis a degeneration of the vertebral body.

SUMMARY

The practice of EMS in the 21st century means treating a growing elderly population. The "Graying of America" has resulted in a greater number of people age 65 and older, many of whom will be in home settings. When treating elderly patients, keep in mind the anatomical, physiological, and emotional changes that occur with age. However, never jump to conclusions based solely on age. Weigh normal age-related changes against abnormal changes—i.e., those resulting from a medical condition or trauma. Recall that elderly patients are much more susceptible to medication side effects and toxicity than younger patients. They also are more susceptible to trauma and environmental stressors. Abuse of the elderly occurs, and you should bear this in mind whenever injuries do not match the history. Any suspected abuse or neglect of an elderly patient should be reported to the emergency department and/or the appropriate governmental authorities.

CHAPTER 44

Abuse and Assault

Objectives

After reading this chapter, you should be able to:

1. Discuss the incidence of abuse and assault. (p. 1853)
2. Describe the categories of abuse. (pp. 1853–1862)
3. Discuss examples of spouse, elder, child, and sexual abuse. (pp. 1853–1864)
4. Describe the characteristics associated with the profile of a typical spouse, elder, or child abuser and the typical assailant of sexual abuse. (pp. 1855, 1857, 1859, 1864)
5. Identify the profile of the "at-risk" spouse, elder, and child.

(pp. 1854–1856, 1856–1857, 1859, 1862–1863)

6. Discuss the assessment and management of the abused patient. (pp. 1856, 1857, 1859–1862, 1864)
7. Discuss the legal aspects associated with abuse situations. (pp. 1853, 1856, 1862, 1864–1865)
8. Identify community resources that are able to assist victims of abuse and assault. (pp. 1856, 1857, 1865)
9. Discuss the documentation necessary when caring for abused and assaulted patients. (pp. 1856, 1862, 1865)

INTRODUCTION

Because of underreporting, it is difficult to provide accurate statistics on the incidence of abuse and assault in the United States today. That makes available figures even more overwhelming in their seriousness. To grasp the magnitude of the problem, consider these facts.

- Nearly three million children suffer abuse each year and more than 1,000 die annually.

- Between two to four million women each year are battered by their partners or spouses.

- Elder abuse occurs at an incidence of between 700,000 to 1.1 million annually.

Abuse and assaults transcend gender, race, age, and socio-economic status. The effects are serious and long-lasting. Victims may die as a result of their injuries or have long-term healthcare problems. No victim ever forgets his or her pain. Even after the physical wounds have healed, the emotional injuries never completely fade.

Unfortunately, the pattern of abuse and assault forms a cycle that is difficult to break. Parents who harm each other are more likely to abuse their children. Children who suffer abuse have a greater likelihood of becoming abusers themselves. At some point in their lives, they may abuse their dates, their partners, their children, their elders, or others.

The EMS system is involved with many cases of abuse. Although law enforcement is not always present, you have a responsibility to identify victims of abuse and initiate some kind of action. In many areas, laws require healthcare personnel to report actual or suspected incidences of abuse. Early detection is critical to breaking the cycle of abuse through social services support and alterations in behavior.

Abuse and assaults transcend gender, race, age, and socio-economic status.

Early detection is critical to breaking the cycle of abuse through social services support and alterations in behavior.

PARTNER ABUSE

The potential for **partner abuse** has existed for as long as couples have interacted. It results when a man or woman subjects a domestic partner to some form of physical or psychological violence. The victim may be a husband or wife, someone who shares a residence, or simply a boyfriend or girlfriend.

* **partner abuse** physical or emotional violence from a man or woman towards a domestic partner.

The most widespread and best known form of abuse involves the abuse of women by men. However, battery is not limited to women. Men can be—and are—abused by women. They suffer the same feelings of guilt, humiliation, and a loss of control. A battered man feels trapped just like a battered woman, but is often even less likely to report the abuse, either out of a sense of shame or a lack of resources for support, or both.

Battery also affects same-sex couples. Abusive relationships between men or between women follow the same patterns and the same conditioning as those seen in heterosexual relationships. What can be said of women battered by men can generally be said of most battery situations, regardless of the gender of the victim or the abuser.

REASONS FOR NOT REPORTING ABUSE

Victims of partner abuse hesitate or fail to report the problem for a number of reasons. Fear presents one of the biggest obstacles to taking action. Most battered partners fear reprisals, either to themselves or to their children. They also fear being humiliated for their powerlessness or inability to stop the violence, especially if the battered partner is a male.

Reporting abuse is usually the last resort. Many partners hope the abusive behavior will simply just end. This hope is fueled when the abuser promises to change—a common reaction after a violent episode. The abused partner may also be in denial—claiming that the situation is less serious than it is or rationalizing that the violence is somehow justified. Some abused women, for example, believe they are the cause of the abusive behavior or that the abuse is part of the marriage and should be endured to preserve the family.

Finally, many victims of abuse lack the knowledge or financial means to seek help. They may not know where to turn or who to trust. They may also lack the money to seek counseling, intervention, or a safe place to live. A partner who lacks job training and/or who must support dependent children may find the prospect of starting life anew more frightening than the abuse. Unfortunately, an abusive situation rarely ceases without some kind of separation or intervention. Escalation of violence is common, with injuries becoming more severe. Over time, abuse becomes more frequent, often occurring without provocation, and more inclusive. If children were not initially involved, they may become victims as the episodes escalate.

IDENTIFICATION OF PARTNER ABUSE

Partner abuse can fall into several categories. The most obvious form is physical abuse, which involves the application of force in ways too numerous to list here. In addition to direct personal injury, physical abuse may exacerbate existing medical conditions, such as hypertension, diabetes, or asthma. These conditions can also be affected by verbal abuse, which consists of words chosen to control or harm a person. Verbal abuse may leave no physical mark, but it damages a person's self-esteem and can lead to depression, substance abuse, or other self-destructive behavior.

Sexual abuse, which is a form of physical abuse, can also occur between partners. It involves forced sexual contact and includes marital or date rape. (For more on sexual abuse and assault, see material later in the chapter.)

In identifying an abusive family situation, keep in mind the ten generic risk factors identified in "Domestic Violence: Cracking the Code of Silence," a source cited in the DOT's National Standard Curriculum. These factors, based on research of battered women, include:

1. Male is unemployed.
2. Male uses illegal drugs at least once a year.

In addition to direct personal injury, physical abuse may exacerbate existing medical conditions, such as hypertension, diabetes, or asthma.

3. Partners have different religious backgrounds.
4. Family income is below the poverty level.
5. Partners are unmarried.
6. Either partner is violent toward children at home.
7. Male did not graduate from high school.
8. Male is unemployed or has a blue-collar job.
9. Male is between 18 and 30 years old.
10. Male saw his father hit his mother.

CHARACTERISTICS OF PARTNER ABUSERS

As already indicated, partner abuse occurs in all demographic groups. However, abuse is more common in lower socio-economic levels in which wage earners have trouble paying bills, holding down jobs, or keeping pace with technological changes that make their job skills outdated or obsolete.

A history of family violence makes a person more likely to repeat the pattern as an adult. Typically the abuser does not like being out of control, but at the same time feels powerless to change. The situation is made worse if both parties do not know how to back down from a conflict. Lacking any alternative, one or both of the partners may turn to physical and/or verbal violence. In some cases, abusers will think they are demonstrating discipline rather than violent behavior.

Abusers usually exhibit overly aggressive personalities—an outgrowth of low self-esteem. They often feel insecure and jealous, flying into sudden and unpredictable rages. Use of alcohol or drugs increases the likelihood that the abuser will lose control and may not even clearly remember his or her actions.

In the aftermath of an abusive incident, the abuser often feels a sense of remorse and shame. The person may seek to relieve his or her guilt by promising to change or even seeking help. For a time, the abuser may appear charming or loving, convincing an abused partner to think that perhaps the pattern has finally been broken. All too often, however, the cycle of violence repeats itself in just a few days, weeks, or months.

CHARACTERISTICS OF ABUSED PARTNERS

It may be difficult to identify the abused partner. As mentioned, the primary risk factor for abuse is a history of violence between parents, a factor that will not be immediately known to you or other EMS providers. However, studies have revealed that abused partners share certain common characteristics. They include:

- *Pregnancy:* Forty-five percent of women suffer some form of battery during pregnancy.
- *Substance abuse:* Abused partners often seek the numbing effect of alcohol and/or drugs.
- *Emotional disorders:* Abused partners frequently exhibit depression, evasiveness, anxiety, or suicidal behavior.

As mentioned earlier, the victim may seek to protect his or her attacker, either by delaying care and/or by providing alternative explanations for injuries. Remain alert to subtle signs that the patient is being less than honest. Many victims, for example, avoid eye contact, exhibit nervous behavior, and/or watch the abuser, if present. The victim may also provide verbal clues, saying such things as "we've been having some problems lately" or "I always seem to be causing some kind of trouble."

APPROACHING THE BATTERED PATIENT

In assessing the battered patient, direct questioning usually works best. Convey an awareness that the person's partner may have caused the harm or created conditions that led to the injury and/or the emotional trauma. Once the subject of abuse has been introduced, exhibit a willingness to discuss it. Remember to avoid both judgmental questions such as "Why don't you leave?" or judgmental statements such as "How awful!"

Throughout the assessment, listen carefully to the patient. Indicate your attention by saying, "I hear what you are telling me." Often victims of abuse feel a sense of relief when someone else knows about the situation. This can be the first step toward seeking help.

When speaking with abused patients, encourage them to regain control over their lives. Do this by helping them to identify what they want for themselves and, in many cases, for their children. Also, be prepared to share your knowledge of community resources, such as shelters and counseling services, that may offer help. Find out about the support services, both for the victim and the abuser, that are available in your area.

Finally, do not leave the scene without advising the patient to take all necessary precautions. Rehearse the quickest way to leave the home. Find out where the patient will go and/or who the patient will call. If the patient drives, suggest carrying the keys to the vehicle at all times. Remind the patient that it is a crime to beat another person and that, depending upon the type of injury, assault is either a misdemeanor or a felony.

Keep in mind that in cases of partner abuse, the abuser may be reported and taken into custody by the police. However, the person may soon be released on his or her own recognizance, sometimes within a matter of hours. The patient may already know this and be reluctant to take any action. If the patient does not know this, it is your duty to inform him or her of this possibility and to tell the person about available protection programs.

ELDER ABUSE

As noted in Chapter 43, elder abuse is a widespread medical and social problem caused by many factors. They include:

- Increased life expectancies
- Increased dependency on others, as a result of longevity
- Decreased productivity in later years
- Physical and mental impairments, especially among the "old old"
- Limited resources for long-term care of the elderly
- Economic factors, such as strained family finances
- Stress on middle-age caretakers responsible for two generations—children and parents

The problem of elder abuse is expected to grow along with the size of the elderly population, which will increase dramatically within the next 20–30 years as baby boomers turn age 65 and older. It is your responsibility to be aware of this situation and to remain alert to signs of elder abuse.

IDENTIFICATION OF ELDER ABUSE

There are basically two types of elder abuse—domestic and institutional. **Domestic elder abuse** takes place when an elder is being cared for in a home-based setting, usually by relatives. **Institutional elder abuse** occurs when an elder is being cared for by a person with a legal or contractual responsibility to provide care, such as paid caregivers, nursing home staff, or other professionals. Both types of abuse can be either acts of commission (acts of physical, sexual, or emotional violence) or acts of omission (neglect).

In some cases, signs of elder abuse are subtle, such as theft of the victim's belongings or loss of freedom. Other signs, such as wounds, untreated decubitus ulcers, or poor hygiene, are more obvious. For additional information on the signs of elder abuse, see Chapter 43.

✱ **domestic elder abuse** physical or emotional violence or neglect when an elder is being cared for in a home-based setting.

✱ **institutional elder abuse** physical or emotional violence or neglect when an elder is being cared for by a person paid to provide care.

THEORIES ABOUT DOMESTIC ELDER ABUSE

There are four main theories about causes of domestic elder abuse. Commonly, caregivers feel stressed and overburdened. They are ill-equipped to provide care or simply lack the knowledge to do the job correctly. Another cause of elder abuse is their physical and/or mental impairment. Elders in poor health are more likely to be abused than elders in good health. This situation results, in part, from their inability to report the abuse. Yet another cause of elder abuse is family history, or the cycle of violence mentioned earlier. Finally, elder abuse increases proportionately with the personal problems of the caregivers. Abusers of the elderly tend to have more difficulties, either financial or emotional, than non-abusers.

CHARACTERISTICS OF ABUSED ELDERS

Like partner abuse, elder abuse cuts across all demographic groups. As a result, it is difficult to outline an accurate profile of the abused elder. The most common cases involve elderly women abused by their sons. However, this pattern is skewed by the fact that women live longer than men. Elder abuse most frequently occurs among people who are dependent upon others for their care, especially among those elders who are mentally or physically challenged. In such cases, elders may be repeatedly abused by relatives who believe the elder will not or cannot ask for help.

In cases of neglect, abused elders most commonly live alone. They may be mentally competent, but fear asking for help because relatives have complained about providing care or have threatened to place them in a nursing home. Like abused partners, they may be reluctant to give information about their abusers for fear of retaliation.

CHARACTERISTICS OF ELDER ABUSERS

It is also difficult to profile the people who are most likely to abuse elders. According to the National Aging Resource Center on Elder Abuse, the percentages in Table 44-1 reflect the reported perpetrators of elder abuse in domestic settings. As you can see, the most typical abusers are adult children, who are either overstressed by care of the elder or who were abused themselves.

As with partner abusers, there are several characteristics commonly found in abusers of the elderly. Often, the perpetrators exhibit alcoholic behavior, drug addiction, or some mental impairment. The abuser may also be dependent upon the income or assistance of the elder—a situation that can cause resentment, anger, and, in some cases, violence.

For more on the management of elder abuse, see Chapter 43.

Table 44-1	PERPETRATORS OF DOMESTIC ELDER ABUSE	
Group		**Percentage**
Adult children		32.5
Grandchildren		4.2
Spouse		14.4
Sibling		2.5
Other relatives		12.5
Friend/neighbor		7.5
All others		18.2
Unknown		2.0

CHILD ABUSE

 child abuse physical or emotional violence or neglect towards a person from infancy to eighteen years of age.

Child abuse can occur from infancy to age 18 and can be inflicted by any number of caregivers.

As pointed out in Chapters 41 and 42, child abuse is one of the most difficult circumstances that you will face as a paramedic. **Child abuse** may range from physical or emotional impairment to neglect of a child's most basic needs (Figure 44-1). It can occur from infancy to age 18 and can be inflicted by any number of caregivers—parents, foster parents, step-parents, babysitters, siblings, step-siblings, or other relatives or friends charged with a child's care.

Although you may be familiar with some of the following information from your training or from earlier chapters in this book, it bears repeating. The damage done to a child can last a lifetime and, as stressed, perpetuate a cycle of violence in generations to come.

FIGURE 44-1   Child abuse comes in many forms. Be alert and report any concerns you may have regarding abuse or neglect.

CHARACTERISTICS OF CHILD ABUSERS

As with other types of abusers, you cannot relate child abuse to social class, income, or education. However, certain patterns do emerge, most notably a history of abuse within their own families. Most child abusers were physically or emotionally abused as children. They often would prefer to use other forms of discipline, but under stress they regress to the earliest and most familiar patterns. Once resorting to physical discipline, the punishments become more severe and more frequent.

In cases of reported physical abuse, perpetrators tend to be men. However, the statistics for men and women even out when neglect is taken into account. As indicated earlier, potential child abusers can include a wide variety of caregivers. In most cases, however, one or both parents are the most likely abusers. Frequent behavioral traits include:

- Use or abuse of drugs and/or alcohol
- Immaturity and preoccupation with self
- Lack of obvious feeling for the child, rarely looking at or touching the child
- Seemingly unconcerned about the child's injury, treatment, or prognosis
- Openly critical of the child, with little indication of guilt or remorse for involvement in the child's condition
- Little identification with the child's pain, whether it be physical or emotional

Any one of these signs should raise suspicion in your mind of possible child abuse. The infant or child will provide other clues, even before you begin your physical examination.

CHARACTERISTICS OF ABUSED CHILDREN

A child's behavior is one of the most important indicators of abuse. Some behavior is age-related. For example, abused children under age six usually appear excessively passive, while abused children over age six seem aggressive. Other behavioral clues include:

- Crying, often hopelessly, during treatment or not crying at all
- Avoiding the parents or showing little concern for their absence
- Unusually wary or fearful of physical contact
- Apprehensive and/or constantly on the alert for danger
- Prone to sudden behavioral changes
- Absence of nearly all emotions
- Neediness, constantly requesting favors, food, or things

In general, use your instincts and knowledge of age-appropriate behavior (see Chapters 41 and 42) to guide your first impression of the child. If the child's behavior is atypical, maintain an index of suspicion throughout your assessment.

IDENTIFICATION OF THE ABUSED CHILD

As you know, children very commonly get injured and not all injured children are abused. If a child volunteers the story of his or her injury without hesitation and if it matches the story told by the parent and the symptoms of injury,

A child's behavior is one of the most important indicators of abuse.

Use your instincts and knowledge of age-appropriate behavior to guide your first impression of a child whom you suspect may have been abused.

Table 44-2	COLOR OF BRUISES AND THEIR AGE*	
Age		**Skin Appearance**
0 to 2 days		tender and swollen, red
0 to 5 days		blue, purple
5 to 7 days		green
7 to 10 days		yellow
10 or more days		brown
2 or more weeks		cleared

*Adapted from Richardson, A.C., "Cutaneous Manifestations of Abuse" in Reece, R.M. *Child Abuse: Medical Diagnosis and Management.*

Content Review

COMMON CONDITIONS MISTAKEN FOR ABUSE
- Car seat burns
- Staphylococcal scalded skin syndrome
- Chicken pox (cigarette burns)
- Hematological disorders that cause easy bruising

Soft-tissue injuries are common indicators of abuse, especially multiple bruises in different places on the body, in different stages of healing, and/or with distinctive shapes.

child abuse is very unlikely. However, in cases in which the behavior of a caregiver and/or child has raised an index of suspicion, you may face a challenge in distinguishing between an intentional injury and an authentic accident. Conditions commonly mistaken for abuse are car seat burns, staphylococcal scalded skin syndrome, chicken pox (cigarette burns), and hematological disorders that can cause bruising. In assessing a child, look for common patterns of physical abuse, evidence of emotional abuse, and/or environmental clues of neglect.

Physical Examination

In most cases, signs of physical mistreatment of a child should be the easiest type of abuse for you to recognize. Soft tissue injuries are the most common indicators, especially multiple bruises in different planes of the body, in different stages of healing, and with distinctive shapes (Table 44-2 and Figure 44-2). Other common warning signs include defensive wounds on the hands and forearms and symmetrical injuries such as bites or burns. Any of these conditions carry a high index of suspicion of abuse.

Burns and Scalds Abusive burns often have distinctive patterns that indicate the implement or source used to injure the child. The burns tend to be in certain common locations—the soles of the feet, palms of the hands, back, or buttocks. They may or may not be found in conjunction with other injuries.

FIGURE 44-2 Severe multiple bruises can lead to death.

Because children have thinner skin than adults (other than elders), they also tend to scald more easily. The temperature of hot water in most residences is about 140°F, which can scald an adult in only about five seconds. (Bath water for children should be kept below 120°F.) When children accidentally get into water that is too hot, you can expect to see "splash" burns—marks created by spattering water as children try to escape. Intentional scalding, however, is characterized by the conspicuous lack of splash burns. Such "dipping injuries" are a common form of child abuse.

Fractures Fractures constitute the second most common form of child abuse. Sites of fractures include the skull, nose, facial structures, and upper extremities. Twisting and jerking fractures result from grabbing a child by an extremity, while neck injuries occur from shaking a child. Because children have soft, pliable ribs, they rarely experience accidental fractures to this region. As a result, you should maintain a high index of suspicion of abuse whenever you encounter a child with fractured ribs.

Head Injuries Over time, injuries from abuse tend to progress from the extremities and trunk to the head. Head injuries commonly found in abused children include scalp wounds, skull fractures, subdural or subgaleal hematomas, and repeated contusions.

Injuries to the head claim the largest number of lives among abused children. They also account for most of the long-term disability associated with child abuse.

Shaken Baby Syndrome Shaken baby syndrome frequently occurs when a parent or caregiver becomes frustrated with a crying infant and all other attempts to quiet the baby have failed. It happens when a person picks up the infant and shakes the baby vigorously. The movement can cause permanent brain damage such as subdural hematomas or diffuse swelling. It may also result in injuries to the neck and spine or retinal hemorrhages, which in turn can lead to blindness. If the infant is shaken hard enough or repeatedly, the baby may die from the injuries.

Abdominal Injuries Although abdominal injuries represent a small proportion of the injuries suffered by abused children, they are usually very serious. Blunt force can result in trauma to the liver, spleen, or mesentery. You should look for pain, swelling, and vomiting, as well as hemodynamic compromise from these injuries.

Signs of Neglect

Some forms of child abuse are less obvious than physical injuries. Abuse may result from neglect. Caregivers simply do not provide children with adequate food, clothing, shelter, or medical care.

As a paramedic, you may be in a unique position to observe and report neglect. Unlike many other healthcare or public-safety workers, EMS personnel get an opportunity to see the child's home environment for themselves. Unhealthy or unclean conditions are clear evidence of a caregiver's inability to provide for a child's safety or well-being.

In examining a child, keep in mind the following common signs of neglect:

- Malnutrition (Neglected children are often underweight, sometimes by up to 30 percent.)
- Severe diaper rash
- Diarrhea and/or dehydration
- Hair loss

Intentional scalding is characterized by the conspicuous lack of splash burns.

Because children have soft, pliable ribs, they rarely experience accidental fractures to this region.

- Untreated medical conditions
- Inappropriate, dirty, or torn clothing
- Tired and listless attitudes
- Near constant demands for physical contact or attention

Signs of Emotional Abuse

Emotional abuse is often the hardest form of abuse to identify. It may take any one of the following six forms:

1. Parents or caregivers simply ignore the child, showing indifference to the child's needs and failing to provide any stimulation.
2. Parents or caregivers reject, humiliate, or criticize the child.
3. The child may be isolated and deprived of normal human contact or nurturing.
4. A child may be terrorized or bullied through verbal assaults and threats, creating feelings of fear and anxiety.
5. A parent or caregiver may encourage destructive or antisocial behavior.
6. The child may be over-pressured by unrealistic expectations of success.

RECORDING AND REPORTING CHILD ABUSE

As with all other forms of abuse, you have a responsibility to report suspected cases of child abuse.

As with all other forms of abuse, you have a responsibility to report suspected cases of child abuse. In some instances, you might have a chance to provide early intervention. An abusive adult may actively seek help or may send out signals for help. For example, a potential abuser may make several calls within a 24-hour period. The person may also summon help for inconsequential symptoms or demonstrate an inability to handle an impeding crisis. These are warning signs and should be duly noted.

When confronted with a case of child abuse, try to conduct the examination with another colleague present.

When confronted with an actual case of child abuse, try to conduct the examination with another colleague present. You must keep your personal reactions to yourself and record only your objective observations. Assumptions must not be included in your report. The final document should be objective, legible, and written with the knowledge that it may be used in a future court or child custody case. At all times, put the child's interest first, treating him or her with utmost kindness and gentleness. (For more on your EMS and legal responsibilities, see material later in the chapter.)

SEXUAL ASSAULT

Anyone can be a victim of sexual violence. Statistics from the National Victims Center and the U.S. Department of Justice reveal that males and females of all backgrounds, from infancy to old age, have reported crimes involving forced or unwanted sexual contact. According to the Bureau of Justice Statistics, over 260,000 rapes and nearly 100,000 sexual assaults are reported each year. However, these figures reflect only a small percentage of cases, with an estimated 63–74 percent of all incidents going unreported.

Although the legal definitions vary from state to state, courts generally interpret **sexual assault** as unwanted sexual contact, whether it be genital, oral, rectal, or manual. **Rape** is usually defined as penile penetration of the genitalia or rectum (however slight) without consent of the victim. Both forms of sexual violence are prosecuted as crimes, with rape constituting a felony offense. As a result, your actions at the scene and the report that you file will in all likelihood impact on the outcome of a trial.

CHARACTERISTICS OF VICTIMS OF SEXUAL ASSAULT/RAPE

It is difficult to profile a victim of sexual assault or rape because of the variety of victims. However, statistics reveal certain patterns. The group most likely to be victimized is made up of adolescent females younger than age 18. Nearly two-thirds of all rapes and sexual assaults take place between the hours of 6 P.M. and 6 A.M. at the victim's home or at the home of a friend, relative, or acquaintance. A woman is raped, on average, every two minutes in the United States and is four times as likely to be raped by someone she knows than by a stranger.

Particularly alarming is the number of children who suffer some form of sexual abuse. According to the Department of Justice, one in two rape victims are under age 18; one in six are under age 12. Other government figures show that approximately one-third of all juvenile victims of sexual abuse are children younger than 6 years of age. Typically, contact involves a male assailant and a female victim, but not always. The contact can range from exposure to fondling to penetration. Although sexual abuse can occur in families of all descriptions, children raised in families where there is domestic violence are eight times more likely to be sexually molested within that family.

Sexual assault and rape carry serious consequences. Victims may be physically injured during the assault or even killed. They commonly suffer internal injuries, particularly if multiple assailants are involved in the attack. Rape can result in infections, sexually transmitted diseases, and unwanted pregnancies. The psychological damage is deep and long-lasting. Shame, anger, and a lack of trust may persist for years—or even a lifetime.

Children, in particular, find it difficult to speak about molestation. It is likely that they know the person and fear reprisal or, in some instances, even seek to protect the individual. In many cases, the assailants physically explore the child without intercourse or force the child to touch or fondle them. Victims, especially very young children, may be confused about the situation or, lacking physical evidence of abuse, fear that nobody will believe them. Symptoms of sexual abuse, regardless of its form, may include:

- Nightmares
- Restlessness
- Withdrawal tendencies
- Hostility
- Phobias related to the offender
- Regressive behavior, such as bed wetting
- Truancy
- Promiscuity, in older children and teens
- Drug and alcohol abuse

* **sexual assault** unwanted oral, genital, rectal, or manual sexual contact.

* **rape** penile penetration of the genitalia or rectum without the consent of the victim.

The legal definition of rape varies from state to state. You should review the appropriate laws in your state pertaining to rape and sexual assault.

CHARACTERISTICS OF SEXUAL ASSAILANTS

Like the victims of sexual assaults, the assailants can come from almost any background. However, the violent victimizers of children are substantially more likely than the victimizers of adults to have been physically or sexually abused as children. Many assailants, particularly adolescents and abusive adults, think domination is part of any relationship. Such thinking can lead to date rape or marital rape. In a significant percentage of all cases, the assailants are under the influence of alcohol or drugs. Nearly 30 percent of all rapists use weapons, underscoring the fact that sexual assaults are violent crimes.

In cases of date rape, the assailant may have drugged the unknowing victim with flunitrazepam (Rohypnol), known by the street names of "roofie," "roche," "rib," or "rope." The victim may exhibit extreme intoxication without a corresponding strong smell of alcohol or may have drug-induced amnesia (a common effect), making questioning difficult or impossible. More often than not, the alleged assailant in such cases lives on a college campus, the location of most EMS calls involving what is known as the "date rape drug."

EMS RESPONSIBILITIES

In calls involving abuse or assault, your primary responsibility is safety—both your own and that of the patient.

Your response to a call involving a sexual assault is in many ways similar to your response to any abusive situation. In both instances, your primary responsibility is safety—both your own and that of the patient. You should never enter a scene if your safety is compromised, and you should leave the scene as soon as you feel unsafe.

You can expect victims of assault or abuse to feel unsafe as a result of the violence they have suffered. One of your primary responsibilities is to provide a safe environment for an already traumatized patient. Sometimes you can provide safety merely by your official presence. Other times, you may have to move the patient to the ambulance where you can lock the doors or move to a different location entirely. In still other instances, you may have to summon additional personnel. (For more on crime scene management, see Chapter 48.)

In many cases, a same-sex paramedic—you or a colleague—should maintain contact with the victim of an alleged sexual assault.

You are also responsible for providing proper psychosocial care for the victims of abuse and assault. Privacy is a major consideration. In many cases, a same-sex paramedic—you or a colleague—should maintain contact with the victim. Although you may need to expose the victim during assessment, you should cover the patient and remove him or her from public view as soon as possible.

When talking with a victim of sexual assault, use open-ended questions to help the patient regain a sense of self-control.

When talking with the patient, use open-ended questions to reestablish a sense of control. You might say, for example, "Would you like to sit on a seat or ride on the stretcher?" Or you might ask, "Is there someone you would like us to call?" As mentioned in earlier sections, remain non-judgmental throughout treatment, avoiding subjective comments both of the patient and the assailant. In a reassuring voice, encourage the patient to report the rape, explaining the importance of preserving evidence.

Medical treatment of victims of abuse and assault is essentially the same as with other patients. However, you should always remember the origins of the patient's injuries and provide appropriate emotional support. Keep in mind that the patient has been harmed by another human being, in many cases a person that they know intimately.

LEGAL CONSIDERATIONS

As noted throughout this chapter, abuse and assault constitute crimes. Although their nature and extent of the crime often depends upon local laws, you have a responsibility to report suspected cases to the appropriate law enforcement officials.

Because the assailants may be detained only a short time, you also have an obligation to find out about the victim and witness protection programs available in your area.

Specialized resources include both private and state or federally funded programs. Make a point of learning about hospital units for the victims of sexual assault, public and private shelters for battered persons, and state agencies responsible for youths and their families. Also acquaint yourself with nurses trained as Sexual Assault Nurse Examiners (SANE). They have completed programs allowing them to perform the physical exam for sexual assaults. They have detailed information on the protection of evidence, something that you must keep in mind throughout the call.

As you have read, your actions can affect the prosecution of a crime. Clothing should only be removed from a patient when necessary for assessment and treatment. All items should then be turned over to the proper authorities.

In the case of rape, patients should not urinate, defecate, douche, bathe, eat, drink, or smoke. Some jurisdictions have specific rules for evidence protection, such as using paper bags to collect evidence or placing bags over the patient's hands to preserve trace evidence. Remember that any evidence that you collect must remain in your custody until you can give it directly to a law enforcement official to preserve the **chain of evidence.**

As indicated, it is important that you carefully and objectively document all your findings. You may end up defending your words in a court of law. Regardless of the emotions evoked by the call, you must remain a professional at all times.

Finally, you should study the local laws and protocols regarding cases of abuse and assault. All 50 states require healthcare workers to report suspected cases of child abuse. Some states require EMS personnel to report even a suspicion of abuse or assault. Some states allow minors to seek medical care for sexual assault without parental consent. The Joint Commission of Accreditation of Healthcare Organizations (JCAHO) mandates that hospital personnel screen incoming patients for abuse. Regardless of where you live, take time to learn the rules and regulations that affect your practice, both for your sake and for the sake of your patients.

✱ chain of evidence legally retaining items of evidence and accounting for their whereabouts at all times to prevent loss or tampering.

Your actions in the case of alleged sexual assaults can affect the prosecution of a crime. Protect the evidence.

Regardless of the emotions evoked by a call involving abuse or assault, you must remain professional at all times.

∫ UMMARY

The incidence of abuse is widespread today, and you will encounter many cases during your paramedic career. You should learn the hallmarks of partner abuse, elder abuse, child abuse, and sexual assaults. You should also learn to recognize significant physical and emotional assessment findings as well as characteristics of the victims and assailants. Proper treatment of victims of abuse and assault includes knowing the legal requirements of your area, protecting evidence, and properly documenting your findings and actions.

CHAPTER 45

The Challenged Patient

Objectives

After reading this chapter, you should be able to:

1. Describe the various etiologies and types of hearing impairments. (pp. 1868–1869)
2. Recognize the patient with a hearing impairment. (p. 1869)
3. Anticipate accommodations that may be needed in order to properly manage the patient with a hearing impairment. (pp. 1869–1870)
4. Describe the various etiologies and types, recognize patients with, and anticipate accommodations that may be needed in order to properly manage each of the following conditions:

   a. visual impairments (pp. 1870–1871)
   b. speech impairments (pp. 1871–1872)
   c. obesity (pp. 1872–1873)
   d. paraplegia/quadriplegia (pp. 1873–1874)
   e. mental illness (p. 1874)
   f. developmentally disabled (pp. 1874–1875)
   g. Down syndrome (pp. 1875–1876)
   h. emotional impairment (p. 1874)

   Continued

INTRODUCTION

Throughout your EMS career, you can expect to encounter a number of patients who live with a variety of impairments or special challenges. Many will have met these challenges so successfully that you may not notice them right away. For example, people with hearing impairments might lip read so well that you may not initially realize they cannot hear. People with more obvious challenges, such as paralysis, may have accepted their impairments and built active and rewarding lives. A patient with a history of polio, for example, may have lived with the problem so long that he or she neglects to tell you about it right away. Instead the patient talks about a more immediate problem—the reason for summoning EMS.

The one thing that challenged patients share is their variety. They might have any number of physical, mental, or emotional impairments. They might have contracted a pathological illness that necessitates a special living or working arrangement. They might be suffering from a terminal illness or a communicable disease. They may come from a cultural or financial situation that dictates medical practices contrary to those of the EMS community. The key to treating the "challenged" patient is to understand and recognize the special condition or situation and to make any accommodations that may be needed for proper patient care.

PHYSICAL CHALLENGES

A number of physical impairments—conditions that limit the use of one or more parts of the body—can affect patient assessment and/or treatment. These impairments may be the result of accidents, birth injuries, chronic illnesses, aging, and more. Impairments can limit the ability of a patient to hear, see, speak, or move. Patients will react to their impairments in different ways—from acceptance, to denial, to anger, to shame. It is important that you quickly recognize the impairment and exhibit knowledge and sensitivity to assure the patient that you understand his or her special needs.

HEARING IMPAIRMENTS

Hearing impairments involve a decrease or loss in the ability to distinguish or hear sounds, particularly those involving speech. An inability to hear is commonly described as **deafness**. A person may be completely deaf or partially deaf. Deafness may be in one ear or both ears. The condition may be present at birth or may occur later in life as a result of an accident, illness, or aging.

Types of Hearing Impairments

There are basically two types of deafness—**conductive deafness** and **sensorineural deafness**. Many forms of conductive deafness may be treated and cured, especially if caught early. Sensorineural deafness, on the other hand, is often incurable.

Conductive Deafness Conductive deafness results from any condition that prevents sound waves from being transmitted from the external ear to the middle or inner ear. The condition can be either temporary or permanent.

If an infant or child does not respond to verbal stimulation or questions, rule out the possibility of conductive deafness when performing your assessment of disability. Congenital malformation of the ear is a possible, but rare cause of conductive deafness in the neonate. A more common cause of conductive deafness in children is **otitis media,** an infection of the middle ear. This condition often arises from various childhood illnesses, particularly those involving the upper respiratory tract. To prevent hearing loss, children under age six who experience recurrent otitis media may need to take daily prophylactic antibiotics or have tympanostomy (myringotomy) tubes placed.

In addition to infection, a number of other conditions can result in a temporary loss of hearing. Anyone can experience conductive deafness during an airline flight, where changes in air pressure can affect hearing. A deep-water dive can have a similar effect. Impacted **cerumen,** or earwax, is yet another common and easily treatable cause of conductive deafness.

Other causes might be the temporary blockage of the ear canal by various irritants such as dust, hair spray, insects, or water ("swimmer's ear"). Patient attempts to clean the canal with cotton applicators may disrupt the ear's natural cleaning process and push the debris deeper into the ear, which sets the stage for bacterial infections and conductive deafness.

Obstructions can also be caused by hematomas, which may result from blunt trauma to the ear. Force to the mandible, such as a fractured jaw, can also produce a temporary loss of hearing and may in fact result in fragments of bone displaced to the ear canal. Although these conditions cannot be treated in the field, they should be taken into account when a trauma patient appears not to respond to, or "hear," your questions.

Sensorineural Deafness Sensorineural deafness arises from the inability of nerve impulses to reach the auditory center of the brain because of damage either to the inner ear or to the brain itself. It is usually a permanent condition.

In the case of infants and children, sensorineural deafness often results from congenital defects or birth injuries. Preterm infants are particularly at risk for sensorineural deafness, especially those with severe asphyxia or recurrent apnea in the neonatal period. Ototoxic drugs, such as furosemide (Lasix) and gentamycin,

It is important that you quickly recognize the impairment and exhibit the knowledge and sensitivity to assure the patient that you understand his or her special needs.

* **deafness** the inability to hear.

* **conductive deafness** deafness caused when there is a blocking of the transmission of the sound waves through the external ear canal to the middle or inner ear.

* **sensorineural deafness** deafness caused by the inability of nerve impulses to reach the auditory center of the brain because of nerve damage either to the inner ear or to the brain.

* **otitis media** middle ear infection.

* **cerumen** ear wax.

can also cause sensorineural deafness if administered to infants in neonatal intensive care units. Finally, many children who develop this type of hearing loss have mothers who contracted rubella (German measles) or cytomegalovirus (cmv), during the first three months of pregnancy.

Diseases, such as bacterial meningitis, or viral illnesses, such as **labrynthitis** (inner ear infection), can lead to sensorineural deafness at any age. Taking high does of ototoxic drugs such as aspirin can also cause sensorineural deafness in both children and adults. A common symptom of aspirin toxicity is "ringing in the ears" (tinnitus). Other causes of sensorineural deafness include tumors of the brain or middle ear, concussion, severe blows to the ear, and repeated loud noises such as chain saws, heavy machinery, gun fire, rock music, or sudden blasts of sound.

Conditions associated with aging can also lead to permanent hearing loss. **Presbycusis** is a progressive sensorineural hearing loss that begins after age 20, but is usually significant only in people over age 65. More common in men than women, this type of hearing loss affects high-frequency sounds first, then low-frequency sounds. Eventually, human voices becomes harder to detect, especially if background noise is present. Elderly people with this condition will often tell others not to "mumble" or will ask them to speak louder.

> ✳ **labrynthitis** inner ear infection that causes vertigo, nausea, and an unsteady gait.

> ✳ **presbycusis** progressive hearing loss that occurs with aging.

Recognition of Deafness

As mentioned, it is important to detect deafness early in your assessment. A partially deaf person may ask questions repeatedly, misunderstand answers to questions, or respond inappropriately. Such reactions can easily be mistaken for head injury, leading to misdirected treatment.

The most obvious sign of deafness is a hearing aid. Unfortunately, hearing aids do not work for all types of deafness. Also, many people do not wear hearing aids, even when they have been prescribed. In addition, deaf people may have poor diction due to partial hearing loss or hearing loss later in life. They might use their hands to gesture or use sign language. As noted, deaf people may ask you to speak louder or they may speak excessively loud themselves. Finally, deaf people will commonly face you so that they can read your lips. Be sure that you are fully facing deaf patients before you speak to them.

> *A partially deaf person may ask questions repeatedly, misunderstand answers to questions, or respond inappropriately. Such reactions can easily be mistaken for head injury, leading to misdirected treatment.*
>

Accommodations for Deaf Patients

When managing a patient with a hearing impairment, you can do several things to ease communication. Begin by identifying yourself and making sure the patient knows that you are speaking to him or her. Get the patient's attention by moving so you can be seen or by gently touching the person, if appropriate. By addressing deaf patients face to face, you give them the opportunity to read your lips and interpret your expression.

When talking with a deaf patient, speak slowly in a normal voice. Never yell or use exaggerated gestures. These techniques often distort your facial and body language, making you seem angry or threatening. Keep in mind that nearly 80 percent of hearing loss is related to high-pitched sounds. As a result, you might use a low-pitched voice to speak directly into the patient's ear. Whatever you do, make sure that background noise is reduced as much as possible, turning off the TV, radio, or other sources of sound.

If you are called to a deaf patient's home during the night, you may need to help find or adjust a hearing aid. If you cannot locate the device, you might put a stethoscope on the patient and try speaking into it. Alternatively, you might make use of an "amplified" listener—e.g., an ear microphone.

> *By addressing deaf patients face to face, you give them the opportunity to read your lips and interpret your expression.*
>

Don't forget one of the most simple and effective means of communication—use of pen and paper. As long as you don't need to move quickly, you can write out notes for the patient to read and wait for the person to respond in the same way. You can also use a pen and paper to draw pictures to illustrate basic needs or procedures. This approach can ease a patient's anxiety, reducing the fear of miscommunication or lack of control over his or her treatment.

Finally, many people with hearing impairments know sign language, usually American Sign Language (ASL). If this is the case, try to utilize an interpreter, often a family member or even a neighbor. Make sure that you document the name of the person who did the interpreting and the information received. Also, notify the receiving hospital of the need to have an interpreter on hand if the person is unable to accompany you.

VISUAL IMPAIRMENTS

When caring for the patient with a visual impairment, it is important to note if the impairment is a permanent disability or if it is a new symptom as a result of the illness or injury for which you were called. It is necessary to understand the causes of blindness before this determination can be made.

Etiologies

Visual impairments can result from a number of causes. Possible etiologies include injury, disease, congenital conditions, infection (such as cytomegalovirus [CMV]), and degeneration of the retina, optic nerve, or nerve pathways. A description of each of the etiologies follows.

Injury A previous injury to the eye can cause a permanent vision loss. An injury to the orbit usually includes injury to the tissue around the orbit as well as to the eye itself. This can cause muscle and nerve damage that may lead to permanent loss of eyesight. Penetrating injuries can result in **enucleation,** which is removal of the eyeball. Chemical and thermal burns to the eye can result in damage to the cornea and can also lead to permanent vision loss if not treated quickly. A temporary loss of vision can result from an injury, such as the chemical burn that may occur with the deployment of an airbag, or from a corneal abrasion. Once treated, these injuries rarely lead to permanent loss of vision.

Disease Visual impairments may also be caused by a disease of the eye, or as a secondary result of the primary disease process. **Glaucoma,** for example, is a group of eye diseases that results in increased intraocular pressure on the optic nerve. If not treated, glaucoma leads to loss of peripheral vision and blindness.

The are two different types of glaucoma, primary and secondary. The cause of primary glaucoma remains unknown. However, secondary glaucoma results from other eye diseases. The incidence of glaucoma is higher in blacks than in whites. A black person between the ages of 45 and 65 is 15 times more likely to have glaucoma than a white person in the same age group.

Diabetic retinopathy is another disease-related visual impairment. It results from diabetes mellitus, which causes disorders in the blood vessels that lead to the retina. Small hemorrhages in these blood vessels leads to a slow loss of vision and possible blindness.

Congenital and Degenerative Disorders A congenital disorder that causes visual disturbances is cerebral palsy. Premature birth can lead to blindness in the

---

Content Review

CAUSES OF VISUAL IMPAIRMENTS

- Injury
- Disease
- Congenital conditions
- Infection
- Degeneration of the retina, optic nerve, or nerve pathways

✱ **enucleation** removal of the eyeball after trauma or illness.

✱ **glaucoma** group of eye diseases that results in increased intraocular pressure on the optic nerve; if left untreated, can lead to blindness.

✱ **diabetic retinopathy** slow loss of vision as a result of damage done by diabetes.

neonate. Degeneration of the eyeball, optic nerve, or nerve pathways is most commonly caused by aging and can slowly lead to loss of vision. Cytomegalovirus (CMV), an opportunistic infection often seen in AIDS patients, can lead to blindness by causing retinitis—an inflammation of the retina.

Recognizing and Accommodating Visual Impairments

Many visually impaired people live independent, active lives (Figure 45–1). Depending upon the degree of impairment and a person's adjustment to the loss of vision, you may or may not recognize the condition right away. In cases of obvious blindness, identify yourself as you approach the patient so that the person knows you are there. Also, describe everything you are doing as you do it.

Many blind people have tools to assist them in their activities of daily living. The most obvious is a seeing eye dog. When approaching a person with a seeing eye dog, DO NOT pet the dog or disturb it while the dog is in its harness. For the dog, the harness means that it is working. Ask permission from the patient to touch the dog. Never grab the leash, the harness, or the patient's arm without asking permission. Doing this may place the dog or the owner—or yourself—in danger.

Accommodation must be made for transporting the guide dog with the patient. Circumstances and local protocols will dictate whether you transport the dog in the ambulance with the patient or have the dog transported in another vehicle.

If your patient does not have a guide dog, inquire about other tools that the person may want brought to the hospital. If the patient is ambulatory, have the person take your arm for guidance rather than taking the patient's arm.

SPEECH IMPAIRMENTS

When performing an assessment, you may come across a patient who is awake, alert, and oriented, but cannot communicate with you due to a speech impairment. Possible miscommunication can hinder both the treatment you administer and the information that you provide to the receiving facility.

Types of Speech Impairments

You may encounter four types of speech impairments—language disorders, articulation disorders, voice production disorders, and fluency disorders. A discussion of each disorder follows.

Language Disorders   A language disorder is an impaired ability to understand the spoken or written word. In children, language disorders result from a number of causes such as congenital learning disorders, cerebral palsy, or hearing impairments. A child who receives inadequate language stimulation in the first year of life may also experience delayed speaking ability.

In an adult patient, language disorders may result from a variety of illnesses or injuries. The person may have experienced a stroke, aneurysm, head injury, brain tumor, hearing loss, or some kind of emotional trauma. The loss of ability to communicate in speech, writing, or signs is known as **aphasia**. Aphasia can manifest itself in the following ways:

- **Sensory aphasia**—a person can no longer understand the spoken word. Patients with sensory aphasia will not respond to your questions because they cannot understand what you are saying.

FIGURE 45-1   Individuals who are visually impaired can still maintain active, independent lives.

✱ **aphasia** occurs when the individual suffers a brain injury due to stroke or head injury and no longer has the ability to speak or read.

✱ **sensory aphasia** occurs when the patient cannot understand the spoken word.

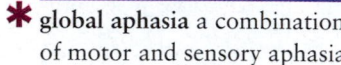

- **Motor aphasia**—a person can no longer use the symbols of speech. Patients with motor aphasia, also known as expressive aphasia, will understand what you say, but cannot clearly articulate a response. They may respond to your questions slowly, use the wrong words, or act out answers. It is important to allow such patients to express their responses in whatever way they can.
- **Global aphasia**—occurs when a person has both sensory and motor aphasia. These patients can neither understand nor respond to your questions. A brain tumor in Broca's region can cause this condition.

Articulation Disorders Articulation disorders, also known as dysarthria, affect the way a person's speech is heard by others. These disorders occur when sounds are produced or put together incorrectly or in a way that makes it difficult to understand the spoken word. Articulation disorders may start at an early age, when the child learns to say words incorrectly or when a hearing impairment is involved. This type of disorder can also occur in both children and adults when neural damage causes a disturbance in the nerve pathways leading from the brain to the larynx, mouth, or lips.

When speaking with someone who has an articulation disorder, you will notice that they pronounce their words incorrectly or that their speech is slurred. They may leave certain sounds out of a word because they are too difficult for them to pronounce. Again, it is important for you to listen carefully and let the person complete a response.

Voice Production Disorders When a patient has a voice production disorder, the quality of the person's voice is affected. This can be caused by trauma due to overuse of the vocal cords or infection. Cancer of the larynx can also cause a speech failure by impeding air from passing through the vocal cords. A patient with a production disorder will exhibit hoarseness, harshness, an inappropriate pitch, or abnormal nasal resonance.

Fluency Disorders Fluency disorders present as stuttering. Although the cause of stuttering is not fully understood, the condition is found more often in men than in women. Stuttering occurs when sounds or syllables are repeated and the patient cannot put words together fluidly. When speaking with patients who stutter, do not interrupt or finish their answers out of frustration. Let patients complete what they have to say, and do not correct how they say it.

Accommodations for Speech Impairments

When speaking to a patient with a speech impairment, never assume that the person lacks intelligence. It will be difficult, if not impossible, to complete a thorough interview if you have insulted the patient. Do not to rush the patient or predict an answer. Try to form questions that require short, direct answers. Prepare to spend extra time during your interview.

When asking questions, look directly at the patient. If you cannot understand what the person has said, politely ask him or her to repeat it. Never pretend to understand when you don't. You might miss valuable information about the patient's chief complaint—the reason for the call. If all else fails, give the patient an opportunity to write responses to your questions.

OBESITY

Over 40 percent of people in the United States are considered obese, while many more are heavier than their ideal body weight. An obese patient can make a difficult job even more difficult for an EMS provider. Besides the obvious difficulty of lifting and moving the obese patient, excess weight can exacerbate the complaint for which you were called. Obesity can also lead to a number of serious medical conditions, including hypertension, heart disease, strokes, diabetes, and joint and muscle problems.

Etiologies

People require a certain amount of body fat in order to metabolize vitamins and minerals. Obesity occurs when a person has an abnormal amount of body fat and a weight 20 to 30 percent heavier than is normal for people of the same age, gender, and height.

Obesity occurs for a number of reasons. In many cases, it happens when a person's caloric intake is higher than the amount of calories required to meet his or her energy needs. In such cases, diet, exercise, and life style choices play a role in the person's condition. Genetic factors may also predispose a patient toward obesity. In rare cases, an obese patient may have a low basal metabolic rate, which causes the body to burn calories at a slower rate. In such cases, the condition may be produced by an illness, particularly hypothyroidism.

Accommodations for Obese Patients

Regardless of the cause of your patient's obesity, your primary responsibility is to provide thorough and professional medical care. Conduct an extensive medical history, keeping in mind the chronic medical conditions commonly associated with obesity.

Obese patients often mistakenly blame signs and symptoms of an untreated illness on their weight. For example, they may quickly dismiss shortness of breath by saying "When you're as heavy as me, you can't expect to walk up a flight of stairs without some extra breathing." Don't accept such an answer. The shortness of breath may be caused by congestive heart failure. Obtain a complete history of the symptoms and the activities the person was doing when they appeared. While the patient usually experiences shortness of breath when climbing stairs, this time the condition may have started while sitting down or may have been more severe than usual.

When doing your patient assessment, you may also have to make accommodations for the person's weight. For example, if the patient's adipose tissue presents an obstruction, you may need to place ECG monitoring electrodes on the arms and thighs instead of on the chest. You may also need to auscultate lung sounds anteriorly on a patient who is too obese to lean forward. In assessing an obese patient, flexibility is the key. Keep in mind that no two patients and no two environments will be just alike.

Positioning an obese patient for transport may prove especially difficult, as many EMS transportation devices are not designed or rated for high weights. Always be sure you have enough lifting assistance for the circumstances. Never compromise your health or safety during the transport process. Another EMS crew or the fire department may be necessary to move your patient safely. Finally, remember to let the emergency department know that extra lifting assistance and special stretchers will be needed upon your arrival.

PARALYSIS

Always expect the unexpected in EMS. During your career, you may respond to a call and find that your patient is paralyzed from a previous traumatic or medical event. You will have to treat the chief complaint while taking into account the accommodations that must be made when treating a patient who cannot move some or all of his or her extremities.

If the adipose tissue on an obese patient presents an obstruction, you may need to place ECG monitoring electrodes on the arms and thighs instead of on the chest.

When transporting an extremely obese patient, summon adequate assistance. Try not to draw excess attention to the patient in order to protect the person from further embarrassment.

Be prepared to be extremely innovative when determining how to transport a morbidly obese patient who will not fit the ambulance stretcher.

A paralyzed patient may be paraplegic or quadriplegic. A paraplegic patient has been paralyzed from the waist down, while a quadriplegic patient has paralysis of all four extremities. In addition, spinal cord injuries in the area of C3 to C5 and above may also paralyze the patient's respiratory muscles and compromise the ability to breathe.

If your patient depends on a home ventilator, it is important to maintain a patent airway and to keep the ventilator functioning. Also, a paralyzed patient may have been breathing through a tracheostomy for some time. Therefore, you should keep suction nearby in case the person experiences an airway obstruction. You may also need to use a bag-valve-mask to transport the patient to the ambulance if the ventilator does not transport easily. If your ambulance is equipped, use the ventilator with an onboard power supply to save the ventilator's batteries. This is an already anxious time for your patient, so you may need to spend some extra time reassuring the person before making any changes in the life-support system.

If the patient has suffered a recent spinal cord injury, halo traction may still be intact. Be sure to stabilize the traction before transport. The patient can probably tell you how to assist with the halo traction; if not, a call to the patient's physician may be necessary.

While performing your physical assessment, you may come across a **colostomy**. This device is necessary when the patient does not have normal bowel function due to paralysis of the muscles needed for proper elimination. Be sure to take any other assisting devices, such as canes or wheelchairs, so the patient can get around once out of your care. (For more on acute interventions for physically disabled and other chronic care patients, see Chapter 46.)

MENTAL CHALLENGES AND EMOTIONAL IMPAIRMENTS

Mental and emotional illnesses present a special challenge to the EMS provider. They may range from the psychoses caused by complex biochemical brain diseases, such as bipolar disorder (manic depression), to the personality disorders related to personality development, to a traumatic experience. Emotional impairments can include such conditions as hysteria, compulsive behavior, or anxiety. For a detailed discussion on the etiologies, assessment, management and treatment of these patients, see Chapter 38.

DEVELOPMENTAL DISABILITIES

People with developmental disabilities are those individuals with impaired or insufficient development of the brain who are unable to learn at the usual rate. In recent years, a large number of people with developmental disabilities have been mainstreamed into the day-to-day activities of life. They hold jobs and live in residential settings, either on their own, with their families, or in group homes.

Developmental disabilities can result from a variety of reasons. They can be genetic, such as in Down syndrome, or they can be the product of brain injury caused by some hypoxic or traumatic event. Such injuries can take place before birth, during birth, or anytime thereafter.

ACCOMMODATIONS FOR DEVELOPMENTAL DISABILITIES

Unless a patient has Down syndrome, it may be difficult to recognize someone with a developmental disability unless the person lives in a group home or other special residential setting. The disability may only become obvious when you start your interview, and even then the person may be able to provide adequate information (Figure 45-2). Remember that a person with a developmental disability can recognize body language, tone, and disrespect just like anyone else. Treat them as you would any other patient, listening to their answers, particularly if you suspect physical or emotional abuse. As mentioned in previous chapters, this group has a higher than average chance of being abused, particularly by someone they know.

If a patient has a severe cognitive disability, you may need to rely on others to obtain the chief complain and history. In this case, plan to spend a little extra time on your physical assessment because the patient may not be able to tell you what is wrong. Also, many children or young people with learning disabilities have been taught to be wary of strangers who may seek to touch them. You will have to establish a basis of trust with the patient, perhaps by making it clear that you are a member of the medical community or by asking for the support of a person the patient does trust. Also, some people with developmental disabilities have been judged "stupid" or "bad" for behavior that results in an accident and they may try to cover up the events that led up to the call.

At all times, keep in mind that a person with a developmental disability may not understand what is happening. The ambulance, special equipment, and even your uniform may confuse or scare them. In cases of severe disabilities, it will be important to keep the primary caregiver with you at all times, even in the back of the ambulance. Talk to disabled patients in terms they will understand and demonstrate what you are doing, as much as possible, on yourself or your partner.

Remember that a person with a developmental disability can recognize body language, tone, and disrespect just like anyone else. Treat them as you would any other patient.

DOWN SYNDROME

Until the mid-1900s, people with Down syndrome lived largely out of public view and tended to die at an early age. Today, however, Down syndrome people attend special schools, hold paid jobs, and, because of improved medical care, can live long lives.

Down syndrome is named after J. Langdon Down, the British physician who studied and identified the condition. It results from an extra chromosome, usually on chromosome 21 or 22. Instead of 46 chromosomes, a person with Down syndrome has 47.

Although the cause is unknown, the chromosomal abnormality increases with the age of the mother, especially after age 40. It also occurs at a higher rate in parents with a chromosomal abnormality, such as the translocation of chromosome 21 to chromosome 14. In such cases, the parent, usually the mother, is phenotypically normal, but has 45 chromosomes. Theoretically the chance is one in three that the mother will have a Down syndrome child.

Typically Down syndrome presents with easily recognized physical features. They include:

- Eyes sloped up at the outer corners
- Folds of skin on either side of the nose that cover the inner corner of the eye
- Small face and features
- Large and protruding tongue
- Flattening on the back of the head
- Short and broad hands

Patients with Down syndrome are often loving and trusting. Be sure to treat them with respect and patience.

In addition to mild to moderate developmental disability, Down syndrome patients may have other physical ailments, such as heart defects, intestinal defects, and chronic lung problems. Down syndrome people are also at risk of developing cataracts, blindness, and Alzheimer's disease at an early age.

When assessing the Down syndrome patient, consider the level of their developmental delay and follow the general guidelines mentioned earlier. Transport to the hospital should be uneventful, especially if the care giver accompanies you.

FETAL ALCOHOL SYNDROME

Fetal Alcohol Syndrome (FAS) is sometimes confused with Down syndrome because of similar facial characteristics. Unlike Down syndrome, FAS is a preventable disorder, caused by excessive alcohol consumption during pregnancy. Children who suffer FAS have characteristic features, including:

- Small head with multiple facial abnormalities
- Small eyes with short slits
- Wide, flat nose bridge
- Lack of a groove between the nose and lip
- Small jaw

FAS patients often exhibit delayed physical growth, mental disabilities, and hyperactivity. Again, follow the preceding general guidelines when treating children with FAS.

PATHOLOGICAL CHALLENGES

As you will learn in Chapter 46, "Acute Interventions for the Chronic-Care Patient," you will encounter a number of challenged patients with chronic conditions. It is important for you to be aware of most common of these conditions, since chronic-care patients require higher-than-average interventions and transport.

Fingers turned
laterally with
joint fusion

Rheumatoid
nodules

FIGURE 45-3 Rheumatoid arthritis causes joints to become painful and deformed.

ARTHRITIS

The three most common types of arthritis include:

- Juvenile rheumatoid arthritis (JRA)—a connective tissue disorder that strikes before age 16
- Rheumatoid arthritis—an autoimmune disorder
- Osteoarthritis—a degenerative joint disease, the most common arthritis seen in elderly patients

All forms of arthritis cause painful swelling and irritation of the joints, making everyday tasks sometimes impossible. Arthritis patients commonly have joint stiffness and limited range of motion. Sometimes the smaller joints of the hands and feet become deformed (Figure 45-3). In addition, children with JRA may suffer complications involving the spleen or liver.

Treatment for arthritis includes aspirin, non-steroidal antiinflammatory drugs (NSAIDS), and/or corticosteroids. It is important for you to recognize the side effects of these medications because you may have been called upon to treat a medication side effect rather than the disease. NSAIDS can cause stomach upset and vomiting, with or without bloody emesis. Corticosteroids, such as prednisone, can cause hyperglycemia, bloody emesis, and decreased immunity. You should also take note of all the patient's medications so that you do not administer a medication that can interact with the ones already taken by the patient.

When transporting arthritis patients, keep in mind their high level of discomfort. Use pillows to elevate affected extremities. The most comfortable patient position might not be the best position to start an IV, but try to make the patient as comfortable as possible. Special padding techniques may be required due to the patient's arthritis.

Most cases of arthritis encountered in emergency medicine are due to osteoarthritis.

When transporting arthritis patients, keep in mind their high level of discomfort.

CANCER

Entire books have been written on the subject of cancer. It is impossible to list all that a health care provider needs to know about cancer in a small part of a single chapter. In fact, "cancer" is really many different diseases, each with its own characteristics. However, there are some basic points that a paramedic should keep in mind when treating the patient with cancer.

Cancer is caused by the abnormal growth of cells in normal tissue. The primary site of origin of the cancer cells determines the type of cancer that the patient has. If the cancer starts in epithelial tissue, it is called a carcinoma. If the cancer forms in connective tissue, it is called a sarcoma. It may be difficult for you to recognize a cancer patient because the disease often has few obvious signs and symptoms. Rather, the treatments for the disease take on telltale signs, such as anorexia leading to weight loss or alopecia (hair loss). Tattoos may be left on the skin by

FIGURE 45-4 Take every effort to protect cancer patients from infection. Keep a mask on yourself and the patient during transport and during transfer at the hospital.

neutropenic a condition that results from an abnormally low neutrophil count in the blood (less than 2000/mm³).

If a person has recently undergone chemotherapy, assume that the patient is neutropenic. For this reason, keep a mask on the patient during transport and during transfer at the emergency department.

radiation oncologists to mark positioning of radiation therapy equipment. In addition, physical changes, such as loss of a breast (mastectomy), may be obvious.

Management of the cancer patient can present a special challenge to the paramedic. Many patients undergoing chemotherapy treatments become **neutropenic.** This is a condition in which chemotherapy creates a dangerously low level of neutrophils—the white blood cells responsible for the destruction of bacteria and other infectious organisms. Frequently during chemotherapy, the neutrophils are destroyed along with the cancer cells, severely increasing the patient's risk for infection.

If patients have recently undergone chemotherapy, assume that they are neutropenic. Decrease their exposure to infection as much as possible. Remember that once infected, a neutropenic patient can quickly go into septic shock, sometimes in a matter of hours. For this reason, keep a mask on a patient both during transport and during transfer at the emergency department (Figure 45-4).

In treating cancer patients, also keep in mind that their veins may have become scarred and difficult to access due to frequent IV starts, blood draws, and caustic chemotherapy transfusions. Cancer patients may also have an implanted infusion port, found just below the skin, with the catheter inserted into the subclavian vein or brachial artery. This port is accessed for infusion of chemotherapy drugs or IV fluids using sterile technique.

You need special training to use these ports and should not attempt to access them unless you have such training. Local protocols usually dictate whether an EMS provider may access one of these devices. The patient may request that you do not start a peripheral IV if their port can be accessed at the hospital. In such cases, you need to consider if your IV is a life-saving necessity that cannot wait or if the patient can indeed wait for access at the emergency department.

Cancer patients may also have a peripheral access device such as a Groshong catheter or Hickman catheter, which have access ports that extend outside the skin. In this situation, it may simply be a matter of flushing the line and then hooking up your IV fluids to this external catheter. Whatever you decide to do, involve the patient in the decision-making process whenever possible. Cancer patients lose much control over their lives during treatment, so it is important for them to maintain as much control over their EMS care as possible.

CEREBRAL PALSY

Cerebral palsy is a group of a disorders caused by damage to the cerebrum *in utero* or by trauma during birth. Prenatal exposure of the mother to German measles can cause cerebral palsy, along with any event that leads to hypoxia in the fetus. Premature birth or brain damage from a difficult delivery can also lead to cerebral palsy. Other causes include encephalitis, meningitis, or head injury from a fall or the abuse of an infant.

Patients with cerebral palsy have difficulty controlling motor functions, causing spasticity of the muscles. This condition may affect a single limb or the entire body. About two thirds of cerebral palsy patients have a below normal intellectual capacity and about half experience seizures. Conversely, a full third of CP patients have normal intelligence and a few are highly gifted.

There are three main types of cerebral palsy—spastic paralysis, athetosis, and ataxia. Spastic paralysis, which is the most common form of cerebral palsy, forces the muscles into a state of permanent stiffness and contracture. When both legs are affected, the knees turn inward, causing the characteristic "scissor gait." Athetosis causes an involuntary writhing movement, usually affecting arms, feet, hands, and legs. If the patient's face is affected, the person may demonstrate drooling or grimacing. Ataxic cerebral palsy is the rarest form of the disease and causes problems with coordination of gait and balance.

In treating patients with cerebral palsy, keep this fact in mind: Many people with atheotoid and diplegic cerebral palsy are highly intelligent. Do not automatically assume that a person with cerebral palsy cannot communicate with you. Also, as you might expect, many cerebral palsy patients rely on special devices to help them with their mobility. Diplegic patients, for example, may be dependent on wheelchairs.

When transporting cerebral palsy patients, make accommodations to prevent further injury. If they experience severe contractions, the patients may not rest comfortably on a stretcher. Use pillows and extra blankets to pad extremities that are not in proper alignment. Have suction available if a patient drools. If a patient has difficulty communicating, make sure that the care giver helps in your assessment. Be alert for cerebral palsy patients who sign. If you do not know sign language, find someone who does and alert the emergency department.

CYSTIC FIBROSIS (MUCOVISCIDOSIS)

Cystic fibrosis (CF) is an inherited disorder that involves the exocrine (mucus producing) glands, primarily in the lungs and the digestive system. Thick mucus forms in the lungs, causing bronchial obstruction and atelectasis, or collapse of the alveoli. In addition, the thick mucus causes blockages in the small ducts of the pancreas, leading to a decrease in the pancreatic enzymes needed for digestion. This results in malnutrition, even for patients on healthy diets.

Obtaining a complete medical history is important to the recognition of a CF patient. A unique characteristic of CF is the high concentration of chloride in the sweat, leading to the use of a diagnostic test known as the "sweat test." A CF patient may also complain of frequent lung infections, clay-colored stools, or clubbing of the fingers or toes.

Recent medical advances have extended the lives of CF patients so that some live well into their thirties. However, because of a poor prognosis, most of the CF patients that you see will be children and adolescents. In treating these patients, remember that they have been chronically ill for their entire life. The last thing they may want is another trip to the hospital. For this reason, transport can be difficult for both the patient and family members. To allay their fears, keep in mind the developmental stage of your patient. A child with cystic fibrosis is still a child. So recall everything you have learned about the treatment of pediatric patients.

Because of the high probability of respiratory distress in a CF patient, some form of oxygen therapy may be necessary. You may need to have a family member or care giver hold blow by oxygen, rather than use a mask, if that is all the patient will tolerate. Suctioning may be necessary to help the patient clear the thick secretions from the airway. CF patients may be taking antibiotics to prevent

Many people with atheotoid and diplegic cerebral palsy are highly intelligent. Do not automatically assume that they cannot communicate with you.

* muscoviscidosis cystic fibrosis of the pancreas resulting in abnormally viscous mucoid secretion from the pancreas.

In treating patients with cystic fibrosis, remember that they have been chronically ill for their entire lives. The last thing they may want is another trip to the hospital.

FIGURE 45-5 Patients with multiple sclerosis and muscular dystrophy may use a cane to aid in ambulation. Be sure to take such devices with you on the ambulance.

infection and using inhalers or Mucomyst to thin their secretions. Make sure that you take along all medications so that the hospital staff can continue with the patient's regimen.

MULTIPLE SCLEROSIS

Multiple sclerosis (MS) is a disorder of the central nervous system that usually strikes between the ages of 20 and 40, affecting women more than men. The exact cause of MS is unknown, but it is considered to be an autoimmune disorder. Characteristically, repeated inflammation of the myelin sheath surrounding the nerves leads to scar tissue, which in turn blocks nerve impulses to the affected area.

The onset of MS is slow. It starts with a slight change in the strength of a muscle and a numbness or tingling in the affected muscle. For example, a patient may start to drop things, blaming it on clumsiness. Doctors encourage MS patients to lead as normal a life as possible, but they become increasingly tired. Their gait may become unsteady, and their speech may slur. MS patients may also develop eye problems, such as double vision due to weakness of the eye muscles or eye pain due to neuritis of the optic nerve.

The initial signs of MS are usually temporary. However, they return and become more frequent and long lasting. As the symptoms progress, they become more permanent, leading to a weak extremity or paralysis. Over time, some patients may become bedridden and lose control of bladder function. Eventually an MS patient may develop a lung or urinary infection, which may lead to death. As with other chronically ill patients, people with MS may experience mood swings and seek medical attention for their feelings.

Transport of an MS patient to the hospital may require supportive care, such as oxygen therapy. Make sure the patient is comfortable and help position the person as necessary. Do not expect patients with MS to walk to the ambulance. Even if normally ambulatory, they may be in a more weakened state than usual. Again, be sure to bring assistive devices, such as a wheelchair or cane so that the patient can maintain as much independence as possible (Figure 45-5).

MUSCULAR DYSTROPHY

Muscular dystrophy (MD) is a group of hereditary disorders characterized by progressive weakness and wasting of muscle tissue. It is a genetic disorder, leading to gradual degeneration of muscle fibers. The most common form of MD is Duchenne muscular dystrophy, which typically affects boys between the ages of 3 and 6. It leads to progressive muscle weakness in the legs and pelvis and to paralysis by age 12. Ultimately, the disease affects the respiratory muscles and heart, causing death at an early age. The other various MD disorders are classified by the age of the patient at onset of symptoms and by the muscles affected.

Since MD is a hereditary disease, you should obtain a complete family history. You should also note the particular muscle groups that the patient cannot move. Again, since MD patients are primarily children; choose age-appropriate language. Respiratory support, such as oxygen, may be needed, especially in the later stages of the disease.

POLIOMYELITIS

Poliomyelitis is a communicable disease that affects the gray matter of the brain and the spinal cord. Although it is highly contagious, immunization has made outbreaks of polio extremely rare in developed nations. However, it is important to know about the disease since many people born before development of the polio vaccination in the 1950s were affected by the disease.

Typically, the polio virus enters the body through the gastrointestinal tract. It circulates through the digestive tract and then enters the blood stream. There, it is carried to the central nervous system where the virus enters the nerve cells and alters them. In cases of paralytic poliomyelitis, patients experience asymmetrical muscle weakness that leads to permanent paralysis.

Although most patients recover from the disease itself, they are left with permanent paralysis of the affected muscles. You may recognize a polio victim by the use of assistive devices for ambulation or by the reduced size of the affected limb due to muscle atrophy. Some patients may have experienced paralysis of the respiratory muscles, requiring assisted ventilation. Patients on long-term ventilators will typically have tracheotomies.

Along with polio, you should know about a related disorder called post-polio syndrome. Post-polio syndrome affects those patients who suffered severely from polio more than 30 years ago. Although the cause of post-polio syndrome remains unknown, researchers think the condition results from the stress of long-term weakness in the affected nerves. Patients with this condition quickly tire, especially after exercise, and develop an intolerance for cold in their extremities.

Many patients with polio or post-polio syndrome try to maintain their independence. They may insist on walking to the ambulance, but should not be encouraged to do so. The idea of hospitalization will frustrate them, since many polio survivors have memories of spending months or even years in hospitals as children. Unlike other chronically ill patients, most do not require frequent trips to the hospital. Therefore, this may be their first time in the back of an ambulance. Try to alleviate their anxiety as much as possible.

PREVIOUS HEAD INJURIES

A patient with a previous head injury may not be easily recognized. You may not notice anything different about the patient until the person starts to speak. A patient with a head injury may display similar symptoms to that of a stroke, without the hemiparesis, or paralysis to one side of the body. The presenting symptoms will be related to the area of the brain that has been injured. The patient may have aphasia, slurred speech, loss of vision or hearing, or may develop a learning disability. Such patients may also exhibit short-term memory loss and may not even have any recollection of their original injury.

Obtaining a medical history from these patients is very important, especially if you are responding to a traumatic event. Note any new symptoms the patient may be having or the recurrence of old ones. Conduct the physical assessment slowly. If the patient cannot speak, look for obvious physical signs of trauma or for facial expressions of pain. Transport considerations will depend upon the condition for which you were called. However, information about the previous head injury should be an important part of the patient's transfer.

SPINA BIFIDA

Spina bifida is a congenital abnormality that falls under the category of neural tube defects. It presents when there is a defect in the closure of the backbone and the spinal canal. In spina bifida occulta, the patient exhibits few outward signs of the deformity. In spina bifida cystica, the failure of the closure allows the spinal cord and covering membranes to protrude from the back, causing an obvious deformity.

Symptoms depend upon which part of the spinal cord is protruding through the back. The patient may have paralysis of both lower extremities and lack of bowel or bladder control. A large percentage of children born with spina bifida have hydrocephalus, which results from the accumulation of fluid in the brain.

Permanent disabilities cannot be assessed until the defect is surgically corrected. If the patient has hydrocephalus, a shunt will need to be inserted to help drain off the excess fluid.

When treating spina bifida patients, keep several things in mind. Recent research has shown that between 18 to 73 percent of children and adolescents with spina bifida have latex allergies. For safety, assume that all patients with spina bifida have this problem. In transporting a spina bifida patient, be sure to take along any devices that aid the patient.

MYASTHENIA GRAVIS

Myasthenia gravis is an autoimmune disease characterized by chronic weakness of voluntary muscles and progressive fatigue. The condition results from a problem with the neurotransmitters, which causes a blocking of nerve signals to the muscles. It occurs most frequently in women between the ages of 20 and 50.

A patient with myasthenia gravis may complain of a complete lack of energy, especially in the evening. The disease commonly involves muscles in the face. You may note eyelid drooping or difficulty in chewing or swallowing. The patient may also complain of double vision. In severe cases, a patient may experience paralysis of the respiratory muscles, leading to respiratory arrest. These patients may need assisted ventilations en route to the emergency facility.

OTHER CHALLENGES

In addition to the challenges described in the preceding sections, you can expect to meet a whole range of special situations that will affect the quality of the patient service that you provide. The following are some of the special situations or conditions that you will encounter, if you have not already done so.

CULTURALLY DIVERSE PATIENTS

As a health care provider, you are ethically required to take care of all patients in the same manner, regardless of their race, religion, gender, ethnic background, or living situation. What may make it difficult for you to treat culturally different patients may not be the differences per se, but your inability to understand them. Do not consider this a reason for refusing treatment. Rather, consider it a learning experience that will prepare you for a similar situation on another run. With United States society becoming more diverse, instead of less diverse, tolerance of cultural differences will become an important part of your career (Figure 45-6).

From time to time, you may encounter a patient who will make a decision about medical care you do not agree with. For example, Christian Scientists do not believe in human intervention in sickness through the use of drugs or other

For safety, assume that all patients with spina bifida have a latex allergy.

As a health care provider, you are ethically required to take care of all patients in the same manner, regardless of their race, religion, gender, ethnic background, and living situation.

Many ethnic groups believe in and practice varying forms of folk medicine. You should respect these beliefs and remember that some folk remedies may interact with traditional medical therapies. If you work in an area populated by a specific ethnic group, learn more about the group's folk medicine beliefs and practices.

FIGURE 45-6 United States society is becoming diverse, with the largest number of immigrants coming from Asia and Latin America.

therapies. You cannot force these patients to accept care. You should, however, obtain a signed document indicating informed refusal of consent.

Accommodation of a culturally diverse population will require patience and, in some cases, ingenuity. If your patient does not speak English, communication may be a problem. You may need to rely on a family member to act as an interpreter or on a translator device, such as telephone language line for non-English speaking people. Notify the receiving facility of the need for an interpreter.

TERMINALLY ILL PATIENTS

Caring for a terminally ill patient can be an emotional challenge. Many times, the patient will choose to die at home, but at the last minute the family compromises those wishes by calling for an ambulance. In other cases, the patient may call for an ambulance so that a newly developed condition can be treated or a medication adjusted. See Chapter 46 for a fuller discussion.

PATIENTS WITH COMMUNICABLE DISEASES

When treating people with communicable diseases, you should withhold all personal judgment. Although you will have to take BSI precautions just as you would with any patient, keep in mind the heightened sensitivity of a person with a communicable disease. Most of these patients are familiar with the health care setting and understand why you must take certain protective measures. However, you should still explain that you take these measures with other patients that have a similar disease. Also, you do not need to take additional precautions that are not required by departmental policy. The patient will generally spot these extra measures, feeling guilt, shame, or anger. For more information on the etiologies and treatment of communicable diseases, see Chapter 37.

PATIENTS WITH FINANCIAL CHALLENGES

One of the exciting parts of a career in EMS is the opportunity to meet people of all backgrounds. You have the opportunity to help and educate people who may not otherwise have access to health care. For example, you may get sent to a street corner where a homeless man has fallen and needs medical attention, but cannot afford to pay the medical bills. It is your job to help the patient understand that he can receive health care regardless of his financial situation (Figure 45-7).

Become familiar with public hospitals and clinics that provide services to people without money or adequate insurance coverage. Calm a patient's fears by discussing this or other information. In providing care, always keep this guideline in mind: Treat the patient, not the financial condition the patient is in.

FIGURE 45-7 Homeless people sometimes refuse care, thinking they cannot afford to pay the medical bills. Become familiar with public hospitals and clinics that provide services to the needy.

Treat the patient, not the financial condition the patient is in.

SUMMARY

It is important to be aware of the pathophysiology of diseases that you may encounter throughout your career. You should also know the characteristics of impairments that are commonly found in the medical setting. They may be the primary reason that your patient seeks help, or they may not be the reason your patient called at all. Whatever the circumstances, it is important to learn the various etiologies of these impairments and illnesses in order to treat your patient with the knowledge and respect that each of your patients deserves every day.

CHAPTER 46

Acute Interventions for the Chronic-Care Patient

Objectives

After reading this chapter, you should be able to:

1. Compare and contrast the primary objectives of the paramedic and the home care provider. (pp. 1886, 1891)
2. Identify the importance of home health care medicine as it relates to emergency medical services. (pp. 1885–1886)
3. Differentiate between the role of the paramedic and the role of the home care provider. (pp. 1886, 1891)
4. Compare and contrast the primary objectives of acute care, home care, and hospice care. (pp. 1886, 1891, 1917)
5. Discuss aspects of home care that enhance the quality of patient care and aspects that have the potential

to become detrimental. (pp. 1885–1900)
6. List pathologies and complications in home care patients that commonly result in ALS intervention. (pp. 1897–1917)
7. Compare the cost, mortality, and quality of care for a given patient in the hospital versus the home care setting. (pp. 1885–1886)
8. Discuss the significance of palliative care programs as related to a patient in a home health care or hospice setting. (pp. 1891, 1917)
9. Define hospice care, comfort care, and DNR/DNAR as they relate to local

Continued

practice, law, and policy. (pp. 1891, 1896, 1917–1919)

10. List and describe the characteristics of typical home care devices related to airway maintenance, artificial and alveolar ventilation, vascular access, drug administration, and the GI/GU tract. (pp. 1889–1890, 1897, 1901–1914)

11. Discuss the complications of assessing each of the devices described above. (pp. 1901–1914)

12. Describe indications, contraindications, and techniques for urinary catheter insertion in the male and female patient in an out-of-hospital setting. (pp. 1910–1911)

13. Identify failure of GI/GU, ventilatory, vascular access, and drain devices found in the home care setting. (pp. 1901–1915)

14. Discuss the relationship between local home care treatment

protocols/SOPs and local EMS Protocols/SOPs. (p. 1891)

15. Discuss differences in the ability of individuals to accept and cope with their own impending death. (p. 1919)

16. List the stages of the grief process and relate them to an individual in hospice care. (p. 1919)

17. Discuss the rights of the terminally ill patient. (pp. 1917–1919)

18. Summarize the types of home health care available in your area and the services provided. (pp. 1885–1891)

19. Given a series of home care scenarios, determine which patients should receive follow-up home care and which should be transported to an emergency care facility. (pp. 1892–1896)

20. Given a series of scenarios, demonstrate interaction and support with the family members/support persons for a patient who has died. (pp. 1917–1919)

INTRODUCTION

One of the major trends in modern health care involves the shifting of patients out of the hospital and back into their homes as soon as possible. The result has been a huge increase in home health care needs and services. In 1963, approximately 1,100 health care agencies existed in the United States. Today, more than 20,000 agencies employ over 665,000 caregivers—nurses, home health aides, physical therapists, occupational therapists, and other health care professionals.

EPIDEMIOLOGY OF HOME CARE

A number of factors have promoted the growth of home care, including enactment of Medicare in 1965, the advent of health maintenance organizations (HMOs), improved medical technology, and studies showing improved recovery rates and lower costs with home care. The shift to home care has important implications for ALS providers. As patients assume greater responsibility for their own treatment and recovery, the likelihood of ALS intervention for the chronic-care patient increases. Calls may come from the patient, the patient's family, or a home health care provider.

The primary driving force in home health care is cost-containment.

In home care settings, you can expect to encounter a sometimes dizzying array of devices, machines, and equipment designed to provide anything from supportive to life-sustaining care. As a paramedic, you should become familiar with the basic functions of the common home care devices and, just as important, recognize

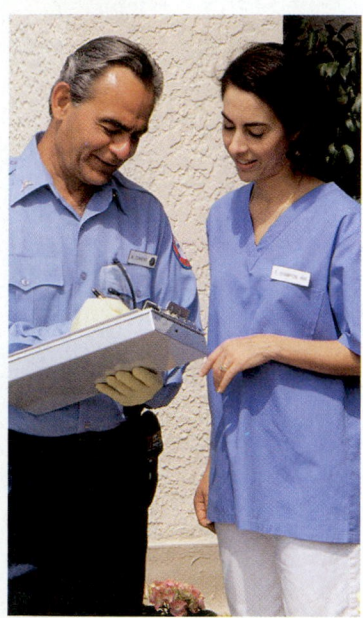

FIGURE 46-1 The home health care provider usually knows the patient better than anyone else and will often spot subtle changes in the patient's condition.

the underlying need for them. The failure or malfunction of this type of equipment has the potential to become a life-threatening or life-altering event. New technologies and machines are being developed constantly. It is your responsibility to stay informed of these changes and the assessment complications that may be involved with the use of each device.

ALS RESPONSE TO HOME CARE PATIENTS

A number of situations may involve you in the treatment of a home care patient—equipment failure, unexpected complications, absence of a caregiver, need for transport, inability of the patient or caregiver to operate a device, and more. As already mentioned, you might also be called upon to provide emotional support or intervention. Taking responsibility for an illness or an ill family member can be a stressful and overwhelming experience. Some people may be ill-equipped to deal with complicated directions, mechanical problems, or the stress of long-term care. Do not minimize their frustrations or allow them to interfere with your care.

Your primary role as an ALS provider is to identify and treat any life-threatening problems. An important source of information is the home care provider—whether it be a nurse, nurse's aid, family member, or friend. Remember that this person usually knows the patient better than anyone else. The provider will often spot subtle changes in the patient's condition that may seem insignificant to the outsider. Listen carefully to what this person says (Figure 46-1).

Home care providers are often health care professionals, but be sensitive in questioning their training or background. You must obtain certain information to care for your patient, and the home care provider may be the only source you have for critical items such as the patient's baseline mental status. If you meet resistance, either from the home care provider's lack of training or a misunderstanding of your needs, try rephrasing your question or using less technical language. You may also find evidence of neglect or improper patient care by the home care provider. Correct any immediate life-threats that you find, and document your findings in your patient report. You should also report the situation to your supervisors for corrective action. However, do not confront the home care worker yourself.

At all times, keep in mind the presence of the patient. Involve him or her in the questioning process. If the caregiver mentions a change or reaction, you might say: "Did you notice this change, too?" "How do you think you reacted?"

Typical Responses

Many of the medical problems that you will encounter in a home care setting are the same as the ones that you will encounter elsewhere in the field. However, you must always keep in mind that the home care patient is in a more fragile state to begin with. A member of the medical community has already decided that the person needs extra help. A home care patient is more likely to decompensate and go into crisis more quickly than the general population. As a result, you need to monitor the home care patient carefully and be ready to intervene at all times. Some of the typical responses involve airway complications, respiratory failure, cardiac decompensation, alterations in peripheral circulation, altered mental status, GI/GU crises, infections and/or septic complications, and equipment malfunction. (For more specific information on examples, see later sections of the chapter.)

Airway Complications The airway is always your paramount concern, and the home care patient is no exception. In the absence of documentation proving the patient's request to withhold intubation and mechanical ventilation, you should protect the airway at all costs. However, even if the patient has a valid Do Not Resuscitate (DNR) order, remember that, in certain situations, you still can use basic airway techniques and suctioning to protect the airway.

Airway compromise can be the result of many different etiologies. Problems that you might encounter include inadequate pulmonary toilet, inadequate alveolar ventilation, and inadequate alveolar oxygenation. (For more on airway problems, see material later in the chapter.)

Respiratory Failure As you will read later in the chapter, any number of respiratory problems can be treated in a home care setting. Some of the most common conditions that will lead to respiratory failure or acute crisis include:

- Emphysema
- Bronchitis
- Asthma
- Cystic fibrosis
- Congestive heart failure
- Pulmonary embolus
- Sleep apnea
- **Guillain-Barré syndrome**
- **Myasthenia gravis**

Cardiac Decompensation Regardless of the setting, cardiac decompensation is a true medical emergency that can lead to life-threatening shock. This condition requires aggressive identification and treatment. Home care patients who have borderline cardiac output may be placed at risk if their cardiac demand increases from stress or illness and their system cannot compensate. Some other common causes of cardiac decompensation include:

- Congestive heart failure
- Acute myocardial infarction (MI) (Home care patients are at higher risk.)
- Cardiac **hypertrophy**
- Calcification or degeneration of the heart's conductive system
- Heart transplant
- Sepsis

Alterations in Peripheral Circulation You already know that the heart circulates blood throughout the body. However, in the case of home care patients, remember that bodily movement also aids in circulation. If a patient has limited mobility, expect the entire circulatory system to be less effective and weaker. As muscle tone declines, so does the flow of blood. When circulation slows, movement becomes more difficult, thus creating a vicious cycle that leads to poorer circulation overall.

Keep in mind that alterations in peripheral circulation can complicate or worsen the course of treatment for a home care patient. Slowed circulation may result in delayed healing, increased risk of infections, or even **gangrene.** Diabetes, a problem that affects some 16 million Americans, commonly results in poor circulation, especially to the extremities. These patients are at high risk of unhealed wounds or ulcers, particularly on the feet.

Altered Mental Status A common ALS response to a home care patient involves some kind of subtle or obvious change in mental status. In the home care patient, always suspect an exacerbation of their condition as well as other causes. Never forget that these patients are at higher risk than the general population of

✱ Guillain–Barré syndrome acute viral infection that triggers the production of autoantibodies, which damage the myelin sheath covering the peripheral nerves; causes rapid, progressive loss of motor function, ranging from muscle weakness to full-body paralysis.

✱ Myasthenia gravis disease characterized by episodic muscle weakness triggered by an autoimmune attack of the acetylcholine receptors.

Regardless of the setting, cardiac decompensation is a true medical emergency that can lead to life-threatening shock.

✱ hypertrophy an increase in the size or bulk of an organ or structure; caused by growth rather than by a tumor.

If a patient has limited mobility, expect the entire circulatory system to be less effective and weaker.

✱ gangrene death of tissue or bone, usually from an insufficient blood supply.

developing new medical problems. Some common causes of altered mental status include:

- Hypoxia (from any number of respiratory or airway problems)
- Hypotension (from any number of cardiac problems or shock)
- Sepsis
- Altered electrolytes or blood chemistries (common in dialysis patients)
- Hypoglycemia (diabetes)
- Alzheimer's disease
- Cancerous tumor or brain lesions
- Overdose
- Stroke (brain attack)

GI/GU Crises EMS personnel find themselves involved in a number of calls involving home care patients with gastrointestinal or genitourinary problems. The problem often revolves around a misplaced or removed catheter, such as a Foley or a percutaneous endoscopic gastrostomy (PEG) tube. This may not seem like an emergency to you, but the inability to eat or urinate for a period of time can easily compromise an already weakened patient. In addition, home interventions such as peritoneal dialysis can alter fluid balances or electrolytes, creating a subtle but life-threatening problem.

Infections and Septic Complications You should always maintain a high index of suspicion for infection in a home care patient with a decreased immune response, either from poor general health or a specific disease. Be particularly alert to infections in patients with indwelling devices such as gastrostomy tubes, peripherally-inserted central catheter (PICC) lines, Foley catheters, or colostomies. Also remember that patients with limited lung function or tracheotomies cannot clear their airway easily, putting them at a higher risk of lung infections.

Patients who have decreased **sensorium** from a variety of conditions may have wounds and ulcers that they are unaware of, especially if they have been bedridden or inactive for long periods of time. Surgically implanted drains or wound closures may become infected without the patient realizing it. A bed-bound patient may also develop decubitus wounds, or bedsores (Figure 46-2). If these problems are not identified or treated, they can progress from a generalized infection to gangrene and sepsis.

In identifying infections, look for the following general signs:

- Redness and/or swelling, especially at the insertion site of an indwelling device
- Purulent discharge at the insertion site
- Warm skin at the insertion site
- Fever

Infection at the cellular level is called **cellulitis** and is not life-threatening. When an infection spreads systemically, however, it can lead to sepsis—a serious medical emergency. This may cause a patient's immune system to fail, resulting in septic shock. Signs and symptoms of sepsis include:

- Redness at an insertion site
- Fever
- Altered mental status
- Poor skin color or **turgor**

You should always maintain a high index of suspicion for infection in a home care patient with a decreased immune response.

sensorium sensory apparatus of the body as a whole; also that portion of the brain that functions as a center of sensations.

cellulitis inflammation of cellular or connective tissue.

turgor ability of the skin to return to normal appearance after being subjected to pressure.

FIGURE 46-2a **Stage 1** Inflammation or redness of the skin that does not return to normal after 15 minutes of removal of pressure. Edema is present. It involves the epidermis. Skin may or may not be broken.

FIGURE 46-2b **Stage 2** Skin blister or shallow skin ulcer. Involves the epidermis. Looks like a shallow crater. Area is red, warm, and may or may not have drainage.

FIGURE 46-2c **Stage 3** Full-thickness skin loss exposing subcutaneous tissue, may extend into the next layer. Edema, inflammation, and necrosis present. Drainage present, which may or may not have an odor.

FIGURE 46-2d **Stage 4** Full-thickness ulcer. Muscle and/or bone can be seen. Infection and necrosis is present. Drainage present, which may or may not have an odor.

FIGURE 46-2 Pressure sores are classified by the depth of tissue destruction.

- Signs of shock
- Vomiting
- Diarrhea

Keep in mind that home care patients may already be receiving treatment for a generalized infection that has in fact worsened or spread. Inquire if a pattern of deterioration has been seen by the caregiver or home care provider. In cases of septic shock, ALS treatment is mainly supportive. Provide fluid for hypotension and necessary airway and oxygen support.

Equipment Malfunction Home care equipment has the normal limitations of any machine. The power may go out and stop the machine from functioning. The machine may break and/or need maintenance. Some machines, if inoperative, can create a life threat to a patient. Common examples include home ventilators, oxygen delivery systems, apnea monitors, and home dialysis machines.

In cases of equipment malfunction, you may be called upon to take the place of a device (such as a ventilator) or to treat problems that have arisen as a result of the malfunction. Even the malfunction of a glucometer for a diabetic can be a difficult situation for some patients to handle, especially if they suspect hypoglycemia. Your job is to assess the problem and take the appropriate actions.

Other Medical Disorders and Home Care Patients As already mentioned, you can expect to find a wide variety of problems treated in the home care setting. They can range from an infant on an apnea monitor to progressive dementia in a family member to psychosocial support of the family of a home care patient.

Some other conditions that may be treated at home include:

- Brain or spinal trauma
- Arthritis
- Psychological disorders
- Cancer
- Hepatitis
- AIDS
- Transplants (including patients awaiting transplants)

Commonly Found Medical Devices

As previously mentioned, home care patients use a vast number of devices. They range from the simplicity of a nasal cannula to the complexity of a home ventilator. If you encounter an unfamiliar device—which may happen at some time in your career—don't panic. Find out what it's used for, and you will then have an idea on how to proceed. Don't be afraid to look foolish by asking questions. You won't. You will be foolish, and endanger the patient, if you pretend to understand a device, but don't. Some commonly used devices include:

You will be foolish, and endanger the patient, if you pretend to understand a device, but don't.

- Glucometers
- IV infusions and in-dwelling IV sites
- Nebulized and aerosolized medication administrators
- Shunts, fistulas, and venous grafts
- Oxygen concentrators, oxygen tanks, and liquid oxygen systems
- Oxygen masks and nebulizers
- Tracheotomies and home ventilators
- G-tubes, colostomies, and urostomies
- Surgical drains
- Apnea monitors, cardiac monitors, and pulse oximeters
- Wheelchairs, canes, and walkers

Spend some time at the hospital talking with health care personnel about new devices being introduced for the home care setting. Study or make copies of the brochures that come with these devices. You might also talk with manufacturers or vendors, the people who commonly deliver equipment to home care patients.

Intervention by a Home Health Care Practitioner or Physician

Most calls involving home care patients will require acute intervention in problems such as inadequate respiratory support, acute respiratory events, acute cardiac events, acute sepsis, or GI/GU crises. Keep in mind, however, that you may not be the first person to provide intervention. If home care patients have a good relationship with their home health care practitioner or physician, they may contact this person first. In fact, they may be required to do so in order to receive reimbursement for medical services.

Remain especially alert to home care patients receiving medications for pain management. They are at risk for pharmacological side effects and possible overdose. The patient may also be taking non-prescription drugs that could interact with prescribed medications. Substance abuse, especially in critically ill patients, is also a possibility.

Hospice patients have unique psychological needs due to the terminal nature of their illness. Although they and their families will have been counseled about the disease process, emotional support is still part of your job. If a call involves a hospice patient, the situation will almost always require intervention by specially trained health care professionals. Find out the names of these people as quickly as possible and determine the advisability of consultation versus rapid transport. (For more on hospice care, see the closing sections of this chapter.)

* **hospice** program of palliative care and support services that addresses the physical, social, economic, and spiritual needs of terminally ill patients and their families.

Injury Control and Prevention

As always, the most effective intervention is prevention. Before the patient comes home, steps should be taken to prepare the home. For example, purchasing a shower chair, raised toilet seat, and grab bars for the bathroom, arranging furniture for free access, having a bedpan or commode chair within patient reach, removing hazards to mobility such as throw rugs and electrical cords, providing a cordless phone. You should also keep in mind the matrix, or strategy, for injury prevention developed by William Haddon in 1972. Its ten steps are:

1. Prevent the creation of hazard to begin with.
2. Reduce the amount of the hazard brought into existence.
3. Prevent the release of the hazard that already exists.
4. Modify the rate of distribution of the hazard from the source.
5. Separate the hazard and that which is to be protected in both time and space.
6. Separate the hazard and that which is to be protected by a barrier.
7. Modify the basic qualities of the hazard.
8. Make that which is to be protected more resistant to the hazard.
9. Counter the damage already done by the hazard.
10. Stabilize, repair, and rehabilitate the object of the damage.

These ten steps can be used to protect paramedics from the hazards they encounter in the workplace or to protect patients from injuries at home. The steps can be seen in such simple areas as BSI precautions (barrier protection), the use of side rails to prevent falls, or the use of home rehabilitation to stabilize or repair a patient's injuries.

GENERAL SYSTEM PATHOPHYSIOLOGY, ASSESSMENT, AND MANAGEMENT

Assessment and management of home care patients can be challenging. You can gain confidence by becoming familiar with the pathophysiology of the diseases most commonly found in home care settings. You must also keep in mind the emotional needs of both the home care patient and the caregivers or family members affected by the patient's condition. Some caregivers love what they do and treat the patient's condition as part of their daily lives. Other households feel constant, unremitting stress, and possibly resentment toward the patient's condition.

Getting a feel for the emotional context of a patient's care should be a part of any call. However, in the case of home care patients, you must exhibit extra sensitivity. The way in which you interact with the patient and family can greatly affect the ease and efficiency with which you assess the patient and gather information. Developing a consistent, comprehensive approach to patient assessment and treatment can be your best strategy for dealing with these sometimes complicated responses. The one thing home care calls have in common is their diversity. Be prepared to draw on all your EMS skills and to think quickly as you figure out the most effective management plan.

The one thing home care calls have in common is their diversity.

ASSESSMENT

Assessment of the home care patient follows the same basic steps as any other patient—scene size-up, initial assessment, focused history and physical examination, ongoing assessment, and continued management. However, you will need to modify your mind set for the home care patient—i.e., observe for conditions that you might not ordinarily look for in the general population. This section highlights some of the points you should keep in mind or emphasize when assessing the home care patient. (For more on assessment, see the Patient Assessment division, Chapters 10 through 15. For information on assessment-based management, see Chapter 47.)

Scene Size-Up

As with any call, your assessment of the scene begins before you get out of your vehicle. In the case of home care patients, note any special equipment you may observe upon entering the home. This will alert you to any possible chronic problems that the patient might have. As you approach the scene, keep the following questions in mind:

- Is there a wheelchair ramp next to the front steps?
- Is there oxygen equipment in view?
- Is there a trail of oxygen tubing that leads into the patient's bedroom?
- Are there infection control supplies on the counter?
- Is there a sharps container present? (This means there are sharps too!)
- Is the patient in a hospital bed?

It is a serious mistake to arrive on the scene with a "take-over" mentality that all but eliminates the home care provider from the assessment process.

Introduce yourself to any other medical personnel on the scene—nurse, aide, hospice worker, and so on. By making personal contact, you will help create a health care team that can pool resources and share information. It is a serious mistake to arrive on the scene with a "take-over" mentality that all but eliminates the home care provider from the assessment process.

Scene Safety After you have identified the scene as a home care situation, remain alert for special hazards that might be present. As mentioned earlier, emotions often run high in a home care situation. Evaluate whether any of the people present have a threatening attitude that could be directed toward you. If at any time you don't feel comfortable, withdraw and seek assistance, either from the police or additional personnel. Ask someone to put any pets in another room and have all sources of sound (TV, radio, etc.) turned off so that you can work in a quiet, focused environment. As in any patient's home, look for weapons that the patient might use for self-defense—firearms, knives, or chemical sprays.

Other special hazards that you may face in a home care situation include infectious wastes, medical supplies such as needles, and potentially dangerous equipment. You would hope that all home care providers are meticulous with the safe disposal of sharps. However, don't take it for granted. You cannot help any patients if you are on disability because you contracted hepatitis or AIDS from a needle stick. Look around carefully.

In responding to any home care situation, keep in mind the following guidelines.

- Any patient with limited movement may be contaminated with feces, urine, or **emesis.**
- Any bed-bound patient may have weeping wounds, bleeding, or decubitus ulcers (bedsores).
- Sharps may be present.
- Collection bags for urine or feces sometimes leak.
- Tracheostomy patients clear mucus by coughing, which can spray.
- Any electrical machine has the potential for electric shock.
- A hospital bed, wheelchair, or walker could be contaminated with body fluid.
- Contaminated medical devices, such as a nebulizer, may be left around unprotected.
- Oxygen in the presence of flame has the potential for fire or explosion.
- Equipment may be in the way and cause you to fall—or it may be unstable and fall on you.
- Medical wastes may not be properly contained or discarded.

✱ **emesis** vomitus.

Don't minimize the impact of any of these hazards. You can always be contaminated by any patient, but treatment of the home care patient has the potential for a broader range of exposures. Be sure to remove any medical waste you generate so the patient does not return to an unsafe environment. If at all possible, you should also remove any medical waste that is already there for the same reason. Always use BSI precautions and be careful!

Be sure to remove any medical wastes that you generate so the patient does not return to an unsafe environment.

Patient Milieu Another important part of the scene size-up involves an evaluation of the patient's environment. Is the house clean or filthy? Is there nutritious food available? Are the sanitary facilities clean? Is the house heated and/or air conditioned? Is there adequate electricity? Is there insect or vermin infestation? The answers to such questions obviously have an impact upon the patient's health and his or her ability to recover.

Also note the condition of the patient's specific medical devices. For example, is the nasal cannula clean? Is the wheelchair in good working order? Is the ventilator well situated for safety and effectiveness? Again, these observations provide important clues to the quality of the home care received by the patient and the ability or willingness of the patient to comply with a prescribed treatment regimen.

Remember that you not only have a responsibility to treat the patient, but to act as an advocate. If a patient is living in a hazardous or unhealthy environment, you have an obligation to notify the proper agency to ensure that the person receives the necessary help. Often hospital social services will be of assistance. The patient's home care agency or the police might also intervene, depending upon the situation.

Remain alert to signs of abuse and/or neglect. In many states, you are required by law to report signs of child or elder abuse. (See Chapters 42, 43, and 44.) Know the laws in your state. Home care patients, whether old or young, may be helpless to improve their situation. It is the responsibility of all health care workers to look out for their safety and well being.

Initial Assessment, Focused History, Physical Exam

At this point in your assessment, you may already have a good base of information without actually having seen the patient! As you approach the patient, begin your initial assessment by observing general appearance, skin color and quality, quality of respiration, and level of distress. Also note any medical equipment that the patient may be currently using.

As you continue to assess the patient for the ABCs, try to ascertain from the primary care provider (if present) a baseline presentation for the patient. Were you called just because his or her condition has gotten worse? Or, are you here for a new problem? For some home care patients, respiratory distress may be a chronic condition. For example, a COPD patient might always have difficulty breathing. Your first impulse may be to reach for your airway supplies only to find that this is the patient's norm and that you were called to treat an unrelated problem. You must be flexible in your judgments and listen carefully to the report provided by the caregiver or family member who summoned EMS.

As with any patient, treat it as you see it! Once you have established the patient's baseline, assess for changes from the norm. Airway and breathing are always your first concern, followed by circulation. If there are any serious threats to the ABCs, you must treat them. If you are unable to stabilize the patient, complete your rapid assessment and transport immediately. In such cases, your detailed and ongoing assessments will be performed en route to the hospital, if possible.

In non-critical patients, you might take the opportunity to compare vital signs to the bedside records, if they are kept. The focus of your exam should be on the chief complaint and how it might relate to the patient's chronic condition. Be meticulous in your exam, especially with the home care patient. As stated earlier, home care patients are more susceptible to complications than most other patients and can deteriorate rapidly—i.e., a non-critical patient can quickly become a critical patient.

In examining a home care patient, be sure to inspect, palpate, and auscultate all potential problem areas. In bed-bound patients, look for decubiti (pressure sores or bed sores) on parts of the body subjected to constant pressure or friction. As mentioned, decubiti pose a significant danger to the patient through infection or sepsis and may require surgical debridement.

Mental Status If your patient has a preexisting altered mental status such as dementia or Alzheimer's disease, you must have a good understanding of his or her normal mentation before transport. This information is vital to the physician evaluating and treating the patient at the receiving facility. As stressed in Chapter 43, depression can mimic senility and senility can mimic organic brain syndrome. Dementia can also be a sign or symptom of a number of other serious medical problems, such as hypoglycemia and AIDS.

In general, assessment of mental status follows the same general procedure as with other patients. However, you must tailor your questions to the home care

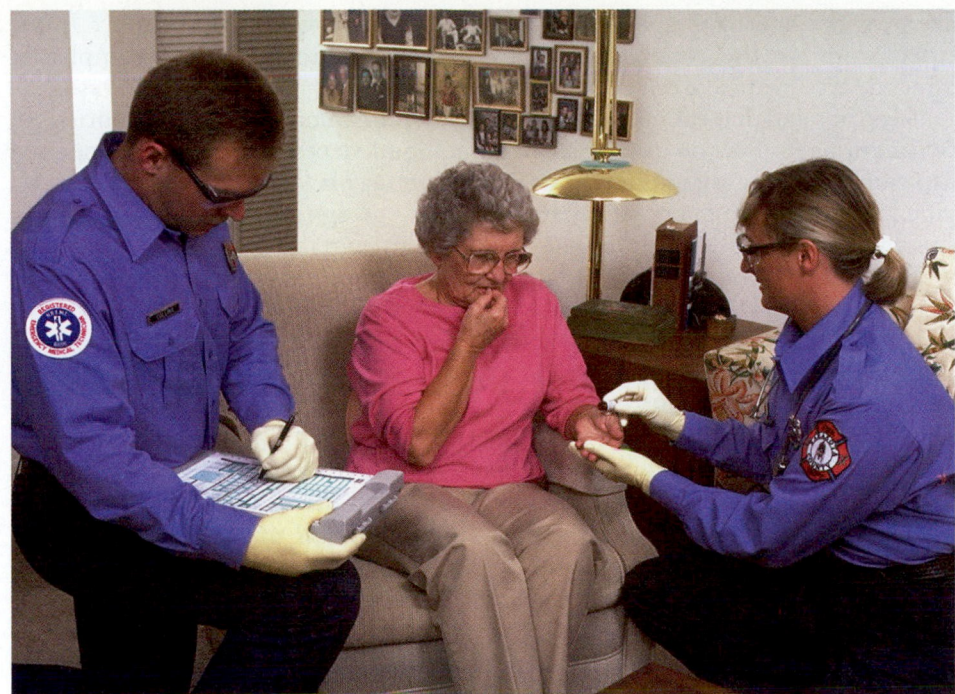

FIGURE 46-3   When assessing a chronic-care patient, tailor your questions to the home-care setting. Remember that the stress in many home-care settings, or fear of removal from the home, can increase patient confusion.

setting (Figure 46-3). For example, a person who does not work may be oriented but not know the date or even the day of the week. Also keep in mind the high level of stress in many home care situations and the effect this may have on patient confusion.

To avoid insulting the patient with what may appear to be childlike questions, preface your assessment by saying, "Since I don't know your condition very well, I need to ask you some very basic questions." If patients understand that you are following a systematic assessment, they usually cooperate in what, for them, is often a tedious process.

If a patient cannot or will not answer questions, rely on family members or health care providers to explain why the patient's current mental status is a departure from the norm. For example, belligerent behavior might be normal for a home care patient. If this is the case, find out what is different this time than other times. Perhaps, as pointed out earlier, nothing may be different—the family member or caregiver has just reached the breaking point and is in need of outside assistance.

Remember that home care patients, especially older or terminal patients, are fearful of being removed from the home environment. This can trigger depression, which in turn worsens a preexisting altered mental status. The key in such cases is tactful questioning combined with your own powers of observation. Pay particular attention to body language and interactions between household members. Note any evidence that the altered mental condition may have been triggered or worsened by a treatable cause and present this information as part of your focused history.

Other Considerations In preparing your history, take into account any long-term medical problems—i.e., the conditions that necessitated home care—and the specific events that led to the current crisis. Use the home health history and written orders from the physician, if available. As mentioned, talk to the health care provider and to the patient. What changes, if any, have taken place in the patient's life in the recent past? Has patient treatment and/or compliance changed? Are medical devices operating correctly?

Keep in mind that eating habits, fluid intake, and minor illnesses or injuries can have a dramatic effect on a seriously ill home-bound patient. Have a high index of suspicion for any new conditions that the patient may be developing. For example, evidence of dementia in an AIDS patient is a serious sign. Correlate this with your physical exam and use this information in developing your treatment plan.

In the case of home care patients, you may more commonly encounter Do Not Resuscitate (DNR) orders, Do Not Attempt Resuscitation (DNAR) orders, living wills, and so on. Ascertain whether these documents are in place before beginning any life-saving treatments. If that information is unavailable, act in the best interests of the patient. Also, keep in mind, that a DNR or DNAR doesn't mean that you have to withhold *all* treatment. For example, if a CHF patient with crackles and shortness of breath has a DNR, you may still be able to start a line, give nitroglycerin, administer an IV diuretic, and/or transport the patient to the hospital. However, you must read the specific instructions contained within the advance directives and consult with medical control.

Advance directives are designed to prevent useless treatment and invasion to the body when natural death or dying occurs. However, many people who have advance directives can be treated in crisis situations and recover. You must use your judgment on a case-by-case basis to determine what qualifies as a resuscitative or life-sustaining measure. (Additional material on advance directives appears later in the chapter.)

TRANSPORT AND MANAGEMENT TREATMENT PLAN

Transport and/or treatment of a home care patient often involves replacing home health treatment modalities with ALS modalities. Airway and ventilatory support should be straightforward, as EMS providers are usually equipped and trained in the use of most necessary supplies. Some home care interventions, such as Foley catheters, can simply be brought along with the patient. Other interventions, such as percutaneous endoscopic gastrostomy (PEG) tubes, must be flushed and capped, which you may not be trained or equipped to do. In this case, the home care provider should assist you.

In some instances, you may be forced to take the support mechanism on your ambulance if you cannot find a suitable replacement. Certain infusion pumps or other devices may be essential to the patient's well-being and you must bring them along. You should critically assess the risks of discontinuing the home care intervention versus transporting the mechanism. Seek advice from your base physician if you are unfamiliar with the intervention and if the home health provider is unable to help.

You should critically assess the risks of discontinuing the home health care intervention versus transporting the mechanism.

When taking a home care patient to a receiving facility, be sure to notify family members and caregivers, if they are not present. Before leaving the scene, secure the home, making sure that doors and windows are locked. In all likelihood, you will need to notify the patient's physician and/or the appropriate health care agency, if you have not already done so.

Document your findings and all care steps carefully. Your run report will become part of the home care patient's record and may in fact suggest modifications in the treatment plan. If the patient is not already using a home care agency, provide names of services in your community or refer the person to the proper social service agency. You might also mention non-medical attendant care such as housekeeping services and Meals-on-Wheels. As mentioned earlier, if you suspect the need for intervention in patient care, report your suspicions to the appropriate agency.

SPECIFIC ACUTE HOME HEALTH SITUATIONS

Although you will undoubtedly intervene in a wide variety of home care situations during your EMS career, you can expect to encounter certain conditions more commonly than others. The chronic-care patients that will most likely require acute ALS intervention include those with respiratory disorders, cardiac problems, vascular access devices (VADs), GI/GU disorders, and acute infections. You may also be called upon to intervene in the home care of mothers and their newborn infants and to provide assistance in hospice settings. A discussion of each of these situations will help you to prepare for your increasing involvement in the home health care system of the 2000s.

Content Review

COMMON ACUTE HOME CARE SITUATIONS
- Respiratory disorders
- Cardiac problems
- Use of VADs
- GI/GU disorders
- Acute infections

RESPIRATORY DISORDERS

Respiratory disorders account for more than 630,000 of the hospital patients discharged for home care each year. Nearly 37 percent of patients with simple pneumonia and pleurisy and more than 50 percent of patients with chronic obstructive pulmonary disease (COPD) often receive home care within one day of their discharge from the hospital.

Some of the most common home care devices used to treat respiratory disorders include oxygen equipment, portable suctioning machines, aerosol equipment and nebulizers, incentive spirometers, various home ventilators, and tracheostomy tubes and collars. In order to provide intervention with these devices, you need to review pertinent respiratory anatomy and physiology as it relates to home oxygen and respiratory therapy. (See Chapter 27, "Pulmonology.") You also need to review the pathophysiology of the disorders that most frequently require home respiratory support.

Select respiratory disorders and the medical therapy used to treat them are discussed in the following sections. As you read this material, keep in mind earlier comments on the increased risk of airway infections and respiratory compromise in the home care patient.

Content Review

COMMON HOME RESPIRATORY EQUIPMENT
- Oxygen equipment
- Portable suctioning machines
- Aerosol equipment and nebulizers
- Incentive spirometers
- Home ventilators
- Tracheostomy tubes and collars

Chronic Diseases Requiring Home Respiratory Support

Many home care patients have a lung capacity that is minimally able to meet their normal requirements. Sometimes even simple activities, such as climbing stairs, can severely stress their system. Unlike patients with normal lung capacities, they simply do not have the ability for any increased workload. Even walking from one room to another may require use of oxygen equipment. The following is a review of some of the conditions you may find in the respiratory compromised patient.

Many home care patients have a lung capacity that is minimally able to meet their normal requirements.

COPD As you know, COPD is a triad of diseases—emphysema, chronic bronchitis, and asthma. Some patients may have one, two, or all three disorders. All three are outflow obstructive diseases, impeding the exhalation of air from the lungs. This causes an increase in carbon dioxide and a decrease in oxygenation.

COPD patients work harder to breathe than healthy people. When that work becomes too much, they tire quickly. If home equipment fails for any reason, they often panic, worsening their situation. As with any COPD patient, direct your treatment toward increasing oxygen flow. Be prepared to take over their breathing as soon as patients can no longer move enough oxygen to sustain themselves.

Figure 46-4 If the home equipment for a COPD patient fails or is insufficient, you may have to replace it with equipment from the ALS unit.

In some cases, this may mean fixing or replacing home respiratory equipment and/or transport to the hospital (Figure 46-4).

In treating the COPD patient, keep in mind the following disease-specific information.

Bronchitis and Emphysema These two diseases go hand-in-hand. Most often they result from smoking, but can have other causes as well. Bronchitis involves the chronic overproduction of mucus, which narrows bronchial passages and restricts air flow. Emphysema typically leads to a stiffening and enlargement of the alveoli. This loss of elasticity and compliance requires higher pressures in the lungs to facilitate gas exchanges at the alveolar level. Usually these patients are thin (because breathing takes up a large portion of their daily caloric intake) and barrel chested (due to the retention of air in the lungs as a result of outflow obstruction).

In cases of acute exacerbation, these patients have a difficult time compensating. They may exhibit wheezing with diminished lung sounds, use of accessory muscles, retractions, tripod positioning, and the inability to speak in full sentences. Home treatments that you may see include oxygen, nebulized or aerosol medications, and possibly a ventilator utilizing **PEEP, CPAP,** or **BiPAP.** PEEP is provided through an endotracheal tube, while CPAP and BiPAP are provided through a tightly fitted mask.

When providing intervention, don't forget that home care patients usually have a high dosing regimen, which may make them less responsive to their medications. Always provide these patients with high flow oxygen. Medications that may be helpful include:

* Nebulized beta-2 specific agonist bronchodilators, such as albuterol or metaproterenol
* IV or oral corticosteroids, such as methylprednisolone (Solu-Medtrol)
* Nebulized anticholinergics (ipratropium)

* **PEEP** positive end expiratory pressure.

* **CPAP** continuous positive airway pressure.

* **BiPAP** bilevel positive airway pressure.

When providing intervention, don't forget that home care patients usually have a high dosing regimen, which may make them less responsive to their medications.

Asthma　Asthma, sometimes referred to as reactive airway disease, can be seen with any age patient. A crisis often occurs when some reactant causes an acute constriction of the bronchial passages. Home care patients with asthma can usually handle these episodes on their own. If the episode becomes severe, however, you may be called by a caregiver or parent. (Asthma in children can be especially stressful for the family, so be sure to review its treatment in Chapter 42.)

With asthmatic patients, look for wheezing with diminished lung sounds, use of accessory muscles, and the inability to speak in full sentences. Head bobbing in children is an ominous sign of impending respiratory failure.

Home treatments you may see include oxygen, oral medications, and a variety of nebulizers and/or inhalers. In providing support, always administer high flow oxygen. Medications that may be helpful include the same ones used to treat bronchitis and emphysema. You may also consider an epinephrine IV or SQ. However, use this medication with caution when treating the elderly or very weak patients.

Long-term care of asthma involves the avoidance or elimination of reactants that can trigger the problem. Try to gather as much information as possible about the cause of the attack so that the physician and patient can take action to avoid future episodes.

Congestive Heart Failure (CHF)

CHF often presents as a respiratory problem. For more information on this condition, see "Cardiac Problems" in Chapter 28, "Cardiology."

Cystic Fibrosis (CF)

Cystic fibrosis is a genetic disorder usually identified during childhood, sometimes in the late teenage years. It is characterized by chronic and copious overproduction of mucus, inflammation of the small airways and hyperinflation of the alveoli, chronic infections, and erosion of the pulmonary blood vessels secondary to infection. CF is an **exocrine** disease that causes other systemic problems, such as GI disturbances, pancreatic disorders, and glucose intolerance.

✶ exocrine disorder involving external secretions.

Treatment of CF typically involves frequent postural drainage of mucus and chest percussion. Some patients may use mechanical vibrators to facilitate the percussions. They usually take medications aimed at mucus reduction and control of bacterial infection.

In the later stages, most CF patients will be colonized with respiratory system pathogens such as Pseudomonas aerugionosa.

CF can be regarded as a terminal disease. Few patients live to the age of 40. Take this fact into account when treating the patient. At all times, remain sensitive to the emotional state of both the patient and any members of the family who may be present.

You may be summoned to help a CF patient for a variety of reasons. The vigorous coughing associated with the disease can result in **hemoptysis** and pneumothorax. Severe or fatal pulmonary hemorrhage can occur at any time. Patients can also suffer **cor pulmonale,** or right ventricular hypertrophy secondary to pulmonary hypertension.

✶ hemoptysis expectoration of blood arising from the oral cavity, larynx, trachea, bronchi, or lungs; characterized by sudden coughing with production of salty sputum with frothy bright red blood.

In treating a CF patient, ascertain the stage of the disease and inquire about any standing medical orders. Also find out if the patient or family has initiated any advance directives. Your treatment will flow from this information and your own assessment. There is no specific in-field treatment for acute problems stemming from CF. As a general rule, you will provide respiratory support, ventilation, and intubation, if indicated. Be sure to counsel the family or summon the proper counselor to do so, especially if the patient is in the terminal stage of the disease.

✶ cor pulmonale congestive heart failure secondary to pulmonary hypertension.

In treating a CF patient, ascertain the stage of the disease and inquire about any standing orders.

Bronchopulmonary Dysplasia (BPD)

This disease primarily affects infants of low birth weight. It is characterized by an ongoing need for mechanical ventilation in newborns who have been treated for respiratory distress of any cause. These infants may simply fail to wean from mandatory ventilation or from O_2. They are also at increased risk of lower respiratory tract infections, especially

Intermittent Mandatory Ventilation (IMV) respirator setting where a patient-triggered breath does not result in assistance by the machine.

Keep in mind that pulmonary congestion and edema may develop in infants with BPD if excessive fluids have been administered.

demylenation destruction or removal of the myelin sheath of nerve tissue; found in Guillain–Barré syndrome.

viral infections, and may require immediate hospitalization if signs of respiratory infection or increased distress develop.

Home care providers will have been advised to wean infants to lower **Intermittent Mandatory Ventillation (IMV)** settings. However, if the process occurs too quickly, the infant may be at risk of becoming hypoxemic. Arterial oxygenation should be maintained at or above 88 to 90 percent saturation and should be monitored continuously with a pulse oximeter.

Keep in mind that pulmonary congestion and edema may develop in BPD infants if excessive fluids have been administered. Question caregivers about fluid intake, which may need to be restricted to about 120 mL/kg per day. Inquire, too, about the use of diuretic therapy, which is sometimes prescribed to these patients.

Even after an infant is weaned from a ventilator, supplemental oxygen may still be required for weeks or even months. In such cases, it is usually delivered by nasal cannula.

Remember that BPD is a serious condition in infants. Reduced lung compliance and increased airway resistance may persist for several years. The best treatment is adequate ventilatory support and prompt transport to the nearest neonatal unit.

Neuromuscular Degenerative Diseases As a group, these diseases affect respiratory action through degeneration of the muscles used for breathing. Patients who suffer from neuromuscular degeneration may at some point require respiratory support. Other problems, particularly an inability to ambulate, will have a huge impact on the patient's life.

Many patients with neuromuscular degenerative diseases will be cared for by family members. However, if the condition worsens, professional home care providers may be involved and ALS may be summoned. In cases of respiratory compromise, there is little that you can do other than provide airway and respiratory support and transport. Expect to see all manner of respiratory home care devices, including oxygen and ventilators.

In treating and transporting these patients, keep in mind the following information on the leading neuromuscular degenerative diseases.

Muscular Dystrophy This genetically inherited disorder causes a defect in the intracellular metabolism of muscle cells. The condition leads to degeneration and atrophy of muscles, which are eventually replaced by fatty and connective tissue. There is no cure as yet, and treatment is multidisciplinary because of the many muscle systems involved. These patients have difficulty moving and may need assistance with daily tasks. ALS involvement would almost certainly be for respiratory failure or accidental injuries, usually related to falls.

Poliomyelitis Poliomyelitis is an infectious disease rarely seen today because of effective vaccines. When it does occur, the disease causes destruction of motor neurons, leading to muscular atrophy, muscle weakness, and paralysis. Patients have difficulty ambulating. However, unless respiratory muscles are involved, there may be no systemic effects. Children who contract the disease may suffer permanent crippling or deformity. But once the disease is resolved, further degeneration will cease.

It has been shown that after polio patients recover normal functioning they sometimes experience a **demylenation** of affected neurons and a return of the disability. This condition is known as post polio syndrome. Its pathophysiology is unknown.

Guillain–Barré Syndrome This syndrome is thought to be an autoimmune response to a viral (rarely bacterial) infection. It is usually preceded by a febrile episode with a respiratory and/or GI infection. The disease is characterized by muscle weakness leading to paralysis caused by nerve demylenation. It usually starts in the distal extremities and progresses proximally.

Progression of this disorder may take several days. Once it reaches the patient's trunk, respiratory involvement becomes an obvious concern. One way to differentiate Guillain–Barré from a spinal injury is the increased motor involvement. In other words, motor deficits are greater than sensory deficits. As a rule, there is no cognitive or CNS involvement with the disease. With supportive ventilatory care, the patient can be expected to recover.

Myasthenia Gravis   Myasthenia gravis is a rare disease that affects the neuronal junction. Due to the breakdown in acetylcholine receptors, nerve impulses are dampened. This disease is characterized by muscle weakness and can be more apparent in muscles proximal to the body than distally.

There is no cure for this disorder, and treatment is aimed at relieving symptoms. If the disease progresses to the diaphragm or intercostal muscles, respiratory compromise can result. Sometimes patients may have an acute exacerbation of the disease brought on by infection or stress. In such cases, intubation or artificial ventilation may be required. These episodes are most commonly preceded by difficulty swallowing or breathing.

Sleep Apnea   Sleep apnea is a complex condition not yet fully understood by experts. It is characterized by long pauses in the respiratory cycle that can be caused by a relaxation of the pharynx or lack of respiratory drive. It can result in hypertension, cardiac arrhythmias, and chronic fatigue.

As a general rule, the muscles of the airway become more relaxed as the mind falls deeper and deeper into sleep. This is what leads to snoring and, in some cases, blockage of the airway. With sleep apnea, decreased oxygen levels cause a partial awakening of the patient. Breathing then resumes and the patient returns to sleep, often with no memory of the incident. Repeated over and over, such interruptions destroy normal sleep patterns and the patient spends much of the sleeping period in a hypoxic state.

People with sleep apnea often suffer alterations in their blood pressure and stroke volume. They lose the normal effect of declining blood pressure as they sleep and their pulse oximetry may fall to 80 percent or less. In patients who have ingested alcohol, the reading can fall to 50 percent.

Treatment of sleep apnea may include surgical alteration of the airway, medications, prescribed loss of weight, avoidance of any CNS depressant or alcohol, or use of a CPAP ventilator.

Patients Awaiting Lung Transplants   Patients receive lung transplants for a variety of cardiopulmonary diseases. Single-lung transplants are performed for pulmonary fibrosis, COPD, or reversible hypertension or cardiac disease. Double-lung transplants are performed for cystic fibrosis, COPD, or **bronchiectasis.** Patients may also receive heart-lung transplants for primary pulmonary hypertension or various congenital diseases. Remember that patients awaiting organ transplants are in the end-stages of their diseases and traditional therapies are unlikely to be effective.

✳ **bronchiectasis** chronic dilation of a bronchus or bronchi, with a secondary infection typically involving the lower portion of the lung.

Medical Therapy Found in the Home Setting

The treatment of chronic respiratory disorders in the home setting requires a wide range of devices. The following are some of the most common types of medical therapy that you can expect to encounter.

Home Oxygen Therapy   Oxygen therapy has many advantages for the home care patient. First, it is relatively simple to manage. Second, most patients tolerate it easily. Third, oxygen therapy can add much to the quality of a patient's life. Studies have shown that long-term oxygen use raises the life expectancy of COPD patients considerably. It also prevents hypoxic states that may result in permanent cognitive damage or degeneration.

A medical equipment supplier usually delivers, sets up, and educates patients on the home oxygen delivery systems that they will use. In most cases, the systems include:

- A source of oxygen—e.g., concentrator, cylinder, or liquid oxygen reservoir
- Regulator-flow meter
- Nasal cannula, face mask, tracheostomy collar, oxygen tubing (large-bore for face tents or tracheostomy collars)
- Humidifier
- Sterile water for respiratory therapy (Make sure it is sterile!)

Very few problems arise from the systems themselves. When they do occur, patients or home care providers can usually correct the situation on their own. However, you may be called upon to provide oxygen while a home system is repaired or to transport the patient to the hospital until the system is replaced. You may also be summoned if a condition unexpectedly worsens and the home oxygen system proves insufficient.

When you arrive at the scene, review the physician's prescription for the type of therapy and the source of the oxygen supply. As already noted, the three sources include:

- *Oxygen concentrators.* These systems supply the lowest concentrations of home oxygen. They extract oxygen from room air and add to the flow received by the patient. Home concentrators usually provide no more than six liters of oxygen per minute.
- *Oxygen cylinders.* Cylinders or tanks are used by patients who may require more than six liters/minute or for some reason cannot have a concentrator. Cylinders involve the same technology that you use on your own portable oxygen systems.
- *Liquid oxygen.* Patients who require constant oxygen may have a liquid oxygen system. This allows much more oxygen to be stored in the home. Patients will use this system as a reservoir to fill portable tanks that they make take outside the home.

Although these systems are relatively safe, any high pressure tank or liquid system has the potential for explosion. In a polite manner, ensure that the patient and home care provider adheres to these safety tips:

- Alert the local fire department to the presence of oxygen in the home.
- Keep a fire extinguisher on hand.
- If a fire does start, turn the oxygen off immediately and leave the house.
- Don't smoke—and do not allow others to smoke—near the oxygen system. (No open flames or smoking within ten feet of oxygen.)
- Do not use electrical equipment near oxygen administration.
- Store the oxygen tank in an approved, upright position.
- Keep a tank or reservoir away from direct sunlight or heat.
- Ground all oxygen cylinders.

In terms of the oxygen therapy itself, keep these guidelines in mind:

- Ensure the ability of the patient/home care provider to administer oxygen.
- Make sure the patient knows what to do in case of a power failure.
- Evaluate sterile conditions, especially disinfection of reusable equipment.
- As with any patient with chronic respiratory problems, remain alert to signs and symptoms of hypoxemia.

Artificial Airways/Tracheostomies Patients who have long-term upper airway problems often have a tracheostomy. A **tracheostomy** is a small surgical opening that a surgeon makes from the anterior neck into the trachea. The tracheostomy may be temporary or permanent. The technique is used on any patient who requires artificial ventilation for a long period of time. (Endotracheal or nasal intubation can only be used on a short-term basis. Pressure on the tracheal tissues, from the inflated cuff, can cause necrosis.) Tracheostomies may also be used on patients who have had damage to their larynx, epiglottis, or upper airway structures from surgery or trauma. They may also be performed on patients who have cancer of the larynx or neck.

The tracheostomy consists of the surgical opening (stoma), an outer cannula, and an inner cannula. The outer cannula keeps the stoma open and is held in place by twill tape or Velcro around the neck. The inner cannula is similar to a mini ET tube and slides down into the trachea a few inches. Due to the small size of the airway, the inner cannula usually has a low pressure cuff at the end to hold it in place and provide a good seal. In the case of infants, there is no inner cannula because of the small size of infant airways. Also, the airways of infants are more pliable than older patients and more susceptible to blockage.

Tracheostomy patients who have had a larygectomy may have some ability for speech, and some may have an air connection to the oropharynx or nasopharynx. Keep this in mind if you need to ventilate a person with a tracheostomy. It may be necessary to block off the nose and mouth to prevent air from escaping upwardly instead of being pushed into the lungs.

Those patients who are unable to speak will use an artificial larynx. This device looks like a small flashlight. It creates an electronic vibration, which the patient manipulates by pressing the device up against the neck and by changing the shape of his or her mouth (much as you do when you speak). If the patient does not have an artificial larynx, you will need to resort to writing or signing for communication. Remember that an inability to communicate can create a lot of stress and frustration for the patient. Try to be part of the solution, not part of the problem.

Routine care of the tracheostomy includes:

- Keeping the stoma clean and dry
- Periodic changing of the outer cannula
- Changing and cleaning the inner cannula from every few weeks to every few months, depending on the patient
- For ventilator patients, routine changing of the ventilator hose connections
- Frequent suctioning, due to increased secretions

It is important to remember that a tracheostomy eliminates a large part of the normal air-filtering process. The trapping of bacteria in the nasopharynx and

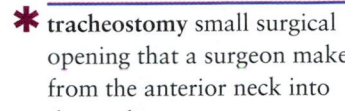
tracheostomy small surgical opening that a surgeon makes from the anterior neck into the trachea.

oropharynx no longer occurs. Neither does the humidification and heating of air by the nasal passages. This means that bacteria have a more direct route to the lungs, and the air received in the lungs is drier and cooler than normal. Therefore, people with a tracheostomy have a higher incidence of lung infections, mucus production, and irritation. Since they have less control over their airway, it is also more difficult for them to clear blocked airways.

If a patient is not currently using a tracheostomy, it may be closed with a Trach-button. This device simply plugs up the opening until it is needed again.

Common Complications   The most common problems faced by tracheostomy patients include blockage of the airway by mucus and a dislodged cannula. The patient can usually clear the obstructing mucus by coughing. (Be careful—the mucus can fly out of the stoma for quite a distance.) Sometimes suctioning, either by the patient or by the caregiver, will suffice. Cannulas can become dislodged by patient movement, or, in the case of children, by their growth. In assessing a child with a cannula problem, find out when it was last changed. Maybe the child is ready for the next size. Children can also have their stoma blocked by foreign objects that enter by accident or are put there by a sibling. Other complications include infection of the stoma, drying of the tracheal mucus leading to crusting or bleeding, and tracheal erosion from an over-inflated cuff (causing necrosis).

Management   If EMS has been called, it means that neither the patient nor the caregiver has been able to solve the problem. If the tracheostomy patient is on a ventilator, you must rapidly determine if the problem is with the ventilator or with the airway itself. If the problem is simply a loose fitting or disconnected tube, fix it. If the problem is not immediately apparent, do not waste time trying to troubleshoot the machine—unless you are qualified to do so. Your bag-valve device will connect directly to where the ventilator tubing connects. Remove the tubing, connect the bag-valve device to the trach connector, and ventilate (Figure 46-5).

If the problem is with the patient's airway, you will need to clear it. If the patient is hypoxic, always hyperventilate before suctioning. Be sure to evaluate any postural or positional considerations. If the patient is slumped over, straighten him or her up. Remember to ensure that ventilations are directed downward into the lungs, not upward into the mouth. (Ask the home care provider if there is a connection from the trachea to the upper airway.)

If you are unable to ventilate, clearing the airway is your first priority. Visualize as much of the airway as possible and check for obstructions. If none are visible, introduce a suction catheter and suction while withdrawing—no more than 10–15 seconds for an adult, 5 seconds for a child. Again, always hyperventilate before and after suctioning.

If it appears that the inner cannula is blocked or dislodged, you may remove it. If cuffed, you must first deflate the cuff. Connect a 10 cc syringe to the cuff

FIGURE 46-5   Artificial ventilation can be accomplished in the patient with a tracheostomy tube by attaching the bag-valve device directly to the tube.

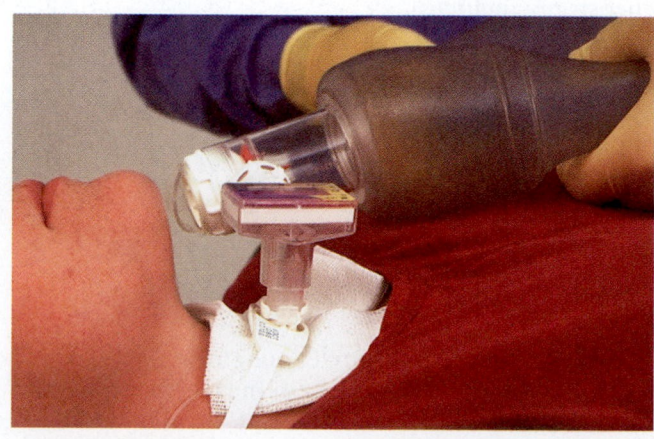

valve and withdraw the air. If a syringe is unavailable, you can cut off the valve and the air will escape. You can then remove the inner cannula, hyperventilate, and continue to suction as needed.

If necessary, you may intubate the stoma. The inner cannula must always be removed first. Use an appropriate sized tube to pass through the outer cannula, and advance so the ET cuff (if a cuffed tube is used) is 1-2 cm inside the trachea. Inflate the cuff and verify placement by auscultating the epigastrum and both lungs. Add an end tidal CO_2 device to the end of the tube. Pulse oximetry should also be used to monitor patient oxygenation.

Once the airway is secure, you may proceed with the rest of your assessment. It is inappropriate to proceed until you have protected the airway.

Home Ventilation Although you will see positive pressure ventilators with most home care patients, you may also encounter negative pressure ventilators. Both devices are used to ventilate patients for a wide variety of diseases and conditions.

Some of the most common reasons patients may be on a ventilator include:

- Decreased respiratory drive
  —spinal cord injury
- Ventilatory muscle weakness
  —muscular dystrophy
  —poliomyelitis
  —myasthenia gravis
  —Guillian–Barré syndrome
- Obstructive Pulmonary Disorders
  —COPD
  —sleep apnea
  —cystic fibrosis
  —bronchopulmonary dysplasia
- Other Disorders
  —pediatric sleep apnea
  —chest wall deformities

Ventilators provide ventilation in several different ways. They also have a number of operating controls and options, depending upon the manufacturer. Volume-cycled ventilation, for example, has long been the standard type of ventilatory support for all forms of severe respiratory failure. All modern ventilators can provide this feature as well as several other modes that vary in ventilatory waveform, method of terminating the machine-aided cycle, and so on.

Positive-Pressure Ventilators According to current practice, positive-pressure ventilation (PPV) is the recommended form of support for acute respiratory disorders. A positive pressure ventilator pushes air into the lungs, either through a face mask, nasal mask, or tracheostomy. Features of this type of ventilator include variations in tidal volume, respiratory rate, flow rate, and pressure. Optional connectors will be available for oxygen and a humidifier.

There are too many types of positive-pressure ventilators to list here. However, any home care provider should be familiar with a patient's particular machine—including the small ventilators that attach to a mobile patient's wheelchair.

Negative Pressure Ventilators Ventilators that apply negative pressure to the chest—tank, cuirass, or poncho-wrap—require a rigid structure to support the vacuum department. When they expand, they pull on the chest, causing it to expand and allowing air to flow into the lungs. This mimics the normal breathing process.

According to current practice, positive-pressure ventilation (PPV) is the recommended form of support for acute respiratory disorders.

The iron lung is one of the best known examples of negative pressure ventilators. However, some home care patients may also be fitted with a poncho-wrap—a suit that is sealed at all openings. Patients most commonly use this device at night.

PEEP, CPAP, and BiPAP These three ventilator options add pressure at various times in the respiratory cycle. They may be used by full-time or part-time ventilator patients. Keep in mind that there is a danger of pneumothorax because of the increased pulmonary pressure. Take this into account during your assessment of PEEP.

PEEP PEEP, or positive end expiratory pressure, is used to keep alveoli from collapsing. It works by providing a little back pressure at the end of expiration. This option can be used for newborns—usually premature—who have insufficient surfactant to keep the alveoli inflated or in adults who have surfactant washout from acute pulmonary edema, **ARDS**, or drowning.

PEEP also has a use in treating COPD. However, due to stiffening and degeneration of the alveoli in emphysema, patients require higher diffusion pressures for gas exchange. If you ever see COPD patients pursing their lips as they exhale, they are providing their own PEEP. By blowing against a slight resistance, they will keep their alveoli open. A COPD patient who is getting worse may deteriorate to the point where he or she needs occasional assistance from a ventilator with PEEP.

CPAP CPAP, or continuous positive airway pressure, is used to keep pharyngeal structures from collapsing at the end of a breath. This option is often prescribed for sleep apnea patients who need help in keeping their airways open. Most of these patients will use nasal CPAP—a mask that encompasses the nose (Figure 46-6). In these cases, patients must learn to keep their mouths closed for the mask to work correctly. Otherwise the pressure will be lost. The idea behind mask CPAP or nasal CPAP is the same as PEEP, except that CPAP is provided by mask, while PEEP is provided by endotracheal tube.

✱ **ARDS** acute respiratory distress syndrome.

Nasal mask with straps

Tubing to the unit

FIGURE 46-6   Sleep apnea patients will often use continuous positive airway pressure—CPAP—to keep their airways open.

BiPAP BiPAP, or bilevel positive airway pressure, provides two levels of pressure—one on inspiration and one on exhalation. This option is used for patients who require more or higher levels of pressure than CPAP. Although the settings on the patient's home ventilator may be useful to the ED or to follow-up patient care, they are not essential to your assessment. Try to gather this information at the scene, but don't let it delay your management of any serious airway or breathing problems.

As you may already have inferred, a home care patient with a chronic respiratory problem might eventually progress from home oxygen, to occasional ventilator support (PEEP, CPAP, BiPAP), to full ventilator dependency. Knowing each stage of the illness and how it relates to the various ventilatory options will give you a more complete understanding of the patient's clinical progress.

General Assessment Considerations Assessment of the respiratory patient should focus on the patient's entire respiratory apparatus. Any deficit found in the system must be rapidly identified and managed.

As you approach the patient, look at the effort required to breathe. Observe for head bobbing, retractions, respiratory rate, tripod posturing, pursed lips, cyanosis, and depth of respiration. Listen for sounds of wheezing or rales. Note any devices or medications that the patient is currently using.

Immediately assess the patient's mental status by talking to him or her as you approach. Patients will indicate understanding with their eyes even if they are unable to speak due to dyspnea. Note the number of words that they can speak without stopping for a breath. Rapidly confirm the patient's baseline respiratory effort and mental status from the home care worker, if present.

Next, auscultate the lungs to identify the type of problem that the patient may be having and to determine tidal volume. Look at the patient's chest to spot any irregularities, retractions, or abdominal breathing. You can use pulse oximetry as an adjunct to your assessment, but don't rely on it alone. If the patient has poor peripheral circulation, it may not give an accurate reading.

Finally, complete your assessment by considering the full range of problems that might have caused the patient's current complaint. Whenever assessing a home care patient, you must remain vigilant for complications other than the chronic medical condition being treated at home. An asthma patient, for example, might be having a myocardial infarction (MI).

General Management Considerations As always, your first considerations when intervening in the care of a chronically ill patient center on the ABCs. In the absence of documentation or a valid prehospital DNR, you must maintain a patent airway or improve on the airway that is already in place. This may be as simple as suctioning secretions from an airway device, such as a tracheostomy tube. You should also assess the placement of airway devices that you did not insert. It is easy for a device to become dislodged, obstructing the airway or failing to ensure patency. You may be forced to remove home airway devices and replace them with your own interventions, such as endotracheal tubes.

Ventilatory problems are traditionally easy to fix in the prehospital environment. If a home ventilator fails, you should begin manual positive pressure ventilation immediately. The failure may be easy to remedy, such as in the case of unplugged power cords or a temporary loss of electricity. If you are familiar with the ventilator, you can adjust the settings to restore or improve ventilations. However, if you are unfamiliar with the ventilator, play it safe and support ventilations with your own equipment.

As with ventilation, oxygenation problems are also generally easy for EMS providers to fix. First, assess the patency of the patient's home oxygen delivery system. The power may be off, the tubing damaged, or the oxygen supply

If you are having problems ventilating patients with their home health equipment, remove it and use equipment from the EMS unit.

If a home ventilator fails, you should begin manual positive pressure ventilation immediately.

depleted. You can adjust the flow rate of an intact home oxygen delivery system or replace it with your own system.

Whatever interventions you choose, you will have to make arrangements for the devices to be transported with you to the hospital. Flexibility is the key to transporting home care patients. You should reassure the patient that you will properly care for their needs, as they will be physically as well as psychologically dependent upon their home care systems.

VASCULAR ACCESS DEVICES

Vascular access devices (VADs) are used to provide any parenteral treatment on a long-term basis. The type of device and treatment depends upon the disease process involved. Patients may have chemotherapy, hemodialysis, peritoneal dialysis, Total Parenteral Nutrition (TPN) feedings, or antibiotic therapy provided through a VAD.

Types of VADs

There are approximately 500,000 long-term therapy catheters inserted each year. Some of the most common VADs that you can expect to find in the home are described in the following sections. Consult your local protocols and procedures for accessing VADs.

Hickman, Broviac, and Groshong Catheters These catheters may be single, double, or triple lumen and can be inserted into any central vein in the trunk of the body. The subclavian vein is the most common anatomical insertion site, as it is usually easy to locate and secure.

Although these catheters have slight differences, each has an external port that looks like a typical intravenous port. The external hub of the catheter is sutured to the skin and has a cuff that promotes fibrous in-growth. This growth helps anchor the catheter to the body and prevents infection from traveling down the catheter. The highest risk of infection or accidental removal of the catheter is during the first two weeks after insertion. Care of these devices consists of keeping the site clean and dry and the administration of anticoagulant therapy to prevent clot formations.

VADs will often be routed through a subcutaneous tunnel to protect the site of venous puncture.

Peripherally Inserted Central Catheters Peripherally inserted central catheters, or PICC lines, are inserted into a peripheral vein, such as the median cubital vein in the antecubital fossa. These veins are easily accessible and allow a physician to thread a catheter from the insertion site into central venous circulation. PICC lines are inserted under fluoroscopy by radiology rather than in an operating room. As a result, the procedure has relatively low complication rate.

Surgically Implanted Medication Delivery Systems Surgically implanted devices, such as the Port-A-Cath or Medi-Port, are similar to Hickman-style catheters. However, the infusion port is implanted completely below the skin. These devices are disc-shaped and have a diaphragm that requires a specially shaped needle, such as the Huber needle, to access. They are typically found in the upper chest and can be felt through the skin.

Never access a surgically implanted port unless local protocols allow you to do so and only if you have the training and equipment to complete the procedure.

Never access a surgically implanted port unless local protocols allow you to do so. If such protocols exist, only properly trained personnel with proper equipment should complete the procedure. A regular intravenous catheter or needle will permanently damage an implanted port. Surgically implanted medication delivery devices should only be accessed using sterile technique.

Dialysis Shunts Dialysis shunts are used for patients undergoing hemodialysis to filter their blood. An A-V shunt is a loop connecting an artery and a vein, usu-

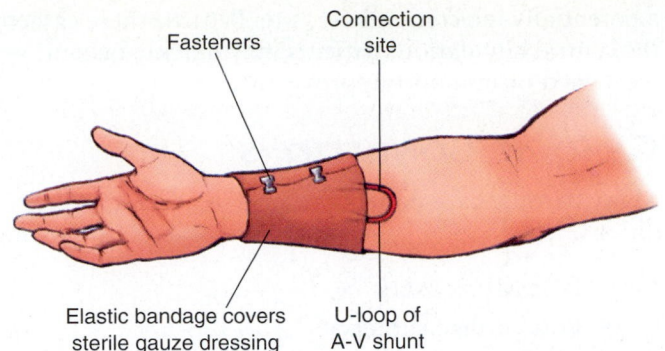

Fasteners

Connection site

Elastic bandage covers sterile gauze dressing

U-loop of A-V shunt

FIGURE 46-7 An A-V shunt is a loop connecting an artery and a vein, usually in the distal arm, where the dialysis apparatus draws and returns blood. It is used in home-care patients requiring dialysis.

ally in the distal arm, where the dialysis apparatus draws out and returns blood (Figure 46-7). A fistula connects an artery and a vein, creating an artificially large blood vessel for access. It is also usually found in the upper extremity.

Both shunts and fistulas are created surgically and are very delicate. As a result, you should avoid vascular access and application of blood pressure cuffs in the extremity where they are located. Some jurisdictions allow shunt access by paramedics during life-threatening emergencies. You will be able to see the shunt in the extremity, and you should be able to auscultate a bruit over the area. Failure to auscultate a bruit over the shunt area may indicate an obstruction, either a thrombus that has formed or an embolus that has lodged there.

Anticoagulant Therapy

Patients with vascular access devices will be on some type of anticoagulant therapy. The most commonly found anticoagulants will be those used to flush the device to prevent clot formation. Some patients may be on systemic anticoagulants as well. Because VADs are artificial, the body's natural clotting mechanism must be suppressed in order to ensure that the devices function properly. As a result, these patients will be much more prone to bleeding disorders. The most common sites for hemorrhage are GI bleeding, strokes, and extremity bruising.

VAD Complications

In treating patients with VADs, keep in mind possible complications. The most common complications result from various types of obstructions. A thrombus may form at the catheter site, or an embolus may lodge there after formation elsewhere in the body. Inactivity increases the risk for clot formation. Other obstructive problems include catheter kinking or catheter tip embolus.

With central venous access devices, you should always be aware of the potential for an air embolus. The devices provide a clear pathway for air to enter central circulation. Signs and symptoms of an air embolus include:

- Headache
- Shortness of breath with clear lungs
- Hypoxia
- Chest pain
- Other indications of myocardial ischemia
- Altered mental status

Of course, any device implanted in the body has a risk of infection or hemorrhage. Look for redness, swelling, tenderness, localized heat, or discharge for

Avoid obtaining vascular access and blood pressure in the extremity where a shunt is located.

It is prudent to have an orientation session on VADs used by the home health agencies in your area. Following this, an assortment of specialized needles and supplies should be carried.

a potentially infected catheter site. Because these catheters provide a channel into the central circulation, patients may quickly become septic, especially if they are weakened or immunosuppressed.

CARDIAC CONDITIONS

Many chronic-care patients receive treatment for a wide variety of cardiac conditions. You may be called to intervene in the following situations:

- Post MI recovery
- Post cardiac surgery
- Heart transplant
- CHF
- Hypertension
- Implanted pacemaker
- Atherosclerosis
- Congenital malformation (pediatric)

Home care for the cardiac patient can consist of oxygen, monitoring devices, and regular visits by a home health care provider. You can expect to find a variety of medications associated with the specific cardiac problem, bedside cardiac monitors (for adults and children), diagnostic devices such as a halter monitor, and possibly a defibrillator. For a review of the assessment, treatment, and management of cardiac problems, see Chapter 28.

GI/GU CRISIS

Patients with various long-term devices to support gastrointestinal or genitourinary functions may need ALS intervention. Your response may be directly related to a problem with the GI or GU device, or you may simply need to be aware of the device and support during transport.

Urinary Tract Devices

There are various medical devices designed to support patients with urinary tract dysfunction. External devices, such as Texas catheters (also called condom catheters), attach to the male external genitalia to collect urine (Figure 46-8). Because these devices are not inserted into the urethra, they reduce the risk of infection. However, they do not collect urine in a sterile manner, nor are they adequate for long-term use.

Internal catheters, such as Foley or indwelling catheters, are the most commonly used devices for urinary tract dysfunction. They are long catheters with a balloon tip that is inserted through the urethra into the urinary bladder. The balloon is then inflated with saline to keep the device in place (Figure 46-9). Internal catheters are well-tolerated for long-term use and are frequently found in hospitals, skilled nursing facilities, or home-care situations.

Suprapubic catheters are similar in purpose to internal catheters. However, they are inserted directly through the abdominal wall into the urinary bladder. Suprapubic catheters may be used instead of indwelling catheters in the event of surgery or other problems with the genitalia or bladder.

Urostomies are a surgical diversion of the urinary tract to a stoma, or hole, in the abdominal wall. A collection device will be attached to the stoma outside the body to collect urine. Urostomies are used when the bladder is unable to effectively collect urine.

Tape

Sheath

Catheter

FIGURE 46-8 An external urinary tract device.

✱ **urostomy** surgical diversion of the urinary tract to a stoma, or hole, in the abdominal wall.

Connection between catheter
and drainage tubing

Urethral
meatus

Connection between
drainage tubing
and bag

Emptying spout

FIGURE 46-9   An internal urinary catheter with balloon. Note sites where bacteria can enter.

Urinary Device Complications

Most complications related to urinary tract support devices result from infection or device malfunctions. Infection is a very common problem with urinary tract devices because the area is rich with pathogens and because the catheter provides a pathway directly into the body. Remain alert to foul-smelling urine or altered urine color, such as "tea" colored, cloudy, or blood-tinged urine. Also look for signs and symptoms of systemic infection, or urosepsis, as urinary infections can quickly spread in the immunocompromised patient. Suprapubic catheters or urostomies may also have infections at the abdominal wall site. You should note redness, swelling, heat, discharge, or loss of skin integrity.

Device malfunctions typically include accidental displacement of the device, obstruction, balloon ruptures in devices that use a balloon as an anchor, or leaking collection devices. Changes in the patient's anatomy, such as a shortened urinary tract or tissue necrosis can also cause malfunctions. Ensure that the collection device is empty and record the amount of urine output. Look for kinks or other obstructions in the device, and make sure that the collection bag is placed below the patient.

Gastrointestinal Tract Devices

You can expect to encounter a wide variety of devices to support the gastrointestinal tract. Nasogastric (NG) tubes are commonly seen by EMS personnel, as they are often used to decompress gastric contents in the prehospital

FIGURE 46-10   A nasogastric feeding tube.

Nasogastric feeding (gavage) liquid food goes into the patient

Nostrils (naso)

Esophagus

Stomach (gastric)

Feeding pump

environment (Figure 46-10). NG tubes may also be used to lavage the GI system in various situations, such as GI bleeding or substance ingestion. NG tubes are not usually long-term devices, as they cause discomfort and may lead to tissue necrosis in the nasal passages if left intact for an extended period.

Feeding tubes are more substantial than NG tubes and come to rest in either the duodenum or jejunum. Often they are weighted to help them pass through the pyloric sphincter and have a steel filament to facilitate insertion. Feeding tubes are used for supplemental nutrition when a person cannot swallow due to dysphagia, paralysis, or unconsciousness.

For longer-term supplemental nutrition, a gastric tube may be inserted through the abdominal wall into the small intestine (Figure 46-11). Indications for a gastrostomy tube include Alzheimer's disease, neurological deficits from strokes or head trauma, or mental retardation. Gastrostomy tubes come in many forms, such as percutaneous endoscopic gastrostomy (PEG) tubes, surgical gastrostomy tubes, and Jejunal tubes, to name a few. These tubes have different means of insertion (surgical vs. endoscopic), location (stomach vs. duodenum), and function (feeding vs. aspiration prevention).

A **colostomy** is used to bypass part of the large intestine and allow feces to be collected outside the body in a collection bag, either on a temporary or permanent basis. Indications for a colostomy include cancer of the bowel or rectum, diverticulitis, Crohn's disease, or trauma. A surgical connection of the bowel to an ostomy created in the skin results in diversion of feces into the collection bag (Figure 46-12).

* **colostomy** opening of a portion of the colon through the abdominal wall, allowing feces to be collected outside the body.

FIGURE 46-11 A gastrostomy feeding tube.

Tube feeding

Feeding pump

Esophagus

Gastrostomy

Stomach

Gastrointestinal Tract Device Complications

Complications from GI tract devices include tube misplacement, obstruction, or infection. Because misplaced tubes can obstruct the airway or GI system, you should always ensure device patency if you have doubts about placement of the tube. First, have the patient speak to you. If he or she cannot speak, the tube may be in the airway and need to be removed. Second, to assure patency of an NG tube, use a 60 mL syringe to insert air into the stomach. Use your stethoscope to listen over the epigastrum for air movement within the stomach. A low-pitched, rumbling should be heard. You may also note stomach contents spontaneously moving up the tube or they may be aspirated with a 60 cc syringe. In such cases, patients may be repositioned to return patency, or the device may be reinserted.

Tubes are also prone to obstructions. Colostomies may become clogged or otherwise obstructed. Feeding tubes can become clogged due to the thick consistency of supplemental feedings or pill fragments. As a result, the tubes may require irrigation with water. In addition, the thick consistency of food may cause bowel obstructions or constipation.

As might be expected, ostomies can become infected (or lose skin integrity from pressure). Look for signs and symptoms of skin or systemic infection. In addition, remember that digestive enzymes may leak from various ostomies and begin to digest the skin and abdominal contents.

A displaced gastrostomy or jeuojenostomy tube must be replaced as soon as possible after dislodgement. Some services train paramedics in G-tube changes and insertions.

Psychosocial Implications

Many patients with GI or GU support devices lead active and otherwise normal lives. These patients may be understandably self-conscious about their conditions

FIGURE 46-12 Examples of colostomy stoma locations.

and many experience embarrassment, avoidance, anger, or discomfort when questioned. You should be sensitive to the patient's emotions during your patient assessment and treatment.

ACUTE INFECTIONS

After physicians or hospital personnel treat open wounds, they typically release patients to home care. These wounds may be surgical wounds or loss of skin integrity for other reasons. In such instances, you may see dressings covering wounds to protect against infection, absorb drainage, or immobilize the wound area. Gauze packing may also be inserted in infected spaces to absorb drainage.

Drains may sometimes be inserted in a wound site to remove blood, serum bile, or pus from the area. Drains are typically soft rubber tubes that have one end in the wound and the other end attached to a bag or suction device. Common drains include the Penrose drain, which is a simple rubber tube, and the Jackson-Pratt drain, which includes a suction bulb.

Wounds are typically closed with sutures, wires, staples, or cyanoacrylate adhesives. The type of closure used depends upon the wound and the preferences of the physician closing it. Sutures are the most common device used to secure a wound, but staples and adhesives are becoming more widespread due to their ease of use. Wires are typically used to secure musculoskeletal structures, such as ribs or the sternum after a sternotomy.

In assessing wounds, always be aware of the potential for improper wound healing. As already mentioned, home care patients are at increased risk of infection. The immunological response and rate of wound healing expected in the general population is compromised in the home care patient by poor peripheral perfusion, a sedentary existence, the presence of percutaneous and implanted medical devices, the existences of chronic diseases, and more.

An infected superficial wound may quickly lead to major infections or sepsis in the immunocompromised or weakened patient. Keep in mind that the chronically ill or homebound patient, particularly the elderly, often have a decreased ability to perceive pain or to perform self-care. Pay particular attention to signs of infection in wounds found in home care patients. If you inspect a wound, be sure to use sterile technique and redress the wound. For more on the treatment of bedsores and shear, see Chapter 43.

Pay particular attention to signs of infection in wounds found in home care patients.

MATERNAL AND NEWBORN CARE

Today, many women who deliver their babies in a hospital will be discharged in 24 hours or less. This trend, fueled by rising health care costs, greatly shortens the transition time from hospital to home. Some parents may not yet be emotionally prepared to care for a new baby, especially first-time parents. Rapid discharge may also leave a mother or newborn with an unrecognized problem or complication stemming from delivery. As a result, you the ALS provider might be summoned to the home and called on to utilize the neonatology and pediatrics skills that you learned in Chapters 39, 40, and 41.

Common Maternal Complications

For the mother, post partum bleeding and embolus (especially after Cesarean) are the most common complications. Management of an embolus would be the same as with any patient with a similar complaint. Post partum bleeding can be a serious condition. Management steps include:

- Massage of uterus, if not already contracted
- Administration of fluids to correct hypotension
- Administration of certain medications, such as Pitocin (if ordered)
- Rapid transport to the hospital, if necessary

Mothers may also experience **post partum depression.** In such cases, women may have difficulty caring for both themselves and their newborn. In extreme cases, babies have been neglected or even harmed.

When entering the home, be sensitive to the needs of the parents. First-time mothers and/or fathers may be inexperienced in childrearing and may call EMS for what a more experienced parent might regard as normal. It is important that you always take any parent's concerns seriously, and if no medical support is needed, provide emotional reassurance. If you suspect neglect or abuse of the newborn, take actions recommended in Chapters 41, 42, and 44.

✱ post partum depression the "let down" feeling experienced during the period following birth occurring in 70–80% of mothers.

Common Infant/Child Complications

As pointed out in Chapter 41, newborns must rapidly adapt to a new environment and may well not have reached a state where they can thrive on their own. Newborns must be positioned properly to breathe, their noses must be clear (newborns are nose breathers), and they must be kept warm because of immature thermoregulation. Newborns also have immature immune systems and can develop rapid, life-threatening infections or septicemia.

Infants with recognized problems may already be receiving home care. They may have cardiac or respiratory abnormalities or other congenital defects. Premature or low birth weight babies—as well as babies with any number of respiratory disorders—are at risk for sleep apnea. Such babies may wear apnea monitors around their chest so that an alarm sounds at any pause in their breathing pattern. Some infants may also be on pulse oximetry. If you are summoned because of an alarm and find a normal breathing pattern, still encourage the parents or caregivers to have the baby examined as soon as possible.

As noted, newborns may also be discharged from the hospital with an undetected cardiac or respiratory condition. Signs and symptoms of cardiac or respiratory insufficiency include:

- Cyanosis
- Bradycardia (< 100 b/m)
- Crackles
- Respiratory distress

In such cases, resuscitation should be initiated immediately. Management should be towards respiratory support with BVM or intubation, as necessary. If any newborn has a heart rate < 80 b/m despite 30 seconds or more of oxygenation, start CPR. Preserve warmth and obtain a record from the parents of feeding intake since birth. If the infant has not been feeding or has been vomiting with diarrhea, it may be dehydrated. In this case, a fluid bolus of 20 mL/kg is indicated. If a peripheral IV cannot be obtained in two attempts or two minutes, obtain access via the intraosseus route. If blood sugar is below 80 mg/dl administer $D_{25}W$ (some experts suggest $D_{10}W$) at a dosage of 0.5 mg/kg.

For a newborn with infection or septicemia, look for fever, tachycardia, and irritability. If septicemia progresses to septic shock, you should initiate resuscitation as previously described.

Children who have serious, long-term health problems are usually cared for by their parents at home—with or without the help of a home care professional. Commonly found medical therapies for children who are home care patients include:

- Mechanical ventilators
- IV medications or nutrition
- Oxygen therapy
- Tracheostomies
- Feeding tubes
- Pulse oximeters
- Apnea monitors

Parents of children with special needs are often highly educated regarding their child's problem. Always listen to them even when their attitude may appear condescending.

Education of the parents or caregivers by doctors and nurses forms a critical component in their ability to deal with a crisis. Some people adapt well to the task and can deal with their child's chronic problems in a professional manner. Others, however, may become panicked or, either through misunderstanding or denial, have little comprehension of the situation. As with any difficult call, maintain a professional demeanor at all times.

When dealing with children, remember to keep the parents or caregivers informed of your assessment and treatment plans. Children quickly pick up on a

Table 46-1	PERCENT OF HOSPICE PATIENTS BY AGE
Age	**Percent**
Under 45 years	8.1
45-54 years	7.9
55-64 years	14.8
65-69 years	8.7
70-74 years	15.6
75-79 years	14.5
80-84 years	12.3
85 years and older	16.4

Source: National Center for Health Statistics

person's emotions. As a result, it is part of your job to act in a supportive and controlled manner. Calming a child could make a huge difference in the long-term effects of the current episode.

HOSPICE AND COMFORT CARE

Today more than 2,250 hospices—and hundreds of volunteer agencies—provide support for the terminally ill and their families. Initially philanthropic, these programs are now covered by Medicare. Some states—such as Florida, Michigan, Kentucky, and New York—also include them under Medicaid. Most programs are home-based, with Medicare and Medicaid stipulating that at least 80 percent of an agency's care be provided to patients in their homes.

Up to 450,000 patients a year receive services from hospices funded by Medicare or Medicaid. (Thousands more receive help from private or volunteer agencies.) Although the majority of Medicare patients are age 70 and older (Table 46-1), children receive benefits, too. Reimbursement is extended to those patients with a life expectancy of six months or less.

The goal of hospices is to provide palliative or comfort care rather than curative care. This is a very different role than most other branches of the health care profession, including EMS. For an ALS team, care is usually geared toward aggressive and life-saving treatment. A hospice team, on the other hand, seeks to relieve symptoms, manage pain, and give patients control over the end of their lives. It is important to remember that these patients have, for the most part, exhausted or declined curative resources.

The goal of hospice care is to provide palliative or comfort care rather than curative care.

ALS Intervention

Involvement in a hospice situation can be a difficult and stressful call. In most cases, family members, caregivers, and health care workers have been instructed to call a hospice rather than EMS. However, you may be summoned for intervention, particularly in situations involving transport. You should always keep in mind that the hospice patient is in an end-stage disease and has already expressed wishes to withhold resuscitation. However, even a valid DNR order should not prevent you from performing palliative and/or comfort care.

FIGURE 46-13   The incidence of AIDS and HIV infection in children is increasing worldwide. These children may be among the patients that you may encounter in a hospice setting.

Common diseases that you can expect to see in hospice include:

- Congestive heart failure (CHF)
- Cystic fibrosis
- COPD
- AIDS (Figure 46-13)
- Alzheimer's
- Cancer

Terminally ill patients may take up to 3,000 milligrams of morphine a day with few side effects other than constipation.

If you are called to the house of a terminally ill patient, it is your responsibility to respect the wishes of the patient and the ideals of hospice care.

In some instances, particularly with cancer, you may also be confronted with patients on high dosages of pain medications. In cases of cancer, for example, morphine is the drug of choice. It is important for you to know that patients, who often take doses of up to 3,000 milligrams a day, will have few side effects other than constipation. They will have grown used to the drug and normal side effects will not be seen. Other drugs that may be administered include Percocet, Oxycontin, or a Duragesic patch. Some patients may also have a portable pump that provides a continuous infusion of medication through a PICC line. The pumps can be small and hidden by clothing.

In a hospice, you need to establish communication with the home health care worker as quickly as possible. Your inclination may be to intubate, start a line, or administer medications. However, as noted, palliative care supersedes curative care. A hospice worker, when faced with the end-stage of a disease, may do nothing in accordance with the patient's wishes. Therefore, it is vital that you gain a clear understanding of these wishes, whether through a family member or a written document. If you are called to the house, it is your responsibility to respect the wishes of the patient and the ideals of hospice care.

In a hospice situation, family members might panic at a patient's imminent death and appropriate care might involve support for the family rather than resuscitation of the patient. Local protocols may also vary in respect to DNRs, DNARs, living wills, and durable power of attorney documents. Be sure that you are familiar with these legal statements and their implications for care of the terminally ill. (See Chapter 2, "Medical/Legal Aspects of Prehospital Care.")

Terminally ill patients who are not involved in a hospice present a potentially gray area. Remember that while hospice prepares families for the impending death of their loved ones, families without hospice may be ill-prepared for the end-stages of life. Don't assume that all terminal patients are under hospice care. A simple question to determine the presence of hospice may alter your course of treatment and approach to the family.

Regardless of whether a patient is in hospice or not, keep in mind the stages of the grief process—denial, anger, depression, bargaining, and acceptance. Remember that both the patient and the family will go through these stages, and, in the case of the terminally ill, the patient may have reached acceptance well ahead of those who remain behind.

Caring for a hospice patient can be a challenge for paramedics as they must act within the scope of the patient's wishes.

Content Review

STAGES OF DEATH AND GRIEF
- Denial
- Anger
- Depression
- Bargaining
- Acceptance

Summary

The shift toward home health care is one of the most important trends of the 2000s and will have a great impact on the ALS profession. You can expect in your career to provide acute intervention for a growing number of chronic-care patients of all ages and in all stages of the disease process. These calls will challenge you to use all of your assessment skills in developing an effective management plan, which in many cases will be based on input from an extended team of home health care workers.

CHAPTER 47

Assessment-Based Management

Objectives

After reading this chapter, you should be able to:

1. Explain how effective assessment is critical to clinical decision making. (pp. 1922–1924)

2. Explain how the paramedic's attitude and uncooperative patients affect assessment and decision making. (pp. 1924–1926)

3. Explain strategies to prevent labeling, tunnel vision, and decrease environmental distractions. (pp. 1923–1927)

4. Describe how personnel considerations and staffing configurations affect assessment and decision making. (pp. 1926–1927)

5. Synthesize and apply concepts of scene management and choreography to simulated emergency calls. (p. 1927)

6. Explain the roles of the team leader and the patient care person. (p. 1927)

Continued

Objectives Continued

7. List and explain the rationale for bringing the essential care items to the patient. (pp. 1927–1928)
8. When given a simulated call, list the appropriate equipment to be taken to the patient. (p. 1928)
9. Explain the general approach to the emergency patient. (pp. 1928–1932)
10. Explain the general approach, patient assessment differentials, and management priorities for patients with various types of emergencies that may be experienced in prehospital care. (pp. 1922–1932)
11. Describe how to effectively communicate patient information face to face, over the telephone, by radio, and in writing. (pp. 1932–1934)
12. Given various preprogrammed and moulaged patients, provide the appropriate scene size-up, initial assessment, focused assessment, and detailed assessment, then provide the appropriate care, ongoing assessments, and patient transport. (pp. 1921–1935)

INTRODUCTION

A paramedic does more than just follow a standard sequence of assessment steps—scene size-up, initial assessment, focused history and physical exam, ongoing assessment, and detailed physical exam. While carrying out the assessment in a systematic way, a paramedic is constantly thinking and reasoning.

The kind of reasoning a paramedic needs to do has been described as an "inverted pyramid"—with the broad end at the top and the narrow point at the bottom (Figure 47-1). As soon as you receive the dispatch and the patient's chief

DIFFERENTIAL DIAGNOSIS Form a mental list of possible causes of the patient's complaint. Consider as many causes as possible. Think broadly. Avoid tunnel vision.

NARROWING PROCESS Use information gathered during the assessment to eliminate some possible causes, support others based on patterns of signs, symptoms, and history. Begin narrowing toward a field diagnosis.

FIELD DIAGNOSIS Form a field diagnosis of the most probable cause or causes of the patient's complaint, based on information gathered during the assessment.

complaint, you try to form a mental list of all the possible causes of the patient's problem. (Such a list is often called a "differential diagnosis.") You want to keep your mind wide open, avoiding tunnel vision.

For example, the victim of an auto crash has an obvious open extremity fracture with associated external blood loss. Serious as it is, the paramedic should resist being distracted by this injury. Suppose the patient had suffered a heart attack or cardiac arrest prior to or following the crash. Suppose the patient had other, more serious injuries, such as blunt abdominal trauma and internal bleeding. What if the paramedic fails to consider these other possibilities, focuses on the obvious leg injury, and spends on-scene time splinting the fracture instead of completing the assessment and initiating rapid transport?

Far better if the paramedic uses inverted-pyramid reasoning skills (which may also be called critical thinking, problem-solving, or clinical decision-making) to assess the patient and prioritize emergency care. The paramedic begins by considering a wide variety of possible medical conditions and injuries. Then, while working through the standard sequence of assessment steps, the paramedic uses the information gathered at each step of the assessment to eliminate some possibilities and support other possibilities. The paramedic considers pertinent negatives (signs that are *not* present, such as paralysis or an erratic pulse) as well as findings that are present (such as reddening and tenderness in one abdominal quadrant) to narrow in on a field diagnosis.

EFFECTIVE ASSESSMENT

Assessment forms the foundation for patient care.

Assessment forms the foundation for patient care. You can't treat or report a problem that is not found or identified. To find a problem, you must gather, evaluate, and synthesize information. Based on this process, you can then make decisions and take appropriate actions—formulate a management plan and determine the priorities for patient care.

A paramedic is entrusted with a great deal of independent judgment and responsibility for performing the correct actions for each individual patient, including such advanced skills as ECG interpretation, rapid sequence intubation,

FIGURE 47–2 If the patient is unable to provide a history, gather information for the patient history from family members or bystanders.

and medication administration. Additionally, the medical director and hospital staff must rely on your experience and expertise as you describe the patient's condition and your conclusions about it. Consequently, the ability to reason and to reach a field diagnosis is critical to paramedic practice.

IMPORTANCE OF ACCURATE INFORMATION

The decisions that you make as a paramedic will only be as good as the information that you collect. To make accurate decisions, you need to gather accurate information.

The decisions you make as a paramedic will only be as good as the information you collect.

The History

A patient's history is a crucial part of the medical record, especially in medical conditions (as contrasted to trauma, where the physical exam takes precedence over the history). Very often, doctors will base 80 percent of their diagnosis upon the history. As a result, it is important for you to question the patient, family members, and bystanders (Figure 47-2). However, you must not allow your knowledge of the disease—or your suspicion of the underlying problem—to affect the quality of the history you gather. Just because a patient has had a heart attack in the past does not mean that the person is having one now. Focus your questioning on the present complaint and associated problems.

The Physical Exam

Never forget, or minimize, the importance of a thorough physical exam, especially when there is the possibility of trauma. Although the physical exam may be compromised by field conditions, it should never be done in a cursory manner. Even when you are dealing with angry family members or are in a bad physical environment, you must perform an effective examination. If field conditions make the exam difficult or nearly impossible, you may have to move the patient into the ambulance or some other controlled environment in order to perform the exam. If the patient is unresponsive or if there is a significant mechanism of injury, perform a complete head-to-toe assessment. If a patient is a responsive medical patient or has suffered minor trauma, focus your exam on the systems associated with the patient's chief complaint.

Pattern Recognition

In assessing a patient, remain alert to patterns. Compare the information that you gather with your knowledge base—what you have learned about the pathophysiology and presentation of various diseases and injuries. For example, a trauma patient with decreased mental status, unequal pupils, swelling or discoloration around the eyes, and bleeding from the ear is presenting a pattern typical of basilar skull fracture. A patient who complains of a cough, gradual onset of breathing difficulty, sharp chest pain, and shaking chills with an elevated temperature is displaying a pattern typical of pneumonia. There may be times when you don't recognize a pattern. Obviously, the greater your knowledge base, the greater the likelihood you will recognize patterns. The ability to recognize patterns also increases with experience, which is why new paramedics are generally assigned to work with experienced paramedics for a time.

Assessment/Field Diagnosis

Sometimes your field diagnosis will be based on a combination of pattern recognition and intuition, which is also based on experience. Once you have determined the problem, your next step is to formulate a plan of action, based upon the patient's condition and the environment.

BLS/ALS Protocols

All EMS systems have protocols devised by the medical director that guide both BLS and ALS patient care. However, protocols and standing orders do not replace the paramedic's judgment. For example, you must exercise judgment, based on your assessment and field diagnosis, to know which protocol to use. You must exercise judgment to know when and how to follow a protocol—and you must also exercise judgment about when to deviate from a protocol. If a patient is allergic to a medication, for example, you do not administer it, even though a protocol calls for its use.

FACTORS AFFECTING ASSESSMENT AND DECISION MAKING

A number of factors—both internal (for example, your personal attitudes) and external (for example, the patient's attitude, distracting injuries, or environmental factors at the scene)—can affect your assessment of the patient and ultimately your decisions on how to manage treatment. By keeping these factors in mind, you can avoid the limitations that they impose on your collection and evaluation of patient information.

Personal Attitudes

You must be as nonjudgmental as possible to avoid "short circuiting" accurate data collection and the recognition of patterns.

Your attitude is one of the most critical factors in performing an effective assessment. You must be as nonjudgmental as possible to avoid "short circuiting" accurate data collection and pattern recognition by leaping to conclusions before completing a thorough assessment. Remember the popular computer mnemonic GIGO—garbage in/garbage out. You can't reach valid conclusions about your patient based on a hasty or incomplete assessment. You will be unable to provide good medical management if, for example, you base decisions on the patient's social standing or "likability."

Seek to identify any preconceived notions that you may have about a group and then work to eliminate them. As mentioned in Chapter 43, for example, a number of signs and symptoms have been mistakenly ascribed to aging when in

FIGURE 47-3   In treating substance abuse patients, maintain a nonjudgmental attitude.

fact they may point to serious medical conditions. A preconception that decreased mental acuity in an elderly patient is "normal" may lead you to miss what is really wrong with this patient and cause you to provide inadequate care.

Uncooperative Patients

Admittedly, uncooperative patients make it difficult to perform good assessments. All too often these patients are perceived as being "high," either on alcohol or drugs. However, you must remember that there are many other possible causes for patient belligerence.

Whenever assessing an uncooperative or restless patient, consider medical causes—hypoxia, hypovolemia, hypoglycemia, or a head injury, such as a concussion or a subdural hematoma. Be careful not to jump to the conclusion that this patient is "just another drunk" or a "frequent flyer." The frequent flyer that you have transported for alcoholic behavior in the past may, this time, be suffering from trauma or a medical emergency.

If the person is in fact a substance abuser, keep in mind that abuse or addiction is an illness. No matter how difficult these patients are to manage, they still deserve the best care that you can provide (Figure 47-3). If you treat every patient in the manner in which you would want your loved ones treated, you will seldom go wrong.

If you treat every patient in the manner in which you would want your loved ones treated, you will never go wrong.

Patient Compliance

Not all patients welcome the sight of an ALS team. Cultural and ethnic barriers—as well as prior negative experiences—may cause a patient to lack confidence in the rescuers. Such situations make it difficult for you to be effective at the scene, and the patients in fact may refuse to provide expressed consent for treatment or transport. It is your job to treat the patients in a way that will increase their confidence. If language is a barrier, try to speak through a friend, relative, or bystander who understands the patient's language, or in the case of deafness, signs. If you live in a community with a large ethnic population, try to become familiar with body language and customs of that culture. For example, some groups consider it rude to make eye contact. (For more on culturally diverse patients, see Chapter 45.) Again, don't permit yourself to make snap judgments about the patient.

Distracting Injuries

Yet another factor that can affect your assessment and decisions involves obvious, but distracting injuries. A nasty-looking tibial fracture might cause the paramedic to overlook the less obvious signs of internal bleeding. Scalp lacerations usually look worse than they really are and could divert your attention from more serious injuries, such as an open chest wound. You must resist the temptation to form a field diagnosis too early. While paramedics often have to rely on their "gut instinct," it may also lead them to make snap judgments. An open, bleeding fracture of the femur may be so distracting that a paramedic rushes to treat it, missing the fact that the patient is also having difficulty breathing. Always take a systematic approach to patient assessment to avoid distractions and to find and prioritize care for all of the patient's injuries and conditions.

Environmental and Personnel Considerations

You've probably already experienced some of the environmental factors that can affect patient assessment and care. Among others, they include scene chaos, violent or dangerous situations, high noise levels, or crowds of bystanders. Even crowds of responders can be a problem, in some instances.

A large number of rescuers moving around can be just as distracting as a large number of bystanders.

While having enough help is crucial, it is also important to use personnel wisely (Figure 47-4). A large number of rescuers moving around can be just as distracting as a large number of bystanders. In such situations, some of the rescuers might be staged nearby and brought to the scene when and if necessary. Some may also be assigned to control bystanders.

As a rule, assessment is best achieved by one rescuer. A single paramedic can gather information and provide treatment sequentially. In the case of two paramedics, one paramedic can assess the patient, while the other provides simultaneous treatment. With multiple responders, however, assessment and history may take place by "committee," which often leads to disorganized management.

FIGURE 47-4 When multiple responders are on the scene, everyone should have a designated task.

ASSESSMENT/MANAGEMENT CHOREOGRAPHY

While too many people, or multiple-tier responders, may make it hard to acquire a patient history and conduct a physical exam, it becomes even more difficult if the responders are all at the same professional level and have no clear direction. It is important to plan for these events so that personnel have predesignated roles. (See Chapter 48 on incident command.) These roles may be rotated among team members so no one is left out, but there must be a plan to avoid "freelancing." If there is only one paramedic, then that person must assume all ALS roles.

In the case of a two-paramedic team, an effective preplan involves the roles of team leader and patient care provider, assigned on an alternating basis. Paramedics who work together regularly may develop their own plan, but a universally understood plan allows for other rescuers to participate in a rescue without interrupting the flow. While the dynamics of field situations may necessitate changes in plans, a general "game plan" can go a long way toward preventing chaos. If field dynamics dictate a change in the preplanned roles, you are still working from a solid base. In setting up a two-person team, keep in mind the following descriptions of team leader and patient care provider roles.

Team Leader

The team leader is usually the person who will accompany the patient through to definitive care. The paramedic charged with this role should establish contact and maintain dialogue with the patient. He or she obtains the history, performs the physical examination, and presents the patient, in both verbal and written reports. During multiple casualty situations, the team leader acts as the initial EMS commander.

The team leader must maintain overall patient perspective and provide leadership to the team by designating tasks and coordinating transportation. While the team leader must actively participate in critical interventions, it is important that this person not fall into the trap of trying to do everything alone. During ACLS calls, for example, the team leader's tasks might include the following: reading the ECG, talking on the radio and giving drug orders, controlling the drug box, and keeping notes on drug administrations and effects. Actual treatment, however, would be left to the designated patient care provider.

Patient Care Provider

The patient care provider should ensure "scene cover"—i.e., watching the team leader's back. This person should gather scene information, talk to relatives and bystanders, and obtain vital signs. The patient care provider performs any skills or interventions requested by the team leader, such as attaching monitoring leads, administering oxygen, obtaining venous access, administering medications, and securing transportation equipment. In multiple casualty situations, the patient care provider acts as the triage group leader. During ACLS calls, he or she administers drugs, monitors tube placement, and oversees BCLS.

THE RIGHT EQUIPMENT

Having the right equipment at the patient's side is essential. As a paramedic, you must be prepared to manage many conditions and injuries or changes in the patient's condition. As already mentioned, assessment and management must usually be done simultaneously. If you do not have the right equipment readily available, then you have compromised patient care and, in fact, the patient may die.

If you do not have the right equipment readily available, you have compromised patient care.

Think of your equipment as items in a backpack. Just like backpacking, you must downsize your equipment to minimum weight and bulk to facilitate rapid movement. At the same time, you need certain essential equipment to ensure survival—in this case, patient survival. The following is a list of the essential equipment for paramedic management of life-threatening conditions. You must bring these items to the side of every patient, regardless of what you initially think you may need:

- Infection Control
  - Infection control supplies—e.g., gloves, eye shields
- Airway Control
  - Oral airways
  - Nasal airways
  - Suction (electric or manual)
  - Rigid tonsil-tip and flexible suction catheters
  - Laryngoscope and blades
  - Endotracheal tubes, stylettes, syringes, tape
- Breathing
  - Pocket mask
  - Manual ventilation bag-valve-mask
  - Spare masks in various sizes
  - Oxygen tank and regulator
  - Oxygen masks, cannulas, and extension tubing
  - Occlusive dressings
  - Large bore IV catheter for thoracic decompression
- Circulation
  - Dressings
  - Bandages and tape
  - Sphygmomanometer, stethoscope
  - Note pad and pen or pencil
- Disability
  - Rigid collars
  - Flashlight
- Dysrhythmia
  - Cardiac monitor/defibrillator
- Exposure and Protection
  - Scissors
  - Space blankets or something to cover the patient

You may also pack some optional "take in" equipment, such as drug therapy and venous access supplies. The method by which these supplies are carried may depend upon how your system is designed—e.g., paramedic ambulances versus paramedics in non-transporting vehicles. It may also depend upon local protocols, flexibility of standing orders, the number of paramedic responders in your area, and the difficulty of accessing patients because of terrain or some other problem.

In most cases, venous access supplies should be carried with the drug box since venous access is required to administer most medications. The drug box should also contain any medications allowed in the formulary.

GENERAL APPROACH TO THE PATIENT

In addition to having the essential equipment, you need to have the essential demeanor to calm or reassure the patient. You must look and act the part of a professional, while exhibiting the compassion and understanding associated with an effective "bedside manner." While patients may not have the ability to rate your medical performance, they can certainly rate your people skills and service. Be aware of your body language and the messages it sends, either intentionally or unintentionally. Think carefully about what you say and how you say it—this includes your conversations with other members of the ALS team and anyone else at the scene.

Once again, it helps to preplan your general approach to the patient. This will prevent confusion and improve the accuracy of your assessment. One team member should engage in an active, concerned dialogue with the patient. This same person should also demonstrate the listening skills needed to collect information and to convey a caring attitude. Taking notes may prevent asking the same question repeatedly, as well as ensure that you acquire and pass on accurate data.

By approaching the patient with the right equipment and the right attitude, you minimize confusion and stand ready to provide effective emergency care.

The following sections briefly review the steps of the assessment that you will perform systematically on all patients. To review the assessment steps in detail, see Chapter 12.

Be aware of your body language and the messages it sends, either intentionally or unintentionally.

SCENE SIZE-UP

The scene size up has the following components:

- Body substance isolation—Be sure you are wearing disposable gloves and are wearing or have available other protective equipment that may be needed such as gown, mask, and eye protection.
- Scene safety—Observe the scene for any hazards to yourself, other rescuers, bystanders, and the patient. This is as important at a medical scene as at a trauma scene.
- Locate all patients, such as those who may have wandered away from a vehicle collision or additional patients in a household where the patient appears to be suffering from carbon monoxide or other toxic exposure.
- Mechanism of injury or nature of the illness—Determine this as well as possible at this stage of the call and remain observant for additional information as the call progresses.

If you determine that you may need additional equipment or support, now is the time to call for help.

INITIAL ASSESSMENT

After you size up the scene, you quickly begin the initial assessment for the purpose of detecting and treating immediate life threats. The components of the initial assessment are:

- Forming a general impression
- Mental status assessment (AVPU)
- Airway assessment
- Breathing assessment
- Circulation assessment
- Determining the patient's priority for further on-scene care or immediate transport

Depending on your findings during the initial assessment, you might determine that one of the following approaches is appropriate for the patient's priority status.

Resuscitative Approach

Take the resuscitation approach whenever you suspect a life-threatening problem, including:

- Cardiac or respiratory arrest
- Respiratory distress or failure
- Unstable dysrhythmias
- Status epilepticus (series of generalized motor seizures without an intervening return of consciousness)
- Coma or altered mental status
- Shock or hypotension
- Major trauma
- Possible C-spine injury

In these cases, you must take immediate resuscitative action (such as CPR and defibrillation and ventilation) or other critical action (such as supplemental oxygen, control of major bleeding, or C-spine immobilization). Additional assessment and care can be performed after resuscitation and the rapid trauma assessment and/or en route to the hospital.

Contemplative Approach

Use the contemplative approach when immediate intervention is not necessary, such as with stable chest pain or a mild allergic reaction. In such situations, the focused history and physical exam, followed by any required interventions, will be performed at the scene, before transport to the hospital.

Immediate Evacuation

In some situations, you will need to immediately evacuate the patient to the ambulance (Figure 47-5). For example, a patient with severe internal bleeding requires life-saving interventions beyond a paramedic's skills. You might also resort to immediate evacuation if the scene is too chaotic for rational assessment or if it is too unsafe or unstable.

FIGURE 47-5 High-priority patients require immediate evacuation, with continued assessment and care done en route.

FOCUSED HISTORY AND PHYSICAL EXAM

Following the initial assessment, you will perform the focused history and physical exam. Based on the patient's chief complaint and the information you have gathered during the initial assessment, you should consider your patient to belong to one of the following four categories:

- Trauma patient with a significant mechanism of injury or altered mental status
- Trauma patient with an isolated injury
- Medical patient who is responsive
- Medical patient who is unresponsive

For a trauma patient with a significant mechanism of injury or altered mental status or for an unresponsive medical patient, perform a complete head-to-toe physical examination (rapid trauma assessment for the trauma patient, rapid medical assessment for the medical patient). For the trauma patient with an isolated injury or for the responsive medical patient, perform a physical exam focused on body systems related to the chief complaint.

For a medical patient, gather the history before performing the physical exam, unless the patient is unable to provide a history and there are no family members or bystanders who can provide information. For a trauma patient, gather the history after you have performed the physical exam. (Of course, elements of the history and the physical exam are often obtained simultaneously if partners are working together or as you talk to the responsive patient while examining him.)

THE ONGOING ASSESSMENT AND THE DETAILED PHYSICAL EXAM

The ongoing assessment must be performed on all patients to monitor and to observe trends in the patient's condition—every 5 minutes if the patient is unstable, every 15 minutes if the patient is stable. Ongoing assessments must be performed until the patient is transferred to the care of hospital personnel. The ongoing assessment includes evaluation of the following:

- Mental status
- Airway, breathing, and circulation (ABCs)
- Transport priorities
- Vital signs
- Focused assessment of any problem areas or conditions
- Effectiveness of interventions
- Management plans

The detailed physical exam is similar to but more thorough than the rapid trauma assessment. It is generally performed only on trauma patients and only if time and the patient's condition permit. The purpose is to find any injuries or conditions that may have been missed during earlier assessments. In a critical patient, continuing ongoing assessments are more important than a detailed physical exam.

IDENTIFICATION OF LIFE-THREATENING PROBLEMS

At all stages of the assessment, from initial assessment through ongoing assessments, from the scene to the ambulance to arrival at the hospital, you must actively and continuously look for and manage any life-threatening problems.

You need to rapidly determine the chief complaint and to assess the distress in a systematic manner. Obtain baseline vital signs along with the focused physical exam, but if partners are working together, one may obtain the baseline vital signs earlier in the assessment. Focus on the relevant portions of the history and the physical findings. For example, a history of appendicitis would be relevant for a patient complaining of right lower quadrant pain, less relevant for a trauma patient with possible spinal injury.

If you have an educated suspicion of what you are looking for, then you will be able to ask more productive questions. However, you are less likely to find something if you don't suspect it. For this reason, throughout your assessment, keep in mind the mechanism of injury and the nature of the illness (as determined, starting with the initial assessment and the patient's chief complaint). Listen carefully to everything the patient says. With experience, you will develop skill at "multi-tasking"—asking questions, listening to answers, and caring for the patient almost simultaneously. However, until you gain that experience, and unless you are actively managing a life-threatening condition, ask questions and just listen. Allow your partner to perform necessary tasks so that you do not miss any important clues.

The ability of a patient to describe symptoms and a paramedic's ability to listen greatly affect the quality and outcome of an assessment. The severity of pain does not always correlate well with the life-threatening potential of a condition. For example, a long splinter jammed under a fingernail will certainly cause pain, but few lives have been lost to such an injury. Conversely, some patients, especially the elderly, suffer myocardial infarctions with only vague symptoms that do not include chest pain. In addition, the location of pain and its source do not always correlate well, especially if it is visceral pain. For example, gall bladder attacks are often characterized by pain that is referred to the shoulder. As a paramedic, you must listen with your ears and then use your knowledge base about various illnesses and diseases to interpret what the patient says.

Basically your role as paramedic is to rapidly and accurately assess the patient and then to treat for the worst case scenario. This is the underlying principle of assessment-based management—your guide for providing effective emergency care.

PRESENTING THE PATIENT

The ability to communicate effectively is the key to transferring patient information, whether in an out-of-hospital setting or within the hospital itself. Although neither basic nor advanced life-support interventions may be required for every patient, a skill that will be used on every single patient is that of effective presentation, whether it is over the radio or telephone, in writing, or in face-to-face transfers at the receiving facility. Despite the frequency with which paramedics present patients, this is often the weakest link in patient care.

ESTABLISHING TRUST AND CREDIBILITY

Effective presentation and communication skills help establish a paramedic's credibility (Figure 47-6). They also inspire the trust and confidence of patients and other medical personnel. If you present your assessment, your findings, and your treatment in a clear, concise manner, you give the impression of a job well done. A poor presentation, on the other hand, implies poor assessment and poor patient care.

FIGURE 47-6 A clear, concise patient report will enable the hospital staff to prepare for the needs of the patient.

Other health care providers have little time or interest in listening to rambling, disjointed presentations that cover unimportant details while omitting vital information. Use the SOAP format or some variation of it. Not only does SOAP help you organize your presentation, most health care providers have become accustomed to listening to it and know what to expect. (SOAP stands for *s*ubjective, *o*bjective, *a*ssessment, and *p*lan. For a detailed description, see Chapter 15.)

The way in which you present the patient has direct implications for the person's care and recovery. Poor presentations compromise patient care. They lead to incomplete or even incorrect medical orders. If you do not communicate a patient's needs or status completely or accurately, a person may be denied some form of treatment based on the information that you have conveyed.

As a paramedic, you will be an extension of the supervisory physician, working under his or her license. No doctor is going to issue orders for medications or other patient care based on guesswork. You are the doctor's eyes and ears at the emergency scene, and it is essential that you provide accurate information about both the patient and the emergency situation.

Poor presentations compromise patient care.

DEVELOPING EFFECTIVE PRESENTATION SKILLS

The most effective oral presentations usually meet these guidelines:

- Last less than one minute
- Are very concise and clear
- Avoid extensive use of medical jargon
- Follow a basic format, usually the SOAP format or some variation
- Include both pertinent findings and pertinent negatives (findings that might be expected, given the patient's complaint or condition, but are absent or denied by the patient)
- Conclude with specific actions, requests, or questions related to the plan

The best way to become proficient at presenting patients is to plan ahead and to practice. Start with an end in mind—know what particular areas of information will be asked for or expected so that you can be ready with that information. As you become more experienced, the flow of information will become second nature to you. Until that time, use a pre-printed form to help you organize your thoughts and information and to take notes during the patient work-up. Practice presenting both simulated and real patients, perhaps at company or unit drills. Listen to other paramedics as they present patients and learn from them. Adopt their good habits and avoid their bad ones.

An ideal presentation should include the following:

- Patient identification, age, sex, and degree of distress
- Chief complaint (why a patient called)
- Present illness/injury
  - Pertinent details about the present problem
  - Pertinent negatives
- Past medical history
  - Allergies
  - Medications
  - Pertinent medical history
- Physical signs
  - Vital signs
  - Pertinent positive findings
  - Pertinent negative findings

Plan ahead. Know what particular areas of information will be asked for or expected so that you can be ready with that information.

- Assessment
  - Paramedic impression
- Plan
  - What has been done
  - Orders requested

Remember, the key to developing presentation skills is repetition and an understanding of the format being used. Once you have mastered this, you can transfer the patient with the satisfaction and confidence of a job well done. (For more detail on this topic, review Chapters 14 and 15 on communications and documentation.)

REVIEW OF COMMON COMPLAINTS

In order to develop as an entry-level practitioner at the paramedic level, it is important to participate in scenario-based reviews of commonly encountered complaints. As mentioned, you might take part in company or unit drills in which you will observe and work with experienced paramedics. You might also participate in laboratory-based simulations.

PRACTICE SESSIONS

The goal of practice sessions is to choreograph the roles and actions of the EMS response team. These sessions will give you the chance to practice assessment and decision making on cases that you are likely to encounter in out-of-hospital situations. They also give you the opportunity to provide intervention based upon your assessment and to reinforce the modalities in local and/or regional treatment protocols. Finally, you can practice patient presentation, both verbally and in written form. At all phases, you get the benefit of feedback from the team members and crew with whom you will be working.

LABORATORY-BASED SIMULATIONS

Laboratory-based simulations require you to assess a pre-programmed patient or mannequin. You will make decisions relative to interventions and transportation. You will also provide interventions, package the patient (or mannequin), and transport. Ideally, you will work as part of a team and practice the various roles assigned to team members, including that of patient.

SELF-MOTIVATION

The chance to practice does not stop at the classroom or at your unit. While a paramedic student or the new member of a team, take advantage of every opportunity to practice your new skills. Recruit family members or friends—or even a teddy bear—as volunteer patients. What is important is to practice, practice, practice until you feel comfortable with as many different situations as possible.

Summary

Assessment forms the basis of patient care. In order to make correct decisions, you must gather information and then evaluate and synthesize it. A variety of factors may affect assessment and the decision-making process itself. Some of these factors include paramedic attitude; uncooperative patients; obvious, but distracting injuries; narrow, or tunnel, vision; the environment; patient compliance; and personnel considerations.

It is important to have the right equipment readily available to treat immediately life-threatening conditions. Effective communication and transfer of patient information—whether done face to face, over the telephone or radio, or in writing—is crucial to presenting the patient and assuring continuation of effective care.

Remember, the best way to develop good assessment skills is to practice until you become comfortable with a wide range of patient complaints.

CHAPTER 48

Operations

Objectives

Part 1: Ambulance Operations (begins on p. 1940)

After reading Part 1 of this chapter, you should be able to:

1. Identify current local and state standards that influence ambulance design, equipment requirements, and staffing of ambulances. (pp. 1940–1942)

2. Discuss the importance of completing an ambulance equipment/supply checklist. (pp. 1942–1943)

3. Discuss factors used to determine ambulance stationing and staffing within a community. (pp. 1943–1944)

4. Describe the advantages and disadvantages of air medical transport and identify conditions/situations in which air medical transport should be considered. (pp. 1949–1952)

Part 2: Medical Incident Command (begins on p. 1953)

After reading Part 2 of this chapter, you should be able to:

1. Explain the need for the incident management system (IMS)/incident command system (ICS) in managing emergency medical services incidents. (pp. 1953, 1954)

2. Define the terms multiple casualty incident (MCI), disaster management, open or uncontained incident, and closed or contained incident. (pp. 1953, 1956, 1969)

Continued

3. Describe essential elements of the scene size-up when arriving at a potential MCI. (p. 1956)
4. Describe the role of the paramedics and EMS system in planning for MCIs and disasters. (pp. 1954–1956, 1970, 1971)
5. Describe the functional components (command, finance, logistics, operations, and planning) of the incident management system. (pp. 1954–1960)
6. Differentiate between singular and unified command and identify when each is most applicable. (p. 1955)
7. Describe the role of command, the need for command transfer, and procedures for transferring it. (pp. 1954, 1955–1956, 1958)
8. Differentiate between incident command structures used at small, medium, and large-scale incidents. (pp. 1954–1955)
9. Explain the local/regional threshold for establishing command and implementation of the incident management system including MCI declaration. (pp. 1954–1955)
10. List and describe the functions of the following groups and leaders in ICS as it pertains to EMS incidents: safety, logistics, rehabilitation/rehab, staging, treatment, triage, transportation, extrication/rescue, disposition of deceased/morgue, and communications. (pp. 1957, 1959–1960, 1962–1969)
11. Describe the methods and rationale for identifying specific functions and leaders for the functions in ICS. (pp. 1954–1955, 1957–1958)
12. Describe the role of both command posts and emergency operations centers in MCI and disaster management. (pp. 1955–1956, 1958, 1960)

13. Describe the role of the on-scene physician at multiple casualty incidents. (p. 1967)
14. Define triage and describe the principles of triage. (pp. 1962–1963, 1964–1966)
15. Describe the START (simple triage and rapid transport) method of initial triage. (pp. 1963–1964)
16. Given color-coded tags and numerical priorities, assign the following terms to each: immediate, delayed, hold, deceased. (pp. 1962–1963, 1964–1965)
17. Define primary and secondary triage and describe when primary and secondary triage techniques should be implemented. (pp. 1962–1963)
18. Describe need for and techniques used in tracking patients during multiple casualty incidents. (pp. 1958, 1963–1965, 1968)
19. Describe techniques used to allocate patients to hospitals and track them. (pp. 1967–1968)
20. Describe modifications of telecommunications procedures during multiple casualty incidents. (pp. 1957, 1968–1969, 1976)
21. List and describe the essential equipment to provide logistical support to MCI operations to include: airway, respiratory, and hemorrhage control; burn management; patient packaging/immobilization. (p. 1966)
22. List the physical and psychological signs of critical incident stress and describe the role of critical incident stress management sessions in MCIs. (pp. 1960, 1968, 1972)
23. Describe the role of table top exercises and small and large MCI drills in preparation for MCIs. (p. 1971)

Part 3: Rescue Awareness and Operations (begins on p. 1972)

After reading Part 3 of this chapter, you should be able to:

1. Define the term rescue, and explain the medical and mechanical aspects of rescue operations. (pp. 1970–1971)
2. Describe the phases of a rescue operation, and the role of the paramedic at each phase. (pp. 1977–1980)
3. List and describe the personal protective equipment needed to safely operate in the rescue environment to

include: head, eye, and hand protection; personal flotation devices; thermal protection/layering systems; high visibility clothing. (pp. 1973–1975)

4. Explain the risks and complications associated with rescues involving moving water, low head dams, flat water, trenches, motor vehicles, and confined spaces. (pp. 1981–1987, 1988–1995)

5. Explain the effects of immersion hypothermia on the ability to survive sudden immersion and self rescue. (pp. 1981–1982)

6. Explain the benefits and disadvantages of water-entry or "go techniques" versus the reach-throw-row-go approach to water rescue. (p. 1982)

7. Explain the self rescue position if unexpectedly immersed in moving water. (pp. 1982, 1985)

8. Describe the use of apparatus placement, headlights and emergency vehicle lighting, cone and flare placement, and reflective and high visibility clothing to reduce scene risk at highway incidents. (pp. 1990–1991)

9. List and describe the design element hazards and associated protective actions associated with autos and trucks, including energy-absorbing bumpers, air bag/supplemental restraint systems, catalytic converters, and conventional and non-conventional fuel systems. (pp. 1991–1992)

10. Given a diagram of a passenger auto, identify the A, B, C, and D posts, fire wall, and unibody versus frame construction. (p. 1993)

11. Explain the difference between tempered and safety glass, identify its locations on a vehicle, and describe how to break it. (p. 1993)

12. Explain typical door anatomy and methods to access through stuck doors. (p. 1993)

13. Describe methods for emergency stabilization using rope, cribbing, jacks, spare tires, and come-a-longs for vehicles found in various positions. (pp. 1992, 1994–1995)

14. Describe electrical and other hazards commonly found at highway incidents (above and below the ground). (pp. 1991–1992)

15. Define low-angle rescue, high-angle rescue, belay, rappel, scrambling, and hasty rope slide. (pp. 1995–1996)

16. Describe the procedure for Stokes litter packaging for low-angle evacuations. (pp. 1996–1997)

17. Explain anchoring, litter/rope attachment, and lowering and raising procedures as they apply to low-angle litter evacuation. (pp. 1996, 1998)

18. Explain techniques used in non-technical litter carries over rough terrain. (p. 1998)

19. Explain non-technical high-angle rescue procedures using aerial apparatus. (p. 1998)

20. Explain assessment and care modifications (including pain medication, temperature control, and hydration) necessary for attending entrapped patients. (pp. 1999–2000)

21. List the equipment necessary for an "off road" medical pack. (pp. 1975, 2000)

22. Explain the different types of "Stokes" or basket stretchers and the advantages and disadvantages associated with each. (pp. 1996–1997)

23. Given a list of rescue scenarios, provide the victim survivability profile and identify which are rescue versus body recovery situations. (pp. 1972–2000)

24. Given a series of pictures, identify those considered "confined spaces" and potentially oxygen deficient. (pp. 1988–1990)

Part 4: Hazardous Materials Incidents (begins on p. 2001)

After reading Part 4 of this chapter, you should be able to:

1. Explain the role of the paramedic/EMS responder at the hazardous material incident. (pp. 2001–2002)

2. Identify resources for substance identification, decontamination, and treatment information. (pp. 2006–2008)

3. Identify primary and secondary decontamination risk. (p. 2011)
4. Describe topical, respiratory, gastrointestinal, and parenteral routes of exposure. (p. 2011)
5. Explain acute and delayed toxicity, local versus systemic effects, dose response, and synergistic effects. (pp. 2011–2012)
6. Explain how the substance and route of contamination alters triage and decontamination methods. (pp. 2014–2015)
7. Explain the employment and limitations of field decontamination procedures. (pp. 2016–2017)
8. Explain the use and limitations of personal protective equipment (PPE) in hazardous material situations. (pp. 2017–2018)
9. List and explain the common signs, symptoms, and treatment of exposures to corrosives, pulmonary irritants, pesticides, chemical asphyxiants, and hydrocarbon solvents. (pp. 2011–2014)
10. Describe the characteristics of hazardous materials and explain their importance to the risk assessment process. (pp. 2001, 2002–2009, 2015–2016)
11. Describe the hazards and protection strategies for alpha, beta, and gamma radiation. (p. 2010)
12. Define the toxicologic terms and their use in the risk assessment process. (p. 2010)
13. Given a specific hazardous material, research the appropriate information about its physical and chemical properties and hazards, suggest the appropriate medical response, and determine the risk of secondary contamination. (pp. 2006–2008)
14. Identify the factors that determine where and when to treat a hazardous material incident patient. (pp. 2008–2009, 2015–2016)
15. Determine the appropriate level of PPE for various hazardous material incidents. (pp. 2017–2018)
16. Explain decontamination procedures including critical patient rapid two-step decontamination and non-critical patient eight-step decontamination. (pp. 2016–2017)
17. Identify the four most common solutions used for decontamination. (p. 2016)
18. Identify the body areas that are difficult to decontaminate. (p. 2016)
19. Explain the medical monitoring procedures for hazardous material team members. (pp. 2018–2019)
20. Explain the factors that influence the heat stress of hazardous material team personnel. (p. 2019)
21. Explain the documentation necessary for hazmat medical monitoring and rehabilitation operations. (pp. 2018–2019)
22. Given a stimulated hazardous substance, use reference material to determine the appropriate actions. (pp. 2006–2008)
23. Integrate the principles and practices of hazardous materials response in an effective manner to prevent and limit contamination, morbidity, and mortality. (pp. 2001–2019)
24. Size up a hazardous material (hazmat) incident and determine: potential hazards to the rescuers, public, and environment and potential risk of primary contamination to patients and secondary contamination to rescuers. (pp. 2002–2009, 2010–2018)
25. Given a contaminated patient, determine the necessary level of decontamination, level of rescuer PPE, decontamination methods, treatment, and transportation and patient isolation techniques. (pp. 2012–2018)
26. Determine the hazards present to the patient and paramedic given an incident involving a hazardous material (pp. 2001–2019)

Part 5: Crime Scene Awareness (begins on p. 2019)

After reading Part 5 of this chapter, you should be able to:

1. Explain how EMS providers are often mistaken for the police. (pp. 2020, 2025)
2. Explain specific techniques for risk reduction when approaching highway encounters, violent street

incidents, residences, and "dark houses." (pp. 2020–2021, 2023–2026)

3. Describe the warning signs of potentially violent situations. (pp. 2020–2021, 2023–2025)

4. Explain emergency evasive techniques for potentially violent situations, including threats of physical violence, firearms encounters, and edged weapons encounters. (pp. 2020–2031)

5. Explain EMS considerations for the following types of violent or potentially violent situations: gangs and gang violence, hostages/sniper situations, clandestine drug labs, domestic violence, and emotionally disturbed people. (pp. 2020–2026)

6. Explain the following techniques: field "contact and cover" procedures during assessment and care, evasive tactics, and concealment techniques. (pp. 2026–2031)

7. Describe police evidence considerations and techniques to assist in evidence preservation (pp. 2031–2033)

8. Given several crime scene scenarios, identify potential hazards and determine if the scene is safe to enter, then provide care preserving the crime scene as appropriate. (pp. 1940–2033)

INTRODUCTION

While patient care is your core responsibility as a paramedic, operations are also a critical part of your job. You are already familiar with many aspects of EMS operations through your prior EMT-Basic training and your experience. However, because the safety of so many people—the EMS team, patients, and bystanders—depends on effective and efficient operations, it is important to review and practice operational procedures regularly so that they become second nature and can be performed smoothly, especially during a high-stress emergency.

This chapter discusses the paramedic responsibilities involved in five aspects of EMS operations: Part 1, Ambulance Operations; Part 2, Medical Incident Command; Part 3, Rescue Awareness and Operations; Part 4, Hazardous Materials Incidents; and Part 5, Crime Scene Awareness.

Part 1: Ambulance Operations

Good ambulance operations depend upon effective ambulance maintenance as well as operations. In addition to the communication and dispatch skills described in Chapter 14, you should be proficient in these five areas: ambulance standards, maintenance of ambulance equipment and supplies, ambulance stationing, safe ambulance operations, and the utilization of air medical transport.

AMBULANCE STANDARDS

Oversight for EMS usually falls to state governments, and state statutes lay out many of the requirements for ambulance service. National standards and trends influence these laws. Typically, state laws are broad, while corresponding regulations provide more specific guidelines or rules. For example, a public health law may authorize the state department of health to issue regulations through its EMS Bureau. These regulations, known as the "state EMS code," might then handle such matters as the **essential equipment** to be carried on ambulances.

Government standards tend to be generic enough so that they are "palatable," affordable, and politically feasible to all EMS agencies in the state. States usually set **minimum standards,** rather than a **gold standard,** for operation. In other words, they establish the lowest level at which units will be allowed to op-

* **essential equipment** equipment/supplies required on every ambulance.

* **minimum standards** lowest or least allowable standards.

* **gold standard** ultimate standard of excellence.

FIGURE 48-1 Four types of ambulances. (a) Type I. (b) Type II. (c) Type III. (d) Medium duty.

erate. The regulations written by local and/or regional EMS systems tend to be much more detailed and often approach a gold standard.

AMBULANCE DESIGN

The U.S. General Services Administration Automotive Commodity Center issues the federal regulations that specify ambulance design and manufacturing requirements. These specs—known as the **DOT KKK 1822D specs**—attempt to influence safety standards as well as standardize the look of ambulances. Over the years, the "KKK specifications" have had a significant influence on ambulance manufacturing. They describe the following three basic ambulance designs:

* *Type I*—conventional truck cab-chassis with modular body.
* *Type II*—standard van, forward control integral cab-body.
* *Type III*—specialty van, forward control integral cab-body.

In addition to these three designs (Figure 48-1), there is also a medium duty ambulance rescue vehicle. It is designed to handle heavier loads and has a gross weight of approximately 24,000 pounds.

The federal specifications provide standards for ambulances used by the federal government and also provide guidelines for the states. Massachusetts, for example, refers to the federal specifications in its state regulations. In such cases, the federal specifications become the state standard. Some states, including Connecticut, Vermont, and New Jersey, have developed their own standards, often

✱ **DOT KKK 1822D specs** the manufacturing and design specifications produced by the Federal General Services Administrative Automotive Commodity Center.

using the federal specifications as the basis. A few states, such as New York, use neither federal nor state specifications. Instead, the decisions for ambulance purchases are made locally or regionally.

Other agencies and organizations also influence standards. Air ambulance standards are designed with input from representatives of the National Flight Nurses Association (NFNA) and the National Flight Paramedics Association (NFPA). The Federal Communications Commission (FCC) specifies radio bands and types of equipment that may be used in ambulances.

MEDICAL EQUIPMENT STANDARDS

As the agency charged with protecting worker safety, the Occupational Safety and Health Administration (OSHA) has helped ensure ambulance equipment lists that include disinfecting agents, sharps containers, red bag, HEPA masks, and personal protective equipment. The National Institute for Occupational Safety and Health (NIOSH) has established similar standards. Other voluntary standards have been set by peer organizations, such as the National Fire Protection Association (NFPA). Often, these standards are incorporated in local ordinances.

Local medical direction boards sometimes list the medications paramedics can carry as well as ALS equipment and supplies that should be on every ambulance. For example, where paramedics are trained to obtain a 12-lead ECG, the board may specify the brand of equipment in order to standardize care.

ADDITIONAL GUIDELINES

At the national level, the Commission on Accreditation of Ambulance Services (CAAS) provides a voluntary "gold standard" for EMS. CAAS requires that onboard medical equipment and supplies comply with state and local guidelines. In the absence of these guidelines, CAAS requires services to develop guidelines that meet or exceed those established by the American College of Surgeons (ACS). The ACS Committee of Trauma issued its first list of "essential equipment" to be carried on ambulances in 1970 and revised it in 1994.

CHECKING AMBULANCES

The shift checklist makes the work environment safer by assuring mechanical maintenance and the availability of personal protection equipment.

On each shift, an essential duty is completion of the ambulance equipment and supply checklist. A typical checklist includes:

- Patient infection control, comfort, and protection supplies
- Initial and focused assessment equipment
- Equipment for the transfer of the patient
- Equipment for airway maintenance, ventilation, and resuscitation
- Oxygen therapy and suction equipment
- Equipment for assisting with cardiac resuscitation
- Supplies and equipment for immobilization of suspected bone injuries
- Supplies for wound care and treatment of shock
- Supplies for childbirth
- Supplies, equipment, and medications for the treatment of acute poisoning, snakebite, chemical burns, and diabetic emergencies
- Advanced Life Support equipment, medications, and supplies
- Safety and miscellaneous equipment
- Information on the operation and inspection of the ambulance itself

Routine, detailed shift checks of the ambulance can minimize risks. Many services, for example, hold a "stretcher day" once a week. Routine preventative maintenance makes it less likely that a faulty stretcher will cause an injury to a patient or paramedic. Medication expiration dates should be checked each shift, and older, unexpired drugs marked so they will be used first. In services that use scheduled medications such as narcotics, paramedics should sign for these medications at the beginning and end of each shift.

As mentioned, the vehicle itself should be regularly checked. If the ambulance or any equipment needs repair, it is your responsibility to report this to your supervisor as prescribed by the SOPs for your service.

To meet OSHA requirements, you must also make sure that the ambulance has been properly disinfected after the transport of any patients with potentially communicable diseases. Most services routinely clean the ambulance after every call, and some agencies document the procedure. All services are required, either by OSHA or the state equivalent of OSHA, to have an exposure control plan that specifies cleaning requirements and the methods of cleaning up blood spills in the ambulance. If there is no specific SOP in your agency, you should document cleaning and disinfecting on the shift checklist.

Finally, you should do all scheduled tests, maintenance, and calibrations on specific medical equipment. Items that should be regularly checked include:

- Automated external defibrillator (AED)
- Glucometer
- Cardiac monitor
- Oxygen systems
- Automated transport ventilator (ATV)
- Pulse oximeter
- Suction units
- Laryngoscope blades
- Lighted stylets
- Penlights
- Any other battery operated equipment

AMBULANCE DEPLOYMENT AND STAFFING

The maneuvering of ambulances and crews to minimize response times is known as **deployment.** Deployment is based upon a number of factors: location of the facilities to house ambulances, location of hospitals, anticipated call volume, and geographic and traffic considerations. Ideally, deployment decisions take into account both past community responses and projected **demographic** changes. The highest volume of calls, or **peak load,** should be described in terms of both day of the week and time of day.

In communities that do not have multiple strategically located stations, services often deploy ambulances to wait for calls at specific high-volume locations. Such stationing locations are known as **primary areas of responsibility (PAR).** These same ambulances may be relocated throughout the day as the population moves—to work or to school—and as other ambulances in the community respond to calls. The size of a PAR may differ from a few city blocks to a larger location, such as "northeast sector of town." Size depends upon the number of ambulances available and the expected call volume. One sophisticated deployment strategy that has become popular is **system status management (SSM).** SSM is a computerized personnel and ambulance deployment system designed to meet service demands with fewer resources and to ensure appropriate response time and vehicle location.

Expiration dates on medications should be checked each shift, and the older, unexpired drugs marked appropriately so that they will be used first.

It is your responsibility to report ambulance/equipment problems or failures to your supervisor in a manner prescribed by the SOPs for your service.

Content Review

DEPLOYMENT FACTORS
Location of facilities to house ambulances
Location of hospitals
Anticipated volume of calls
Local geographic and traffic considerations

✱ **deployment** strategy used by an EMS agency to maneuver its ambulances and crews in an effort to reduce response times.

✱ **demographic** pertaining to population makeup or changes.

✱ **peak load** the highest volume of calls at a given time.

✱ **primary area of responsibility (PAR)** stationing of ambulances at specific high-volume locations.

✱ **system status management (SSM)** a computerized personnel and ambulance deployment system.

TRAFFIC CONGESTION

In deployment, traffic congestion must be taken into account as well as special situations such as a grade-level railroad. Some communities, for example, station ambulances on both sides of the tracks. Other special considerations include daily activities such as commuter traffic and school bus schedules. Other considerations include sporting events, VIP appearances, and public gatherings.

National guidelines help communities set the standards. For example, a cardiac arrest victim should receive defibrillation within the first four minutes and ALS within eight minutes. A system's standards for reliability must take into account the time frames for such calls. An example of such a standard might be response within four minutes to 90% of the priority one calls (cardiac arrests, respiratory complaints, and motor vehicle collisions).

To meet reliability standards, many communities use a **tiered response system** in which public safety personnel trained as first responders carry an AED to a patient's side within four minutes. This first tier of response is followed by a second tier that brings an ALS unit to the patient within eight minutes. Some communities add a third tier by separating their paramedics from their ambulances. The ideal system for your area will depend upon such considerations as available personnel, available training, and many other factors.

* **tiered response system** system that allows multiple vehicles to arrive at an EMS call at different times, often providing different levels of care or transport.

OPERATIONAL STAFFING

How many paramedics should be assigned to a unit? This is a complex decision. Clearly, when two paramedics are assigned to an ambulance, there is a reduced ability to provide ALS response to simultaneous additional emergencies. As a result, some communities combine an EMT-Intermediate with a paramedic to make an ALS unit. Other communities, such as New York City, specify that an ALS unit must have two paramedics so they can back each other up in on-scene decisions. Because community needs and resources vary so widely, unit staffing will in all likelihood continue to be settled locally.

In general, ambulance staffing should take peak load into account. Some services vary shift times to assure ample coverage for the busiest days and times of day. Services should also take into account the need for **reserve capacity**—the ability to muster additional crews when all ambulances are on call or when resources are taxed by a multiple casualty incident. Some services fulfill this need by asking off-duty personnel to carry pagers or to volunteer for backup.

Finally, standards for ambulance operators (drivers) and for driving the vehicle itself are usually determined at the local service level.

* **reserve capacity** the ability of an EMS agency to respond to calls beyond those handled by the on-duty crews.

SAFE AMBULANCE OPERATIONS

Patients, family members, motorists, and other EMS providers are injured—sometimes fatally—in ambulance collisions. In addition to personal injuries, ambulance collisions exact a high toll: vehicle repair or replacement, lawsuits, down time from work, increased insurance premiums, and damage to your agency's reputation in the community.

EDUCATING PROVIDERS

The first part of any education program is recognizing and defining the problem. There are no national statistics on ambulance collisions. However, some states do keep data, and their example can provide a starting point. The following statistics come from an analysis of 22 years of **reportable collisions**—accidents involving over $1,000 in vehicle damage or a personal injury—in New York State.

* **reportable collisions** collisions that involve over $1,000 in damage or a personal injury.

During the years 1974–1996, New York recorded 7,756 reportable ambulance collisions involving 64 fatalities and 10,636 injuries. The first rule in medical practice is "do no harm," and yet these collisions by emergency vehicles harmed a considerable number of people.

The data collected by New York provides a profile of the typical ambulance collision. Inclement weather accounted for a relatively small number of the accidents. About 18% occurred on rainy days, 16% on cloudy days, and 6% on days with snow, sleet, hail, or freezing rain. The majority (55%) took place on clear days. Some 67% took place during daylight hours. Head-on collisions accounted for only 1% of the collisions. The largest number (41%) occurred when the ambulance struck another vehicle or was itself struck laterally or at a right angle. Approximately 21% resulted from side-swiping or overtaking another vehicle. Another 12% occurred during a right or left turn.

Probably the most important observation from the data is that nearly three-quarters (72%) of all collisions took place at intersections. Most safety-minded ambulance operators agree that the days of "blowing through" an intersection at high speeds with lights blazing and siren blasting have come and gone. Yet nearly half of all collisions took place at locations with a traffic control device. Another third took place at locations with no traffic device or sign at all.

Based on the New York statistics, the profile of a typical ambulance collision might be: *a lateral collision that takes place on a dry road during daylight hours on a clear day in an intersection with a traffic light.* Typically, when ambulance operators respond in poor weather conditions, they try to drive with a bubble of safety around the vehicle. Maybe the bubble should be there all the time!

Most safety-minded ambulance operators agree that the days of "blowing through" an intersection at high speeds with lights blazing and siren blasting have come and gone.

REDUCING AMBULANCE COLLISIONS

If you have the opportunity to develop programs to reduce ambulance collisions in your community, consider implementing the following actions or standards:

- Routine use of driver qualification checklists and driver's license checks, either through the local police or the Department of Motor Vehicles

- Demonstrated driver understanding of preventive mechanical maintenance, including a vehicle operator checklist and a procedure for reporting any problems found during the check or while driving the vehicle

- Provision of plenty of hands-on driver training, using experienced and qualified field officers. (A 10,000–24,000 pound ambulance has a much longer stopping distance than the 2,500 pound pickup truck that an operator drove to work. The goal is to prevent an inexperienced driver from being stopped by a light pole—or another car—after sliding through an intersection.

- Implementation of a slow-speed course to assure that operators know how to use mirrors, back up, park, and handle ambulance-sized vehicles—including accurate estimation of braking distance and turn radius

- Training that ensures that operators know how to react to emergency situations such as the loss of brakes, loss of power steering, a stuck accelerator, a blown-out tire, or vehicle breakdown

- Demonstrated driver knowledge of both the primary and back-up routes to all hospitals in your service response area

- Demonstrated driver understanding of the rules, regulations, and laws that your Department of Motor Vehicles has established, for drivers in general and for ambulance operators in particular

FIGURE 48-2 Use of a spotter.

STANDARD OPERATING PROCEDURES

Each EMS agency should have standard operating procedures (SOPs) pertaining to the operation of its vehicles. At a minimum, they should spell out:

* Procedure for qualifying as an ambulance operator
* Procedure for handling and reporting an ambulance collision
* Process for investigating and reviewing each collision
* Process for implementing quality assurance in the aftermath of a collision
* Method for using a **spotter** when backing up a vehicle (Figure 48-2)
* Use of seat belts in the ambulance, and the procedure for transporting a child passenger under 40 pounds
* Guidelines on what constitutes an emergency response and the exemptions that may be taken under state laws
* Guidelines on prudent speed; proper travel in, and the circumstances for using, oncoming lanes; and safe negotiation of intersections
* Circumstances and procedures for use of escorts
* A policy of zero tolerance for driving the vehicle under the influence of alcohol or any drugs

* **spotter** the person behind the left rear side of the ambulance who assists the operator in backing up the vehicle.

THE DUE REGARD STANDARD

State laws pertaining to ambulance operation tend to be similar and to include the legal concept of **due regard.** Essentially, due regard exempts ambulance drivers from certain laws but at the same time holds them to a higher standard.

State laws typically exempt ambulance drivers who are operating in an emergency from posted speed limits, posted directions of travel, parking regulations, and requirements to wait at red lights. However, ambulances are rarely or never exempt from prohibitions against passing over a railroad crossing with the gates down and passing a school bus with flashing red lights.

While the laws are often liberal in their exemptions, they place the responsibility for use of these exemptions squarely on the shoulders of the drivers. The laws often say, for example, "the foregoing exemptions do not relieve the operator of an emergency vehicle from acting with due regard for the safety of all persons." Such language sets a higher standard for ambulance operators than for almost any other driver. Nowhere else in the motor vehicle laws are drivers held accountable for the safety of all other motorists!

* **due regard** legal terminology found in the motor vehicle laws of most states that sets up a higher standard for the operators of emergency vehicles.

Ambulances are rarely or never exempt from prohibitions against passing over a railroad crossing with the gates down or passing a school bus with flashing lights.

The moral is this: As an ambulance driver, you will always be held to a higher standard than other drivers. You must be attentive and prepared to shoulder the responsibilities that come with the profession that you have chosen.

LIGHTS AND SIREN: A FALSE SENSE OF SECURITY

As a general rule, do not rely solely on lights and siren to alert other motorists of your approach. Studies have shown that most motorists do not see or hear your ambulance until it is within 50 to 100 feet of their vehicles. Even so, the siren is the most commonly used—and abused—audible warning device. Before you decide to turn on the siren, consider the following points:

- Motorists are less inclined to yield to an ambulance when the siren is continually sounded.
- Many motorists feel that the right-of-way privileges given to ambulances are abused when sirens are sounded.
- Inexperienced motorists tend to increase their driving speeds by 10 to 15 miles per hour when a siren is sounded.
- The continuous sound of a siren can possibly worsen sick or injured patients by increasing their anxiety.
- Ambulance operators may also develop anxiety from sirens used on long runs, not to mention the possibility of hearing problems.

Some states and services have specific laws and/or SOPs that address the use of sirens. Some useful guidelines include:

- Use the siren sparingly and only when you must.
- Never assume all motorists will hear your siren.
- Assume that some motorists will hear your siren, but choose to ignore it.
- Be prepared for panic and erratic maneuvers when drivers do hear your siren.
- Never use the siren to scare someone.

Whenever the ambulance is on the road, day or night, turn on the headlights to increase its visibility. Alternating headlamps should only be used at night if they are installed in a secondary lamp. Probably the most useful light is the one in the center of the cowling on the front hood. This light can usually be easily seen in the rear view mirror of the car in front of you.

Each corner of the ambulance should have large flashers that blink in tandem or unison to help oncoming vehicles identify the location and size of the ambulance. Consider the latest research when designing or picking the lighting on your ambulance. At present, recommendations lean toward the use of single beam bulbs and strobes instead of relying on one type of lighting system. The most important point is visibility. The vehicle must be clearly visible from 360 degrees to all other motorists and pedestrians.

ESCORTS/MULTI-VEHICLE RESPONSES

Use of a police escort for ambulances is rarely recommended—except when the ambulance needs guidance in an unfamiliar district. Ambulances and police cars have different braking distances. If an ambulance follows a police car too closely, it can easily rear end the car. Also, the vehicles have different acceleration speeds. An ambulance may have trouble keeping up with a police car. A gap

As a general rule, do not rely solely on lights and siren to alert other motorists of your approach.

The role of lights and siren in the modern emergency response situation has diminished. Recent data has shown that lights and siren shave only a few seconds off response time but significantly increase the possibility of injury to the responding crew.

often develops, allowing other vehicles to pull in between. Finally, other motorists may not realize that the two vehicles are traveling together. After the police car speeds by, a vehicle may pull in front of an ambulance.

Multi-vehicle responses pose similar dangers. Additional danger occurs when two emergency vehicles approach an intersection at the same time. Besides totally confusing motorists and pedestrians, the potential for an intersection collision increases dramatically. Often motorists fail to yield the right of way to the first emergency vehicle, the second, or both.

Even if you pay attention to other calls in your district, do not assume you are aware of them all. To avoid warning perpetrators, for example, the police often respond to incidents without announcing their approach. Always negotiate an intersection assuming that you may meet another emergency vehicle.

PARKING AND LOADING THE AMBULANCE

Whenever you arrive first at the site of a motor vehicle collision, size up the scene for potential hazards. Establish a danger zone, parking at least 100 feet from the wreckage upwind and uphill (if possible) to avoid fire or any escaping hazardous liquids or fumes. If there is no fire or escaping liquids or fumes, park at least 50 feet from the wreckage. If possible, assign a crew member to handle traffic until the police arrive to take control of the task.

If your ambulance is the first emergency vehicle on the scene, park in front of the wreckage so your warning lights can alert approaching motorists. Then set up flares or non-incendiary warning devices as quickly as possible. If the scene has already been secured, park beyond the wreckage to avoid being exposed to traffic. If command has already been established by an on-scene EMS unit, you may receive pre-arrival instructions.

Always be aware of potential traffic hazards. Many EMS providers have been seriously injured or killed when struck by passing motorists. As much as possible, try not to expose your crew or your patient to traffic. Keep in mind that rear ambulance doors often obstruct warning lights when they are opened to load the patient. Also, studies have shown that red revolving lights attract drunk or tired drivers. Consider pulling off the road, turning off your headlights, and using just the amber rear sealed blinkers that flash in tandem or in unison to help oncoming motorists identify the size and location of your vehicle.

THE DEADLY INTERSECTION

Recall that New York statistics reveal 72% of all ambulance collisions occur in intersections. Exercise extreme caution whenever you approach an intersection. Keep in mind the braking distance of your ambulance, the effectiveness of lights and siren, the rules of the road, the SOPs of your service, the acceleration needed to get through the intersection safely, and more. Helpful tips include:

- Stop at all red lights and stop signs and then proceed with caution.
- Always proceed through an intersection slowly.
- Make eye contact with other motorists to assure they understand your intentions.
- If you are using any of the exemptions offered to you as an emergency vehicle, such as passing through a red light or a stop sign, make sure you warn motorists by appropriately flashing your lights and sounding the siren.
- Remember that lights and siren only "ask" the public to yield the right of way. If the public does not yield, it may be because they misunderstand your intentions, cannot hear the siren due to noise in

their own vehicles, or cannot see your lights. Never assume that other motorists have a clue to what you plan on doing at the intersection.

- Always go around cars stopped at the intersection on their left (driver's) side. In some instances, this may involve passing into the oncoming lane, which should be done slowly and very cautiously. You invite trouble when you use a clear right lane to sneak past a group of cars at an intersection. If motorists are doing what they should do under motor vehicle laws, they may pull into the right lane just as you attempt to pass.

- Know how long it takes for your ambulance to cross an intersection. This will help you judge whether you have enough time to pass through safely.

- Watch pedestrians at an intersection carefully. If they all seem to be staring in another direction, rather than at your ambulance, they may well be looking at the fire truck headed your way.

- Remember that an ambulance may weigh over 10,000 pounds, a medium duty vehicle 24,000 pounds. Even at speeds as slow as 30 miles per hour, these vehicles will not stop on a dime. When negotiating an intersection, consider "covering the brake" to shorten stopping distance.

UTILIZING AIR MEDICAL TRANSPORT

Air medical transport involves fixed-wing aircraft and rotorcraft. Air rescues are commonly referred to as **aeromedical evacuations,** or medevac.

> **✱ aeromedical evacuations** transport by helicopter or fixed-wing aircraft.

FIXED-WING AIRCRAFT

Fixed-wing aircraft generally are employed when patients require transport over distances of more than 100 miles, primarily in remote regions, such as parts of Alaska and Canada. They may also be used to bring patients injured far from their homes to hospitals nearer to where they live. EMS units may also respond to medical emergencies aboard commercial aircraft that have been forced to land. Most major airlines now carry AEDs as part of their first aid equipment, so you can expect to find almost anything when called to a landing strip.

ROTORCRAFT

The type of air transport that you will most likely encounter as a paramedic will involve rotorcraft, or helicopters. The use of helicopters for medical rescue grew out of their proven benefit during the Korean War and the conflict in Vietnam. Today there are over 200 hospital-based air medical transport programs in the United States (Figure 48-3). Many agencies now have the ability to order medically equipped helicopters to traumatic incidents requiring rapid response. They also use helicopters to transport patients from the field, especially in rural areas, to specialized hospitals. Finally, helicopters can provide quick inter-hospital transport of critically ill or injured patients.

ADVANTAGES AND DISADVANTAGES OF AIR TRANSPORT

Aeromedical transport offers a number of advantages and disadvantages. Advantages include more rapid transport in many situations, access to remote areas, access to specialty units (e.g., neonatal intensive care units, replantation units, transplant

FIGURE 48-3 A hospital-based helicopter.

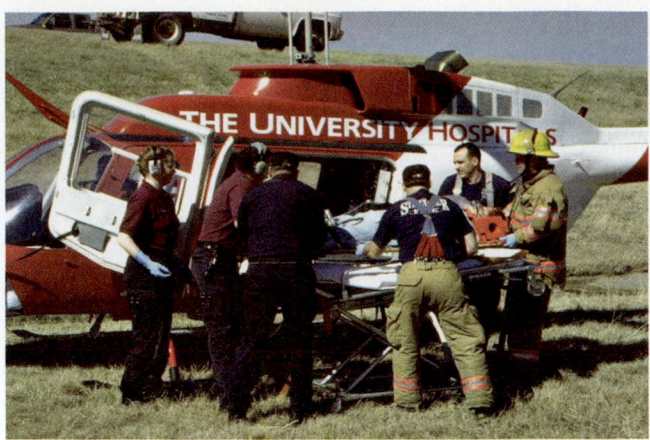

centers, burn centers), access to personnel with specialized skills (e.g., surgical airway, thoracotomy, rapid sequence intubation, critical care), and access to specialty supplies (e.g., aortic balloon pumps).

Disadvantages of aeromedical evacuation include weather and environmental restrictions to flying, altitude limitations, and airspeed limitations. Depending on the specific aircraft, cabin size can also restrict the number of crew members, the amount of equipment carried onboard, and the configuration of the stretcher. In smaller aircraft, such as the commonly used Bell LongRanger®, size limits the crew to the pilot and one flight medic and/or flight nurse. It also restricts the procedures that can be done on the patient during flight.

In the case of helicopter transport, in-flight climate control systems may not meet with your normal expectations. The thin walls of the fuselage do not allow much space for thermal insulation. Expect the "ship" to be hot in summer and cool in winter. Inside lighting is limited, otherwise the glare might enter the pilot's compartment, severely affecting his or her vision. Even though there is a curtain between the patient's compartment and the pilot, the lights still must be kept low, making ongoing patient assessment a challenge for the flight crew.

Finally, helicopter transport costs a lot of money. Some communities simply cannot afford to have a program.

ACTIVATION

Local and/or state guidelines may exist for the use of air medical transport in your area. Just as the public should access EMS by a single point (i.e., 911), ideally there should be a single access point for air medical transport in your region. To be effective, the need for medevac should be considered as early as possible. The decision should take into consideration the pilot's input, particularly regarding the safety of weather conditions, potential landing sites, and terrain.

INDICATIONS FOR USE

The indications for patient transport by helicopter include medical emergencies, trauma emergencies, and search and rescue missions. Factors that may warrant the need for air medical transport include:

Clinical Criteria

- Trauma score < 12
- Glasgow Coma Scale < 10
- Penetrating trauma to abdomen, pelvis, chest, neck, or head

Consider the need for medevac as early as possible.

Stable patients who are accessible to ground vehicles are best transported by ground vehicles.

- Spinal cord or spinal column injury or any injury producing paralysis or lateralizing signs
- Partial or total amputation or an extremity (excluding digits)
- Two or more long bone fractures or pelvis fracture
- Crush injury to abdomen, chest, or head
- Major burns or burns to face, hands, feet, or perineum; burns with respiratory involvement; electrical or chemical burns
- Patients in serious traumatic event < 12 or > 55 years of age
- Patients with near-drowning injuries
- Adult patients with:
  —Systolic BP < 90 mmHg
  —Respiratory rate < 10 or > 35 per minute
  —Heart rate < 60 or > 120 per minute
  —Unresponsive to verbal stimuli

The mechanism of injury may also indicate the need for air transport. However, keep in mind that a number of local programs require physiological abnormalities in addition to MOI findings:

Mechanism of Injury

- Vehicle roll-over with unbelted passengers
- Vehicle striking pedestrian > 20 mph
- Falls > 10 feet
- Motorcycle victim ejected at > 20 mph
- Multiple victims

Difficult Access

- Wilderness rescue
- Ambulance egress or access impeded by road conditions, weather, or traffic

Time/Distance Factors

- Transport to trauma center > 15 minutes by ground ambulance
- Transport time to local hospital by ground ambulance greater than transport time to trauma center by helicopter
- Patient extrication time > 20 minutes
- Utilization of local ground ambulance results in absence of ground ambulance coverage for local community

The Federal Aviation Agency (FAA) does not license commercial operators to do rescue missions involving special means of access, such as rappelling out of a helicopter. Such missions are usually undertaken by highly trained teams who respond with police agencies under a state or local public safety regulation.

It is important to weigh the risks versus benefits before using a helicopter for EMS patient transport.

PATIENT PREPARATION AND TRANSFER

Be familiar with any special considerations that must be taken into account prior to loading the patient. For example, you may need to immobilize the patient on a specific type of backboard. Smaller helicopters might accept only a certain size backboard, while larger helicopters might accommodate an entire stretcher. Also, some helicopter services limit the length of the patient when supine, which could alter your method of immobilizing a fractured femur. In this instance, a standard bipolar splint may extend the leg too far to fit inside the ship.

Some agencies specify procedures to limit the spread of bloodborne pathogens in the helicopter. You might, for instance, be required to wrap the packaged patient in a disposable blanket or to place the patient in a body bag. It will also be necessary to convert IV bags to pressure infuser bags. The patient may need to be intubated prior to flight due to the limited area around the airway once the patient is onboard. Depending on altitude, you may find it useful to put fluid in the air cuffs of tubes such as Foley catheters or endotracheal tubes, since the fluid will not expand or contract as gases do at varying altitudes. A PASG may also be affected by pressure changes. Remember to maintain the pressure in the device as the plane or helicopter lands.

Since it is difficult to assess a patient's lungs sounds in a helicopter, ensure tube placement by visualization, observation of symmetrical chest expansion and condensation in the ET tube, positive color changes, or a reading with an end-tidal carbon dioxide detector. Pulse oximeter readings will also be useful.

> *Remember that air pressure is changed by altitude, which affects IV bags, air cuffs of tubes, and the use of a PASG.*
>
>

SCENE SAFETY AND THE LANDING ZONE

The medical helicopter industry has suffered a number of very serious crashes, especially in the mid 1980s. Recently, great strides have been made in improving the safety of helicopter transport. An important factor in bringing about these changes has been the focus on safety among flight personnel. The Commission on Accreditation of Air Medical Services (CAAMS), for example, was developed as a voluntary agency dedicated to ensuring the safety of the air transport environment and to promoting the highest quality of patient care.

Flight crews should familiarize all EMS personnel in their region with their procedures and expectations. This will go a long way toward maintaining a safe scene and defining a safe landing zone (LZ) for the incoming helicopter. All paramedics should be able to select an appropriate LZ. As a rule, a helicopter requires an LZ of approximately 100 by 100 feet (about 30 large steps on each side) on ground with less than an eight-degree slope. Paramedics should also be able to describe the terrain, major landmarks, estimated distance to the nearest town, and other pertinent information to the pilot on a designated frequency.

The LZ, as well as the approach and departure path, should be clear of wires, towers, vehicles, people, and loose objects. Most flight crews suggest that EMS crews mark the LZ with a single flare in an upwind position. During night operations, never shine a light into the pilot's eyes. This could cause temporary blindness or interfere with depth perception.

Once the aircraft has landed, approach it with extreme caution and only upon approval of the flight crew. Make sure all loose objects, such as pillows and linens, are secured on the stretcher. Allow the flight crew to direct loading of the patient. Stay clear of the tail rotor at all times. Approach in crouch. A sudden gust of wind can cause the main rotor to dip to a point as close as four feet from the ground. If the helicopter has landed on an incline, approach from the downhill side. Keep all vehicles at least 100 feet away from the helicopter. Do not allow anyone to smoke within 200 feet of the aircraft.

Part 2: Medical Incident Command

Occasionally, paramedics are called upon to treat more than one patient at a time. The multi-patient incident may result from a motor vehicle collision (MVC), an apartment fire, a gang fight, or any number of other scenarios. During your career, you can also expect to respond to a much larger **multiple casualty incident (MCI)**, also known as a mass casualty incident (Figure 48-4). The MCI can involve "everyday" incidents such as a bus vs. tractor-trailer collision, disasters such as tornadoes, train wrecks, airline crashes, or even a terrorist event. Some districts define an MCI as any incident involving three or more patients. Others set the level for an MCI at five, seven, or more patients. In a disaster, the number of patients can reach into the hundreds or thousands.

ORIGINS OF THE INCIDENT MANAGEMENT SYSTEM

Based on the confusion surrounding several major fires in the 1970s, the fire service took the lead in organizing responses to large-scale emergencies. The result was several versions of the Incident Command System (ICS)—a management program designed for controlling, directing, and coordinating emergency response resources. In recent years, the various ICS systems have been merged into the comprehensive, standardized **Incident Management System (IMS)**. It is a national system used for the management of multiple casualty incidents, involving assumption of responsibility for command and designation and coordination of such elements as triage, treatment, transport, and staging. Although the Incident Command System was originally developed for use at major fires, the standardized IMS has been adopted by law enforcement, EMS, hospitals, and industry.

* **multiple casualty incident (MCI)** incident that generates large numbers of patients and that often makes traditional EMS response ineffective because of special circumstances surrounding the event; also known as a mass casualty incident.

The same techniques and tools used to respond to a multiple-patient MVC will be used to manage a major MCI.

* **Incident Management System (IMS)** national system used for the management of multiple casualty incidents, involving assumption of responsibility for command and designation and coordination of such elements as triage, treatment, transport, and staging; sometimes called the Incident Command System.

FIGURE 48-4 At a multiple casualty incident, the first on-scene unit must assume command.

REGULATIONS AND STANDARDS

The only federal requirement for use of IMS falls under the OSHA regulations requiring "the use of a site-specific ICS" during an emergency response to the release of hazardous substances. Regulations by the Environmental Protection Agency (EPA), however, have picked up this wording so that even non-OSHA states must comply with this requirement.

National consensus standards, or widely agreed upon guidelines, have been developed by the National Fire Protection Association. These standards are not laws or regulations, but they recommend MCI practices. Some of the standards with which you should be familiar include the ones that relate to hazardous materials incidents, health and safety IMS, and disaster management. In addition, various states have passed laws requiring the use of IMS. Become familiar with the laws in your state. Pay particular attention to any **scene-authority law**—a statute specifying who has ultimate authority at an MCI.

The national standard curriculum for implementing the Incident Management System is taught by the National Fire Academy in Emmitsburg, Maryland. However, California Firescope and several major urban fire departments have also developed programs. Become familiar with the specific type of IMS used within your jurisdiction.

A UNIFORM, FLEXIBLE SYSTEM

With its uniform terminology and approach, the Incident Management System has a number of advantages. First, an IMS can supersede jurisdictional and geographic boundaries to provide a well-organized response to routine and large-scale emergencies. Second, an IMS has the flexibility to respond to emergencies in both the public and the private sectors.

The following sections focus on the major functional areas of IMS. Use the mnemonic **C-FLOP** to keep these areas in mind:

C   command
F   finance/administration
L   logistics
O   operations
P   planning

COMMAND AT MASS-CASUALTY INCIDENTS

The most important functional area in the Incident Management System is **command.** The Incident Commander (IC)—also known as the Officer in Command (OIC) or the Incident Manager (IM)—is the individual who runs the incident (Figure 48-5). Establishing command at a multi-agency, multi-jurisdictional incident can be complicated. If state or local law does not decide the issue, the decision should be part of a preexisting MCI plan.

The ultimate authority for decision making rests with the Incident Commander. Because it would be too confusing or impossible for all on-scene personnel to report directly to the IC, the IC delegates certain functions and responsibilities to others. In this way, the IC maintains a reasonable **span of control,** or number of people or tasks that a single individual can monitor. Depending upon the scope of the incident, the span of control may range from three to seven people with an average of five.

---

* scene-authority law state or local statute specifying who has ultimate authority at an MCI.

* C-FLOP mnemonic for the main functional areas with the IMS—command, finance/administration, logistics, operations, and planning.

* command the individual or group responsible for coordinating all activities and who makes final decisions on the emergency scene; often referred to as the Incident Commander (IC) or Officer in Charge (OIC).

The ultimate authority for decision making rests with the Incident Commander.

* span of control number of people or tasks that a single individual can monitor.

SINGULAR VS. UNIFIED COMMAND

At small incidents with limited jurisdictions, **singular command** usually works best. For example, a traffic accident may involve the local fire department, EMS, and police. The three agencies might agree that the fire department should assume overall command, thus creating a singular command situation. In incidents with overlapping responsibilities or jurisdictions—such as terrorist attacks, explosions, sniper or hostage situations, and large-scale disasters—a **unified command** will be established. In these cases, law enforcement, fire, and EMS from several jurisdictions will coordinate their activities.

In establishing a unified command, the co-managers try to achieve balanced decision making. Together, they identify and access the agencies or organizations that might be needed at the scene, such as the American Red Cross, health department, public works, and so on. They select sector leaders and establish reasonable and unified spans of control. Finally, the commanders determine the need for public information officers and liaison with the media.

When the Incident Management System is expanded or the scene is large, co-managers set up a **command post** (CP) where command officers from various agencies can meet and confer. Because a command post may operate for weeks, the site should be selected carefully. Access to telephones, restrooms, and shelters should be taken into account. Also, the command post should be close enough to the scene so officers can monitor operations but far enough away so that they are outside the direct operational area. Persons operating on the scene, members of the media, and bystanders should not have routine access to the CP.

ESTABLISHING COMMAND

An MCI may be declared when an incident produces multiple patients, has circumstances that make scene management challenging, or significantly taxes the available resources of a system. Generally, when two or more units respond to an emergency or when casualties include two or more patients, you should implement the Incident Management System.

As a rule, the first arriving unit establishes command. If you are the first to arrive, depending on the scope of the incident and local protocols, you and your partner will most likely fill the roles of Incident Commander and Triage Officer— at least until other units arrive. Never forget the importance of assigning command early in an incident. Most MCIs are won or lost in the first ten minutes.

* **singular command** process where a single individual is responsible for coordinating an incident; most useful in single-jurisdictional incidents.

* **unified command** process in which managers from different jurisdictions—law enforcement, fire, EMS—coordinate their activities and share responsibility for command.

* **command post** (CP) place where command officers from various agencies can meet with each other and select a management staff.

Generally, when two or more units respond to an emergency or when casualties include two or more patients, you should implement the Incident Management System.

Never forget the importance of assigning command early in an incident.

Without incident command, emergency personnel may freelance. They may fail to prioritize patients, underestimate the severity of the incident, or delay requesting additional resources. Successful handing of any MCI involves coordination of all key personnel—whether it be two people, twenty, or more.

INCIDENT SIZE-UP

Scene size-up is an integral part of establishing command. Survey the scene through the windshield of your vehicle as you arrive on-scene. Do not exit the vehicle until you have identified all the elements of the incident and noted any potential hazards. At an MVC, for example, do not miss the vehicle partially hidden in the woods or the pool of gasoline near your vehicle. Once you have determined the visible scope of an incident and any obvious hazards, relay this information to dispatch.

In managing an MCI, you must keep in mind three main priorities: life safety, incident stabilization, and property conservation.

Life Safety

Life safety is always your top priority. If you arrive first on the scene, you must observe and protect all rescuers, including yourself, from hazards. Then, and only then, will you attend to patients with immediate life threats. Keep in mind, however, that the needs of the many usually outweigh the needs of the few. If you commit to caring for the first patient that you encounter, you may neglect ten other critical patients lying nearby. If you are the Incident Commander, remember that responsibility for triage belongs to the Triage Officer. At a small-scale incident, the IC may end up triaging some patients. Even so, the Triage Officer assumes the main responsibility for sorting patients into categories based upon the severity of their injuries.

Incident Stabilization

Your second priority is incident stabilization. To achieve this goal, quickly identify whether the situation is an **open incident** or a **closed incident.** An open incident, also known as an uncontained incident, has the potential to generate more patients at any time. A fire that traps people inside an office building is an example. You may find only several patients when you arrive on-scene. However, other patients—including fire fighters—may soon appear. As a result, the Incident Commander must anticipate the need for additional resources. Whenever you command an open incident, remember this point: It's better to call too many resources than too few.

In the case of a closed or contained incident, such as a multi-vehicle collision, the injuries have usually already occurred by the time you arrive. Yet even a so-called closed incident carries the potential for additional hazards such as an undetected gas leak or further injury to patients wandering about the scene. Stabilizing the incident to prevent further injuries helps ensure a smoother and more successful management of an MCI.

* **open incident** an incident that has the potential to generate additional patients; also known as an uncontained incident or an unstable incident.

* **closed incident** an incident that is not likely to generate any further patients; also known as a contained incident or a stable incident.

Whenever you command an open incident, remember this point: It's better to call too many resources than too few.

Property Conservation

The third priority is conservation of property. Rescue personnel must never damage property unless it is absolutely necessary for achieving the first two priorities, life safety and incident stabilization. Property conservation includes protection of the environment where operations are staged.

IDENTIFYING A STAGING AREA

Identification of a staging area is part of scene assessment. At MCIs involving hazardous materials or structural fires, for example, you must note wind speed and direction. The staging area and command post must lie well beyond the reach of any fumes, smoke, water, chemicals, or other hazardous materials.

Once you establish command of an MCI, choose both a primary and a secondary staging area. Keep in mind the main purpose of a staging area—organization of resources in one place for quick and easy deployment. Position the primary staging area as close to the scene as possible without compromising safety. Make sure the site has good access and exit points to ensure the flow of emergency vehicles. The secondary staging area should ideally lie in a different direction. This will provide you with a contingency plan in case the primary staging area becomes unusable. Conditions that may force a change in staging areas include altered traffic patterns, shifts in wind direction, or restricted access due to the deployment of fire hoses or other special equipment.

INCIDENT COMMUNICATIONS

Communications are the cornerstone of the Incident Management System. Once command is established, the Incident Commander has a responsibility to relay this information to dispatch. Then, as soon as possible, the IC should transmit a preliminary report that includes the following data: type of incident, approximate number of patients by priority, request for additional resources, staging instructions, and a plan of action. If a fixed command post is required, the IC should communicate the location of this site as well.

Once an MCI has been declared, further communications should be moved to a secondary, or tactical, channel. The Incident Commander must be able to supply the information necessary to coordinate resources. That is the whole purpose of the Incident Management System. Use of a secondary channel will also prevent an Incident Commander from interfering with the communications by other jurisdictions or from overwhelming the primary EMS channel.

Remember that communications will involve units from different jurisdictions and perhaps different districts. One of the foundations of incident management is the use of a common terminology. Eliminate all radio codes, which may have different meanings in different places, and use only plain English. In fact, it may be preferable to avoid radio codes even in routine operations. Then there will be no need to even think about switching to plain English when you assume command of an MCI.

Communications are the cornerstone of the Incident Management System.

RESOURCE UTILIZATION

Most EMS units will require additional ambulances, personnel, equipment, and medical supplies. In many cases, they will also require specialized equipment and perhaps the help of public or private agencies.

The primary role of an Incident Commander is the strategic deployment of all necessary resources at an incident, which means setting goals and determining the tactics needed to accomplish these goals. The Incident Commander must continually assess the effectiveness of a given strategy or plan.

To ensure flexibility, an Incident Commander should radio a brief progress report approximately every ten minutes until the incident has been stabilized. The report should state established goals, tactics, and resources and any progress or lack of progress. This forces an Incident Commander to monitor an operation, adapt to changing circumstances, and/or to eliminate ineffective tactics entirely. Subordinates should deliver similar reports to the Incident Commander so that he or she can properly evaluate the overall operation.

The primary role of an Incident Commander is the strategic deployment of all necessary resources at an incident.

COMMAND PROCEDURES

Several procedures help an Incident Commander to manage an MCI. First and foremost, all personnel must be able to recognize the IC. The Incident Management System calls for the IC and other officers to wear special reflective vests. The vests can be color-coded to functional areas and may have the officer's title on the front and back. Such vests should be worn whenever IMS is utilized, even at smaller incidents. By making a basic set of vests available on every response unit, especially for command and triage, personnel will get in the habit of wearing and/or recognizing the vests prior to a major incident.

An Incident Commander can also benefit from the use of a worksheet or clipboard. An IMS worksheet should include basic information on the incident, a small area to sketch the scene, and a checklist of important items to remember. It might also include a section to record on-scene units and personnel, their assignments, and relevant patient information, particularly transport data. Many commercial paper and computer products are available for this purpose.

You will find a worksheet especially useful when transferring command, as often happens when higher-ranking officers arrive on scene. Command is only transferred face-to-face, with the current Incident Commander conducting a short but complete briefing on the incident status. A higher-ranking officer does not become IC simply by his or her arrival—a briefing must take place. The worksheet serves as an outline for the briefing.

TERMINATION OF COMMAND

As the incident progresses, resources will be reassigned or released. For example, an Incident Commander who transfers command to a higher-ranking officer may become an aide to the new IC or be assigned to a totally new IMS role. Eventually resources will be **demobilized,** or released for use elsewhere in the EMS system. Once the incident has progressed to the point where the IMS is no longer needed, command should be terminated. A final progress report should be delivered to the communications center. All units will then return to routine rules of operation.

The point at which command terminates depends upon the incident. Some high-impact incidents, such as natural disasters or terrorist events, may last for weeks. However, not all agencies may have a significant presence for the long-term. EMS may have a strong initial response, for example, but may simply have a single ambulance stand by for the long term. Other agencies may be released entirely from the incident if their services are no longer needed.

SUPPORT OF INCIDENT COMMAND

Incident command is supported by four sections or functional areas: finance/administration, logistics, operations, and planning. Each section has a place within the Incident Management System and is headed by a **Section Chief.** However, all four areas may not be established at every incident. At small- or medium-sized incidents, for example, operations may be the only section implemented. At large-scale or long-term incidents, finance/administration, logistics, and planning may be activated. These sections may not be staffed with EMS personnel. However, they may help coordinate some EMS activities.

In addition, officers handling public information, safety, outside liaisons, and critical stress debriefing may report to the Incident Commander. Together they are known as the **Management Staff,** or Command Staff. Management Staff and Section Chiefs comprise and carry out **Staff Functions.**

As a paramedic, it is more important for you to know how the Incident Management System works than to be an expert in specific job functions. Figure 48-6

Command is only transferred face to face, with the current Incident Commander conducting a short but complete briefing on the incident status.

* **demobilized** resources—personnel, vehicles, and equipment—released for use outside the incident when they are no longer needed at the scene.

* **Section Chief** officer who supervises major functional areas or sections; reports to the Incident Commander.

* **Management Staff** officers that handle public information, safety, outside liaisons, and critical stress debriefing; also known as the Command Staff.

* **Staff Functions** officers who perform supervisory roles in the IMS rather than actually performing a task.

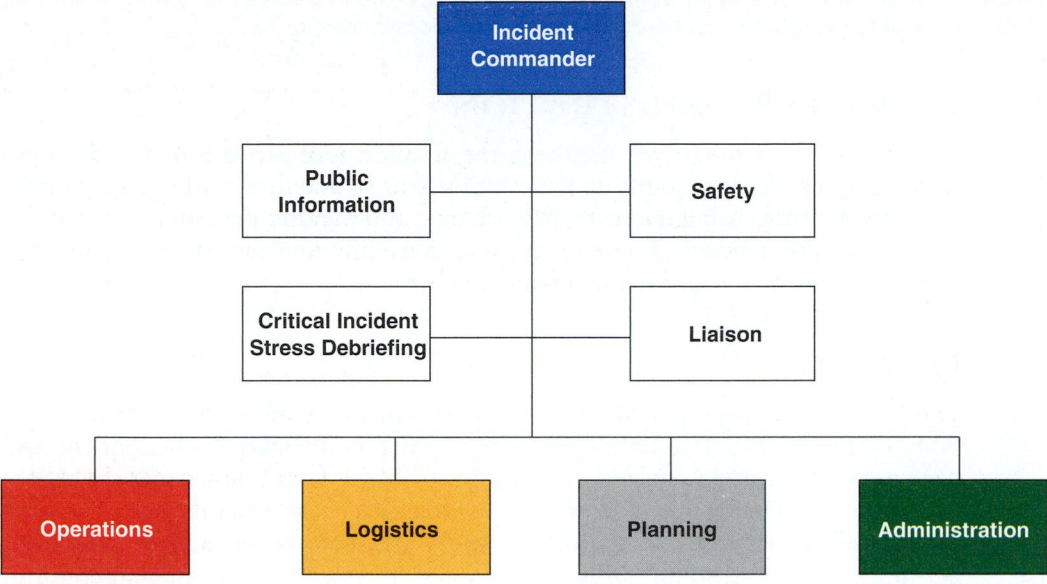

IMS LINE POSITIONS AND COMMAND STAFF

- Incident Commander
  - Public Information
  - Safety
  - Critical Incident Stress Debriefing
  - Liaison
  - Operations
  - Logistics
  - Planning
  - Administration

FIGURE 48-6 Basic elements of the Incident Management System.

and the following sections give you a quick overview of the basic elements of the Incident Command System.

MANAGEMENT STAFF

The Management Staff can play an important role in supporting the Incident Commander, particularly at major incidents or disasters.

Safety Officer

The **Safety Officer** may hold the most important role at an MCI. This person—or, in some cases, team of people—monitors all on-scene actions and ensures that they do not create any potentially harmful conditions. Some of the areas that must be monitored include infection control, use of personal protective equipment, crowd control, lifting of patients and equipment, and quality of scene lighting. Under the Incident Management System, the Safety Officer has the authority to stop any action that is deemed an immediate life threat.

> ✱ Safety Officer monitors all on-scene actions and ensures that they do not create any potentially harmful conditions.

Liaison Officer

The **Liaison Officer** coordinates all incident operations that involve outside agencies such as other emergency services, disaster support networks, private industry representatives, government agencies, and more. The Liaison Officer makes sure these outside resources are connected with the appropriate functional areas and are deployed effectively.

> ✱ Liaison Officer coordinates all incident operations that involve outside agencies.

Public Information Officer (PIO)

Although you may not have a preexisting relation with the media in your community, a major incident will put your unit in the public spotlight. The **Public Information Officer** collects data about the incident and releases it to the press.

> ✱ Public Information Officer (**PIO**) collects data about the incident and releases it to the press.

* Critical Incident Stress Management (CISM) Team monitors the emotional status of all on-scene personnel and provides the necessary support.

* Finance/Administration responsible for maintaining records for personnel, time, and costs of resources/procurement; reports directly to the IC.

* Logistics supports incident operations, coordinating procurement and distribution of all medical resources.

* Medical Supply Unit coordinates procurement and distribution of equipment and supplies at an MCI.

* Facilities Unit selects and maintains areas used for rehabilitation and command.

* Operations carries out directions from command and does the actual work at an incident.

* branches functional levels within the IMS based upon primary roles and geographic locations.

* Planning provides past, present, and future information about an incident.

* mutual aid agreements or plans for sharing departmental resources.

Critical Incident Stress Management (CISM) Team

The **CISM Team** monitors the emotional status of all on-scene personnel. The CISM Team will support these workers and attempt to reduce the stress. They may also conduct on-scene debriefings, if necessary.

FINANCE/ADMINISTRATION

On large-scale or long-term incidents the **finance/administration** staff assumes responsibility for all accounting and administrative activities. It keeps personnel and time records, estimates costs, pays claims, and handles procurement of items required at the incident. These functions are usually performed by the jurisdictional government where the incident has occurred.

LOGISTICS

The **logistics** section supports incident operations. One of its most critical functions is staffing the **Medical Supply Unit,** which coordinates procurement and distribution of equipment and supplies at an MCI. Other units may be established as well. The **Facilities Unit,** for example, selects and maintains areas used for rehabilitation and command. It assures adequate food, water, restrooms, lighting, power, and so on. Other units might be set up to manage field communications, on-scene medical care for workers, and so on.

OPERATIONS

Whatever work needs to be performed at an incident takes place under **Operations.** This section carries out tactical objectives, directs front-end activities, participates in planning, modifies the action plan, maintains discipline, and accounts for personnel. In short, Operations gets the job done.

As will be explained later, Operations may have many **branches**—functional levels based upon primary roles or geography. Branches organized by role might include sections within EMS, rescue, fire, law enforcement, and so on. Branches based on geography might include the Operations at various locations.

PLANNING

Planning helps formulate the overall action plan and oversees changes in that plan. It collects information such as weather reports, documents incident actions, and develops contingency plans. It ensures that written SOPs for **mutual aid**—agreements for sharing departmental resources—are activated or fulfilled. The Planning section operates according to the principle of "anything that can go wrong will go wrong," using past incidents to anticipate troubles that might arise at the current incident. When Command and Operations must switch tactics, Planning provides the necessary strategic support.

DIVISION OF FUNCTIONS

There are several ways to divide functions at an incident. The choice depends on the scope of an MCI, the structure of your department, the implementation of singular or unified command, and so on. If you are an Incident Commander, one of your jobs will be to organize line functions—i.e., Operations—in the most effective manner. Figure 48-7, for example, shows the functional levels within a typical EMS branch.

IMS EMS BRANCH

FIGURE 48-7   Example of branches that may operate in a major incident.

BRANCHES

Command may establish any number of branches organized by primary role or geography. Branches are supervised by Branch Directors, who report to the Section Chief for their functional area. The EMS Branch Director supervises all patient care and transportation operations. Rescue may be an independent branch or may report to the director of EMS or fire.

GROUPS AND DIVISIONS

Branches may be further organized into groups or divisions. Groups are based upon function, while divisions are based upon geography. As an example, think of Triage as a group and the responders working on the third floor of a multi-floor incident as a division. The supervisors of groups and divisions in turn report to the Branch Director.

UNITS

Groups and divisions can be broken into task-specific groups called units, supervised by Unit Leaders, who report to the group or division supervisor.

SECTORS

Depending on the type of Incident Management System in your area, you may hear the term Sectors. **Sector** is an interchangeable name for a branch, group, or division. However, it does not designate a functional or geographic area. Individuals who supervise a sector are often called Sector Officers.

FUNCTIONAL GROUPS WITHIN AN EMS BRANCH

The flexibility of the Incident Management System is founded on the ability to implement only the areas that are needed at an incident.

The Incident Management System operates under the "tool box" theory. Do not remove a tool from the toolbox unless you actually need it. The flexibility of IMS is founded on the ability to implement only the areas needed at an incident. This holds for all areas of IMS, including branches, groups, sectors, divisions, and specific areas where EMS operates. At many EMS incidents, the basic IMS organization in Figure 48-8 will provide all the "tools" you need.

TRIAGE

✱ **triage** act of sorting patients based upon the severity of their injuries.

All personnel should be trained in triage techniques and all response units should carry triage equipment.

Triage is the act of sorting patients based upon the severity of their injuries. In order to do the most good for the most people, you need to determine which patients need immediate care to live, which will live despite delays in care, and which will die despite receiving medical care. Because triage will direct subsequent operations, it is one of the first functions performed at an MCI. Therefore, all personnel should be trained in triage techniques and all response units should carry triage equipment. The Triage Group Supervisor may act independently or may supervise the Triage Group/Sector.

✱ **primary triage** triage that takes place early in the incident, usually upon first arrival.

Primary and Secondary Triage

Triage occurs in phases. **Primary triage** takes place early, when you first contact patients and provides a basic categorization of sustained injuries. It must be done

FIGURE 48-8   Organization for a small to medium-sized incident.

quickly and efficiently so command can determine on-site treatment needs and resources. Universally recognized triage categories include:

Category	Color	Priority
Immediate	Red	Priority-1 (P-1)
Delayed	Yellow	Priority-2 (P-2)
Hold	Green	Priority-3 (P-3)
Deceased	Black	Priority-0 (P-0)

Secondary triage takes place throughout the incident as patients are collected, moved to treatment areas, and receive care. A patient's condition may change, requiring you to upgrade or downgrade the triage category.

The START System

The most widely used triage system is **START,** an acronym for Simple Triage and Rapid Transport, a system developed at Hoag Memorial Hospital in Newport Beach, California. START's easy procedures allow for rapid sorting of patients into the preceding categories. START does not require a specific diagnosis. Instead it focuses on these signs or symptoms (Figure 48-9):

- Ability to walk
- Respiratory effort
- Pulses/perfusions
- Neurological status

Ability to Walk You initiate the START system by asking patients who can walk to get up and come to you. Any patients who can comply, despite their injuries, is categorized "green" and the appropriate tag is placed on the patient. Because patients who can walk will walk, you should make every effort to confine them to one site. There is enough confusion at an MCI without having the "walking wounded" wandering around the scene.

Respiratory Effort Next, you begin to triage the non-walking patients. Remember to keep the focus on tagging patients. Your only treatment effort should be directed toward correction of airway problems and severe bleeding. Begin by assessing breathing. If patients are not breathing, open their airway manually. Tag patients who start to breathe spontaneously "red," those who fail to respond "black." For those who are breathing, quickly assess respiratory rate. Patients with respirations above 30/minute should be tagged "red." If respirations are less than 30/minute, go to the next assessment step.

Pulse/Perfusion Assessment of circulatory status can be accomplished in two ways: radial pulses and capillary refill. Delayed capillary refill (over 2 seconds) is a poor indicator of perfusion in adults. It can be compromised by cold weather or be normally delayed in certain people. Therefore, the preferred method of assessing perfusion is the radial pulse. The presence of a radial pulse indicates a systolic blood pressure of at least 90 mmHg. Patients with absent radial pulses will be triaged "red." If patients have respirations less than 30/minute and a present radial pulse, go to the next assessment step.

Neurological Status You now quickly assess mental status. Use this quick test: Ask patients to grip both of your hands. If they can perform this simple task, categorize them Priority-2 or "yellow." If they cannot follow such simple commands, categorize them Priority-1 or "red."

* **secondary triage** triage that takes place after patients are moved to a treatment area to determine any change in status.

* **START** acronym for the most widely used disaster triage system; stands for Simple Triage and Rapid Transport.

Content Review

SIGNS AND SYMPTOMS IN START

Can get up and walk
Open airway
Respirations over 30/minute
Follows commands

START TRIAGE SYSTEM

WALKING WOUNDED?

MINOR

RESPIRATIONS?

NO
Open Airway!
RESPIRATIONS?

Yes

No
DECEASED

Yes
IMMEDIATE

Under 30/min?

Over 30/min?
IMMEDIATE

PERFUSION?

Absent Radial Pulse
or Cap Refill > 2 sec
IMMEDIATE

Radial Pulse Present
or Cap Refill < 2 sec

Control Bleeding!

MENTAL STATUS

Cannot Follow
Simple Commands
IMMEDIATE

Can Follow
Simple Commands
DELAYED

FIGURE 48-9   Operation of the START system, the most widely used triage system.

Triage Tagging/Labeling

As already mentioned, you should attach a color-coded tag to each patient that you have triaged. Tagging offers these advantages:

- Alerts care providers to patient priorities—i.e., provides organization of treatment
- Prevents re-triage of the same patient
- Serves as a tracking system during transport and/or treatment

Commercial tags are available, such as the METTAG (Figure 48-10). However, you can also use colored surveyor's tape. Each has its advantages and disadvantages. Tags provide tear-off strips that help you count patients in each triage category. Tags also make it easier to track patients, record treatment information, and indicate a patient's location in a transportation accident. But tags

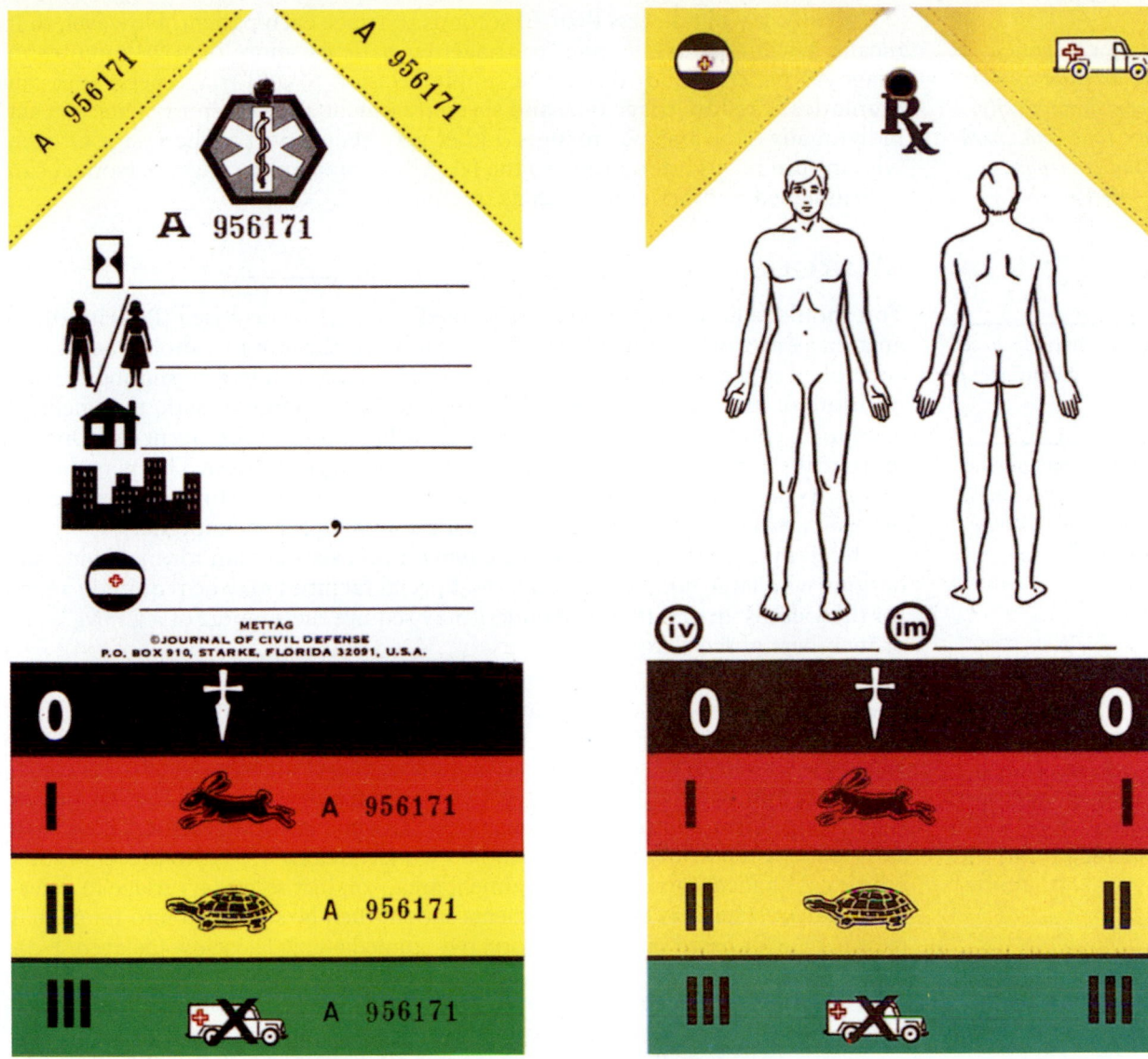

FIGURE 48-10   The METTAG.

can be damaged in wet weather, and tear-off strips can make it difficult to change patient categories. Surveyor's tape costs less money, but does not allow you to count patients during triage. Also, black tape cannot be easily seen at night.

Some systems combine use both tags and tape. Others use tags only when immediate transport is unavailable and/or when patients need to be sorted into separate treatment areas. Whatever tagging method you use, it must (1) be easy to use and (2) provide rapid visual identification of priorities.

The Need for Speed

While you must not become committed to single-patient care during triage, that does not mean you do nothing. Simple care—opening airways and direct pressure on profuse bleeding—can save lives early in an incident. So the Triage Officer should carry infection control supplies, oral airways, and trauma dressings as well as tags or tape, a portable radio to communicate with the Incident Commander, a command vest, and flashlight (at night).

Ideally, it will take less than 30 seconds to triage each patient. However, that means it will take five minutes to triage ten patients, more than 20 minutes to triage 40 patients, and so on. The simple decision to add triage personnel can dramatically reduce triage time and speed treatment and transport. They can act individually or be assigned to units. Either way, they report to the Triage Officer, who in turn relays information to the IC. After completing triage, personnel can be reassigned to other units, such as treatment.

MORGUE

You should collect patients who are triaged "black," or deceased (Priority-0), in an area away from treatment. This area, known as the **morgue,** should be access-controlled so that bystanders or the media cannot enter it. In determining the disposition of the deceased, you will need to work closely with the medical examiner, coroner, law enforcement, and other appropriate agencies. Once a morgue is established, it will be supervised by a **Morgue Officer.** This person may report to the Triage Officer or the Treatment Officer. In many cases, these supervisors will assist in selecting and securing an area for the morgue.

Keep in mind the importance of having a preexisting plan for managing situations with large numbers of fatalities. Special facilities may be required to care for the victims. In addition, responders may require the support of a CISM Team or members of the clergy.

TREATMENT

When the number of patients exceeds the number of ambulances available for transportation, you will need to collect patients into treatment areas. The **Treatment Group Supervisor** controls all actions in the Treatment Group/Sector. Those who carry patients to the treatment area should work in teams of four to prevent lifting injuries. As patients arrive in the treatment area, conduct secondary triage to determine if their status has changed. Patients should then be separated into functional treatment areas based on their category: red (immediate, P-1), yellow (delayed, P-2), or green (hold, P-3).

Essential equipment for a treatment area includes airway maintenance supplies, oxygen and delivery devices, bleeding control supplies, and burn management supplies as well as immobilization and transportation devices such as stretchers, spine boards, or other equipment to move patients.

Red Treatment Unit

This area provides care for all critical patients. As a result, Command and/or Logistics will assign the bulk of medical resources to this unit. Providers with ALS skills usually report to the red treatment area so they can stabilize patients and prepare them for transport. Because medical resources can be quickly used, a supply system is necessary to support this operation. Finally, this is the place where any on-scene physicians or nurses should be utilized.

Yellow Treatment Unit

Teams of responders carry all non-critical patients to this unit for stabilization. Although these patients are not as critical as those in the red area, ALS procedures may still be necessary. A patient with an isolated femur fracture, for example, will probably be categorized yellow. Although this patient does not require immediate intervention or transport, he or she may still require an intravenous line and eventual surgical intervention.

Green Treatment Unit

Ambulatory patients report to the green area, where they are prepared for transport. Very little care is necessary in this area, but these patients still require monitoring in case their condition deteriorates. In such instances, they will be triaged and moved to the appropriate treatment area.

Supervision of Treatment Units

Each of the preceding units is supervised by a **Treatment Unit Leader,** who reports to the Treatment Group Supervisor. The leader's job requires extreme flexibility to ensure that patients receive adequate care. Patient conditions can change and responders, equipment, or supplies may not be available in the sub-area. As a result, communications must be carefully coordinated. The Treatment Group Supervisor must be apprised of activities in each sub-area. He or she must also help coordinate operations with other functional areas, particularly command, triage, and transport.

✱ **Treatment Unit Leaders** EMS personnel who manage the various treatment units and who report to the Treatment Group Supervisor.

ON-SCENE PHYSICIANS

At some high-impact or long-term incidents, physicians may support EMS. For example, they may be better able to make difficult triage decisions, perform advanced triage and treatment, or perform emergency surgery to extricate a patient as a last resort. Physicians also provide direct supervision and medical direction over paramedics in the treatment area, removing the need to operate under standing orders or radio contact. A contingency plan should outline when and how physicians respond to and operate at an MCI.

STAGING

Ambulances may be the most precious resource at a mass casualty incident. As a result, ambulances must be staged as they arrive to allow proper access to the scene and, more important, egress with the patients. If ambulances arrive before they are needed to treat patients, they should be kept in a **staging** area under a **Staging Officer.** This area may be a roadway, a parking lot, or some other site where the units can wait until they are deployed by command.

Depending on local protocols, drivers or crew members will be required to wait with the vehicles until they are needed for transport. A staging pool keeps personnel from "freelancing" and ensures their availability for quick deployment. It also prevents premature commitment of resources. If ambulances are required for immediate transport, the staging area can serve as a loading area for patients.

✱ **Staging** locations where ambulances, personnel, and equipment are kept in reserve for use at an incident.

✱ **Staging Officer** supervises the staging area and guards against premature commitment of resources and freelancing by personnel; reports to the branch director.

TRANSPORT

The **Transportation Supervisor** coordinates operations with the Staging Officer and the Treatment Supervisor. His or her job is to get patients into the ambulances and routed to hospitals. If you are assigned to this role, you will need to be flexible in determining the order in which patients are packaged and loaded. You may, for example, elect to place two critical patients in one ambulance for transport to a trauma center. If you decide that the ambulance provider cannot adequately care for two critical patients, you may instead decide to transport one critical and one non-critical patient. You may also take into account the facilities at a given hospital and avoid overwhelming its resources with critical patients.

✱ **Transportation Supervisor** coordinates operations with the Staging Officer and the Transportation Supervisor; gets patients into the ambulances and routed to the hospitals.

The routing of patients to hospitals is as important as getting them into the ambulances. Early in the incident, your communications center should contact local hospitals and determine how many patients in each triage category they can handle. You must also consider any specialties that a hospital may have—trauma centers, burn units, neurological teams, and so on. Keep in mind, too, that many patients may have left the scene before the arrival of EMS and transported themselves to the closest hospital.

A Transportation Supervisor needs to implement some type of tracking system or destination log, which ideally will include each patient's triage tag number; triage priority; age, gender, and major injuries; transporting unit; hospital destination; departure time; and patient's name, if possible. The tracking sheet not only helps to organize activities at an MCI, it also proves invaluable in reconstructing the incident later. In addition, this record will help document on-scene patient care.

EXTRICATION/RESCUE

Extrication, or Rescue, may be a branch or a group. If it is considered an EMS function, it will be a group (sector) under the EMS branch. If it is a fire department function, it may be under the fire branch. If the rescue is extensive or long-term, the operation may be its own branch. The Extrication/Rescue group removes patients from entanglements and arranges for them to be carried to treatment areas. The operation has many facets and may require specialized personnel and equipment. During extended operations, treatment personnel will need to work in this area and begin patient care prior to removal.

Depending on the circumstances, personnel operating in this area will need personal protective equipment, including helmets, eye protection, gloves, breathing apparatus, and/or protective clothing. Some of the rescue tools may also require specific support materials, such as gasoline, electricity, or compressed air. Extrication/rescue is a very dangerous area, and all efforts should be taken to ensure that operations are well supervised and safe.

REHABILITATION

At extended operations, a special rehabilitation area should be established to support on-scene responders. Arrangements should be made with Logistics to ensure the necessary food, water, and medical monitoring supplies.

Ideally, rescuers should regularly rotate through a dedicated rehabilitation area away from the incident. The site should provide thermal control and shelter from fumes, crowds, or the media. In this environment, rescuers can rest and hydrate themselves. Medical personnel operating in this area will take the vital signs of rescuers and watch for signs of fatigue or incident stress. A predetermined threshold should be established so that rescuers with abnormal vitals are removed from the operation. This is especially important during extremely hot or cold conditions.

Provision should also be made for a **Rapid Intervention Team.** If possible, an ambulance and crew should be dedicated to stand by outside the staging area in case a rescuer becomes ill or injured. Unfortunately, the demands of a large-scale MCI sometimes prevent implementation of this aspect of the IMS.

COMMUNICATIONS

It cannot be said too often that communications forms the cornerstone of the Incident Management System. Therefore, it helps to review some basic rules.

First, think about what you are going to say before you say it. Does the message really need to be transmitted over the radio? Remember that the frequencies at an MCI will already be congested with messages. As a result, you should try to prevent as much unnecessary radio traffic as possible.

Second, key up your radio before transmitting. Wait one second after pressing the button to speak. This allows your radio to begin transmitting effectively—and all other radios to begin listening—before you begin your message. Keep in mind that missed messages mean missed chances at increased coordination and efficiency.

Third, acknowledge each message with feedback to ensure that you understood it. For example, the message "Staging from Transport, send two ambulances" should not be acknowledged with "Staging received." It should be answered with "Staging received, send two ambulances."

Other rules include points already covered: the use of plain English instead of radio codes; the need for a common radio channel between command, groups (sectors), divisions, and units; face-to-face communications when appropriate; and respect for the lines of communication established by the IMS. In other words, report to the person you are supposed to report to.

EMS Communications Officer

At large-scale incidents, the Incident Management System provides for an EMS **Communications Officer,** also known as the EMS COM or the MED COM. This person works closely with the Transportation Supervisor to notify hospitals of incoming patients. A dedicated radio channel works best for this purpose. The EMS COM will not deliver complete patient reports, which would increase the communications traffic. Instead, he or she will transmit the basic information collected by the Transportation Supervisor, such as the number of Priority 1 patients en route to a hospital, the expected arrival time, and so on.

* EMS Communications Officer notifies hospitals of incoming patients from an MCI; reports to the Transportation Officer and may also be called the EMS COM or MED COM.

Alternative Means of Communication

Remember that your primary radio system may not always work at an MCI. Disasters can knock out radio towers and power. Frequencies can be overwhelmed. Telephone lines can be down. Radio batteries can fail. As a result, alternative means of communication should be included in every MCI preplan and should be practiced regularly. You might use cellular phones, mobile data terminals, alphanumeric pagers, fax machines, or other technology to overcome the failure of your primary radio system. When all else fails, runners can be used to hand deliver messages around the incident scene. Although there are obvious limitations to this method, it may be your last resort. So know how to use it.

DISASTER MANAGEMENT

Disasters can alter the routine operating procedures used at high-impact events. For example, disasters can damage a region's infrastructure, preventing the operation of railroads, hospitals, radio systems, and so on. If a disaster occurs in your jurisdiction, you will be a victim as much as a responder, which is why outside assistance is often required. As a rule, **disaster management** occurs in the following four stages: mitigation, planning, response, and recovery.

* disaster management management of incidents that generate large numbers of patients, often overwhelming resources and damaging parts of the infrastructure.

MITIGATION

Mitigation involves the prevention or limiting of disasters in the first place. For example, the public safety community tries to prevent people from building houses on flood plains or from putting up structures unable to withstand the impact of natural phenomena or terrorist attacks. In addition, most communities today have early warning systems to alert people to emergencies such as hurricanes, tornadoes, volcanic eruptions, or earthquakes.

PLANNING

As already indicated, planning is integral to the successful management of all high-impact emergencies. Every community should take part in a hazard analysis and then rate these hazards according to their likelihood, then devise relocation plans and/or evacuation procedures as needed. When possible, every effort should be made to keep people in their natural social groupings. That is, provide home-based relocation instead of removing people to hospitals and clinics when they are not injured. If you must evacuate people, use whatever means you have to spread the message frequently and with urgency. Alert people to the nature of the disaster, estimated time of impact, and expected severity. Advise people of safe routes out of the area and appropriate destinations.

Critical to any successful disaster plan will be provision for an efficient communication system in case the primary system fails. Decide, for example, where a central communications center might be established for people needing help. Set up guidelines on the use of radios by all EMS personnel. Make arrangements for portable radios and recorders as necessary.

RESPONSE

In a disaster, there is a great disparity between casualties and resources. The event overwhelms the natural order and causes a great loss of property and/or life. A disaster almost always requires outside assistance and alternative operating plans. In general, you will follow Incident Management System guidelines.

RECOVERY

Recovery involves the return of your department, your jurisdiction, and your community to normal as soon as possible. Actions taken will vary with the nature of the disaster and/or the disaster plan. You may be involved with the reunion of families, follow-up care, and support of the personnel charged with handling potential hazards such as collapsed buildings, highways, and so on.

MEETING THE CHALLENGE OF MASS CASUALTY INCIDENTS

As implied by the preceding sections, you will never be more challenged in your EMS career than when you respond to an MCI. The routine actions that you do every day will suddenly become more difficult or, in some cases, impossible because of the stress of the incident. For this reason, you should anticipate various problems and work to overcome them.

COMMON PROBLEMS

Things can—and do—go wrong at MCIs and disasters. One way to avert or minimize complications is to anticipate them. As the saying goes, "Forewarned is forearmed." Studies of past incidents have revealed the following common problems, any of which can hinder the success of the operation.

- Lack of recognizable EMS command in the field
- Failure to provide adequate widespread notification of an event

- Failure to provide proper triage
- Lack of rapid "initial" stabilization of patients
- Failure to move, collect, and organize patients rapidly into a treatment area
- Overly time-consuming patient care
- Premature transportation of patients
- Improper or inefficient use of in-field personnel
- Improper distribution of patients to medical facilities
- Failure to establish an accurate patient-tracking system
- Inability to communicate with on-scene units, regional EMS agencies, or other personnel
- Lack of command vests for all IMS officers or supervisors
- Lack of adequate training and/or practice of rescuers at an MCI
- Lack of drills among regional agencies involved in the IMS
- Lack of proper community assessment, preplanning, and contingency plans

PREPLANNING, DRILLS, AND CRITIQUES

Anticipate any problems that may occur and work toward removing them. Anything that can be planned in advance should be planned in advance.

The first step is a complete assessment of the potential hazards—both natural and human—that could occur in your area. If you live in Kansas, for example, you might not worry about hurricanes, but tornadoes are a very real possibility. Sites of potential incidents in almost any community include chemical or nuclear plants, factories or mines, schools, jails, sporting arenas, entertainment centers, railroads, airports, and so on.

Then develop a plan that outlines the SOPs and protocols for potential incidents. You will not, of course, be able to plan for every possible scenario. If you develop 100 preplans, for example, you can expect to be summoned to scenario 101 or 102—i.e., the unscripted event. For this reason, you must develop contingency plans for worst-case scenarios. For example, how would you communicate with ambulances if something or someone knocked out the dispatch center? What would you do if the local hospital suddenly became unusable because of chemical contamination?

Then test the preplan. Start small. Tabletop drills, for example, are a good place to begin. Once you have worked out the wrinkles, distribute the plan to everyone in your department, surrounding departments, local police, fire departments, hospitals—in short, to anyone who could be involved. Ensure that the necessary mutual aid agreements are in place and that the appropriate personnel know about these agreements.

Then make sure that all personnel who could show up at an MCI have received proper training in use of the IMS. As you have learned, the first responders on the scene will often determine the course of an event. Run or take part in drills so that you can gain practice in MCI operations and large-scale use of the Incident Management System. Again, start small. Use local drills within your department to help familiarize personnel with the system. Then, aim for large-scale drills that involve outside agencies.

Finally, never say "It will never happen here." Experience has proven time and again that mass casualty incidents and disasters can occur almost anywhere and at any time. Make it part of your professional training to be ready to act as an Incident Commander—the person charged running the IMS.

Never say, "It will never happen here."

CRITICAL INCIDENT STRESS MANAGEMENT

As you already know, every EMS professional faces the possibility of critical incident stress (CIS)—the powerful emotional response to a catastrophic event. The response can begin during the event or immediately after. There can also be a delayed response, such as a flashback during a later call. Reactions can be physical, emotional, behavioral, or a combination of all three.

For this reason, you or your agency should make provisions for use of specially trained Critical Incident Stress Management (CISM) Teams of a local chapter of **Trauma Intervention Programs (TIP)**. Such resources will provide access to mental health workers or other specially trained personnel who are familiar with emergency operations. CISM team members should circulate around the scene of a high-impact incident to spot anyone exhibiting a stress reaction. Others should be available for debriefing after an event.

At smaller incidents, a CISM team will probably not be activated. For this reason, you and other members of your crew should be aware of the signs or symptoms of a stress reaction. Be ready to help each other. For more on the management of stress within an EMS agency or unit, see Chapter 1.

∗ Trauma Intervention Programs (TIP) a national non-profit organization that establishes and operates local chapters of citizen volunteers specially trained to provide assistance to anyone emotionally traumatized by a crisis event.

Part 3: Rescue Awareness and Operations

What do you do when your patient is pinned beneath a vehicle, trapped in a collapsed building, or injured climbing a rock face or crawling into a cave. When people get injured or stranded in such situations, often somebody must first rescue the patient before emergency medical care can even begin.

ROLE OF THE PARAMEDIC

It is not practical to train every paramedic in every rescue specialty (Figure 48-11). It is possible, though, to train all paramedics to an "awareness level." Awareness training teaches recognition of hazards and understanding of the need for additional expertise at the scene. Failing to train paramedics in rescue awareness will end in the injury or death of EMS personnel, patients, or both.

Rescue involves a combination of medical and mechanical skills. If a rescue unit does not have medical training, your unit provides the balance. In any rescue situation, treatment begins at the site of the incident. If the patient can be accessed in any way, treatment may start before the patient is actually released from entrapment. Once medical care begins, it continues throughout the incident. The

FIGURE 48-11 It is impossible for an individual paramedic to be highly trained in all types of rescue. Instead, specialized rescue teams should be utilized.

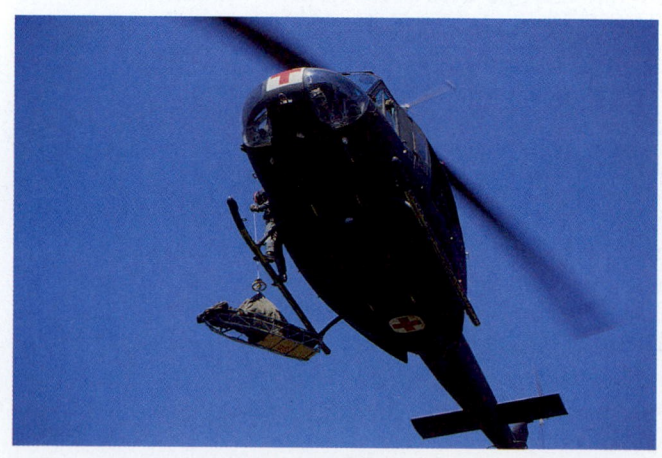

trick is to balance the medical and mechanical rescue skills. Teams must coordinate efforts to meet both medical and physical needs of the patient.

The role of EMS in a rescue operation varies from area to area. Some localities, for example, may require additional training beyond the awareness level. In general, however, all paramedics should have the proper training and personal protective equipment (PPE) to allow them to access the patient, provide assessment, and establish incident command.

As first responders, paramedics should understand the hazards associated with various environments—e.g., extreme heat or cold, potentially toxic atmospheres, unstable structures, and so on. They should also be able to recognize when it is safe and unsafe to access the patient or attempt a rescue. If you deem an environment safe and if you have the training to effect a rescue, you should at least participate in the rescue under the guidance of individuals with additional expertise. You should also understand the rescue process so that you can decide when various treatments are indicated or contraindicated.

The following pages focus on considerations that apply to most rescue situations—rescuer PPE and safety, the seven general phases of a rescue operation, and a "rescue awareness level" for the following environments:

- Surface water—e.g., "low head" dams, flat water, moving water
- Hazardous atmospheres—e.g., confined spaces, trenches, hazmat incidents
- Highway operations—e.g., unstable vehicles, hazardous cargoes, volatile fuels
- Hazardous terrains—e.g., high-angle cliffs, off-road wilderness areas

PROTECTIVE EQUIPMENT

Personal and patient safety equipment are paramount in any rescue. Some of the equipment discussed here has application in many rescue situations. Other pieces of gear are appropriate to specific environments or conditions.

RESCUER PROTECTION

In all rescues, EMS personnel should wear highly visible clothing. Ideally, PPE should fit the situation, but gear can be adapted. In fact, most PPE has not been specifically designed for EMS use. Instead, it has been borrowed from other fields, such as firefighting, mountaineering, caving, occupational safety, and more. The use of adapted gear has resulted from the lack of a national uniform reporting system to identify risk-related exposures for EMS personnel. Future risk management and PPE design should be driven by such data. At a minimum, the following equipment should be available:

- **Helmets:** The best helmets have a four-point, non-elastic suspension system, most of which are designed to withstand a greater impact than the two-point system in construction hard hats. Avoid helmets with non-removable "duck bills" in the back, which often cannot be worn in tight spaces. A compact firefighting helmet that meets NFPA standards is adequate for most vehicle and structural applications, climbing helmets for confined space and technical rescues, padded rafting or kayaking helmets for water rescues.
- **Eye Protection:** Two essential pieces of eye gear are goggles, vented to prevent fogging, and industrial safety glasses. These should be ANSI approved. Do not rely on the face shields found in fire helmets. They usually provide inadequate eye protection.

The application of safety equipment—both to the rescuers and to the patient—is paramount in any rescue situation.

FIGURE 48-12 Full protective gear, including turnout gear, eye protection, helmet, and gloves.

- **Hearing Protection:** High-quality earmuff styles provide the best hearing protection. However, you must also think about practicality, convenience, availability, and environmental considerations. In high-noise areas, for example, you might use the multi-baffled rubber earplugs used by the military or the sponge-like disposable earplugs.

- **Respiratory Protection:** Surgical masks or commercial dust masks prove adequate for most occasions. These should be routinely carried on all EMS units.

- **Gloves:** Leather gloves usually protect against cuts and punctures. They allow free movement of the fingers and ample dexterity. Heavy, gauntlet-style gloves are too awkward for most rescue work.

- **Foot Protection:** The best general boots for EMS work are high-top, steel-toed and/or shank boots with a coarse lug sole to provide traction and prevent slipping. For rescue operations, lace-up boots offer greater stability and better ankle support and don't come off as easily as pull-on boots when walking through deep mud. Insulation may be useful in colder working environments.

- **Flame/Flash Protection:** Every service should have an SOP calling for the use of flame/flash protection whenever the potential for fire exists. Turnout gear, coveralls, or jump suits all offer some arm and leg protection and help prevent damage to your uniform (Figure 48-12) and are quick and easy to apply. For protection against the sharp, jagged metal or glass at motor vehicle collisions or structural collapses, turnout gear generally works best. For limited flash protection, choose gear made from Nomex®, PBI®, or flame-retardant cotton. For high visibility, pick bright colors such as orange or lime and reflective trim or symbols. Some services use highly visible gear and/or orange safety vests at all highway operations—day and night. Insulated gear or jumpsuits are helpful in cold environments, but they can also increase heat stress during heavy work or in high ambient temperatures.

- **Personal Flotation Devices (PFDs):** If your service includes areas where water emergencies can result, your unit should carry PFDs that meet the U.S. Coast Guard standards for flotation. They should be worn whenever operating on or around water. The Type III PFD is preferred for rescue work. Attach an easily accessible knife, strobe light, and whistle to the PFD.

- **Lighting:** Many rescuers carry at least a flashlight or, better yet, a headlamp that can be attached to a helmet for hands-free operation. Consider the long-burning headlamps commonly worn by mountaineers and found through catalogs, the internet, or climbing/camping stores.

- **Hazmat Suits or SCBA (self-contained breathing apparatus):** These should only be made available to the personnel trained to use them. Most services or regions have special hazmat units to provide the highly specialized support for rescues involving toxic substances.

- **Extended, Remote, or Wilderness Protection:** If your unit provides service to a remote or wilderness area, you would be advised to have a backcountry survival pack as pre-loaded with PPE for inclement weather (cold, rain, snow, wind), provisions for personal drinking water (iodine tablets/water filter), snacks for a few hours (energy gels or bars), temporary shelter (tent/tarp/bivouac ["bivy"] sack), butane lighter, and some redundancy in lighting in case of light source failure.

PATIENT PROTECTION

Many of the considerations for rescuer safety also apply to patients, with several significant differences. A patient protective equipment cache should include:

- **Helmets:** Patients usually do not require the same heavy-duty helmets as rescuers. Less expensive, construction-style hard hats provide adequate protection against minor hazards. However, if you anticipate greater danger, as in climbing or caving rescues, outfit patients with the same high-grade helmets as rescuers would use.

- **Eye Protection:** Vented goggles, held in place by elastic bands, are ideal. They are not as easily dislodged as safety glasses. You might also use workshop face shields.

- **Hearing and Respiratory Protection:** Apply the same considerations as for yourself. Earplugs are usually adequate for hearing protection.

- **Protective Blankets:** You should have a variety of protective blankets. Inexpensive vinyl tarps do a good job of protecting patients from water, weather, and most debris. Aluminized rescue blankets protect from fire, heat, or glass dust. Commercially available wool blankets provide excellent insulation from the cold. Plastic shielding (the kind used by landscapers) and plastic trash bags of many sizes and weights are also very useful. One 55-gallon-drum liner is large enough to cover a single patient. It can serve as a disposable blanket, poncho, vapor barrier, or, in a wilderness situation, bivy sack.

- **Protective Shielding:** Circumstances may call for more substantial protective equipment. All rescue teams should be trained to use backboards and other commonly found equipment as shields to protect patients from fire, weather, falling rock or debris, glass, or other sharp-edged objects. Shields specifically designed for a Stokes basket should be available. Keep in mind, however, that a device that shields a patient from debris or the elements may also limit rescuers' access to the patient.

Personal flotation devices should be worn whenever operating on or around water.

Content Review

CHECKLIST FOR BACKCOUNTRY SURVIVAL PACK

PPE for inclement weather
Provisions for drinking water
Snacks for a few hours
Temporary shelter
Butane lighter
Redundant light sources

Always be sure to avoid covering the patient's mouth and nose during rescue operations.

SAFETY PROCEDURES

As you already know, safety—your own and that of your crew—is your first priority. Yet, in rescue situations a number of factors prod you to take action—your own desire to access the patient for treatment, the urging of people to "do something," the patient's cries for help, the presence of media, frustration at rescuers' lack of medical experience, and more. However, one mistake can spell disaster for you, your crew, and/or the entrapped victim. One way to curb "heroics" is by establishing rescue SOPs, determining crew assignments, and, above all else, preplanning scenarios well in advance of actual rescues.

RESCUE SOPs

Standard operating procedures (SOPs) are the nuts and bolts of effective EMS practice. At rescue situations, all teams should have written safety procedures familiar to everyone. Contents should include sections on all types of anticipated rescues. Each section should specify required safety equipment, required or prohibited actions, and any rescue-specific modifications in assignments. SOPs should include a statement requiring a Safety Officer and an explanation of that person's relationship to Incident Command. Ideally, the Safety Officer should be someone with the knowledge and authority to intervene in unsafe situations. This person makes the "go/no go" decision in the operation.

CREW ASSIGNMENTS

EMS units must anticipate crew assignments and special needs before the rescue operation takes place.

Search-and-rescue planners often use personnel screening to determine the participants. Programs exist to identify the physical capabilities of crew members. In addition, psychological testing is recommended. It may even be desirable to screen for specific traits, such as phobias. For example, a rescuer's inordinate fear of heights or small spaces should be taken into account when assigning duties. There must be regular practice of any dangerous rescue techniques that members of a unit may be trained to perform (Figure 48-13).

FIGURE 48-13 Dangerous rescue techniques, such as vertical rescue, should be frequently practiced to ensure utmost safety.

PREPLANNING

Preplanning starts with identification of potential rescue locations, structures, or activities within your area, then evaluates the training and equipment needed to manage each event. The preplan considers efficient use of existing resources and anticipates the need for additional equipment, rescuers, and/or expertise.

Due to the intensity and length of many rescue operations, provisions must be made for the maintenance and rotation of rescue personnel, as discussed earlier for multiple casualty events. On-scene diets should be high in complex carbohydrates and low in sugars and fats. Fluid replacement should consist of diluted (at least 50%) electrolyte solutions such as those found in sports drinks. The classic coffee-and-donuts regimen should be avoided altogether.

Preplanning should be part of a broader regional emergency rescue plan, to be tested and modified in practice exercises. When possible, specialized groups, such as high-angle teams, should take part. These "test-runs" will provide ample opportunity to practice the IMS as it applies to rescue situations.

RESCUE OPERATIONS

As already mentioned, many types of rescue operations include technically difficult procedures, very specialized equipment, or both. *They should be attempted only by personnel with special training and experience in these areas.* Some of these special rescue operations will be examined later. But first you need to be aware of the general approach to most rescue situations. Although procedures vary from area to area and rescue to rescue, most calls go through seven general phases: arrival and size-up, hazard control, patient access, medical treatment, disentanglement, patient packaging, and removal/transport.

PHASE 1: ARRIVAL AND SIZE-UP

Size-up begins with the dispatcher's call. Although the dispatcher's message may indicate a rescue situation, you must still evaluate the environment and potential risks. Upon arrival, you or another paramedic must quickly establish Medical Command and appoint a Triage Officer. You must also conduct a rapid scene-size up, determine the number of patients, and notify dispatch of the magnitude of the event. Now is the time to implement the IMS, any mutual-aid agreements, and the procedures for contacting off-duty personnel or backup ALS units.

Prompt recognition of a rescue situation and identification of the specific type are essential. You may be summoned to a structural collapse, vehicle rollover, or climbing accident. Each holds the potential for entrapment and the need for specialized crews and equipment. Be careful not to overestimate your capability to handle a rescue. Individual acts of courage may be called for, but safety comes first. If in doubt, err on the side of safety.

In calling for backup, *don't undersell overkill.* Remember that it is always easier to send back a rescue crew than to rectify a tragedy caused by too few rescuers or hasty heroics. Realistically evaluate the time needed to access and evacuate a patient. Use the IMS to shave off valuable response minutes.

PHASE 2: HAZARD CONTROL

Identify on-scene hazards quickly and clearly. You must often deal with these hazards before even attempting to reach the patient to avoid risk to yourself and other crew members. Control as many of hazards as possible, but don't attempt to go beyond your training or skills. Some situations, for example, involve chemical

Practice exercises with specialized rescue teams will give you and your unit ample opportunity to utilize the IMS as it applies to rescue situations.

Rescue operations should only be attempted by personnel with special training and experience in these areas.

Content Review

PHASES OF A RESCUE OPERATION

Arrival and size-up
Hazard control
Patient access
Medical treatment
Disentanglement
Patient packaging
Removal/transport

Be careful not to overestimate your capability to handle a rescue situation. In calling for backup, follow this precaution: "Don't undersell overkill."

spills, radiation, gas leaks, explosives, or other dangerous substances. You will need to employ a hazmat team and confine your actions to a safe area. Electric wires hold a "double threat" for fire and shock.

The very environment in which you stand can be risk filled. Look around to determine the possibility of lightning, avalanches, rock slides, cave-ins, and so on. Ensure that all personnel wear appropriate PPE, and never forget traffic hazards. The following list is just a sampling of other potential hazards.

- Poisonous or caustic substances
- Biological agents or germ-infected materials
- Swift moving currents, floating debris, or contaminated water
- Confined spaces such as vessels, trenches, mines, or caves
- Extreme heights or icy rock faces, especially in mountainous areas
- Possible psychological instability, as often experienced in hostage crises, urban violence, mass hysteria, or individual emotional trauma on the part of either the patient or the crew

PHASE 3: PATIENT ACCESS

After controlling hazards, you will then attempt to gain access to the patient or patients. First formulate a plan. Determine the best method to gain access and deploy personnel. Take steps to stabilize the patient's location. For example, look for threats of structural collapse, cave-ins, or vehicle rollover.

Access triggers the technical beginning of the rescue.

Access is the technical beginning of the rescue. This is the point when you and/or the Command and Safety Officer must honestly evaluate the training and skills needed to access the patient. Untrained, poorly equipped, or inexperienced rescue personnel must not put their safety—and the safety of others—at risk by attempting foolhardy, heroic rescues.

Key medical, technical, and command personnel must confer with the Safety Officer on strategy. To assure that everyone understands and supports the plan, a formal briefing should be held for rescuers before the operation begins. Even with well-trained personnel and adequate equipment, rescue efforts can be poorly executed because team members do not understand the "big picture" or do not know what is expected of each member of the team.

PHASE 4: MEDICAL TREATMENT

After devising a plan, medical personnel can begin to make patient contact (Figure 48-14). A paramedic has three general responsibilities during this phase:

- Initiation or patient assessment and care as soon as possible
- Maintenance of patient care procedures during disentanglement
- Accompaniment of the patient during removal and transport

FIGURE 48-14 Assessment and care may need to be modified, depending upon the on-scene environment and any special hazards.

If you are treating the patient, as conditions allow, quickly conduct an initial assessment (MS-ABC and C-spine status). The next critical steps include rapid trauma assessment for the patient with a significant MOI and medically oriented recommendations to the evacuation team.

A patient's condition may change dramatically during disentanglement and removal. Therefore, first, identify and care for existing problems. Second, anticipate changing patient conditions and the assistance and equipment needed to cope with them. Continually evaluate risks to both rescuers and patient. In many situations, the best overall patient care requires rapid stabilization and immediate removal. Final positive patient outcome may depend upon initial sacrifice of definitive patient care so that the patient and rescuers can be removed from imminent danger. Examples of such situations include:

- Injured, stranded high-rise window cleaners; workers on water, radio, or TV towers; high-rise construction workers
- Workers or bystanders involved in a trench cave-in
- Persons stranded in swift-running, rising water
- Patients entrapped in vehicles with an associated fire
- Patients overcome by life-threatening atmospheres
- Victims entrapped with unstable and/or volatile hazardous materials

In such cases, rapid transport of a non-stabilized patient to a safer location may be justified by the risk of injury to the rescuers and exposure of the patient to even greater complications. Rapid movement might be required even though the transport will aggravate existing patient injuries. Generally, management for the entrapped patient has the same foundation as all emergency care:

- Initial assessment of the MS-ABCs
- Management of life-threatening airway, breathing, and circulation problems
- Immobilization of the spine
- Splinting of major fractures
- Packaging with consideration to patient injuries, **extrication** requirements, and environment conditions
- Ongoing reassessment during the transport phase

Patient management during a rescue often follows the same protocols used "on the street." However, some specifics may be, or should be, significantly different. Differences result mainly from the lengthy time periods often required to access, disentangle, and/or evacuate the patient. EMS personnel are trained in rapid stabilization and transport, particularly with trauma patients. However, during a rescue mission, the desire to achieve speedy transport, as well as to obey the "Golden Hour" rule, may be impossible to fulfill. As a result, you must be able to "shift gears" mentally to an extended-care situation.

In addition to extended field time, you must be prepared to provide more in-depth psychological support for rescue patients than usual. This is especially true when a patient has already been entrapped for a considerable amount of time. Establish a solid rapport with the patient, striking up a constant and reassuring conversation. In quieting the fears, keep in mind the following tips:

- Learn and use the patient's name and tell the patient your name.
- Be sure other team members know and use the patient's name.
- Be sure the patient knows that you will not abandon him or her.
- Avoid negative or fearful comments regarding the operation, its cause, or the patient's condition within earshot of the patient.
- Explain all delays to the patient and identify steps that will be taken to remedy the situation.
- Ask special rescue teams to explain any technical aspects of the operation that could frighten or impact upon the patient's condition. Translate these operations into clear, simple terms for the patient.
- Don't lie to the patient. If something may hurt, acknowledge it. If the patient suspects an unstable environment, acknowledge that

Content Review

GOALS OF RESCUE ASSESSMENT

Identify and care for existing patient problem
Anticipate changing patient conditions and determine in advance the assistance and equipment needed

✱ **extrication** use of force to free a patient from entrapment.

In responding to rescues, you must be prepared to "shift gears" mentally to an extended-care situation.

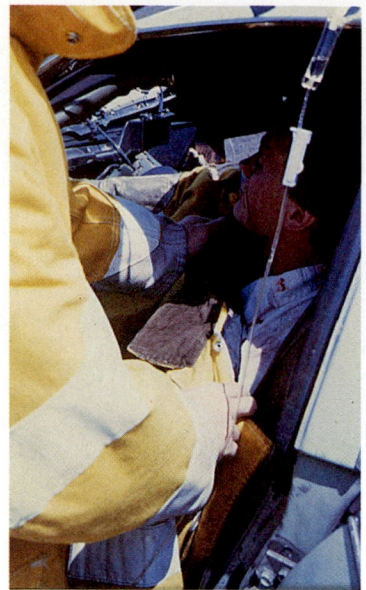

FIGURE 48-15 Disentanglement can be prolonged, as in the case of auto entrapment.

✱ **disentanglement** process of freeing a patient from wreckage to allow for proper care, removal, and transfer.

Disentanglement may be the most technical and time-consuming portion of the rescue.

✱ **active rescue zone** area where special rescue teams operate; also known as the "hot zone" or "inner circle."

It is paramount that the rescuer know how to properly package the patient to prevent further injury.

too. However, be sure to explain what will be done to mitigate the situation.

- Above all else, stay calm and professional. If you don't know the answer to a question, find somebody who does. Remember: Rescues are driven by patient needs.

PHASE 5: DISENTANGLEMENT

Disentanglement involves the actual release from the cause of entrapment, such as the dashboard of a wrecked automobile, a concrete slab from a structural collapse, or the blocked entry to a cave. This phase may be the most technical and time-consuming portion of the rescue (Figure 48-15). If assigned to patient care during this phase of the rescue, you have three responsibilities. They are:

- Confidence and the technical expertise and gear needed to function effectively in the **active rescue zone** ("hot zone" or "inner circle")
- Readiness to provide prolonged patient care
- Ability to call for and/or use special rescue resources

If you or another member of the rescue team cannot fulfill these requirements, reassess available rescue personnel and call for backup. Disentanglement is not a time for the claustrophobic or the squeamish.

Methods used to disentangle the patient must be constantly analyzed on a risk-to-benefit basis. You and other members of the rescue team must balance the patient's medical needs with such concerns as the time it will take to perform treatment, the safety of the environment, and so on. If a patient has a severely crushed extremity and it will take an inordinate amount of time to release the extremity, the patient may bleed to death without an amputation. This is only one of the hard treatment decisions that may be faced during disentanglement.

PHASE 6: PATIENT PACKAGING

After disentanglement, a patient must be appropriately packaged. You must consider such things as the means of egress—e.g., a litter carry through the woods versus walking a patient out. You must also factor time based upon the patient's medical conditions—e.g., rapid extrication techniques versus application of a Kendrick Extrication Device (KED). Some specialized rescue techniques require complex forms of packaging—e.g., being lifted out of a hole in a Stokes basket by a ladder truck, being vertically hauled through a manhole in a Sked® stretcher, and so on. In situations where the patient may be vertical or suspended in a Stokes, the rescuer must know how to properly package the patient to prevent additional injury.

PHASE 7: REMOVAL/TRANSPORT

Removal of the patient may be one of the most difficult tasks (Figure 48-16) or it may be as easy as placing the person on a stretcher and wheeling it to a nearby ambulance. Transportation to a medical facility should be planned well in advance, especially if you anticipate any delays. Decisions regarding patient transport—by ground vehicle, aircraft, or physical carry-out—should be based on advice from medical direction. En route to the hospital, perform ongoing assessment and administer additional therapy per medical direction.

FIGURE 48-16 Packaging and removal can be a time-consuming process, as in the case of a vertical rescue.

SURFACE WATER RESCUES

Water emergencies are among the most common rescue situations, because people are attracted to water in such great numbers and for such a wide variety of activities. Most water rescues are resolved without the involvement of EMS personnel—e.g., bystanders jump into a pool to pull out a struggling swimmer, other boaters rescue someone whose canoe has overturned, and so on. However, some water emergencies require special training and equipment. In such cases, the temperature and dynamics of flat or moving water place both the victim and the rescuer at high risk. Although all the possible scenarios for water rescue training cannot be covered here, the following are some general concepts.

GENERAL BACKGROUND

Water rescues may involve pools, rivers, streams, lakes, canals, flooded gravel pits, or the ocean. Some communities have drainage systems that remain dry until flash floods turn them into raging rivers. Most people who get injured or drown in these bodies of water never intended to get into trouble. But one or more factors conspire to create an emergency—the weather changes, swimmers underestimate the water's power, non-swimmers neglect to wear a PFD and fall in, people develop a muscle stitch or cramp while in the water, submerged debris knocks waders off their feet, boats collide, and more.

Nearly all incidents in and around water are preventable. Become familiar with safe aquatic practices. First, know how to swim and make swimming part of your physical exercise. Second, remember that even the strongest swimmer can get into trouble. Therefore, always carry PFDs aboard your unit and always wear a PFD whenever you are around water or ice. (Make sure your crew does the same.) Third, consider taking a basic water rescue course.

Water Temperature

Human body temperature is normally 98.6°F. Almost any body of water is colder and will cause heat loss. Water temperature in smaller bodies of water varies widely with the seasons and the amount of runoff. Yet, even on warm days, water temperature can be quite cold in most places. As a result, water temperature and heat loss figure in the demise of most victims and ill-equipped rescuers.

As implied, immersion can rapidly lead to hypothermia, a condition discussed in Chapter 36. As a rule, people cannot maintain body heat in water that is less than 92°F. The colder the water, the faster the loss of heat. In fact, water causes heat loss 25 times faster than air. Immersion in 35°F water for 15 to 20 minutes is likely to kill a person. Factors contributing to the demise of a hypothermic patient include:

- Incapacitation and an inability to self rescue
- Inability to follow simple directions
- Inability to grasp a line or flotation device
- Laryngospasm (caused by sudden immersion in cold water), thus a greater likelihood of drowning

A number of actions can delay the onset of hypothermia in water rescues. The use of PFDs slows heat loss and lessens the energy required for flotation. If people suddenly become submerged, they can also assume the **Heat Escape Lessening Position (HELP)**—floating with the head out of water and the body in a fetal tuck. Researchers estimate that someone who has practiced with HELP can reduce heat loss by almost 60%, as compared to the heat expended when treading water. If a group of victims find themselves in the water, researchers also suggest huddling together. This technique not only prevents heat loss, but provides a better target for members of a rescue team.

Basic Rescue Techniques

Basic rescue techniques vary with the dynamics of the water—i.e., moving water versus non-moving (flat) water. If your unit responds to frozen bodies of water, you may also add techniques for ice rescue and include the proper cold water entry dry suits as part of your PPE cache (Figure 48-17).

The water rescue model is REACH-THROW-ROW-GO. All paramedics should be trained in reach-and-throw techniques. A PFD is useless if it is not worn. So all EMS personnel should put it on, even for shore-based rescues. If at first you are unable to talk the patient into a self-rescue, then reach with a pole or long rescue device. If this is not effective or if the victim is too far out, try throwing a flotation device. All paramedics should become proficient with a water-throw bag for shore-based operations. Remember: Boat-based techniques require specialized rescue training. Water-entry ("go") is the last resort—and is an action best left to specialized water rescuers.

MOVING WATER

By far the most dangerous water rescues involve water that is moving. Competency at handling the power and dynamics of swift-water rescues comes only with extensive training and experience. The force of moving water can be very deceptive. The hydraulics of moving water change with a number of variables, including water depth, velocity, obstructions to flow, changing tides, and more. Only specially trained rescuers can readily recognize these factors.

To train for swift-water entry, rescuers must develop a proficiency in many specialized skills. In preparation for technical rope rescues, they must master the skills required for high-angle rope rescues. They must also become well-practiced in such skills as crossing moving water bodies, defensive swimming, use of throw bags and boogy boards, shore-based swimming, boat-based rescue techniques, management of water-specific emergencies, the capability to package the patient with water-related injuries, and more.

Content Review

ACTIONS TO DELAY HYPOTHERMIA
Use of PFDs
Use of HELP
Huddling together

✱ **Heat Escape Lessening Position (HELP)** an in-water, head-up tuck or fetal position designed to reduce heat loss by as much as 60%.

The water rescue model is REACH-THROW-ROW-GO.

Water entry is a last resort—and is an action best left to specialized water rescuers.

Four swift-water rescue scenarios present a special challenge and danger to rescuers. They include recirculating currents ("drowning machines"), strainers, foot/extremity pins, and dams or hydroelectric intakes.

Recirculating Currents

Recirculating currents result from water moving over a uniform obstruction to flow such as a large rock or low head dam. The movement of currents can create what is known as a "drowning machine" (Figure 48-18).

Upon first appearance, recirculating currents can look very tame. Anglers, for example, often fish on the downstream portion of a low head dam, casting their lines into the recirculating waters. This is a good place to catch fish because they can often be seen just below the dam. But think about it. If fish with their natural ability to swim get stuck in the recirculating currents, imagine what would happen to humans if they got too close to the dam. Once caught in the re-circulating currents, people find it very difficult to escape. The resulting rescue can be extremely hazardous—even for specially trained rescuers.

Strainers

When moving water flows through obstructions such as downed trees, grating, or wire mesh, an unequal force is created on the two sides of the so-called "strainers" (Figure 48-19). Currents can literally force a person up against a strainer, making it difficult to be removed due to the power of the current. In some cases, the current might be flowing into a drainage pipe under the surface, which is in turn covered by a rebar (metal) grate. Victims can get sucked into the grate and are then pinned against it.

✳ **recirculating current** movement of currents over a uniform obstruction; also known as a "drowning machine."

✳ **strainer** a partial obstruction that filters, or strains, the water, such as downed trees or wire mesh, causing an unequal force on the two sides.

FIGURE 48-18   When water flows over a large uniform object, it can create a hydraulic or hole with a recirculating current that moves against the river's flow and can trap people.

FIGURE 48-19   Strainers are objects that allow water to flow through them but that will trap other objects—and people.

This too can be a hazardous rescue. If you are floating downstream and see the potential of getting pinned against a strainer, attempt to swim over the object. Whatever you do, don't put your feet on the bottom—your feet could get stuck or you could get swept off your feet and slammed into the obstruction.

Foot/Extremity Pins

It is always unsafe to walk in fast-moving water over knee depth because of the danger of entrapping a foot or extremity. When this occurs, the weight and force of the water can knock you below the surface. To remove the foot or extremity, it must be extracted the same way it went in. Water currents often make this extremely difficult. Again, this is a hazardous rescue because of the need to work below the surface of already dangerous water conditions.

It is always unsafe to walk in fast-moving water over knee depth because of the danger of entrapping a foot or extremity.

Dams/Hydroelectric Intakes

Yet another dangerous situation involves dams and hydroelectric intakes, such as those often found along rivers. The height of the dam is no indication of the degree of hazard. As already indicated, low head dams can create powerful drowning machines. Assume that all dams have the ability to form recirculating currents. Hydroelectric intakes serve as dangerous strainers.

Self-Rescue Techniques

Some water survival techniques have already been mentioned—such as wearing PFDs and the use of HELP. However, if you suddenly fall in swift-running water (or flat for that matter), keep these suggestions in mind:

- Cover your mouth and nose during entry.
- Protect your head and, if possible, keep your face out of the water.
- Do not attempt to stand up in moving water.
- Float on your back, with your feet pointed downstream.
- Steer with your feet, and point your head toward the nearest shore at a 45-degree angle or continue to float downstream until you come to an area where the water slows enough for you to swim to the edge.
- If the water turns a bend, remember that the outside of the curve moves faster that the inside of the curve.
- Look for large objects, such as rocks, that can block the water and cause recirculating currents or strainers.
- Learn to identify **eddies**—water that flows around especially large objects and, for a time, flows upstream around the downside of the obstruction. These back currents move more slowly and can actually sweep you toward the edge—and safety.
- Above all else, take precautions not to fall into the water in the first place. Remember: reach-throw-row-go, with "go" being the absolutely last resort.

✳ eddies water that flows around especially large objects and, for a time, flows upstream around the downside of an obstruction; provides an opportunity to escape dangerous currents.

FLAT WATER

The greatest problem with flat water is that it looks so calm. Yet, a large proportion of drowning or near-drowning incidents take place in flat or slow-moving water. Some of the factors in these deaths were mentioned earlier. In a significant number of cases, alcohol plays a role. Nearly 50% of boating fatalities, for example, result from intoxication or impairment by alcohol—a drug that impairs the ability to think, reason, and survive in a water accident.

Factors Affecting Survival

A number of factors help determine the demise or survival of a patient. A person's "survivability profile" is affected by age, posture, lung volume, water temperature, and more. Two especially important factors, are the presence of PFDs and what is known as the "cold-protective response."

Content Review

FACTORS AFFECTING SURVIVAL

Age
Posture
Lung volume
Water temperature
Use of PFDs
Mammalian diving reflex

Personal Flotation Devices Many recreational water users associate "life preservers" with rough water or people who can't swim. But PFDs should be essential items for all water-related activities. One study, for example, linked nearly 89% of all boating fatalities to the lack of a PFD.

Every system should have a strict SOP mandating the use of PFDs for all EMS personnel. Even services in arid regions can be involved in water rescues. They can be called to swimming pool accidents or river-rafting accidents. In some places, especially in the southwest, they can respond to flash-flooding in canyons that can trap or kill hikers or "canyoneers." The same flash flooding can overload drainage systems, creating hazardous conditions for the public and rescuers alike.

Cold Protective Response The same cold water that can kill people also triggers a protective response known as the "mammalian diving reflex." This is how it works: When the face of a human, or any mammal, is plunged into water less than 68°F, the parasympathetic nervous system is stimulated. The heart rate rapidly decreases to a bradycardic rhythm. Meanwhile, blood pressure drops and vasoconstriction occurs throughout the body. Blood is shunted from less vital organs to the heart and brain, temporarily delivering life-sustaining oxygen. As a general rule, the colder the water, the more oxygen is diverted.

The mammalian reflex, along with the length of time the head was above water during the cooling process, can significantly delay death. Some patients have been resuscitated after 45 minutes under water. As a rule, the reflex is more pronounced in children than in adults.

Location of Submerged Victims

Because of protective physiologic responses, rescuers must make every effort to locate submerged victims. Interview witnesses to establish a relative location. Ask each witness to locate an object across the water to form a line. Repeat this process with each witness. Use the point of convergence among lines to target the most accurate "last seen" location. Start searching from this point and fan out in larger and larger circles, forming a radius equal to the depth of the water.

Rescue Versus Body Recovery

A number of conditions determine when a rescue turns into a body recovery. Some factors are length of time submerged, any known or suspected trauma, age and physical condition of the victim, water temperature and environmental conditions, and estimated time for rescue or removal.

Once a patient is recovered, you should attempt resuscitation on any hypothermic and/or pulseless, nonbreathing patient who has been submerged in cold water. (Some experts advise providing resuscitation to every drowning patient, regardless of water temperature, even those who have been in the water for some time.) A patient must be rewarmed before an accurate assessment can be made. Remember: water-rescue patients are never dead until they are warm and dead. (For more on drowning and near-drowning, see Chapter 36.)

Remember: Water-rescue patients are never dead until they are warm and dead.

In-Water Patient Immobilization

In flat water where you are able to safely stand, it is important that you know how to perform in-water immobilization. In general, the procedure mirrors the application of a long board, with the following modifications:

- **Phase One: In-Water Spinal Immobilization**
  1. Apply the head-splint technique. (There are other techniques, but they do not work as well because of the use of PFDs by the rescuers.)
  2. Approach the patient from the side.
  3. Move the patient's arms over the head.
  4. Use the patient's arms as a "splint" to hold the head in place.
  5. If the patient was found face down, perform steps 1–4, then rotate the patient toward the rescuer in a face-up position.
  6. Assure an open airway.
  7. Maintain this position until a cervical collar is applied.

- **Phase Two: Rigid Cervical Collar Application**
  1. A second rescuer determines the proper collar size.
  2. This second rescuer then holds the open collar under the victim's neck.
  3. The primary rescuer maintains immobilization and a patent airway.
  4. The second rescuer brings the collar up to the back of the patient's neck. The primary rescuer allows the second rescuer to bring the collar around the patient's neck and secure the fastener on the collar while the primary rescuer maintains the airway.
  5. The second rescuer secures the patient's hands at the waist.

- **Phase Three: Back Boarding and Extrication from the Water**
  1. Secure the necessary personnel—two rescuers in the water and additional rescuers at the water's edge—and the correct equipment. It is strongly urged that rescuers use a floating backboard for water rescue.
  2. Submerge the board under the patient's waist.
  3. Never lift the patient to the board. Instead, allow the board to float up to the victim. (If the board does not float, lift it gently to the victim.)
  4. Secure the patient with straps, cravats, or other devices.
  5. Move the patient to an extrication point along the shore or boat.
  6. Always extricate the patient head first, so the body weight does not compress possible spinal trauma.
  7. If possible, avoid extrication of the patient through surf, as the board could capsize and dump the patient back into the water. Consider using bystanders who can swim as a breakwall behind the patient.
  8. Maintain airway management during extrication.

HAZARDOUS ATMOSPHERE RESCUES

Confined-space rescues present any number of potentially fatal threats, but one of the most serious is an oxygen-deficient environment. At first glance, most confined spaces appear relatively safe. Here's where rescue awareness comes in. According to NIOSH, nearly 60% of all fatalities associated with confined spaces are people attempting to rescue a victim.

While "confined space" can have a variety of interpretations, OSHA regulation CFR 1910.146 interprets the term to mean any space with limited access/egress that is not designed for human occupancy or habitation. In other words, confined spaces

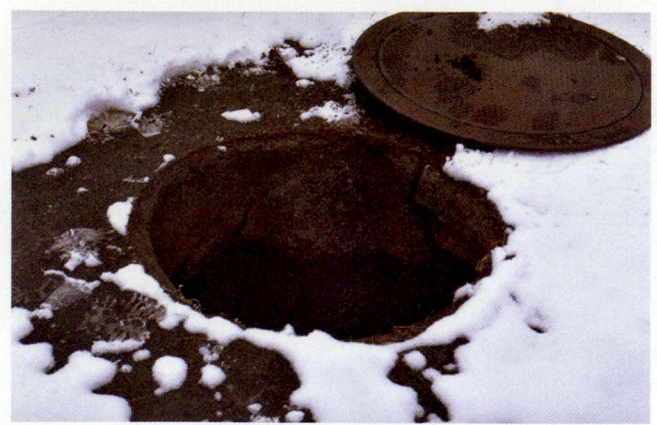

FIGURE 48-20A Manholes provide access to underground utility vaults. The vault may have a limited or hazardous atmosphere and may offer the potential for entrapment.

FIGURE 48-20B Rescuers should never be permitted to enter confined spaces, such as silos, unless they have training, equipment, and experience in this environment.

are not safe for people to enter for any sustained period of time. Examples of confined spaces are transport or storage tanks, grain bins and silos, wells and cisterns, manholes and pumping stations, drainage culverts, pits, hoppers, underground vaults, and mine or cave shafts (Figures 48-20A–B).

CONFINED-SPACE HAZARDS

Some of the most common risks in confined-space rescues include:

Confined-space rescues carry a high risk of oxygen deficiency.

FIGURE 48-21 Rescuers exposed to toxic or hazardous materials will need to go through decontamination.

- **Oxygen-Deficient Atmospheres:** Untrained rescuers may not readily think of oxygen deficiency. It simply is not a "visible" threat. Special entry teams know otherwise. Before going into a confined space, they monitor the atmosphere to determine oxygen concentration, levels of hydrogen sulfide, explosive limits, flammable atmosphere, or toxic contaminants. They are also aware that increases in oxygen content for any reasons—e.g., a gust of wind—can give atmospheric monitoring meters a false reading.

- **Toxic or Explosive Chemicals:** Many chemicals found in confined spaces can be toxic, especially if inhaled (Figure 48-21). Some of the poisonous fumes contain gases that displace oxygen in the red blood cells. Other chemicals are highly explosive. Dangerous chemical gasses commonly found in confined spaces include hydrogen sulfide (H_2S), carbon dioxide (CO_2), carbon monoxide (CO), exceptionally low or high oxygen concentrations, Chlorine (Cl_2), ammonia (NH_3), and nitrogen dioxide (NO_2).

- **Engulfment:** Some confined spaces contain grain, coal, sand, or other substances that can bury a patient or rescuer. Dust from these materials can also create a highly explosive atmosphere.

- **Machinery Entrapment:** Confined spaces come with all sorts of machinery or equipment that can entrap a person, including augers or screws.

- **Electricity:** Confined spaces often contain electric-powered equipment. In addition to the risk of shock or electrocution, these machines potentially contain stored energy. To ensure safe entry, it may first be necessary to blank out all power into the site. Second, stored energy should be dissipated, following lock out/tag out procedures. Third, the space may need to be ventilated to ensure against oxygen deficiency or explosive dust particles. Remember: It takes only one spark to trigger an explosion.

- **Structural Concerns:** Structure supports and shapes further complicate confined-space rescues. Some confined spaces have "I" beams that can cause injury due to limited light and height. Other confined spaces have non-cylindrical shapes that present difficult extrication problems. Confined spaces can be shaped in the form Ls, Ts, Xs, and any combination thereof. Because of limited access, rescuers may find it difficult or even impossible to use standard SCBA. They may have to resort to supplied air breathing apparatus—i.e., oxygen lines. They may also need to be lowered into the space with a full-body harness or other system to make retrieval easier in case something goes wrong.

It only takes one spark to trigger an explosion. Be careful of all potential sources of electricity.

CONFINED-SPACE PROTECTIONS IN THE WORKPLACE

Fortunately, state and federal laws require most industries to develop a confined-space rescue program. This means that employers must provide a training program for all employees who work in or around confined spaces. These employees may be called upon to perform on-site rescues and may indeed be an important part of the emergency response.

OSHA also requires a permit process before workers may enter a confined space such as a trench. In addition, most industries must fulfill strict requirements such as ongoing atmospheric monitoring, posted warnings, and work-site permits with detailed data on hazard management. The area must be made safe or workers must don PPE. Retrieval devices must also be in place whenever workers enter the spaces. Non-permitted sites are the most likely locations for emergencies because of inadequate atmospheric monitoring.

The types of confined-space emergencies most commonly encountered in the workplace include falls, medical emergencies (often hazmat-related), oxygen deficiencies or asphyxia, explosions, and entrapment. You should never allow untrained rescuers into a confined space. You will almost always summon outside specialized agencies for support.

CAVE-INS AND STRUCTURAL COLLAPSES

Collapsed trenches or cave-ins can occur almost anywhere. In fact, most trench collapses occur in trenches less than 12 feet deep and 6 feet wide, particularly in trenches that do not comply with OSHA regulations. To understand the medical magnitude of a collapsed trench, consider these facts. A typical cubic foot of soil weights 100 pounds. As a result, just two feet of soil on the chest or back can weigh between 700 to 1,000 pounds. People are literally buried alive. Unless uncovered quickly, they suffer death by asphyxiation.

Reasons for Collapses/Cave-Ins

Trenches collapse or cave in for a number of reasons, including:

- Contractors disregard safety regulations. (Federal law requires either shoring or a trench box for excavations deeper than 5 feet.)
- The lip of one or both sides of the trench caves in.

- The wall shears away or falls in entirely.
- The "spoil pile," or removed dirt, is placed too close to the edge.
- Water seepage, ground vibrations, intersecting trenches, or previously disturbed soil weaken the structural integrity.

Rescue from Trenches/Cave-Ins

If a collapsed trench or cave-in has caused a burial, a secondary collapse is likely.

If a collapse has caused burial, a secondary collapse is likely. Therefore, your initial actions should be geared toward safety. Secure the scene, establish command, secure a perimeter, and immediately summon a team specializing in trench rescue. Meanwhile, do not allow entry in the area surrounding the trench or cave-in. Safe access can take place only when proper shoring is in place.

HIGHWAY OPERATIONS AND VEHICLE RESCUES

As you know, the most common rescue situations for EMS personnel involve motor vehicle collisions. These generally go through the phases covered earlier. However, certain modifications must be made to meet the special hazards associated with traffic control and the extrication from wrecked vehicles.

HAZARDS IN HIGHWAY OPERATIONS

To prepare for highway rescues, you must size up the scene, identify all hazards, and assure scene safety. With highway operations, this means reducing traffic-related hazards and identifying hazards related to the vehicle crash itself.

Traffic Hazards

Traffic flow is the largest single hazard associated with EMS highway operations.

Traffic flow is the largest single hazard associated with EMS highway operations. You may have to respond to incidents on roads with limited access and to incidents on highways with unlimited access. In either situation, you will need to work closely with police to avoid unnecessary congestion and further collisions. Remember: back-ups impede the flow both to and from the scene.

An even bigger personal danger results from the risk of vehicles hitting EMS apparatus or personnel. Studies have shown that drivers who are tired, drunk, or drugged actually drive right into the emergency lights. Spectators can worsen the situation by getting out of their cars to watch or even "help."

At this point in your career, you probably already know some of the things you can do to reduce traffic hazards. Here are a few tried-and-tested techniques:

- **Staging:** Staging is critical at any MCI but has an added importance on limited-access highways. Always consider staging emergency vehicles away from the scene and have Command bring the vehicles in whenever there is an appropriate place and/or assignment for the crews. The staging area should be within a minute or two of the scene, ideally in a large parking area. Some situations simply cannot accommodate the entire response at once.
- **Positioning of Apparatus:** When apparatus does arrive, ensure that it causes the minimum reduction of traffic flow. As much as possible, position apparatus to protect the scene. The ambulance loading area should NOT be directly exposed to traffic. Also, DO NOT rely solely on ambulance lights to warn traffic away. These lights are often obstructed when medics open the doors for loading.

DO NOT rely solely on ambulance lights to warn traffic away.

- **Emergency Lighting:** Use only a minimum of warning lights to alert traffic of a hazard and to define the actual size of your vehicle. Too many lights can confuse or blind drivers, causing yet other accidents. Experts strongly advise that you turn off all headlights when parked at the scene and rely instead on amber scene lighting.
- **Redirection of Traffic:** Be sure traffic cones and flares are placed early in the incident. If the police are not already on scene, this is your responsibility. As a first responder, you must redirect traffic away from the collision and away from all emergency workers. In other words, you need to create a safety zone. Make sure that you do not place lighted flares too near any sources of fuel or brush, otherwise you risk an explosion or fire. Once you light the flares, allow them to burn out. DO NOT try to extinguish them. Attempting to pick up a flare can cause a very severe thermal burn.
- **High Visibility:** Make sure all rescuers are dressed in highly visible clothing. Don a brightly colored turnout coat or vest with reflective tape. You can apply the tape at the scene.

Other Hazards

Other, non-traffic hazards at highway operations include:

- **Fire and Fuel:** Spilled fuel increases the chances of fire. Be very careful whenever you smell or see pools of liquid at a collision. Bystanders who are smoking can cause a bigger problem than the original crash if they flick lighted ashes into a fuel leak. DO NOT drive your emergency vehicle over a fuel spill—or worse yet, park on one! Remember that all automobiles manufactured since the 1970s have catalytic converters. They run at a temperature of around 1,200°F— hot enough to heat fuel to the point of ignition. Be especially careful when a vehicle has gone off the road into dry grass or brush. The debris can be just as dangerous as spilled fuel, especially when brought into contact with a blazing hot catalytic converter.

  Bystanders who are smoking can cause a bigger problem than the original crash if they flick ashes into a fuel leak.

- **Alternative Fuel Systems:** Be equally cautious of vehicles powered by alternative fuel systems. High-pressure tanks, especially if filled with natural gas, are extremely volatile. Even vehicles powered by electricity can be dangerous. The storage cells possess the energy to spark, flash, and more.
- **Sharp Objects:** Automobile collisions mean lots of sharp objects— glass, metal, plastic, or fiberglass. Be sure to wear appropriate protective gear, such as heavy leather gloves and eyewear.
- **Electric Power:** Contact with downed power lines (Figure 48-22) or underground electrical feeds can be lethal. If a vehicle is in contact with electrical lines, consider it to be "charged" and call the power company immediately. In most newer communities, electric lines run underground. However, a vehicle can still run onto a transformer or an electric feed box. Make sure you look under the car and all around it during your scene size up. DO NOT touch a vehicle until you have ruled out all electrical hazards.

  DO NOT touch a vehicle until you have ruled out all electrical hazards.

- **Energy-Absorbing Bumpers:** The bumpers on many vehicles come with pistons and are designed to withstand a slow-speed collision. Sometimes these bumpers become "loaded" in the crushed position. When exposed to fire or even just tapped by rescue workers, the pistons can suddenly unload their stored energy. Some bumpers have been thrown a hundred

Downed Lines

In accidents involving downed electrical wires and damaged utility poles, the danger zone should extend beyond each intact pole for a full span and to the sides for the distance that the severed wires can reach. Stay out of the danger zone until the utility company has deactivated the wires, or until trained rescuers have moved and anchored them.

FIGURE 48-22 Establish a danger zone in motor vehicle collisions involving electrical hazards.

feet from the vehicle when they unload. As a result, you must examine bumpers for loading. Stay away from a loaded bumper unless you are specially trained to deal with this hazard.

- **Supplemental Restraint Systems (SRS)/Air Bags:** Air bags also have the potential to release stored energy. If they have not deployed during the collision, they may do so during an extrication. These devices must be deactivated prior to disentanglement. Auto manufacturers can provide information about power removal or power dissipation for their particular brand. Also, keep in mind that many new-model vehicles come equipped with side impact bags.

- **Hazardous Cargoes:** An incredible amount of hazardous materials travel across the highways of North America. For your personal safety, suspect hazmat at any scene involving commercial vehicles.

- **Rolling Vehicles:** As you already know, you must size up the position of a vehicle. You might arrive on the scene and see the vehicle on all four wheels and consider it stable. Then a crew member jumps into the rear to stabilize the patient's neck manually. Suddenly the vehicle starts rolling down the street. This situation is not only embarrassing, it is dangerous! So always check that the transmission is in park. Make sure the parking brake is on, the ignition is off, and any key rings with remote ignition starters are removed.

- **Unstable Vehicles:** Motor vehicles can land in all kinds of unstable positions. They can roll onto their side or roof. They can stop on an incline or unstable terrain. They can be suspended over a cliff or river. They can come to rest on a patch of ice or an on-site spill or leak. In such situations, you need to request the necessary stabilization crews or equipment. You should also know how to apply proper techniques for temporary stabilization, using ropes, chocks, or a come-a-long. Under no circumstances should you allow rescuers to access the patient until the vehicle is stabilized.

For your personal safety, suspect hazmat at any scene involving commercial vehicles.

AUTO ANATOMY

You must know some basics of automobile construction or "anatomy." Obviously, vehicles can differ greatly, both in terms of manufacture and design. However, most recent automobiles have certain features in common that can guide you in simple access situations.

Basic Constructions

Vehicles can have either a unibody or a frame construction. Most automobiles today have a unibody design, while older vehicles and light-weight trucks have a frame construction. For unibody vehicles to maintain their integrity all the following features must remain intact: roof posts, floor, firewall, truck support, and windshield.

Both types of construction have roof supports. The support posts are lettered from front to back. The first post, which supports the roof at the windshield, is called the "A" post. The next post is the "B" post. The third post is the "C" post. Station wagons have an additional rear "D" post. If you remove the plastic molding on the posts, the remaining steel can be easily cut with a hacksaw. Application of power steering fluid helps reduce the heat produced by cutting. Remember that cutting a post will interrupt the unibody vehicle's construction.

Firewall and Engine Compartment

The firewall separates the engine and occupant compartments. Frequently, the firewall can collapse on a patient's legs. Sometimes, a patient's feet may go through the firewall. Movement on other parts of the vehicle, such as cutting a rocker panel or roof support post, can place additional pressure on the feet. The engine compartment usually contains the battery. This can cause a fire hazard, so many rescue teams cut the battery cables. Before disconnecting the power, it's a good idea to move back electric seats and lower power windows.

Glass

Vehicles have two types of glass: safety glass and tempered glass. Safety glass is made from three layers of fused materials: glass–plastic laminate–glass. It is found in windshields and designed to stay intact when shattered or broken. However, safety glass can still produce glass dust or fracture into long shards. These materials can easily get into a patient's eyes, nose, or mouth or create cuts. Therefore, be sure to cover a patient whenever you remove this type of glass.

Tempered glass has high tensile strength. However, it does not stay intact when shattered or broken. It fractures into many small beads of glass, all of which can cause injuries and cuts.

Doors

The doors of most newer vehicles contain a reinforcing bar to protect the occupant in side-impact collisions. They also have a case-hardened steel "Nader" pin. Named after consumer advocate Ralph Nader, these pins help keep the doors from blowing open and ejecting the occupants. If the Nader pin has been engaged, it will be difficult to pry open the door. You must first disengage the latch or use hydraulic jaws.

Before attempting to assist a patient through a door, you should be trained in proper extrication techniques. In general you should follow these steps:

- Try all four doors first—a door is the easiest means of access.
- Otherwise, gain access through the window farthest from the patient(s).
- Alternatively, use simple hand tools to peel back the outer sheet of metal on the door, exposing the lock mechanism. Unlock the lock and pry the cams from around the Nader pin. Then pry out the door.

RESCUE STRATEGIES

In managing highway operations or vehicle rescues, you should use the following general strategies:

- **Initial Scene Size-Up:** Establish command, call for appropriate backup, locate and triage the patients. Triage may be delayed until hazards are controlled.

- **Control Hazards:** This topic has already been covered. But always remember this point: Traffic can be your worst enemy at a collision.

- **Assess the Degree of Entrapment and Fastest Means of Extrication:** Try all doors. If they can't be opened, decide whether it is advisable and/or necessary to break glass. Although you may not have the training or responsibility to use extrication equipment, you should observe their use so you know what technical skills are available should you need them (Figure 48-23). Be aware of the considerations and techniques for door removal, roof removal, dashboard or firewall rollup, and construction of a new door.

- **Establish Circles of Operation:** Set up two circles of operation early in the incident. The inner circle is the area where the actual rescue takes place. Limit the number of workers in this area to team members operating rescue tools and/or charged with actual patient care. If two different units must work in the inner circle—e.g., a fire department and an EMS crew—you will need to maintain a good working balance between the crews to avoid "over rescuing." The outer circle is where staging takes place. Hold all additional equipment and personnel in this area until they are assigned a duty.

- **Treatment, Packaging, Removal:** As a rule, the role of EMS personnel in vehicle stabilization and removal is that of patient care provider. Once specialized rescue personnel assure you that the vehicle is stable and the scene is safe to enter, you may approach the patient, initiate assessment, and administer emergency care. Patient care always precedes removal from the vehicle unless delay would endanger the life of the patient, EMS personnel, or others. Again, work with rescuers in any way possible to minimize risk, both to the patient and to on-scene personnel. You should be well-practiced in the application of long spineboards for rapid removal of the patient through the doors or vertical extrication through removed roofs.

Patient care always precedes removal from the vehicle unless delay would endanger the life of the patient, EMS personnel, or others.

RESCUE SKILLS PRACTICE

Depending upon local protocols, you should practice or observe the use of the various disentanglement or extrication skills commonly used with vehicle rescues, many of which have already been mentioned. Know how to gain access using hand tools through non-deformed doors, deformed doors, safety and tempered glass, trunks, and floors. Become familiar with the use of heavy hydraulic equipment employed by special rescue teams in your area and take part in practice scenarios to build agency cooperation.

HAZARDOUS TERRAIN RESCUES

In recent years, outdoor activities—mountain, rock, and ice climbing, mountain biking, cross-country skiing, snowboarding, and hiking—have drawn more and more people into rugged areas. Inevitably accidents happen in places that can be hard to reach. You don't have to live in the wilderness to take part in a hazardous terrain rescue. For example, a mountain biker can get injured on trails that run along power lines or a rock climber can get injured on an outcropping in a relatively populated area. Some climbers even scale buildings!

As a paramedic, you must know how to take part in rugged terrain rescues. At a minimum, you should know how to perform litter evacuations without causing additional injury to patients. Even more important, you should develop a "rescue awareness" so that you know when to call specialized teams and how to work with those teams once they arrive on scene.

TYPES OF HAZARDOUS TERRAIN

In general, there are three types of hazardous terrain: steep slope or "low-angle" terrain, vertical or "high-angle" terrain, and flat terrain with obstructions. Low-angle terrains typically can be accessed by walking or **scrambling**—climbing over boulders or rocks using both hands and feet. Footing can be difficult, and it may be hazardous to carry a litter even with multiple rescuers. As a result, low-angle teams use ropes to counteract gravity and/or may set a rope to act as a hand line. Any error can result in a fall or tumble.

High-angle terrain usually involves a cliff, gorge, side of a building, or terrain so steep that hands must be used when scaling it. Crews depend on rope and/or aerial apparatus for access and litter movement. Errors are likely to cause serious, life-threatening injuries or death.

Flat terrain with obstructions includes trails, paths, or creek beds. Obstructions can take many forms such as downed trees, rocks, slippery leaves or pine needles, and **scree**—the loose pebbles or rock debris that can form on the slopes or bases of mountains. Although this is the least hazardous type of rugged terrain, it is still possible to slip while carrying a patient, causing injury.

PATIENT ACCESS IN HAZARDOUS TERRAIN

Unless you have been trained in high-angle or low-angle rescue, patient access and removal should be left to specialized teams. Even if you have the skills to perform the rescue, you will in all likelihood need additional resources to provide the necessary balance of technical and medical support for the patient.

High-Angle Rescues

High-angle, or vertical, rescuers must constantly contend with the effects of gravity. Any organization that could be assigned a vertical technical rescue must have

Develop the "rescue awareness" to know when to call specialized rescue teams and how to work with those teams when they arrive on scene.

✱ **scrambling** climbing over rocks and/or downed trees on a steep trail without the aid of ropes. This can be especially dangerous when the surface is icy.

✱ **scree** loose pebbles or rock debris that can form on the slopes or bases of mountains; sometimes used to describe debris in sloping dry stream beds.

FIGURE 48-24A High-angle rescue is dangerous and difficult and should be deferred to those with special high-angle training and equipment.

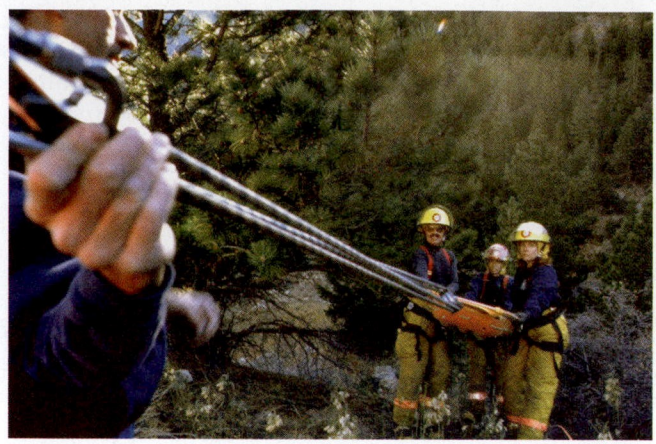

FIGURE 48-24B Low-angle situations are less difficult than high-angle situations. Many EMS agencies have trained their paramedics in the skills of low-angle rescue.

extensive training and top-of-the-line equipment (Figure 48-24A). Each member of a high-angle team must have complete competency in knot tying, use of ladders and/or ropes to ascend and descend a steep face, ability to rig a hauling system, and the skills for packaging a patient for evacuation by litter and rope.

Low-Angle Rescues

Many EMS systems have trained their paramedics in the skills of low-angle or "off-the-road" rescue. Like high-angle rescues, crews require rope, harnesses, hardware, and the necessary safety systems (Figure 48-24B). Low-angle rescues may be up to 40°, except if the face is overly smooth. Then a high-angle team will be better able to handle the more technical access and evacuation.

Each member of a low-angle crew must know how to assemble a hasty harness tied from two-inch tubular webbing (or don a climbing harness), rappel and ascend by rope, package a patient in a litter, and rig a simple hauling system to assist the litter team up the embankment. Teams must also know how to set up a hasty rope slide to assist with balance and footing on rough terrain. Although low-angle rescues involve less technical skill than high-angle rescues, they still require ongoing practice and proper equipment.

PATIENT PACKAGING FOR ROUGH TERRAIN

The Stokes basket stretcher is the standard litter for rough terrain evacuation (Figures 48-25A–B). It provides a rigid frame for patient protection and is easy to carry with an adequate number of personnel. Alternative spinal immobilizers can be used in a Stokes basket such as the KED, "halfback" backboard (extrication/rescue vest), or the Sked®. As a last resort, the Stokes itself can be used as spinal immobilizer.

Stokes baskets came in wire, tubular, and plastic styles. The older "military style" wire mesh Stokes will not accept a backboard. Newer models, however, offer several advantages including greater strength, less expense, better air/water flow through the basket, and better flotation in water rescues.

FIGURE 48-25A   A basket stretcher.

FIGURE 48-25B   A basket stretcher is often used to carry patients over rough terrain.

Plastic basket stretchers are usually weaker than wire mesh types. They are often rated for only 300 to 600 pounds. However, they tend to offer better patient protection. In general, Stokes baskets with plastic bottoms and steel frames are best. These versatile units can also be slid in snow, when necessary.

Most Stokes baskets, regardless of their style, are not equipped with adequate restraints. As a result, they require additional strapping or lacing for rough terrain. A plastic litter shield can be used to protect the patient from dust and falling objects. When moving across flat terrain, lace the patient into the Stokes basket to limit movement. When using a Stokes basket for high-angle or low-angle evacuation, take the following additional steps:

- Apply a harness to the patient.
- Apply leg stirrups to the patient.
- Secure the patient to a litter to prevent movement.
- Tie the tail of one litter line to the patient's harness.
- Use a helmet or litter shield to protect the patient.
- Administer fluids (IV or orally).
- Allow accessibility for taking BP, performing suction, and assessing distal perfusion.
- Ensure adequate padding—a crucial consideration.
- Consider use of a patient heating/cooling system, especially for prolonged evacuations.
- Provide for an airway clearing system via a gravity "tip line," if necessary.

PATIENT REMOVAL FROM HAZARDOUS TERRAIN

When removing the patient from a hazardous terrain, a non-technical evacuation is usually faster. In other words, when possible, walk the patient out. Remember: carrying a patient on a litter can be a strenuous task even under ideal conditions. The rougher the terrain, the more demanding the litter carry.

Carrying a patient on a litter over flat ground can be a strenuous task even under ideal conditions.

Flat Rough Terrain

When removing a patient in a litter from a flat rough terrain, make sure you have enough litter carriers to "leapfrog" ahead of each other to save time and to rotate rescuers. An adequate number of litter bearers would be two or three teams of six. Litter bearers should be approximately the same height.

Several devices exist to ease the difficulty of a litter carry. For example, litter bearers can run webbing straps over the litter rails, across their shoulders, and into their free hands. This will help distribute the weight across the bearers' backs. Another helpful device is the litter wheel. It attaches to the bottom of a Stokes basket frame and takes most of the weight of the litter. Bearers must keep the litter balanced and control its motion.

Low-Angle/High-Angle Evacuation

Before beginning patient removal, rescuers must ensure that all anchors are secure. They must check their own safety equipment and recheck patient packaging. They must also have the necessary lowering and hauling systems in place, again doing the recommended safety checks.

Materials, especially ropes, should never be used if there is any question of their safety. If you see a frayed rope or any stressed or damaged equipment, do not hesitate to point it out to the rescuers in a polite, but professional manner. Also, because hauling sometimes requires many "helpers," you may be asked to assist. Make sure you understand all directions given by the rescuers.

Some high-angle units, especially fire departments, make use of aerial apparatus such as tower-ladders or bucket trucks to assist in the removal of a patient in a Stokes basket. These units are usually employed in structural environments but can be adapted to hazardous terrain if there is room for a truck.

When using aerial apparatus, it is necessary to provide a litter belay during movement to a bucket. Litters, of course, must then be correctly attached to the bucket. Use of aerial ladders can be difficult because upper sections are usually not wide enough to slot the litter. The litter must always be properly belayed if being slid down the ladder. Finally, ladders or other aerial apparatus should NOT be used as a crane to move a litter. They are neither designed nor rated for this work. Serious stress can cause accidents resulting in patient death.

Use of Helicopters

Helicopters can be useful in hazardous terrain rescues, especially when hospitals lie at a distant location. Be aware of the difference in mission, crew training, and capabilities of helicopters that do air medical care versus helicopters that do rescue. You should be familiar with the advantages, disadvantages, and local restrictions for each of the following practices or techniques BEFORE you summon a helicopter from the field:

- Boarding and deboarding practices
- Restrictions on carrying non-crew members
- Use of cable winches for rescues
- Weight restrictions
- Restrictions on hovering rescues
- Use and practice of one-skids and toe-ins
- Use of **short hauls** or sling loads of equipment and/or personnel, as opposed to the more dangerous rappel-based rescues

Evacuation is a team effort.

Ladders or other aerial apparatus should NOT be used as a crane to move a litter.

Be aware of the difference in mission, crew training, and capabilities of helicopters that do air medical care versus helicopters that do rescue.

✱ short haul a helicopter extrication technique where a person is attached to a rope that is, in turn, attached to a helicopter. The aircraft lifts off with the person attached to it. Obviously this means of evacuation requires highly specialized skills.

Packaging/Evacuation Practice

Depending upon local protocols, you should practice the packaging and evacuation techniques expected of EMS personnel in your region. You should familiarize yourself with the specific types of basket stretchers and litters available to your unit and the proper packaging, immobilization, and restraint techniques for use with each type. Also practice with other equipment used for rough-terrain rescues, including the Sked® and appropriate half-spine devices.

Practice or observe the skills required for low-angle and high-angle rescues. When possible, take part in exercises with the rescue units that you would summon to perform these evacuations. By fully understanding the capabilities of the rescue response teams in your area, you will circumvent any "turf" issues and know how to work together when a multi-jurisdictional event occurs.

EXTENDED CARE ASSESSMENT AND ENVIRONMENTAL ISSUES

Environmental emergencies can present their own special challenges. For rescue operations, at least some personnel should have formal training in managing patients whose injuries have been aggravated by prolonged lack of treatment, often under extreme conditions. If SOPs do not already exist, procedures adopted from wilderness medical research will prove useful. Position papers written by the Wilderness Medical Society or the National Association for Search and Rescue can serve as guidelines for protocols.

Regardless of the source, you will discover that many protocols for extended care vary substantially from standard EMS procedures. If your agency anticipates involvement in some of the rescue situations described in this chapter, you should consider protocols that at least address the following areas:

- Long-term hydration management
- Repositioning of dislocations
- Cleansing and care of wounds
- Removal of impaled objects
- Non-pharmacological pain management—utilizing proper splinting, distracting the patient by talking or asking questions, scratching or creating sensory stimuli when doing painful procedures
- Pharmacological pain management—utilizing pharmacological agents with isolated trauma such as amputation or fracture or with multiple trauma such as crushing or pinning of more than an extremity
- Assessment and care of head and spinal injuries
- Management of hypothermia or hyperthermia
- Termination of CPR
- Treatment of crush injuries and compartment syndromes.

A number of environmental issues can affect your assessment during a rescue situation. Some of the most important issues include the following:

- **Weather/Temperature Extremes:** Extreme weather or temperature conditions increase the risk of patient hypo/hyperthermia. These conditions also make it difficult or impossible to expose the patient completely for full assessment and treatment.
- **Limited Patient Access:** Parts of the patient may not be accessible for examination. Cramped space and low-lighting conditions also make

assessment difficult. For this reason, it is important that you carry a headlamp with extended battery packs.

- **Difficulty Transporting Street Equipment:** Hazardous terrain often makes it difficult to transport typical street equipment to the patient. As a result, equipment usually must be downsized. Often you will utilize a backpack to keep your hands free for carrying. Essential equipment includes:
  - *Airway*—oral and nasal airways, manual suction, intubation equipment
  - *Breathing*—thoracic decompression equipment, small oxygen tank/regulator, masks/cannulas, pocket mask/BVM
  - *Circulation*—bandages/dressings, triangular bandages, occlusive dressings, IV administration equipment, BP cuff and stethoscope
  - *Disability*—extrication collars
  - *Expose*—scissors
  - *Miscellaneous*—headlamp/flashlight, space blanket, padded aluminum splint (SAM® splint), PPE (leather gloves, latex gloves, eye shields)

- **Cumbersome PPE:** Necessary, but cumbersome, PPE can restrict rescuer mobility. In certain instances, some of the PPE might be removed to perform care steps. For example, heavy outer gloves might be taken off during administration of an IV but reapplied as soon as possible.

- **Patient Exposure:** Patients should be quickly covered to assure thermal protection. During the extrication, place hard protection, such as a spine board, and take steps to prevent patient contact with sharp objects or debris. For example, use an aluminized blanket to protect against glass shards.

- **Use of ALS Skills:** Good BLS skills are mandatory in hazardous terrains, but limit ALS skills to those that are really essential. More wires and tubing complicate the extrication process. Continuous oxygenation and definitive airway control and volume may be essential. However, rescuers can't carry lots of oxygen tanks into rugged terrains. As a result, you may have to use your tank at a slower flow rate so that it will last longer.

- **Patient Monitoring:** Hazardous terrain can alter your use of monitoring equipment. In high noise areas, for example, you may have to take BP by palpation or use a compact pulse oximetry unit. An ECG monitor can be cumbersome during extrication and more difficult to use than in a street situation.

- **Improvisation:** Improvisation is common in rescue situations. To minimize the amount of equipment carried over hazardous terrain, you may want to consider such techniques as tying upper extremity fractures to the torso or tying lower extremity fractures to the uninjured leg. Lightweight SAM® splints can be very useful in the backwoods and should be part of your downsized medical gear. Whatever you do, continue talking to the patient and explain exactly what is happening. The patient is already frightened by the entrapment. Don't worsen the situation by making the patient feel even more out of control.

Good BLS skills are mandatory in hazardous terrains, but limit ALS skills to those that are really needed. Do not complicate any already complicated operation.

Part 4: Hazardous Materials Incidents

Hazardous materials (hazmats) are all around us. American companies manufacture more than 50 billion tons of hazardous materials a year. Some 4 billion tons are shipped throughout the United States by truck, pipeline, railroad, and tanker (Figure 48-26). You learned about some hazardous materials in Chapters 34 and 36 on toxicology and environmental emergencies. This chapter deals with hazardous materials spilled or released as a result of an accident, equipment failure, human error, or intentional violation of laws and regulations.

Also keep in mind the definition of a hazardous material offered by the U.S. Department of Transportation (DOT). A hazardous material can be regarded as "any substance which may pose an unreasonable risk to health and safety of operating or emergency personnel, the public, and/or the environment if not properly controlled during handling, storage, manufacture, processing, packaging, use, disposal, or transportation."

✳ **hazardous material (hazmat)** any substance that causes adverse health effects upon human exposure.

Even a small-scale hazmat incident almost always turns into a multi-jurisdictional event, thus triggering use of the IMS.

ROLE OF THE PARAMEDIC

Even a small-scale hazardous material incident is almost always a multi-jurisdictional event. All EMS personnel should be trained in how to respond to hazmat incidents and how to interact with other agencies that might respond. Traditionally, paramedics do not perform containment and control functions at a hazamt response. As first responders, they may size up the incident, assess the toxicological risk, and activate the Incident Management System. They will also be called upon to evaluate decontamination methods, treatment and transport of exposed patients, and medical monitoring of hazmat teams.

REQUIREMENTS AND STANDARDS

Two federal agencies—the Occupational Safety and Health Administration (OSHA) and the Environmental Protection Agency (EPA)—have set forth regulations and standards for dealing with hazmat emergencies. The most important are in OSHA publication CFR 1910.120, "Hazardous Waste Operations and Emergency Response Standard (1989)." This standard provides specific response

Content Review

EMS HAZMAT FIRST RESPONDER TASKS

Size up incident
Assess toxicological risk
Activate the IMS
Establish command

Content Review

HAZMAT REQUIREMENTS/ STANDARDS

OSHA publication CFR 1910.120
EPA regulation 40 CFR 311
NFPA standard 473

procedures, including use of an Incident Management System (IMS), personal protective equipment (PPE), a Safety Officer, and training requirements. The EPA has published a mirror regulation, 40 CFR 311, that applies to agencies that fall outside of OSHA. In addition, the National Fire Protection Association (NFPA) has published NPFA 473, *Standard for Competencies for EMS Personnel Responding to Hazardous Materials Incidents*. This standard, along with two other NPFA standards for hazmat response, deals with the training standards for EMS personnel assigned to hazmat incidents.

LEVELS OF TRAINING

The above documents set forth three levels of training appropriate to EMS response at hazmat incidents—Awareness Level, EMS Level 1, and EMS Level 2. The Awareness Level applies to responders who may arrive first at a scene and discover a toxic substance. Training focuses on recognition of hazmat incidents, basic hazmat identification techniques, and individual protection from involvement in the incident. All EMS personnel, as well as police officers and firefighters, need to be trained to the Awareness Level.

EMS Level 1 training, or the "operations level," is required for those who may perform patient care in the cold zone on patients who do NOT present a significant risk of secondary contamination. This training focuses on hazard assessment, patient assessment, and patient care for previously contaminated patients. EMS Level 2 training, or the "technician level," is required for those who may perform patient care in the warm zone on patients who still present a significant risk of secondary contamination. This training focuses on personal protection, decontamination procedures, and treatment for patients who are beginning or undergoing decontamination.

The level of training required for each individual depends on their role in the hazmat response system. All systems require some individuals trained in both the EMS Level 1 and Level 2 standards. In this way, patient care can begin during decontamination and continue after the patient has been cleaned of contaminants.

INCIDENT SIZE-UP

Sizing up a hazardous materials incident is a very difficult task. You often receive inaccurate or incomplete information, and events tend to develop very quickly. As already indicated, you can also expect a number of agencies to be involved, and you should practice the Incident Management System regularly with the other agencies that typically respond to a hazmat call.

IMS AND HAZMAT EMERGENCIES

You should be prepared for the special circumstances surrounding most hazmat emergencies. Some incidents, for example, will require immediate evacuation of patients from a contaminated area. Other incidents will have ambulatory contaminated patients who seek out EMS personnel as soon as you arrive on scene. Never compromise scene safety during the early phase of a hazmat operation. Otherwise, you risk becoming a contaminated patient.

Quickly determine whether the hazmat emergency is an open or a closed incident—that is, whether it has the potential for generating more patients. As you learned regarding the IMS system, the answer to this question will determine the resources that you request, how you stage them, and how you deploy personnel. In reaching your decision, remember that some chemicals have delayed effects. Triage must be ongoing, as patient conditions can change rapidly.

Priorities for a hazmat incident are the same as for any other major incident: life safety, incident stabilization, and property conservation.

Never compromise scene safety during the early phase of a hazmat operation. Otherwise, you risk becoming a patient yourself.

Hazardous Materials Threatened by Fire
When hazardous materials are either involved in or threatened by fire, the size of the danger zone is dictated by the nature of the materials. Use binoculars to read the placard on the truck and refer to the Emergency Response Guidebook for a safe distance to establish your command post.

DANGER
HAZARDOUS MATERIALS

Refer to D.O.T. Emergency Response Guidebook

WIND

Refer to D.O.T. Emergency Response Guidebook

CHEMICALS

Hazardous Materials
Leaking containers of dangerous chemicals may produce a health as well as a fire hazard. When chemicals have been spilled, whether fumes are evident or not, the ambulance should be parked upwind. If the hazardous material is known, seek advice from experts through the dispatcher or CHEMTREC.

FIGURE 48-27   Transportation incidents may involve hazardous materials.

Finally, keep in mind that the best site for deploying resources will be uphill and upwind. This will help prevent contamination from ground-based liquids, high vapor density gases, run-off water, and vapor clouds (Figure 48-27).

Basic IMS at a hazmat incident will require a command post, a staging area, and a decontamination corridor. Depending upon the event, the Incident Commander may also establish separate areas—such as treatment areas and personnel staging areas—to prevent unnecessary exposure to contamination. A backup plan for areas of operations must be determined early in the event. For example, what would you do if the wind direction suddenly shifted and a cloud of chlorine gas headed toward your staging area?

INCIDENT AWARENESS

Virtually, every emergency site—residential, business, or highway—has the potential for hazardous materials. For example, most households keep ammonia and liquid bleach in the kitchen or laundry. When combined, these substances produce a toxic gas. Homes with kerosene heaters or blocked flues can be filled with carbon monoxide. Always keep the possibility of dangerous substances in mind when you approach the scene. Binoculars can help you survey many scenes from a safe distance (Figure 48-28).

One of the most critical aspects of any hazmat response is the simple awareness that a dangerous substance is present.

Transportation

Any transportation accident—automobile, truck, or railroad—should raise a suspicion of hazardous materials. Maintain a high degree of hazmat awareness whenever you are summoned to collisions involving commercial vehicles, pest

FIGURE 48-28 Don't take any chances. Use binoculars to make a visual inspection of a potentially hazardous situation—such as a suspicious storage tank—from a safe distance.

Do not rule out the presence of a hazmat at an MVC just because you do not see a warning placard.

* **warning placard** diamond-shaped graphic placed on vehicles to indicate hazard classification.

* **weapons of mass destruction (WMD)** variety of chemical, biological, nuclear, or other devices used by terrorists to strike at government or high-profile targets, designed to create a maximum number of casualties.

Content Review

POTENTIAL TERRORIST TARGETS

Public buildings
Multinational headquarters
Shopping centers
Workplaces
Sites of assembly

control vehicles, tanker trucks, tractor-trailers, or cars powered by alternative fuels. Do not rule out hazardous materials just because you do not see a **warning placard.** Hospitals and laboratories, for example, routinely and legally transport medical radioactive isotopes in unmarked passenger cars. You might look in the back seat and see a container with a label indicating radioactive contents. Railroad accidents merit special attention. A railroad tank car can carry up to 34,000 gallons, and there may be several tank cars hitched together. Fortunately, railroads run along fixed lines, which means you can preplan your response.

Fixed Facilities

Hazmat incidents can also take place at fixed facilities. Chemical plants and all manufacturing operations have tanks, storage vessels, and pipelines used to transport products and/or wastes. Additional fixed sites with possible hazardous materials include warehouses, hardware or agricultural stores, water treatment centers, and loading docks. A farm or ranch may have hazardous materials stored in silos, barns, greenhouses, and other locations. Finally, remember that pipelines can be damaged by earthquakes, construction crews, or, if above ground, vehicle crashes. A ruptured gas or oil line can spell disaster, especially if ignited.

Terrorism

Terrorists can also create hazmat incidents, using a variety of chemical, biological, nuclear, or other devices to strike at government or high-profile targets. These **weapons of mass destruction (WMD)** can be manufactured from materials as simple as those found on most farms, as in the Oklahoma City bombing in 1993, or can be as unexpected as the use of hijacked commercial airliners to attack the World Trade Center and the Pentagon in 2001, with the concomitant release of jet fuel and other substances.

Terrorists usually select their targets by activity, particularly government or industrial, and by the number of people present. Potential targets include public buildings, multinational headquarters, shopping centers, workplaces, and sites of assembly such as arenas, stadiums, and transportation centers, or places of worship. All of these locations should be identified in any mass casualty or disaster plan for your community.

FIGURE 48-29 Vehicles carrying hazardous materials are required to display placards indicating the nature of their contents. You should regularly review the symbols, color codes, and hazard class numbers so that you can identify dangerous materials.

In responding to a suspected terrorist incident, look for clues. Patients in a closed environment, such as a subway or an office building, will exhibit similar symptoms if they have been exposed to a chemical or biological WMD. In the case of an explosion, remember that a secondary device may exist. Take every precaution not to fall victim to a terrorist attack yourself. Make full use of the Incident Management System and all specialized.

At terrorist incidents, remember that a secondary device may be present.

RECOGNITION OF HAZARDS

To aid in the visual recognition of hazardous materials, two simple systems have been developed. The Department of Transportation (DOT) has implemented placards to identify dangerous substances in transit, while the National Fire Protection Association (NFPA) has devised a system for fixed facilities.

Placard Classifications

Many vehicles are required by law to carry diamond-shaped placards (Figure 48-29) indicating hazmat classification through a color code and hazard-class number. Some also carry a four-digit **UN number** specific to the chemical. Placards also use symbols to indicate hazard types. For example, a flame symbol indicates a flammable substance, a ball-on-fire symbol indicates an oxidizer, a propeller symbol indicates a radioactive substance, and a skull-and-crossbones symbol indicates a poisonous substance.

Combined, these colors, numbers, and symbols help you to recognize the specific nature of the hazardous material. For instance, a red placard with the number 2 and a flame symbol means that the vehicle is carrying a flammable gas. Over time, you will become more familiar with these and other important symbols such as a "W" with a line through it, which means "reacts with water."

Keep in mind several shortcomings of the placard system. Although some substances need to be placarded in all quantities, others need to be placarded only if they are transported in large quantities. This means that there may be hazardous materials onboard a truck, but they fall below the quantity required for placarding. Also, the "Dangerous" placard means that there are two or more substances onboard between 1,000 and 5,000 pounds total weight. However, the generic placard tells you nothing about the nature of the materials. Finally, people can remove placards or fail to apply them in the first place.

✳ **UN number** a four-digit number specific to a given chemical; some UN numbers are assigned to a group of related chemicals, but with different characteristics, such as the UN 1203 designation for diesel fuel, gasohol, gasoline, motor fuels, motor spirits, and petrol. (The letters *UN* stand for "United Nations." Sometimes the letters *NH* for "North American" appear with or instead of the UN designation.)

Placards may only provide minimal information about a hazardous substance. Some materials, when shipped in smaller quantities, may not require a placard at all.

FIGURE 48-30A NFPA 704 hazardous materials classifications.

FIGURE 48-30B NFPA 704 labeling on a tank.

NFPA 704 System

The NFPA 704 System places placards on tanks and storage vessels at fixed facilities. On these placards, the diamond shape is divided into four color-coded sections (Figures 48-30A–B). The top, red segment indicates flammability. The left, blue segment indicates health hazard. The right, yellow segment indicates reactivity. The bottom, white segment indicates special information such as water reactivity, oxidizer, or radioactivity. Flammability, health hazard, and reactivity are measured on a scale of 0 to 4. A designation of 0 indicates no hazard, while a designation of 4 indicates extreme hazard.

> *Identification of a specific hazardous substance forms the "crux," or most problematic part, of a hazmat incident.*

IDENTIFICATION OF SUBSTANCES

Once you have determined that an incident involves hazardous materials, you must next try to identify the particular substance. This is the crux of dealing with a hazmat incident. You will often lack adequate on-scene information to make a positive identification, or you will get conflicting preliminary information. Therefore, you must be familiar with the resources that can assist you. To prevent dangerous misinterpretations, try to locate two or more concurring reference sources. Do not take action or treat patients until you find this information.

Emergency Response Guidebook (ERG)

Suppose you see a tanker truck bearing a red (3) placard with the UN number 1203 in the middle. Based on what you already know, you can determine that the incident involves a flammable liquid. To identify the specific liquid, you will need the *North American Emergency Response Guidebook*.

The ERG—published by the U.S. Department of Transportation, Transport Canada, and the Secretary of Communications and Transportation of Mexico—should be carried on every emergency vehicle. It lists more than a thousand hazardous materials, along with placards, UN numbers, and chemical names. It also cross-references each identification number to specific emergency procedures related to the chemical. The ERG includes, for example, a list of evacuation distances for the most hazardous substances. It is revised every three years.

When using the ERG, keep in mind two shortcomings. First, the reference provides only basic, generic information on medical treatment. Second, more than one chemical can have the same UN number. For example, UN 1203 may be diesel fuel, gasohol, gasoline, motor fuels, motor spirits, or petrol. The difference between a gasoline leak and a diesel fuel leak is dramatic, highlighting the need to use other methods of positive identification.

Shipping Papers

The most accurate information about a transported substance can be found in the **shipping papers,** or bill of lading. Trucks, boats, airplanes, and trains routinely carry these documents. Ideally, they should list the specific substances and quantities carried. However, drivers, pilots, or engineers may not take these papers when they exit the vehicle or craft, and you may find the scene too unstable to retrieve them. In some cases, the papers may be incomplete or inadequate, requiring location of additional sources of identification.

Material Safety Data Sheets (MSDS)

Fixed facility employers are required by law to post **material safety data sheets** (**MSDS**), containing detailed information about all potentially hazardous substances on site. The sheets typically list the following data: the names and characteristics of the materials; what types of health, fire, and reactivity dangers the materials pose; any specific equipment or techniques required for safe handling of the materials; and suggested emergency first-aid treatment.

Monitors and Testing

If you are unable to secure positive identification using the preceding sources, you may have to rely on monitors and other means of testing. If you do not have the training and equipment to do the reconnaissance, leave testing to the hazmat team.

Other Sources of Information

Once you have identified the hazardous substance, you will need to determine its specific chemical or physical properties. You can consult textbooks, handbooks, or technical specialists. You might also make use of a computerized database such as **CAMEO®**—Computer-Aided Management of Emergency Operations. Developed by the Environmental Protection Agency (EPA) and the National Oceanic and Atmospheric Administration (NOAA), this web site provides answers to technical questions, opportunities for skills practice, copies of software, links for networking, and more. Yet another source of information is your local or regional poison control center.

Two other sources of information are **CHEMTREC**—the Chemical Transportation Emergency Center—and **CHEMTEL, Inc.** Established by the Chemical Manufacturer's Association, CHEMTREC maintains a 24-hour, toll-free hotline. It provides information on the chemical properties of a substance and explains how the material should be handled. If necessary, CHEMTREC will even contact shippers and manufacturers to find out more detailed information

* **shipping papers** documents routinely carried aboard vehicles transporting hazardous materials; ideally should identify specific substances and quantities carried; also known as bills of lading.

* **material safety data sheets** (**MSDS**) easily accessible sheets of detailed information about chemicals found at fixed facilities.

* **CAMEO®** Computer-Aided Management of Emergency Operations; website developed by the EPA and NOAA as a source of information, skills, and links related to hazardous substances.

* **CHEMTREC** Chemical Transportation Emergency Center; maintains a 24-hour toll-free hotline at 800-424-9300; for collect calls and calls from other points of origin, dial 703-527-3887.

* **CHEMTEL, Inc.** Chemical Telephone, Incorporated; maintains a 24-hour, toll-free hotline at 800-255-3024; for collect calls and calls from other points of origin, dial 813-979-0626.

about the incident and provide field assistance. In the United States and Canada, the toll-free number for CHEMTREC is 800-424-9300. For collect calls and calls from other points of origin, contact 703-527-3887. CHEMTREC can also refer you to the proper agencies for emergencies involving radioactive materials.

CHEMTEL, Inc. maintains another 24-hour, toll-free emergency response communications center for the United States and Canada. In addition to providing support for chemical emergencies, CHEMTEL also supplies the names of state and federal authorities for dealing with radioactive incidents. For toll-free calls, dial 800-255-3024. For collect calls and calls from other points of origin, contact 813-979-0626.

HAZARDOUS MATERIALS ZONES

While waiting for additional help, keep a bad situation from becoming worse by evacuating uncontaminated people from the area around the incident.

As noted, your main priority at a hazmat incident is safety—in order of priority your own safety, then the safety of your crew, patient(s), and the public. Request expert help right away, just as you would under the IMS. Establish command and hold it until relieved by somebody higher in the chain of command. Keep a bad situation from becoming worse by evacuating people from the area around the incident. Do not risk anyone's safety by allowing "heroic" rescues. The result can only be more contaminated patients. Prepare for the arrival of additional resources by setting up the following control zones (Figure 48-31):

FIGURE 48-31 The three zones typically established at a hazmat incident.

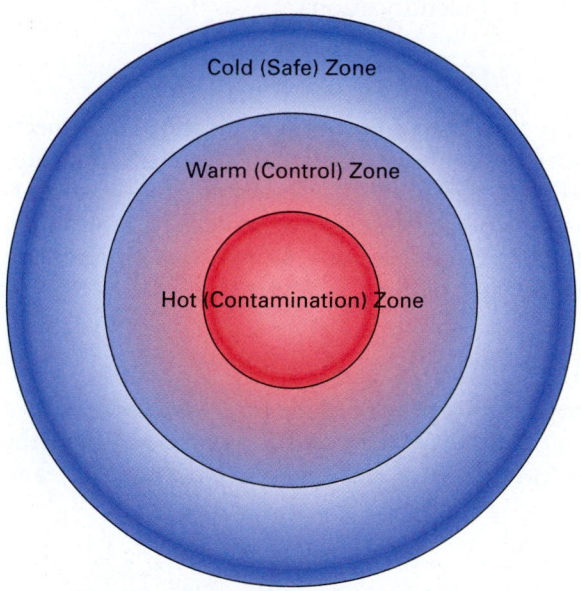

Hot (Contamination) Zone
- Contamination is actually present.
- Personnel must wear appropriate protective gear.
- Number of rescuers limited to those absolutely necessary.
- Bystanders never allowed.

Warm (Control) Zone
- Area surrounding the contamination zone.
- Vital to preventing spread of contamination.
- Personnel must wear appropriate protective gear.
- Life-saving emergency care is performed.

Cold (Safe) Zone
- Normal triage, stabilization, and treatment are performed.
- Rescuers must shed contaminated gear before entering the cold zone.

- *Hot (red) zone:* The hot zone, or "exclusionary zone," is the site of contamination. Prevent anyone without appropriate high-level personal protection equipment (PPE) from entering this area. Hold any patients who escape from this zone in the warm zone.
- *Warm (yellow) zone:* The warm zone, also called the contamination reduction zone, abuts the hot zone. It is a "buffer zone" with a decontamination corridor for patients and EMS personnel leaving the hot zone. The corridor has "hot" end and a "cold" end.
- *Cold (green) zone:* The cold zone, or "safe zone," is the area where the incident operation takes place. It includes the command post, medical monitoring and rehabilitation, treatment areas, and apparatus staging. The cold zone must be free of any contamination. You and your crew should remain inside this zone unless you have the necessary training, equipment, and support to enter other areas.

SPECIALIZED TERMINOLOGY

To prevent conflicts between the personnel or departments working at a hazmat incident, everyone should use the same terminology.

TERMS FOR MEDICAL HAZMAT OPERATIONS

The following are general terms relevant to chemical and/or radioactive materials that you may encounter during a hazmat operation.

- *Boiling point*—temperature at which a liquid becomes a gas.
- *Flammable/explosive limits*—range (upper and lower) of vapor concentration in the air at which an ignition will initiate combustion. The lower explosive limit (LEL) is the lowest concentration of chemical that will burn in the air. Below the LEL, there is not enough chemical to support combustion. The upper explosive limit (UEL) is the highest concentration of chemical that will burn in the air. Above the UEL, there is too much chemical and not enough oxygen to support combustion.
- *Flash point*—lowest temperature at which a liquid will give off enough vapors to ignite.
- *Ignition temperature*—lowest temperature at which a liquid will give off enough vapors to support combustion; slightly higher than the flash point.
- *Specific gravity*—the weight of a volume of liquid compared with an equal volume of water. Chemicals with a specific gravity greater than one will sink in water, while chemicals with a specific gravity less than one will float on water.
- *Vapor density*—the weight of a vapor or gas compared with the weight of an equal volume of air. Chemicals with a vapor density greater than one will fall to the lowest point possible, while chemicals with a vapor density less than one will rise.
- *Vapor pressure*—pressure of a vapor against the inside walls of a container. As temperatures increase, so do vapor pressures.
- *Water solubility*—ability of a chemical to dissolve into solution in water.

✳ **hot zone** location at a hazmat incident where the actual hazardous material and highest levels of contamination exist; also called the red zone or the exclusionary zone.

✳ **warm zone** location at a hazmat incident adjacent to the hot zone; area where a decontamination corridor is established; also called the yellow zone or contamination reduction zone.

✳ **cold zone** location at a hazmat incident outside the warm zone; area where incident operations take place; also called the green zone or the safe zone.

- *Alpha radiation*—neutrons and protons released by the nucleus of a radioactive substance. This is a very weak particle and will only travel a few inches in the air. Alpha particles are stopped by paper, clothing, or intact skin. They are hazardous if inhaled or ingested.
- *Beta radiation*—electrons released with great energy by a radioactive substance. Beta particles have more energy than alpha particles and will travel 6 to 10 feet in the air. Beta particles will penetrate a few millimeters of skin.
- *Gamma radiation*—high-energy photons, such as x-rays. Gamma rays have the ability to penetrate most substances and to damage any cells within the body. Heavy shielding is needed for protection against gamma rays. Because gamma rays are electromagnetic (instead of particles), no decontamination is required.

TOXICOLOGICAL TERMS

It is equally important to learn the terminology related to the toxic effects of hazardous materials. Here are the most important toxicological terms used in the field:

- *Threshold limit value/time weighted average (TLV/TWA)*—maximum concentration of a substance in the air that a person can be exposed to for eight hours each day, forty hours per week, without suffering any adverse health effects. The lower the TLV/TWA, the more toxic the substance. The Permissible Exposure Limit (PEL) is a similar measure of toxicity.
- *Threshold limit value/short-term exposure limit (TLV/STEL)*—maximum concentration of a substance that a person can be exposed to for 15 minutes (time-weighted); not to be exceeded or repeated more than four times daily with 60-minute rests between each of the four exposures.
- *Threshold limit value/ceiling level (TLV-CL)*—maximum concentration of a substance that should never be exceeded, even for a moment.
- *Lethal concentration/lethal doses (LCt/LD)*—concentration (in air) or dose (if ingested, injected, or absorbed) that results in the death of 50% of the test subjects. Also referred to as the LCt50 or LD50.
- *Parts per million/parts per billion (ppm/ppb)*—representation of the concentration of a substance in the air or a solution, with parts of the substance expressed per million or billion parts of the air or solution.
- *Immediately dangerous to life and health (IDLH)*—level of concentration of a substance that causes an immediate threat to life. It may also cause delayed or irreversible effects or interfere with a person's ability to remove himself or herself from the contaminated area.

CONTAMINATION AND TOXICOLOGY REVIEW

You have studied some of the following material in Chapter 34. The following is a review, highlighting topics relevant to hazmat situations.

TYPES OF CONTAMINATION

When people or equipment come in contact with a toxic substance, they are considered to be contaminated. **Primary contamination** occurs with direct exposure. **Secondary contamination** takes place when a contaminated person or object contacts an uncontaminated person or object. Touching a contaminated patient, for example, can result in a contaminated care provider. Gas exposure rarely results in secondary contamination. Liquid and particulate matter are much more likely to be transferred.

Consider this example. A pipeline ruptures and sprays several people with a hazardous substance. This is primary contamination. One of these patients walks out of the area and calls an ambulance. When this patient climbs into the back of the ambulance, he exposes the paramedics and ambulance. This is secondary contamination. As a member of the EMS crew, you must make every effort not to become part of the incident through such secondary contamination.

ROUTES OF EXPOSURE

As you know, there are four routes of exposure to a hazardous substance: inhalation, absorption, injection, and ingestion. The most common is inhalation. Once substances enter the bronchial tree, they can be quickly absorbed, especially in oxygen-deficient atmospheres. The substance then enters the central circulation and is distributed throughout the body. As a result, inhaled substances often trigger a rapid onset of symptoms.

Toxic substances may also be taken in through the skin, by either topical absorption or parenteral injection via a laceration, burn, or puncture. The least common route of exposure to hazmats is gastrointestinal. However, in occupations involving hazardous materials, people ingest poisons by eating, drinking, or smoking around deadly substances. People can also forget to wash their hands and introduce the substance in their mouths.

CYCLES AND ACTIONS OF POISONS

Absorption—the rate at which a substance is delivered into the blood stream—varies with the type and dosage. In general, the higher the dose, the greater the effect. Resources mentioned earlier provide information on a given substance's actions, distribution to target organs, likely areas of deposit, and so on.

Effects may be acute or delayed. **Acute effects** manifest themselves immediately or shortly after exposure. **Delayed effects** may not become apparent for hours, days, weeks, months, or even years. A person exposed to chlorine gas, for example, immediately develops shortness of breath—an acute effect. A person exposed to a carcinogen, on the other hand, may develop a malignancy years later—a delayed effect. Some substances, such as mustard gas cause immediate damage, but victims do not develop symptoms for many hours.

Once a substance is introduced into the body, it is distributed to target organs. Effects may be local or systemic. **Local effects** involve areas around the immediate site and should be evaluated based upon the burn model. You can usually expect some skin irritation (topical) or perhaps acute bronchospasm (respiratory). An acid sprayed on the skin, for example, creates immediate skin damage at the point of contact. **Systemic effects** occur throughout the body. They can affect the cardiovascular, neurologic, hepatic, and/or renal systems. Although hydrofluoric acid may cause local skin burns upon contact, for example, it can also trigger hypocalcemia and dysrhythmias, making it potentially fatal.

---

* **primary contamination** direct exposure of a person or item to a hazardous substance.

* **secondary contamination** transfer of a hazardous substance to a non-contaminated person or item via contact with someone or something already contaminated by the substance.

Although gas exposure rarely results in secondary contamination, liquid and particulate matter can be easily transferred.

Content Review

COMMON ROUTES OF HAZMAT EXPOSURE

Respiratory inhalation
Topical absorption
Parenteral injection
Gastrointestinal ingestion

In hazmat situations, the least common route of exposure is through gastrointestinal ingestion. The most common routes are inhalation and topical absorption.

* **acute effects** signs and/or symptoms rapidly displayed upon exposure to a toxic substance.

* **delayed effects** signs, symptoms, and/or conditions developed hours, days, weeks, months, or even years after the exposure.

* **local effects** effects involving areas around the immediate site; should be evaluated based upon the burn model.

* **systemic effects** effects that occur throughout the body after exposure to a toxic substance.

Before administering any medication to a hazmat patient, be sure to obtain at least two independent sources of agreement. Also consult with medical direction or the poison control center on possible synergistic effects or treatments.

The organs mostly commonly associated with toxic substances are the liver and kidneys. The liver metabolizes most substances by chemically altering them, a process known as **biotransformation.** The kidneys can usually excrete the substances through the urine. However, both the liver and kidneys may be adversely affected by chemicals, as are other organs, losing their ability to eliminate the toxic substances and creating a life-threatening situation.

When treating patients exposed to toxic substances, keep in mind that two substances or drugs may work together to produce an effect that neither can produce on its own. This is called **synergism.** Before administering any medication, be sure to consult medical direction or the poison control center on possible synergistic effects of treatments.

TREATMENT OF COMMON EXPOSURES

After ensuring your own safety, all toxic-exposure patients should receive the necessary supportive measures—airway support and suctioning, respiratory support, supplemental oxygen, circulatory support, and intravenous access. Before you administer specific pharmacological treatment, at least two sources should agree on the medication, and you should confer with medical direction.

The following are several of the most common classifications of chemicals to which patients may be exposed. A brief overview of effects and treatment procedures is provided for each circumstance. This is a generic discussion, not intended to replace the specific resources already described.

Corrosives

Corrosives—acids and alkalis (bases)—can be found in many everyday materials, for example the alkali sodium hydroxide found in most drain cleaners. Corrosives can be inhaled, ingested, absorbed, or injected. Primary effects include severe skin burns and respiratory burns and/or edema. Some may have systemic effects.

When decontaminating a patient exposed to solid corrosives, brush off dry particles. In the case of liquid corrosives, flush the exposed area with large quantities of water. Tincture of green soap may help in decontamination. Irrigate eye injuries with water, possibly using a topical ophthalmic anesthetic such as tetracaine to reduce eye discomfort. In patients with pulmonary edema, consider the administration of furosemide (Lasix) or albuterol. If the patient has ingested a corrosive, DO NOT induce vomiting. If the patient can swallow and is not drooling, you may direct the person to drink 5cc/kg water up to 200 cc. As with other injuries, maintain and support the ABCs.

If a patient has ingested a corrosive, DO NOT induce vomiting.

Pulmonary Irritants

Many substances can be pulmonary irritants, including fumes from chlorine and ammonia. When inhaled, chlorine mixes with respiratory secretions to produce hydrochloric acid. Ammonia mixes with respiratory secretions to produce ammonium hydroxide, an alkali. In addition to tissue damage, these chemicals can cause pulmonary edema. The substances can also injure intact skin.

Primary respiratory exposure cannot be decontaminated. However, you should remove the patient's clothing to prevent any trapped gas from being contained near the body. You should also flush any exposed skin with large quantities of water. Irrigate eye injuries with water, possibly using tetracaine to reduce eye discomfort. Treat pulmonary edema with furosemide, if indicated. Again, treatment includes maintaining and supporting the ABCs.

Primary respiratory exposure cannot be decontaminated. However, you should remove the patient's clothing to release any trapped gases.

Pesticides

Toxic pesticides or insecticides primarily include carbamates and organophosphates. Exposure may occur through all four routes of exposure—inhalation, absorption, ingestion, or injection. The substances can act to block **acetylcholinesterase (AChE)**—an enzyme that stops the action of acetylocholine, a neurotransmitter. The result is overstimulation of the muscarinic receptors and the SLUDGE syndrome: salivation, lacrimation, urination, diarrhea, gastrointestinal distress, and emesis. Stimulation of the nicotinic receptor may also trigger involuntary muscle contraction and pinpoint pupils.

These chemicals will continue to be absorbed as long as they remain on the skin. As a result, decontamination with large amounts of water and tincture of green soap is essential. Remove all clothing and jewelry to prevent the chemical from being trapped against the skin. Maintain and support airway, breathing, and circulation. Secretions in the airway may need to be suctioned.

The primary treatment for significant exposure to pesticides is atropinization. The dose should be increased until the SLUDGE symptoms start to resolve. For carbamates, Pralidoxime is NOT recommended. If an adult patient presents with seizures, administer 5 to 10 mg of diazepam. Do NOT induce vomiting if the patient has ingested the chemical. However, if the patient can swallow and has an intact gag reflex, you can administer 5 cc/kg up to 200 ml of water.

Chemical Asphyxiants

The most common chemical asphyxiants include carbon monoxide (CO) and cyanides such as bitter almond oil, hydrocyanic acid, potassium cyanide, wild cherry syrup, prussic acid, and nitroprusside. Keep in mind that both CO and cyanides are byproducts of combustion, so patients who present with smoke inhalation may need to be assessed for these substances as well. Most patients are exposed to CO and cyanides through inhalation. However, keep in mind that cyanides can also be ingested, absorbed, or injected.

These two chemicals have different actions once inhaled. Carbon monoxide has a very high affinity for hemoglobin—approximately 200 times greater than oxygen. As a result, it displaces oxygen in the red blood cells. Cyanides, on the other hand, inhibit the action of **cytochrome oxidase.** This enzyme complex, found in cellular mitochondria, enables oxygen to create the adenosine triphosphate (ATP) required for all muscle energy. Primary effects of CO exposure include changes in mental status and other signs of hypoxia such as chest pain, loss of consciousness, or seizures. Primary effects of cyanides include rapid onset of unconsciousness, seizures, and cardiopulmonary arrest.

Decontamination of patients exposed to CO and cyanide asphyxiants is usually unnecessary. However, they must be removed from the toxic environment without exposing rescuers to inhalation. Take off the patient's clothing to prevent entrapment of any toxic gases, while maintaining airway, breathing, and circulatory support. Definitive treatment for CO inhalation is oxygenation. In some cases, it may be provided through hyperbaric therapy.

Definitive treatment for cyanide exposure can be provided by several interventions carried in a cyanide kit. First, administer amyl nitrite. This short-acting vasodilator has the ability to convert hemoglobin to methemoglobin, which forms a nontoxic complex with cyanide ions. Wrap an ampule in gauze or cloth and crush it between your fingers. Then place it in front of a spontaneously

* **acetylcholinesterase (AchE)** enzyme that stops the action of acetylocholine, a neurotransmitter.

Most pesticides will continue to be absorbed as long as they are on the skin. Decontamination with large of amounts of water and tincture of green soap is essential.

The primary pharmacological treatment of significant exposure to pesticides is atropinization. The dose should be increased until the SLUDGE symptoms start to resolve.

Assess patients who present with smoke inhalation for the presence of carbon monoxide and cyanides—two byproducts of combustion.

* **cytochrome oxidase** enzyme complex, found in cellular mitochondria, that enables oxygen to create the adenosine triphosphate (ATP) required for all muscle energy.

Definitive treatment for CO inhalation is oxygenation.

Keep in mind that amyl nitrite is volatile and highly flammable. When mixed with air or oxygen, it can be easily ignited.

breathing patient for 15 seconds. Repeat at one-minute intervals until an infusion of sodium nitrite is ready. Keep in mind that amyl nitrite is volatile and highly flammable when mixed with air or oxygen.

Next, administer the sodium nitrite, 300 mg IV push over 5 minutes. (Sodium nitrite also produces methemoglobin.) Quickly follow the sodium nitrite with an infusion of sodium thiosulfate, 12.5 g. IV push over 5 minutes. The sodium thiosulfate converts the cyanide/methemoglobin complexes into thiocyanate, which can be excreted by the kidneys. If the signs and symptoms reappear, the process should be repeated at half the original doses.

Hydrocarbon Solvents

Many chemicals can act as solvents, including xylene and methylene chloride. Usually found in liquid form, they give off easily inhaled vapors. Primary effects include dysrhythmias, pulmonary edema, and respiratory failure. Delayed effects include damage to the central nervous system and the renal system. Exposure to these chemicals may be intentional, such as among drug abusers seeking the CNS effects (euphoria) produced by the fumes. If the patient ingests the chemical and vomits, aspiration may lead to pulmonary edema.

Treatment varies with the route of exposure. In cases of topical contact, decontaminate the exposed area with large quantities of warm water and tincture of green soap. If the patient has ingested the solvent, DO NOT induce vomiting. If the adult patient presents with seizures, administer 5–10 mg diazepam. In the case of inhalation, maintain and support the ABCs.

APPROACHES TO DECONTAMINATION

Decontamination (decon) attempts to reduce or remove hazardous substances from people and/or equipment to prevent adverse health effects. It can be accomplished by physical or chemical means. Physical decontamination involves the removal of chemicals, while chemical decontamination focuses on changing the hazardous substance into something less harmful.

There are several purposes for performing decon. First, decon reduces the dosage of the material to which patients are exposed. Second, it reduces the risk of secondary contamination of rescuers, on-scene personnel, bystanders, hospital personnel, families of rescuers, and the general public.

METHODS OF DECONTAMINATION

There are four methods of decontamination—dilution, absorption, neutralization, and isolation. The method used depends upon the type of hazardous substance and the route of exposure. In many instances, rescuers will use two or more of these methods during the decontamination process.

- *Dilution* involves the application of large quantities of water. Water is considered the universal decon solution, especially for reducing topical absorption. It may be aided by use of a soap, such as tincture of green soap. Note that a few chemicals should never be mixed with water.
- *Absorption* entails the use of pads or towels to "blot" up the hazardous material. The process is usually applied after washing with water to dry the patient or object. Absorption is not usually a primary decon method.

- *Neutralization* occurs when one substance reduces or eliminates the toxicity of another, such as adding an acid to a base. This method is almost never used by EMS personnel because, in a field setting, it is difficult to identify the exact substance and proper neutralizing agent. Also, neutralization often produces an exothermic reaction, or release of large quantities of heat, which can be as or more damaging than the original chemical.
- *Isolation* is separating the patient or equipment from the hazardous substance. It begins as hazmat teams remove patients from the hot zone to the warm zone. Further, any items that might contain or trap a hazardous substance are removed, including clothing and jewelry. All contaminated items should be properly disposed of or stored.

Neutralization is almost never used by EMS personnel as a method of decontamination. Be aware of its risks—possible misidentifcation of the chemical or neutralizing agent and potential for exothermic reactions

DECONTAMINATION DECISION MAKING

The priorities of incident management—life safety, incident stabilization, and property conservation—should guide your decision making throughout a hazmat incident. For example, you should try to prevent any run-off waters used for decontamination from damaging the environment. However, environmental considerations form a major concern only when are no life threats—i.e., patients are stable and not expected to deteriorate during the decon process. If life threats exist, patients come first, environmental considerations last.

If life threats exist, the patients come first, environmental considerations last.

Modes of Operation

In general, there are two modes of EMS operation at hazmat incidents: "fast-break" and long-term decision making. Fast-break decision making occurs when immediate action is needed to prevent contamination and handle life threats. Long-term decision making takes place at extended events with hazmat teams.

Fast-Break Decision Making Contaminated victims will often self-rescue. They will walk themselves from the primary incident site to the EMS units. In such cases, you must make fast-break decisions to prevent rescuer contamination. It may take time for a hazmat team to arrive and set up operations. In the interim, contaminated patients may try to leave the scene entirely. As a result, all EMS units must be prepared for gross decontamination. Basic personal protective equipment should be on board and all personnel should be familiar with the two-step decontamination procedures covered later.

All EMS units must be prepared for gross decontamination procedures.

Implement this mode of decision making at all incidents with critical patients and unknown or life-threatening materials. Fire apparatus often respond very quickly and carry large quantities of water that can be used for decon. Remove patient clothing, treat life-threatening problems, and wash with water. While it is preferable to use warm water to prevent hypothermia, this option is not always available. Please remember that the first rule of EMS is NOT TO BECOME A PATIENT! At no time should you or other crew members expose yourselves to contaminants—even to rescue a critically injured patient. Instead, contain and isolate the patient as best possible until the proper support arrives.

At no time should you or other crew members expose yourselves to contaminants—even to rescue a critically injured patient.

When treating critically injured hazmat patients, it is important to perform a rapid risk-to-benefit assessment. Ask yourself these questions: How much risk of exposure will I incur by intubating a patient during decon? Does the patient really need an intravenous line established right now? Few ALS procedures will truly make a difference if performed rapidly, but one mistake can make any rescuer into a patient. Take a few moments, and think before you act.

At incidents where patients are non-critical, rescuers can take a more contemplative approach, especially if they can identify the substance. Decontamination and treatment proceed simultaneously, following the general steps already

Content Review

**ADVANTAGES OF LONG-
TERM DECISION MAKING**

More complete
  decontamination
Better PPE
Less secondary
  contamination
Greater property
  conservation
More thorough substance
  research
Less room for error

*Self-rescued patients often
decide the mode of operation at
a hazmat incident. Be prepared
for fast-break operations
whenever you suspect the
presence of a toxic substance.*

Content Review

**FOUR MOST COMMON
DECONTAMINATION
SOLVENTS**

Water
Tincture of green soap
Isopropyl alcohol
Vegetable oil

Content Review

TWO-STEP DECON

Removal of clothing and
  personal effects
Gross decontamination (two
  times)

mentioned. However, depending upon whether the substance has been identified and the type of substance involved, you may be able to give special attention to other matters. For example, you might contain run-off water. You might better protect patient privacy, grossly decontaminating ambulatory patients in a more controlled setting. You might also spend time on patient monitoring, reclothing patients, isolating or containing patients, and so on.

Long-Term Decision Making At more extended events, you will engage in long-term decision making. This mode of operation most often occurs when patients remain in the hot zone and have not self rescued. Traditionally, EMS personnel have not been trained or equipped to enter the hot zone to retrieve these patients. Instead, a hazmat team is summoned promptly, and the EMS crew awaits the team's arrival. The team will not make their entry until you or members of your crew perform the necessary medical monitoring and establish a decontamination corridor. It often takes 60 minutes or more for actual team deployment.

This mode of operation provides a number of advantages: a better opportunity for thorough decontamination, better PPE, less chance of secondary decontamination, greater consideration of the environment, and more detailed research of the actual hazardous substance. Obviously, long-term decision making presents less opportunity for error and is preferable to fast-break decision making. Unfortunately, self-rescued patients often decide the mode of operation the minute you arrive on the scene. So always be prepared for fast-break operations.

FIELD DECONTAMINATION

As mentioned, the decontamination method and type of PPE depend upon the substance involved. If in doubt, assume the worst-case scenario. When dealing with unknowns, do not attempt to neutralize. Brush dry particles off the patient before the application of water to prevent possible chemical reactions. Next, wash with great quantities of water—the universal decon agent—using tincture of green soap if possible. Isopropyl alcohol is an effective agent for some isocyanates, while vegetable oil can be used to decon water-reactive substances.

Two-Step Process

Use the two-step decon process for gross decontamination of patients who cannot wait for a more comprehensive decon process, usually patients at a fast-break incident. As noted, remove all clothing, including shoes, socks, and jewelry. (Remember to have some method of accounting for personal effects BEFORE hazmat incidents occur.) Wash and rinse the patients with soap and water, making sure that they do not stay in the run-off. Repeat the process, allowing the fluid to drain away each time. Pay special attention to difficult contamination areas such as the scalp and hair, ears, nostrils, axilla, fingernails, naval, genitals, groin, buttocks, behind the knees, between the toes, and toenails.

Eight-Step Process

The eight-step process takes place in a complete decontamination corridor and is much more thorough. To leave the hot zone, the rescuers follow these steps:

- **Step 1:** Rescuers enter the decon area at the hot end of the corridor and mechanically remove contaminants from the victims.
- **Step 2:** Rescuers drop equipment in a tool-drop area and remove outer gloves.
- **Step 3:** Decon personnel shower and scrub all victims and rescuers, using gross decontamination. As surface decontamination is

removed, the dilution is conducted into a contained area. Victims may be moved ahead to Step 6 or Step 7.

- **Step 4:** Rescuers remove and isolate their SCBA. If re-entry is necessary, the team dons new SCBA from a non-contaminated side.
- **Step 5:** Rescuers remove all protective clothing. Articles are isolated, labeled for disposal, and placed on the contaminated side.
- **Step 6:** Rescuers remove all personal clothing. Victims who have not had their clothing removed have it taken off here. All items are isolated in plastic bags and labeled for later disposal or storage.
- **Step 7:** Rescuers and victims receive a full-body washing, using soft scrub brushes or sponges, water, and mild soap or detergent. Cleaning tools are bagged for later disposal.
- **Step 8:** Patients receive rapid assessment and stabilization before being transported to hospitals for further care. EMS crews medically monitor rescuers, complete exposure records, and transport rescuers to hospitals as needed.

These procedures are not set in stone. Small variations may exist from system to system. Know the procedures in your jurisdiction.

Transportation Considerations

No patient who undergoes field decontamination is truly decontaminated. Field-decontaminated patients, sometimes called **semi-decontaminated patients,** may still need to undergo a more invasive decon process at a medical facility. Depending on the type of exposure, wounds may need debridement, hair or nails may need to be trimmed or removed, and so on. However, it is always better to deliver a grossly decontaminated living patient to the hospital than a perfectly decontaminated corpse. Just make sure that field-decontaminated patients are transported to facilities capable of performing more thorough decon procedures.

When transporting field-decontaminated patients, always recall that they may still have some contamination in or on them. For example, a patient may have ingested a chemical, which can be expelled if the patient coughs or vomits. As a result, use as much disposable equipment as possible. Keep in mind that any airborne hazard will not only incapacitate the crew in the back of the ambulance, but will affect the driver as well. Although it is not practical to line the ambulance in plastic, you can isolate the patient using a stretcher decon pool. The pool can help contain any potentially contaminated body fluids. Plastic can also be used to cover the pool, adding yet another protective barrier.

HAZMAT PROTECTION EQUIPMENT

Personal protective equipment for a hazmat incident is specifically designed for such incidents. There are basically four levels of hazmat protective equipment, from Level A (highest) to Level D (minimum).

- *Level A*—provides the highest level of respiratory and splash protection. This hazmat suit offers a high degree of protection against chemical breakthrough time and fully encapsulates the rescuer, even covering the SCBA. The sealed, impermeable suits are typically used by hazmat teams entering hot zones with an unknown substance and a significant potential for both respiratory and dermal hazards.
- *Level B*—offers full respiratory protection when there is a lower probability of dermal hazard. The Level B suit is non-encapsulating

No patient who undergoes field decontamination is ever truly decontaminated.

✱ **semi-decontaminated patient** another term for field-decontaminated patient.

It is always better to deliver a grossly decontaminated living patient to the hospital than a perfectly decontaminated corpse.

When possible, protect the crew from secondary decontamination by placing a semi-decontaminated patient in a stretcher decon pool.

air-purifying respirator (APR)
system of filtering a normal environment for a specific chemical substance using filter cartridges.

but chemically resistant. Seams for zippers, gloves, boots, and mask interface are usually sealed with duct tape. The SCBA is worn outside the suit, allowing increased maneuverability and ease in changing SCBA bottles. The decon team typically wear Level B protection.

- *Level C*—includes a non-permeable suit, boots, and gear for protecting eyes and hands. Instead of SCBA, Level C protective equipment uses an **air-purifying respirator (APR)**. The APR relies on filters to protect against a known contaminant in a normal environment. The canisters in the APR must be specifically selected and are not usually implemented in a hazmat emergency response. Level C clothing is usually worn during transport of patients with the potential for secondary contamination.
- *Level D*—consists of structural firefighter, or turn-out, gear. Level D gear is usually not suitable for hazmat incidents.

The level of hazmat protective gear depends on the substance involved. Ideally, the chemical should be identified so a permeability chart can be consulted to determine breakthrough time. No single material is suitable to all hazmats. Some materials are resistant to certain chemicals, non-resistant to others.

When chemicals can be identified, consult a permeability chart to determine the breakthrough time on a hazmat suit.

EMS personnel should not become involved in any hazmat situation without PPE. All ambulances carry some level of PPE, even if not ideal. If the situation is emergent and the chemical unknown, use as much barrier protection as possible. Full turnout gear (Level D) or a Tyvek suit is better than no gear at all. HEPA filter masks and double or triple gloves offer good protection against some hazards. Latex gloves are not chemically resistant. Instead, use nitrile gloves, which have a high resistance to most chemicals. Also, leather boots will absorb chemicals permanently, so be sure to don rubber boots.

If the situation is emergent and the chemical is unknown, use as much barrier protection as possible, even if less than ideal.

MEDICAL MONITORING AND REHABILITATION

One of the primary roles of EMS personnel at a hazmat incident is the medical monitoring of entry personnel. All hazmat team members should undergo regular annual physical examinations, with baseline vital signs placed on file.

ENTRY READINESS

Prior to entry, you or other EMS crew members will assess rescuers and document the following information: blood pressure, pulse, respiratory rate, temperature, body weight, ECG, and mental/neurologic status. If you observe anything abnormal, do not allow the hazmat team member to attempt a rescue.

Hazmat team members will enter the hot zone only in groups of two, with two more members in PPE remaining outside as a backup team. The PPE used at hazmat incidents can cause significant stress and dehydration. As a result, entry team personnel should prehydrate themselves with 8 to 16 ounces of water or sport drink. Because sport drinks are more effective at half strength, dilute them with 50% water when possible.

If you observe anything abnormal during pre-entry medical monitoring, do not allow the hazmat team member to attempt a rescue.

AFTER-EXIT "REHAB"

After the hazmat entry team exits the hot zone and completes decontamination, they should report back to EMS for post-entry monitoring. Measure and document the same parameters as before entry. Rehydrate the team with more water or diluted sports drink. You can use weight changes to estimate any fluid losses.

Check with medical direction or protocols to determine fluid replacement by means of PO or IV. Entry team members should not be allowed to re-enter the hot zone until they are alert, non-tachycardic, normotensive, and within a reasonable percentage of their normal body weight.

HEAT STRESS FACTORS

In evaluating heat stress, primary considerations include temperature and humidity. Prehydration, duration and degree of activity, and the team member's overall physical fitness will also have a bearing on your evaluation. Keep in mind that Level A suits protect a rescuer but prevent cooling. A rescuer essentially works inside an encapsulated sauna. Therefore, place heat stress at the top of your list of tasks for post-exit medical monitoring.

IMPORTANCE OF PRACTICE

Practice the skills that you can expect to use at a hazmat incident in most EMS systems. Put on and take off Level B hazmat protective equipment. Set up a rapid two-step decontamination process and an eight-step decontamination process, preferably with the help of the local hazmat team. With a crew member, identify a simulated chemical, determine the correct PPE, and establish the proper decontamination methods. Practice pre-entry and post-exit medical monitoring and documentation. Prepare a patient and ambulance for transport. As these skills may be rarely used except in the busiest EMS systems, you should work closely with your local hazmat team to practice these skills on a regular basis.

Part 5: Crime Scene Awareness

Regardless of where you work as a paramedic—the inner city, suburbs, or rural America—you can be affected by violence. It can take all forms, from interpersonal abuse in the home to gang activities in the street and can involve weapons ranging from fists to guns to explosives. While people of all ages and backgrounds commit acts of violence, according to the Division of Violence Prevention at the National Center for Injury Prevention and Control arrest rates for homicide, rape, robbery, and aggravated assault are consistently higher for ages 15 to 34 than for all other age groups.

Approximately one of six victims of violent crimes requires medical attention, often by the emergency medical services. Many victims fail to report the violence to the police. As a result, the EMS may be a victim's only contact with professionals who can intervene to prevent further harm.

EMS providers find it almost impossible to predict exactly when and where a violent incident will occur. Nearly all calls that a paramedic handles on a given day will progress without any threat of danger. In fact, you have a higher risk of being injured by oncoming traffic than by a violent act. Even so, you cannot let down your "crime scene awareness." Otherwise, you risk becoming a victim or hostage of a violent situation. Your most important safety tactic is an ability to identify potentially violent situations as soon as possible. Also be aware of local issues that hold a potential for violence, such as the presence of street gangs or a known area of drug activity.

Equally as important, familiarize yourself with standard operating procedures (SOPs) for handling violent situations and/or the specialized resources that you can call upon for backup. Find out, for example, whether your unit has access to a **Tactical Emergency Medical Service (TEMS)**—a unit that provides on-site medical support to law enforcement. If so, know how and when to access it.

* Tactical Emergency Medical Services (TEMS) a specially trained unit that provides on-site medical support to law enforcement.

Above all else, remain alert to the signs of danger from the start of a call to the time you return your ambulance to service.

APPROACH TO THE SCENE

Your safety strategy begins as soon as you are dispatched on a call.

Your safety strategy begins with dispatch. Emergency medical dispatchers try to keep callers on the line to obtain as much information as possible, remaining alert to background noises such as fighting or intoxicated persons, and warn incoming units of these dangers. Modern computer aided dispatch (CAD) programs provide instant information on previous calls at a location and display "caution indicators" to notify dispatchers when a location has a history of violence.

Even in the age of computers, however, some of your best information can still come from your own experience and that of other crews. Your memory of previous calls can serve as an important indicator of trouble. For example, if a bar or club has a reputation for fights and you are summoned there, you will already have a high suspicion of danger before you arrive.

POSSIBLE SCENARIOS

There are three possible scenarios for violence during a call. The dispatcher may advise you of a potentially violent scene en route to the call and you will be alert to danger from the start. In other cases, you may not spot danger until you arrive on the scene and begin your size-up and approach. In yet a third scenario, you may not face danger until the start of patient care or transport.

Advised of Danger En Route

Never follow police units to the scene. To do so might place you at the center of violence.

When the dispatcher reports possible danger, do not approach the scene until it is secured by law enforcement. Remember that lights and sirens can draw a crowd and/or alert the perpetrator of a crime, so use them cautiously or not at all. Never follow police units to the scene. To do so might place you at the center of violence. If you arrive first, keep the ambulance out of sight so that the rig does not attract the attention of bystanders or parties involved in the incident. While you wait for police to secure the scene, set up a staging area.

Management of the incident requires interagency cooperation. Communicate with the police—you are in this together. Be sure you understand any differences in dispatch terminology. For example, what is a code 1 emergency for police units may be a code 3 emergency for EMS units. Work with police to determine if and when you should approach the scene.

Keep in mind that violence can occur or resume even with the police present. Furthermore, depending upon your uniform colors and the use of badges, people might mistake you for the police—especially if you exit from a vehicle with flashing lights and siren. They might expect you to intervene in a violent situation, or they might direct aggression toward you as an authority figure. If the scene cannot be made safe, retreat immediately (Figure 48-32).

Observing Danger upon Arrival

Even if dispatch has not alerted you to danger, you must still keep this possibility in mind once you arrive. One of the main purposes of the scene size-up is to search for any possible hazards such as downed power lines or hazmats. As you look for these, observe for other signs of trouble such as crowds gathering on the street, an unusual silence, or a darkened residence. Obviously, you will adopt a different approach for a confirmed medical emergency than for an "unknown problem, caller hang-up." Even so, do not exit the vehicle until you have ruled out all immediate hazards.

FIGURE 48-32   Never approach the scene until you are advised that the scene is secure. Remember, even if a scene has been declared secure, violence may still erupt.

If you have any doubts about a call, park away from the scene. If you must park in view of the location, take an unconventional approach to the door (Figure 48-33). People will expect you to use the sidewalk, so approach from the side, the lawn, or flush against the house. Avoid getting between a residence and the lighted ambulance so you do not "backlight" yourself. Hold your flashlight to the side rather than in front of you (Figure 48-34). Assailants often fire at the light.

Before announcing your presence, observe for signs of danger. If you can, look into windows for evidence of fighting, weapons, or the use of alcohol or

FIGURE 48-33   Approach potentially unstable scenes single file along an unconventional path.

FIGURE 48-34   Hold a flashlight to the side of your body, not in front of it. Armed assailants usually aim at the light.

FIGURE 48-35 Stand to the side of the door when knocking. Do not stand directly in front of a door or window, making yourself an unwitting target.

drugs. Gradually make your way to the doorknob side of the door or the side opposite the hinges (Figure 48-35). Listen for any signs of danger such as loud noises, items breaking, incoherent speech, or the lack of any sounds at all.

If you spot danger at any time during your approach, immediately stop and reevaluate the situation. Decide whether it is in the interest of your own safety to continue or retreat until law enforcement officials can be summoned. Rather than risk becoming injured or killed, err on the side of safety.

Rather than risk becoming injured or killed, err on the side of safety.

Eruption of Danger during Care or Transport

Remain alert throughout a call, especially in areas with a history of violence. You may enter the scene and spot weapons or drugs. Additional combative people may arrive on scene. The patient or bystanders may become agitated or threatening. Even if treatment has begun, you must place your own safety first. You now have two tactical options: (1) quickly package the patient and leave the scene with the patient or (2) retreat without the patient.

In most cases, you can legally leave a patient behind when there is a documented danger.

Your choice of action depends upon the level of danger. Abandonment is always a concern. However, in most cases, you can legally leave a patient behind when there is a documented danger. As discussed later, keep accurate records of incidents involving violence. If you must defend yourself, use the minimum amount of force necessary. Immediately summon police and retreat as needed.

Regardless of the situation, always have a way out. Failure to plan will eventually get you into trouble. Make sure SOPs include an escape plan. Then adhere to this plan so you do not become a victim of violence yourself.

SPECIFIC DANGEROUS SCENES

Most out-of-hospital services were developed to meet the needs of individual patients in controlled situations. However, in recent years, EMS personnel trained for this limited role have been pressed increasingly into service in potentially hazardous situations. The following are some of the known dangers that you may face "on the street." (Tactical safety strategies are discussed later.)

HIGHWAY ENCOUNTERS

The preceding examples of known dangers have focused largely on residences. However, EMS units frequently report to roadside calls involving motor vehicle collisions, disabled vehicles, or sick and/or unresponsive people inside a car—e.g., "man slumped over wheel" calls. Dangers of highway operations and the steps that you should take to protect yourself were discussed earlier in the chapter. However, highway operations also hold the risk of violence from occupants who may be fleeing felons, intoxicated or drugged, or in possession of weapons. Some potential warning signs of danger include:

- Violent or abusive behavior
- An altered mental state
- Grabbing or hiding items inside the vehicle
- Arguing or fighting among passengers
- Lack of activity where activity is expected
- Physical signs of alcohol or drug abuse—e.g., liquor bottles, beer cans, or syringes
- Open or unlatched trunks—a potential hiding spot for people or weapons
- Differing stories told by occupants

To make a safe approach to a vehicle at a roadside emergency, follow these steps:

- Park the ambulance in a position that provides safety from traffic.
- Notify dispatch of the situation, location, the vehicle make and model, and the state and number of the license plate.
- Use a one-person approach. The driver should remain in the ambulance, which is elevated and provides greater visibility.
- The driver should remain prepared to radio for immediate help and to back or drive away rapidly once the other medic returns.
- At nighttime, use the ambulance lights to illuminate the vehicle. However, do not walk between the ambulance and the other vehicle. You will be backlighted, forming an easy target.
- Since police approach vehicles from the driver's side, you should approach from the passenger's side—an unexpected route.
- Use the A, B, and C door posts for cover.
- Observe the rear seat. Do not move forward of the C post unless you are sure there are no threats in the rear seat or foot wells.
- Retreat to the ambulance (or another strategic position of cover) at the first sign of danger.
- Make sure you have mapped out your intended retreat and escape with the ambulance driver.

VIOLENT STREET INCIDENTS

The following are some of the dangerous street situations that you may face at some point in your EMS career.

Murder, Assault, Robbery

Violent acts take place at residences, schools, and commercial establishments. However, according to the U.S. Department of Justice, the most common location is on the streets. In order of occurrence, the most frequent crimes are simple assaults, aggravated assaults, rapes and sexual assaults, robberies, and homicides. In one-quarter of violent crimes, offenders used or threatened the use of a weapon. Homicides are most commonly committed with handguns, but knives, blunt objects, and other types of guns or weapons may also be used. About one in five violent victimizations involve the use of alcohol.

While motives vary, there has been a recent rise in **hate crimes**—crimes committed against a person solely on the basis of the individual's actual or perceived race, color, national origin, ethnicity, gender, disability, or sexual orientation. A number of states or communities have passed legislation on the management of hate crimes, including the steps to be taken on scene. Determine whether these laws exist in your area, and establish protocols that your agency should follow. Crew assignments, for example, should be well thought out in advance of the response to a hate crime. You should also know the specific type of information that must be documented for later use by the courts.

In responding to the scene of any violent crime, keep these points in mind:

* Dangerous weapons may have been used in the crime.
* Perpetrators may still be on-scene or could return to the scene.
* Patients may sometimes exhibit violence toward EMS, particularly if they risk criminal penalties as a result of the original incident.

Dangerous Crowds and Bystanders

Crowds can quickly become large and volatile, especially in the case of a hate crime. Violence can be directed against anyone or anything in the path of an angry crowd. Your status as an EMS provider does not give you immunity. Whenever a crowd is present, look for these warning signs:

* Shouts or increasingly loud voices
* Pushing or shoving
* Hostilities toward anyone on scene, including the perpetrator of a crime, the victim, police, and so on
* Rapid increase in the crowd size
* Inability of law enforcement officials to control bystanders

Constantly monitor the crowd and retreat if necessary. If possible, take the patient with you. Rapid transport may require limited or tactical assessment at the scene with more in-depth assessment done inside the safety of the ambulance. Be sure to document reasons for the quick assessment and transport.

Street Gangs

Street gangs can be found in big cities, suburban towns, and lately in rural America. In fact, some organized gangs have purposely branched out into smaller towns in an effort to escape surveillance and expand their illicit businesses. Gangs account for a disproportionate amount of youth violence. Gang activity is associated with high levels of delinquency, illegal drug use, physical violence,

---

* **hate crimes** crimes committed against a person wholly on the basis of the individual's actual or perceived race, color, national origin, ethnicity, gender, disability, or sexual orientation.

Crew assignments should be well thought out in advance of the response to a hate crime.

and weapons possession. Young people from all demographic backgrounds report some knowledge of gangs or gang activity.

Some of the largest and best-known gangs include the Crips, Bloods, Almighty Latin King Nation (Latin Kings), Hell's Angels, Outlaws, Pagans, and Banditos. Local variations can be found throughout the country. In some places, gangs have used firebombs, Molotov cocktails, and, on a limited basis, hand grenades as weapons of revenge and intimidation. Links have been drawn between street gangs and the sale of drugs, which finances gang activities.

Commonly observed gang characteristics include the following:

- Appearance—Gang members frequently wear unique clothing specific to the group. Because the clothing is often a particular color or hue, it is referred to as the gang's "colors." Wearing a color, even a bandana, can signify gang membership. Within the gang, members sometimes wear different articles to signify rank.
- Graffiti—Gangs have territories, or "turfs." Members often mark their turf with graffiti of the gang's logo, warning away intruders, bragging about crimes, insulting rival gangs, or taunting police.
- Tattoos—Many gang members wear tattoos or other body markings to identify their gang affiliation. Some gangs even require these tattoos. The tattoos will be in the gang's colors and often contain the gang's motto or logo.
- Hand signals/language—Gangs commonly create their own methods of communication. They give gang-related meanings to everyday words or create codes. Hand signs provide quick identification among gang members, warn of approaching law enforcement, or show disrespect to other gangs. Gang members often perform signals so quickly that an uninformed outsider may not spot them, much less understand them.

EMS units venturing into gang territory must be extremely cautious. Danger is increased if your uniform looks similar to the uniform worn by police. Gangs with a history of arrest may in fact make every effort to prevent you from transporting one of their members to a hospital or any other place beyond the reach of the gang. Do not force the issue if your safety is at stake.

EMS uniforms should not resemble law enforcement uniforms.

DRUG-RELATED CRIMES

The sale of drugs goes hand-in-hand with violence. Hundreds of people die each year in drug deals gone bad. In addition, drug dealers protect their drug stashes and "shooting galleries" with booby traps, weapons, and attack dogs. The combination of a high cash flow, addiction, and automatic weapons threatens anyone who unwittingly walks onto the scene of a drug deal or threatens to uncover an illicit drug operation.

Signs that can alert you to involvement of drugs at an EMS call include:

- Prior history of drugs in the neighborhood of the call
- Clinical evidence that the patient has used drugs of some kind
- Drug-related comments by bystanders
- Drug paraphernalia visible at the scene such as the following:
  - Tiny zip-top bags or vials
  - Sandwich bags with the corners torn off (indicating drug packaging) or untied corners of sandwich bags (indicating drug use)
  - Syringes or needles
  - Glass tubes, pipes, or homemade devices for smoking drugs
  - Chemical odors or residues

Whenever you observe any of the preceding items, assume the use or presence of drugs at the scene. Even if the patient is not involved, others at the scene may still pose a danger. Keep in mind that not all patients who use drugs will be seeking to harm you. Some may, in fact, be looking for help. Evaluate each situation carefully. Above all else, remember to retreat and/or request police backup at the earliest sign of danger.

CLANDESTINE DRUG LABORATORIES

Drug dealers often set up "laboratories" to manufacture controlled substances or to otherwise refine or convert a substance to another more profitable or useable form such as tablets. One of the most common substances manufactured in drug laboratories is methamphetamine, also known by street names such as "crank," "speed," or "crystal." Other drugs include LSD, "crack," and more.

Clandestine drug laboratories, or "clan labs," have three requirements: privacy, utilities, and equipment such as glassware, chemical containers, and heating mantles or burners. Most clan labs are uncovered by neighbors who report suspicious odors or activities. Raids on clan labs have a way of turning into hazmat operations. All too often, the labs contain toxic fumes and volatile chemicals. The people on scene complicate matters by fighting or shooting at the rescuers who come to extricate them from the toxic environment. As they retreat, drug dealers may also trigger booby traps or wait for police or EMS personnel to trigger them. If you ever come upon a clan lab, take these actions:

- Leave the area immediately.
- Do not touch anything.
- Never stop any chemical reactions already in progress.
- Do not smoke or bring any source of flame near the lab.
- Notify the police.
- Initiate ICS and hazmat procedures.
- Consider evacuation of the area.

Laboratories can be found anywhere—on farms, in trailers, in city apartments, and more. They may be mobile, roaming from place to place in a camper or truck. Or they may be disassembled and stored in a variety of locations. The job of raiding clan labs belongs to specialized personnel—not EMS crews.

DOMESTIC VIOLENCE

Domestic violence may be physical, emotional, sexual, verbal, or economic. It may be directed against a spouse or partner, or it may involve children and/or older relatives. When you go to the scene of domestic violence, the abuser may turn on you or other crew members. You have two main concerns: the safety of yourself and your crew and protection of the patient from further harm.

TACTICAL CONSIDERATIONS

As mentioned on several occasions, your best tactical response to violence is observation. Know the warning signs and stay out of danger in the first place. If the dispatcher alerts you to hazards, resort to staging until the appropriate authorities can resolve the situation. That said, you still may find yourself in situations with a potential for danger. In such instances, you must have a "game plan" in place. This section presents some of the actions you can take to protect your own safety while attempting to provide tactical patient care.

SAFETY TACTICS

Dangerous situations mean extreme stress. As a result, your response to danger will be most effective if you practice tactical options frequently. Even on routine calls, think about safety, contact and cover, escape routes, and other strategies that can help you make a better decision when you are faced with actual danger. Borrowing a phrase from professional sports: "You will play the game the way you practice." If you have rehearsed the responses to danger before you actually need them, you will be more likely to use them successfully. The following sections describe some proven methods for EMS safety in dangerous situations.

Retreat

The prudent strategy is to retreat whenever you spot indicators of violence or potential physical confrontations, particularly with fleeing criminals or emotionally disturbed people. Retreat in a calm, but decisive manner. Be aware that the danger is now at your back and integrate cover into your retreat. Ideally you will retreat to the ambulance so you can summon help. However, if a dangerous obstacle—such as a crowd—blocks access to your rig, retreat by foot or by any means possible. Nothing in the ambulance is worth your life.

In deciding how far to retreat, your primary goal is to protect. You must be out of the immediate line of sight. You must also seek cover from gunfire. Finally, you must allow enough distance to react if a person or crowd attempts to move toward you again. You need time and space to respond to changing situations. As soon as possible, notify other responding units and agencies of the danger. Activate appropriate codes, SOPs, and/or interagency agreements, particularly with law enforcement. Be sure to document your observations of danger and your specific responses. Include information such as:

- Actions taken while on scene
- Reasons you retreated
- Time at which you left and/or returned to the scene
- Personnel or agencies contacted

Keep in mind that retreat does not mean the end of a call. As already mentioned, you should seek to stage at a safe area until police secure the scene and you can respond again. Staging, along with thorough documentation, will reduce liability and provide evidence to refute charges of abandonment.

Nothing in the ambulance is worth your life. Retreat by foot or by whatever means possible to avoid violence that threatens your life.

Cover and Concealment

When faced with danger, two of your most immediate and practical strategies are cover and concealment (Figures 48-36A–B). **Concealment** hides your body, such as when you crouch behind bushes or vehicle doors. However, most common objects do not stop bullets. During armed encounters, seek **cover** by hiding your body behind solid and impenetrable objects such as brick walls, rocks, large trees or telephone poles, or a vehicle engine block.

In applying these safety tactics, keep in mind these general rules:

- As you approach any scene, remain aware of the surroundings and any potential sources of protection in case you must retreat or are "pinned down."
- Choose your cover carefully. You may have only one chance to pick your protection. Select the item that hides your body adequately while shielding you against ballistics.

✱ **concealment** hiding the body behind objects that shield a person from view but that offer little or no protection against bullets or other ballistics.

✱ **cover** hiding the body behind solid and impenetrable objects that protect a person from bullets.

FIGURE 48-36A Concealing yourself means placing your body behind an object that can hide you from view.

FIGURE 48-36B Taking cover is finding a position that both hides you and protects your body from projectiles.

- Once you have made your choice of cover, conceal as much of your body as possible. Be conscious of any reflective clothing that you may be wearing. Armed assailants can use it as a target, especially at night.
- Constantly look to improve your protection and location.

Distraction and Evasion

Distraction and evasion can be integrated into any retreat. Some specific techniques to avoid physical violence include:

- Throwing equipment to trip, slow, or distract an aggressor
- Wedging a stretcher in a doorway to block an attacker
- Using an unconventional path while retreating
- Anticipating the moves of the aggressor and taking counter moves
- Overturning objects in the path of the attacker
- Using preplanned tactics with your partner to confuse or "throw off" an aggressor

Key to the success of these tactics is your own physical condition. Regular exercise and good health ensure that you will have the strength to outrun or, if necessary, defend yourself against an attacker. Some units provide basic training in self-defense or have protocols on its use. Make sure you take advantage of the training and know the protocols related to application of force.

Contact and Cover

The concept of contact and cover comes from a police procedure developed in San Diego, California, where several officers were injured or killed while interviewing suspects. Studies of the incidents revealed that the officers focused directly on the suspect, reducing their ability to observe the "big picture." This left them exposed to violence. To solve this problem, the San Diego police adopted an interview approach in which one officer "contacts" the suspect while another stands 90 degrees to the side. By standing at a different angle, the second officer can provide "cover" to the officer dealing with the suspect.

When adapted to EMS practice, the procedure assigns the roles shown in Table 48-1. As with any tactic adopted from another discipline, contact and cover has obvious correlations and drawbacks for EMS. The tactic is ideal for

Table 48-1   CONTACT AND COVER

Contact Provider	Cover Provider
Initiates and provides direct patient care.	Observes the scene for danger while the "contact" provider cares for the patient.
Performs patient assessment.	Generally avoids patient care duties that would prevent observation of the scene.
Handles most interpersonal scene contact.	In small crews, may perform limited functions such as handling equipment.

street encounters with intoxicated persons or subjects acting in a suspicious manner. An obvious drawback is that two medics working on a cardiac arrest will not be able to designate one person to act solely as a "cover" medic.

Perhaps the best application of this police procedure to EMS is its emphasis on the importance of observation and teamwork. A crew that works well together will assign roles—formally or informally—to guarantee safety and patient care. In its most basic form, contact and cover means that you will watch your partner's back while your partner watches yours.

Warning Signals and Communication

In the case of "street survival," communication is an invaluable tool. Every team or crew should develop methods of alerting other providers to danger without alerting the aggressor. Devise prearranged verbal and nonverbal clues and then practice them. Be sure to involve dispatch in the process. Choose signals that will indicate a variety of circumstances while sounding harmless to an attacker. This can be a life-saving technique in situations where you find yourself, the crew, and/or the patient held hostage. Your so-called "routine" radio reports can spell out the nature of the trouble and summon help from a **Special Weapons and Tactics (SWAT) Team**—a trained police unit equipped to handle hostage holders or other difficult law enforcement situations.

✳ **Special Weapons and Tactics (SWAT) Team** a trained police unit equipped to handle hostage holders and other difficult law enforcement situations.

TACTICAL PATIENT CARE

The increased involvement of care providers in violent situations has raised discussion and debate over the tactical training and protection offered to the EMS community. Interagency planning is essential, especially for clarifying the duties and roles of EMS and law enforcement agencies at crime scenes, riots, or terrorist events. Other aspects of tactical patient care include the use of body armor by EMS providers and the training of special tactical EMS personnel.

Body Armor

Several years ago few EMS providers would have considered wearing **body armor,** or bullet-proof vests, while on duty. Today more and more providers are taking "tactical patient care" seriously. An increasing number of EMS agencies have chosen to supply body armor or to provide a sum of cash toward its purchase. Body armor manufacturers have responded by designing and marketing vests specifically for the EMS community.

Unlike conventional armor, body armor is soft. Fibers such as Kevlar® are woven tightly together to form the vest. The tight weave and strength of the material offer protection from many handgun bullets, most knives, and blunt trauma. The number of layers of fiber determine the rating or "stopping power" of a vest. Most body armor is rated from level 1 (least protective) to level 3 (most

✳ **body armor** vest made of tightly woven, strong fibers that offer protection against handgun bullets, most knives, and blunt trauma; also known as "bullet-proof vests."

protective). Specialty vests with steel inserts and other materials are available for use by the military or by SWAT teams.

Some critics of body armor claim that wearers may feel a false sense of security. They point out that body armor offers reduced protection when wet and that it provides little or no protection against high-velocity bullets, such as those fired by a rifle, or from thin or dual-edged weapons. An ice pick, for example, can penetrate between the fibers of most vests. Supporters of body armor feel it should be viewed just like any other PPE. They point to the new threats faced by emergency responders, such as paramilitary groups, terrorists, drug-related violence, and the widespread possession of handguns.

Whether you purchase or wear body armor is a personal decision. However, for it to be effective, you must follow several guidelines. They include:

- Keep in mind the limitations of body armor. Never do anything you wouldn't do without it.

- Remember that body armor doesn't cover the whole body. You can still get seriously injured or killed.

- Even though body armor can prevent many types of penetration, you can still experience severe cavitation.

- For body armor to work, it must be worn. The temptation not to wear it—especially in hot temperatures—can render even the best body armor useless.

Tactical EMS

As already mentioned, the provision of care in violent or tactically "hot" zones such as sniper situations necessitates risks far beyond those found on most EMS calls. Medical personnel assigned to such incidents require special training and authorization. Like hazmat teams, they must don special equipment, function with compact gear, and, in most cases, work as medical adjuncts to the police or military.

The patient care offered by a Tactical Emergency Medical Service (TEMS) differs from routine EMS care in several ways. Differences include these:

- A major priority is extraction of the patient from the hot zone.
- Care may be modified to meet tactical considerations.
- Trauma patients outnumber medical patients.
- Treatment and transport interventions must almost always be coordinated with an incident commander.
- Patients must be moved to tactically cold zones for complete assessment, care, and transport.
- Metal clipboards, chemical agents, and other tools may be used as defensive weapons.

* **EMT-Tacticals (EMT-Ts)** EMS personnel trained to serve with a Technical Emergency Medical Service or a law enforcement agency.

* **CONTOMS** Counter-Narcotics Tactical Operations; program that manages the training and certification of EMT-Ts and SWAT-Medics.

Local protocols, standing orders, and issues of medical direction must be resolved before employment of a TEMS unit, which may be composed of EMTs, paramedics, and/or physicians who operate as part of a tactical law enforcement team. Certification of SWAT-Medics and **EMT-Tacticals (EMT-Ts)** is offered by several organizations including the **CONTOMS**—Counter-Narcotics Tactical Operations—program and the National Tactical Officers Association (NTOA). The training required of EMT-Ts or SWAT-Medics involves strenuous physical activity under a variety of conditions. In a CONTOMS program, medics may be exposed to scenarios or skills such as:

- Raids on clandestine drug laboratories
- Emergency medical care in barricade situations
- Wounding effects of weapons and booby traps
- Special medical gear for tactical operations
- Use of CS, OC or other riot-control agents
- Blank-firing weapons
- Helicopter operations
- Pyrotechnics (smoke and distraction devices)
- Operation under extreme conditions, darkness, and psychological stress
- Fire fighting and hazmat operations

In summoning or working with a TEMS unit, follow the same general approaches and procedures recommended in Parts 2, 3, and 4 of this chapter. If you have not had exposure to such a unit, find out more about EMT-Ts or SWAT-Medics from local law enforcement officials or from sites sponsored by CONTOMS on NTOA on the Internet.

EMS AT CRIME SCENES

The goal of performing EMS at a crime scene is to provide high-quality patient care while preserving evidence. NEVER jeopardize patient care for the sake of evidence. However, do not perform patient care with disregard of the criminal investigation that will follow.

NEVER jeopardize patient care for the sake of evidence.

EMS AND POLICE OPERATIONS

Often police and EMS personnel respond to the same crisis but for different purposes. The EMS crew is there to treat patients and save lives. Law enforcement officers have come to protect the public and to solve a crime. These two goals sometimes create tensions between the two teams. For example, police and paramedics often work under different time constraints. As a paramedic, you have a limited time at the scene. The police, on the other hand, spend much more time at the location of a crime. In some major cases, police can remain on the scene for days or weeks as they methodically look for evidence.

The key to cooperation between EMS and law enforcement personnel is communication. You should become aware of the nature and significance of physical evidence at a crime scene and, if possible, keep that evidence intact. Police, on the other hand, should be aware that your responsibility is to save a life. However, police and paramedics can usually reach a common ground. By preserving evidence, you can help the police to lock up a criminal before the person hurts or kills someone else. Remember: EMS personnel and law enforcement are really on the same side. Talk to each other.

Remember: EMS personnel and law enforcement are really on the same side. Talk to each other.

PRESERVING EVIDENCE

Be aware that anything on and around the patient may be evidence. You never know when a seemingly unimportant item may in fact be evidence that could help solve a crime. Whenever in doubt, save or treat an object as evidence.

Whenever in doubt, save or treat an object as evidence.

Anything you touch, walk on, pick up, cut, wipe off, or move could be evidence. Developing an awareness of evidence can affect the way you treat patients. For example, if clothing must be removed, never cut through a gunshot or knife hole. Instead, try to cut as far away from the wound as possible. Instead of placing the cut cloth or garment in a plastic bag, put it in a brown paper bag so condensation does not build up and destroy body fluid evidence.

Also, when examining a patient, remember that you may be at risk. The victim may have a concealed weapon, such as a knife or gun. Or the person who committed the crime may be intent on finishing it and reappear to attack the patient. As always, your first responsibility is to protect yourself. If you have any suspicions at all about the patient or the safety of the scene, wait for the police to frisk the patient and/or secure the scene.

Types of Evidence

While it is unrealistic to train EMS personnel in the details of police work, it is not unrealistic to ask them to develop an awareness of the general types of evidence that they may expect to encounter at a crime scene. Some of the main categories of evidence include: prints, blood and body fluids, particulate evidence, and your own observations at the scene.

Prints Prints include fingerprints, footprints, and tire prints. Of the three, fingerprints can be the most valuable source of evidence. As a paramedic, try not to disturb any fingerprint evidence that may be present. Second, do not leave behind your own fingerprints at a crime scene. The only way to preserve fingerprints is simply not to touch anything. Of course, this is impossible when treating a patient. However, you can and should minimize what you touch. If you must touch or move an item, remember to tell the police.

You will be wearing disposable gloves as a part of infection control. These gloves prevent you from leaving your own fingerprints, but they will not prevent you from smudging existing prints. Again, touch as little as possible. Bring in only necessary equipment. The more equipment you have, the more evidence you have to disturb, including fingerprints. Also, scan the approach to the scene and the scene itself for footprints or tire prints and avoid disturbing them.

Blood and Body Fluids Blood and body fluids also give police a lot of information about a crime. Matching the DNA found in blood samples or other body fluids to the DNA of a suspect is nearly 100% accurate. Technologists need only a small sample to ascertain the genetic code. The way in which blood is splattered or dropped at the scene (called **blood spatter evidence**) provides yet other clues for police.

Preserving blood evidence can be performed in the following ways:

- Avoid mixing samples of blood whenever possible. Cross-contamination of blood will render blood evidence useless.
- Avoid tracking blood on your shoes. You will leave your own footprints, plus risk contaminating other blood evidence.
- If you must cut bloody clothing from a victim, place each piece in a separate brown paper bag. If the garment is wet, gently roll it in the paper bag to layer it. Place the entire contents in a second paper bag and then in a plastic bag for body fluid protection.
- Do not throw clothes stained with blood or other body fluids in a single pile or in a puddle of blood.

Brown paper bags allow evaporation and prevent mold from forming. This makes them ideal for crime scene evidence collection.

Content Review

TYPES OF EVIDENCE

Prints—fingerprints, footprints, tire prints
Blood and blood splatter
Body fluids
Particulate evidence
On-scene EMS observations

If you must touch or move an item, remember to tell the police.

* **blood spatter evidence** the pattern that blood forms when it is splattered or dropped at the scene of a crime.

- Do not clean up or smudge blood spatters left at a scene.
- If you leave behind blood from a venipuncture, notify police.
- Because blood can be a biohazard, ask police whether the scene should be secured for evidence collection.

Particulate Evidence Particulate evidence, also known as microscopic or trace evidence, refers to evidence that cannot be readily seen by the human eye such as hairs or carpet and clothing fibers. Minimal handling of a victim's clothes by EMS personnel may help to preserve this evidence.

On-Scene Observations Everything that you and other members of the EMS crew see and hear can serve as evidence. Your observations of the scene will become part of the police record—and ultimately part of the court record. Be sure to look for and record the following information:

- Conditions at the scene—absence or presence of lights, locked or unlocked doors, open or closed curtains, and so on
- Position of the patient/victim
- Injuries suffered by the patient/victim
- Statements of persons at the scene
- Statements by the patient/victim
- Dying declarations
- Suspicious persons at, or fleeing from, the scene
- Presence and/or location of any weapons

If the victim is deceased by the time you arrive, any staff not immediately needed on the scene should leave to minimize the risk of disturbing evidence. If a gun is seen or found on the deceased victim, do not touch or move it unless it must be secured for the safety of others. Pick it up only as a last resort, and only touch it by the side grips or handles. The grips are coarse and will not generally leave good fingerprints. NEVER put anything into the barrel of the gun to lift or move it. The barrel of a gun can house the majority of the evidence used by the police—traces of gun powder, rifling patterns, and even flesh or blood.

Documenting Evidence

Record only the facts at the scene of a crime, and record them accurately. Use quotation marks to indicate the words of bystanders and any remarks made by the patient. Avoid opinions not relevant to patient care. If the patient has died, do not offer any judgments that might contradict later findings by the medical examiner. For example, a knife wound is not a knife wound until it is proven that a knife caused the laceration. Instead, describe the shape and anatomical location of the puncture or cut.

Also keep in mind the protocols, local laws, and ethical considerations in reporting certain crimes such as child abuse, rape, geriatric abuse, or domestic violence. (For more on reporting abuse and assault see Chapter 44.) Finally, follow local policies and regulations regarding confidentiality surrounding any criminal case. Any offhand remarks that you make might later become testimony in a courtroom along with documents that you prepare at the scene.

SUMMARY

As a paramedic, you should be familiar with standards that influence ambulance design, equipment requirements, and staffing. You should also regularly complete all checklists regarding onboard equipment and essential supplies. Be aware of items that require routine maintenance or calibration as well as the expiration dates on all drugs. Keep in mind OSHA safety requirements and know how to report equipment problems or failures. Be familiar with the profile of a typical ambulance collision and to develop strategies for preventing it from occurring. Also be aware of the issues policies surrounding the staging and staffing of ambulances. Appreciate the conditions or situations that merit air medical transport and the safety issues involved in packaging the patient, selecting a landing site, and approaching the aircraft.

Every paramedic should be thoroughly familiar with the procedures used in a typical Incident Management System. You should be able follow these procedures at every multi-patient, multi-unit response—from the smallest incident to the largest. Expect to respond to several MCIs during your EMS career. A good preplan, regular use of the IMS, and MCI training will allow you to handle each event calmly and professionally.

Whenever you function in any phase of a rescue, you must be properly outfitted with protective equipment. You must also have training specific to the type of rescue. During the operational phases of a rescue, you must provide direct patient care and work with technical teams to assure optimal patient management. Any paramedic assigned to rescue duties should have training in the care of patients who may require prolonged management.

Every member of an EMS team should be prepared to face the challenges of the hazmat incident. As with any EMS operation, the primary consideration is your own safety. You become useless at a hazmat incident if you become contaminated yourself.

Similarly, your first priority at any crime scene is your own safety. To protect your life and the lives of others, you need to develop a "crime scene awareness." Do not needlessly expose yourself to dangers better left to professional emergency medical personnel such as SWAT-Medics or EMT-Ts. When you do treat the victim(s) at a crime scene, keep in mind that police and EMS personnel must work together to preserve the evidence. Touch only those items or objects that pertain directly to patient care.

Further Reading

GENERAL

Bledsoe, B.E, R.S. Porter, and R.A. Cherry. *Paramedic Care: Principles and Practice,* 5-volume set (Vol. 1, *Introduction to Advanced Prehospital Care;* Vol. 2, *Patient Assessment;* Vol. 3, *Medical Emergencies;* Vol. 4, *Trauma Emergencies;* Vol. 5, *Special Considerations/Operations*). Upper Saddle River, NJ: Brady/Prentice-Hall Health, 2000/2001.

EMT-Paramedic National Standard Curriculum. Washington, DC: U.S. Department of Transportation, National Highway Traffic Safety Administration, 1998.

DIVISION ONE: INTRODUCTION TO ADVANCED PREHOSPITAL CARE

Barkin, R.M., et. al. *Pediatric Emergency Medicine.* 2nd ed. Philadelphia: W.B. Saunders, 1997.

Beauchamp, T. and J.E. Childress, eds. *Principles of Biomedical Ethics.* New York: Oxford University Press, 2001.

Bledsoe, B.E. *Atlas of Paramedic Skills.* Upper Saddle River, NJ: Brady/Prentice Hall Health, 1987.

Bledsoe, B.E., D.E. Clayden, and F.J. Papa. *Prehospital Emergency Pharmacology.* 5th edition. Upper Saddle River, NJ: Brady/Prentice Hall Health, 2001.

Brody, H. *Ethical Decisions in Emergency Medicine.* 2nd. ed. Tucson, AZ: Galen Press, 1995.

Cherry, R.A. and B.E. Bledsoe. *Drug Guide for Paramedics.* Upper Saddle, NJ: Brady/Prentice Hall Health, 2001.

Chung, M.B. *Math Principles and Practice: Preparing for Health Career Success.* Upper Saddle River, NJ: Prentice Hall, 1999.

Cohn, B.M. and A.J. Azzara. *Legal Aspects of Emergency Medical Services.* Philadelphia: W.B. Saunders, 1998.

Dacey, J. and J. Travers. *Human Development Across the Lifespan.* Dubuque, IA: Wm. C. Brown Publishers, 1991.

Dernocoeur, K.B. *Streetsense: Communication, Safety, and Control.* 3rd ed. Redmond, WA: Laing Research Services, 1996.

Guyton, A.C. and J.E. Hall. *Textbook of Medical Physiology.* 10th ed. Philadelphia: W.B. Saunders, 2001.

Iserson, K.V., et. al. *Ethics in Emergency Medicine.* Baltimore: Waverly Press, 1986.

Katz, J. and E. Green. *Managing Quality: A Guide to System-Wide Performance Management in Health Care.* 2nd ed. St. Louis: Mosby, 1997.

Kübler-Ross, E. *On Death and Dying.* New York: Macmillan, 1969.

Kumar, V., R. Cotran, S. Robbins. *Basic Pathology.* 6th ed. Philadelphia: W.B. Saunders, 1997.

Louisell, D. and H. Williams. *Medical Malpractice.* New York: Matthew Bender, 1995.

Martini, F.H., E.F. Bartholomew, and B.E. Bledsoe. *Anatomy and Physiology for Emergency Care.* Upper Saddle River, NJ: Brady/Prentice Hall Health, 2002.

McCance, K.L and S.E. Heuther. *Pathophysiology: The Biologic Basis for Disease in Adults and Children.* 3rd ed. St. Louis: Mosby, 1998.

Mikolaj, A.A. *Drug Dosage Calculations for the Emergency Care Provider.* Upper Saddle River, NJ: Brady/Prentice Hall, 1997.

Mitchell, J. and G. Bray. *Emergency Services Stress: Guidelines for Preserving the Health and Careers of Emergency Services Personnel.* Englewood Cliffs, NJ: Prentice Hall, 1990.

National Academy of Sciences, National Research Council. *Accidental Death and Disability: The Neglected Disease of Modern Society.* Washington, DC: U.S. Department of Health, Education, and Welfare, 1966.

Page, J.O. *The Paramedics.* Morristown, NJ: Backdraft Publications, 1976.

Roberts, J.R. and J.R. Hedges. *Clinical Procedures in Emergency Medicine.* 3rd ed. Philadelphia: W.B. Saunders, 1997.

Roush, W.R. *Principles of EMS Systems.* 2nd ed. American College of Emergency Physicians, 1994.

Shannon, M.T., B.A. Wilson, and C.L. Stang. *Health Professional's Drug Guide 2002.* Upper Saddle River, NJ: Prentice Hall, 2002.

Veatch, R. and H. Flack. *Case Studies in Allied Health Ethics.* Upper Saddle River, NJ: Prentice Hall, 1997.

DIVISION TWO: PATIENT ASSESSMENT

Bates, B., L.S. Bickley, and R.A. Hoekelman. *A Guide to Physical Examination and History Taking.* 7th ed. Philadelphia: J.B. Lippincott, 1999.

Bevelacqua, A.S. *Prehospital Documentation: A Systematic Approach.* Upper Saddle River, NJ: Brady/Prentice Hall, 1992.

Chameides, L. and M.F. Hazinski, eds. *Textbook of Pediatric Advanced Life Support.* Dallas: American Heart Association, 1994.

Clawson, J.J. "Emergency Medical Dispatch" in *Principles of EMS Systems.* 2nd ed. W.R. Roush, ed. Dallas: American College of Emergency Physicians, 1994.

Clawson, J.J. and K.B. Dernocoeur. *Principles of Emergency Medical Dispatch.* Englewood Cliffs, NJ: Prentice Hall, 1986.

Coulehan, J.L. and M.R. Block. *The Medical Interview: Mastering Skills for Clinical Practice.* 4th ed. Philadelphia. F.A. Davis, 2001.

Delbridge, T.R. and P. Paris. "EMS Communications" in *Principles of EMS Systems.* 2nd ed. W.R. Roush, ed. Dallas: American College of Emergency Physicians, 1994.

DeLorenzo, R. "Sneezes, Wheezes, and Breezes—Listening to the Chest" in *JEMS 20* (October 1995).

Dickinson, E. *Fire Service Emergency Care.* Upper Saddle River, NJ: Brady/Prentice Hall, 1999.

Epstein, O., et. al. *Clinical Examination.* St. Louis: Mosby, 1997.

Foltin, G., et. al. *Teaching Resource for Instruction in Prehospital Pediatrics.* New York: Center for Pediatric Medicine, 1998.

Janing, J. "Critical Thinking: Incorporation into the Paramedic Curriculum" in *Prehospital and Disaster Medicine 9* (October–November 1994).

Lipkin, M., Jr., S.M. Putnam, and A. Lazare. *The Medical Interview: Clinical Care, Education, and Research.* New York: Springer, 1994.

Martini, F.H., E.F. Bartholomew, and B.E. Bledsoe. *Anatomy and Physiology for Emergency Care.* Upper Saddle River, NJ: Brady/Prentice Hall Health, 2002.

Seidel, H.M., et. al. *Mosby's Guide to Physical Examination.* St. Louis: Mosby, 1999.

Stanford, T.M. *EMS Report Writing: A Pocket Reference.* Englewood Cliffs, NJ: Brady/Prentice Hall, 1992.

Willms, J.L., H. Schneiderman, and P.S. Algranati. *Physical Diagnosis: Bedside Evaluation of Diagnosis and Function.* Baltimore: Williams & Wilkins, 1994.

DIVISION THREE: TRAUMA EMERGENCIES

American College of Surgeons, Committee on Trauma, *Advanced Trauma Life Support Course: Student Manual*. Chicago: American College of Surgeons, 1997.

American College of Surgeons, Committee on Trauma. *Resources for Optimal Care of the Injured Patient*. Chicago: American College of Surgeons, 1998.

Bledsoe, B.E., D.E.Clayden, and F.J. Papa. *Pocket Reference for EMTs and Paramedics*. 2nd edition. Upper Saddle River, NJ: Prentice Hall, 1998.

Butman, A., S. Martin, R. Vomacka, and N. McSwain. *Comprehensive Guide to Pre-Hospital Skills: A Skills Manual for EMT-Basic, EMT-Intermediate, and EMT-Paramedic*. St. Louis: Mosby, 1996.

Campbell, J.E. and the Alabama Chapter of the American College of Emergency Physicians. *Basic Trauma Life Support for Paramedics and Advanced EMS Providers*, 4th. ed. Upper Saddle River, NJ: Brady/Prentice Hall, 2000.

De Lorenzo, R.A. and R.S. Porter. *Tactical Emergency Care: Military and Operational Out-of-Hospital Medicine*. Upper Saddle River, NJ: Prentice Hall, 1999.

DiMaio, V.J. *Gunshot Wounds: Practical Aspects of Firearms, Ballistics, and Forensic Techniques*. 2nd ed. New York: CRC Press, 1999.

Ivatury, R.R. and G.C. Cayten, eds. *Textbook of Penetrating Trauma*. Media, PA: Williams & Wilkins, 1996.

Mattox, K.L., et. al. *Trauma*. 4th ed. Appleton & Lange, Norwalk, CT, 2000.

Maull, K.K. and J. and D. Dennis. *Trauma Update for the EMT*. Upper Saddle River, NJ: Prentice Hall, 1998.

Paturas, J., E. Wertz, and N. McSwain. *PHTLS: Prehospital Trauma Life Support*. 4th ed. St. Louis: Mosby, 1998.

Rosen, P and R.M. Barkin, eds. *Emergency Medicine: Concepts and Clinical Practice*. 5th ed. St. Louis: Mosby, 2002.

Uman, M.A. *All About Lightning*. Mineola, NY: Dover, 1996.

DIVISION FOUR: MEDICAL EMERGENCIES

American Heart Association. *Guidelines 2000 for Cardiopulmonary Resuscitation and Emergency Cardiovascular Care*. Dallas: American Heart Association, 2000.

American Heart Association. *Textbook of Advanced Cardiac Life Support*. 4th ed. Dallas: American Heart Association, 1997.

American Psychiatric Association. *Diagnostic and Statistical Manual of Mental Disorders*. 4th ed. (DSM-IV-TR). Washington, DC.: American Psychiatric Press, 2000.

Andreoli, T.E., et. al. *Cecil Essentials of Medicine*. 5th ed. Philadelphia: W.B. Saunders, 2001.

Auerbach, P.S., ed. *Wilderness Medicine: Management of Wilderness and Environmental Emergencies*. 3rd ed. St. Louis: Mosby, 1995.

Barrett, J.T. *Textbook of Immunology: An Introduction to Immunochemistry and Immunobiology*. 4th ed. St. Louis: Mosby, 1983.

Beasley, B.M. *Understanding 12 Lead EKGs: A Practical Approach*. Upper Saddle River, NJ: Brady/Prentice Hall Health, 2001

Beasley, B.M. *Understanding EKGs: A Practical Approach*. Upper Saddle River, NJ: Brady/Prentice Hall Health, 1999

Benenson, A.S., ed. *Control of Communicable Diseases Manual*. 17th ed. Washington, DC: American Public Health Association, 2000.

Brillman, J.C. and R.W. Quenzer. *Infectious Disease in Emergency Medicine*. 2nd ed. Philadelphia: Lippincott, Williams, and Wilkins, 1998.

Canan, S., C.D. Miller, and M. Taigman. *Taigman's Advanced Cardiology (In Plain English)*. Upper Saddle River, NJ: Brady/Prentice Hall, 1995.

Conover, M.B. *Understanding Electrocardiography*. 7th ed. St. Louis: Mosby, 1996.

Cotran, R.S., V. Kumar, and T. Collins. *Robbins Pathological Basis of Disease*. 6th ed. Philadephia: W.B. Saunders, 1998.

Cunningham, F.G., et. al. *Williams Obstetrics*. 21st ed. New York: McGraw Hill, 2001.

Dalton, A.L., D. Limmer, J.J. Mistovich, and H.A. Werman. *Advanced Medical Life Support*. Upper Saddle River, NJ: Brady/Prentice Hall, 1999.

Ewald, P.W. *Evolution of Infectious Disease*. New York: Oxford University Press, 1997.

Fauci, A.S., et. al. *Harrison's Principles of Internal Medicine*, 15th ed. New York: McGraw Hill, 2001.

Goldfrank, L.W., ed. and N.E. Flamenbau, contributor. *Goldfrank's Toxicologic Emergencies*. 6th ed. New York: McGraw Hill, 1998.

Gorbach, S., J. Bartlett, and N. Blacklow. *Infectious Diseases*. 2nd ed. Philadelphia: W.B. Saunders, 1998.

Greenspan, F.S. and G. J. Strewler. *Basic & Clinical Endocrinology. 6th ed*. New York: McGraw Hill, 2001.

Isada, C.M., et. al. *Infectious Diseases Handbook*. 3rd ed. Hudson, OH: Lexi-Comp Inc., 1999.

Mistovich, J.J., R.W. Benner, and G. Margolis. *Advanced Cardiac Life Support*. Upper Saddle River, NJ: Prentice Hall, 1998.

National Institute of Neurological Disorders and Stroke. *Rapid Identification and Treatment of Acute Stroke*. Bethesda, MD: National Institutes of Health, 1997.

Rosen, P. and R.M. Barkin, eds. *Emergency Medicine: Concepts and Clinical Practice*. 5th ed. St. Louis: Mosby, 2002.

Saunders, C.E. and M.T. Ho. *Current Emergency Diagnosis and Treatment*. 5th ed. Norwalk, CT: Appleton & Lange, 2000.

Taylor, M. *Gastrointestinal Emergencies*. 2nd ed. Baltimore: Williams and Wilkins, 1997.

Tintinelli, J.E., et. al. *Emergency Medicine: A Comprehensive Study Guide*. 5th ed. New York: McGraw Hill, 1999.

Walraven, G. *Basic Arrhythmias*. 5th ed. Upper Saddle River, NJ: Brady/Prentice Hall, 1999.

DIVISION FIVE: SPECIAL CONSIDERATIONS/OPERATIONS

American Heart Association and American Academy of Pediatrics. *Textbook of Neonatal Resuscitation*. 4th ed. Dallas: American Heart Association, 2000.

American Heart Association and American Academy of Pediatrics. *Textbook of Pediatric Advanced Life Support*. 4th ed. Dallas: American Heart Association, 2000.

American Heart Association. *Guidelines 2000 for Cardiopulmonary Resuscitation and Emergency Cardiovascular Care*. Dallas: American Heart Association, 2000.

American Nurses Associations. *Culturally Competent Assessment for Family Violence*. Washington, DC: American Nurses Publishing, 1998.

Auf der Heide, E. *Disaster Response: Principles of Preparation and Coordination*. St. Louis: Mosby, 1989.

Balinsky, W. *Home Care: Current Problems and Future Solutions*. San Francisco: Mossey-Bass Publishers, 1994.

Beers, M.H., et. al., eds. *The Merck Manual of Geriatrics*. 3rd ed. Whitehouse Station, NJ: Merck & Co., Inc., 2001.

Behrman, R.E., et. al. *Nelson Textbook of Pediatrics*. 16th ed. Philadelphia: W.B. Saunders, 2000.

Browner, B.D., ed., et. al. *Emergency Care and Transport of the Sick and Injured*. 7th ed. Sudbury, MA: Jones & Bartlett Publishers, 1999.

Christen, H. and P. Maniscalco. *The EMS Incident Management System: EMS Operations for Mass Casualty and High-Impact Incidents*. Upper Saddle River, NJ: Brady/Prentice Hall, 1998.

Cohn, B.M. and A.J. Azzara. "EMS and Law Enforcement," in *Legal Aspects of Emergency Medical Services*. Philadelphia: W.B. Saunders, 1998.

De Lorenzo, R.A. and R.S. Porter. *Weapons of Mass Destruction: Emergency Care*. Upper Saddle River, NJ: Prentice Hall, 2000.

Eichelberger, MR., et. al. *Pediatric Emergencies*. 2nd ed. Upper Saddle River, NJ: Prentice Hall, 1997.

Elling, R. and R. Guerin. *Ambulance Accident Prevention Seminar Student Workbook*. Albany, NY: Health Education Services, 1988.

Fitch, J., R. Keller, et. al. *EMS Management: Beyond the Street*. 2nd ed. Carlsbad, CA: JEMS Publishing, 1993.

Hamburger, L.K. and C. Renzetti. *Domestic Partner Abuse*. New York: Springer Publishing, 1996.

Hobbs, C.J. and J.M. Wynne. *Physical Signs of Child Abuse: A Color Atlas*. London: W.B. Saunders, 1996.

Kaplan, S.J. *Family Violence: A Clinical and Legal Guide*. Washington, DC. American Psychiatric Press, 1996.

Lesak, D.M. *Hazardous Materials: Strategies and Tactics*. Upper Saddle River, NJ: Brady/Prentice Hall, 1999.

Markenson, D.S. *Pediatric Prehospital Care*. Upper Saddle River, NJ: Brady/Prentice Hall 2002.

Merrick, C., ed. *Rescue Technician: Operational Readiness for Rescue Providers*. St. Louis: Mosby, 1998.

Moore, R.E. *Vehicle Rescue and Extrication*. St. Louis: Mosby, 1991.

Noll, G.G., M.S. Hildebrand, and J.G. Yvorra. *Hazardous Materials: Managing the Incident*. Stillwater, OK: Fire Protection Publications, 1995.

Peto, G.J. and W.J. Medve. *EMS Driving: The Safe Way*. Upper Saddle River, NJ: Prentice Hall, 1996.

Phipps, W., et. al. *Medical-Surgical Nursing: Concepts and Clinical Practice*. 6th ed. St. Louis: Mosby, 1999.

Ray, S. *Swiftwater Rescue: A Manual for the Rescue Professional*. Asheville, NC: CPS Press, 1997.

Reece, R.M. *Child Abuse: Medical Diagnosis and Management*. Philadelphia: Lea & Febiger, 1994.

Samuels, D., et. al. *Air-Medical Crew National Standard Curriculum Instructor Manual*. Pasadena: ASHBEAMS, 1998.

Smith, D.S. and S.J. Smith. *Water Rescue: Basic Skills for Emergency Responders*. St. Louis: Mosby, 1994.

Spratt, S.J., et. al., eds. *Home Health Care: Principles and Practices*. Delray Beach, FL: GR/St. Lucie Press, 1997.

Stutz, D.R. and S. Ulin. *Haztox: EMS Response to Hazardous Materials Incidents*. Miramar, FL: GDS Communications, 1994.

Tilton, B. and F. Hubbell. *Medicine for the Backcountry*. 3rd ed. Globe Pequot Press, 2000.

Vines, T. *High-Angle Rescue Techniques*. 2nd ed. St. Louis: Mosby, 1999.

Wilkerson, J.A. *Medicine for Mountaineering & Other Wilderness Activities*. 5th ed. Merced, CA: Mountaineers Books, 2002.

Glossary

2,3-diphosphoglycerate (2,3-DPG) chemical in the red blood cells that affects hemoglobin's affinity for oxygen.

abandonment termination of the paramedic-patient relationship without assurance that an equal or greater level of care will continue.

ABCs airway, breathing, and circulation.

abduction movement of a body part away from the midline.

aberrant conduction conduction of the electrical impulse through the heart's conductive system in an abnormal fashion.

ABO blood group two antigens known as A and B. A person may have either (type A or type B), both (type AB), or neither (type O).

abortion termination of pregnancy before the 20th week of gestation. The term "abortion" refers to both miscarriage and induced abortion.

abrasion scraping or abrading away of the superficial layers of the skin.

abruptio placentae a condition in which the placenta separates from the uterine wall.

absence seizure type of generalized seizure with sudden onset, characterized by a brief loss of awareness and rapid recovery.

absolute refractory period the period of the cardiac cycle when the myocardial cells have not completely repolarized and stimulation will not produce any depolarization whatever.

absorption see surface absorption.

acceleration the rate at which speed or velocity increases.

acclimatization the reversible changes in body structure and function by which the body becomes adjusted to a change in environment.

acetylcholinesterase (AChE) enzyme that stops the action of acetylocholine, a neurotransmitter.

acid a substance that liberates hydrogen ions ($H+$) when in solution.

acidosis a high concentration of hydrogen ions; a pH below 7.35.

ACLS advanced cardiac life support.

acquired immunity protection from infection or disease that is (a) developed by the body after exposure to an antigen (active acquired immunity) or (b) transferred to the person from an outside source such as from the mother through the placenta or as a serum (passive acquired immunity).

acquired immunodeficiency syndrome see AIDS.

acrocyanosis cyanosis of the extremities.

action potential the stimulation of myocardial cells, as evidenced by a change in the membrane electrical charge, that subsequently spreads across the myocardium.

activated charcoal a powder, usually pre-mixed with water, that will adsorb (bind) some poisons and help prevent them from being absorbed by the body.

active immunity acquired immunity that occurs following exposure to an antigen and results in the production of antibodies specific for the antigen; immunity developed after birth as a result of a direct exposure to an antigen or disease.

active listening the process of responding to your patient's statements with words or gestures that demonstrate your understanding.

active rescue zone area where special rescue teams operate; also known as the *hot zone* or *inner circle.*

active transport movement of a substance through a cell membrane against the osmotic gradient; that is, from an area of lesser concentration to an area of greater concentration, opposite to the normal direction of diffusion; requires the use of energy.

actual damages refers to compensable physical, psychological, or financial harm.

acuity the severity or acuteness of your patient's condition.

acute arterial occlusion the sudden occlusion of arterial blood flow.

acute effects signs and/or symptoms rapidly displayed upon exposure to a toxic substance.

acute gastroenteritis sudden onset of inflammation of the stomach and intestines.

acute myocardial infarction (AMI) see myocardial infarction.

acute pulmonary embolism blockage that occurs when a blood clot or other particle lodges in a pulmonary artery.

acute renal failure (ARF) the sudden-onset of severely decreased urine production.

acute respiratory distress syndrome (ARDS) respiratory insufficiency marked by progressive hypoxemia, due to severe inflammatory damage and fluid accumulation in the alveoli of the lungs. Also called *adult respiratory distress syndrome.*

acute retinal artery occlusion a non-traumatic occlusion of the retinal artery resulting in a sudden, painless loss of vision in one eye.

acute tubular necrosis a particular syndrome characterized by the sudden death of renal tubular cells.

addendum addition or supplement to an original report.

addiction compulsive and overwhelming dependence on a drug; an addiction may be physiological, psychological, or both.

Addison's disease endocrine disorder characterized by adrenocortical insufficiency. Symptoms may include weakness, fatigue, weight loss, and hyperpigmentation of skin and mucous membranes.

Addisonian crisis form of shock associated with adrenocortical insufficiency and characterized by profound hypotension and electrolyte imbalances.

adduction movement of a body part toward the midline.

adenosine triphosphate (ATP) a high-energy compound present in all cells, especially muscle cells; when split by enzyme action it yields energy.

adhesion union of normally separate tissue surfaces by a fibrous band of new tissue.

adjunct medication agent that enhances the effects of other drugs.

administration tubing flexible, clear plastic tubing that connects the solution bag to the IV cannula.

administrative law law that is enacted by governmental agencies at either the federal or state level. Also called *regulatory law.*

adrenergic pertaining to the neurotransmitter norepinephrine.

adrenocorticotropic hormone hormone secreted by the anterior lobe of the pituitary gland that is essential to the function of the adrenal cortex, including production of glucocorticoids.

adult respiratory distress syndrome *see* acute respiratory distress syndrome.

advance directive a document created to ensure that certain treatment choices are honored when a patient is unable to express his choice of treatment.

advanced life support (ALS) advanced life-saving procedures such as intravenous therapy, drug therapy, intubation, and defibrillation.

aerobic with oxygen or requiring oxygen.

aerobic metabolism the stage of metabolism requiring the presence of oxygen, in which the breakdown of glucose (in a process called the Krebs or citric acid cycle) yields a high amount of energy.

aeromedical evacuations transport by helicopter.

affect visible indicators of mood.

afferent carrying impulses toward the central nervous system. Sensory nerves are afferent nerves.

affinity force of attraction between a drug and a receptor.

afterbirth the placenta and accompanying membranes that are expelled from the uterus after the birth of a child.

afterload the resistance a contraction of the heart must overcome in order to eject blood; in cardiac physiology,

defined as the tension of cardiac muscle during systole (contraction).

against medical advice (AMA) when a patient refuses medical care after being advised that he needs it.

ageism discrimination against aged or elderly people.

aggregate to cluster or come together.

agonist drug that binds to a receptor and causes it to initiate the expected response.

agonist-antagonist drug that binds to a receptor and stimulates some of its effects but blocks others; also called *partial agonist.*

AIDS acquired immunodeficiency syndrome, a group of signs, symptoms, and disorders that often develop as a consequence of HIV infection.

air embolism air in the vein.

airbags inflatable high-pressure pillows that when inflated can lift up to 20 tons, depending upon the make.

airborne transmitted through the air by droplets or particles.

air-purifying respirator (APR) system of filtering a normal environment for a specific chemical substance using filter cartridges.

albumin a protein commonly present in plant and animal tissues. In the blood, albumin works to maintain blood volume and blood pressure and provides colloid osmotic pressure, which prevents plasma loss from the capillaries.

aldosterone hormone secreted by the adrenal cortex that increases sodium reabsorption by the kidneys; it plays a part in regulation of blood volume, blood pressure, and blood levels of potassium, chloride, and bicarbonate.

algorithm schematic flow chart that outlines appropriate care for specific signs and symptoms.

alkali a substance that liberates hydroxyl ions (OH^-) when in solution; a strong base.

alkalosis a low concentration of hydrogen ions; a pH above 7.45.

allergen a substance capable of inducing allergy of specific hypersensitivity.

allergic reaction an exaggerated response by the immune system to a foreign substance.

allergy exaggerated immune response to an environmental antigen.

allied health professions ancillary health-care professions, apart from physicians and nurses.

alloimmunity *see* isoimmunity.

alpha radiation low level form of nuclear radiation; a weak source of energy that is stopped by clothing or the first layers of skin.

ALS *see* advanced life support.

alveoli microscopic air sacs where most oxygen and carbon dioxide gas exchanges take place.

Alzheimer's disease a degenerative brain disorder; the most common cause of dementia in the elderly.

amniotic fluid clear, watery fluid that surrounds and protects the developing fetus.

amniotic sac the membranes that surround and protect the developing fetus throughout the period of intrauterine development.

ampere basic unit for measuring the strength of an electric current.

amphiarthrosis joint that permits a limited amount of independent motion.

ampule breakable glass vessel containing liquid medication.

amputation severance, removal, or detachment, either partial or complete, of a body part.

amyotrophic lateral sclerosis (ALS) progressive degeneration of specific nerve cells that control voluntary movement characterized by weakness, loss of motor control, difficulty speaking, and cramping. Also called *Lou Gehrig's disease.*

anabolism the constructive phase of metabolism in which cells convert nonliving substances into living cytoplasm.

anaerobic metabolism the stage of metabolism that does not require oxygen, in which the breakdown of glucose (in a process called glycolysis) produces pyruvic acid and yields very little energy.

anaerobic able to live without oxygen.

analgesia the absence of the sensation of pain.

analgesic medication that relieves the sensation of pain.

anaphylactic shock *see* anaphylaxis.

anaphylaxis a life-threatening allergic reaction; also called *anaphylactic shock.*

anastomosis communication between two or more blood vessels.

anatomy the structure of an organism; body structure.

anchor time set of hours when a night-shift worker can reliably expect to rest without interruption.

anemia a reduction in the hemoglobin content in the blood to a point below that required to meet the oxygen requirements of the body.

anesthesia the absence of all sensation.

anesthetic medication that induces a loss of sensation to touch or pain.

aneurysm a weakening or ballooning in the wall of a blood vessel.

anger hostility or rage to compensate for an underlying feeling of anxiety.

angina pectoris chest pain that results when blood supply's oxygen demands exceed the heart's.

angiocatheter *see* over-the-needle catheter.

angioneurotic edema marked edema of the skin that usually involves the head, neck, face, and upper airway; a common manifestation of severe allergic reactions and anaphylaxis.

angiotensin a vasopressor hormone that causes contraction of the smooth muscles of arteries and arterioles, produced when renin is released from the kidneys; angiotensin I is a physiologically inactive form, while angiotensin II is an active form.

anion an ion with a negative charge—so called because it will be attracted to an anode, or positive pole.

anithyperlipidemic drug used to treat high blood cholesterol.

anorexia nervosa psychological disorder characterized by voluntary refusal to eat.

anorexia absence of appetite.

anoxia the absence or near-absence of oxygen.

anoxic hypoxemia an oxygen deficiency due to disordered pulmonary mechanisms of oxygenation.

antacid alkalotic compound used to increase the gastric environment's pH.

antagonist drug that binds to a receptor but does not cause it to initiate the expected response.

antepartum before the onset of labor.

anterior cord syndrome condition that is caused by bony fragments or pressure compressing the arteries of the anterior spinal cord and resulting in loss of motor function and sensation to pain, light touch, and temperature below the injury site.

anterior medial fissure deep crease along the ventral surface of the spinal cord that divides the cord into right and left halves.

anterograde amnesia inability to remember events that occurred after the trauma that caused the condition.

antibiotics substances that destroy or inhibit microorganisms; agents that kill or decrease the growth of bacteria.

antibody a substance produced by B lymphocytes in response to the presence of a foreign antigen that will combine with and control or destroy the antigen, thus preventing infection.

anticipatory thinking ahead.

anticoagulant drug that inhibits blood clotting.

antidiuresis formation and passage of a concentrated urine, preserving blood volume.

antidiuretic hormone (ADH) hormone released by the posterior pituitary that induces an increase in peripheral vascular resistance and causes the kidneys to retain water, decreasing urine output, and also causes splenic vascular constriction.

antidote a substance that will neutralize a specific toxin or counteract its effect on the body.

antidysrhythmic drug used to treat and prevent abnormal cardiac rhythms.

antiemetic medication used to prevent vomiting.

antigen processing the recognition, ingestion, and breakdown of a foreign antigen, culminating in production of an antibody to the antigen or in a direct cytotoxic response to the antigen.

antigen protein on the surface of a donor's red blood cells that the patient's body recognizes as "self" or "not self."

antigen-antibody complex the substance formed when an antibody combines with an antigen to deactivate or destroy it; also called *immune complex*.

antigen-presenting cells (APCs) cells, such as macrophages, that present (express onto their surfaces) portions of the antigens they have digested.

antihyperlipidemic drug used to treat high blood cholesterol.

antihypertensive drug used to treat hypertension.

antineoplastic agent drug used to treat cancer.

antiplatelet drug that decreases the formation of platelet plugs.

antiseptic cleansing agent that is not toxic to living tissue.

antitussive medication that suppresses the stimulus to cough in the central nervous system.

anuria no elimination of urine.

anxiety disorder condition characterized by dominating apprehension and fear.

anxiety state of uneasiness, discomfort, apprehension, and restlessness.

anxious avoidant attachment a type of bonding that occurs when an infant learns that his caregivers will not be responsive or helpful when needed.

anxious resistant attachment a type of bonding that occurs when an infant learns to be uncertain about whether or not his caregivers will be responsive or helpful when needed.

aortic dissection a degeneration of the wall of the aorta.

APGAR scoring a numerical system of rating the condition of a newborn. It evaluates the newborn's heart rate, respiratory rate, muscle tone, reflex irritability, and color.

aphasia absence or impairment of the ability to communicate through speaking, writing, or signing as a result of brain dysfunction; occurs when the individual suffers brain damage due to stroke or head injury.

apnea absence of breathing.

apneustic respiration breathing characterized by a prolonged inspiration unrelieved by expiration attempts, seen in patients with damage to the upper part of the pons.

apoptosis response in which an injured cell releases enzymes that engulf and destroy itself; one way the body rids itself of damaged and dead cells.

appendicitis inflammation of the vermiform appendix at the juncture of the large and small intestines.

appendicular skeleton bones of the extremities, shoulder girdle, and pelvis (excepting the sacrum).

aqueous humor clear fluid filling the anterior chamber of the eye.

arachnoid membrane middle layer of the meninges.

ARDS *see* acute respiratory distress syndrome.

arrhythmia the absence of cardiac electrical activity; often used interchangeably with dysrhythmia.

arterial gas embolism (AGE) an air bubble, or air embolism, that enters the circulatory system from a damaged lung.

arteries vessels that carry blood from the heart to the body tissues.

arteriole a small artery.

arteriosclerosis a thickening, loss of elasticity, and hardening of the walls of the arteries from calcium deposits.

arthritis inflammation of a joint.

articular surface surface of a bone that moves against another bone.

artifact deflection on the ECG produced by factors other than the heart's electrical activity.

ascending loop of Henle the part of the nephron tubule beyond the descending loop of Henle.

ascending reticular activating system a series of nervous tissues keeping the human system in a state of consciousness.

ascending tracts bundles of axons along the spinal cord that transmit signals from the body to the brain.

ascites bulges in the flanks and across the abdomen, indicating edema caused by congestive heart failure.

asepsis a condition free of pathogens.

asphyxia a decrease in the amount of oxygen and an increase in the amount of carbon dioxide as a result of some interference with respiration.

aspiration inhaling foreign material such as vomitus into the lungs.

assault an act that unlawfully places a person in apprehension of immediate bodily harm without his consent.

assay test that determines the amount and purity of a given chemical in a preparation in the laboratory.

asthma a condition marked by recurrent attacks of dyspnea with wheezing due to spasmodic constriction of the bronchi, often as a response to allergens, or by mucous plugs in the arterial walls.

ataxic respiration poor respirations due to CNS damage, causing ineffective thoracic muscular coordination.

atelectasis alveolar collapse; collapse of a lung or part of a lung.

atherosclerosis a progressive, degenerative disease of the medium-sized and large arteries.

atrophy a decrease in cell size resulting from a decreased workload.

atypical angina *see* Prinzmetal's angina.

augmented limb leads another term for unipolar limb leads, reflecting the fact that the ground lead is disconnected, which increases the amplitude of deflection on the ECG tracing.

auscultation listening with a stethoscope for sounds produced by the body.

authoritarian a parenting style that demands absolute obedience without regard to a child's individual freedom.

authoritative a parenting style that emphasizes a balance between a respect for authority and individual freedom.

autoimmune disease condition in which the body makes antibodies against its own tissues.

autoimmunity an immune response to self antigens, which the body normally tolerates.

automaticity pacemaker cells' capability of self-depolarization.

autonomic dysfunction an abnormality of the involuntary aspect of the nervous system.

autonomic ganglia groups of autonomic nerve cells located outside the central nervous system.

autonomic hyperreflexia syndrome condition associated with the body's adjustment to the effects of spinal shock; presentations include sudden hypertension, bradycardia, pounding headache, blurred vision, and sweating and flushing of the skin above the point of injury.

autonomic nervous system part of the nervous system controlling involuntary bodily functions. It is divided into the sympathetic and the parasympathetic systems.

autonomic neuropathy condition that damages the autonomic nervous system, which usually senses changes in core temperature and controls vasodilation and perspiration to dissipate heat.

autonomy a competent adult patient's right to determine what happens to his own body.

autoregulation process that controls blood flow to tissue by causing alterations in the tissue.

avulsion forceful tearing away or separation of body tissue; an avulsion may be partial or complete.

axial loading application of the forces of trauma along the axis of the spine; this often results in compression fractures of the spine.

axial skeleton bones of the head, thorax, and spine.

axis deviation *see* left axis deviation, right axis deviation.

axon extension of a neuron that serves as a pathway for transmission of signals to and from the brain; major component of white matter.

B lymphocytes white blood cells that, in response to the presence of an antigen, produce antibodies that attack the antigen, develop a memory for the antigen, and confer long-term immunity to the antigen.

Babinski response big toe dorsiflexes and the other toes fan out when sole is stimulated.

bacteria (singular *bacterium*) single-cell organisms with a cell membrane and cytoplasm but no organized nucleus.

bacterial tracheitis bacterial infection of the airway, subglottic region; in children, most likely to appear after episodes of croup.

bactericidal capable of killing bacteria.

bacteriostatic capable of inhibiting bacterial growth or reproduction.

bag-valve mask ventilation device consisting of a self-inflating bag with two one-way valves and a transparent plastic face mask.

ballistics the study of projectile motion and its interactions with the gun, the air, and the object it contacts.

baroreceptor sensory nerve ending, found in the walls of the atria of the heart, vena cava, aortic arch, and carotid sinus, that is stimulated by changes in pressure.

barotrauma injury caused by pressure within an enclosed space; when occuring during a diving descent is commonly called *the squeeze.*

basal metabolic rate (BMR) rate at which the body consumes energy just to maintain stability; the basic metabolic rate (measured by the rate of oxygen consumption) of an awake, relaxed person 12 to 14 hours after eating and at a comfortable temperature.

basic life support (BLS) refers to basic life-saving procedures such as artificial ventilation and cardiopulmonary resuscitation (CPR).

basophil type of white blood cell that participates in allergic responses.

battery the unlawful touching of another individual without his consent.

Battle's sign black and blue discoloration over the mastoid process.

behavior a person's observable conduct and activity.

behavioral emergency situation in which a patient's behavior becomes so unusual that it alarms the patient or another person and requires intervention.

Bell's palsy one-sided facial paralysis with an unknown cause characterized by the inability to close the eye, pain, tearing of the eyes, drooling, hypersensitivity to sound, and impairment of taste.

bend fractures fractures characterized by angulation and deformity in the bone without an obvious break.

benign prostatic hypertrophy a noncancerous enlargement of the prostate associated with aging.

bereavement death of a loved one.

beta radiation medium-strength radiation that is stopped with light clothing or the uppermost layers of skin.

bilateral periorbital ecchymosis black-and-blue discoloration of the area surrounding the eyes. It is usually associated with basilar skull fracture. Also called *raccoon eyes.*

bioassay test to ascertain a drug's availability in a biological model.

bioavailability amount of a drug that is still active after it reaches its target tissue.

bioequivalence relative therapeutic effectiveness of chemically equivalent drugs.

bioethics the application of ethics to the life sciences.

biologic half-life time the body takes to clear one half of a drug.

biological/organic related to disease processes or structural changes.

biotransformation changing a substance in the body from chemical to another; in the case of hazardous materials, the body tries to create less toxic materials.

BiPAP bilevel positive airway pressure.

bipolar disorder condition characterized by one or more manic episodes, with or without periods of depression.

bipolar limb leads electrocardiogram leads applied to the arms and legs that contain two electrodes of opposite (positive and negative) polarity; leads I, II, and III.

birth injury avoidable and unavoidable mechanical and anoxic trauma incurred by the newborn during labor and delivery.

blast wind the air movement caused as the heated and pressurized products of an explosion move outward.

blepharospasm twitching of the eyelids.

blood pressure force of blood against arteries' walls as the heart contracts and relaxes.

blood spatter evidence the pattern that blood forms when it is spattered or dropped at the scene of a crime.

blood tube glass container with color-coded, self-healing rubber top.

blood tubing IV administration tubing that contains a filter to prevent clots or other debris from entering the patient.

bloodborne transmitted by contact with blood or body fluids.

blood-brain barrier tight junctions of the capillary endothelial cells in the central nervous system vasculature through which only non-protein-bound, highly lipid-soluble drugs can pass.

blunt trauma injury caused by the collision of an object with the body in which the object does not enter the body.

BLS *see* basic life support.

body armor vest made of tightly woven, strong fibers that offer protection against handgun bullets, most knives, and blunt trauma; also known as a *bullet-proof vest*.

body language *see* nonverbal communication.

body substance isolation (BSI) a strict form of infection control that is based on the assumption that all blood and other body fluids are infectious.

body surface area (BSA) amount of a patient's body affected by a burn.

Bohr effect phenomenon in which a decrease in pCO_2/acidity causes an increase in the quantity of oxygen that binds with the hemoglobin and, conversely, an increase in pCO_2/acidity causes the hemoglobin to give up a greater quantity of oxygen.

bolus concentrated mass of medication.

bonding the formation of a close personal relationship (as between mother and child), especially through frequent or constant association.

borborygmi loud, prolonged, gurgling bowel sounds indicating hyperperistalsis.

bowel obstruction blockage of the hollow space within the intestines.

Bowman's capsule the hollow, cup-shaped first part of the nephron tubule.

bradycardia a slow heart rate; a heart rate less than 60 beats per minute.

bradypnea slow respiration.

brain abscess a collection of pus localized in an area of the brain.

brain ischemia injury to brain tissues caused by an inadequate supply of oxygen and nutrients.

brainstem part of the brain connecting the cerebral hemispheres with the spinal cord. It is comprised of the mesencephalon (midbrain), the pons, and the medulla oblongata.

branch functional level within the Incident Management System based upon primary roles and geographic locations. Also called *sector*.

breach of duty an action or inaction that violates the standard of care expected from a paramedic.

bronchi tubes from the trachea into the lungs.

bronchiectasis chronic dilation of a bronchus or bronchi, with a secondary infection typically involving the lower portion of the lung.

bronchiolitis viral infection of the medium-sized airways, occurring most frequently during the first year of life.

bronchophony abnormal clarity of patient's transmitted voice sounds.

Broselow tape a measuring tape for infants that provides important information regarding airway equipment and medication doses based on your patient's length.

Brown-Séquard's syndrome condition caused by partial cutting of one side of the spinal cord resulting in sensory and motor loss to that side of the body.

Brudzinkis's sign physical exam finding in which flexion of the neck causes flexion of the hips and knees.

bruit sound of turbulent blood flow around a partial obstruction.

bubble sheet scannible run sheet on which boxes or "bubbles" are filled in to record information.

buccal between the cheek and gums.

buckle fractures fractures characterized by a raised or bulging projection at the fracture site.

buffer a substance that tends to preserve or restore a normal acid-base balance by increasing or decreasing the concentration of hydrogen ions.

bulimia nervosa recurrent episodes of binge eating.

bundle branch block a kind of interventricular heart block in which conduction through either the right or left bundle branches is blocked or delayed.

bundle of Kent an accessory AV conduction pathway that is thought to be responsible for the ECG findings of pre-excitation syndrome.

burette chamber calibrated chamber of Berutrol IV administration tubing that enables precise measurement and delivery of fluids and medicated solutions.

burnout occurs when coping mechanisms no longer buffer job stressors, which can compromise personal health and well-being.

bursa sac containing synovial fluid that cushions adjacent structures.

bursitis acute or chronic inflammation of the small synovial sacs.

CAGE questionnaire a questionnaire designed to determine the presence of alcoholism.

calcaneus the largest bone of the foot; the heel.

caliber the diameter of a bullet expressed in hundredths of an inch. (.22 caliber = 0.22 inches); the inside diameter of the barrel of a handgun, shotgun, or rifle.

callus thickened area that forms at the site of a fracture as part of the repair process.

CAMEO® Computer-Aided Management of Emergency Operations; website developed by the EPA and NOAA as a source of information, skills, and links related to hazardous substances.

cancellous having a lattice-work structure, as in the spongy tissue of a bone.

cannula hollow needle used to puncture a vein.

cannulation *see* intravenous access.

capillary one of the minute blood vessels that connect the ends of arterioles with the beginnings of venules; where oxygen is diffused to body tissue and products of metabolism enter the bloodstream.

capnography the measurement of exhaled carbon dioxide concentrations.

carbon dioxide waste product of the body's metabolism.

cardiac arrest the absence of ventricular contraction.

cardiac contractile force the strength of a contraction of the heart.

cardiac cycle the period of time from the end of one cardiac contraction to the end of the next.

cardiac depolarization a reversal of charges at a cell membrane so that the inside of the cell becomes positive in relation to the outside; the opposite of the cell's resting state in which the inside of the cell is negative in relation to the outside.

cardiac monitor machine that displays and records the electrical activity of the heart.

cardiac output the amount of blood pumped by the heart in one minute (computed as stroke volume × heart rate).

cardiac tamponade accumulation of excess fluid inside the pericardium.

cardioacceleratory center a sympathetic nervous system center in the medulla oblongata, controlling the release of epinephrine and norepinephrine.

cardiogenic shock shock caused by insufficient cardiac output; the inability of the heart to pump enough blood to perfuse all parts of the body.

cardioinhibitory center a parasympathetic center in the medulla oblongata, controlling the vagus nerve.

cardiovascular disease (CVD) disease affecting the heart, peripheral blood vessels, or both.

carina the point at which the trachea bifurcates into the right and left mainstem bronchi.

carpal bones bones of the wrist.

carrier mediated diffusion process in which carrier proteins transport large molecules across the cell membrane; also called *facilitated diffusion*.

cartilage connective tissue providing the articular surfaces of the skeletal system.

catabolism the destructive phase of metabolism in which cells break down complex substances into simpler substances with release of energy.

cataracts medical condition in which the lens of the eye loses its clearness.

catatonia condition characterized by immobility and stupor, often a sign of schizophrenia.

catecholamine a hormone, such as epinephrine or norepinephrine, that strongly affects the nervous and cardiovascular systems, metabolic rate, temperature, and smooth muscle.

catheter inserted through the needle Teflon catheter inserted through a large metal stylet; also called *intracatheter*.

catheter a tube passed into or through the body.

cation an ion with a positive charge—so called because it will be attracted to a cathode, or negative pole.

cavitation the outward motion of tissue due to a projectile's passage, resulting in a temporary cavity and vacuum.

cell membrane also *plasma membrane;* the outer covering of a cell.

cell the basic structural unit of all plants and animals; a membrane enclosing a thick fluid and a nucleus. Cells are specialized to carry out all of the body's basic functions.

cell-mediated immunity the short-term immunity to an antigen provided by T lymphocytes, which directly attack the antigen but do not produce antibodies or memory for the antigen. Also called *cellular immunity*.

cellular swelling swelling of a cell caused by injury to or change in permeability of the cell membrane with resulting inability to maintain stable intra- and extracellular fluid and electrolyte levels.

cellular telephone system telephone system divided into regions, or cells, that are served by radio base stations.

cellulitis inflammation of cellular or connective tissue.

central cord syndrome condition usually related to hyperflexion of the cervical spine that results in motor weakness, usually in the upper extremities and possible bladder dysfunction.

central IV line intravenous line placed into the superior vena cava for the administration of long-term fluid therapy.

central nervous system the brain and the spinal cord.

central neurogenic hyperventilation hyperventilation caused by a lesion in the central nervous system, often characterized by rapid, deep, noisy respirations.

central pain syndrome condition resulting from damage or injury to the brain, brainstem, or spinal cord characterized by intense, steady pain described as burning, aching, tingling, or a "pins and needles" sensation.

central venous access surgical puncture of the internal jugular, subclavian, or femoral vein.

cerebellum portion of the brain located dorsally to the pons and medulla oblongata. It plays an important role in the fine motor movement, posture, equilibrium, and muscle tone.

cerebral perfusion pressure (CPP) the pressure moving blood through the brain.

cerebrospinal fluid fluid surrounding and bathing the brain and spinal cord.

cerebrum largest part of the brain, consisting of two hemispheres. The cerebrum is the seat of consciousness and the center of the higher mental functions such as memory, learning, reasoning, judgement, intelligence, and the emotions.

certification the process by which an agency or association grants recognition to an individual who has met its qualifications.

cerumen ear wax.

C-FLOP mnemonic for the main functional areas within the IMS—command, finance/administration, logistics, operations, and planning.

chain of evidence legally retaining items of evidence and accounting for their whereabouts at all times to prevent loss or tampering.

chancroid highly contagious sexually transmitted ulcer.

chemoreceptor sense organ or sensory nerve ending located outside the central nervous system that is stimulated by and reacts to chemical stimuli.

chemotactic factors chemicals released by white blood cells that attract more white blood cells to an area of inflammation.

chemotaxis the movement of white blood cells in response to chemical signals.

CHEMTEL, Inc. Chemical Telephone, Incorporated; maintains a 24-hour, toll-free hotline at 800-255-3024; for collect calls and calls from other points of origin, dial 813-979-0626.

CHEMTREC Chemical Transportation Emergency Center; maintains a 24-hour, toll-free hotline at 800-424-9300; for collect calls and calls from other points of origin, dial 703-527-3887.

Cheyne-Stokes respiration a breathing pattern characterized by a period of apnea lasting 10-60 seconds, followed by gradually increasing depth and frequency of respirations; respiratory pattern of alternating periods of apnea and tachypnea.

chief complaint the pain, discomfort, or dysfunction that caused your patient to request help.

child abuse physical or emotional violence or neglect towards a person from infancy to eighteen years of age.

chlamydia group of intracellular parasites that cause sexually transmitted diseases.

choanal atresia congenital closure of the passage between the nose and pharynx by a bony or membranous structure.

cholinergic pertaining to the neurotransmitter acetylcholine.

chronic gastroenteritis non-acute inflammation of the gastric mucosa.

chronic obstructive pulmonary disease (COPD) a disease characterized by a decreased ability of the lungs to perform the function of ventilation.

chronic renal failure permanently inadequate renal function due to nephron loss.

chronotropy pertaining to heart rate.

chyme semifluid mixture of ingested food and digestive secretions found in the stomach and small intestine.

circadian rhythms physiological phenomena that occur at approximately 24-hour intervals.

circulation assessment evaluating the pulse and skin and controlling hemorrhage.

circulatory overload overload that occurs if too much medication is administered for the patient's condition.

circumcision the surgical removal of the foreskin of the penis.

circumduction movement at a synovial joint where the distal end of a bone describes a circle but the shaft does not rotate.

cirrhosis degenerative disease of the liver.

civil law division of the legal system that deals with noncriminal issues and conflicts between two or more parties.

claudication severe pain in the calf muscle due to inadequate blood supply. It typically occurs with exertion and subsides with rest.

clavicle bone that holds the scapula and shoulder joint at a fixed distance from the sternum.

cleaning washing an object with cleaners such as soap and water.

cleft lip congenital vertical fissure in the upper lip.

cleft palate congenital fissure in the roof of the mouth, forming a passageway between oral and nasal cavities.

clinical judgment the use of knowledge and experience to diagnose patients and plan their treatment.

clitoris highly innervated and vascular erectile tissue anterior to the labia minora.

clonal diversity the development, by B lymphocyte precursors in the bone marrow, of receptors for every possible type of antigen.

clonal selection the process by which a specific antigen reacts with the appropriate receptors on the surface of immature B lymphocytes, thereby activating them and prompting them to proliferate, differentiate, and produce antibodies to the activating antigen.

clonic phase phase of a seizure characterized by alternating contraction and relaxation of muscles.

closed fracture a broken bone in which the bone ends or the forces that caused it do not penetrate the skin.

closed incident an incident that is not likely to generate any further patients; also known as a *contained incident* or a *stable incident*.

closed pneumothorax *see* pneumothorax.

closed stance a posture or body position that is tense and suggests negativity, discomfort, fear, disgust, or anger.

closed-ended questions questions that ask for specific information and require only very short or yes-or-no answers. Also called *direct questions*.

clotting the body's three-step response to stop the loss of blood.

coagulation necrosis the process in which an acid, while destroying tissue, forms an insoluble layer that limits further damage.

coagulation the third step in the clotting process, which involves the formation of a protein called fibrin that forms a network around a wound to stop bleeding, ward off infection, and lay a foundation for healing and repair of the wound.

cold zone location at a hazmat incident outside the warm zone; area where incident operations take place; also called the *green zone* or the *safe zone*.

colic acute pain associated with cramping or spasms in the abdominal organs.

collagen tough, strong protein that comprises most of the body's connective tissue.

collecting duct the larger structure beyond the distal nephron tubule into which urine drips.

colloid osmotic pressure *see* oncotic force.

colloids substances, such as proteins or starches, consisting of large molecules or molecule aggregates that disperse evenly within a liquid without forming a true solution; intravenous solutions containing large proteins that cannot pass through capillary membranes.

colostomy a surgical diversion of the large intestine through an opening in the skin where the fecal matter is collected in a pouch; may be temporary or permanent.

coma a state of unconsciousness from which the patient cannot be aroused.

command post (CP) place where command officers from various agencies can meet with each other and select a management staff.

command the individual or group responsible for coordinating all activities and who makes final decisions on the emergency scene; often referred to as the Incident Commander (IC) or Officer in Charge (OIC).

comminuted fracture fracture in which a bone is broken into several pieces.

common law law that is derived from society's acceptance of customs and norms over time. Also called *case law* or *judge-made law*.

communicable period time when a host can transmit an infectious agent to someone else.

communicable capable of being transmitted to another host.

communication the exchange of common symbols— written, spoken, or other kinds such as signing and body language; the process of exchanging information between individuals.

community-acquired infection an infection occurring in a nonhospitalized patient who is not undergoing regular medical procedures, including the use of instruments such as catheters.

comorbidity having more than one disease at a time.

compartment syndrome condition that occurs when circulation to a portion of the body is cut off; muscle ischemia that is caused by rising pressures within an anatomic fascial space.

compensated shock early stage of shock during which the body's compensatory mechanisms are able to maintain normal perfusion.

compensatory pause the pause following an ectopic beat where the SA node is unaffected and the cadence of the heart is uninterrupted.

competent able to make an informed decision about medical care.

competitive antagonism one drug binds to a receptor and causes the expected effect while also blocking another drug from triggering the same receptor.

complex partial seizure type of partial seizure usually originating in the temporal lobe characterized by an aura and focal findings such as alterations in mental status or mood.

compliance the stiffness or flexibility of the lung tissue.

concealment hiding the body behind objects that shield a person from view but that offer little or no protection against bullets or other ballistics.

concentration weight per volume.

concussion a transient period of unconsciousness. In most cases, the unconsciousness will be followed by a complete return of function.

conduction moving electrons, ions, heat, or sound waves through a conductor or conducting medium.

conductive deafness deafness caused when there is a blocking of the transmission of the sound waves through the external ear canal to the middle or inner ear.

conductivity ability of cells to propagate the electrical impulse from one cell to another.

confidentiality the principle of law that prohibits the release of medical or other personal information about a patient without the patient's consent.

confusion state of being unclear or unable to make a decision easily.

congenital present at birth.

congestive heart failure (CHF) condition in which the heart's reduced stroke volume causes an overload of fluid in the body's other tissues. *See also* heart failure.

congregate care living arrangement in which the elderly live in, but do not own, individual apartments or rooms and receive select services.

conjuctiva mucous membrane that lines the eyelids.

connective tissue the most abundant body tissue; it provides support, connection, and insulation. Examples: bone, cartilage, fat, blood.

consent the patient's granting of permission for treatment.

constitutional law law based on the U.S. Constitution.

contamination presence of an agent only on the surface of the host without penetrating it.

continuous quality improvement (CQI) a program designed to refine and improve an EMS system, emphasizing customer satisfaction.

CONTOMS Counter-Narcotics Tactical Operations; program that manages the training and certification of EMT-Ts and SWAT-Medics.

contractility ability of muscle cells to contract, or shorten.

contraction inward movement of wound edges during healing that eventually brings the wound edges together.

contrecoup injury occurring on the opposite side; an injury to the brain opposite the site of impact.

contusion closed wound in which the skin is unbroken, although damage has occurred to the tissue immediately beneath.

convection transfer of heat via currents in liquids or gases.

conventional reasoning the stage of moral development during which children desire approval from individuals and society.

convergent focusing on only the most important aspect of a critical situation.

cor pulmonale hypertrophy of the right ventricle resulting from disorders of the lung; congestive heart failure secondary to pulmonary hypertension.

core temperature the body temperature of the deep tissues, which usually does not vary more than a degree or so from its normal 37° C (98.6° F).

cornea thin, delicate layer covering the pupil and the iris.

coronary heart disease (CHD) a type of CVD; the single largest killer of Americans.

cortex the outer tissue of an organ such as the kidney.

cortisol a steroid hormone released by the adrenal cortex that regulates the metabolism of fats, carbohydrates, sodium, potassium, and proteins and also has an anti-inflammatory effect.

coup injury an injury to the brain occurring on the same side as the site of impact.

coupling interval distance between the preceding beat and a premature ventricular contraction (PVC).

cover hiding the body behind solid and impenetrable objects that protect a person from bullets.

CPAP continuous positive airway pressure.

crackles light crackling, popping, nonmusical sounds heard usually during inspiration.

cramping muscle pain resulting from overactivity, lack of oxygen, and accumulation of waste products.

cranial nerves twelve pairs of nerves that extend from the lower surface of the brain.

cranium vault-like portion of the skull encasing the brain.

creatinine a waste product caused by metabolism within muscle cells.

crepitation (or crepitus) crunching sounds of unlubricated parts in joints rubbing against each other.

cribbing wooden slates used to shore up heavy equipment.

cricothyroid membrane membrane between the cricoid and thyroid cartilages of the larynx.

cricothyrostomy the introduction of a needle or other tube into the cricothyroid membrane, usually to provide an emergency airway.

cricothyrotomy a surgical incision into the cricothyroid membrane, usually to provide an emergency airway.

criminal law division of the legal system that deals with wrongs committed against society or its members.

critical incident stress debriefing (CISD) a process used to help rescuers work through their responses to a critical incident within 24 to 72 hours after the event.

critical incident stress management (CISM) a system of related interventions usually performed by regional, non-partisan, multi-disciplinary teams composed of EMS peers and specifically trained mental health workers.

critical incident an event that has a powerful emotional impact on a rescuer that can cause an acute stress reaction.

critical thinking thought process used to analyze and evaluate.

Crohn's disease idiopathic inflammatory bowel disorder associated with the small intestine.

croup viral illness characterized by inspiratory and expiratory stridor and a seal-bark-like cough.

crowning the bulging of the fetal head past the opening of the vagina during a contraction. Crowning is an indication of impending delivery.

crumple zone the region of a vehicle designed to absorb the energy of impact.

crush injury mechanism of injury in which tissue is locally compressed by high-pressure forces.

crush syndrome systemic disorder of severe metabolic disturbances resulting from the crush of a limb or other body part.

crystalloids substances capable of crystallization. In solution, unlike colloids, they can diffuse through a membrane, such as a capillary wall; intravenous solutions that contain electrolytes but lack the larger proteins associated with colloids.

Cullen's sign discoloration around the umbilicus suggestive of intra-abdominal hemorrhage.

cultural imposition the imposition of one's beliefs, values, and patterns of behavior on people of another culture.

current the rate of flow of an electric charge.

Cushing's reflex a collective change in vital signs (increased blood pressure and temperature and decreased pulse and respirations) associated with increasing intracranial pressure.

Cushing's syndrome pathological condition resulting from excess adrenocortical hormones. Symptoms may include changed body habitus, hypertension, vulnerability to infection.

cyanosis bluish discoloration of the skin due to reduced hemoglobin in the blood.

cystic medial necrosis a death or degeneration of a part of the wall of an artery.

cystitis an infection and inflammation of the urinary bladder.

cytochrome oxidase enzyme complex, found in cellular mitochondria, that enables oxygen to create the adenosine triphosphate (ATP) required for all muscle energy.

cytokines proteins, produced by white blood cells, that regulate immune responses by binding with and affecting the function of the cells that produced them or of other, nearby cells.

cytoplasm the thick fluid, or *protoplasm*, that fills a cell.

cytotoxic toxic, or poisonous, to cells.

deafness the inability to hear.

debridement the cleaning up or removal of debris, dead cells, and scabs from a wound, principally through phagocytosis.

deceleration the rate at which speed or velocity decreases.

decerebrate posture sustained contraction of extensor muscles of the extremities resulting from a lesion in the brainstem. The patient presents with stiff and extended extremities and retracted head.

decode to interpret a message.

decompensated shock advanced stages of shock when the body's compensatory mechanisms are no longer able to maintain normal perfusion; also called *progressive shock*.

decompression illness development of nitrogen bubbles within the tissues due to a rapid reduction of air pressure when a diver returns to the surface; also called *the bends*.

decontaminate to destroy or remove pathogens.

decontamination the process of minimizing toxicity by reducing the amount of toxin absorbed into the body.

decorticate posture characteristic posture associated with a lesion at or above the upper brainstem. The patient presents with the arms flexed, fists clenched, and legs extended.

deep frostbite freezing involving epidermal and subcutaneous tissues resulting in a white appearance, hard (frozen) feeling on palpation, and loss of sensation.

deep venous thrombosis a blood clot in a vein.

defamation an intentional false communication that injures another person's reputation or good name.

defibrillation the process of passing an electrical current through a fibrillating heart to depolarize a "critical mass" of myocardial cells. This allows them to depolarize uniformly, resulting in an organized rhythm.

defusing a short, informal type of debriefing held within hours of a critical incident.

degenerative neurological disorders a collection of diseases that selectively affect one or more functional systems of the central nervous system.

degloving injury avulsion in which the mechanism of injury tears the skin off the underlying muscle, tissue, blood vessels, and bone.

degranulation the emptying of granules from the interior of a mast cell into the extracellular environment.

dehydration excessive loss of body fluid.

delayed effects signs, symptoms, and/or conditions developed hours, days, weeks, months, or even years after exposure to a toxic substance.

delayed hypersensitivity reaction a hypersensitivity reaction that takes place after the elapse of some time following reexposure to an antigen. Delayed hypersensitivity reactions are usually less severe than immediate reactions.

DeLee suction trap a suction device that contains a suction trap connected to a suction catheter. The negative pressure that powers it can come either from the mouth of the operator or, preferably, from an external vacuum source.

delirium tremens (DTs) disorder found in habitual and excessive users of alcoholic beverages after cessation of drinking for 48–72 hours. Patients experience visual, tactile, and auditory disturbances. Death may result in severe cases.

delirium condition characterized by relatively rapid onset of widespread disorganized thought.

delusions fixed, false beliefs not widely held within the individual's cultural or religious group.

demand valve device a ventilation device that is manually operated by a push button or lever.

dementia a deterioration of mental status that is usually associated with structural neurological disease.

demobilization establishment and staffing of a transition point with the object of providing crews time to regroup between a large-scale critical stress situation and going off duty or back to regular duty.

demobilized release of resources—personnel, vehicles, and equipment—for use outside the incident when they are no longer needed at the scene.

demographic pertaining to population makeup or changes.

demylenation destruction or removal of the myelin sheath of nerve tissue; found in Guillain–Barré syndrome.

denature alter the usual substance of something.

depersonalization feeling detached from oneself.

deployment strategy used by an EMS agency to maneuver its ambulances and crews in an effort to reduce response times.

depression a mood disorder characterized by hopelessness and malaise.

dermatome topographical region of the body surface innervated by one nerve root.

dermis true skin, also called the *corium*. It is the layer of tissue producing the epidermis and housing the structures, blood vessels, and nerves normally associated with the skin.

descending loop of Henle the part of the nephron tubule beyond the proximal tubule.

descending tracts bundles of axons along the spinal cord that transmit signals from the brain to the body.

desired dose specific quantity of medication needed.

detailed physical exam careful, thorough process of eliciting the history and conducting a physical exam.

devascularization loss of blood vessels from a body part.

diabetes insipidus excessive urine production caused by inadequate production of antidiuretic hormone.

diabetes mellitus disorder of inadequate insulin activity, due either to inadequate production of insulin or to decreased responsiveness of body cells to insulin.

diabetic ketoacidosis complication of Type I diabetes due to decreased insulin intake. Marked by high blood glucose, metabolic acidosis, and, in advanced stages, coma. Ketoacidosis is often called diabetic coma.

diabetic retinopathy slow loss of vision as a result of damage done by diabetes.

dialysate the solution used in dialysis that is hypo-osmolar to many of the wastes and key electrolytes in blood.

dialysis a procedure that replaces some lost kidney functions.

diaphoresis sweatiness.

diaphragmatic hernia protrusion of abdominal contents into the thoracic cavity through an opening in the diaphragm.

diaphysis hollow shaft found in long bones.

diarthrosis a synovial joint.

diastole the period of time when the myocardium is relaxed and cardiac filling and coronary perfusion occur.

diastolic blood pressure force of blood against arteries when ventricles relax.

diencephalon portion of the brain lying beneath the cerebrum and above the brainstem. It contains the thalamus, the hypothalamus, and the limbic system.

differential field diagnosis the list of possible causes for your patient's symptoms.

difficult child an infant, who can be characterized by irregularity of bodily functions, intense reactions, and withdrawal from new situations.

diffuse axonal injury type of brain injury characterized by shearing, stretching, or tearing of nerve fibers with subsequent axonal damage.

diffusion the movement of molecules through a membrane from an area of greater concentration to an area of lesser concentration.

digestive tract internal passageway that begins at the mouth and ends at the anus.

digital communications data or sounds are translated into a digital code for transmission.

dilation enlargement. In reference to the heart, an abnormal enlargement resulting from pathology.

diplopia double vision.

direct pressure method of hemorrhage control that relies on the application of pressure to the actual site of the bleeding.

direct questions *see* closed-ended questions.

disaster management management of incidents that generate large numbers of patients, often overwhelming resources and damaging parts of the infrastructure.

disease period the duration from the onset of signs and symptoms of disease until the resolution of symptoms or death.

disentanglement process of freeing a patient from wreckage, to allow for proper care, removal, and transfer.

disinfectant cleansing agent that is toxic to living tissue.

disinfecting cleaning with an agent that can kill some microorganisms on the surface of an object.

dislocation complete displacement of a bone end from its position in a joint capsule.

dissecting aortic aneurysm aneurysm caused when blood gets between and separates the layers of the arterial wall.

disseminated intravascular coagulation (DIC) a disorder of coagulation caused by systemic activation of the coagulation cascade.

dissociate separate; break down. For example, sodium bicarbonate, when placed in water, dissociates into a sodium cation and a bicarbonate anion.

dissociative disorder condition in which the individual avoids stress by separating from his core personality.

distal tubule the part of the tubule beyond the ascending loop of Henle.

distributive shock shock that results from mechanisms that prevent the appropriate distribution of nutrients and removal of metabolic waste products; Examples include septic shock, neurogenic shock, and anaphylactic shock.

diuresis formation and passage of a dilute urine, decreasing blood volume; secretion of large amounts of urine.

diuretic a medication that stimulates the kidneys to excrete excess water.

diuretic an agent that increases urine secretion and elimination of body water; drug used to reduce circulating blood volume by increasing the amount of urine.

divergent taking into account all aspects of a complex situation.

diverticula small outpouchings in the mucosal lining of the intestinal tract.

diverticulitis inflammation of diverticula.

diverticulosis presence of diverticula, with or without associated bleeding.

Do Not Resuscitate (DNR) order legal document, usually signed by the patient and his physician, that indicates to medical personnel which, if any, life-sustaining measures should be taken when the patient's heart and respiratory functions have ceased.

domestic elder abuse physical or emotional violence or neglect when an elder is being cared for in a home-based setting.

dosage on hand the amount of drug available in a solution.

dose packaging medication packages that contain a single dose for a single patient.

DOT KKK 1822D specs the manufacturing and design specifications produced by the Federal General Services Administrative Automotive Commodity Center.

down time duration from the beginning of the cardiac arrest until effective CPR is established. *see also* total down time.

down-regulation binding of a drug or hormone to a target cell receptor that causes the number of receptors to decrease.

drag the forces acting on a projectile in motion to slow its progress.

drip chamber clear plastic chamber that allows visualization of the intravenous drip rate.

drip rate pace at which the fluid moves from the intravenous bag into the patient.

dromotropy pertaining to the speed of cardiac impulse transmission.

drop former device in a drip chamber that regulates the size of drops.

drowning asphyxiation resulting from submersion in liquid with death occurring within 24 hours of submersion.

drug overdose poisoning from a pharmacological substance in excess of that usually prescribed or that the body can tolerate.

drug chemical used to diagnose, treat, or prevent disease.

drug-response relationship correlation of different amounts of a drug to clinical response.

ductus arteriosus channel between the main pulmonary artery and the aorta of the fetus.

due regard legal terminology found in the motor vehicle laws of most states that sets up a higher standard for the operators of emergency vehicles.

duplex communication system that allows simultaneous two-way communications by using two frequencies for each channel.

dura mater tough layer of the meninges firmly attached to the interior of the skull and the spinal column.

duration of action length of time the amount of drug remains above its minimum effective concentration.

duty to act a formal contractual or informal legal obligation to provide care.

dynamic steady state homeostasis; the tendency of the body to maintain a net constant composition although the components of the body's internal environment are always changing.

dysmenorrhea painful menstruation.

dyspareunia painful sexual intercourse.

dysphagia inability to swallow or difficulty swallowing.

dysphoria an exaggerated feeling of depression or unrest, characterized by a mood of general dissatisfaction, restlessness, discomfort, and unhappiness.

dysplasia a change in cell size, shape, or appearance caused by an external stressor.

dyspnea an abnormality of breathing rate, pattern, or effort; the sensation of having difficulty in breathing.

dysrhythmia any deviation from the normal electrical rhythm of the heart.

dystonias a group of disorders characterized by muscle contractions that cause twisting and repetitive movements, abnormal postures, or freezing in the middle of an action.

dysuria painful urination often associated with cystitis.

easy child an infant, who can be characterized by regularity of bodily functions, low or moderate intensity of reactions, and acceptance of new situations.

ecchymosis blue-black discoloration of the skin due to leakage of blood into the tissues.

echo procedure immediately repeating each transmission received during radio communications.

ectopic beat cardiac depolarization resulting from depolarization of ectopic focus.

ectopic focus nonpacemaker heart cell that automatically depolarizes; *pl.* ectopic foci.

ectopic pregnancy the implantation of a developing fetus outside of the uterus, often in fallopian tubes.

eddies water that flows around especially large objects and, for a time, flows upstream around the downside of an obstruction; provides an opportunity to escape dangerous currents.

edema excess fluid in the interstitial space.

effacement the thinning of the cervix during labor.

efferent carrying impulses away from the brain or spinal cord to the periphery. Motor nerves are efferent nerves.

efficacy a drug's ability to cause the expected response.

egophony abnormal change in tone of patient's transmitted voice sounds.

Einthoven's triangle the triangle around the heart formed by the bipolar limb leads.

ejection fraction ratio of blood pumped from the ventricle to the amount remaining at end of diastole.

elder abuse *see* domestic elder abuse; institutional elder abuse.

elderly a person age 65 or older.

electrical alternans alternating amplitude of the P, QRS, and T waves on the ECG rhythm strip as the heart swings in a pendulum-like fashion within the pericardial sac during tamponade.

electrocardiogram (ECG) the graphic recording of the heart's electrical activity. It may be displayed either on paper or on an oscilloscope.

electrolyte a substance that, in water, separates into electrically charged particles.

emancipated minor a person under 18 years of age who is married, pregnant, a parent, a member of the armed forces, or financially independent and living away from home.

embolus undissolved solid, liquid, or gaseous matter in the bloodstream that may cause blockage of blood vessels; *pl.* emboli.

emergency doctrine *see* implied consent.

emergency medical dispatcher (EMD) EMS person responsible for assignment of emergency medical resources to a medical emergency.

emergency medical services (EMS) system a comprehensive network of personnel, equipment, and resources established for the purpose of delivering aid and emergency medical care to the community.

Emergency Medical Services for Children (EMSC) federally funded program aimed at improving the health of pediatric patients who suffer from life-threatening illnesses and injuries.

emergent phase first stage of the burn process that is characterized by a catecholamine release and pain-mediated reaction.

emesis vomitus.

empathy identification with and understanding of another's situation, feelings, and motives.

EMT-Tacticals (EMT-Ts) EMS personnel trained to serve with a tactical Emergency Medical Services or a law enforcement agency.

encephalitis acute infection of the brain, usually caused by a virus.

encode to create a message.

endocrine gland gland that secretes chemical substances directly into the blood; also called a *ductless gland*.

endometriosis condition in which endometrial tissue grows outside of the uterus.

endometritis infection of the endometrium.

endometrium the inner layer of the uterine wall where the fertilized egg implants.

endotoxin toxic products released when bacteria die and decompose.

endotracheal intubation passing a tube into the trachea to protect and maintain the airway and to permit medication administration and deep suctioning.

end-stage renal failure an extreme failure of kidney function due to nephron loss.

enema a liquid bolus of medication that is injected into the rectum.

energy the capacity to do work in the strict physical sense.

enteral route delivery of a medication through the gastrointestinal tract.

enterotoxin an exotoxin that produces gastrointestinal symptoms and diseases such as food poisoning.

enucleation removal of the eyeball after trauma or illness.

environmental emergency a medical condition caused or exacerbated by the weather, terrain, atmospheric pressure, or other local factors.

epicardium serous membrane covering the outer surface of the heart; the visceral pericardium.

epidemiology the study of factors that influence the frequency, distribution, and causes of injury, disease, and other health-related events in a population.

epidermis outermost layer of the skin composed of dead or dying cells.

epididymis a saclike duct adjacent to a testis that stores sperm cells.

epidural hematoma accumulation of blood between the dura mater and the cranium.

epiglottitis infection and inflammation of the epiglottis.

epiphyseal fracture disruption in the epiphyseal plate of a child's bone.

epiphyseal plate area of the metaphysis where cartilage is generated during bone growth in childhood.

epiphysis end of a long bone, including the epiphsyeal or growth plate, and supporting structures underlying the joint.

epistaxis nosebleed.

epithelial tissue the protective tissue that lines internal and external body tissues. Examples: skin, mucous membranes, the lining of the intestinal tract.

epithelialization early stage of wound healing in which epithelial cells migrate over the surface of the wound.

erythema general reddening of the skin due to dilation of the superficial capillaries.

erythrocyte red blood cell.

erythropoiesis the process of producing red blood cells.

erythropoietin a hormone produced by kidney cells that stimulates maturation of red blood cells in the bone marrow.

eschar hard, leathery product of a deep full thickness burn; it consists of dead and denatured skin.

Esophageal Tracheal CombiTube dual-lumen airway with a ventilation port for each lumen.

esophageal varicies enlarged and tortuous esophageal veins.

essential equipment equipment/supplies required on every ambulance.

estimated date of confinement (EDC) the approximate day the infant will be born. This date is usually set at 40 weeks after the date of the mother's last menstrual period (LMP).

ethics the rules or standards that govern the conduct of members of a particular group or profession.

ethnocentrism viewing one's own life as the most desirable, acceptable, or best, and acting in a superior manner to another culture's way of life.

ETT endotracheal tube.

eustachian tube a tube that connects the ear with the nasal cavity.

evaporation change from liquid to a gaseous state.

evisceration a protrusion of organs from a wound.

excitability ability of cells to respond to an electrical stimulus.

exertional metabolic rate rate at which the body consumes energy during activity. It is faster than the basic metabolic rate.

exocrine gland gland that secretes chemical substances to nearby tissues through a duct; also called a *ducted gland.*

exotoxin a soluble poisonous substance secreted during growth of a bacterium.

expectorant medication intended to increase the productivity of cough.

exposure any occurrence of blood or body fluids coming in contact with non-intact skin, mucous membranes, or parenteral contact (needle stick).

expressed consent verbal, nonverbal, or written communication by a patient that he wishes to receive medical care.

exsanguination the draining of blood to the point at which life cannot be sustained.

extension tubing IV tubing used to extend a macrodrip or microdrip setup.

extension bending motion that increases the angle between articulating elements.

external immune system *see* secretory immune system.

extracellular fluid (ECF) the fluid outside the body cells. Extracellular fluid is comprised of intravascular fluid and interstitial fluid.

extrapyramidal symptoms (EPS) common side effects of antipsychotic medications, include muscle tremors and parkinsonism-like effects.

extrauterine outside the uterus.

extravasation leakage of fluid or medication from the blood vessel that is commonly found with infiltration.

extravascular space the volume contained by all the cells (intracellular space) and the spaces between the cells (interstitial space).

extravascular outside the vein.

extrication use of force to free a patient from entrapment.

extubation removing a tube from a body opening.

facilitated diffusion diffusion of a substance such as glucose through a cell membrane that requires the assistance of a "helper," or carrier protein; *see also* carrier mediated diffusion.

facsimile machine device for electronically transmitting and receiving printed information.

factitious disorder condition in which the patient feigns illness in order to assume the sick role.

fallopian tubes thin tubes that extend laterally from the uterus and conduct eggs from the ovaries into the uterine cavity.

false imprisonment intentional and unjustifiable detention of a person without his consent or other legal authority.

fascia a fibrous membrane that covers, supports, and separates muscles and may also unite the skin with underlying tissue.

fasciculations involuntary contractions or twitchings of muscle fibers.

fasciculus small bundle of muscle fibers.

fatigue fracture break in a bone associated with prolonged or repeated stress.

fatigue condition in which a muscle's ability to respond to stimulation is lost or reduced through overactivity.

fatty change a result of cellular injury and swelling in which lipids (fat vesicles) invade the area of injury; occurs most commonly in the liver.

fear feeling of alarm and discontentment in the expectation of danger.

febrile seizures seizures that occur as a result of a sudden increase in temperature; occur most commonly between ages 6 months and 6 years.

fecal-oral route transmission of organisms picked up from the gastrointestinal tract (e.g., feces) into the mouth.

Federal Communications Commission agency that controls all nongovernmental communications in the United States.

feedback a response to a message.

femur large bone of the proximal lower extremity.

fibrin protein fibers that trap red blood cells; the end product of the coagulation cascade that forms an intertwined "net" that traps blood elements and thickens blood.

fibrinolysis the process through which plasmin dismantles a blood clot.

fibroblasts cells that secrete collagen, a critical factor in wound healing.

fibrosis the formation of fiber-like connective tissue, also called *scar tissue* in an organ.

fibula the small bone of the lower leg.

field diagnosis prehospital evaluation of the patient's condition and its causes.

filtrate the fluid produced in Bowman's capsule by filtration of blood.

filtration movement of water out of the plasma across the capillary membrane into the interstitial space; movement of molecules across a membrane from an area of higher pressure to an area of lower pressure.

FiO₂ concentration of oxygen in inspired air.

first-pass effect the liver's partial or complete inactivation of a drug before it reaches the systemic circulation.

flail chest one or more ribs fractured in two or more places, creating an unattached rib segment. Breathing will cause paradoxical chest wall motion.

flanks the part of the back below the ribs and above the hip bones.

flat affect appearance of being disinterested, often lacking facial expression.

flechettes arrow-shaped projectiles found in some military ordnance.

flexion bending motion that reduces the angle between articulating elements.

fluid shift phase stage of the burn process in which there is a massive shift of fluid from the intravascular to the extravascular space.

focused history and physical exam problem-oriented assessment process based on initial assessment and chief complaint.

food poisoning nonspecific term often applied to gastroenteritis that occurs suddenly and that is caused by the ingestion of food containing preformed toxins.

foreign body airway obstruction (FBAO) blockage or obstruction of the airway by an object that impairs respiration.

Frank-Starling mechanism process by which an increase in cardiac output occurs in proportion to the diastolic stretch of the heart muscle fibers.

free drug availability proportion of a drug available in the body to cause either desired or undesired effects.

French unit of measurement approximately equal to one-third millimeter.

frostbite environmentally induced freezing of body tissues causing destruction of cells.

fugue state condition in which an amnesiac patient physically flees.

full thickness burn burn that damages all layers of the skin; characterized by areas that are white and dry; also called *third-degree burn.*

functional impairment decreased ability to meet daily needs on an independent basis.

fungus plant-like microorganism.

gag reflex mechanism that stimulates retching, or striving to vomit, when the soft palate is touched.

galea aponeurotica connective tissue sheet covering the superior aspect of the cranium.

gamma radiation powerful electromagnetic radiation emitted by radioactive substances with powerful penetrating properties; it is stronger than alpha and beta radiation.

gangrene death of tissue or bone, usually from an insufficient blood supply; deep space infection usually caused by the anaerobic bacterium *Clostridium perfringens.*

gastric lavage removing an ingested poison by repeatedly filling and emptying the stomach with water or saline via a gastric tube; also known as *pumping the stomach.*

gastroenteritis nonacute inflammation of the gastrointestinal mucosa. Generalized disorder involving nausea, vomiting, gastrointestinal cramping or discomfort, and diarrhea. *See also* acute gastroenteritis.

gauge the size of a needle's or tube's diameter.

general adaptation syndrome (GAS) a sequence of stress response stages: stage I, alarm; stage II, resistance or adaptation; stage III, exhaustion.

general impression your initial, intuitive evaluation of your patient.

generalized seizures seizures that begin as an electrical discharge in a small area of the brain but spread to involve the entire cerebral cortex, causing widespread malfunction.

genitourinary system the male organ system that includes reproductive and urinary structures.

geriatric abuse a syndrome in which an elderly person is physically or psychologically injured by another person.

geriatrics the study and treatment of diseases of the aged.

German measles *see* rubella.

gerontology scientific study of the effects of aging and of age-related diseases on humans.

Glasgow Coma Scale scoring system for monitoring the neurological status of patients with head injuries.

glaucoma group of eye diseases that results in increased intraocular pressure on the optic nerve; if left untreated, can lead to blindness.

global aphasia a combination of motor and sensory aphasia.

glomerular filtration rate (GFR) the volume per day at which blood is filtered through capillaries of the glomerulus.

glomerular filtration the removal from blood of water and other elements, which enter the nephron tubule.

glomerulonephritis a form of nephritis, or inflammation of the kidneys; primarily involves the glomeruli, one of the capillary networks that are part of the renal corpuscles in the nephrons.

glomerulus a tuft of capillaries from which blood is filtered into a nephron.

glottic function opening and closing of the glottic space.

glottis lip-like opening between the vocal cords.

glucagon hormone that increases the blood glucose level by stimulating the liver to change stored glycogen to glucose.

glucocorticoids hormones released by the adrenal cortex that increase glucose production and reduce the body's inflammation response.

glucometer tool used to measure blood glucose level.

gluconeogenesis conversion of protein and fat to form glucose.

glucose intolerance the body cells' inability to take up glucose from the bloodstream.

glycogen a polysaccharide; one of the forms in which the body stores glucose.

glycogenolysis the breakdown of glycogen to glucose, primarily by liver cells.

glycolysis the first stage of the process in which the cell breaks apart an energy source, commonly glucose, and releases a small amount of energy.

glycosuria glucose in urine, which occurs when blood glucose levels exceed the kidney's ability to reabsorb glucose.

gold standard ultimate standard of excellence.

Golden Hour the 60 minute period after a severe injury; it is the maximum acceptable time between the injury and initiation of surgery for the seriously injured trauma patient.

gomphosis a joint that connects a tooth to the jaw.

gonorrhea sexually transmitted disease caused by a gram-negative bacterium.

Good Samaritan laws laws that provide immunity to certain people who assist at the scene of a medical emergency.

gout inflammation of joints and connective tissue due to build-up of uric acid crystals.

Gram stain method of differentiating types of bacteria according to their reaction to a chemical stain process.

granulation filling of a wound by the inward growth of healthy tissues from the wound edges.

granulocytes white blood cells charged with the primary purpose of neutralizing foreign bacteria.

granuloma a tumor or growth that forms when foreign bodies that cannot be destroyed by macrophages are surrounded and walled off.

Graves' disease endocrine disorder characterized by excess thyroid hormones resulting in body changes associated with increased metabolism; primary cause of thyrotoxicosis.

gray matter areas in the central nervous system dominated by nerve cell bodies; central portion of the spinal cord.

Gray a unit of absorbed radiation dose equal to 100 rads.

great vessels large arteries and veins located in the mediastinum that enter and exit the heart.

greenstick fracture partial fracture of a child's bone.

Grey-Turner's sign discoloration over the flanks suggesting intra-abdominal bleeding.

growth hormone hormone secreted by the anterior pituitary gland that promotes the uptake of glucose and amino acids in the muscle cells and stimulates protein synthesis.

growth plate the area just below the head of a long bone in which growth in bone length occurs in the epiphyseal plate.

gtts drops (Latin *guttae*, drops [*gutta*, drop]).

guarding protective tensing of the abdominal muscles by a patient suffering abdominal pain; may be a voluntary or involuntary response.

Guillain–Barré syndrome acute viral infection that triggers the production of autoantibodies, which damage the myelin sheath covering the peripheral nerves; causes rapid, progressive loss of motor function, ranging from muscle weakness to full-body paralysis.

gynecology the branch of medicine that deals with the health maintenance and the diseases of women, primarily of the reproductive organs.

hairline fracture small crack in a bone that does not disrupt its total structure.

half-life time required for half of the nuclei of a radioactive substance to lose activity by undergoing radioactive decay. In biology and pharmacology, the time required by the body to metabolize and inactivate half the amount of a substance taken in.

hallucinations sensory perceptions with no basis in reality.

hantavirus family of viruses that are carried by the deer mouse and transmitted by ticks and other arthropods.

haptens molecules that do not trigger an immune response on their own but can become immunogenic when combined with larger molecules.

hate crimes crimes committed against a person solely on the basis of the individual's actual or perceived race, color, national origin, ethnicity, gender, disability, or sexual orientation.

haversian canals small perforations of the long bones through which the blood vessels and nerves travel into the bone itself.

hazardous material (hazmat) any substance that causes adverse health effects upon human exposure.

health-care professionals properly trained and licensed or certified providers of health care.

heart failure clinical syndrome in which the heart's mechanical performance is compromised so that cardiac output cannot meet the body's needs. *See also* congestive heart failure.

heat cramps acute painful spasms of the voluntary muscles following strenuous activity in a hot environment without adequate fluid or salt intake.

heat escape lessening position (HELP) developed by Dr. John Hayward. It is an in-water, head-up tuck or fetal position designed to reduce heat loss by as much as 60%.

heat exhaustion a mild heat illness; an acute reaction to heat exposure.

heat illness increased core body temperature due to inadequate thermolysis.

heatstroke acute, dangerous reaction to heat exposure, characterized by a body temperature usually above 105° F (40.6° C) and central nervous system disturbances. The body usually ceases to perspire.

HEENT head, eyes, ears, nose, and throat.

hematemesis vomiting blood.

hematochezia passage of stools containing red blood.

hematocrit the percentage of the blood consisting of the red blood cells, or erythrocytes.

hematology the study of blood and blood-forming organs.

hematoma collection of blood beneath the skin or trapped within a body compartment.

hematopoiesis the process through which pluripotent stem cells differentiate into various types of blood cells.

hematuria blood in the urine.

hemoconcentration elevated numbers of red and white blood cells.

hemocytoblasts *see* stem cells.

hemodialysis a dialysis procedure relying on vascular access to the blood and on an artificial membrane.

hemoglobin an iron-based compound found in red blood cells that binds with oxygen and transports it to body cells.

hemolysis destruction of red blood cells.

hemophilia a blood disorder in which one of the proteins necessary for blood clotting is missing or defective.

hemopneumothorax condition where air and blood are in the pleural space.

hemoptysis coughing up blood.

hemorrhage an abnormal internal or external discharge of blood.

hemorrhoid small mass of swollen veins in the anus or rectum.

hemostasis the body's natural ability to stop bleeding, the ability to clot blood.

hemothorax accumulation in the pleural cavity of blood or fluid containing blood.

HEPA high-efficiency particulate air.

heparin lock peripheral IV port that does not use a bag of fluid.

hepatic alteration change in a medication's chemical composition that occurs in the liver.

hepatitis inflammation of the liver characterized by diffuse or patchy tissue necrosis.

hepatomegaly enlarged liver.

hernia protrusion of an organ through its protective sheath.

herniation protrusion or projection of an organ or part of an organ through the wall of the cavity that normally contains it.

herpes simplex virus organism that causes infections characterized by fluid-filled vesicles, usually in the oral cavity or on the genitals.

herpes zoster an acute eruption caused by a reactivation of latent varicella virus (chicken pox) in the dorsal root ganglia; also known as *shingles*.

hiatal hernia protrusion of the stomach upward into the mediastinal cavity through the esophageal hiatus of the diaphragm.

high-pressure regulator regulator used to transfer oxygen at high pressures from tank to tank.

hilum the notched part of the kidney where the ureter and other structures join kidney tissue.

histamine substance released during the degranulation of mast cells and basophils that increases blood flow to the injury site due to vasodilation and increased permeability of capillary walls.

HIV human immunodeficiency virus, a virus that breaks down the immune defenses, making the body vulnerable to a variety of infections and disorders. *See also* AIDS.

HLA antigens antigens the body recognizes as self or non-self; present on all body cells except the red blood cells.

hollow-needle catheter stylet that does not have a Teflon tube but is itself inserted into the vein and secured there.

homeostasis the natural tendency of the body to maintain a steady and normal internal environment.

hookworm parasite that attaches to the host's intestinal lining.

hormone chemical substance released by a gland that controls or affects processes in other glands or body systems.

hospice program of palliative care and support services that addresses the physical, social, economic, and spiritual needs of terminally ill patients and their families.

hot zone location at a hazmat incident where the actual hazardous material and highest levels of contamination exist; also called the *red zone* or the *exclusionary zone*.

Huber needle needle that has an opening on the side of the shaft instead of the tip.

human immunodeficiency virus *see* HIV.

humerus the single bone of the proximal upper extremity.

humoral immunity the long-term immunity to an antigen provided by antibodies produced by B lymphocytes.

hydrolysis the breakage of a chemical bond by adding water, or by incorporating a hydroxyl (OH^-) group into one fragment and a hydrogen ion (H^+) into the other.

hydrostatic pressure blood pressure or force against vessel walls created by the heart beat. Hydrostatic pressure tends to force water out of the capillaries into the interstitial space.

Hymenoptera any of an order of highly specialized insects such as bees and wasps.

hyperbaric oxygen chamber recompression chamber used to treat patients suffering from barotrauma.

hyperbilirubinemia an excessive amount of bilirubin—the orange-colored pigment associated with bile—in the blood. In newborns, the condition appears as jaundice. Precipitating factors include maternal Rh or ABO incompatibility, neonatal septis, anoxia, hypoglycemia, and congenital liver or gastrointestinal defects.

hypercarbia excessive pressure of carbon dioxide in the blood.

hyperglycemia excessive blood glucose.

hyperglycemic hyperosmolar nonketotic (HHNK) coma complication of type II diabetes due to inadequate insulin activity. Marked by high blood glucose, marked dehydration, and decreased mental function.

hypermetabolic phase stage of the burn process in which there is increased body metabolism in an attempt by the body to heal the burn.

hyperosmolar a solution that has a concentration of the substance greater than that of a second solution.

hyperplasia an increase in number of cells resulting from an increased workload.

hypersensitivity an exaggerated and harmful immune response; an umbrella term for allergy, autoimmunity, and isoimmunity. *Syn.* allergy.

hypertension blood pressure higher than normal.

hypertensive emergency an acute elevation of blood pressure that requires the blood pressure to be lowered within one hour; characterized by end-organ changes such as hypertensive encephalopathy, renal failure, or blindness.

hypertensive encephalopathy a cerebral disorder of hypertension indicated by severe headache, nausea, vomiting, and altered mental status. Neurological symptoms may include blindness, muscle twitches, inability to speak, weakness, and paralysis.

hyperthermia unusually high core body temperature.

hyperthyroidism excessive secretion of thyroid hormones resulting in an increased metabolic rate.

hypertonic state in which a solution has a higher solute concentration on one side of a semi-permeable membrane than on the other side; one solution may be hypertonic to another.

hypertrophy an increase in cell size or organ size resulting from an increased workload.

hyphema blood in the anterior chamber of the eye, in front of the iris.

hypnosis instigation of sleep.

hypochondriasis an abnormal concern with one's health, with the false belief of suffering from some disease, despite medical assurances to the contrary; commonly known as *hypochondria*.

hypodermic needle hollow metal tube used with syringe to administer medications.

hypoglycemia deficiency of blood glucose. Sometimes called *insulin shock*.

hypoglycemic seizure seizure that occurs when brain cells aren't functioning normally due to low blood glucose.

hypo-osmolar a solution that has a concentration of the substance lower than that of a second solution.

hypoperfusion inadequate perfusion of the body tissues, resulting in an inadequate supply of oxygen and nutrients to the body tissues, also called *shock*.

hypotension lower than normal systolic and diastolic blood pressure.

hypothalamus portion of the brain important for controlling certain metabolic activities, including regulation of body temperature.

hypothermia decrease in body's core temperature.

hypothyroidism inadequate secretion of thyroid hormones resulting in a decreased metabolic rate.

hypotonic state in which a solution has a lower solute concentration on one side of a semi-permeable membrane than on the other side; one solution may be hypotonic to another.

hypoventilation reduction in breathing rate and depth.

hypovolemia reduced volume in the cardiovascular system.

hypovolemic shock shock caused by a loss of intravascular fluid volume.

hypoxemia decreased partial pressure of oxygen in the blood.

hypoxia state in which insufficient oxygen is available to meet the oxygen requirements of the cells.

hypoxic drive mechanism that increases respiratory stimulation when P_aO_2 falls and inhibits respiratory stimulation when P_aO_2 climbs.

iliac crest lateral bony ridge that is a landmark of the pelvis.

ilium large, flat innominate bone.

immediate hypersensitivity reaction a hypersensitivity reaction that occurs swiftly following reexposure to an antigen. Immediate hypersensitivity reactions are usually more severe than delayed reactions. The swiftest and most severe of such reactions is anaphylaxis.

immune complex *see* antigen-antibody complex.

immune response the body's reactions that inactivate or eliminate foreign antigens.

immune senescence diminished vigor of the immune response to the challenge and rechallenge by pathogens.

immune system the body system responsible for combating infection.

immunity (1) exemption from legal liability. (2) a long-term condition of protection from infection or disease; the body's ability to respond to the presence of a pathogen.

immunogens antigens that are able to trigger an immune response.

immunoglobulins antibodies; proteins, produced in response to foreign antigens, that destroy or control the antigens.

impacted fracture break in a bone in which the bone is compressed on itself.

impaled object foreign body embedded in a wound.

impetigo infection of the skin caused by staphylococci or streptococci.

implied consent consent for treatment that is presumed for a patient who is mentally, physically, or emotionally unable to grant consent. Also called *emergency doctrine*.

impulse control disorder condition characterized by the patient's failure to control recurrent impulses.

impulsive acting instinctively without stopping to think.

incendiary an agent that combusts easily or creates combustion.

Incident Management System (IMS) national system used for the management of multiple-casualty incidents, involving assumption of responsibility for command and designation and coordination of such elements as triage, treatment, transport, and staging; sometimes called the *Incident Command System*.

incision very smooth or surgical laceration, frequently caused by a knife, scalpel, razor blade, or piece of glass.

incontinence inability to retain urine or feces because of loss of sphincter control or cerebral or spinal lesions.

incubation period the time between contact with a disease organism and the appearance of the first symptoms.

index case the individual who first introduced an infectious agent to a population.

index of suspicion the anticipation of injury to a body region, organ, or structure based on analysis of the mechanism of injury.

induced active immunity immunity achieved through vaccination given to generate an immune response that results in the development of antibodies specific for the injected antigen; also called *artificially acquired immunity*.

inertia tendency of an object to remain at rest or remain in motion unless acted upon by an external force.

infarction area of dead tissue caused by lack of blood.

infection presence of an agent within the host, without necessarily causing disease.

infectious disease any disease caused by the growth of pathogenic microorganisms, which may be spread from person to person.

infestation presence of parasites that do not break the host's skin.

inflammation the body's response to cellular injury; also called the *inflammatory response*. In contrast to the immune response, inflammation develops swiftly, is nonspecific (attacks all unwanted substances in the same way), and is temporary, leading to healing.

inflammatory process a nonspecific defense mechanism that wards off damage from microorganisms or trauma.

inflammatory response *see* inflammation.

influenza disease caused by a group of viruses.

informed consent consent for treatment that is given based on full disclosure of information.

infusion controller gravity-flow device that regulates fluid's passage through an electromechanical pump.

infusion pump device that delivers fluids and medications under positive pressure.

infusion rate speed at which a medication is delivered intravenously.

infusion liquid medication delivered through a vein.

ingestion entry of a substance into the body through the gastrointestinal tract.

inhalation entry of a substance into the body through the respiratory tract; drawing of medication into the lungs along with air during breathing.

initial assessment prehospital process designed to identify and correct life-threatening airway, breathing, and circulation problems.

injection entry of a substance into the body through a break in the skin; placement of medication in or under the skin with a needle and synringe.

injury current *see* current of injury.

injury risk a real or potentially hazardous situation that puts people in danger of sustaining injury.

injury intentional or unintentional damage to a person resulting from acute exposure to thermal, mechanical, electrical, or chemical energy or from the absence of such essentials as heat and oxygen.

injury-surveillance program the ongoing systematic collection, analysis, and interpretation of injury data essential to the planning, implementation, and evaluation of public health practice.

innominate one of the structures of the pelvis.

inotropy pertaining to cardiac contractile force.

insertion attachment of a muscle to a bone that moves when the muscle contracts.

inspection the process of informed observation.

institutional elder abuse physical or emotional violence or neglect when an elder is being cared for by a person paid to provide care.

insufflate to blow into.

insulin pancreatic hormone needed to transport simple sugars from the interstitial spaces into the cells; substance that decreases blood glucose level.

integumentary system skin, consisting of the epidermis, dermis, and subcutaneous layers.

intercalated discs specialized bands of tissue inserted between myocardial cells that increase the rate in which the action potential is spread from cell to cell.

intermittent claudication intermittent calf pain while walking that subsides with rest.

intermittent mandatory ventillation (IMV) respirator setting where a patient-triggered breath does not result in assistance by the machine.

interpolated beat a premature ventricular contraction (PVC) that falls between two sinus beats without effectively interrupting this rhythm.

interstitial fluid the fluid in body tissues that is outside the cells and outside the vascular system.

interstitial nephritis an inflammation within the tissue surrounding the nephrons.

interstitial space space between cells.

intervener physician a licensed physician, professionally unrelated to patients on scene, who attempts to assist EMS providers with patient care.

intervertebral disk cartilaginous pad between vertebrae that serves as a shock absorber.

intracatheter *see* catheter inserted through the needle.

intracellular fluid (ICF) the fluid inside the body cells.

intracerebral hemorrhage bleeding directly into the tissue of the brain.

intracranial pressure (ICP) pressure exerted on the brain by the blood and cerebrospinal fluid.

intractable resistant to cure, relief, or control.

intradermal within the dermal layer of the skin.

intramuscular within the muscle.

intraosseous within the bone.

intrapartum occurring during childbirth.

intrarenal abscess a pocket of infection within kidney tissue.

intravascular fluid the fluid within the circulatory system; blood plasma.

intravascular space the volume contained by all the arteries, veins, capillaries, and other components of the circulatory system.

intravenous access surgical puncture of a vein to deliver medication or withdraw blood; also called *cannulation*.

intravenous fluid chemically prepared solution tailored to the body's specific needs.

intubation passing a tube into a body opening.

intussusception condition that occurs when part of an intestine slips into the part just distal to itself.

involuntary consent consent to treatment granted by the authority of a court order.

ion a charged particle; an atom or group of atoms whose electrical charge has changed from neutral to positive or negative by losing or gaining one or more electrons.

ionization the process of changing a substance into separate charged particles (ions).

ionize to become electrically charged or polar.

ionizing radiation electromagnetic radiation (e.g., x-ray) or particulate radiation (e.g., alpha particles, beta particles, and neutrons) that, by direct or secondary processes, ionizes materials that absorb the radiation. Ionizing radiation can penetrate the cells of living organisms, depositing an electrical charge within them. When sufficiently intense, this form of energy kills cells.

iris pigmented portion of the eye; the muscular area that constricts or dilates to change the size of the pupil.

irreversible antagonism a competitive antagonist permanently binds with a receptor site.

irreversible shock shock that has progressed so far that no medical intervention can reverse the condition and death is inevitable.

ischemia a blockage in the delivery of oxygenated blood to the cells.

ischial tuberosity one of the bony knobs of the posterior hip.

ischium irregular innominate bone.

isoimmunity an immune response to antigens from another member of the same species, for example Rh reactions between a mother and infant or transplant rejections; also called *alloimmunity*.

isolette also known as an *incubator*; a clear plastic enclosed bassinet used to keep prematurely born infants warm.

isometric exercise active exercise performed against stable resistance, where muscles are exercised in a motionless manner.

isosthenuria the inability to concentrate or dilute urine relative to the osmolarity of blood.

isotonic exercise active exercise during which muscles are worked through their range of motion.

isotonic state in which solutions on opposite sides of a semi-permeable membrane are in equal concentration; solutions may be isotonic to each other.

J wave ECG deflection found at the junction of the QRS complex and the ST segment. It is associated with hypothermia and seen at core temperatures below 32° C, most commonly in leads II and V_6; also called an *Osborn wave*.

Jackson's theory of thermal wounds explanation of the physical effects of thermal burns.

jargon language used by a particular group or profession.

joint capsule the ligaments that surround a joint; *synovial capsule*.

joint area where adjacent bones articulate.

Joule's law principle identifying that the rate of production of heat by a constant direct current is directly proportional to the resistance of the circuit and the square of the current.

justice the obligation to treat all patients fairly.

keloid a formation resulting from overproduction of scar tissue.

Kernig's sign inability to fully extend the knee with hips flexed.

ketone bodies compounds produced during the catabolism of fatty acids, including acetoacetic acid, b-hydroxybutyric acid, and acetone.

ketosis the presence of significant quantities of ketone bodies in the blood.

kidney transplantation implantation of a kidney into a person without functioning kidneys.

kidney an organ that produces urine and performs other functions related to the urinary system.

kinetic energy the energy an object has while it is in motion. It is related to the object's mass and velocity.

kinetics the branch of physics that deals with motion, taking into consideration mass and force.

Korotkoff sounds sounds of blood hitting arterial walls.

Korsakoff's psychosis psychosis characterized by disorientation, muttering delirium, insomnia, delusions, and hallucinations. Symptoms include painful extremities, bilateral wrist drop (rarely), bilateral foot drop (frequently), and pain on pressure over the long nerves.

Kreb's cycle process of aerobic metabolism that uses carbohydrates, proteins, and fats to release energy for the body; also known as the *citric acid cycle.*

Kussmaul's respiration rapid, deep respirations caused by severe metabolic and CNS problems.

kyphosis exaggeration of the normal posterior curvature of the spine.

labia structures that protect the vagina and urethra, including the *labia majora* and the *labia minora.*

labor the time and processes that occur during childbirth; the physiologic and mechanical process in which the baby, placenta, and amniotic sac are expelled through the birth canal.

labrynthitis inner ear infection that causes vertigo, nausea, and an unsteady gait.

laceration an open wound, normally a tear with jagged borders.

lacrimal fluid liquid that lubricates the eye.

lactic acid compound produced from pyruvic acid during anerobic glycolysis.

laminae posterior bones of a vertebra that help make up the foramen, or opening, of the spinal canal.

laryngoscope instrument for lifting the tongue and epiglottis in order to see the vocal cords.

larynx the complex structure that joins the pharynx with the trachea.

latent period time when a host cannot transmit an infectious agent to someone else.

laxative medication used to decrease stool's firmness and increase its water content.

Le Fort criteria classification system for fractures involving the maxilla.

leading questions questions framed to guide the direction of a patient's answers.

legislative law law created by law-making bodies such as Congress and state assemblies. Also called *statutory law.*

lesion any disruption in normal tissue.

leukemia a cancer of the hematopoietic cells.

leukocyte white blood cell.

leukocytosis too many white blood cells.

leukopenia too few white blood cells.

leukopoiesis the process through which stem cells differentiate into the white blood cells' immature forms.

leukotrienes also called *slow-reacting substances of anaphylaxis (SRS-A);* substances synthesized by mast cells during inflammatory response that cause vasoconstriction, vascular permeability, and chemotaxis; mediators released from mast cells upon contact with allergens.

leur lock adapter with a rubber-covered needle used to puncture a blood tube's self-healing top.

leur-sampling needle long, exposed needle that screws into the vacutainer and is inserted directly into the vein.

liability legal responsibility.

libel the act of injuring a person's character, name, or reputation by false statements made in writing or through the mass media with malicious intent or reckless disregard for the falsity of those statements.

lice parasitic infestation of the skin of the scalp, trunk, or pubic area.

licensure the process by which a governmental agency grants permission to engage in a given occupation to an applicant who has attained the degree of competency required to ensure the public's protection.

life expectancy based on the year of birth, the average number of additional years of life expected for a member of a population.

life-care community communities that provide apartments/homes for independent living and a range of services, including nursing care.

ligament of Treitz ligament that supports the duodenojejunal junction.

ligament connective tissue that connects bone to bone and holds joints together.

ligamentum arteriosum cord-like remnant of a fetal vessel connecting the pulmonary artery to the aorta at the aortic isthmus.

liquefaction necrosis the process in which an alkali dissolves and liquefies tissue.

living will a legal document that allows a person to specify the kinds of medical treatment he wishes to receive should the need arise.

local effects effects involving areas around the immediate site; should be evaluated based upon the burn model.

local limited to one area of the body.

lock-out/tag-out locking off of a machinery switch, then placing a tag on the switch stating why it is shut off; method of preventing equipment from being accidentally restarted.

lower gastrointestinal bleeding bleeding in the gastrointestinal tract distal to the ligament of Treitz.

lumen opening, or space, within a needle, artery, vein, or other hollow vessel.

Lyme disease recurrent inflammatory disorder caused by a tick-borne spirochete.

lymph overflow circulatory fluid in spaces between tissues.

lymphangitis inflammation of the lymph channels, usually as a result of a distal infection.

lymphatic system secondary circulatory system that collects overflow fluid from the tissue spaces and filters it before returning it to the circulatory system.

lymphocyte a type of leukocyte, or white blood cell, that attacks foreign substances as part of the body's immune response.

lymphokine a cytokine released by a lymphocyte.

lymphoma a cancer of the lymphatic system.

maceration process of softening a solid by soaking in a liquid.

macrodrip tubing administration tubing that delivers a relatively large amount of fluid.

macrophage immune system cell that has the ability to recognize and ingest foreign antibodies.

Magill forceps scissor-style clamps with circular tips.

major basic protein (MBP) a larvacidal peptide.

major histocompatibility complex (MHC) a group of genes on chromosome 6 that provide the genetic code for HLA antigens.

major trauma patient person who has suffered significant mechanism of injury.

malfeasance a breach of duty by performance of a wrongful or unlawful act.

malleolus the protuberance of the ankle.

Mallory-Weiss tear esophageal laceration, usually secondary to vomiting.

mammalian diving reflex a complex cardiovascular reflex, resulting from submersion of the face and nose in water, that constricts blood flow everywhere except to the brain.

mandible the jawbone.

manic characterized by excessive excitement or activity (mania).

manometer pressure gauge with a scale calibrated in millimeters of mercury (mmHg).

Marfan's Syndrome hereditary condition of connective tissue, bones, muscles, ligaments, and skeletal structures characterized by irregular and unsteady gait, tall lean body type with long extremities, flat feet, stooped shoulders. The aorta is usually dilated and may become weakened enough to allow an aneurysm to develop.

mask a device for protecting the face. *See also* respirator.

mass a measure of the matter that an object contains; the property of a physical body that gives the body inertia.

mast cell specialized cell of the immune system which contains chemicals that assist in the immune response.

material safety data sheets (MSDS) easily accessible sheets of detailed information about chemicals found at fixed facilities.

maturation continuing processes of wound reconstruction that may occur over a period of years after initial healing, as scar tissue is remodeled and strengthened.

maxilla bone of the upper jaw.

maximum life span the theoretical, species-specific, longest duration of life, excluding premature or "unnatural" death.

McBurney's point common site of pain from appendicitis, one to two inches above the anterior iliac crest in a direct line with the umbilicus.

measles highly contagious, acute viral disease characterized by a reddish rash that appears on the fourth or fifth day of illness.

measured volume administration set IV setup that delivers specific volumes of fluid.

mechanism of injury the processes and forces that cause trauma.

meconium dark green material found in the intestine of the full-term newborn. It can be expelled from the intestine into the amniotic fluid during periods of fetal distress.

medical direction medical policies, procedures, and practices that are available to providers either on-line or off-line.

medical director a physician who is legally responsible for all of the clinical and patient-care aspects of an EMS system. Also referred to as *medical direction*.

medically clean careful handling to prevent contamination.

medicated solution parenteral medication packaged in an IV bag and administered as an IV infusion.

medication injection port in an intravenous administration set, a self-healing membrane into which a hypodermic needle is inserted for drug administration.

medications foreign substances placed into the human body. *See also* drug.

medulla oblongata lower portion of the brainstem, connecting the pons and the spinal cord. It contains major centers for control of respiratory, cardiac, and vasomotor activity.

medulla the inner tissue of an organ such as the kidney.

medullary canal cavity within a bone that contains the marrow.

melena dark, tarry, foul smelling stool resulting from gastrointestinal bleeding.

memory cells cells produced by mature B lymphocytes that "remember" the activating antigen and will trigger a stronger and swifter immune response if reexposure to the antigen occurs.

menarche the onset of menses, usually occurring between ages 10 and 14.

Meniere's disease a disease of the inner ear characterized by vertigo, nerve deafness, and a roar or buzzing in the ear.

meninges three membranes that surround and protect the brain and spinal cord: the dura mater, pia mater, and arachnoid membrane.

meningitis inflammation of the meninges, usually caused by an infection.

meningomyelocele hernia of the spinal cord and membranes through a defect in the spinal column.

menopause the cessation of menses and ovarian function due to decreased secretion of estrogen.

menorrhagia excessive menstrual flow.

menstruation sloughing of the uterine lining (endometrium) if a fertilized egg is not implanted. It is controlled by the cyclical release of hormones. Menstruation is also called a *period*.

mental status examination (MSE) a structured exam designed to quickly evaluate a patient's level of mental functioning.

mental status the state of the patient's cerebral functioning.

mesencephalon portion of the brain connecting the pons and cerebellum with the cerebral hemispheres; also called the *midbrain*. It controls motor coordination and eye movement.

mesenteric infarct death of tissue in the peritoneal fold (mesentery) that encircles the small intestine; a life-threatening condition.

mesentery double fold of peritoneum that supports the major portion of the small bowel, suspending it from the posterior abdominal wall.

metabolic acidosis acidity caused by an increase in acid, often because of increased production of acids during metabolism or from causes such as vomiting, diarrhea, diabetes, or medication.

metabolic alkalosis alkalinity caused by an increase in plasma bicarbonate resulting from causes including diuresis, vomiting, or ingestion of too much sodium bicarbonate.

metabolism the total changes that take place in an organism during physiological processes; the sum of cellular processes that produce the energy and molecules needed for growth and repair.

metacarpals bones of the palm.

metaphysis growth zone of a bone, active during the development stages of youth. It is located between the epiphysis and the diaphysis.

metaplasia replacement of one type of cell by another type of cell that is not normal for that tissue.

metatarsal one of the bones forming the arch of the foot.

metered dose inhaler handheld device that produces a medicated spray for inhalation.

microangiopathy a disease affecting the smallest blood vessels.

microcirculation blood flow in the arterioles, capillaries, and venules.

microdrip tubing administration tubing that delivers a relatively small amount of fluid.

midbrain portion of the brain connecting the pons and cerebellum with the cerebral hemispheres.

minimum effective concentration minimum level of drug needed to cause a given effect.

minimum standards lowest or least allowable standards.

minor depending on state law, this is usually a person under the age of 18.

minute volume amount of gas inhaled and exhaled in one minute.

miscarriage commonly used term to describe a pregnancy which ends before 20 weeks gestation; may also be called spontaneous abortion.

misfeasance a breach of duty by performance of a legal act in a manner that is harmful or injurious.

mitosis cell division with division of the nucleus; each daughter cell contains the same number of chromosomes as the mother cell.

mittelschmerz abdominal pain associated with ovulation.

Mix-o-Vial *see* nonconstituted drug vial.

mobile data terminal vehicle-mounted computer keyboard and display.

modeling a procedure whereby a subject observes a model perform some behavior and then attempts to imitate that behavior.

monoclonal antibody an antibody that is very pure and specific to a single antigen.

monokine a cytokine released by a macrophage.

mononucleosis acute disease caused by the Epstein-Barr virus.

mons pubis fatty layer of tissue over the pubic symphysis.

mood disorder pervasive and sustained emotion that colors a person's perception of the world.

morals social, religious, or personal standards of right and wrong.

morgue area where deceased victims of an incident are collected.

Moro reflex occurring when a newborn is startled, arms are thrown wide, fingers spread, and a grabbing motion follows. Also called *startle reflex*.

motion the process of changing place; movement.

motor aphasia occurs when the patient cannot speak but can understand what is said.

mucolytic medication intended to make mucus more watery.

mucosal immune system *see* secretory immune system.

mucous membrane lining in body cavities that handle air transport; usually contains small, mucus-secreting cells.

mucus slippery secretion that lubricates and protects airway surfaces.

multiple casualty incident (MCI) incident that generates large numbers of patients and that often makes traditional EMS response ineffective because of special circumstances surrounding the event; also known as a *mass casualty incident.*

multiple myeloma a cancerous disorder of plasma cells.

multiple organ dysfunction syndrome (MODS) progressive impairment of two or more organ systems resulting from an uncontrolled inflammatory response to a severe illness or injury.

multiple personality disorder manifestation of two or more complete systems of personality.

multiple sclerosis disease that involves inflammation of certain nerve cells followed by demyelination, or the destruction of the myelin sheath, which is the fatty insulation surrounding nerve fibers.

multiplex duplex system that can transmit voice and data simultaneously.

mumps acute viral disease characterized by painful enlargement of the salivary glands.

Murphy's sign pain caused when an inflamed gallbladder is palpated by pressing under the right costal margin.

muscle tissue tissue that is capable of contraction when stimulated. There are three types of muscle tissue: *cardiac* (myocardium, or heart muscle), *smooth* (within intestines, surrounding blood vessels), and *skeletal*, or *striated* (allows skeletal movement). Skeletal muscle is mostly under voluntary, or conscious, control; smooth muscle is under involuntary, or unconscious, control; cardiac muscle is capable of spontaneous, or self-excited, contraction.

muscoviscidosis cystic fibrosis of the pancreas resulting in abnormally viscous mucoid secretion from the pancreas.

muscular dystrophy a group of genetic diseases characterized by progressive muscle weakness and degeneration of the skeletal or voluntary muscle fibers.

mutual aid agreements or plans for sharing departmental resources.

myesthania gravis disease characterized by episodic muscle weakness triggered by an autoimmune attack of the acetylcholine receptors.

myocardial infarction (MI) death and subsequent necrosis of the heart muscle caused by inadequate blood supply; also *acute myocardial infarction (AMI)*.

myocardium the cardiac muscle tissue of the heart.

myoclonus temporary, involuntary twitching or spasm of a muscle or group of muscles.

myometrium the thick middle layer of the uterine wall made up of smooth muscle fibers.

myotome muscle and tissue of the body innervated by spinal nerve roots.

myxedema coma life-threatening condition associated with advanced myxedema, with profound hypothermia, bradycardia, and electrolyte imbalance.

myxedema condition that reflects long-term exposure to inadequate levels of thyroid hormones with resultant changes in body structure and function.

nares the openings of the nostrils.

nasal cannula catheter placed at the nares.

nasal flaring excessive widening of the nares with respiration.

nasal medication drug administered through the mucous membranes of the nose.

nasal septum cartilage that separates the right and left nasal cavities.

nasogastric tube/orogastric tube a tube that runs through the nose or mouth and esophagus into the stomach; used for administering liquid nutrients or medications or for removing air or liquids from the stomach.

nasolacrimal duct narrow tube that carries into the nasal cavity tears and debris that have drained from the eye.

nasopharyngeal airway uncuffed tube that follows the natural curvature of the nasopharynx, passing through the nose and extending from the nostril to the posterior pharynx.

nasotracheal route through the nose and into the trachea.

natural immunity inborn protection against infection or disease that is part of the person's or species' genetic makeup; genetically predetermined immunity that is present at birth; also called *innate immunity*.

naturally acquired immunity immunity that begins to develop after birth and is continually enhanced by exposure to new pathogens and antigens throughout life.

nature of illness a patient's general medical condition or complaint.

near-drowning an incident of potentially fatal submersion in liquid which did not result in death or in which death occurred more than 24 hours after submersion.

nebulizer inhalation aid that disperses liquid into aerosol spray or mist.

necrosis cell death; a pathological cell change; the sloughing off of dead tissue. Four types of necrotic cell change are *coagulative, liquefactive, caseous,* and *fatty. Gangrenous necrosis* refers to tissue death over a wide area.

needle adapter rigid plastic device specifically constructed to fit into the hub of an intravenous cannula.

needle cricothyrotomy surgical airway technique that inserts a 14-gauge needle into the trachea at the cricothyroid membrane.

negative feedback a mechanism of response that serves to maintain a state of internal constancy, or homeostasis. Changes in the internal environment trigger mechanisms that reverse or negate the change, hence the term "negative feedback."

negligence deviation from accepted standards of care recognized by law for the protection of others against the unreasonable risk of harm.

neonatal abstinence syndrome (NAS) a generalized disorder presenting a clinical picture of CNS hyperirritability, gastrointestinal dysfunction, respiratory distress, and vague autonomic symptoms. It may be due to intrauterine exposure to heroin, methadone, or other less potent opiates. Non-opiate central nervous system depressants may also cause NAS.

neonate an infant from the time of birth to one month of age.

neoplasm literally meaning "new form"; a new or abnormal formation; a tumor.

neovascularization new growth of capillaries in response to healing.

nephrology the medical specialty dealing with the kidneys.

nephron a microscopic structure within kidney that produces urine.

nerve tissue tissue that transmits electrical impulses throughout the body.

net filtration the total loss of water from blood plasma across the capillary membrane into the interstitial space. Normally, hydrostatic pressure forcing water out of the capillary is balanced by oncotic force pulling water into the capillary for a net filtration of zero.

neuroeffector junction specialized synapse between a nerve cell and the organ or tissue it innervates.

neurogenic shock shock resulting from brain or spinal cord injury that causes an interruption of nerve impulses to the arteries with loss of arterial tone, dilation, and relative hypovolemia.

neuroleptanesthesia anesthesia that combines decreased sensation of pain with amnesia while the patient remains conscious.

neuroleptic antipsychotic (literally, *affecting the nerves*).

neuron nerve cell.

neurotransmitter chemical messenger that conducts a nervous impulse across a synapse. Examples include acetylcholine, norepinephrine, and dopamine.

neutron radiation powerful radiation with penetrating properties between that of beta and gamma radiation.

neutropenia a reduction in the number of neutrophils; a low neutrophil count.

neutrophil the most common phagocytic white blood cell.

newborn a baby in the first few hours of its life, also called a *newly born infant*.

nitrogen narcosis a state of stupor that develops during deep dives due to nitrogen's effect on cerebral function; also called *raptures of the deep*.

nocturia excessive urination during the night.

noncardiogenic shock types of shock that result from causes other than inadequate cardiac output.

noncompensatory pause pause following an ectopic beat where the SA node is depolarized and the underlying cadence of the heart is interrupted.

noncompetitive antagonism the binding of an antagonist causes a deformity of the binding site that prevents an agonist from fitting and binding.

nonconstituted drug vial/Mix-o-Vial vial with two containers, one holding a powdered medication and the other holding a liquid mixing solution.

nonfeasance a breach of duty by failure to perform a required act or duty.

nonmaleficence the obligation not to harm the patient.

nonverbal communication gestures, mannerisms, and postures by which a person communicates with others; also called *body language*.

normal flora organisms that live inside our bodies without ordinarily causing disease.

normal sinus rhythm the normal heart rhythm.

nosocomial acquired while in the hospital.

nucleus the organelle within a cell that contains the DNA, or genetic material; in the cells of higher organisms, the nucleus is surrounded by a membrane.

obligate intracellular parasite organism that can grow and reproduce only within a host cell.

oblique fracture break in a bone running across it at an angle other than 90 degrees.

oblique having a slanted position or direction.

obstetrics the branch of medicine that deals with the care of women throughout pregnancy.

obstructive shock shock resulting from interference with the blood flowing through the cardiovascular system.

ocular medication drug administered through the mucous membranes of the eye.

off-line medical direction refers to medical policies, procedures, and practices that medical direction has set up in advance of a call.

ohm basic unit for measuring the strength of electrical resistance.

Ohm's law the physical law identifying that the current in amperes in an electrical circuit is directly proportional to the voltage and inversely proportional to the resistance.

old-old an elderly person age 80 or older.

oliguria decreased urine elimination to 400-500 ml or less per day.

omphalocele congenital hernia of the umbilicus.

oncotic force a form of osmotic pressure exerted by the large protein particles, or colloids, present in blood plasma. In the capillaries, the plasma colloids tend to pull water from the interstitial space across the capillary membrane into the capillary. Oncotic force is also called *colloid osmotic pressure*.

on-line medical direction occurs when a qualified physician gives direct orders to a prehospital care provider by either radio or telephone.

onset of action the time from administration until a medication reaches its minimum effective concentration.

open cricothyrotomy surgical airway technique that places an endotracheal or tracheostomy tube directly into the trachea through a surgical incision at the cricothyroid membrane.

open fracture a broken bone in which the bone ends or the forces that caused it penetrate the surrounding skin.

open incident an incident that has the potential to generate additional patients; also known as an *uncontained incident* or an *unstable incident*.

open pneumothorax *see* pneumothorax.

open stance a posture or body position that is relaxed and suggests confidence, ease, warmth, and attentiveness.

open-ended questions questions that permit unguided, spontaneous answers.

ophthalmoscope handheld device used to examine interior of eye.

opportunistic pathogen ordinarily nonharmful bacterium that causes disease only under unusual circumstances.

opposition pairing of muscles that permits extension and flexion of limbs.

oral drug administration the delivery of any medication that is taken by mouth and swallowed into the lower gastrointestinal tract.

orbit the eye socket.

ordnance military weapons and munitions.

organ system a group of organs that work together. Examples: the cardiovascular system, formed of the heart, blood vessels, and blood; the gastrointestinal system, comprising the mouth, salivary glands, esophagus, stomach, intestines, liver, pancreas, gall bladder, rectum, and anus.

organ a group of tissues functioning together. Examples: heart, liver, brain, ovary, eye.

organelles structures that perform specific functions within a cell.

organic *see* biological.

organism the sum of all the cells, tissues, organs, and organ systems of a living being. Examples: the human organism, a bacterial organism.

organophosphates phosphorus-containing organic pesticides.

origin attachment of a muscle to a bone that does not move (or experiences the least movement) when the muscle contracts.

orogastric tube *see* nasogastric tube/orogastric tube.

oropharyngeal airway semicircular device that follows the palate's curvature.

orthopnea difficulty in breathing while lying supine.

orthostatic hypotension a decrease in blood pressure that occurs when a person moves from a supine or sitting to an upright position.

osmolality the concentration of solute per kilogram of water. *See also* osmolarity.

osmolarity the concentration of solute per liter of water (often used synonymously with *osmolality*).

osmosis the passage of a solvent such as water through a membrane; movement of solvent in a solution from an area of lower solute concentration to an area of higher solute concentration.

osmotic diuresis greatly increased urination and dehydration due to high levels of glucose that cannot be reabsorbed into the blood from the kidney tubules, causing a loss of water into the urine.

osmotic gradient the difference in concentration between solutions on opposite sides of a semipermeable membrane.

osmotic pressure the pressure exerted by the concentration of solutes on one side of a membrane that, if hypertonic, tends to "pull" water (cause osmosis) from the other side of the membrane.

osteoarthritis a degenerative joint disease, characterized by a loss of articular cartilage and hypertrophy of bone.

osteoblast cell that helps in the creation of new bone during growth and bone repair.

osteoclast bone cell that absorbs and removes excess bone.

osteocyte bone-forming cell found in the bone matrix that helps maintain the bone.

osteoporosis weakening of bone tissue due to loss of essential minerals, especially calcium.

otitis media middle ear infection.

otoscope handheld device used to examine interior of ears and nose.

ovaries the primary female sex glands, which secrete estrogen and progesterone and produce eggs for reproduction.

overdrive respiration positive pressure ventilation supplied to a breathing patient.

overhydration the presence or retention of an abnormally high amount of body fluid.

overpressure a rapid increase then decrease in atmospheric pressure created by an explosion.

over-the-needle catheter semi-flexible catheter enclosing a sharp metal stylet; also called *angiocatheter*.

ovulation the release of an egg from the ovary.

oxidation the loss of hydrogen atoms or the acceptance of an oxygen atom. This increases the positive charge (or lessens the negative charge) on the molecule.

oxidizer an agent that enhances combustion of a fuel.

oxygen gas necessary for energy production.

PA alveolar partial pressure.

Pa arterial partial pressure.

pack/year history a way to quantify your patient's smoking history by multiplying number of packs smoked per day by the number of years smoking.

pallor paleness.

palmar grasp a reflex in the newborn, which is elicited by placing a finger firmly in the infant's palm.

palpation using your sense of touch to gather information.

pancolitis ulcerative colitis spread throughout the entire colon.

panic attack extreme period of anxiety resulting in great emotional distress.

papilla the tip of a pyramid; it juts into the hollow space of the kidney.

paradoxical breathing assymetrical chest wall movement that lessens respiratory efficiency.

parasite organism that lives in or on another organism.

parasympathetic nervous system division of the autonomic nervous system that is responsible for controlling vegetative functions. Parasympathetic nervous system actions include decreased heart rate and constriction of the bronchioles and pupils. Its actions are mediated by the neurotransmitter acetylcholine.

parasympatholytic drug or other substance that blocks or inhibits the actions of the parasympathetic nervous system. Also called *anticholinergic*.

parasympathomimetic drug or other substance that causes effects like those of the parasympathetic nervous system. Also called *cholinergic*.

parenchyma principle or essential parts of an organ.

parent drug *see* prodrug.

parenteral route delivery of a medication outside of the gastrointestinal tract, typically using needles to inject medications into the circulatory system or tissues.

Parkinson's disease chronic and progressive motor system disorder characterized by tremor, rigidity, bradykinesia, and postural instability.

paroxysmal nocturnal dyspnea (PND) a sudden episode of difficult breathing that occurs after lying down; most commonly caused by left heart failure.

partial pressure the pressure exerted by each component of a gas mixture.

partial seizures seizures that remain confined to a limited portion of the brain, causing localized malfunction. Partial seizures may spread and become generalized.

partial thickness burn burn in which the epidermis is burned through and the dermis is damaged; characterized by redness and blistering; also called a *second-degree burn*.

particulate evidence evidence such as hairs or fibers that cannot be readily seen with the human eye; also known as *microscopic evidence* or *trace evidence*.

partner abuse physical or emotional violence from a man or woman towards a domestic partner.

passive transport movement of a substance without the use of energy.

pathogens microorganisms capable of producing infection or disease, such as bacteria and viruses.

pathology the study of disease and its causes.

pathophysiology the study of how diseases alter normal physiology.

patient assessment problem-oriented evaluation of patient and establishment of priorities based on existing and potential threats to human life.

patient interview interaction with a patient for the purpose of obtaining in-depth information about the emergency and the patient's pertinent medical history.

peak load the highest volume of calls at a given time.

pedicles thick, bony struts that connect the vertebral bodies with the spinous and transverse processes and help make up the opening for the spinal canal.

PEEP *see* positive end-expiratory pressure.

peer review an evaluation of the quality of emergency care administered by an individual, which is conducted by that individual's peers (others of equal rank). Also, an evaluation of articles submitted for publication.

pelvic inflammatory disease (PID) an acute infection of the reproductive organs that can be caused by a bacteria, virus, or fungus.

pelvic space division of the abdominal cavity containing those organs located within the pelvis.

pelvis skeletal structure where the lower extremities attach to the body.

penetrating trauma injury caused by an object breaking the skin and entering the body.

penis the male organ of copulation.

peptic ulcer erosion caused by gastric acid.

percussion the production of sound waves by striking one object against another.

perforating canals structures through which blood vessels enter and exit the bone shaft.

perfusion the supplying of oxygen and nutrients to the body tissues as a result of the constant passage of blood through the capillaries.

pericardial tamponade filling of the pericardial sac with fluid, which in turn limits the filling and function of the heart.

pericardium fibrous sac that surrounds the heart.

perimetrium the serosal peritoneal membrane which forms the outermost layer of the uterine wall.

perinephric abscess a pocket of infection in the layer of fat surrounding the kidney.

perineum muscular tissue that separates the vagina and the anus.

periorbital ecchymosis black and blue discoloration surrounding the eye sockets.

periosteum the tough exterior covering of a bone.

peripheral arterial atherosclerotic disease a progressive degenerative disease of the medium-sized and large arteries.

peripheral nervous system part of the nervous system that extends throughout the body and is composed of the cranial nerves arising from the brain and the peripheral nerves arising from the spinal cord. Its subdivisions are the somatic and the autonomic nervous systems.

peripheral neuropathy any malfunction or damage of the peripheral nerves. Results may include muscle weakness, loss of sensation, impaired reflexes, and internal organ malfunctions.

peripheral vascular resistance the resistance of the vessels to the flow of blood: increased when the vessels constrict, decreased when the vessels relax.

peripheral venous access surgical puncture of a vein in the arm, leg, or neck.

peripherally inserted central catheter (PICC) line threaded into the central circulation via a peripheral site.

peristalsis wavelike muscular motion of the esophagus and bowel that moves food through the digestive system.

peritoneal dialysis a dialysis procedure relying on the peritoneal membrane as the semipermeable membrane.

peritoneal space division of the abdominal cavity containing those organs or portions of organs covered by the peritoneum.

peritoneum fine fibrous tissue surrounding the interior of most of the abdominal cavity and covering most of the small bowel and some of the abdominal organs.

peritonitis inflammation of the peritoneum caused by chemical or bacterial irritation.

permissive a parenting style that takes a tolerant, accepting view of a child's behavior.

persistent fetal circulation condition in which blood continues to bypass the fetal respiratory system, resulting in ongoing hypoxia.

personal protective equipment (PPE) equipment used by EMS personnel to protect against injury and the spread of infectious disease.

personal-care home living arrangement that includes room, board, and some supervision.

personality disorder condition that results in persistently maladaptive behavior.

pertussis disease characterized by severe, violent coughing.

pH abbreviation for *potential of hydrogen*. A measure of relative acidity or alkalinity. Since the pH scale is inverse to the concentration of acidic hydrogen ions, the lower the pH the greater the acidity and the higher the pH the greater the alkalinity. A normal pH range is 7.35 to 7.45.

phagocytes cells that have the ability to ingest other cells and substances, such as bacteria and cell debris.

phagocytosis process in which white blood cells engulf and destroy an invader.

phalanges bones of the fingers.

pharmacodynamics how a drug interacts with the body to cause its effects.

pharmacokinetics how a drug is absorbed, distributed, metabolized (biotransformed), and excreted; how drugs are transported into and out of the body.

pharmacology the study of drugs and their interactions with the body.

pharyngitis infection of the pharynx and tonsils.

pharyngo-tracheal lumen airway PtL is a two-tube airway system.

pharynx a muscular tube that extends vertically from the back of the soft palate to the superior aspect of the esophagus.

phobia excessive fear that interferes with functioning.

phototherapy exposure to sunlight or artificial light for therapeutic purposes.

physiological stress a chemical or physical disturbance in the cells or tissue fluid produced by a change in the external environment or within the body.

physiology the functions of an organism; the physical and chemical processes of a living thing.

pia mater inner and most delicate layer of the meninges. It covers the convolutions of the brain and spinal cord.

Pierre Robin syndrome unusually small jaw, combined with a cleft palate, downward displacement of the tongue, and an absent gag reflex.

pill-rolling motion an involuntary tremor, usually in one hand or sometimes in both, in which fingers move as if they were rolling a pin back and forth.

pinna outer, visible portion of the ear.

pinworm parasite that is 3-10 mm long and lives in the distal colon.

pitting depression that results from pressure against skin when pitting edema is present.

placenta the organ that serves as a lifeline for the developing fetus. The placenta is attached to the wall of the uterus and the umbilical cord.

placental barrier biochemical barrier at the maternal/fetal interface that restricts certain molecules.

plasma membrane *see* cell membrane.

plasma thick, pale yellow fluid that makes up the liquid part of the blood.

plasma-level profile describes the lengths of onset, duration, and termination of action, as well as the drug's minimum effective concentration and toxic levels.

platelet phase a step in the clotting process in which platelets adhere to blood vessel walls and to each other.

platelet one of the fragments of cytoplasm that circulate in the blood and work with components of the coagulation system to promote blood clotting. Platelets also release serotonin, a vasoconstrictive substance.

pleura membranous connective tissue covering the lungs.

pleural friction rub the squeaking or grating sound of the pleural linings rubbing together.

pleuritic sharp or tearing, as a description of pain.

pluripotent stem cell a cell from which the various types of blood cells can form.

pneumatic anti-shock garment (PASG) garment designed to produce uniform pressure on the lower extremities and abdomen; used with shock and hemorrhage patients in some EMS systems.

pneumomediastinum the presence of air in the mediastinum.

pneumonia acute infection of the lung, including alveolar spaces and interstitial tissue.

pneumothorax a collection of air in the pleural space, causing a loss of the negative pressure that binds the lung to the chest wall. In an *open pneumothorax*, air enters the pleural space through an injury to the chest wall. In a *closed pneumothorax*, air enters the pleural space through an opening in the pleura that covers the lung. A *tension pneumothorax* develops when air in the pleural space cannot escape, causing a build-up of pressure and collapse of the lung. *See also* hemothorax, spontaneous pneumothorax.

Poiseuille's law a law of physiology stating that blood flow through a vessel is directly proportional to the radius of the vessel to the fourth power.

poliomyelitis (polio) infectious, inflammatory viral disease of the central nervous system that sometimes results in permanent paralysis.

polycythemia an excess of red blood cells.

polymorphonuclear cells *see* granulocytes.

polypharmacy multiple drug therapy in which there is a concurrent use of a number of drugs.

polyuria excessive urination.

pons process of tissue responsible for the communication interchange between the cerebellum, the cerebrum, midbrain, and the spinal cord.

portal system a venous subsystem that collects blood, fluids, and nutrients absorbed by the bowel and transports them to the liver.

positive end-expiratory pressure (PEEP) a method of holding the alveoli open by increasing expiratory pressure. Some bag-valve units used in EMS have PEEP attachments. Also EMS personnel sometimes transport patients who are on ventilators with PEEP attachments.

post partum depression the "let down" feeling experienced during the period following birth occurring in 70–80% of mothers.

post-conventional reasoning the stage of moral development during which individuals make moral decisions according to an enlightened conscience.

posterior medial sulcus shallow longitudinal groove along the dorsal surface of the spinal cord.

post-ganglionic nerves nerve fibers that extend from the autonomic ganglia to the target tissues.

postrenal acute renal failure acute renal failure due to obstruction distal to the kidney.

posttraumatic stress syndrome reaction to an extreme stressor.

posture position, attitude, or bearing of the body.

PPD purified protein derivative, the substance used in a test for tuberculosis.

prearrival instructions dispatcher's instructions to caller for appropriate emergency measures.

pre-conventional reasoning the stage of moral development during which children respond mainly to cultural control to avoid punishment and attain satisfaction.

precordial (chest) leads electrocardiogram leads applied to the chest in a pattern that permits a view of the horizontal plane of the heart; leads V1, V2, V3, V4, V5, and V6.

precordium area of the chest wall overlying the heart.

prefilled syringe syringe packaged in a tamper-proof container with the medication already in the barrel; also called *preloaded syringe*.

pre-ganglionic nerves nerve fibers that extend from the central nervous system to the autonomic ganglia.

prehospital care report (PCR) the written record of an EMS response.

preload the pressure within the ventricles at the end of diastole; commonly called the end-diastolic volume.

preloaded syringe *see* prefilled syringe.

premenstrual syndrome (PMS) a variety of signs and symptoms, such as weight gain, irritability, or specific food cravings associated with the changing hormonal levels that precede menstruation.

prerenal acute renal failure acute renal failure due to decreased blood perfusion of kidneys.

presbycusis progressive hearing loss that occurs with aging.

pressure ulcer ischemic damage and subsequent necrosis affecting the skin, subcutaneous tissue, and often the muscle; result of intense pressure over a short time or low pressure over a long time; also known as *pressure sore* or *bedsore*.

pressure wave area of overpressure that radiates outward from an explosion.

preventive strategy a management plan to minimize further damage to vital tissues.

primary area of responsibility (PAR) stationing of ambulances at specific high-volume locations.

primary care basic health care provided at the patient's first contact with the health-care system.

primary contamination direct exposure of a person or item to a hazardous substance.

primary immune response the initial development of antibodies in response to the first exposure to an antigen in which the immune system becomes "primed" to produce a faster, stronger response to any future exposures.

primary intention simple healing of a minor wound without granulation or pus formation.

primary prevention keeping an injury from ever occurring.

primary problem the underlying cause for your patient's symptoms.

primary triage triage that takes place early in the incident, usually upon first arrival.

Prinzmetal's angina variant of angina pectoris caused by vasospasm of the coronary arteries; not blockage per se. Also called *vasopastic angina* or *atypical angina*.

prions particles of protein, folded in such a way that protease enzymes cannot act upon them.

priority dispatching system using medically-approved questions and predetermined guidelines to determine the appropriate level of response.

proactive acting to prevent or deal with potential problems before they occur.

proctitis ulcerative colitis limited to the rectum.

prodrug medication that is not active when administered, but whose biotransformation converts it into active metabolites; also called *parent drug*.

profession refers to the existence of a specialized body of knowledge or skills.

professionalism refers to the conduct or qualities that characterize a practitioner in a particular field or occupation.

profile the size and shape of a projectile as it contacts a target; it is the energy exchange surface of the contact.

prognosis the anticipated outcome of a disease or injury.

prolonged QT interval QT interval greater than .44 seconds.

prompt care facilities hospital agencies that provide limited care and non-emergent medical treatment.

prostaglandins substances synthesized by mast cells during inflammatory response that cause vasoconstriction, vascular permeability, and chemotaxis and also cause pain. Prostaglandins also act to control inflammation by suppressing histamine release and releasing lysosomal enzymes.

prostate a gland that surrounds the male bladder neck and the first portion of urethra; it produces fluid that mixes with sperm to make semen.

prostatitis infection and inflammation of the prostate gland.

protocols the policies and procedures for all components of an EMS system; principles for managing certain patient conditions.

prototype drug that best demonstrates the class's common properties and illustrates its particular characteristics.

protozoan single-celled parasitic organism with flexible membranes and the ability to move.

proximal tubule the part of the nephron tubule beyond Bowman's capsule.

proximate cause action or inaction of the paramedic that immediately caused or worsened the damage suffered by the patient.

pruritus itching; often occurs as a symptom of some systemic change or illness.

PSAP public safety access point.

pseudo-instinctive learned actions that are practiced until they can be done without thinking.

psychogenic amnesia failure to recall, as opposed to inability to recall.

psychoneuroimmunological regulation the interactions of psychological, neurological/endocrine, and immunological factors that contribute to alteration of the immune system as an outcome of a stress response that is not quickly resolved.

psychosis extreme response to stress characterized by impaired ability to deal with reality.

psychosocial related to a patient's personality style, dynamics of unresolved conflict, or crisis management methods.

psychotherapeutic medication drug used to treat mental dysfunction.

pubis irregular innominate bone.

puerperium the time period surrounding the birth of the fetus.

pulmonary embolism blood clot that travels to the pulmonary circulation and hinders oxygenation of the blood.

pulmonary hilum central medial region of the lung where the bronchi and pulmonary vasculature enter the lung.

pulmonary over-pressure expansion of air held in the lungs during ascent. If not exhaled, the expanded air may cause injury to the lungs and surrounding structures.

pulse oximeter noninvasive device that measures the oxygen saturation of blood.

pulse oximetry a measurement of hemoglobin oxygen saturation in the peripheral tissues.

pulse pressure difference between the systolic and diastolic blood pressures.

pulse quality strength, which can be weak, thready, strong, or bounding.

pulse rate number of pulses felt in one minute.

pulse rhythm pattern and equality of intervals between beats.

pulsus paradoxus drop in blood pressure of greater than 10 torr during inspiration.

puncture specific soft-tissue injury involving a deep, narrow wound to the skin and underlying organs that carries an increased danger of infection.

pupil dark opening in the center of the iris through which light enters the eye.

pus a liquid mixture of dead cells, bits of dead tissue, and tissue fluid that may accumulate in inflamed tissues.

pyelonephritis an infection and inflammation of the kidney.

pyramids the visible tissue structures within the medulla of a kidney.

pyrexia fever, or above-normal body temperature.

pyrogen any substance causing a fever, such as viruses and bacteria or substances produced within the body in response to infection or inflammation.

QRS axis reduction of all the heart's electrical forces to a single vector represented by an arrow moving in a single plane. Also called *vector*.

QT interval period from the beginning of the QRS to the end of the T wave.

quality assurance (QA) a program designed to maintain continuous monitoring and measurement of the quality of clinical care delivered to patients.

quality improvement (QI) an evaluation program that emphasizes service and uses customer satisfaction as the ultimate indicator of system performance.

quality of respiration depth and pattern of breathing.

rabies viral disorder that affects the nervous system.

rad basic unit of absorbed radiation dose.

radiation transfer of energy through space or matter. *See also* ionizing radiation.

radio band a range of radio frequencies.

radio frequency the number of times per minute a radio wave oscillates.

radius bone on the thumb side of the forearm.

rape Penile penetration of the genitalia or rectum without the consent of the victim.

rapid sequence intubation giving medications to sedate (induce) and temporarily paralyze a patient and then performing orotracheal intubation.

rapid trauma assessment quick check for signs of serious injury.

reabsorption the movement of a substance from a nephron tubule back into the blood.

reactive acting on problems after they occur.

reasonable force the minimal amount of force necessary to ensure that an unruly or violent person does not cause injury to himself or others.

rebound tenderness pain on release of the examiner's hands, allowing the abdominal wall to return to its normal position; associated with peritoneal irritation.

receptor specialized protein that combines with a drug resulting in a biochemical effect.

reciprocal in an ECG, a mirror image seen typically on the opposite wall of the injured area.

reciprocity the process by which an agency grants automatic certification or licensure to an individual who has comparable certification or licensure from another agency.

recirculating currents movement of currents over a uniform obstruction; also known as a *drowning machine*.

recompression resubmission of a person to a greater pressure so that gradual decompression can be achieved; often used in the treatment of diving emergencies.

red bone marrow tissue within the internal cavity of a bone responsible for manufacture of erythrocytes and other blood cells.

reduced nephron mass the decrease in number of functional nephrons that causes chronic renal failure.

reduced renal mass the decrease in kidney size associated with chronic renal failure.

reduction returning of displaced bone ends to their proper anatomic orientation.

referred pain pain that is felt at a location away from its source.

reflective acting thoughtfully, deliberately, and analytically.

refractory period the period of time when myocardial cells have not yet completely repolarized and cannot be stimulated again. *See also* absolute refractory period, relative refractory period.

regeneration regrowth through cell proliferation.

registration the process of entering one's name and essential information within a particular record.

regulatory law *see* administrative law.

relative refractory period the period of the cardiac cycle when, although the myocardial cells have not completely repolarized, a sufficiently strong stimulus may produce depolarization.

remodeling stage in the wound healing process in which collagen is broken down and relaid in an orderly fashion.

renal acute renal failure ARF due to pathology within kidney tissue itself.

renal calculi kidney stones.

renal dialysis artificial replacement of some critical kidney functions.

renal pelvis the hollow space of the kidney at the junction with a ureter.

renal pertaining to the kidneys.

renin an enzyme produced by kidney cells that plays a key role in controlling arterial blood pressure.

repair healing of a wound with scar formation.

repolarization return of a muscle cell to its pre-excitation resting state.

reportable collisions collisions that involve over $1,000 in damage or a personal injury.

res ipsa loquitur a legal doctrine invoked by plaintiffs to support a claim of negligence, it is a Latin term that means "the thing speaks for itself."

reserve capacity the ability of an EMS agency to respond to calls beyond those handled by the on-duty crews.

reservoir any living creature or environment (water, soil, etc.) that can harbor an infectious agent.

resiliency the connective strength and elasticity of an object or fabric.

resistance (1) a host's ability to fight off infection. (2) property of a conductor that opposes the passage of an electric current.

resolution the complete healing of a wound and return of tissues to their normal structure and function; the ending of inflammation with no scar formation.

respiration the exchange of gases between a living organism and its environment; exchange of oxygen and carbon dioxide during inhalation and exhalation in the lungs and at the cellular level.

respirator an apparatus worn that cleanses or qualifies the air.

respiratory acidosis acidity caused by abnormal retention of carbon dioxide resulting from impaired ventilation.

respiratory alkalosis alkalinity caused by excessive elimination of carbon dioxide resulting from increased respirations.

respiratory effort how hard patient works to breathe.

respiratory rate number of times a person breathes in one minute.

respiratory shock shock resulting from failure of the respiratory system to supply oxygen to the alveoli or remove CO_2 from them.

respiratory syncytial virus (RSV) common cause of pneumonia and bronchiolitis in children.

response time time elapsed from when a unit is alerted until it arrives on the scene.

resting potential the normal electrical state of cardiac cells.

restraint asphyxia death from positioning that prevents sufficient intake of oxygen.

resuscitation provision of efforts to return a spontaneous pulse and breathing.

reticular activating system the system responsible for consciousness. A series of nervous tissues keeping the human system in a state of consciousness.

reticuloendothelial system (RES) the cells involved in the immune response.

retina light- and color-sensing tissue lining the posterior chamber of the eye.

retinal detachment condition that may be of traumatic origin and present with patient complaint of a dark curtain obstructing a portion of the field of view.

retinopathy any disorder of the retina.

retroauricular ecchymosis black-and-blue discoloration over the mastoid process (just behind the ear) that is characteristic of a basilar skull fracture. Also called *Battle's sign.*

retrograde amnesia inability to remember events that occurred before the trauma that caused the condition.

retroperitoneal space division of the abdominal cavity containing those organs posterior to the peritoneal lining.

return of spontaneous circulation resuscitation results in the patient's having a spontaneous pulse.

review of systems a list of questions categorized by body system.

Rh blood group a group of antigens discovered on the red blood cells of rhesus monkeys that is also present to some extent in humans.

Rh factor an antigen in the Rh blood group that is also known as *antigen D*. About 85% of North Americans have the Rh factor (are Rh positive) while about 15% do not have the Rh factor (are Rh negative). Rh positive and Rh negative blood are incompatible.

rhabdomyolysis acute disease that involves the destruction of skeletal muscle.

rheumatoid arthritis chronic disease that causes deterioration of peripheral joint connective tissue.

rhonchi continuous sounds with a lower pitch and a snoring quality.

rhythm strip electrocardiogram printout.

rooting reflex occurring when an infant's cheek is touched by a hand or cloth, the hungry infant turns his head to the right or left.

rotation turning along the axis of a bone or joint.

rouleaux group of red blood cells that are stuck together.

rubella (German measles) systemic viral disease characterized by a fine pink rash that appears on the face, trunk, and extremities and fades quickly.

rule of nines method of estimating amount of body surface area burned by a division of the body into regions, each of which represents approximately 9 percent of total BSA (plus 1 percent for the genital region).

rule of palms method of estimating amount of body surface area burned that sizes the area burned in comparison to the patient's palmar surface.

rules of evidence guidelines for permitting a new medication, process, or procedure to be used in EMS.

rust out an inability to keep abreast of new technologies and standards.

Ryan White Act federal law that outlines the rights and responsibilities of agencies and health care workers when an infectious disease exposure occurs.

scabies skin disease caused by mite infestation and characterized by intense itching.

scaffolding a teaching/learning technique in which one builds on what has already been learned.

scapula triangular bone buried within the musculature of the upper back.

scene safety doing everything possible to ensure a safe environment.

scene-authority law legal state or local statute specifying who has ultimate authority at an MCI.

schizophrenia common disorder involving significant change in behavior often including hallucinations, delusions, and depression.

sclera the "white" of the eye.

scope of practice range of duties and skills paramedics are allowed and expected to perform.

scrambling climbing over rocks and/or downed trees on a steep trail without the aid of ropes. This can be especially dangerous when the surface is wet or icy.

scree loose pebbles or rock debris that can form on the slopes or bases of mountains; sometimes used to describe debris in sloping dry stream beds.

scrotum a muscular sac outside of the abdominal cavity that contains the testes, epididymis, and vas deferens.

scuba abbreviation for self-contained underwater breathing apparatus. Portable apparatus that contains compressed air which allows the diver to breathe underwater.

sebaceous glands glands within the dermis secreting sebum.

sebum fatty secretion of the sebaceous gland; it helps keep the skin pliable and waterproof.

second messenger chemical that participates in complex cascading reactions that eventually cause a drug's desired effect.

secondary contamination transfer of a hazardous substance to a non-contaminated person or item via contact with someone or something already contaminated by the substance.

secondary immune response the swift, strong response of the immune system to repeated exposures to an antigen.

secondary intention complex healing of a larger wound involving sealing of the wound through scab formation, granulation or filling of the wound, and constriction of the wound.

secondary prevention medical care after an injury or illness that helps to prevent further problems from occurring.

secondary triage triage that takes place after patients are moved to a treatment area to determine any change in status.

secretion the movement of a substance from the blood into a nephron tubule.

secretory immune system lymphoid tissues beneath the mucosal endothelium that secrete substances such as sweat, tears, saliva, mucus, and breast milk; also called the *external immune system* or the *mucosal immune system.*

sector *see* branch.

secure attachment a type of bonding that occurs when an infant learns that his caregivers will be responsive and helpful when needed.

sedation state of decreased anxiety and inhibitions.

seizure a temporary alteration in behavior due to the massive electrical discharge of one or more groups of neurons in the brain. Seizures can be clinically classified as generalized or partial.

Sellick's maneuver pressure applied in a posterior direction to the anterior cricoid cartilage, occludes the esophagus.

semantic related to the meaning of words.

semen male reproductive fluid.

semicircular canals the three rings of the inner ear. They sense the motion of the head and provide positional sense for the body.

semi-decontaminated patient another name for field-decontaminated patient.

semi-Fowler's position sitting up at 45°.

semipermeable able to allow some, but not all, substances to pass through. Cell membranes are semipermeable.

Sengstaken-Blakemore tube three-lumen tube used in treating esophageal bleeding.

senile dementia general term used to describe an abnormal decline in mental functioning seen in the elderly; also called *organic brain syndrome* or *multi-infarct dementia*.

sensitization initial exposure of a person to an antigen that results in an immune response.

sensorineural deafness deafness caused by the inability of nerve impulses to reach the auditory center of the brain because of nerve damage either to the inner ear or to the brain.

sensorium sensory apparatus of the body as a whole; also that portion of the brain that functions as a center of sensations.

sensory aphasia occurs when the patient cannot understand the spoken word.

septic shock shock that develops as the result of infection carried by the bloodstream, eventually causing dysfunction of multiple organ systems.

septicemia the systemic spread of toxins through the bloodstream. Also called *sepsis*.

septum cartilage that separates the right and left nasal cavities.

sequestration the trapping of red blood cells by an organ such as the spleen.

seroconversion creation of antibodies after exposure to a disease.

serotonin a substance released by platelets that, through constriction and dilation of blood vessels, affects blood flow to an injured or affected site.

serous fluid a cellular component of blood, similar to plasma.

serum solution containing whole antibodies for a specific pathogen.

sesamoid bone bone that forms in a tendon.

sexual assault Unwanted oral, genital, rectal, or manual sexual contact.

sexually transmitted disease (STD) illness most commonly transmitted through sexual contact.

sharps container rigid, puncture resistant container clearly marked as a biohazard.

shipping papers documents routinely carried aboard vehicles transporting hazardous materials; ideally should identify specific substances and quantities carried; also known as *bills of lading*.

shock a state of inadequate tissue perfusion. *See also* hypoperfusion.

short haul a helicopter extrication technique where a person is attached to a rope that is, in turn, attached to a helicopter. The aircraft lifts off with the person attached to it.

shunt surgical connection that runs from the brain to the abdomen for the purpose of draining excess CNS fluid and preventing increased intracranial pressure.

Shy-Drager syndrome chronic orthostatic hypotension caused by a primary autonomic nervous system deficiency.

sick sinus syndrome a group of disorders characterized by dysfunction of the sinoatrial node in the heart.

sickle cell anemia an inherited disorder of red blood cell production so named because the red blood cells become sickle-shaped when oxygen levels are low. Also called *sickle cell disease*.

side effect unintended response to a drug.

silent myocardial infarction a myocardial infarction that occurs without exhibiting obvious signs and symptoms.

silo gas toxic fumes (oxides of nitrogen) produced by the fermentation of grains in a silo.

simple diffusion the random motion of molecules from an area of high concentration to an area of lower concentration.

simple partial seizure type of partial seizure that involves local motor, sensory, or autonomic dysfunction of one area of the body. There is no loss of consciousness.

simplex communication system that transmits and receives on the same frequency.

singular command process where a single individual is responsible for coordinating an incident; most useful in single-jurisdictional incidents.

sinus air cavity that conducts fluids from the eustachian tubes and tear ducts to and from the nasopharynx.

sinusitis inflammation of the paranasal sinuses.

slander act of injuring a person's character, name, or reputation by false or malicious statements spoken with malicious intent or reckless disregard for the falsity of those statements.

slow-reacting substance of anaphylaxis (SRS-A) substance released from basophils and mast cells that causes spasm of the bronchiole smooth muscle, resulting in an asthma-like attack and occasionally asphyxia. *See also* leukotrienes.

sociocultural related to the patient's actions and interactions within society.

solvent a substance that dissolves other substances, forming a solution.

somatic nervous system part of the nervous system controlling voluntary bodily functions.

somatic pain sharp, localized pain that originates in walls of the body such as skeletal muscles.

somatoform disorder condition characterized by physical symptoms that have no apparent physiological cause and are attributable to psychological factors.

span of control number of people or tasks that a single individual can monitor.

spasm intermittent or continuous contraction of a muscle.

Special Weapons and Tactics (SWAT) Team a trained police unit equipped to handle hostage holders and other difficult law enforcement situations.

sperm cell male reproductive cell.

sphygmomanometer blood pressure measuring device comprising a bulb, a cuff, and a manometer.

spike sharp-pointed device inserted into the IV solution bag's administration set port.

spina bifida (SB) a neural defect that results from the failure of one or more of the fetal vertebrae to close properly during the first month of pregnancy.

spinal canal opening in the vertebrae that accomodates the spinal cord.

spinal cord central nervous system (CNS) pathway responsible for transmitting sensory input from the body to the brain and for conducting motor impulses from the brain to the body muscles and organs.

spinal nerves 31 pairs of nerves that originate along the spinal cord from anterior and posterior nerve roots.

spinous process prominence at the posterior part of a vertebra.

spiral fracture a curving break in a bone as may be caused by rotational forces.

spondylosis a degeneration of the vertebral body.

spontaneous pneumothorax a pneumothorax (collection of air in the pleural space) that occurs spontaneously, in the absence of blunt or penetrating trauma.

spotter the person behind the left rear side of the ambulance who assists the operator in backing up the vehicle.

sprain tearing of a joint capsule's connective tissues.

staging location where ambulances, personnel, and equipment are kept in reserve for use at an incident.

standard of care the degree of care, skill, and judgment that would be expected under like or similar circumstances by a similarly trained, reasonable paramedic in the same community.

standing orders preauthorized treatment procedures; a type of treatment protocol.

Starling's law of the heart law of physiology stating that the more the myocardium is stretched, up to a certain amount, the more forceful the subsequent contraction will be.

START acronym for *simple triage and rapid transport*, the most widely used disaster triage system.

startle reflex *see* Moro reflex.

status epilepticus prolonged seizure or multiple seizures with no regaining of consciousness between them.

status epilepticus series of two or more generalized motor seizures without any intervening periods of consciousness.

statutory law *see* legislative law.

stem cells undifferentiated cells in the bone marrow from which all blood cells, including thrombocytes, erythrocytes, and various types of leukocytes, develop; stem cells are also called *hemocytoblasts*.

stenosis narrowing or constriction.

sterile free of all forms of life.

sterilizing use of a chemical or physical method such as pressurized steam to kill all microorganisms on an object.

stethoscope tool used to auscultate most sounds.

stock solution standard concentration of routinely used medications.

Stokes-Adams syndrome a series of symptoms resulting from heart block, most commonly syncope.

stoma opening in the anterior neck that connects the trachea with ambient air; a permanent surgical opening in the neck through which the patient breathes.

strain injury resulting from overstretching of muscle fibers.

strainers a partial obstruction that filters, or strains, the water such as downed trees or wire mesh; causes an unequal force on the two sides.

stress response changes within the body initiated by a stressor.

stress a hardship or strain; a state of physical or psychological arousal to stimulus.

stressor a stimulus that causes stress.

stridor predominantly inspiratory wheeze associated with laryngeal obstruction.

stroke volume the amount of blood ejected by the heart in one cardiac contraction.

stroke injury or death of brain tissue resulting from interruption of cerebral blood flow and oxygenation; also known as a *cerebral vascular accident* or *brain attack*.

stylet plastic-covered metal wire used to bend the endotracheal tube into a J or hockey-stick shape.

subarachnoid hemorrhage bleeding that occurs between the arachoid and dura mater of the brain.

subcutaneous emphysema presence of air in the subcutaneous tissue; the resulting crackling sensation or sound.

subcutaneous tissue body layer beneath the dermis; the layer of loose connective tissue between the skin and muscle.

subdural hematoma collection of blood directly beneath the dura mater.

subendocardial infarction myocardial infarction that affects only the deeper levels of the myocardium; also called *non-Q-wave infarction* because it typically does not result in a significant Q wave in the affected lead.

subglottic referring to the lower airway.

sublingual beneath the tongue.

subluxation partial displacement of a bone end from its position in a joint capsule.

substance abuse use of a pharmacological substance for purposes other than medically defined reasons.

sucking reflex occurring when an infant's lips are stroked.

suction to remove with a vacuum-type device.

sudden death death within one hour after the onset of symptoms.

sudden infant death syndrome (SIDS) illness of unknown etiology that occurs during the first year of life, with the peak at ages 2–4 months.

sudoriferous glands glands within the dermis that secrete sweat.

superficial burn a burn that involves only the epidermis; characterized by reddening of the skin; also called a *first-degree burn.*

superficial frostbite freezing involving only epidermal tissues resulting in redness followed by blanching and diminished sensation; also called *frostnip.*

suppository medication packaged in a soft, pliable form, for insertion into the rectum.

supraglottic referring to the upper airway.

surface absorption entry of a substance into the body directly through the skin or mucous membrane.

surfactant substance that decreases surface tension.

survival when a patient is resuscitated and survives to be discharged from the hospital.

sutures pseudo-joints that join the various bones of the skull to form the cranium.

sympathetic nervous system division of the autonomic nervous system that prepares the body for stressful situations. Sympathetic nervous system actions include increased heart rate and dilation of the bronchioles and pupils. Its actions are mediated by the neurotransmitters epinephrine and norepinephrine.

sympatholytic drug or other substance that blocks the actions of the sympathetic nervous system. Also called *antiadrenergic.*

sympathomimetic drug or other substance that causes effects like those of the sympathetic nervous system. Also called *adrenergic.*

synapse space between nerve cells.

synarthrosis a joint that doesn't permit movement.

synchronized cardioversion the passage of an electric current through the heart during a specific part of the cardiac cycle to terminate certain kinds of dysrhythmias.

syncope transient loss of consciousness due to inadequate flow of blood to the brain with rapid recovery of consciousness upon becoming supine; fainting.

syncytium group of cardiac muscle cells that physiologically function as a unit.

synergism a standard pharmacological principle in which two substances or drugs work together to produce an effect that neither of them can produce on its own.

synovial fluid substance that lubricates synovial joints.

synovial joint type of joint that permits the greatest degree of independent motion.

syphilis blood-borne sexually transmitted disease caused by the spirochete *Treponema pallidum.*

syringe plastic tube with which liquid medications can be drawn up, stored, and injected.

system status management (SSM) a computerized personnel and ambulance deployment system

systemic effects effects that occur throughout the body after exposure to a toxic substance.

systemic throughout the body.

systole the period of the cardiac cycle when the myocardium is contracting.

systolic blood pressure force of blood against arteries when ventricles contract.

T cell receptor (TCR) a molecule on the surface of a helper T cell that responds to a specific antigen. There is a specific TCR for every antigen to which the human body may be exposed.

T lymphocytes white blood cells that do not produce antibodies but, instead, attacks antigens directly.

tachycardia pulse rate higher than 100.

tachycardia rapid heart rate; a heart rate greater than 100 beats per minute.

tachypnea rapid respiration.

Tactical Emergency Medical Service (TEMS) specially trained unit that extracts patients from tactically hot zones; provides on-site medical support to law enforcement personnel.

tactile fremitus vibratory tremors felt through the chest by palpation.

teachable moments the time shortly after an injury when patients may be more receptive to teaching about how similar injury or illness could be prevented in the future.

ten-code radio communications system using codes that begin with the word ten.

tenderness pain that is elicited through palpation.

tendinitis inflammation of a tendon and/or its protective sheath.

tendons long, thin, very strong collagen tissues that connect muscles to bones.

tension lines natural patterns in the surface of the skin revealing tensions within.

tension pneumothorax buildup of air under pressure within the thorax. The resulting compression of the lung severely reduces the effectiveness of respirations. *See* pneumothorax.

teratogenic drug medication that may deform or kill the fetus.

terminal-drop hypothesis a theory that death is preceded by a five-year period of decreasing cognitive functioning.

termination of action time from when the drug's level drops below its minimum effective concentration until it is eliminated from the body.

tertiary prevention rehabilitation after an injury or illness that helps to prevent further problems from occurring.

testes primary male reproductive organs, which produce hormones responsible for sexual maturation and sperm; singular *testis*.

tetanus acute bacterial infection of the central nervous system.

thalamus switching station between the pons and the cerebrum in the brain.

therapeutic index the maximum tolerated dose divided by the minimum curative close of a drug; the range between curative and toxic dosages; also called *therapeutic window*.

therapy regulator pressure regulator used for delivering oxygen to patients.

thermal gradient the difference in temperature between the environment and the body.

thermogenesis the production of heat, especially within the body.

thermoregulation the maintenance or regulation of a particular temperature of the body.

thoracoabdominal pump process by which respirations assist blood return to the heart.

thrill vibration or humming felt when palpating the pulse.

thrombocyte blood platelet.

thrombocytopenia an abnormal decrease in the number of platelets.

thrombocytosis an abnormal increase in the number of platelets.

thrombolytic drug that acts directly on thrombi by breaking them down.

thrombophlebitis inflammation of the vein.

thrombosis clot formation in coronary arteries or cerebral vasculature.

thrombus blood clot.

thyrotoxic crisis toxic condition characterized by hyperthermia, tachycardia, nervous symptoms, and rapid metabolism; also known as *thyroid storm*.

thyrotoxicosis condition that reflects prolonged exposure to excess thyroid hormones with resultant changes in body structure and function.

tibia the larger bone of the lower leg that articulates with the femur.

tidal volume average volume of gas inhaled or exhaled in one respiratory cycle.

tiered response system system that allows multiple vehicles to arrive at an EMS call at different times, often providing different levels of care or transport.

tilt test drop in the systolic blood pressure of 20 mmHg or an increase in the pulse rate of 20 beats per minute when a patient is moved from a supine to a sitting position; a finding suggestive of a relative hypovolemia.

tinnitus the sensation of ringing in the ears.

tissue a group of cells that perform a similar function.

tocolysis the process of stopping labor.

tolerance the need to progressively increase the dose of a drug to reproduce the effect originally achieved by smaller doses.

tone state of slight contraction of muscles that gives them firmness and keeps them ready to move.

tonic phase phase of a seizure characterized by tension or contraction of muscles.

tonic-clonic seizure type of generalized seizure characterized by rapid loss of consciousness and motor coordination, muscle spasms, and jerking motions.

tonicity solute concentration or osmotic pressure relative to the blood plasma or body cells.

topical medications material applied to and absorbed through the skin or mucous membranes.

tort a civil wrong committed by one individual against another.

total body water (TBW) the total amount of water in the body at a given time.

total down time duration from the beginning of the arrest until the patient's delivery to the emergency department.

total lung capacity maximum lung capacity.

touch pad computer on which you enter data by touching areas of the display screen.

tourniquet a constrictor used on an extremity to apply circumferential pressure on all arteries to control bleeding.

toxicology study of the detection, chemistry, pharmacological actions, and antidotes of toxic substances.

toxidrome a toxic syndrome; a group of typical signs and symptoms consistently associated with exposure to a particular type of toxin.

toxin any chemical (drug, poison, or other) that causes adverse effects on an organism that is exposed to it; any poisonous chemical secreted by bacteria or released following destruction of the bacteria.

trachea 10–12 cm long tube that connects the larynx to the mainstem bronchi.

tracheal deviation any position of the trachea other than midline.

tracheal tugging retraction of the tissues of the neck due to airway obstruction or dyspnea.

tracheobronchial tree the structures of the trachea and the bronchi.

tracheostomy a surgical incision that a surgeon makes from the anterior neck into the trachea; held open by a metal or plastic tube.

trajectory the path a projectile follows.

transdermal absorbed through the skin.

transection a cutting across a long axis; a cross-sectional cut.

transient ischemic attack (TIA) temporary interruption of blood supply to the brain; often seen as a precursor to a stroke.

transmural infarction myocardial infarction that affects the full thickness of the myocardium and almost always results in a pathological Q wave in the affected leads.

transverse fracture a break that runs across a bone perpendicular to the bone's orientation.

transverse process bony outgrowth of the vertebral pedicle that serves as a site for muscle attachment and articulation with the ribs.

trauma center medical facility that has the capability of caring for the acutely injured patient. Trauma centers must meet strict criteria to use this designation.

Trauma Intervention Programs (TIP) a national non-profit organization that establishes and operates local chapters of citizen volunteers specially trained to provide assistance to anyone emotionally traumatized by a crisis event.

trauma registry a data retrieval system for trauma patient information, used to evaluate and improve the trauma system.

trauma triage criteria guidelines to aid prehospital personnel in determining which trauma patients require urgent transportation to a trauma center.

trauma a physical injury or wound caused by external force or violence.

trench foot a painful foot disorder resembling frostbite and resulting from exposure to cold and wet, which can eventually result in tissue sloughing or gangrene; also called *immersion foot*.

triage tag a tag containing vital information, affixed to a patient during a multi-patient incident.

triage a method of sorting patients by the severity of their injuries.

trichinosis disease resulting from an infestation of *Trichinella spriralis*.

trichomoniasis sexually transmitted disease caused by the protozoan *Trichomonas vaginalis*.

trocar a sharp, pointed instrument.

trunking communication system that pools all frequencies and routes transmissions to the next available frequency.

trust vs. mistrust refers to a stage of psychosocial development that lasts from birth to about 1 1/2 years of age.

tuberculosis (TB) disease caused by a bacterium known as *Mycobacterium tuberculosis* that primarily affects the respiratory system.

tunica adventitia outer fibrous layer of the blood vessels that maintains their maximum size.

tunica intima smooth interior layer of the blood vessels that provides for the free flow of blood.

tunica media the middle, muscular layer of the blood vessels that controls the vessels' lumen size.

turgor normal tension in a cell; the resistance of the skin to deformation.

turgor normal tension in the skin.

turnover the continual synthesis and breakdown of body substances that results in the dynamic steady state or homeostasis.

two-pillow orthopnea the number of pillows—in this case, two—needed to ease the difficulty of breathing while lying down; a significant factor in assessing the level of respiratory distress.

ulna bone on the little finger side of the forearm.

ultrahigh frequency radio frequency band from 300 to 3,000 megahertz.

umbilical cord structure containing two arteries and one vein that connects the placenta and the fetus.

UN number a four-digit identification number specific to a given chemical; some UN numbers are assigned to a group of related chemicals, but with different characteristics, such the UN 1203 designation for diesel fuel, gasohol, gasoline, motor fuels, motor spirits, and petrol. (The letters *UN* stand for "United Nations." Sometimes the letters *NA* for "North America" appear with or instead of the UN designation.)

unified command process in which managers from different jurisdictions—law enforcement, fire, EMS—coordinate their activities and share responsibility for command.

unipolar limb leads electrocardiogram leads applied to the arms and legs, consisting of one polarized (positive) electrode and a nonpolarized reference point that is created by the ECG machine combining two additional electrodes; also called *augmented limb leads*; leads aVR, aVL, and aVF.

unit predetermined amount of medication or fluid.

upper airway obstruction an interference with air movement through the upper airway.

upper gastrointestinal bleeding bleeding within the gastrointestinal tract proximal to the ligament of Treitz.

up-regulation a drug causes the formation of more receptors than normal.

urea waste derived from ammonia produced through protein metabolism.

uremia the syndrome of signs and symptoms associated with chronic renal failure.

ureter a duct that carries urine from kidney to urinary bladder.

urethra the duct that carries urine from the bladder out of the body; in men, it also carries reproductive fluid (semen) to the outside of the body.

urethritis an infection and inflammation of the urethra.

urinary bladder the muscular organ that stores urine before its elimination from the body.

urinary stasis a condition in which the bladder empties incompletely during urination.

urinary system the group of organs that produces urine, maintaining fluid and electrolyte balance for the body.

urinary tract infection (UTI) an infection, usually bacterial, at any site in the urinary tract.

urine the fluid made by the kidney and eliminated from the body.

urology the surgical specialty dealing with the urinary/genitourinary system.

urosepsis septicemia originating from the urinary tract.

urostomy surgical diversion of the urinary tract to a stoma, or hole, in the abdominal wall.

urticaria the raised areas, or wheals, that occur on the skin, associated with vasodilation due to histamine release; commonly called *hives*.

uterus hollow organ in the center of the abdomen that provides the site for fetal development.

vaccine solution containing a modified pathogen that does not actually cause disease but still stimulates the development of antibodies specific to it.

vacutainer device that holds blood tubes.

vagal response stimulation of the vagus nerve causing a parasympathetic response.

vagina canal that connects the external female genitalia to the uterus.

vagus nerve the 10th cranial nerve that monitors and controls the heart, respiration, and much of the abdominal viscera.

vallecula depression between the epiglottis and the base of the tongue.

valsalva maneuver forced exhalation against a closed glottis, such as with coughing. This maneuver stimulates the parasympathetic nervous system via the vagus nerve, which in turn slows the heart rate.

varicella viral disease characterized by a rash of fluid-filled vesicles that rupture, forming small ulcers that eventually scab.

varicose veins dilated superficial veins, usually in the lower extremity. Also called *varicosities*.

vas deferens the duct that carries sperm cells from epididymis to urethra.

vascular phase a step in the clotting process in which smooth blood vessel muscle contracts, reducing the vessel lumen and the flow of blood through it.

vasculitis inflammation of blood vessels.

vasomotor center center in the medulla oblongata that controls arterial and, to a degree, venous tone.

vasopastic angina *see* Prinzmetal's angina.

vector a force that has both magnitude and direction. *See also* QRS axis.

vein a blood vessel that carries blood toward the heart.

velocity the rate of motion in a particular direction in relation to time.

venous access device surgically implanted port that permits repeated access to central venous circulation.

venous constricting band flat rubber band used to impede venous return and make veins easier to see.

ventilation the mechanical process of moving air in and out of the lungs.

ventricular filling the forcing of blood into the ventricle by the contraction of the atrium.

Venturi mask high-flow face mask that uses a venturi system to deliver relatively precise oxygen concentrations.

vertebra one of 33 bones making up the vertebral column.

vertebral body short column of bone that forms the weight-bearing portion of a vertebra.

vertigo the sensation of faintness or dizziness; may cause a loss of balance.

very high frequency radio frequency band from 30 to 300 megahertz.

vial plastic or glass container with a self-healing rubber top.

virulence an organism's strength or ability to infect or overcome the body's defenses.

virus disease-causing organism that can be seen only with an electron microscope.

visceral pain dull, poorly localized pain that originates in the walls of hollow organs.

visual acuity wall chart/card wall chart or handheld card with lines of letters used to test vision.

vital statistics height and weight.

vitreous humor clear watery fluid filling the posterior chamber of the eye. It is responsible for giving the eye its spherical shape.

voltage the difference of electric potential between two points with different concentrations of electrons.

volume on hand the available amount solution containing a medication.

volvulus twisting of the intestine on itself.

von Willebrand's disease condition in which the vWF component of factor VIII is deficient.

warm zone location at a hazmat incident adjacent to the hot zone; area where a decontamination corridor is established; also called the *yellow zone* or the *contamination reduction zone*.

warning placard diamond-shaped graphic placed on vehicles to indicated hazard classification.

washout release of accumulated lactic acid, carbon dioxide (carbonic acid), potassium, and rouleaux into the venous circulation.

weapons of mass destruction (WMD) variety of chemical, biological, or nuclear devices used by terrorists to strike at government or high-profile targets; designed to create a maximum number of casualties.

Wernicke's syndrome condition characterized by loss of memory and disorientation, associated with chronic alcohol intake and a diet deficient in thiamine.

wheezes continuous, high-pitched musical sounds similar to a whistle.

whispered pectoriloquy abnormal clarity of patient's transmitted whispers.

white matter material that surrounds gray matter in the spinal cord; made up largely of axons.

whole bowel irrigation administration of polyethylene glycol continuously at 1–2 L/hr through a nasogastric tube until the effluent is clear or objects are recovered.

window phase time between exposure to a disease and seroconversion.

withdrawal referring to alcohol or drug withdrawal in which the patient's body reacts severely when deprived of the abused substance.

wrap points mechanisms of injury in which an appendage gets caught and significantly twisted.

xiphisternal joint union between xiphoid process and body of the sternum.

yaw swing or wobble around the axis of a projectile's travel.

years of productive life a calculation made by subtracting the age at death from 65.

yellow bone marrow tissue that stores fat in semi-liquid form within the internal cavities of a bone.

Zollinger-Ellison syndrome condition that causes the stomach to secrete excessive amounts of hydrochloric acid and pepsin.

zone of coagulation area in a burn nearest the heat source that suffers the most damage and is characterized by clotted blood and thrombosed blood vessels.

zone of hyperemia area peripheral to a burn that is characterized by increased blood flow.

zone of stasis area in a burn surrounding the zone of coagulation and characterized by decreased blood flow.

zygoma the cheekbone.

Index

Autonomy, 61
Autoregulation, 158
AV blocks. *See* Atrioventricular blocks
AV junction. *See* Atrioventricular junction
Avoidance language, 583
Avoidant personality disorder, 1621
AVPU (Alert, Verbal stimuli, Painful stimuli, Unresponsive), 714–715
Avulsions, 918–919
Axial loading, 837
Axial skeleton, 134
Axial stress, 1072–1073
Axons, 177

Babinski response, 687
Back boarding, 1985
Back pain, 1374–1377
Back safety, 35–37
Bacteria, 296–297, 1558–1559
Bacterial tracheitis, 1760
Bactericidal, 1559
Bacteriostatic, 1559
Bag-valve devices, 569–570
Bag-valve mask, 569
Balance, 182
Ballistics, 860–863
Bandage materials, for soft-tissue trauma, 929–931
Bandaging
    anatomical considerations for, 940–943
    complications, 943
    objectives of, 937–940
Barbiturates, 1491
Bare lymphocyte syndrome, 309
Bargaining, 42
Baroreceptors, 102
Barotrauma, 322, 554, 1540, 1542
Barton, Clara, 10
Basal metabolic rate (BMR), 1519
Base, 207
Baseline vital signs, 733, 740
Basic life support (BLS), 9, 1290, 1532, 1924
Basophil, 124, 1399
Battery, 88–89
Battle's sign, 744
B cells, 1396
Behavior
    cardiovascular patients, 1284
    confusing, 604–605
    definition of, 1607
    evaluation of, 676
    facilitating, 762
    professional, 576–577
    sexual, 405
Behavioral disorders, 1843–1845
Behavioral emergencies, 1607–1608
    assessment, 1609–1613
    management, 1624–1626
    violent patients and restraints, 1626–1629
    See also Psychiatric disorders
Beliefs, 599
Bell's palsy, 1373
Bend fractures, 1788
Beneficence, 61
Benevolence, 61
Benign prostatic hypertrophy, 1433
Benign tumors, 1369

Benzodiazepines, 1491
Bereavement, 1617
Beta$_2$ specific agents, 391–392
Beta adrenergic antagonists, 383
Beta adrenergic receptors, 102
Beta agonists, 1403
Beta blockers, 380, 1521, 1840
Beta particles, 1550
Beta radiation, 960, 2010
Biaxial joints, 133
Bicarbonate, 109
Bicarbonate buffer system, 113–114
Biceps, reflex testing of, 687
Bigeminy, 1264
Bilateral periorbital ecchymosis, 1030
Bilevel positive airway pressure (BIPAP), 1898, 1906, 1907
Bioassay, 344
Bioavailability, 350
Bioequivalence, 344
Bioethics, 61
Biological conditions, and psychiatric disorders, 1608–1609
Biologic half-life, 358
Biot's respirations, 503, 1160
Biotransformation, 351–352, 2010
BIPAP (bilevel positive airway pressure), 1898, 1906, 1907
Bipolar disorder, 283, 1618
Bipolar limb leads, 1207
Birth injuries, 1709–1710
Births, multiple, 1676
Bites
    black widow spider, 1483–1484
    brown recluse spider, 1481–1482
    snake, 1484–1487
Black widow spider bites, 1483–1484
Blankets, protective, 1973
Blast injuries, 848–854
Blastocyst, 1644
Blast wind, 850
Bleeding, vaginal, 1636, 1655, 1659
Blepharospasm, 982
Blind patients, 585, 606
Blood, 119–120
    carbon dioxide concentration in, 237–238
    circulatory system and, 224
    components of, 120–127
    hemostasis, 127–130
    high altitude sickness and, 1547
    as intravenous fluid, 452
    oxygen concentration in, 236–237
    pathophysiology, 272–273
Bloodborne, 1562
Blood-brain barrier, 158, 346, 351
Blood clotting, 880–882
Blood clotting abnormalities, 1511–1512
Blood components, 272–273
Blood evidence, 2032–2033
Blood flow, 210
Blood glucometer, 1353
Blood glucose, 629, 741, 1382–1383
Blood group antigens, 301–302
Blood loss, response to, 897–898
Blood pressure, 223, 616–618
    arterial, 251–252
    general survey and, 624–625
    head, facial, and neck injuries, 1059–1060

Coma, 1342
    diabetic, 1384–1386
    hyperglycemic hyperosmolar nonketotic, 1386–1387
    myxedema, 1390
Combative patients. *See* Uncooperative patients
Comfort care, 1917–1919
Command, 1954. *See also* Medical incident command
Command post (CP), 1955
Command staff, and stress, 50
Comminuted fracture, 993
Common cold, 1586–1587
Common law, 74
Common pathway, 129
Communicable diseases, 1563, 1881. *See also* Infectious diseases
Communicable period, 1564
Communication, 12, 15–16, 575, 772
    basic elements of, 575–577
    cardiovascular emergencies, 1306
    crime scenes, 2027
    degenerative neurological disorders and, 1374
    documentation and, 797–798
    elderly people, 1805, 1808–1810
    emergency medical dispatcher, 16
    EMS dispatch, 16
    EMS response, 775–778
    general guidelines, 577–580
    history taking, 592–593
    interview techniques, 580–583
    mass-casualty incidents, 1957
    medical incident command, 1968–1969
    patients with special needs, 584–587
    pediatric emergencies, 1716–1717
    regulation, 786–787
    reporting procedures, 783–786
    skills, 31
    street gangs, 2025
    technology, 779–783
    transferring patient care, 587
    verbal, 773–774
    written, 774
Communications hardware, 16
Communications software, 16
Community, illness and injury prevention for, 56–59
Community-acquired infection, 1452
Community involvement, 27
Community needs assessment, 58–59
Community resources, 58
Co-morbidity, 1100, 1801
Companions, dying, 337
Comparative negligence, 81
Compartment syndrome
    indicators of, 1001
    management of, 948–949
    muscular injury, 989
    soft-tissue trauma, 926
Compensated hypothermia, 1528
Compensated shock, 287, 898–899, 1764
Compensation, 287
Compensatory pause, 1254
Competent, 84
Competitive antagonism, 356
Complaints
    answering, 75
    filing of, 75
    review of, 1932
Complete block, 1252–1253

Complete insertion, 486
Completeness, 799
Complex partial seizure, 1363
Compliance, 505, 1925–1926
Complications
    bandaging, 943
    burns, 966–969
    cricothyrotomy, 558
    endotracheal intubation, 522–524
    soft-tissue trauma, 925–927
Comprehensive Drug Abuse Prevention and Control
    Act, 343
Compression, 1074
Computers, 782
Concealment, 2027–2028
Concentration, 434, 490
Concept formation, 765–766
Conception, 1647
Concretions, 1477
Concussion, 1034, 1074
Conduction, 1517
Conduction disorders, 1276–1279
Conductive deafness, 1868
Conductivity, 99, 217, 1205
Confidentiality, 65–67, 83–84
Confined space explosions, 850
Confined space hazards, 1988–1989
Conflict resolution, 62–63
Confrontation, 582
Confusing behaviors and histories, 604–605
Confusion, 1610
Congenital anomalies, 1684–1685
Congenital disorders, 1870–1871
Congenital heart disease, 1768
Congenital immune deficiencies, 309
Congestive heart failure (CHF), 1319, 1899
Conjunctiva, 163
Connective tissue, 100
Connective tissue injuries, 869, 1010, 1018–1019
Consciousness
    cardiovascular patients, 1283
    pediatric patients, 1727
    physical examination, 622
    seizures and, 1362
    urinary system, 1437
Consent, 67, 84–89
Conservation of energy, 826
Consolidated Omnibus Budget Reconciliation Act (COBRA),
    11–12
Consolidation, 1582
Constipation, drugs used for, 396
Constitutional law, 74
Constricting band, 464
Contact and cover, 2028–2029
Contagion, 1562–1564
Contaminated equipment, disposal of, 416
Contamination, 1563, 2010–2014
Contemplative approach, 1930
Continence, 1805–1806
Continuing education, 32, 1712–1713
Continuous positive airway pressure (CPAP), 1898,
    1906, 1907
Continuous quality improvement (CQI), 22
CONTOMS (Counter Narcotics Tactical Operations),
    2030–2031
Contraceptives, oral, 404

Cytotoxic, 98
Cytotoxin, 98

D$_5$W, 275, 451
Daily life, and patient history, 599
Dalton's Law, 1539
Damage pathway, 866–868
Dams, 1985
Dangerous crowds and bystanders, 2025
Data
    interpretation of, 766
    preliminary, 594
    trauma registry and, 823
Data collection, 54
Date rape drug, 1492
DCAP-BTLS, 725
Dead space volume, 239
Deafness, 586, 605, 1868–1870
Death, 41–45, 92, 337, 1920
Debridement, 306
Debriefing, 50
Deceleration, 827
Decerebrate posture, 1350
Decision, 76
Decision making
    decontamination, 2015–2016
    ethical, 60
    factors affecting, 1924–1926
    patient transport, 821, 822
    See also Clinical decision making
Decode, 575
Decompensated shock, 899–900, 1764–1765
Decompensation, 103, 287–288
Decompression illness, 1541, 1542–1544
Decontamination, 1459, 1569
    equipment, 40–41
    hazardous materials incidents, 2014–2017
Decorticate, 714
Decorticate posture, 1350
Decubitus ulcers. *See* Pressure ulcers
Deep frostbite, 1534
Deep venous thrombosis, 1334–1335
Defamation, 83–84
Defendant, 75
Defenses, to negligence charges, 81
Defensive strategies, 45
Defibrillation, 1297–1299, 1300–1301
Defibrillator, 1297
Deflection, 1209
Defusing, 50
Degenerative disorders
    musculoskeletal trauma, 995–996
    neurological, 1371–1374
    neuromuscular, 1900–1901
    visual impairments and, 1870–1871
Degloving injury, 918
Degranulation, 304–305, 1399
Dehydration, 106–107, 1525
Delayed effects, 2011
Delayed healing, 926
Delayed hypersensitivity reactions, 1398–1399
Delayed sensitivity reaction, 308
DeLee suction trap, 1684
Delirium, 604, 1614, 1829–1830
Delirium tremens (DTs), 1494
Delivery
    abnormal situations, 1672–1676

    complications, 1676–1679
    field, 1666–1668
    precipitous, 1674–1675, 1676
Delta wave, 1279
Deltoid muscle injections, 444
Delusions, 1614
Demand pacemakers, 1274
Demand valve device, 571–572
Demargination, 123
Dementia, 604, 1614, 1829, 1830
Demobilization, 50, 1958
Demographics
    ambulance operations and, 1943
    geriatric patients, 1800–1802
Demylenation, 1900
Denature, 955
Dendrites, 177
Denial, 41
Dental system, 327
Dependence, 1488
Dependent personality disorder, 1621
Depersonalization, 1620
Deployment, ambulance, 1943–1944
Depolarization, 177, 214, 215–216, 1204–1205
Deposition, 75
Depression, 42, 331, 604, 1617–1618, 1844, 1915
Dermatones, 187
Dermis, 118
Descending loop of Henle, 249
Descending tracts, 185
Descent injuries, 1540
Design, ambulance, 1941–1942
Desired dose, 490
Detailed physical examination, 744–750
    general approach, 1931
    head, facial, and neck injuries, 1052
    musculoskeletal trauma, 1001
    shock, 902
    soft-tissue trauma, 935
Detection, 775–776
Devascularization, 131
Development. *See* Life-span development
Developmental disabilities, 1874–1876
Dextran, 274, 451
Dextrose, 1064
Diabetes, 1651
Diabetes insipidus, 201
Diabetes mellitus, 280, 1380–1384, 1831–1832
Diabetic coma, 1384–1386
Diabetic ketoacidosis, 1384–1386, 1777
Diabetic retinopathy, 1870
Diabetogenic effect of pregnancy, 1662
Diagnosis, field, 1924. *See also* Assessment
Diagnostic testing, respiratory system assessment, 1170–1172
Dialysate, 1447
Dialysis, 1432
    peritoneal, 1448
    renal, 1446–1447
Dialysis shunts, 1908–1909
Diapedesis, 123
Diaphoresis, 1163, 1283
Diaphragm, 173
    traumatic rupture/perforation, 1118
    ventilation and, 1159
Diaphragmatic hernia, 1684, 1702–1703
Diaphysis, 131
Diarrhea, 397, 1709, 1775

ECG leads, 1207, 1217
ECG monitoring. *See* Electrocardiographic
    monitoring
Echo procedure, 785
Eclampsia, 1659–1660, 1661
Ecstasy, 1492
Ectopic beat, 1221
Ectopic focus, 1221
Ectopic pregnancy, 1636, 1656–1657
Ectopic tachycardia, 1230, 1231
Eddies, 1985
Edema, 271, 464, 1284
    airway obstruction and, 499
    angioneurotic, 1399
    pulmonary, 1174–1176, 1822
    soft-tissue trauma and, 940
Education
    ambulance operations, 1944–1945
    certification levels, 17–18
    continuing, 32
    EMS providers, 54
    initial, 17
    National Registry of Emergency Medical Technicians, 18
    pediatric patients, 1714–1715
    professional journals, 19
    professional organizations, 18–19
    public, 12, 14–15
Effacement, 1663
Effector, 103
Efficacy, 355
Egophony, 651
Eight-step decontamination, 2016–2017
Einthoven's triangle, 1207
Ejection, 837
Ejection fraction, 222, 1203
Elapidae, 1485
Elastic bandages, 931
Elbows, 137–139
    bandaging, 942–943
    injuries, 1017
    physical examination of, 662, 664, 665
Elderly patients. *See* Geriatric patients
Electrical activity, pulseless, 1770
Electrical alternans, 1116
Electrical burns, 956–958, 978–980, 985
Electrical lines, downed, 1992
Electrical therapy, 1751–1752
Electricity, 1988–1989
Electrocardiogram (ECG), 1206–1210, 1349
Electrocardiographic (ECG) monitoring, 1206
    electrical events in heart, 1210–1217
    electrocardiogram, 1206–1210
    field, 1291–1294
    prehospital, 1336–1339
    rhythm strips, 1217–1219
Electrodes, 1207
Electrolytes, 107–110, 409
    electrocardiogram and, 1279
    role of, 214
    tubular handling of, 250–251
Electromechanical infusion devices, 475–476
Electromechanical pump tubing, 454–455
Electrons, 1550
Electrophysiology, 214, 1204–1205
Elimination, 352, 1806
Elixirs, 354, 427

Elongation of the QT interval, 281
Emancipated minor, 86
Emboli, 466, 853. *See also* Pulmonary embolism
Embolic strokes, 1357
Embryonic stage, 1647
EMD. *See* Emergency medical dispatcher
Emergency lighting, 1975, 1991
Emergency medical dispatcher (EMD), 16,
    776–777
Emergency medical services (EMS), 9
    communications, 15–16, 775–778
    crime scenes, 2031–2033
    education and certification, 17–19
    history of, 9–12
    illness and injury prevention, 52–56
    local and state level agencies, 12–13
    medical direction, 13–14
    mutual aid and mass-casualty preparation, 21
    patient transport, 19–20
    public information and education, 14–15
    quality assurance and improvement, 21–23
    receiving facilities, 20–21
    research, 23
    responsive medical patients, 741–742
    system financing, 23–24
    tactical, 8, 2019, 2026–2031
Emergency Medical Services for Children (EMSC), 1715–1716
Emergency Medical Services Systems Act, 11
Emergency medical technician-basic (EMT-B), 18
Emergency medical technician-intermediate (EMT-I), 18
Emergency medical technician-paramedic (EMT-P), 18. *See also*
    Paramedics
Emergency medical technician-tactical (EMT-T), 2030
Emergency response, and communications, 775–778
Emergency Response Guidebook (ERG), 2006–2007
Emergency synchronized cardioversion, 1299, 1302, 1303
Emergent phase, 955
Emesis, 397–398, 1893
Emotional abuse, of children, 1862
Emotional disorders, 1855, 1874
Emotional support, for head, facial, and neck injuries, 1065
Empathy, 30, 575, 582
Emphysema, 1167, 1177–1179, 1898
EMS. *See* Emergency medical services
EMS Communications Officer, 1969
Emulsions, 354, 427
Encephalitic phase, 1595
Encephalitis, 1594
Encephalomyelitis, 1595
Encode, 575
End-diastolic volume, 222
Endobroncheal intubation, 523–524
Endocardium, 207, 1202
Endocrine disorders, 280–281, 1831–1832
Endocrine glands, 102, 1379
Endocrine signaling, 102
Endocrine system, 101, 103–104, 195–199
    adrenal glands, 204–205
    drugs used for, 399–405
    geriatric patients, 1814
    gonads, 205–206
    hypothalamus, 200
    late adulthood, 333
    pancreas, 203–204
    parathyroid glands, 203
    pineal gland, 206

Judgment, 1612
    clinical, 757
    evaluation of, 677–678
    nervous system assessment, 1345
Jugular vein. *See* External jugular vein
Jugular venous distention (JVD), 1349
Junctional escape complex and rhythm, 1256–1257
Justice, 61
J waves, 1530

Keloid, 926
Kernig's sign, 1585
Ketoacidosis, diabetic, 1384–1386
Ketone bodies, 1382
Ketosis, 1382
Kidney failure, 282
Kidneys, 246–252
Kidney stones, 282, 1432, 1449–1451
Kidney transplantation, 1432
Kinetic energy, 826–827
Kinetics, of blunt trauma, 826–827
Klebsiella pneumoniae, 1416
Kleptomania, 1622
Knees, 143–145
    bandaging, 942–943
    injuries, 1015–1016
    physical examination of, 665, 668, 669
Knives, 865–866
Knowledge, fundamental, 761–762
Korotkoff sounds, 616
Korsakoff's psychosis, 1356
Kübler-Ross, Elizabeth, 41–42, 337
Kussmaul's respirations, 503, 1160, 1349, 1385
Kyphosis, 1814

Labeling, triage, 1964–1965
Labels, 452
Labia, 254
Labia majora, 254
Labia minora, 254
Labor
    active, 1652
    false, 1663
    management, 1666
    maternal complications, 1677–1679
    preterm, 1663–1664
    stages of, 1665–1666
Laboratory-based simulations, 1934
Labrynthitis, 1869
Lacerations
    soft-tissue, 522, 915–917
    spinal cord, 1074–1075
Lacrimal fluid, 163
Lactated Ringer's, 275, 451
Lactic acid, 883
Lactose intolerance, 282
Laminae, 168
Landing zone, 1952
Language
    avoidance, 583
    communication and, 586–587
    history taking, 592–593, 605
    physical examination and, 676–677
    street gangs, 2023
Language disorders, 1871–1872
Lanoxin, 1841

Large cell carcinoma, 1187
Larrey, Jean, 10
Laryngeal mask airway (LMA), 549, 550
Laryngeal spasm, 499
Laryngopharynx, 228
Laryngoscope, 516–517
Laryngoscopy, 552–553
Laryngotracheobronchitis, 1591, 1757–1758
Larynx, 228–229
Late adulthood, 321, 332–337
Latent period, 1564
Latent syphilis, 1599
Lateral impacts, 834, 838–839
Lateral marginal veins, 211
Law
    categories of, 75
    EMS-related and paramedic-related, 76–78
    ethics and, 60
    sources of, 74
    See also Legal issues
Lawsuits, 75–76
Lawyers, documentation for, 791
Laxatives, 396
Lead (metal), 1478
Leader, team, 1927
Leadership, 29–30
Leading questions, 580, 581
Leads, 1207, 1217
LeChetalier's Principle, 115
Le Fort criteria, 1040
Left atrium, 1203
Left bundle branch, 217–218, 1205
Left coronary artery, 211, 1203
Left ventricular failure, 1318
Leg, intravenous access in, 458–460. *See also* Extremities
Legal accountability, 78–82
Legal duties, 74–78
Legal issues
    documentation for, 791
    pharmacology, 343–344
    sexual assault, 1864–1865
    See also Law
Legal system, 74–75
Legibility, 799, 801
Legislative law, 74
Leisure activities, and patient history, 599
Lesions, 623, 631–633
Lethal concentration/lethal doses (LCt/LD), 2010
Leukemia, 1509–1510
Leukemoid reaction, 1509
Leukocytes, 98, 123, 272
Leukocytosis, 1509
Leukopenia, 1509
Leukopoiesis, 123
Leukotriene antagonists, 393
Leukotreines, 305
Leur lock, 478
Leur-sampling needle, 479
Liability, 74
    medical, 78–81
    special concerns, 81–82
Liaison Officer, 1959
Libel, 84, 783, 802
Lice, 1602
Licensure, 17, 77

urinary system, 1433–1436
    visceral, 1408, 1434
Pain control, for soft-tissue trauma, 940
Pain disorder, 1619
Painful stimuli, 714
Pain medications, non-prescription, 1476–1477
Pallor, 1163
Palmar grasp, 323
Palpation, 505, 611–612
    cardiovascular patients, 1289–1290
    respiratory system assessment, 1167
    soft-tissue trauma, 936
    thoracic trauma, 1121–1122
Palpitations, 1284
Pancolitis, 1420
Pancreas, 203–204, 401–403
Pancreas disorders, 1380–1388
Pancreatitis, 1427–1428
Pancuronium, 1062
Panic attacks, 1615–1616
Paper bag syndrome, 835, 836
Papilla, 247
Papillary muscles, 209
Para-aminophenol derivatives, 362
Paracrine signaling, 102
Paradoxical breathing, 501
Paralysis, 1873–1874
Paralytics, 1062
Paralytic shellfish poisoning, 1479
Paramedic-patient relationships, 82–90
Paramedics
    characteristics, 7
    clinical decision making, 757–759
    crime and accident scenes, 92
    death and dying, 41–45
    disease protection, 37–41
    documentation, 92–93
    ethics and, 64–70
    hazardous materials incidents, 2001–2002
    legal accountability, 78–82
    legal duties and ethical responsibilities, 74–78
    pediatric care, 1714–1716
    physical fitness, 33–37
    professionalism, 7–8, 28–32
    profession description, 6–7
    rescue awareness and operations, 1972–1973
    responsibilities, 25–28
    resuscitation issues, 90–92
    safety considerations, 50–52
    scope of practice, 8
    stress and stress management, 45–50
    trauma care and, 819–823
Paranoid personality disorder, 1621
Paranoid schizophrenia, 1615
Parasites, 298, 1561
Parasympathetic nervous system, 177, 194–195, 372–375
Parasympatholytics, 372
Parasympathomimetics, 372
Parathyroid glands, 203, 399–400
Parathyroid hormone (PTH), 203
Parenchyma, 231
Parental-separation reactions, 326
Parent drug, 351
Parenteral administration
    calculating dosages for, 492
    medication packaging, 433–439

    routes of, 353–354, 440–448
    syringes and needles, 432–433
Parenting styles, 328
Parents, communication and psychological support
    for, 1715
Parietal pericardium, 207
Parity, 1632, 1648
Parking, of ambulances, 1948
Parkinson's disease, 369–371, 1372, 1831
Paroxysmal junctional tachycardia, 1259–1261
Paroxysmal nocturnal dyspnea (PND), 601, 1165, 1319
Paroxysmal phase, 1589
Paroxysmal supraventricular tachycardia (PSVT), 1236–1239,
    1259
Paroxysms, 1259
Partial agonist, 356
Partial pressure, 235
Partial pressure of oxygen, 225
Partial rebreather mask, 567
Partial seizures, 1362, 1363
Partial thickness burn, 965, 975–977
Particulate evidence, 2031
Partner abuse, 1853–1857
Parts per million/parts per billion (ppm/ppb), 2010
Passive acquired immunity, 300
Passive immunity, 1397
Passive transport, 349
Pathogenesis
    HIV, 1573
    tuberculosis, 1579–1580
Pathogens, 37–38, 267, 408, 1396, 1557, 1558
Pathological challenges, 1876–1882
Pathological fractures, 994, 1513
Pathological gambling, 1622
Pathological Q wave, 1314
Pathologic state, 359
Pathology, 264
Pathophysiology, 24, 264
    abdominal trauma, 1135–1143
    acid-base derangements, 275–277
    acute renal failure, 1439–1441
    Addison's disease, 1393
    adult respiratory distress syndrome, 1175
    allergies, 1398–1399
    anaphylaxis, 1399
    asthma, 1181–1182, 1761
    burns, 954–969
    carbon monoxide inhalation, 1189
    cellular adaptation, injury, and death, 265–271
    central nervous system dysfunction, 1194
    chronic bronchitis, 1179–1180
    chronic renal failure 1443–1444
    Cushing's syndrome, 1392
    diabetic ketoacidosis, 1385
    diving emergencies, 1540
    drowning and near-drowning, 1535–1537
    emphysema, 1177–1178
    facial injuries, 1026–1027, 1039–1044
    fluids and fluid imbalances, 271–275
    gastroenterology, 1408–1409
    genetics and other causes, 277–283
    geriatric patients, 1803–1806, 1807–1808, 1812–1818
    Graves' disease, 1389
    head injuries, 1026–1039
    hyperglycemic hyperosmolar nonketotic coma, 1387
    hyperventilation syndrome, 1193

Pulse deficit, 1243
Pulse oximeter, 625
Pulse oximetry, 505–507, 625, 628
  nervous system assessment and, 1353
  pediatric patients, 1731–1732
  respiratory system assessment and, 1170–1171
  responsive medical patients, 741
Pulse pressure, 617, 887
Pulse quality, 614, 753
Pulse rate, 614, 753
Pulse rhythm, 614
Pulse, 614–615, 624, 1289, 1770, 1963
Pulseless electrical activity, 1276, 1770
Pulseless ventricular tachycardia, 1770
Pulsus alternans, 1320
Pulsus paradoxus, 503, 1116, 1169, 1320
Pump failure, 1313
Punctures, 917
Pupils, 163, 1733
Pure Food and Drug Act, 343
Purified protein derivative (PPD), 1566
Purkinje system, 217, 1205
Pus, 306
P waves, 1210, 1219
Pyelonephritis, 1452
Pyramids, 247
Pyrexia, 1526
Pyrogenic reaction, 465–466
Pyrogens, 1526
Pyromania, 1622

QRS complex, 1210, 1219
QRS interval, 1215
QT interval, 281, 1215
Quadriceps, reflex testing of, 687
Quadrigeminy, 1264
Quality assurance (QA), 21–23
Quality factor (QF), 1551
Quality improvement (QI), 12, 21–23, 823
Questioning, 577, 580–581, 1121
Quiet, 504
Q wave, 1210

Rabies, 1594–1596
Race, osteoporosis, 1836
Rad, 961
Radiation
  heat loss, 1517–1518
  nuclear, 1549–1553
Radiation absorbed dose (RAD), 1551
Radiation burns, 959–962, 983–984, 985
Radio band, 774
Radio communication, 779–781, 784–785
Radio frequency, 774
Radioisotope, 1549, 1550
Radionuclide, 1549
Radius fractures, 1013–1014
Railroad accidents, 2001–2002
Rales, 1168
Rape, 1863
Rapid extrication, 1092–1093
Rapid Intervention Team, 1969
Rapid sequence induction (RSI), 537
Rapid sequence intubation (RSI), 535, 537–540, 1056, 1747
Rapid trauma assessment, 724–733, 998
  abdominal trauma, 1146–1148

head, facial, and neck injuries, 1048–1052
hemorrhage, 891–892
shock, 901–902
soft-tissue trauma, 933–934
spinal trauma, 1079–1082
thermal burns, 972–974
thoracic trauma, 1120–1124
Rapport, 576, 591–594, 690
Reabsorption, 249
Reactive decision making, 763
Rear-end impacts, 834, 840–841
Reasonable force, 89
Reasoning, 330
Reassurance, 603
Re-bleeding, 926
Rebound tenderness, 1140
Receiving facilities, 12, 20–21
Receptor, 355
Receptor sites, drug actions and, 355–356
Reciprocal socialization, 324–325
Reciprocity, 17
Recirculating currents, 1983
Recompression, 1543
Recording
  child abuse, 1862
  detailed physical examination findings, 750
  incident, 777–778
  physical examination findings, 695–696
Recovery, 1567–1569, 1970
Recreation hazards, 57
Recreational vehicle accidents, 846–848
Rectal administration, 353, 430–432
Rectum, 748
Rectus femoris muscle injections, 446
Red blood cells, 121–123, 1506–1509
Red bone marrow, 132
Red treatment unit, 1966
Reduced nephron mass, 1444
Reduced renal mass, 1444
Reduction, 1009
Red zone, 2007
Reentry, 1221
Reevaluation, 765
Reference materials, 341–342
Referrals
  musculoskeletal trauma, 1021–1022
  soft-tissue trauma, 951
Referred pain, 596, 1408, 1434
Reflection, 582, 593, 767
Reflective decision making, 763
Reflexes
  detailed physical examination, 750
  infancy, 323
  testing, 685–689
Reflex hammer, 618, 621
Refractory period, 1216
Reframing, 49
Refusal of service. *See* Patient refusals
Regeneration, 306
Registry, trauma, 823
Regulations, 12
  communications, 786–787
  Incident Management System, 1954
Rehabilitation, 1968, 2018–2019
Relative level, 578
Relative refractory period, 1216

K
**Interceptive guidance
Serial extraction**

MR
1 vs 4

L
Edgewise treatment

MR
4 vs 5

M
Total treatment

MR
1 2 3 4 5

Fig. 6-133 Patient M.R. **A,** At initial examination. The primary canines have been extracted. **B,** After extraction of the primary first molars. **C,** Before extraction. **D,** Following extraction of the first premolars. **E,** During emergence of the permanent canines and exfoliation of the primary second molars. **F,** During emergence of the seconds premolars. **G,** Before, and **H,** Following multibanded treatment. **I,** Two years after retention. **J,** Fifteen years after treatment (lateral and anterior view). **K,** Response during interceptive guidance. **L,** Considerably less of response during edgewise treatment. **M,** Response as indicated by the five cephalometric tracings *(1, 2, 3, 4, 5)* that were taken at each step in the treatment: *(1)* Before treatment; *(2)* After the extraction of the primary canine; *(3)* After the extraction of the primary first molars; *(4)* After the extraction of the first premolars; and *(5)* After the edgewise treatment.

Fig. 6-134 Facial appearance of patient M.R. **A** and **B,** Before, and **C** and **D,** following serial extraction. **E** and **F,** After the multibanded treatment. *Continued.*

G   H   I

Fig. 6-134, cont'd   **G, H,** and **I,** Fifteen years after treatment.

for 3° during the serial extraction period and for one more degree during the active period of treatment. Throughout total treatment the A-N-B was reduced from 3° to 1°, indicating a modest improvement in the jaw relationship (Fig. 6-135).

It was important in *M.R.'s* case that the tooth-size jaw-size discrepancy not be corrected by extension of the teeth posteriorly, anteriorly, laterally, or vertically. If this had been done in such a relatively high angle facial pattern, the molar extrusion would have resulted in an unfavorable downward and backward rotation of the mandible. With extrusion of the molars and the *dumping* forward of the incisors, the occlusal plane would have been tipped unfavorably and the alveolodental protrusion worsened. With the mandibular rotation and the tipped occlusal plane the maxillary incisor would have been rabbited downward and backward, revealing more gingival tissue. Concomitantly the posterior molars would have been impacted; the dental arches would have been expanded; the mandibular incisors would have been tipped off basal bone, creating an unstable situation that required prolonged retention; and the harmony and balance of the facial profile would have been worsened considerably.

The total space analysis indicated an anterior and posterior space discrepancy (Table 6-6). The anterior discrepancy was corrected by serial extraction and extraction of the permanent first premolars. The posterior discrepancy was corrected by extraction of the permanent third molars.

Often high angle facial patterns are associated with an open bite relationship of the anterior teeth. To preface the discussion of this type of Class I malocclusion, the characteristic features of a true hereditary open bite malocclusion as described by Subtelny[62] will now be outlined:

1. An excessively steep mandibular plane angle or a high angle facial configuration

2. A retrognathic mandible relative to cranial base
3. A significantly greater anterior vertical dimension of the skeletal face, especially in the lower portion
4. A maxillary mandibular alveolodental protrusion
5. A relatively short ramus height
6. A relatively large gonial angle
7. A relative overeruption of the maxillary molars and incisor teeth (this is an extremely important observation and must be considered when planning treatment)
8. A relatively shorter posterior cranial base
9. A relatively obtuse angle between the posterior and anterior cranial bases
10. A relatively distal maxillary alveolar process in relation to the anterior cranial base

A word of caution is important relative to Subtelny's remarks with regard to the overeruption of the maxillary molars, which contributes to the open bite relationship. It is quite possible that extraction of the permanent molars would be preferable to extraction of the premolars in an attempt to correct this malocclusion. Molar extraction has the same effect as molar intrusion: it encourages the mandible to rotate up and forward, which, in turn, reduces the steep mandibular plane angle, the long lower anterior face height, the retrognathism of the mandible, and the anterior open bite.

A typical example of the treatment plan preferred for the severe high angle Class I discrepancy malocclusion is illustrated in the case of *patient J.L.* (Fig. 6-136). Before treatment the patient's cephalometric analysis indicated that he had an FMA of a whopping 47°. Throughout the course of multibonded treatment, which followed extraction of the permanent first molars, this angle was reduced to 43°—indicating a favorable upward and forward rotation of the mandible. His IMPA before treatment was 68° and his FMIA

FMA	31°
IMPA	91°
FMIA	58°
OP	13°
Z	57°
SNA	78°
SNB	75°
ANB	3°

FMA	27°
IMPA	88°
FMIA	65°
OP	8°
Z	71°
SNA	80°
SNB	78°
ANB	2°

FMA	25°
IMPA	86°
FMIA	69°
OP	7°
Z	75°
SNA	80°
SNB	79°
ANB	1°

Fig. 6-135   Cephalometric analyses of patient M.R. **A,** Before serial extraction. **B,** Following serial extraction. **C,** Following multibanded treatment.

65°. Both these figures denote that the mandibular incisors had a favorable axial inclination. In addition, the alignment of these teeth was favorable as indicated by the study models. The S-N-A was 75°, the S-N-B, 73°, and the A-N-B, 2°. This implies that the maxilla was well related to the mandible but that both were in a retrognathic position. The OP angle was steep, and the Z angle was small. Throughout treatment the mandibular incisors were maintained in a favorable relationship as indicated by the IMPA. The S-N-A remained constant but the S-N-B increased by 2°, suggesting a favorable forward rotation of the mandible. It has been said that an extremely high angle facial pattern is a potential Class III malocclusion. This statement is substantiated by the reduction of the A-N-B from 2° to 0° during treatment.

Throughout the first year of mechanotherapy, no attachments were placed on the mandibular dentition. The mandibular molars were allowed to drift mesially. As a result the mandible rotated favorably, and the occlusal plane angle was reduced from 17° to 13°. This further improved the Z angle and the soft tissue profile.

Fig. 6-136   Patient J.L. Facial configuration before, **A** and **B,** and after, **C** and **D,** treatment. Study models of the dentition before, **E,** and after, **F,** treatment.   *Continued.*

FMA	47
IMPA	68
FMIA	65
OP	17
Z	60
SNA	75
SNB	73
ANB	2

Fig. 6-136, cont'd   Cephalometric analyses before, **G**, and after, **H**, treatment.

FMA	43
IMPA	68
FMIA	69
OP	13
Z	73
SNA	75
SNB	75
ANB	0

The favorable axial inclination and alignment of the mandibular incisors was reflected in a 0 mm deficit in the anterior arch area of the total space analysis. The 16 mm deficit in the middle area reflected a mesial migration of the mandibular molars, causing a crowded condition of the premolar teeth. The deficit of 9 mm in the posterior arch area reflected a severe high angle configuration. The total deficit of 25 mm, which was primarily toward the posterior area, was relieved by extraction of the permanent first molars. To bring about a more favorable relationship, the mandibular curve of occlusion was not completely leveled (Table 6-6).

CLASS II TREATMENT

Serial extraction can be an important part of Class II treatment; however, if extreme caution is not exercised, the malocclusion can be aggravated. The orthodontist should always inform the parents that appliances will be required to treat the Class II discrepancy when all the permanent teeth have emerged. Again, it must be stressed, that serial extraction does not replace mechanotherapy, particularly in Class II malocclusions. Nevertheless, in a rewarding number of instances, it does reduce it significantly at the *difficult* age of adolescence.

Treatment procedure B—interceptive treatment, interceptive guidance, active treatment

Initial period of interceptive treatment. During this period, which may extend 1 to 1½ years, the primary first molars and maxillary first premolars are extracted as early as possible. This provides space for retraction of the permanent maxillary anterior teeth. Appliances are placed on the four permanent maxillary incisors and first molars and on the primary second molars. With a maxillary edgewise arch and an anterior high pull headgear, the maxillary incisors are retracted, intruded, and torqued. This reduces the overjet and overbite.

The primary objective of the initial period of interceptive treatment is to decrease the vulnerability of and possible injury to the maxillary incisors. In the mandible the primary canines are extracted to relieve the permanent incisor crowding. Later the primary first molars and the premolars are extracted. To prevent collapse of the mandibular incisors and accentuation of the curve of occlusion, appliances are placed on the permanent incisors and first molars and on the primary second molars. Progress is made from round leveling arches to ideal edgewise arches.

In the interceptive phase, the method of treatment used to correct a Class II malocclusion is determined by the type of Class II. It can be seen from the proportional facial analysis that there are several types. With this analysis and with the total space analysis, the treatment of Class II malocclusions may involve nonextraction or one of the following series of extractions: (1) maxillary first premolars, (2) four first premolars, (3) maxillary first premolars and mandibular second premolars, (4) permanent maxillary first molars and mandibular third molars, (5) permanent maxillary second molars and mandibular third molars, (6) third molars, (7) four premolars plus permanent maxillary first molars and mandibular third molars, (8) four premolars plus permanent maxillary second molars and mandibular third molars, or (9) four first premolars and four third molars. Or jaw surgery may be performed. Since serial extraction usually culminates in the extraction of the first premolars, it is obvious from this list that it is not indicated in the treatment of all Class II malocclusions.

Period of interceptive guidance. During this period retention appliances are worn and serial extraction is continued. The parents are informed that appointments will be required every 3 months for assessment of growth and development with the aid of diagnostic records and that teeth will be extracted periodically as indicated.

Second period of active treatment. When all the permanent teeth have emerged, a multibonded appliance is placed and the Class II is corrected, adhering to the principles of Tweed edgewise mechanotherapy.

Patient J.O. (Figs. 6-137 through 6-139) is a good example of a Class II malocclusion treated by serial extraction and edgewise mechanotherapy.

A relatively high angle facial pattern, a prognathic maxilla and retrognathic mandible, a skeletal discrepancy, and a maxillary mandibular alveolodental protrusion with open bite relationship of the anterior teeth are present.

Fig. 6-137, *A,* illustrates the malocclusion before serial extraction. Note the Class II intercuspation of the molars and the open bite relationship of the anterior teeth. *B* shows the dental relationship after serial extraction and before multibonded appliance therapy. Significant improvement has been made in both the incisor and the molar relationships. To this point no mechanotherapy has been used. *C* shows the complete multibonded appliance with edgewise arches during final space closure. *D* shows the final occlusion after treatment, and *E* and *F,* the 2-year appearance.

The soft tissue profile and facial appearance before and after serial extraction, and after treatment, are illustrated in Fig. 6-138. Note the prognathic maxilla, retrognathic mandible, and moderately high angle facial pattern before serial extraction. Improvement may be seen as treatment progresses, particularly in the mandible and in the smile.

Before serial extraction the FMA was 32°, indicating a relatively high angle facial pattern; this improved to 30° during serial extraction and to 29° during active treatment. Reduction in the FMA suggests a favorable upward and forward rotation of the mandible. During serial extraction the IMPA was reduced 5° (from 96° to 91°) and the FMIA increased 6° (from 53° to 59°), both signifying a reduction in the alveolodental protrusion and an uprighting of the mandibular incisors. Further improvement took place during active treatment, with the IMPA decreasing to 89° and the FMIA to 62°. Throughout treatment the skeletal discrepancy improved: A-N-B was reduced from 9° to 3°; the maxilla became less prognathic (from 86° to 82°); and the mandible became less retrognathic (from 77° to 79°). The occlusal plane remained fairly constant, indicating good control throughout treatment. The Z angle increased from 64° to 76°, denoting improvement in the facial harmony and balance (Fig. 6-139).

In the total space analysis the anterior arch area had a deficit of 15.4 mm. Two thirds of this was cephalometric correction, indicating an alveolodental protrusion. The middle arch area had a surplus of 1.5 mm, and the posterior arch area a deficit of 15.0 mm. The anterior deficit was corrected by extraction of four first premolars, and the posterior deficit was corrected by extraction of the four third molars (Table 6-6).

Mechanotherapy

The treatment objectives after the serial extraction phase are (1) closure of residual extraction spaces, (2) improvement of the axial inclination of individual teeth, (3) correction of rotations, (4) correction of midline discrepancy, (5) correction of a residual overbite, (6) correction of a residual overjet, (7) correction of crossbites, (8) refinement of the intercuspation of individual teeth, (9) improvement and coordination of arch form, and (10) correction of the Class II relationship in some Class II patients.

When the serial extraction phase has been completed, the

Fig. 6-137 Patient J.O. **A,** Before, and **B,** following serial extraction. **C,** Final stage of over-treatment. **D,** End of treatment. **E** and **F,** Two years after retention. **G** and **H,** Seven years after retention. Note chipped enamel on the maxillary incisors, caused by a blow while playing football without a mouth guard.

A, B, C

D, E, F

G   H

Fig. 6-138   Facial configuration of patient J.O. **A** and **B,** Before, and **C** and **D,** after serial extraction. **E** and **F,** Following active treatment. **G** and **H,** Seven years after treatment.

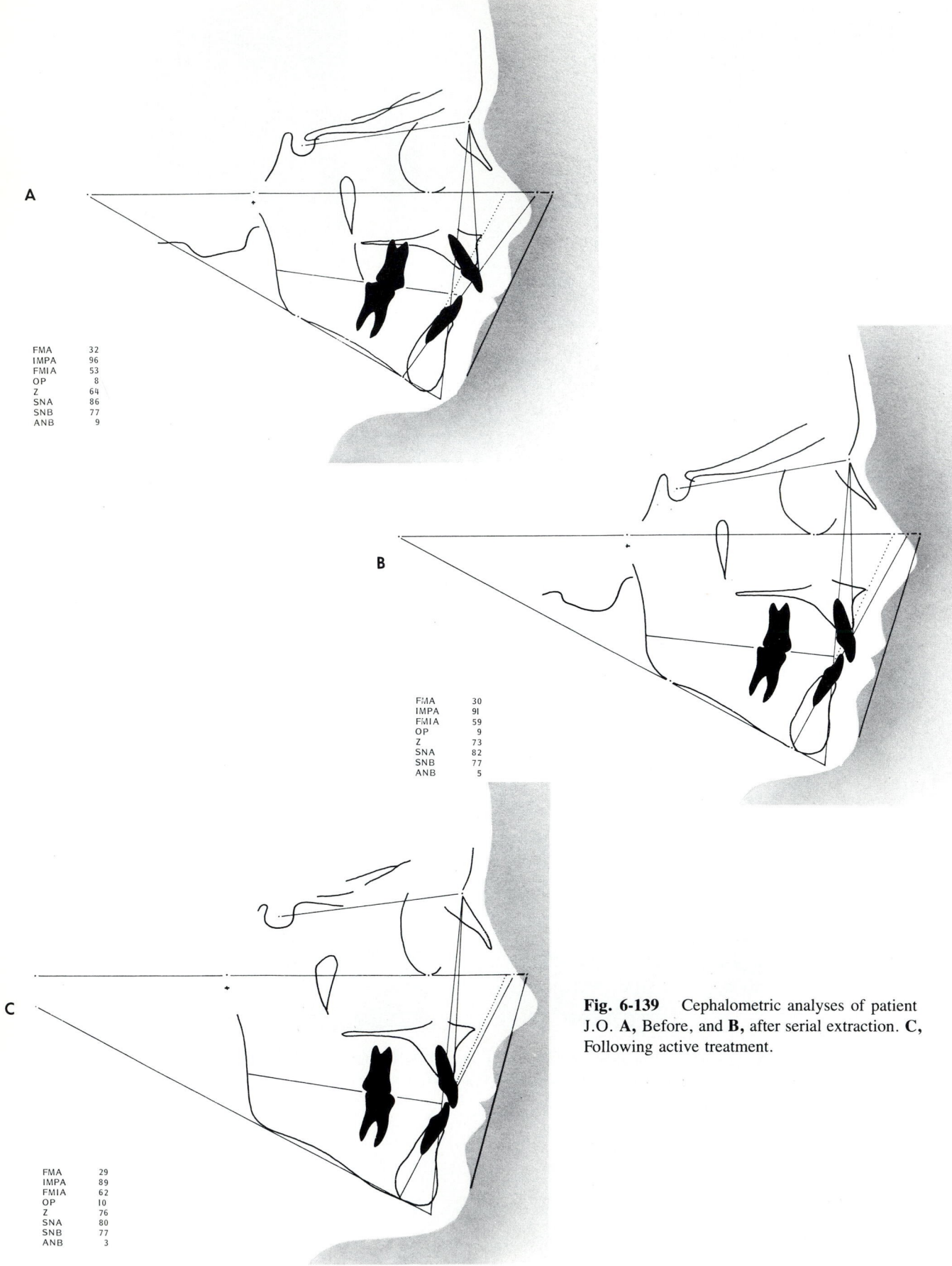

A	
FMA	32
IMPA	96
FMIA	53
OP	8
Z	64
SNA	86
SNB	77
ANB	9

B	
FMA	30
IMPA	9I
FMIA	59
OP	9
Z	73
SNA	82
SNB	77
ANB	5

C	
FMA	29
IMPA	89
FMIA	62
OP	I0
Z	76
SNA	80
SNB	77
ANB	3

Fig. 6-139   Cephalometric analyses of patient J.O. **A,** Before, and **B,** after serial extraction. **C,** Following active treatment.

multibonded appliance is placed and treatment is initiated using the traditional concepts of the Tweed philosophy. The modern concepts of The Charles H. Tweed International Foundation for Orthodontic Research can be summarized as follows[44,46] (see Chapter 11):

Directional force systems

10-2 Anchorage

Readout

Prescription arches

Performance testing

Dr. Tweed's primary objectives in treatment included a healthy dentition, stability, optimal function, healthy supporting tissues and optimal facial esthetics. These are excellent treatment goals; nevertheless, they are too general:

The *directional force* technique is a group of force systems using directional control to position the teeth precisely in both the maxilla and the mandible so they will be in optimum harmony with their environment.

The *10-2* concept is a sequential anchorage system wherein the archwire stabilizes 10 teeth while 2 teeth receive the active force. Instead of 12 teeth being involved in the anchorage preparation at one time, only 2 are receiving active force. The sequence begins with the second molars and is completed with the second premolars. When this type of improved anchorage preparation is used, there is less risk that the dentition will move unfavorably downward and forward and patient cooperation is not as crucial.

With *readout* the objectives of orthodontic treatment can be defined by accurate measurement. Tooth movements can be predetermined, monitored during treatment, and checked for accuracy of final placement.

Prescription arches include the tabulation of second-order angulation associated with *10-2 anchorage* and *readout*. They also permit the precise measurement and tabulation of buccolinguoaxial inclinations of teeth so third-order bends can be incorporated in the archwire. Finally, they include the horizontal first-order bends. These prescription arches are designed specifically for individual malocclusions.

Performance testing is a relatively recent development that involves the serial measurement of tooth movement and dental relationships so treatment progress can be evaluated. This particular edgewise appliance, originally designed by Tweed and modified by Merrifield and his associates, is the precision instrument used in achieving treatment goals. It is characterized by simplicity, efficiency, and comfort; it is hygienic and esthetic; and, above all, it has a wide range of versatility.

When the appliance is removed and retainers are placed—a critical stage in the correction of the malocclusion occurs. This is referred to as the *period of recovery*. If the corrective procedures barely achieve the normal relationship of teeth, there will be an inevitable relapse. Any change that occurs will be away from ideal occlusion. However, if treatment is completed by overcorrection, all changes that take place

Fig. 6-140   The smile that makes it all worthwhile.

during the recovery period will be toward the ideal relationship. This provides the ideal circumstances for obtaining the original objectives: health of the dentition and the supporting structures, optimal function, stability, and beautiful facial esthetics (Fig. 6-140).

When facial deformity has been corrected and mental anguish eliminated, a dull and unhappy facial expression becomes bright and happy. What greater reward could any orthodontist want or expect.

Charles H. Tweed

I would add . . . the earlier this occurs the better.

REFERENCES

1. American Board of Orthodontics: *Specific instructions for candidates,* St Louis, 1993, American Board of Orthodontics.
2. Angle EH: *Malocclusion of the teeth,* ed 7, Philadelphia, 1907, SS White Dental.
3. Arita M, Iwagaki H: *Studies on the serial observations of dento-facial region in the Japanese children,* Tokyo, 1963, Nihon University School of Dentistry.
4. Baker C: Development of the occlusion of the teeth, *J Am Dent Assoc* 31:1470, 1944.
5. Baume LJ: Physiological tooth migration and its significance for the development of occlusion. I. The biogenetic course of the deciduous teeth, *J Dent Res* 29:123, 1950.
6. Baume LJ: Physiological tooth migration and its significance for the development of occlusion. II. The biogenesis of accessional dentition, *J Dent Res* 29:331, 1950.
7. Baume LJ: Physiological tooth migration and its significance for the development of occlusion. III. The biogenesis of the successional dentition, *J Dent Res* 29:338, 1950.
8. Baume LJ: Physiological tooth migration and its significance for the development of occlusion. IV. The biogenesis of overbite, *J Dent Res* 29:440, 1950.
9. Baume LJ: Developmental and diagnostic aspects of the primary dentition. *Int Dent J* 9:349, 1959.
10. Bilkey ER: Is there writing on the wall? [Editorial.] *Oral Health* 71:4, 1981.

11. Björk A: Variations in the growth pattern of the human mandible; longitudinal radiographic study by the implant method, *J Dent Res* 42:400, 1963.
12. Black GV: *Descriptive anatomy of the human teeth*, ed 5, Philadelphia, 1902, SS White Dental.
13. Brodie A: Late growth changes in the human face, *Angle Orthod* 23:146, 1953.
14. Bunon R: *Essay sur les maladies des dents; ou I'on propose les moyens de leur procurer une bonne confirmation dès la plus tendre enfance, et d'en assurer la conservation pendant tout le cours de la vie*, Paris, 1743.
15. Burlington Orthodontic Research Project, University of Toronto, Faculty of Dentistry, Report no 3, 1957.
16. Dale JG, Rushton JS et al: *A half century of care, a future of caring*, Tucson, Ariz, 1982, The Charles H. Tweed International Foundation.
17. DeKock WJ: Dental arch depth and width studies longitudinally from 12 years of age to adulthood, *Am J Orthod* 62:56, 1972.
18. Delabarre CF: *Traité de la second dentition et méthode naturelle de la diriger suivis d'un apercu de séméiotique buccale*, Paris, 1918.
19. Enlow DH: *The human face; an account of the postnatal growth and development of the craniofacial skeleton*, New York, 1968, Paul B Hoeber.
20. Enlow DH: *Handbook of facial growth*, ed 2, Philadelphia, 1982, WB Saunders.
21. Fanning EA: Effect of extraction of deciduous molars on the formation and eruption of their successors, *Angle Orthod* 32:44, 1962.
22. Fanning EA: Longitudinal study of tooth formation and root resorption, *NZ Dent J* 57:202, 1961.
23. Fanning EA, Hunt EE: Linear increments of growth in the roots of permanent mandibular teeth, *J Dent Res* 43(suppl):981, 1964.
24. Franke G: *Ueber Wachstum und Verbildungen des Kiefers und der Nasenscheidewand auf grund vergleichender Kiefer-messungen und experimenteller Untersuchungen über Knochenwachstum*, Leipzig, 1921, Curt Kabitzsch.
25. Garcia-Hernandez J, Dale JG: "Facial considerations in mixed-dentition analysis in preparation for guidance of occlusion." Postgraduate Thesis, Department of Paedodontics, University of Toronto, Faculty of Dentistry, 1979.
26. Garn SM, Lewis AB: The gradient and the pattern of crown-size reduction in simple hypodontia, *Angle Orthod* 40:51, 1970.
27. Grøn AM: Prediction of tooth emergence, *J Dent Res* 41:573, 1962.
28. Hixon EH, Oldfather RE: Estimation of the sizes of unerupted cuspid and bicuspid teeth, *Angle Orthod* 28:236, 1958.
29. Horowitz SL, Hixon EH: *The nature of orthodontic diagnosis*, St Louis, 1966, Mosby, Chapter 16.
30. Hotz R: Guidance of eruption versus serial extraction, *Am J Orthod* 58:1, 1970.
31. Huckaba GW: Arch size analysis and tooth size prediction, *Dent Clin North Am* p 431, 1964.
32. Hurme VO: Ranges in normalcy in eruption of permanent teeth, *J Dent Child* 16:11, 1949.
33. Jacobi A: Course of lectures on dentition and its derangements, *Am Med Times* 1:416, 1860.
34. Kjellgren B: Serial extraction as a corrective procedure in dental orthopedic therapy, *Eur Orthod Soc Trans* p. 134, 1947-1948.
35. Lebret L: Personal communications.
36. Lewis SM, Lehman IA: A quantitative study of the relation between certain factors in the development of the dental arch and the occlusion of the teeth, *Int J Orthod* 18:1015, 1932.
37. Lo RT, Moyers RE: Studies in the etiology and prevention of malocclusion. I. The sequence of eruption of the permanent dentition, *Am J Orthod* 39:460, 1953.
38. Lundt RC, Law DB: A review of the chronology of calcification of deciduous teeth, *J Am Dent Assoc* 89:599, 1974.
39. Mayne WR: *Serial extraction*. In Graber TM, editor: *Current orthodontic concepts and techniques*, Philadelphia, 1969, WB Saunders, Chapter 4.
40. McNamara J: Components of Class II malocclusion in children 8-10 years of age, *Angle Orthod* 51:177, 1981.
41. Meredith HV: Order and age of eruption for the deciduous dentition, *J Dent Res* 25:43, 1946.
42. Meredith HV, Knott V: *Childhood changes of head, face, and dentition—a collection of research reports*, Iowa City, 1973, Iowa Orthodontic Society.
43. Merrifield LL: The profile line as an aid in critically evaluating facial esthetics, *Am J Orthod* 52:804, 1966.
44. Merrifield LL: Differential diagnosis with total space analysis, *J Charles H Tweed Int Found* 6:10, 1978.
45. Harris GS: Graphic display of total space analysis, *J Tweed Foundation* 13:128-152, 1985.
46. Merrifield LL: The systems of directional force, *J Charles H Tweed Int Found* 10:15, 1982.
47. Moorrees CFA: Growth changes of the dental arches—a longitudinal study, *J Can Dent Assoc* 24:449, 1958.
48. Moorrees CFA: *The dentition of the growing child; a longitudinal study of dental development between 3 and 18 years of age*, Cambridge, Mass, 1959, Harvard University Press.
49. Moorrees CFA: Dental development—a growth study based on tooth eruption as a measure of physiologic age, *Eur Orthod Soc Trans* 40:92, 1964.
50. Moorrees CFA: Changes in dental arch dimensions expressed on the basis of tooth eruption as a measure of biologic age, *J Dent Res* 44:129, 1965.
51. Moorrees CFA: Normal variation in dental development determined with reference to tooth eruption statistics, *J Dent Res* 44:161, 1965.
52. Moorrees CFA, Chadha JM: Crown diameters of corresponding tooth groups in deciduous and permanent dentition, *J Dent Res* 41:466, 1962.
53. Moorrees CFA, Chadha JM: Available space for the incisors during dental development; a growth study based on physiological age, *Angle Orthod* 35:12, 1965.
54. Moorrees CFA, Kent RL Jr: *Patterns of dental maturation*. In McNamara JA editor: *The biology of occlusal development, Monograph 6, Craniofacial growth series*, Ann Arbor, 1978, Center for Human Growth and Development, University of Michigan.
55. Moorrees CFA, Kent RL Jr: A step function model using tooth counts to assess the developmental timing of the dentition, *Ann Hum Biol* 5:55, 1978.
56. Moorrees CFA, Thomsen S et al: Mesiodistal crown diameters of the deciduous and permanent teeth in individuals, *J Dent Res* 36:39, 1957.
57. Robinow M, Richards TW, Anderson M: The eruption of deciduous teeth, *Growth* 6:127, 1942.
58. Schudy FF: The rotation of the mandible resulting from growth; its implications in orthodontic treatment, *Angle Orthod* 35:36, 1965.
59. Sillman JH: Dimensional changes of the dental arches; longitudinal study from birth to 24 years, *Am J Orthod* 50:824, 1964.
60. Steiner C: Cephalometrics in clinical practice, *Angle Orthod* 29:8, 1959.
61. Stone I: *The origin*, Garden City, NY, 1980, Doubleday.
62. Subtelny JD, Sakuda M: Openbite, diagnosis and treatment, *Am J Orthod* 50:337, 1964.
63. Ten Cate AR, et al: *Oral histology: development, structure, and function*, St Louis, 1980, Mosby.
64. Tweed CH: Treatment planning and therapy in the mixed-dentition, *Am J Orthod* 49:900, 1963.
65. Tweed CH: *Clinical orthodontics*, St Louis, 1966, Mosby.
66. Tweed CH: The diagnostic facial triangle in the control of treatment objectives, *Am J Orthod* 55:651, 1969.
67. Virel A: *Decorated man*, New York, 1980, Harry N. Abrams.
68. Wagers LE: Preorthodontic guidance and the corrective mixed-dentition treatment concept, *Am J Orthod* 69:1, 1976.
69. Zsigmundy O: Ueber die Veränderungen des Zahnbogens bei der zweiten Dentition, *Arch Anat* p 367, 1890.

ADDITIONAL READINGS

Bolton WA: The clinical application of a tooth size analysis, *Am J Orthod* 48:504, 1962.

Clifton OW: Lower first premolar extraction: a viable alternative? *Am J Orthod Dentofac Orthop* 90(2):158-163, 1986.

Dale J: J.C.O. interviews: Dr. Jack G. Dale on serial extraction, *J Clin Orthod* 10:44, 116, 196, 1976.

Dewel BF: Serial extractions in orthodontics; indications, objections, and treatment procedures, *Int J Orthod* 40:906, 1954.

Dewel BF: A critical analysis of serial extraction in orthodontic treatment, *Am J Orthod* 45:424, 1959.

Dewel BF: Serial extraction, its limitations and contraindications in orthodontic treatment, *Am J Orthod* 53:904, 1967.

Dibbets JM et al: Long-term effects of orthodontic treatment, including extraction, on signs and symptoms attributed to CMD, *Eur J Orthod* 14(1):16-20, 1992.

Garfinkle RL, Artese A et al: Effect of extraction in the late mixed-dentition on the eruption of the first premolar in Macaca nemestrina, *Angle Orthod* 50:23, 1980.

Gianelly AA et al: Condylar position and extraction treatment, *Am J Orthod Dentofac Orthop* 93(3):201-205, 1988.

Gianelly AA et al: Longitudinal evaluation of condylar position in extraction and nonextraction treatment, *Am J Orthod Dentofac Orthop* 100(5):416-420, 1991.

Gilmore CA et al: Mandibular incisor dimensions and crowding, *Am J Orthod* 86(6):493-502, 1984.

Greer GW, Artese A et al: Effect of extraction in the early mixed-dentition on the eruption of the first premolar in Macaca pemestrina, *Angle Orthod* 50:34, 1980.

Hägg U, Taranger J: Maturation indicators and the pubertal growth spurt, *Am J Orthod* 82:299, 1982.

Heath J: The interception of malocclusion by planned serial extraction, *N Z Dent J* 49:77, 1953.

Heath J: Dangers and pitfalls of serial extraction, *Eur Orthod Soc Trans* 37:60, 1961.

Hotz R: Active supervision of the eruption of teeth by extraction, *Eur Orthod Soc Trans* p. 34, 1947-1948.

Jacobs SG: A re-assessment of serial extraction, *Aust Orthod J* 10(2):90-97 (15 ref), 1987.

Jegou I: Indication and limits on the choice of extraction of 14-24 and 35-45 in treating Angle class-II malocclusion by a Tweed-Merrifield analysis of the total space, *Orthod Fr* 55(2):485-494, 1984.

Jones O et al: Orthodontic management of a patient with Class I malocclusion and severe crowding, *Am J Orthod Dentofac Orthop* 98(3):189-196, 1990.

Klapper L et al: The influence of extraction and nonextraction orthodontic treatment on brachyfacial and dolichofacial growth patterns, *Am J Orthod Dentofac Orthop* 101(5):425-430, 1992.

Krogman WM: Biological timing and dento-facial complex, *J Dent Child* 35:175, 328, 377, 1968.

Leighton BC, Hunter WS: Relationship between lower arch spacing/crowding and facial height and depth, *Angle Orthod* 82:418, 1982.

Little, R.M.: The effects of eruption guidance and serial extraction on developing dentition, *Pediatr Dent* 9(1):65-70, 1987.

Little RM, Riedel RA, Årtun J: An evaluation of changes in mandibular anterior alignment from 10-20 years post retention, *Am J Orthod Dentofac Orthop* 93:423-428, 1988.

Little RM, Waller TR, Riedel RA: Stability and relapse of mandibular anterior alignment—first premolar extraction cases treated by traditional edgewise orthodontics, *Am J Orthod* 80:349-365, 1981.

Little RM et al: Serial extraction of first premolars—postretention evaluation of stability and relapse, *Angle Orthod* 60(4):255-262, 1990.

Lloyd ZB: Serial extraction as a treatment procedure, *Am J Orthod* 42:728, 1956.

McNamara JA, Brudon WL: *Orthodontic and orthopedic treatment in the mixed dentition,* ed 1, Ann Arbor, 1993, Needham Press.

McReynolds DC et al: Mandibular second premolar extraction—postretention evaluation of stability and relapse, *Angle Orthod* 6(2):133-144, 1991.

Moorrees CFA: Variability of dental and facial development, *Ann NY Acad Sci* 134:846, 1966.

Moorrees CFA, Fanning EA, Grøn AM: Consideration of dental development in serial extraction, *Angle Orthod* 33:44, 1963.

Moorrees CFA, Fanning EA, Grøn AM, Lebret J: Timing of orthodontic treatment in relation to tooth formation, *Eur Orthod Soc Trans* 38:87, 1962.

Moorrees CFA, Fanning EA, Hunt EE Jr: Age variation of formation stages for ten permanent teeth, *J Dent Res* 42:1490, 1963.

Moorrees CFA, Fanning EA, Hunt EE Jr: Formation and resorption of three deciduous teeth in children, *Am J Phys Anthropol* 21:99, 1963.

Moorrees CFA, Reed RB: Biometrics of crowding and spacing of the teeth in the mandible, *Am J Phys Anthropol* 12:77, 1954.

Moorrees CFA, Reed RB: Correlations among crown diameters of human teeth, *Arch Oral Biol* 9:685, 1964.

Moorrees CFA, Reed RB, Chadha JM: Growth changes of the dentition defined in terms of chronologic and biologic age, *Am J Orthod* 50:789, 1964.

Ortial JP: The Tweed technic. Choice of extraction and treatment strategy. I. *Attual Dent* 3(16):10-1, 13-5, 17-21 *passim,* 1987.

Renfoe EW: The philosophy of extraction in orthodontics: 1966 (classified article), *Int J Orthod* 27(1-2):3-8, 1989.

Richardson ME: Late lower arch crowding in relation to primary crowding, *Angle Orthod* 52:300, 1982.

Richardson ME: The effect of mandibular first premolar extraction on third molar space, *Angle Orthod* 59(4):291-294, 1989.

Sanin C, Savara B, Sekiguchi T: Longitudinal dentofacial changes in untreated persons, *Am J Orthod* 55:135, 1969.

Tanner JM: *Growth at adolescence,* ed 2, Cambridge, Mass, 1962, Blackwell Scientific Publications.

Toshniwal NG: A review of serial extraction, *J Indian Dent Assoc* 61(12):291-293, 1990.

Tweed CH: The Frankfort-mandibular plane angle in orthodontic diagnosis, classification, treatment planning, and prognosis, *Am J Orthod Oral Surg* 32:175, 1946.

Tweed CH: The Frankfort-mandibular incisor angle in orthodontic diagnosis treatment planning and prognosis, *Angle Orthod* 24:121, 1954.

Tweed CH: *Pre-orthodontic guidance procedure, classification of facial growth trends, treatment timing.* In Kraus BS, Reidel RA, editors: *Vistas in orthodontics,* Philadelphia, 1962, Lea & Febiger, Chapter 8.

Yamaguchi K et al: The effects of extraction and nonextraction treatment on the mandibular position, *Am J Orthod Dentofac Orthop* 100(5):443-452, 1991.

SECTION II

Techniques and Treatment

CHAPTER 7

Functional Appliances

THOMAS M. GRABER

THE ANDRESEN ACTIVATOR

Origin. Theories on bone plasticity may be traced back to Roux[165] and Wolff,[213] who believed that form was intimately related to function. Changes in functional stresses produced changes in internal bone architecture and external shape. Although Robin[164] introduced a *monobloc* early in the twentieth century, which effectively postured the mandible forward, it was not intended to effect structural change or guide jaw growth. Rather, it was used as a passive positioning device in neonates with micromandible and cleft lip and palate (later referred to as the Pierre Robin syndrome) to prevent glossoptosis, or literally swallowing of the tongue. For Viggo Andresen,[7] however, who was unaware of the Robin appliance, the possible effect of function on bone shape, size, and position offered hope in correcting sagittal malrelationships, primarily Class II, division 1 malocclusions, in the growing child, by changing the functional pattern of the stomatognathic system. The working hypothesis was tested on his daughter, who went away to camp during the summer. Andresen removed the fixed labiolingual appliances and placed a modified Hawley-type retainer on the maxillary arch, but he added a lower lingual horseshoe flange that guided the mandible forward some 3 to 4 mm when the teeth were brought into maximum interarch contact (Fig. 7-1). This was done to prevent any relapse over the 3-month vacation period.[7] On his daughter's return from camp, Andresen was pleasantly surprised to see that the nighttime wearing of the appliance had produced a complete sagittal correction and a significantly improved facial profile. The result was stable. Trying this on numerous other

patients who were going away for the summer and then on patients under routine care, Andresen observed a significant sagittal basal bone and neuromuscular improvement that he could not produce with conventional fixed appliances.[8,9]

Rationale. The explanation behind the sagittal changes is that the appliance activated or increased the activity of the

Fig. 7-1 Andresen-Häupl activator. No tooth-moving parts. The original appliances were made of Vulcanite. In this appliance, being used to treat a Class II, division 1, malocclusion, the palatal acrylic has been cut out and a heavy Coffin spring laid across the palate for stability. The loops at the canine region stand away from the teeth, allowing maxillary intercanine development. These loops are the forerunner of the Balters Bionator loops, which extended to the distal of the deciduous second molars, holding off cheek pressure—also a forerunner of the Fränkel buccal shields. (From Andresen V, Häupl K: *Funktionskieferorthopädie. Die Grundlagen des "norwegischen Systems,"* ed 2, Leipzig, 1939, H. Meusser.)

Special credit is given to the late Professor Olav Slagsvold and to WB Saunders Company for permission to use some of the illustrations and factual material from *Activator development and philosophy*, in Graber TM, and Neumann B: *Removable orthodontic appliances*, ed 1, Philadelphia, 1977, WB Saunders.

Fig. 7-2   Construction bite. Correcting the buccal segment relationship from Class II to Class I, or approximately a 6 mm advancement. Note that the overjet is still excessive in this case, probably because of labial malposition of the upper incisor segment. This would be corrected after the sagittal relationship was normalized. There is a 3 to 4 mm vertical opening to allow the mandible to come forward sufficiently to correct the anteroposterior buccal intercuspation. (From Andresen V, Häupl K: *Funktionskieferorthopädie. Die Grundlagen des "norwegischen Systems,"* ed 2, Leipzig, 1939, H. Meusser.)

protractor and elevator muscles, with concomitant relaxation and stretching of the retractors. Eliminating the abnormal perioral muscle function by mandibular protraction prevented deforming and restrictive action by the lower lip trap and hyperactivity of the mentalis and the submandibular muscle groups (Figs. 7-2 and 7-3). The change in muscle pattern thus would produce not only a new and more favorable muscle pattern but also a change in bony structures as they adapted to the new functional stresses[8] (Fig. 7-4). The intermittent forces produced by the loose appliance were thought to create favorable tooth position changes, even though the appliance was worn only at night. Like Robin's monobloc, the appliance used by Andresen was passive, with no intrinsic force systems.[8-10] The extrinsic force came from the loose appliance's stimulating the elevators and protractors to contract as the patient bit into the appliance. It was hypothesized that growth increments were greater at night, providing optimal tissue response.

The original name used by Andresen for this type of treatment was biomechanical orthodontics, and only later after further work on the concepts and technique refinements with Karl Häupl was it changed to *functional jaw orthopedics,* which was more descriptive.[11-13] The concepts were broadened to include the potential of altering skeletal relationships, depending on the amount and direction of jaw growth. The forward posturing of the construction bite activated the muscles, which in turn enhanced a sagittal skeletal change, harnessing the growth potential—hence the functional orthopedic connotation. To much of the orthodontic world, however, it became known as *the Norwegian system,* despite the fact that Andresen was a Dane and Häupl a German (both were teaching at the dental school in Oslo, Norway).

THE BITE-OPENING CONTROVERSY

Whereas the sagittal construction bite advancement concept was generally accepted by most clinicians in Europe (it varied from 3 to 6 mm, depending on the severity of the anteroposterior malrelationship and resultant abnormal buc-

Fig. 7-3   Lateral view of study models of severe Class II, division 1, malocclusion (Fig. 7-2) shown in habitual occlusion and in a proper construction bite. In this case the lingual inclination of the lower incisor segment is a favorable characteristic, as is the deeper than normal overbite, improving the treatment prognosis. (From Andresen V, Häupl K: *Funktionskieferorthopädie. Die Grundlagen des "norwegischen Systems,"* Leipzig, 1942, J.A. Barth.)

cal segment interdigitation), the functional jaw orthopedic concepts elicited considerable controversy, even among Norwegian orthodontists, over the amount of vertical opening and the effect produced by the appliance on the muscles. Selmer-Olsen,[176] who became professor of orthodontics at the University of Oslo after World War II, felt that muscles could not actually be stimulated or activated during sleep, since Nature had designed them to rest at night and swallowing took place only 4 to 8 times an hour. He interpreted the activator action as a stretching of the muscles, fascial sheets, and ligaments when the mandible was opened beyond postural resting position. The activator was, in truth, a foreign body and the tooth-moving force produced was due not to the kinetic energy of muscle function but to the potential energy of stretched tissues. Woodside[214,215] and Woodside et al.[216] were to refer to this later as the *viscoelastic* properties of the tissue. Current debate on the exact nature of the activator effect still reflects this dichotomy of opinion. Condylar unloading seems to be a factor.

Andresen's interpretation presupposed freedom for the mandible to assume rest position. Slagsvold[179] noted that it did not appear from the literature and his own observations that Andresen considered the degree of mandibular displacement in relation to this position. Nevertheless, it would mean a violation of his principles to displace the mandible beyond it. Andresen had only a 2 mm interocclusal clearance between the upper and lower jaw, or the thickness of a match. Even later when changed to 2 to 4 mm, it would still be within the freeway space limits of most patients, particularly for sleeping individuals.[14] Too wide an opening made compliance more difficult and could introduce potentially depressing action on the posterior teeth.

The Selmer-Olsen, Harvold,[81,82] and Woodside interpretations are based on the fact that in most activators, as modified from the original appliance, the interocclusal separation did, indeed, exceed the postural rest position if for no other reason than to keep the appliance in place at night during sleep to maintain a sagittal corrective stimulus.[158] The cognitive interpretations of Selmer-Olsen were subsequently corroborated by Ahlgren,[1-5] Thompson,[188] Witt,[209,210] Witt and Komposch,[211] and Witt and Meyer.[212]

Rolf Grude,[74,75] an associate and disciple of Andresen, believed that the appliance worked best only if the vertical dimension established did not exceed postural resting position. If it was increased beyond that, the action became fundamentally changed. Fränkel[56] and Fränkel and Reiss[59] concurred in this assessment.

The concepts and explanations of Paul Herren[93,94] had a significant impact on activator use and philosophy. He stated that the traditional nighttime loose-fitting appliance did not work as claimed. (Reitan[161] had already questioned the Roux *shaking of the bone* theory espoused by Andresen and Häupl with his monumental doctoral dissertation on tissue reactions in 1951.) Herren came to the conclusion that the activator did not increase the frequency of closing movements, even if the freeway space was not exceeded. Tooth movement forces thus were not created by nocturnal functional movements stimulated by the activator. The Herren interpretation was as follows:

Various forces acting on the mandible are in equilibrium by virtue of constant adjustments between them. Gravity and air pressure are dominant independent variables, and muscle tonus and tension are dominant dependent variables. When there is a gravity component change or an intraoral air pressure change, the mandible is moved or pulled to a new position wherein the initial changes are compensated for by reactive changes in muscle tension and tonus. Also changes in muscle tonus are compensated for by a change in muscle tension as the mandible tends to relocate. The mandibular position determined by the activator is the desired postural position rather than a momentary rest position that is free of appliance guidance. The activator limits mandibular movement in all planes of space except an opening or vertical movement. When the mandible would normally have a number of rest positions during sleep (depending on body position), the activator tends to prevent it from moving to these positions, splinting the lower jaw

Fig. 7-4   Profile with the jaw in habitual Class II occlusion, **A,** and protracted into Class I sagittal relationship, **B,** A good clinical test for demonstrating the dramatic change possible in the profile.

Fig. 7-5 Various forces acting on the upper and lower arches. In this instance the influence of gravity is quite different when the head is erect, **A,** from what it is when the patient is sleeping with the head turned to one side or the other, **B,** The activator then tends to prevent the normal change or adaptation to varying postural and gravitational forces, which elicits a positive reaction from the buccinator mechanism and the protractor and retractor muscles. Since a patient swallows only four to eight times an hour during sleep, this action would more likely be responsible for the changes produced by the activator. (From Herren P: *Am J Orthod* 45:512, 1959.)

in the desired centric relationship regardless of sleeping posture (Fig. 7-5). The muscle forces that would normally be acting at night to maintain mandibular postural equilibrium with changing body positions are thus transmitted to the appliance, which in turn exerts force on the teeth and alveolar bone, causing the resultant movement. Any mandibular movements that occur are of minor importance.

Head posture during sleep. Since head position changes many times during sleep, the direction of the resultant force on the activator also changes. At any particular moment the rest position depends on head and body posture, so the restriction of muscle movement that would create the desired mandibular position change without the activator in place varies constantly, involving different muscle groups and creating different force vectors on the activator. The plane of sleep (light or deep), the intraoral air pressure, the dream cycle, and the state of mind are additional conditioning factors, all uncontrolled by the orthodontist. Only the mandibular position held by the appliance is determined by the clinician; however, this splinting effect on the mandible is such that it can help predetermine the net effect of the variable forces. If the activator is designed properly and worn as prescribed, the resultant of all the controlled and uncontrolled forces is usually to enhance adaptation to the position created by the appliance (Figs. 7-6 and 7-7).

Herren[93] attempted to assess the magnitude of the resultant forces acting on the mandible, as well as the interaction between them. He pointed out that the weight of the mandible, tongue, and appliance are constant, averaging about 250 g. Muscle tonus and tensions vary, depending on the degree of stretching, the control from the central nervous system, the relation with the bed or pillow, whether the head is prone or supine, etc. If the patient is dorsally recumbent while sleeping and the head is upright, then the muscle forces must balance the weight of the lower jaw, associated soft tissue structures, and appliance. It is clear that the forces

active are entirely different in multiple prone, supine, rotated combinations from what they are in an alert, awakened, upright head posture. Over a prolonged period the duration that a particular position is held and the resultant forces would be factors to consider. The forces created are basically intermittent, however, even though some teeth or groups of teeth may be subject to pressure for a protracted time. The loose appliance is responsible for some of the intermittent action. Removal of the appliance during the day also produces a net intermittent action, calling up a new muscle engram to establish the neuromuscular engram consistent with diurnal postural changes and activities. Hence the same conclusion was reached by Herren as by Selmer-Olsen but with a different basis for reasoning.

Working hypotheses. Thus for the conventional nighttime wear of the passive Andresen activator, there are two working hypotheses as far as the effect on the teeth themselves is concerned:

Fig. 7-6 Instead of the postural alterations evoked by changes in body position, **A,** as shown in Fig. 7-5, the activator splints the jaws in a more normal transverse, sagittal, and vertical relationship when it is worn, **B,** (From Herren P: *Schweiz Monatsschr Zahnheilkd* 63:829, 1953.)

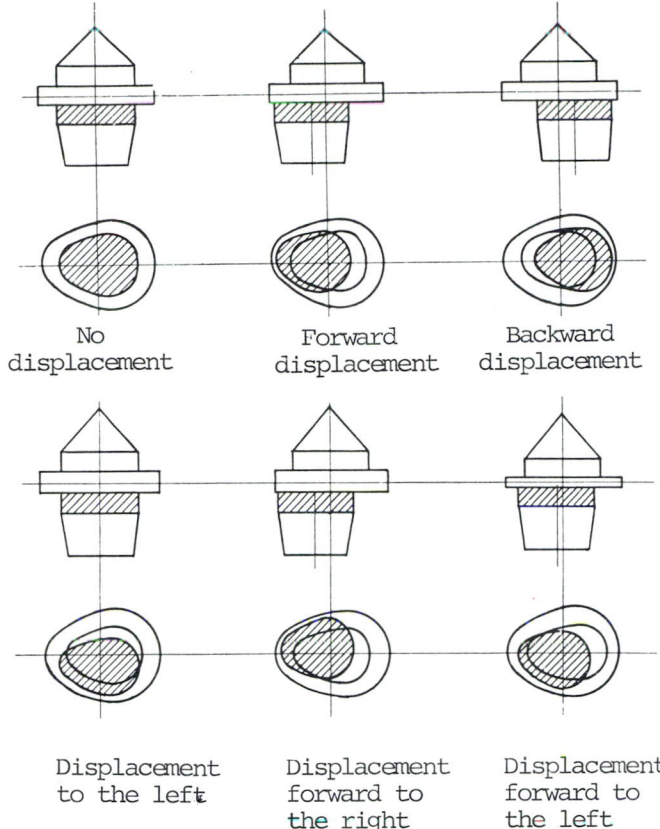

No
displacement

Forward
displacement

Backward
displacement

Displacement
to the left

Displacement
forward to
the right

Displacement
forward to
the left

Fig. 7-7   The direction of force acting on the activator at any particular moment depends on the spatial relationships between the posture induced by the activator and the momentary rest position. The view is from the top of the head with the face to the left of the ovoid outline. (From Herren P: *Schweiz Monatsschr Zahnheilkd* 63:829, 1953.)

1. The original Andresen-Häupl theory[14] attributed tooth movement to a loose-fitting functionally generated mobility providing intermittent forces created by the elevator and protractor muscles, as well as by elements of the buccinator mechanism, that jolted or shook the teeth, pushing the appliance back into position on the maxillary teeth when it dropped away. A prerequisite was that the bite opening could not exceed the normal interocclusal clearance or freeway space.[14] This approach, using nocturnal wear of a loosely fitting appliance, is espoused by Ahlgren.[1-5]

2. The second hypothesis,[178] as described previously and closely following the Herren analysis, denied the nocturnal functional activity during sleep. Rather, it suggested that the activator at rest moves the teeth and creates the desired changes. The appliance is squeezed between the jaws most of the time, splinting them in the *ought to be* sagittal relationship and preventing compensatory postural changes that would normally occur without the activator in place. The resultant forces created vary from time to time and change in magnitude. They are intermittent, but the net result is that they are transmitted to the activator, which distributes them to the teeth and alveolar bone, enhancing the adaptive process. The action is still considered to be primarily interrupted or intermittent in nature. The forces produce a strain in the tissues and are a mechanical phenomenon, whether the strain is due to muscles directly or whether it acts indirectly through the appliance* (Fig. 7-8).

---

*References, 2, 13, 48, 72, 81-83, 98-101, 168-173, 187, 211, 215, 216.

A   B

Fig. 7-8   When the patient is awake and upright, **A,** muscle tonus, muscle tension, and atmospheric pressure balance the weight of the mandible and associated tissues plus the activator. If the mouth is open, then the weight and gravitational effect are balanced by the muscles alone. If the patient sleeps reclined while wearing the activator, **B,** then muscle tension, muscle tonus, and gravity all act in the same direction. When the patient is asleep, the lips drop open; then *function,* as far as any appliance is concerned, is minimal.

Sagittal change. The desired sagittal change needed to correct the anteroposterior malrelationship is produced by the forward posturing of the mandible in the construction bite. This was recognized as dependent on growth guidance to achieve the skeletal alteration required, as well as favorable dentoalveolar adjustment. Controversy still surrounds this working hypothesis, despite definitive research by Petrovic et al.[151-157] on rats and the primate studies by Elgoyhen et al.,[45] Graber,[64] Graber,[68] McDougall et al.,[123] McNamara,[127-130] McNamara et al.,[131,132] and Stutzmann et al.[186,187]

Their studies indicate that mandibular growth enhancement occurs as well as redirection of condylar growth and maxillary horizontal growth with forward posturing appliances, worn during a growing period (a headgear effect). A number of studies on treated patients* also indicate that when treated Class II patients are compared with nontreated controls, mandibular length is enhanced by functional appliances. The results are variable, as Graber[64] has shown in a study of 58 completed Fränkel appliance patients, but the potential for change seems to be there. The *unloading* of the condyle is considered a potentially significant factor by Johnston.[111]

The same philosophy is applicable for the Herbst appliance. The working hypothesis is that all growth restrictions are removed (Fig. 7-9). This is in spite of articles by Creekmore and Radney,[38] Gianelly et al.,[63] and Ricketts[162] that do not find enhanced mandibular growth specifically attributable to functional appliances. But then these clinicians have had limited experience with functionals.

The net effect is that patients attain the *achievable optimum,* with the most favorable functional environment, freed of any restrictive neuromuscular aberrations resulting from compensatory, adaptive, or homeostatic activity. The correct comparison should be with similar malocclusions, not so-called normals. This means controls matched for sex, age, pattern of growth direction, or morphology.

Vertical opening variations. A number of modifications of the original Andresen activator have been introduced. This is because of the ongoing controversy over the amount of vertical opening and degree of forward posturing created by the activator, as well as the differing views regarding nocturnal wear versus full-time wear (which would provide potentially active functional stimulus and predictable forces from relatively constant head posture), and the arguments for loose appliances versus functional appliances *anchored* to the maxilla.

Whereas Andresen and his disciples recommended an opening of no more than 4 mm within the confines of the freeway space, as do Fränkel, Fleischer, and others, many clinicians* have turned to varying degrees of mandibular advancement and larger vertical openings of the construction bite (ranging from 4 to 15 mm). Some[14,51,187,211] recommend a specific intermolar clearance, varying from the Andresen

---

*References 21, 22, 39, 40, 55, 60, 71, 84-88, 115, 122, 128, 131, 140-142, 149-151, 154-158.

*References 2, 14, 48, 72, 81-83, 98-101, 133, 170-172, 174, 187, 211, 215-217.

Fig. 7-9 Immediate effect of placing a functional appliance that postures the mandible forward. The condyle is brought forward in the fossa, which removes the usual functional stresses and constraints. The retractor muscles of the mandible are activated, and the resultant force is directed against the maxillary arch. (From Bimler P: In Graber TM, Neumann B: *Removable orthodontic appliances,* ed 2, Philadelphia, 1984, WB Saunders.)

recommendation by different amounts. Others* prefer to open the construction bite a specific amount beyond the postural rest position (Fig. 7-10).

A definite problem exists in rest position determination. Day and night rest positions are usually significantly different, mainly because of change in body and head posture and spatial relationships. Experience has shown that postural resting position varies from morning to night in the same individual depending on posture, mental anxiety, and fatigue.[67] The variability is greater at night, and the variation is great among individuals, even with normal occlusions. Thus any formula that recommends a specific distance for all patients is arbitrary and unrealistic. Even the most precise orthodontic interocclusal measurements in the dental chair are hardly likely to be replicated at night when the activator is worn. With malocclusions, vertical intermolar distance determinations must depend on relative infraclusion or supraclusion of buccal segment teeth. Differential eruption may be needed in some cases but should be avoided in others. As long as the original 2 to 4 mm opening recommended by Andresen and Häupl[13] was observed, it was probable that the activator construction bite would be within the limits of the freeway space and would not impinge on rest position, except in anterior open bite malocclusions, with overeruption of buccal segments. However, most appliance modifications subsequently introduced have had larger vertical openings and displace the mandible beyond the muscularly determined daytime postural resting position part of the time or all of the time they are worn.[172] It is

*References 2, 3, 77-80, 84, 85, 98-101, 160-162, 214-216.

Fig. 7-10 A number of activators require a larger vertical opening. The Herren, Harvold, Hamilton, Woodside, and L.S.U. activators all exceed the freeway space or postural rest position, eliciting the viscoelastic properties of the associated tissues. In this illustration there is an 8 mm opening between the first molars. The lower incisors are capped by the acrylic to provide more stability and reduce the tendency to procline these teeth.

emphasized again that nocturnal rest position is usually different, with a greater interocclusal clearance, and is modifiable by various head positions during sleep.

As Slagsvold and Kolstad[180] ask, can such appliances logically be called activators in the true sense? What do they activate if they call on stretch reflex or viscoelastic properties of the tissues?

This is not to question that many so-called activator modifications work, regardless of the vertical opening or variations in the amount of horizontal mandibular advancement. Part of this is a testimony to the great adaptability of the human organism. Normal is a range and seldom a point. The success of these modifications may be due to different combinations of muscle force, elastic tissue reaction, horizontal versus vertical displacement, age at time of use, length of wear, sleeping posture, and choice of cases to be treated based on growth intensity, direction, and amount left. The justification of each approach by the various proponents of different construction bites makes interesting reading. One unanswered question is, "What is the role of nocturnal parafunctional activity (bruxing and clenching)?"

Egil Harvold,[81-83] one of the foremost proponents of a high construction bite, feels that the wider jaw opening enlists the elastic properties in the elevator and retractor muscles (the "viscoelastic force of the associated soft tissues," as Woodside[214] terms it). This force is transmitted to the teeth; and the appliance, which is worn at night, is more likely to stay in place, producing the desired changes.

As previously noted Paul Herren[93,94] subscribes to this philosophy; and Robert Shaye[178] does the same.

Herren based his observations on patients who wore activators that displaced the mandible 2 or 3 mm below intercuspal position. Even with this relatively small interocclusal distance, he felt that the activator was literally squeezed between the jaws most of the time that it was worn. Since he believed that the same status existed for activators that opened the bite much beyond rest position, he concluded that the action was the same for all activators, regardless of the amount of vertical displacement. However, the forces are more continuous in action and constant in direction when the bite is opened more widely. In addition, their magnitude is greater, with one exception. When the mouth is open, the rest vertical dimension is modified to a more caudal position and the pressure of the closing muscles thus decreases with adaptation to the appliance being worn.

Ahlgren[1] concurred with Herren, basing his conclusions on considerable electromyographic and neurophysiologic research. As long as the appliance is in place, with a vertical opening exceeding the postural rest vertical dimension, the muscles are subject to stretch. Being elastically extensible, they respond similarly to a rubber band, with the tension increasing exponentially as the amount of vertical opening increases. The action also elicits a phenomenon referred to by Sherrington as stretch reflex—either the tonic or the phasic type. A maintained stretch incites a long-lasting tonic stretch reflex contraction whereas a momentary stretch elicits a transient phasic stretch reflex response. Hence the activator produces a tonic stretch reflex in most instances. The tonic reflex response varies inversely with each level of sleep. It is greatest during the wakeful state, active but less intense during the rapid eye light plane of sleep, and non-existent in the deep phase of sleep.

When the activator is worn during the day, the frequency of deglutition is enhanced while the activator is in place and there is increased phasic muscle activity; but during sleep, even in the deep plane of sleep, phasic muscle contractions can be discerned in the tongue and contiguous jaw musculature. During the deep sleep phase, when the muscles are atonic, myoclonic twitches of the tongue and associated musculature push the activator into place against the teeth, creating intermittent forces. This is in contradistinction to the effect during daytime wear, when the passive tension and tonus of the stretched muscles exert a more continuous force on the teeth and investing tissues.

Schwarz,[174] in his wider open activator studies, noted that the force created varied with the changing magnitude of the blood pressure and the tetanic oscillations of the muscle contractions. He did not observe an increase in the frequency of mandibular movements when the appliance was worn. Again, the vertical opening was beyond postural resting position, eliciting a stretch reflex and viscoelastic tissue response (in contradistinction to the small vertical opening recommended by Andresen, to stay within the confines of the interocclusal clearance and permit optimal forward posturing for the needed sagittal correction).

Eschler[48,52] became quite prominent in the functional orthopedic field and wielded considerable influence with his research and deductions. He developed a working hypothesis, based on his own electromyographic studies, that varied from those previously cited. To him the response was primarily a stretch reflex. When the appliance is in the mouth, it elicits isotonic contractions in the elevator muscles. These are replaced by tonic (isometric) proprioceptively oriented contractions after the mandibular teeth are fully seated in the appliance. Since the mandible is prevented by the appliance from achieving a normal postural rest position, the muscles remain stretched. They fatigue in due course, relax, and allow the mandible to drop. The cycle is repeated when the muscles recover. Eschler saw no evidence of direct activation of the protractor muscles. The therapeutic effect was attributed to the stretch reflex. Hence the effect was proportionate to the opening, with a recommendation of 4 to 6 mm for optimum patient tolerance and cooperation. His research indicated increased frequency of mandibular movements with activator wear, confirming Andresen's observations. Thilander and Filipsson[187] also conducted electromyographic studies on patients wearing activators, but conducted the studies during waking hours. They found only insignificant muscle activity when the activator was at rest. During mandibular movements, however, an increased activity was seen, especially in the retracting muscles. There was also an increased swallowing activity, probably caused by increased saliva flow.

Fig. 7-11   Transducer placement in the interproximal space of an activator worn at night. Note the contact with the lower left molar. Long periods of transducer activity were observed during sleep. (From Witt E, Komposch G: *Fortschr Kieferorthop* 32:345, 1971.)

Clearly although there is essential agreement between Ahlgren,[3] Harvold,[81] Herren,[93] Selmer-Olsen,[176] and Thilander and Filipsson,[187] differences of opinion by Eschler[48] and Schwarz[174] could be a matter more of interpretation than of actual findings. Eschler is actually in partial agreement with both broad hypotheses.

Nocturnal activity. Elucidating the arguments on the exact effect of the vertical opening of the activator construction bite are studies by Komposch and Hockenjos,[114] Schmuth,[170-172] and Witt and Komposch.[211] These authors used transducers at night to assess the type and amount of force generated by activators opened beyond postural resting position (Fig. 7-11). They found long periods of continuous pressure from the mandibular teeth against the activator when the intermolar distance exceeded 4 to 6 mm (Figs. 7-12 and 7-13). This pressure consisted of three components[114,209-212]:

1. A basic pressure varying with the amount of mandibular displacement, head position, and plane of sleep
2. Oscillations synchronized with breathing rhythm
3. Oscillations synchronized with blood pulse

When the vertical displacement was 4 to 6 mm and the horizontal forward posturing half the width of a premolar (3 to 5 mm), the mean sagittal forces ranged from 315 to 395 g for a group of sleeping adults (Fig. 7-13). With the same amount of vertical opening but with no forward posturing the means were much less: between 145 and 270 g. The mean vertical forces ranged from 70 to 175 g. In most subjects the forces were greater when the mandible was displaced downward and forward than when displaced downward only, but this tendency was not statistically significant. However, Ahlgren[1] has observed that the stretch reflex activity of temporal and masseter muscles correlates positively with the amount of mandibular opening (Figs. 7-14 and 7-15).

Witt and Komposch[211] also confirmed that forces exerted on the teeth and supporting structures varied with the plane of sleep and head position (Fig. 7-16). Relatively small depressing forces were found in patients sleeping on their back, while sagittal forces were relatively strong. During the initial stages of sleep the forces were varied but stronger.

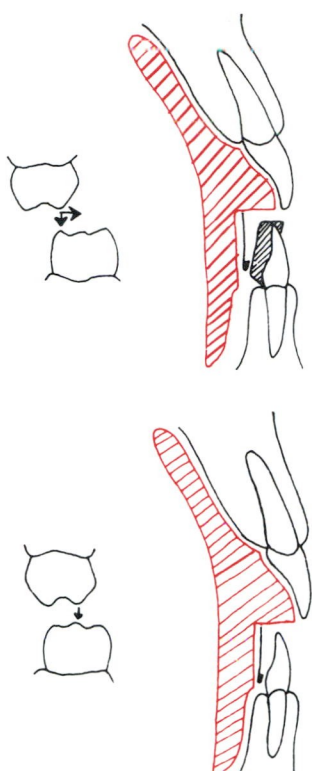

Fig. 7-12 Transducer placement for registration of posterior forces against the activator and anterior forces against the lower incisors and activator during activator therapy. The forward posturing of the mandible was increased by addition of a splint on the linguo-incisal aspect of the lower incisors. (From Witt E, Komposch G: *Fortschr Kieferorthop* 32:345, 1971.)

As the plane of sleep became deeper, the variability was less but the magnitude was significantly reduced.

Recent experiments by Sander[167,168] have shed additional light on functional appliance action. Schmuth[170,172] and Sander separately measured the forces produced between the upper and lower jaws with different construction bites and found that the amount of force was dependent on the vertical height and sagittal position of the lower jaw. Sander[167] also measured the interocclusal clearance in patients with and without activators worn during sleep, since it is important in determining the vertical construction bite, as previously indicated. He showed that in patients who have large horizontal displacements, there was a tendency to disclude the lower jaw from the appliance to avoid the large forces produced. With vertical opening there was less of an effect.

However, a study of mandibular activity patterns in controls not wearing an activator showed a broad range of activity. At the beginning of the night, frequent mandibular movements, including wide-open movements, could be seen. These frequently occurred with tooth contact. After the first sleep phase the lower jaw slowly opened, probably under the influence of gravity, although some closing movements could still be seen. In one control there was an open-

Fig. 7-13 Charting of force increments in grams for downward *(dotted line)* and downward and forward *(solid line)* displacement in 30 adult activator patients. Based on means of individual registrations every 5 minutes. (From Witt E, Komposch G: *Fortschr Kieferorthop* 32:345, 1971.)

Fig. 7-14 Variation of posterior forces exerted against the activator over a 2-hour period for both downward and downward and forward displacement. (From Witt E, Komposch G: *Fortschr Kieferorthop* 32:345, 1971.)

Fig. 7-15 Variation in vertical forces exerted against the activator during a 2-hour period. (From Witt E, Komposch G: *Forstchr Kieferorthop* 32:345, 1971.)

Fig. 7-16 Variations in the amount of force exerted by an activator over a 15-minute period of restless sleep with changes in body posture: *1*, Body and head on the right side; *2*, sleeping on the back; *3*, head turned to rest on the right side; *4*, head turned to rest on the left side; *5*, body and head both turned to rest on the left side. (From Witt E, Komposch G; *Fortschr Kieferorthop* 32:345, 1971.)

ing movement that preceded the closing movement. As time passed, the interocclusal clearance increased. Long periods of muscle inactivity were interrupted by active periods during the night. Closing movements reached maximum intercuspation only briefly. The lower jaw would then open, sometimes actively and sometimes passively, because of gravity. Experimental results confirmed that a nocturnal rest position exists that does not mimic the diurnal registration. Near maximum or maximum occlusal contact was recorded less than 0.8% of the total sleep time.[167,168] The implications again stress the time-linked variability of mandibular position and function, making it difficult to assess the exact role of the activator when it is worn.

The mode of action of activators that have a vertical opening of 4 to 6 mm below intercuspal position is well documented. The teeth are subject to almost continuous force when the activator is in place, although the force magnitude varies considerably from patient to patient, as well as within the same patient, depending on the factors just listed. The inescapable conclusion is that these are not functional jaw orthopedic appliances in the truest sense. Perhaps the term suggested by Slagsvold[179] would be more appropriate. He calls them tools for *the muscle stretch method*. Thus the term *monobloc* originally used by Robin and preferred by Hotz is semantically more correct[98]; however, usage has made *activator* the preferred term.

REACTION TO ACTIVATOR THERAPY

As with the range of recommendations on the amount of vertical and sagittal opening for the activator, so there are variations on the theme of tissue response. Since activators are used primarily on Class II, division 1 and Class II,

division 2 problems, most of the literature and case reports are directed to treatment results in these categories. Remarkable results are shown in some cases; in others, poor or partial correction; and in still others, actual detrimental exacerbation of the malocclusion. Conditioning factors are the morphogenetic pattern, severity of the malocclusion, growth increments, growth direction, growth timing, patient cooperation, design of the appliance, amount of vertical or sagittal displacement, and original inclination of the teeth. A correct diagnosis is clearly a prerequisite for successful activator therapy, no less than for fixed appliances.

Expansion. Expansion of the maxillary arch with activator therapy has been demonstrated routinely.[74] Slagsvold and Kolstad[180] found increased molar width in all cases studied (Fig. 7-17).

Overbite. Reduction of excessive overbite is to be expected in most patients properly chosen and treated (Fig. 7-18). One prerequisite for case selection is a deep bite condition. The vertical change must be documented by careful studies.[3,160] Cephalometric analyses[83,107,181] have shown that with eruption may also come a posterior mandibular rotation, as the bite is opened. A significant part of this change is due to differential eruption of the lower molar teeth; however, elimination of a functional retrusion may offset this potentially deleterious effect. In addition, some withholding of maxillary incisor eruption is likely with activator wear, although actual depression is not to be expected, except with wide construction bites. Clark actually allows free eruption of lower molars with twin block therapy.

Sagittal change. Sagittal changes have been the primary objective and have been studied extensively. Variation is perhaps greatest in the accomplishment of this vector of change, whose conditioning factors have already been

Fig. 7-17 Because most Class II, division 1, malocclusions have a narrow maxillary arch, particularly in the canine region, expansion has been an accepted procedure in activator therapy. This can be done ahead of time (as with the Clark twin block and Hamilton Expansion-Activator approach) or afterward. Use of buccal shielding wires, as with the Bionator, or buccal shields of the Fränkel appliance permits significant expansion without *pushing out from within*. However, many activators have been designed with jackscrews or Coffin springs in midpalate to expand the buccal segments, allowing retraction of the maxillary incisors with the labial wire. Note the expansion achieved by a common type of activator. (From Slagsvold O: In Graber TM, Neumann B: *Removable orthodontic appliances*, Philadelphia, 1977, WB Saunders.)

Fig. 7-18 Treatment of a Class II, division 2, malocclusion with an activator. The elimination of the deep overbite, with correction of the sagittal malrelationship was accomplished in less than 2 years. (From Slagsvold O: In Graber TM, Neumann B: *Removable orthodontic appliances*, Philadelphia, 1977, WB Saunders.)

listed. However, successful apical base change can be achieved, as documented in the literature;* retardation of anterior maxillary growth or an actual lingual tipping of the maxillary anterior teeth may contribute part of this.† Of course there are many‡ who believe that mandibular growth is stimulated by the activator. The research of McNamara,[124,125,127-130] McNamara et al.,[126,131,132] Petrovic,[151-153] Petrovic et al.,[154-157] and Stutzmann et al.[185,186] has clearly shown the potential for this effect on experimental animals. Enhanced condylar growth, selective areas of change (usually the posterosuperior condylar aspect), and change in trabecular alignment all are documented. Changed orofacial muscle activity also occurs, with an increase in lateral pterygoid contractions (Fig. 7-19). A skeletal adaptation to the new position and a gradual disappearance of the modified neuromuscular pattern have been observed.

Condylar response. The unique nature of the phylogenetically and ontogenetically secondary cartilage status of the condyle makes it physiologically different from primary cartilage seen in epiphyses and diaphyses, cranial base cartilages, and the nasal septum. It grows by division of undifferentiated cells, the prechondroblasts, and its growth is regulated to a greater extent by local factors than by growth hormones[152] (Fig. 7-20). Petrovic et al.[157] have concluded from their extensive studies that condylar growth is an expression of locally structured homeostasis for the establishment and maintenance of a functionally coordinated stomatognathic system. The growth depends on continuous information from the teeth (periodontal mechanoreceptors),

---

*References 39, 42, 55, 60, 64, 65, 88, 89, 130, 140, 181, 189.
†References 39, 42, 79, 88, 89, 107, 140, 181, 189, 214-216.
‡References 21, 22, 45, 53-59, 87, 95, 123-132, 151-157, 184, 186.

Fig. 7-19 Example of the sagittal and vertical change possible with activator treatment. Before, **A** and **C,** and after, **B** and **D,** facial and intra-oral views show a significant improvement in facial balance, with elimination of the excessive overjet and overbite and establishment of normal perioral muscle function. The treatment was aided for a short time with a cervical extra-oral appliance. Treatment time was 16 months. (From Slagsvold O: In Graber TM, Neumann B: *Removable orthodontic appliances,* Philadelphia, 1977, WB Saunders.)

as well as from the muscles and TMJ itself. A strong role for lateral pterygoid activity is described.[154] In experiments in which the lateral pterygoid was excised, significantly reduced condylar growth was observed. According to Petrovic,[151] activation of the muscles is the key to condylar growth enhancement. Appliances that merely splint the mandible in an anterior position do not activate these muscles and therefore do not stimulate condylar growth. Thus muscle tonus and monosynaptic and polysynaptic reflexes must be maintained. In the deep plane of sleep the activator has little effect on mitotic activity of the prechondroblasts. Growth hormone, although less effective on the condylar cartilage than local factors, does enhance activator effectiveness. It is suggested that the lateral pterygoids, which supply the functional stimulus and also the blood and nutritional supply, are a major pathway to the cartilage metabolism.[24,157]

The question exists, however, about stimulation of condylar growth by an appliance that is worn only during sleeping hours. Gerber[62] and, as pointed out earlier, Herren[93,94] found no increase in muscle activity when the activator was worn. However, Witt[210] studied the Bionator, a modified

activator worn during the day, and did observe increased activity, with the mandible being moved reflexly forward, substantiating the high mitotic activity in the prechondroblasts seen by Stutzmann et al.[185] when appliances are worn during waking hours. So it is questionable whether there is optimal condylar growth stimulation with activator wear limited to sleeping hours only. Other adjustive factors must be present—dental response, possible maxillary horizontal growth restriction, change in the condylar trabecular orientation (Stutzmann angle), remodeling of the articular fossa itself, and elimination of a posterior condylar displacement so often seen with Class II, division 2 deep overbite problems and less frequently, but still of concern, with many Class II, division 1 malocclusions.

Tooth movement. A number of investigators* have studied activator-related anteroposterior dental arch changes with casts and cephalograms. Björk[28] and Parkhouse[150] observed forward displacement of the lower anterior teeth and alveolar bone. Jacobsson[107] observed bodily movement of the lower incisors. Ascher,[16] Dietrich,[42] and Trayfoot and

---

*References 16, 28, 39, 42, 76, 83, 107.

Fig. 7-20 **A,** Primary cartilage growth centers (e.g., in the epiphyses of long bones, in the nasal septum) have a columnar arrangement. **B,** In contrast, the secondary cartilage of the condyle grows by division of the undifferentiated prechondroblast cells. Secondary cartilage is regulated to a lesser extent by hormones and to a greater extent by local factors than is primary cartilage. (From Petrovic A, Stutzmann J, Oudet C: In McNamara JA, Carlson DS, Ribbens KA, editors: *The effect of surgical intervention on craniofacial growth, Monograph 12, Craniofacial growth series,* Ann Arbor, 1982, Center for Human Growth and Development, University of Michigan.)

Richardson[191] reported labial tipping of the lower incisors; yet Moss[140] reported lingual tipping in at least half of his material. Demisch[40] observed accelerated mesial drift of the lower buccal segments whereas Harvold and Vargervik[83] and Softley[181] concluded that the lower dental arch remained stable on its base. Hagerström[76] and Slagsvold and Kolstad[180] saw increased spacing in the lower dental arch.

From the wealth of material studied, it seems likely that the lower dental arch does come forward some during activator treatment. If the lower incisors are already labially inclined initially, or if such reaction is not acceptable, some other form of therapy may be indicated. Conditioning factors also are the direction and amount of growth, length of appliance wear, and (most important) design of the activator—whether there is incisal capping, whether forward posturing involves labial pressure on the teeth and alveolar bone or alveolar bone only, and the degrees of forward advancement and vertical opening that are needed for the construction bite.

Many case reports show that the maxillary anterior teeth can be retracted with activators.* The axial inclination of

---

*References 83, 107, 159, 181, 190.

these teeth may also be improved. The primary action is lingual tipping, however, and this can be undesirable because overbite is increased with the uprighting of maxillary incisors and premature contact may be created in the incisal region, restricting optimum forward mandibular posturing for basal sagittal correction, as well as eliminating functional retrusion. Torque or bodily movement of incisors is difficult if not impossible to achieve, even with a modified activator.

The question of distalization of maxillary posterior segments by activator treatment is not completely answered. Withholding of the fullest potential of maxillary horizontal growth is accepted by most investigators. Clinically, a space can frequently be seen, particularly in young patients. A distal tipping of buccal segment teeth can also be seen in many cases. Demisch[40] has concluded that the maxillary molars either are stopped in their normal path of eruption or move distally. Woodside[214,215] and Woodside et al.[216] strive to withhold the normal eruption of maxillary molars while allowing the mandibular molars to move mesially and superiorly. Harvold and Vargervik[83] could not confirm distalization. McNamara[129] has reported practically no maxillary change in his Fränkel appliance studies; but Lee Graber[64] has shown a headgear distalization effect in some Fränkel

Fig. 7-21 In this untreated Class II, division 2, malocclusion there is a strong upward and forward rotation of the mandibular growth pattern leading to a marked mentolabial sulcus, decreased anterior face height, and enhancement of the original overbite problem. Correction with any type of conventional orthodontic therapy is difficult. Vertical correction is as important as sagittal. Activator therapy here would attempt to stimulate all possible upward and forward eruption of lower posterior segments. (From Björk A: *Nord Klin Odontol* 1:1, 1966.)

Fig. 7-22 This downward and backward rotational growth pattern does not respond well to activator therapy. Short ramus height, excessive anterior face height, compensatory tongue posture, and function all team up to aggravate the original open bite malocclusion. (From Björk A: *Nord Klin Odontol* 1:1, 1966.)

case reports and a wide variation of reaction in patients. Again, growth amounts, growth direction, growth timing, appliance design, appliance wear, selective grinding, and use of the eruptive potential of posterior teeth all can affect the degree of correction (Figs. 7-21 and 7-22). Nocturnal parafunctional activity could also be a consideration. Patient cooperation and full-time wear versus nighttime-only wear obviously will qualify the final result.

APPLIANCE DESIGN

Andresen appliance. The traditional one-piece appliance, involving both dental arches, is passive and has no active parts like springs, jackscrews, or elastics (Fig. 7-23). The maxillary labial arch is passive but can be activated if necessary to tip upper incisors lingually. It is worn only at night and has a vertical opening within the limits of the freeway space, or 2 to 4 mm at most, with an average mandibular advancement of 3 to 5 mm. Generally it is used for less severe Class II malocclusions, with deeper than normal overbite and upright or lingually inclined lower incisors. Lower incisors were not capped with acrylic in the original appliance, although most current use of this appliance incorporates indexing or capping, or a lower labial wire, to reduce the labial tipping tendency of the lower anterior segment. Since the purpose of this chapter is to

Fig. 7-23 The classical Andresen activator for nighttime wear. It is passive in the sense that there are no tooth-moving parts. (Courtesy Johan Ahlgren.)

present the philosophy and general details and tissue reactions, the appliances mentioned are not discussed in detail. Refer to books by the author[67] together with Bedrich Neumann,[70] Thomas Rakosi,[160] and Alexandre Petrovic[151-157] for construction minutiae.[70,71] Current use by clinicians such as Johan Ahlgren[3-5] carefully documents the response.

Activator modifications. A number of changes have been introduced through the years to attempt to achieve different treatment objectives. The most common is the incorporation of one or more jackscrews to expand the upper, lower, or both dental arches. Modification of the labial archwire to extend posteriorly in the Bionator, opposing the posterior teeth, serves to relieve cheek pressure. Finger springs have been added for limited tooth movement. Acrylic capping of the lower incisors is generally incorporated to increase resistance of the lower incisors to labial tipping. The bulk of the original appliance has been reduced by many clinicians—notably Balters,[18] Bimler,[25-27] Fleischer and Fleischer-Peters,[53] Fränkel,[54-57] Fränkel and Fränkel,[58] Fränkel and Reiss,[59] Klammt,[113] Schmuth,[170,172] and Stockfisch.[182,183] A cross-palatal wire or Coffin spring has been substituted for the acrylic. Of course, the original sagittal and vertical mandibular displacements have been varied, mostly by increasing the vertical bite opening. These will be discussed in more detail in the section on construction bite.

The Bionator, as developed by Balters,[18] is the most frequently used activator modification today (Fig. 7-24). Significant success has been achieved by Fleischer, with his Bio-Modulator modification of the Balters Bionator (Figs. 7-25, 7-26, and 7-30 to 7-35). Reversing the transpalatal loop, replacing the single labial arch with upper and lower labial arches, reducing the acrylic bulk significantly, enhancing maxillary anchorage by the addition of interprox-

imal spurs and C-stops at the mesial of the first permanent molars and canines, and using a thin metal plate between the upper and lower occlusal surfaces to serve as functional occlusal plane permit both horizontal and vertical control[53] (Fig. 7-26). The metal plate is used for selective retardation or guidance of eruption to establish a normal vertical and horizontal relationship. For a fuller discussion of this important modification of the Bionator, in addition to other appliances used by Shaye, Janson, Hamilton, and Schmuth, refer to the second edition of *Removable Orthodontic Appliances* by Graber and Neumann,[70] as well as *Dentofacial Orthopedics with Functional Appliances* by Graber, Rakosi, and Petrovic.[71]

The development of various other skeleton activators has also allowed full-time wear, day and night. The advantages, as far as tissue response is concerned, have already been described.

The Fränkel appliance. A fundamental activator modification is the Fränkel function regulator[54-59] (Fig. 7-27). It resorts to the same basic forward posturing of the mandible for sagittal correction but postures by steps instead of all at once. A critical requirement is that the appliance be fixed to the maxillary arch, anchored by interproximal wires in the molar and canine area to enhance maxillary anchorage, rather than left loose or free-floating, as recommended by Andresen and Häupl. With the exception of a maxillary molar rest to prevent maxillary molar eruption, the remainder of the appliance has minimal tooth contact. As a passive exercise device there are no active parts.

A unique characteristic is the incorporation of buccal shields and anterior lip pads, which serve to relieve cheek and lip pressure and to break up abnormal perioral muscle habits. They are extended into the depths of the vestibule to exert a stretch effect on the vestibular mucosa and underlying periosteal layer, in an attempt to enhance basal

Fig. 7-24 The Bionator, as modified from the original activator by Balters, uses a heavy Coffin-type transpalatal wire instead of an acrylic cover. The labial wire is not a tooth-moving adjunct but a screening wire, holding the lip away from the teeth and extending into the buccal sulcus as far as the distal of the deciduous second molars. To enhance eruption in the desired direction, the acrylic is removed and trimmed in the interdental area. The construction bite is usually taken in an end-to-end incisal relationship if this permits passage of interocclusal wiring. The appliance is an effective adjunct in many TMJ problems requiring forward posturing of the mandible.

Fig. 7-25 The basic Bio-Modulator of Fleischer. The labial wire is similar to its progenitor, the Bionator; but the lower labial wire (lip bumper), which intercepts the abnormal lower lip trap, screens the lower incisors to allow autonomous improvement with the release of the abnormal perioral muscle deforming action. No acrylic is interposed between the occlusal surfaces so as not to impede eruption. (Courtesy Erich Fleischer.)

Fig. 7-26 The Fleischer Bio-Modulator, with the stainless metal interocclusal plane. This allows proprioceptive contact of selected teeth that do not need to erupt while stimulating teeth that are in infraclusion and not touching the metal plane. The skeleton appliance is easier to wear than the conventional activator and does not require the precise and sometimes arduous selective trimming of the acrylic for control of guided eruption. (Courtesy Erich Fleischer.)

Fig. 7-27 The Fränkel function regulator makes maximum use of the vestibule as its area of operation, screening away abnormal lip and cheek pressures. **A,** Labial model. *a,* Labial bow; *b,* canine loop; *c,* buccal shield; *d,* lip pads. **B,** Lingual model. *a,* Palatal bow; *b,* protrusion bow; *c,* lower lingual wires; *d,* buccal shield; *e,* lower lip pads; *f,* lower lingual plate. The wire assemblage anchors the FR on the maxillary arch. There is no interocclusal acrylic or interference with eruption of the mandibular teeth with either the FR I or the FR II. The lingual acrylic pad and its passive wires, which lie lingual to the lower anterior teeth, are the only contact in the lower arch since the construction bite maintains the lower jaw in a forward position in the trough formed by the lingual acrylic pad and the labial lip pads. For optimum tissue reaction and patient acceptance and cooperation, the 6 mm sagittal change is usually accomplished in two stages of 3 mm each. The posturing trough is advanced by a simple adjustment with the same appliance. (Courtesy Rolf Fränkel.)

bone development. The concepts are based on well-reasoned and well-researched philosophies. The work of Enlow,[46] Hoyte and Enlow,[102] Moffett,[138] and Moffett and Koskinen-Moffett[139] shows that stimulation of bone growth is possible with periosteal pull. Recent studies by L. W. Graber[64] and T. M. Graber[68] confirm the enhanced transverse maxillary growth induced by the buccal shields, both on primates and in human patients.

Whereas Andresen and Häupl looked for autonomous neuromuscular function and improvement resulting from nocturnal activator wear, Fränkel demands full-time wear and a rigorous program of oral gymnastics. The FR is truly an exercise device and achieves optimum results only if so used. Again, diagnosis, case selection, growth amounts and direction, growth timing, and patient cooperation are qualifying factors in the ultimate treatment result. There can be no denying the dramatic sagittal basal bone, dental, and profile improvement, as well as the restoration of normal perioral muscle function in the properly selected and treated cases (Fig. 7-28). Unlike the activator, however, which can be modified many ways and still produce an acceptable response, the Fränkel appliance demands a rigid discipline of fabrication, fitting, and patient wear for the best possible

correction.[70,71] Some recent reports that attempt to assess the efficacy of the appliance are unfortunately tainted by poor case selection, improper fabrication, improper use, lack of anchoring the appliance on the maxilla (letting it float free in the mouth), and itinerant patient cooperation. Misuse of the appliance negates any conclusions drawn.[38,63,162] Oral exercises are a critical part of the Fränkel regimen but are largely ignored by many American orthodontists. This cannot produce the best results, for a truly functional appliance requires elimination of abnormal perioral function, muscle adaptation to an optimal sagittal jaw relationship, and neuromuscular reinforcement of the new and improved jaw relationship. Of all the so-called functional appliances, the Fränkel is the one that relies most on function. The reader is again referred to books by the author on these appliances for a more extensive discussion of all aspects of use.

THE CONSTRUCTION BITE

One of the most important aspects of activator fabrication is the establishment of proper horizontal and vertical mandibular displacement before construction of the appliance.

A   B   C

Fig. 7-28   Plaster casts. **A,** Type of treatment result to be expected by correct use of the Fränkel appliance in a properly selected Class II, division 1, malocclusion. **B,** Autonomous expansion caused by screening of aberrant muscle activity by the buccal shields and lip pads, which occupy the vestibule. The expansion is stable in the great majority of cases. **C,** Three and one half years posttreatment with no appliance control. (**A** to **C** courtesy Rolf Fränkel.)

There is no one *cookbook* for determining the relationships. Much depends on the type of activator used, the case selection, the dentofacial morphology, the growth pattern, the desired result, and the need for other therapeutic assists (e.g., fixed appliances, extraoral force, extraction). Since the Bionator, or skeleton activator, and its modifications are currently the most frequently used functional appliances, this section will be devoted to a discussion of the construction bite for that appliance.

A complete diagnostic discipline is essential before selecting a patient for the functional appliance. As Rakosi[160] stresses, it is no less important to do a thorough cephalometric, cast, and functional analysis for the functional orthopedic regimen than it is to do these for a full fixed appliance problem. Facial pattern is important; growth amounts and growth direction are equally important. Only if the case analysis satisfies the demanding criteria for a functional appliance, and *only if patient cooperation is likely to be good*, should such an appliance be used. The operator should always keep in mind that this is primarily an interceptive appliance, seldom capable of achieving full correction and complete dental detailing, and an interceptive appliance should be considered a first-phase effort in the total treatment planning. In this short survey chapter the concern is primarily with the use of functional appliances in Class II mandibular retrusion problems. The reader is referred to *Removable Orthodontic Appliances* by Graber and Neumann[70] and to *Dentofacial Orthopedics with Functional Appliances* by Graber et al.[71] for management of Class III malocclusions with functional appliances.

Anterior Mandibular Posturing

Generally, for the conventional activator and modifications like the Bionator, if the severity of the malocclusion is not too great, the protraction is planned to achieve an end-to-end incisal contact relationship. For practical purposes it should not exceed 4 to 6 mm in most cases (Fig. 7-29). Patient acceptance is likely to be less, and the danger of lower incisor procumbency is greater with larger amounts. As a general rule the anterior positioning should always be 3 mm or more posterior to the most protrusive mandibular position possible. This measurement is checked by having the patient move the jaw forward as much as possible and then drop back 3 to 4 mm. When there is severe lingual inclination of the lower anterior segment, a larger anterior repositioning may be used, with the objective of allowing the lower incisors to tip labially to a better inclination, increasing canine space and reducing the excessive overjet. However, this must still follow the 3 mm drop-back from extreme functional protrusion. Usually in severe problems it is better to bring the mandible forward in two or three steps of 2 to 3 mm each. Research by Petrovic et al.[157]

Fig. 7-29 Bionator functional appliance on working models. The mandible is postured forward for correction of the sagittal discrepancy. The lower incisors are capped with acrylic. Minimal bite opening is used for this appliance, which strives for an end-to-end incisal relationship in the construction bite; this is not true of the Woodside, Herren, L.S.U., or Hamilton activators.

and Shaye[178] has shown that tissue response and reactivation are better in the condyle with this procedure. Patient adjustment and cooperation are enhanced. Such a staged mandibular protraction is recommended by Fränkel[56] and his disciples in the use of the function regulator (FR).

Since the maxillary incisors are frequently tipped labially and are often spaced, it may be preferrable to use an active plate (or limited fixed appliances) to retract and rotate the incisors first for a short time and then use the activator; or the construction bite may disclose the need for incisor retraction during functional appliance wear, and a forward position can be established that is 2 or 3 mm less than end-to-end incisal contact.

In most routine cases, however, when adequate growth increments are expected and the growth direction is favorable, an advancement of 4 to 6 mm to establish the supportive, proprioceptively desirable, end-to-end incisal relationship is standard operating procedure and is likely to produce the desired result, with proper patient compliance (Fig. 7-29). Many of these patients have a 1.0 to 1.5 mm posterior condylar displacement associated with mandibular overclosure, so this retruded habitual occlusion position is also eliminated by the forward posturing. The vertical opening is within interocclusal space limits, resulting in a thin construction bite. Both elevator and protractor muscles are activated; and there is a greater hyoid musculature compensation or retractive force, which is distributed against the maxillary arch. This slightly inhibits normal anterior maxillary dentoalveolar relocation. Biting into the appliance and swallowing enhance the neuromuscular and osseous adaptation to the new posture. No effect is expected on the inclination of the maxillary base, and usually it is not necessary to construct more than one appliance in moderate sagittal discrepancy cases.

Vertical mandibular posturing

The opening of the bite varies with the severity of the malocclusion, the amount of anterior displacement, the growth amounts and direction projections, and the type of appliance used. The following general considerations will guide the clinician in most problems, however, recognizing that there is variance in vertical opening used by different authors and clinicians (Fleischer and Fleischer-Peters,[53] Fränkel,[55-57] Fränkel and Fränkel,[58] Fränkel and Reiss,[59] Hamilton,[79] Moss,[140-142] Rakosi,[160] Schmuth,[170-172] Shaye,[178] Woodside,[214,215] and Woodside et al.[216]

1. Mandibular postural displacement is essential to creating the neuromuscular activation required for correction in sagittal or vertical directions, or both.
2. The greater the anterior mandibular displacement for the construction bite, the less the vertical opening should be. For example, in extreme sagittal protraction (6 to 7 mm) the vertical opening should just clear the cusps, or 2 to 3 mm at most. The treatment objective in such cases is to achieve the greatest possible horizontal correction of the anteroposterior discrepancy. Such positioning is recommended when there is likely to be a more horizontal growth vector. Only enough opening is created to permit interocclusal wires, rests, or the metal plate of the Fleischer Bio-Modulator. This is true for the Fränkel appliance as well. The vertical opening is usually within the limits of the postural resting position, as used by Andresen and his followers. Witt[209] measured the forces produced by such a maneuver and found a range of 315 to 395 g for the horizontal force and a variance from 70 to 175 g for the vertical component. In an attempt to eliminate the need for more than one appliance, the clinician is again cautioned against attempting extreme change in the sagittal mandibular posture. Shaye[178] and others have introduced jackscrew adjustments to allow progressive forward posturing or reactivating, which is better from both tissue reaction and patient cooperation aspects.

3. When there is the probability of a more vertical growth direction for the mandible, the vertical opening can be more extensive, beyond the postural rest position. Such opening elicits both stretch reflex and viscoelastic response from the mandibular elevator muscles and soft tissues. Although less sagittal mandibular response can be expected from this construction bite, the wider vertical opening is more effective in controlling the inclination of the maxillary base, withholding maxillary posterior face height enhancement, and allowing the anterior end of the maxillary plane to tip downward and help compensate for the vertical mandibular growth pattern. Woodside[216] has discussed this changing of palatal and occlusal planes and particularly the desirable therapeutic effects achieved by tipping down of the occlusal plane.

The interocclusal vertical relationship is achieved by having a thicker wax wafer for the construction bite. Too large a vertical opening, however, makes patient acceptance more difficult, as does too large a sagittal correction. In most cases the mandible should not be opened more than 4.0 mm beyond the postural rest position. Fränkel has stressed many times that the vertical opening should not be so great as to prevent the patient from doing lip seal exercises; and if any oral gymnastics are to be prescribed, the same admonition applies to the activator. With the results shown by Fränkel for the FR and his strong reliance on this appliance as an exercise device, it seems logical that lip seal exercises should be beneficial with Bionator wear also. The elimination of lip incompetence and enhancement of nasal breathing are firstline treatment objectives.

In wider open vertical construction bites, dentoalveolar compensation is usually greater. Maxillary incisors are likely to be inclined more to the lingual, and mandibular incisors are more labially tipped.

4. In open bite problems, when little or no sagittal change is desired, the more extreme vertical opening of the bite is essential. The thick interocclusal acrylic wafer elicits both stretch reflex and viscoelastic depressive response

on the posterior teeth, interfering with normal eruption. Woodside et al.[216] have shown dramatic results using the posterior bite block effect, which allows upward and forward rotation of the mandible, closing down the anterior open bite. Repelling magnets in a twin block appliance or Dellinger appliance may enhance posterior tooth depression. The effect is similar to the changes produced by the Milwaukee brace (but of much lesser magnitude, of course). This effect is combined with the downward tipping of the anterior maxillary base and occlusal plane to produce the ultimate correction. The efficacy of the activator in deep overbite cases has been documented in metric studies, but the effect varies from patient to patient in open bite problems.[179] In a study of 30 severe open bite cases treated with a function regulator, Fränkel and Fränkel[58] showed significant improvement in the anterior/posterior height ratio, a change in the direction of mandibular rotation, a closing down of the bite, and a real improvement in the soft tissue profile.

MECHANISMS OF CLASS II CORRECTION WITH FUNCTIONAL ORTHOPEDICS

Thousands of case reports attest to the beneficial changes produced by functional appliances. Dramatic facial changes seldom seen with conventional fixed appliances not only are possible but also are fairly routine (Figs. 7-30 through 7-35). The reasons for these changes, however, are more obscure and they vary from patient to patient. The oversimplistic assignment of the change to *condylar growth stimulation* has clouded the picture. We are dealing with a cybernetic process. A number of the conditioning factors have already been discussed. Morphogenetic pattern, growth timing, amounts and direction of sagittal and vertical discrepancies, neuromuscular patterns, functional displacement, dentoalveolar compensation, type of appliance used, and patient compliance are the most important variables; but the list is incomplete.[160] Such nebulous entities as *tissue response* or *rate of fibroblast turnover* may be as important although more difficult to assess. (See Chapters 2, 3.) The controversy over the effect on condylar growth has not been resolved, yet the fact is that sagittal change of major magnitude is achieved. How does this happen? A listing of probable components responsible for the change has been developed by the author. The millimetric values assigned are arbitrary and vary from case to case. The response and interrelationship of the various components are equally variable. (Compensation is the name of the game.) The reader is referred to the discussion of this question by Stöckli and Teuscher in Chapter 8 (p. 446).

Class II correction, the likely scenario*

The amount of sagittal correction needed is 6 to 7 mm. The following anticipated growth increments and other changes are typical:

---

*The varying amounts of each component depend on growth increments, direction, timing, and length of treatment.

Fig. 7-30 Boy with a Class II, division 1, malocclusion treated by a modified Bionator (Bio-Modulator). Typical hypotonic upper lip, mouth breathing, marked mentolabial sulcus, and hypertonic mentalis activity were in evidence. (Courtesy Erich Fleischer.)

1. Condylar growth amounts, 1.0 to 3.0 mm (mandible outgrows maxilla 1 to 5 mm)
2. Fossa growth and adaptation, 0.5 to 1.0 mm
3. Eliminating functional retrusion, 0.5 to 1.5 mm
4. More favorable growth direction (trabecular angle), 0.5 to 1.0 mm

5. Withholding of downward and forward maxillary arch movement, 1.0 to 2.0 mm
6. Differential upward and forward eruption of lower buccal segments, 1.5 to 2.5 mm
7. Headgear effect, 1.0 to 2.0 mm

Fig. 7-31   Despite a severe mandibular retrusion, **A** to **C** show a marked facial improvement during treatment. **D** shows eruption of the premolars with the establishment of a normal occlusion, normal muscle activity, and good facial balance. Fleischer often uses a thin stainless steel bite rim interocclusally (like Cervera) for selective guidance of eruption. This obviates the need for selective grinding of acrylic, as is done with most activators. (Courtesy Erich Fleischer.)

Fig. 7-32 Class II, division 1, malocclusion in a 11-year-old boy with a retained infantile swallowing habit. **A** to **C,** Initial success with the Bionator was limited because of lack of patient cooperation. After 2 years of intermittent success, the patient's attitude changed and cooperation improved and remained at a high level till the end of treatment. (**A** to **F** courtesy Erich Fleischer.)

Fig. 7-32, cont'd   **D** to **F,** After 4 years of treatment. Satisfactory results and harmonious facial relationships are shown in Fig. 7-33 taken before and after treatment. Only the modified Bionator (Bio-Modulator) appliance was used.

A

B

Fig. 7-33   Cephalograms of the patient in Fig. 7-32 treated with the Fleischer modified Bionator. The original deep bite and shallow mandibular plane are favorable characteristics for functional appliance treatment. **A,** Before treatment, age 10 years 3 months. **B,** After treatment, age 12 years 9 months. (**A** to **C** courtesy Erich Fleischer.)

	10 yr 3 mo	12 yr 9 mo
S-N-A	84°	83°
S-N-B	76°	78°
A-N-B	8°	5°
A to N (perp)	1 mm	−1 mm
1̲ to A	+5 mm	+2 mm
1̅ to Pog	+5 mm	+6 mm
Pog to N (perp)	−10 mm	−8 mm
Max length	90 mm	91 mm
Mand length	107 mm	114 mm
Skel diff	17 mm	23 mm
Saddle angle	125°	127°
Ar to Ptm	31 mm	31 mm
Mand pl angle	19°	20°
Ant face height	68 mm	69 mm
Post face height	51 mm	56 mm
Ant cranial base length	70 mm	71 mm
1̲ to S-N	110°	102°
1̅ to Mand pl	104°	108°

C

Fig. 7-33, cont'd   C, Cephalometric summary.

Fig. 7-34   Lateral study cast of a boy 9 years 7 months old with a severe Class II, division 1, malocclusion. (Courtesy Erich Fleischer.)

Fig. 7-35 Cephalograms of the patient in Fig. 7-34. **A,** Severe overbite and overjet are exacerbated by abnormal perioral muscle function. **B,** At the end of treatment (13 years 7 months). Normal muscle function. **C,** At 16 years 2 months (about 3 years out of treatment). Result still stable. The modified Bionator was used to achieve this result. Full-time wear during active treatment, rather than nighttime only, is a major requirement, as opposed to requirements of the conventional Andresen activator. The appliance can then be used at night only as a retainer. (**A** to **D** courtesy Erich Fleischer.)

	9 yr 7 mo	13 yr 7 mo	16 yr 2 mo
S-N-A	82°	83°	80°
S-N-B	75°	78°	79°
A-N-B	7°	5°	1°
A to N (perp)	+3 mm	+4 mm	+1 mm
1̲ to A	+7 mm	+2 mm	+6 mm
1̄ to Pog	0 mm	+5 mm	+1 mm
Pog to N (perp)	−3 mm	−1 mm	+4 mm
Max length	89 mm	95 mm	92 mm
Mand length	107 mm	102 mm	126 mm
Skel diff	18 mm	25 mm	34 mm
Saddle angle	130°		128°
Ar to Ptm	34 mm	35 mm	35 mm
Mand pl angle	17°	20°	15°
1̲ to S-N	115°	95°	98°
1̄ to mand pl	99°	103°	98°
Ant facial height	55 mm	67 mm	70 mm
Post facial height	43 mm	49 mm	55 mm
Ant cranial base length	66 mm	69 mm	72 mm

Fig. 7-35, cont'd   D, Cephalometric summary.

Recognizing that skeletal malocclusions are three-dimensional, with the majority of Class II malocclusions demonstrating a narrow maxillary arch and a sagittal discrepancy, with changed tongue position and function, Hamilton introduced his expansion activator approach. The first generation of appliances was removable and yet achieved fairly stable results. Many activators have incorporated jackscrews for expansion purposes, with development of the dental arches during sagittal correction a valid treatment objective. The latest advance has been his bonded activator, which achieves rapid and dramatic correction with a truly functional appliance. If it is worn all the time, after being bonded to the maxillary arch, there is no compliance problem and the young patients adapt to the forward posturing functional position quickly. As shown some years ago by Melanson and Van Dyken[133] at Michigan in their study on primates, unloading the temporomandibular joint actually stimulated optimal growth and adaptation. The bonded Herbst appliance enlists the same approach (see "Mixed Dentition Treatment," in Chapter 9) with comparable results. With the Hamilton bonded expansion activator, however, forward guidance of the mandible is achieved primarily by proprioceptive guidance from the lingual flanges of the bonded appliance. There is no actual joining of maxillary and mandibular arches, as there is with the bonded Herbst appliance (Fig. 7-36). That this approach is an excellent adjunct for mixed dentition treatment or even deciduous dentition interception in severe cases, eliminating abnormal, deforming perioral muscle function, has been shown in many cases by Hamilton (Figs. 7-37 through 7-40). Similar results are shown by Joho and colleagues.

Hamilton points out, as does Graber and others, that most of these functional appliance cases ultimately require bonded, bracketed, tooth-borne appliances to complete the detailing, to achieve correct individual tooth positions, and to eliminate rotations. With bonding this phase is relatively easy and usually completed in well under a year.

Controversy continues as to whether the traditional activator or even the bionator or Fränkel function regulator are really what the name implies: functional appliances—if worn only at bedtime (the recommendation made by so many orthodontists). It is more likely that the appliance

Fig. 7-36 **A,** Hamilton bonded activator from below. Lingual flanges in dark extend toward the viewer. The palatal jackscrew is partly open. The impressions of the lower posterior teeth are imbedded in the occlusal extensions in a forward postured relationship. **B,** Hamilton appliance, bonded to maxillary arch, jackscrew in center of palate. The lingual flanges that guide the mandible forward extend toward the viewer. **C,** Bonded Hamilton expansion-activator on maxillary arch. Lingual guiding flanges extend toward the lower arch and tongue.

Fig. 7-37   Hamilton bonded expansion activator case. Girl (5 years, 2 months) with severe Class II, division 1 malocclusion with constricted maxilla and retruded mandible. Perioral muscle activity was compensatory and enhancing the malocclusion. The tentative treatment plan was to institute the primary stage of treatment immediately, with defined options of treatment in either/or mixed dentition and permanent dentition. Bonded activator was placed and the malocclusion was over-treated in an 8-month period. Upper and lower removable acrylic retainers were worn for an additional 6 months. The current state at 7 years is a Class I relationship with excellent skeletal and dental relations. No additional therapy is contemplated. **A** and **B,** Beginning facial views. **C** and **D,** Facial photos 2 years later.

serves as a transient posturing splint. Since the average person swallows only 4 to 8 times an hour during sleep and probably only twice that when wearing a functional appliance, this is a small percentage of time for any stimulating or unloading effect to occur from forward posturing. Petrovic and Stutzmann[156] have shown that there is an excitation of the retrodiskal pad (posterior disk attachment) and some lateral pterygoid activity which would enhance metabolism of the temporomandibular joint in a growing child. However, for the appliance to be optimally effective, it would have to provide continual and repeated functional stimuli. To achieve this objective, some proponents require daytime wear. It has always been a major thesis of Rolf Fränkel[57] that function regulators should be worn both day and night. He refers to his appliance as an exercise device. His impressive results seem to achieve maximum stimulation of optimal condylar growth and direction. The problem is that most functional appliances such as activator, monobloc, LSU activator, and Fränkel appliance, are bulky, thereby making it difficult to speak. With allergies and respiratory problems, patients complain about breathing difficulties. Initial adjustment is not easy, and some young patients find the appliances relatively uncomfortable and remove them as soon as the parent is out of the room. Patient compliance is a continuing problem. Thus many clinicians,

who have tried functional appliances because of the demonstrated results and biologic justification, have given up because of a lack of continued patient cooperation, as well as the clinician's inability to determine just how much the patient has worn the appliance (protestations to the contrary notwithstanding).

Martin Schwarz recognized the compliance difficulties when he made his double plate[173]; it consisted of upper and lower removable appliances that were held by suitable retention wires and that had opposing occlusal acrylic guiding ramps that postured the mandible forward on complete closure. With half the bulk of a monobloc, it is easier to wear such appliances; minor tooth movement can actually be accomplished at the same time with wire appurtenances.

William Clark has emulated Schwarz' thinking with his twin blocks, which are modified Schwarz' double plates. His success with occlusal guide planes has been well documented. And now, with the incorporation of rare earth magnets in the attraction mode, the success is enhanced and more rapid (Figs. 7-41 through 7-58). Like Hamilton, Clark recognizes the need to restore normal maxillary width and does this in his arch development stage of treatment, before sagittal correction with the twin-block appliance and using fixed or removable expansion appliances, such as the jackscrew or quad helix fixed appliance (Figs. 7-41 and 7-51).

Text continued on p. 420.

Fig. 7-38 Intraoral views of beginning and end of treatment for Hamilton bonded expansion activator patient in Fig. 7-37. No appliances are being worn now. **A** and **B** at 5 years and 2 months. **C** and **D,** 21 months later.

Fig. 7-39   Severe mixed dentition Class II, division 1 (8 year, 1 month girl). Moderate prognathism of restricted maxillary arch. The tentative treatment plan called for a bonded Hamilton expansion activator for 7 months, a rapid palatal expansion appliance for 3 months. Comprehensive treatment and arch length enhancement was to be carried out with partial fixed appliances as needed for detailing. A functional retainer with built-in overtreatment was to be worn as needed. In actuality, the first stage was carried out with highly satisfactory results and no additional care was necessary. **A** and **B,** Facial views at 8 years, 1 month. **C** and **D,** Final facial views at 13 years, 9 months.

Fig. 7-40 Intra-oral views of patient in Fig. 7-39 at beginning and end of treatment, as well as post-treatment observation period. No appliances have been worn for some time.

Standard twin blocks (Clark)

Class II, division 1 malocclusion
Permanent dentition

Fig. 7-41 **A,** Drawing of Clark twin block appliances. Attracting rare earth magnets can be embedded in the small 70 degree angulated inclined planes *(hash-marked areas)*, *A.* The occlusal acrylic surfaces, *B,* do not cap the buccal cusps. The lower appliance terminates at the distal of the lower second premolar to allow for upward and forward lower molar eruption. The heavily shaded occlusal cover in the maxillary appliance is trimmed later for controlled eruption. The jackscrew, *C,* in the maxillary appliance can be used as needed for arch width changes. Retention wires and clasps, *D,* provide intra-arch stability. **B,** Twin block on models. Note inclined forward posturing planes, with imbedded attracting rare earth magnets.

Fig. 7-42 *Case J.C.* **A** and **B,** Boy (8 years, 9 months,) with disfiguring Class II, division 1, malocclusion. Perioral musculature is abnormal, with a lower lip trap that further enhances the overjet. Lower incisors occlude in palatal tissue. Other sequelae are a narrow maxillary arch and a *gummy* smile. **C** and **D,** Profile views taken before and immediately after insertion of forward posturing functional magnetic appliances. **E, F, G,** Intra-oral views before therapy.

Fig. 7-43 *Case J.C.* Intraoral views, after 8 months of magnetic twin block treatment.

Fig. 7-44 *Case J.C.* Facial views 8 months after start of treatment.

Fig. 7-45   *Case J.C.* **A,** Upper retainer with inclined ramp behind maxillary incisors, worn until fixed appliance phase. **B, C, D,** Intra-orals before second phase fixed appliance detailing.

Fig. 7-46   *Case J.C.* **A** and **B,** Bonded brackets and intruding adjustments on incisor segments to eliminate excessive overbite and reduce excessive gingival display. **C** and **D,** Intra-oral views 1 year out of retention.

Fig. 7-47 *Case J.C.* Facial views, 1 year out of retention.

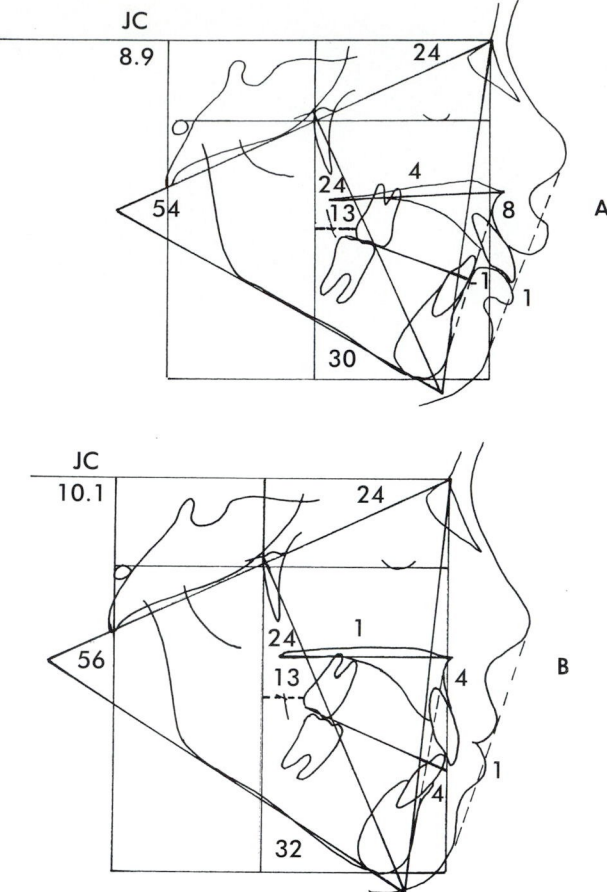

Fig. 7-48 *Case J.C.* Cephalometric tracings before and after twin block therapy (approximately a 14 month interval).

If only mild expansion is needed, it can be accomplished by the palatal jackscrew in the bonded maxillary twin block element and will also improve alignment as needed.

The orthopedic phase with the twin blocks recognizes the need for eruption of lower molars to eliminate excessive overbite. By not covering the mandibular molars they are free to erupt in an upward and forward vector, aiding the Class II correction. The occlusal acrylic does not cover the

buccal cusps of both upper and lower posterior teeth (Figs. 7-41 and 7-43). It should be emphasized that functional appliances resort to reciprocal dental Class II correction in a noninvasive manner, avoiding the potential iatrogenic sequelae of periodontal involvement, gingival inflammation, crestal bone loss, root resorption, or dilaceration. This reciprocal upper and lower arch dental adjustment must be controlled, of course. Too often it has not been controlled with conventional functional appliances, because the mandibular incisors are excessively proclined. It is not maltreatment, however, to obtain dental correction with biocompatible measures.

For Phase I of twin block therapy the magnets in attraction mode are embedded in the 70 degree inclines of the upper and lower appliances (Fig. 7-41, *A*) to enhance functional activity and inter-arch contact in the protrusive relationship (Fig. 7-41, *B*). The patient is instructed to wear the appliances all the time, removing them only for cleaning. Note the positions of the inclines differ in the upper and lower appliances (anterior, upper; posterior, lower). Moss and Shaw (1990) have reported using repelling magnets in a different configuration on upper and lower appliances, again

Text continued on p. 428.

Fig. 7-49   *Case J.C.* Cephalometric superimpositions of **A** tracings in Fig. 7-48, and **B,** beginning treatment and an additional year after previous examination (comparing age 8.9 and 11.1).

Fig. 7-50   *Case F.H.* **A, B, C,** At initial examination (14 years, 11 months), with a full Class II, division 1, malocclusion, complicated by crowding in both arches. Overjet was 10 mm, with a deep impinging overbite. A chronic labial gingival inflammation existed in the lower right central incisor area. The first phase of arch development treatment was with an upper quad helix and lower fixed lingual appliances for 6 months. The following twin magnetic block phase was for 5 months only because of minimal skeletal involvement. The full fixed bioprogressive phase took 20 months. The labially compromised lower left central incisor was torqued back into the alveolar process, the lower labial frenum resected and the labial gingival infection eliminated. Retention was for 1 year.

Fig. 7-51 *Case F.H.* Arch development phase, **A, B, C,** using quad helix appliance.

Fig. 7-52 *Case F.H.* Lower arch development with looped lingual arch: **A, B,** and **C.**

Fig. 7-53 *Case F.H.* Intraorals before twin block magnetic phase.

Fig. 7-54 *Case F.H.* Magnetic twin blocks with magnets in contact on upper and lower occlusal inclined planes in protrusive relationship, **A, B,** and **C.**

Continued.

Fig. 7-54, cont'd   Occlusion 2 months later, **D, E,** and **F.** Upper and lower appliances, showing magnets on inclined planes. Note maxillary jackscrew for any needed expansion. Lower molars are free to erupt, **G** and **H.**

Fig. 7-55   *Case F.H.* **A** and **B,** Profile changes after magnetic twin block therapy (1 year interval).

Fig. 7-56 *Case F.H.* Fixed appliance phase, **A, B, C,** and **D.** After treatment, age 17 years, 8 months, **E, F, G,** and **H.**

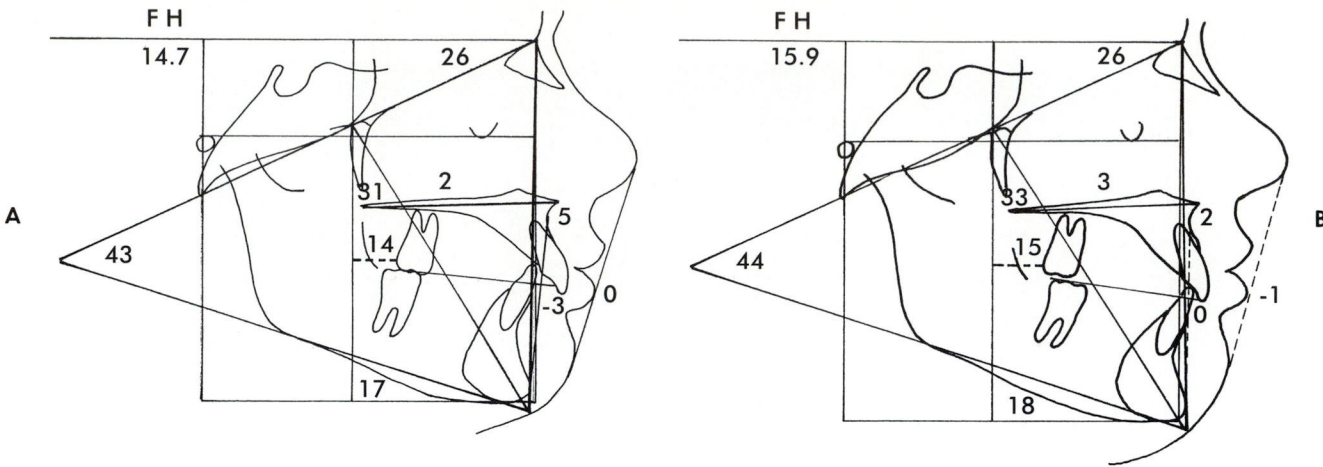

Fig. 7-57 *Case F.H.* Cephalometric tracings, at beginning of treatment and after twin block therapy (1 year interval).

Fig. 7-58 *Case F.H.* Cephalometric superimpositions. **A,** 14′7″ and 15′9″. **B,** 14′7″ and 17′8″, after fixed appliances. Major change occurred in magnetic twin block phase.

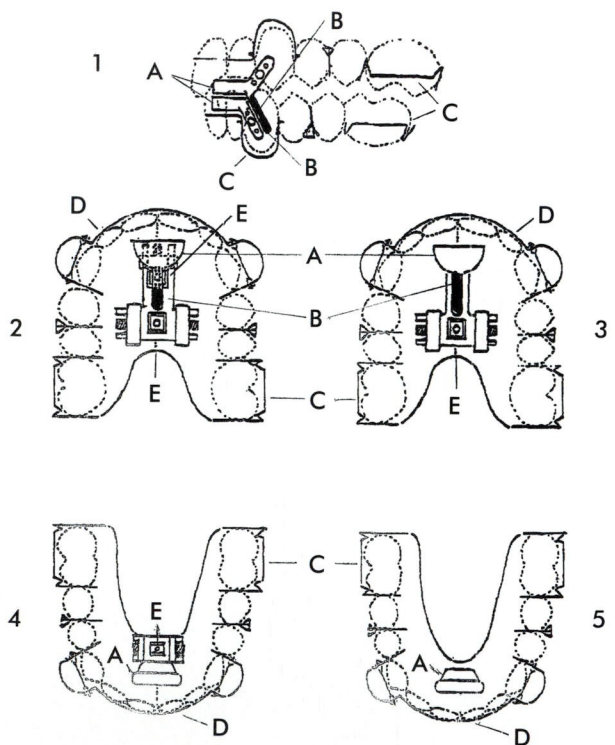

Fig. 7-59 Functional Magnetic Appliance (FMA) **1.** Lateral view with magnets together in protrusive relationship. **2.** Maxillary appliance, with jackscrews for both expansion and incisor segment protraction. **3,** Maxillary appliance, with expansion screw only. Note guidance prongs in maxillary appliances. **4.** Mandibular appliance with expansion jackscrew. **5.** Mandibular appliance with magnet only imbedded in lingual acrylic. *A,* Miniaturized rare earth magnets. *B,* Maxillary forward guidance prong. *C,* Retention clasps. *D,* Labial arch wire, *E,* Jackscrew.

Fig. 7-60 FMA of Vardimon. Upper and lower modified Schwarz plates, similar to the Clark twin block functional approach. Instead of bilateral angled magnetic inclines, lingual midline magnets are imbedded in the acrylic. A maxillary guiding prong which slides on the lingual acrylic of the lower appliance during closure brings the mandible forward into the desired protrusive relationship as the magnets come into contact. This unloads the condyles, much the same as conventional functional appliances—only the functional stimulus of the two-part system is significantly more frequent and apparently greater. Patient compliance is better than with a single *monobloc* appliance. Jackscrews may be incorporated in both appliances as needed for transverse control. In top view, magnets, *A*, approach each other, along lingual guidance prong. *B*, Retention tags, *C*, insert in acrylic of upper and lower appliances. In middle view, note magnet, *A*, and guidance prong, *B*, imbedded in palatal acrylic. Retention clasps, *D*, may be supplemented by small elastics, hooking over bonded brackets, *E*. This increases resistance to dislodgement by magnetic action. Either single or double magnets, *A*, round or oblong, may be used in lower appliance, bottom view.

to aid in forward posturing. Repelling magnets require a different orientation of the inclines.

Following the rapid and desired sagittal correction, the twin blocks are worn for an additional 2 to 3 months to stabilize the occlusion and allow for needed posterior eruption, which occurs more slowly. The acrylic is trimmed away from the maxillary occlusal surfaces of the maxillary molars and premolars gradually to allow for their downward and forward eruption. The lower appliance is discarded and an inclined plane is added to the maxillary appliance, which serves as a short term retainer for Phase II to continue stabilization and allow posterior segment eruption that is needed.

Vardimon and associates,* as well as Joho and Derendelilier,[111a] have been aware of the potential of the use of rare earth magnets in orthodontics and dentofacial orthopedics for some time and have produced a series of research reports on the efficacy and specific applications of rare earth magnets. Blechman[30a,30b] has been a pioneer in the magnetic field, albeit not with functional appliances. Taking advantage of the miniaturization of these powerful and small permanent magnets made of samarium cobalt and neodymium-iron-boron, both upper and lower removable appliances may have strategically placed magnets, delivering attracting or repelling force that is extremely effective and rapid. Considerable experimentation has been done on the size, shape,

*References 194-203.

and placement of the magnet. If the magnets are too strong, they clamp the two appliances together, effecting a monobloc, which defeats the purpose. If they are too strong, they tend to dislodge the removable appliances from their respective jaws. If the magnets are too small, they do not have a stimulating effect on jaw position. The correct size, shape, and angulation of opposing magnets are all-important, as shown by Vardimon (Figs. 7-59 through 7-61).

After continuing experimentation on animals and human patients, a technique has now evolved that satisfies the criteria needed to maintain sufficient stability of the appliance in each arch and the demands for constant functional stimulation of forward and backward movement, yet reasonably retains the facility of speaking and swallowing. These appliances serve as functional, loading and unloading, repetitive mechanisms, not only during swallowing but also innumerable times during the waking hours. Appliances should be removed for eating and cleaning. They are considered effective tools in the functional appliance armamentaria. A good example of mixed dentition, Phase One FMA therapy, is seen in Figs. 7-62 through 7-65. Eight months of functional guidance at the right time greatly reduces sagittal basal discrepancy; eliminates deforming perioral muscle function and speech problems; and makes Phase Two fixed mechanotherapy much shorter, easier, and more likely to be successful without premolar extraction and undue reliance on prolonged extra-oral force.

Current research is exploring the use of light bonded

Fig. 7-61 Upper and lower FMA, using jackscrews for expansion. Small double magnets, *A,* are imbedded in palatal acrylic immediately anterior to guidance prong, *B,* and jackscrew, *C.* Lower oblong magnet, *A,* is attached to jackscrew, *C,* so as not to interfere with widening process. Maxillary guidance prong slides down the magnetic surface during closure.

Fig. 7-62 *Patient S.D.* Severe Class II, division 1 (8 year old girl), lip trap compensation, lower incisors forced lingually, with premature deciduous lower canine loss.

Fig. 7-63 *Patient S.D.* Magnet functional therapy, phase I. **A,** Anterior view at beginning of mixed dentition stage one. **B,** Eight months later with marked reduction of overjet and elimination of abnormal lip habit. **C,** Narrow maxillary arch caused by abnormal lip and tongue function and posture. **D,** Eight months of magnetic functional, combined with jackscrew slow palatal expansion.

acrylic upper and lower appliances, which incorporate angulated attraction magnets to optimize sagittal correction. Magnets may also be used in the palatal midline of the upper appliance at the same time to achieve the desired expansion.[197] Following this phase of treatment, brackets are bonded on individual teeth as needed to complete the detailing.

Blechman has been involved in medical use of electromagnetic fields and has pioneered in orthodontic usage.[30b] He hypothesized that static magnetic fields may have some electric field effect that potentiates tissue response. In vitro orthodontic research on this hypothesis has produced mixed results thus far. Clinically, however, in magnet deimpaction of palatally malposed maxillary canines, the eruption into the mouth is as little as one third of the time required by conventional appliances.[203] However, it is not likely that magnets in functional appliances would have any electric field effect on the condyle. Magnetic functional appliances, of course, cannot be any more effective in a nongrowing child than any other functional appliance. Improperly designed magnetic appliances or improper case selection can result in proclination of the lower incisors, even as it does with other types of activators. At present, the buccal shields

of the Fränkel appliance or the buccal loops of the bionator have not been incorporated in magnetic functionals. Since they seem to relieve pressure from the buccinator mechanism and tend to enhance autonomous expansion, there is no reason why they could not be added in the future without unduly jeopardizing speech and patient cooperation. Today, magnets seem to offer an exciting advance in achieving better functional efficiency and stimulation of optimal growth amounts and direction with minimum bulk. At last, functional appliances can truly live up to their name.

ADVANTAGES OF FUNCTIONAL APPLIANCES

It is pertinent to ask, "Why functional appliances? Do they have any advantages over fixed appliances?" The answer is not absolute and is couched in probabilities, but it is definitive enough to accept for the majority of cases.

The activator allows more effective oral prophylaxis and maintenance of better hard and soft tissue integrity. Of particular concern are the potential for root resorption, sheared alveolar crests, decalcification of enamel surfaces, gingival hypertrophy, chronic inflammation, and the potential fibrotic

Fig. 7-64 *Patient S.D.* **A,** Upper and lower FMA in place with magnets in contact in attractive mode. This is a transient position, repeated countless times during the day and night, with swallowing breathing, kinetic action. **B,** Angulated oblong magnet in maxillary appliance, with acrylic customized guidance ramp at approximately 70 degrees—similar to Clark twin block. Jackscrew has already been opened. **C,** Mandibular oblong magnet seen in mirror image of lingual surface of lower appliance. Lower brackets may be bonded to labial surfaces of lower incisors, for labial wire to snap below, enhancing retention during continuing functional exercises.

Fig. 7-65 *Patient S.D.* Lateral cephalograms at beginning of treatment. **A,** Note severe overjet and lingually inclined lower incisors. **B,** Upper and lower FMA appliances in place. Arrow shows opposing angulated attractive mode brackets, imbedded in acrylic lingual to incisors. **C,** Lateral cephalogram after 8 months of FMA treatment. Second phase of fixed appliances is planned in permanent dentition, but basal dysplasia and abnormal deforming perioral muscle function have largely been eliminated.

changes too often seen with fixed appliances that have not been taken care of properly by the patient. When there is periodontal disease or a hormonal problem, removable appliances are kinder to the tissue. The problems of decalcification associated with fixed appliances need not be elaborated; they are well known, whether full bands or direct bonded attachments are used. Trapping of acidogenic debris is a real hazard. Too often the question has been, "What price orthodontics?" These are the cases that appear in litigation.

To the question of elimination of abnormal perioral muscle function that is an associated factor in most Class II, division 1 malocclusions, the answer is also in favor of functional appliances. Regardless of where the clinician stands on the question of the relationship of form and function, and the potentially deleterious effects of the hyperactive mentalis and hyoid musculature and the *lip trap,* there is little doubt that elimination of abnormal muscle activity is beneficial (Figs. 7-30 to 7-35). Many fixed appliance regimens now use lip bumpers and shields, emulating functional appliances, in appreciating this aspect.

The answer to the crucial question of whether functional appliances can stimulate condylar growth beyond normal pattern is still open to discussion and needs more clinical research on actual patients to have any air of finality. Animal experiments have produced overwhelming evidence of the possibilities, however, and cephalometric measurements on properly selected and treated patients show a variable response but produce many examples of enhanced mandibular growth during functional appliance wear.[64] Is this *catch-up* growth? Is it due merely to the elimination of restrictive abnormal perioral muscle function and functional retrusion? Or is it merely fortuitous timing with a growth spurt?

The research of Graber[64] and Graber[68] on humans and nonhuman primates and Stutzmann et al.[185] on rats shows that the trabecular angle can be changed by forward advancement of the mandible, producing a change in growth direction that would help reduce the sagittal discrepancy. However, trabecular changes are temporary and actual changes in mandibular morphology caused by them are hard to measure. Until we know more, the best that can be said is that functional appliances do eliminate factors that may stand in the way of accomplishing the most favorable growth pattern and they permit the attainment of the achievable optimum. When we realize the adaptability of the living organism, and recognize the range of normal response, and when we see that the Japanese people are, on the average, 4 inches taller now than they were before World War II largely because of diet (Americans are taller, too, though by not as much), we cannot deny the potential for change.

The question of change in sagittal position is a corollary to condylar response. Firm clinical evidence exists of a large number of Class II, division 1 malocclusions with deep bite that also have a most retruded condylar position in the fossa on habitual occlusion. Functional appliances are capable of eliminating the functional retrusions effectively, particularly in Class II, division 2 malocclusions. As our *most likely scenario* shows, the total sagittal change is the result of multiple factors, no one of which is responsible for the major change. Modified functional appliances are an important tool in TMD cases. They may also prevent development of TMD problems.

Animal experimentation shows significant remodeling of the articular fossa in subjects with mandibular advancement. Although this is one area of lesser potential for significant change, it is a membranous bone region and is adaptable to normal and abnormal function. The changes induced in the articular eminence and condylar path after the eruption of the deciduous incisor teeth show the potential for functional effect on these structures. It is likely that functional appliances are more effective than fixed appliances in producing any such changes.

The potential for slight restriction of horizontal maxillary growth exists for functional appliances. Redirection of maxillary growth or relocation of the maxilla in a more vertical direction is demonstrated in selected cases. However, fixed appliance orthopedic procedures are more effective than functional appliances in this regard—which leads to the obvious conclusion that a combination of fixed and functional appliances could produce the best possible of all orthodontic worlds, using each component of the appliance for the effect it produces best. The following chapter, by Stöckli and Teuscher, as well as Chapter 9 by McNamara, makes this philosophy a practical reality.

REFERENCES

1. Ahlgren J: An electromyographic analysis of the response to activator (Andresen-Häupl) therapy, *Odontol Rev* 11:125, 1960.
2. Ahlgren J: The neurophysiologic principles of the Andresen method of functional jaw orthopedics. A critical analysis and new hypothesis, *Sven Tandlak Tidskr* 63:1, 1970.
3. Ahlgren J: A longitudinal clinical and cephalometric study of 50 malocclusion cases treated with activator appliances, *Trans Eur Orthod Soc* p. 285, 1973.
4. Ahlgren J: Changes in length and torque of the masticatory muscles produced by the activator appliance, *Swed Dent J* (suppl 15), 1982.
5. Ahlgren J: Munskärmaktivator: en modifierad Andresen-plät, *Tandläkartidningen* 75:300, 1983.
6. Altuna G, Niegel S: Bionators in Class II treatment. *J Clin Orthod* 19:185, 1985.
7. Andresen V: Beitrag zur Retention, *Z Zahnaertzl Orthop* 3:121, 1910.
8. Andresen V: Bio-mekanisk ortodonti: et ortodontisk system for privatpraksis og skoletannklinikker, *Nor Tannlaegeforen Tid* 41:71, 161, 442, 1931.
9. Andresen V: Bio-mekanisk ortodonti: et ortodontisk system for privatpraksis og skoletannklinikker, *Nor Tannlaegeforen Tid* 42:131, 215, 295, 1932.
10. Andresen V: Ueber das sogenannte "norwegische System der Funktions-Kiefer-Orthopädie," *Dtsch Zahnaerztl Wochenschr* 39:235, 283, 1936.
11. Andresen V, Häupl K: *Funktionskieferorthopädie. Die Grundlagen des "norwegischen Systems,"* ed 2, Leipzig, 1939, H. Meusser.
12. Andresen V, Häupl K: *Funktionskieferorthopädie. Die Grundlagen des "norwegischen Systems,"* ed 3, Leipzig, 1942, JA Barth Verlag.
13. Andresen V, Häupl K: *Funktionskieferorthopädie. Die Grundlagen des "norwegischen Systems,"* ed 4, Leipzig, 1945, JA Barth Verlag.
14. Andresen V, Häupl K, Petrik L: *Funktionskieferorthopädie,* ed 6, Munich, 1957, JA Barth.

15. Arat M, Iseri H: Orthodontic and orthopaedic approach in the treatment of skeletal open bite, *Eur J Orthod* 14:207, 1992.

16. Ascher F: Kontrollierte Ergebnisse der Rückbissbehandlung mit funktionskieferorthopädischen Geräten, *Fortscher Kieferorthop* 32:149, 1971.

17. Ballard CF: A consideration of the physiological background of mandibular posture and movement. *Dent Pract Dent Rec* 6:80, 1955.

18. Balters W: *Eine Einführung in die Bionatorheilmethode: ausgewählte Schriften und Vorträge,* Heidelberg, 1973, C Herrmann.

19. Barbre RE, Sinclair PM: A cephalometric evaluation of anterior openbite correction with the magnetic active vertical corrector, *Angle Orthod* 6:93, 1991.

20. Battagel JM: The relationship between hard and soft tissue changes following treatment of Class II, division 1 malocclusion using Edgewise and Fränkel appliance techniques, *Eur J Orthod* 12:154, 1990.

21. Baume LJ: Cephalo-facial growth patterns and the functional adaptation of the temporomandibular joint structures, *Eur Orthod Soc Rep Congr,* p 79, 1969.

22. Baume LJ, Derichsweiler H: Is the condylar growth center responsive to orthodontic therapy? An experimental study in *Macaca mulatta, Oral Surg* 14:347, 1961.

23. Bierbaek L, Melsen B, Terp S: A laminagraphic study of the alterations in the temporo-mandibular joint following activator treatment, *Eur J Orthod* 6:157, 1984.

24. Biggerstaff RH: "The condylar plexus." Personal communication, July 1983.

25. Bimler HP: Die elastischen Gebissformer, *Zahnaerztl Welt* 4:499, 1949.

26. Bimler HP: JCO/interviews Dr. H.P. Bimler on functional appliances, *J Clin Orthod* 17:39, 1983.

27. Bimler HP: *The Bimler appliance.* In Graber TM, Neumann B: *Removable orthodontic appliances,* ed 2, Philadelphia, 1984, WB Saunders.

28. Björk A: The principle of the Andresen method of orthodontic treatment, a discussion based on cephalometric x-ray analysis of treated cases, *Am J Orthod* 37:437, 1951.

29. Björk A: Prediction of mandibular growth rotation, *Am J Orthod* 55:585, 1969.

30. Björk A, Palling M: Adolescent age changes in sagittal jaw relation, alveolar prognathy, and incisal inclination, *Acta Odontol Scand* 12:201, 1954-1955.

30a. Blechman AM: Magnetic force systems in orthodontics: clinical results of a pilot study, *Am J Orthod* 87:201-210, 1985.

30b. Blechman AM, Smiley H: Magnetic force in orthodontics, *Am J Orthod* 79:435-443, 1978.

31. Bolmgren GA, Moshiri F: Bionator treatment in Class II, division 1, *Angle Orthod* 56:255, 1986.

32. Bondevik O: How effective is the combined activator-headgear treatment? *Eur J Orthod* 13:482, 1991.

33. Breitner C: Experimentelle Veränderung der mesiodistalen Beziehungen der oberen und unteren Zahnreihen, *Z Stomatol* 28:134, 620, 1930.

34. Brieden CM, Pangrazio-Kulbersh V, Kulbersh R: Maxillary skeletal and dental change with Fränkel appliance therapy—an implant study, *Angle Orthod* 54:226, 1984.

35. Chabre C: Vertical control with a headgear-activator combination, *J Clin Orthod* 24:618, 1990.

36. Chang HF, Wu KM et al: Effects of activator treatment on Class II, division 1 malocclusion, *J Clin Orthod* 23:560, 1989.

37. Charlier JP, Petrovic A, Herrmann-Stutzmann J: Effect of mandibular hyperpulsion on the prechondroblastic zone of young rat condyle, *Am J Orthod* 55:71, 1969.

38. Creekmore TD, Radney LJ: Fränkel appliance therapy: orthopedic or orthodontic? *Am J Orthod* 83:89, 1983.

39. Demisch A: Effects of activator therapy on the craniofacial skeleton in Class II, Division 1, malocclusion, *Eur Orthod Soc Rep Congr,* p 295, 1972.

40. Demisch A: *Herren's dentofacial orthopedics.* In Graber TM, Neumann B, editors: *Removable orthodontic appliances,* ed 2, Philadelphia, 1984, WB Saunders.

41. Dermaut LR, van den Eynde F, de Pauw G: Skeletal and dentoalveolar changes as a result of headgear activator therapy related to different vertical growth patterns, *Eur J Orthod* 14:140, 1992.

42. Dietrich UC: Aktivator-mandibuläre Reaktion, *Schweiz Monatsschr Zahnheilkd* 83:1092, 1973.

43. Drage KJ, Hunt NP: Overjet relapse following functional appliance therapy, *Br J Orthod* 17:205, 1990.

44. Eirew HL, McDowell F, Phillips JG: The Fraenkel appliance—avoidance of lower incisor proclination, *Br J Orthod* 8:189, 1981.

45. Elgoyhen JC, Moyers RE, et al: Craniofacial adaptation to protrusive function in young rhesus monkeys, *Am J Orthod* 62:469, 1972.

46. Enlow DH: *The dynamics of skeletal growth and remodelling.* In *Scientific foundations of orthopedic surgery,* London, 1981, Heinemann Medical.

47. Enlow DH, DiGangi D, McNamara JA Jr, Mina M: An evaluation of the morphogenic and anatomic effects of the functional regulator utilizing the counterpart analysis, *Eur J Orthod* 10:192, 1988.

48. Eschler J: Wesen und Möglichkeiten der Verwendung von kontinuierlicher und intermittierenden Kräften im Rahmen des Andresen-Häupl'schen Behandlungssystems, *Oesterr Z Stomatol* 47:53, 1950.

49. Eschler J: *Die funktionelle Orthopädie des Kausystems.* Munich, 1952, C Hanser.

50. Eschler J: Die muskuläre Wirkungsweise des Andresen-Häuplschen Apparates, *Oesterr Z Stomatol* 49:79, 1952.

51. Eschler J: Elektrophysiologische und pathologische Untersuchungen des Kausystems. IV. Mitteilung: Elektromyographische Untersuchungen über die Wirksamkeit muskeltonussteigernder Medikamente bei Anwendung des Andresen-Häupl Apparates, *Dtsch Zahnaerztl Z* 10:1421, 1955.

52. Eschler J: Die Kieferdehnung mit funktionskieferorthopädischen Apparaten: der Funktionator, *Zahnaertzl Welt* 63:203, 1962.

53. Fleischer E, Fleischer A: *Bionator modification; the Bio-M-S therapy.* In Graber TM, Neumann B: *Removable orthodontic appliances,* ed 2, Philadelphia, 1984, WB Saunders.

54. Fränkel R: Concerning recent articles on Fränkel appliance therapy (letter), *Am J Orthod* 85:441, 1984.

55. Fränkel R: *Technik und Handhabung der Funktionsregler,* Berlin, 1973, VEB Verlag Volk und Gesundheit.

56. Fränkel R: *Biomechanical aspects of the form/function relationship in craniofacial morphogenesis: a clinician's approach.* In McNamara JA, Ribbens KA, Howe RP, editors: *Clinical alteration of the growing face, Monograph 14, Craniofacial growth series,* Ann Arbor, 1983, Center for Human Growth and Development, University of Michigan.

57. Fränkel R: "The functional strategy in the orofacial area." Presented at the 83rd annual session, American Association of Orthodontists, Boston, May 1983.

58. Fränkel R, Fränkel C: A functional approach to treatment of skeletal open bite, *Am J Orthod* 84:54, 1983.

59. Fränkel R, Reiss W: Problematik der Unterkiefernachentwicklung bei Distalfällen, *Fortschr Kieferorthop* 31:345, 1970.

60. Freunthaller P: Cephalometric observations in Class II, division 1 malocclusions treated with the activator, *Angle Orthod* 37:18, 1967.

61. Gaumond G: Hyperpropulsor activator, *J Clin Orthod* 20:405, 1986.

62. Gerber M: Beobachtungen an schlafenden Aktivatorträgern, *Fortschr Kieferorthop* 18:205, 1957.

63. Gianelly AA, Brosnan P, Martignoni M, Bernstein L: Mandibular growth, condyle position, and Fränkel appliance therapy, *Angle Orthod* 53:131, 1983.

64. Graber LW: "Results of Fränkel appliance therapy on Class II, division 1 malocclusion patients: clinical research with functional appliances." Presented at the 83rd annual session, American Association of Orthodontists, Boston, May 1983.

65. Graber TM: Postmortems in posttreatment adjustment, *Am J Orthod* 52:331, 1966.

66. Graber TM: Maxillary second molar extraction in Class II malocclusion, *Am J Orthod* 56:331, 1969.

67. Graber TM: *Orthodontics; principles and practice*, ed 3, Philadelphia, 1972, WB Saunders.

68. Graber TM: "The effect of buccal shields on the maxillary dental arch width in the squirrel monkey *(Saimiri sciureus)*." Presented at the 83rd annual session, American Association of Orthodontists, Boston, May 1983.

69. Graber TM: *Physiological principles of functional appliances*, St Louis, 1985, Mosby.

70. Graber TM, Neumann B: *Removable orthodontic appliances*, ed 2, Philadelphia, 1984, WB Saunders.

71. Graber TM, Rakosi T, Petrovic A, editors: *Dentofacial orthopedics with functional appliances*, St Louis, 1986, Mosby.

72. Grohs R, Petrik L: Die Funktionskieferorthopädie als Helferin der Prothetik, *Z Stomatol* 42:160-178, 1944.

73. Grossman WJ, Greenfield BE, Timms DJ: Electromyography as an aid in diagnosis and treatment analysis, *Am J Orthod* 47:481, 1961.

74. Grude R: Myofunctional therapy. A review of various cases some years after their treatment by the Norwegian system had been completed, *Nor Tannlaegeforen Tid* 62:1, 1952.

75. Grude R: Ortodontisk terapi med avtagbar apparatur, *Nord Klin Odont* 3/15(6):1, 1966.

76. Hagerström L: Sex fall av distalbett med retruderade överkäksinsisiver behandlade med expansion *Sven Tandlaekarforeb Tidn* 61:826, 1969.

77. Hale LR, Tonge EA: A long-term follow-up of four cases treated with the Andreasen appliance, *Br J Orthod* 13:195, 1986.

78. Hamano Y, Ahlgren J; A cephalometric study of the construction bite of the activator, *Eur J Orthod* 9:305, 1987.

79. Hamilton, DC: "Integration of functional and fixed appliances. The expansion activator system." Presented at the 83rd annual session, American Association of Orthodontists, Boston, May 1983.

80. Hansen K, Pancherz H: Long-term effects of Herbst treatment in relation to normal growth development: a cephalometric study, *Eur J Orthod* 14:285, 1992.

81. Harvold EP: *Distalokklusjon, Behandlingsmetodik, Tandlaegebladet* 50:146, 1946.

82. Harvold EP: *The activator in interceptive orthodontics*, St Louis, 1974, Mosby.

83. Harvold EP, Vargervik K: Morphogenetic response to activator treatment, *Am J Orthod* 60:478, 1971.

84. Hasund A: The use of activators in a system employing fixed appliances, *Eur Orthod Soc Rep Congr*, p 329, 1969.

85. Häupl K: *Gewebsumbau und Zahnverdrängung in der Funktionskieferorthopädie: eine funktionell-histologische Studie*, Leipzig, 1938, JA Barth.

86. Häupl K: Transformation of the temporomandibular joint during orthodontic treatment, *Am J Orthod* 47:151, 1961 (Abstract).

87. Häupl K, Psansky R: Experimentelle Untersuchungen über Gelenkstransformation bei Verwendung der Methoden der Funktionskieferorthopädie, *Dtsch Zahn Mund Kieferheilkd* 6:439, 1939.

88. Hausser E: Wachstum und Entwicklung unter dem Einfluss funktionskieferorthopädischer Therapie, *Fortschr Kieferorthop* 24:310, 1963.

89. Hausser E: Functional orthodontic treatment with the activator, *Trans Eur Orthod Soc* p. 427, 1973.

90. Hausser E: Funktionskieferorthopädische Behandlung mit dem Aktivator, *Fortschr Kieferorthop* 36:1, 1975.

91. Haynes S: Anterior vertical changes in function regulator therapy, *Eur J Orthod* 5:219, 1983.

92. Haynes S: Profile changes in modified functional regulator therapy, *Angle Orthod* 56:309, 1986.

93. Herren P: Die Wirkungsweise des Aktivators, *Schweiz Monatsschr Zahnheilkd* 63:829, 1953.

94. Herren P: The activator's mode of action, *Am J Orthod* 45:512, 1959.

95. Hoffer O: Les modifications de l'articulation temporomandibulaire par l'action des moyens orthopédiques, *Orthod Fr* 29:97, 1958.

96. Hollender L, Lindahl L: Radiographic study of articular remodeling in the temporomandibular joint after condylar fractures, *Scand J Dent Res* 82:462, 1974.

97. Hopkins JB, Murphy J: Variations in good occlusions, *Angle Orthod* 41:55, 1971.

98. Hotz R: Die funktionelle Beurteilung der Bisslage als Ausgangspunkt für die Prognose und die Begrenzung des Behandlungs, *Fortschr Kieferorthop* 16:255, 1955.

99. Hotz RP: Application and appliance manipulation of functional forces, *Am J Orthod* 58:459, 1970.

100. Hotz R: *Orthodontics in daily practice: possibilities and limitations in the area of children's dentistry*, Bern, 1974, H Huber.

101. Hotz R, Mühlemann H: Die Funktion in der Beurteilung und Therapie von Bissanomalien, *Schweiz Monatsschr Zahnheilkd* 62:592, 1952.

102. Hoyte DAN, Enlow DH: Wolff's law and the problem of muscle attachment on resorptive surface of bone, *Am J Phys Anthropol* 24:205, 1966.

103. Humerfelt A, Slagsvold O: Changes in occlusion and craniofacial pattern between 11 and 25 years of age. A follow-up study of individuals with normal occlusion, *Eur Orthod Soc Rep Congr* p. 113, 1972.

104. Ingervall B: Relation between retruded contact, intercuspal, and rest positions of the mandible in children with Angle Class II, division 2 malocclusions, *Odontol Rev* 19:1, 1968.

105. Ingervall B, Bitsanis E: Function of masticatory muscles during the initial phase of activator treatment, *Eur J Orthod* 8:172, 1986.

106. Isaacson KG, Reed RT, Stephens CD: The Harvold activator: simplified construction and use, *J Clin Orthod* 17:845, 1984.

107. Jacobsson SO: Cephalometric evaluation of treatment effect on Class II, division 1 malocclusions, *Am J Orthod* 53:446, 1967.

108. Jacobsson SO, Paulin G: The influence of activator treatment on skeletal growth in Angle Class II: 1 case: a roentgenocephalometric study, *Eur J Orthod* 12:174, 1990.

109. Johannesen B: "Overjet and labio-lingual position of incisor teeth in treated Class II, division 1 malocclusions." Thesis. University of Oslo, 1972.

110. Johannesen B: A critical evaluation of treatment planning Class II, division 1, malocclusions, *Studieweek* p. 112, 1975.

111. Johnston LE: Seminar at the University of Chicago, November 1979.

111a. Joho JP, Derendeliler MA: Magnetic activator device II (MAD II) for correction of Class II, division 1 malocclusions, *Am J Orthod Dentofac Orthop* 103:223-239, 1993.

112. Kerr WJ, TenHave TR, McNamara JA, Jr: A comparison of skeletal and dental changes produced by function regulators (FR-2 and FR-3), *Eur J Orthod* 11:235, 1989.

113. Klammt G: Der offene Aktivator, *Dtsch Stomat* 5:322, 1955.

114. Komposch G, Hockenjos C: Die Reaktionsfähigkeit des Temporomandibularen, *Fortschr Kieferorthop* 38:121, 1977.

115. Korkhaus G: Ein kieferorthopädisch interessantes Zwillingpaar, *Fortschr Kieferorthop* 32:257, 1971.

116. Koski K: Cranial growth centers: facts or fallacies? *Am J Orthod* 54:566, 1968.

117. Lehman R, Hulsink JH: Treatment of Class II malocclusion with a headgear-activator combination, *J Clin Orthod* 23:430, 1989.

118. Lehman R, Romuli A, Bakker V: Five-year treatment results with a headgear-activator combination, *Eur J Orthod* 10:309, 1988.

119. Loh MK, Kerr WJ: The function regulator III: effects and indications for use, *Br J Orthod* 12:153, 1985.

120. Lund K: Mandibular growth and remodelling processes after condylar fracture: a longitudinal roentgencephalometric study, *Acta Odontol Scand* 32 (suppl 64), 1974.

121. Madone G, Ingervall B: Stability of results and function of the masticatory system in patients treated with the Herren type of activator, *Eur J Orthod* 6:92, 1984.

122. May FJ: "A laminagraphic and cephalometric evaluation of dental and skeletal changes occurring during activator treatment." Thesis, University of Minnesota. Cited in Hirzel HC, Grewe JM: Activators; a practical approach, *Am J Orthod* 66:557, 1974.

123. McDougall PD, McNamara JA, Dierkes JM: Arch width development in Class II patients with the Fränkel appliance, *Am J Orthod* 82:10, 1982.

124. McNamara JA, Jr: The functional regulator (FR-3) of Fränkel, *Am J Orthod* 88:409,1985.

125. McNamara JA, Jr: Dentofacial adaptations in adult patients following functional regulator therapy, *Am J Orthod* 85:57, 1984.

126. McNamara JA, Jr, Bookstein FL, Shaughnessy TG: Skeletal and dental changes following functional regulator therapy on Class II patients, *Am J Orthod* 88:91, 1985.

127. McNamara JA: Neuromuscular and skeletal adaptations to altered function in the orofacial region, *Am J Orthod* 64:578, 1973.

128. McNamara JA: Functional determinants of craniofacial size and shape, *Eur J Orthod* 2:131, 1980.

129. McNamara JA: Components of Class II malocclusions in children 8-10 years of age, *Angle Orthod* 51:177, 1981.

130. McNamara JA: *A method of cephalometric analysis*. In McNamara JA, Ribbens KA, Howe HP, editors: *Clinical alteration of the growing face, Monograph 14, Craniofacial growth series*, Ann Arbor, 1983, Center for Human Growth and Development, University of Michigan.

131. McNamara JA, Graber LW: Mandibular growth in the rhesus monkey *(Macaca mulatta)*, *Am J Phys Anthropol* 42:15, 1975.

132. McNamara JA, Hinton RJ, Hoffman DL: Histologic analysis of temporomandibular joint adaptation to protrusive function in young adult rhesus monkeys, *Am J Orthod* 82:288, 1982.

133. Melanson E, Van Dyken C: "Studies in condylar growth." Thesis, University of Michigan, Ann Arbor, 1972.

134. Mills JR: The effect of functional appliances on the skeletal pattern, *Br J Orthod* 18:267, 1991.

135. Mills JRE: The stability of the lower labial segment, *Dent Pract Dent Rec* 18:293, 1968.

136. Mills JRE: *Clinical control of craniofacial growth: a skeptic's viewpoint*. In McNamara JA, Ribbens KA, Howe RP, editors: *Clinical alteration of the growing face, Monograph 14, Craniofacial growth series*, Ann Arbor, 1983, Center for Human Growth and Development, University of Michigan.

137. Mills JRE: A clinician looks at facial growth, *Br J Orthod* 10:58, 1983.

138. Moffett BC: *Responses of the craniofacial skeleton to mechanical forces*. In *Symposium on clinical and bioengineering aspects of dentofacial orthopedics*, University of Connecticut, October 1981.

139. Moffett BC, Koskinen-Moffett L: *A biologic look at mandibular growth rotation*. In Carlson DS, editor: *Craniofacial biology, Monograph 10, Craniofacial growth series*, Ann Arbor, 1981, Center for Human Growth and Development, University of Michigan.

140. Moss JP: Cephalometric changes during functional appliance therapy, *Eur Orthod Soc Trans*, p 327, 1962.

141. Moss JP: Function—fact or fiction? *Am J Orthod* 67:625, 1975.

142. Moss JP: An investigation of the muscle activity of patients with a Class II, division 2, malocclusion and the changes during treatment, *Trans Eur Orthod Soc* p. 87, 1975.

143. Neumann B: Funktionskieferorthopädie. Rückblick und Ausblick, *Fortschr Kieferorthop* 36:73, 1975.

144. Nielsen IL: Facial growth during treatment with the function regulator appliance, *Am J Orthod* 85:401, 1985.

145. Orton HS, Noble PM: Fixed-removable approach to presurgical orthodontic treatment, *J Clin Orthod* 24:296, 1990.

146. Owen AH III: Frontal facial changes with the Fränkel appliance, *Angle Orthod* 58:257, 1988.

147. Owen AH III: Clinical management of the Fränkel FR II appliance, *J Clin Orthod* 17:605, 1983.

148. Owen AH III: Clinical application of the Fränkel appliance, case reports, *Angle Orthod* 53:29, 1983.

149. Ozerovic B: Some changes in occlusion and craniofacial pattern obtained during treatment with removable orthodontic appliances, *Eur Orthod Soc Rep Congr* p. 329, 1972.

150. Parkhouse RC: A cephalometric appraisal of cases of Angle's Class II, division 1 malocclusion treated by the Andresen appliance, *Dent Pract Dent Rec* 19:425, 1969.

151. Petrovic A: Recherches sur les mécanismes histophysiologiques de la croissance osseuse cranio-faciale, *Ann Biol* 9:303, 1970.

152. Petrovic AG: Mechanisms and regulation of mandibular condylar growth, *Acta Morphol Neerl Scand* 10:25, 1972.

153. Petrovic AG: "Experimental investigation on the modus operandi of various orthopedic appliances." Continuing education course, American Dental, Association, GV Black Institute and Kenilworth Research Foundation, Chicago, March 1983.

154. Petrovic A, Gasson N, Oudet C: Wirkung der übertriebenen posturalen Vorschubstellung des Unterkiefers auf das Kondylenwachstum der normalen und der mit Wachstumshormon behandelten Ratte, *Fortschr Kieferorthop* 36:86, 1975.

155. Petrovic A, Oudet C, Gasson N: Unterkieferpropulsion durch eine im Oberkiefer fixierte Vorbissführung mit seitlicher Biss-sperre von unterschiedlicher Höhe. Auswirkungen bei Ratten während der Wachstumsperiode und bei erwachsenen Tieren, *Fortschr Kieferorthop* 43:243, 1982.

156. Petrovic A, Stutzmann J: Le muscle ptérygoïdienne externe et al croissance du condyle mandibulaire. Recherches expérimentales chez le jeune rat, *Orthod Fr* 43:271, 1972.

157. Petrovic A, Stutzmann J, Oudet C: *Defects in mandibular growth resulting from condylectomy and resection of the pterygoid and masseter muscles*. In McNamara JA, Carlson, DS, Ribbens KA, editors: *The effect of surgical intervention on craniofacial growth, Monograph 12, Craniofacial growth series*, Ann Arbor, 1982, Center for Human Growth and Development, University of Michigan.

158. Pfeiffer JP, Grobéty D: Simultaneous use of cervical appliance and activator: an orthopedic approach to fixed appliance therapy, *Am J Orthod* 61:353, 1972.

159. Qwarnström KE, Sarnäs KV: Röntgenkefalometriska studier av förändringar vid funktionskäkortopedisk behandling av distalbett, 7 fall av Angle Klass II:1, *Odontol Rev* 5:118, 1954.

160. Rakosi T: *Biomechanics of functional orthopedic appliances*. In McNamara JA, Ribbins KA, Howe RP, editors: *Clinical alteration of the growing face, Monograph 14, Craniofacial growth series*, Ann Arbor, 1983, Center for Human Growth and Development, University of Michigan.

161. Reitan K: "The initial tissue reaction incident to orthodontic tooth movement as related to the influence of function. An experimental histological study on animal and human material." Thesis, University of Oslo, 1951.

162. Ricketts RM: *Orthopedics in the eyes of the clinician*. In *Symposium on clinical and bioengineering aspects of dentofacial orthopedics*, University of Connecticut, October 1981.

163. Righellis EG: Treatment effects of Fränkel, activator and extraoral traction appliances, *Angle Orthod* 53:107, 1983.

164. Robin P: Observation sur un nouvel appareil de redressement, *Rev Stomatol* 9:423, 1902.

165. Roux W: *Gesammelte Abhandlungen über Entwicklungsmechanik der Organismen*, Leipzig, 1895, W. Engelmann.

166. Sahm G, Bartsch A, Witt E: Micro-electronic monitoring of functional appliance wear, *Eur J Orthod* 12:297, 1990.

167. Sander FG: *Zur Frage der Biomechanik des Aktivators—Entwicklung und Erprobung neuer Unterrrsuchungsmethoden*, Wiesbaden, 1980, Westdeutscher Verlag GmbH.

168. Sander FG: *The effects of functional appliances and Class II elastics on masticatory patterns*. In McNamara JA, Ribbins KA, Howe RP, editors: *Clinical alteration of the growing face, Monograph 14, Craniofacial growth series*, Ann Arbor, 1983, Center for Human Growth and Development, University of Michigan.

169. Schmuth GPF: Milestones in the development and practical application of functional appliances, *Am J Orthod* 84:48, 1983.

170. Schmuth GPF: Untersuchungen über die auf das FKO-Gerät einwirkende Kaumuskeltätigkeit während des Schlafes, *Fortschr Kieferorthop* 16:327, 1955.

171. Schmuth GPF: Muskeltätigkeit und Muskelwirkung im Bahmen der Funktionskieferorthopädie, *Dtsch Zahn Mund Kieferheilkd* 32:4, 1960.

172. Schmuth GPF: Behandlungszeit—Retentionszeit—Rezidive, *Fortschr Kieferorthop* 27:22, 1966.

173. Schwarz AM: Grundsätzliches über die heutigen kieferorthopädischen Behandlungsverfahren, *Oesterr Z Stomatol* 47:400, 448, 1950.

174. Schwarz AM: Die Wirkungsweise des Aktivators, *Fortschr Kieferorthop* 13:117, 1952.

175. Scott JH: The growth of the human face, *Proc R Soc Med* 47:91, 1954.

176. Selmer-Olsen R: En kritisk betraktning over "Det norske system," *Nor Tannlaegefor Tid* 47:85, 134, 176, 1937.

177. Sergl HG: Changes in craniofacial pattern caused by functional adaptation—an experimental study in young rabbits, *Eur Orthod Soc Rep Congr*, p. 197, 1972.

178. Shaye R: J.C.O. interviews: Dr. Robert Shaye on functional appliances, *J Clin Orthod* 17:330, 1983.

179. Slagsvold O: *Activator development and philosophy.* In Graber TM, Neumann B: *Removable orthodontic appliances,* ed 1, Philadelphia, 1977, WB Saunders Co.

180. Slagsvold, O, Kolstad I: "Class II, division 1 malocclusions treated with activators: a study of posttreatment stability." Unpublished.

181. Softley JW: Cephalometric changes in seven "post normal" cases treated by the Andresen method, *Dent Rec* 73:485-494, 1953.

182. Stockfisch H: *Der Kinetor in der Kieferorthopädie. Die Praxis des polyvalenten bimaxillären Apparates und seine rationelle Technik mit Plastik—Fertigteilen,* Heidelberg, 1966, A. Hüthig.

183. Stockfisch H: Possibilities and limitations of the Kinetor, *Trans Eur Orthod Soc* p. 457, 1973.

184. Stöckli PW, Willert HG: Tissue reactions in the temporomandibular joint resulting from anterior displacement of the mandible in the monkey, *Am J Orthod* 60:142, 1971.

185. Stutzmann J, Petrovic A, Graber TM: Auswirkungen seitlicher Vestibularsschilder nach Fränkel auf das maxillare Breitwachstum der Ratte, *Stomatol DDR* 33:753, 1983.

186. Stutzmann J, Petrovic A, Malan A: Seasonal variations of human alveolar bone turnover. A quantitative evaluation in organ culture, *J Interdiscipl Cycle Res* 12:177, 1981.

187. Thilander B, Filipsson R: Muscle activity related to activator and intermaxillary traction in Angle Class II, division 1 malocclusions. An electromyographic study of the temporal, masseter and suprahyoid muscles, *Acta Odontol Scand* 24:241, 1966.

188. Thompson JR: The rest position of the mandible and its significance to dental science, *J Am Dent Assoc* 33:151, 1946.

189. Tonge EA, Heath JK, Meikle M: Anterior mandibular displacement and condylar growth, *Am J Orthod* 82:277, 1982.

190. Trayfoot J, Richardson A: Angle Class II, division 1 malocclusions treated by the Andresen method, *Br Dent J* 124:516, 1968.

191. Trenouth MJ: A functional appliance system for the correction of Class II relationships, *Br J Orthod* 16:169, 1989.

192. Tryti T: "Angle Kl. II, 1 malokklusjoner korrigert med fasialbue og aktivator." Thesis, University of Oslo, 1974.

193. Tulley WJ: The scope and limitations of treatment with the activator, *Am J Orthod* 61:562, 1972.

194. Vardimon AD, Graber TM: Expansion of palatal sutures in diverse force magnitude and application, *J Dent Res* 66:347-348, 1987, (abstract).

195. Vardimon AD, Graber TM, Voss LR: Splitting and remodelling of circum-maxillary sutures with conventional versus magnetic appliances, *Society* p. 78, 1987.

196. Vardimon AD, Graber TM et al: Magnetic versus mechanical expansion with different force thresholds and points of force application, *Am J Orthod Dentofac Orthop* 92:455-466, 1987.

197. Vardimon AD, Mueller HG et al: Effects of Teflon coating on corrosion and magnetic forces in neodymium-iron-boron rare earth magnets, *Br J Dent Res* 69:312, 1988, (abstract).

198. Vardimon AD, Graber TM, Voss LR: Stability of magnetic versus mechanical palatal expansion, *Eur Orthod Jour* 11:107-115, 1989.

199. Vardimon AD, Stutzmann JJ et al: Functional orthopedic magnetic appliance (FOMA)—modus operandi, *Am J Orthod Dentofac Orthop* 97:371-387, 1989.

200. Vardimon AD, Graber TM et al: Functional orthopedic magnetic appliance (FOMA) III—modus operandi, *Am J Orthod Dentofac Orthop* 97:135-148, 1990.

201. Vardimon AD, Graber TM: Determinants controlling iatrogenic external root resorption during and after palatal expansion, *Angle Orthod* 61:113-124, 1991.

202. Vardimon AD, Graber TM, Pitaru S: Ursachen und Reparaturvorgänge der externen Wurzelresorption nach Gaumennahterweiterung mit magnetischen und konventionellen Dehnapparaten, *Festschrift GPF Schmuth Fortschritte f Kieferorthop* 52:193-203, 1991.

203. Vardimon AD, Graber TM et al: Rare earth magnets and impaction, *Am J Orthod* 100:494-512, 1991. (Dewel Award for best clinical article in the *AJO/DO* for 1991. Presented May, 1992, St Louis.)

204. Vardimon AD, Graber TM, Pitaru S: Repair process of external root resorption subsequent to palatal expansion treatment, *AJO/DO* 103, February 1993.

205. Vargervik K, Harvold EP: Response to activator treatment in Class II malocclusions, *Am J Orthod* 88:242, 1988.

206. Watson WG: Functional appliances questioned, *Am J Orthod* 82:519, 1982.

207. Williams S, Melsen B: Condylar development and mandibular rotation and displacement during activator treatment, *Am J Orthod* 81:322, 1982.

208. Williams S, Melsen B: The interplay between sagittal and vertical growth factors—an implant study of activator treatment, *Am J Orthod* 81:327, 1982.

209. Witt E: Investigations into orthodontic forces of different appliances, *Eur Orthod Soc Rep Congr*, p 391, 1966.

210. Witt E: Muscular physiological investigations into the effect of bimaxillary appliances, *Trans Eur Orthod Soc* p. 448, 1973.

211. Witt E, Komposch G: Intermaxilläre Kraftwirkung bimaxillärer Geräte, *Fortschr Kieferorthop* 32:345, 1971.

212. Witt E, Meyer U: Indications for and working action of bimaxillary appliances, *Eur Orthod Soc Rep Congr*, p. 321, 1972.

213. Wolff J: *Das Gesetz der Transformation der Knochen,* Berlin, 1892, Hirschwald.

214. Woodside DG: Some effects of activator treatment on the mandible and the midface, *Trans Eur Orthod Soc* p 443, 1973.

215. Woodside DG: *The activator.* In Graber TM, Neumann B: *Removable orthodontic appliances,* ed 1, Philadelphia, 1977, WB Saunders Co.

216. Woodside DG, Altuna G et al: Primate experiments in malocclusion and bone induction, *Am J Orthod* 83:460, 1983.

CHAPTER 8

Combined Activator Headgear Orthopedics

PAUL W. STÖCKLI
ULLRICH M. TEUSCHER

BASIC CONSIDERATIONS OF FACIAL GROWTH AND DEVELOPMENT

To be able to adapt treatment to the growth processes in an optimal manner, the clinician must respect the relationships between the displacement trends of the different facial units. The movement of the mandibular symphysis relative to the rest of the face is of paramount importance. The superimposition in Fig. 8-1, representing average growth expression during a 3-year interval, shows that the symphysis moves downward, as well as forward. This is also illustrated by the displacement of gnathion along the Y-axis of Downs or, in a similar manner, along the facial axis of Ricketts. A growth axis of this kind represents nothing more than the result of vertical and sagittal displacement. In average facial growth (Fig. 8-1) the basis for the constancy of pattern must be a balance of displacements among the several components of the facial mosaic.

Vertical factors exert a dominant influence on the anteroposterior displacement of the symphysis.* Pathologic conditions (e.g., the longitudinally documented case of congenital muscular dystrophy published by Kreiborg et al.[68]) exemplify the impact of excessive vertical development with utmost clarity (Fig. 8-2). As a consequence of the missing vertical control—in this case related to the marked atrophy of the mandibular elevator muscles—the symphysis was drastically displaced downward and backward during the 8-year growth period.

Counterpart analysis

In an average growth pattern (Fig. 8-1) with downward and forward displacement of the mandibular symphysis along the Y-axis, the descent of the glenoid fossae and the vertical growth of the condyles balance the vertical down-

ward movement of the maxillary body and upper alveolar process plus the upward movement of the lower alveolar process (Fig. 8-3). If the vertical development of the maxilla and of the upper plus the lower alveolar processes is less than the vertical contribution of fossae and condyles, the symphysis will move predominantly forward. Thus the sagittal greatly surpasses the vertical fraction, as expressed by a closing reaction of the Y-axis (Fig. 8-4). However, if the vertical development of the maxilla and of the alveolar processes is greater than the vertical contribution of fossae and

Fig. 8-1 Average displacement of maxillary and mandibular structures during a 3-year period. Superimposition on the anterior cranial base. Point of registration at sella.

---

*References 22, 23, 26, 34, 61, 62, 107-109, 119, 136, 137.

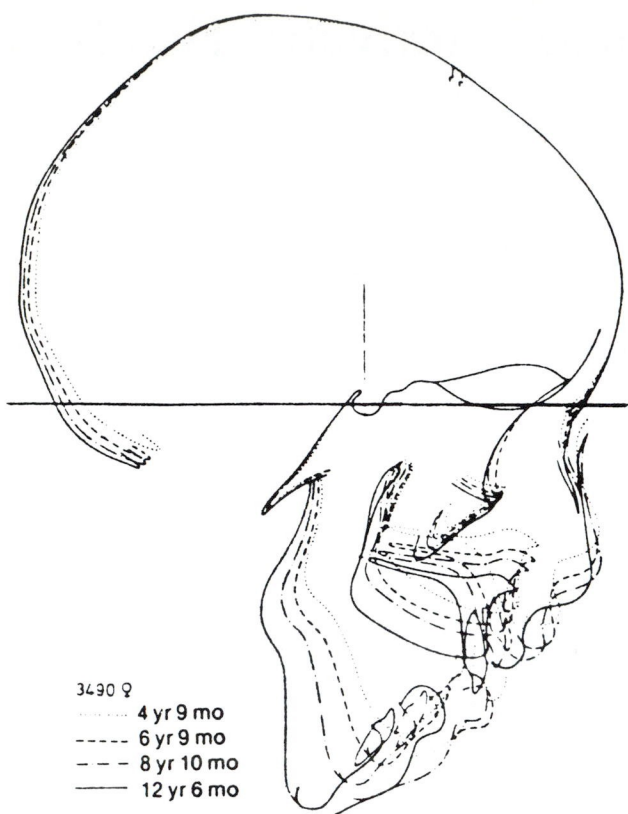

3490 ♀
.... 4 yr 9 mo
----- 6 yr 9 mo
--- 8 yr 10 mo
——— 12 yr 6 mo

Fig. 8-2 Excessive vertical development of the facial structures with backward rotation of the mandible in a child with congenital muscular dystrophy. (From Kreiborg S et al: *Am J Orthod* 74:207, 1978.)

Fig. 8-3 The vertical growth of the mandibular condyles *(CO)* and the descent of the glenoid fossae *(FO)* balance the vertical downward movement of the maxilla *(MA)* and upper alveolar process *(UA)* plus the upward movement of the lower alveolar process *(LA)*. Average growth pattern with downward and forward displacement of the mandibular symphysis (gnathion) along the Y-axis.

condyles, then the symphysis will move almost exclusively downward, thereby opening the Y-axis (Fig. 8-5). In conclusion, if the growth factors of fossae and condyles are maintained at a constant level, the vertical components of maxilla plus upper and lower alveolar processes will strongly influence the inferior displacement of the mandibular symphysis and thereby its anteroposterior position.

The order of magnitude of these natural growth processes is highly relevant in appraising treatment concepts. Approximate calculations, based on the studies of Björk and Skieller,[24,25] Luder,[71] Riolo et al.,[105] Teuscher,[123] and others, indicate a descent of the maxillary complex of about 0.7 mm* per year relative to the cranial base (Fig. 8-6) with a dentoalveolar height gain of almost 1 mm in the upper (Fig. 8-7) and around 0.75 mm in the lower (Fig. 8-8) jaw. Thus vertical development of the maxillary complex measured in the molar region amounts to some 1.5 to 2 mm per year. If the lower dentoalveolar increase is included, an overall vertical development of between 2 and 3 mm can be expected. As a counterpart the movement of the glenoid fossa and the amount of condylar growth must be taken into account. The

vertical downward movement of the fossa is estimated to be only about 0.25 to 0.5 mm per year[14,21,105,123] (Fig. 8-9). By far the greatest annual change in this interplay is in the condylar region, where on the average an addition of more than 2.5 mm can be registered[71,103,123] (Fig. 8-10). Comparing the vertical contribution of the glenoid fossae and the mandibular condyles with the vertical contributions of the maxilla and the upper and lower alveolar processes reveals that the stated equilibrium is also quantitatively apparent within biologic limits. Basically the condylar element must compensate for the vertical development of three facial components, each of which is relatively small. This equilibrium of displacements can be easily disturbed when orthodontic and/or orthopedic treatment is superimposed. In most treatment procedures the tendency is to increase the vertical dimension of the dentoalveolar regions or even of the midfacial structures. The fact that the extrusive mechanical aspect present in most devices does not result in a biologic response in all cases can be attributed to the control effect of the occlusal forces deriving from the adductor muscles. In many instances, however, the efficacy of orthodontic appliances prevails over the antagonistic occlusal forces. In view of the mere 2.5 mm annual growth increase in the

*25.4 mm = 1 inch.